Cardiac Arrest

The Science and Practice of Resuscitation Medicine

Second edition

Cardiac Arrest is the definitive and most comprehensive reference in advanced life support and resuscitation medicine.

This new edition brings the reader completely up-to-date with developments in the field, focusing on practical issues of decision making, clinical management and prevention, as well as providing clear explanations of the science informing the practice. The coverage includes information on the latest pharmacotherapeutic options, the latest chest compression techniques and airway management protocols, all backed by clearly explained, evidence-based scientific research. The content is consistent with the latest guidelines for practice in this area, as detailed by the major international governing organizations.

This volume is essential reading for all those working in the hospital environments of emergency medicine, critical care, cardiology and anesthesia, as well as those providing care in the pre-hospital setting, including paramedics and other staff from the emergency services.

Norman A. Paradis is Adjunct Professor of Surgery, University of Colorado Health Sciences Center.

Henry R. Halperin is Professor of Medicine, Radiology, and Biomedical Engineering at the Johns Hopkins University School of Medicine, Baltimore, USA.

Karl B. Kern is Professor of Medicine at the Sarver Heart Center, University of Arizona, USA.

Volker Wenzel is Associate Professor of Anesthesiology and Critical Care Medicine in the Department of Anesthesiology and Critical Care Medicine of Innsbruck Medical University, Innsbruck, Austria.

Douglas A. Chamberlain CBE is Honorary Professor of Resuscitation Medicine at the School of Medicine, Cardiff University, Wales and Visiting Professor of Cardiology at the University of Brighton, Sussex, UK.

From reviews of the first edition:

. . . It is a tribute to the editors of this book, and the contributors they have selected, that they have managed to produce a book of enormous quality on the science of resuscitation medicine.   *The Lancet*

The excellent book, the first of its kind in the field of cardiac arrest, provides a balance of theoretical and clinical information. It achieves a level of authority and sophistication well beyond that of the advanced cardiac life support guidelines and will be of considerable use to all those practicing or teaching clinical resuscitation.
                          The New England Journal of Medicine

The book has virtually everything one would ever want to know about the causes of cardiac arrest, the applied physiology, and its treatment. Physicians and nurses involved in the management of critically ill or injured patients should have Cardiac Arrest in their personal libraries for ready reference.   *Resuscitation*

Cardiac Arrest

The Science and Practice of Resuscitation Medicine

Second edition

Editors

Norman A. Paradis, M.D.
University of Colorado, Denver, USA

Henry R. Halperin, M.D., M.A.
Johns Hopkins University School of Medicine, Baltimore, MD, USA

Karl B. Kern, M.D.
University of Arizona, Sarver Heart Center, Tucson, AZ, USA

Volker Wenzel, M.D., M.Sc.
Innsbruck Medical University, Innsbruck, Austria

Douglas A. Chamberlain CBE, M.D.
School of Medicine, Cardiff University, Wales, UK

Senior Associate Editor

Max Harry Weil, M.D.
Weil Institute of Critical Care Medicine, Rancho Mirage, CA, USA

Associate Editors

Scott M. Eleff, M.D.
William Beaumont Hospital, Royal Oak, MI, USA

Terry L. Vanden Hoek, M.D.
University of Chicago, IL, USA

Vinay M. Nadkarni, M.D.
Children's Hospital of Philadelphia, PA, USA

Development Editor

Pamela Talalay, Ph.D.
Johns Hopkins University School of Medicine, Baltimore, MD, USA

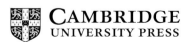

CAMBRIDGE
UNIVERSITY PRESS

CAMBRIDGE UNIVERSITY PRESS
Cambridge, New York, Melbourne, Madrid, Cape Town, Singapore, São Paulo

CAMBRIDGE UNIVERSITY PRESS
The Edinburgh Building, Cambridge CB2 8RU, UK

Published in the United States of America by Cambridge University Press, New York

www.cambridge.org
Information on this title: www.cambridge.org/9780521847001

First published 2007

Printed in Malaysia by Imago

A catalogue record for this book is available from the British Library

ISBN 978-0-521-84700-1 hardback

In memory of Harold Paradis, M.D., without whose inspiration this effort would never have been undertaken, and for Christine, without whose patience it would never have been completed. **N.A.P.**

To my wife, Sharon Tusa Halperin, and children, Victoria and Eric Halperin, whose patience and support inspired me to complete my contributions to this work. In memory of Victor Halperin, D.D.S., who inspired me to undertake a career in academic medicine and complete this work. **H.R.H.**

To Martha, my wife, who always understood that the most worthwhile books are written with friends, and that true friendship develops best while fly fishing, and to Matt, my youngest son, who has helped me keep my perspective that each day is wonderful and full of promise. **K.B.K.**

To my daughter Katharina, whose love from Innsbruck to the moon and back keeps me going on good days and especially on bad days, and in memory of Gunther and Ute Wenzel. And to my friends worldwide providing ideas, critique, encouragement, and hard work. **V.W.**

To my wife Jennifer, who continues to be incredibly tolerant of a husband who is forever ensconced in his study and who offers no help with the washing up. **D.A.C.**

Contents

†Deceased

Part VII Special issues in resuscitation

Contributors

Mark G. Angelos
Department of Emergency Medicine
The Ohio State University
146 Means Hall
1654 Upham Drive
Columbus OH 43220
USA

Charles Antzelevitch
Masonic Medical Research laboratory
2150 Bleecker Street
Utica NY 13501–1787, USA

Dan E. Arking
McKusick-Nathans Institute of Genetic Medicine
Johns Hopkins University School of Medicine
Baltimore
MD
USA

Hans-Richard Arntz
Division of Cardiology
Humboldt University
Campus Benjamin Franklin
Charité Berlin
Hindenburgdamm 30
Berlin D-12200
Germany

M. Dominique Ashen
Blalock 524 C – Cardiology
The Johns Hopkins Ciccarone
Preventive Cardiology Center
600 North Wolfe Street
Baltimore MD 21287
USA

Dianne L. Atkins
Division of Pediatric Cardiology
Children's Hospital of Iowa
Department of Pediatrics
Carver College of Medicine
University of Iowa
Iowa City
USA

James L. Atkins
Division of Military Casualty Research
Walter Reed Army Institute of Research
Silver Spring
MD
USA

Tom P. Aufderheide
Department of Emergency Medicine
Medical College of Wisconsin
9200 West Wisconsin Avenue
FEH Room 1870
Milwaukee WI 53266
USA

Thomas Aversano
Johns Hopkins University
Baltimore
MD
USA

Iyad M. Ayoub
Medical Service
North Chicago VA Medical Center
3001 Green Bay Road
North Chicago IL 60064
USA

David Baker
University of Washington
Clinical Trial Center 1107 NE 45th Street
Suite 505
Seattle, WA 98105
USA

Gad Bar-Joseph
Pediatric Intensive Care
Meyer Children's Hospital
Rambam Medical Center
PO Box 9602
Haifa 31096
Israel

Peter Baskett
Formerly Department of Anaesthesia
Frenchay Hospital and the Royal Infirmary
Bristol UK

Michael Baubin
Department of Anaesthesia and Critical Care Medicine
Innsbruck Medical University
Anichstrasse 35
Innsbruck A-6020
Austria

Wilhelm Behringer
Department of Emergency Medicine
Vienna General Hospital
Waehringer Guertel 18–20
1090 Vienna
Austria

Dave Beiser
Department of Emergency Medicine
University of Chicago
5841 South Maryland Avenue MC5068
Chicago IL 60637
USA

Bjørn Bendz
Department of Cardiology
Rikshospitalet University Hospital
Oslo 0027
Norway

Robert A. Berg
University of Arizona College of Medicine
Department of Pediatrics
P O Box 245017
Tucson AZ 85721-5017
USA

Ronald D. Berger
Johns Hopkins Medical Institutions
Carnegie 592
600 North Wolfe Street
Baltimore MD 21287
USA

Stephen Bernard
Department of Epidemiology and Preventive Medicine
Monash University
St Kilda Road
Prahran VIC 3181
Australia

Joost Bierens
Department of Anesthesiology
VU University Medical Centre
P O Box 7057
Amsterdam 1007 MB
The Netherlands

Joseph Bisera
Institute of Critical Care Medicine
35–100 Bob Hope Drive
Rancho Mirage CA 92270
USA

Roger S. Blumenthal
Blalock 524 C – Cardiology
The Johns Hopkins Ciccarone
Preventive Cardiology Center
600 North Wolfe Street
Baltimore MD 21287
USA

Bernd W. Böttiger
Department of Anaesthesiology
University of Heidelberg
Im Neuenheimer Feld 110
D-69120 Heidelberg
Germany

Allan Braslow
45 Greenwich Hill Drive
Greenwich
CT 06831, USA

David Burris
Norman M Rich Department of Surgery
Uniformed Services University of the Health Sciences
Bethesda MD
USA

Hugh G. Calkins
Carnegie 520
Johns Hopkins University
600 North Wolfe Street
Baltimore MD 21287-0409
USA

Catherine Campbell
Blalock 524 C – Cardiology
The Johns Hopkins Ciccarone
Preventive Cardiology Center
600 North Wolfe Street
Baltimore MD 21287
USA

Erga L. Cerchiari
Department of Anaesthesiology and Intensive Therapy
Maggiore Hospital
Largo Nigrisoli 2
40131 Bologna
Italy

Douglas Chamberlain
Prehospital Research Unit
School of Medicine
Cardiff University
UK

Alan Cheng
Johns Hopkins Hospital
Carnegie 568
600 North Wolfe Street
Baltimore MD 21287
USA

Ulrik Juul Christensen
Sophus Medical ApS
Copenhagen
Denmark

Leonard A. Cobb
Medic One Support Group
Harborview Medical Center
325 9th Avenue
Box 359748
Seattle WA 98112
USA

Mick Colquhoun
Resuscitation Council
5th Floor
Tavistock House North
Tavistock Square
London WC1H 9HR
UK

Michelle Cretikos
Simpson Centre for Health Services Research
Liverpool Health Service
University of New South Wales
Sydney
Australia

Carys Sian Davies
Department of Health
Area 407
133–155 Waterloo Road
London SE1 8UG
UK

Charles D. Deakin
Shackleton Department of Anesthesia
Southampton University Hospitals NHS Trust
Tremona Road
Southampton SO16 6YD
UK

Paul Dorian
Division of Cardiology
St Michael's Hospital
Rm 7051, Queen Wing
30 Bond Street
Toronto ON M5B 1W8
Canada

Martin W. Dünser
Department of Anesthesiology and Critical Care Medicine
Innsbruck Medical University
Anichstrasse 35
Innsbruck 6020
Austria

Uwe Ebmeyer
Klinic for Anaesthesiologie und Intensivtherapie
Otto-von-Guericke University
Magdeburg
Leipsiger Str 44
Magdeburg D-39120
Germany

Trygve Eftestøl
Department of Electrical and Computer Engineering
Stavanger University College
Stavanger N-4036
Norway

Mickey S. Eisenberg
Department of Medicine
University of Washington, Seattle,
WA, USA
King County EMS
999 Third Avenue, Suite 700
Seattle WA 98104
USA

Philip Eisenburger
Universitatsklinik fur
Notfallmedizin
Allgemeines Krankenhaus der Stadt
Wien
Wahringer Gurtel 18–20/6/D
Wien A-1090
Austria

Scott M. Eleff
Department of Emergency Medicine
William Beaumont Hospital
Royal Oak
MI
USA

Gordon A. Ewy
Sarver Heath Center Department of Cardiology
University of Arizona
Tucson
AZ
USA

P.B. Fenwick
Consciousness Research Group
University of Southampton
Southampton
UK
and
Critical Care Department
Hammersmith Hospitals NHS Trust
London
UK

Alastair Fischer
St. George's Hospital
University of London
Cranmer Terrace
London SW17 0RE
UK

Matthias Fischer
Department of Anaesthesiology and Intensive Care
   Medicine
Klinik am Eichert
Eichertstrasse 3
Göppingen 73035
Germany

Michael P. Frenneaux
Department of Cardiovascular Medicine
The Medical School
University of Birmingham
Edgbaston
Birmingham B15 2TT
UK

David A. Gabbott
Department of Anaesthetics
Gloucester Royal Hospital
Great Western Road
Gloucester CL1 3NN
UK

Andrea Gabrielli
Division of Critical Care Medicine
University of Florida
1600 SW Archer Road
Gainesville FL 32610-0254
USA

Luis García-Castrillo Riesgo
Universidad de Cantabria
Hospital Universitario Marqués de Caldecilla
Santander
Spain

Raúl J. Gazmuri
Medical Service
North Chicago VA Medical Center
3001 Green Bay Road
North Chicago IL 60064
USA

Romergryko G. Geocadin
Department of Neurology
The Johns Hopkins Hospital
Meyer 8-140
600 North Wolfe Street
Baltimore MD 21287
USA

Ty J. Gluckman
Blalock 524 C – Cardiology
The Johns Hopkins Ciccarone
Preventive Cardiology Center
600 North Wolfe Street
Baltimore MD 21287
USA

Alan D. Guerci
Department of Medicine,
St. Francis Hospital
100 Port Washington Blvd.
Roslyn, New York 11576, USA

Henry R. Halperin
Johns Hopkins University
Blalock 524A
Bayview Campus
600 North Wolfe Street
Baltimore MD 21287
USA

Kimm Hamann
Department of Emergency Medicine
University of Chicago
5841 South Maryland Avenue MC5068
Chicago IL 60637
USA

Michael T. Handrigan
Department of Resuscitation Medicine
Naval Medical Research Center
Silver Spring MD 20910
USA

Daniel F. Hanley
Department of Neurology
Neurosurgery and Anesthesiology-Critical Care
   Medicine
Johns Hopkins University School of Medicine
Baltimore MD
USA

Jason S. Haukoos
Department of Emergency Medicine
Denver Health Medical Center
777 Bannock Street
Mail Code 0108
Denver CO 80204
USA

Kenneth Heard
University of Colorado School of Medicine, Department
   of Surgery (Emergency Medicine)
4200 E 9th Avenue, 4215
Denver CO 80262
USA

Charles Henrikson
Blalock 425 C – Cardiology
The Johns Hopkins Ciccarone
Preventive Cardiology Center
600 North Wolfe Street
Baltimore MD 21287
USA

Holger Herff
Department of Anesthesiology and
   Critical Care Medicine
Innsbruck Medical University
Anichstr. 35, 6020 Innsbruck,
Austria

Johan Herlitz
Department of Metabolism and Cardiovascular Research
Sahlgrenska University Hospital
SE-413 45 Goteborg
Sweden

Quinn H. Hogan
Medical College of Wisconsin
Department of Anesthiology
8701 Watertown Plank Road
Milwaukee, WI 53226-0509, USA

Robert Hoke
Department of Cardiology-Angiology
University of Leipzig
Johannisallee 32
04103 Leipzig
Germany

Michael Holzer
University Klinik fur Notfallmedizin
AKH Wien
Waehringer Guertel 18–20
Vienna A-1090
Austria

Benjamin Honigman
Emergency Medicine B215
4200 East 9th Avenue
Denver CO 75390-8579
USA

Ahamed H. Idris
University of Texas Southwestern
Medical Center at Dallas
5323 Harry Hines Boulevard
Dallas TX 75390-8579
USA

Stefan Jochberger
Department of Anesthesiology and Critical Care Medicine
Innsbruck Medical University
Anichstrasse 35
6020 Innsbruck
Austria

Janice Jones
Department of Physiology and Biophysics
Georgetown University
Washington
DC
USA

Lesley A. Kane
Department of Biological Chemistry
Johns Hopkins University
Bayview Campus
Mason F Lord Building
Center Tower, Room 601
Baltimore MD 21224
USA

Laurence M. Katz
Department of Emergency Medicine
University of North Carolina School of Medicine
Neuroscience Hospital
Ground Floor
101 Manning Drive
Chapel Hill NC 27599
USA

Michael J. Kellum
Department of Emergency
Mercy Walworth Medical Center
Lake Geneva
WI
USA

Karl B. Kern
Sarver Heart Center
University of Arizona
1501 North Campbell Avenue
Tucson AZ 85724
USA

Thomas Kerz
Department of Neurosurgery Intensive Care Unit
Johannes Gutenberg-Universität Klinikum
Langenbeckstr 1
Mainz D-55131
Germany

Fulvio Kette
Emergency Department and Intensive Care Unit
S. Vito al Tagliamento Hospital
Via Savorgnano 2
33078 San Vito al Tagliamento
Italy

Walter Kloeck
72 Sophia Street
Fairland
2195 Johannesburg
South Africa

Peter Kohl
University Laboratory of Physiology
The Cardiac Mechano-Electric Feedback Lab
Oxford OX1 3PT

Julieta Kolarova
21730 Boschome Drive
Kildeer IL 60047
USA

Ronald J. Korthuis
Department of Medical Pharmacology and Physiology
School of Medicine
One Hospital Drive, MA415
University of Missouri-Columbia
Columbia MO 65212
USA

Rudolph W. Koster
Department of Cardiology
Academic Medical Center
University of Amsterdam
Room F-239
Meibergdreef 9
Amsterdam 1105 AZ
The Netherlands

Thomas Krafft
Geographisches Institut
Universitat Köln
Albertus-Magnus-Platz
D-50923 Köln
Germany

Gary S. Krause
Department of Emergency Medicine
Wayne State University
550 East Canfield Avenue
51.2 Lande Building
Detroit MI 48201
USA

Anette C. Krismer
Department of Anesthesiology and Critical Care Medicine
Innsbruck Medical University
Anichstrasse 35
Innsbruck A-6020
Austria

Peter Kudenchuk
University of Washington Medical Center
Campus Box 356422
1959 NE Pacific Street
Seattle WA 98195
USA

Todd M. Larabee
Division of Emergency Medicine
UCHSC B215
4200 East 9th Avenue
Denver CO 80262
USA

Wolfgang Lederer
Department of Anaesthesiology and Critical Care
    Medicine
University of Innsbruck
Anichstrasse 25
A-6020 Innsbruck
Austria

Howard R. Levin
Department of Surgery
Division of Cardiothoracic Surgery
College of Physicians and Surgeons
Columbia University
New York, NY 10032, USA

Karl H. Lindner
Department of Anesthesiology and Critical Care Medicine
Innsbruck Medical University
Anichstrasse 35
Innsbruck A-6020
Austria

Mark Link
Tufts University School of Medicine
NEMC Box #197
750 Washington Street
Boston MA 02111
USA

Freddy Lippert
Copenhagen Hospital Corporation
Copenhagen University Hospital
Denmark

Peter Mair
Department of Anaesthesia and Intensive Care Medicine
Innsbruck Medical University
Anichstrasse 35
Innsbruck A-6020
Austria

James Mennegazzi
University of Pittsburgh School of Medicine
Pittsburgh PA
USA

William H. Montgomery
Department of Anesthesiology
Straub Clinic and Hospital
University of Hawaii School of Medicine
888 South King Street
Honolulu
Hawaii 96813
USA

Peter Morley
Intensive Care Unit
Royal Melbourne Hospital
Grattan Street
Parkville VIC 3050
Australia

Stephen Morris
Department of Anaesthesia
Llandough Hospital
Penarth
Cardiff CF64 2XX
UK

Arthur J. Moss
University of Rochester Medical Center
Department of Medicine
Rochester, New York, USA

Vinay M. Nadkarni
Departments of Anesthesia, Critical Care and Pediatrics
The Children's Hospital of Philadelphia
34th Street and Civic Center Blvd
Philadelphia PA 19104-4399
USA

Carlo Napolitano
Department of Medicine and Department of Biomedical
    Engineering
Johns Hopkins University
Baltimore
USA

Robert W. Neumar
Department of Emergency Medicine
University of Pennsylvania School of Medicine
Hospital of the University of Pennsylvania
3400 Spruce Street
Philadelphia PA 19104-4283
USA

Graham Nichol
University of Washington
Clinical Trial Center
1107 NE 45th Street
Suite 505
Seattle WA 98105
USA

James T. Niemann
Department of Emergency Medicine
Harbor-UCLA Medical Center
1000 West Carson Street, Box 21
Torrance CA 90509
USA

Susan Niermeyer
Division of Neonatology
University of Colorado
School of Medicine
The Children's Hospital
4200 East 9th Avenue
Denver, CO 80218, USA

Marko Noc
University Ljubljana Medical Center
Center for Intensive Internal Medicine
Zaloska Cesta 7
Ljubljana 1000
Slovenia

Jerry P. Nolan
Anaesthesia and Intensive Care Medicine
Royal United Hospital
Combe Park
Bath BA1 3ND
UK

Brian J. O'Neil
Department of Emergency Medicine
William Beaumont Hospital
3601 W Thirteen Mile Road
Royal Oak MI 48073
USA

Joseph P. Ornato
Department of Emergency Medicine
Virginia Commonwealth University
401 N 12th Street
Richmond, VA 23298
USA

Jerry Overton
Richmond Ambulance Authority
Richmond VA
USA

Norman A. Paradis
University of Colorado
Denver
Colorado
USA

Gideon Paret
Department of Pediatric Critical Care
The Chaim Sheba Medical Center
Safra Children's Hospital
Tel Hashomer, Israel

Sam Parnia
Consciousness Research Group
University of Southampton
Southampton
UK
and
Critical Care Department
Hammersmith Hospitals NHS Trust
London
UK

Richard Pawl
Department of Emergency Medicine
Medical College of Georgia
1120 15th Street
AF 2014
Augusta GA 30912-2800
USA

Mary Ann Peberdy
Department of Medicine and Emergency Medicine
Virginia Commonwealth University Health System
1200 East Broad Street,
West Hospital, 10th Floor
Room 1042, P O Box 980204
Richmond VA 23298
USA

Tommaso Pellis
Cardiac Mechano-Electric Feedback Lab
The University Laboratory of Physiology
Oxford OX1 3PT

Gavin Perkins
26 Hollie Lucas Road
Kings Heath
Birmingham
B13 0QL, UK

Edward Platia
Cardiac Arrhythmia Center
Washington Hospital Center DC
110 Irving Street
Washington DC 2010
USA

Kees Polderman
Department of Intensive Care
VU University Medical Center
Amsterdam
The Netherlands

Andreas W. Prengel
Department of Anesthesiology, Critical Care Medicine,
    and Pain Therapy
Ruhr University Hospital Bochum
In der Schornau 23–25
44892 Bochum
Germany

Silvia G. Priori
Department of Molecular Cardiology
IRCCS Fondazione Salvatore Maugeri
Via Maugeri 10 / 10a
27100 Pavia
Italy

Richard Pumphrey
Department of Immunology
Manchester Royal Infirmary
Manchester M13 9WL
UK

Walter Rabl
Institute of Legal Medicine
Innsbruck Medical University
Muellerstrasse 44
Innsbruck A-6020
Austria

Jeejabai Radhakrishnan
Department of Medicine
Rosalind Franklin University of Medicine and Science
3333 Green Bay Road
North Chicago IL
USA

Barry K. Rayburn
School of Medicine
University of Alabama
Tinsley Harrison Tower THT 321
1530 3rd Avenue S
Birmingham AL 35294-0006
USA

Robert Roach
Division of Neonatology
University of Colorado School of Medicine
The Children's Hospital
4200 East 9th Avenue
Denver, CO 80218, USA

Colin Robertson
Department of Accident and Emergency
The Royal Infirmary of Edinburgh
51 Little France Crescent
Edinburgh EH16 4SA
Scotland
UK

Iain Robertson-Steel
West Midlands Ambulance Service NHS Trust
Dudley
West Midlands
UK

Risto O. Roine
Department of Neurology, Turku University Hospital,
Finland

Peter Safar
deceased

Arthur B. Sanders
Department of Emergency Medicine
University of Arizona
P O Box 245057
1501 N Campbell Avenue
Tucson AZ 85724-5057
USA

Birgit Schwarz
Department of Anaesthesia and Intensive Care Medicine
Innsbruck Medical University
Anichstrasse 35
Innsbruck A-6020
Austria

Michael Shuster
Department of Emergency Medicine
Mineral Springs Hospital
Box 1050
Banff AB T1L 1H7
Canada

Tom Silfvast
Department of Anaesthesia and Intensive Care Medicine
Meilhati Hospital
Helsinki University Hospital
P O Box 340
FIN-00029
Helsinki
Finland

Michiel Sinaasappel
Laser Center
Academic Medical Center
University of Amsterdam
Meibergdreef 9
1105 AZ
Amsterdam
The Netherlands

Sunil K. Sinha
The Johns Hopkins Hospital
Carnegie 530
600 North Wolfe Street
Baltimore MD 21287-1345
USA

Jasmeet Soar
Anaesthetics and Intensive Care
Southmead Hospital
N. Bristol NHS Trust
Westburg-on-Trym
Bristol BS10 5NB
UK

Eldar Soreide
Intensive Care Unit
Division of Acute Care Medicine
Stavanger University Hospital
PB 8100
4068 Stavanger
Norway

K. Spearpoint
Department of Anaesthetics and Intensive Care
5th Floor, Hammersmith House
Hammersmith Hospital
Du Cane Road
London W12 0HS
UK

Fabian Spöhr
Department of Anaesthesiology
University of Heidelberg
Im Neuenheimer Feld 110
D-69120 Heidelberg
Germany

Mark Stacey
Anaesthetics Department
Llandough Hospital
Penarth
Cardiff CF64 2XX
UK

Karl-Heinz Stadlbauer
Department of Anesthesiology and Critical Care Medicine
Innsbruck Medical University
Anichstrasse 35
Innsbruck A-6020
Austria

Edward R. Stapleton
Department of Emergency Medicine
080, Level 4, Health Science Center
State University of NY
    at Stony Brook,
Stony Brook
New York 11794-8350
USA

Petter Andreas Steen
Department of Anaesthesiology
Ulleval University Hospital
Oslo N-0407
Norway

Stig Steen
Department of Cardiothoracic Surgery
University Hospital of Lund
Lund University
Box 117
Lund S-22100
Sweden

Hans-Ulrich Strohmenger
Department of Anaesthesiology and Critical Care
    Medicine
Medical University Innsbruck
Anichstrasse
6020 Innsbruck
Austria

Peter H. Sugden
Imperial College London
NHLI Division (Cardiac Medicine)
Flowers Building (4th Floor)
Armstrong Road
London SW7 2AZ
UK

Shijie Sun
Weil Institute of Critical Care Medicine
1696 North Sunrise Way
Building 3
Palm Springs CA 92262
USA

David Szpilman
Intensive Care Unit
Hospital Miguel Couto
Av das Americas 3555
Bloco 2, Sala 302
Barra da Tijuca
Rio de Janeiro 22631-004
Brazil

Willis A. Tacker Jr
Basic Medical Sciences
Purdue University
625 Harrison Street
West Lafayette IN 47907-2006
USA

Wanchun Tang
Weil Institute of Critical Care Medicine
1696 North Sunrise Way
Building 3
Palm Springs CA 92262
USA

Marjaana Tiainen
Department of Neurology, Helsinki University
    Hospital, Finland
Finland

Sergio Timerman
Resuscitation Department
Heart Institute of Sao Paolo
Av Dr Eneas de Carvalho
Aguiar 44
Sao Paulo 05403-900
Brazil

Gordon F. Tomaselli
Cardiovascular Clinical Research Center
Johns Hopkins University School of Medicine
600 North Wolfe Street
Baltimore MD 21287
USA

Wolfgang Ummenhofer
Department of Anaesthesia
University Hospital
21 Spital Strasse
CH-4031 Basel
Switzerland

Anouk Van Alem
Department of Cardiology
Academic Medical Center
Room B2-238
Meibergdreef 9
1105 AZ Amsterdam
The Netherlands

Terry L. Vanden Hoek
Department of Emergency Medicine
University of Chicago
5841 South Maryland Avenue MC 5068
Chicago IL 60637
USA

Jennifer E. Van Eyk
Johns Hopkins University – Bayview Campus
5200 Eastern Avenue
Mason F Lord Building
Center Tower, Room 602
Baltimore MD 21224
USA

Wolfgang Voelckel
Department of Anaesthesiology and Critical Care
Innsbruck Medical University
Anichstrasse 35
Innsbruck A-6020
Austria

Martin von Planta
Department of Internal Medicine
University of Basel
St Johanns-Vorstadt 44
CH-4056 Basel
Switzerland

Beat Walpoth
Cardiovascular Research
Service of Cardiovascular Surgery
University Hospital
Geneva 1211
Switzerland

Kevin R. Ward
Department of Emergency Medicine
Virginia Commonwealth University
401 N 12th Street
Richmond VA 23298
USA

David S. Warner
Departments of Anesthesiology, Neurobiology and
    Surgery
Duke University Medical Center
Box 3094
Durham NC 27710
USA

Karl Wegscheider
Institute for Statistics and Econometry
University of Hamburg
Von-Melle-Park 5
20146 Hamburg
Germany

Max Harry Weil
Weil Institute of Critical Care Medicine
35-100 Bob Hope Drive
Rancho Mirage CA 92270
USA

Myron Weisfeldt
Johns Hopkins University Medical Center
Department of Medicine
1830 E. Monument St., 9th Floor
Baltimore, MD 21287, USA

Volker Wenzel
Department of Anesthesiology and Critical Care Medicine
Innsbruck Medical University
Anichstrasse 35
Innsbruck A-6020
Austria

Roger D. White
Mayo Clinic College of Medicine
200 First Street SW
Rochester Minn
USA

Lars Wiklund
Department of Surgical Sciences
Uppsala University Hospital
75185 Uppsala
Sweden

Wei Xiong
Cardiovascular Clinical Research Center
Johns Hopkins University School of Medicine
600 North Wolfe Street
Baltimore MD 21287
USA

Markus Zabel
Division of Cardiology
University of Göttingen
Germany

Mathias Zuercher
Department of Anaesthesia
University Hospital
21 Spital Strasse
CH-4031 Basel
Switzerland

Menekhem Zviman
Cardiovascular Clinical Research Center
Johns Hopkins University School of Medicine
600 N. Wolfe St.
Baltimore, MD 21287, USA

Foreword

Myron L. Weisfeldt, M.D.

This monograph on cardiac resuscitation medicine is the standard reference in the field. This Second Edition a decade later presents an entirely changed and dynamic field. Advances in resuscitative medicine encompass the basic science understanding of physiology and pathophysiology as well as advances in understanding of the causal mechanisms involved in successful or non-successful resuscitation. There are new programs and approaches at a practical and real-world level that improve survival and the quality of survival from cardiac arrest. I would maintain that these prerequisites relate to the need for this updated monograph. It is important that this text be acquired and used by providers of emergency cardiac care in both the out-of-hospital and in-hospital settings. It will be of value universally in the emergency departments. Clinical investigators will find this text of tremendous value when pursuing the improvement of survival from cardiac arrest, as well as laboratory-based clinical investigators attempting to identify and justify approaches to improving the outcome of cardiac arrest. As the underlying science of resuscitation deepens, basic scientists will value these state-of-the-art discussions. Resuscitation Science has broadened the focus from mechanics to reperfusion injury, post-resuscitation inflammation and programmed cell death.

To substantiate my statements about this update and its value to the medical and resuscitative community, I have identified what I consider to be the eight major advances in resuscitative medicine over the last decade.

1. *The advent of inexpensive, easy-to-use Automatic External Defibrillators (AEDs) for use by the lay public.* Ten years ago, industry was just beginning to produce these revolutionary devices. The FDA considered use of these AEDs by other than physicians, nurses and trained Emergency Medical Technicians (EMTs) as "illegal," off label, over-the-counter use of an approved

device. Ten years ago, only one or two states referred to defibrillation as being covered by the Good Samaritan law. Now all states consider such resuscitative efforts by members of the lay public to be encompassed by the Good Samaritan statutes. Ten years ago there were no convincing data that AEDs are effective in improving the outcome of resuscitation. Perhaps the most remarkable result was in the casinos of Las Vegas where Terry Valenzuela and his colleagues measured time from collapse to defibrillation precisely (on video cameras). Security guards could defibrillate with an average time of 4.4 minutes and survival of 59% in 90 subjects. If defibrillation was performed within 3 minutes ($n = 20$), survival was over 70%. As well, in the Public Access Defibrillation study (PAD), we now have data to support the value of the AEDs in the public arenas when added to CPR instruction. Ten years ago we had no conscientious programs to implement AEDs in full public view in airports and other transportation facilities, on-board airlines, in exercise facilities, or recently by government mandate in large public buildings. Although these programs clearly have had little impact on the overall public health survival rate from cardiac arrest, they have produced some of the most rewarding survivals because of the promptness of resuscitation and the clear ability of those resuscitated very quickly to recover fully and rapidly.

2. *Change in the characteristics of the population suffering cardiac arrest.* Ten years ago, broad population studies showing that 70% or so of people suffering cardiac arrest have ventricular fibrillation (or ventricular tachycardia) as the first documented electrocardiographic rhythm. Now, multiple large population studies note that 20% to 30% of those suffering a cardiac arrest have ventricular tachycardia (VT) or ventricular fibrillation (VF) as their initial rhythm. The majority now have an absence of electrical activity, or occasionally will have electromechanical dissociation. The reason for this major change, one can only speculate. One possibility is that, in fact, modern drug treatment of coronary disease and heart failure combined with implantation of automatic defibrillators in their target population has led to this change. For survivors of cardiac arrest caused by ventricular tachycardia or fibrillation, implantation of defibrillators has provided an increasing standard of care. This is also true for patients with congenitally inherited causes of sudden death, and many individuals with reduced left ventricular function due to previous myocardial infarction or cardiomyopathy. It is possible that we are implanting defibrillators currently at sufficient rate to have an impact in the

United States on the overall public health's incidence of cardiac arrest from these arrhythmias. Drug and procedural treatment strategies for chronic coronary disease and heart failure may also be impacting on the incidence of sudden death from VT/VF. It is very clear that, in these broad populations, beta-blocking agents as well as angiotensin II receptor blockers, and antiplatelet drugs (for coronary disease), and aldosterone antagonist improve survival from these chronic cardiac states. It is less clear that they reduce the incidence of sudden death particularly sudden death from VF or VT. That is a likely possibility. A final speculation is that cardiac arrest in advanced age is more likely not VT/VF. With the striking decline in age-adjusted mortality from cardiovascular disease, we have less incidence of death and perhaps less sudden death from VT/VF in younger individuals on a population basis.

This change in the initial arrhythmia has a number of significant impacts. First, survival of this group of patients who do not have VT/VF is much lower and we know little about what are effective ways of resuscitating this population. We also know less about the long-term management and care of these patients that may result in their survival since it is likely that placing automatic implantable defibrillators in these patients will not improve their long-term outcome even if they survive their initial arrest. These, and a whole host of other theoretical and practical problems, emanate from this change in population suffering cardiac arrest.

3. *In recent years there has been recognition of the need to extend animal data on CPR performance and effectiveness from the laboratory into the clinical arena.* It is very clear from animal studies that all interruptions of chest compressions are detrimental to the hemodynamics of CPR, particularly coronary blood flow. It has long been recognized that indices of coronary blood flow are very closely related to human survival. Interruptions from repeated looks at the electrocardiogram, multiple defibrillation attempts, or procedures such as inefficient intubation, have been minimized on the basis of these data. In addition, it has been demonstrated in animal models very convincingly that hyperventilation or even "usual" ventilation during resuscitation is too much ventilation and is detrimental. Related to these issues, performance of cardiopulmonary resuscitation in the real-world situation, both in the hospital by healthcare professionals and out-of-the hospital by EMTs, is characterized by multiple, prolonged and repeated interrupts of chest compression and hyperventilation. Monitoring systems, feedback systems, and other systems for controlling or at least documenting the way resuscitation is

performed, are beginning to change the policies and practices of CPR performance. It is very clear that, from point "2" above, we come to the realization that in 70% of arrest in which the initial electrocardiogram is not VT/VF, it is only the quality of CPR and its performance that can lead to return of spontaneous circulation and ultimately the possibility of survival.

4. *In VT/VF Arrest, Dr. Lance Becker and I proposed a three-phase model to integrate and characterize specifically the time relationships of the value of rapid defibrillation, the performance of cardiopulmonary resuscitation, and the need for other measures focused on the metabolic factors that decrease survival after prolonged cardiac arrest.* Phase 1 of the three-phase model identifies the first 4 or 5 minutes as a time when initial defibrillation has a remarkable survival benefit. It next identifies that between 4 minutes and 10 minutes, optimal survival is very poor if there is no CPR performed. Shock at this time may be detrimental in addition to the time wasted. During Phase 2 from 4 to 10 minutes after arrest, it may be critical to perform cardiopulmonary resuscitation to achieve even a 20–30% survival rate. Finally in Phase 3, after 10 minutes without resuscitation, the model identifies the possibility that drugs and pharmacological agents as well as subsequent treatment strategies such as hypothermia may be required to reach reasonable survival.

5. *We are beginning to see devices that may improve perfusion during cardiopulmonary resuscitation and thus may improve survival.* It is understood that the hemodynamics of CPR are not excellent with regard to restoring and maintaining brain and particularly myocardial blood flow. Fluctuating intra-thoracic pressure to a greater degree (both positive during compression or the "systolic" phase of the CPR cycle and increasing negative intra-thoracic pressure during the "diastolic" phase) in animal models seems to show very convincing benefit in improving blood flow as well as animal survival. There are initial studies in man suggesting favorable hemodynamic changes occur. To date, the vest-like devices that increase intra-thoracic pressure during the systolic phase are cumbersome. Motivation to use devices is important. There have been variable results in humans – none that are convincing. A small airway valve device that decreases intra-thoracic pressure between compression cycles improves blood flow in animals and humans. This device is associated with improved short-term survival and we await larger studies which are ongoing to see whether this device will improve long-term and meaningful survival.

6. *Moderate hypothermia may be useful in patients who*

after out-of-hospital cardiac arrest have not awakened when they reach the emergency department. Two studies appear to show benefit of 12 to 24 hours of 32° to 33 °C, hypothermia in terms of improving survival and brain function following such episodes of out-of-hospital cardiac arrest. This benefit has been accepted in AHA guidelines, but is not accepted by the FDA. Much is happening in the experimental arena to develop devices that induces easy controllable hypothermia. There are initial studies to potentially bring hypothermia earlier in the course of resuscitation. Again, animal studies suggest that broad implementation of early hypothermia after cardiac arrest may improve survival remarkably.

7. *Registry-based information on in-hospital and out-of-hospital CPR.* Detailed performance data with results are now available for thousands of in-hospital resuscitations. There are also increasing numbers of epidemiological studies and other out-of-hospital registry studies that have identified correlates of survival from cardiac arrest as related to resuscitation strategies, maneuvers and approaches. We are beginning to define "best" practices and (if you will) the "worst" practices.

8. *There is a new horizon of technology that will certainly impact on resuscitation* This technology revolution I predict will include patient sensors that identify futility of cardiac resuscitation. Diagnosis of death is inadequately made in many individuals with current clinical criteria. Perhaps more importantly, we will use sensors that will identify patient status from the point of view of metabolism blood flow and oxygen delivery. They will provide an assessment of the current status of the patient and/or what the resuscitative maneuvers have accomplished. This type of information will dictate care patterns and strategies to improve survival from the point of view of drug administration as well as device and hemodynamic strategies. The strategies are likely to be complex and therefore it is highly likely that devices will integrate the clinical status of the patient with the information obtained with sensors into a care and management. These will emerge particularly as metabolic phase markers lead to specific therapeutic strategies. Information will likely be used at the scene and in the emergency department that is ultimately going to receive the patient. Similar devices and approaches will almost certainly change in-hospital and ED management of the arrest occurring in that circumstance.

9. In summary, this new volume on the science and practice of resuscitative medicine is extraordinarily timely. The depth and breadth of new material and chapters are remarkable and valuable. The new authors include

the current generation of the most contributory and thoughtful leaders of the field. The text should be embraced by a broad and deep audience of those interested in this exciting and forward-moving field and branch of medicine. The worldwide authorship reflects the fact that sudden death is a worldwide problem that is increasingly gaining true worldwide attention!

July 12, 2006

Preface to the first edition

O, that I could but call these dead to life!

King Henry VI
William Shakespeare

There is a no more frightening experience for a clinician than a patient's sudden and complete loss of vital signs. The need to initiate multiple complex therapies, all the while knowing that each minute that passes dramatically decreases the chances for a good outcome, makes sudden death the penultimate medical emergency.

Premature death is the adversary of physicians. For millennia, the loss of life signs was considered the victory of death. Students were taught that once patients had succumbed they were beyond the healing arts. Only relatively recently have physicians regularly attempted to wrest such patients back from death.

Accurate numbers are difficult to obtain. It is said that more than 300,000 persons die each year from sudden cardiac death in the United States alone. Worldwide the figure is in the millions. Sudden death is not, however, caused by coronary artery disease alone. Hemorrhage and asphyxiation, among others, can kill physiologically competent patients without warning. Sudden death is not defined by etiology; it is the circumstance of cardiopulmonary arrest in a person with functional vital organ systems. It is death in the midst of life, and it is always tragic.

We are just beginning to appreciate the magnitude of this problem and the potential for therapy. Just a 5% improvement in outcome – something that could be achieved in many communities by better application of standard care – would save more lives than therapies that have received far more attention. The potential for good is astounding; the relationship of cost to benefit compelling.

Sudden cardiopulmonary arrest is the most difficult disease state to treat. Remarkable improvement in the quality of care has been achieved in a relatively short time by the American Heart Association's and the European Resuscitation Council's guidelines to therapy. Their efforts define the standard; this text is an attempt to delineate state-of-the-art. Our efforts are complementary. One cannot hope to individualize therapy to the patient's benefit without excellent basic care, and international consensus provides this basis.

Our difficulty in treating cardiopulmonary arrest reflects a limited understanding of the pathophysiology of global ischemia and reperfusion. Physicians are naturally uncomfortable in using therapies that are poorly understood and that have not been clearly demonstrated effective. However, these patients do not allow us the luxury of waiting for more definite knowledge. We must apply all our skill and limited knowledge immediately if persons with "hearts and brains too good to die" are not to be lost forever.

This text is for clinicians who wish to practice both the science and the art of resuscitation. Every physician will at some time attempt to resuscitate a patient from sudden death, but few will have had the opportunity to learn from teachers dedicated to this skill. That is the purpose of this book. In each chapter, a recognized authority has been asked not only to review present knowledge, but also to describe the state of their art. Cardiac arrest patients do not have the luxury of seeking out experts. You must bring that expertise to the bed or curb side.

This is intended to be a comprehensive text incorporat-ing critical analysis of material not readily available else-where. The text begins with chapters that place our current knowledge into context, describing the magnitude of the problem. The next two sections describe the basic science of ischemia and reperfusion at the cellular, organ system, and organismal levels and the pathophysiology of cardio-pulmonary arrest and resuscitation. The fourth and fifth sections focus on state-of-the-art therapy for cardiopul-monary arrest, first without respect to etiology and then under specific circumstances. Contributors were asked to provide insights that complement widely disseminated guidelines. The sixth section focuses on the pathophysiol-ogy and therapy of postresuscitation syndrome, a complex disease state that is increasingly believed to underlie the morbidity and death following resuscitation. The therapy sections conclude with summaries intended to bring together concepts discussed throughout the chapters on cardiopulmonary resuscitation and postreperfusion syn-drome.

We are at the beginning of what will be a rapid expansion in our knowledge of the pathophysiology and therapy of sudden death, global ischemia, and reperfusion injury. This text is intended not only to reflect the field, but also to affect it. We hope to convince the reader that there is art even in the management of this, the most dire medical emergency. "Life is short and the art is long." Considering the millions of lives that are cut short and the limits of our knowledge, the art must be very long indeed.

The Editors

Preface to the second edition

O, that I could but call these dead to life!

King Henry VI
William Shakespeare

Death in the midst of life is the adversary of physicians. For millennia the loss of signs of life was considered the victory of death. Students were taught, and people believed, that once patients had succumbed they were beyond the healing arts. On a historical time frame, only relatively recently have physicians regularly attempted to wrest such patients back from death. We believe that the second edition of this text represents yet another step in resuscitative medicine's coming of age.

There is a no more frightening experience for clinicians than a patient's sudden loss of vital signs. The need to initiate multiple complex therapies, knowing that each minute that passes dramatically decreases the chances for a good outcome, makes sudden death the penultimate medical emergency.

It is difficult to obtain accurate numbers, but it is said that more than 300 000 persons die each year from sudden cardiac death in the United States alone. Worldwide the number is in the millions. Sudden death is not, however, caused by coronary artery disease alone. Hemorrhage and asphyxiation, among others, can kill physiologically competent patients without warning. Sudden death is not defined by etiology, but rather by the setting in which it occurs in a person with functional vital organ systems. It is not the natural ending of life, but death in the midst of life, and it is always tragic.

We are just beginning to appreciate the magnitude of this problem and the potential for therapy. Even a small improvement in outcomes of these patients – something that could be achieved in many communities by better application of established interventions-would save more lives than therapies that have received far more attention.

The potential for good is astounding; the relationship of benefit to cost for some interventions is compelling.

If we acknowledge that sudden cardiopulmonary arrest may be among the most difficult conditions that confront rescuers, then remarkable improvement in the standardization of care has been achieved in a relatively short time through the efforts of national organizations which have developed evidence-based guidelines for resuscitative therapy. Their efforts have defined the current standard. This text is an attempt to disseminate the state-of-the-art. We believe that these efforts are complementary, as one cannot hope to enhance therapy to the patient's benefit without international consensus on excellent basic care.

Remarkable progress has been made since the first edition. It has become clear that the treatment of lost hemodynamics is optimized by good and uninterrupted chest compression. A number of studies now indicate that simply removing interruptions can dramatically improve the rate of return of spontaneous circulation. At the same time, it appears that the application of mild hypothermia initiated after restoration of circulation can improve the neurologic outcome of cardiac arrest patients to a degree unanticipated only a few years ago. The combination of the improved chest compression and mild hypothermia has led to preliminary reports of intact survival in more than 50% of patients suffering out-of-hospital sudden death. We must admit that, even as enthusiasts of resuscitation medicine, we did not dream that improvements of this magnitude would occur for decades to come. Confirmation of this improvement in well-controlled clinical trials would mark an important event in medical history.

Our continued difficulty in treating cardiopulmonary arrest reflects ongoing limitations in our understanding of the pathophysiology of global ischemia and reperfusion. Yet the past few years have seen remarkable progress. Better understanding of the reperfusion event, reflected in delineation of phenomena such as programmed cell death, and the genomic and proteomic patterns during reperfusion, can only lead to even greater improvements in outcome. But we really do not understand fully the pathological processes that are taking place in these patients, and physicians are naturally uncomfortable in using therapies that are not fully understood and have not been clearly demonstrated to be effective. Nonetheless, the precarious status of these patients does not allow us the luxury of waiting for more definitive knowledge. We must apply all our skills, and our limited knowledge, immediately if persons with "hearts and brains too good to die" are not to be lost forever.

This text is for clinicians who wish to practice both the science and the art of resuscitation medicine. Every physician will at some time attempt to resuscitate a patient from sudden death, but few will have had the opportunity to learn from teachers dedicated to this skill. That, ultimately, is the purpose of this book. In each chapter, recognized authorities have been asked to review present knowledge, and describe the state of their art. Cardiac arrest patients do not have the luxury of seeking out experts. They must rely on the basic knowledge of all physicians.

This is intended to be a comprehensive text incorporating critical analysis of material not readily available elsewhere. The text begins with chapters that place our current knowledge into context, describing the magnitude of the problem. The next sections describe the basic science of ischemia and reperfusion at the cellular, organ system, and organismal levels and the pathophysiology of cardiopulmonary arrest and resuscitation. The final sections focus on state-of-the-art therapy for cardiopulmonary arrest, first without respect to etiology and then under specific circumstances. Contributors were asked to provide insights that complement widely disseminated guidelines. The last section focuses on the pathophysiology and therapy of postresuscitation syndrome, a complex disease state that underlies much of the morbidity and death in these patients.

The last few years have seen acceleration in publications related to resuscitation. We may be at the end of the beginning of what may be looked back upon as a rapid expansion in our knowledge of sudden death, global ischemia, and reperfusion injury. We hope that the second edition of the text not only accurately reflects the field, but provides a foundation upon which it may advance.

The Editors

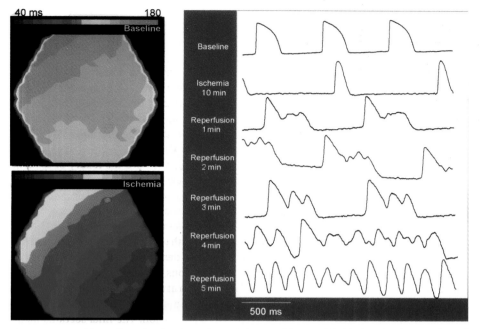

Plate 6.3 Optical map of conduction in a guinea pig heart subject to global ischemia. The crowding of conduction isochrones indicates substantial slowing of conduction with ischemia and during early reperfusion. Optical APs during ischemia and reperfusion reveals AP shortening with ischemia and relengthening with reperfusion that is spatially and temporally heterogeneous and is associated with afterdepolarization-mediated triggered activity.

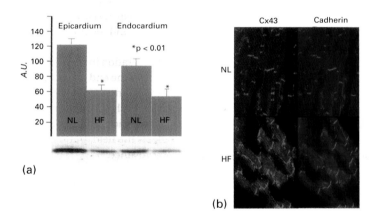

Plate 6.6 Decreased expression and redistribution of Cx43 protein in the failing heart. (a) Western blot shows a reduction in Cx43 protein in the failing heart (HF) in both the endocardial and epicardial regions of the left ventricle compared with normal heart (NL). (b) Immunohistochemical staining demonstrates redistribution of Cx43 from the cell ends to the lateral margins of the cell. Cx43 co-localizes with the intercalated disc protein N-cadherin in the normal but not the failing ventricle. Modified from Akar et al.[151] reproduced with permission.

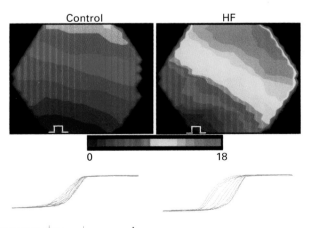

Plate 6.7 Slowed conduction in the failing heart. Optical maps from wedges of left ventricular myocardium stained with a voltage-sensitive dye. Isochronal maps reveal crowding of isochronal lines in the failing tissue preparation. Below the maps are the upstrokes of the action potentials from several regions in the imaging window; the separation of the upstrokes confirms the conduction slowing in the failing heart.

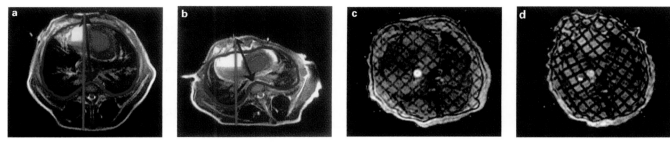

Plate 9.10 Axial MRI images of pig thorax during CPR. Left panels (a and c) are images during relaxed phase. Right panels (b and d) are at peak compression. Panels a and b illustrate the type of measurements that can be performed. The light blue line demonstrates the anterior-posterior distance of the sternum. Areas of the sections through the left ventricle (red) and the intrathoracic cavity (green) can be readily calculated. The image in panel A was taken before compression and panel b at the peak compression (20% AP distance). Deformation of the chest wall, the heart and other organs is clearly visible. Also visible is that the direction of compression was not through the sternum-spine axis (blue arrow), thus shortening at this axis cannot be calculated simply from the AP distance. Panels c and d illustrate the use of tagging. MRI images are acquired during multiple phases of the compression-release cycle. Recording the movement of the tagged grid produces a strain map. The complex features of deformations during the circumferentially compressed phase are clear (panel d).

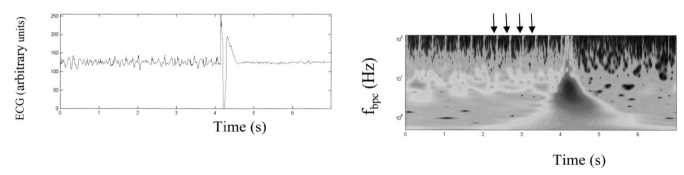

Plate 21.2 Attempted defibrillation of human ventricular fibrillation. *Left:* 7 seconds of human ECG exhibiting VF containing a defibrillation shock event. *Right:* Scalogram corresponding to the ECG signal. Notice the high frequency spiking prior to the shock evident in the scalogram – indicated by arrows. (After Addison *et al., IEEE Eng. Med. Biol.* (2002) © IEEE 2002.)

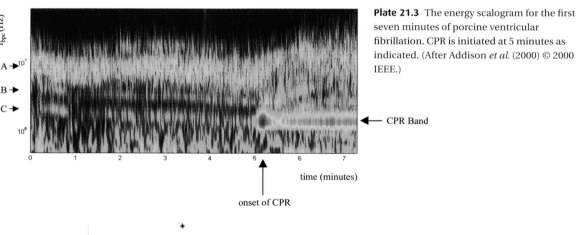

Plate 21.3 The energy scalogram for the first seven minutes of porcine ventricular fibrillation. CPR is initiated at 5 minutes as indicated. (After Addison *et al.* (2000) © 2000 IEEE.)

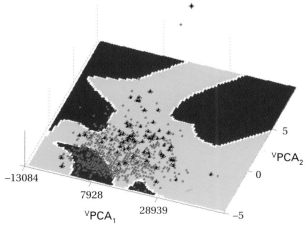

Plate 21.4 Defibrillation outcome prediction. Decision regions corresponding to the ROSC/noROSC prediction problem. The classes are identified by the following color scheme: yellow = decision region for ROSC (restoration of spontaneous circulation), blue = decision region for noROSC. The coordinate corresponding to ROSC outcomes are shown as stars (*) and noROSC as points (.). To predict the outcome of an ECG tracing, the features vPCA1 and vPCA2 are computed from the tracing. If the coordinate point corresponding to (vPCA1,vPCA2) is mapped into the yellow decision area, an ROSC outcome is predicted. If it is found to be in the blue area, a noROSC outcome is predicted. (After Eftestøl *et al. Resuscitation* (2005) © Elsevier 2005.)

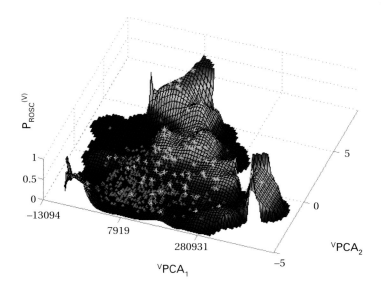

Plate 21.5 The probability of ROSC. A functional relationship between the feature representations of all the VF waveforms extracts and corresponding ROSC/NO ROSC outcome with the feature representation coordinates from Fig. 21.4 superimposed. This can be explained as a division of the feature space defined by vPCA1 and vPCA2 into equal-sized cells. In each cell the PROSC value is estimated as the number of ROSC coordinates divided by the total number of coordinates in the cell. To compute the probability of successful outcome of an ECG tracing, the features vPCA1 and vPCA2 are computed from the tracing. The coordinate point corresponding to (vPCA1,vPCA2) is mapped onto the PROSC function surface, where the probability value can be read directly. (After Eftestøl *et al. Expert Rev. Cardiovasc. Ther.* (2003) © Future Drugs 2003.)

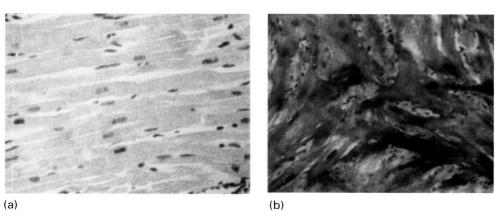

(a)　　　　　　　　　　(b)

Plate 65.11 Histopathology of hypertrophic and dilated cardiomyopathy. (a) The normal architecture of healthy myocardium shows orderly alignment of myocytes with minimal interstitial fibrosis. (b) Hypertrophic cardiomyopathy, demonstrating marked enlargement and disarray of myocytes (red) with increased interstitial fibrosis (blue). Stains: (a), hematoxylin and eosin; (b), Masson trichrome. (With permission from ref. 32.)

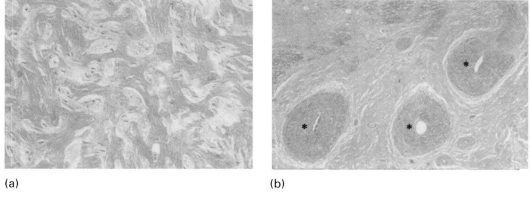

(a)　　　　　　　　　　(b)

Plate 65.12 Histological specimen of hypertrophic cardiomyopathy in a 13-year-old showing (a) marked cellular disarray with hypertrophied cells arranged in a chaotic pattern; (b) several abnormal intramural coronary arteries, with markedly thickened walls and narrowed lumina. RV = right ventricle; hematoxylin and eosin stain in (b) and (c); original magnifications ×50. (With permission from ref. 40.)

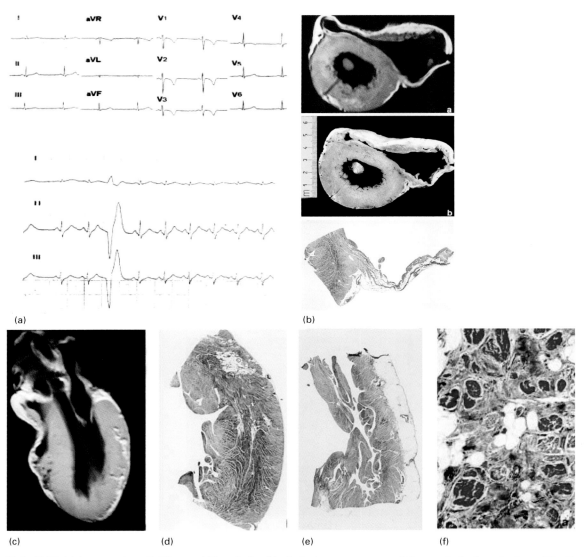

Plate 65.13 (a) An asymptomatic 17-year-old boy died suddenly during a soccer game. Retrospectively, the only signs of the disease were basal ECG showing T-wave inversion in right precordial leads up to V4 and isolated premature ventricular beat of left bundle-branch block morphology during step test. (b) Same case, in vitro NMR cross-sectional view showing a uniformly whitish right ventricular free wall with anterior and inferior aneurysms (note a spotty involvement of the posterolateral wall of the left ventricle); also, corresponding cross section of the heart specimen with infundibular and inferior subtricuspidal aneurysms, and panoramic histological view of the inferior aneurysm showing wall thinning with fibrofatty replacement. (c) In vitro NMR scan in the long-axis view showing extensive involvement of the anterior free wall of the right ventricle and patchy involvement of the posterior wall of the left ventricle; the interventricular septum is spared. (d) Corresponding panoramic histological view of the left ventricle showing a spot of fibrofatty replacement of the myocardium. (e) Control heart from a 20-year-old man who died in a motor vehicle accident. Panoramic histological view of the lateral free wall of the right ventricle: the fatty tissue is limited to the subepicardium and only slightly infiltrates the myocardium. (f) Myocardial atrophy with fibrous and fatty tissue replacement (Azan stains; original magnification, (a) (b) (e) and (f) ×2.5). (With permission from ref. 65.)

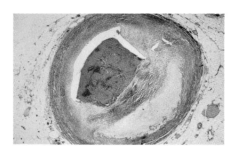

Plate 65.20 Fresh occlusive thrombosis of the proximal anterior descending coronary artery superimposed by an eccentric atheromatous plaque with a large lipid core in a 33-year-old man who died suddenly. Azan stain, original magnification ×25. (With permission from ref. 18.)

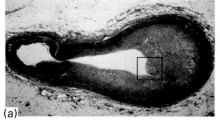
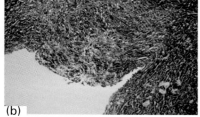

Plate 65.21 Proximal left anterior descending coronary artery of a 30-year-old man who died suddenly. (a) Histology showing an obstructive eccentric fibrous plaque at the origin of the first diagonal branch. Note the preserved tunica media. Azan stain, original magnification × 25. (b) Close-up of the boxed area showing a layer of intimal cell hyperplasia. Azan stain, original magnification × 200. (With permission from ref. 18.)

Part I

Introduction

A history of cardiopulmonary resuscitation

Mickey S. Eisenberg[1], Peter Baskett[2], and Douglas Chamberlain[3]

[1] Department of Medicine, University of Washington, Seattle, WA, USA
[2] Formerly Department of Anaesthesia, Frenchay Hospital and the Royal Infirmary, Bristol, UK
[3] Prehospital Research Unit, School of Medicine, Cardiff University, UK

For much of recorded history, humans have viewed death as irreversible. For religious and scientific reasons it was considered impossible, or even blasphemous, to attempt to reverse death. It was not until the latter part of the eighteenth century that humans began to believe that resuscitation was possible. Another 200 years passed before the skills for resuscitation were developed to a degree that made the reversibility of cardiac arrest a practical reality in the 1960s. Many important observations and much real progress had nevertheless been made during the intervening years. But the clinical problems were poorly understood, the implications of new discoveries were not always appreciated, single components of life-saving were attempted in isolation, procedures that were potentially effective were often displaced by those of no value, and suitable technology was lacking. Resuscitation had to await its time. Nevertheless, its history is of interest and has important lessons for us today.

The earliest years

The first written account of a resuscitation attempt is that of Elijah the prophet. The story in the Bible tells of a grief-stricken mother who brought her lifeless child to Elijah and begged for help. Elijah stretched himself upon the child three times and, with the assistance of God, brought the child back to life. An even more detailed account of a resuscitation attempt is that of the prophet Elisha, a disciple of Elijah. The child of a Shunemite couple whom Elisha had befriended suffered from a severe headache. He cried out, "*Oh, my head, my head!*" and collapsed. Was this a subarachnoid bleed? The Bible gives no further clues. The boy

died several hours later. The frantic mother found Elisha who entered the house and:

> . . . placed himself over the child. He put his mouth on his mouth, his eyes on his eyes, and his hands on his hands, as he bent over him. And the body of the child became warm. He stepped down, walked once up and down the room, then mounted and bent over him. Thereupon, the boy sneezed seven times, and the boy opened his eyes.

Some authorities speculate that the weight of Elisha compressed the child's chest and that Elisha's beard tickled the child's nose and caused subsequent sneezing! Perhaps this is the origin of the phrase "*God bless you*" following a sneeze.[1]

From biblical times until the Middle Ages, several people stand out in the quest to reverse sudden death. Among these is Galen (AD 130 to 200), who lived in Greece. His writings – more than 22 volumes – influenced medicine for the next 1300 years: until the sixteenth century he was considered the final authority on all matters related to health and disease. His experiments, conducted mostly on pigs and monkeys (human vivisection was taboo!), constituted a fund of anatomical and physiological knowledge. Throughout the Middle Ages, there could be no divergence from the "truth of Galen" – however wrong he may have been in some of his writings.[2] Galen taught that the innate heat of life was produced in the furnace of the heart. It was turned on at birth and extinguished at death, never to be lit again. This strongly held belief, passed on through the centuries, is one reason why no one believed that death could be reversed. A non-breathing person was not receiving pneuma; the heart's furnace became permanently cooled.

Cardiac Arrest: The Science and Practice of Resuscitation Medicine. 2nd edn., ed. Norman Paradis, Henry Halperin, Karl Kern, Volker Wenzel, Douglas Chamberlain. Published by Cambridge University Press. © Cambridge University Press, 2007.

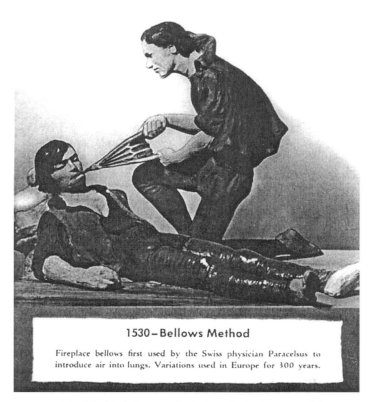

1530 – Bellows Method

Fireplace bellows first used by the Swiss physician Paracelsus to introduce air into lungs. Variations used in Europe for 300 years.

Fig. 1.1. The bellows method of ventilation (courtesy of the Chicago Museum of Science and Industry).

With the end of the Western Roman Empire in AD 476, Western culture entered a millennium of intellectual stagnation that influenced every aspect of society, including medicine. The first stirring of modern scientific inquiry occurred during the Renaissance and reached fruition in the Enlightenment of the eighteenth century. The work of the two great anatomists of the Renaissance, Andreas Versalius and William Harvey, finally began to erode the inviolable "truth of Galen."

In 1543 Andreas Versalius (1514 to 1564), at 28 years of age, published *De Humani Corporis Fabrica*,[3] a remarkable treatise on human anatomy which began to discard the ancient Galenic superstitions. Versalius' ability to refute the statements of Galen was due largely to the availability of cadavers. The judge of the Padua criminal court became interested in Versalius' early work and in 1539 made the bodies of executed criminals available, apparently delaying executions for his convenience.[4] Although, strictly, he was not the first in the sixteenth century to describe artificial ventilation, he described how the lungs of animals collapsed after the chest was opened and that the heart was then affected.[3] But then:

. . . that life may. . . be restored to the animal, an opening must be attempted in the . . trachea, into which a tube of reed or cane should be put; you will then blow into this, so that the lungs may rise again and the animal take in air. . . I have seen none. . . that has afforded me greater joy!

Versalius must be considered the true father both of modern anatomy and of resuscitation. Sadly, his heterodox views were widely condemned. To avoid execution, allegedly for conducting an autopsy on a nobleman whose heart was seen to be beating, he set out on a pilgrimage to the Holy Land but died before he was able to return.[4–6]

As is so often the case, a new idea emerges almost simultaneously from more than one source. The illustration on the use of bellows for artificial ventilation (Fig. 1.1) is from the frontispiece of the 1974 American Heart Association publication on standards for cardiopulmonary resuscitation;[7] it has a notation that the method dates from 1530. It was in that year, 13 years before the publication of Versalius' great work, that Paracelsus[8] was said to have used the technique in an apnoeic patient. But he, too, was a controversial figure, driven out of Basel to wander through Europe, eventually to meet a violent death.[9,10] He had much less influence on subsequent events than did Versalius. Indeed, no firm evidence exists to confirm the belief that Paracelsus was responsible for the use of bellows for ventilation or indeed wrote on the topic at all![2]

In the following century, the pace of progress quickened. The English physician William Harvey, who had studied in Padua 60 years after Versalius, was the first to provide a definitive description of the circulatory system in *Exercitatio Anatomica de Motu Cordis et Sanguinis in Animalibus*.[11] *De Motu Cordis*, as it is commonly known, wrought a revolution in medicine and biology after it was published in 1628 with only 17 brief chapters and 72 pages. Robert Hooke was among a group of gifted all round British scientists in the latter part of the seventeenth century, which included Robert Boyle, Isaac Newton, Thomas Willis, and Christopher Wren.[12] He was a prominent member and Curator of the Royal Society which had been founded in 1660. In October 1667, Hooke demonstrated to the members of the Society – using a dog – that the movements of the heart and lungs were independent of each other but that the action of the heart was entirely dependent on lung inflation with air.[13] Hooke also experimented with combustion and showed that fresh air was essential for burning charcoal and that "satiated air" would not support combustion. One hundred years before the discovery of oxygen, Hooke drew the analogy between fresh and "satiate" in combustion and in respiration in animals "*who live no longer than they have fresh air to breath.*"[14]

By the eighteenth century, the stage was set for an explosion of experimentation and growth in knowledge about the human body. This burgeoning of scientific discovery and the development of the scientific method occurred during the period known as the Enlightenment. Its leaders claimed that the means to discover truth was through the scientific method. The rise of secularism and the concomitant rise of science allowed the first attempts at resuscitation to be made. In the mid 1700s the four main components of resuscitation (artificial ventilation, artificial circulation, electricity, and emergency medical services) began to emerge. They would eventually develop and coalesce, giving us the ability to reverse death.

The search for artificial ventilation

Deaths during the eighteenth century must be placed in their medical context. People did not generally die from cardiovascular disease; they died principally from accidents, infectious disease, drowning, and smoke inhalation from fires. One of the first accounts of mouth-to-mouth resuscitation appeared in 1744,[15,16] although the event actually took place in 1732. A Scottish surgeon named William Tossach was called to a man overcome by

nauseous steam arising from coals set on fire in the pit. His skin was cold, there was not the least pulse in either heart or arteries and not the least breathing could be observed. I applied my mouth close to his and blowed my breath as strong as I could, but having neglected to stop all his nostrils, all the air came out of them, wherefore taking hold of them with one hand . . . I blew again my breath as strong as I could, raising his chest fully with it and immediately I felt six or seven beats of the heart.

Tossach added that the man had walked home 4 hours later. Tossach modestly commented that his technique "*is at least very simple, and absolutely safe, and therefore can at least be no harm, if there is not an advantage in acquainting the publick of it.*" John Fothergill, a London practitioner, did feel when he learned of the incident in 1745[17] that for facts of such great importance it is the duty of everyone "*to render them as extensively public as it is possible.*" And so indeed he did, with a list of indications for its use that included suffocation in water.

Drowning was by then a matter of great and growing concern. Fothergill, together with wealthy and benevolent gentlemen in Holland, was influential in the formation in 1767 of a Society for the Recovery of Drowned Persons in Amsterdam (*Maatschappy tot Redding van Drenkelingen*), later called the Humane Society (Fig. 1.2a). One year after its establishment, magistrates in Milan and Venice began

similar societies. In 1769, the city of Hamburg passed an ordinance providing notices to be read in churches describing assistance to be given to drowned, strangled, and frozen persons and those overcome by noxious gases. Paris began a rescue society in 1771, followed by London (Fig. 1.2b) and St. Petersburg in 1774.[18] Within 4 years of its founding, the society in Amsterdam claimed that 150 persons were saved by their recommendations.[19] The members of the society recommended: (*a*) warming the victim; (*b*) removing swallowed or aspirated water by positioning the victim's head lower than feet, applying manual pressure to the abdomen, and tickling the victim's throat; (*c*) stimulating the victim by such means as rectal and oral fumigation with tobacco smoke; (*d*) using a bellows or mouth-to-mouth method (mouth-to-mouth or mouth-to-nostril respiration is described including the advice that "*a cloth or handkerchief may be used to render the operation less indelicate*"); and (*e*) bloodletting. In general, 6 or more hours were considered a reasonable duration for a resuscitative effort.[19,20]

Unfortunately, mouth-to-mouth ventilation was soon discouraged by the Royal Humane Society of London. This was partly on aesthetic grounds, a consideration even today, but also because Priestley had discovered by 1774 that the composition of expired air was different from that which was inhaled – and therefore "*unfit to enter any lungs again.*"

Although some recommendations for mouth-to-mouth ventilation continued through the nineteenth and early twentieth centuries,[21] it was well out of fashion and virtually forgotten. William Hunter considered it to be "*a method practised by the vulgar.*"[22] So it was that the Royal Humane Society in 1782, less than 10 years after it had been formed, recommended bellows once again in preference to mouth-to-mouth ventilation.[18] By this time, the technique had been developed and refined. In 1776, John Hunter (the brother of William Hunter who guided his early career) had presented to the Society the results of experiments in which bellows were designed to be introduced into one nostril, while at the same time the other nostril and the mouth were occluded. Its mechanism generated both positive and negative pressure.[23] It is noteworthy that John Hunter had also gained considerable experience in humans and made attempts to revive persons who had been hanged as a judicial process.[24]

But using bellows to blow into the nose was clearly not satisfactory, nor universally accepted. The Versalius technique of tracheal intubation was becoming fashionable again, even while bellows and the mouth-to-mouth methods were still in vogue. There were very full details of the technique in a letter from Dr William Cullen[25] dated 1776: "*Dr. Monro informs me, it is very practicable to introduce directly into the glottis and trachea a crooked tube such*

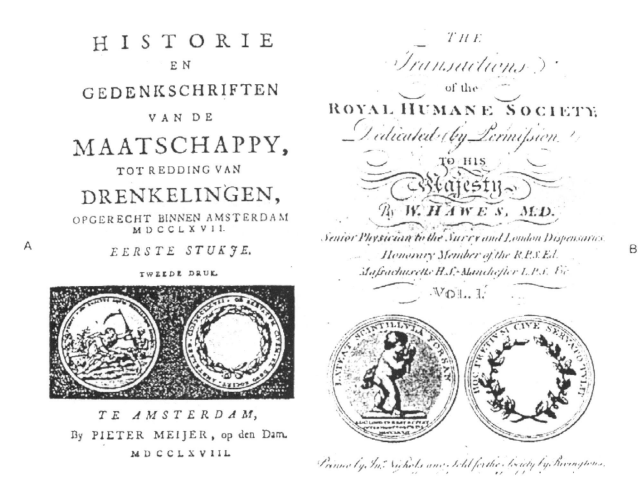

Fig. 1.2. (a) An account of the founding of the Amsterdam Rescue Society in 1767.
(b) Cover of *Royal Humane Society of London Transactions,* showing medals awarded to rescuers (by courtesy of the Society).

as a catheter used for a male adult." Dr. Monro, a professor of anatomy, had other prescient views, for in the same letter we read:

Whether blowing in is done by a person's mouth or by bellows, Dr. Munro opines that the air is ready to pass by the gullet into the stomach, but that this may be prevented by pressing the lower part of the larynx backwards upon the gullet. To persons of little knowledge of anatomy it is to be observed that the pressure should be only on the cricoid cartilage, by which the gullet may be flattened, while the passage through the lungs is not obstructed.

Cricoid pressure became accepted in anesthesia and in resuscitation 185 years later after its description by Sellick,[26] but he and others subsequently became aware of Dr. Munro's earlier recommendation.[27]

Despite all the shortcomings and ill-advised notions on treatment, efforts to prevent death from drowning were

nevertheless effective. Herholdt and Rafn[28] reported in a landmark publication of 1796 that 990 lives had been saved by 1793, with a survival rate over the previous 9 years of 50%. The efforts showed commitment and ingenuity. The amphibious craft illustrated in Herholdt and Rafn's book (Fig. 1.3) was used to move quickly over rough ice to reach drowning victims; if the ice gave way, the rescuer himself would not be at risk because he had a safe haven all around him. The value of postural drainage to empty the lungs was, however, more controversial, especially as it was recognized that the lungs even in fatal cases might remain relatively dry.

By this time, interest had been aroused not only in resuscitation but also in the numbers being treated. Charles Kite was an active member of the London Humane Society who wrote an Essay on the Recovery of the Apparently Dead in 1778 describing the epidemiology of drowning for which he

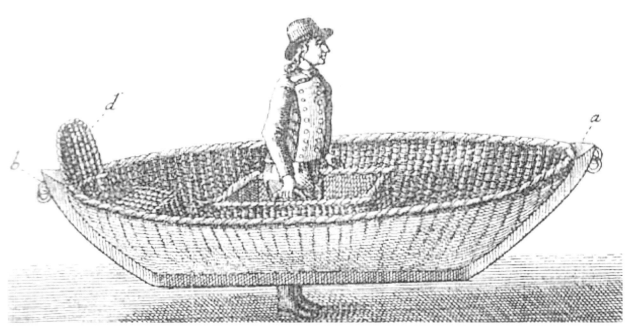

Fig. 1.3. An amphibious rescue craft designed for work on ice.

was awarded the Silver Medal of the Society.[29] He has been described as the father of resuscitation epidemiology.[30] He emphasized the need to keep accurate records and the need for speedy intervention. He advocated artificial ventilation with warm air or "*dephlogisticated air*" (see below) and suggested cricoid pressure and treatment of cardiac arrest with electric shocks. He was a methodical person and designed a pocket resuscitation kit in a case with "*a collection that comprehends every article except an electrical machine*" and also a description of the correct way to use these instruments[31] "*. . .it will prove a very considerable acquisition to the resuscitation air.*" He practiced his theories and describes vividly his experience of a remarkable recovery from drowning in a soldier with a head injury.[32]

At this time, the concepts of fresh and satiated air, set down by Versalius and Hooke two and one centuries earlier, were refined by three scientists working in different countries and more or less independently, although they had some contact. Although the credit for discovering oxygen is usually given to Priestley (1775)[33] from England and Lavoisier from France (1775),[34] it is now agreed that Carl Scheele, a Swedish chemist working in Germany was the first to isolate "*fire air*" in 1772 and 1773. He demonstrated that this was essential for plants to live but could not make an accurate analogy with human respiration. He was slow to publish his findings and his paper of 1777[35] followed that of Priestley who had published his work 2 years earlier in 1775.[33]

Priestley was a Yorkshireman who had trained as a priest and a teacher but had a passion for the composition and chemistry of gases.[36] In 1774, while acting as librarian to the Earl of Sherborne, Priestley had collected a colorless odorless gas from heating red mercuric oxide with sunlight focused through a 12-inch burning lens. He had isolated oxygen but did not call it that – he called it "*dephlogisticated air*" and recorded that it supported combustion vigorously and that a mouse survived in a sealed container filled with this gas for much longer than in atmospheric air. He inhaled the gas himself and "*I fancied that my breast felt peculiarly light and easy for some time afterwards.*"[37]

Lavoisier was born in Paris and studied both law and a wide spectrum of scientific subjects, including geology, mineralogy, electricity, anatomy, biology, chemistry, botany, and weather forecasting.[36] In 1766, he was awarded a Gold Medal by the King for the design of a new form of street lighting for Paris. Lavoisier was aware of the work of Scheele and Priestley but branched out further. He was able to demonstrate that "*air eminently respirable*" or "*fire air*" or "*dephlogisticated air*" was an element, and that when combined with hydrogen it formed water. This newly discovered element was renamed oxygen. He undertook a number of experiments that showed that oxygen was consumed during respiration and carbon dioxide and heat were produced, especially during exercise and after a robust meal.

Both Priestley and Lavoisier were liberals and supported the French Revolution. This was not to stand them in good stead. Priestley was vilified in England and had to emigrate to the United States where he died in Pennsylvania in 1804. Lavoisier was beheaded in public (immediately after his father-in-law). Joseph-Louis Lagrange is quoted by Wilkinson[36] as having said "*It took only an instant to cut off that head but it is unlikely that a hundred years will suffice to produce a better one.*"

In the middle of the nineteenth century, a major change occurred in artificial respiration. Marshall Hall (1790 – 857), a physician in London, advocated the use of mechanical expansion and compression of the chest wall. In his paper *Asphyxia, its rationale and its remedy* of 1856,[38] he criticized the Royal Humane Society's techniques, and recognized that in a supine position the victim's tongue and larynx fell back and blocked the airway. His method involved repeatedly shifting the victim's position from prone (expiratory) to side (inspiratory) 15 times a minute.[39] Over the next 100 years, dozens of other mechanical methods were promoted. Henry Silvester, a London physician, advocated raising the victim's arms above the head to expand the upper rib cage and then placing them on the chest and applying pressure to cause exhalation.[40] A New York physician, Benjamin Howard, described what he called the direct method in which the victim was placed on his or her back while a bystander held the tip of the tongue.[41] The rescuer knelt astride the patient's hips and pushed into the upper abdomen and squeezed the ribs at a rate of 15 times per minute. In 1890, the Royal Medical and Chirurgical Society in England formed a committee under the chairmanship of Sir Edward Sharpey-Shafer to evaluate current methods but concluded that they were all inadequate.[42] (Schafer has caused confusion by adding Sharpey to his name in honor of his teacher in anatomy and physiology, William Sharpey.) Although essentially an histologist and the author of the standard textbook of the time, *Essentials of Histology*, which had appeared in 1899 and continued through 17 editions until 1953,[43] Shafer also had a profound interest in artificial respiration. He developed a new method[44] with intermittent pressure on the back of the prone victim which he believed not only achieved adequate gas exchange, but also maintained an open airway, allowed water and mucus to drain away, posed no other risk to other organs, was easy to learn, and could be performed without fatigue. Schafer did comparative experiments on his laboratory assistant using each of the methods devised by Hall, Silvester, Howard, and himself and claimed that his own method produced by far the best expired minute volumes (6.76 L). Although this method faced considerable opposition (and some said that perhaps Schafer's laboratory assistant was too keen to please his professor[45]), it gradually became a standard, both throughout much of Europe and in the United States, and

was not dropped from the First Aid Textbook of the American Red Cross until 1959 when the whispers of its detractors rose to a clamor.[46]

The methods used for mechanical artificial respiration did vary, however, on a geographical basis. Silvester's method was followed in Germany,[47] Holland, and Russia, whereas Schafer's method was followed in the United States, England, France, and Belgium.[48] Colonel Holger Nielsen, in Denmark, believed that the best solution to the controversy was to develop yet another method that combined the best features of both the popular techniques. His original plan was to have two rescuers: one was to perform prone pressure on the lower back to cause exhalation, whilst the other rescuer was to lift the arms above the victim to facilitate inhalation. The Danish Red Cross rejected this proposal in 1930 because it could not be performed by a single person. Nielsen went back to the drawing board. Apparently, his breakthrough came when he visited a masseur for relief from rheumatic pains in his shoulders. Nielsen noticed that when the masseur pressed down on his shoulder blades he experienced a forceful expiration. This personal experience led him to suggest in 1932 that a single rescuer be positioned at the head of the victim, alternating pressure on the upper back for expiration with arm lifting for inhalation. He presented physiological data to support the superiority of his prone back pressure–arm lift method over Schafer's or Silvester's techniques. Acceptance of Nielsen's method by Red Cross societies was rapid. Instruction in the new artificial respiration spread throughout Europe and to the United States.[48]

Frank Eve, a physician who practiced in Hull in Yorkshire, adopted a different approach.[49] He regarded the thorax as a cylinder with a piston, the diaphragm. He noted that the cylinder wall is often rigid, especially in elderly men and in victims of drowning. He believed it was better to exploit the piston element

Essentially the method consists of laying the patient on a stretcher which is pivoted about its middle on a trestle and rocking up and down rhythmically so that the weight of the viscera pushes the flaccid diaphragm up and down.

Eve produced case reports in 1932[50] to support his rocking method and experimental evidence in 1933[51] claiming tidal volumes of 650 ml – much greater than the various chest compression and arm lift methods. His technique was officially adopted and endorsed in the United Kingdom by the Royal Navy during the Second World War, before being superseded by the expired air method.

In 1949, Archer S. Gordon began evaluating different methods of artificial respiration to determine which was most effective. Gordon's research included measurements on fresh corpses from the adult wards of Cook County Hospital in Chicago. With no research funds available at first, Gordon worked with no salary and, since he was on-call 24 hours, slept in his supervisor's office. He later recalled: *"When I received a call that a patient had expired, I rushed across the street, got my cart of equipment, rushed to the ward, moved the corpse to a secluded examining room, and proceeded with my studies."* Gordon would insert a tube into the trachea and connect it to a respirometer; it was long before the days of sophisticated electronic measurement devices. He measured the results of his experiments on the smoked drums of a kymograph. Not only did he smoke the paper for the drums himself, but also after each case he would shellac the tracing in order to preserve the record. Gordon's early results were published in 1950.[52]

Meanwhile, the US Defense Department became interested in his work; some form of manual resuscitation might help soldiers stricken by nerve gas. At the instigation of the military, Gordon began working with live subjects. He anesthetized medical student volunteers and paralyzed them with curare in order to carry out procedures similar to those used on corpses. By 1951, his considerable bank of data had shown that a modified Holger Nielsen method of manual respiration surpassed all others that he had tested, in terms of efficacy and ease of performance learning. In a subsequent paper,[53] Gordon alluded to mouth-to-mouth and mouth-to-nose artificial respiration, but stated that because of the "*difficulties involved in studying and teaching the method, it has not been included in these tests.*" It was a missed opportunity. Had Gordon included mouth-to-mouth ventilation in his tests, he would have found it to be far superior to any of the manual methods.

Gordon's research came after 200 years of experiments in artificial respiration. In 1953, Karpovich was able to list 105 published methods recommended for adults and 12 for infants.[1] With the cacophony caused by the advocates of so many methods, and with none being truly effective, it is no wonder that confusion, argument, and controversy ruled. Many of the experiments by Gordon and others were done with tracheal tubes in place, thanks to the inventiveness of Kuhn,[54] Magill,[55,56] and Mackintosh[57] and thus the problem of obstructed airway was never taken into account. Even if the airway was not obstructed, these techniques resulted in air exchanges well below that which was needed to sustain life. In the early 1950s, the world awaited a better method.

The kiss of life

James Elam was the first contemporary investigator to prove that expired air was sufficient to maintain adequate oxygenation, when he used mouth-to-nose breathing on patients with acute poliomyelitis paralysis during an epidemic in Minnesota in 1946.[58] These episodes invariably occurred at times of equipment failure or when patients arrived in the hospital with acute respiratory paralysis.

Elam chose mouth-to-nose ventilation because he believed it was the obvious thing to do in such emergencies. He described his first experience in detail:[59]

I had just gotten to Minneapolis . . . and I was browsing around to get acquainted with the ward when along the corridor came a gurney racing – a nurse pulling it and two orderlies pushing it and the kid on it was blue. I went into total reflex behavior. I stepped out in the middle of the corridor, stopped the gurney, grabbed the sheet, wiped the copious mucous [sic] off his mouth and face, tilted his head back, took a big breath, sealed my lips around his nose, and inflated his lungs. In four breaths. I kept on because they had to do a tracheostomy. He was just totally unable to swallow; he had bulbar polio.

With a zealot's passion he spoke of the value of mouth-to-nose ventilation whenever he could, drawing attention to the ineffectiveness of the Holger Nielsen method. To prove that exhaled air was adequate to oxygenate a non-breathing person, Elam obtained permission to do studies on postoperative surgical patients before they recovered from ether anesthesia. The tracheal tube was left in place and succinyl choline was continued as a drip. Elam found by blowing into the tube with his expired air that normal arterial oxygen saturation could be maintained in the patients. After he had published his results in 1954,[60] the US Army Chemical Center in Edgewood, Maryland, recognized the potential value of Elam's findings as a method for ventilating victims of nerve gas (anticholinesterase) poisoning. Although impressed by a successful technique that required no respiration equipment, the Army could not endorse the technique without the blessing of the National Research Council. The Red Cross, meanwhile, was unconvinced that expired air resuscitation was superior to other techniques: manual methods continued to prevail.[61]

By good fortune, Peter Safar joined James Elam on a long car journey from an anesthesia meeting in Kansas City to their homes in Baltimore in October 1956; their 2 days together led to a collaboration that was to change resuscitation practice for ever. Safar was stimulated to become involved in resuscitation research and began a series of experiments on curarized volunteers to see if mouth-to-mouth artificial respiration was effective. By the spring of 1957, he had proved conclusively three essential points in relation to artificial ventilation:[62] first, simply tilting a person's head backward would usually open the airway; second, most existing manual ventilation techniques provided little air, whereas mouth-to-mouth provided excellent artificial ventilation; third, mouth-to-mouth resuscitation could be performed easily and effectively.

Review (ethics) committees did not exist at the time of Safar's experiments on human subjects; the chief investigator was responsible for ensuring the safety of subjects and for the ethical conduct of research. Safar was well aware of the potential risks. He went to great lengths to explain the experiment to the subjects, instituted multiple safeguards to ensure their safety, and supervised each experiment himself. The volunteers were heavily sedated and thus were not conscious of their paralysis, which generally lasted 1 to 3 hours. All subjects breathed a combination of 50% oxygen and 50% nitrous oxide and were closely monitored. No one was allowed to remain in a non-breathing state for more than 90 seconds, and the high oxygen content of the blood (from breathing 50% oxygen) made this safe.[62]

Within a year, Elam, Safar, and Gordon convinced the world to switch from manual to mouth-to-mouth methods.[63] A 1958 issue of *J. Am. Med. Assoc.* contains the following endorsement:[64]

Skilful performance of expired air breathing is an easily learned, lifesaving procedure. It has revived many victims unresponsive to other methods and has been proved in real emergencies under field conditions. Information about expired air breathing should be disseminated as widely as possible.

The invention of the self-inflating bag valve mask by Ruben in 1957 provided a key advance in artificial ventilation that was independent of compressed gas and the aesthetic drawbacks of the mouth to mouth method.[65,66] It became, and remains, the optimal method for healthcare professionals to provide artificial ventilation in the emergency situation.

The search for artificial circulation

Probably the first mention of chest compression to treat cardiac arrest appeared in a dental journal – written by John Hill, an English surgeon, in 1868.[67] He treated patients aged 72, 12, and 8 – all of whom were recognized as having lost both respiration and circulation as a result of chloroform. The front of the chest was compressed forcibly three times each 15 seconds, and the inspiration that followed a rapid release was used to administer ammonia (now known to be a potent venoconstrictor!). All survived; the younger child regained a pulse only after 15 minutes of treatment and relapsed once – but nevertheless made a slow recovery over several days. Better known is the 1883 recommendation of Professor Franz Koenig to use

sternal compression for artificial ventilation.[68] Eight years later, Dr. Friedrich Maass, one of his assistants, performed compressions in two patients intentionally to counter chloroform-induced cardiac arrest.[69] One case involved an 18-year-old man who had lost his pulse during induction of anesthesia and was regarded as dead. Maass initially tried a slow rate of chest compressions to simulate respirations, but, when the situation did not improve, he increased the rate to 120 compressions per minute and noted a carotid pulse. Within 25 minutes the patient achieved a spontaneous pulse and blood pressure. After the man recovered Maass operated on him without complications. Maass concluded: "*So long as compression is applied at the speed of the patient's breathing, slow deterioration. When compression is speeded up, gradual improvement follows. . .*" Maass later described his technique thus:

One steps to the left side of the patient facing his head, and presses deep in the heart region with strong movements . . . The frequency of compression is 120 or more per minute. The effectiveness of the efforts is recognized from the artificially produced carotid pulse and the constriction of the pupils.

External chest compressions survived, predominantly in Germany, for several more decades,[70] but it was used in association with the inefficient methods of artificial ventilation by then in vogue and failed to become well established. Case reports were not widely available because they were published only in German or French, but more importantly the technique could not be successful in most cases of cardiac arrest until defibrillation was developed. No therapy, regardless how innovative, was likely to gain widespread acceptance if it rarely or ever succeeded. Moreover, the relationship between heart disease, ventricular fibrillation, and sudden death was not appreciated until well into the twentieth century. As a result, the role of chest compression to support an artificial circulation was largely ignored until it was rediscovered in 1960.

Open chest cardiac massage was also introduced relatively late, despite the cardiac arrests that occurred during anesthesia. Although Moritz Schiff had practiced and described the technique under experimental conditions and chloroform anesthesia in 1874,[71,72] the first recorded attempt in man was by Niehans in Berne – recorded by a colleague in 1903.[73] But the first definite success had occurred 2 years earlier in Tromsø: it was described only after Igelsrud told a colleague of it when he visited the USA.[74] Interest in open cardiac massage continued for a while. Green in 1906[75] described 40 cases that were by then in the literature, of which nine had been "entirely successful" and eight others had shown transient recovery of pulse and respiration. But it was never a procedure that, by itself, would have a high success rate, nor could it be widely applied.

The accidental rediscovery of artificial circulation occurred in William Kouwenhoven's laboratory at Johns Hopkins University in Baltimore.[76] Kouwenhoven and Guy Knickerbocker were studying fibrillation in the hearts of anesthetized dogs. In one series of experiments they wanted to determine how long they could leave a dog's heart fibrillating and still achieve defibrillation successfully. On this particular occasion they had taken an anesthetized dog and inserted a catheter into the femoral artery to measure its arterial blood pressure. While observing the dog's fallen arterial pressure, Knickerbocker applied the defibrillator's paddles to the animal. He noticed a blip on the blood pressure indicator. The force of the application of the paddles to the dog's chest had caused a pulsation of blood and a momentary increase in arterial pressure apparently. Knickerbocker called Kouwenhoven over, and they both observed the phenomenon. By repeatedly applying the paddles, they were able to extend the period of time the dog's heart was in fibrillation from approximately 1 minute to several minutes and still successfully achieve defibrillation.

Several weeks after the initial observation, James Jude, a surgical resident at the time, joined the team. All three soon realized that they could use their hands to apply pressure to the chest and achieve artificial circulation. At first it was not at all evident where to compress the chest. Should it be side to side? front to back? on the upper chest? lower chest? Through a series of experiments in late 1958 the team discovered that the best procedure was to apply rhythmic pressure on the lower part of the sternum and press straight down using the heel of the hand. Other locations led to higher rates of complications, including lacerations of the liver, stomach, or lungs. They repeatedly measured actual arterial pressures and through trial and error discovered that the optimal depth of compression should be 1 to 2 inches and the best rate of compression was approximately 60 to 80 per minute.[61] Their success with dogs led the three experimenters to consider trying the technique on humans. Jude and other residents began applying the experimental results to living patients. The first person to have this lifesaving procedure, recalled Jude, was described as follows:[77,78]

. . . rather an obese female who was having a cholecystectomy and was being held in the emergency room just before surgery. The patient went into cardiac arrest as a result of fluothane anesthetic . . . This woman had no blood pressure, no pulse, and ordinarily we would have opened up her chest and done direct cardiac massage. Instead, since we weren't in the operating room, we applied external cardiac massage and they immediately switched back to

straight oxygen in ventilation. Her blood pressure and pulse came back at once. We didn't have to open up her chest. They went ahead and did the operation on her, and she recovered completely.

In 1960 the three investigators reported their findings on 20 cases of in-hospital cardiac arrest.[76,79] Fourteen of the 20 patients (70%) survived and were discharged from the hospital. Many of the patients were in cardiac arrest as a result of anesthesia. Three patients were documented to be in ventricular fibrillation. The duration of chest compression varied from less than 1 minute to 65 minutes. The article was very clear: chest compression buys time until the external defibrillator arrives on the scene. As the authors write in the article: "*Anyone, anywhere, can now initiate cardiac resuscitative procedures. All that is needed is two hands.*" However, respiration or ventilation received relatively little attention in the 1960 article. Many of the patients had been intubated. Soon, however, chest compression formally 'married' mouth-to-mouth ventilation: the couple's new name was CPR.

The birth of cardiopulmonary resuscitation

Ventilation and compression combined

Between 1958 and 1961 artificial respiration was combined with artificial circulation to create CPR. The period began with demonstrations that mouth-to-mouth ventilation was effective for artificial respiration and chest compression was effective for artificial circulation. Now all that was needed was the formal connection of the two techniques to create CPR as it is practiced today. And that took place at the scientific level when Safar, Hackett, Jude, and Kouwenhoven presented their findings at the Maryland Medical Society meeting held on September 16, 1960 in Ocean City. In the opening remarks the moderator said: "*Our purpose today is to bring to you, then, this new idea.*" It was so new that it was still without a name. The moderator stated that the two techniques "*cannot be considered any longer as separate units, but as parts of a whole and complete approach to resuscitation.*"[80] In his remarks Safar stressed the importance of combining ventilation and circulation. He presented convincing data that chest compression alone did not provide effective ventilation; that required mouth-to-mouth respiration.

To promote CPR, Jude, Knickerbocker, and Safar began a world speaking tour. In 1962 Gordon, along with David Adams, produced a 27-minute training film called *The Pulse of Life*. The film was used in CPR classes and viewed by millions of students. For the film, Gordon and Adams devised the easy to remember mnemonic of A, B, and

C standing for the sequence of steps in CPR: airway, breathing, circulation. In 1963, the American Heart Association formally endorsed CPR. Three years later, the National Research Council of the National Academy of Sciences convened an *ad hoc* conference on cardiopulmonary resuscitation. The conference was the direct result of requests from the American National Red Cross and other agencies to establish standardized training and performance standards for CPR. Over 30 national organizations were represented at the conference; its recommendations were reported in *J. Am. Med. Assoc.*[81]

From electrical therapy to defibrillation

The discovery of electricity is obscured by antiquity, but the ancient Greek and Chinese civilizations were aware of magnetic properties of lodestones. But for 2000 years no progress occurred in the understanding of magnetism or electricity. Superstition and the occult ruled. The Renaissance allowed scientific inquiry to begin, and superstitions slowly began to crumble. William Gilbert (1544 to 1603), physician to Queen Elizabeth I, performed the first experiments that clarified the properties of magnets and electrostatic charges and published *De Magnete* in 1600.[82] Gilbert gave us the word electricity.

By the middle of the eighteenth century, electricity was thought to be so pervasive that it was considered to be the fifth element after fire, water, earth, and air. In 1743, Johann Gottlob Kruger who was Professor of Medicine at the University of Halle wrote omnisciently: "... .*through electrification, changes in the deepest regions of the human body can be brought forth.*" Electricity, he claimed, would be *"a new kind of cur,"* and he called for experiments to demonstrate its effect on life. Kruger predicted a benefit of electricity in the treatment of paralyzed limbs. Electricity would function "*just as one uses flagellation with nettles to restore sensation and reestablish the power of motion.*" Kruger's lecture and subsequent publication on the application of electricity to medicine earned him the title of founding father of electrotherapy.[83]

Kruger's contemporaries soon began to recommend electricity for many different ailments. A student of Kruger's named Christian Gottlieb Kratzenstein reported the successful use of electrotherapy in paralysis in 1744. He wrote of "*a woman who lost the paralysis in her small finger within one quarter of an hour by electrification.*"[84] This unknown woman may have been the first person to benefit from electrotherapy. It was a humble beginning to a journey that would culminate 200 years later in Cleveland, Ohio, with the first successful defibrillation of a human heart.

An account of what was purported to be a human resuscitation by electricity had already been described in 1774 in the Register of the Royal Humane Society of London in relation to a child who had fallen out of a window and appeared to be dead:[85]

Mr. Squires tried the effects of electricity. Twenty minutes elapsed before he could apply the shock, which he gave to various parts of the body in vain; but, upon transmitting a few shocks through the thorax, he perceived a small pulsation; in a few minutes the child began to breathe with great difficulty. . .

Kite provides an illustration of the device likely to have been used by Mr. Squire to resuscitate the child (Fig. 1.4).[86] Kite's device may properly be called a proto-defibrillator. All of the elements of a modern defibrillator are there: it had a source of energy in a Leyden jar that served as a capacitor; an electrometer functioned as the energy setting; brass knobs served as the electrodes; metallic strings were equivalent to the cables; and glass or wooden tubes served as insulators to prevent the operator from being shocked. Or as Kite so delicately put it, "*In this manner, shocks may be sent through any part of the body . . . without a probability of the assistants receiving any inconvenience.*" But with the delays that had occurred and the nature of the event, it is hard to credit that fibrillation and defibrillation had occurred in this instance.

The history of true defibrillation may well go back to 1775, the year after Dr. Squires's experience. Abildgaard, a remarkable Danish veterinarian does not seem to be well known and deserves better recognition. An excellent account of his role in defibrillation and a translation from Latin of his relevant writings were published to commemorate the bicentennial of his experiments.[87] He wrote:

I took a hen, which I knocked down with the first shock directed to the head. . . it lay without feeling as if completely dead and was unable to be aroused by any stimulus. . . I tried an electric shock directed through the chest to the spine . . . it rose up and, set loose on the ground, walked about quietly on its feet. . . after the experiment was repeated rather often, the hen was completely stunned, walked with some difficulty, and did not eat for a day and night; then later it was very well and even laid an egg.

Why did he do such an experiment, and indeed was the hen really dead? His two further quotes seem to address these questions satisfactorily:

. . . all reports of men, slain by a bolt of lightning, state that nothing in such bodies, when dissected, was found which was sufficient to be called the cause of death. . . I took a different hen, along with the same cock, upon which I had conducted the second experiment. I left both on the ground. . . made lifeless by one shock. . . But on the next morning I found them completely dead and very cold, and I

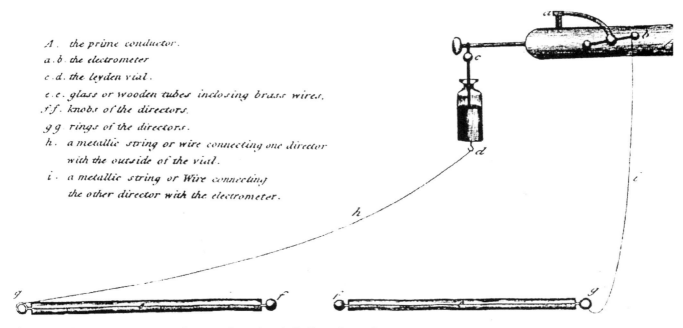

A. the prime conductor.
a.b. the electrometer
c.d. the leyden vial.
e.e. glass or wooden tubes inclosing brass wires.
f.f. knobs of the directors.
g.g. rings of the directors.
h. a metallic string or wire connecting one director
   with the outside of the vial.
i. a metallic string or wire connecting
   the other director with the electrometer.

Fig. 1.4. Kite's apparatus containing elements of a modern defibrillator (from ref. 6).

was unable to revive them with the electrical machine with any amount of trying.

It is noteworthy that, while the capacitor discharge to the head was capable of killing a chicken, revival needed a discharge across the thorax. His work did not go unnoticed at the time, with at least two subsequent references in the literature including an anonymous comment in 1779[88] that was particularly prescient: that Dr. Abidgaard's experiments may lead to conjectures "*as to the cause of death from lightning, but also, perhaps, to important discoveries with respect to the means of recovery in such a case.*"

The potential of capacitors is limited. But in 1799, Alessandro Volta, Professor of Physics at the University of Pavia, used the principle of two dissimilar metals to generate electricity by creating the world's first electrochemical battery.[89] This followed from Galvani's discovery that the leg of a frog twitched when in contact with both iron and brass.[90]

Galvani's work made it obvious that electricity led to muscle contractions. Starting a stilled heart with electricity became an important goal of medical science. Physicians still had little understanding of the heart's electrical conduction system, but they knew it was a muscle. What was not clear, however, was whether an arrested heart could be restarted. The ability to restart a non-beating heart was essential if death were to be reversed. Many studies took place at the beginning of the 19th century, but the results

were contradictory and inconclusive. During the French Revolution, the French anatomist and physiologist, Xavier Bichat, realized the advantages of studying the issues of electricity and the heart on the bodies of victims of the guillotine. Bichat received permission from the revolutionary authorities to conduct electrical experiments on freshly decapitated bodies. He tried to stimulate the muscles and the heart using galvanism and chemical stimulants. He concluded that the heart could be excited reliably only by direct contact with electric stimulation.[82] Other French scientists performed similar experiments and reached somewhat contradictory conclusions. The time interval from death to the performing of the experiments, which was the most important factor explaining the heart's responsiveness, was often not taken into account. The importance of time was intensively studied in a special commission formed by the Academy of Turin in Italy. The conclusion of the committee was that the heart lost its ability to contract in response to electrostimulation 40 minutes after death.[82]

In 1804, Aldini, who was Galvani's nephew, wrote about the need to integrate artificial respiration and electric therapy. According to Aldini, electricity should be used immediately and not after a long period of artificial ventilation, the sequence recommended by most other scientists. Aldini wrote: "*Artificial respiration ought to be attempted but it should be accompanied by the application of Galvanic power externally to the diaphragm and to the region of the heart.*" He may thus have been the first to advocate a combination that presaged modern CPR and defibrillation. Aldini freely admitted to ignorance about how electricity affects the heart, but "*. . that it does affect (the heart) has, I trust, been sufficiently demonstrated by experiments.*"[91]

The use of electricity for resuscitation and the need to apply it rapidly were evident in the advice of Richard Reece, a London physician. In *The Medical Guide* in 1820,[92] Reece described the optimal means of resuscitation. He wrote:

> In cases of suspended animation what is necessary to be done should be done quickly; therefore, on the first alarm of any person being drowned or suffocated, while the body is searching for, or conveying to the nearest house, the following articles should be got ready: viz. warm blankets, flannels, a large furnace of warm water, heated bricks, a pair of bellows, warming-pan, sal volatile, clyster pipes, and an electrifying machine.

His book provides an example of such an electric machine and a description of the device by its inventor, de Sanctis. The device, called a *reanimation chair*, consists of a voltaic battery, a bellows to ventilate the lungs and a metal tube to be inserted in the esophagus for delivery of stimulating vapors. The three resuscitation items were packaged in a carrying case and available for purchase in a medical supply store in London. The bellows was to be inserted in the mouth and the nose clamped shut. An assistant was to press on the ribs to cause expiration after each ventilation with the bellows. The voltaic pile was to be suspended from a hook attached to the back of a chair. One wire from the battery was attached to the metal tube in the oesophagus, and the second wire was to be successively touched to "*the regions of the heart, the diaphragm and the stomach . . .*"[92] There is no record of anyone being resuscitated successfully by use of the reanimation chair. Nevertheless, the pathway of electric stimulation advocated by de Sanctis was not totally bizarre. Stimulation with an esophageal electrode was explored in 1956 as a means of achieving cardiac pacing; and in 1979 the first automatic external defibrillator was designed with a posterior pharynx–anterior chest pathway of current flow.[93]

Which route of electricity – chest, neck, or total body stimulation – was best for treating heart conditions provided a common source for debate in the nineteenth century. Many scientists and physicians claimed that total body electrification was most beneficial for cardiovascular disease and gave names to these types of therapy that sounded more scientific than they were. Electrohydriatics or electrobalneotherapy referred to immersion in a tub of electrified water. For a static bath with cephalic douche the patient sat in a dry tub with sparks applied to the head. Autoconduction, also known as inductothermia, involved standing inside a large circular solenoid cage, which used

a high-frequency electricity of several hundred thousand oscillations per second. According to the inventor of such a device, "*These currents can be very powerful. They produce no pain or conscious phenomenon in the person treated. The current, nevertheless, acts very energetically on the tissues.*"[92] This treatment was similar in principle to microwaving the entire body! High-frequency treatments were especially popular in France from 1890 to 1930 and were used to treat diabetes, gout, obesity, and many other conditions.[82] Virtually every disease and malady, according to some authority, could benefit from electricity.

Little progress could be made in using electricity to counter sudden death until the most frequent underlying cause had been discovered. A lethal arrhythmia that we now know as ventricular fibrillation was first described in 1850 by Hoffa and Ludwig in Germany.[94] They demonstrated that strong galvanic or faradic currents applied directly to the ventricles of a dog's heart caused a disordered and ineffective action. This was given a variety of names: tremulations fibrillaires, delirium cordis, intervermiform (wormlike) movements, fibrillar contractions, herz-delirium, undulatory movements, and intervermicular actions. Ludwig was also known for his development of the kymograph (which became the direct precursor of the electrocardiogram), although he did not specifically use his kymograph to record ventricular fibrillation. It was considered only a curiosity with little relevance to humans.

John MacWilliam in a series of articles from 1887 to 1889 published in the *British Medical Journal*, made the first detailed descriptions of ventricular fibrillation. Until that time, it had been assumed that sudden cardiac failure took the form of quiet standstill. Experiments that MacWilliam performed on dogs refuted this idea. He described how tumultuous activity could have an effect similar to that of a motionless heart:[95]

> In many of these cases the fatal issue is determined or ensured by the occurrence of fibrillar contraction in the ventricles. . . . A sudden, unexpected, and irretrievable cardiac failure may, even in the absence of any prominent exciting cause, present itself in the form of an abrupt onset of fibrillar contraction (ventricular delirium). The cardiac pump is thrown out of gear, and the last of its vital energy is dissipated in a violent and prolonged turmoil of fruitless activity in the ventricular walls.

McWilliam[96] was the first to speculate that fibrillation is the most common mode of sudden death in humans, including those induced by anesthetics. No one picked up on his theory until 1913, when Levy showed convincingly the relationship between chloroform and fibrillation.[82] He was also aware that defibrillation is more difficult to induce in a healthy heart than in a diseased or weakened heart.

McWilliam never investigated the effect of electricity to stop the fibrillations of a heart muscle, nor is it certain that he even thought of this possibility. He did, however, appreciate the value of electrical pacing. The concept was not new. Steiner[97] had successfully paced a variety of animals with chloroform-arrested hearts using direct current via needles thrust into the heart, and even tried it in a patient! Green[98] was later successful in man using hand-held external electrodes, whilst McWilliam[99] described a path from the back to over the cardiac apex. But we had to wait until 1952 for external pacing to be accepted[100] and until 1959[101] for acceptable intracardiac pacing.

It was not anesthesia, which could cause all forms of cardiac arrest, but rather accidental electrocutions, that led to further work on ventricular fibrillation. Many Western nations began to use electricity during the last two decades of the nineteenth century, and accidental deaths from electrocution entered the scientific community's consciousness. Investigators in the 1880s believed that death from electrocution was caused by respiratory paralysis secondary to overwhelming trauma to the central nervous system: "...*the condition after the shock is merely one of suspended animation in which respiratory function is suspended.*"[82]

Final proof that electrocution caused ventricular fibrillation came at the turn of the century. Jean Louis Prevost and Frederic Battelli, both physiologists, reported in the year 1899[102] that a weak current passed through the heart or through the intact chest fibrillated the heart. But their interest was not only in the induction of fibrillation: crucially, they also took a major interest in the restoration of the heart beat by electricity and were the first to show unequivocally that it was possible:

... we asked ourselves what would be the effect of applying a high voltage current on a dog whose heart had just been put into a state of ventricular tremulation. We worked on 6 dogs, in three of which we noticed that the heart that had been paralysed with ventricular tremulation started to beat again and the pressure rose and stayed up after the application for 1–2 s of a 4800 volt current applied from the head to the feet.

It does seem, however, that they did not appreciate the importance of their findings in relation to sudden death, despite McWilliam's earlier speculations. Three decades passed before others came to appreciate the significance of Prevost and Battelli's work and its relevance to humans.

Even when the problem of ventricular fibrillation was widely understood, no one believed that anything could be done to alleviate it. In 1913 the Electric Light Association of Chicago commissioned a report addressing resuscitation from electric shock. The report acknowledged ventricular fibrillation as a cause of death in linemen but stated "*a*

solution of the problem in a manner permitting the life of the individual to continue may be impracticable."[103]

During the first two decades of the twentieth century, researchers pursued non-electrical interests related to chemical fibrillation when the real solution should have been within their grasp. Chemical defibrillation was investigated in the hope that a regular heartbeat would resume or could be started with another chemical agent. It was also advocated erroneously to stop defibrillation so that heart massage could be more effective. Salts of potassium chloride were the most common agents used for chemical defibrillation, but calcium chloride was also used to start an arrested heart.[104] The connection between electricity and defibrillation was picked up again in 1926, when the Consolidated Electric Company of New York City sought advice from the Rockefeller Institute on how to deal with the alarming number of fatal electric accidents among its workers. The institute in turn funded research at several universities, including Johns Hopkins University, which was also supported later by the New York Edison Power Company.

In 1930, Donald Hooker, William Kouwenhoven, and Orthello Langworthy, with funding from Edison Power, began to study the direct effects of electricity on the heart.[105] They confirmed that electric shocks, even small ones, could induce ventricular fibrillation in the heart and that more powerful shocks could eliminate the fibrillation. Moreover, after inducing ventricular fibrillation in dogs they were then able to defibrillate the heart without opening the chest.[106] Their closed-chest defibrillation was effective only if the fibrillatory contractions were vigorous and the period of absent circulation or breathing did not exceed several minutes: longer periods required openheart massage for electric shocks to be successful. Since an initial shock was required to place the heart in ventricular fibrillation, it was only logical to call the subsequent shock that defibrillated the heart the countershock. The term *countershock* was used synonymously for many years to mean attempted defibrillation. They were by then close to developing effective defibrillation in humans.

But it was a surgeon who achieved this breakthrough. Claude Beck had worked for years in Cleveland, Ohio on a technique for defibrillation of the human heart. He witnessed a cardiac arrest while an intern in 1922: the anesthetist announced that the patient's heart had stopped during a urological procedure. To the amazement of Beck, the surgical resident removed his gloves and went to a telephone in a corner of the room and called the fire department.[107] He remained in total bewilderment as the fire department rescue squad rushed into the operating room 15 minutes later and applied oxygen-powered resuscitators to the patient's face. The patient died, but the episode left an indelible impression on Beck. Twenty years later he wrote, "*. . . surgeons should not turn these emergencies over to the care of the fire department. We should take care of them ourselves. . . And so I prepared myself to handle it.*"[108] Beck would go on to develop techniques to take back the management of cardiac arrest from the fire department and place it in the hands of surgeons. Ironically, 20 years after his accomplishment the management of most cardiac arrests in the USA once again returned to the fire department.

Cardiac surgeons during the 1930s were well aware that ventricular fibrillation, when it occurred during an operation, was fatal. Beck and his colleague Mautz[109] quoted case reports, but believed that drugs together with electricity could potentially stop ventricular fibrillation in man as had been shown in dogs. They believed that "surgeons should be equipped to use this method." But 10 more years were to pass before long-term success was achieved.

On the basis of the work of Hooker and Kouwenhoven, Beck decided to construct an alternating current (AC) internal defibrillator. He achieved his first successful resuscitation in 1947.[110] A 14-year-old boy was undergoing surgery for a severe congenital funnel chest. The 3-hour operation was uneventful except for a 45-minute period of a rapid heart rate of 160 beats/min for which digitalis was used. During the closure of the large incision in the chest, the pulse suddenly stopped and the blood pressure fell to zero. The boy had gone into cardiac arrest. Dr. Beck immediately reopened the chest and began manual heart massage that was continued for 35 minutes. Another 10 minutes passed before the defibrillator arrived in the operating room. The first shock using electrode paddles placed directly on the sides of the heart was unsuccessful. Beck gave a second successful shock after administering procainamide, and in a very few seconds a feeble, regular, and fast contraction of the heart occurred. The blood pressure rose from zero to 50 mm Hg. Twenty minutes after the successful defibrillation, the chest wound was closed. After 3 hours the child awoke and was able to answer questions. He suffered no neurological damage and his exercise tolerance was considerably improved. What started as a straightforward operation led to 45 minutes of cardiac arrest before resuscitation with the first successful defibrillation in a human. Beck thus earned a place in medical history.

Eight years later, in 1955, another medical "first" was achieved when an out-of-hospital cardiac arrest, that occurred just outside the door of the University Hospital in Cleveland, was treated successfully.[111] Dr. Albert T. Ransone – who was 65 – had had an ECG taken in the hospital following chest pain the night before. As he was leaving, he collapsed and was rushed to the emergency department, pulseless, cyanotic, and with dilated pupils. A subsequent review of the cardiogram revealed an acute posterolateral myocardial infarction. Beck and his colleague David Leighninger immediately opened his chest, not even delaying to remove his shirt or prepare the skin. They compressed his heart by hand for 25 minutes until the electrical defibrillator, which was located in a laboratory far distant from the emergency department, was brought. Defibrillation was achieved after the third AC shock of 3 A lasting 2 full seconds. Ransone left the hospital 11 days later and returned to practice before retiring in Florida. He died in February 1984 at 93 years of age. Beck's defibrillator added 28 years of life to someone whose heart "*was too good to die,*" a phrase that was first used in relation to this case.[112]

Although Kouwenhoven's paper mentioned the ability to defibrillate the heart internally, no one at that time, including Kouwenhoven, pursued the possibility of closed-chest defibrillation in humans. The work of his group had been brought to a halt by the Second World War. The research resumed afterwards under the sponsorship of the Department of Surgery at Johns Hopkins and again was funded by the Edison Electric Institute, which had not given up hope that a means of closed-chest defibrillation could be developed for accidental electrocution of linemen.[113] They built a device that was to evolve into the Hopkins AC defibrillator[114] which underwent a long series of tests in dogs. After 52 successful tests, Kouwenhoven, who was an engineer without medical qualifications, approached Dr Blalock with whom he was cooperating but was frustrated to be told that this was not enough: he should run additional tests. While the tests were under way, Kouwenhoven visited Dr Paul Zoll in Boston who was also developing a closed-chest defibrillator.

For Paul Zoll the development of an external defibrillator was a natural extension of his earlier work with an external cardiac pacemaker. Like the other researchers in the field, Zoll had spent several years perfecting the procedure in a series of animal experiments and by 1955 he was ready to try it on humans. On August 22 of that year a 64-year-old woman admitted 5 days earlier for a serious heart attack collapsed with ventricular fibrillation. Zoll and his colleagues applied a single 360-volt countershock using electrodes across the woman's chest.[115] The ventricular fibrillation stopped at once, but her heart did not start beating normally and she died. The next two patients also died following successful external defibrillation, but Zoll remained undaunted. Finally, on November 17, a 67-year-old man survived several episodes of ventricular fibrillation after treatment with Zoll's external defibrillator, and was discharged a month later. Over a period of 4 months,

Zoll had treated ventricular fibrillation 11 times successfully in four different patients. The energy required ranged from 240 to 720 volts. Zoll had worried about the potential damage such high energy could cause but was able later to write: "*The complete recovery in Case 4 after repeated countershock indicates that external defibrillation can be accomplished without ill effect to the patient.*"

The defibrillator Zoll designed, as well as earlier versions invented by Kouwenhoven and Beck, used AC and were run from line (mains) current, the electricity from the wall sockets. These AC defibrillators were very large and heavy, mainly because they contained a transformer to step up the line current from 110 volts to approximately 1000 volts, which was required to defibrillate the heart. The major limitation of AC defibrillators thus was their lack of portability. They could be packaged in a large cabinet, and wheels attached to the bottom would allow some maneuverability, but basically it was difficult to bring them to the patient. Even in the hospital this was time-consuming, and the possibility of transportation to a patient's home was out of the question. Not many lives would be saved unless the inherent non-portability of AC defibrillators could be solved.

Bernard Lown is credited with solving the portability problem in the 1960s. Years later he would win the Nobel Prize for Peace, but another major contribution to humanity was the development of a defibrillator that used DC instead of AC; this allowed battery operation and eliminated the need for a heavy transformer.[116] A capacitor could store energy until it was released in one massive jolt to the chest wall.

In recent years, biphasic waveforms have been shown to have advantages over the simpler monophasic shocks. They could have been available much earlier. Kouwenhoven, Becker, and Knickerbocker had produced a portable defibrillator in 1963 that used a discharge that had been derived by progressively reducing the number of cycles of alternating current until it became "diphasic" – or biphasic as we would now call it. It could be operated using 6- or 12-volt dry batteries. Again this group was well ahead, but had the frustration once more that their progress had escaped wide medical notice, possibly because the device was described only in an engineering journal (Fig. 1.5).[117]

With the development of portable DC defibrillators, prehospital resuscitation had become a practical possibility. Not only could a defibrillator reach a patient more rapidly, but mouth-to-mouth ventilation and chest compression were now available to buy precious minutes of time.

Prehospital resuscitation

The concept of using ambulances to bring aid to the victim rather than the other way around emerged during the Napoleonic war, and the honor of developing the first emergency medical service probably belongs to Baron Dominique-Jean Larrey. In 1792, the Baron – Napoleon's

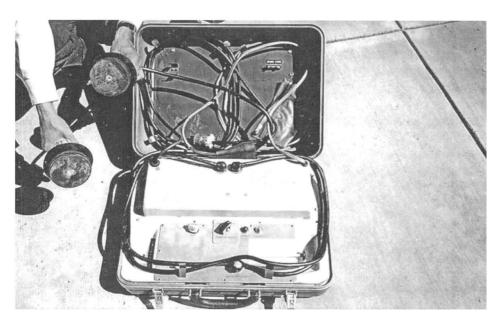

Fig. 1.5. Kouwenhoven's "Mine" biphasic portable defibrillator of 1963.

chief army surgeon – devised the first ambulance service to bring aid directly to the injured soldier. When Larrey first entered the military, the only medical care was well to the rear of the army. After the fighting was over, fallen soldiers would be picked up, and those still alive were taken to field hospitals. Larrey was shocked by the delays in providing even minimal care to soldiers. His indignation led him to design a lightweight, two-wheeled ambulance that allowed the surgeon to be mobile and work directly on the battlefield. The vehicles were called *voitures d'ambulance* because they travelled with the "flying artillery" on the field of battle.[118,119] The term "ambulance" referred at the time to a hospital, not a vehicle, but no doubt it was from this that the more familiar use of the word derives. Civilians were not to benefit from ambulances for many years, although the need had been recognized – especially during times of plague so that "*all possible care should be taken to provide such means of conveyance for the sick that they may receive no injury.*"[120]

Urban ambulance services for civilians first appeared in Cincinnati (in 1865 and in New York City in 1866). Within 15 years every urban area in the USA had some form of ambulance service.[121] Other countries lagged behind. In 1881 a volunteer ambulance service was set up in Vienna after a disastrous fire in a theatre[121a] and Dr. James Cantlie, who had written one of the first English books on first aid, gave a public demonstration that was attended by physicians from Germany, Spain, and Russia – leading to the introduction of civilian ambulances in those countries. In the same year, Reginald Harrison from Liverpool visited the USA to investigate the services and subsequently set up a horse-drawn ambulance managed by the police. In 1903, a steam ambulance was available in London and 1905 a motor ambulance was established in Scotland.[122]

For civilians, ambulance services were for many years merely a means to bring the patient to the hospital but provided no medical care at the scene. In 1914 Cantlie set up a College in London to train attendants with considerable initial success:[123] 14 000 students attended in the first 3 years. But the initiative was not well supported and the College closed in 1923. During the 1930s and 1940s municipal fire departments in some cities of the USA (including Los Angeles, Columbus, Baltimore, and Seattle) began to provide rescue, first aid, and resuscitation care. In 1966 the United States National Academy of Sciences and the President's Commission on Highway Safety issued reports decrying the unevenness of ambulance personnel competency and the lack of standard procedures. The commission described the carnage resulting from traffic accidents as the neglected disease of society. The subsequent National Highway Safety and Traffic Act of 1966[124] authorized the Department of Transportation to establish a national curriculum for prehospital personnel, which led to the training of emergency medical technicians. In the same year, a similar scheme for advanced first aid training began in the UK.[125] But nowhere in the West was there any definitive treatment for prehospital cardiac arrest.

In 1965 Frank Pantridge turned his attention to this vexing problem of heart attacks and sudden cardiac death. His sensitivity to the problem came from two sources. First, personnel in the emergency department of the Royal Victoria Hospital in Belfast frequently commented on the number of patients who were dead on arrival. Second, Pantridge was aware of an epidemiological study in Belfast that indicated that, among middle-aged or younger men with acute myocardial infarction, more that 60% died within 1 hour of the onset of symptoms.[126] Thus the problem of death from acute MI had to be solved outside the hospital, not in the emergency room or the coronary care unit. He wrote:

The majority of deaths from coronary attacks were occurring outside the hospital, and nothing whatever was being done about them. It became very clear to me that a coronary care unit confined to the hospital would have a minimal impact on mortality.

He wanted his coronary care unit in the community.

Pantridge's solution was to develop the world's first mobile coronary care unit, or MCCU. He staffed it with an ambulance driver, a junior physician, and a nurse. Pantridge encountered several obstacles to the creation of the MCCU. He dealt with them in his typical fashion: head-on, with bulldog determination to succeed and transparent contempt for politicians and other authorities who opposed him. A modest grant was obtained, and an old disused ambulance was resuscitated. There were, of course, various other problems. "*My non-cardiological medical colleagues in the hospital were totally unconvinced and totally uncooperative,*" Pantridge said. "*It was considered unorthodox, if not illegal, to send junior hospital personnel, doctors, and nurses outside the hospital.*" But despite all obstacles, Pantridge's new programme began service on January 1, 1966.

Of ground-breaking importance in the 1967 *Lancet* publication by Pantridge and Geddes[127] was the reported outcome in ten patients who had cardiac arrest. All had ventricular fibrillation; six arrests occurred after the arrival of the MCCU, and four occurred before arrival of the ambulance. All ten patients were resuscitated and admitted to the hospital. Five were subsequently discharged. But the system reacted too slowly to resuscitate persons who fibrillated before a call was placed.

When the unit was established, it was assumed that most sudden cardiac deaths in the community were the result of acute myocardial infarction. It was not appreciated that ventricular fibrillation can occur without new infarction and with only seconds of warning – or none at all. Today we know that the mechanisms of sudden death in the community are diverse and complex. The Belfast system was ideal for patients whose hearts fibrillated after the ambulance was at the scene or *en route*. But the article has historical importance because it served to stimulate prehospital emergency cardiac care programs throughout the world. It is noteworthy that August 1967 is 200 years to the month from the founding of the Amsterdam Rescue Society.

Although the concept of mobile coronary care was introduced only in the 1960s, the concept that the doctor should go out to the patient was not new for victims of trauma. Kirschner in Germany had recommended this practice as early as 1938.[128] By 1957 there was a mobile operating unit in Heidelberg with another well equipped system in Cologne.

Paramedic-staffed mobile intensive care units

The extensive international readership of the *Lancet* helps explain why Pantridge's idea spread so rapidly to other countries. Within 2 years, similar programs that included physicians in the MCCU began in Australia and Europe. The first programme in the USA was started in 1968 by William Grace at St. Vincent's Hospital in Greenwich Village in New York City. It was soon followed by a programme in Charlottesville, Virginia, begun by Richard Crampton. Both programs were models of the Belfast programme. They used specially equipped ambulances and placed physicians on board to provide advanced resuscitation care directly at the scene of cardiac emergencies.

William Grace had visited Pantridge in Belfast and spent 10 days learning about the program. Shortly after returning to New York City, Grace set about establishing an MCCU patterned after the Belfast unit. The ambulance operated in the catchment area of a large area in the lower west side of Manhattan. Calls for medical emergencies in which chest pain was a complaint were passed on from the police emergency call number to the hospital. Among the first group of patients seen by the MCCU were three patients treated for ventricular fibrillation of whom one survived.[129]

Like the Belfast program, the St. Vincent's MCCU was not established to provide primary response for sudden cardiac arrest, but rather was designed to treat the early period of acute MI. Ventricular fibrillation, if it occurred after arrival, could be managed, but patients suffering ventricular fibrillation before the MCCU's arrival could seldom be resuscitated. Although the first in the USA to

bring advanced resuscitation directly to the scene of a life-threatening emergency, it was nevertheless limited in vision and was not nationally applicable. An evolution in prehospital emergency care was needed. Pantridge and Geddes had broken the conceptual block that resuscitation was restricted to hospitals. Now someone had to break a conceptual block that kept resuscitation in the hands of physicians. This happened in the USA and in Ireland but with different international impact.

The evolution from physician-staffed mobile intensive care units to paramedic-staffed units in the USA occurred independently and almost simultaneously in six communities. The innovators were Eugene Nagel in Miami, Leonard Cobb in Seattle, Leonard Rose in Portland, Michael Criley in Los Angeles, James Warren in Columbus Ohio, and Costas Lambrew in Nassau County New York. These six programs took a different approach to the problem of cardiac emergencies. Not only were paramedics used instead of physicians, but also from their inception the programs were established to deal with the problem of sudden cardiac arrest that may have already occurred before a call for help was received. Four of the six programs had a strong base of a fire department ambulance service in their communities. Thus it was fire fighters who took on the additional role of paramedics.

Nagel understood that the model of the physician-staffed prehospital MCCU could never become accepted in the USA. Physicians were too expensive to await calls in fire stations, and help would take too long to arrive on scene if they had to be picked up from hospitals. But he moved incrementally, taking radio and telemetry as his first step. Before he could sell the need for defibrillation and medications, he had to prove that not only was ventricular fibrillation a major prehospital problem, but also that the ECG signal could be sent from the field to the hospital. The decision to use telemetry was, however, more than a proving exercise and scientific data gathering. For Nagel it was the Trojan horse that gained him access through the legal impediments that were stopping fire fighters from defibrillating patients and administering medications. He hoped to find support for his innovative approach from the medical community; instead he only encountered discouragement. Nagel recalled this opposition:

It was a rare doctor that favored us doing any of this stuff – very rare. We had incidents in the street when we were just sending an EKG, where doctors on the scene would tell the firemen to quit fooling around and haul the victim in. There were some strange orders out in the field from doctors on the scene. The second big force against our doing anything was from emergency department nurses.[130]

Eventually, opposition was overcome and paramedics were given permission to undertake some emergency procedures without radio contact. Nagel vividly recalled the first save of the Miami paramedic program.

There was a guy named Dan Jones who was then about 60 years old, who was a wino who lived in a fleabag in the bad part of town. Jones was well known to rescue. In June of '69 they got a call – man down – it was Jones. They put the paddles on him, he was in VF, started CPR, zapped him, he came back to sinus rhythm, brought him in to ER and three days later he was out and walking around. In gratitude, about a week later, he came down to Station 1, which he had never done before, and he said he would like to talk to the man who saved his life. They told me they had never seen Dan Jones in a clean shirt and sober, both of which he was that day. He would periodically come to the fire house and just say hello and he seemed to be sober. In my talks in those days I said this was the new cure for alcoholism. That was our first true save.[130]

Pantridge's article also motivated Leonard Cobb in Seattle. He knew the Seattle Fire Department was already involved in first aid and therefore approached the Fire Chief, Gordon Vickery, to propose a new training program to treat cardiac arrest. The fire department already had one of the first computerized systems in the USA for documenting first aid runs. Cobb realized that this system could provide scientific documentation for the efficacy (or lack thereof) of Pantridge's suggestions and suggested to Vickery that they pool their knowledge and resources. Cobb and his colleagues then provided instruction and training in cardiac emergencies including cardiac arrest to volunteer fire fighters. The program became operational in March 1970, 9 months after Nagel's first save in Miami. The mobile unit – and there was only one at first – was stationed outside the Harborview Hospital emergency department. As Cobb himself points out, the mobile unit was not the real innovation. Rather, it was the concept of a tiered response to medical emergencies. The idea was "*that we would get someone out there quickly*" – via the fire department's already existing mobile first aid units – "*and then a secondary response would come from the mobile intensive coronary care unit.*" The beauty of the tiered response system was the efficient use of fire department personnel, which allowed aid personnel to reach the scene quickly (on an average of 3 minutes) to start CPR. Then a few minutes later the paramedics arrived to provide more definitive care such as defibrillation. In this way the brain could be kept alive until the electric shock converted the heart to a normal rhythm. After stabilization the paramedics would transport the patient to the hospital.

The Seattle paramedic program did more than pioneer paramedics and develop a tiered response system. It was the first program in the world to make citizens part of the emergency system. Cobb knew from data the program had collected that the sooner CPR was started, the better the chances of survival. He reasoned that the best way to ensure early initiation of CPR was to train the bystanders. Thus Cobb, with the support of Vickery, began a program in 1972 called Medic 2. Its goal was to train over 100 000 people in Seattle how to do CPR. Cobb recalled how the idea was first proposed:

One day he [Vickery] said, "Look, if it's so important to get CPR started quickly and if firemen come around to do it, it can't be that complicated that other folks couldn't also learn – firemen are not created by God to do CPR. You could train the public." I said, "That sounds like a very good idea." Shortly afterwards things started.[130]

By the twentieth anniversary of the Medic 2 program, over half a million people in Seattle and the surrounding suburbs had received training in CPR in a course of approximately 3 hours. But some people were sceptical about mass citizen training in CPR; indeed, many felt the potential for harm was too great to allow such a procedure in the hands of laypersons. The sceptics also had the support of national medical organizations. The alarmist voices were stilled by some fortunate saves. Cobb recalled one resuscitation soon after the Medic 2 program began involving a man who was indeed in ventricular fibrillation:

In March 1973 there were these kids playing golf at Jackson Park. They came across a victim a quarter of a mile from the clubhouse. But these kids had taken the CPR course over at the local high school. Two or three of them started doing CPR and the other kid ran off and phoned the fire department. Shortly they came with the aid car and Medic 1 screaming over the fairways. They got him started up again. He survived; he's alive today (1990). That was a very convincing story. I didn't mind it being written up in the *Reader's Digest*.[130]

In early 1969 Michael Criley wondered if Nagel's scheme could be set up in the Los Angeles area using the services of existing Fire Department rescue squads, which were, as Criley later put it, "*busy doing things like rescuing cats from trees.*" The mobile units began responding to emergency calls in August 1969, 2 months after the units in Miami. Leonard Rose in Portland developed a slightly different system, one that used private ambulance drivers as paramedics. Having overcome legal difficulties in relation to training, the unit was working by September 1969. In Columbus, Ohio, Warren had long been interested in the problem of sudden cardiac death and had set up the region's first in-hospital cardiac care unit in 1955. He had been deeply impressed by Pantridge's work and, in association with Richard Lewis, set up a scheme with the Fire Department that became operational in October 1969. The

Nassau County program was unique in that police officers were trained as paramedics. A police department-based paramedic service also began in Grand Rapids, Michigan, although this model was not widely imitated. Thus, the decade of the 1960s that had started with the development of CPR had, by its end, effective paramedic programs in six major American cities.

The American systems were not, however, the first to have non-medical personnel using defibrillators for prehospital cardiac arrest. It was the Irish Heart Foundation that led the way,[131] although their pioneering work went largely unnoticed. Two private ambulances in Dublin were equipped with defibrillators and the ambulance staff were trained to use them. From December 1967 to November 1971, 20 patients who suffered a cardiac arrest either immediately before, or after, the arrival of an ambulance were defibrillated by ambulance staff; 11 survived to hospital discharge.

Other schemes were set up in the UK independently of events elsewhere, but were operational effectively only after those in Ireland and the USA. In 1968, encouraged by the success of the Belfast mobile coronary care unit, a pilot coronary ambulance scheme was set up in Brighton under the direction of William Parker, the local Medical Officer of Health. It relied on general practitioners and medical staff from one of the hospitals to provide medical expertise. It responded to few calls, usually without the promised medical cover, and the specialized equipment was rarely used. After one unsuccessful attempt at defibrillation – due primarily to equipment failure – the decision was made to train ambulance personnel who manned the ordinary emergency ambulances. These were operational from 1971 and by the end of the following decade over 40 patients per year were being discharged alive after prehospital cardiac arrest from a population of 300 000.[132] A second initiative was set up in Gloucester and Bristol in the South West of England providing a service from 1972.[133] Originally the emphasis was on effective pain control and ventilation, but soon ambulances were available that were manned by paramedics equipped with mechanical ventilators, intravenous fluids, electrocardiographs with telemetry, and defibrillators. The success of these schemes in Brighton and the South West of England led eventually to a national system of paramedics within the UK.

In mainland Europe, the same motivation to bring treatment to patients with cardiac arrest of life-threatening conditions took a different path. In most countries, the decision was made to have mobile intensive care units that were manned by physicians. The differences between the systems in the USA and the UK on the one hand and France and Germany (with most of Europe) have been described by Dick.[128]

The quest continues

By the early 1970s, CPR, defibrillation, and a rapid means to provide prehospital care were all in place. The structure to resuscitate sudden death victims had been built and was proving successful. That most of the world did not have this structure in place in the 1970s was largely due to lack of diffusion and spread of the ideas, combined with reactionary local inertia, rather than the impossibility of carrying them out.

However, the story of resuscitation does not stop with paramedic defibrillation. By 1975, Diack had already realized that electronic pattern recognition of the waveforms of ventricular fibrillation could be used in the logic of a defibrillator to permit or withhold the electrical discharge.[93] The human role could therefore be reduced to the simple task of recognizing the possible need for defibrillation, applying electrodes, and activating the machine. The first automated unit was used successfully by paramedics in Brighton in 1980,[134] and the first successful randomized trial of their efficacy was published from Seattle in 1989.[135] The introduction of AEDs expanded the possibility for prehospital resuscitation from cardiac arrest enormously, because defibrillation could now be undertaken by laypersons with modest or even no training. They have proved successful when used in fixed sites where cardiac arrest might be expected[136,137] or where access to conventional help is unavailable as in aircraft.[138] They are also being used within the community in so-called first responder schemes[139] and within the homes of vulnerable patients.[140]

Provision of speedy defibrillation was, however, recognized to be only part of the answer in the battle against unexpected sudden cardiac death. Whilst community instruction in CPR can reach many citizens and thus widen the time frame for successful defibrillation, inevitably many calls for help will come from individuals who have not been instructed or lack the confidence to perform poorly remembered skills. There is a role for providing instruction during the emergency itself. In 1981 a programme to provide telephone instructions in CPR began in King County, Washington. This programme used the emergency dispatchers to give instant directions while the fire department EMT personnel were *en route* to the scene.[141] This demonstration project increased the rate of bystander-provided CPR by 50%. Dispatcher-assisted CPR is now standard care for dispatcher centers in many parts of the world.

Guidelines for best practice techniques in basic and advanced life support have been produced by the American Heart Association, the European Resuscitation

Council, and by Resuscitation Councils in other parts of the world. Increasingly, cooperation between organizations and individuals proved valuable. The International Liaison Committee on Resuscitation (ILCOR) was set up in 1992,[142] and now provides a forum for a consensus on the science of resuscitation that permits identical or similar evidence-based practices to be used the world over.

Nonetheless, the last 20 years have not seen a fundamental breakthrough. CPR is basically unchanged since it was first integrated into an effective system in 1960. Defibrillation is also largely unchanged, although further sophistication over and above those of waveform analysis can be expected. The pharmacological management of cardiac arrest has not demonstrated real progress over several decades, and emergency medical services in the twenty-first century are similar to those of the 1970s. The quest to reverse sudden death has not stopped, but it has also not led to a new scientific or historical breakthrough. Increasingly, it must be accepted that cardiac arrest that occurs in the community is a community problem and that emergency services cannot usually be available in time to provide successful definitive treatment. Wider involvement of responders within the community has to be a key strategy. Other significant advances are likely to require a more complete understanding of heart and brain physiology, and perhaps one day we will be able to counter very much more effectively than at present both ischemic heart disease and sudden cardiac death. Future chapters are still to be written.

REFERENCES

1. Karpovich, P.V. *Adventures in Artificial Respiration.* New York: Association Press, 1953.
2. Baker, A.B. Artificial respiration, the history of an idea. *Med. Hist.* 1971; **15**: 336–346.
3. Versalius, A. De humani corporis fabrica. *Libri Septum 1543,* Cap XIX, p.658, Basel. (See Safar, P. History of cardiopulmonary–cerebral resuscitation. In Kaye, W. & Bircher, N.G., eds. *Cardiopulmonary Resuscitation,* New York: Churchill Livingstone, 1989.)
4. *Gillispie's Dictionary of Scientific Biography.* New York: Scribner, 1970.
5. Silverman, M.E. Andreas Versalius and De Humana Corporis Fabrica. *Clin Cardiol.* 1991; **14**: 276–279.
6. Vellejo-Manzur, F., Perkins Y., Varon, J., & Baskett, P. *Resuscitation great*: Andreas Versalius, the concept of an artificial airway. *Resuscitation* 2003; **56**: 3–7.
7. Standards for Cardiopulmonary Resuscitation (CPR) and Emergency Cardiac Care (ECC). *J. Am. Med. Assoc.* 1974; 227(Suppl.): 833–868.

8. Davis, J.E., Sternbach, G.L., Varon, J., & Froman, R.E. Jr. *Resuscitation great*: Paracelsus and mechanical ventilation. *Resuscitation* 2000; **47**: 3–5.
9. Garrison, F.H. *History of Medicine,* 4th edn. Philadelphia: W.B. Saunders, 1929.
10. Gravenstein, J.S. Paracelsus and his contribution to anesthesia. *Anesthesiology* 1956; **26**: 805–811.
11. Harvey, W. Exercitatio anatomica de motu cordis et sanguinis in animalibus. Francofurti, 1628. *The Keynes English Translation,* 1928. Classics of Medicine Library, Birmingham, 1987.
12. Baskett, T.F. *Resuscitation great*: Robert Hooke and the origins of artificial respiration. *Resuscitation* 2004; **60**: 125–127.
13. Hooke, R. An account of an experiment made by M. Hook, of preserving animals alive by blowing into their lungs with bellows. *Phil. Trans.* 1667; **2**: 539–540.
14. Middleton, W.S. The medical aspects of Robert Hooke. *Ann. Med. Hist.* 1927; **9**: 227–243.
15. Tossach, W.A. A man dead in appearance recovered by distending the lungs with air. *Med. Essays Observations* 1744; **5**: 605–608.
16. Bartecchi, C.E. Cardiopulmonary resuscitation – an element of sophistication in the 18th century. *Am. Heart J.* 1980; **100**(4): 580–581.
17. Fothergill, J. Observations on a case published in the last volume of the medical essays, etc. of recovering a man dead in appearance, by distending the lungs with air. *Phil. Trans. Roy. Soc. Lond.* 1745; **43**: 275–281.
18. Bishop, P.J. *A Short History of the Royal Humane Society to Mark its 200th Anniversary.* London: Royal Humane Society, 1974.
19. Cary, F.J. A brief history of the methods of resuscitation of the apparently drowned. *Johns Hopkins Hosp. Bull.* 1918; **270**: 243–251.
20. Lee, R.V. Cardiopulmonary resuscitation in the eighteenth century. A historical perspective on present practice. *J. Hist. Med. Allied Sci.* 1972; **27**: 418–433.
21. Woods, R.H. On artificial respiration. *Trans. Roy. Acad. Med. Ir.* 1906; **24**: 137–141.
22. Hunter, W. Quoted by Keith, A. Three Huntarian lectures on the mechanism underlying the various methods of artificial respiration (Lecture I). *Lancet* 1909; **i**: 745–749.
23. Hunter, J. Proposals for the recovery of people apparently drowned. *Phil. Trans. Roy. Humane Soc.* London, 1776.
24. Moore, W. *Resuscitation great*: John Hunter – Surgeon and resuscitator. *Resuscitation* 2005; **66**: 3–5.
25. Cullen, W.A. A letter to Lord Cathcart, President of the Board of Police in Scotland, concerning the recovery of persons drowned and seemingly dead. *Med. Tracts,* London, 1776.
26. Sellick, B.A. Cricoid pressure to control regurgitation of stomach contents during induction or anaesthesia. *Lancet* 1961; **ii**: 2404–2406.
27. Saliem, M.R., Sellick, B.A., & Elam, J.O. The historical background of cricoid pressure in anaesthesia and resuscitation. *Anaesth. Analg.* 1974; **53**: 230–232.

28. Herholdt, J.D., & Rafn, C.G. *An Attempt at an Historical Survey on Life-saving Measures for Drowning Persons and Information on the Best Means by which They can Again be Brought Back to Life*. Printed H. Tikiob's, Bookseller, with M. Seest. 1796. Reprinted 1960. Scandinavian Society of Anaesthesiologists.

29. Kite, C. An essay on the recovery of the apparently dead (p.146), London. C. Dilly in the *Poultry*, 1788.

30. Eisenberg, M.S. Charles Kite's essay on the recovery of the apparently dead: the first scientific study of sudden death. *Ann. Emerg. Med.* 1994; **23**: 1049–1053.

31. Alzaga, A.G., Varon, J., & Baskett, P. *Resuscitation great*: Charles Kite: the clinical epidemiology of sudden cardiac death and the origin of the early defibrillator. *Resuscitation* 2005; **64**: 7–12.

32. Kite, C. Essays and observations, physiological and medical on the submersion of animals. London, 1795. 377–385.

33. Priestley, J. On different kinds of air. *Phil. Trans.* 1775, London.

34. Lavoisier, A.L. Oeuvres, publiées par les soins de son Excellence le Ministre de l'Instruction Publique et des Cultes, sous la direction de M. Dumas et E Grimaux, Paris, Imprimerie National. (6 vols) 1864–1893.

35. Scheele, C.W. *Chemische Abhandling von der Luft und den Feuer*. Liepzig, 1777.

36. Wilkinson, D.J. *Resuscitation great*: The contributions of Lavoisier, Scheele and Priestley to the early understanding of respiratory physiology in the eighteenth century. *Resuscitation* 2004; **61**: 249–255.

37. Priestley, J. Experiments and observations on different kinds of air. *Philo. Trans.* (6 vols) 1774–86. 1772: **61**: 216.

38. Hall, M. Asphyxia, its rationale and its remedy. *Lancet* 1856; **i**: 393–394.

39. Hall, M. On a new mode of effecting artificial respiration. *Lancet* 1856; **i**: 229.

40. Silvester, H.R. A new method of resuscitating stillborn children and of restoring persons apparently dead or drowned. *Bri. Med. J.* 1858; **ii**: 576.

41. Howard, B. The more usual methods of artificial respiration. *Lancet* 1877; **iii**: 193–196.

42. Writer, D. *Resuscitation great*: Sir Edward Sharpey-Schafer and his simple and efficient method of performing artificial respiration. *Resuscitation* 2004; **61**: 113–116.

43. Talbott, J.H. Sir E.A. Sharpey-Shafer (1850–1935) In *A Biographical History of Medicine*. New York: Grune and Stratton, 1970: 953–956.

44. Shafer, E.A. Description of a simple and efficient method of performing artificial respiration in the human subject, to which is appended instructions for the treatment of the apparently drowned. *Med. Chir. Trans.* 1904; **87**: 609–614. (Also discussion: 615–623).

45. Comroe, J.H. Jr. In comes the good air. Part I. Rise and fall of the Schafer method. *Am. Rev. Resp. Dis.* 1979; **119**: 803–809.

46. Gordon, A.S., Sadove, M.S., Raymon, F., & Ivy, A.C. Critical survey of manual artificial respiration. *J. Am. Med. Assoc.* 1951; **147**: 1444–1453.

47. Keith, A. The mechanism underlying the various methods of artificial respiration. *Lancet* 1909; **i**: 895–900.

48. Brooks, D.K. Historical outline to resuscitation. In Arnold, E., ed. *Resuscitation, Care of the Critically Ill*. London, 1986: chapter 1.

49. Baskett, T.F. *Resuscitation great*: Eve's rocking method of artificial respiration. *Resuscitation* 2005; **65**: 245–247.

50. Eve, F.C. Actuation of the inert diaphragm by a gravity method. *Lancet* 1932; **i**: 995–997.

51. Killick, E.M., & Eve, F.C. Physiological investigation of the rocking method of artificial respiration. *Lancet* 1933; **ii**: 740–742.

52. Gordon, A.S., Raymon, F., Sadove, M., & Ivy, A.C. Manual artificial respiration. *J. Am. Med. Assoc.* 1950; **14**: 1447–1452.

53. Wright-St Clair, R.E. The development of resuscitation. *NZ Med. J.* 1985; **8**: 339–341.

54. Kuhn, F. *Die perorale Intubation*. Berlin: S. Karger,1911.

55. Magill, I.W. Endotracheal anaesthesia. *Proc. Roy. Soc. Med.* 1929; **22**: 83–87 (also reproduced in *Anaesthesia* 1978; **33**: 580–586.

56. Baskett, P.J.F. *Resuscitation great*: Sir Ivan Whiteside Magill KCVO DSc (Hon). *Resuscitation* 2003; **59**: 159–162.

57. Macintosh, R.R. A new laryngoscope. *Lancet* 1943; **i**: 485.

58. Elam, J.O. Rediscovery of expired air methods for emergency ventilation. In Safar, P., & Elam J.O. eds. *Advances in Cardiopulmonary Resuscitation*. New York: Springer-Verlag, 1977: 263–265.

59. Personal interview with author (ME), August 1990.

60. Elam, J.O., Brown, E.S. & Elder Jr. Artificial ventilation by the mouth-to-mask method. A study of the respiratory gas exchange of paralysed patients ventilated by the operator's expired air. *N. Eng L.J Med.* 1954; **250**: 749–754.

61. Safar, P. History of cardiopulmonary-cerebral resuscitation. In Kaye, W., & Bircher, N,, eds. *Cardiopulmonary Resuscitation*. New York: Livingstone, 1989: Chapter 1.

62. Safar, P. Ventilatory efficacy of mouth-to-mouth artificial respiration; airway obstruction during manual and mouth-to-mouth artificial respiration. *J. Am. Med. Assoc.* 1958; **167**: 335–341.

63. Safar, P. & Elam, J.O. Manual versus mouth-to-mouth methods of artificial respiration. *Anesthesiology* 1958; **19**: 111–112.

64. Dill, D.B. Symposium on mouth-to-mouth resuscitation (expired air inflation). Council on Medical Physics. *J. Am. Med. Assoc.* 1958; **167**: 317–319.

65. Ruben, H. A new apparatus for artificial ventilation, (in Danish). *Ugeskr Laeger* 1957: **119**: 14–16.

66. Baskett, P.J.F. & Zorab, J.S.M. *Resuscitation great*: Henning Ruben – The Ruben Valve and the Ambu bag. *Resuscitation* 2003; **56**: 123–129.

67. Hill, J.D. Observations on some of the dangers of choloroform in surgical practice, and a successful mode of treatment. *Br. J. Dent. Sci.* 1868; **11**: 335–338.

68. Koenig, F. *Lehrbuch der allgemeinen Chirurgie*, Erste Abthuilung. Berlin. August Hirchwald, 1883; 60–61.

69. Maass, D. Die methode der wiederbelebung bei herztod nach chloroformeinathmung. *Berl. Klin. Wschr.* 1892; **12**: 265–268.

70. Böhrer, H. & Goerig, M. Early proponents of cardiac massage. *Anaesthesia* 1995; **50**: 869–871.

71. Hake, T.G. Studies on ether and chloroform from Professor Schiff's physiological laboratory. *Practitioner* 1874; **12**: 241–250.

72. Vallejo- Manzur, F., Varon, J., Fromm, R., & Baskett, P.J.F. *Resuscitation great*: Moritz Schiff and the history of open-chest massage. *Resuscitation* 2002; **53**: 3–5.

73. Zesas, D.G. Über Massage des freigelegten Herzens beim Chloroformkollaps. *Zentralbl Chir.* 1903; **30**: 452–464.

74. Keen, W.G. A case of total laryngectomy (unsuccessful) and a case of abdominal hysterectormy) successful) in both of which massage of the heart for chloroform collapse was employed, with notes of 25 other cases of cardiac massage. *Ther. Gaz.* 1904; **20**(third series): 217–230.

75. Green, T.A. Heart massage as a means of restoration in cases of apparent sudden death, with a synopsis of 40 cases. *Lancet* 1906; **ii**: 1708–1714.

76. Kouwenhoven, W.B., Jude, J.R., & Knickerbocker, C.G. Closed-chest cardiac massage. *J Am. Med. Assoc.* 1960; **173**: 1064–1067.

77. Personal interview with author (ME), November 1990.

78. Jude, J.R. Personal reminiscences of the origin and history of cardiopulmonary resuscitation (CPR). *Am. J. Cardiol.* 2003; **92**: 956–963.

79. Jude, J.R., Kouwenhoven, W.B., & Knickerbocker, G.G. Clinical and experimental application of a new treatment for cardiac arrest. *Surg. Forum* 1960; **11**: 252–254.

80. Symposium. Recent advances in emergency resuscitation. *Md State Med. J.* 1961; **10**: 398–411.

81. Cardiopulmonary Resuscitation Committee on CPR of the Division of Medical Sciences, National Academy of Sciences–National Research Council. *J. Am. Med. Assoc.* 1966; **198**: 138–145, 372–409.

82. Schechter, D.C. *Exploring the Origins of Cardiac Electrical Stimulation.* Minneapolis: Medtronic, Inc, 1983.

83. Fink, K.J. Johann Kruger on electricity: "Cui bono," for whom to what good? *Electr. Quart.* Part 1. 1990; **1**: 12.

84. Licht, S. History of electrotherapy. In *Therapeutic Electricity and Ultraviolet Radiation.* Waverley Press, 1967.

85. Stillings, D. The first defibrillation? *Med. Instrum.* 1976; **10**: 168.

86. Schechter, D.C. Early experience with resuscitation by means of electricity. *Surgery* 1971; **69**: 360–372.

87. Abildgaard, P.C. Tentamina electrica in animalibus instituta. *Societatis Medicae Havniensis Collectanea* 1775; **2**: 157–61. Translation in Driscol, T.E., Ratnoff, O.D., & Nygaard, O.F. The remarkable Dr. Abildgaard and countershock. The bicentennial of his electrical experiments on animals. *Ann. Int. Med.* 1975; **83**: 872–882.

88. Anonymous. *Medical and Philosophical Commentaries by a Society in Edinburgh* (p. 255). London. J. Murray, 1779; **6**: 252–255.

89. Volta, A. On the electricity excited by the mere contact of conducting substances of different kinds. *Phil. Trans.* 1800; Part 2; 405.

90. Galvani, L. De viribus electricitatis in motu musculare commentarius. *De Bononiensi Scientarium, et Artium Instituto atque Atademia Commentarii.* 1791; **7**: 363–418.

91. Aldini, J. *General Views on the Application of Galvanism to Medical Purposes; Principally in Cases of Suspended Animation.* London: Royal Humane Society, 1819. p. 97.

92. Reece, R. Electroresuscitation. In *The Medical Guide.* London, 1820.

93. Diack, A.W., Welborn, W.S., Rullman, R.G., Walter, C.W., & Wayne, M.A. An automatic cardiac resuscitator for emergency treatment of cardiac arrest. *Med. Instrum.* 1979; **13**: 78–83.

94. Hoffa, M., & Ludwig, C. Einige neue versuche über Herzbewegung. *Z. Rat. Med.* 1850; **9**: 107–144.

95. McWilliam, J.A. Cardiac failure and sudden death. *Br. Med. J.* 1889; **i**: 6–8.

96. McWilliam, J.A. Fibrillar contraction of the heart. *J. Physiol.* 1887; **8**: 296–310.

97. Steiner, F. Ueber die Electropunctur des Herzens als Wiederbelebungsmittel in der Chloroformsyncope. *Arch. Klin. Chir.* 1871; **12**: 748–790.

98. Green, T. On death from chloroform: its prevention by galvanism. *Br. Med. J.* 1872; **i**: 551–553.

99. McWilliam, J.A. Electrical stimulation of the heart in man. *Br. Med. J.* 1889; **i**: 348–350.

100. Zoll, P.M. Resuscitaton of the heart in ventricular standstill by external electric stimulation. *N. Engl. J. Med.* 1952; **247**: 768–771.

101. Furman, S., & Schwedel, JB. An intracardiac pacemaker for Stokes–Adams seizures. *N. Engl. J. Med.* 1959; **261**: 943–948.

102. Prevost, J-L., & Battelli, F. La mort par les courants électriques – courants alternatifs a haute tension. *J. Physiol. Path. Gen.* 1899; **ii**: 427–442.

103. Report of the Commission on Resuscitation from Electric Shock. Read before the National Electric Light Association, Chicago, June 1913.

104. Hooker, D.R. On the recovery of the heart in electric shock. *Am. J. Physiol.* 1930; **91**: 305–328.

105. Hooker, D.R., Kouwenhoven, W.B., & Langworthy, C.R. The effect of alternating electrical currents on the heart. *Am. J. Physiol.* 1933; **103**: 444–454.

106. Kouwenhoven, W.B., & Hooker, R.D. Resuscitation by countershock. *Electr. Eng.* 1933 (July); 475–477.

107. Meyer, J.A. Claude Beck and cardiac resuscitation. *Ann. Thorac. Surg.* 1988; **45**: 103–105.

108. Leighninger, D.S. Contributions of Claude Beck. In Safar, P., ed. *Advances in Cardiopulmonary Resuscitation.* New York: Springer-Verlag, 1975: 259–262.

109. Beck, C.S., & Mautz, F.R. The control of the heart beat by the surgeon: with special reference to ventricular fibrillation occurring during operation. *Ann. Surg.* 1937; **106**: 525–537.

110. Beck, C.S., Pritchard, W.H., & Feil, H.S. Ventricular fibrillation of long duration abolished by electric shock. *J. Am. Med. Assoc.* 1947; **135**: 985–986.

111. Beck, C.S., Weckesser, E.C., & Barry, F.M. Fatal heart attack and successful defibrillation. New concepts in coronary heart disease. *J. Am. Med. Assoc.* 1956; **161**: 434–436.

112. Weckesser, E.C. 29–year survival after myocardial infarction with ventricular fibrillation treated by electrical countershock. [Letter]. *N. Engl. J. Med.* 1985; **312**: 248.

113. Sladen, A. Closed-chest massage: Kouwenhoven, W.B. Jude, Knickerbocker, G.C. *J. Am. Med. Assoc.* 1984; **251**: 3137–3140.

114. Kouwenhoven, W.B. The development of the defibrillator. *Ann. Intern. Med.* 1969; **71**: 449–458.

115. Zoll, P.M., Linenthal, A.J., Gibson, W., *et al.* Termination of ventricular fibrillation in man by externally applied electric countershock. *N. Engl. J. Med.* 1956; **254**: 727–732.

116. Lown, B., Amarasingham, R., & Neuman, J. New method for terminating cardiac arrhythmias; use of synchronized capacitor discharge. *J. Am. Med. Assoc.* 1962; **182**: 548–555.

117. Kouwenhoven, W.B., Knickerbocker, G.C., & Becker, E.M. Portable defibrillator. *IEEE Trans. Power Appar Syst.* 1963; **69**: 1089–1093.

118. Larrey, D. *Memoires de chirurgerie et campagnes.* Paris. Remanences, 1982 (5 vols).

119. Baker, D., Cazalaa, J.-B., & Carli, P. *Resuscitation great:* Larrey and Percy – a tale of two Barons. *Resuscitation* 2005; **66**: 259–262.

120. Mead, R. *A Short Discourse Concerning the Pestilence Contagion.* 8th edn, London. (Quoted in ref. 122).

121. Haller, S.J. The beginnings of urban ambulance service in the United States and England. *J. Emerg. Med.* 1990; **8**: 743–755.

121a. Figl, M. & Pelinka, L.E. *Resuscitation great:* Jaromir Baron von Mundy – founder of the Vienna ambulance service. *Resuscitation* 2005; **66**: 121–125.

122. Burr, M.L. A concise history of ambulance services in Britain. *Med. Officer* 1969; **121**: 228–235.

123. Cantlie, N., & Seaver, G. *Sir James Cantlie*, London, 1939. (Quoted in ref. 122.)

124. Highway Safety Act of 1966. http://www.nhtsa.dot.gov/nhtsa/whatsup/tea21/GrantMan/HTML/07_Sect402Leg23USC_Chap4.html Accessed August 30, 2005.

125. Ministry of Health 1966. *Report by a working party on ambulance training and equipment, Part 1* – Training. London: HMSO.

126. McNeilly, R.H., & Pemberton, J. Duration of last attack in 998 fatal cases of coronary aftery disease and its relation to possible cardiac resuscitation *Br. Med. J.* 1968; **iii**: 139–142.

127. Pantridge, J.F., & Geddes, J.S. A mobile intensive-care unit in the management of myocardial infarction. *Lancet* 1967; **ii**: 271–273.

128. Dick, W.F. Ango-American vs. France–German EMSS. *Prehosp. Disaster Med.* 2003; **18**: 29–37.

129. Grace, W.J., & Chadbourn, J.A. The mobile coronary care unit. *Dis. Chest* 1969; **55**: 452–455.

130. Personal interview with author (ME), March to July 1989.

131. Gearty, G.F., Hickey, N., Bourke, G.J., & Mulcahy, R. Prehospital coronary care service. *Br. Med. J.* 1971; **iii**: 33–35.

132. White, N.M., Parker, W.S., Binning, R.A., Kimber, E.R., Ead, H.W., & Chamberlain, D.A. Mobile coronary care provided by ambulance personnel. *Br. Med. J.* 1973; **iii**: 618–622.

133. Baskett, P.J.F., Diamond, A.W., & Cochrane, D.F. Urban mobile resuscitation – training and service. *Br. J. Anaesth.* 1976; **48**: 377–385.

134. Jaggarao, N.S.V., Heber, M., Grainger, R., Vincent, R., Chamberlain, D.A., & Aronson, A.L. Use of an automated external defibrillator–pacemaker by ambulance staff. *Lancet* 1982; **ii**: 73–75.

135. Cummins, R.O., Eisenberg, M.S., Litwin, P.E., Graves, J.R., Hearne, T.R., & Hallstrom, A.P. Automatic external defibrillators used by emergency medical technicians. A controlled clinical trial. *J. Am. Med. Assoc.* 1987; **257**: 1605–1610.

136. Valenzuela, T.D., Roe, D.J., Nichol, G., Clark, L.L., Spaite, D.W., & Hardman, R.G. Outcomes of rapid defibrillation by security officers after cardiac arrest in casinos. *N. Engl. J. Med.* 2000; **343**: 1206–1209.

137. Whitfield, R., Colquhoun, M., Chamberlain, D., Newcombe, R., Davies, C.S., & Boyle, R. The Department of Health National defibrillator programme: analysis of downloads from 250 deployments of public access defibrillation. *Resuscitation* 2005; **64**: 269–277.

138. Page, R.L., Joglar, J.A., Kowal, R.C. *et al.* Use of automated external defibrillators by a U.S. airline. *N. Engl. J. Med.* 2000; **343**: 1210–1216.

139. White, R.D., & Vokov, L.F. Early defibrillation by police: initial experience with measurement of critical time intervals and patient outcomes. *Ann. Emerg. Med.* 1994; **23**: 1009–1013.

140. Home Automatic External Defibrillator Trial – HAT. http://www.clinicaltrials.gov/ct/gui/show/NCT00047411 Accessed August 30, 2005.

141. Culley, L.L., Clark, J.J., Eisenberg, M.S., & Larsen, M.P. Dispatcher assisted CPR: common delays and time standards for delivery. *Ann. Emerg. Med.* 1991; **20**: 362–366.

142. The International Liaison Committee on Resuscitation (ILCOR) – Past, present and future: compiled by the Founding Members. *Resuscitation* 2005; **67**: 157–161.

2

The epidemiology of sudden death

Graham Nichol and David Baker

University of Washington Clinical Trial Center, Seattle, WA, USA

Epidemiology is the study of the distribution and determinants of health-related states or events in specified populations and the application of this study to the control of health problems.[1] Although much has been learned from epidemiologic studies of cardiac arrest, this broad definition should be tempered by the recognition that death can be deferred but not prevented.

Epidemiology and the study of cardiac arrest

Much of what we understand today about the basic pathophysiology of cardiac arrest has been gained through observational rather than randomized studies of patients at risk for or in a state of cardiac arrest. This is only natural since sudden death is a relatively unpredictable event that usually occurs out-of-hospital and the victim is initially treated by emergency medical services providers, then transported to hospital for further triage and treatment in the emergency department. The epidemiologic study of cardiac arrest not only provides information about risk factors for the onset of arrest, the current status of treatment of the condition, but also suggests how to improve treatment and directs physicians toward future studies of resuscitation.

In broad terms, epidemiologic data are used to identify cellular (e.g., gene mutations that predispose to arrhythmias), environmental, social, educational, behavioral (e.g., activity level, smoking), clinical (e.g., atherosclerosis, reduced ventricular function, diabetes), or health system risk factors that predispose individuals to cardiac arrest or particular outcomes after its onset. By identifying risk factors that are amenable to modification, such as diet or smoking, physicians have attempted to improve survival through prevention. By identifying favorable interventional factors for survival, such as early cardiopulmonary resuscitation (CPR), physicians have improved the acute treatment of sudden death. By identifying individuals who have survived cardiac arrest, physicians have improved secondary prevention by implanting devices to treat recurrent events. The declining rates of cardiovascular disease observed in high-income countries[2–4] suggests that there has been some success in applying these strategies but that there is still a long way to go.

This chapter considers the definition, the nature, and magnitude of cardiac arrest. It describes some of the methods used to study cardiac arrest, incidence and survival statistics, as well as particular concepts important to understanding the literature in this field.

Definition of sudden death

An international consensus workshop classified cardiac arrest as the "cessation of cardiac mechanical activity, as confirmed by the absence of signs of circulation."[5] This definition emphasizes that cardiac arrest is a clinical syndrome that involves the sudden (usually less than 1 hour from onset of first symptoms until death) loss of detectable pulse, or cessation of spontaneous breathing. If an EMS provider or physician did not witness the event, then it may be uncertain as to whether a cardiac arrest has occurred. The World Health Organization proposed an alternate definition that acknowledges that many cardiac arrests are not witnessed: for those patients without an identifiable non-cardiac etiology, sudden cardiac death includes death within 1 hour of symptom onset for witnessed events or within 24 hours of having been observed alive and symptom-free for unwitnessed events.[6]

Such definitions have several limitations despite their widespread use. First, "presumed cardiac etiology" is frequently used as an inclusion or a priori subgroup criterion, but can only accurately be determined by conducting a postmortem examination. Since it is impractical to perform an autopsy on every fatal arrest, classification must rely on limited information that is available to emergency providers in the out-of-hospital setting or physicians in the emergency room.[7] It is frequently difficult for emergency providers to ascertain whether and how long the patient had symptoms beforehand when they are trying to provide acute resuscitation in the field. In the absence of precise definitions, use of the etiology of arrest as an inclusion criterion will create bias. Therefore, episodes should be included in epidemiologic studies regardless of their etiology.

Since the likelihood of underlying disease is uncertain, many studies presume that an arrest is of cardiac origin unless there is another obvious cause: specifically, unless the episode is known or likely to have been caused by trauma, submersion, drug overdose, asphyxia, exsanguinations, or any other non-cardiac cause as determined by the rescuers.(5) Such classifications are important especially for out-of-hospital cardiac arrest studies, but remain inexact because they are subject to ascertainment bias due to incomplete assessment on the basis of information at the scene, or toxicology tests ordered selectively on patients successfully transferred to hospital, and the frequent lack of autopsy data.

Second, many epidemiologic studies of cardiac arrest use emergency medical services as the sampling frame, so unwitnessed deaths that did not result in a call for aid are difficult to ascertain and therefore are not included. The exclusion of such patients from a study would underestimate episode incidence and overestimate survival compared to a study that included them.

Third, there is geographic variation in the frequency of "do not attempt resuscitation" declarations by individuals and family members and whether EMS providers can choose not to initiate or to cease efforts in the field. The inclusion or exclusion of such patients in different epidemiologic studies makes it difficult to compare the incidence and outcome of cardiac arrest in different jurisdictions.

Reasonable alternative definitions that address these limitations are unexpected cardiac death without any reference to duration of symptoms, and EMS-treated cardiac arrest. The latter might include any persons evaluated by organized EMS personnel who: a) receive attempts at external defibrillation (by lay responders or emergency personnel), or receive chest compressions by organized EMS personnel; or b) are pulseless but do not receive attempts to defibrillate or CPR by EMS personnel. This would include those with "do not attempt resuscitation" directives, a history of terminal illness or intractable disease, or a request from the patient's family to "not treat."

Unexpected cardiac death generally occurs in persons with known or previously unrecognized ischemic heart disease.[8,9] Other causes of sudden death include non-ischemic heart disease (especially arrhythmic including ventricular fibrillation, Wolff-Parkinson-White syndrome, long QT syndrome, Brugada syndrome, short-coupled torsade de pointes and catecholamine-induced polymorphic ventricular tachyarrhythmia), pulmonary diseases including embolus, cerebral nervous system disease, vascular catastrophes including ruptured aneurysms, as well as drugs and poisons. Patients without identifiable abnormalities are categorized as idiopathic. Although routine cardiac imaging may seem normal in such patients, discrete genetic or anatomic abnormalities are sometimes identified by more sophisticated tools such as magnetic resonance imaging, positron emission tomography, or genetic testing. Traumatic sudden death is usually considered separately from unexpected cardiac death, because the treatment and prognosis of traumatic and non-traumatic arrest differ so much from each other.

Global burden of illness

Globally, cardiovascular disease contributes 30.9% of global mortality and 10.3% of the global burden of disease.[10–12] It is responsible for more deaths than any other disease in industrialized countries, and three-quarters of mortality due to non-communicable diseases in developing countries. Eighty percent of deaths due to cardiovascular disease occur in low- and middle-income countries.

In the United States, cardiovascular disease is the leading cause of death among individuals aged greater than 65 years, the second leading cause of death among individuals aged 0 to 14 years and 45 to 64 years, and the fourth leading cause of death among individuals aged 15 to 24 years (www.americanheart.org/downloadable/heart/1103834819155FS23LCD5.pdf accessed on March 2, 2005). Cardiovascular disease is estimated to have cost $368 billion in the United States in 2004 (http://nhlbi.nih.gov/about/03factbka.pdf accessed on October 22, 2004).

About half of coronary heart deaths are sudden.[13] Since there were 7.2 million coronary heart deaths worldwide in

2002.(http://www3.who.int/whosis/ accessed on August 28, 2005), this implies there were 3.6 million unexpected cardiac arrests. About 2/3 of these occur without prior recognition of cardiac disease.[14] About 60% of unexpected cardiac deaths may be treated by EMS.[15] Although the proportion of those treated by EMS is likely less in those countries that have limited access to emergency services, this implies that as many as 2.2 million cardiac arrests are treated by EMS worldwide annually.

Incidence vs. survival

The wide variation in incidence and outcome after unexpected cardiac death is attributable in part to several factors in addition to differences in clinical risk factors and EMS care. Considering some of these factors requires clarification of some epidemiologic concepts.

First, it is important to distinguish between two common epidemiologic measures: incidence and survival rate. The incidence of cardiac arrest is the attack rate of cardiac arrest in the community. Risk factors for increased incidence of cardiac arrest include previous health, age, race, and gender. Early identification of modifiable risk factors can reduce an individual's risk of cardiac arrest.

The survival rate is the complement of the case-fatality rate, and is defined as the number of survivors divided by the number of individuals who experienced unexpected cardiac death. The latter requires a specific and measurable definition.[16] For example, subjects who inadvertently are treated in the field, such as a person with syncope who receives bystander CPR, should not be included. Stratification of the denominator for a survival calculation can distort an assessment of the quality of a community's EMS system. For example, survival can be expressed relative to the total number of deaths in a community, the number of 911 dispatch calls to the area, or those who received field interventions such as CPR or defibrillation. Each of these groups has a particular sensitivity and specificity for detecting true cardiac arrest. If a surveillance system reports as cardiac arrest an episode that was not, then incidence and survival are overestimated (the latter only if the patient lives). If the system misses a true cardiac arrest, then incidence and survival are underestimated (the latter if the patient dies.) Therefore, a surveillance system must assess all events in a consistent and comprehensive manner. EMS systems that habitually monitor their episodes sometimes utilize multiple methods of ascertainment to do so. A process of adjudication is useful to differentiate possible cardiac arrest from definite cases.

By changing the definition of a "case," the denominator is adjusted, thereby altering the apparent survival rate. For example, Eisenberg et al. demonstrated a two-fold range in survival rates in the same population depending on the subgroup or denominator chosen.[17] Therefore, studies should clearly state the criteria for inclusion in the study or registry. An alternate approach in settings where complete ascertainment of episodes is likely to be challenging is to compare the absolute number of survivors rather than the proportion of survivors.[16]

The risk factors for survival (or mortality) after a person has suffered a cardiac arrest can be considered separately from those affecting incidence. These factors become important for predicting and improving survival. Many of these factors relate to the timeliness[18,19] and quality of resuscitation at the scene of arrest.[20] Some confusion between incidence and survival is understandable, because some, but not all, factors that affect incidence also affect survival. Other factors that increase incidence, however, may not affect survival. For example, male sex is a risk factor for incidence of sudden death, but survival rates for men and women are similar. The following section explores factors that influence the *incidence* of sudden death, and those that predict *survival* from cardiac arrest.

Data sources

Data to describe out-of-hospital cardiac arrest can be obtained from a variety of sources, each of which has particular advantages and disadvantages. Some population-based studies use death certificates or International Classification of Diseases (ICD) coded hospital discharge data. Such data are frequently accessible from a central location or computer. Moreover, such data are quite complete since a death certificate is filed for all deaths. Nonetheless, assignment of causation is inaccurate on death certificates for several reasons. Many patients are classified as having cardiac arrest for lack of a better diagnosis. Certificates can be completed hours to days after the event, by a physician not in attendance at the time of death. Confounding diseases, such as stroke or drug intoxications, present much like cardiac arrest and are likely to be misclassified. Estimates of the incidence of unexpected cardiac death that are based on death certificates overestimate the true incidence by as much as 47%.[21]

Hospital discharge data are another inaccurate method of estimating cardiac arrest because there is no specific ICD code for cardiac arrest. Instead, several non-specific cardiac codes are combined (e.g., ICD-9 code 390 to 398, 402, or 404 to 429) and it is assumed that these cases represented sudden cardiac arrest if the death was reported as occurring out of hospital or in the emergency room or as "dead on arrival."[22] Such an approach has good sensitivity (most people dying from "cardiac arrest" will have ceased cardiac mechanical activity!) but poor specificity (not every person reported as dying from "cardiac arrest" actually died *primarily* from cardiac arrest).

An alternate approach to studying cardiac arrest relies on data collated from EMS patient care records. Such databases usually have a more precise description of what happened to the patient immediately before and after the onset of the episode and consequently may be more accurate than death certificates. EMS databases accumulate large numbers of patients in relatively short time periods because they usually encompass the entire community, thus covering a larger population than patients presenting to a single hospital. One weakness as a data source, however, is that they do not necessarily identify all victims of cardiac arrest. They may miss patients treated by other EMS providers, or not treated by EMS, or those who are transported by the family or suffer cardiac arrest in the emergency department or elsewhere in the hospital.

The study of in-hospital cardiac arrest has some advantages over that of out-of-hospital arrest.[23] There is usually a shorter response interval until treatment, more highly trained providers able to respond in a timely manner, better information about events leading to the arrest, and more complete follow-up. Critics of in-hospital studies, however, argue that because of co-morbid illness and other factors, the in-hospital setting fails to simulate the out-of-hospital patient experience. To the extent that these patients were sick enough to require hospital admission, any cardiopulmonary arrest may not be sudden and hence not classifiable as sudden death.

Some countries or regions have developed registries that include detailed information on cardiac arrest victims. For example, Sweden,[24] Norway, Scotland,[25] and Western Australia have large registries of cardiac arrest data. Recently a pilot study demonstrated the feasibility of collating process and outcome data related to consecutive cases of out-of-hospital cardiac arrest in multiple countries by using secure and confidential web-based methods.[26] Also, the American Heart Association and National Institutes of Health are supporting an out-of-hospital cardiac arrest registry in the catchment areas of EMS agencies that are participating in the Resuscitation Outcomes Consortium (www.uwctc.org accessed on September 16, 2005). Collectively, these large registries will contribute to a better understanding of the incidence and outcome of unexpected cardiac death especially if they are able to migrate towards using common definitions of eligibility and covariates.

Accuracy of data

Epidemiologists' ability to interpret research results is limited by the accuracy of the data collected. It is unfortunate that although the technology now exists to collect accurate information, these methods have generally not been incorporated into EMS care and research. Time is the most critical factor during cardiac arrest treatment, yet determining accurate times remains a serious obstacle. Accurate assessment of the duration of time since the onset of arrest has taken on increased importance since the recognition that therapy may need to be tailored to the duration of this interval.[27] A few studies have determined the moment of cardiac arrest or collapse with precision by video recording of public-use areas[28] or telemetry monitoring integrated into a defibrillator.[29] Estimates of the time of onset of cardiac arrest are used[30,31] but are subject to bias.[32] An alternate approach to increasing the accuracy of response time intervals is to synchronize all EMS-related time pieces to an atomic clock.[33]

The time of the call to 911 and the time rescuers get to the victim's address are standard time points in most systems, because these are collected by a central dispatcher rather than estimated by the rescuers. Although some dispatch centers interpret the time of call to be the time the call was received at the dispatch center, some interpret it as the time the call was answered, and others interpret it as the time that EMS providers were sent to respond. Another potential cause of variation in dispatch times is that some EMS agencies use a single dispatch center, whereas others use an initial public safety answering point that then transfers medical calls to an EMS dispatch center for disposition. Although response time intervals are not always included in resuscitation registries,[5] epidemiologic studies that assess these intervals should ensure that they are measured in a consistent manner within each EMS agency. The length of time for rescuers to get from the vehicle to each patient's side can be an additional source of uncertainty and delay in some systems.[34,35] The interval from call to EMS until defibrillation may be a better measure of the performance of EMS systems when compared to the interval from call to arrival on scene.[35] Few studies have accurately recorded the moment of all treatment time points, including defibrillation, intubation, and drug administration.

Technological solutions avoid some of these problems. Monitor/defibrillators can record time and treatments with precision to the second. Audio or ECG recordings of the actual arrest can be reviewed after the event to relate the process of care to timing intervals.[36,37] Electronic patient records can capture field data and transmit it to a central receiving station for verification, analysis, and interpretation. These methods may increase the accuracy of measurements of response time intervals.

The physiologic characteristics of a patient in cardiac arrest may also be used to estimate time or response to treatment. Ventricular fibrillation has an underlying organized rhythm that is influenced by the underlying mechanism of arrhythmia[38] and predicts the duration of VF as well as the response to treatment.[39] Various morphologic characteristics of ventricular fibrillation correlate with successful defibrillation in animal models[40–42] and observational human data.[42–44] To date, there are no prospective or controlled studies that demonstrate that defibrillation guided by waveform characteristics improves outcomes.

Elevation of the level of carbon dioxide in tissue or exhaled air is another possible marker of duration or severity of circulatory shock.[45–47] An important limitation of using end-tidal carbon dioxide, however, is that it correlates poorly with tissue levels in the absence of cardiac output. To date, there are no published prospective or controlled studies that demonstrate that resuscitation guided by carbon dioxide levels improves outcomes.

Another source of potential inaccuracy is the interpretation of the initial recorded rhythm. One study found that paramedics could reliably differentiate large-amplitude VF from flat-line asystole, but were not consistent in differentiating fine VF from coarse asystole.[48] Another identified errors in rhythm analysis by automated external defibrillators.[49] Such inconsistencies may affect survival rates by significantly changing the subgroup identified as having VF and hence changing the denominator, as well as by changing the likelihood of successful resuscitation. In summary, accurate data collection during a cardiac arrest is not a trivial matter, and development and implementation of newer methods will be crucial to future studies.

Incidence of cardiac arrest

The true incidence of out-of-hospital cardiac arrest is unknown. Its reported incidence in the United States is 1.9/1000 person years among those aged 50 to 79 years.[14] Since the US population aged 50 to 79 is 67 667 031 (http://www.census.gov/ accessed on Aug 28 2005), this implies 130 000 out-of-hospital cardiac arrests. The reported incidence of EMS-treated cardiac arrest is 36/100 000 to 81/100 000 total population.[15,50] Since the total US population is 297 227 385 (http://www.census.gov/ accessed on Sep 21 2005), this implies 107 000 to 240 000 treated arrests occur in the United States annually. Of these, 20 to 38% have ventricular fibrillation or ventricular tachycardia as the first recorded rhythm.[14,50] This implies

21 000 to 91 000 treated ventricular fibrillation arrests annually.

The reported incidence of unexpected cardiac arrest in Europe is 1/1000 population.[51] Since the European population is 455 489 113 (http://www.populationdata.net/ accessed on Aug 28 2005), this implies 450 000 out-of-hospital arrests occur annually in Europe.

During the early twentieth century, the incidence of coronary artery disease in the United States and other high-income countries increased dramatically. In the 1940s, cardiovascular disease became the leading cause of death, overtaking deaths caused by infectious agents. In the early twenty-first century, cardiovascular disease has become a ubiquitous cause of morbidity in most countries.[52] This epidemiologic transition reflects increased longevity in low and middle income countries, and thereby increased exposure to cardiovascular risk factors. It also reflects adverse lifestyle changes, including increased inactivity, obesity, tobacco use, and consumption of fats. Nonetheless, there has been a steady decline in morbidity and mortality from most cardiovascular diseases in high-income countries over the last 30 years.[2–4] Much of this reduction has been attributed to modification of risk factors.[53] Although the incidence of ventricular fibrillation and cardiac arrest with any first initial rhythm is decreasing over time,[50] there has been little improvement in survival from cardiac arrest.[54,55]

Unexpected cardiac death in children

Unexpected cardiac death in children merits special consideration in the field of acute resuscitation, because its incidence, etiology, prognosis, and treatment differ from those of out-of-hospital adult episodes. The reported incidence of out-of-hospital pediatric unexpected cardiac death is 2.6 to 19.7 annual cases per 100 000.[56] Unexpected death in the pediatric patient is usually due to trauma, sudden infant death syndrome, respiratory causes or submersion,[57] but ventricular fibrillation is still commonly observed.[58] The reported average survival to discharge is 6.7%. Children with submersion or traumatic injury have a poorer prognosis.

Unexpected cardiac death in hospital

Unexpected cardiac death in hospital also merits special consideration because of its unique characteristics. A large multicenter cohort study of in-hospital cardiopulmonary arrest events excluded events that occur out-of-hospital to avoid double counting.[59] For adults, the reported incidence of unexpected cardiac death in hospital was 0.174 ± 0.087 per bed per year. The commonest causes of these events were arrhythmia, respiratory distress, hypotension, or myocardial infarction. The average survival to discharge was 17%.

High-risk subgroups

The patients at highest risk for cardiac arrest account for only a small portion of arrests in the community.[60] The largest number of cardiac arrests in the community occur in the low-risk general public simply because there are so many more of these individuals than those in the high-risk subgroups.

Witnessed VF is commonly used to assess the efficacy of an EMS agency, because it provides a homogeneous population for analysis that is readily responsive to timely intervention.[61] It is to be hoped that survival figures may become more closely comparable among communities by use of such a definition; but this may not be true because VF is correlated with response time.[62] A potential limitation to this approach is that as the subgroup becomes smaller, the results become less applicable to the larger population. Also, focusing on a subgroup of patients with a particular initial rhythm rather than all treated cardiac arrests may give a biased sense of outcomes. By considering only patients with ventricular fibrillation, one may underestimate the burden of illness and improvements in treatment, because the incidence has decreased and rates of survival to hospital admission or discharge have been static over time for ventricular fibrillation but not pulseless electrical activity or asystole.[50] The updated Utstein template and recommendations offer some logical guidelines for investigators reporting on subgroups.[5]

Calculating incidence of cardiac arrest

Incidence is the occurrence rate per year for a disease within a population at risk. It is usually calculated by taking a ratio of the number of persons developing a disease each year divided by the population at risk. This "simple" measurement becomes quite complicated when applied to cardiac arrest because of the effect of age on the incidence. Many cardiac arrest studies reported incidence as the number of cardiac arrests per year divided by the population within the region. If we use Seattle with a census population of 460 000 aged 20 years or older as an example, there were 372 cardiac arrests within the metropolitan area during 2000, an incidence of 372/460 000/yr or 0.81 cardiac arrests/1000/yr. Focusing on the adult population in this manner is common, and underestimates the total number of arrests slightly, but not the incidence since cardiac arrest is uncommon in the pediatric population.

A separate but related issue is that incidence rates are usually based on the census population of the catchment area of the EMS agency even though the number of individuals fluctuates by time of day and day of week. A city that has a large population ingress during the working week may appear falsely to have an elevated rate of unexpected cardiac death.

If large unaccountable differences in incidence are present, there are important public health questions that require investigation and may prove critical for efforts to improve survival. Likewise, this information may be useful for comparing survival statistics from different communities. Therefore incidence should be routinely reported in cardiac arrest studies.

Risk factors for incidence of cardiac arrest

Despite considerable study, the real causes of sudden death remain obscure. Predicting how a complex system with multiple interrelated elements responds to a variation in an individual component is a general problem in systems biology. Atherosclerosis is likely a factor in the majority of cases; structural and congenital abnormalities, fibrosis, and conditions such as myocarditis contribute to most of the rest.[15] Many risk factors for cardiac arrest, such as hypertension and hypercholesterolemia, are present for long periods of time and are likely to be identified any time an individual is evaluated. Others are evanescent, difficult to document, and less understood. Here, risk factors are classified as cellular, phenotypic, environmental, social, educational, behavioral, clinical, or health system risk factors. A combination of these factors is usually present. In each group, risk factors can be divided into those that are fixed (so-called "fate" factors) and those that can be modified to some extent. The latter may evolve over time or be transient. Evolving factors that may modify the risk of lethal arrhythmia include cell membrane levels of polyunsaturated fatty acids,[63] ion channel function,[64] and local or systemic inflammation.[65] Transient factors that may suddenly trigger a lethal arrhythmia include transient ischemia and reperfusion, transient systemic factors, transient autonomic and neurohumoral factors, and toxic/proarrhythmic effects.[13] The interplay of these factors is complex, as socioeconomic gradients exist in some circulating factors that are not fully explained by health-related behaviors or risk factors for coronary heart disease.[66] Efforts should be made to modify risk whenever feasible. A caveat to this approach is that population stratification approaches, such risk factors derived from the Framingham Heart Study, predict well the risk of events in large community groups, but less well the risk of specific asymptomatic individuals.

Cellular

Animal experimental, cell biology, genetic, nutritional, and epidemiologic studies demonstrate that cellular constituents such as cell membrane and free fatty acid levels of n-3 polyunsaturated fatty acids (PUFAs) alter cardiac ion channel function, modify cardiac action potential and reduce myocardial vulnerability to ventricular fibrillation.[67] These findings have important clinical and public health implications, because n-3 PUFA levels can be altered by inexpensive changes in dietary intake. Specifically, ingestion of one fatty fish meal a week is associated with a marked reduction in sudden cardiac death.

Elevations in plasma non-esterified fatty acid (NEFA) levels[68] and high-sensitivity C-reactive protein (CRP) levels[65] or decreased long-chain n-3 fatty acid levels are independently associated with elevated risk of unexpected cardiac death. It remains unclear whether elevation of CRP indicates an underlying inflammatory pathological process or whether it is directly proarrhythmic.

Genetically based risk factors for cardiac arrest may include factors that facilitate the onset of ischemia and infarction, including activators of plaque rupture and thrombogenesis; alterations in neuroendocrine signaling, including differences in transmitter pathways that contribute to sympathetic–parasympathetic imbalance; and potential triggers or attenuators of cardiocyte membrance excitability and transcellular conduction.[69,70] Molecular genetic analysis has identified an inherited disease and likely cause of death in 40% of families with at least one member who had unexplained cardiac death at age 40 years or less.[71] A caveat to the potential role of genetic screening to identify mutations that predispose to arrhythmia is that familial clustering of cardiac death may reflect shared environmental or genetically transmittable abnormalities. Regardless of which of these is correct, familial risks for sudden death are separable from familial risks for myocardial infarction.[68,72]

Identification of cellular and genetic risk factors for cardiac arrest may have therapeutic implications. For example, KvLTQ1 gene mutations are predisposed to arrhythmias that may be more responsive to beta-blockers;[73] carriers of SCN5A gene mutations are predisposed to arrhythmias that may be more responsive to electrical defibrillation.[74]

Environment

The incidence and outcome of cardiac arrest vary by time of day, day of week, or season.[75–80] Data from the Framingham study show that the highest risk for MI is on awakening and it decreases progressively during the day. Various physiologic processes have been considered to explain this phenomenon, such as increased clotting or increased parasympathetic instability. Some researchers have suggested that part of the morning peak in cardiac arrest may be due to a reporting artifact (i.e., the patients really die during the night but are not discovered until early morning). Potential interventions to reduce periodic variation in unexpected cardiac death include resource allocation of EMS and hospital resources to match anticipated need.

Social

Disparities in incidence of cardiac arrest are observed across socioeconomic gradients as well as across geographic region.[81–87] Cardiovascular disease is the leading cause of income-related differences in premature mortality in the United States,[88] and Canada.[89] Non-hispanic blacks bear a disproportionate burden of morbidity and mortality due to cardiovascular disease.[90] These disparities may be caused by differences in genetic risk, health behaviors, educational attainment, socioeconomic disadvantage, access to preventive care, or other yet to be identified variables. As understanding of the magnitude and cause of these disparities increases, potential interventions include culturally appropriate public health initiatives, community support, and equitable access to quality care.

Behavioral

Cigarette smoking is thought to be the single most important cause of preventable death in the United States. An estimated 438 000 persons in the United States die prematurely each year due to exposure to tobacco smoke.[91] The deleterious effects of smoking may be mediated through increased plasma catecholamines, heart rate, and arterial blood pressure; production of coronary spasm; and increases in myocardial work and oxygen demand with concomitant reduction in oxygen supply.[92] Collectively, these effects lower ventricular fibrillation thresholds. In patients who successfully quit smoking, rates of sudden death return to near normal over time. Of great concern is the effect of "passive smoking," which has been associated with an increase in smoking-related disease, primarily heart disease.[93]

Exercise, much like weight loss, can be both good and bad. Persons who exercise regularly have a decreased incidence of coronary artery disease compared to persons who are sedentary,[94] and decreased mortality in those with that disease who exercise compared to those who do not.[95] Nevertheless, the heavy exertion with exercise is associated with an increase in acute events, such as MI. A period of strenuous activity was associated with a temporary increase in the risk of having an MI for about 1 hour after the exertion.[96] Heavy exertion in persons who do not exercise regularly was associated with the highest risk.

Use of street drugs is associated with unexpected cardiac death. Cocaine use is associated with severe and catastrophic heart disease in many individuals. It increases adrenergic stimulation by blocking the presynaptic reuptake of norepinephrine and dopamine, thus causing an increased sensitivity to catecholamines. The combined effect of cocaine and cigarette smoke is worse than either one alone.[97] Opioids are also associated with cardiac arrest.[98] Both cocaine and methadone prolong QT intervals, predisposing to ventricular arrhythmias.[99]

Moderate alcohol intake is associated with reduced cardiovascular mortality compared to no alcohol intake, although the mechanisms by which alcohol is protective remain unclear. This effect is thought to be mediated through increased levels of HDL.[100] Nevertheless, heavy consumption is associated with increased mortality, an effect sometimes referred to as "holiday heart" because it is often associated with binge drinking in otherwise healthy people during weekends.[101] In the Physicians' Health Study, after controlling for multiple confounders, men who consumed two to six drinks per week had a 60 to 80% reduced risk of unexpected cardiac death compared to those who rarely or never consumed alcohol.[102] In the British Regional Heart Study, the relative risk of unexpected cardiac death in those who drank more than six drinks per day was twice as high as occasional or light drinkers.[103]

Emotional factors influence the occurrence of cardiac disease. Characteristics such as anger, chronic stress, aggressiveness, anxiety, and hostility are difficult to measure objectively, however, and there are many confounding issues. Educational attainment moderates the risk of acute infarction due to anger.[104] Studies have yet to confirm a definite relationship between emotional factors and cardiac arrest.

Clinical

Sudden death has been associated with all forms of cardiac disease. The rates of sudden death parallel the prevalence of risk factors for coronary artery disease. Known coronary artery disease or a previous episode of sudden death remains the greatest risk factor for sudden death.

Cardiac arrest is particularly common in patients with established cardiovascular disease. Patients with acute coronary syndromes (ACS) or myocardial infarction (MI) are at high risk of dying (i.e., >5%) within 30 days of presentation, regardless of whether ST-segment elevation is present or absent.[105] The risk of death remains elevated for at least 6 months in patients with ACS,[106] and for at least 1 year in patients with MI.[107] Patients with ventricular dysfunction are at higher risk than those without.[108] At least one-half of these deaths are suspected to have an arrhythmic mechanism.[109] Several non-invasive diagnostic tests may identify patients who are at high risk of cardiac arrest, but have low sensitivity and specificity,[110] and are generally available only in tertiary care centers. More than 1 000 000 patients are discharged with MI, and more than 780 000 patients are discharged with a primary diagnosis of ACS in the United States each year.(http://www.cdc.gov/nchs, accessed on June 9, 2002) Since more than 16% of these have a left ventricular ejection fraction (EF) < 40%,[111] thousands of individuals are annually at increased risk of cardiac arrest.

Ischemia and reperfusion, which occur commonly during the early phases of MI, are clearly associated with arrhythmias. Because only 20% of sudden cardiac death victims have acute infarction, it is assumed that transient ischemia rather than infarction has a major role in triggering sudden death. Transient systemic factors, such as hypoxia, hypotension, acidosis, or electrolyte abnormalities, can affect electrophysiologic stability and susceptibility to arrhythmias. A vigilant search should be made for an underlying cause of arrhythmia even in the setting of electrolyte abnormalities, however, as hypokalemia may be a cause or consequence of cardiac arrest.[112]

Congenital or acquired arrhythmias are a known risk factor for cardiac arrest. Unfortunately, the severity of risk is not well defined because of the many associated factors that may confound evaluation of a particular patient. Deaths in athletes have drawn considerable public interest to this problem. Although known arrhythmias increase the chance of cardiac arrest, the degree to which various arrhythmias increase the chance of cardiac arrest is difficult to predict precisely. Screening of athletes for risk of arrhythmia lacks sensitivity and specificity.[113]

The rate of cardiac arrest increases exponentially with increasing age. The rates for cardiac arrest are substantially higher at any given age for men than for women. Since more women in the population are older than men, the overall incidence by gender are similar, although women are at less risk at any particular age.

Race is an important risk factor for many cardiovascular diseases. Blacks have a higher rate of hypertension, left ventricular hypertrophy, renal disease, and diabetes compared to whites. As a consequence of these differences in the distribution of risk factors, the incidence of cardiac arrest is significantly higher in blacks than in whites.[81]

Hypertension predisposes patients to develop CAD, cardiac hypertrophy, congestive heart failure, stroke, renal disease, and sudden death. The risk is continuous, without evidence of a threshold, down to blood pressures as low as 115/75.[114] Twofold to threefold increases in CAD are seen in patients with systolic blood pressure above 160 or diastolic blood pressures above 95.[115] Hypertension affects about 65 million persons in the United States,[116] and may affect more than 90% of individuals during their lifetime.[117] As many as two-thirds of affected Americans are untreated or undertreated.[118] This care gap has important public health implications since randomized trials have definitively shown that treatment of hypertension reduces the risk of cardiovascular events and mortality.[119]

Elevations of serum cholesterol and triglycerides are known risk factors for cardiac death. The risk of CAD increases as total cholesterol increases, with low-density lipoprotein (LDL) cholesterol associated with elevated risk and high-density lipoprotein (HDL) cholesterol associated with decreased risk.[120] Elevated triglycerides are especially of concern for women.[121] The levels of lipids are thought to be mediated through an unclear combination of hereditary predisposition and diet. Strict control of diet (less than 10 g of fat per day) can even cause regression of preexisting CAD.[122] Reduction of dietary saturated fat and partial replacement by unsaturates for at least 2 years reduces cardiovascular events, and cardiovascular and all-cause mortality.[123]

Obesity is an independent risk factor for cardiac disease. The prevalence of obesity among adults aged 20 to 74 years has risen from 13% to 31% during the past 25 years,[124–126] despite a decrease in the prevalence of all other risk factors except diabetes over time across all body mass index groups in the United States.[127] Similar increases in obesity have been observed in other high-income countries.

Diabetes is associated with increased CAD. The prevalence of diabetes is increasing over time in the United States.[128] About 10% of the population have diagnosed or undiagnosed diabetes. Diet, exercise, and tighter control over glucose levels may lower the increased risk of CAD associated with diabetes. Since diabetics have an elevated incidence of hypertension, control of blood pressure will also reduce the risk of CAD and renal failure. Renal failure is associated with an increased incidence of cardiac arrest.[129]

Male patients presenting with impotence related to vascular disease are at high risk for sudden death.[130] More than two-thirds of males admitted with acute MI were found to have had significant complaints of sexual dysfunction before infarction.[131] Therefore physicians evaluating patients with non-cardiac vascular disease should ensure that these patients are evaluated for cardiac risk as well.

Health system

There is incontrovertible evidence that implantable cardioverter defibrillators reduce the risk of unexpected cardiac death in those with elevated risk of arrest or those who have survived an initial event.[132] Implantation of these devices shortly after an acute cardiovascular event is deleterious,[133] but non-invasive alternatives exist.[134] Nonetheless, antiarrhythmic devices are potentially underutilized in some settings.[135]

A variety of prescription and non-prescription pharmaceutical agents increase or decrease the risk of arrhythmia or cardiac arrest (Table 2.1). Drugs that have the most significant impact on mortality due to cardiac arrest lack direct electrophysiological effects on myocardial excitability.[136] This implies that these agents act on proximate events that can predispose to lethal arrhythmias (e.g., ischemia, fibrosis). Other agents decrease cardiovascular or all-cause mortality, but have not been demonstrated to decrease cardiac arrest. The latter outcome likely reflects lack of statistical power to detect a difference in an event that is infrequent compared with events or mortality. Nevertheless, lack of demonstrated benefit specific to cardiac arrest should not be interpreted as lack of need to prescribe agents that are otherwise effective in those with cardiovascular disease.

Pharmaceutical agents act via diverse mechanisms to modify the risk of arrhythmia or arrhythmic death. Angiotensin-converting enzyme (ACE) inhibitors decrease the incidence of ventricular tachycardia independent of changes in ejection fraction in humans with heart failure.[137] ACE inhibitors may block remodeling by cardiac myocytes,[138] or reduce ventricular fibrillation in the setting of acute coronary occlusion and reperfusion.[139] Randomized trials demonstrate that ACE inhibitors reduce the risk of sudden cardiac death by 20% in patients after myocardial infarction.[140] Aldosterone antagonists decrease cardiac deaths including those due to sudden events in patients with heart failure, perhaps due to blunting of myocardial fibrosis and hypokalemia that predispose to arrhythmias.[141] Beta-blockers attenuate the toxic effects of norepinephrine upon cardiac myocytes,[142]

Table 2.1. Effect of drugs on long-term risk of cardiovascular death and cardiac arrest

Drug	Effect on Cardiovascular Mortality	Effect on Cardiac Arrest Mortality
Angiotensin-converting enzyme inhibitors	−	−
Aldosterone antagonist	−	−
Beta-blockers	−	−
HMB coreductase inhibitors	−	−
Amiodarone	−	−
Angiotensin-receptor blockers	±	±
Thrombolytic therapy	−	−
Low molecular weight heparin	±	±
Iib/IIIa receptor antagonists	±	±
Clopidogrel	−	±
ASA	−	±
Warfarin	−	±
Digoxin	±	±
Drugs that prolong QT interval[a]	±	+
Vaughan-Williams Class IC[b]	+	+
Vaughan-Williams Class III[c]	+	+
Inotropes	+	+
Cyclooxygenase inhibitors	+	+

[a] Includes, but not limited to: selected antiarrhythmic agents, terfenadine, astemizole, cocaine, methadone.
[b] Flecainide, Encainide.
[c] D-Sotalol, dofetilide.

improve systolic function and reverse statistics,[143] and reduce death due to cardiac arrest in patients with heart failure.[144–148]

Disorders of endothelial function, inflammatory responses, plaque stability, and thrombus formation predispose to cardiovascular events.[149–151] Statins reduce serum cholesterol but also modify these factors. Randomized trials have demonstrated that statins reduce all-cause mortality and sudden cardiac death in those with and without coronary artery disease.[152,153] Although there is some evidence that elevated cholesterol is not an independent risk factor for cardiac death,[65] "statin" inhibitors of hydroxyglutaryl-CoA reductase reduce CRP expression levels.

Although observational studies suggested that digoxin was associated with increased risk of cardiac arrest,[154] a large randomized trial demonstrated that digoxin therapy does not increase this risk in patients with symptomatic heart failure and reduced ventricular function.[155]

To date, all drugs that enhance cardiac contractility, regardless of mechanism, have been shown to increase mortality among those with symptomatic heart failure and decreased ventricular function.[156–159] This increased mortality is attributable to sudden death, presumably

due to lethal ventricular arrhythmias. Class IC antiarrhythmic agents (e.g., flecainide, encainide, and moricizine) suppress ventricular arrhythmias but are associated with increased mortality due to cardiac arrest.[160,161] Pure class III agents have also been evaluated as antiarrhythmic agents. D-Sotalol was associated with significantly increased mortality and sudden arrhythmic death compared to placebo.[162] Dofetilide reduced atrial fibrillation, but not total mortality, ventricular tachycardia, or ventricular fibrillation in patients with heart failure and reduced ventricular function, and was associated with a 3% incidence of torsade de pointes.[163]

Amiodarone has little proarrhythmic effect and does not worsen heart failure.[164,165] It reduces modestly arrhythmic death in patients with heart failure or previous myocardial infarction.[166–171] Amiodarone reduced the composite cardiovascular endpoint of death, recurrent ventricular tachycardia or fibrillation, or syncopal ICD shocks by 44% compared to conventional therapy guided by electrophysiological testing or Holter monitoring in survivors of ventricular fibrillation.[172] There was an important but non-significant reduction in recurrence of potentially lethal arrhythmia after 2 years of therapy. The lack of a placebo arm in this trial limits its generalizability, as it is unclear whether the benefit is due to amiodarone or the harmful effects of conventional antiarrhythmic drugs (mainly class I agents in this case.)

Angiotensin receptor blocker agents (ARBs) decrease serum inflammatory markers[173] and decrease thrombosis via increased tissue-plasminogen activator (t-PA) and decreased plasminogen activator inhibitor-1 (PAI-1)[174] in patients with heart failure. Randomized trials of ARBs have demonstrated heterogeneous effects on reduction of all-cause mortality and sudden cardiac death compared to captopril in patients with heart failure or acute infarction.[175–177]

Coronary plaque rupture precipitates thrombosis, infarction, and thereby sudden death. Successful reperfusion on an infarct-related artery increases electrical stability at the edge of the infarcted area, and reduces the subsequent risk of ventricular arrhythmias.[178] Thrombolytic therapy reduces the risk of all-cause mortality and to a variable degree sudden cardiac death in patients with acute myocardial infarction.[179] There are inconclusive trial data regarding the effect of low-molecular weight heparin,[180] platelet glycoprotein IIb/IIIa receptor antagonists,[181] or clopidogrel[182] upon all-cause mortality and unexpected cardiac death in patients with acute infarction or acute coronary syndromes. Chronic antiplatelet therapy with aspirin reduces the odds of vascular death in high-risk individuals, but the benefit is smaller and not significant in low-risk individuals.[183] Warfarin reduces all-cause mortality in patients with coronary artery disease but is associated with increased risk of bleeding.[184]

Drugs such as quinidine, erythromycin, psychotropic drugs, cocaine, and terfenadine that produce proarrhythmic side effects can be associated with prolongation of the Q-T interval and an increased risk of sudden death.

Variation in process and outcome after unexpected cardiac death

There is a wide geographic variation in outcomes after the onset of cardiac arrest.[185,186] This is attributable in part to regional differences in the availability of out-of-hospital and hospital-based emergency cardiac care.[185] Potential interventions for out-of-hospital cardiac arrest include: bystander CPR, lay responder defibrillation programs,[187] experienced EMS providers,[188] and interventions provided by EMS providers[189,190] or at receiving hospitals.[191,192] Only lay responder defibrillation and therapeutic hypothermia, however, have been shown in randomized trials to improve significantly outcomes to hospital discharge after cardiac arrest.

Also there is regional variation in EMS processes such as EMS service level provided, number of EMS providers responding, use of procedures or drugs in the field, training, quality assurance/feedback, and response time intervals. Some of these factors have been associated with differences in survival or quality of life after resuscitation,[186,193–196] although no analysis has had adequate power to detect independent effects of all factors.

The median reported rate of survival to discharge after out-of-hospital unexpected cardiac death with any first recorded rhythm is only 6.4%.[186] It is likely that this overestimates the actual rate of survival in many communities because of publication bias. In many large urban areas the rate is less than 2%,[34,197,198] and it is even lower in some cities and rural areas. Most communities are not aware of their own survival rates as cardiac arrest data are not routinely tracked. Yet a city with an organized emergency medical service (EMS) system and dedicated quality assurance can achieve survival of 15 to 20%[50] (and Unpublished data, Seattle Medic One program, August 28, 2005). If the average survival could be improved from 5 to 20% by optimizing the chain of survival, the premature deaths of 16 000 to 36 000 in North America, or 67 500 in Europe could be prevented each year.

There are several challenges to improving survival from cardiac arrest. Successful treatment depends more on when treatment is done than on what is done. The most crucial treatment takes place outside the hospital by citizens and trained rescuers. Treatment crosses medical disciplines, with EMS providers, emergency physicians, cardiologists, anesthesiologists, critical care physicians, and primary care physicians all involved in delivering care and contributing to research. Treatments are relatively standardized, but what generates considerable controversy is the timely delivery of care. The latter depends on the implementation and maintenance of an integrated, community-wide, emergency cardiac care system that has been referred to as the chain of survival.[199,200]

The chain includes early access, early CPR, early defibrillation, and early ACLS. The strength of the chain of survival is the strongest predictor of survival for victims of cardiac arrest. It is not measured directly in studies as a single variable because it includes many interlinked factors. During treatment of cardiac arrest, single factors are less important than how and how quickly all the treatments are put together. Communities that have effective chains of survival will have good survival rates; conversely, communities that have even one weak link in the chain will suffer poor survival rates.

Identification, monitoring, and comparison of outcomes after EMS care among communities is desirable because it aids development of better systems. Since treatment of cardiac arrest is generally initiated by the EMS system, it is crucial for system managers to make decisions about what system or set of protocols works best. Difficulties in reporting survival rates and comparing results among communities make it difficult to determine how much survival benefit can be obtained from a particular intervention, such as upgrading equipment or changing the CPR protocol. The Utstein guidelines are an important step to improving uniformity in reporting survival rates. These guidelines aim for use of clear standardized definitions in an effort to facilitate comparison of community survival rates and logical subgroup analysis.

As already indicated, the primary obstacle to effective treatment is time. Whereas it is relatively easy to know the best treatment for victims of cardiac arrest, the difficulty lies in providing that treatment rapidly. It is the extended time until defibrillation and treatment that is responsible for most deaths from cardiac arrest. Since time relates primarily to the structure of the emergency cardiac care system within the community, changes that reduce the response time intervals should improve survival.

The multiple factors that affect survival after cardiac arrest are described below: risk factors are classified as social, educational, behavioral, clinical, or health system risk factors.

Risk factors affecting survival from sudden death

Social

Socioeconomic status is an important factor in predicting survival from cardiac arrest.[201] In Seattle, high socioeconomic status estimated was associated with a 1.6-fold increase in survival rate, after adjustments for age, witnessed collapse, bystander-initiated cardiopulmonary resuscitation, time from call to paramedic arrival, activity, location of collapse, and chronic morbidity. Part of the challenge of separating socioeconomic status from associated factors (e.g., race or geography) is the need to assess the validity of the surrogate estimate of socioeconomic status. It is unclear whether a single value (the socioeconomic status surrogate) reflects an individual's cumulative lifetime experience with the health care system, diet, exercise, smoking, stress, and the factors thought to be mediators of socioeconomic status. Determining the role of socioeconomic status in incidence and survival from cardiac arrest is a worthy but complex analytic task.

Location

A large proportion of cardiac arrests occur in the patient's home.[24,202] Such patients are older, less often witnessed, less often receive bystander CPR, and have a longer interval between collapse and the arrival of EMS providers.[203,204] Even when these factors are accounted for, arrest in the home is an independent predictor of adverse outcomes. Persons who venture into public places are unlikely to be healthy.

Witnessed cardiac arrest

Witnessed cardiac arrest has been consistently observed to be an important predictor of successful resuscitation.[205] It is only logical that people who suffer unwitnessed cardiac arrest will not fare well. Those with witnessed arrest who are treated promptly have a particularly good prognosis. Extended resuscitation efforts on some of these individuals may be futile.[206–208] Criteria exist for field termination of resuscitation, as ongoing efforts may not be justifiable in those who do not achieve restoration of circulation, because of the cost and risks of speeding ambulances to both rescuers and citizens. Yet successful resuscitation is occasionally observed after prolonged CPR.[209,210–213] These discordant results reflect a need to tailor therapy to the duration of time since the onset of arrest.[27]

Clinical

Initial cardiac rhythm

Which cardiac rhythm is present upon arrival of EMS providers is an important predictor of outcome. The likelihood that the initial recorded rhythm will be ventricular fibrillation depends on the time interval since the onset of arrest.[62] Patients in VT or VF are several times more likely to survive than are patients with asystole and PEA. But patients who are not in ventricular fibrillation are indeed resuscitated with ACLS treatment. For example, 13% of those who survived cardiac arrest in Seattle, WA in 1999–2000 were initially in one of the poor prognostic rhythms (asystole or PEA).[50] Although the rate of survival to discharge remains low in these latter groups, the proportion of patients admitted to hospital has increased over time. Thus, resuscitation attempts and further research are warranted for these patients.

Age

Age is an independent factor in survival from cardiac arrest, but is not as strong a predictor as many other factors. Although some controversy exists with respect to resuscitation in elderly persons, studies so far show that many older persons do quite well after cardiac arrest. Nevertheless, elderly patients have lower survival and quality of life after resuscitation compared to the non-elderly.[214] Some of these differences reflect the presence or absence of prior comorbid illness.[215] A 10-year increase in age resulted in a decrease in survival rate of 10 to 50%.[81,201]

Gender

The effect of gender upon outcomes after cardiac arrest is unclear. A single-center observational study suggested that survival to discharge rates for women and men are about the same.[216] However a large community-based cohort study suggested that women had markedly reduced rates of ventricular fibrillation (VF), slightly older age, fewer witnessed arrests, and fewer arrests in public locations than men.[217] Unadjusted survival rates were lower in women than in men (11% vs. 15%, $P < 0.0001$). Women had similar survival after adjustment for VF (OR, 0.97; 95% CI, 0.85 to 1.11) and after adjustment for VF plus additional factors (OR, 1.09; 95% CI, 0.93 to 1.27).

Race

Race is an significant and important independent predictor for survival from cardiac arrest.[81,218] In Chicago, the survival rate for blacks was 0.8% compared to 2.6% for whites. Blacks were found to have significantly fewer witnessed cardiac arrests or favorable initial rhythms, were less likely to receive bystander CPR, and to be admitted to the hospital. When they were admitted, blacks were half as likely to survive. There was no important difference in the response time for EMS. In Seattle, the initial resuscitation rate was low in black victims (17.1% vs. 40.7%), and rates of survival to hospital discharge were also lower in blacks (9.4% vs 17.1%). The differences in outcomes were not fully explained by features of the collapse or relevant EMS factors. Possible explanations for the racial gap in outcomes after cardiac arrest include less bystander-initiated cardiopulmonary resuscitation, poorer levels of health, and differences in the underlying cardiac disorders. Improving survival for blacks could be accomplished by a general strengthening of the chain of survival for all citizens. In addition, problems in the chain of survival specific to the black community need to be sought and targeted for improvement.

Health system

Bystander cardiopulmonary resuscitation

Since its rediscovery by Kouwenhoven, Jude, and Knickerbocker in 1954,[219] external chest compressions coupled with ventilation (CPR) have been shown to be life-saving, in numerous studies conferring a twofold to three-fold increase in survival rate.[205,220,221] Despite such benefit, many members of the general public are not well trained in this technique. The elderly and minorities are less likely to be trained, to be familiar with what CPR is or how to be trained to perform it,[222] and less likely to perform it at the time of arrest.[81,82] Teaching CPR to citizens can be substantially improved. An effective program for training older people, who are more likely to be present at an arrest, to perform CPR has not been developed. Most communities have rates of bystander CPR around 20 to 30% of arrests. Short video-based, self-instruction programs of CPR training, however, have achieved initial competency equivalent to standard CPR.[223] Broad implementation of such programs may improve the likelihood of bystander CPR in the next decade.

Lay responder defibrillation

Lay responder or public access defibrillation is a strategy that consists of training and equipping lay volunteers to use defibrillation while awaiting arrival of emergency medical services (EMS) providers. A large randomized trial evaluated the effectiveness of public access defibrillation.[224] Participating sites were communities served by EMS systems that provided advanced life support. Each site identified distinct units within their service area (e.g., office buildings, public areas). Volunteer lay responders in both control and intervention units were trained to: (a) recognize cardiac arrest, (b) dial 911, and (c) perform CPR. Units randomized to intervention also received training in application of an AED. The intervention was designed to place a trained lay responder, with an AED in CPR+AED units, at the side of an individual experiencing arrest within 3 minutes of event identification.

The study population comprised individuals with out-of-hospital sudden cardiac arrest. More than 19 000 volunteer responders in 24 North American regions participated. There were more survivors to hospital discharge in the units assigned to have volunteers trained in CPR plus the use of AEDs (30 survivors among 128 arrests) than there were in the units assigned to have volunteers trained only in CPR (15 among 107; $P = 0.03$; relative risk, 2.0; 95 percent confidence interval, 1.07 to 3.77); there were only two survivors in residential complexes. This trial confirmed that training and equipping volunteers to attempt early defibrillation within a structured response system can increase the number of survivors to hospital discharge after out-of-hospital cardiac arrest in public locations. Trained laypersons can use AEDs safely and effectively.

Paramedic-witnessed cardiac arrest

Cardiac arrest witnessed by paramedics deserves special attention. This includes all patients who suffer arrest after the arrival of rescuers; they or others have called for help from 911 before arrest, usually for chest pain or shortness of breath.[225] They account for less than 15% of cardiac arrests in most series. These patients may have an underlying pathologic condition that is somewhat different from that in sudden death since they have symptoms longer (and are able to call for help). Of note, not all of these patients have an initial recorded rhythm of ventricular fibrillation or ventricular tachycardia. In addition, because their cardiac arrest has occurred in the presence of paramedics, they may provide a better indication of how well the EMS performs than the overall community-wide survival rate. Patients who are witnessed by paramedics have a two- to threefold increase in survival rate compared with those not witnessed by paramedics.

Short treatment intervals

The chance of survival diminishes with each passing minute without CPR, defibrillation, or advanced cardiac life support.[186,205,226,227] In an EMS system staffed by highly trained, experienced EMS providers who treat a high volume of calls and perform a high volume of procedures each year, with independent medical oversight and quality assurance in Seattle, WA, survival was predicted by time to CPR and defibrillation.[205] In patients with witnessed ventricular fibrillation before EMS arrival, survival decreased by 3% with each minute until CPR was started, and by 4% with each minute to first shock after CPR has been started. In a similar mature EMS system in King County, Washington, survival was predicted by three time intervals: time to CPR, defibrillation, and advanced cardiac life support (ACLS) care.[226] In patients with witnessed ventricular fibrillation before EMS arrival, survival decreased by 3% for each minute to first shock after CPR has been started, and by 2% for each minute to advanced care after the first shock. Although not all communities have these exact findings, modeling survival provides the best data currently available on the effect of interventions such as CPR or defibrillation. In other EMS systems staffed by less experienced EMS providers who have a lower call volume each year, provision of CPR and defibrillation, but not advanced cardiac life support, significantly improved survival to discharge.[135] Collectively, these studies emphasize the importance of timely intervention and of considering differences in EMS structure and function when comparing results across EMS systems.

Rescuer performance

The training and performance of rescuers in the EMS predicts outcome after cardiac arrest.[188] Physician involvement in training, supervision, evaluation, and leadership is likely to be a substantial ingredient of successful systems and is currently not measured.[228] The use of quality assurance in EMS is infrequent and immature, but can have significant and important effects on outcome. When quality assurance is performed, it sometimes assesses factors such as education rather than performance or outcome indicators. Recent studies have demonstrated that CPR is frequently not performed according to evidence-based guidelines in the out-of-hospital and in-hospital setting.[37,229,230] Although these studies lacked power to detect a significant relationship between CPR process and patient outcome, a related study demonstrated that a greater rate of chest compressions was associated with a greater likelihood of achieving restoration of spontaneous circulation.[231] Collectively, these studies reemphasize the importance of medical oversight to assure and improve the quality of prehospital emergency care.

Future directions

In the future, significant changes in resuscitation are likely to occur. Observational studies will continue to improve the field of resuscitation. New epidemiologic data are desperately needed to answer the following questions:

- What is the current incidence and survival rate of out-of-hospital cardiac arrest? Why has the survival rate after cardiac arrest remained static?
- Can the proportion of cases that receive bystander CPR be increased?
- Can outcomes be improved by broad implementation of quality assurance of EMS care?
- Is training and equipping family members of those at risk for cardiac arrest an effective method of reducing time to defibrillation and increasing survival?

- Can differences in incidence and survival according to race and socioeconomic status be reduced?

To find answers to these questions and to test future therapies, more accurate and larger quantities of data are needed than are currently available. National or international databases offer the best opportunities to do so. Data accuracy must be improved so that real verifiable time intervals can be measured. A critical step towards improving outcomes is for every community to monitor and improve its rate of survival after out-of-hospital cardiac arrest. Finally, new therapies must be developed to improve treatment.

REFERENCES

1. Last, J.M. ed. *A Dictionary of Epidemiology*. Oxford, England: International Epidemiological Association, 2000.

2. Gillum, R.F. Sudden coronary death in the United States: 1980–1985. *Circulation* 1989; **79**: 756–765.

3. Higgins, M.W., & Luepker, R.V. *Trends in Coronary Heart Disease Mortality: The Influence of Medical Care*. New York: Oxford University Press, 1988.

4. Rosamond, W.D., Chambless, L.E., Folsom, A.R. *et al*. Trends in the incidence of myocardial infarction and in mortality due to coronary heart disease, 1987 to 1994. *N. Engl. J. Med.* 1998; **339**: 861–867.

5. Jacobs, I., Nadkarni, V., Bahr, J. *et al*. Cardiac arrest and cardiopulmonary resuscitation outcome reports: update and simplification of the Utstein templates for resuscitation registries: a statement for healthcare professionals from a task force of the International Liaison Committee on Resuscitation (American Heart Association, European Resuscitation Council, Australian Resuscitation Council, New Zealand Resuscitation Council, Heart and Stroke Foundation of Canada, InterAmerican Heart Foundation, Resuscitation Councils of Southern Africa). *Circulation* 2004; **110**(21): 3385–3397.

6. Working Group on Ischemic Heart Disease Registers. Report of A Working Group. Parts I and II. Copenhagen, Denmark: Regional Office for Europe, World Health Organization, 1969.

7. Kurkciyan, I., Meron, G., Behringer, W. *et al*. Accuracy and impact of presumed cause in patients with cardiac arrest. *Circulation* 1998; **98**(8): 766–771.

8. Uretsky, B.F., Thygesen, K., Armstrong, P.W. *et al*. Acute coronary findings at autopsy in heart failure patients with sudden death: results from the assessment of treatment with lisinopril and survival (ATLAS) trial. *Circulation* 2000; **102**(6): 611–616.

9. Soo, L.H., Gray, D., & Hampton, J.R. Pathological features of witnessed out-of-hospital cardiac arrest presenting with ventricular fibrillation. *Resuscitation* 2001; **51**(3): 257–264.

10. Yusuf, S., Reddy, S., Ounpuu, S., & Anand, S. Global burden of cardiovascular diseases: part I: general considerations, the epidemiologic transition, risk factors, and impact of urbanization. *Circulation* 2001; **104**(22): 2746–2753.

11. Anonymous. *World Health Report 2002: Reducing Risks and Promoting Healthy Life*. Geneva: World Health Organization, 2002.

12. Mathers, C.D., Stein, C., Fat Ma, D. *et al*. *Global Burden of Disease 2000*. Version 2: *Methods and Results*. Geneva: World Health Organization, 2002.

13. Myerburg, R.J., Kessler, K.M., & Castellanos, A. Sudden cardiac death: epidemiology, transient risk, and intervention assessment. *Ann. Intern. Med.* 1993; **119**(12): 1187–1197.

14. Rea, T.D., Pearce, R.M., Raghunathan, T.E. *et al*. Incidence of out-of-hospital cardiac arrest. *Am. J. Cardiol.* 2004; **93**(12): 1455–1460.

15. Chugh, S.S., Jui, J., Gunson, K. *et al*. Current burden of sudden cardiac death: multiple source surveillance versus retrospective death certificate-based review in a large U.S. community. *J. Am. Coll. Cardiol.* 2004; **44**(6): 1268–1275.

16. Sayre, M.R., Travers, A.H., Daya, M. *et al*. Measuring survival rates from sudden cardiac arrest: the elusive definition. *Resuscitation* 2004; **62**(1): 25–34.

17. Eisenberg, M.S., Cummins, R.O., & Larsen, M.P. Numerators, denominators and survival rates: reporting survival from out-of-hospital cardiac arrest. *Am. J. Emerg. Med.* 1991; **9**: 544–546.

18. Martens, P., Mullie, A., Calle, P., Van Hoeyweghen, R., & Group, B.C.R.S. Influence on outcome after cardiac arrest of time elapsed between call for help and start of bystander basic CPR. *Resuscitation* 1993; **25**: 227–234.

19. Valenzuela, T.D., Spaite, D.W., Meislin, H.W., Clark, L.L., Wright, A.L., & Ewy, GA. Emergency vehicle intervals versus collapse-to-CPR and collapse-to- defibrillation intervals: monitoring emergency medical services system performance in sudden cardiac arrest. *Ann. Emerg. Med.* 1993; **22**(11): 1678–1683.

20. Wik, L., Steen, P., & Bircher, N. Quality of bystander cardiopulmonary resuscitation influences outcome after prehospital cardiac arrest. *Resuscitation* 1994; **28**: 195–203.

21. Fox, C.S., Evans, J.C., Larson, M.G. *et al*. A comparison of death certificate out-of-hospital coronary heart disease death with physician-adjudicated sudden cardiac death. *Am. J. Cardiol.* 2005; **95**(7): 856–859.

22. Zheng, Z.J., Croft, J.B., Giles, W.H., & Mensah, G.A. Sudden cardiac death in the United States, 1989 to 1998. *Circulation* 2001; **104**(18): 2158–2163.

23. Cummins, R.O., & Graves, J.R. Cardiopulmonary resuscitation: clinics in critical care medicine. In Kaye, W., & Bircher, N., eds. *Cardiopulmonary Resuscitation: Clinics in Critical Care Medicine*. New York: Churchill-Livingstone, 1989.

24. Holmberg, M., Holmberg, S., Herlitz, J., & Gardelov, B. Survival after cardiac arrest outside hospital in Sweden. Swedish Cardiac Arrest Registry. *Resuscitation* 1998; **36**(1): 29–36.

25. Cobbe, S.M., Redmond, M.J., Watson, J.M., Hollingworth, J., & Carrington, D.J. "Heartstart Scotland" – initial experience of a national scheme for out of hospital defibrillation. *Br. Med. J.* 1991; **302**(6791): 1517–1520.

26. Nichol, G., Steen, P., Herlitz, J. *et al.* International Resuscitation Network Registry: design, rationale and preliminary results. *Resuscitation* 2005; **65**(3): 265–277.

27. Weisfeldt, M.L., & Becker, L.B. Resuscitation after cardiac arrest: a 3-phase time-sensitive model. *J. Am. Med. Assoc.* 2002; **288**(23): 3035–3038.

28. Valenzuela, T.D., Roe, D.J., Nichol, G., Clark, L.L., Spaite, D.W., & Hardman, R.G. Outcomes of rapid defibrillation by security officers after cardiac arrest in casinos. *N. Engl. J. Med.* 2000; **343**(17): 1206–1209.

29. Martinez-Rubio, A., Kanaan, N., Borggrefe, M. *et al.* Advances for treating in-hospital cardiac arrest: safety and effectiveness of a new automatic external cardioverter-defibrillator. *J. Am. Coll. Cardiol.* 2003; **41**(4): 627–632.

30. Morrison, L.J., Dorian, P., Long, J. *et al.* Out-of-hospital cardiac arrest rectilinear biphasic to monophasic damped sine defibrillation waveforms with advanced life support intervention trial (ORBIT). *Resuscitation* 2005; **66**(2): 149–157.

31. van Alem, A.P., Vrenken, R.H., de Vos, R., Tijssen, J.G., & Koster, R.W. Use of automated external defibrillator by first responders in out of hospital cardiac arrest: prospective controlled trial. *Br. Med. J.* 2003; **327**(7427): 1312.

32. Hallstrom, A.P. Should time from cardiac arrest until call to emergency medical services (EMS) be collected in EMS research? *Crit. Care Med.* 2002; **30**(4 Suppl): S127–S130.

33. Ornato, J.P., Doctor, M.L., Harbour, L.F. *et al.* Synchronization of timepieces to the atomic clock in an urban emergency medical services system. *Ann. Emerg. Med.* 1998; **31**(4): 483–487.

34. Lombardi, G., Gallagher, J., & Gennis, P. Outcome of out-of-hospital cardiac arrest in New York City. The Pre-Hospital Arrest Survival Evaluation (PHASE) Study. *J. Am. Med. Assoc.* 1994; **271**(9): 678–683.

35. Valenzuela, T.D., Spaite, D.W., Meislin, H.W., Wright, A.L., & Ewy, G.A. Emergency vehicle intervals versus collapse-to-CPR and collapse-to-defibrillation intervals: monitoring emergency medical services system performance in sudden cardiac arrest. *Ann. Emerg. Med.* 1993; **22**: 1678–1683.

36. Sunde, K., Eftestol, T., Askenberg, C., & Steen, P.A. Quality assessment of defibrillation and advanced life support using data from the medical control module of the defibrillator. *Resuscitation* 1999; **41**(3): 237–247.

37. Valenzuela, T.D., Kern, K.B., Clark, L.L. *et al.* Interruptions of chest compressions during emergency medical systems resuscitation. *Circulation* 2005; **112**(9): 1259–1265.

38. Everett, T.H.4th., Wilson, E.E., Foreman, S., & Olgin, J.E. Mechanisms of ventricular fibrillation in canine models of congestive heart failure and ischemia assessed by in vivo noncontact mapping. *Circulation* 2005; **112**(11): 1532–1541.

39. Brown, C.G., Dzwonczyk, R., & Martin, D.R. Physiologic measurement of the ventricular fibrillation ECG signal: estimating the duration of ventricular fibrillation. *Ann. Emerg. Med.* 1993; **22**(1): 70–74.

40. Lightfoot, C.B., Nremt, P., Callaway, C.W. *et al.* Dynamic nature of electrocardiographic waveform predicts rescue shock outcome in porcine ventricular fibrillation. *Ann. Emerg. Med.* 2003; **42**(2): 230–241.

41. Berg, R.A., Hilwig, R.W., Kern, K.B., & Ewy, G.A. Precountershock cardiopulmonary resuscitation improves ventricular fibrillation median frequency and myocardial readiness for successful defibrillation from prolonged ventricular fibrillation: a randomized, controlled swine study. *Ann. Emerg. Med.* 2002; **40**(6): 563–570.

42. Callaway, C.W., Sherman, L.D., Mosesso, V.N., Jr., Dietrich, T.J., Holt, E., & Clarkson, M.C. Scaling exponent predicts defibrillation success for out-of-hospital ventricular fibrillation cardiac arrest. *Circulation* 2001; **103**(12): 1656–1661.

43. Jekova, I., Dushanova, J., & Popivanov, D. Method for ventricular fibrillation detection in the external electrocardiogram using nonlinear prediction. *Physiol. Meas.* 2002; **23**(2): 337–345.

44. Eftestol, T., Sunde, K., & Steen, P.A. Effects of interrupting precordial compressions on the calculated probability of defibrillation success during out-of-hospital cardiac arrest. *Circulation* 2002; **105**(19): 2270–2273.

45. Maldonado, F.A., Weil, M.H., Tang, W. *et al.* Myocardial hypercarbic acidosis reduces cardiac resuscitability. *Anesthesiology* 1993; **78**(2): 343–352.

46. Jin, X., Weil, M.H., Tang, W. *et al.* End-tidal carbon dioxide as a noninvasive indicator of cardiac index during circulatory shock. *Crit. Care Med.* 2000; **28**(7): 2415–2419.

47. Pernat, A., Weil, M.H., Tang, W. *et al.* Effects of hyper- and hypoventilation on gastric and sublingual PCO_2. *J. Appl. Physiol.* 1999; **87**(3): 933–937.

48. Pirrallo, R.G., Swor, R.A., & Maio, R.F. Inter-rater agreement of paramedic rhythm labeling. *Ann. Emerg. Med.* 1993; **22**(11): 1684–1687.

49. Macdonald, R.D., Swanson, J.M., Mottley, J.L., & Weinstein, C. Performance and error analysis of automated external defibrillator use in the out-of-hospital setting. *Ann. Emerg. Med.* 2001; **38**(3): 262–267.

50. Cobb, L.A., Fahrenbruch, C.E., Olsufka, M., & Copass, M.K. Changing incidence of out-of-hospital ventricular fibrillation, 1980–2000. *J. Am. Med. Assoc.* 2002; **288**(23): 3008–3013.

51. de Vreede-Swagemakers, J.J., Gorgels, A.P., Dubois-Arbouw, W.I. *et al.* Out-of-hospital cardiac arrest in the 1990's: a population-based study in the Maastricht area on incidence, characteristics and survival. *J. Am. Coll. Cardiol.* 1997; **30**(6): 1500–1505.

52. Reddy, K.S., & Yusuf, S. Emerging epidemic of cardiovascular disease in developing countries. *Circulation* 1998; **97**(6): 596–601.

53. Tillinghast, S.J., Doliszny, K.M., Gomez-Marin, O., Lilja, G.P., & Campion, B.C. Change in survival from out-of-hospital cardiac arrest and its effect on coronary heart disease mortality – Minneapolis-St. Paul: the Minnesota Heart Survey. *Am. J. Epidemiol.* 1991; **134**(8): 851–861.

54. Rea, T.D., Eisenberg, M.S., Becker, L.J., Murray, J.A., & Hearne, T. Temporal trends in sudden cardiac arrest: a 25-year emergency medical services perspective. *Circulation* 2003; **107**(22): 2780–2785.

55. Herlitz, J., Bang, A., Gunnarsson, J. *et al.* Factors associated with survival to hospital discharge among patients hospitalised alive after out of hospital cardiac arrest: change in outcome over 20 years in the community of Goteborg, Sweden. *Heart* 2003; **89**(1): 25–30.

56. Donoghue, A., Nadkarni, V., Berg, R.A. *et al.* Out-of-hospital pediatric cardiac arrest: an epidemiologic review and assessment of current knowledge. *Ann. Emerg. Med.* 2005; **46**(6): 512–522.

57. Young, K.D., Gausche-Hill, M., McClung, C.D., & Lewis, R.J. A prospective, population-based study of the epidemiology and outcome of out-of-hospital pediatric cardiopulmonary arrest. *Pediatrics* 2004; **114**(1): 157–164.

58. Mogayzel, C., Quan, L., Graves, L., Teidman, D., Fahrenbruch, C., & Herndon, P. Out-of-hospital ventricular fibrillation in children and adolescents: causes and outcomes. *Ann. Emerg. Med.* 1995; **25**: 484–491.

59. Peberdy, M.A., Kaye, W., Ornato, J.P. *et al.* Cardiopulmonary resuscitation of adults in the hospital: a report of 14, 720 cardiac arrest from the National Registry of Cardiopulmonary Resuscitation. *Resuscitation* 2003; **58**: 297–308.

60. Huikuri, H.V., Castellanos, A., & Myerburg, R.J. Sudden death due to cardiac arrhythmias. *N. Engl. J. Med.* 2001; **345**(20): 1473–1482.

61. Eisenberg, M.S., Cummins, R.O., Damon, S., Larsen, M.P., & Hearne, T.R. Survival rates from out-of-hospital cardiac arrest: recommendations for uniform definitions and data to report. *Ann. Emerg. Med.* 1990; **19**: 1249–1259.

62. Holmberg, M., Holmberg, S., & Herlitz, J. An alternate estimate of the disappearance rate of ventricular fibrillation in out-of-hospital cardiac arrest in Sweden. *Resuscitation* 2001; **49**: 219–220.

63. Leaf, A., Kang, J.X., Xiao, Y.F., & Billman, G.E. Clinical prevention of sudden cardiac death by n-3 polyunsaturated fatty acids and mechanism of prevention of arrhythmias by n-3 fish oils. *Circulation* 2003; **107**(21): 2646–2652.

64. Roden, D.M., & Yang, T. Protecting the heart against arrhythmias: potassium current physiology and repolarization reserve. *Circulation* 2005; **112**(10): 1376–1378.

65. Albert, C.M., Ma, J., Rifai, N., Stampfer, M.J., & Ridker, P.M. Prospective study of C-reactive protein, homocysteine, and plasma lipid levels as predictors of sudden cardiac death. *Circulation* 2002; **105**(22): 2595–2599.

66. Kumari, M., Marmot, M., & Brunner, E. Social determinants of von willebrand factor: the Whitehall II study. *Arterioscler. Thromb. Vasc. Biol.* 2000; **20**(7): 1842–1847.

67. Siscovick, D.S., Lemaitre, R.N., & Mozaffarian, D. The fish story: a diet-heart hypothesis with clinical implications: n-3 polyunsaturated fatty acids, myocardial vulnerability, and sudden death. *Circulation* 2003; **107**(21): 2632–2634.

68. Jouven, X., Desnos, M., Guerot, C., & Ducimetiere, P. Predicting sudden death in the population: the Paris Prospective Study I. *Circulation* 1999; **99**(15): 1978–1983.

69. Spooner, P.M., Albert, C., Benjamin, E.J. *et al.* Sudden cardiac death, genes, and arrhythmogenesis: consideration of new population and mechanistic approaches from a National Heart, Lung, and Blood Institute workshop, Part II. *Circulation* 2001; **103**(20): 2447–2452.

70. Spooner, P.M., Albert, C., Benjamin, E.J. *et al.* Sudden cardiac death, genes, and arrhythmogenesis : consideration of new population and mechanistic approaches from a national heart, lung, and blood institute workshop, part I. *Circulation* 2001; **103**(19): 2361–2364.

71. Tan, H.L., Hofman, N., van Langen, I.M., van der Wal, A.C., & Wilde, A.A. Sudden unexplained death: heritability and diagnostic yield of cardiological and genetic examination in surviving relatives. *Circulation* 2005; **112**(2): 207–213.

72. Friedlander, Y., Siscovick, D.S., Weinmann, S. *et al.* Family history as a risk factor for primary cardiac arrest. *Circulation* 1998; **97**(2): 155–160.

73. Priori, S.G., Barhanin, J., Hauer, R.N. *et al.* Genetic and molecular basis of cardiac arrhythmias: impact on clinical management parts I and II. *Circulation* 1999; **99**(4): 518–528.

74. Schwartz, P.J., Priori, S.G., Spazzolini, C. *et al.* Genotype–phenotype correlation in the long-QT syndrome: gene-specific triggers for life-threatening arrhythmias. *Circulation* 2001; **103**(1): 89–95.

75. Page, R.L., Zipes, D.P., Powell, J.L. *et al.* Seasonal variation of mortality in the antiarrhythmics versus implantable defibrillators (AVID) study registry. *Heart Rhythm* 2004; **1**(4): 435–440.

76. Anonymous. Fall-related injuries during the holiday season – United States, 2000–2003. *Morb. Mortal. Wkly Rep.* 2004; **53**(48): 1127–1129.

77. Crawford, J.R., & Parker, M.J. Seasonal variation of proximal femoral fractures in the United Kingdom. *Injury* 2003; **34**(3): 223–225.

78. Allegra, J.R., Cochrane, D.G., Allegra, E.M., & Cable, G. Calendar patterns in the occurrence of cardiac arrest. *Am. J. Emerg. Med.* 2002; **20**(6): 513–517.

79. Herlitz, J., Eek, M., Holmberg, M., & Holmberg, S. Diurnal, weekly and seasonal rhythm of out of hospital cardiac arrest in Sweden. *Resuscitation* 2002; **54**(2): 133–138.

80. Gruska, M., Gaul, G.B., Winkler, M. *et al.* Increased occurrence of out-of-hospital cardiac arrest on Mondays in a community-based study. *Chronobiol. Int* 2005; **22**(1): 107–120.

81. Becker, L.B., Han, B.H., Meyer, P.M. *et al.* Racial differences in the incidence of cardiac arrest and subsequent survival. The CPR Chicago Project. *N. Engl. J. Med.* 1993; **329**(9): 600–606.

82. Iwashyna, T.J., Christakis, N.A., & Becker, L.B. Neighborhoods matter: a population-based study of provision of cardiopulmonary resuscitation. *Ann. Emerg. Med.* 1999; **34**(4 Pt 1): 459–468.

83. Sampson, R.J., Raudenbush, S.W., & Earls, F. Neighborhoods and violent crime: a multilevel study of collective efficacy. *Science* 1997; **277**(5328): 918–924.

84. Sampson, R.J., Morenoff, J.D., & Raudenbush, S. Social anatomy of racial and ethnic disparities in violence. *Am. J. Public. Health* 2005; **95**(2): 224–232.

85. Dunn, L., Henry, J., & Beard, D. Social deprivation and head injury: a national study. *J. Neurol. Neurosurg. Psychiatry* 2003; **74**(8): 1060–1064.

86. Cubbin, C., LeClere, F.B., & Smith, G.S. Socioeconomic status and the occurrence of fatal and nonfatal injury in the United States. *Am. J. Public Health* 2000; **90**(1): 70–77.

87. Cubbin, C., LeClere, F.B., & Smith, G.S. Socioeconomic status and injury mortality: individual and neighbourhood determinants. *J. Epidemiol. Commun. Hlth.* 2000; **54**(7): 517–524.

88. Singh, G.K., & Siahpush, M. Increasing inequalities in all-cause and cardiovascular mortality among US adults aged 25–64 years by area socioeconomic status, 1969–1998. *Int. J. Epidemiol.* 2002; **31**(3): 600–613.

89. Wilkins, R., Berthelot, J.-M., & Ng, E. Trends in mortality by neighbourhood income in urban Canada from 1971 to 1996. *Health Reports* 2002(Dec. 11).

90. Anonymous. Health disparities experienced by black or African Americans – United States. *Morb. Mortal. Wkly Rep.* 2005; **54**(1): 1–3.

91. Anonymous. Annual smoking-attributable mortality, years of potential life lost, and productivity losses – United States, 1997–2001. *Morb. Mortal. Wkly Rep.* 2005; **54**(25): 625–628.

92. Mehta, M.C., Jain, A.C., Mehta, A., & Billie, M. *Cardiac arrhythmias following intravenous nicotine: experimental study in dogs. J. Cardiovasc. Pharmacol. Ther.* 1997; **2**(4): 291–298.

93. Jamrozik, K. Estimate of deaths attributable to passive smoking among UK adults: database analysis. *Br. Med. J.* 2005; **330**(7495): 812.

94. Berlin, J.A., & Colditz, G.A. A meta-analysis of physical activity in the prevention of coronary heart disease. *Am. J. Epidemiol.* 1990; **132**(4): 612–628.

95. Taylor, R.S., Brown, A., Ebrahim, S. *et al.* Exercise-based rehabilitation for patients with coronary heart disease: systematic review and meta-analysis of randomized controlled trials. *Am. J. Med.* 2004; **116**(10): 682–692.

96. Mittleman, M.A., Maclure, M., Tofler, G.H., Sherwood, J.B., Goldberg, R.J., & Muller, J.E. Triggering of acute myocardial infarction by heavy physical exertion. Protection against triggering by regular exertion. Determinants of Myocardial Infarction Onset Study Investigators. *N. Engl. J. Med.* 1993; **329**(23): 1677–1683.

97. Moliterno, D.J., Willard, J.E., Lange, R.A. *et al.* Coronary-artery vasoconstriction induced by cocaine, cigarette smoking, or both. *N. Engl. J. Med.* 1994; **330**(7): 454–459.

98. Paredes, V.L., Rea, T.D., Eisenberg, M.S. *et al.* Out-of-hospital care of critical drug overdoses involving cardiac arrest. *Acad. Emerg. Med.* 2004; **11**(1): 71–74.

99. Krantz, M.J., Rowan, S.B., & Mehler, P.S. Cocaine-related torsade de pointes in a methadone maintenance patient. *J. Addict. Dis.* 2005; **24**(1): 53–60.

100. Gaziano, J.M., Buring, J.E., Breslow, J.L. *et al.* Moderate alcohol intake, increased levels of high-density lipoprotein and its subfractions, and decreased risk of myocardial infarction. *N. Engl. J. Med.* 1993; **329**(25): 1829–1834.

101. Kupari, M., & Koskinen, P. Alcohol, cardiac arrhythmias and sudden death. *Novartis Found Symp.* 1998; **216**: 68–79.

102. Albert, C.M., Manson, J.E., Cook, N.R., Ajani, U.A., Gaziano, J.M., & Hennekens, C.H. Moderate alcohol consumption and the risk of sudden cardiac death among US male physicians. *Circulation* 1999; **100**(9): 944–950.

103. Wannamethee, G., & Shaper, A.G. Alcohol and sudden cardiac death. *Br. Heart J.* 1992; **68**(5): 443–448.

104. Mittleman, M.A., Maclure, M., Nachnani, M., Sherwood, J.B., & Muller, J.E. Educational attainment, anger, and the risk of triggering myocardial infarction onset. The Determinants of Myocardial Infarction Onset Study Investigators. *Arch. Intern. Med.* 1997; **157**(7): 769–775.

105. Anonymous. A comparison of recombinant hirudin with heparin for the treatment of acute coronary syndromes. The Global Use of Strategies to Open Occluded Coronary Arteries (GUSTO) IIb investigators. *N. Engl. J. Med.* 1996; **335**(11): 775–782.

106. Alexander, J.H., Sparapani, R.A., Mahaffey, K.W. *et al.* Association between minor elevations of creatine kinase-MB level and mortality in patients with acute coronary syndromes without ST-segment elevation. PURSUIT Steering Committee. Platelet Glycoprotein IIb/IIIa in Unstable Angina: Receptor Suppression Using Integrilin Therapy. *J. Am. Med. Assoc.* 2000; **283**(3): 347–353.

107. Califf, R.M., Pieper, K.S., Lee, K.L. *et al.* Prediction of 1-year survival after thrombolysis for acute myocardial infarction in the global utilization of streptokinase and TPA for occluded coronary arteries trial. *Circulation* 2000; **101**(19): 2231–2238.

108. Pinski, S.L., Yao, Q., Epstein, A.E. *et al.* Determinants of outcome in patients with sustained ventricular tachyarrhythmias: the antiarrhythmics versus implantable defibrillators (AVID) study registry. *Am. Heart J.* 2000; **139**(5): 804–813.

109. Moss, A.J., DeCamilla, J., & Davis, H. Cardiac death in the first 6 months after myocardial infarction: potential for mortality reduction in the early posthospital period. *Am. J. Cardiol.* 1977; **39**(6): 816–820.

110. Bailey, J.J., Berson, A.S., Handelsman, H., & Hodges, M. Utility of current risk stratification tests for predicting major arrhythmic events after myocardial infarction. *J. Am. Coll. Cardiol.* 2001; **38**(7): 1902–1911.

111. La Rovere, M.T., Bigger, J.T., Jr., Marcus, F.I., Mortara, A., & Schwartz, P.J., for the ATRAMI Investigators. Baroflex sensitivity and heart-rate variability in prediction of total cardiac mortality after myocardial infarction. *Lancet* 1998; **351**: 478–484.

112. Thompson, R.G., & Cobb, L.A. Hypokalemia after resuscitation from out-of-hospital ventricular fibrillation. *J. Am. Med. Assoc.* 1982; **248**(21): 2860–2863.

113. Estes, N.A., 3rd, Link, M.S., Cannom, D. *et al.* Report of the NASPE policy conference on arrhythmias and the athlete. *J. Cardiovasc. Electrophysiol.* 2001; **12**(10): 1208–1219.

114. Lewington, S., Clarke, R., Qizilbash, N., Peto, R., & Collins, R. Age-specific relevance of usual blood pressure to vascular mortality: a meta-analysis of individual data for one million

adults in 61 prospective studies. *Lancet* 2002; **360**(9349): 1903–1913.

115. Castelli, W.P. Epidemiology of coronary heart disease: the Framingham study. *Am. J. Med.* 1984; **76**(2A): 4–12.

116. Fields, L.E., Burt, V.L., Cutler, J.A., Hughes, J., Roccella, E.J., & Sorlie, P. The burden of adult hypertension in the United States 1999 to 2000: a rising tide. *Hypertension* 2004; **44**(4): 398–404.

117. Vasan, R.S., Beiser, A., Seshadri, S. *et al.* Residual lifetime risk for developing hypertension in middle-aged women and men: the Framingham Heart Study. *J. Am. Med. Assoc.* 2002; **287**(8): 1003–1010.

118. Hajjar, I., & Kotchen, T.A. Trends in prevalence, awareness, treatment, and control of hypertension in the United States, 1988–2000. *J. Am. Med. Assoc.* 2003; **290**(2): 199–206.

119. Psaty, B.M., Lumley, T., Furberg, C.D. *et al.* Health outcomes associated with various antihypertensive therapies used as first-line agents: a network meta-analysis. *J. Am. Med. Assoc.* 2003; **289**(19): 2534–2544.

120. Stamler, J., Wentworth, D., & Neaton, J.D. Is relationship between serum cholesterol and risk of premature death from coronary heart disease continuous and graded? Findings in 356 222 primary screenees of the Multiple Risk Factor Intervention Trial (MRFIT). *J. Am. Med. Assoc.* 1986; **256**(20): 2823–2828.

121. Castelli, W.P. The triglyceride issue: a view from Framingham. *Am. Heart J.* 1986; **112**(2): 432–437.

122. Gould, K.L., Ornish, D., Kirkeeide, R. *et al.* Improved stenosis geometry by quantitative coronary arteriography after vigorous risk factor modification. *Am. J. Cardiol.* 1992; **69**(9): 845–853.

123. Hooper, L., Summerbell, C.D., Higgins, J.P.T. *et al.* Reduced or modified dietary fat for preventing cardiovascular disease. *Cochrane Database Syst. Rev.* 2005(3).

124. Flegal, K.M., Carroll, M.D., Kuczmarski, R.J., & Johnson, C.L. Overweight and obesity in the United States: prevalence and trends, 1960–1994. *Int. J. Obes. Relat. Metab. Disord.* 1998; **22**(1): 39–47.

125. Flegal, K.M., Carroll, M.D., Ogden, C.L., & Johnson, C.L. Prevalence and trends in obesity among US adults, 1999–2000. *J. Am. Med. Assoc.* 2002; **288**(14): 1723–1727.

126. Mokdad, A.H., Serdula, M.K., Dietz, W.H., Bowman, B.A., Marks, J.S., & Koplan, J.P. The spread of the obesity epidemic in the United States, 1991–1998. *J. Am. Med. Assoc.* 1999; **282**(16): 1519–1522.

127. Gregg, E.W., Cheng, Y.J., Cadwell, B.L. *et al.* Secular trends in cardiovascular disease risk factors according to body mass index in US adults. *J. Am. Med. Assoc.* 2005; **293**(15): 1868–1874.

128. Mokdad, A.H., Bowman, B.A., Ford, E.S., Vinicor, F., Marks, J.S., & Koplan, J.P. The continuing epidemics of obesity and diabetes in the United States. *J. Am. Med. Assoc.* 2001; **286**(10): 1195–1200.

129. Karnik, J.A., Young, B.S., Lew, N.L. *et al.* Cardiac arrest and sudden death in dialysis units. *Kidney Int.* 2001; **60**(1): 350–357.

130. Michal, V. Arterial disease as a cause of impotence. *Clin. Endocrinol. Metab.* 1982; **11**(3): 725–748.

131. Wabrek, A.J., & Burchell, R.C. Male sexual dysfunction associated with coronary heart disease. *Arch. Sex Behav.* 1980; **9**(1): 69–75.

132. Connolly, S.J., Hallstrom, A.P., Cappato, R. *et al.* Meta-analysis of the implantable cardioverter defibrillator secondary prevention trials. *Eur. Heart J.* 2000; **21**(24): 2071–2078.

133. Hohnloser, S.H., Kuck, K.H., Dorian, P. *et al.* Prophylactic use of an implantable cardioverter-defibrillator after acute myocardial infarction. *N. Engl. J. Med.* 2004; **351**(24): 2481–2488.

134. Feldman, A.M., Klein, H., Tchou, P. *et al.* Use of a wearable defibrillator in terminating tachyarrhythmias in patients at high risk for sudden death: results of the WEARIT/BIROAD. *Pacing Clin. Electrophysiol.* 2004; **27**(1): 4–9.

135. Parkash, R., Tang, A., Wells, G. *et al.* Use of implantable cardioverter defibrillators after out-of-hospital cardiac arrest: a prospective follow-up study. *CMAJ.* 2004; **171**(9): 1053–1056.

136. Alberte, C., Zipes, D.P. Use of nonantiarrhythmic drugs for prevention of sudden cardiac death. *J. Cardiovasc. Electrophysiol.* 2003; **14**(9 Suppl): S87–S95.

137. Fletcher, R.D., Cintron, G.B., Johnson, G., Orndorff, J., Carson, P., & Cohn, J.N. Enalapril decreases prevalence of ventricular tachycardia in patients with chronic congestive heart failure. The V-HeFT II VA Cooperative Studies Group. *Circulation* 1993; **87**(6 Suppl): VI49–VI55.

138. Schrier, R.W., & Abraham, W.T. Hormones and hemodynamics in heart failure. *N. Engl. J. Med.* 1999; **341**(8): 577–585.

139. Elfellah, M.S., & Ogilvie, R.I. Effect of vasodilator drugs on coronary occlusion and reperfusion arrhythmias in anesthetized dogs. *J. Cardiovasc. Pharmacol.* 1985; **7**(5): 826–832.

140. Domanski, M.J., Exner, D.V., Borkowf, C.B., Geller, N.L., Rosenberg, Y., & Pfeffer, M.A. Effect of angiotensin converting enzyme inhibition on sudden cardiac death in patients following acute myocardial infarction. A meta-analysis of randomized clinical trials. *J. Am. Coll. Cardiol.* 1999; **33**(3): 598–604.

141. Pitt, B., Zannad, F., Remme, W.J. *et al.* The effect of spironolactone on morbidity and mortality in patients with severe heart failure. *N. Engl. J. Med.* 1999; **341**(10): 709–717.

142. Mann, D.L., Kent, R.L., Parsons, B., & Cooper, G.4th. Adrenergic effects on the biology of the adult mammalian cardiocyte. *Circulation* 1992; **85**(2): 790–804.

143. Eichhorn, E.J., & Bristow, M.R. Medical therapy can improve the biological properties of the chronically failing heart. A new era in the treatment of heart failure. *Circulation* 1996; **94**(9): 2285–2296.

144. Anonymous. Randomised, placebo-controlled trial of carvedilol in patients with congestive heart failure due to ischaemic heart disease. Australia/New Zealand Heart Failure Research Collaborative Group. *Lancet* 1997; **349**(9049): 375–380.

145. Packer, M., Bristow, M.R., Cohn, J.N. *et al.* The effect of carvedilol on morbidity and mortality in patients with chronic heart failure. *N. Engl. J. Med.* 1996; **334**: 1349–1355.

146. Anonymous. Effect of metoprolol CR/XL in chronic heart failure: Metoprolol CR/XL Randomised Intervention Trial in Congestive Heart Failure (MERIT-HF). *Lancet* 1999; **353**(9169): 2001–2007.

147. Anonymous. The Cardiac Insufficiency Bisoprolol Study II (CIBIS-II): a randomised trial. *Lancet* 1999; **353**(9146): 9–13.

148. Domanski, M.J., Krause-Steinrauf, H., Massie, B.M. *et al.* A comparative analysis of the results from 4 trials of beta-blocker therapy for heart failure: BEST, CIBIS-II, MERIT-HF, and COPERNICUS. *J. Card. Fail.* 2003; **9**(5): 354–363.

149. Dimmeler, S., Haendeler, J., Galle, J., & Zeiher, A.M. Oxidized low-density lipoprotein induces apoptosis of human endothelial cells by activation of CPP32-like proteases. A mechanistic clue to the 'response to injury' hypothesis. *Circulation* 1997; **95**(7): 1760–1763.

150. Hassall, D.G., Owen, J.S., & Bruckdorfer, K.R. The aggregation of isolated human platelets in the presence of lipoproteins and prostacyclin. *Biochem J.* 1983; **216**(1): 43–49.

151. Ridker, P.M., & Haughie, P. Prospective studies of C-reactive protein as a risk factor for cardiovascular disease. *J. Investig. Med.* 1998; **46**(8): 391–395.

152. LaRosa, J.C., He, J., & Vupputuri, S. Effect of statins on risk of coronary disease: a meta-analysis of randomized controlled trials. *J. Am. Med. Assoc.* 1999; **282**(24): 2340–2346.

153. Anonymous. MRC/BHF Heart Protection Study of cholesterol lowering with simvastatin in 20 536 high-risk individuals: a randomised placebo-controlled trial. *Lancet* 2002; **360**(9326): 7–22.

154. Sweeney, M.O., Moss, A.J., & Eberly, S. Instantaneous cardiac death in the posthospital period after acute myocardial infarction. *Am. J. Cardiol.* 1992; **70**(18): 1375–1379.

155. Anonymous. The effect of digoxin on mortality and morbidity in patients with heart failure. The Digitalis Investigation Group. *N. Engl. J. Med.* 1997; **336**(8): 525–533.

156. Packer, M., Carver, J.R., Rodeheffer, R.J. *et al.* Effect of oral milrinone on mortality in severe chronic heart failure. *N. Engl. J. Med.* 1991; **325**: 1468–1475.

157. Kubo, S.H., Gollub, S., Bourge, R. *et al.* Beneficial effects of pimobendan on exercise tolerance and quality of life in patients with heart failure. Results of a multicenter trial. The Pimobendan Multicenter Research Group. *Circulation* 1992; **85**(3): 942–949.

158. Massie, B.M., Berk, M.R., Brozena, S.C. *et al.* Can further benefit be achieved by adding flosequinan to patients with congestive heart failure who remain symptomatic on diuretic, digoxin, and an angiotensin converting enzyme inhibitor? Results of the flosequinan-ACE inhibitor trial (FACET). *Circulation* 1993; **88**(2): 492–501.

159. Cohn, J.N., Goldstein, S.O., Greenberg, B.H. *et al.* A dose-dependent increase in mortality with vesnarinone among patients with severe heart failure. Vesnarinone Trial Investigators. *N. Engl. J. Med.* 1998; **339**(25): 1810–1816.

160. Anonymous. Preliminary report: effect of encainide and flecainide on mortality in a randomized trial of arrhythmia suppression after myocardial infarction. The Cardiac Arrhythmia Suppression Trial (CAST) Investigators. *N. Engl. J. Med.* 1989; **321**(6): 406–412.

161. Anonymous. Effect of the antiarrhythmic agent moricizine on survival after myocardial infarction. The Cardiac Arrhythmia Suppression Trial II Investigators. *N. Engl. J. Med.* 1992; **327**(4): 227–233.

162. Waldo, A.L., Camm, A.J., deRuyter, H. *et al.* Effect of d-sotalol on mortality in patients with left ventricular dysfunction after recent and remote myocardial infarction. The SWORD Investigators. Survival With Oral d-Sotalol. *Lancet* 1996; **348**(9019): 7–12.

163. Torp-Pedersen, C., Moller, M., Bloch-Thomsen, P.E. *et al.* Dofetilide in patients with congestive heart failure and left ventricular dysfunction. Danish Investigations of Arrhythmia and Mortality on Dofetilide Study Group. *N. Engl. J. Med.* 1999; **341**(12): 857–865.

164. Doval, H.C., Nul, D.R., Grancelli, H.O., Perrone, S.V., Bortman, G.R., & Curiel, R. Randomised trial of low-dose amiodarone in severe congestive heart failure. Grupo de Estudio de la Sobrevida en la Insuficiencia Cardiaca en Argentina (GESICA). *Lancet* 1994; **344**(8921): 493–498.

165. Nicklas, J.M., McKenna, W.J., Stewart, R.A. *et al.* Prospective, double-blind, placebo-controlled trial of low-dose amiodarone in patients with severe heart failure and asymptomatic frequent ventricular ectopy. *Am. Heart J.* 1991; **122**(4 Pt 1): 1016–1021.

166. Cairns, J.A., Connolly, S.J., Roberts, R., & Gent, M. Randomised trial of outcome after myocardial infarction in patients with frequent or repetitive ventricular premature depolarisations: CAMIAT. Canadian Amiodarone Myocardial Infarction Arrhythmia Trial Investigators [published erratum appears in *Lancet* 1997 Jun 14; **349**(9067): 1776] [see comments]. *Lancet* 1997; **349**(9053): 675–682.

167. Julian, D.G., Camm, A.J., Frangin, G. *et al.* Randomised trial of effect of amiodarone on mortality in patients with left-ventricular dysfunction after recent myocardial infarction: EMIAT. European Myocardial Infarct Amiodarone Trial Investigators. *Lancet* 1997; **349**(9053): 667–674.

168. Burkart, F., Pfisterer, M., Kiowski, W., Follath, F., & Burckhardt, D. Effect of antiarrhythmic therapy on mortality in survivors of myocardial infarction with asymptomatic complex ventricular arrhythmias: Basel Antiarrhythmic Study of Infarct Survival (BASIS). *J. Am. Coll. Cardiol.* 1990; **16**(7): 1711–1718.

169. Ceremuzynski, L., Kleczar, E., Krzeminska-Pakula, M. *et al.* Effect of amiodarone on mortality after myocardial infarction: a double-blind, placebo-controlled, pilot study. *J. Am. Coll. Cardiol.* 1992; **20**(5): 1056–1062.

170. Pfisterer, M., Kiowski, W., Burckhardt, D., Follath, F., & Burkart, F. Beneficial effect of amiodarone on cardiac mortality in patients with asymptomatic complex ventricular arrhythmias after acute myocardial infarction and preserved but not impaired left ventricular function. *Am. J. Cardiol.* 1992; **69**(17): 1399–1402.

171. Anonymous. Effect of prophylactic amiodarone on mortality after acute myocardial infarction and in congestive heart

failure: meta-analysis of individual data from 6500 patients in randomised trials. Amiodarone Trials Meta-Analysis Investigators. *Lancet* 1997; **350**(9089): 1417–1424.

172. Greene, H.L. The CASCADE Study: randomized antiarrhythmic drug therapy in survivors of cardiac arrest in Seattle. CASCADE Investigators. *Am. J. Cardiol.* 1993; **72**(16): 70F–74F.

173. Tsutamoto, T., Wada, A., Maeda, K. *et al.* Angiotensin II type 1 receptor antagonist decreases plasma levels of tumor necrosis factor alpha, interleukin-6 and soluble adhesion molecules in patients with chronic heart failure. *J. Am. Coll. Cardiol.* 2000; **35**(3): 714–721.

174. Goodfield, N.E., Newby, D.E., Ludlam, C.A., & Flapan, A.D. Effects of acute angiotensin II type 1 receptor antagonism and angiotensin converting enzyme inhibition on plasma fibrinolytic parameters in patients with heart failure. *Circulation* 1999; **99**(23): 2983–2985.

175. Pitt, B. Evaluation of Losartan in the Elderly (ELITE) Trial: clinical implications. *Eur. Heart J.* 1997; **18**(8): 1197–1199.

176. Pitt, B., Poole-Wilson, P.A., Segal, R. *et al.* Effect of losartan compared with captopril on mortality in patients with symptomatic heart failure: randomised trial – the Losartan Heart Failure Survival Study ELITE II. *Lancet* 2000; **355**(9215): 1582–1587.

177. Dickstein, K., & Kjekshus, J. Effects of losartan and captopril on mortality and morbidity in high-risk patients after acute myocardial infarction: the OPTIMAAL randomised trial. Optimal Trial in Myocardial Infarction with Angiotensin II Antagonist Losartan. *Lancet* 2002; **360**(9335): 752–760.

178. Marcus, F.I., Cobb, L.A., Edwards, J.E. *et al.* Mechanism of death and prevalence of myocardial ischemic symptoms in the terminal event after acute myocardial infarction. *Am. J. Cardiol.* 1988; **61**(1): 8–15.

179. Anonymous. Indications for fibrinolytic therapy in suspected acute myocardial infarction: collaborative overview of early mortality and major morbidity results from all randomised trials of more than 1000 patients. Fibrinolytic Therapy Trialists' (FTT) Collaborative Group. *Lancet* 1994; **343**: 311–322.

180. Cohen, M., Demers, C., Gurfinkel, E.P. *et al.* A comparison of low-molecular-weight heparin with unfractionated heparin for unstable coronary artery disease. Efficacy and Safety of Subcutaneous Enoxaparin in Non-Q-Wave Coronary Events Study Group. *N. Engl. J. Med.* 1997; **337**(7): 447–452.

181. Kong, D.F., Califf, R.M., Miller, D.P. *et al.* Clinical outcomes of therapeutic agents that block the platelet glycoprotein IIb/IIIa integrin in ischemic heart disease. *Circulation* 1998; **98**(25): 2829–2835.

182. Yusuf, S., Zhao, F., Mehta, S.R., Chrolavicius, S., Tognoni, G., & Fox, K.K. Effects of clopidogrel in addition to aspirin in patients with acute coronary syndromes without ST-segment elevation. *N. Engl. J. Med.* 2001; **345**(7): 494–502.

183. Anonymous. Collaborative overview of randomised trials of antiplatelet therapy – I: Prevention of death, myocardial infarction, and stroke by prolonged antiplatelet therapy in various categories of patients. Antiplatelet Trialists' Collaboration. *Br. Med. J.* 1994; **308**(6921): 81–106.

184. Anand, S.S., & Yusuf, S. Oral anticoagulant therapy in patients with coronary artery disease: a meta-analysis. *J. Am. Med. Assoc.* 1999; **282**(21): 2058–2067.

185. Eisenberg, M.S., Horwood, B.T., Cummins, R.O., Reynolds-Haertle, R., & Hearne, T.R. Cardiac arrest and resuscitation: a tale of 29 cities. *Ann. Emerg. Med.* 1990; **19**: 179–186.

186. Nichol, G., Stiell, I.G., Laupacis, A., Pham, B., De Maio, V., & Wells, G.A. A cumulative metaanalysis of the effectiveness of defibrillator-capable emergency medical services for victims of out-of-hospital cardiac arrest. *Ann. Emerg. Med.* 1999; **34**(4): 517–525.

187. Anonymous. Public-access defibrillation and survival after out-of-hospital cardiac arrest. *N. Engl. J. Med.* 2004; **351**(7): 637–646.

188. Soo, L.H., Gray, D., Young, T., Skene, A., & Hampton, J.R. Influence of ambulance crew's length of experience on the outcome of out-of-hospital cardiac arrest. *Eur. Heart J.* 1999; **20**(7): 535–540.

189. Kudenchuk, P.J., Cobb, L.A., Copass, M.K. *et al.* Amiodarone for resuscitation after out-of-hospital cardiac arrest due to ventricular fibrillation. *N. Engl. J. Med.* 1999; **341**(12): 871–878.

190. Dorian, P., Cass, D., Schwartz, B., Cooper, R., Gelaznikas, R., & Barr, A. Amiodarone as compared with lidocaine for shock-resistant ventricular fibrillation. *N. Engl. J. Med.* 2002; **346**(12): 884–890.

191. Bernard, S.A., Gray, T.W., Buist, M.D. *et al.* Treatment of comatose survivors of out-of-hospital cardiac arrest with induced hypothermia.[comment]. *N. Engl. J Med.* 2002; **346**(8): 557–563.

192. Anonymous. Mild therapeutic hypothermia to improve the neurologic outcome after cardiac arrest. The Hypothermia after Cardiac Arrest Study Group.[erratum appears in *N. Engl. J. Med.* 2002 May 30; **346**(22): 1756]. *N. Engl. J. Med.* 2002; **346**(8): 549–556.

193. van der Hoeven, J., de Koning, J., van der Weyden, P., & Meinders, A. Improved outcome for patients with a cardiac arrest by supervision of the emergency medical services system. *Netherlands J. Med.* 1995; **46**: 123–130.

194. Bergner, L., Bergner, M., Hallstrom, A.P., Eisenberg, M.S., & Cobb, L.A. Service factors and health status of survivors of out-of-hospital cardiac arrest. *Am. J. Emerg. Med.* 1983; **1**(3): 259–263.

195. Frandsen, F., Nielsen, J.R., Gram, L. *et al.* Evaluation of intensified prehospital treatment in out-of-hospital cardiac arrest: survival and cerebral prognosis. The Odense Ambulance Study. *Cardiology* 1991; **79**: 256–264.

196. Stiell, I.G., Wells, G.A., Field, B.J. *et al.* Improved out-of-hospital cardiac arrest survival through the inexpensive optimization of an existing defibrillation program: OPALS study phase II. Ontario Prehospital Advanced Life Support. *J. Am. Med. Assoc.* 1999; **281**(13): 1175–1181.

197. Becker, L.B., Ostrander, M.P., Barrett, J., & Kondos, G.T. Outcomes of CPR in a large metropolitan area – where are the survivors? *Ann. Emerg. Med.* 1991; **20**(4): 355–361.

198. Eckstein, M., Stratton, S.J., & Chan, L.S. Cardiac arrest resuscitation evaluation in Los Angeles: CARE-LA. *Ann. Emerg. Med.* 2005; **45**(5): 504–509.

199. Cummins, R.O., Ornato, J.P., Thies, W.H., & Pepe, P.E. Improving survival from sudden cardiac arrest: The "chain of survival" concept. *Circulation* 1991; **83**: 1832–1847.

200. Jacobs, I., Callanan, V., Nichol, G. *et al.* The chain of survival. *Ann. Emerg. Med.* 2001; **37**(4 Pt 2): S5–S16.

201. Hallstrom, A., Boutin, P., Cobb, L., & Johnson, E. Socioeconomic status and prediction of ventricular fibrillation survival. *Am. J. Public Health* 1993; **83**(2): 245–248.

202. Pell, J.P., Sirel, J., Marsden, A.K., & Cobbe, S.M. Sex differences in outcome following community-based cardiopulmonary arrest. *Eur. Heart J.* 2000; **21**(3): 239–244.

203. Litwin, P.E., Eisenberg, M.S., Hallstrom, A.P., & Cummins, R.O. The location of collapse and its effect on survival from cardiac arrest. *Ann. Emerg. Med.* 1987; **16**(7): 787–791.

204. Herlitz, J., Eek, M., Holmberg, M., Engdahl, J., & Holmberg, S. Characteristics and outcome among patients having out of hospital cardiac arrest at home compared with elsewhere. *Heart* 2002; **88**(6): 579–582.

205. Weaver, W.D., Cobb, L.A., Hallstrom, A.P. *et al.* Considerations for improving survival from out-of-hospital cardiac arrest. *Ann. Emerg. Med.* 1986; **15**: 1181–1186.

206. Gray, W.A., Capone, R.J., & Most, A.S. Unsuccessful emergency medical resuscitation – are continued efforts in the emergency department justified? *N. Engl. J. Med.* 1991; **325**(20): 1393–1398.

207. Kellermann, A., Hackman, B., & Somes, G. Predicting the outcome of unsuccessful prehospital advanced cardiac life support. *J. Am. Med. Assoc.* 1993; **270**: 1433–1436.

208. Bonnin, M.J., Pepe, P.E., Kimball, K.T., & Clark, P.S. Distinct criteria for termination of resuscitation in the out-of-hospital setting. *J. Am. Med. Assoc.* 1993; **270**: 1457–1462.

209. Beyersdorf, F., Kirsh, M., Buckberg, G.D., Allen, B.S., Bonchek, L.I., & Arom, K.V. Warm glutamate/aspartate-enriched blood cardioplegic solution for perioperative sudden death. *J. Thorac. Cardiovasc. Surg.* 1992; **104**(4): 1141–1147.

210. Plaisance, P., Lurie, K.G., & Payen, D. Inspiratory impedance during active compression-decompression cardiopulmonary resuscitation: a randomized evaluation in patients in cardiac arrest. *Circulation* 2000; **101**(9): 989–994.

211. Wolcke, B.B., Mauer, D.K., Schoefmann, M.F. *et al.* Comparison of standard cardiopulmonary resuscitation versus the combination of active compression-decompression cardiopulmonary resuscitation and an inspiratory impedance threshold device for out-of-hospital cardiac arrest. *Circulation* 2003; **108**(18): 2201–2205.

212. Thayne, R.C., Thomas, D.C., Neville, J.D., & van Dellen, A. Use of an impedance threshold device improves short-term outcomes following out-of-hospital cardiac arrest. *Resuscitation* 2005; **67**(1): 103–108.

213. Aufderheide, T., Pirallo, R.G., Provo, T.A., & Lurie, K.G. Clinical evaluation of an inspiratory impedance threshold device during standard cardiopulmonary resuscitation in patients with out-of-hospital cardiac arrest. *Crit. Care Med.* 2005; **33**(4):

214. Bunch, T.J., White, R.D., Khan, A.H., & Packer, D.L. Impact of age on long-term survival and quality of life following out-of-hospital cardiac arrest. *Crit. Care Med.* 2004; **32**(4): 963–967.

215. Hallstrom, A.P., Cobb, L.A., & Yu, B.H. Influence of comorbidity on the outcome of patients treated for out-of-hospital ventricular fibrillation. *Circulation* 1996; **93**(11): 2019–2022.

216. Mahapatra, S., Bunch, T.J., White, R.D., Hodge, D.O., & Packer, D.L. Sex differences in outcome after ventricular fibrillation in out-of-hospital cardiac arrest. *Resuscitation* 2005; **65**(2): 197–202.

217. Kim, C., Fahrenbruch, C.E., Cobb, L.A., & Eisenberg, M.S. Out-of-hospital cardiac arrest in men and women. *Circulation* 2001; **104**(22): 2699–2703.

218. Cowie, M.R., Fahrenbruch, C.E., Cobb, L.A., & Hallstrom, A.P. Out-of-hospital cardiac arrest: racial differences in outcome in Seattle. *Am. J. Public Health* 1993; **83**(7): 955–959.

219. Kouwenhoven, W.B., Jude, J.R., & Knickerbocker, G.G. Closed-chest cardiac massage. *J. Am. Med. Assoc.* 1960; **173**: 1064–1067.

220. Thompson, R.G., Hallstrom, A.P., & Cobb, L.A. Bystander-initiated cardiopulmonary resuscitation in the management of ventricular fibrillation. *Ann. Intern. Med.* 1979; **90**(5): 737–740.

221. Herlitz, J., Ekstrom, L., Wennerblom, B., Axelsson, A., Bang, A., & Holmberg, S. Effect of bystander initiated cardiopulmonary resuscitation on ventricular fibrillation and survival after witnessed cardiac arrest outside hospital. *Br. Heart J.* 1994; **72**: 408–412.

222. Demirovic, J. Cardiopulmonary resuscitation programs revisited: results of a community study among older African Americans. *Am. J. Geriatr. Cardiol.* 2004; **13**(4): 182–187.

223. Lynch, B., Einspruch, E.L., Nichol, G., Becker, L.B., Aufderheide, T.P., & Idris, A. Effectiveness of a 30-min CPR self-instruction program for lay responders: a controlled randomized study. *Resuscitation* 2005; **67**(1): 31–43.

224. Hallstrom, A.P., Ornato, J.P., Weisfeldt, M. *et al.* Public-access defibrillation and survival after out-of-hospital cardiac arrest. *N. Engl. J. Med.* 2004; **351**(7): 637–646.

225. De Maio, V.J., Stiell, I.G., Wells, G.A., & Spaite, D.W. Cardiac arrest witnessed by emergency medical services personnel: descriptive epidemiology, prodromal symptoms, and predictors of survival. OPALS study group. *Ann. Emerg. Med.* 2000; **35**(2): 138–146.

226. Larsen, M.P., Eisenberg, M.S., Cummins, R.O., & Hallstrom, A.P. Predicting survival from out-of-hospital cardiac arrest: a graphic model. *Ann. Emerg. Med.* 1993; **22**(11): 1652–1658.

227. Valenzuela, T., Roe, D.J., Cretin, S., Spaite, D.W., & Larsen, M.P. Estimating effectiveness of cardiac arrest interventions: a logistic regression survival model. *Circulation* 1997; **96**: 3308–3313.

228. Pepe, P.E., Mattox, K.L., Duke, J.H., Fisher, P.B., & Prentice, F.D. Effect of full-time, specialized physician supervision on the success of a large, urban emergency medical services system. *Crit. Care Med.* 1993; **21**(9): 1279–1286.

229. Wik, L., Kramer-Johansen, J., Myklebust, H. *et al.* Quality of cardiopulmonary resuscitation during out-of-hospital cardiac arrest. *J. Am. Med. Assoc.* 2005; **293**(3): 299–304.

230. Abella, B.S., Alvarado, J.P., Myklebust, H. *et al.* Quality of cardiopulmonary resuscitation during in-hospital cardiac arrest. *J. Am. Med. Assoc.* 2005; **293**(3): 305–310.

231. Abella, B.S., Sandbo, N., Vassilatos, P. *et al.* Chest compression rates during cardiopulmonary resuscitation are suboptimal: a prospective study during in-hospital cardiac arrest. *Circulation* 2005; **111**(4): 428–434.

Part II

Basic science

3

Global cellular ischemia/reperfusion during cardiac arrest: critical stress responses and the postresuscitation syndrome

Kimm Hamann, Dave Beiser, and Terry L. Vanden Hoek

Department of Emergency Medicine, University of Chicago, USA

Cardiac arrest is the most lethal disease of ischemia/reperfusion (I/R) with only 5%–7% of out-of-hospital cardiac arrest (OHCA) victims surviving to hospital discharge.[1] Why a patient passes from full human function to "death" within minutes to hours, often despite an initially successful resuscitation and restoration of normal vital signs, is unclear. Certainly compared with the focal tissue ischemia of stroke or myocardial infarction the ischemic interval of cardiac arrest is measured in minutes rather than hours; yet, the establishment of reperfusion following cardiac arrest resuscitation, unlike that following focal ischemia, cannot be considered definitive therapy. Indeed, out of every 100 cardiac arrest victims, about 30 will achieve return of spontaneous circulation (ROSC) but only 5 survive the postresuscitation period to hospital discharge.[1–6] Thus, postresuscitation deaths contribute significantly to overall out-of-hospital cardiac arrest mortality as most patients who are initially "saved" die during a lethal post-resuscitation syndrome often during the first 24–72 hours, characterized by early cardiovascular collapse with multi-organ failure [7–9] *and* subsequent *failure of central nervous system recovery*.[10–12] If we could successfully treat or prevent reperfusion injury it would result in an estimated 6–10 fold improvement in survival following cardiac arrest. Efforts to improve post-resuscitation care are well justified since 75% of patients who are discharged alive return to their communities with intact neurological function and a good quality of life.[13–15]

The extent of such post-resuscitation injury is likely to be associated with the time of ischemia. Weisfeldt and Becker proposed a "three-phase time-sensitive" model of cardiac arrest highlighting the need for different treatments at specific ischemia times of cardiac arrest.[16] The model suggests optimal treatment of cardiac arrest should be phase-specific: (1) the electrical phase (from onset to ~4 minutes), where ideal treatment is defibrillation; (2) the circulatory phase (from ~4 to ~10 minutes), which requires high quality CPR prior to defibrillation; and (3) the metabolic phase (after ~10 minutes of ischemia), which likely requires therapies directed at the modulation of oxidants, immune system mediators, microvascular injury, apoptosis, and energy substrate depletion.[7,9,17–21] This chapter will focus on events likely to occur with greatest severity in those cardiac arrest patients resuscitated from the metabolic phase.

The post-resuscitation period represents a critical therapeutic window for improving outcomes through interruption of death pathways and abrogation of ongoing end-organ ischemic injury. Proof of this assertion comes from recent clinical studies demonstrating that therapeutic hypothermia, induced during the immediate post-resuscitation period, significantly improves clinical outcomes.[22–25] Unfortunately, hypothermia is one of the only examples of an effective post-resuscitation intervention. It also stands out as particularly non-specific therapy that is likely to act in a somewhat "global" fashion to modulate entire classes of fundamental intracellular processes mediating post-resuscitation disease. A deeper understanding of the cellular mechanisms of post-resuscitation injury, through the development of new clinical biomarkers and measures, is vital to optimizing the delivery of therapeutic hypothermia and developing therapies targeted at specific pathways or subclasses of cardiac arrest patients. In addition, similarities between the post-resuscitation and sepsis syndromes[20,26] suggest opportunities for the development of new therapies targeted at specific mediators of post-resuscitation injury. Hypothermia, and the achievement of

Cardiac Arrest: The Science and Practice of Resuscitation Medicine. 2nd edn., ed. Norman Paradis, Henry Halperin, Karl Kern, Volker Wenzel, Douglas Chamberlain. Published by Cambridge University Press. © Cambridge University Press, 2007.

core body temperature goals, might simply be one component of a larger protocol of "early-goal-directed therapy"[27] directed at the molecular level toward modulating critical post-resuscitation events.

This chapter reviews the clinical and basic science features of the post-resuscitation syndrome, with particular focus on the cardiovascular system, cellular stress-responses, and mechanisms of cell injury and death following cardiac arrest and resuscitation. In particular, the role of oxidants and critical stress responses including inflammation, apoptosis, and death pathways will be highlighted. An improved understanding of these cellular mechanisms will likely be vital to optimizing the clinical application of therapeutic hypothermia. In addition, new therapies targeted at modulation of cytokines and oxidants have great promise for the treatment of cardiac arrest. Similar to the treatment of electrical phase patients by using defibrillation, such therapies could some day routinely resuscitate patients in the metabolic phase – the sickest of cardiac arrest patients – back to previous human function.

The post-resuscitation syndrome

The post-resuscitation syndrome is characterized by systemic inflammation, myocardial dysfunction,[7,9,17,18] circulatory collapse and multi-organ failure leading often to either death during the first 24–72 hours or subsequent failure of central nervous system recovery.[10–12] The post-resuscitation and sepsis syndromes share many similar features including endothelial dysfunction, thrombosis, impairment of fibrinolysis, marked elevation of inflammatory mediators, and mild hyperthermia.[20,25,28–30] Recent clinical studies have noted the appearance of peripheral markers of this inflammatory cascade such as cytokines/chemokines (e.g., IL-1ra, IL-6, IL-8, IL-10) and other inflammatory mediators including activated polymorphonuclear leukocytes, endothelial adhesion molecules, and complement following out-of-hospital cardiac arrest (OHCA) – findings similar to those seen during sepsis.[20,31–35] In cardiac arrest patients, non-survivors demonstrate plasma IL-6 concentrations that are 20-fold greater than these of survivors, and approximately 50-fold greater than baseline values from normal humans.[20,36]

Why a sepsis-like syndrome would be seen in the context of a non-infectious disease is intriguing. Cardiac arrest involves sudden, global, multi-organ ischemia. Reperfusion occurs during cardiopulmonary resuscitation (CPR) and more fully at return of spontaneous circulation (ROSC). The changes in oxidant stress and redox state associated with these critical transitions during whole-body ischemia/reperfusion likely activate a host of cellular stress responses at the transcription and protein level. These critical stress responses throughout multiple organs could explain the simultaneous triggering of cytokines, chemokines, activated complement and polymorphonuclear leukocytes, and endothelial cell adhesion molecules. Interestingly, such stress responses could be quite adaptive when localized to tissue injured by trauma or microbial invasion, local events that can also cause localized changes in oxidant stress and altered redox state. When they become simultaneously global throughout the body as may occur during cardiac arrest, however, these same stress responses could become overly amplified with devastating and lethal consequences.

Regarding post-resuscitation myocardial injury, while much work has focused on neurological injury after resuscitation, less is known about the earlier cardiovascular injury and collapse that is often seen in these patients. In a small clinical study of post-resuscitation hemodynamic instability, survivors of out-of-hospital cardiac arrest usually demonstrated improvement of cardiac index (CI) by 24 hours, with persistently low CI at 72 hours associated with death by multi-organ failure.[9] Nevertheless, this study did not include those patients who died early after ROSC prior to reaching the cardiac catheterization laboratory; that is, those exhibiting the most acute and severe postresuscitation cardiovascular injury. Postresuscitation cardiac dysfunction has been associated with elevated plasma TNF-alpha levels in swine models.[37] In addition, TNF-alpha-induced caspase-3 activation has been shown to mediate cardiac dysfunction in response to endotoxin challenge in mice.[38] Understanding such cardiovascular post-resuscitation injury is important as it represents the most accelerated and lethal form of three distinct post-resuscitation phenotypes: intact survival, neurological impairment, or in-hospital death due to cardiovascular collapse.

Redox-mediated intracellular stress responses

The list of potential mediators of post-resuscitation injury is legion and includes both the intracellular and extracellular expression of multiple reactive oxidant species; pro-inflammatory mediators of the innate immune system such as cytokines/chemokines (e.g., IL-6, IL-8), endothelial adhesion factors, activated complement and leukocytes; and other pro-apoptotic signaling molecules. We will begin by discussing the intracellular mechanisms of redox-signaling.

During the global ischemia of cardiac arrest, the myocardial intracellular environment is characterized by striking changes in myocardial oxygen tension (PO_2), carbon dioxide tension (PCO_2), and pH. Following the onset of ventricular fibrillation, intramyocardial PO_2 levels rapidly plummet, while PCO_2 and hydrogen ion concentrations increase.[39–41] After only 4 minutes of ventricular fibrillation in swine, myocardial PCO_2 may increase to well over 200 torr with a corresponding drop in pH to 6.0 and below.[41] Indeed, increased myocardial CO_2 during cardiac arrest may negatively affect the heart's ability to be successfully defibrillated.[42] Furthermore, hypercarbic acidosis has been shown to worsen myocardial contractility in an isolated rat heart preparation[43] and worsen outcomes in a swine model of cardiac arrest.[44] The myocardial intracellular environment undergoes another transformation as these trends are reversed with the initiation of effective cardiopulmonary resuscitation (i.e., partial-flow reperfusion). Finally, upon return of spontaneous circulation, the myocardium undergoes a third transition as reperfusion leads to the rapid normalization of these parameters within 30 minutes post-resuscitation.[40,41]

These striking shifts in the cellular microenvironment have the potential for radical alteration of the potential for oxidant signaling, ROS-mediated damage, and eventual cell dysfunction or death. Oxygen, for example, is essential for life; as an acceptor of electrons from the mitochondrial electron transport chain it allows concurrent synthesis of adenosine triphosphate (ATP) through oxidative phosphorylation. Control of oxygen delivery at the tissue and cellular level thus is critical for survival. Changes in redox state precipitated by sudden drops in tissue O_2 tension can trigger adaptive oxidant signaling responses that attempt to restore metabolic homeostasis. Although there are numerous sources of oxidant signaling molecules in the cardiovascular system, mitochondria appear to be critical oxygen biosensors capable of acting as first responders to the PO_2 changes associated with cardiac arrest.[45–49]

Our own studies of I/R in cardiomyocytes suggest that oxidant stress is generated within seconds to minutes of ischemia onset. This increase in oxidant stress is seen both at the cardiomyocyte level[45] and at a systemic level within minutes of CPR in swine models of cardiac arrest.[50,51] Prolonged ischemia can induce superoxide generation and lipid peroxidation; alter cardiolipin and affect the integrity of the mitochondrial electron transport chain. Reducing equivalents present at the time of resuscitation fuel a burst of lethal oxidant generation as a result of electron transfer from complexes I and II into the intermitochondrial membrane space via complex III, with subsequent cytochrome c release and apoptosis.[48]

Recent work demonstrates the existence of a "pH paradox," a worsening of cardiomyocyte survival after ischemia despite rapid normalization of pH during reperfusion. Acidotic reperfusion of ischemic cardiomyocytes by using hypercarbia has been reported to improve cell survival.[52] The mechanism of this protective effect is not entirely clear, however. Hypercarbia may act as a mitochondrial inhibitor; indeed, recently researchers from our laboratory have demonstrated that a brief transient period of mitochondrial inhibition during the reperfusion of chick cardiomyocytes *in vitro* abrogated the generation of ROS and improved cell survival through a mitochondrial complex III-dependent mechanism.[53] Thus, even though the rapid normalization of O_2, CO_2, and pH is an implied intermediate goal of CPR, an uncontrolled overly rapid transition might worsen mitochondrial recovery and post-resuscitation oxidant injury. The conditions for a more controlled reperfusion (e.g., temperature, transitions in tissue O_2 and CO_2) that minimize post-resuscitation injury are not known, but likely vary depending on time of ischemia (i.e., they are phase specific).

The type of oxidant species generated in the heart during cardiac arrest and reperfusion likely are numerous, with many species (particularly superoxide, H_2O_2, and nitric oxide) capable of both good and bad effects depending upon redox state, tissue CO_2 levels and pH, and other species present. The formation of intracellular ROS and that of nitric oxide are interrelated, with one species affecting and regulating the other.[54] We have previously utilized a nitric oxide synthase inhibitor (NOS), NG-nitro-L-arginine methyl ester (L-NAME), to block the formation of nitric oxide in our cardiomyocyte model during conditions of hypoxia,[55] supporting the notion that cardiac cells can generate significant amounts of NO within minutes of onset of cardiac arrest-like conditions. In turn NO can interact with superoxide to form peroxynitrite, with concurrent oxidant damage. Indeed, inhibition of NOS has been shown to reduce myocardial O_2 consumption in an intact dog preparation and improve coronary perfusion pressure and rate of ROSC in a swine model of cardiac arrest.[56,57] While NO can play a deleterious role in reperfusion injury, depending upon timing and concurrent generation of other oxidants, it can also exert highly protective effects.[54]

Other oxidase systems such as NADPH oxidase, xanthine oxidase, and cytochrome P450 systems would likely be affected by this initial oxidant stress response by mitochondria and could further amplify oxidant stress via increased generation of ROS. The underlying mechanism of oxygen sensing by mitochondria may involve redox regulation of nitrite and nitric oxide homeostasis in the inner mitochondrial membrane[58], with inhibition of cytochrome c oxidase by nitric oxide as well as superoxide generation from complex III.[59] In addition, mitochondrial membrane and cell membrane anion channels may be sensitive to redox state and control the release of superoxide into the cytosol and possibly the extracellular space.[45]

The oxidant tipping point

Such oxidant and inflammatory stress responses can play both adaptive and deleterious roles in the organism, depending upon the threshold that is reached during conditions of ischemia/reperfusion. Indeed, the importance of oxidant stress for adaptive cardiovascular responses is suggested by recent findings that high-dose antioxidants taken chronically may actually increase cardiovascular disease mortality.[60] Although such stress responses are necessary for survival against local traumatic injury or infection, when quickly generalized to a multi-organ level during cardiac arrest, these same critical stress responses could result in amplification of oxidant and inflammatory stress that shifts the balance from survival to activation of the death pathway.

Such an oxidant "tipping point" may be seen at the molecular level. For example, Stamler and Hausladen have proposed a continuum of nitric oxide- and ROS-mediated Cys-SH oxidant modifications that progresses from SNO (S-nitrosylation) to SOH (sulfenic acid), disulfide (SS), sulfinic (SO_2^-), and sulfonic (SO_3^-) acids.[61] This continuum may define how a cell or tissue "ramps up" its response to changes in redox state, eventually crossing the oxidant stress threshold from adaptive signaling to irreversible damage. In addition, the timing of adaptive oxidant modifications of Cys-SH is important, such that adaptive oxidation to disulfide linkages can protect against subsequent oxidant damage by more lethal oxidants if induced early. Protective strategies such as intra-ischemic hypothermia could conceivably be mediated by such oxidant modulation, with induction of protein protection prior to the increased oxidant stress of ROSC.

Circulating messengers of I/R injury: extracellular oxidants and cytokines/chemokines

Extracellular expression of pro-inflammatory and oxidant molecules amplifies the magnitude and local extent of the original I/R injury through both autocrine and paracrine effects, which promote increased oxidant production and release of cytokines/chemokines.[62–64] For example, both serum and tissue levels of the oxidant stress marker F2-isoprostane increase significantly within minutes of cardiopulmonary resuscitation after swine cardiac arrest,

reaching a peak within 30 minutes after ROSC.[50,51,65] Such molecules also play an important role in communicating the original insult to distal/remote tissues by promoting microvascular injury through the recruitment, activation and/or diapedesis of a variety of circulating cell types (e.g., leukocytes, platelets); and increased fibrin clot formation with decreased fibrinolysis,[30] the end result being poor capillary tissue perfusion, tissue ischemia and multi-organ dysfunction.[62–64] Evidence for such distal amplification of injury through microvascular injury comes from several mouse models of I/R injury of gut or liver. Such models can generate significant injury "at a distance," with splanchnic organ ischemia producing increased pulmonary sequestration of circulating leukocytes, increased levels of pulmonary tissue in chemokines related to human IL-8 such as MIP-2 and KC, and microvascular permeability.[66–68] Cardiac arrest conceivably amplifies this "injury at a distance" many fold, since multiple organs experience I/R conditions simultaneously.

I/R-induced oxidant and inflammatory protein signaling pathways have been shown to have an impact on distal tissues through direct endocrine pathways as well.[63] These direct endocrine pathways may initially represent adaptive homeostatic responses to I/R that then become amplified in a maladaptive manner long after the initial injury.[63] Such a direct oxidant pathway has been postulated in part to mediate post-ischemic myocardial stunning.[64] Isolated hepatic I/R injury has been shown to inactivate mitochondrial superoxide dismutase (MnSOD), a mitochondrial antioxidant enzyme, within pulmonary endothelial cells.[69] Pro-inflammatory cytokines, such as TNF-alpha, have also been shown to have direct negative inotropic effects on myocardium.[70] In a murine model of resuscitated hemorrhagic shock (a related state of global I/R,[71]) infusion of a soluble TNF-alpha receptor antagonist (etanercept) significantly attenuates post-resuscitation LV dysfunction.[72] Another example of direct organ–organ communication of I/R injury comes from recent work in a model of focal intestinal I/R.[73] In this model, *Tnfrsf1a–/–* mice showed decreased pulmonary infiltration of polymorphonuclear cells, decreased NF-kB activation and decreased mRNA expression in several NF-kB target genes encoding pro-inflammatory cytokines/chemokines.

Transcriptional pathways of critical stress response

As noted in the above mouse model, I/R can alter gene expression.[73] A recent transcriptome analysis of rat myocardium after focal I/R demonstrated increased expression of mRNA of pro-inflammatory proteins such as IL-6 and IL-18 at 2 days post-reperfusion with later transcription of genes encoding pro-apoptotic caspases.[74] Such transcriptional alterations may be triggered by changes in oxidant stress and redox state via stress-sensitive transcription factors such as NF-kB.[75,76]

Similar transcriptional stress responses are likely to occur following global I/R. For example, in murine models of unresuscitated hemorrhagic shock (HS), a brief, but profound, period of HS rapidly leads to hepatic NF-kB activation, TNF-alpha mRNA expression, as well as increases in plasma TNF-alpha concentration.[77,78] In a separate murine model, unresuscitated HS leads to upregulation of NF-kB gene expression at 1 hour and an associated sustained NF-kB activation lasting 24 hours, suggesting the possibility of a sustained period of pro-inflammatory transcription.[79] Such rapid and sustained activation of NF-kB-mediated responses, in contrast to episodic activation and spontaneous resolution, has been associated with induction of cell death pathways.[80]

Reperfusion during resuscitation also appears to trigger activation of transcription factors and early gene-expression of cytokines/chemokines and prostaglandins within multiple vital organs, including the liver, spleen, lung, and muscle after whole-body ischemia due to hemorrhagic shock.[81] Such transcriptional changes appear to be modulated by the severity of hemorrhage and the timing and choice of therapeutic intervention.[82–84]

Such a rapid multi-organ activation of innate immune response by NF-kB signaling has already been modeled in non-cardiac arrest patients exposed to non-toxic doses of endotoxin.[85] Genomic systems biology approaches suggest that innate immune responses in humans evolve quickly, and the stress responses seen within 4–6 hours of initiation may be critical for successful return to a normal human phenotype.[85] Factors that both initiate and limit innate immune responses evolve significantly between time of onset and at 4–6 hours, with their balance and trend likely to be critical for successful resolution of both "pro-inflammatory" and "counter-inflammatory" stress response phases.

Post-resuscitation syndrome: the connection among oxidant stress, inflammation, and apoptosis

In addition to microvascular and direct inhibitory effects, oxidant stress and inflammation are thought to trigger proapoptotic pathways. For example, I/R has been shown to trigger apoptotic cell death through the Fas/Fas ligand pathway leading to caspase activation.[48,86] Fas (also known as CD95) is a membrane-bound receptor in the tumor necrosis family expressed in a variety of cells including heart and lung. Researchers from our laboratory have demonstrated the expression of both Fas and FasL in human epithelium.[87] Cytokines may play an important role in activating metalloproteinases which can cleave membrane-bound Fas and FasL to its soluble form that then can be released into the circulation.[88] Although the role of apoptosis following cardiac arrest is not entirely known, it is conceivable that such high circulating levels of cytokines could induce myocardial apoptosis and play an important role in cardiovascular dysfunction and collapse. This notion is consistent with some pathology studies involving heart tissue from cardiac arrest patients. A case series of pathology specimens taken from postmortem heart tissue showed widespread uptake of apoptosis markers throughout the myocardium of patients after sudden death.[89]

Programmed cell death in the heart

If injury to a cell is too great, or if its "usefulness" has expired, a cell or neighboring cells may signal its removal. Physiological removal of cells has been termed programmed cell death (PCD) because a genetic program consisting of a sequence of molecular signaling and biochemical events is initiated to dismantle the affected cell. Apoptosis, a specialized form of cell death, was originally equated with PCD; however, it is becoming clear that there are many forms of PCD and that even necrotic cell death may be regulated in many tissues,[90] including the heart,[91] particularly after ischemic injury.[92,93]

Necrosis/oncosis

The terms "necrosis" or "oncosis" traditionally have been used to refer to an unregulated cell death morphologically typified by cellular swelling and plasma membrane rupture. While historically viewed as a pathological or "accidental" form of cell death resulting from acute cellular injury, or as a result of bioenergetic catastrophe,[94,95] recent evidence suggests that necrosis/oncosis may be a substitute, or alternate pathway, for myocardial cell death and loss of cardiac function,[91] – particularly when apoptosis is blocked, for example, by caspase inhibition.[96,97] Regulated or "programmed" forms of necrosis have been described recently in a number of cell types (see reviews[90,95,98]), and may involve a number of molecular mediators or regulators normally associated with apoptosis, such as certain members of the Bcl-2 family (see below). Such regulated forms of necrosis have not yet been described specifically in cardiac arrest, but in light of the numerous descriptions of "necrotic," "oncotic," or generally "non-apoptotic" cell death in the heart, it is likely that continued dissection of death mechanisms in the heart after arrest or infarction will elucidate such mechanisms and their potential role in myocardial damage. Interestingly, an atypical pathway of cardiomyocyte cell death caused by hypoxia and acidosis has recently been described, which seems to involve a combination of features of apoptosis and necrosis.[99] A pro-apoptotic member of the Bcl-2 family (see below), BNip3, and its actions on the mitochondrial permeability pore were implicated in this death mechanism, but activation of the apoptotic proteases, caspases, was not. On the other hand, the involvement of specific caspases in additional, perhaps intermediate, forms of cell death, have been linked to non-apoptotic forms of PCD recently termed "parapto-sis" and "pyroptosis."

Paraptosis and pyroptosis – caspase-associated non-apoptotic cell death

Another form of PCD distinct from apoptosis has been termed paraptosis (for "next to" or "related to" apoptosis) and is characterized morphologically by cytoplasmic vacuolation and late mitochondrial swelling.[100] Although this death is not blocked by either the anti-apoptotic protein, Bcl-x_L, or by certain caspase inhibitors, this form of cell death is driven by an alternative activity of caspase-9, perhaps related to phosphorylation of caspase-9 by specific kinases.[101] Caspase-9 has been associated with ischemia/reperfusion (I/R)-induced cell death in a number of models of cardiomyocyte injury,[102–104] but the potential role of paraptosis-like cell death in myocardial injury is unknown.

Recently, the term pyroptosis (for "fire or fever," Greek) was proposed to describe a cell death that is uniquely dependent on caspase-1. Although caspase-1 is classified as a member of the inflammatory caspase subfamily (see below) and has been dissociated from certain physiological pathways of apoptosis[105,106] recent evidence suggests that caspase-1 can interact with multiple pathways of both inflammation and cell death.[107,108] Of particular note are recent descriptions of key roles for caspase-1 in ischemia-induced cell death.[108–110] In a murine model of myocardial ischemia, caspase-1 acts in synergy with hypoxia to stimulate caspase-3-mediated apoptosis[108] and inhibition of caspase-1 in a suprafused human myocardium model of I/R reduced ischemia dysfunction at least in part by inhibiting proinflammatory cytokines, IL-18 and IL-1β.[111]

The latter study is particularly interesting in light of the previously discussed connection between post-resuscitation disease and the sepsis syndrome.[20,26]

Whereas pyropposis as originally described[112] may be a novel form of cell death induced by infection with *Salmonella* and *Shigella* species, pyroptosis as a process likely plays a physiological role in a variety of tissues,[113] and growing evidence of the participation of caspase-1 and inflammation in the post-ischemic myocardium suggests that this pathway is important in cardiac arrest. Like the involvement of the extrinsic apoptotic pathway described below, thus far the participation of caspase-1 has been examined specifically in cardiac arrest from a perspective of global ischemia and damage to "outlying" tissues such as the brain.[114] Nonetheless, the significance of caspase-1 activation to potential inflammatory or "pyroptosis-like" responses following cardiac arrest in either the brain or heart remains to be more thoroughly investigated.

Autophagy

Before we consider apoptosis and several of its well-characterized molecular mediators and regulators, another potential form of cell death has attracted a great deal of attention for its role in physiological homeostatic processes, including processes of cell death and survival in the myocardium.[115] Autophagy ("to eat oneself," Greek) is a regulated process by which a cell carries out lysosomal degradation of its own constituents, including cytoplasm (microautophagy) and larger cytoplasmic proteins and organelles such as mitochondria (macroautophagy). Chaperone-mediated autophagy is a third form of the process largely confined to mammalian systems, involving the formation of a complex between cytosolic protein substrates and protein chaperones and subsequent translocation into the lysosome. There is some disagreement as to whether autophagy truly represents an initiated form of cell death or a cellular response to stress from which a cell may or may not recover. It is clear that autophagic processes can occur in the heart, however, and (macro)autophagy has been described recently in the chronically ischemic myocardium.[116] In the latter study, autophagy was hypothesized as a homeostatic process utilized for the turnover of unnecessary or dysfunctional organelles and cytoplasmic proteins in the ischemic myocardium, which could protect against further ischemia.[116] Recently, in a murine model of autophagy[117] the pro-death function of autophagy was examined in mouse heart muscle.[118] Transgenic expression of cardiac Bcl-2 (and its subsequent interaction with the autophagy protein, Beclin-1) helped maintain levels of autophagy that were compatible with cell survival, rather than cell death.[118] Selective or preferential autophagy of the mitochondria has been termed mitophagy,[119] and is thought to occur as a process of mitochondrial quality control, or as a cellular response to overwhelming numbers of damaged mitochondria.[120] In I/R injury, oxidative damage to mitochondrial membrane proteins can lead to opening of the mitochondrial permeability transition (MPT) pore.[121] At one extreme, MPT opening can lead to necrosis through ATP depletion or to apoptosis via cytochrome c release (see below) and cell death.[119] MPT pore formation under less severe stress can promote autophagy, however, or more specifically mitophagy, and the removal of ROS-producing mitochondria may be a survival mechanism.[119] Thus, a greater understanding of the occurrence and extent of autophagy in the stressed myocardium will be important in considering future therapeutic approaches to the management and treatment of cardiac disease,[115] and post-resuscitation survival.

Apoptosis

Of the known forms of PCD, apoptosis is by far the best characterized at the molecular level. Morphologically, apoptosis is characterized by nuclear condensation and fragmentation and by cell shrinkage. Indeed, J.F.R Kerr, the originator of the term "apoptosis,"[122] initially described this cell death as "shrinkage necrosis."[123] DNA fragmentation or "laddering" is another characteristic of apoptosis, and this, along with many of the morphological aspects, is due a subclass of proteases called caspases (*c*ysteinyl *asp*artate-specific prote*ases*), although there are now recognized forms of apoptosis that may be caspase-independent processes.

A number of excellent reviews of apoptosis in the heart exist[124–128] and the reader is referred to these and others for more comprehensive and detailed reviews of molecular mechanisms of apoptotic pathways of cell death in cardiomyocytes. Here, we will briefly consider the major pathways and molecular participants of apoptosis and the evidence for their involvement in I/R-induced injury in the myocardium, particularly with regard to the involvement of the mitochondria. Recently, there has been recognition that apoptosis of cardiomyocytes (and perhaps other cell types, such as endothelial cells[129,130]) can occur in various pathologies of the human heart, including heart failure,[131,132] I/R injury in myocardial infarction,[133,134] and in ischemic injury during cardiosurgical procedures.[135,136] Most recently, evidence of apoptotic death of cardiomyocytes in the global

I/R following cardiac arrest and resuscitation has been studied and related directly to cardiac function and survival.

Caspases

As implied above, caspases are central to the dismantling of a cell via the major pathways of apoptosis (discussed below). Fourteen mammalian caspases have been identified to date,[137] and the apoptotic caspases can be grouped into two general categories: (i) initiator or "upstream" caspases, including caspases-2, -8, -9, and -10, and (ii) "executioner" or apoptosis effectors, caspases-3, -6 and –7 (Fig.3.1). The remaining caspases make up a third group and are often referred to as "inflammatory" caspases. These are involved in the maturation of certain cytokines, such as IL-1β. All caspases exist as zymogens or "procaspases" and generally are activated by proteolytic cleavage, either through autolytic cleavage or activation via induced proximity or dimerization/oligomerization[138–140] or, for the executioner caspases, by cleavage by other (upstream) caspases. The initiator caspases possess specialized prodomains (CARD = *ca*spase *r*ecruitment *d*omain or DED = *d*eath *e*ffector *d*omain) involved in their activation, and generally speaking, once activated, these initiator caspases activate the effector caspases via cleavage of their pro-forms (e.g., procaspase-3). On the basis of specific sequence preferences, caspases perform distinct roles in the apoptotic process, although in caspase-deficient cells, one or more caspases may substitute for the missing caspase.[125] Literally hundreds of caspase substrates have been identified, and these include major structural elements of the cell, cell cycle proteins, protein kinases and phosphatases, transcription factors, and components of the DNA repair machinery, as well as apoptotic regulators, such as members of the Bcl-2 family.[141,142] As outlined below, the activation of several different caspases has been observed in I/R-induced apoptosis in isolated cardiomyocytes and in intact myocardium.

In addition to control of initiating events of apoptosis pathways discussed below, regulation of caspase activity also is accomplished directly via endogenous inhibitors of the caspases known as inhibitors of apoptosis proteins (IAPs) (Fig. 3.1) An extended discussion of IAPs is not possible here, and the reader is referred to several recent reviews of this protein family.[143–146] Briefly, IAPs were first identified in baculoviruses, (see reviews[143,147]); and in mammals there are at least seven IAP family members, each of which contains one or more baculoviral repeat (BIR) domains, through which they interact with certain caspases. Specific interactions between caspases and BIR

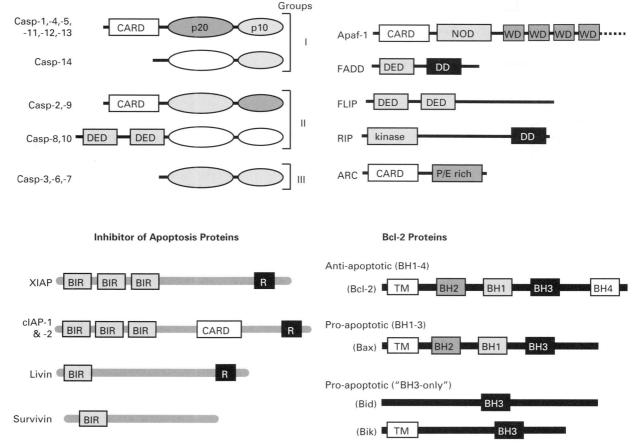

Fig. 3.1. Primary structures and diverse interacting domains of major protein groups associated with apoptosis. Examples in each of the major families and groups of apoptotic proteins and regulators are shown, including critical functional and interacting domains: CARD = caspase recruitment domain; p20 = large caspase subunit; plO = small caspase subunit; DED = death effector domain; BIR = Baculovirus IAP domain; R = Ring zinc finger domain; NOD = nucleotide-binding oligomerization or "ATPase" domain; P/E-rich = proline/glutamine-rich domain;WD = tryptophan-aspartate repeats; DD = death domain; TM = transmembrane domain; BH1-4 = Bel-2 homology domains 1–4. Mammalian caspases have been organized into three major groups: group I containing the inflammatory or "cytokine maturation" caspases; group II comprised of initiators of apoptosis containing CARD or DED prodomains; and group III containing the effector caspases. (Caspases -11 and -12 are of mouse origin; caspase-13 described from bovine cells {Shi, 2002 #1943}) The Bcl-2 protein family has also been subdivided into three major groups, including the anti-apoptotic proteins, such as Bcl-2 and BCI-XL, which act to block the release of cytochrome c and other apoptogenic mitochondrial proteins. The proapoptotic members of the family are further divided into two subfamilies: the multi-domain proapoptotic proteins, represented by Bax and Bak; and the BH3-only subfamily containing at least 10 members. The WD domains in Apaf-1 are thought to be responsible for binding cytochrome c, while the NOD domains are involved in binding ATP/dATP and analogs driving conformational changes, which are critical for apoptosome formation (see Fig. 3.2, text and cited reviews for additional details regarding these and other molecular interactions).

domains have been elucidated recently, and XIAP (the most studied of the IAPs), inhibits the effector caspases-3 and -7 and the initiator caspase-9 through BIR2 and BIR3 regions, respectively.[148,149] These caspase inhibitors can be inhibited themselves by the mitochondrial proteins Smac/DIABLO (second mitochondria-derived activator of caspase/direct IAP-binding protein with low pI)[150,151] and Omi/HtrA2.[152–154] The involvement of IAPs, Smac, and Omi in I/R-induced apoptosis is not well studied, particularly in the heart, but recently a deficiency of XIAP expression was

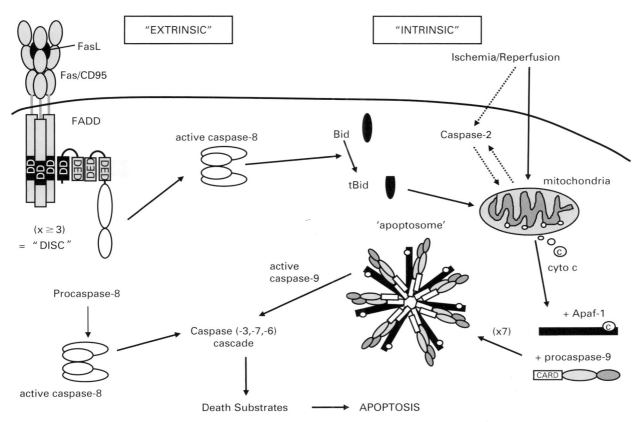

Fig. 3.2. Diagrammatic summary of the two major pathways of apoptosis in mammalian cells. The extrinsic pathway is initiated by the binding of a death ligand/cytokine trimer such as FasL (Fas ligand) to its trimerized receptor (here, Fas/CD95). This leads to the recruitment of adaptors such as FADD and, in turn, procaspase-8 (or-10). Oligomerization of these proteins comprises the death-inducing signaling complex (DISC) and leads to the activation of caspase-8. Caspase-8 initiates the caspase cascade and/or cleaves Bid (to truncated or "tBid") for cross-talk to the mitochondrial pathway. The mitochondrial or intrinsic pathway can be initiated by a number of stress factors, including ischemia/reperfusion, and may involve caspase-2 activation and direct effects on the mitochondria and/or activation of pro-apoptotic Bcl-2 proteins, such as Bax and Bak. Details of these mitochondrial interactions and models of cytochrome c (and other apoptogenic proteins, e.g., Smac/DIABLO, Omi/HtrAl, AIF, & EndoG) release are summarized in Fig. 3.3. Cytochrome c forms a complex with Apaf-1, which in the presence of ATP/dATP, induces formation of a heptameric, wheel-like structure to which procaspase-9 molecules are recruited. Activation of caspase-9 leads to initiation of the caspase cascade involving effector caspases-3, -7 and -6, and to DNA fragmentation and caspase-mediated dismantling of the cell.

found in post-infarction hearts in a murine model,[155] and increased ratios of XIAP to Smac were associated with minocycline-induced cardioprotection in a rat model of I/R injury.[156] A novel "CARD-carrying" caspase inhibitor (see Fig. 3.1), ARC (*a*poptosis *r*epressor with *C*ARD domain) has been identified recently, which interacts with at least two initiator caspases, caspases-2 and -8.[157] ARC appears to be expressed primarily in skeletal and cardiac muscle cells, and recent evidence indicates that ARC can protect a myogenic cell line from oxidant stress by preserving mitochondrial function.[158] This protection is likely a result, at least in part, of ARC's ability to interact with and prevent the activation of the pro-apoptotic Bax protein[159]

(see below). In addition, the calcium-binding activity of ARC also has been implicated in its anti-apoptotic activities.[160]

Pathways of caspase activation

There are two major pathways of caspase activation in mammalian cells: the "extrinsic" or death receptor-mediated pathway and the "intrinsic" or mitochondria-mediated pathway (Fig. 3.2). The extrinsic pathway is mediated by specific membrane receptors, primarily of the tumor necrosis factor receptor (TNFR) superfamily, and the most well-characterized death receptor besides TNFR itself, is Fas (CD95). The binding of the death ligand trimer, FasL, to the preformed Fas surface receptor homotrimer results in the formation of a death-inducing signaling complex (DISC), involving the adaptor protein FADD (*Fas-asscocated protein with a death domain*), which is recruited via its death domain (DD), and in turn recruits procaspase-8 (or-10) via death effector domains (DED), resulting in activation of caspase-8 (see review[161]). If only small amounts of caspase-8 are activated, the pathway may proceed through the cleavage of Bid and the pro-apoptotic effects of truncated Bid (tBid) on the mitochondria. Direct activation of caspase-3 by larger amounts of DISC formation and active caspase-8, however, can bypass the mitochondria to lead directly to the caspase cascade and apoptotic death (Fig. 2).[162] FADD and RIP (*receptor-interacting protein*) levels are increased in hearts of TNF-? transgenic mice,[163] whereas the levels of another protein, FLIP (*FLICE (caspase-8)-inhibitor protein*), are decreased in rat cardiomyoctes following hypoxia.[164] Both conditions can sensitize cardiomyocytes and other myocardial cells to death receptor-mediated killing. FADD and RIP have also been associated with innate immunity,[165,166] and in light of the potential role of such responses in post-resuscitation disease, future investigations of these molecules may have important implications beyond their roles in apoptosis. There are several recent reports of Fas/caspase-8 involvement in I/R-induced apoptosis in myocardium, mostly from isolated cells or isolated heart models of myocardial infarction.[167–170] These reports also suggest that a significant portion of the infarct is due to activation of the Fas-mediated pathway, but that blockade of the pathway in Fas-deficient mice,[167,170] or in cells expressing a dominant negative FADD,[168] only partially reduced infarct size. These data suggest that the initiating infarct persists, and that initiation of the injury is Fas-independent. It is possible, therefore, that the mitochondrial pathway plays a critical role in the early stages of I/R injury. Indeed, our data[102,103] and those of others[171] support an initiating role for the mitochondrial pathway in I/R injury and place Fas/caspase-8 activation downstream in amplification or post-infarction roles.[172]

As the name suggests, the mitochondrial or intrinsic pathway centers on the mitochondria and mitochondrial proteins, but can involve other organelles as well.[173] Details of this pathway of apoptosis in cardiomyocytes have been reviewed recently and elegantly[126,127] and because of space restrictions, we will limit our discussion to a brief consideration of critical pathway mechanisms and what is known about the major players in I/R-induced injury in the heart. As mentioned above, several studies have implicated mitochondria in the initiation of I/R-induced apoptosis (see recent review[174]). Mitochondria in cardiomyocytes depolarize during ischemia and a central role for generation of mitochondrial reactive oxygen species (ROS) has been implicated in this depolarization.[175] At reperfusion, a burst of ROS production can lead to the release of cytochrome c from the mitochondria, which in turn initiates formation of the wheel-like, heptad structure known as the apoptosome, ultimately resulting in the activation of caspase-9 and the caspase cascade (Fig. 3.2). Release of cytochrome c, and perhaps other apoptogenic molecules such as Smac/DIABLO, Omi/HtrA2, as well as AIF (*apoptosis-inducing factor*) and Endo G (*endonuclease G*) (see below), involves the permeabilization of the outer mitochondrial membrane. There have been several mechanistic models of this permeabilization (see reviews[126,176,177]), and while still poorly understood, most include critical roles for the Bcl-2 family of proteins (see Fig. 3.3).[126,178,179] Recent demonstrations of potential roles of Bcl-2 family proteins in the regulation of ROS production[180] strengthens this association and generates numerous important questions on the specific roles of Bcl-2 proteins in I/R-induced apoptosis.

The Bcl-2 family

The Bcl-2 family of proteins includes more than 20 members all of which share at least one of four conserved Bcl-2 homology (BH) domains (Fig. 3.1). These proteins are grouped into at least three different interacting classes or subfamilies: (1) the anti-apoptoptic proteins, including Bcl-2, Bcl-x_L and at least two others, (2) the pro-apoptotic proteins, which include Bax and Bak as the most characterized members, and (3) the so-called "BH3-only" proteins, including Bid, Bad, Bim, BNip3, PUMA and Noxa, among others. The interactions among these proteins can modulate critical steps early in the sequence of apoptotic events through their initimate associations with the mitochondria. Regulation of the activity of many Bcl-2 proteins is posttranslational, and both cleavage and conformational changes are among such regulatory mechanisms.[181–183] Regulation of mitochondrial permeabilization by homo- and heterotypic interactions between Bcl-2 proteins is importantly, but not exclusively, involved in I/R-induced apoptosis.[127] Direct interactions of Bcl-2 proteins with the outer mitochondrial membrane and disruption of normal mitochondrial respiratory function appear to be key to the intrinsic pathway.[127]

Of the Bcl-2 family members, Bid and Bax are two pro-apoptotic members, which have been centers of attention with regard to ischemia-induced cell death in the heart.

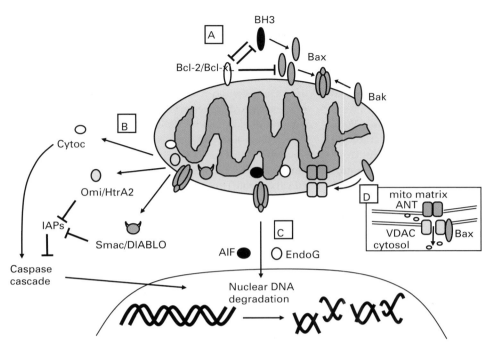

Fig. 3.3. Simplified diagram of apoptotic mitochondrial events.(a) Following an apoptotic insult, the activation of BH3-only proteins leads to the release of cytochrome c (cyto c), as well as LAP inhibitors, Smac/DIABLO and Omi/HtrA2 (b), from the inner membrane and intermembrane space. BH3 proteins may directly activate Bax and Bak or inactivate their antagonists, the anti-apoptotic proteins, such as Bcl-2 and BCI-XL. Bax is cytosolic and must translocate to the mitochondrial to exert its effects, while Bak possesses a transmembrane domain (see Fig. 3.l) and is normally found in the outer mitochondrial membrane. In one model, following an apoptotic signal, Bax and/or Bak can oligomerize and may form channels large enough for cyto c and other proteins to escape into the cytosol. As shown in Fig. 3.2, cyto c induces the formation of the apoptosome, initiating the caspase cascade. (c) Two other mitochondrial proteins, AIF and EndoG, can also be released. While their release from the mitochondria may be associated with caspase activity in some cells, their direct participation in DNA degradation appears to be caspase-independent (d). Another model of apoptogenic protein release involve the putative mitochondrial permeability transition (MPT) pore thought to consist of the adenine nucleotide translocase (ANT), the voltage-dependent anion channel (VDAC) and other unknown constituents. This model also involves Bax (or Bak) and proposes that Bax binds VDAC, inducing conformational changes which permit apoptogenic protein release.

For example, through the use of Bax knockout mice, the participation of Bax in I/R injury in isolated murine hearts also was elucidated recently; functional and apoptotic parameters examined in this study showed reduced damage in the Bax-/- hearts and moderate levels of damage markers in the heterozygote (Bax+/−) mice.[184] In healthy cells, Bid is located in the cytosol; it has been well studied as a "cross-talker" between the death receptor (e.g., Fas)/caspase-8 pathway and the mitochondrial pathway via caspase-8 cleavage to truncated Bid (tBid)[185] (see Fig. 3.2) Caspase-8-mediated Bid processing was recently observed (only during reperfusion) in a model of I/R-induced apoptosis in rat cardiomyocytes.[169] A role for Bid in I/R injury was also demonstrated in additional rat and rabbit models.[186,187] While a detailed discussion is beyond the scope of this chapter, there are several other BH3 proteins, such as BNip3, Bad, and Puma, for which there is also now evidence supporting roles in I/R injury in the heart.[188–193]

AIF and EndoG – caspase-independent apoptosis?

Although caspases have been traditionally associated with apoptosis as initiators, there are at least two factors released by the permeabilized mitochondrion, namely AIF and Endo G, which translocate to the nucleus (Fig. 3.3) and may separately or in conjunction[194] initiate chromatin condensation and DNA fragmentation, two hallmarks of apoptosis. Mammalian AIF is a flavoprotein with an oxidoreductase domain, and overexpression of AIF can cause caspase-independent cell death in some systems.[195] There is some evidence, however, that endogenous AIF release from the mitochondria requires caspase activity,[196] and this represents a requirement for caspase-2 activity, which has been shown to act on the mitochondria following certain apoptogenic stimulation of some cells,[197–199] including I/R induction of cardiomyocytes.[103] Both EndoG and AIF are expressed in the mammalian heart,[200–202] but their roles in ischemic injury to the myocardium, particularly during and after cardiac arrest, are not yet clear. Nevertheless, there is evidence of AIF participation in experimental infarcts in rat hearts,[203] and protective treatments in perfused hearts blocked the I/R-induced release of AIF.[204] On the other hand, AIF has also been shown to have a potential *anti*-apoptotic role through its activity as a free radical scavenger.[205] Furthermore, recent evidence shows that AIF may function as a vital mitochondrial respiratory enzyme in the myocardium[206] and that its loss may lead to oxidative stress in the myocardium and the development of mitochondrial dysfunction, dilated cardiomyopathy, and heart failure.[207,208] Much work remains to be done before we understand the mechanistic and, in some cases dualistic, roles of apoptotic molecules in I/R-injury in general, and in the post-arrest heart in particular.

Apoptosis as an anti-inflammatory strategy

One major feature of apoptotic removal of damaged cells is the avoidance of inflammation, but apoptosis may also function to resolve ongoing inflammation. In light of the recent view that the resuscitated, post-arrest condition is similar to one of sepsis or inflammation,[209] this potential anti-inflammatory role for apoptosis takes on new meaning and significance. I/R injury can activate the transcription factor NF-kB, and although this factor can regulate the transcription of protective, anti-apoptotic genes, it also initiates gene programs leading to innate immune responses and the promotion of inflammation (see review[210]). Recent data suggest that the innate immune system may play an important role in cardiovascular diseases,[211] including ischemic injury in which these responses may be beneficial in the short term, but maladaptive if not resolved.[212] The extent and duration of the innate immune response is regulated by factors such as cytokines, which help limit and resolve the response. One such cytokine, IL-6, recently has been identified as a critical factor in resolving innate immune responses (see review[213]). In general, resolution of inflammation is thought to involve apoptosis of inflammatory leukocytes,[214,215] and IL-6 may be intimately involved in this process.[213] Much of the activity of IL-6 in resolution of inflammatory leukocytes can be attributed to signaling through an endogenous soluble IL-6 receptor (sIL-6R), a process referred to as IL-6 trans-signaling. While certain cell types can be rescued *in vitro* by IL-6,[216,217] IL-6 trans-signaling promotes caspase-3-mediated apoptosis of neutrophils.[218] The precise regulation of these IL-6 activities is not clear, but the data support a central role for this cytokine and its effects on apoptosis of inflammatory cells in the induction and control or limitation of the innate response, such as that seen following cardiac arrest and resuscitation.[209,219]

Conclusion

Developing a better understanding of the molecular pathophysiology of the post-resuscitation injury phenotype – ranging from early cardiovascular collapse and death, to minimal cardiovascular dysfunction, to neurological impairment at hospital discharge – is the first step towards developing other post-resuscitation therapies beyond therapeutic hypothermia. Common cell responses throughout the body (i.e., global responses) that occur during the ischemia of cardiac arrest and the reperfusion of CPR and ROSC likely involve oxidant stress and inflammation. Both can be highly adaptive and protective in moderation, but when a threshold of oxidant injury and circulating inflammatory mediators is surpassed, post-resuscitation injury ensues. Apoptosis plays a critical dual role in both containing inflammation (i.e., apoptosis of leukocytes) and amplifying injury (e.g., apoptosis of cardiac myocytes and other vital tissue). Treating these critical events by using new cytokine, oxidant and apoptosis modulation strategies will be necessary to resuscitate patients fully from the Metabolic Phase of cardiac arrest.

REFERENCES

1. Nichol, G., Stiell, I.G. Laupacis, A. Pham, B. De Maio, V.J., & Wells, G.A. A cumulative meta-analysis of the effectiveness of defibrillator-capable emergency medical services for victims of out-of-hospital cardiac arrest. *Ann. Emerg. Med.* 1999; **34**(4 Pt 1): 517–525.
2. Eisenberg, M.S., Bergner, L., & Hallstrom, A. Cardiac resuscitation in the community. Importance of rapid provision and implications for program planning. *J. Am. Med. Assoc.* 1979; **241**(18): 1905–1907.

3. Becker, L.B., Ostrander, M.P. Barrett, J., & Kondos, G.T. Outcome of CPR in a large metropolitan area – where are the survivors?[comment]. *Ann. Emerg. Med.* 1991; **20**(4): 355–361.

4. Schoenenberger, R.A., von Planta, M., & von Planta, I. Survival after failed out-of-hospital resuscitation. Are further therapeutic efforts in the emergency department futile? *Arch. Intern. Med.,* 1994; **154**(21): 2433–2437.

5. Becker, L.B., Han, B.H. Meyer, P.M. *et al.* Racial differences in the incidence of cardiac arrest and subsequent survival. The CPR Chicago Project.[comment]. *N. Engl. J. Med.* 1993; **329**(9): 600–606.

6. Becker, L.B. The epidemiology of sudden death. In Paradis, N.A., Halperin, H.R., & Nowak, R.M. eds. *Cardiac Arrest: The Science and Practice of Resuscitation Medicine.* Baltimore: Williams & Wilkins, 1996: 28–47.

7. Kern, K.B., Hilwig, R.W. Rhee, K.H., & Berg, R.A. Myocardial dysfunction after resuscitation from cardiac arrest: an example of global myocardial stunning. *J. Am. Coll. Cardiol.* 1996; **28**(1): 232–240.

8. Berg, R.A., Sanders, A.B. Kern, K.B. *et al.* Adverse hemodynamic effects of interrupting chest compressions for rescue breathing during cardiopulmonary resuscitation for ventricular fibrillation cardiac arrest. *Circulation* 2001; **104**(20): 2465–70.

9. Laurent, I., Monchi, M. Chiche, J.D. *et al.* Reversible myocardial dysfunction in survivors of out-of-hospital cardiac arrest. *J. Am. Coll. Cardiol.* 2002; **40**(12): 2110–2116.

10. Anonymous. Barbiturate therapy for the ischemic brain. *N. Engl. J. Med.* 1986; **315**(6): 397–398.

11. Edgren, E., Hedstrand, U. Kelsey, S. Sutton-Tyrrell, K., & Safar, P. Assessment of neurological prognosis in comatose survivors of cardiac arrest. BRCT I Study Group. *Lancet* 1994; **343**(8905): 1055–1059.

12. Gueugniaud, P.Y., Mols, P. Goldstein, P. *et al.* A comparison of repeated high doses and repeated standard doses of epinephrine for cardiac arrest outside the hospital. European Epinephrine Study Group. *N. Engl. J. Med.* 1998; **339**(22): 1595–1601.

13. Jorgensen, E.O. & Holm, S. Prediction of neurological outcome after cardiopulmonary resuscitation. *Resuscitation* 1999; **41**(2): 145–152.

14. Pearn, J. Successful cardiopulmonary resuscitation outcome reviews. *Resuscitation* 2000; **47**(3): 311–316.

15. Grubb, N.R. Managing out-of-hospital cardiac arrest survivors: 1. Neurological perspective. *Heart* 2001; **85**(1): 6–8.

16. Weisfeldt, M.L. & Becker, L.B. Resuscitation after cardiac arrest: a 3-phase time-sensitive model.[comment]. *J. Am. Med. Assoc.* 2002; **288**(23): 3035–3038.

17. Tang, W., Weil, M.H. Sun, S. Gazmuri, R.J., & Bisera, J. Progressive myocardial dysfunction after cardiac resuscitation. *Crit. Care Med.* 1993; **21**(7): 1046–1050.

18. Gazmuri, R.J., Weil, M.H. Bisera, J. Tang, W. Fukui, M., & McKee, D. Myocardial dysfunction after successful resuscitation from cardiac arrest. *Crit. Care Med.* 1996; **24**(6): 992–1000.

19. Weil, M.H. & Tang, W. Cardiopulmonary resuscitation: a promise as yet largely unfulfilled. *Dis. Mon.* 1997; **43**(7): 429–501.

20. Adrie, C., Adib-Conquy, M. Laurent, I. *et al.* Successful cardiopulmonary resuscitation after cardiac arrest as a "sepsis-like" syndrome. *Circulation* 2002; **106**(5): 562–568.

21. El-Menyar, A.A. The resuscitation outcome: revisit the story of the stony heart. *Chest* 2005; **128**(4): 2835–2846.

22. Bernard, S., Buist, M. Monteiro, O., & Smith, K. Induced hypothermia using large volume, ice-cold intravenous fluid in comatose survivors of out-of-hospital cardiac arrest: a preliminary report. *Resuscitation* 2003; **56**(1): 9–13.

23. Bernard, S.A., Gray, T.W. Buist, M.D. *et al.* Treatment of comatose survivors of out-of-hospital cardiac arrest with induced hypothermia. *N. Eng. J. Med.* 2002; **346**(8): 557–563.

24. Bernard, S.A., Jones, B.M., & Horne, M.K. Clinical trial of induced hypothermia in comatose survivors of out-of-hospital cardiac arrest. *Ann. Emerg. Med.* 1997; **30**(2): 146–153.

25. Anonymous. Therapeutic hypothermia after cardiac arrest. The hypothermia after Cardiac Arrest (HACA) Group. *N. Engl. J. Med.* 2002; **347**(1): 63–65.

26. Adrie, C., Laurent, I. Monchi, M. Cariou, A. Dhainaou, J.F., & Spaulding, C. Postresuscitation disease after cardiac arrest: a sepsis-like syndrome? *Curr. Opin. Crit. Care* 2004; **10**(3): 208–212.

27. Rivers, E., Nguyen, B. Havstad, S. *et al.* Early goal-directed therapy in the treatment of severe sepsis and septic shock. *N. Engl. J. Med.* 2001; **345**(19): 1368–1377.

28. Bottiger, B.W., Motsch, J. Bohrer, H. *et al.* Activation of blood coagulation after cardiac arrest is not balanced adequately by activation of endogenous fibrinolysis. *Circulation* 1995; **92**(9): 2572–2578.

29. Gando, S., Kameue, T. Nanzaki, S., & Nakanishi, Y. Massive fibrin formation with consecutive impairment of fibrinolysis in patients with out-of-hospital cardiac arrest. *Thromb. Haemost.* 1997; **77**(2): 278–282.

30. Adrie, C., Monchi, M. Laurent, I. *et al.* Coagulopathy after successful cardiopulmonary resuscitation following cardiac arrest: implication of the protein C anticoagulant pathway. *J. Am. Coll. Cardiol.* 2005; **46**(1): 21–28.

31. Mussack, T., Biberthaler, P. Kanz, K.G. Wiedemann, E. Gippner-Steppert, C., & Jochum, M. S-100b, sE-selectin, and sP-selectin for evaluation of hypoxic brain damage in patients after cardiopulmonary resuscitation: pilot study. *World J. Surg.* 2001; **25**(5): 539–543.

32. Shyu, K.G., Chang, H. Lin, C.C. Huang, F.Y., & Hung, C.R. Concentrations of serum interleukin-8 after successful cardiopulmonary resuscitation in patients with cardiopulmonary arrest. *Am. Heart J.* 1997; **134**(3): 551–556.

33. Gando, S., Nanzaki, S. Morimoto, Y. Kobayashi, S., & Kemmotsu, O. Alterations of soluble L- and P-selectins during cardiac arrest and CPR.[see comment]. *Intens. Care Med.* 1999; **25**(6): 588–593.

34. Gando, S., Nanzaki, S. Morimoto, Y. Kobayashi, S., & Kemmotsu, O. Out-of-hospital cardiac arrest increases

soluble vascular endothelial adhesion molecules and neutrophil elastase associated with endothelial injury. *Intens. Care Med.* 2000; **26**(1): 38–44.

35. Bottiger, B.W.M.D., Motsch, J.M.D. Braun, V.M.D. Martin, E.M.D., & Kirschfink, M.D.V.M.P. Marked activation of complement and leukocytes and an increase in the concentrations of soluble endothelial adhesion molecules during cardiopulmonary resuscitation and early reperfusion after cardiac arrest in humans. *Crit. Care Med.* 2002; **30**(11): 2473–2480.

36. Vgontzas, A.N., Bixler, E.O. Lin, H.M. Prolo, P. Trakada, G., & Chrousos, G.P. IL-6 and its circadian secretion in humans. *Neuroimmunomodulation* 2005; **12**(3): 131–140.

37. Niemann, J., Garner, D., & Lewis, R. Tumor necrosis factor-[alpha] is associated with early postresuscitation myocardial dysfunction. *Crit. Care Med.* 2004; **32**(8): 1753–1758.

38. Carlson, D.L., Willis, M.S. White, D.J. Horton, J.W., & Giroir, B.P. Tumor necrosis factor-alpha-induced caspase activation mediates endotoxin-related cardiac dysfunction. *Crit. Care Med.* 2005; **33**(5): 1021–1028.

39. Magovern, G.J., Jr., Flaherty, J.T. Kanter, K.R. Schaff, H.V. Gott, V.L., & Gardner, T.J. Assessment of myocardial protection during global ischemia with myocardial gas tension monitoring. *Surgery* 1982; **92**(2): 373–379.

40. Kette, F., Weil, M.H. Gazmuri, R.J. Bisera, J., & Rackow, E.C. Intramyocardial hypercarbic acidosis during cardiac arrest and resuscitation. *Crit. Care Med.* 1993; **21**(6): 901–906.

41. Johnson, B.A., Weil, M.H. Tang, W. Noc, M. McKee, D., & McCandless, D. Mechanisms of myocardial hypercarbic acidosis during cardiac arrest. *J. Appl. Physiol.* 1995; **78**(4): 1579–1584.

42. Maldonado, F.A., Weil, M.H. Tang, W. *et al.* Myocardial hypercarbic acidosis reduces cardiac resuscitability. *Anesthesiology* 1993; **78**(2): 343–352.

43. Tang, W.C., Weil, M.H. Gazmuri, R.J. Bisera, J., & Rackow, E.C. Reversible impairment of myocardial contractility due to hypercarbic acidosis in the isolated perfused rat heart. *Crit. Care Med.* 1991; **19**(2): 218–224.

44. Idris, A.H., Wenzel, V. Becker, L.B. Banner, M.J., &. Orban, D.J. Does hypoxia or hypercarbia independently affect resuscitation from cardiac arrest? *Chest* 1995; **108**(2): 522–528.

45. Vanden Hoek, T.L., Becker, L.B. Shao, Z. Li, C., & Schumacker, P.T. Reactive oxygen species released from mitochondria during brief hypoxia induce preconditioning in cardiomyocytes. *J. Biol. Chem.* 1998; **273**(29): 18092–18098.

46. Duranteau, J., Chandel, N.S. Kulisz, A. Shao, Z., & Schumacker, P.T. Intracellular signaling by reactive oxygen species during hypoxia in cardiomyocytes. *J. Biol. Chem.* 1998; **273**(19): 11619–11624.

47. Agani, F.H., P. Pichiule, J.C. Chavez, and J.C. LaManna, The role of mitochondria in the regulation of hypoxia-inducible factor 1 expression during hypoxia. *J. Biol. Chem.* 2000; **275**(46): 35863–35867.

48. Vanden Hoek, T.L., Qin, Y. Wojcik, K. *et al.* Reperfusion, not simulated ischemia, initiates intrinsic apoptosis injury in chick cardiomyocytes. *Am. J. Physiol. – Heart Circ. Physiol.* 2003; **284**(1): H141–H150.

49. Schumacker, P.T. Hypoxia-inducible factor-1 (HIF-1). *Crit. Care Med.* 2005; **33**(12 Suppl): S423–S425.

50. Idris, A.H., Roberts, L.J. 2nd, Caruso, L. *et al.* Oxidant injury occurs rapidly after cardiac arrest, cardiopulmonary resuscitation, and reperfusion.[see comment]. *Crit. Care Med.* 2005; **33**(9): 2043–2048.

51. Basu, S., Liu, X. Nozari, A. Rubertsson, S. Miclescu, A., & Wiklund, L. Evidence for time-dependent maximum increase of free radical damage and eicosanoid formation in the brain as related to duration of cardiac arrest and cardio-pulmonary resuscitation. *Free Rad. Res.* 2003; **37**(3): 251–256.

52. Bhatti, S., Zimmer, G., & Bereitier-Hahn, J. Enzyme release from chick myocytes during hypoxia and reoxygenation: dependence on pH. *J. Mol. Cell Cardiol.* 1989; **21**: 995–1008.

53. State-specific mortality from sudden cardiac death – United States, 1999. *Morb. Mortal. Wkly Rep.* 2002; **51**(6): 123–126.

54. Lebuffe, G., Schumacker, P.T. Shao, Z.H. Anderson, T. Iwase, H., & Vanden Hoek, T.L. ROS and NO trigger early preconditioning: relationship to mitochondrial KATP channel. *Am. J. Physiol. – Heart Circ. Physiol.* 2003; **284**(1): H299–H308.

55. Lavani, R., Chang, W. Anderson, T. *et al.* Controlled reperfusion of ischemic cardiomyocytes by altering CO_2 modifies mitochondrial oxidant injury. Submitted.

56. Sherman, A.J., Davis, C.A. 3rd, Klocke, F.J. *et al.* Blockade of nitric oxide synthesis reduces myocardial oxygen consumption in vivo. *Circulation* 1997; **95**(5): 1328–1334.

57. Krismer, A.C., Lindner, K.H. Wenzel, V. Rainer, B. Mueller, G., & Lingnau, W. Inhibition of nitric oxide improves coronary perfusion pressure and return of spontaneous circulation in a porcine cardiopulmonary resuscitation model.[see comment]. *Crit. Care Med.* 2001; **29**(3): 482–486.

58. Shiva, S., Brookes, P.S. Patel, R.P. Anderson, P.G., & Darley-Usmar, V.M. Nitric oxide partitioning into mitochondrial membranes and the control of respiration at cytochrome c oxidase. *Proc. Natl. Acad. Sci. U S A* 2001; **98**(13): 7212–7217.

59. Chandel, N.S., McClintock, D.S. Feliciano, C.E. *et al.* Reactive oxygen species generated at mitochondrial complex III stabilize hypoxia-inducible factor-1 alpha during hypoxia: a mechanism of O2 sensing. *J. Biol. Chem.* 2000; **275**(33): 25130–25138.

60. Miller, E.R., 3rd, Pastor-Barriuso, R. Dalal, D. Riemersma, R.A. Appel, L.J., & Guallar, E. Meta-analysis: high-dosage vitamin E supplementation may increase all-cause mortality. *Ann. Intern. Med.* 2005; **142**(1): 37–46.

61. Stamler, J.S. & Hausladen, A. Oxidative modifications in nitrosative stress. *Nat. Struct. Biol.* 1998; **5**(4): 247–249.

62. Mann, D.L. Stress activated cytokines and the heart. *Cytokine Growth Factor Revi.* 1996; **7**(4): 341–354.

63. Mann, D.L. Stress-activated cytokines and the heart: from adaptation to maladaptation. *Ann. Revi. Physiol.* 2003; **65**: 81–101.

64. Lefer, D.J. & Granger, D.N. Oxidative stress and cardiac disease. *Am. J. Med.* 2000; **109**(4): 315–323.

65. Basu, S., Nozari, A. Liu, X.L. Rubertsson, S., & Wiklund, L. Development of a novel biomarker of free radical damage in reperfusion injury after cardiac arrest. *FEBS Lett.* 2000; **470**(1): 1–6.

66. Waisman, D., Brod, V. Wolff, R. *et al.* Effects of hyperoxia on local and remote microcirculatory inflammatory response after splanchnic ischemia and reperfusion. *Am. J. Physiol. – Heart Circ. Physiol.* 2003; **285**(2): H643–H652.

67. Colletti, L.M., Kunkel, S.L. Walz, A. *et al.* Chemokine expression during hepatic ischemia/reperfusion-induced lung injury in the rat. The role of epithelial neutrophil activating protein. *J. Clin. Invest.* 1995; **95**(1): 134–141.

68. Yoshidome, H., Lentsch, A.B. Cheadle, W.G. Miller, F.N., & Edwards, M.J. Enhanced pulmonary expression of CXC chemokines during hepatic ischemia/reperfusion-induced lung injury in mice. *J. Surg. Res.* 1999; **81**(1): 33–37.

69. Gray, K.D., MacMillan-Crow, L.A. Simovic, M.O. Stain, S.C., & May, A.K. Pulmonary MnSOD is nitrated following hepatic ischemia-reperfusion. *Surg. Infec.* 2004; **5**(2): 166–173.

70. Yokoyama, T., Vaca, L. Rossen, R.D. Durante, W. Hazarika, P., & Mann, D.L. Cellular basis for the negative inotropic effects of tumor necrosis factor-alpha in the adult mammalian heart. *J. Clin. Invest.* 1993; **92**(5): 2303–2312.

71. Becker, L.B., Weisfeldt, M.L. Weil, M.H. *et al.* The PULSE initiative: scientific priorities and strategic planning for resuscitation research and life saving therapies. *Circulation* 2002; **105**(21): 2562–2570.

72. Vallejo, J.G., Nemoto, S. Ishiyama, M. *et al.* Functional significance of inflammatory mediators in a murine model of resuscitated hemorrhagic shock. *Am. J. Physiol. Heart Circ. Physiol.* 2005; **288**(3): H1272–1277.

73. Chen, L.W., Egan, L. Li, Z.W. Greten, F.R. Kagnoff, M.F., & Karin, M. The two faces of IKK and NF-kappaB inhibition: prevention of systemic inflammation but increased local injury following intestinal ischemia-reperfusion. *Nat. Med.* 2003; **9**(5): 575–581.

74. Roy, S., Khanna, S. Kuhn, D.E. *et al.* Transcriptome analysis of the ischemia-reperfused remodeling myocardium: temporal changes in inflammation and extracellular matrix. *Physiol. Genom.* 2006; **25**(3): 364–374.

75. Marshall, H.E., Merchant, K., & Stamler, J.S. Nitrosation and oxidation in the regulation of gene expression. *Faseb J.* 2000; **14**(13): 1889–1900.

76. Kabe, Y., Ando, K. Hirao, S. Yoshida, M., & Handa, H. Redox regulation of NF-kappaB activation: distinct redox regulation between the cytoplasm and the nucleus. *Antioxid. Redox Signal.* 2005; **7**(3–4): 395–403.

77. Altavilla, D., Saitta, A. Guarini, S. *et al.* Oxidative stress causes nuclear factor-kappaB activation in acute hypovolemic hemorrhagic shock. *Free Rad. Biol. Med.* 2001; **30**(10): 1055–1066.

78. Altavilla, D., Saitta, A. Squadrito, G. *et al.* Evidence for a role of nuclear factor-kappaB in acute hypovolemic hemorrhagic shock. *Surgery* 2002; **131**(1): 50–58.

79. Sundar, S.V., Li, Y.Y. Rollwagen, F.M., & Maheshwari, R.K. Hemorrhagic shock induces differential gene expression and apoptosis in mouse liver. *Biochem. Biophys. Res. Commun.* 2005; **332**(3): 688–696.

80. Ortis, F., Cardozo, A.K. Crispim, D. Storling, J. Mandrup-Poulsen, T., & Eizirik, D.L. Cytokine-induced pro-apoptotic gene expression in insulin-producing cells is related to rapid, sustained and non-oscillatory NF-{kappa}B activation. *Mol. Endocrinol.* 2006.

81. Hierholzer, C. & Billiar, T.R. Molecular mechanisms in the early phase of hemorrhagic shock. *Langenbecks Arch. Surg.* 2001; **386**(4): 302–308.

82. Alam, H.B., Stegalkina, S. Rhee, P., & Koustova, E. cDNA array analysis of gene expression following hemorrhagic shock and resuscitation in rats. *Resuscitation* 2002; **54**(2): 195–206.

83. Brundage, S.I., Schreiber, M.A. Holcomb, J.B. *et al.* Amplification of the proinflammatory transcription factor cascade increases with severity of uncontrolled hemorrhage in swine. *J. Surg. Res.* 2003; **113**(1): 74–80.

84. Chen, H., Alam, H.B. Querol, R.I. Rhee, P. Li, Y., & Koustova, E. Identification of expression patterns associated with hemorrhage and resuscitation: integrated approach to data analysis. *J. Trauma* 2006; **60**(4): 701–724.

85. Calvano, S.E., Xiao, W. Richards, D.R. *et al.* A network-based analysis of systemic inflammation in humans. *Nature* 2005; **437**(7061): 1032–1037.

86. Gottlieb, R.A., Burleson, K.O. Kloner, R.A. Babior, B.M., & Engler, R.L. Reperfusion injury induces apoptosis in rabbit cardiomyocytes. *J. Clin. Invest.* 1994; **94**(4): 1621–1628.

87. Hamann, K.J., Dorscheid, D.R. Ko, F.D. *et al.* Expression of Fas (CD95) and FasL (CD95L) in human airway epithelium. *Am. J. Resp. Cell Molec. Biol.* 1998; **19**(4): 537–542.

88. Kayagaki, N., Kawasaki, A. Ebata, T. *et al.* Metalloproteinase-mediated release of human Fas ligand. *J. Exp. Med.* 1995; **182**(6): 1777–1783.

89. Edston, E., Grontoft, L., & Johnsson, J. TUNEL: a useful screening method in sudden cardiac death. *Int. J. Legal Med.* 2002; **116**(1): 22–26.

90. Yuan, J., Lipinski, M., & Degterev, A. Diversity in the mechanisms of neuronal cell death. *Neuron* 2003; **40**(2): 401–413.

91. McCully, J.D., Wakiyama, H. Hsieh, Y.J. Jones, M., & Levitsky, S. Differential contribution of necrosis and apoptosis in myocardial ischemia-reperfusion injury. *Am. J. Physiol. Heart Circ. Physiol.* 2004; **286**(5): H1923–H1935.

92. Jaeschke, H. & Lemasters, J.J. Apoptosis versus oncotic necrosis in hepatic ischemia/reperfusion injury. *Gastroenterology* 2003; **125**(4): 1246–1257.

93. Degterev, A., Huang, Z. Boyce, M. *et al.* Chemical inhibitor of nonapoptotic cell death with therapeutic potential for ischemic brain injury. *Nat. Chem. Biol.* 2005; **1**(2): 112–119.

94. Zong, W.X., Ditsworth, D. Bauer, D.E. Wang, Z.Q., & Thompson, C.B. Alkylating DNA damage stimulates a regulated form of necrotic cell death. *Genes Dev* 2004; **18**(11): 1272–1282.

95. Zong, W.X. & Thompson, C.B. Necrotic death as a cell fate. *Genes Dev.* 2006; **20**(1): 1–15.

96. Kern, J.C. & Kehrer, J.P. Acrolein-induced cell death: a caspase-influenced decision between apoptosis and oncosis/necrosis. *Chem. Biol. Interact.* 2002; **139**(1): 79–95.

97. Jaattela, M. & Tschopp, J. Caspase-independent cell death in T lymphocytes. *Nat. Immunol.* 2003; **4**(5): 416–423.

98. Assuncao Guimaraes, C. & Linden, R. Programmed cell deaths. Apoptosis and alternative deathstyles. *Eur. J. Biochem.* 2004; **271**(9): 1638–1650.

99. Graham, R.M., Frazier, D.P. Thompson, J.W. *et al.* A unique pathway of cardiac myocyte death caused by hypoxia-acidosis. *J. Exp. Biol.* 2004; **207**(18): 3189–3200.

100. Sperandio, S., de Belle, I. & Bredesen, D.E. An alternative, nonapoptotic form of programmed cell death. *Proc. Natl Acad. Sci. U S A* 2000; **97**(26): 14376–14381.

101. Sperandio, S., Poksay, K. de Belle, I. *et al.* Paraptosis: mediation by MAP kinases and inhibition by AIP-1/Alix. *Cell Death Differ.* 2004; **11**(10): 1066–1075.

102. Vanden Hoek, T.L., Qin, Y. Wojcik, K. *et al.* Reperfusion, not simulated ischemia, initiates intrinsic apoptosis injury in chick cardiomyocytes. *Am. J. Physiol. Heart Circ. Physiol.* 2003; **284**(1): H141–H150.

103. Qin, Y., Vanden Hoek, T.L. Wojcik, K. *et al.* Caspase-dependent cytochrome c release and cell death in chick cardiomyocytes after simulated ischemia-reperfusion. *Am. J. Physiol. Heart Circ. Physiol.* 2004; **286**(6): H2280–H2286.

104. Lundberg, K.C. & Szweda, L.I. Initiation of mitochondrial-mediated apoptosis during cardiac reperfusion. *Arch. Biochem. Biophys.* 2004; **432**(1): 50–57.

105. Li, P., Allen, H. Banerjee, S. *et al.* Mice deficient in IL-1 beta-converting enzyme are defective in production of mature IL-1 beta and resistant to endotoxic shock. *Cell* 1995; **80**(3): 401–411.

106. Li, P., Allen, H. Banerjee, S. & Seshadri, T. Characterization of mice deficient in interleukin-1 beta converting enzyme. *J. Cell. Biochem.* 1997; **64**(1): 27–32.

107. Gottlieb, R. ICE-ing the heart. *Circ. Res.* 2005; **96**(10): 1036–1038.

108. Syed, F.M., Hahn, H.S. Odley, A. *et al.* Proapoptotic effects of caspase-1/interleukin-converting enzyme dominate in myocardial ischemia. *Circ. Res.* 2005; **96**(10): 1103–1109.

109. Frantz, S., Ducharme, A. Sawyer, D. *et al.* Targeted deletion of caspase-1 reduces early mortality and left ventricular dilatation following myocardial infarction. *J. Mol. Cell. Cardiol.* 2003; **35**(6): 685–694.

110. Zhang, W.H., Wang, X. Narayanan, M. *et al.* Fundamental role of the Rip2/caspase-1 pathway in hypoxia and ischemia-induced neuronal cell death. *Proc. Natl Acad. Sci. U S A* 2003; **100**(26): 16012–16017.

111. Pomerantz, B.J., Reznikov, L.L. Harken, A.H. & Dinarello, C.A. Inhibition of caspase 1 reduces human myocardial ischemic dysfunction via inhibition of IL-18 and IL-1beta. *Proc. Natl Acad. Sci. U S A* 2001; **98**(5): 2871–2876.

112. Brennan, M.A. & Cookson, B.T. Salmonella induces macrophage death by caspase-1-dependent necrosis. *Mol. Microbiol.* 2000; **38**(1): 31–40.

113. Fink, S.L. & Cookson, B.T. Apoptosis, pyroptosis, and necrosis: mechanistic description of dead and dying eukaryotic cells. *Infect. Immun.* 2005; **73**(4): 1907–1916.

114. Katz, L.M., Lotocki, G. Wang, Y. Kraydieh, S. Dietrich, W.D., & Keane, R.W. Regulation of caspases and XIAP in the brain after asphyxial cardiac arrest in rats. *Neuroreport* 2001; **12**(17): 3751–3754.

115. Terman, A. & Brunk, U.T. Autophagy in cardiac myocyte homeostasis, aging, and pathology. *Cardiovasc. Res.* 2005; **68**(3): 355–365.

116. Yan, L., Vatner, D.E. Kim, S.J. *et al.* Autophagy in chronically ischemic myocardium. *Proc. Natl Acad. Sci. U S A* 2005; **102**(39): 13807–13812.

117. Mizushima, N., Yamamoto, A. Matsui, M. Yoshimori, T. & Ohsumi, Y. In vivo analysis of autophagy in response to nutrient starvation using transgenic mice expressing a fluorescent autophagosome marker. *Mol. Biol. Cell.* 2004; **15**(3): 1101–1111.

118. Pattingre, S., Tassa, A. Qu, X. *et al.* Bcl-2 antiapoptotic proteins inhibit Beclin 1-dependent autophagy. *Cell* 2005; **122**(6): 927–939.

119. Lemasters, J.J. Selective mitochondrial autophagy, or mitophagy, as a targeted defense against oxidative stress, mitochondrial dysfunction, and aging. *Rejuvenation Res.* 2005; **8**(1): 3–5.

120. Priault, M., Salin, B. Schaeffer, J. Vallette, F.M. di Rago, J.P., & Martinou, J.C. Impairing the bioenergetic status and the biogenesis of mitochondria triggers mitophagy in yeast. *Cell Death Differ.* 2005.

121. He, L. & Lemasters, J.J. Regulated and unregulated mitochondrial permeability transition pores: a new paradigm of pore structure and function? *FEBS Lett.* 2002; **512**(1–3): 1–7.

122. Kerr, J.F., Wyllie, A.H., & Currie, A.R. Apoptosis: a basic biological phenomenon with wide-ranging implications in tissue kinetics. *Br. J. Cancer* 1972; **26**(4): 239–257.

123. Kerr, J.F. Shrinkage necrosis: a distinct mode of cellular death. *J. Pathol.* 1971; **105**(1): 13–20.

124. Bishopric, N.H., Andreka, P. Slepak, T., & Webster, K.A. Molecular mechanisms of apoptosis in the cardiac myocyte. *Curr. Opin. Pharmacol.* 2001; **1**(2): 141–150.

125. Clerk, A., Cole, S.M. Cullingford, T.E. Harrison, J.G. Jormakka, M., & Valks, D.M. Regulation of cardiac myocyte cell death. *Pharmacol. Ther.* 2003; **97**(3): 223–261.

126. Crow, M.T., Mani, K. Nam, Y.J., & Kitsis, R.N. The mitochondrial death pathway and cardiac myocyte apoptosis. *Circ. Res.* 2004; **95**(10): 957–970.

127. Regula, K.M. & Kirshenbaum, L.A. Apoptosis of ventricular myocytes: a means to an end. *J. Mol. Cell. Cardiol.* 2005; **38**(1): 3–13.

128. Logue, S.E., Gustafsson, A.B. Samali, A. & Gottlieb, R.A. Ischemia/reperfusion injury at the intersection with cell death. *J. Mol. Cell. Cardiol.* 2005; **38**(1): 21–33.

129. Vinten-Johansen, J., Zhao, Z.Q. Zatta, A.J. Kin, H. Halkos, M.E., & Kerendi, F. Postconditioning – A new link in nature's armor against myocardial ischemia-reperfusion injury. *Basic Res. Cardiol.* 2005; **100**(4): 295–310.

130. Winn, R.K. & Harlan, J.M. The role of endothelial cell apoptosis in inflammatory and immune diseases. *J. Thromb. Haemost.* 2005; **3**(8): 1815–1824.

131. Olivetti, G., Abbi, R. Quaini, F. *et al.* Apoptosis in the failing human heart. *N. Engl. J. Med.* 1997; **336**(16): 1131–1141.

132. Abbate, A., Scarpa, S. Santini, D. *et al.* Myocardial expression of survivin, an apoptosis inhibitor, in aging and heart failure. An experimental study in the spontaneously hypertensive rat. *Int. J. Cardiol.* 2005.

133. Saraste, A., Pulkki, K. Kallajoki, M. Henriksen, K. Parvinen, M., & Voipio-Pulkki, L.M. Apoptosis in human acute myocardial infarction. *Circulation* 1997; **95**(2): 320–323.

134. Abbate, A., Melfi, R. Patti, G. *et al.* Apoptosis in recent myocardial infarction. *Clin Ter.* 2000; **151**(4): 247–251.

135. Anselmi, A., Abbate, A. Girola, F. *et al.* Myocardial ischemia, stunning, inflammation, and apoptosis during cardiac surgery: a review of evidence. *Eur. J. Cardiothorac. Surg.* 2004; **25**(3): 304–311.

136. Yeh, C.H., Chen, T.P. Wu, Y.C. Lin, Y.M., & Jing Lin, P. Inhibition of NFkappaB activation with curcumin attenuates plasma inflammatory cytokines surge and cardiomyocytic apoptosis following cardiac ischemia/reperfusion. *J. Surg. Res.* 2005; **125**(1): 109–116.

137. Shi, Y. Mechanisms of caspase activation and inhibition during apoptosis. *Mol. Cell* 2002; **9**(3): 459–470.

138. Chang, D.W., Ditsworth, D. Liu, H. Srinivasula, S.M. Alnemri, E.S., & Yang, X. Oligomerization is a general mechanism for the activation of apoptosis initiator and inflammatory pro-caspases. *J. Biol. Chem.* 2003; **278**(19): 16466–16469.

139. Shi, Y. Caspase activation: revisiting the induced proximity model. *Cell* 2004; **117**(7): 855–858.

140. Chao, Y., Shiozaki, E.N. Srinivasula, S.M. Rigotti, D.J. Fairman, R., & Shi, Y. Engineering a dimeric caspase-9: a re-evaluation of the induced proximity model for caspase activation. *PLoS Biol* 2005; **3**(6): e183.

141. Earnshaw, W.C., Martins, L.M., & Kaufmann, S.H. Mammalian caspases: structure, activation, substrates, and functions during apoptosis. *Annu. Rev. Biochem.* 1999; **68**: 383–424.

142. Fischer, U., Janicke, R.U., & Schulze-Osthoff, K. Many cuts to ruin: a comprehensive update of caspase substrates. *Cell Death Differ.* 2003; **10**(1): 76–100.

143. Vaux, D.L. & Silke, J. Mammalian mitochondrial IAP binding proteins. *Biochem. Biophys. Res. Commun.* 2003; **304**(3): 499–504.

144. Vaux, D.L. & Silke, J. IAPs, RINGs and ubiquitylation. *Nat. Rev. Mol. Cell. Biol.* 2005; **6**(4): 287–297.

145. Schimmer, A.D. & Dalili, S. Targeting the IAP family of caspase inhibitors as an emerging therapeutic strategy. *Hematology* (Am. Soc. Hematol. Educ. Program), 2005: 215–219.

146. Ni, T., Li, W., & Zou, F. The ubiquitin ligase ability of IAPs regulates apoptosis. *IUBMB Life* 2005; **57**(12): 779–785.

147. Liston, P., Fong, W.G., & Korneluk, R.G. The inhibitors of apoptosis: there is more to life than Bcl2. *Oncogene* 2003; **22**(53): 8568–8580.

148. Bratton, S.B., Walker, G. Srinivasula, S.M. *et al.* Recruitment, activation and retention of caspases-9 and -3 by Apaf-1 apoptosome and associated XIAP complexes. *EMBO J* 2001; **20**(5): 998–1009.

149. Deveraux, Q.L., Roy, N. Stennicke, H.R. *et al.* IAPs block apoptotic events induced by caspase-8 and cytochrome c by direct inhibition of distinct caspases. *EMBO J* 1998; **17**(8): 2215–2223.

150. Du, C., Fang, M. Li, Y. Li, L., & Wang, X. Smac, a mitochondrial protein that promotes cytochrome c-dependent caspase activation by eliminating IAP inhibition. *Cell* 2000; **102**(1): 33–42.

151. Verhagen, A.M. & Vaux, D.L. Cell death regulation by the mammalian IAP antagonist Diablo/Smac. *Apoptosis* 2002; **7**(2): 163–166.

152. Suzuki, Y., Imai, Y. Nakayama, H. Takahashi, K. Takio, K., & Takahashi, R. A serine protease, HtrA2, is released from the mitochondria and interacts with XIAP, inducing cell death. *Mol. Cell.* 2001; **8**(3): 613–621.

153. Verhagen, A.M., Silke, J. Ekert, P.G. *et al.* HtrA2 promotes cell death through its serine protease activity and its ability to antagonize inhibitor of apoptosis proteins. *J. Biol. Chem.* 2002; **277**(1): 445–454.

154. Yang, Q.H., Church-Hajduk, R. Ren, J. Newton, M.L., & Du, C. Omi/HtrA2 catalytic cleavage of inhibitor of apoptosis (IAP) irreversibly inactivates IAPs and facilitates caspase activity in apoptosis. *Genes Dev.* 2003; **17**(12): 1487–1496.

155. Lyn, D., Bao, S. Bennett, N.A. Liu, X. & Emmett, N.L. Ischemia elicits a coordinated expression of pro-survival proteins in mouse myocardium. *Sci. World J* 2002; **2**: 997–1003.

156. Scarabelli, T.M., Stephanou, A. Pasini, E. *et al.* Minocycline inhibits caspase activation and reactivation, increases the ratio of XIAP to smac/DIABLO, and reduces the mitochondrial leakage of cytochrome C and smac/DIABLO. *J. Am. Coll. Cardiol.* 2004; **43**(5): 865–874.

157. Koseki, T., Inohara, N. Chen, S., & Nunez, G. ARC, an inhibitor of apoptosis expressed in skeletal muscle and heart that interacts selectively with caspases. *Proc. Natl Acad. Sci. U S A* 1998; **95**(9): 5156–5160.

158. Neuss, M., Monticone, R. Lundberg, M.S. Chesley, A.T. Fleck, E., & Crow, M.T. The apoptotic regulatory protein ARC (apoptosis repressor with caspase recruitment domain) prevents oxidant stress-mediated cell death by preserving mitochondrial function. *J. Biol. Chem.* 2001; **276**(36): 33915–33922.

159. Nam, Y.J., Mani, K. Ashton, A.W. *et al.* Inhibition of both the extrinsic and intrinsic death pathways through nonhomotypic death-fold interactions. *Mol. Cell.* 2004; **15**(6): 901–912.

160. Jo, D.G., Jun, J.I. Chang, J.W. *et al.* Calcium binding of ARC mediates regulation of caspase 8 and cell death. *Mol. Cell. Biol.* 2004; **24**(22): 9763–9770.

161. Ashkenazi, A. & Dixit, V.M. Apoptosis control by death and decoy receptors. *Curr. Opin. Cell. Biol.* 1999; **11**(2): 255–260.

162. Scaffidi, C., Schmitz, I. Zha, J. Korsmeyer, S.J. Krammer, P.H. & Peter, M.E. Differential modulation of apoptosis sensitivity in CD95 type I and type II cells. *J. Biol. Chem.* 1999; **274**(32): 22532–22538.

163. Kubota, T., Miyagishima, M. Frye, C.S. *et al.* Overexpression of tumor necrosis factor- alpha activates both anti- and pro-apoptotic pathways in the myocardium. *J. Mol. Cell. Cardiol.* 2001; **33**(7): 1331–1344.

164. Yaniv, G., Shilkrut, M. Lotan, R. Berke, G. Larisch, S., & Binah, O. Hypoxia predisposes neonatal rat ventricular myocytes to apoptosis induced by activation of the Fas (CD95/Apo-1) receptor: Fas activation and apoptosis in hypoxic myocytes. *Cardiovasc. Res.* 2002; **54**(3): 611–623.

165. Balachandran, S., Thomas, E., & Barber, G.N. A FADD-dependent innate immune mechanism in mammalian cells. *Nature* 2004; **432**(7015): 401–405.

166. Meylan, E. & Tschopp, J. The RIP kinases: crucial integrators of cellular stress. *Trends Biochem. Sci.* 2005; **30**(3): 151–159.

167. Jeremias, I., Kupatt, C. Martin-Villalba, A. *et al.* Involvement of CD95/Apo1/Fas in cell death after myocardial ischemia. *Circulation* 2000; **102**(8): 915–920.

168. Chao, W., Shen, Y. Li, L., & Rosenzweig, A. Importance of FADD signaling in serum deprivation- and hypoxia-induced cardiomyocyte apoptosis. *J. Biol. Chem.* 2002; **277**(35): 31639–31645.

169. Scarabelli, T.M., Stephanou, A. Pasini, E. *et al.* Different signaling pathways induce apoptosis in endothelial cells and cardiac myocytes during ischemia/reperfusion injury. *Circ. Res.* 2002; **90**(6): 745–748.

170. Lee, P., Sata, M. Lefer, D.J. Factor, S.M. Walsh, K., & Kitsis, R.N. Fas pathway is a critical mediator of cardiac myocyte death and MI during ischemia-reperfusion in vivo. *Am. J. Physiol. Heart Circ. Physiol.* 2003; **284**(2): H456–H463.

171. Gomez, L., Chavanis, N. Argaud, L. *et al.* Fas-independent mitochondrial damage triggers cardiomyocyte death after ischemia-reperfusion. *Am. J. Physiol. Heart Circ. Physiol.* 2005; **289**(5): H2153–H2158.

172. Li, Y., Takemura, G. Kosai, K. *et al.* Critical roles for the Fas/Fas ligand system in postinfarction ventricular remodeling and heart failure. *Circ. Res.* 2004; **95**(6): 627–636.

173. Ferri, K.F. & Kroemer, G. Organelle-specific initiation of cell death pathways. *Nat. Cell Biol.* 2001; **3**(11): E255–E263.

174. Borutaite, V. & Brown, G.C. Mitochondria in apoptosis of ischemic heart. *FEBS Lett.* 2003; **541**(1–3): 1–5.

175. Levraut, J., Iwase, H. Shao, Z.H. Vanden Hoek, T.L., & Schumacker, P.T. Cell death during ischemia: relationship to mitochondrial depolarization and ROS generation. *Am. J. Physiol. Heart Circ. Physiol.* 2003; **284**(2): H549–H558.

176. van Gurp, M., Festjens, N. van Loo, G. Saelens, X., & Vandenabeele, P. Mitochondrial intermembrane proteins in cell death. *Biochem. Biophys. Res. Commun.* 2003; **304**(3): 487–497.

177. Orrenius, S. Mitochondrial regulation of apoptotic cell death. *Toxicol. Lett.* 2004; **149**(1–3): 19–23.

178. Green, D.R. & Kroemer, G. The pathophysiology of mitochondrial cell death. *Science* 2004; **305**(5684): 626–629.

179. Festjens, N., van Gurp, M. van Loo, G. Saelens, X., & Vandenabeele, P. Bcl-2 family members as sentinels of cellular integrity and role of mitochondrial intermembrane space

proteins in apoptotic cell death. *Acta Haematol.* 2004; **111**(1–2): 7–27.

180. Chen, J., Graham, S.H. Nakayama, M. *et al.* Apoptosis repressor genes Bcl-2 and Bcl-x-long are expressed in the rat brain following global ischemia. *J. Cereb. Blood Flow Metab.* 1997; **17**(1): 2–10.

181. Reed, J.C., Jurgensmeier, J.M., & Matsuyama, S. Bcl-2 family proteins and mitochondria. *Biochim. Biophys. Acta* 1998; **1366**(1–2): 127–137.

182. Gross, A., McDonnell, J.M., & Korsmeyer, S.J. BCL-2 family members and the mitochondria in apoptosis. *Genes Dev.* 1999; **13**(15): 1899–1911.

183. Kuwana, T. & Newmeyer, D.D. Bcl-2-family proteins and the role of mitochondria in apoptosis. *Curr. Opin. Cell. Biol.* 2003; **15**(6): 691–699.

184. Hochhauser, E., Kivity, S. Offen, D. *et al.* Bax ablation protects against myocardial ischemia-reperfusion injury in transgenic mice. *Am. J. Physiol. Heart Circ. Physiol.* 2003; **284**(6): H2351–H2359.

185. Li, H., Zhu, H. Xu, C.J., & Yuan, J. Cleavage of BID by caspase 8 mediates the mitochondrial damage in the Fas pathway of apoptosis. *Cell* 1998; **94**(4): 491–501.

186. Chen, M., He, H. Zhan, S. Krajewski, S. Reed, J.C. & Gottlieb, R.A. Bid is cleaved by calpain to an active fragment in vitro and during myocardial ischemia/reperfusion. *J. Biol. Chem.* 2001; **276**(33): 30724–30728.

187. Chen, M., Won, D.J. Krajewski, S., & Gottlieb, R.A. Calpain and mitochondria in ischemia/reperfusion injury. *J. Biol. Chem.* 2002; **277**(32): 29181–29186.

188. Kubasiak, L.A., Hernandez, O.M. Bishopric, N.H., & Webster, K.A. Hypoxia and acidosis activate cardiac myocyte death through the Bcl-2 family protein BNIP3. *Proc. Natl Acad. Sci. U S A* 2002; **99**(20): 12825–12830.

189. Webster, K.A., Graham, R.M., & Bishopric, N.H. BNip3 and signal-specific programmed death in the heart. *J. Mol. Cell. Cardiol.* 2005; **38**(1): 35–45.

190. Murriel, C.L., Churchill, E. Inagaki, K. Szweda, L.I., & Mochly-Rosen, D. Protein kinase Cdelta activation induces apoptosis in response to cardiac ischemia and reperfusion damage: a mechanism involving BAD and the mitochondria. *J. Biol. Chem.* 2004; **279**(46): 47985–47991.

191. Uchiyama, T., Engelman, R.M. Maulik, N., & Das, D.K. Role of Akt signaling in mitochondrial survival pathway triggered by hypoxic preconditioning. *Circulation* 2004; **109**(24): 3042–3049.

192. Lee, S.D., Kuo, W.W. Wu, C.H. *et al.* Effects of short- and long-term hypobaric hypoxia on Bcl2 family in rat heart. *Int. J. Cardiol.* 2006; **108**(3): 376–384.

193. Toth, A., Jeffers, J.R. Nickson, P. *et al.* Targeted Deletion of Puma Attenuates Cardiomyocyte Death and Improves Cardiac Function during Ischemia/reperfusion. *Am. J. Physiol. Heart Circ. Physiol.* 2006; **291**(1): H52–H60.

194. Wang, X., Yang, C. Chai, J. Shi, Y., & Xue, D. Mechanisms of AIF-mediated apoptotic DNA degradation in *Caenorhabditis elegans*. *Science* 2002; **298**(5598): 1587–1592.

195. Wu, M., Xu, L.G. Li, X. Zhai, Z. & Shu, H.B. AMID, an apoptosis-inducing factor-homologous mitochondrion-associated protein, induces caspase-independent apoptosis. *J. Biol. Chem.* 2002; **277**(28): 25617–25623.

196. Arnoult, D., Gaume, B. Karbowski, M. Sharpe, J.C. Cecconi, F., & Youle, R.J. Mitochondrial release of AIF and EndoG requires caspase activation downstream of Bax/Bak-mediated permeabilization. *EMBO J.* 2003; **22**(17): 4385–4399.

197. Lassus, P., Opitz-Araya, X., & Lazebnik, Y. Requirement for caspase-2 in stress-induced apoptosis before mitochondrial permeabilization. *Science* 2002; **297**(5585): 1352–1354.

198. Guo, Y., Srinivasula, S.M. Druilhe, A. Fernandes-Alnemri, T. & Alnemri, E.S. Caspase-2 induces apoptosis by releasing proapoptotic proteins from mitochondria. *J. Biol. Chem.* 2002; **277**(16): 13430–13437.

199. Robertson, J.D., Enoksson, M. Suomela, M. Zhivotovsky, B., & Orrenius, S. Caspase-2 acts upstream of mitochondria to promote cytochrome c release during etoposide-induced apoptosis. *J. Biol. Chem.* 2002; **277**(33): 29803–29809.

200. Cummings, O.W., King, T.C. Holden, J.A., & Low, R.L. Purification and characterization of the potent endonuclease in extracts of bovine heart mitochondria. *J. Biol. Chem.* 1987; **262**(5): 2005–2015.

201. Daugas, E., Nochy, D. Ravagnan, L. *et al.* Apoptosis-inducing factor (AIF): a ubiquitous mitochondrial oxidoreductase involved in apoptosis. *FEBS Lett.* 2000; **476**(3): 118–123.

202. Xie, Q., Lin, T. Zhang, Y. Zheng, J., & Bonanno, J.A. Molecular cloning and characterization of a human AIF-like gene with ability to induce apoptosis. *J. Biol. Chem.* 2005; **280**(20): 19673–19681.

203. Kim, G.T., Chun, Y.S. Park, J.W., & Kim, M.S. Role of apoptosis-inducing factor in myocardial cell death by ischemia-reperfusion. *Biochem. Biophys. Res. Commun.* 2003; **309**(3): 619–624.

204. Varbiro, G., Toth, A. Tapodi, A. *et al.* Protective effect of amiodarone but not N-desethylamiodarone on postischemic hearts through the inhibition of mitochondrial permeability transition. *J. Pharmacol. Exp. Ther.* 2003; **307**(2): 615–625.

205. Klein, J.A., Longo-Guess, C.M. Rossmann, M.P. *et al.* The harlequin mouse mutation downregulates apoptosis-inducing factor. *Nature* 2002; **419**(6905): 367–374.

206. Vahsen, N., Cande, C. Briere, J.J. *et al.* AIF deficiency compromises oxidative phosphorylation. *EMBO J.* 2004; **23**(23): 4679–4689.

207. Joza, N., Oudit, G.Y. Brown, D. *et al.* Muscle-specific loss of apoptosis-inducing factor leads to mitochondrial dysfunction, skeletal muscle atrophy, and dilated cardiomyopathy. *Mol. Cell. Biol.* 2005; **25**(23): 10261–10272.

208. van Empel, V.P., Bertrand, A.T. van der Nagel, R. *et al.* Downregulation of apoptosis-inducing factor in harlequin mutant mice sensitizes the myocardium to oxidative stress-related cell death and pressure overload-induced decompensation. *Circ Res.* 2005; **96**(12): e92–e101.

209. Adrie, C., Adib-Conquy, M. Laurent, I. *et al.* Successful cardiopulmonary resuscitation after cardiac arrest as a "sepsis-like" syndrome. *Circulation* 2002; **106**(5): 562–568.

210. Valen, G. Signal transduction through nuclear factor kappa B in ischemia-reperfusion and heart failure. *Basic Res. Cardiol.* 2004; **99**(1): 1–7.

211. Frantz, S., Bauersachs, J. & Kelly, R.A. Innate immunity and the heart. *Curr. Pharm. Des.* 2005; **11**(10): 1279–1290.

212. Taqueti, V.R., Mitchell, R.N. & Lichtman, A.H. Protecting the Pump: Controlling Myocardial Inflammatory Responses. *Annu. Rev. Physiol.* 2005; **175**(6): 3463–3468.

213. Jones, S.A. Directing transition from innate to acquired immunity: defining a role for IL-6. *J. Immunol.* 2005; **175**(6): 3463–3468.

214. Haslett, C. Granulocyte apoptosis and inflammatory disease. *Br. Med. Bull.* 1997; **53**(3): 669–683.

215. Serhan, C.N. & Savill, J. Resolution of inflammation: the beginning programs the end. *Nat. Immunol.* 2005; **6**(12): 1191–1197.

216. Teague, T.K., Marrack, P. Kappler, J.W., & Vella, A.T. IL-6 rescues resting mouse T cells from apoptosis. *J. Immunol.* 1997; **158**(12): 5791–5796.

217. Narimatsu, M., Maeda, H. Itoh, S. *et al.* Tissue-specific autoregulation of the stat3 gene and its role in interleukin-6-induced survival signals in T cells. *Mol. Cell. Biol.* 2001; **21**(19): 6615–6625.

218. McLoughlin, R.M., Witowski, J. Robson, R.L. *et al.* Interplay between IFN-gamma and IL-6 signaling governs neutrophil trafficking and apoptosis during acute inflammation. *J. Clin. Invest.* 2003; **112**(4): 598–607.

219. Adrie, C., Laurent, I. Monchi, M. Cariou, A. Dhainaou, J.F., & Spaulding, C. Postresuscitation disease after cardiac arrest: a sepsis-like syndrome? *Curr. Opin. Crit. Care* 2004; **10**(3): 208–212.

4

Genetics, genomics and proteomics in sudden cardiac death

Lesley A. Kane[1], Silvia G. Priori[2,3], Carlo Napolitano[2], Dan E. Arking[4], and Jennifer E. Van Eyk[1,5]

[1] Department of Biological Chemistry, Johns Hopkins University, Baltimore, USA,
[2] Molecular Cardiology, IRCCS Fondazione Salvatore Maugeri, Pavia, Italy and
[3] Department of Cardiology, University of Pavia, Pavia, Italy
[4] McKusick-Nathans Institute of Genetic Medicine, Johns Hopkins University School of Medicine, Baltimore, USA
[5] Department of Medicine and Department of Biomedical Engineering, Johns Hopkins Universtiy, Baltimore, USA

Introduction

Sudden cardiac death (SCD) is an enigma: despite an overall decrease in cardiac mortality, SCD rates appear to be rising along with the concomitant increase in prevalence of coronary disease and heart failure. Even with decades of research, the underlying cellular mechanisms and stimulus/triggers are not well understood. This chapter addresses the application of large scale "omic" strategies to this critical clinical problem. First, is a discussion of the steps currently underway using genetic strategies to characterize several inherited arrhythmogenic diseases. The final two sections focus on two newer strategies, the technologies of genomics and proteomics.

Genetics, genomics and proteomics are complementary technologies. Figure 4.1 shows the flow from genes to proteins and emphasizes the increasing complexity at each step. Genetics strategies concentrate on identifying and characterizing a small number of candidate genes, informed by our understanding of the relevant biology, and are largely focused on analyzing sequence variants. Genomics looks more globally, with new approaches using unbiased whole-genome scans to examine both sequence variants and other genomic alterations, such as copy number polymorphism. Analysis of expressed genes, mRNA, is performed using the technologies of transcriptomics. Finally, the expressed proteins are studied using proteomics. This includes potential mutations (seen as amino acid changes) as well as post-translational modification (such as glycosylation or phosphorylation). It is only through the combined application of these technologies that we will be able to elucidate the underlying mechanisms of SCD, with the ultimate goal of both predicting individual risk and improving therapeutic intervention.

Genetics of cardiac ion channel diseases causing sudden death

Introduction

The inherited diseases of the heart occurring in the absence of structural abnormalities are the so-called "primary electrical disorders" or "inherited arrhythmogenic diseases." They typically manifest with peculiar electrocardiographic features, syncope and sudden death in young, otherwise healthy, individuals. The common denominator of these disorders is the abnormality of proteins controlling the excitability of myocardial cells and their response, but the spectrum of genes and mechanisms underlying these disorders is remarkable and progressively expanding.

This section will summarize current understanding of the genetic determinants of cardiac instability and the abnormalities predisposing to sudden cardiac death in the absence of structural cardiac abnormalities. We will also briefly review the role of molecular genetics for management and risk stratification.

Strategies for genetic analysis

The common denominator of all Mendelian (monogenic) disorders associated with a risk of cardiac arrhythmia and sudden death is the remarkable genetic heterogeneity. With the exception of a few mutational hot spots

Cardiac Arrest: The Science and Practice of Resuscitation Medicine. 2nd edn., ed. Norman Paradis, Henry Halperin, Karl Kern, Volker Wenzel, Douglas Chamberlain. Published by Cambridge University Press. © Cambridge University Press, 2007.

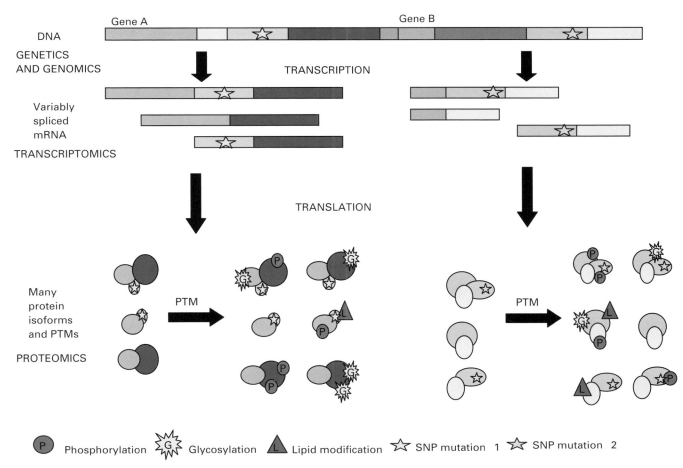

Fig. 4.1. Genetics, genomics, transcriptomics and proteomics. DNA can contain a variety of mutations and/or SNPs, that have the potential to be correlated to disease phenotypes. Such mutations may or may not be passed on to the mRNA during transcription; they can be left out either if they are not present in the transcribed region of the gene or by alternate splicing of the mRNA. The mRNA is then translated into proteins whose amino acid sequences could be affected by the original DNA mutation. Proteins often undergo post-translational modifications (PTMs), resulting in even greater complexity. Combining genetic, genomic and proteomic data allows for the examination of all the steps along the way to the final cellular makeup.

identified in long QT syndrome, the vast majority of probands carry a private (i.e., nonrecurrent) mutation. Obviously, this has profound impact on the choice of strategies for testing, because it implies that the screening for known mutations is not feasible. Systematic screening of the complete open reading frame (ORF) of known genes by denaturing high-performance liquid chromatography (DHPLC) (or similar techniques allowing detection of PCR fragment mobility anomalies) with subsequent DNA sequencing of the abnormal migration patterns, is the most widely used approach. Other laboratories perform direct ORF sequencing. At present there are no robust sensitivity analyses performed to suggest which approach is superior.

The success rate of genetic testing varies greatly according to the different diseases. Approximately 70% of clinically affected patients are successfully genotyped for long QT syndrome (five genes) and catecholaminergic polymorphic ventricular tachycardia (CPVT) (two genes), while this percentage drops to 20%–25% for Brugada syndrome patients. No data are available for other conditions such as Familial Atrial fibrillation, Progressive AV block and sick sinus syndrome since they have been only recently characterized.

LQT4 and LQT7 variants of LQTS (see below) are considered rare and present peculiar phenotypes. Therefore, systematic analysis in all patients of this gene is not indicated. Finally LQT8 usually arises *de novo* and all the reported

Table 4.1. Genetic loci and genes causing Long QT syndrome

Locus name	Chromosomal locus	Inheritance	Gene symbol	Protein	Phenotype[a]	OMIM ID
LQT1	11p15.5	AD	KCNQ1	I_{Ks} potassium channel alpha subunit (KvLQT1)	Long QT	192500
LQT2	7q35–q36	AD	KCNH2	I_{Kr} potassium channel alpha subunit (HERG)	Long QT	152427
LQT3	3p21	AD	SCN5A	Cardiac sodium channel alpha subunit (Nav 1.5)	Long QT	603830
LQT4	4q25–q27	AD	ANK2	Ankyrin B, anchoring protein	Long QT, atrial fibrillation	600919
LQT5	21q22.1–q22.2	AD	KCNE1	I_{Ks} potassium channel beta subunit (MinK)	Long QT	176261
LQT6	21q22.1–q22.2	AD	KCNE2	I_K potassium channel beta subunit (MiRP)	Long QT	603796
AND/LQT7	17q23.1–q24.2	AD	KCNJ2	I_{K1} potassium channel (Kir2.1)	Long QT, potassium-sensitive periodic paralysis, dysmorphic features	170390
LQT8/TS	12p13.3	AD[b]	CACNA1c	Voltage-gated calcium channel, CaV1.2	Long QT, syndactyly, septal defect, patent foramen ovale, mental retardation	601005
JLNS1	11p15.5	AR	KCNQ1	I_{Ks} potassium channel alpha subunit (KvLQT1)	Long QT, deafness	220400
JLNS2	21q22.1–q22.2	AR	KCNE1	I_{Ks} potassium channel beta subunit (MinK)	Long QT, deafness	176261

AD = autosomal dominant; AR = autosomal recessive; RBBB = right bundle branch block; LQT1 to LQT6 also defined as Romano-Ward; JLNS = Jervell and Lange–Nielsen syndrome; TS = Timothy syndrome; [a] syncope and sudden death are additional manifestations possibly occurring in all variants; [b] parental mosaicism was demonstrated.

patients in whom genetic analysis was performed have the same *CACNA1c* gene mutation (see below).

Long QT syndrome

Clinical presentation

The Long QT syndrome (LQTS) is an inherited arrhythmogenic disease in the structurally normal heart characterized by abnormally prolonged QT interval with peculiar mor-

phological abnormalities of the T wave. LQTS manifests with syncope and/or cardiac arrest with a mean age of onset of symptoms (syncope or sudden death) of 12 years. Two major phenotypic variants have been described in the early 1960s: one autosomal dominant (Romano–Ward syndrome)[1] and one rare autosomal recessive (Jervell and Lange–Nielsen syndrome) also presenting with sensorineural deafness[2] (Table 4.1). Another rare LQTS variant presenting with syndactyly and congenital heart defects has been recently linked to a specific cardiac calcium channel mutation (see below).

Genetic bases and pathophysiology

Seven LQTS genes have been identified as of March 2005 (Table 4.1). Isolated QT interval prolongation with or without syncope/cardiac arrest (Romano–Ward syndrome) may be due to mutations in five different genes while two variants display QT interval prolongation in the context of a multiorgan disease (Andersen syndrome, Timothy syndrome). All but one (LQT4) LQTS genetic subtypes are caused by cardiac ion channels encoding genes.

These share the typical features of the different genetic variants of LQTS by grouping them according to their common pathophysiological substrate.

Defective I_{Ks} (LQT1, LQT5, JLN1 and JLN2)

KCNQ1 (causing LQT1 and JLN1) and KCNE1 (causing LQT5 and JLN2) encode respectively for the alpha (KvLQT1) and the beta (MinK) subunit of the potassium channel conducting the I_{Ks} current, the slow component of the delayed rectifier current (I_K), the major repolarizing current during phase 3 of the cardiac action potential. In order to form a functional channel, KvLQT1 proteins form homotetramers and co-assemble with (probably two) Mink subunits.

LQT1 is the most prevalent genetic form of LQTS, accounting for approximately 50% of genotyped patients. Hundreds of different mutations have been reported and in vitro expression of mutated proteins suggested multiple biophysical consequences but all of them ultimately causing a loss of function through haploinsufficiency or dominant negative effect.[3] Homozygous or compound heterozygous mutations of KCNQ1 also cause the Jervell and Lange-Nielsen form of LQTS (JLN1).

KCNE1 (LQT5) mutations are rather infrequent accounting approximately for 2%–3% of genotyped LQTS patients and they may cause both Romano–Ward (LQT5) and, if homozygous, Jervell and Lange-Nielsen (JLN2).[4]

Defective I_{Kr} (LQT2 and LQT6)

KCNH2 (LQT2) and KCNE2 (LQT6) genes encode for the alpha (HERG) and the beta (MiRP) subunit of the potassium channel conducting the I_{Kr} current, the rapid component of the cardiac delayed rectifier. The KCNH2-encoded protein, HERG, is a six transmembrane-segment protein that forms homotetramers in the plasmalemma in order to make up functional channels. The physiological role of MiRP protein to recapitulate fully the current has been postulated,[5] although co-assembly of MiRP with other voltage-gated potassium channels such as KvLQT1 has

been also reported.[6] LQT2 is the second most common variant of LQTS, accounting for 35%–40% of mutations. Functional expression studies have demonstrated that KCNH2 mutations cause a reduction of I_{Kr} current, but, similar to LQT1 mutations, this effect may arise from different biophysical mechanisms.[7] LQT2 is characterized by higher penetrance and severity than LQT1.[8] Mutations in the KCNE2 gene[9] cause the LQT6 variant of LQTS, which has a very low relative prevalence (<1%) and the associated phenotypes are characterized by incomplete penetrance and very mild manifestations.

Defective I_{Na} (LQT3)

SCN5A encodes for cardiac sodium channel conducting the sodium inward current (I_{Na}). At variance with KvLQT1 and HERG protein mutations, a single SCN5A transcript forms a fully functional channel protein (Nav1.5). Several allelic variants have been reported and functional expression studies showed that, at variance with LQT1 and LQT2-associated mutations, LQT3 defects cause a gain of function with an increased I_{Na} (7). This final effect may originate from altered current kinetic (delayed inactivation) or single channel properties abnormalities (disperse reopenings, bursting). The prevalence of LQT3 among LQTS patient is estimated to be 10%–15%.

Defective Ankyrin B (LQT4)

The phenotype of the LQT4 patients differs from the typical LQTS:[10] QT interval is only mildly prolonged, but they also present with sinus bradycardia, paroxysmal atrial fibrillation (detected in >50% of the patients), and with polyphasic T waves. Recently, a missense mutation in the ANK2 gene was identified in one family.[11] ANK2 encodes for an intracellular protein (Ankyrin B) that regulates the proper intracellular localization of plasmalemmal ion channels (calcium channel, sodium channel, sodium/calcium exchanger) and sarcoplasmic reticulum channels (ryanodine receptor, inositol triphosphate receptor). The paucity of LQT4 patients genotyped so far prevents gathering further insights on the phenotypic features of this variant of LQTS.

Defective I_{Ca} (LQT8 – Timothy syndrome)

LQT8, also called Timothy syndrome, is a rare and severe disorder in which severe QT interval prolongation is invariably associated with cutaneous syndactyly (hands and feet) and a plethora of additional phenotypes (some still poorly defined) occurring with variable incidence among the affected subjects. The markedly prolonged and abnormal ventricular repolarization (QT interval duration often exceeds 600 ms) frequently causes the appearance of a 2:1

functional atrioventricular block and macroscopic T wave electrical alternans.

A high proportion of LQT8 patients have congenital heart defects, mental retardation and autism. Furthermore, severe hypoglycemia and immunologic (recurrent infections) disturbances are present in approximately 40% of cases.

The therapeutic approach to LQT8 is unavoidably empiric because of the limited clinical experience. The effectiveness of beta-blockers or other drugs is unknown and primary prevention with ICD may be considered. It appears also important to monitor closely glucose metabolism (intractable fatal hypoglycemia has been reported), and to consider seriously any hyperpyrexia event.

The gene for Timothy syndrome has been recently identified as *CACNA1c* encoding for the cardiac voltage-gated calcium channel (CaV1.2) (Table 4.1).[12] Interestingly, the same mutation G408R was found in all the 13 probands in whom the analysis was performed. In vitro functional characterization showed a net increase of calcium inward current and prolonged duration of action potential duration.[12]

Genotype–phenotype correlation

In the last few years several studies have outlined the distinguishing features of the three most common genetic variants of LQTS (LQT1, LQT2, LQT3), which account for approximately 97% of all genotyped patients.

Locus-specific repolarization morphology and locus-specific triggers for cardiac events have been described.[13] LQT1 patients usually develop symptoms during physical activity; conversely, LQT3 have events at rest. Auditory stimuli and arousal are relatively specific triggers for LQT2 patients while swimming is a predisposing setting for cardiac events in LQT1 patients.[13]

Locus-specific differences of the natural history of LQTS have also been demonstrated and, combined with the QT interval duration, allow genotype-based risk stratification:[8] a QTc >500 ms, and a LQT2 or LQT3 genotype are the strongest predictors of outcome. Gender further modulates the outcome according to the underlying genetic defect: the LQT3 males and LQT2 females are the highest risk subgroups. Preliminary evidence in small patients populations suggests that risk stratification be further refined when the position of a mutation on the predicted protein topology is taken into consideration: LQT2 patients with mutation in the pore-region are at greater risk of cardiac events.[14,15]

Finally, a recent study by Priori *et al.* has demonstrated that the response to beta-blocker therapy is also modulated by the underlying genotype with a satisfactory response among LQT1 but only partial protection afforded by this therapy for LQT2 and LQT3 patients.[16]

Brugada syndrome

Clinical presentation

Brugada syndrome (BrS) is characterized by ST segment elevation in the right precordial leads (V1 to V3), right bundle branch block, and susceptibility to ventricular tachyarrhythmia. The typical age of onset of clinical manifestations (syncope or cardiac arrest) is the third to fourth decade of life, even though malignant forms with earlier onset and even with neonatal manifestations have been reported.[17] Cardiac events typically occur during sleep or at rest.[18] The disease is inherited as an autosomal dominant trait, but there is a striking unbalanced male to female ratio of 8:1 for clinical manifestations. The lack of effective pharmacological treatments makes the risk stratification a primary issue in BrS. Available evidence attributes the highest risk for events to patients with a spontaneously abnormal ECG and a history of syncope. More debated is the usefulness of programmed electrical stimulation (PES).[19]

Genetic basis and pathophysiology

The initial report of *SCN5A* mutations in BrS was published in 1998[20] and, as of today, tens of different mutations have been reported. Unfortunately, *SCN5A* accounts for no more than 20% of clinical cases.[21] Therefore, genetic testing is not conclusive in 80% of BrS patients. Another BrS locus was mapped in a 5 cM region on chromosome 3p22-25 but the corresponding gene has not been identified yet (Table 4.2). Genetic testing, when successful, allows confirmation of the diagnosis in borderline cases, identification of silent carriers, and assessment of reproductive risk. Several electrophysiological abnormalities have been identified all leading to a loss of sodium current:[7] reduced current density, slower recovery of inactivation, shift of voltage dependence of inactivation, enhancement in the intermediate inactivation, altered interaction with the sodium channel β-subunit, and altered trafficking due to loss of ankyrin G binding.[22]

Progressive cardiac conduction defect

Clinical presentation

Progressive cardiac conduction defect (PCCD) is a common disorder in the elderly population. It is characterized by progressive slowing of cardiac conduction through the His-Purkinje system with right or left bundle branch block and widening of QRS complexes. In the majority of cases, it develops as a sporadic trait and is

Table 4.2. Genetic loci and genes involved in Brugada syndrome, Short QT syndrome, atrial fibrillation, conduction block, and sinus node disease

Locus name	Chromosomal locus	Inheritance	Gene symbol	Protein	Phenotype[a]	OMIM ID
BrS1	3p21	AD	SCN5A	Cardiac sodium channel alpha subunit (Nav 1.5)	ST segment elevation, RBBB	601144
BrS2	3p22–25	AD	unknown	unknown	ST segment elevation, RBBB	–
PFHB1	19q13.2–q13.3, 3p21	AD	unknown	unknown	Progressive cardiac conduction defect (PCCD)	113900
PFHB2	3p21	AD	SCN5A	Cardiac sodium channel alpha subunit (Nav 1.5)	Conduction defect, long QT (in some cases)	113900
SSS1	3p21	AD	SCN5A	Cardiac sodium channel alpha subunit (Nav 1.5)	Sinus bradycardia, sinus arrest, and/or sinoatrial block, atrial tachycardias	608567
SQTS1	7q3p2135–q36	AD	KCNH2	I_{Kr} potassium channel alpha subunit (HERG)	Short QT interval	–
SQTS2	11p15.5	AD	KCNQ1	I_{Ks} potassium channel alpha subunit (KvLQT1)	Short QT interval	–
SQTS3	17q23.1–q24.2	AD	KCNJ2	I_{K1} potassium channel (Kir2.1)	Short QT interval	–
ATFB1	11p15.5	AD	KCNQ1	I_{Ks} potassium channel alpha subunit (KvLQT1)	Atrial fibrillation	607554
ATFB2	10q22–q24	AD	unknown	unknown	Atrial fibrillation chronic or paroxysmal	608583
ATFB3	21q22.1–q22.2	AD	KCNE2	I_K potassium channel beta subunit (MiRP)	Atrial fibrillation	–

AD = autosomal dominant; AR = autosomal recessive; [a] syncope and sudden death are additional manifestations possibly occurring in all variants.

considered degenerative of aging. Familial cases have been reported in some instances, thus suggesting a genetic predisposition.

Genetic defects and pathophysiology
The first identified PCCD locus (also defined as progressive familial heart block, PFHB) locus maps to 19q13.3 with an autosomal dominant inheritance (Table 4.2). The linkage with this region was subsequently confirmed by other authors, but the corresponding gene is yet to be identified. Conversely, by candidate gene screening, after the exclusion of the 19q locus, Schott et al.[23] described two families with a SCN5A co-segregating with conduction defects (Table 4.2). Few other mutations have been reported thereafter and in vitro assays suggest a loss of function effect.[7]

Given the low number of reported mutations/patients, at present it is not possible to estimate the prevalence of SCN5A-PCCD, nor the success rate of genotyping.

Sick sinus syndrome

Clinical presentation
Sick sinus syndrome (SSS) manifests with bradycardia, syncope, dizziness, and fatigue. In some cases, sinus node dysfunction and cardiac conduction defect may co-exist. As for PCCD, the majority of SSS cases occur among elderly subjects and are thought to represent a manifestation of aging. Familial recurrence of SSS has been anecdotally reported, although this is considered an "exceptional finding."

Genetic defects and pathophysiology

In 2003, Benson et al.[24] described five affected children from 3 kindreds with congenital SSS, and identified compound heterozygosity (two different mutations, one from paternal and one from maternal origin) for six distinct mutations in the SCN5A gene (Table 4.2). Two of these mutations had previously been associated with Brugada syndrome. Heterozygous carriers were asymptomatic, but showed subclinical cardiac conduction disease, particularly first-degree heart block, suggesting a close relationship between PCCD and SSS. As for PCCD and BrS, in vitro expression of the SSS mutation is consistent with a loss of function.

Familial atrial fibrillation

Clinical presentation

Atrial fibrillation is the most common sustained arrhythmia encountered in clinical practice. It is not life-threatening *per se*, but it is the most frequent cause of embolic stroke. In 3% to 31% of cases no underlying cardiovascular disease can be detected and in some of them a familial inheritance is evident.[25]

Genetic bases and pathophysiology

Brugada et al.[26] mapped the first familial atrial fibrillation (FAF) locus to the long arm of chromosome 10 (10q22–q24) in three families (Table 4.2). The gene located in this region has not been discovered yet. Chen et al.[27] mapped a large family on the short arm of chromosome 11 (11p15.5), however, and identified a missense mutation of KCNQ1, causing a gain-of-function effect on the KvLQT1/MinK channel (see LQT1). The authors speculated that the KCNQ1-FAF mutation is likely to initiate and maintain the arrhythmia by reducing duration of the action potential and the effective refractory period in atrial myocytes.

Very recently, another FAF mutation has been reported in the KCNE2 gene causing an arginine-to-cysteine mutation at position 27 (R27C).[6] This mutation was found in 2/28 probands of families with FAF in whom a systematic screening of cardiac ion channel encoding genes was carried out. Functional study revealed that the mutation had a gain-of-function effect on the KCNQ1-KCNE2 channel; unlike long QT syndrome-associated KCNE2 mutations, it did not alter KCNH2-KCNE2 current.

Unfortunately, despite these anecdotal reports, the genetic determinants of FAF remain poorly characterized. Therefore, at the present time the clinical applicability of genetic testing for FAF is limited to research.

Short QT syndrome

Clinical presentation

The first report of a clinical condition characterized by abnormally short repolarization was from Gussak et al. in 2000.[28] They described two siblings and their mother all of whom displayed persistently short QT interval (260–275 ms). Thereafter few additional unrelated cases have been reported. SQTS is also characterized by the absence of structural heart disease, a quite remarkable familial history of sudden cardiac death and a typical, hyperkalemic-like T wave pattern at the resting ECG. No effective treatment for this disease has been identified so far.

Genetic bases and pathophysiology

One KCNH2 missense mutation was initially identified in two SQTS families.[29] By means of in vitro expression the authors observed a complete loss of the I_{Kr} rectification, resulting in a large increase of current and a gain of function that may explain the abbreviated action potential and therefore the QT interval.

Bellocq et al.[30] reported another gain of function mutation that affected the KCNQ1 gene in a 70-year-old male presenting with idiopathic ventricular fibrillation and short QT intervals (Table 4.2). This mutation causes an increase in transmembrane current and a faster current kinetic, resulting in a reduction of action potential duration.

The third SQTS gene has been recently identified by Priori et al.[31] who reported a gain of function mutation in the KCNJ2 gene, the same as that causing LQT7 (Andersen syndrome) when loss of function is present.

The recent findings on the genetic defects underlying the SQTS phenotype together with the data on LQT3, BrS and FAF, demonstrate that at least five genes encoding cardiac ion channels and involved in the inherited arrhythmogenic diseases (KCNQ1, KCNH2, SCN5A, KCNE2, KCNJ2) may carry both gain and loss of function mutations. According to their primary biophysical consequence they originate different, and sometimes opposite, phenotypes. Whereas the electrocardiographic manifestations diverge, the common denominator of these different clinical entities is the electrically unstable substrate that leads to cardiac arrhythmias and sudden death.

Catecholaminergic polymorphic ventricular tachycardia

Clinical presentation

Catecholaminergic polymorphic ventricular tachycardia (CPVT)[32] is characterized by exercise- or acute emotion-induced polymorphic ventricular arrhythmias, often

Table 4.3. Genetic loci and genes causing catecholaminergic polymorphic ventricular tachycardia

Locus name	Chromosomal locus	Inheritance	Gene symbol	Protein	Phenotype	OMIM ID
CPVT1	1q42.1–q43	AD	*RyR2*	Cardiac Ryanondine receptor	Exercise-induced arrhythmias, normal resting ECG, bradycardia, sudden death	604772
CPVT2	1p13.3–p11	AR	*CASQ 2*	Cardiac Calsequestrin	Exercise-induced arrhythmias, normal resting ECG, bradycardia, sudden death	114251

causing syncope, a normal resting electrocardiogram, and the absence of structural cardiac abnormalities. Symptoms usually develop during childhood or adolescence, although anecdotal reports of first symptoms during adulthood have been reported. In approximately 13%, cardiac arrest is the first manifestation of the disease and familial history of sudden deaths is present in 30% of cases.[33] The resting electrocardiogram is unremarkable[33] and the diagnosis relies upon the reproducible pattern of arrhythmias during graded exercise, in which a ventricular tachycardia with an alternating 180° QRS axis on a beat-to-beat basis (the so-called bidirectional VT) is observed. In some patients irregular polymorphic VT is observed but the correlation with exercise remains striking.[33]

Genetic bases and pathophysiology

CPVT1: autosomal dominant

The first locus was identified by Swan *et al.* who mapped the disease to chromosome 1q42–43.[34] In late 2000, Priori *et al.* identified mutations in four families and demonstrated that the CPVT gene on chromosome 1 is the cardiac Ryanodine receptor (*RyR2*).[35] Additional mutations have been reported thereafter (Table 4.3).[36,37]

The Ryanodine receptor is a large protein that tetramerizes across the membrane of sarcoplasmic reticulum (SR) and is a major player in the regulation of the intracellular calcium fluxes and the excitation-contraction coupling. The identification of *RyR2* mutations in CPVT points to the pivotal role of intracellular Ca^{2+} handling in arrhythmogenesis. RyR2 mutant proteins have been expressed in different in vitro models (lipid bilayer, HEK293 cells, HL1-cardiomyocytes) and the results consistently showed that *RYR2* defects cause a Ca^{2+} "leakage" from the SR in conditions of sympathetic (catecholamines) activation,[38,39] while the basal channel activity appears normal.

CPVT2: Autosomal recessive

Lahat *et al.*[40] in 2001 mapped the autosomal recessive variant of CPVT on chromosome 1p23–21 (Table 4.3). Subsequently, the same group identified *CASQ2* as the gene for this locus (Table 4.3).[41] *CASQ2* encodes the cardiac calsequestrin, the Ca^{2+}-binding/buffering protein localized in the terminal cisternae of the SR. Calsequestrin is bound physically and functionally to the Ryanodine receptor and cooperates with control of the excitation contraction coupling.

One experimental study[42] has investigated (in rat myocytes) the *CASQ2* mutation previously identified by Lahat *et al.* This study showed that *CASQ2*-D307H mutation impairs the SR Ca^{2+} storing and release functions, and destabilizes the Ca^{2+}-induced Ca^{2+} release mechanism via reduced Ca^{2+} buffering inside the SR and/or altered responsiveness of the Ca^{2+} release channel complex to luminal Ca^{2+}.

Taken together, the experimental data demonstrated that both genes involved in CPVT pathogenesis affect the amount of Ca^{2+} released from the SR during adrenergic stimulation. Such an effect may create an electrically unstable substrate, probably through triggered activity-mediated arrhythmogenesis.

Conclusions

Many ion channels highly expressed in the heart and controlling the depolarization-repolarization process have been implicated in cardiac arrhythmias and sudden death. Molecular genetics has revealed such a high level of genetic and functional heterogeneity that the classification of diseases based on their clinical phenotype is compellingly challenged. The same protein, resulting from an altered genetic program, may outcrop a variety of apparently unrelated (sometimes opposite) clinical phenotypes, depending

on the specific functional consequences of the single mutations. Despite this apparently impenetrable complexity,
thanks to these studies, our understanding of cardiac physiology and pathophysiology has improved substantially.
Translation into clinical benefits is a laborious and complex
process that is only recently achieving partial success, with
progressively more informative management algorithms
derived from genotype-phenotype correlations. In the
years to come this process will eventually lead to the development of individualized approaches for prevention and
therapy of cardiac arrhythmias and sudden death.

Genomics and sudden cardiac death

Introduction

While a great deal of progress has been made identifying
the genetic variants underlying monogenic long and short
QT syndromes, little to no progress had been made with
respect to the common forms of SCD. Indeed, the only reliable association reported for a relatively common variant
is with a single nucleotide sequence variant in the SCN5A
Na⁺ channel gene, found only in African-Americans,
which has a small enhancement of arrhythmia risk.[43] With
one-third of SCD events occurring as a first clinical event,
and fully two-thirds of SCD events occurring in individuals
in clinical circumstances that do not provide sufficiently
accurate prediction to warrant preventive intervention,[44]
the ability to identify genetic susceptibility markers for
SCD is critical.

The limitation of linkage studies

Traditional genomic approaches to identifying genetic susceptibility loci have relied upon family-based studies and
linkage analyses. These techniques have proven particularly well-suited to monogenic diseases, which are generally due to rare variants in which carriers are likely to have
disease (high penetrance). In a complex phenotype like
SCD, multiple genes are likely to be involved and the susceptibility variants are likely to be common ("common
disease, common variant" hypothesis),[45,46] and thus the
penetrance for any individual susceptibility variant is likely
to be low. In addition, the ability to collect DNA from families with SCD is extremely limited, as SCD occurs at later
ages, in which collecting DNA from parents is difficult.
Similarly, collecting samples for alternate family-based
strategies, such as affected sibpair analyses, are difficult,
DNA would need to be collected from a huge number of
individuals in the hope of identifying families that will have

a second SCD event. Given these limitations, researchers
have begun to focus on population-based case-control
association studies, in which unrelated affected individuals are compared to appropriate unaffected populations.

Association studies

Association studies: in theory

The association between a specific sequence variant and a
phenotype can arise in two ways. The mutation can occur
multiple times during the course of human history, as in
achondroplasia,[47] each time occurring on a different
genetic background, or haplotype (i.e., it will have different
neighboring polymorphisms each time it occurs). Under
this scenario, whereas the mutation itself will be associated
with disease, neighboring markers will not. More commonly, a mutation may occur once or a few times during
evolution, such as with the ΔF508 mutation in cystic fibrosis,[48] therefore arising on a distinct haplotype. If this
second model holds true for SCD, we can use a property
known as linkage disequilibrium (LD) to identify a region
harboring the underlying functional variant associated
with the phenotype, even in the absence of knowing the
functional variant itself. LD describes the non-random
association of neighboring polymorphisms with each
other. When a mutation occurs on a specific haplotype, it
will be transmitted to offspring along with its neighboring
polymorphisms, which can then serve as surrogates for
the mutation itself. Nevertheless, meiotic recombination
events occurring between a neighboring polymorphism
and the mutation will decrease the association, or LD,
between that marker and the mutation, and thus markers
closer to the mutation will have stronger associations with
the phenotype.

Association studies: past and present

The model for conducting association studies has been the
"candidate gene" approach, in which a list of genes based
on our current understanding of the biology are mined for
single nucleotide polymorphisms (SNPs) that may be associated with SCD. A summary of the studies published to
date is given in Table 4.4. Notably, none of the positive
findings have been replicated in a second study, the gold
standard for validation. In addition, these studies have not
really screened the gene, *per se*, for association with SCD,
but only a specific variant in the gene. There could be additional variants that influence the risk for SCD, but that are
not in LD with the screened SNPs, and thus are missed by
this approach. The revolution in genotyping technologies,
both reducing cost and increasing throughput, has largely
eliminated the single gene/single SNP approach. Indeed,

Table 4.4. Summary of SCD association studies

Gene	Variant	Cases/controls	Association	Reference
Platelet glycoprotein	P1$^{A1/A2}$	98/249	yes	Mikkelsson *et al.* (2000)
α2B-adenoreceptor	in/del	288/412	yes	Snapir *et al.* (2003)
PAI-1	4G/5G	97/113	yes	Anvari *et al.* (2001)
Factor V	Leiden	145/592	no	Reiner *et al.* (2002)
Prothrombin	G20210A	145/592	no	Reiner *et al.*(2002)

there are numerous platforms in which tens of SNPs in hundreds of genes can be screened in a single assay. We can thus start to think about comprehensively screening a gene, using multiple SNPs distributed across the gene. By measuring the LD between our marker SNPs, we can get some measure of our power to identify an unscreened functional variant anywhere in the gene. Although this approach is markedly superior to the single gene/single SNP strategy, and indeed allows for the exploration of genetic pathways (i.e., a series of genes that influence a common outcome), it is still limited by our current understanding of both the biology underlying SCD and of the genome itself.

Association studies: extending the search

Despite the remarkable progress we have made in understanding the human genome, we know the function of fewer than half the identified genes, and have recently discovered non-genic regulatory elements, such as miRNAs. In addition, regulatory elements that are distant from the known structural gene have been identified.[49] Thus, any candidate gene approach has an *a priori* exclusion of more than half of the relevant genome. The remarkable scale-up of genotyping technologies has now reached the point where, with current platforms, we can conduct unbiased whole-genome association studies, screening >500 000 SNPs per sample.[50,51] Thus we can use a high-resolution map of SNPs distributed throughout the genome to identify regions associated with SCD (see Fig. 4.2). Indeed, Ozaki *et al.*[52] have successfully used this approach to identify the lymphotoxin-α gene as a susceptibility locus for myocardial infarction. They screened 92 788 SNPs in 1133 cases and 1006 controls, and identified a functional variant contributing to the observed association.

Assessment of genomic structure

The search for genetic susceptibility loci for complex disease has been limited to looking for a sequence alteration at a particular site. The existence of common copy number polymorphisms, however, in which individuals have heritable amplifications or deletions of specific genomic regions, have now been reported.[53–55] The role of somatic copy number variation in cancer has long been established, but has not been explored with regards to complex disease. These copy number polymorphisms make intriguing candidates for a complex phenotype like SCD, as they may affect multiple genes and be dosage-dependent across individuals. Until recently, detection of changes has been limited to >1 Mb; however, recent advances have allowed for detection of much smaller changes (> 10 kb), including "genome tiling" BAC arrays, digital karyotyping, optical mapping, and oligonucleotide-arrays.[56–59]

Conclusions

The rapid advancement in genomic technologies has opened new avenues of research for identifying susceptibility loci for SCD. Not only can we perform whole-genome scans for sequence variants, eliminating the bias due to our incomplete knowledge of both the genome and biology underlying SCD, but we can also scan for the role of a new class of variants, copy number polymorphisms. The real limitation now is the availability of well-phenotyped samples and appropriate controls. In recognition of this, several projects are currently underway to generate large cohorts for future study,[60,61] giving significant hope that we will be able to identify genetic risk factors for SCD in the near future.

Proteomics and sudden cardiac death

Overview of proteomics strategies

Genetic and genomic strategies as described in this chapter are exceptionally useful for understanding the genotype of diseased individuals. However, although they are powerful, they do not tell the whole story. To understand fully the cellular disease phenotype, it is important to examine not only the genes and mRNA, but also the end

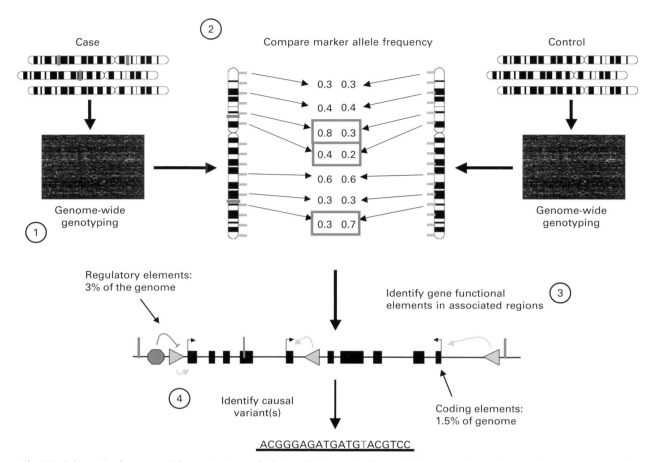

Fig. 4.2. Schematic of genome-wide association study design. (1) Appropriately matched cases and controls are subject to genome-wide SNP genotyping (shown here using Affymetrix chips); (2) SNP allele frequencies are compared to identify regions associated with disease; (3) disease-associated regions are scanned for known functional elements, and cross-species comparisons can be used to identify unknown regulatory elements; (4) direct sequencing of functional elements to identify causal variants.

products – the proteins. Proteomics is the scientific discipline that examines global protein expression (the proteome) in cells. The proteome is dynamic and flexible; proteins are constantly being produced, degraded and modified. Therefore, proteomics strives to quantify proteins as well as to determine the specific isoforms, SNPs and post-translational modifications (PTMs) (eg., phosphorylation, glycosylation, and acetylation) that comprise the proteome. As such, information obtained from proteomic studies is complementary to that obtained from genetics and genomics.

Tissue or serum samples are highly complex mixtures of proteins, and this complexity must be reduced before further analysis. Complexity reduction can be accomplished by attempting to separate all the proteins in the original sample, or by first subfractionating the sample into several less complex mixtures. Often samples are divided based on subcellular organelles, for instance the mitochondria or myofibrils from cardiac myocardium or extracted on the basis of a shared chemical characteristic, such as hydrophobicity, which can be exploited with various detergents. Once appropriately prepared, the sample can be analyzed by a variety of separation technologies (outlined in Table 4.5). Protein separation is based on using one or more of the intrinsic properties of proteins or peptides: pI (charge), mass (size) or hydrophobicity (water/oil solubility). A greater number of parameters/ dimensions used in the separation adds exponential improvements in resolution/separation. The protein separation technologies can be broken down into three main categories: gel electrophoresis; liquid chromatography; and mass spectrometry (MS). In most cases, a combination of these must be used for thorough coverage of the proteome or subproteome.

Table 4.5. Outline of popular proteomic techniques

Technology	Method	Application
Gel electrophoresis		
one-dimensional	– low-moderate separation based on molecular weight	– moderate separation – good for high molecular weight or very hydrophobic proteins
Two-dimensional	– high degree separation based on isoelectric point and molecular weight	– excellent separation and potential for PTM discovery – limited use for very large or very hydrophobic proteins
Two-dimensional-differential gel electrophoresis (DIGE)	– fluorescently tag proteins prior to IEF – tag separate samples with different fluorophores and combine for 2DE	– allows comparison of different samples in the same gel – decreases variability (from gel to gel variation)
Liquid chromatography		
One-dimensional	– affinity columns – based on affinity of proteins to antibodies or other binding ligands – RP-HPLC – based on hydrophobicity – size exclusion columns – based on protein molecular size and shape – ion exchange columns – based on protein charge	– allows moderate separation of proteins or peptides based on a wide variety of properties
Two-dimensional (2DLC)	– IEF-based column followed by RP-HPLC	– combination of two columns for high degree of separation
Mass spectrometry		
MALDI-TOF MS	– protein identification based on peptide mass fingerprint (PMF)	– capable of high through-put analysis of large scale samples – not effective if sample is a mixture of proteins
MS/MS	– protein identification based on peptide fragmentation and amino acid masses	– analysis of more complex mixtures of proteins is possible – requires higher skill level and more time than MALDI-TOF
Immobilized metal affinity column (IMAC)	– chromatographic enrichment for phosphopeptides followed by MS/MS analysis	– enrichment of phosphopeptides allows for greater analysis of this PTM in the MS
Isotope labeling	– Isotope-coded affinity tag (ICAT)-peptides are labeled with heavy and light isotope tags prior to MS stable isotope labeling with amino acids in cell culture (SILAC) – proteins are labeled in cell culture with amino acids containing either heavy or light N or O^{18} labeling – peptides are labeled with either heavy or light oxygen during enzymatic digestion	– all of these procedures allow for accurate relative quantification of peptides between samples – ICAT and O^{18} labeling are good for samples that cannot be obtained from cell culture – SILAC is excellent for quantification since whole protein can be labeled, not just peptides

First described in 1975,[62] two-dimensional gel electrophoresis (2DE) has become one of the most widespread techniques used in proteomics. 2DE separates proteins first by isoelectric point (pI) by a process known as isoelectric focusing (IEF), then in the second dimension by molecular weight. Currently, 2DE has the potential to resolve upwards of 5000 protein spots per gel.[63] Over time, there have been continued improvements in both the first[64,65] and second dimension.[66] With this depth of separation, a significant number of proteins can be analyzed concurrently for changes in both expression level and PTM. Liquid chromatography techniques are similar in that they are used to achieve separation of the proteome on the basis of one or more of the physical properties of proteins.[67,68] The most commonly used is single dimension chromatography, such as reversed phase chromatography. In particular, reversed phase chromatography is often found online with MS, not as a means not to separate proteins, but rather to spread out the resulting peptides to allow for more coverage by the MS, which is especially advantageous when separating peptides from a complex mixture. A movement towards separating proteins by using two- and three-dimensional chromatographic separations is occurring, and often entails combining isochromatographic focusing (pI), ion exchange (charge) or size exclusion (mass) columns with reversed phase HPLC (hydrophobicity).

Once the proteins have been separated into individual or small groups of proteins, MS, which measures extremely accurate masses of proteins (whole mass) or peptides, is used to identify them. MS identification from gels or liquid chromatography techniques involves enzymatic digestion of the protein with the profile of peptide masses compared to a theoretical profile from a known protein database (termed protein mass fingerprinting). A single peptide fragment can be selected in the mass spectrometer and fragmented into its amino acid residues (tandem MS or MS/MS). From these mass spectra, again by homology, the amino acid sequence can be obtained, which allows for unambiguous protein identification. There are many different types of MS analysis each with unique advantages (some of these are listed in Table 4.5). An exhaustive explanation of these technologies is beyond the scope of this chapter, an in-depth review of this material can be found in refs. 69 and 70.

Searching for answers to sudden cardiac death using proteomics

Proteomic analysis of human diseases such as SCD can address a wide variety of biological questions. These technologies can be used to deduce mechanisms of disease through protein alterations or to search for predictive biomarkers of disease. For cardiac diseases there are typically two choices of samples to analyze: either direct analysis of heart tissue or indirect analysis through patient serum or plasma. The advantages and disadvantages as well as appropriate strategies for each are discussed below.

Heart tissue (Fig. 4.3)

The clinical goal of studies on heart tissue is to translate tissue-specific differences into tailored treatment strategies of arrhythmias that target the origin of the malfunction. It is a long process from proteomics and the identification of unique protein changes to identification of a therapeutic target or pathway. It starts with the direct analysis of the protein phenotype of the diseased heart through the analysis of cardiac tissue. This creates a problem when dealing with human heart diseases because of limited tissue availability, although with the appropriate study design it can be possible and compelling.[71] However, owing to tissue limitations, preliminary studies often start with an appropriate and translatable animal model system. Sudden cardiac death presents an even more unique problem since such animal systems are very difficult to develop. Nevertheless, there are fundamental questions about the heart proteome that once answered could lead the way to a greater understanding of cardiac mechanisms and thus SCD. For example, one fundamental question considers the global proteome differences between the conducting tissues of the heart. Although the functions of the ventricles, atria, SA node and AV node are well understood, there are gaps in our knowledge of the similarity or differences of these areas of the heart at the post-translational (protein) level. SCD has primarily been linked to arrhythmic events and as such many of the drugs associated with the prevention of SCD focus on controlling such events. This highlights the extraordinary importance of understanding the conducting regions in the heart. An additional limitation of this kind of study is the purity of the cell preparations. The SA node preparations must not be highly contaminated by the surrounding atrial tissue. Proteomic analysis of SA node as compared to the atrial tissue is underway in our laboratory (JVE) on a rabbit model (Fig. 4.3). It is hoped that this study will reveal differences in expression or PTMs of proteins in these essential tissues. A further advantage of proteomic analysis is the discovery of novel proteins, that were not previously known to be located in these tissues, to exist in mammals, or to exist at all (a hypothetical protein or homology). Often these proteins have no known function. Coupled with the discovery of novel PTMs of proteins, these data represent a wealth of

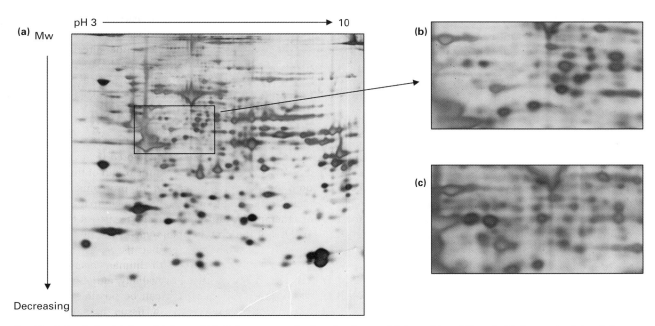

Fig. 4.3. 2-D gel of atrial tissue (a) from rabbit. Enlargements of gel section from atrial tissue (b) and SA node (c) show potential variation in protein content represented by the different spot patterns.

possibilities toward understanding the protein-based mechanisms of these important cell types.

In contractile tissues, membrane channels that conduct the currents and allow the heart to contract are of key significance, and proteomic technology gives a unique ability to look at the status of multiple channels in these special tissues, although very hydrophobic proteins are still somewhat problematic.[72–74] Development of new detergents (eg., ASB-14[75] and C8φ[76]) coupled with one-dimensional (1D) gel electrophoresis or gel-free separation methods that are amenable to detergents are leading the way in adapting traditional proteomic techniques to membrane proteins. Furthermore, initial enzymatic digestion of membrane-enriched subproteomes enables the analysis of "more soluble" peptides. While proteomics technology is developing quickly, there is not yet a "perfect" proteomic method for these troublesome, but important, proteins that provides all desired information.

After the completion of an in-depth proteomics study, candidate proteins that are associated with the treatment or disease remain. It is then imperative to continue the study with more traditional biochemical or molecular biological techniques to validate the proteomics findings and explain the function of the protein phenotype. Such techniques often include the use of transgenic animals, adenoviral gene transfer, or RNAi of isolated myocytes to overexpress or knockout the protein of interest. Candidate proteins can also be further investigated by

analyzing the cellular localization by microscopy techniques. Localization provides key information toward understanding how a protein change may cause or reflect disease phenotypes. Proteomics is very powerful for uncovering the proteins involved in disease processes, but it takes collaboration with other biochemical disciplines to understand fully how protein changes affect phenotype.

Serum

The goals of serum or plasma proteomic studies are most often the identification of biomarkers for a specific disease. Although preferred, these biomarkers do not have directly to be involved in the underlying mechanism of the disease but rather the biomarkers need only reflect or correlate with the disease process. Although analysis of human diseases through blood samples is much more convenient for sample collection, serum has the limitation of being indirect, studying the disease only through the release of proteins from the heart into the blood. Biomarkers of this nature can be used as a predictive index of disease or as a diagnostic marker of the specific disease type or disease progression. For SCD it is possible that heart damage before an event releases proteins or peptides into the blood, producing a predictive proteomic profile and this profile could be used to screen high risk patients for the likelihood of an imminent cardiac event.

Although serum has the advantage of being readily available, it has a major drawback when it comes to proteomic study. The dynamic range of proteins within serum is extremely high, with about 90% of the protein content resulting from only the 10 most abundant proteins.[77] Consequently, the low abundant proteins (often the proteins of interest) are present in such low amounts that it is very difficult to study them. This has led to the development of systems to reproducibly deplete serum of its most abundant proteins.[78,79] An example of this dynamic range problem and potential solution is shown in Fig. 4.4(a) where the same amount of protein is loaded on to a 1-D gel from normal serum (Lane 1) and from IgGs and albumin-depleted serum (Lane 2). Figure 4.4(b) shows a 2-D gel of the fully depleted serum. Clearly, the depleted serum allows visualization of many more low abundant proteins. This depletion technique can be applied to all types of proteomics analysis, in addition to gel-based systems. Figure 4.5 demonstrates the necessity of this depletion applied to 2DLC.

Once the problem of dynamic range has been resolved, the other main problem is developing an appropriate patient cohort for the analysis. One example of a current study (Reynolds Foundation, Johns Hopkins University) cohort is that of patients with implanted ICDs (Implantable Cardioverter Defibrillators). The study involves regularly collecting serum samples and monitoring the arrhythmic incidents recorded by the ICD. Thus, such events can be correlated to the time that serum was taken, and through characterization of the serum, patient's conditions can be correlated with the proteomic phenotype of the serum. A complicating factor is that the proteome is dynamic and there is large biological variation among even control individuals. This variation as well as other factors, such as time course of collection, clotting time, and sex differences must be taken into account in such studies. The overall goal of such large scale serum screens is to allow researchers to predict and potentially prevent SCD.

Findings of such proteomic studies must always be carefully validated against secondary and much larger cohorts. This requires the development of much higher throughput validation technologies that would allow faster validation of potential targets across very large cohorts. This is a quickly developing area of research that has mostly focused on the use of antibody arrays or protein chips. There are several technologies on the market that include A[2] (Beckman), Luminex (BioRad) and the S+S FastQuant (Millipore). Figure 4.6 illustrates how the A[2] array is assembled (Fig. 4.6(a)) and the assay methodology (Fig. 4.6(b)).

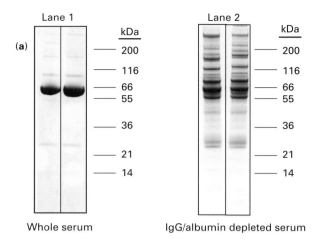

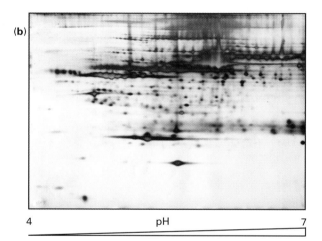

Fig. 4.4 Serum depletion. Depletion of highly abundant proteins is essential for analysis of serum. It is clear from (a) 1-DE of whole serum and IgG/albumin-depleted serum proteins that many more proteins are visible in the depleted sample (Lane 2) than are in the whole serum sample (Lane 1) when both lanes are loaded with the same overall amount of serum protein. (b) A representative 2-D gel of IgG and albumin-depleted serum proteins.

Future prospects

Proteomics is a rapidly evolving field. The technological leaps that have been made since the first two-dimensional gels were described in 1975 are astonishing. Researchers are now capable of separating, identifying, quantifying, and characterizing PTMs of proteins in a much shorter time scale. This ability has almost limitless potential not just for the understanding of disease mechanisms at the cellular level, but equally important, for the discovery of biomarkers to predict and prevent disease progression.

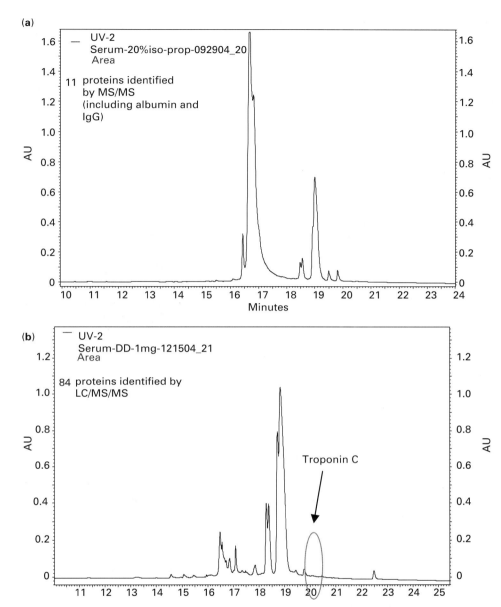

Fig. 4.5. Serum depletion for 2DLC. Depletion of highly abundant proteins from serum is also a requirement for proteomic technologies other than 2DE. Whole serum does not allow for as many proteins to be analyzed as, depleted serum does. (a) 2nd dimension RP-HPLC of whole serum fraction 20 (pH 5.4–5.69) from the 1st dimension (not shown) yields only 11 proteins that were identified by LC MS/MS. (b) 2nd dimension IgG and albumin-depleted serum illustrate that an equivalent 1st dimension fraction (21, pH 5.49–5.56) of depleted serum allows for almost eight times as many identifications (84) from the depleted serum by LC MS/MS.

Conclusions

Advances in our understanding of SCD through the study of inherited arrhythmogenic diseases have been significant. However, there is much left to learn before target therapeutic and diagnostic/prognostic markers are developed. The three scientific strategies discussed in this chapter can work in synchrony to uncover the mysteries behind SCD. Genetics and genomics will continue to provide vital evidence for mutations that predispose patients to arrhythmogenic

(**a**) Generating A² antibody array

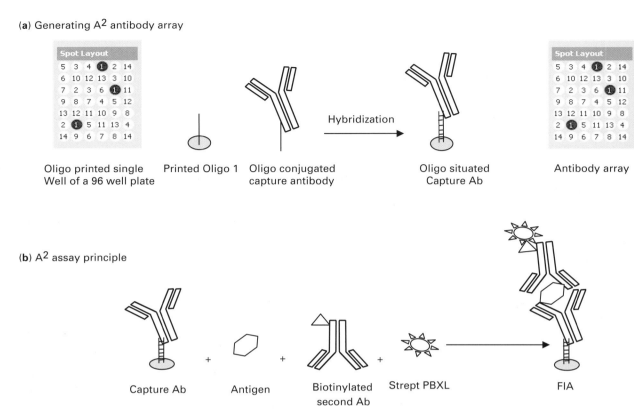

Fig. 4.6 The A² protein array. (a) the A² antibody array is assembled by first printing oligonucleotides on to a 96-well plate. Antibodies are conjugated with complementary oligonucleotides to the ones printed. The antibodies are then hybridized to the plate in a specific pattern corresponding to the oligonucleotides. (b) Antibody pairs are used for capture and detection of proteins to minimize non-specific binding. The binding is assessed by fluorescence of the secondary antibody.

events and proteomics will strive to provide better understanding of the proteins involved and how they are modified to produce a SCD-susceptible phenotype.

Acknowledgments

Genetics and SCD: This work was supported by the following grants: Telethon GGP04066, Ricerca Finalizzata 2003/180, Fondo per gli Investimenti della Ricerca di Base RBNE01XMP4_006, COFIN 2001067817_003.

Genomics and SCD: Dan E. Arking is supported by the Donald W. Reynolds Foundation Clinical Cardiovascular Research Center Grant to Johns Hopkins University.

Proteomics and SCD: The authors would like to thank Qin Fu, Simon Sheng and Steve Elliott for help with several figures as well as Brian Stanley for editing assistance. This work was supported by the Daniel P. Amos Family Foundation, the Donald W. Reynolds Foundation and the NHLBI proteomics grant (contract#HV-28180).

REFERENCES

Genetics

1. Romano, C., Gemme, G., & Pongiglione, R. Aritmie cardiache rare in eta' pediatrica. *Clin. Ped.* 1963; **45**: 656–657.
2. Jervell, A., & Lange-Nielsen, F. Congenital deaf mutism, functional heart disease with prolongation of the QT interval and sudden death. *Am. Heart J.* 1957; **54**: 59–61.
3. Keating, M.T., & Sanguinetti, M.C. Molecular and cellular mechanisms of cardiac arrhythmias. *Cell* 2001; **104**: 569–580.
4. Splawski, I., Tristani-Firouzi, M., Lehmann, M.H., Sanguinetti, M.C., & Keating, M.T. Mutations in the hminK gene cause long QT syndrome and suppress IKs function. *Nat. Genet.* 1997; **17**: 338–340.
5. Abbott, G.W., Sesti, F., Splawski, I. *et al.* MiRP1 forms IKr potassium channels with HERG and is associated with cardiac arrhythmia. *Cell* 1999; **97**: 175–187.
6. Yang, Y., Xia, M., Jin, Q. *et al.* Identification of a KCNE2 gain-of-function mutation in patients with familial atrial fibrillation. *Am. J. Hum. Genet.* 2004; **75**: 899–905.

7. Priori, S.G., Rivolta, I., & Napolitano, C. Genetic of Long QT. Brugada. and other channellopathies. In Zipes, D.P., & Jalife, J., eds. *Cardiac Electrophysiology From Cell to Bedside.* Philadelphia: Saunders, 2004: 462–470.

8. Priori, S.G., Schwartz, P.J., Napolitano, C., *et al.* Risk stratification in the long-QT syndrome. *N. Engl. J. Med.* 2003; **348**: 1866–1874.

9. Abbott, G.W., Sesti, F., Splawski, I. *et al.* MiRP1 forms IKr potassium channels with HERG and is associated with cardiac arrhythmia. *Cell* 1999; **97**: 175–187.

10. Schott, J.J., Charpentier, F., Peltier, S. *et al.* Mapping of a gene for long QT syndrome to chromosome 4q25–27. *Am. J. Hum.Genet.* 1995; **57**: 1114–1122.

11. Mohler, P.J., Schott, J.J., Gramolini, A.O. *et al.* Ankyrin-B mutation causes type 4 long-QT cardiac arrhythmia and sudden cardiac death. *Nature* 2003; **421**: 634–639.

12. Splawski, I., Timothy, K., Sharpe, M.L. *et al.* Cav 1.2 calcium channel dysfunction causes a multisistem disorder including arrhythmia and autism. *Cell* 2004; **119**: 1–20.

13. Priori, S.G., Napolitano, C., & Vicentini, A. Inherited arrhythmia syndromes: applying the molecular biology and genetic to the clinical management. *J. Interv. Cardiol. Electrophysiol.* 2003; **9**: 93–101.

14. Moss, A.J., Zareba, W., Kaufman, E.S. *et al.* Increased risk of arrhythmic events in long-QT syndrome with mutations in the pore region of the human ether-a-go-go-related gene potassium channel. *Circulation* 2002; **105**: 794–799.

15. Shimizu, W., Horie., M., Ohno, S. *et al.* Mutation site-specific differences in arrhythmic risk and sensitivity to sympathetic stimulation in the LQT1 form of congenital long QT syndrome; Multicenter study in Japan. *J. Am. Coll. Cardiol.* 2004; **44**: 117–125.

16. Priori, S.G., Napolitano, C., Schwartz, P.J. *et al.* Association of Long QT syndrome loci and cardiac events among patients treated with beta-blockers. *J. Am. Med. Assoc.* 2004; **292**: 1341–1344.

17. Priori, S.G., Napolitano, C., Giordano, U., Collisani, G., & Memmi, M. Brugada syndrome and sudden cardiac death in children. *Lancet* 2000; **355**: 808–809.

18. Brugada, J., Brugada, R., Antzelevitch, C., Towbin, J.A., Nademanee, K., & Brugada, P. Long-term follow-up of individuals with the electrocardiographic pattern of right bundle-branch block and ST-segment elevation in precordial leads V1 to V3. *Circulation* 2002; **105**: 73–78.

19. Priori, S.G., Aliot, E., Blomstrom-Lundqvist, C. *et al.* Task force on sudden cardiac death of the European Society of Cardiology. *Eur.Heart J.* 2001; **22**: 1374–1450.

20. Chen, Q., Kirsch, G.E., Zhang, D. *et al.* Genetic basis and molecular mechanism for idiopathic ventricular fibrillation. *Nature* 1998; **392**: 293–296.

21. Priori, S.G., Napolitano, C., Gasparini, M. *et al.* Natural history of Brugada syndrome. Insights for risk stratification and management. *Circulation* 2002; **105**: 1342–1347.

22. Mohler, P.J., Rivolta, I., Napolitano, C. *et al.* Nav1.5 E1053K mutation causing Brugada syndrome blocks binding to ankyrin-G and expression of Nav1.5 on the surface of cardiomyocytes. *Proc.Natl Acad Sci USA* 2004; **101**: 17533–17538.

23. Schott, J.J., Alshinawi, C., Kyndt, F. *et al.* Cardiac conduction defects associate with mutations in SCN5A. *Nat.Genet.* 1999; **23**: 20–21.

24. Benson, D.W., Wang, D.W., Dyment, M. *et al.* Congenital sick sinus syndrome caused by recessive mutations in the cardiac sodium channel gene (SCN5A). *J. Clin. Invest.* 2003; **112**: 1019–1028.

25. Wolff, L. Familial auricular fibrillation. *N.Engl.J. Med.* 1943; **229**: 396–397.

26. Brugada, R., Tapscott, T., Czernuszewicz, G.Z. *et al.* Identification of a genetic locus for familial atrial fibrillation. *N.Engl.J.Med.* 1997; **336**: 905–911.

27. Chen, Y.H., Xu, S.J., Bendahhou, S. *et al.* KCNQ1 gain-of-function mutation in familial atrial fibrillation. *Science* 2003; **299**: 251–254.

28. Gussak, I., Brugada, P., Brugada, J. *et al.* Idiopathic short QT interval: a new clinical syndrome? *Cardiology* 2000; **94**: 99–102.

29. Brugada, R., Hong, K., Dumaine, R. *et al.* Sudden death associated with short-QT syndrome linked to mutations in HERG. *Circulation* 2004; **109**: 30–35.

30. Bellocq, C., van Ginneken, A.C., Bezzina, C.R. *et al.* Mutation in the KCNQ1 gene leading to the short QT-interval syndrome. *Circulation* 2004; **109**: 2394–2397.

31. Priori, S.G., Pandit, S.V., Rivolta, I. *et al.* A novel form of short QT syndrome (SQT3) is caused by a mutation in the KCNJ2 gene. *Cir. Res.* 2005; **96**(7): 800–807.

32. Coumel, P., Fidelle, J., Lucet, V., Attuel, P., & Bouvrain, Y. Catecholaminergic-induced severe ventricular arrhythmias with Adams-Stokes syndrome in children: report of four cases. *Br. Heart J.* 1978; **40**: 28–37.

33. Napolitano, C., & Priori, S.G. Genetics of ventricular tachycardia. *Curr.Opin.Cardiol.* 2002; **17**: 222–228.

34. Swan, H., Piippo, K., Viitasalo, M. *et al.* Arrhythmic disorder mapped to chromosome 1q42–q43 causes malignant polymorphic ventricular tachycardia in structurally normal hearts. *J. Am.Coll.Cardiol.* 1999; **34**: 2035–2042.

35. Priori, S.G., Napolitano, C., Tiso, N. *et al.* Mutations in the cardiac ryanodine receptor gene (hRyR2) underlie catecholaminergic polymorphic ventricular tachycardia. *Circulation* 2001; **103**: 196–200.

36. Laitinen, P.J., Brown, K.M., Piippo, K. *et al.* Mutations of the cardiac ryanodine receptor (RyR2) gene in familial polymorphic ventricular tachycardia. *Circulation* 2001; **103**: 485–490.

37. Priori, S.G., Napolitano, C., Memmi, M. *et al.* Clinical and molecular characterization of patients with catecholaminergic polymorphic ventricular tachycardia. *Circulation* 2002; **106**: 69–74.

38. Wehrens, X.H., Lehnart, S.E., Huang, F. *et al.* FKBP12.6 deficiency and defective calcium release channel (ryanodine receptor) function linked to exercise-induced sudden cardiac death. *Cell* 2003; **113**: 829–840.

39. George, C.H., Higgs, G.V., & Lai, F.A. Ryanodine receptor mutations Associated with stress-induced ventricular

tachycardia mediate increased calcium release in stimulated cardiomyocytes. *Circ. Res.* 2003; **93**: 531–540.

40. Lahat, H., Eldar, M., Levy-Nissenbaum, E. *et al.* Autosomal recessive catecholamine- or exercise-induced polymorphic ventricular tachycardia. *Circulation* 2001; **103**: 2822–2827.

41. Lahat, H., Pras, E., Olender, T., *et al.* A missense mutation in a highly conserved region of CASQ2 is associated with autosomal recessive catecholamine-induced polymorphic ventricular tachycardia in Bedouin families from Israel. *Am. J. Hum.Genet.* 2001; **69**: 1378–1384.

42. Viatchenko-Karpinski, S., Terentyev, D., Gyorke, I. *et al.* Abnormal calcium signaling and sudden cardiac death associated with mutation of calsequestrin. *Circ. Res.* 2004; **94**: 471–477.

Genomics

43. Splawski, I., Timothy, K.W., Tateyama, M. *et al.* Variant of SCN5A sodium channel implicated in risk of cardiac arrhythmia. *Science* 2002; **297**(5585): 1333–1336.

44. Myerburg, R.J. Scientific gaps in the prediction and prevention of sudden cardiac death. *J. Cardiovasc. Electrophysiol.* 2002; **13**(7): 709–723.

45. Cargill, M., Altshuler, D., Ireland, J. *et al.* Characterization of single-nucleotide polymorphisms in coding regions of human genes. *Nat. Genet.* 1999; **22**(3): 231–238. Erratum in: Nat. Genet. 1999; **23**(3): 373.

46. Halushka, M.K., Fan, J.B., Bentley, K. *et al.* Patterns of single-nucleotide polymorphisms in candidate genes for blood-pressure homeostasis. *Nat. Genet.* 1999; **22**(3): 239–247.

47. Shiang, R., Thompson, L.M., Zhu, Y.Z. *et al.* Mutations in the transmembrane domain of FGFR3 cause the most common genetic form of dwarfism, achondroplasia. *Cell* 1994; **78**(2): 335–342.

48. Kerem, B., Rommens, J.M., Buchanan, J.A. *et al.* Identification of the cystic fibrosis gene: genetic analysis. *Science* 1989; **245**(4922): 1073–1080.

49. Lettice, L.A., Horikoshi, T., Heaney, S.J. *et al.* Disruption of a long-range cis-acting regulator for Shh causes preaxial polydactyly. *Proc. Natl Acad. Sci. USA* 2002; **99**(11): 7548–7553.

50. Gunderson, K.L., Steemers, F.J., Lee, G., Mendoza, L.G., & Chee, M.S. A genome-wide scalable SNP genotyping assay using microarray technology. *Nat. Genet.* 2005; **37**(5): 549–554. Epub 2005 Apr 17.

51. Matsuzaki, H., Dong, S., Loi, H. *et al.* Genotyping over 100,000 SNPs on a pair of oligonucleotide arrays. *Nat. Methods* 2004; **1**(2): 109–111.

52. Ozaki, K., Ohnishi, Y., Iida, A. *et al.* Functional SNPs in the lymphotoxin-alpha gene that are associated with susceptibility to myocardial infarction. *Nat. Genet.* 2002; **32**(4): 650–654. Epub 2002 Nov 11. Erratum in: *Nat. Genet.* 2003; **33**(1): 107.

53. Sebat, J., Lakshmi, B., Troge, J.*et al.* Large-scale copy number polymorphism in the human genome. *Science* 2004; **305**(5683): 525–528.

54. Iafrate, A.J., Feuk, L., Rivera, M.N. *et al.* Detection of large-scale variation in the human genome. *Nat. Genet.* 2004; **36**(9): 949–951. Epub 2004 Aug 1.

55. Sharp, A.J., Locke, D.P., McGrath, S.D. *et al.* Segmental duplications and copy-number variation in the human genome. *Am. J. Hum. Genet.* 2005 **77**(1): 78–88. Epub 2005 May 25.

56. Buckley, P.G., Mantripragada, K.K., Benetkiewicz, M. *et al.* A full-coverage, high-resolution human chromosome 22 genomic microarray for clinical and research applications. *Hum. Mol. Genet.* 2002; **11**(25): 3221–3229.

57. Wang, T.L., Maierhofer, C., Speicher, M.R. *et al.* Digital karyotyping. *Proc. Natl Acad. Sci. USA* 2002; **99**(25): 16156–16161.

58. Giacalone, J., Delobette, S., Gibaja, V. *et al.* Optical mapping of BAC clones from the human Y chromosome DAZ locus. *Genome Res.* 2000; **10**(9): 1421–1429.

59. Bignell, G.R., Huang, J., Greshock, J. *et al.* High-resolution analysis of DNA copy number using oligonucleotide microarrays. *Genome Res.* 2004; **14**(2): 287–295.

60. Fried, L.P., Borhani, N.O., Enright, P. *et al.* The Cardiovascular Health Study: design and rationale. *Ann. Epidemiol.* 1991; **1**: 263–276.

61. ARIC-Investigators. The atherosclerosis risk in communities (ARIC) study: design and objectives. *Am. J. Epidemiol.* 1989; **129**: 687–702.

Proteomics

62. O'Farrell, P.H. High resolution two-dimensional electrophoresis of proteins. *J. Biol. Chem.* 1975; **250**(10): 4007–4021.

63. Gorg, A., Weiss, W., & Dunn, M.J. Current two-dimensional electrophoresis technology for proteomics. *Proteomics* 2004; **4**(12): 3665–3685.

64. Bjellqvist, B., Ek, K., Righetti, P.G. *et al.* Isoelectric focusing in immobilized pH gradients: principle, methodology and some applications. *J. Biochem. Biophys. Methods* 1982; **6**(4): 317–339.

65. Gorg, A., Obermaier, C., Boguth, G. *et al.* The current state of two-dimensional electrophoresis with immobilized pH gradients. *Electrophoresis* 2000; **21**(6): 1037–1053.

66. Graham, D.R., Garnham, C.P., Fu, Q., Robbins, J., & Van Eyk, J.E. Improvements in two-dimensional gel electrophoresis by utilizing a low cost "in-house" neutral pH sodium dodecyl sulfate-polyacrylamide gel electrophoresis system. *Proteomics* 2005 May 11; [Epub ahead of print]

67. Neverova, I., & Van Eyk, J.E. Role of chromatographic techniques in proteomic analysis. *J. Chromatogr. B Analyt. Technol. Biomed. Life Sci.* 2005; **815**(1–2): 51–63.

68. Shi, Y., Xiang, R., Horvath, C., & Wilkins, JA. The role of liquid chromatography in proteomics. *J. Chromatogr. A.* 2004; **1053**(1–2): 27–36.

69. Yates, J.R. 3rd Mass spectral analysis in proteomics. *Annu. Rev. Biophys. Biomol Struct.* 2004; **33**: 297–316.

70. Koomen, J., Hawke, D., & Kobayashi, R. Developing an understanding of proteomics: an introduction to biological mass spectrometry. *Cancer Invest.* 2005; **23**(1): 47–59.

71. McDonough, J.L., Neverova, I., & Van Eyk, J.E. Proteomic analysis of human biopsy samples by single two-dimensional electrophoresis: coomassie, silver, mass spectrometry, and Western blotting. *Proteomics* 2002; **2**(8): 978–987.

72. Molloy, M.P. Two-dimensional electrophoresis of membrane proteins using immobilized pH gradients. *Anal. Biochem.* 2000; **280**(1): 1–10.

73. Santoni, V., Molloy, M., & Rabilloud, T. Membrane proteins and proteomics: un amour impossible? *Electrophoresis* 2000; **21**(6): 1054–1070.

74. McDonald, TG, Van Eyk, JE. Mitochondrial proteomics. Undercover in the lipid bilayer. *Basic Res. Cardiol.* 2003; **98**(4): 219–227.

75. Chevallet, M., Santoni, V., Poinas, A. *et al.* New zwitterionic detergents improve the analysis of membrane proteins by two-dimensional electrophoresis. *Electrophoresis* 1998; **19**(11): 1901–1909.

76. Santoni, V., Rabilloud, T., Doumas, P. *et al.* Towards the recovery of hydrophobic proteins on two-dimensional electrophoresis gels. *Electrophoresis*. 1999; **20**(4–5): 705–711.

77. Anderson, N.L & Anderson, N.G. The human plasma proteome: history, character, and diagnostic prospects. *Mol. Cell. Proteomics* 2002; **1**(11): 845–867.

78. Fu, Q., Garnham, C.P., Elliott, S.T., Bovenkamp, D.E., & Van Eyk, J.E. A robust, streamlined, and reproducible method for proteomic analysis of serum by delipidation, albumin and IgG depletion, and two-dimensional gel electrophoresis. *Proteomics* 2005 May 27; [Epub ahead of print]

79. Bjorhall, K., Miliotis, T., & Davidsson, P. Comparison of different depletion strategies for improved resolution in proteomic analysis of human serum samples. *Proteomics* 2005; **5**(1): 307–317.

5

Intracellular signaling during myocardial ischemia

Peter H. Sugden

National Heart and Lung Institute Division, Faculty of Medicine, Imperial College London, UK

Introduction

There are several general points to be considered with respect to the perturbations in intracellular signaling that are induced by ischemia and any subsequent reperfusion, and these apply equally to the myocardium and to other tissues. First, what are the changes in the activities of signaling pathways wrought by prolonged periods of ischemia and are these related to any subsequent pathologies? Second, what are the mediators that lead to activation of these signaling pathways and what are the cellular sensors of these mediators? Third, what are the changes that allow short periods of ischemia to be protective against a subsequent period of ischemia that would normally inevitably lead to irreversible myocardial damage (the phenomenon known as ischemic conditioning)? Finally, what are the pharmacological options for intervention so that the damaging effects of ischemia and ischemia–reperfusion can be moderated or the protective effects of conditioning be stimulated? These questions are especially pertinent to the myocardium because the contractile cells (the cardiac myocytes) are terminally differentiated in the adult (i.e., they are incapable of undergoing a complete cycle of cell division), having withdrawn from the cell cycle during the perinatal period. This renders the heart particularly vulnerable to myocyte death such as that occurring during ischemic heart disease because the myocytes that are lost cannot be replaced, and the only palliative alternative is the regional expansion of the pre-existing myocyte pool, i.e., cardiac remodeling.[1]

Ischemia and ischemia–reperfusion are associated with gross disturbances in ionic balance and metabolic activity, and increases in the production of reactive oxygen species (ROS).[2,3] ROS are purposely produced by a number of enzymes (e.g., NAD(P)H oxidases, the xanthine dehydrogenase/oxidase system, various peroxidases) and play important biological roles (e.g., phagocyte-mediated killing of infecting bacteria),[4] but they are also produced as a byproduct of mitochondrial oxidative phosphorylation.[3,5] Even under arobic conditions, incomplete reduction of the end electron acceptor, molecular O_2, gives rise to superoxide anion radicals, hydroxyl radicals, and H_2O_2 (as much as 1%–2% of O_2 is incompletely reduced), and this is exacerbated during ischemia and worsened further during reperfusion.[3,5]

The stress-activated protein kinases (SAPKs)

Classification of SAPKs

Many signaling events involve reversible protein phosphorylation and dephosphorylation (Fig. 5.1). Signaling in ischemia–reperfusion is no exception. One group of signaling proteins that is strongly activated by ischemia and ischemia–reperfusion is the so-called stress-activated protein kinases (SAPKs).[6–8] These are closely related to the bona fide mitogen-activated protein kinases (MAPKs) that regulate cell growth, cell division, and cell survival (i.e., the extracellular signal-regulated kinases 1 and 2 (ERK1/2), or p44-MAPK and p42-MAPK, respectively[9]). Indeed, in spite of attempts to clarify the terminology to render it more logical,[6] SAPKs are still often considered by many to be MAPKs. The general hierarchy of activation of MAPKs/SAPKs is similar in that a MAPK/SAPK kinase kinase phosphorylates and activates a MAPK/SAPK kinase, which then

Cardiac Arrest: The Science and Practice of Resuscitation Medicine. 2nd edn., ed. Norman Paradis, Henry Halperin, Karl Kern, Volker Wenzel, Douglas Chamberlain. Published by Cambridge University Press. © Cambridge University Press, 2007.

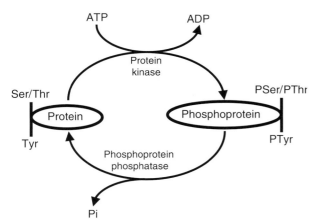

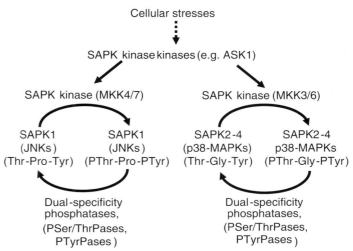

Fig. 5.1. Reversible protein phosphorylation and dephosphorylation. Proteins can be phosphorylated on the hydroxyl groups of Ser-/Thr-residues and/or Tyr-residues by protein kinases, with ATP as the phosphate donor. There are up to about 500 protein kinases encoded in the human genome, of which the largest group phosphorylate Ser-/Thr-residues. In some (though probably not all) cases, the phosphorylation(s) will change the biological activity or properties of the protein concerned. Phosphoproteins are dephosphorylated by phosphoprotein phosphatases (about 100 encoded in the human genome) which hydrolyze the phosphoester bond to release inorganic phosphate (Pi). Notably, these cycles are unidirectional (i.e., operate only in the clockwise direction in Fig. 4.1) but are biologically-reversible (though requiring energy from ATP). All possess a level of activity that is altered by biological signaling events to change the proportions of the dephosphoprotein: phosphoprotein. Because of the cyclical nature, alteration of either the protein kinase activity or the phosphoprotein phosphatase activity (or of both in the opposite direction) changes the dephosphoprotein:phosphoprotein balance.

Fig. 5.2. The stress-activated protein kinase (SAPK) cascades. Activation of the SAPKs [which include the c-Jun N-terminal kinases (JNKs or SAPK1) and p38-mitogen-activated protein kinases (p38-MAPKs, SAPK2–4)], is the last step of a three-tiered protein kinase cascade. SAPK kinase kinases (which are likely themselves to be phosphorylated and dephosphorylated) phosphorylate and activate SAPK kinases, which then phosphorylate and activate the SAPKs. Activation of these cascades is reversed by dual-specificity phosphoprotein phosphatases which act on all three phosphorylated residues (at the SAPK stage only), protein Tyr-phosphatases (PTyrPases, at the SAPK stage only) and/or protein Ser-/Thr-phosphatases (PSer/PThrPases, at all three stages). For simplicity, the SAPK5 (or ERK5) cascade, which is also activated by cellular stresses, is not shown.

phosphorylates and activates a MAPK/SAPK (Fig. 5.2). Such a "cascade" of protein kinases allows signal amplification and integration. An equally important consideration is how activation is reversed and a variety of classes of phosphoprotein phosphatases is responsible for this. A detailed consideration of such phosphatases, however, is outside the scope of this chapter.

The phosphorylation of MAPKs/SAPKs by MAPK/SAPK kinases is unusual in that a Thr- and a Tyr- residue in a Thr-Xaa-Tyr tripeptide activation loop sequence are phosphorylated, and phosphorylation of both residues is necessary for activation. Furthermore, both phosphorylations are carried out by the dual-function (catalyzing both Ser-/Thr- and Tyr- phosphorylations) MAPK/SAPK kinases. The identity of the variable amino acid (Xaa) in the tripeptide sequence is one criterion used for classification of MAPKs/SAPKs. There is specificity upstream in terms of the protein

kinase activators of SAPKs. Thus, the SAPK kinases for the SAPK1 group are different from those for the SAPK2 group. The SAPK kinase kinases constitute a fairly diverse group of kinases and it is still not clear whether there is specificity in terms of their SAPK kinase substrates at this level, because the SAPK1 and SAPK2 families are frequently activated in an apparently concerted manner.

SAPK1

The SAPK1 group (Fig. 5.2), or the c-Jun N-terminal kinases (JNKs), were first identified in livers of rats exposed *in vivo* to the stress of administration of the protein synthesis inhibitor, cycloheximide.[10] In SAPK1, Xaa is Pro-. Their best defined substrate is the transcription factor c-Jun which is phosphorylated in its N-terminal transactivation domain (residues Ser-63 and Ser-73) to increase the ability of the protein to activate transcription. A further effect of these phosphorylations is increased stability of the protein towards proteolytic degradation.[11,12] In *Homo sapiens*, there are three *JNK* genes which give rise to multiple alternatively spliced transcripts.[13] In non-neuronal tissues (including heart), transcripts encoding proteins of approximately 46 kDa and 54 kDa originate from both the *JNK1* and *JNK2* genes. (It is possibly a fairly common misconception that the *JNK1* gene encodes the 46 kDa JNK species and the *JNK2* gene encodes the 54 kDa JNK species: however, as Gupta *et al.*[13] demonstrate, this is not the case.)

SAPK2, SAPK3, and SAPK4

SAPK2, SAPK3, and SAPK4 (Fig. 5.2) are also known as the p38-MAPKs, and the identity of Xaa- is Gly-. The four members of the SAPK2 group (p38-MAPKα and p38MAPKβ) originate from two genes, both of which are alternatively spliced.[14–16] They are inhibited by pyridinylimidazoles such as SB203580 and SB202190,[14] and probably play a role in inflammatory diseases such as rheumatoid arthritis. SAPK3 (p38-MAPKγ, also confusingly termed ERK6) and SAPK4 (p38-MAPKδ) are less well characterized than the SAPK2 group and are not inhibited by SB203580.[14] There is still discussion about the diversity of expression of p38-MAPK isoforms in heart,[17,18] though work in this system has probably concentrated on those which are inhibited by SB203580, i.e., the SAPK2 group.[14] The best-characterized substrates of the SAPK2 group are themselves protein kinases, namely MAPK-activated protein kinases (MAPKAPK) 2 and 3, which phosphorylate the Hsp25/27 small heat shock proteins and their orthologs (e.g., α_B-crystallin).[19,20] Small heat shock proteins are molecular chaperones involved in the control of the stability of the cytoskeleton and possibly apoptosis.[21,22] Whilst the biological role of their phosphorylation is not entirely understood, their phosphorylation state may modulate their ability to regulate cytoskeletal stability.[21] Over-expression of these molecular chaperones protects the heart against ischemia,[23–25] and their phosphorylation during myocardial ischemia or stress has been detected.[26,27] Nevertheless, some doubt remains as to whether the phosphorylation event *per se* is cardioprotective.[28]

SAPK5

The final well-defined member of the SAPK group is SAPK5, also known as extracellular signal-regulated kinase 5 (ERK5) or "big" MAPK 1 (BMK1).[29] The identity of the Xaa-residue is Glu-. Although classified as an ERK on the basis of its Xaa- residue, it appears to be very different from the "classical" ERKs (ERK 1/p44-MAPK and ERK2/p42-MAPK) which, as bona fide MAPKs, regulate cell growth, division, and survival, and which are activated by peptide growth factors and other anabolic mediators. Again, a kinase

distinct from those activating SAPK1–4 is involved in the activation of SAPK5. Regulation of SAPK5 in the heart and cardiac myocytes has not been studied extensively (probably because assessment of its activation is not technically simple), although it is activated by cytotoxic stresses.[30] In other cells, probably the best-defined SAPK5 substrates are the myocyte enhancer factor 2 group of transcription factors,[29] suggesting a role of SAPK5 in regulation of gene expression.

Effects of ischemia and ischemia–reperfusion on SAPK activities

In the isolated heart, global ischemia activates SAPK2 (p38-MAPKα/β) and this probably increases on reperfusion.[31,32] Furthermore, it is possible that the classical SAPK kinase kinase/SAPK kinase cascade is not responsible for this activation, which is instead mediated by SAPK2 autophosphorylation involving an ancillary protein known as TAB1, and the AMP-activated protein kinase.[33,34] In contrast, SAPK1 (JNKs) are not activated by ischemia, but are strongly activated on reperfusion.[31] This is one of the few well-documented examples of differential regulation of SAPK1 and SAPK2 which, as mentioned above, are normally activated *pari passu*. It implies that SAPK1 and SAPK2 are regulated by different upstream activators in this instance. Ischemia and ischemia–reperfusion promote apoptotic and/or necrotic cell death, but it is not clear whether the activation of SAPKs promotes cell death or whether their activation represents a pro-survival response in the face of a cytotoxic insult. The field has been reviewed by both camps recently.[35,36] Resolution of this controversy has not proved simple partly because, although there are relatively selective inhibitors for the SAPK2 cascade (i.e., SB203580 and SB202190), there are no analogous inhibitors of the SAPK1 cascade. Inhibition of SAPK2 with SB203580 does appear to reduce cell death in the myocardium exposed to ischemia–reperfusion[32] an effect that is also seen with "dominant-negative" approaches where activation of SAPK2 is prevented by blocking the SAPK2 cascade with mutated SAPK/SAPK kinase.[37] Furthermore, activation of SAPK1 and SAPK2 is also seen in human hearts in failure following ischemic heart disease.[38]

What are the mediators of ischemia–reperfusion-induced activation of SAPKs?

ROS represent the most likely mediators of ischemia–reperfusion-induced activation of SAPKs. SAPKs are strongly activated by exogenous ROS in the myocardium,[26,39] and the effects of ischemia–reperfusion on activation of SAPKs can be reduced by antioxidants.[39-41] It is not clear how ROS might activate the SAPKs. As with all cyclical processes, it could be through increased positive signaling (activation of SAPK kinases/SAPK kinase kinases) or decreased negative signaling (inhibition of phospho-protein phosphatases). The SAPK kinase ASK1 (apotosis signal-regulated kinase 1) is activated by ROS in a relatively complex manner, the description of which is beyond the scope of this chapter.[42,43] Equally, the dual-specificity phosphoprotein phosphatases are particularly import-ant in dephosphorylating and inactivating SAPKs (and MAPKs).[43,44] These phosphatases are Cys-dependent and contain a reactive sulphydryl group in their active sites which is susceptible to inactivating and possibly irre-versible oxidation.[45]

How might SAPKs induce myocardial death?

Given that it is not clear how ischemia induces the death of cardiac myocytes, then an obvious corollary is that it is not clear how SAPKs might bring this about. In simple terms, cells die by necrosis (unregulated cell death), apoptosis (regulated cell death), or a combination of these. Necrosis of cardiac myocytes probably involves swelling of the cell itself and of subcellular organelles (because of decreased ATP production and hence disturbances in ionic and metabolic balance), ultimately resulting in cell burst-ing. Necrosis does not require energy in the form of ATP, whereas apoptosis is an energy-requiring process. Apoptosis has been detected in hearts exposed to ischemic and ischemia–reperfusion, and probably occurs in vivo as a consequence of ischemic heart disease.[46–49] There are two pathways of apoptosis, the extrinsic (receptor-mediated) pathway and the intrinsic (mitochondrial) pathway.[50] Ultimately, both lead to the activation of proteolytic effec-tor caspases (e.g., caspase 3) with regulated demolition of cellular contents, nuclear and cellular condensation, and resorption of cellular components into neighboring cells. In the mitochondrial pathway, leakage of mitochondrial proteins such as cytochrome c leads to formation of the apoptosome and activation of the initiator caspase, caspase 9.[51] Individuals of a group of proteins (the Bcl2 proteins) either prevent or promote mitochondrial leakage,[51] and these are involved in SAPK1- or SAPK2-mediated apoptosis. An extensive literature in this area now exists (see, for example,[52–58]) though a consensus view has not been reached, probably because different mech-anisms apply to different cell types. For example, activa-tion of the pro-apoptotic Bax or Bad proteins or inhibition of the antiapoptotic activity of Mcl-1 may be essential in SAPK1/SAPK2-activated apoptosis.[52,53,55,59] Further details

are beginning to emerge. Thus, pro-apoptotic Bim is subject to a SAPK1-dependent upregulation at the level of transcription and/or a SAPK1-dependent phosphorylation that may allow it to dissociate from microtubules and either to activate pro-apoptotic Bax/Bak or to inhibit anti-apoptotic Bcl2 in the mitochondrial outer membrane.[54,60] Studies are, as usual, less advanced in cardiac sytems though recent publications suggest that SAPK1 stimulates the mitochondrial pathway of apoptosis,[61] and that migra-tion of Bax (and pro-apoptotic cleaved Bid) to mitochon-dria during simulated ischemia/ischemia–reperfusion may be mediated by an (AMP-activated protein kinase-dependent?) activation of SAPK2.[56,57] A putative scheme of ischemia–reperfusion-induced cell death is shown in Fig. 5.3.

Activation of additional signaling pathways by ischemia–reperfusion

Protein kinase Cδ (PKCδ)

The PKC family are phospholipid-dependent kinases that translate signaling events in the plasma membrane further downstream.[62–64] Although certain members of the PKC family are the cellular receptors for tumor-promoting phorbol esters (and are hence potentially involved in cell division and/or inhibition of apoptosis), PKCδ, even though activated by phorbol esters, appears to promote apoptosis.[65–68] The ROS-mediated pro-apoptotic effects of PKCδ involve its translocation to mitochondria and other subcellular organelles,[65,69] and may additionally involve the non-receptor protein tyro-sine kinase c-Abl (which is activated by ROS), SAPK2 and the pro-apototic Bcl2 proteins, Bax and Bak.[58,70] Alternatively, in neuronal cells, ischemia or ROS causes a caspase-3-dependent cleavage of PKCδ to release its (unregulated and active) catalytic domain.[67,71–73] These two pathways of activation are not necessarily distinct because phosphorylation of a Tyr-residue (Tyr-311) close to the caspase-3-cleavage site in PKCδ appears to enhance the cleavage. Again, analogous studies in myocardial systems are relatively unadvanced, but have still found a focus in PKCδ. Thus, PKCδ has been reported to signal preferentially to the SAPK1 and SAPK2 cascades and to potentiate ischemia-induced damage.[74,75] Furthermore, ROS promote phosphorylation of Tyr-311 (and other Tyr-residues) in PKCδ.[76] These Tyr-phosphory-lations are associated with release of PKCδ into the soluble phase of the cell from the particulate fraction and increased (lipid-independent) catalytic activity.[76] Other

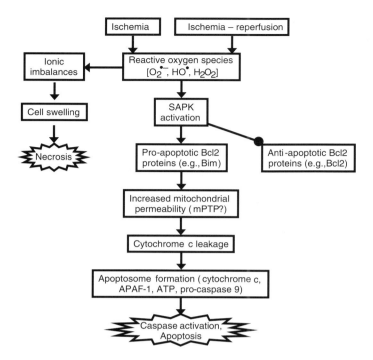

Fig. 5.3. A putative signaling scheme for the death of the cardiac myocyte in ischemia and ischemia–reperfusion. Ischemia and any subsequent reperfusion lead to the formation of reactive oxygen species (ROS, superoxide anion radicals, hydroxyl radicals, H_2O_2) which activate the SAPKs. This leads to phosphorylation of Bcl2 family proteins, increasing the pro-apoptic activity of some and diminishing the anti-apoptotic activity of others. Bcl2 proteins regulate the permeability of the outer mitochondrial membrane, which is increased. The mitochondrial permeability transition pore (mPTP) may also be involved, but this is not regulated through Bcl2 proteins and is in the inner mitochondrial membrane. Cytochrome *c* present in the intermembrane space of the mitochondria leaks out of the mitochondria into the cytoplasm. This leads to the assembly of the apoptosome complex which includes the protein APAF-1, ATP, and inactive initiator pro-caspase 9. Pro-caspase 9 has a low basal activity but, when assembled in the apoptosome, this is sufficient for the transautopeptidase of pro-caspase 9 to occur, cleaving neighboring pro-caspase 9 molecules in the apoptosome. The caspase cascade is triggered, leading ultimately to the activation (by cleavage) of effector caspases such as caspase 3, and cell demolition is initiated. In addition, ROS-induced changes in ionic homeostasis, for which opening of the mPTP may be partly responsible, leads to cell swelling and bursting (necrotic cell death). For a given cell, death can result though apoptosis, necrosis, or a mixture of the two, depending on the signals it receives.

studies have suggested that translocation of PKCδ to the mitochondria following ischemia-reperfusion in the intact heart may induce cell death in the heart by stimulating the mitochondrial pathway of apoptosis.[77]

The endoplasmic reticulum (ER) stress response

The ER stress response (or the unfolded protein response, UPR) embraces a complex series of events that is initially cytoprotective but which, if unrestrained, leads to apoptosis.[50,78] The ER is a complex subcellular organelle that is intimately involved with translation of mRNA species into immature proteins and in their subsequent post-translational processing (polypeptide folding, disulfide bond formation, glycosylation) into mature proteins. The ER is rich in molecular chaperones (proteins that function in these folding processes) such as Grp78. In non-muscle cells, the ER is also the principal intracellular store of Ca^{2+}, although, in cardiac and skeletal muscle myocytes, a specialized form of the ER, the sarcoplasmic reticulum (SR), assumes this role. Disturbances in Ca^{2+} homeostasis (e.g., depletion of ER Ca^{2+} stores) and other stresses (inhibition of glycosylation, oxidative stress, viral infection) trigger the UPR and this involves the release of signaling proteins that are normally tethered to the ER by Grp78 into the cytoplasm. Depletion of SR/ER Ca^{2+} stimulates the UPR in cardiac myocytes.[79] The UPR consists of multiple parallel events, some of which (ASK1, SAPK1/2) have been mentioned earlier. Others include the release of the trans-ER membrane ATF6 transcription factor from its Grp78 tether in the ER, proteolytic cleavage of ATF6 at a juxtamembrane site, and migration of ATF6 to the nucleus where it drives expression of mRNA species encoding proteins (e.g., XBP1, Grp78) which perpetuate the UPR. Induction of the UPR in response to ischemia–reperfusion has not been examined extensively in the heart. Its activation has been detected in ischemic heart disease,[80] however, and conditional activation of a cardiospecifically expressed, cleaved (i.e., activated) ATF6 in transgenic mice protects hearts against ex vivo ischemia-reperfusion injury.[81] Activation of the UPR in a myocardial context will potentially have important implications in cardioprotection.

Ischemic conditioning

In certain settings, controlled myocardial ischemia can confer cardioprotection. Thus, repeated (1–6 times) short periods (5 min) of ischemia interspersed with short periods of reperfusion (5 min) protect the heart against a subsequent period of ischemia which would otherwise be lethal.[82–84] This phenomenon is known as ischemic preconditioning and it was recognized in the heart over 20 years ago.[85] The initial period of protection lasts for only 1 or 2 hours but, in vivo, a "second window of protection" occurs over the 24–72-hour period. Recently, it has been recognized that the heart can also be protected if intermittent ischemia–reperfusion is applied after the period of damaging ischemia, a phenomenon known as ischemic postconditioning.[83,84] Ischemic preconditioning may occur either naturally or unintentionally in certain circumstances, for example during "warm-up" angina or during certain surgical procedures (e.g., percutaneous transluminal coronary angioplasty).[82]

Thus, it would potentially be therapeutically useful if ischemic conditioning could be induced pharmacologically and this provides the motivation for the elucidation of its mechanisms. Nonethelesss, a consensus on the mechanisms of ischemic conditioning is still lacking. Multiple initiating stimuli have been identified and include oxidative stress, vasoactive compounds (adenosine, bradykinin, endothelin, NO, and others) and narcotics such as opioids.[82] Intracellular signaling studies have suggested a role for PKC isoforms (especially PKCε)[75,86] and the mitochondrial K^+_{ATP} channel.[87] More recently, a role for "prosurvival" protein kinases such as ERK1/2 and protein kinase B (PKB, also known as Akt) has been proposed.[83] These are described in more detail in the subsequent section. The suggestion is that ERK1/2 and/or PKB/Akt prevent the opening of the mitochondrial permeability transition pore (mPTP) at the time of reperfusion. The mPTP is a non-selective ion pore in the inner mitochondrial membrane and its opening leads to mitochondrial uncoupling, inhibition of mitochondrial ATP regeneration and loss of ion homeostasis, followed ultimately by cell death.[88] Recent evidence from transgenic mouse studies has indicated that inactivation of mPTP opening caused by targetted gene deletion of one of its components (cyclophilin D) protects the heart against ischemia.[89–91] Furthermore, targeting cyclophilin D with cyclosporin A or sanglifehrin A or inhibition of its other components (the adenine nucleotide translocase) has suggested a strategy for protection,[88] though the current agents available are probably unsuited for routine use in vivo because of their wider effects (e.g., cyclosporin A is an established immunosuppressant that also exhibits renal toxicity).

Potential for therapeutic intervention in ischemia–reperfusion injury

With respect to cell signaling, there are two options for strategies of reduction of the damaging effects of ischemia and ischemia–reperfusion, inhibition of cytotoxic pathways or activation of cytoprotective pathways. Allusions have been made earlier in this chapter of how this may be achieved. For example, inhibition of SAPK1 (JNKs) and SAPK2 (p38-MAPKα/β) during ischemia would be predicted to be cytoprotective and ex vivo evidence to this effect has been presented.[32,36,37] In vivo, the SAPK2 inhibitors appear to improve cardiac viability and performance in a hamster model of dilated cardiomyopathy, though a SAPK1 inhibitor (SP600125) was deleterious.[92] (Note, however, that SP600125 is not particularly selective for SAPK1 and it inhibits a number of potentially prosurvival protein kinases in addition to inhibiting SAPK1.[93]) This is clearly an area for future development.

Two cytoprotective pathways have received attention, the PKB/Akt and the ERK1/2 pathways (Fig. 5.4). PKB/Akt is classically activated by peptide growth factors such as insulin-like growth factor 1 and insulin acting at their transmembrane receptor protein tyrosine kinases. A detailed description of the activation of PKB/Akt activation is outside the scope of this article, though an extensive literature exists.[94–96] In the heart, experimental studies have shown that activation of PKB/Akt is cardioprotective.[97] The ERK1/2 cascade is also activated in the cardiac myocyte by a less-extensive range of peptide growth factors (e.g., epidermal growth factor and platelet-derived growth factor, which also act at receptor protein tyrosine kinases) than PKB/Akt. In cardiac myocytes, however, agonists such as endothelin and α1-adrenergic agonists (which act at a separate class of transmembrane receptors, the Gq/11 protein-coupled receptors) activate ERK1/2.[98,99] This activation probably occurs through a PKC-dependent pathway and hence tumor-promoting phorbol esters are powerful activators of ERK1/2 in cardiac myocytes.[98,99] Again, a detailed description of the ERK1/2 cascade lies outside the scope of this chapter.[9,100] Suffice it to say that the organization of the ERK1/2 cascade is analogous to that of the SAPK cascades. Thus a MAPK kinase kinase (c-Raf, A-Raf or B-Raf) activates MAPK kinases (MKK1/2) which then activate ERK1/2. As with PKB/Akt, there is now extensive evidence that activation of ERK1/2 protects against the damaging effects of myocardial ischemia.[101,102] The mechanisms of cardioprotection are, at least in part, dependent on the abilities of PKB/Akt and ERK1/2 to activate signaling which leads

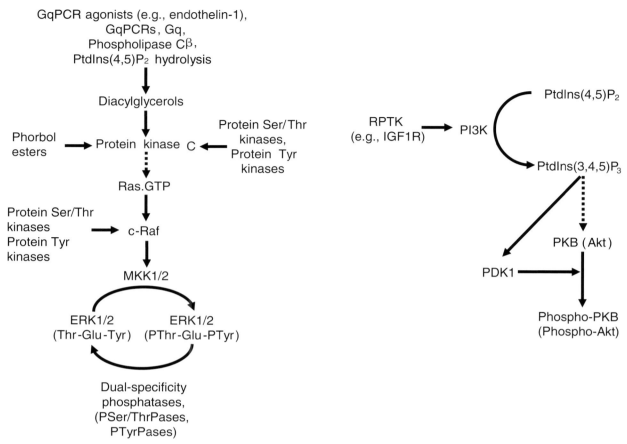

Fig. 5.4. Pro-survival protein kinases. The extracellular signal-regulated kinase 1/2 (ERK1/2) cascade is the archetypical mitogen-activated protein kinase (MAPK) cascade. Activation of upstream signaling events (not described) leads to activation of the guanine nucleotide binding protein Ras by stimulation of exchange of GTP with Ras-bound GDP increases Ras.GTP loading. The Raf isoforms (c-Raf is shown), which are the MAPK kinase kinases for the ERK1/2 cascade, have a high affinity for Ras.GTP and translocate to the membrane. In the case of c-Raf, phosphorylations and probably dephosphorylations occur at this location, and c-Raf becomes fully activated. c-Raf then phosphorylates two Ser-residues on the MAPK kinases, MKK1 and MKK2, to activate them. MKK1/MKK2 then phosphorylate ERK1 and ERK2 on a Tyr- and a Thr-residue to activate them in turn. Activation of c-Raf is reversed by Ras-mediated hydrolysis of the bound GTP and presumably by changes in its phosphorylation state. MKK1/2 are dephosphorylated by protein Ser-/Thr-phosphatases (PSer/ThrPases). ERK1/2 are dephosphorylated on both Tyr- and Thr-residues by the Cys-dependent dual-specificity protein phosphatases. There are at least 13 dual-specificity phosphatases with differential specificity towards the various MAPKs, and they are either constitutively or inducibly expressed. Alternatively, protein Ser-/Thr-phosphatases or Cys-dependent protein Tyr-phosphatases (PTyrPases) dephosphorylate their respective sites individually. The mechanisms of activation of the ERK1/2 cascade by Gq protein-coupled receptor (GqPCR) agonists such as endothelin-1 are incompletely understood. These agonists (or phorbol esters) activate the diacylglycerol-sensitive protein kinase C isoforms and this probably leads to activation of Ras, though the nature of the connections is unclear (indicated by the dashed arrow). Certain receptor protein Tyr-kinases (e.g., the epidermal growth factor receptor, EGFR) will also activate the ERK1/2 cascade in the heart and are thus potentially prosurvival, but these have been omitted for the sake of simplicity.

In the protein kinase B/Akt (PKB/Akt) signaling pathway, activation of receptor protein tyrosine kinases (RPTKs, e.g., the insulin-like growth factor 1 receptor, IGF1R or the IGFR) by their individual extracellular ligands (e.g., IGF1, EGF) leads to their autophosphorylation on specific Tyr-residues. This increased Tyr-phosphorylation promotes binding of phosphoinositide 3-kinase (PI3K) to these phospho-Tyr- (PTyr-) residues. This event places the PI3K catalytic subunit in the plane of the membrane where it phosphorylates phosphatidylinositol 4,5-bisphosphate [PtdIns(4,5)P$_2$] to PtdIns(3,4,5)P$_3$. In the unstimulated state, a proportion of the Ser-/Thr-protein kinase 3-phosphoinositide-dependent kinase 1 (PDK1) is bound to the membrane through its phospholipid-binding domain by the basal levels of PtdIns(3,4,5)P$_3$ present. When PI3K is activated, PtdIns(3,4,5)P$_3$ levels in the plane of the membrane increase and protein kinase B (PKB) translocates to this locale by binding to PtdIns(3,4,5)P$_3$. The juxtapositioning of PDK1 and PKB allows PDK1 to phosphorylate and activate PKB/Akt.

to a reduction in apoptosis. This is mediated in a number of ways–phosphorylation and inhibition of pro-apoptotic Bcl2 proteins and repression of genes encoding proapoptotic protein mediators representing two of them.[103,104] Why then is there not more emphasis on promoting the activation of PKB/Akt and ERK1/2 in the treatment of myocardial ischemia? The problem is that unregulated activation of these pathways in cells capable of division would potentially induce malignancy, and so systemic delivery of such agents would be potentially harmful. Indeed, mutants of a number of the components of the cell survival pathways (c-Raf, B-Raf, PKB/Akt) are established oncogenes.

Conclusions

Understanding of the signaling processes involved in ischemia–reperfusion injury and myocardial cell death has increased dramatically recently and this understanding has led to the formulation of protective strategies. Nevertheless, complicating factors (the problems of toxicity of known inhibitors of cytotoxic signaling pathways, the possibility of malignant transformation in the case of activation of cytoprotective pathways) have so far precluded informed clinical application. It is likely that future refinements (e.g., localized targetting of therapeutic interventions) will eventually bring benefits.

REFERENCES

1. Opie, L.H., Commerford, P.J., Gersh, B.J., & Pfeffer, M.A. Controversies in ventricular remodelling. *Lancet* 2006; **367**: 356–367.
2. Neely, J.R. & Feuvray, D. Metabolic products and myocardial ischemia. *Am. J. Pathol.* 1981; **102**: 282–291.
3. Solaini, G. & Harris, D.A. Biochemical dysfunction in heart mitochondria exposed to ischaemia and reperfusion. *Biochem. J.* 2005; **390**: 377–394.
4. Lambeth, J.D. NOX enzymes and the biology of reactive oxygen. *Nat. Rev. Immunol.* 2004; **4**: 181–189.
5. Giordano, F.J. Oxygen, oxidative stress, hypoxia, and heart failure. *J. Clin. Invest.* 2005; **115**: 500–508.
6. Cohen, P. The search for physiological substrates of MAP and SAP kinases in mammalian cells. *Trends Cell Biol.* 1997; **7**: 353–361.
7. Sugden, P.H. & Clerk, A. "Stress-responsive" mitogen-activated protein kinases (c-Jun N-terminal kinases and p38 mitogen-activated protein kinases) in the myocardium. *Circ. Res.* 1998; **83**: 345–352.
8. Kyriakis, J.M. & Avruch, J. Mammalian mitogen-activated protein kinase signal transduction pathways activated by stress and inflammation. *Physiol. Rev.*, 2001; **81**: 807–869.
9. Chen, Z., Gibson, T.B., Robinson, F. *et al.* MAP kinases. *Chem. Rev.* 2001; **101**: 2449–2476.
10. Kyriakis, J.M., & Avruch, J. pp54 Microtubule-associated protein 2 kinase. A novel serine/threonine kinase regulated by phosphorylation and stimulated by poly-L-lysine. *J. Biol. Chem.* 1990; **265**: 17355–17363.
11. Musti, A.M., Treier, M., & Bohmann, D. Reduced ubiquitin-dependent degradation of c-Jun after phosphorylation by MAP kinases. *Science* 1997; **275**: 400–402.
12. Clerk, A., Kemp, T.J., Harrison, J.G., Mullen, A.J., Barton, P.J., & Sugden, P.H. Up-regulation of c-*jun* mRNA in cardiac myocytes requires the extracellular signal-regulated kinase cascade, but c-Jun N-terminal kinases are required for efficient up-regulation of c-Jun protein. *Biochem, J.* 2002; **368**: 101–110.
13. Gupta, S., Barrett, T., Whitmarsh, A.J. *et al.* Selective interaction of JNK protein kinase isoforms with transcription factors. *EMBO J.* 1996; **15**: 2760–2770.
14. Kumar, S., McDonnell, P.C., Gum, R.J., Hand, A.T., Lee, J.C., & Young, P.R. Novel homologues of CSBP/p38 MAP kinase: activation, substrate specificity and sensitivity to inhibition by pyridinyl imidazoles. *Biochem. Biophys. Res. Commun.* 1997; **235**: 533–538.
15. Lee, J.C., Laydon, J.T., McDonnell, P.C. *et al.* A protein kinase involved in the regulation of inflammatory cytokine biosynthesis. *Nature* 1994; **372**: 739–746.
16. Sanz, V., Arozarena, I., & Crespo, P. Distinct carboxy-termini confer divergent characteristics to the mitogen-activated protein kinase p38α and its splice isoform Mxi2. *FEBS Lett.* 2000; **474**: 169–174.
17. Court, N.W., dos Remedios, C.G., Cordell, J., & Bogoyevitch, M.A. Cardiac expression and subcellular localization of the p38 mitogen-activated protein kinase member, stress-activated protein kinase-3 (SAPK3). *J. Mol. Cell. Cardiol.* 2002; **34**: 413–426.
18. Lemke, L.E., Bloem, L.J., Fouts, R., Esterman, M., Sandusky, G., & Vlahos, C.J. Decreased p38 MAPK activity in end-stage failing human myocardium: p38 MAPK α is the predominant isoform expressed in human heart. *J. Mol. Cell. Cardiol.* 2001; **33**: 1527–1540.
19. Rouse, J., Cohen, P., Trigon, S. *et al.* A novel kinase cascade triggered by stress and heat shock that stimulates MAPKAP kinase-2 and phosphorylation of the small heat shock proteins. *Cell* 1994; **78**: 1027–1037.
20. Ito, H., Okamoto, K., Nakayama, H., Isobe, T., & Kato, K. Phosphorylation of αB-crystallin in response to various types of stress. *J. Biol. Chem.* 1997; **272**: 29934–29941.
21. Landry, J. & Huot, J. Regulation of actin dynamics by stress-activated protein kinase 2 (SAPK2)-dependent phosphorylation of heat-shock protein of 27 kDa (Hsp27). *Biochem. Soc. Symp.* 1999; **64**: 79–89.
22. Beere, H.M. Stressed to death: regulation of apoptotic signaling pathways by heat shock proteins. *Sci. STKE.* 2001; **2001**(93): RE1:

23. Martin, J.L., Mestril, R., Hilal-Dandan, R., Brunton, L.L., & Dillmann, W.H. Small heat shock proteins and protection against ischemic injury in cardiac myocytes. *Circulation* 1997; **96**: 4343–4348.

24. Ray, P.S., Martin, J.L., Swanson, E.A., Otani, H., Dillmann, W.H., & Das D.K. Transgene overexpression of αB-crystallin confers simultaneous protection against cardiomyocyte apoptosis and necrosis during myocardial ischemia and reperfusion. *FASEB J.* 2001; **15**: 393–402.

25. Kumarapeli, A.R., & Wang, X. Genetic modification of the heart: chaperones and the cytoskeleton. *J. Mol. Cell. Cardiol.* 2004; **37**: 1097–1109.

26. Clerk, A., Michael, A., & Sugden, P.H. Stimulation of multiple mitogen-activated protein kinase sub-families by oxidative stress and phosphorylation of the small heat shock protein, HSP25/27, in neonatal ventricular myocytes. *Biochem. J.* 1998; **333**: 581–589.

27. Shu, E., Matsuno, H., Akamastu, S. *et al.* αB-crystallin is phosphorylated during myocardial infarction: involvement of platelet-derived growth factor-BB. *Arch. Biochem. Biophys.* 2005; **438**: 111–118.

28. Martin, J.L., Hickey, E., Weber, L.A., Dillmann, W.H., & Mestril, R. Influence of phosphorylation and oligomerization on the protective role of the small heat shock protein 27 in rat adult cardiomyocytes. *Gene Expr.* 1999; **7**: 349–355.

29. Hayashi, M. & Lee, J.-D. Role of the BMK1/ERK5 signaling pathway: lessons from knockout mice. *J. Mol. Med.* 2004; **82**: 800–808.

30. Kennedy, R.A., Kemp, T.J., Sugden, P.H., & Clerk, A. Using U0126 to dissect the role of the extracellular signal-regulated kinase 1/2 (ERK1/2) cascade in the regulation of gene expression by endothelin-1 in cardiac myocytes. *J. Mol. Cell. Cardiol.* 2006; **41**: 236–247.

31. Bogoyevitch, M.A., Gillespie-Brown, J., Ketterman, A.J. *et al.* Stimulation of the stress-activated mitogen-activated protein kinases subfamilies in perfused heart. p38/RK mitogen-activated kinases and c-Jun N-terminal kinases are activated by ischemia–reperfusion. *Circ. Res.* 1996; **79**: 161–173.

32. Ma, X.L., Kumar, S., Gao, F. *et al.* Inhibition of p38 mitogen-activated protein kinase decreases cardiomyocyte apoptosis and improves cardiac function after myocardial ischemia and reperfusion. *Circulation* 1999; **99**: 1685–1691.

33. Tanno, M., Bassi, R., Gorog, D.A. *et al.* Diverse mechanisms of myocardial p38 mitogen-activated protein kinase activation: evidence for MKK-independent activation by a TAB1-associated mechanism contributing to injury during myocardial ischemia. *Circ. Res.* 2003; **93**: 254–261.

34. Li, J., Miller, E.J., Ninomiya-Tsuji, J., Russel, R.R., 3rd., & Young, L.H. AMP-activated protein kinase activates p38 mitogen-activated protein kinase by increasing recruitment of p38 MAPK to TAB1 in the ischemic heart. *Circ. Res.* 2005; **97**: 872–879.

35. Bishopric, N.H., Andreka, P., Slepak, T., & Webster, K.A. Molecular mechanisms of apoptosis in the cardiac myocyte. *Curr. Opin. Pharmacol.* 2001; **1**: 141–150.

36. Baines, C.P. and Molkentin, J.D. STRESS signaling pathways that modulate cardiac myocyte apoptosis. *J. Mol. Cell. Cardiol.* 2005; **38**: 47–62.

37. Kaiser, R.A., Bueno, O.F., Lips, D.J. *et al.* Targeted inhibition of p38 mitogen-activated protein kinase antagonizes cardiac injury and cell death following ischemia–reperfusion *in vivo.* *J. Biol. Chem.* 2004; **279**: 15524–15530.

38. Cook, S.A., Sugden, P.H., & Clerk, A. Activation of c-Jun N-terminal kinases and p38-mitogen-activated protein kinases in human heart failure secondary to ischemic heart disease. *J. Mol. Cell. Cardiol.* 1999; **31**: 1429–1434.

39. Clerk, A., Fuller, S.J., Michael, A., & Sugden, P.H. Stimulation of "stress-regulated" mitogen-activated protein kinases (stress-activated protein kinases/c-Jun N-terminal kinases and p38-mitogen-activated protein kinases) by oxidative and other stresses. *J. Biol. Chem.* 1998; **273**: 7228–7234.

40. Kyaw, M., Yoshizumi, M., Tsuchiya, K., Kirima, K., & Tamaki, T. Antioxidants inhibit JNK and p38 MAPK activation but not ERK 1/2 activation by angiotensin II in rat aortic smooth muscle cells. *Hypertens. Res.* 2001; **24**: 251–261.

41. Pimentel, D.R., Amin, J.K., Xiao, L. *et al.* Reactive oxygen species mediate amplitude-dependent hypertrophic, and apoptotic responses to mechanical stretch in cardiac myocytes. *Circ. Res.* 2001; **89**: 453–460.

42. Sumbayev, V.V. & Yasinska, I.M. Regulation of MAP kinase-dependent apoptotic pathway: implication of reactive oxygen and nitrogen species. *Arch. Biochem. Biophys.* 2005; **436**: 406–412.

43. Sugden, P.H. & Clerk, A. Oxidative stress and growth-regulating intracellular signalling pathways in cardiac myocytes. *Antioxid. Redox Signal.* 2006; in press.

44. Farooq, A. & Zhou, M.M. Structure and regulation of MAPK phosphatases. *Cell Signal.* 2004; **16**: 769–779.

45. Salmeen, A. & Barford, D. Functions and mechanisms of redox regulation of cysteine-based phosphatases. *Antioxid. Redox Signal.* 2005; **7**: 560–577.

46. Kang, P.M. & Izumo, S. Apoptosis and heart failure: A critical review of the literature. *Circ. Res.* 2000; **86**: 1107–1113.

47. Kang, P.M. & Izumo, S. Apoptosis in the heart: basic mechanisms and implications in cardiovascular diseases. *Trends Mol. Med.* 2003; **9**: 177–182.

48. Scarabelli, T.M. & Gottlieb, R.A. Functional and clinical repercussions of myocyte apoptosis in the multifaceted damage by ischemia/reperfusion injury: old and new concepts after 10 years of contributions. *Cell Death Differ.* 2004; **11** Suppl. 2: S144–S152.

49. Scarabelli, T.M., Knight, R., & Stephanou, A. Clinical implications of apoptosis in ischemic myocardium. *Curr. Probl. Cardiol.* 2006; **31**: 181–264.

50. Danial, N.N. & Korsmeyer, S.J. Cell death: critical control points. *Cell* 2004; **116**: 205–219.

51. Scorrano, L. & Korsmeyer, S.J. Mechanisms of cytochrome *c* release by proapoptotic BCL-2 family members. *Biochem. Biophys. Res. Commun.* 2003; **304**: 437–444.

52. Donovan, N., Becker, E.B., Konishi, Y., & Bonni, A. JNK

phosphorylation and activation of BAD couples the stress-activated signaling pathway to the cell death machinery. *J. Biol. Chem.* 2002; **277**: 40944–40949.

53. Inoshita, S., Takeda, K., Hatai, T. *et al.* Phosphorylation and inactivation of myeloid cell leukemia 1 by JNK in response to oxidative stress. *J. Biol. Chem.* 2002; **277**: 43730–43744.

54. Lei, K. & Davis, R.J. JNK phosphorylation of the Bim-related members of the Bcl2 family induces Bax-dependent apoptosis. *Proc. Natl Acad. Sci. USA* 2003; **100**: 2432–2437.

55. Lei, K., Nimnual, A., Zong, W.X. *et al.* The Bax family of Bcl2-related proteins is essential for apoptotic signal transduction by c-Jun NH$_2$-terminal kinase. *Mol. Cell. Biol.* 2003; **22**: 4929–4942.

56. Brady, N.R., Hamacher-Brady, A., & Gottlieb, R.A. Proapoptotic BCL-2 family members and mitochondrial dysfunction during ischaemia/reperfusion injury, a study employing cardiac HL-1 cells and GFP biosensors. *Biochim. Biophys. Acta* 2006; **1757**: 667–678.

57. Capano, M. & Crompton, M. Bax translocates to mitochondria of heart cells during simulated ischaemia: involvement of AMP-activated and p38 mitogen-activated protein kinases. *Biochem. J.* 2006; **395**: 57–64.

58. Choi, S.-Y., Kim, M.-J., Kang, C.-M. *et al.* Activation of Bak and Bax through c-Abl-protein kinase Cδ-p38 MAPK signaling in response to ionozing radiation in human non-small cell lung cancer cells. *J. Biol. Chem.* 2006; **28**: 7049–7059.

59. Van Laethem, A., van Kelst, S., Lippens, S. *et al.* Activation of p38 MAPK is required for Bax translocation to mitochondria, cytochrome c release and apoptosis induced by UVB irradiation in human keratinocytes. *FASEB J.* 2004; **18**: 1946–1948.

60. Ley, R., Ewings, K.E., Hadfield, K., & Cook, S.J. Regulatory phosphorylation of Bim: sorting out the ERK from the JNK. *Cell Death Differ.* 2005; **12**: 1008–1014.

61. Aoki, H., Kang, P.M., Hampe, J. *et al.* Direct activation of mitochondrial apoptosis machinery by c-Jun N-terminal kinase in adult cardiac myocytes. *J. Biol. Chem.* 2002; **277**: 10244–10250.

62. Newton, A.C. Protein kinase C: structural and spatial regulation by phosphorylation, cofactors, and macromolecular interactions. *Chem. Rev.* 2001; **101**: 2353–2364.

63. Newton, A.C. Regulation of the ABC kinases by phosphorylation: protein kinase C as a paradigm. *Biochem J.* 2003; **370**: 361–371.

64. Parker, P.J. & Murray-Rust, J. PKC at a glance. *J. Cell. Sci.* 2004; **117**: 131–132.

65. Brodie, C. & Blumberg, P.M. Regulation of cell apoptosis by protein kinase c δ. *Apoptosis* 2003; **8**: 19–27.

66. Gutcher, I., Webb, P.R., & Anderson, N.G. The isoform-specific regulation of apoptosis by protein kinase C. *Cell. Mol. Life Sci.* 2003; **60**: 1061–1070.

67. Kanthasamy, A.G., Kitazawa, M., Kanthasamy, A., & Anantharam, V. Role of proteolytic activation of protein kinase Cδ in oxidative stress-induced apoptosis. *Antioxid. Redox Signal.* 2003; **5**: 609–620.

68. Murriel, C.L. & Mochly-Rosen, D. Opposing roles of δ and εprotein kinase C in cardiac ischemia and reperfusion: tar-geting the apoptotic machinery. *Arch. Biochem. Biophys.* 2003; **420**: 246–254.

69. Majumder, P.K., Mishra, N.C., Sun, X. *et al.* Targeting PKC δ to mitochondria in the oxidative stress response. *Cell Death Differ.* 2001; **12**: 465–470.

70. Lasfer, M., Davenne, L., Vadrot, N. *et al.* Protein kinase C delta and c-Abl are required for mitochondrial apoptosis by geno-toxic shock in the absence of p53, p73 and Fas receptor. *FEBS Lett.* 2006; **580**: 2547–2552.

71. Kaul, S., Anantharam, V., Yang, Y., Choi, C.J., Kanthasamy, A., & Kanthasamy, A.G. Tyrosine phosphorylation regulates the proteolytic activation of protein kinase Cδ in dopaminergic neuronal cells. *J. Biol. Chem.* 2005; **280**: 28721–28730.

72. Perez-Pinzon, M.A., Dave, K.R., and Raval, A.P. Role of reactive oxygen species and protein kinase C in ischemic tolerance in the brain. *Antioxid. Redox Signal.* 2005; **7**: 1150–1157.

73. Raval, A.P., Dave, K.R., Prado, R. *et al.* Protein kinase C delta cleavage initiates and aberrant signal transduction pathway after cardiac arrest and oxygen glucose deprivation. *J. Cereb. Blood Flow Metab.* 2005; **25**: 730–741.

74. Heidkamp, M.C., Bayer, A.L., Martin, J.L., & Samarel, A.M. Differential activation of mitogen-activated protein kinase cascades and apoptosis by protein kinase C ε and δ in neo-natal rat ventricular myocytes. *Circ. Res.* 2001; **89**: 882–890.

75. Chen, L., Hahn, H., Wu, G. *et al.* Opposing cardioprotective actions and parallel hypertrophic effects of δPKC and εPKC. *Proc. Natl Acad. Sci. USA* 2001; **98**: 11114–11119.

76. Rybin, V.O., Guo, J., Sabri, A., Elouardighi, H., Schaefer, E., & Steinberg, S.F. Stimulus-specific differences in protein kinase Cδ localization and activation mechanisms in cardiomy-ocytes. *J. Biol. Chem.* 2004; **279**: 19350–19361.

77. Murriel, C.L., Churchill, E., Inagaki, K., Szweda, L.I., & Mochly-Rosen, D. Protein kinase Cδ activation induces apoptosis in response to cardiac ischemia and reperfusion damage: a mechanism involving BAD and the mitochondria. *J. Biol. Chem.* 2004; **279**: 47985–47991.

78. Xu, C., Bailly-Maitre, B., & Reed, J.C. Endoplasmic reticulum stress: cell life and death decisions. *J. Clin. Invest.* 2005; **115**: 2656–2664.

79. Thuerauf, D.J., Hoover, H., Meller, J. *et al.* Sarco/endoplasmic reticulum calcium ATPase-2 expression is regulated by ATF6 during the endoplasmic reticulum stress response. *J. Biol. Chem.* 2001; **276**: 48309–48317.

80. Azfer, A., Niu, J., Rogers, L.M., Adamski, F.M., & Kolattukudy, P.E. Activation of the endoplasmic reticulum stress response during the development of ischemic heart disease. *Am. J. Physiol. Heart Circ. Physiol.* 2006; E-pub (April 14):

81. Martindale, J.J., Fernandez, R., Thuerauf, D. *et al.* Endoplasmic reticulum stress gene induction and protection from ischaemia/reperfusion injury in transgenic mice with a tamoxifen-regulated form of ATF6. *Circ. Res.* 2006; **98**: 1186–1193.

82. Edwards, R.J., Saurin, A.T., Rakhit, R.D., & Marber, M.S. Therapeutic potential of ischaemic preconditioning. *Br. J. Clin. Pharmacol.* 2000; **50**: 87–97.

83. Hausenloy, D.J., Tsang, A., & Yellon, D.M. The reperfusion injury salvage kinase pathway: a common target for both ischemic preconditioning and postconditioning. *Trends Cardiovasc. Med.* 2005; **15**: 69–75.

84. Yellon, D.M. & Hausenloy, D.J. Realizing the clinical potential of ischemic preconditioning and postconditioning. *Nat. Clin. Pract. Cardiovasc. Med.* 2005; **2**: 568–575.

85. Murry, C.E., Jennings, R.B., & Reimer, K.A. Preconditioning with ischemia: a delay of lethal cell injury in ischemic myocardium. *Circulation* 1986; **74**: 1124–1136.

86. Saurin, A.T., Pennington, D.J., Raat, N.J., Latchman, D.S., Owen, M.J., & Marber, M.S. Targeted disruption of the protein kinase C epsilon gene abolishes the infarct size reduction that follows ischaemic preconditioning of isolated buffer-perfused mouse hearts. *Cardiovasc. Res.* 2002; **55**: 672–680.

87. Hanley, P.J. & Daut, J. K_{ATP} channel and preconditioning: a re-examination of the role of mitochondrial K_{ATP} channels and an overview of alternative mechanisms. *J. Mol. Cell. Cardiol.* 2005; **39**: 17–50.

88. Halestrap, A.P., Clarke, S.J., & Javadov, S.A. Mitochondrial permeability transition pore opening during myocardial reperfusion – a target for cardioprotection. *Cardiovasc. Res.* 2004; **61**: 372–385.

89. Baines, C.P., Kaiser, R.A., Purcell, N.H. *et al.* Los of cyclophilin D reveals a critical role for mitochondrial permeability transitin in cell death. *Nature* 2005; **434**: 658–662.

90. Nakagawa, T., Shimizu, S., Watanabe, T. *et al.* Cyclophilin D-dependent mitochondrial permeability transition regulates some necrotic but not apoptotic cell death. *Nature* 2005; **434**: 652–658.

91. Schneider, M.D. Cyclophilin D: knocking on death's door. *Sci STKE*. 2005; 2005(287)pe26:

92. Kyoi, S., Otani, H., Matsuhisa, S. *et al.* Opposing effect of p38 MAP kinase and JNK inhibitors on the development of heart failure in the cardiomyopathic hamster. *Cardiovasc. Res.* 2006; **69**: 888–898.

93. Bain, J., McLauchlan, H., Elliott, M., & Cohen, P. The specificities of protein kinase inhibitors: an update. *Biochem. J.* 2003; **371**: 199–204.

94. Vanhaesebroeck, B. & Alessi, D.R. The PI3K-PDK1 connection: more than just a road to PKB. *Biochem. J.* 2000; **346**: 561–576.

95. Brazil, D.P. & Hemmings, B.A. Ten years of protein kinase B signalling: a hard Akt to follow. *Trends Biochem. Sci.* 2001; **26**: 657–664.

96. Brazil, D.P., Yang, Z.Z., & Hemmings, B.A. Advances in protein kinase B signalling: AKTion on multiple fronts. *Trends Biochem. Sci.* 2004; **29**: 233–242.

97. Matsui, T. & Rosenzweig, A. Convergent signal transduction pathways controlling cardiomyocyte survival and function: the role of PI 3-kinase and Akt. *J. Mol. Cell. Cardiol.* 2005; **38**: 63–71.

98. Bogoyevitch, M.A., Glennon, P.E., & Sugden, P.H. Endothelin-1, phorbol esters and phenylephrine stimulate MAP kinase activities in ventricular cardiomyocytes. *FEBS Lett.* 1993; **317**: 271–275.

99. Bogoyevitch, M.A., Glennon, P.E., Andersson, M.B. *et al.* Endothelin-1 and fibroblast growth factors stimulate the mitogen-activated protein kinase signaling cascade in cardiac myocytes. The potential role of the cascade in the integration of two signaling pathways leading to myocyte hypertrophy. *J. Biol. Chem.* 1994; **269**: 1110–1119.

100. Wellbrock, C., Karasarides, M., & Marais, R. The RAF proteins take centre stage. *Nat Rev. Mol. Cell. Biol.* 2004; **5**: 875–885.

101. Bueno, O.F., De Windt, L.J., Tymitz, K.M. *et al.* The MEK1-ERK1/2 signaling pathway promotes compensated cardiac hypertrophy in transgenic mice. *EMBO J.* 2000; **19**: 6341–6350.

102. Bueno, O.F. & Molkentin, J.D. Involvement of extracellular signal-regulated kinases 1/2 in cardiac hypertrophy and cell death. *Circ. Res.* 2002; **91**: 776–781.

103. Valks, D.M., Cook, S.A., Pham, F.H., Morrison, P.R., Clerk, A., & Sugden, P.H. Phenylephrine promotes phosphorylation of Bad in cardiac myocytes through the extracellular signal-regulated kinases 1/2 and protein kinase A. *J. Mol. Cell. Cardiol.* 2002; **34**: 749–763.

104. Greer, E.L. & Brunet, A. FOXO transcription factors at the interface between longevity and tumor suppression. *Oncogene* 2005; **24**: 7410–7425.

Electrophysiology of ventricular fibrillation and defibrillation

Wei Xiong and Gordon F. Tomaselli

Department of Medicine, Division of Cardiology, Donald W. Reynolds Cardiovascular Clinical Research Center, Johns Hopkins University School of Medicine, Baltimore, MD, USA

Introduction

Sudden cardiac death remains a major public health problem in the United States. Despite extensive study and effective treatments for malignant ventricular arrhythmias more than a quarter of a million people die suddenly each year in this country.[1] Sudden death accounts for more than half of all deaths related to cardiovascular disease, coronary artery disease is the most common pathological condition found in patients who die suddenly, and ventricular fibrillation is the most common immediate cause of death.[2]

In the last decade a decline in the incidence of out-of-hospital ventricular fibrillation and a measurable improvement in the long-term survival of patients who have been resuscitated have been documented in the most well-studied communities.[3,4] Despite these gains and perhaps because of the changing etiology of cardiac arrest, the overall survival of cardiac arrest victims has not changed in the past two decades.[3] In communities with the most sophisticated emergency medical services, the maximal survival rate for out-of-hospital ventricular fibrillation is about 30%.[3,5] Understanding the mechanism of ventricular fibrillation is critical to making a meaningful impact on the incidence of this arrhythmia and improving the survival of sudden death victims.

Ventricular fibrillation was described by Ludwig and Hoffa in 1849 as an incoordinate heart action that produced a high metabolic rate of the myocardium but no useful contractions.[6] The hemodynamic consequences of the disordered cardiac contraction and the fundamental electrophysiologic basis of ventricular fibrillation were understood by the turn of the century. Porter, in 1898, stated that the essential nature of fibrillatory contractions is the result of abnormalities in impulse conduction.[7] Observations by several investigators supported the concept that a critical mass of tissue was required to maintain ventricular fibrillation, spontaneous recovery being common in the fibrillating hearts of small animals such as cats, rabbits, mice, and fowl, while spontaneous recovery in canine, bovine, and human hearts is rare.[8]

By the 1930s a contemporary understanding of ventricular fibrillation was established with only rudimentary electrocardiographic and hemodynamic measurements. This included the concepts that the electrophysiological mechanism is re-entry,[8] anoxia develops with cessation of coronary blood flow, and the progressive decline in the strength of contractions is due to substrate deprivation and accumulation of metabolic byproducts.[9] The last 70 years have seen considerable refinement of our understanding of the electrophysiology, hemodynamics, and metabolic consequences of ventricular fibrillation. Despite intensive study, however, our understanding of the pathophysiology of this lethal ventricular arrhythmia is far from complete.[10,11]

In this chapter we will review the electrophysiological mechanisms of ventricular fibrillation, the resultant mechanical and metabolic derangements associated with this arrhythmia, and the clinical circumstances under which ventricular fibrillation occurs with particular emphasis on the most common precipitant, myocardial ischemia. Finally, a brief perspective on the prevention and treatment of ventricular fibrillation will be presented.

Cardiac Arrest: The Science and Practice of Resuscitation Medicine. 2nd edn., ed. Norman Paradis, Henry Halperin, Karl Kern, Volker Wenzel, Douglas Chamberlain. Published by Cambridge University Press. © Cambridge University Press, 2007.

Basic science

Electrophysiology of ventricular fibrillation

Ventricular fibrillation is a dynamic arrhythmia changing electrically, mechanically, and mechanistically over time. The changing nature of fibrillating myocardium was first summarized by Wiggers who described four phases of ventricular fibrillation.[6] The first or undulatory stage of ventricular fibrillation is characterized by comparatively large wavefronts of excitation when induced by a premature stimulus in the vulnerable period. The undulatory stage is short-lived, lasting 1 to 2 seconds. The second or convulsive stage lasts from 10 to 30 seconds and the hallmark of this phase is the division of the initial wavefronts of activation into smaller segments that activate the ventricle more rapidly. The third stage could last minutes and was termed the tremulous stage, the heart having this appearance as the result of a large number of segments of reentry. In the final stage contractions become progressively weaker as a result of anoxia.[6]

More recent studies that utilize high density mapping of the myocardium have focused on the mechanisms of initiation of ventricular fibrillation (stages 1 and 2) and maintenance (stage 3) of this arrhythmia. The mechanisms of initiation of ventricular fibrillation may differ from the electrophysiologic mechanisms that maintain this tachycardia. Moreover, no single mechanism suffices to explain the initiation of all clinical and experimental ventricular fibrillation, which is critically dependent on the myocardial substrate. Independent of the mechanism initiating fibrillation, the maintenance of this arrhythmia requires a critical mass of fibrillating myocardium, and the appropriate relationship between conduction velocity and refractoriness of the ventricle.[2]

On the surface ECG, ventricular fibrillation appears as an extremely irregular, almost random process of electrical activation. This apparent turbulent pattern of cardiac activity has led to a traditional belief that ventricular fibrillation is the consequence of total disorganized activity; however, on closer examination there is organization in ventricular fibrillation. The multiple wavelet hypothesis,[12,13] initially developed for atrial fibrillation, was proposed by Moe in 1962. Two years later, the first computer model of cardiac fibrillation demonstrated that heterogeneity of refractory periods accounted for the degeneration of periodic re-entrant activity to fibrillation.[14] It was not until 20 years later, however, that firm experimental support for the multiple wavelet hypothesis was provided by Allessie and colleagues.[15] Using high-resolution mapping technology, they demonstrated that multiple propagating wavelets caused fibrillatory activity in the canine atrium.[15]

A related but alternative theory explaining fibrillation in the heart is spiral wave re-entry. This theory posits that fibrillation is the result of activation of the heart by meandering spiral waves (2D) or scroll waves or rotors (3D). Like leading circle re-entry, spiral wave re-entry does not require the presence of an inexcitable anatomical obstacle. The nature of spiral waves produces the conditions necessary for re-entry. The curvature of an activation wavefront creates a spiral of activation with the core of the spiral conducting slowly due to current source-sink mismatch and the distal activation wavefront conducting more rapidly. Although the core of the spiral is excitable, it remains unexcited by the extreme curvature of the wavefront; thus, the location of the core is free to move or drift. Fibrillation produced by scroll waves may be the result of movement or meandering of one or a small number of rotors or the propagation of smaller meandering rotors from a stable mother rotor. In optical mapping studies in isolated perfused canine hearts, transiently erupting rotors, frequent wavefront collisions, and wavebreak generation were easily detected in the fibrillating ventricle.[16] Ventricular fibrillation arises from breakup of a single spiral wave or a pair of counter-rotating spiral waves into multiple smaller wavelets.

In contrast to the multiple wavelet hypothesis, in which constant formation of new wavelets via disintegration of a spiral wave leads to multiple wavelet fibrillation, the mother rotor hypothesis proposes that a single stable high-frequency firing rotor is the driving force of ventricular fibrillation.[17] The multiple wavelets result from the failure of 1:1 conduction originating from the rapid mother rotor to the surrounding myocardium and are merely epiphenomena. In a normal Langendorff-perfused rabbit heart, a single drifting spiral wave was associated with rapid polymorphic ventricular tachycardia that was indistinguishable from ventricular fibrillation.[18] Jalife and colleagues have proposed that the rapid firing rotor with its dominant frequency is the fundamental source that maintains the overall activity. The fast moving wave front originating from a stable focal source propagates across neighboring myocardial tissue and collides with the obstacles along the wavefront, produced by both functional and anatomical heterogeneities, resulting in breakup of the spiral wave and formation of multiple wavelets. The anatomical heterogeneities include the normal atrial and ventricular structures, such as coronary arteries, papillary muscles, atrioventricular rings, orifices of aortic and pulmonary vessels, and changes in orientation of transmural muscle fibers. These unstable wavelets produce the fibrillatory pattern of the ECG.

Heterogeneities of repolarization and conduction in the heart are important contributors to the genesis of ventricular fibrillation. Restitution is a property of cardiac myocytes that explains the changes in action potential duration (APD) with changes in the timing or coupling of activation during a rhythm at steady state. Thus the APD of an extrasystolic beat is determined by the coupling interval of that beat and the APD of the preceding beats. The restitution hypothesis suggests that large oscillations of the APD of the wavefront lead to breakup of spiral waves into multiple wavelets. This process requires that the slope of the action potential restitution curve, the ratio of APD to the preceding diastolic interval, is ≥ 1, indicating that small changes in diastolic intervals lead to dramatic changes in APD. Indeed, the slope of the APD restitution curve is a target for antifibrillatory therapy. Investigators have demonstrated through experiments and simulations that flattening of the restitution curve is antifibrillatory.[19] The dynamic changes in repolarization may further exaggerate existing temporal and spatial heterogeneities in repolarization that constitute an important component of the substrate for ventricular fibrillation (Fig. 6.1). Restitution is a property of conduction as well and recent reports similarly suggest that steep restitution of conduction may be profibrillatory.[20] Importantly, restitution curves for both repolarization and conduction are multiphasic so that simply changing the shape of a portion of the curve may not produce the anticipated effects on predisposition to fibrillation.

The ion channels that participate in the perpetuation of ventricular fibrillation have been debated. Depolarization of the membrane potential during fibrillation would imply that the action potential generated in myocardial cells during this rhythm should be so-called "slow" action potentials, whose upstrokes are mediated by Ca^{2+} channels. There is general agreement that in the later stages after several minutes of fibrillation, Na^+ channels that underlie the upstroke of the "fast" action potential are inactive.[21-23] The role of the Na^+ channel in early ventricular fibrillation is less clear. Recent evidence in a non-ischemic model of VF in an intact canine heart has demonstrated the participation of both Na^+ channels and Ca^{2+} channels in the electrical activation of the fibrillating heart.[21] The rate of the rapid upstroke of the action potential and the inability of either verapamil or the Na^+ channel-specific toxin tetrodotoxin (TTX) to prevent ventricular fibrillation supports a role for

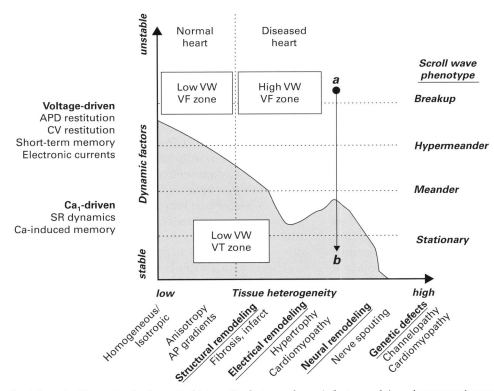

Fig. 6.1. A plot illustrating the theoretical interaction between dynamic factors and tissue heterogeneity responsible for producing ventricular fibrillation. The therapeutic objective is to move the patient from the vulnerable window (white) to the zone of reduced tissue heterogeneity or more stable dynamic factors (gray). Reprinted with permission.[262]

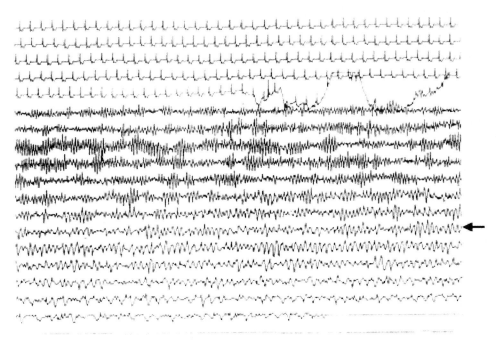

Fig. 6.2. Long-term recordings from a patient who developed ventricular fibrillation. At the onset the surface ECG morphology is consistent with type I ventricular fibrillation. After some time the activation slows and the surface ECG is consistent with type II ventricular fibrillation which ultimately terminates with asystole. Reprinted with permission.[263]

both of these channels in the early stages of the arrhythmia. Identifying the molecular participants in fibrillation during its early stages may provide insights into the mechanism of maintenance of ventricular fibrillation and the mechanism of defibrillation. The latter is particularly relevant to ventricular fibrillation that is treated immediately by implanted defibrillators.

Recent studies have suggested an important role of the inward rectifier potassium current (I_{K1}) in rotor stabilization during ventricular fibrillation.[24,25] In isolated perfused guinea pig hearts, a stable high frequency rotor is always found in the anterior left ventricle maintaining ventricular fibrillation. Cellular experiments with voltage clamp recording have demonstrated that the current density of the outward component of I_{K1} was larger in myocytes isolated from left ventricles than that from right ventricles. Computer simulations further suggested that larger I_{K1} is associated with shorter APD, faster activation, and more stable rotors. On the other hand, a different study of ventricular fibrillation in guinea pig hearts did not find the fastest activation rate or sustained rotors in the anterior left ventricular epicardium.[26] Instead, they observed that the maintained ventricular fibrillation was characterized by the presence of multiple wavelets. The faster activation

rates were located in the apex and slower activation rates were found at the base of the heart, which might be related to the spatial gradient of the rapid component of the delayed rectifier current (I_{Kr}). An alternative explanation for the two competing hypotheses of ventricular maintenance is provided by different types of ventricular fibrillation (type I and type II, Fig. 6.2). In large mammalian hearts, however, mother rotors have not been convincingly demonstrated.[27,28] Thus, it appears that at least at the initial stages of ventricular fibrillation in large mammalian hearts, dynamic wavebreak is a prominent mechanism.

Structural heart disease and sudden death

The mechanism(s) of sudden cardiac death, and ventricular fibrillation in particular, have been described in terms of a biological model by Myerburg and colleagues, where functional alterations initiate a common electrogenic pathway that permits otherwise benign electrical events to initiate lethal arrhythmias in the setting of structural heart disease.[29] There are numerous specific pathological conditions that can provide the appropriate substrate for ventricular fibrillation, which can be divided into four general classes: myocardial infarction, hypertrophy, cardiomyopathy, and structural electrical abnormalities.[29] The overwhelming majority of structural abnormalities are the result of coronary artery disease, with ischemia and reperfusion providing a major adverse modulatory influence that may predispose to VF.

Pathological examination of the hearts of patients who die suddenly reveals prior myocardial infarction in up to 75% of cases,[30,31] although acute myocardial infarction occurs in the minority of cases.[32] The presence of mural thrombus in the coronary arteries is common in pathological examination of hearts of sudden cardiac death victims and may be responsible for transient ischemia or reperfusion of the myocardium that triggers ventricular tachycardia or fibrillation.[33] Such transient functional changes in the setting of any structural disease are likely to have adverse electrophysiological consequences that can be associated with sudden death.[29] Other such modulatory functional influences include metabolic and hemodynamic changes, neurohumoral influences, and the presence of toxins and drugs such as antiarrhythmics.

There is a strong epidemiological association between ventricular hypertrophy and sudden cardiac death that holds true for both primary[34] and secondary[35–37] causes of ventricular hypertrophy. The clinical data available suggest that the majority of sudden deaths in patients with left ventricular hypertrophy are related to malignant ventricular arrhythmias, although adverse hemodynamic consequences of SVT or severe bradyarrhythmias are likely to play a role in some high-risk patients.[38,39] Because of the heterogeneity of this group the appropriate diagnostic and therapeutic strategies for sudden death prevention, short of prevention of ventricular hypertrophy, are controversial and should be tailored for each patient.

Patients with dilated cardiomyopathy of any cause are at high risk of sudden death. The mechanism(s) of death may vary depending on the subgroup of patients selected,[40] but all subgroups are likely to include a significant proportion who die as a result of malignant ventricular arrhythmias. The anatomic and electrophysiogical heterogenity that characterizes the myopathic ventricle provides a suitable substrate for ventricular arrhythmias, which is the probable mechanism of sudden death in the majority of these patients. Unfortunately, identification of those at highest risk and the optimal therapeutic approaches remain elusive.[41]

Other structural and electrical cardiac abnormalities may predispose to ventricular fibrillation in the absence of fibrosis or scar. These include accessory pathways with rapid anterograde conduction[42] and abnormalities of repolarization such as that associated with the long QT syndrome.[43,44] Both substrates are subject to functional modulation by endogenous (e.g., neurohumoral) and

Table 6.1. Factors enhancing the vulnerability of the myocardium to fibrillate

Intrinsic	Extrinsic
Hypertrophy	Increased sympathetic nervous system activity
Ischemia	Vagal stimulation
Myocardial failure	Metabolic abnormalities
Enhanced AV conduction	hypokalemia
bypass tracts	hypomagnesemia
"fast" AV node	Antiarrhythmics and other drugs
Abnormal repolarization	psychotropics
(congenital or acquired)	digitalis
Bradycardia	sympathomimetics
	terfenidate, hisminal
	Environmental (electrocution)

exogenous (e.g., antiarrhythmic drugs) factors that could alter the electrophysiological state of the heart and predispose to ventricular tachycardia and/or fibrillation.

Modulation of a myocardial substrate may lower the ventricular fibrillation threshold, dramatically enhancing the tendency of the heart to fibrillate. The major endogenous factors include myocardial ischemia, autonomic nervous system tone, and metabolic and electrolyte disturbances (Table 6.1). The state of the autonomic nervous system is particularly relevant to sudden cardiac death due to ventricular arrhythmias in patients with myocardial infarction and patients with congenital or acquired QT prolongation. Regeneration of cardiac sympathetic nerves (nerve sprouting) can produce heterogeneous sympathetic innervation and a predisposition to ventricular fibrillation and sudden cardiac death.[45–47] After myocardial infarction there is a region of viable but denervated myocardium that may exhibit arrhythmogenic hypersensitivity to catecholamines.[48] This may contribute to the increased risk of sudden death in patients with heightened sympathetic tone after MI, as assessed by studies of heart rate variability[49] and the efficacy of beta-blocking drugs in reducing mortality after infarction.[50,51] Other possible salutary effects of beta-blockers include: prevention of myocardial ischemia, prevention of catecholamine-induced hypokalemia, and antagonizing catecholamine effects on platelet aggregation.[52] Interestingly, intravenous magnesium chloride, which has many cellular effects, also blocks catecholamine release[53] and may reduce mortality in myocardial infarction.[54]

Metabolic and electrolyte disturbances also modulate potentially arrhythmogenic substrates, increasing the likelihood of ventricular fibrillation. Diuretic usage with its associated hypokalemia and hypomagnesemia has been associated with ventricular fibrillation and sudden cardiac death in patients with acute MI,[55,56] hypertensive heart disease,[57] and heart failure.[58] Changes in serum K^+ may influence the electrophysiological substrate in a number of ways, including altering automaticity, changing excitability, and altering the function of repolarizing currents.

Antiarrhythmic drugs have received much attention recently, not for their efficacy but for their potential for arrhythmia aggravation.[59,60] The propensity of drugs that prolong the QT to produce polymorphic VT and ventricular fibrillation is well known.[61-65] Agents without substantial effects on repolarization may also cause arrhythmia aggravation and increase mortality in patients with structural heart disease.[59,60] In addition to the possibility of arrhythmia aggravation, these agents may interfere with definitive therapy for ventricular fibrillation by increasing the threshold for defibrillation (see below).

The problem of ventricular fibrillation in patients without structural heart disease is a vexing but fortunately uncommon problem.[66] A recent review of 19 studies with a total of 54 patients defined the demographics of patients with apparently normal hearts and ventricular fibrillation. The patients are predominantly middle-aged males, only a quarter have a prior history of syncope, and non-invasive electrocardiographic studies are generally unrewarding. Spontaneous reversion of ventricular fibrillation in this group was uncommon (less than 10%) consistent with the findings of ventricular fibrillation in the presence of structural heart disease.[67] In the absence of an exogenous agent that alters the electrophysiology of the myocardium, the mechanism of ventricular fibrillation and sudden death is poorly defined since there are no strategies to identify these patients prospectively. It is possible that transient functional disturbances that interact with abnormal myocardium, as described previously, may under extreme circumstances produce electrophysiological changes of sufficient magnitude to initiate ventricular arrhythmias in normal hearts. The role of abnormalities of repolarization and, specifically, dispersion and inhomogeneity of repolarization has recently received attention as a mechanism of arrhythmias in normal hearts.

Increasing evidence suggests that genetic factors contribute to the risk of sudden death independent of the risk for coronary artery or other structural heart disease. Two population-based studies suggest that there is a significant genetic influence in the risk of SCD by virtue of the familial clustering of events.[68,69] In a population-based case-control study from Seattle, the rate of cardiac arrest in first-degree relatives of arrest victims was 50% greater than the rate in control subjects, independent of other risk factors for SCD.[68]

In the Paris Prospective study of male municipal employees, a history of SCD in one parent increased risk by 80%; a history of SCD in both parents led to an extraordinary 880% increase in the risk of SCD for the offspring. Again this was independent of other known risk factors for coronary or other structural heart disease.[69] Thus, independent of the presence or risk of myocardial disease, a significant component of the risk for cardiac arrest often resulting from ventricular fibrillation, is genetically determined.

Myocardial substrates for ventricular fibrillation

The development of ventricular fibrillation requires an initiating stimulus and a susceptible myocardium that interact in a complex, incompletely understood fashion. There are many factors that can enhance the vulnerability of the myocardium to fibrillate and thus lower the ventricular fibrillation threshold (Table 6.1). Some are intrinsic to the heart, such as myocardial mass and the existence of bypass tracts, others are the result of cardiac pathology producing local depolarization and abnormal automaticity, and still others can result from altered neurohumoral input to the heart generating increased non-uniformity of refractoriness or altered automaticity.[2,70,71] We will focus on recent findings concerning the induction of fibrillation, with emphasis on the mechanisms that may be operative in patients with common forms of structural heart disease. For a comprehensive discussion of some of the previous literature the reader is referred to several excellent reviews.[2,70,72,73]

Ventricular fibrillation in myocardial ischemia

Ischemic myocardium is one of the most studied and complex models of ventricular fibrillation, providing an appropriate substrate for re-entry, abnormal automaticity, or triggered arrhythmias. For a comprehensive treatment of the mechanisms of arrhythmogenesis in acute and chronic coronary artery disease, the reader is referred to a review by Janse and Wit.[74]

In ischemic tissue, ventricular tachycardia often precedes, and subsequently degenerates into fibrillation.[75] It is clear that arrhythmogenic conditions in ischemic myocardium are dynamic and predispose to the slowed conduction and unidirectional conduction block required to support re-entry. Ischemia also enhances automaticity of Purkinje fibers, promotes abnormal automaticity of muscle fibers, and is associated with alterations in Ca^{2+} homeostasis and enhanced endogenous catecholamine release associated with non-re-entrant arrhythmias.

Ventricular arrhythmias appear in two distinct phases in the first 30 minutes after complete occlusion of a coronary

Table 6.2. Ventricular arrhythmias associated with experimental ischemia

	Phase Ia	Phase Ib
Onset	2–10 minutes	15–20 minutes
Abnormal electrograms	+ + + +	+
Prevention by sympathetic nervous system block	No	Yes
Mechanism	Re-entry	? Automaticity, triggered

artery in an experimental animal (Table 6.2). The first phase occurs immediately after occlusion of the vessel (2–10 minutes) and is called phase Ia; the second or phase Ib occurs 15–20 minutes after coronary occlusion. Experimental evidence suggests that the mechanisms of phase Ia and Ib arrhythmias are different. Phase Ia arrhythmias occur in the setting of marked conduction slowing and delayed activation of the subepicardial muscle.[76] Ventricular electrograms recorded from the epicardial surface of the heart at this time are fractionated and reduced in amplitude, consistent with depolarization of the membrane and slowed conduction.[77] High density mapping has confirmed that during this phase ischemic ventricular arrhythmias are primarily re-entrant. Phase Ib arrhythmias are characterized by less abnormal electrocardiograms[76] and these arrhythmias can be effectively prevented by beta-blockers or prior catecholamine depletion of the myocardium.[78] It seems most likely that phase Ib ventricular arrhythmias are related to the release of endogenous catecholamines that increase the likelihood of non-re-entrant mechanisms such as abnormal automaticity and/or triggered activity.

Reperfusion of ischemic myocardium may also be arrhythmogenic.[79] Indeed, in some species VF occurs more frequently with reperfusion than after ligation of a coronary artery.[80] In humans, reperfusion-associated arrhythmias are frequent, the most common being accelerated idioventricular rhythms, but ventricular fibrillation is decidedly rare.[81] Experimental evidence suggests that macrore-entry is not a common mechanism of ventricular arrhythmias during reperfusion.[82,83] High density mapping of reperfused ischemic myocardium fails to reveal diastolic electrical activity during ventricular tachycardia, and tachycardia is initiated from discrete sites in the subendocardial border zone that lack conduction delay or inexcitable segments.[82–84] Reperfusion-induced ventricular arrhythmias may be due to delayed afterdepolarization-mediated triggered activity.[85] Indirect evidence for this assertion is suppression of these arrhythmias by Ca^{2+} channel block-

ers[85] and α-adrenergic blocking agents,[86] both of which would suppress the rise in intracellular Ca^{2+} during reperfusion and suppress delayed afterdepolarizations (DADs).

The incidence of experimentally induced reperfusion arrhythmias is dependent on the duration of preceding ischemia. In the canine model, at least 3 minutes and less than 30–60 minutes of coronary occlusion are associated with reperfusion-induced ventricular fibrillation.[87] The rate of restoration of coronary flow also influences the arrhythmogenicity of reperfusion. Upon reperfusion of ischemic myocardium, differential recovery of refractoriness, tissue resistance, and conduction establish exaggerated heterogeneity of electrophysiological properties of the myocardium and create a highly arrhythmogenic substate that is particularly pronounced in the border zone, where action potentials are normal.[74] Longer periods of ischemia, similar to that occurring in patients with acute myocardial infarction who receive thrombolytic therapy, are associated with irreversible cell damage and are generally not associated with the malignant ventricular rhythms seen after shorter periods of ischemia (Figs. 6.2, 6.3).

The cellular and molecular mechanisms of arrhythmias associated with myocardial ischemia are incompletely understood. Accumulation of extracellular K^+ occurs in early ischemia and is related to a net K^+ efflux from myocytes resulting in potentially arrhythmogenic changes in excitability.[88,89] Several mechanisms have been proposed to explain the accumulation of extracellular K^+, including inhibition of Na^+–K^+ ATPase, increased K^+ efflux coupled to the efflux of anions generated during ischemia, or modulation of sarcolemmal K^+ channels. Among the K^+ channels most likely to participate in K^+ efflux from ischemic myocytes is the ATP-sensitive K^+ channel, $I_{K(ATP)}$. This current is a time-independent, K^+-selective current that is blocked by ATP and sulfonylureas (e.g., glibenclamide). The conductance and activity of the channel are regulated in a complex fashion by a variety of factors, including internal Mg^{2+},[90,91] ADP,[92] GDP,[93] stimulation of adenosine A1 receptors,[94] and lactate.[95] Modulation of the sensitivity of $I_{K(ATP)}$ to ATP by other byproducts of ischemia has been proposed to account for the apparent increase in channel activity despite very modest reductions in intracellular ATP in early ischemia. Excised patches of membrane from cardiac cells containing $I_{K(ATP)}$ are inhibited with high affinity by sulfonylurea drugs. In intact myocardium, ischemia-induced shortening of the action potential and extracellular K^+ accumulation are only incompletely blocked by higher doses of sulfonylureas. Similarly, if $I_{K(ATP)}$ is activated in isolated heart cells by metabolic inhibition, these agents are not as effective channel blockers as in excised membrane patches.[93,96,97] Modulation of the affinity of these

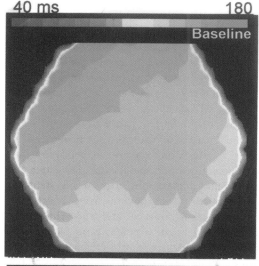

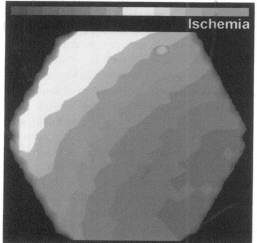

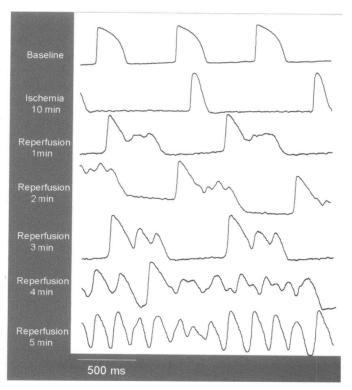

Fig. 6.3. Optical map of conduction in a guinea pig heart subject to global ischemia. The crowding of conduction isochrones indicates substantial slowing of conduction with ischemia and during early reperfusion. Optical APs during ischemia and reperfusion reveals AP shortening with ischemia and relengthening with reperfusion that is spatially and temporally heterogeneous and is associated with afterdepolarization-mediated triggered activity. (See Plate 6.3.)

blockers by other substances produced during myocardial ischemia has been suggested as the cause of this discrepancy.[93,97] Although $I_{K(ATP)}$ is likely to mediate extracellular K$^+$ accumulation during ischemia, activation of other K$^+$ conductances such as Na$^+$-activated[98] or arachidonic acid-activated K$^+$ channels[99] cannot be excluded. Current experimental evidence supports the hypothesis that anion countertransporters and $I_{K(ATP)}$ play a major role in ischemia-induced K$^+$ accumulation, and modulation of these currents may have therapeutic importance in prevention of ischemia-associated arrhythmias and preservation of ischemic myocardium.

Other electrophysiologic and metabolic consequences of ischemia may conspire to produce arrhythmias. Ischemic cells are depolarized at rest and have a different action potential contour from normally polarized cells. These voltage differences support an injury current that has been implicated as an arrhythmogenic substrate in ischemic tissue.[100] Computer modeling of the ischemic border zone has suggested that injury current flowing through an inexcitable gap may be responsible for increased spontaneous diastolic depolarization of latent pacemakers, producing automatic arrhythmias or generating a trigger for a re-entrant tachycardia.[101] Instability and collapse of the mitochondrial membrane potential mediated by inner mitochondrial anion channels (IMAC), leads to release of reactive oxygen species and arrhythmogenic oscillations of the cell membrane potential. Inhibition of the collapse of the mitochondrial membrane potential with blockers of the mitochondrial benzodiazepine receptors (e.g., 4-chlorodiazepam) that regulate IMAC reduce the incidence of VF in experimental ischemia and reperfusion.[102]

Analysis of spiral wave breakup during ventricular fibrillation in a regionally ischemic heart has shown that ischemia causes an increase of wavebreaks in the ischemic border zone and a decrease of wavebreaks in the ischemic zone.[103] Ischemia-induced alterations in APD dynamics may also predispose to the development of ventricular fibrillation; flattened APD restitution slope and reduced conduction velocity in ischemic myocardium sets the stage for type II ventricular fibrillation.[104] In contrast, steepened APD restitution and only modestly changed excitability in the non-ischemic zone facilitates the development of type I ventricular fibrillation.[104] Whether the non-ischemic zone plays a role in ventricular fibrillation, however, remains uncertain.[103,105] Furthermore, the ischemic border zone could be important in initiating ventricular fibrillation, but it may not necessarily be critical in the maintenance of ventricular fibrillation.[106]

The Purkinje network may participate in the initiation of arrhythmias in ischemic myocardium. The differential effect of coronary occlusion on more superficial and deeper endocardial Purkinje fibers may set up the conditions for microre-entry or reflection.[107] Additionally, afterdepolarizations have been observed in Purkinje fibers exposed to potentially toxic byproducts of ischemia such as lysophosphoglycerides.[108] It is conceivable that injury currents or currents induced by myocardial stretch could induce afterdepolarizations and triggered arrhythmias that originate in the Purkinje fibers. These fibers may also be subject to enhanced automaticity, which is a proposed mechanism of delayed arrhythmias in ischemic myocardium.[109,110]

The Purkinje network may also be important in maintaining malignant ventricular arrhythmias associated with ischemia. Intracavitary application of phenol in a canine model of ischemia prevented the production of ventricular fibrillation, but did not eliminate premature ventricular contractions or slower re-entrant ventricular arrhythmias in the ischemic zone. These data suggest that ectopic activity need not originate in the subendocardial Purkinje system, and that the absence of VF in this model may be related to the failure of re-entrant waves in the ischemic territory to be transmitted throughout the ventricles via the Purkinje network.[111]

Sympathetic nervous system activation plays an important role in the genesis of arrhythmias during myocardial ischemia. Much of the evidence for this assertion is indirect but compelling and includes increased catecholamine levels during ischemia at times when ventricular arrhythmias are most likely,[112] reduction in the frequency and severity of arrhythmias in the presence of denervation or beta-blockade,[50,51] and the arrhythmogenic effects of enhanced sympathetic activity during ischemia[113] The mechanism by which activation of the sympathetic nervous system exerts its effects has not been defined, although many possibilities exist. Catecholamines can restore the resting membrane potential in depolarized ischemic myocardium through K^+ channel-mediated effects[114,115] and enhanced activity of the Na^+–K^+ ATPase.[116] The change in resting membrane potential in the presence of catecholamines will affect other electrophysiological properties such as action potential upstroke and duration. Other potential arrhythmogenic mechanisms are catecholamine-induced increases in the rate of rise of phase 4 diastolic depolarization and similarly induced increases in the amplitude of DADs, important prerequisites for the production of automatic and triggered arrhythmias, respectively.

Chronic arrhythmias that persist for years after myocardial infarction may cause ventricular tachycardia, fibrillation, and sudden cardiac death. Ventricular mapping and the induction and termination of ventricular tachycardia by programmed stimulation suggests that these arrhythmias are re-entrant. The substrate and mechanisms of ventricular tachycardia and ventricular fibrillation in chronic coronary artery disease are fundamentally different from those in acute ischemia, where depressed membrane potentials are a prominent cause of conduction slowing and block. In chronic arrhythmias the substrate consists of viable myocardial cells intermixed with fibrosis, with tissue anisotropy being a major cause of conduction slowing.[74]

The pathogenesis of ventricular fibrillation in chronically ischemic myocardium has been limited by the absence of an animal model with sufficiently high rates of ventricular fibrillation. Recently, Canty and coworkers have demonstrated the importance of hibernating but not infarcted myocardium in the development of VF and SCD in a swine model of coronary artery occlusion. SCD in these animals occurred independently of the severity of LAD stenosis, the presence of myocardial necrosis, or scar.[117] Studies of tissue and cellular electrophysiology demonstrate features that may contribute to SCD, including myocyte hypertrophy,[118] defective SR calcium uptake,[119] interstitial fibrosis, and heterogeneous SNS innervation. Importantly, the diurnal variation of SCD is similar to that observed in humans and seems to be modulated by sympathetic tone. This link may result from inhomogeneity in myocardial repolarization during sympathetic activation, because regional reductions in presynaptic norepinephrine uptake are found in hibernating myocardium.[120] These changes may be germane to human studies, which have demonstrated that revascularization has a positive effect on mortality in patients with chronic ischemia.

Studies in humans have provided insight into the pathogenesis of conduction slowing in hibernating myocardium. In biopsy samples taken from chronically ischemic, functionally downregulated ventricular myocardium, as assessed by thallium scanning and MR imaging, biopsy samples from hibernating, reversibly ischemic, and normal myocardium exhibited significant differences in the

density of Cx43, a major intercellular ion channel in the ventricle and an important mediator of cell-to-cell conduction. In addition to decrease in density, the morphology of GJ plaques on immunohistochemical staining changes with a reduction in the plaque size.[121]

Ventricular fibrillation in cardiomyopathy

The mechanism of sudden death and ventricular arrhythmias is less certain in non-ischemic cardiomyopathy, but recent evidence suggests abnormal repolarization of the ventricle may be important. Myocardial cells possess a characteristically long action potential (Fig. 6.4): after an initial rapid upstroke, there is a plateau of maintained

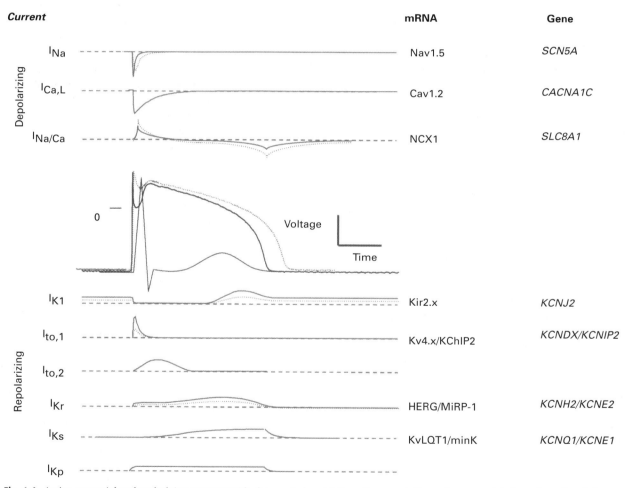

Fig. 6.4. Action potential and underlying currents with changes in heart failure. Representative action potentials from the epicardial surface of a normal (thick line) and failing (dotted line) ventricle. The surface QRST complex is shown overlying the action potentials. The left hand column shows the currents that underlie the ventricular action potential. The right hand columns are the message and gene names for the major subunits that encode the currents. Schematics of the trajectories of the currents during the action potential are shown in the center of the slide, the thick lines represent the normal currents and the dotted lines the currents in failing hearts.

depolarization before repolarization. In cells from failing hearts, animal and human studies consistently reveal a significant prolongation of action potentials compared to those in normal hearts, independent of the mechanism of heart failure.[122–125] The plateau of the action potential is known to be quite labile; this is a time of high membrane resistance, during which small changes in current can easily tip the balance either towards repolarization or towards maintained depolarization. As a rule, the longer the action potential, the more labile is the repolarization process. Maintained or secondary depolarizations that occur before termination of the action potential called early after depolarizations (EADs) can initiate arrhythmias including torsades des pointes ventricular tachycardia and ventricular fibrillation (Fig. 6.5). A variety of conditions common in patients with heart failure can affect either outward (repolarizing) or inward (depolarizing) currents resulting in EADs. Such factors include hypokalemia, hypocalcemia, hypomagnesemia, acidosis, or antiarrhythmic drugs. Increasing inward current will also favor the production of EAD-mediated triggered activity, as might occur with β-adrenergic stimulation or after endogenous release of lipid metabolites that interfere with Na[+] channel inactivation.[126] Stretch-responsive channels have been described in ventricular myocardium[127,128] and proposed to contribute to EADs and enhanced susceptibility to arrhythmia in heart failure.[129]

The ability to isolate viable human ventricular myocytes has enabled the dissection of the changes in membrane current that occur in myocardial failure. The inward Na[+] and Ca[2+] currents do not appear to be altered, at least under basal conditions. Sakaibara et al.[130] found no disease-related changes in gating or permeation of Na[+] currents in human ventricular cells. Measurement of both dihydropyridine binding sites[131] and inward Ca[2+] current in ventricular myocytes from failing hearts also reveal no differences compared to non-failing control cells.[124,132] Nevertheless, there are reports of changes in Ca[2+] channel gating in failing ventricular myocytes,[133] perhaps mediated by changes in auxiliary subunit expression.[134] Human ventricular myocytes contain at least two distinct classes of voltage-dependent K[+] channels. The inward rectifier K[+] current, I_{K1}, sets the resting membrane potential and contributes to the terminal phase of repolarization. The density of I_{K1} is reduced by nearly 40% in cells from myopathic ventricles compared with controls.[125] Another important K[+] current is the transient outward current, I_{to}. Unlike the inward rectifier, I_{to} is expressed in heart cells in a species- and cell type-specific fashion. This current plays a crucial role in the early phases of repolarization and in setting the potential of the plateau of the action potential, which in turn influences all currents

that are active during the remainder of the action potential. Ventricular myocytes from the mid-portion of the ventricular wall have a substantial I_{to} that is blocked by 4-aminopyridine (4-AP). This 4-AP-sensitive current is also significantly reduced (35%–40%) in cells from failing ventricles.[125] Similar changes in I_{to} have been noted in diseased human atria,[135] chronically infarcted canine ventricle,[136] and hypertrophied rat ventricle,[137] all of which are arrhythmogenic substrates. Prolongation of the action potential alone would not necessarily suffice to produce ventricular arrhythmias, particularly if the prolongation were homogeneous. Variations in APD in the failing heart, however, create increases in the dispersion of repolarization and refractoriness that are arrhythmogenic.[138,139] Regional differences in the density of K[+] currents, particularly I_{to}, have been described in several experimental animal models.[140] Spatial inhomogeneity of repolarization in heart failure may be explained by exaggerated regional variability in K[+] currents; however, the role that functional downregulation of K[+] currents plays in potentiating the spatial dispersion of repolarization in heart failure is controversial. For example, in rapid-pacing canine heart failure, induced by rapid pacing, transmural K[+] currents such as I_{K1}, I_{to1}, and the slow component of the delayed rectifier K[+] current (I_{Ks}) were

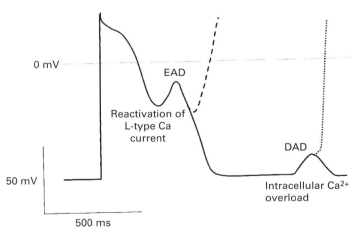

Fig. 6.5. Interruptions of repolarization called afterdepolarizations may mediate the initiation of polymorphic ventricular tachycardia and ventricular fibrillation. Early afterdepolarizations (EADs) occur before the completion of repolarization and result from reactivation of L-type calcium current during phase 3 of the action potential. Delayed afterdepolarizations (DADs) occur after completion of repolarization and result from oscillatory release of calcium from the sarcoplasmic reticulum with activation of depolarizing currents. If either EADs or DADs are of sufficient amplitude a subsequent action potential may ensue ("triggered" action potential).

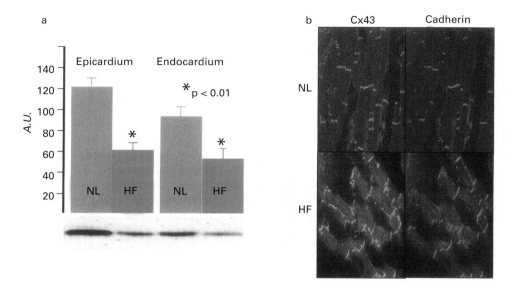

Fig. 6.6. Decreased expression and redistribution of Cx43 protein in the failing heart. (a) Western blot shows a reduction in Cx43 protein in the failing heart (HF) in both the endocardial and epicardial regions of the left ventricle compared with normal heart (NL). (b) Immunohistochemical staining demonstrates redistribution of Cx43 from the cell ends to the lateral margins of the cell. Cx43 co-localizes with the intercalated disc protein N-cadherin in the normal but not the failing ventricle. Modified from Akar *et al.*[151] reproduced with permission. (See Plate 6.6.)

homogeneously decreased across the left ventricular wall.[141] Other ionic currents contribute to repolarization in the heart; alterations in Ca^{2+} handling have electrogenic consequences that may contribute to temporally and spatially labile repolarization. In the same heart failure model, transmural NCX currents were most prominently increased in endocardial myocytes but were not changed in the epicardial cells,[142] disrupting the transmural heterogeneity of NCX and potentially leading to enhanced vulnerability to cardiac arrhythmias. Another plausible contributor involves the influence of the autonomic nervous system, which has a prominent role in heart failure. Additionally, heterogeneity of sympathetic nervous system innervation is well-described in cardiomyopathy patients[143] and has been correlated with heterogeneity of recovery of excitability.[144]

Abnormalities of APD and afterdepolarizations may produce arrhythmias by triggered mechanisms or may predispose the myocardium to re-entry by inhomogeneous changes in APD and dispersion of refractoriness.[145] Spontaneous ventricular tachycardia in a rabbit model of non-ischemic heart failure was attributed to repetitive non-re-entrant activation at subendocardial sites.[146] Furthermore, in patients with end-stage idiopathic cardiomyopathy, spontaneous and induced ventricular arrhythmias occur primarily in the subendocardium by a focal non-re-entrant mechanism, which may result from EADs or DADs.[147]

Significant changes in the network properties of the heart characterize heart failure. In particular, conduction velocity slowing is a prominent feature of the failing ventricle and restitution of conduction is altered (Fig. 6.6). In some models of HF, reductions in Na current density contribute to conduction slowing.[148] Fibrosis is characteristic of human and a number of animal models of heart failure contributing to conduction slowing and block.[149,150] Intercellular ion channels are also remodeled in the failing heart. This remodeling includes a downregulation of Cx43 and aberrations in the subcellular location of the channel, with increased expression on the lateral cell borders (Fig. 6.6). Morphological changes in gap junctions have been described. All of these changes are associated with profound regional changes in conduction in the failing compared with the normal heart. (Fig. 6.7)[151]

Experimental evidence supporting re-entry for initiation of arrhythmias in non-ischemic cardiomyopathy is scarce, even in settings where inhomogeneities of APD or refractoriness have been defined.[152,153] The failure of programmed stimulation of the ventricle in either animal models or humans also argues against an excitable-gap re-entry mechanism for ventricular arrhythmia production in non-ischemic cardiomyopathy. This does not preclude the possibility that VF due to multiple wavelet re-entry is induced by other mechanisms in cardiomyopathy.

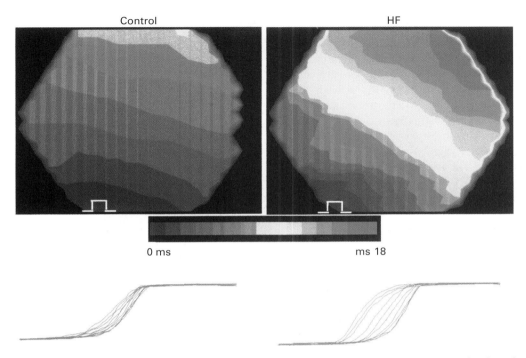

Fig. 6.7. Slowed conduction in the failing heart. Optical maps from wedges of left ventricular myocardium stained with a voltage-sensitive dye. Isochronal maps reveal crowding of isochronal lines in the failing tissue preparation. Below the maps are the upstrokes of the action potentials from several regions in the imaging window; the separation of the upstrokes confirms the conduction slowing in the failing heart. (See Plate 6.7.)

Ventricular fibrillation is less well studied in hypertrophic cardiomyopathy (HCM) but clinical data support a strong association between left ventricular hypertrophy and ventricular arrhythmias and sudden death. As has just been outlined for dilated cardiomyopathy, abnormalities in refractoriness and repolarization are important in arrhythmogenesis in this form of heart disease. Experimental animal models of hypertrophic heart disease have demonstrated an increase in duration of action potentials and, more important, an increase in spatial dispersion of repolarization, without significant changes in impulse conduction.[153] In the dog model with chronic complete atrioventricular block (AVB), there is biventricular hypertrophy.[154] Although systolic function is maintained during 9 weeks of AVB, the APD of the left, but not the right, ventricle is significantly prolonged in chronic AVB compared to that of the control, thereby leading to increased interventricular dispersion of repolarization that is particularly prominent at slow pacing rates. This model is more susceptible to torsades de pointes (TdP), which are associated with increased dispersion of repolarization, afterdepolarizations, and triggered arrhythmias.[154,155] In the heart with biventricular hypertrophy, the slow component of delayed rectifier K^+ current, I_{Ks}, is downregulated[156] and NCX is upregulated.[157] The changes in dispersion of repolarization have been associated with lower ventricular fibrillation thresholds, and both the dispersion of repolarization and reduction in ventricular fibrillation threshold were reversed with K^+ channel antagonists.[153] Patients with primary hypertrophic cardiomyopathy have also been reported to have dispersion and inhomogeneity of conduction, which has been attributed to the histologic disarray of myofibrils in this disease.[158] Inhomogeneities of both repolarization and conduction would be expected to increase the risk of potential lethal arrhythmias in patients with HCM.

Ventricular fibrillation in normal hearts

Re-entry may be initiated by electrical stimulation of normal myocardium, producing fibrillation. In many pathophysiological circumstances, heterogeneous recovery of excitability occurs and may enhance ventricular vulnerability, particularly in the earlier phases of recovery.

It has been demonstrated recently, however, that inhomogeneous dispersion of refractoriness or recovery is not a necessary precondition for electrical induction of VF in normal myocardium.[159,160] In a normal canine heart an appropriately timed suprathreshold stimulus can generate re-entry around a critical point where the field of the stimulus intersects myocardium in the terminal phases of recovery.[160] High density mapping in the region of the stimulus confirmed the presence of a re-entry circuit in the shape of a figure-of-eight prior to the development of VF. These data suggest that regions of the myocardium that are adjacent to the area directly depolarized by the suprathreshold stimulus are not activated, but undergo a graded prolongation of their refractory period.[161] This establishes functional unidirectional conduction block in normal tissue with homogeneous dispersion of refractoriness, a mechanism that may be operative in ventricular fibrillation that is the result of electrical injury.[159]

Inhomogeneities in recovery may exist in normal myocardium, particularly at the junction of ventricular muscle and the specialized conducting system, tissues that have well documented differences in APD that are exaggerated by premature stimulation.[162] Mapping during suprathreshold extrastimulation failed to reveal any participation of the Purkinje fiber network in this model of initiation of ventricular fibrillation, although participation of the specialized conducting system in the maintenance of ventricular fibrillation or its initiation in other models certainly cannot be excluded.[159]

These studies have important implications for the mechanism of initiation of fibrillation, but similarly they also suggest explanations for the concept of the upper limit of vulnerability,[163] and postshock reinitiation of fibrillation as a cause of failed defibrillation.[164] A shock strength above the upper limit of vulnerability will not induce ventricular fibrillation regardless of when it is delivered in the cardiac cycle. The upper limit of vulnerability tends to move in parallel with the defibrillation threshold. Although many electrophysiological mechanisms exist to explain the initiation and maintenance of ventricular fibrillation, the exact mechanism(s) in a given clinical situation are generally unknown. It is most likely that several of the potential offending conditions conspire to produce fibrillation in humans. Using high-resolution optical mapping and computer simulations, Jalife and colleagues[17,18,165,166] have suggested that, in the structurally normal heart, monomorphic ventricular tachycardia results from stationary rotors, but polymorphic ventricular tachycardia and ventricular fibrillation are caused by a single or paired ("figure-of-eight") non-stationary rotors.

Primary electrical diseases of the heart

Fortunately, sustained ventricular tachycardia and ventricular fibrillation rarely occur in structurally normal human hearts; however, primary electrical diseases of the heart such as long[167] and short QT syndromes,[168] catecholaminergic polymorphic VT(CPVT),[169] and Brugada syndrome[170,171] are associated with life-threatening ventricular arrhythmias. (See Chapter 52 for additional discussion of primary electrical diseases of the heart.)

The long QT syndrome is characterized by the prolonged QT interval on the surface ECG, frequent episodes of syncope, and a high incidence of sudden death resulting from ventricular tachycardias especially TDP. There are two clinical forms of congenital long QT syndrome: the Romano–Ward syndrome[172,173] is transmitted as an autosomal dominant trait, and the Jervell and Lange–Nielsen syndrome[174] as an autosomal recessive trait, associated with sensoneurinal deafness. Romano-Ward syndrome is associated with gene mutations of different channels: LQT1(*KCNQ1* encoding KvLQT1), LQT2 (*KCNH2* encoding HERG), LQT3 (*SCN5A*), LQT5 (KCNE1), and LQT6 (*KCNE2*) generates mutants I_{Ks}, I_{Kr}, I_{Na}, mink (combined with KvLQT1 generates I_{Ks}), and MiRP1 (combined with HERG generates I_{Kr}), respectively.[167,175–180] The Jervell and Lange-Nielsen syndrome is very rare and almost exclusively linked to I_{Ks}. The delayed activation or incomplete inactivation of the Na^+ channel or reduction in function of K^+ channels is responsible for the prolonged QT interval. Acquired forms of LQTS are far more common than congenital forms. Acquired LQTS may occur in subjects with subclinical inherited mutations in cardiac ion channels often made clinically manifest by extrinsic factors such as exposure to drugs, structural heart disesase, or electrolyte abnormalities. Certain drugs, such as Class IA and III antiarrhythmics, antihistamines, antimicrobials, and antifungals can alter cardiac ion channel function and/or interfere with the metabolism of other drugs that impair repolarization, resulting in prolongation of the QT intervals and increased risk of sudden death. The short QT syndrome (SQTS) is a more recently described clinical entity characterized by the presence of a short QT interval (QTc < 320 ms) associated with cardiac tachyarrhythmias, syncope, and sudden death. It has been linked to mutations in I_{Kr}, I_{Ks}, and I_{K1} (encoded by *KCNJ2*).[168,181–183] It has been speculated that the arrhythmogenic mechanism is related to heterogeneous abbreviation of the APD and significant transmural dispersion of repolarization setting the stage for ventricular fibrillation.

Catecholaminergic polymorphic ventricular tachycardia (CPVT) is an early-onset, inherited and malignant arrhythmogenic disorder characterized by exercise- or stress-induced ventricular arrhythmias in the absence of structural alterations of the heart. This disorder has been linked to mutations of the *RyR2* (cardiac ryanodine receptor gene)[184,185] and *CASQ2* (calsequestrin gene)[186,187] with autosomal dominant and recessive transmission, respectively. The precise molecular pathogenesis of CPVT is not entirely clear, but it is associated with a leaky RyR2 channel due to a defect in binding to its associated protein FKBP12.6 (calstabin 2) or impaired sarcoplasmic reticulum Ca^{2+} storage.

Brugada syndrome is an autosomal dominant form of idiopathic ventricular fibrillation characterized by ST-segment elevation in right precordial leads V1 to V3 and often with apparent right bundle-branch block.[170,171] The distribution of Brugada syndrome is worldwide, but it is particularly prominent in southeast Asia where it accounts for a significant minority of sudden deaths in the young. Causative mutations have been discovered in the alpha subunit of the cardiac sodium channel gene *SCN5A*.[188] Since the original description, numerous other *SCN5A* mutations have been described. There are other cohorts that are not linked to SCN5A, consistent with genetic heterogeneity of the syndrome.[189] The disease-causing mutations generally result in a loss of function or reduced sodium current due to accelerated inactivation of the sodium channel.

Therapy of ventricular fibrillation

Therapeutic interventions in the management of ventricular fibrillation can be divided into those designed to prevent the arrhythmia or those designed to treat established fibrillation. Strategies to prevent ventricular fibrillation include preventing triggers for induction of fibrillation and reducing the tendency of the myocardium to fibrillate, thus raising the ventricular fibrillation threshold. Treatment of established ventricular fibrillation is prompt defibrillation, most often requiring the delivery of a transthoracic or transmyocardial shock of sufficient strength to terminate the fibrillation.

In communities with the best emergency medical services, survival rates for patients with out-of-hospital ventricular fibrillation is only 25%–33%,[3] emphasizing the importance of identifying patients at risk and implementing strategies to prevent this problem. The only definitive treatment of ventricular fibrillation is expeditious defibrillation. Failing this, efforts should be made to protect the fibrillating myocardium by limiting the adverse metabolic consequences of ongoing fibrillation.

Prevention of ventricular fibrillation

One of the most common circumstances in which ventricular fibrillation is encountered and effectively treated is acute myocardial infarction. Since the inception of the coronary care unit, a major emphasis of the management of the acute myocardial infarction patient has been prevention or prompt treatment of lethal ventricular arrhythmias. The early observation of frequent ventricular arrhythmias complicating acute myocardial infarction[190] and the effectiveness of intravenous lidocaine in prevention of these arrhythmias led to the widespread use of prophylactic lidocaine in this and many other clinical settings. More recent data call into question this approach. Meta-analyses of the use of prophylactic lidocaine in acute MI do support a reduction in the incidence of ventricular tachyarrhythmias, but patients treated with lidocaine experienced a slightly increased overall mortality.[191,192] Another meta-analysis of the incidence of primary ventricular fibrillation complicating acute MI revealed a steep decline in the incidence of fibrillation over the past three decades; indeed, the incidence of primary ventricular fibrillation in 1990 was so low that it was estimated that 400 patients would have to be treated with lidocaine to prevent a single episode.[193] The reason for the decline in ventricular fibrillation is not clear and may be related to several factors, including the more widespread use of beta-blocking drugs, aggressive correction of electrolyte abnormalities, the use of thrombolytic agents, early percutaneous coronary interventions for revascularization, more liberal use of analgesics, and less restrictive criteria for entry into a coronary care unit. Regardless of the etiology of the reduced incidence of ventricular fibrillation, these data make the routine use of lidocaine in acute myocardial infarction an unsupportable strategy.[191–193] The only agents thus far shown both to reduce the incidence of ventricular fibrillation and mortality in acute myocardial infarction are the beta-adrenergic blocking drugs.[50,194]

The problem of prevention of ventricular fibrillation and sudden death in the absence of an acute myocardial infarction has proven to be intractable. Among the many reasons for our inability to prevent sudden death in patients with heart disease, are an incomplete understanding of the mechanism of sudden death, inability to risk-stratify patients accurately, and the limited efficacy of pharmacotherapy for prevention of ventricular tachyarrhythmias. A review of the all the clinical and diagnostic tools available to risk-stratify patients is beyond the scope of this chapter. The evaluation of patients with cardiovascular disease who are at risk must be individualized, and implicit in this statement is a thorough understanding of the nature and extent of heart disease in a given patient. In patients with coronary artery disease the most consistent indicator of risk of mortality is left ventricular dysfunction.[195,196] The role of other diagnostic procedures remains controversial in patients who have not experienced an arrhythmic event but are considered to be at risk. The signal averaged electrocardiogram (SAECG) is a method of identifying low amplitude signals at the body surface by averaging many time-aligned ECG complexes. The SAECG can identify regions of slowed conduction that are manifest as "late potentials" or a prolonged signal-averaged QRS duration. These abnormalities of conduction are indicative of the presence of the substrate for ventricular tachyarrhythmias, but have a low positive predictive value.[197–199] The role of electrophysiological testing is also unclear; inducible ventricular tachycardia in patients with non-sustained ventricular tachycardia and reduced left ventricular function identifies a group of patients at high risk for sudden death, but even in this group the positive predictive value of electrophysiologic testing is low (20%–30%).[200,201] Risk stratification is more problematic in the absence of coronary artery disease, although recent reports of the utility of the SAECG have identified patients at risk in one series, although the predictive value of a positive test is low.[202] Even if risk stratification were optimized, there are very few clincal situations where ventricular fibrillation can be effectively prevented. In the case of ventricular fibrillation associated with coronary artery disease, attempts at prevention of sudden death by using antiarrhythmic drugs have been a dismal failure thus far. The hypothesis tested by the Cardiac Arrhythmia Suppression Trial,[59,60] that is, prevention of premature ventricular contractions will prevent ventricular tachycardia and fibrillation and thus reduce sudden death in patients with a prior myocardial infarction, was not only unproven, but patients treated with the agents used in this trial had an increased mortality. Either the hypothesis is faulty or the agents used in this study were not well chosen in that they reduced the frequency of less malignant ventricular arrhythmias but increased the $$ prevalence of more serious or compromising arrhythmias. The only drugs at present that have been shown to reduce the mortality after myocardial infarction are beta-blockers.[50,51] The mechanism by which these drugs reduce mortality is unknown, but at the concentrations used in the postmyocardial infarction trials they do not have substantial local anesthetic antiarrhythmic effects. The actions of beta-blockers that are relevant to prevention of sudden death and ventricular fibrillation include prevention of

ischemia, antagonism of serum catecholamine effects on the heart, prevention of catecholamine-induced platelet aggregation, hemodynamic improvement, and restoration of inhibitory GTP-binding protein levels in heart failure patients.[52] Studies examining the effect of antiarrhythmics such as amiodarone on mortality in the postinfarction period have revealed mixed results; a meta-analysis of the major trials of amiodarone suggests an overall reduction in mortality by the drug in post-MI and HF patients,[203] which contrasts with most other antiarrhythmic drugs that have at best a neutral effect on overall mortality in this setting.

Other clinical circumstances where effective preventive strategies exist in the management of ventricular fibrillation include the use of calcium channel antagonists in coronary vasospasm,[204] left stellate ganglion resection or beta-blockers and pacing in the long QT syndrome,[43,44] and catheter or surgical ablation of rapidly conducting manifest accessory pathways in the Wolff-Parkinson-White syndrome.[42] In the absence of effective prevention of ventricular fibrillation, implantable defibrillators are the best therapeutic option in the high-risk patient.

Patients resuscitated from ventricular fibrillation in the absence of an acute transmural myocardial infarction[205] are at high risk for recurrence of this arrhythmia and sudden death.[206–208] The evaluation of these patients should be directed at determining the etiology of sudden death and the nature and extent of any underlying heart disease. In the majority of cases a standard cardiac evaluation is supplemented by cardiac catheterization with coronary angiography and left ventriculography and electrophysiologic study. Therapy is individualized based on the evaluation; for example, patients with ischemia, no inducible ventricular arrhythmias, and retained left ventricular function may be treated with surgical myocardial revascularization alone.[209–211] Patients who have an inducible tachycardia may require therapy directed at the arrhythmic substrate such as surgical ablation, antiarrhythmic drugs, or implantation of a cardioverter-defibrillator.[212]

Recently the identification and ablation of triggers for VF has proven to be an effective strategy in selected patients.[213–218] In patients with structurally normal hearts, ventricular fibrillation and monomorphic ventricular premature beats with fixed coupling intervals, localization by endocardial mapping, and ablation eliminated the premature beats and ventricular fibrillation.[213] Similar reports in patients with LQTS and Brugada syndrome[215] and recurrent ventricular fibrillation postmyocardial infarction[217] have appeared.

Defibrillation

Definitive treatment of ventricular fibrillation requires timely correction of the arrhythmia by delivery of an electrical shock to the heart. Defibrillation has been utilized clinically for decades, but its mechanism remains obscure. Recent advances, in particular the refinement of voltage mapping with optical dyes, has allowed the study of electrical events immediately after a shock to the heart. Several hypotheses on the mechanism of defibrillation have been elaborated. The critical mass hypothesis states that defibrillation is achieved when a critical mass of myocardium is depolarized by the shock, and activation waves are extinguished. In such circumstances, the critical mass is considered to be about 75% of the ventricular myocardium[219] and unsuccessful defibrillation results from a failure to depolarize a sufficient amount of the fibrillating myocardium. Alternatively, the observation of an isoelectric window or period of electrical silence, and a different pattern of ventricular activation in the postshock period has suggested that failed defibrillation may be the result of reinitiation of fibrillation by the defibrillating shock.[164] This theory of defibrillation states that in order to defibrillate the myocardium reliably, the shock strength must exceed the upper limit of vulnerability throughout the myocardium. The upper limit of vulnerability is that shock strength above which fibrillation cannot be induced regardless of when it is delivered during the cardiac cycle. The correlation between the defibrillation threshold and the upper limit of vulnerability in animal models,[220] and the similar pattern of ventricular activation after failed defibrillation or when shocks below the upper limit of vulnerability are delivered during sinus rhythm, are in direct support of this hypothesis.[164] In either case, delivery of an insufficient amount of energy will result in failure to terminate or reinitiation of ventricular fibrillation. This is to be distinguished from the ventricular fibrillation threshold, which is irrelevant in ongoing fibrillation, and is the energy necessary to induce the arrhythmia in the non-fibrillating myocardium. Another hypothesis of the mechanism of defibrillation that has recently gained traction is the virtual electrode polarization hypothesis (VEP).[221,222] The VEP hypothesis states that monophasic shocks to the myocardium result in depolarization and repolarization of adjacent regions of the heart. If the voltage gradient between these regions is optimal, activation wavefronts from the depolarized regions may activate the hyperpolarized regions leading to re-entry and re-initiation of ventricular fibrillation.[221] Adjacent areas of differentially polarized myocardium create phase singularities, a tissue substrate for the initiation of functional re-entry.[222] The

unifying requirements for successful defibrillation according to any of these hypotheses are that the shock must be of sufficient strength to extinguish fibrillation and must not generate a new arrhythmia.

The energy required to defibrillate the heart reliably depends on many factors, including the nature of the shocking waveform, the configuration of the defibrillating electrodes, the duration of ventricular fibrillation, and the presence and extent of underlying heart disease. Many other variables that have not been well-characterized may also influence the energy requirement for defibrillation. Motivated by the development of automatic internal defibrillators, the duration of fibrillation and the effect of subthreshold shocks on the ability to defibrillate the heart have been closely examined. Data in humans are scarce, particularly for patients who experience out-of-hospital ventricular fibrillation. Studies that have attempted to evaluate the effect of the duration of ventricular fibrillation on resuscitation have generally shown that survival is worse if fibrillation is of longer duration[223] and if the electrocardiographic appearance of fibrillation is "finer" on the ECG.[224] The success of transthoracic defibrillation in patients experiencing in-hospital cardiac arrest was improved with shorter delays to defibrillation and in the absence of hypoxia and acidosis.[225] More recently such studies have been extended to defibrillation by internal defibrillating systems.

Several notable advances in clinical defibrillation have been made in recent decades. Biphasic waveforms have been shown to be superior to monophasic waveforms in reducing the energy requirement for defibrillation.[226–230] Biphasic waveforms with lower energies provide the additional benefit of reducing postshock myocardial dysfunction and improving cerebral perfusion.[231–233] Public access defibrillation programs improve the outcomes of patients with out-of-hospital cardiac arrest.[234,235] The automated external defibrillator (AED), which can automatically analyze cardiac rhythms, has been an important component of public access defibrillation initiatives.[236,237]

The development and clinical utilization of the internal cardioverter defibrillator (ICD) has dramatically altered the management of patients who survive episodes of sudden death secondary to ventricular tachyarrhythmias.[238] The ICD provides a mechanism for correction of potentially lethal ventricular arrhythmias, regardless of the underlying cause. In view of the limitations in our ability to prevent ventricular tachycardia and fibrillation and sudden death recurrences in patients with structural heart disease, the importance of this therapeutic modality is difficult to overstate. Since their development, ICDs have become more versatile with the ability to pace, cardiovert, defibrillate, and resynchronize cardiac contraction. The increase in versatility has made these devices more complex and has increased the possibility that definitive therapy for ventricular fibrillation could be delayed by attempts at antitachycardia pacing and low energy cardioversion. In general, the longer the duration of ventricular fibrillation, the greater the energy required for defibrillation, both in experimental animals[239] and humans.[240–242] This effect of the delay to defibrillation shock delivery is less important with shock energies near the maximal output of implanted defibrillators (30–35 J) and with times to shock delivery that are within 30 seconds of the onset of ventricular fibrillation.[240,242]

A major confounding influence on the efficacy of defibrillation is the use of antiarrhythmic drugs. The effects of these agents have been studied in both animal models and humans with implanted defibrillators. There is not a consistent correlation between the animal and human data and conflicting results with use of the same preparation and different experimental conditions complicate the interpretation of these results. The assumption that any antiarrhythmic agent can adversely affect the defibrillation threshold is prudent. Despite the variance in the data, several consistent effects of certain antiarrhythmic agents on defibrillation energy have been observed. Sodium-channel-blocking drugs, particularly those with slower unblocking kinetics (i.e., class IC effects) such as flecainide and propafenone will raise both defibrillation and pacing threshold energy requirements,[243–245] and chronically administered amiodarone has similar effects.[246–248] Studies in an anesthetized canine model suggest that agents that block Na^+ channels without a substantial effect on the action potential duration (e.g., lidocaine, mexiletine, tocainide) tend to increase the energy requirements for defibrillation; conversely, agents that prolong the APD tend to decrease this energy.[249] There are no systematic studies in humans to support this hypothesis, but anecdotal reports of increases in defibrillation requirements by Na^+ channel-blocking drugs do not contradict this paradigm.[247,248,250,251]

In addition to successful defibrillation, successful resuscitation is determined by the recovery of spontaneous circulation. Until defibrillation is possible, artificial support of the circulation is the essential goal of CPR. Several clinical studies have shown that the likelihood of successful termination of ventricular fibrillation and survival is inversely related to the duration of cardiac arrest.[252–254] The importance of CPR in improving the aortic-right atrial pressure gradient and therefore coronary perfusion has been demonstrated in several animal models of cardiac arrest.[255–257]

The improvement of coronary blood flow in these studies has been associated with improved efficacy of resuscitation.[255–257] The issue of what is "optimal" CPR, the role of chest compressions prior to defibrillation during prolonged arrests, and advanced life support is discussed elsewhere in this volume.

The typical clinical situation of out-of-hospital cardiac arrest does afford the possibility of prompt defibrillation; in most cases patients have had no circulatory support during prolonged ventricular fibrillation. Immediate defibrillation in this circumstance terminates ventricular fibrillation, but often asystole or electromechanical dissociation follows the shock and is associated with a very high mortality.[258–260] More recent data suggest that after prolonged unsupported ventricular fibrillation, administration of epinephrine and CPR may improve the chances of defibrillation to a life-sustaining rhythm.[261]

Conclusions and future directions

Ventricular fibrillation is the most common cause of sudden cardiac death. If untreated, this arrhythmia is rapidly and uniformly fatal. There are many factors that predispose to VF in patients with structural heart disease, but our ability to identify patients who will experience VF is limited. In the absence of effective pharmacotherapy to prevent VF the only reliable treatment strategy is prompt defibrillation. In the patients at highest risk this is performed automatically by the internal cardioverter defibrillator. It is likely that in the near term these devices will be used more frequently in patients at high-risk, particularly with the recent introduction of non-thoracotomy defibrillating lead systems and the development of smaller, pectorally implanted pulse generators. Further refinements including the development of "leadless" defibrillators may further reduce the risk of implantation, but at the cost of some limitations in the therapeutic flexibility of these devices. The ICD is likely to be the mainstay of therapy of ventricular fibrillation until our strategies for defining who is at greatest risk of developing it are more complete.

Our understanding of the mechanism of the initiation and perpetuation of ventricular fibrillation has been advanced by elegant mapping studies and more recently, investigation of the molecular participants in this arrhythmia has complemented the mapping data. Despite this, our understanding of ventricular fibrillation is quite rudimentary and more complete elucidation of the basic mechanisms of ventricular fibrillation has the potential benefit of the development of preventive and treatment strategies, as well as more effective protection of the heart in fibrillation.

REFERENCES

1. Zheng, Z.J., Croft, J.B., Giles, W.H., & Mensah, G.A. Sudden cardiac death in the United States, 1989 to 1998. *Circulation* 2001; **104**: 2158–2163.
2. Surawicz, B. Ventricular fibrillation. *J. Am. Coll. Cardiol.* 1985; **5**: 43B–54B.
3. Cobb, L.A., Weaver, W.D., Fahrenbruch, C.E., Hallstrom, A.P., & Copass, M.K. Community-based interventions for sudden cardiac death. Impact, limitations, and changes. *Circulation* 1992; **85**: 198–102.
4. Cobb, L.A., Fahrenbruch, C.E., Olsufka, M., & Copass, M.K. Changing incidence of out-of-hospital ventricular fibrillation, 1980–2000. *J. Am. Med. Assoc.* 2002; **288**: 3008–3013.
5. Myerburg, R.J., Kessler, K.M., Estes, D. *et al.* Long-term survival after prehospital cardiac arrest: analysis of outcome during an 8 year study. *Circulation* 1984; **70**: 538–546.
6. Wiggers, C. The mechanism and nature of ventricular fibrillation. *Am. Heart J.* 1940; **20**: 399–412.
7. Porter, W. Recovery of the heart from fibrillary contractions. *Am. J. Physiol.* 1898; **1**: 71–82.
8. Garrey, W. The nature of fibrillatory contraction of the heart. Its relation to tissue mass and form. *Am. J. Physiol.* 1914; **33**: 397–414.
9. Hooker, D., & Kehar, D. Carbohydrate metabolism of the heart during ventricular fibrillation. *Am. J. Physiol.* 1933; **105**: 246–249.
10. Zipes, D.P. Mechanisms of clinical arrhythimas. *J. Cardiovasc. Electrophysiol.* 2003; **14**: 902–912.
11. Jalife, J., & Berenfeld, O. Molecular mechanisms and global dynamics of fibrillation: an integrative approach to the underlying basis of vortex-like reentry. *J. Theor. Biol.* 2004; **230**: 475–487.
12. Mines, G. On circulating excitations in heart muscels and their possible relation to tachycardia and fibrillation. *Trans. R. Soc. Can.* 1914; **4**: 43–52.
13. Moe, G. On the multiple wavelet hypothesis of atrial fibrillation. *Arch. Int. Pharmacodyn.CXL.* 1962: 183–188.
14. Moe, G.K., Rheinboldt, W.C., & Abildskov, J.A. A Computer Model of Atrial Fibrillation. *Am. Heart J.* 1964; **67**: 200–220.
15. Allessie, M., Lammers, W.E.J.E.P., Bonke, F.I.M., & Hollen, J. Experimental evaluation of Moe's multiple wavelet hypothesis of atrial fibrillation. In Zipes, D.P. JJ, ed. *Cardiac Electrophysiology and Arrhythmias.* Orlando, FL: Grune & Stratton, 1985: 265–275.
16. Witkowski, F.X., Leon, L.J., Penkoske, P.A. *et al.* Spatiotemporal evolution of ventricular fibrillation. *Nature* 1998; **392**: 78–82.
17. Gray, R.A., Jalife, J., Panfilov, A. *et al.* Nonstationary vortexlike reentrant activity as a mechanism of polymorphic ventricular tachycardia in the isolated rabbit heart. *Circulation* 1995; **91**: 2454–2469.
18. Gray, R.A., Jalife, J., Panfilov, A.V. *et al.* Mechanisms of cardiac fibrillation. *Science* 1995; **270**: 1222–1223; author reply 1224–1225.
19. Garfinkel, A., Kim, Y.H., Voroshilovsky, O. *et al.* Preventing ventricular fibrillation by flattening cardiac restitution. *Proc. Natl Acad. Sci. USA* 2000; **97**: 6061–6066.
20. Weiss, J.N., Chen, P.S., Wu, T.J., Siegerman, C., & Garfinkel, A. Ventricular fibrillation: new insights into mechanisms. *Ann. NY Acad. Sci.* 2004; **1015**: 122–132.
21. Zhou, X., Guse, P., Wolf, P.D., Rollins, D.L., Smith, W.M., & Ideker, R.E. Existence of both fast and slow channel activity during the early stages of ventricular fibrillation. *Circ. Res.* 1992; **70**: 773–786.
22. Akiyama, T. Intracellular recording of in situ ventricular cells during ventricular fibrillation. *Am. J. Physiol.* 1981; **240**: H465–H471.
23. Merillat, J.C., Lakatta, E.G., Hano, O., & Guarnieri, T. Role of calcium and the calcium channel in the initiation and maintenance of ventricular fibrillation. *Circ. Res.* 1990; **67**: 1115–1123.
24. Warren, M., Guha, P.K., Berenfeld, O. *et al.* Blockade of the inward rectifying potassium current terminates ventricular fibrillation in the guinea pig heart. *J. Cardiovasc. Electrophysiol.* 2003; **14**: 621–631.
25. Samie, F.H., Berenfeld, O., Anumonwo, J. *et al.* Rectification of the background potassium current: a determinant of rotor dynamics in ventricular fibrillation. *Circ. Res.* 2001; **89**: 1216–1223.
26. Choi, B.R., Liu, T., & Salama, G. The distribution of refractory periods influences the dynamics of ventricular fibrillation. *Circ. Res.* 2001; **88**: E49–E58.
27. Rogers, J.M., Huang, J., Melnick, S.B., & Ideker, R.E. Sustained reentry in the left ventricle of fibrillating pig hearts. *Circ. Res.* 2003; **92**: 539–545.
28. Valderrabano, M., Yang, J., Omichi, C., *et al.* Frequency analysis of ventricular fibrillation in Swine ventricles. *Circ. Res.* 2002; **90**: 213–222.
29. Myerburg, R.J., Kessler, K.M., & Castellanos, A. Sudden cardiac death. Structure, function, and time-dependence of risk. *Circulation* 1992; **85**: I2–I10.
30. Friedman, M., Manwaring, J.H., Rosenman, R.H., Donlon, G., Ortega, P., & Grube, S.M. Instantaneous and sudden deaths. Clinical and pathological differentiation in coronary artery disease. *J. Am. Med. Assoc.* 1973; **225**: 1319–1328.
31. Reichenbach, D.D., Moss, N.S., & Meyer, E. Pathology of the heart in sudden cardiac death. *Am. J. Cardiol.* 1977; **39**: 865–872.
32. Newman, W.P., 3rd, Tracy, R.E., Strong, J.P., Johnson, W.D., & Oalmann, M.C. Pathology on sudden coronary death. *Ann. N Y Acad. Sci.* 1982; **382**: 39–49.
33. Davies, M.J. Anatomic features in victims of sudden coronary death. Coronary artery pathology. *Circulation* 1992; **85**: I19–I24.
34. Spirito, P., Chiarella, F., Carratino, L., Berisso, M.Z., Bellotti, P., & Vecchio, C. Clinical course and prognosis of hypertrophic cardiomyopathy in an outpatient population. *N. Engl. J. Med.* 1989; **320**: 749–755.
35. Kannel, W.B., Gordon, T., & Offutt, D. Left ventricular hypertrophy by electrocardiogram. Prevalence, incidence, and

mortality in the Framingham study. *Ann. Intern. Med.* 1969; **71**: 89–105.

36. Cupples, L.A., Gagnon, D.R., & Kannel, W.B. Long- and short-term risk of sudden coronary death. *Circulation* 1992; **85**: I11–I18.

37. Sullivan, J.M., Vander Zwaag, R.V., el-Zeky, F., Ramanathan, K.B., & Mirvis, D.M. Left ventricular hypertrophy: effect on survival. *J. Am. Coll. Cardiol.* 1993; **22**: 508–513.

38. McKenna, W.J., & Camm, A.J. Sudden death in hypertrophic cardiomyopathy. Assessment of patients at high risk. *Circulation* 1989; **80**: 1489–1492.

39. Maron, B.J., & Fananapazir, L. Sudden cardiac death in hypertrophic cardiomyopathy. *Circulation* 1992; **85**: I57–I63.

40. Luu, M., Stevenson, W.G., Stevenson, L.W., Baron, K., & Walden, J. Diverse mechanisms of unexpected cardiac arrest in advanced heart failure. *Circulation* 1989; **80**: 1675–1680.

41. Packer, M. Lack of relation between ventricular arrhythmias and sudden death in patients with chronic heart failure. *Circulation* 1992; **85**: I50–I56.

42. Klein, G.J., Bashore, T.M., Sellers, T.D., Pritchett, E.L., Smith, W.M., & Gallagher, J.J. Ventricular fibrillation in the Wolff-Parkinson–White syndrome. *N. Engl. J. Med.* 1979; **301**: 1080–1085.

43. Schwartz, P.J., Locati, E.H., Moss, A.J., Crampton, R.S., Trazzi, R., & Ruberti, U. Left cardiac sympathetic denervation in the therapy of congenital long QT syndrome. A worldwide report. *Circulation* 1991; **84**: 503–511.

44. Moss, A.J., Schwartz, P.J., Crampton, R.S. *et al.* The long QT syndrome. Prospective longitudinal study of 328 families. *Circulation* 1991; **84**: 1136–1144.

45. Cao, J.M., Chen, L.S., KenKnight, B.H., *et al.* Nerve sprouting and sudden cardiac death. *Circ. Res.* 2000; **86**: 816–821.

46. Chen, P.S., Chen, L.S., Cao, J.M., Sharifi, B., Karagueuzian, H.S., & Fishbein, M.C. Sympathetic nerve sprouting, electrical remodeling and the mechanisms of sudden cardiac death. *Cardiovasc. Res.* 2001; **50**: 409–416.

47. Zhou, S., Cao, J.M., Tebb, Z.D. *et al.* Modulation of QT interval by cardiac sympathetic nerve sprouting and the mechanisms of ventricular arrhythmia in a canine model of sudden cardiac death. *J. Cardiovasc. Electrophysiol.* 2001; **12**: 1068–1073.

48. Inoue, H., & Zipes, D.P. Results of sympathetic denervation in the canine heart: supersensitivity that may be arrhythmogenic. *Circulation* 1987; **75**: 877–887.

49. Kleiger, R.E., Miller, J.P., Bigger, J.T., Jr., & Moss, A.J. Decreased heart rate variability and its association with increased mortality after acute myocardial infarction. *Am. J. Cardiol.* 1987; **59**: 256–262.

50. A randomized trial of propranolol in patients with acute myocardial infarction. I. Mortality results. *J. Am. Med. Assoc.* 1982; **247**: 1707–1714.

51. Ryden, L., Ariniego, R., Arnman, K. *et al.* A double-blind trial of metoprolol in acute myocardial infarction. Effects on ventricular tachyarrhythmias. *N. Engl. J. Med.* 1983; **308**: 614–618.

52. Pitt, B. The role of beta-adrenergic blocking agents in preventing sudden cardiac death. *Circulation* 1992; **85**: I107–I111.

53. von Euler, U.S., & Lishajko, F. Effects of Mg^{2+} and Ca^{2+} on noradrenaline release and uptake in adrenergic nerve granules in differential media. *Acta Physiol. Scand.* 1973; **89**: 415–422.

54. Teo, K.K., Yusuf, S., Collins, R., Held, P.H., & Peto, R. Effects of intravenous magnesium in suspected acute myocardial infarction: overview of randomised trials. *B. Med. J.* 1991; **303**: 1499–1503.

55. Nordrehaug, J.E., & von der Lippe, G. Hypokalaemia and ventricular fibrillation in acute myocardial infarction. *Br. Heart J.* 1983; **50**: 525–529.

56. Solomon, R.J., & Cole, A.G. Importance of potassium in patients with acute myocardial infarction. *Acta Med. Scand. Suppl.* 1981; **647**: 87–93.

57. Lumme, J.A., & Jounela, A.J. Cardiac arrhythmias in hypertensive outpatients on various diuretics. Correlation between incidence and serum potassium and magnesium levels. *Ann. Clin. Res.* 1986; **18**: 186–190.

58. Hulting, J. In-hospital ventricular fibrillation and its relation to serum potassium. *Acta Med. Scand. Suppl.* 1981; **647**: 109–116.

59. The cardiac arrhythmia suppression trial. *N. Engl. J. Med.* 1989; **321**: 1754–1756.

60. Effect of the antiarrhythmic agent moricizine on survival after myocardial infarction. The Cardiac Arrhythmia Suppression Trial II Investigators. *N. Engl. J. Med.* 1992; **327**: 227–233.

61. Kerr, W., & Bender, W. Paroxsmal ventricular fibrillation with cardiac recovery in a case of auricular fibrillation and complete heart block while under quinide sulfate therapy. *Heart* 1921; **9**: 269–281.

62. Selzer, A., & Wray, H.W. Quinidine syncope. Paroxysmal ventricular fibrillation occurring during treatment of chronic atrial arrhythmias. *Circulation* 1964; **30**: 17–26.

63. Keren, A., Tzivoni, D., Gavish, D. *et al.* Etiology, warning signs and therapy of torsade de pointes. A study of 10 patients. *Circulation* 1981; **64**: 1167–1174.

64. Koster, R.W., & Wellens, H.J. Quinidine-induced ventricular flutter and fibrillation without digitalis therapy. *Am. J. Cardiol.* 1976; **38**: 519–523.

65. Sclarovsky, S., Lewin, R.F., Kracoff, O., Strasberg, B., Arditti, A., & Agmon, J. Amiodarone-induced polymorphous ventricular tachycardia. *Am. Heart J.* 1983; **105**: 6–12.

66. Wellens, H.J., Lemery, R., Smeets, J.L. *et al.* Sudden arrhythmic death without overt heart disease. *Circulation* 1992; **85**: I92–I97.

67. Viskin, S., & Belhassen, B. Idiopathic ventricular fibrillation. *Am. Heart J.* 1990; **120**: 661–671.

68. Friedlander, Y., Siscovick, D.S., Weinmann, S. *et al.* Family history as a risk factor for primary cardiac arrest. *Circulation* 1998; **97**: 155–160.

69. Jouven, X., Desnos, M., Guerot, C., & Ducimetiere, P. Predicting sudden death in the population: the Paris Prospective Study I. *Circulation* 1999; **99**: 1978–1983.

70. Surawicz, B. Ventricular fibrillation. *Am. J. Cardiol.* 1971; **28**: 268–287.

71. Han, J. M.G. Nonuniform recovery of excitability in ventricular muscle. *Circ. Res.* 1964; **14**: 44–60.

72. Gettes, L. Ventricular fibrillation. In Surawicz, B. R.C, Prystowsky, E, ed. *Tachycardias.* Boston: Martinus Nijhoff Publishing, 1984: 37–54.

73. Jalife, J. Ventricular fibrillation: mechanisms of initiation and maintenance. *Annu. Rev. Physiol.* 2000; **62**: 25–50.

74. Janse, M.J., & Wit, A.L. Electrophysiological mechanisms of ventricular arrhythmias resulting from myocardial ischemia and infarction. *Physiol. Rev.* 1989; **69**: 1049–1169.

75. Pogwizd, S.M., & Corr, P.B. Reentrant and nonreentrant mechanisms contribute to arrhythmogenesis during early myocardial ischemia: results using three-dimensional mapping. *Circ. Res.* 1987; **61**: 352–371.

76. Kaplinsky, E., Ogawa, S., Balke, C.W., & Dreifus, L.S. Two periods of early ventricular arrhythmia in the canine acute myocardial infarction model. *Circulation.* 1979; **60**: 397–403.

77. Boineau, J.P., & Cox, J.L. Slow ventricular activation in acute myocardial infarction. A source of re-entrant premature ventricular contractions. *Circulation* 1973; **48**: 702–713.

78. Penny, W.J. The deleterious effects of myocardial catecholamines on cellular electrophysiology and arrhythmias during ischaemia and reperfusion. *Eur. Heart J.* 1984; **5**: 960–973.

79. Goldberg, S., Greenspon, A.J., Urban, P.L. *et al.* Reperfusion arrhythmia: a marker of restoration of antegrade flow during intracoronary thrombolysis for acute myocardial infarction. *Am. Heart J.* 1983; **105**: 26–32.

80. Stephenson, S.E. CR, Parridh, T.F., Bauer, F.M. *et al.* Ventricular fibrillation after coronary artery occlusion. Incidence and protection afforded by several drugs. *Am. J. Cardiol.* 1960; **5**: 77–87.

81. Rentrop, P., Blanke, H., Karsch, K.R., Kaiser, H., Kostering, H., & Leitz, K. Selective intracoronary thrombolysis in acute myocardial infarction and unstable angina pectoris. *Circulation* 1981; **63**: 307–317.

82. Pogwizd, S.M., & Corr, P.B. Electrophysiologic mechanisms underlying arrhythmias due to reperfusion of ischemic myocardium. *Circulation* 1987; **76**: 404–426.

83. Ideker, R.E., Klein, G.J., Harrison, L. *et al.* The transition to ventricular fibrillation induced by reperfusion after acute ischemia in the dog: a period of organized epicardial activation. *Circulation* 1981; **63**: 1371–1379.

84. Anzelevitch, C. D.J, Shen, X., & Moe, G.K. Reflected reentry. In Zipes, D.P. JJ, ed. *Cardiac Electrophysiology and Arrhythmias.* New York: Grune and Stratton, 1985: 253–264.

85. Ribeiro, L.G., Brandon, T.A., Debauche, T.L., Maroko, P.R., & Miller, R.R. Antiarrhythmic and hemodynamic effects of calcium channel blocking agents during coronary arterial reperfusion. Comparative effects of verapamil and nifedipine. *Am. J. Cardiol.* 1981; **48**: 69–74.

86. Sheridan, D.J., Penkoske, P.A., Sobel, B.E., & Corr, P.B. Alpha adrenergic contributions to dysrhythmia during myocardial ischemia and reperfusion in cats. *J. Clin. Invest.* 1980; **65**: 161–171.

87. Corbalan, R., Verrier, R.L., & Lown, B. Differing mechanisms for ventricular vulnerability during coronary artery occlusion and release. *Am. Heart J.* 1976; **92**: 223–230.

88. Kleber, A.G. Extracellular potassium accumulation in acute myocardial ischemia. *J. Mol. Cell Cardiol.* 1984; **16**: 389–394.

89. Kleber, A.G., Riegger, C.B., & Janse, M.J. Extracellular K^+ and H^+ shifts in early ischemia: mechanisms and relation to changes in impulse propagation. *J. Mol. Cell Cardiol.* 1987; **19** Suppl 5: 35–44.

90. Lederer, W.J., & Nichols, C.G. Nucleotide modulation of the activity of rat heart ATP-sensitive K^+ channels in isolated membrane patches. *J. Physiol.* 1989; **419**: 193–211.

91. Horie, M., Irisawa, H., & Noma, A. Voltage-dependent magnesium block of adenosine-triphosphate-sensitive potassium channel in guinea-pig ventricular cells. *J. Physiol.* 1987; **387**: 251–272.

92. Venkatesh, N., Lamp, S.T., & Weiss, J.N. Sulfonylureas, ATP-sensitive K^+ channels, and cellular K^+ loss during hypoxia, ischemia, and metabolic inhibition in mammalian ventricle. *Circ. Res.* 1991; **69**: 623–637.

93. Nichols, C.G., & Lederer, W.J. The regulation of ATP-sensitive K^+ channel activity in intact and permeabilized rat ventricular myocytes. *J. Physiol.* 1990; **423**: 91–110.

94. Kirsch, G.E., Codina, J., Birnbaumer, L., & Brown, A.M. Coupling of ATP-sensitive K^+ channels to A1 receptors by G proteins in rat ventricular myocytes. *Am. J. Physiol.* 1990; **259**: H820–H826.

95. Keung, E.C., & Li, Q. Lactate activates ATP-sensitive potassium channels in guinea pig ventricular myocytes. *J. Clin. Invest.* 1991; **88**: 1772–1777.

96. Kameyama, M., Kakei, M., Sato, R., Shibasaki, T., Matsuda, H., & Irisawa, H. Intracellular Na^+ activates a K^+ channel in mammalian cardiac cells. *Nature* 1984; **309**: 354–356.

97. Kim, D., & Clapham, D.E. Potassium channels in cardiac cells activated by arachidonic acid and phospholipids. *Science* 1989; **244**: 1174–1176.

98. Wilde, A.A., Escande, D., Schumacher, C.A. *et al.* Potassium accumulation in the globally ischemic mammalian heart. A role for the ATP-sensitive potassium channel. *Circ. Res.* 1990; **67**: 835–843.

99. Tung, R.T., & Kurachi, Y. On the mechanism of nucleotide diphosphate activation of the ATP-sensitive K^+ channel in ventricular cell of guinea-pig. *J. Physiol.* 1991; **437**: 239–256.

100. Katzung, B.G., Hondeghem, L.M., & Grant, A.O. Letter: Cardiac ventricular automaticity induced by current of injury. *Pflugers Arch.* 1975; **360**: 193–197.

101. Janse, M.J., & van Capelle, F.J. Electrotonic interactions across an inexcitable region as a cause of ectopic activity in acute regional myocardial ischemia. A study in intact porcine and canine hearts and computer models. *Circ. Res.* 1982; **50**: 527–537.

102. Akar, F.G., Aon, M.A., Tomaselli, G.F., & O'Rourke, B. The mitochondrial origin of postischemic arrhythmias. *J. Clin. Invest.* 2005; **115**: 3527–3535.

103. Zaitsev, A.V., Guha, P.K., Sarmast, F. *et al.* Wavebreak formation during ventricular fibrillation in the isolated, regionally ischemic pig heart. *Circ. Res.* 2003; **92**: 546–553.

104. Liu, Y.B., Pak, H.N., Lamp, S.T. *et al.* Coexistence of two types of ventricular fibrillation during acute regional ischemia in rabbit ventricle. *J. Cardiovasc. Electrophysiol.* 2004; **15**: 1433–1440.

105. Rankovic, V., Patel, N., Jain, S. *et al.* Characteristics of ischemic and peri-ischemic regions during ventricular fibrillation in the canine heart. *J. Cardiovasc. Electrophysiol.* 1999; **10**: 1090–1100.

106. Ideker, R.E., Rogers, J., & Huang, J. Types of ventricular fibrillation: 1,2,4,5, or 3000,000? *J. Cardiovasc. Electrophysiol.* 2004; **15**: 1441–1443.

107. Wilensky, R.L., Tranum-Jensen, J., Coronel, R., Wilde, A.A., Fiolet, J.W., & Janse, M.J. The subendocardial border zone during acute ischemia of the rabbit heart: an electrophysiologic, metabolic, and morphologic correlative study. *Circulation* 1986; **74**: 1137–1146.

108. Pogwizd, S.M., Onufer, J.R., Kramer, J.B., Sobel, B.E., & Corr, P.B. Induction of delayed afterdepolarizations and triggered activity in canine Purkinje fibers by lysophosphoglycerides. *Circ. Res.* 1986; **59**: 416–426.

109. Friedman, P.L., Stewart, J.R., Fenoglio, J.J., Jr., & Wit, A.L. Survival of subendocardial Purkinje fibers after extensive myocardial infarction in dogs. *Circ. Res.* 1973; **33**: 597–611.

110. Lazzara, R., el-Sherif, N., & Scherlag, B.J. Electrophysiological properties of canine Purkinje cells in one-day-old myocardial infarction. *Circ. Res.* 1973; **33**: 722–734.

111. Janse, M.J., Kleber, A.G., Capucci, A., Coronel, R., & Wilms-Schopman, F. Electrophysiological basis for arrhythmias caused by acute ischemia. Role of the subendocardium. *J. Mol. Cell Cardiol.* 1986; **18**: 339–355.

112. Schomig, A., Dart, A.M., Dietz, R., Mayer, E., & Kubler, W. Release of endogenous catecholamines in the ischemic myocardium of the rat. Part A: Locally mediated release. *Circ. Res.* 1984; **55**: 689–701.

113. Schwartz, P., & Priori, S. Sympathetic nervous system and cardiac arrhythmias. In Zipes, D.P. JJe, ed. *Cardiac Electrophysiology from Cell to Bedside.* Philadelphia: W.B. Saunders, 1990: 330–342.

114. Boyden, P.A., Gardner, P.I., & Wit, A.L. Action potentials of cardiac muscle in healing infarcts: response to norepinephrine and caffeine. *J. Mol. Cell Cardiol.* 1988; **20**: 525–537.

115. Tromba, C., & Cohen, I.S. A novel action of isoproterenol to inactivate a cardiac K^+ current is not blocked by beta and alpha adrenergic blockers. *Biophys. J.* 1990; **58**: 791–795.

116. Desilets, M., & Baumgarten, C.M. Isoproterenol directly stimulates the Na^+–K^+ pump in isolated cardiac myocytes. *Am. J. Physiol.* 1986; **251**: H218–H25.

117. Canty, J.M., Jr., Suzuki, G., Banas, M.D., Verheyen, F., Borgers, M., & Fallavollita, J.A. Hibernating myocardium: chronically adapted to ischemia but vulnerable to sudden death. *Circ. Res.* 2004; **94**: 1142–1149.

118. Lim, H., Fallavollita, J.A., Hard, R., Kerr, C.W., & Canty, J.M., Jr. Profound apoptosis-mediated regional myocyte loss and compensatory hypertrophy in pigs with hibernating myocardium. *Circulation* 1999; **100**: 2380–2386.

119. Fallavollita, J.A., Jacob, S., Young, R.F., & Canty, J.M., Jr. Regional alterations in SR $Ca^{(2+)}$-ATPase, phospholamban, and HSP-70 expression in chronic hibernating myocardium. *Am. J. Physiol.* 1999; **277**: H1418–H1428.

120. Luisi, A.J., Jr., Fallavollita, J.A., Suzuki, G., & Canty, J.M., Jr. Spatial inhomogeneity of sympathetic nerve function in hibernating myocardium. *Circulation* 2002; **106**: 779–781.

121. Kaprielian, R.R., Gunning, M., Dupont, E. *et al.* Down-regulation of immunodetectable connexin43 and decreased gap junction size in the pathogenesis of chronic hibernation in the human left ventricle. *Circulation* 1998; **97**: 651–660.

122. Aronson, R.S. Characteristics of action potentials of hypertrophied myocardium from rats with renal hypertension. *Circ. Res.* 1980; **47**: 443–454.

123. Scamps, F., Mayoux, E., Charlemagne, D., & Vassort, G. Calcium current in single cells isolated from normal and hypertrophied rat heart. Effects of beta-adrenergic stimulation. *Circ. Res.* 1990; **67**: 199–208.

124. Beuckelmann, D.J., Nabauer, M., & Erdmann, E. Intracellular calcium handling in isolated ventricular myocytes from patients with terminal heart failure. *Circulation* 1992; **85**: 1046–1055.

125. Beuckelmann, D.J., Nabauer, M., & Erdmann, E. Alterations of K^+ currents in isolated human ventricular myocytes from patients with terminal heart failure. *Circ. Res.* 1993; **73**: 379–385.

126. Undrovinas, A.I., Fleidervish, I.A., & Makielski, J.C. Inward sodium current at resting potentials in single cardiac myocytes induced by the ischemic metabolite lysophosphatidylcholine. *Circ. Res.* 1992; **71**: 1231–1241.

127. Hansen, D.E., Borganelli, M., Stacy, G.P., Jr., & Taylor, L.K. Dose-dependent inhibition of stretch-induced arrhythmias by gadolinium in isolated canine ventricles. Evidence for a unique mode of antiarrhythmic action. *Circ. Res.* 1991; **69**: 820–831.

128. Morris, C.E., & Sigurdson, W.J. Stretch-inactivated ion channels coexist with stretch-activated ion channels. *Science* 1989; **243**: 807–809.

129. Aronson, R. & Ming, Z. Cellular mechanisms of arrhythmias in hypertrophied and failing myocardium. *Circulation* 1993; **87** (VII): 76–83.

130. Sakakibara, Y., Furukawa, T., Singer, D.H. *et al.* Sodium current in isolated human ventricular myocytes. *Am. J. Physiol.* 1993; **265**: H1301–H1309.

131. Rasmussen, R.P., Minobe, W., & Bristow, M.R. Calcium antagonist binding sites in failing and nonfailing human ventricular myocardium. *Biochem. Pharmacol.* 1990; **39**: 691–696.

132. Beuckelmann, D.J., Nabauer, M., & Erdmann, E. Characteristics of calcium-current in isolated human ventricular myocytes from patients with terminal heart failure. *J. Mol. Cell Cardiol.* 1991; **23**: 929–937.

133. Schroder, F., Handrock, R., Beuckelmann, D.J. *et al.* Increased availability and open probability of single L-type calcium

channels from failing compared with nonfailing human ventricle. *Circulation* 1998; **98**: 969–976.

134. Hullin, R., Khan, I.F., Wirtz, S. *et al.* Cardiac L-type calcium channel beta-subunits expressed in human heart have differential effects on single channel characteristics. *J. Biol. Chem.* 2003; **278**: 21623–21630.

135. Mansourati, J., & Le Grand, B. Transient outward current in young and adult diseased human atria. *Am. J. Physiol.* 1993; **265**: H1466–H1470.

136. Lue, W.M., & Boyden, P.A. Abnormal electrical properties of myocytes from chronically infarcted canine heart. Alterations in Vmax and the transient outward current. *Circulation* 1992; **85**: 1175–1188.

137. Xu, X.P., & Best, P.M. Decreased transient outward K$^+$ current in ventricular myocytes from acromegalic rats. *Am. J. Physiol.* 1991; **260**: H935–H942.

138. Brugada, P., & Wellens, H.J. Early afterdepolarizations: role in conduction block, "prolonged repolarization-dependent reexcitation," and tachyarrhythmias in the human heart. *Pacing Clin. Electrophysiol.* 1985; **8**: 889–896.

139. Akar, F.G., & Rosenbaum, D.S. Transmural heterogeneities of cellular repolarization underlie polymorphic ventricular tachycardia in failing myocardium. *Circulation* 2001; **104**: 25.

140. Antzelevitch, C., Sicouri, S., Litovsky, S.H. *et al.* Heterogeneity within the ventricular wall. Electrophysiology and pharmacology of epicardial, endocardial, and M cells. *Circ. Res.* 1991; **69**: 1427–1449.

141. Li, G.R., Lau, C.P., Ducharme, A., Tardif, J.C., & Nattel, S. Transmural action potential and ionic current remodeling in ventricles of failing canine hearts. *Am. J. Physiol. Heart Circ. Physiol.* 2002; **283**: H1031–H1041.

142. Xiong, W., Tian, Y., Akar, F., & Tomaselli, G. Differential transmural heterogeneity of Na$^+$–Ca^{2+} exchange in normal and failing hearts. *Circulation* 2004; **110**: III–163A.

143. Henderson, E.B., Kahn, J.K., Corbett, J.R. *et al.* Abnormal I–123 metaiodobenzylguanidine myocardial washout and distribution may reflect myocardial adrenergic derangement in patients with congestive cardiomyopathy. *Circulation* 1988; **78**: 1192–1199.

144. Calkins, H., Allman, K., Bolling, S. *et al.* Correlation between scintigraphic evidence of regional sympathetic neuronal dysfunction and ventricular refractoriness in the human heart. *Circulation* 1993; **88**: 172–179.

145. Kuo, C.S., Munakata, K., Reddy, C.P., & Surawicz, B. Characteristics and possible mechanism of ventricular arrhythmia dependent on the dispersion of action potential durations. *Circulation* 1983; **67**: 1356–1367.

146. Pogwizd, S.M. Nonreentrant mechanisms underlying spontaneous ventricular arrhythmias in a model of nonischemic heart failure in rabbits. *Circulation* 1995; **92**: 1034–1048.

147. Pogwizd, S.M., Schlotthauer, K., Li, L., Yuan, W., & Bers, D.M. Arrhythmogenesis and contractile dysfunction in heart failure: Roles of sodium-calcium exchange, inward rectifier potassium current, and residual beta-adrenergic responsiveness. *Circ. Res.* 2001; **88**: 1159–1167.

148. Undrovinas, A.I., Maltsev, V.A., Kyle, J.W., Silverman, N., & Sabbah, H.N. Gating of the late Na$^+$ channel in normal and failing human myocardium. *J. Mol. Cell Cardiol.* 2002; **34**: 1477–1489.

149. Weber, H.S., & Myers, J.L. Maternal collagen vascular disease associated with fetal heart block and degenerative changes of the atrioventricular valves. *Pediatr. Cardiol.* 1994; **15**: 204–206.

150. Shinagawa, K., Shi, Y.F., Tardif, J.C., Leung, T.K., & Nattel, S. Dynamic nature of atrial fibrillation substrate during development and reversal of heart failure in dogs. *Circulation* 2002; **105**: 2672–2678.

151. Akar, F.G., Spragg, D.D., Tunin, R.S., Kass, D.A., & Tomaselli, G.F. Mechanisms underlying conduction slowing and arrhythmogenesis in nonischemic dilated cardiomyopathy. *Circ. Res.* 2004; **95**: 717–725.

152. Cameron, J.S., Myerburg, R.J., Wong, S.S., *et al.* Electrophysiologic consequences of chronic experimentally induced left ventricular pressure overload. *J. Am. Coll. Cardiol.* 1983; **2**: 481–487.

153. Kowey, P.R., Friechling, T.D., Sewter, J. *et al.* Electrophysiological effects of left ventricular hypertrophy. Effect of calcium and potassium channel blockade. *Circulation* 1991; **83**: 2067–2075.

154. Volders, P.G., Sipido, K.R., Vos, M.A., Kulcsar, A., Verduyn, S.C., & Wellens, H.J. Cellular basis of biventricular hypertrophy and arrhythmogenesis in dogs with chronic complete atrioventricular block and acquired torsade de pointes. *Circulation* 1998; **98**: 1136–1147.

155. Vos, M.A., de Groot, S.H., Verduyn, S.C. *et al.* Enhanced susceptibility for acquired torsade de pointes arrhythmias in the dog with chronic, complete AV block is related to cardiac hypertrophy and electrical remodeling. *Circulation* 1998; **98**: 1125–1135.

156. Volders, P.G., Sipido, K.R., Vos, M.A. *et al.* Downregulation of delayed rectifier K$^+$ currents in dogs with chronic complete atrioventricular block and acquired torsades de pointes. *Circulation* 1999; **100**: 2455–2461.

157. Sipido, K.R., Volders, P.G., de Groot, S.H. *et al.* Enhanced Ca(2$^+$) release and Na/Ca exchange activity in hypertrophied canine ventricular myocytes: potential link between contractile adaptation and arrhythmogenesis. *Circulation* 2000; **102**: 2137–2144.

158. Saumarez, R.C., Camm, A.J., Panagos, A. *et al.* Ventricular fibrillation in hypertrophic cardiomyopathy is associated with increased fractionation of paced right ventricular electrograms. *Circulation* 1992; **86**: 467–474.

159. Chen, P.S., Wolf, P.D., Dixon, E.G. *et al.* Mechanism of ventricular vulnerability to single premature stimuli in open-chest dogs. *Circ. Res.* 1988; **62**: 1191–1209.

160. Frazier, D.W., Wharton, J.M., Wolf, P.D., Smith, W.M., & Ideker, R.E. Mapping the electrical initiation of ventricular fibrillation. *J. Electrocardiol.* 1989; **22** Suppl: 198–199.

161. Kao, C.Y., & Hoffman, B.F. Graded and decremental response in heart muscle fibers. *Am. J. Physiol.* 1958; **194**: 187–196.

162. Gettes, L.S., Morehouse, N., & Surawicz, B. Effect of premature depolarization on the duration of action potentials in Purkinje and ventricular fibers of the moderator band of the pig heart. Role of proximity and the duration of the preceding action potential. *Circ. Res.* 1972; **30**: 55–66.

163. Orias, O., Gilbert, J.L., Siebens, A.A., Suckling, E.E., & Brooks, C.M. Effectiveness of single rectangular electrical pulses of known duration and strength in evoking auricular fibrillation. *Am. J. Physiol.* 1950; **162**: 219–225.

164. Chen, P.S., Wolf, P.D., Melnick, S.D., Danieley, N.D., Smith, W.M., & Ideker, R.E. Comparison of activation during ventricular fibrillation and following unsuccessful defibrillation shocks in open-chest dogs. *Circ. Res.* 1990; **66**: 1544–1560.

165. Jalife, J. & Gray, R. Drifting vortices of electrical waves underlie ventricular fibrillation in the rabbit heart. *Acta Physiol. Scand.* 1996; **157**: 123–131.

166. Pertsov, A.M., Davidenko, J.M., Salomonsz, R., Baxter, W.T., & Jalife, J. Spiral waves of excitation underlie reentrant activity in isolated cardiac muscle. *Circ. Res.* 1993; **72**: 631–650.

167. Keating, M., Atkinson, D., Dunn, C., Timothy, K., Vincent, G.M., & Leppert, M. Linkage of a cardiac arrhythmia, the long QT syndrome, and the Harvey ras-1 gene. *Science* 1991; **252**: 704–706.

168. Gaita, F., Giustetto, C., Bianchi, F. *et al.* Short QT Syndrome: a familial cause of sudden death. *Circulation* 2003; **108**: 965–970.

169. Leenhardt, A., Lucet, V., Denjoy, I., Grau, F., Ngoc, D.D., & Coumel, P. Catecholaminergic polymorphic ventricular tachycardia in children. A 7-year follow-up of 21 patients. *Circulation* 1995; **91**: 1512–1519.

170. Brugada, P., & Brugada, J. Right bundle branch block, persistent ST segment elevation and sudden cardiac death: a distinct clinical and electrocardiographic syndrome. A multicenter report [see comments]. *J. Am. Coll. Cardiol.* 1992; **20**: 1391–1396.

171. Martini, B., Nava, A., Thiene, G. *et al.* Ventricular fibrillation without apparent heart disease: description of six cases. *Am. Heart J.* 1989; **118**: 1203–1209.

172. Romano, C., Gemme, G., & Pongiglione, R. [Rare cardiac arrythmias of the pediatric age. Ii. Syncopal attacks due to paroxysmal ventricular fibrillation. (Presentation of 1st case in Italian pediatric literature)]. *Clin. Pediatr. (Bologna).* 1963; **45**: 656–683.

173. Ward, O.C. A new familial cardiac syndrome in children. *J. Ir. Med. Assoc.* 1964; **54**: 103–106.

174. Jervell, A., & Lange-Nielsen, F. Congenital deaf-mutism, functional heart disease with prolongation of the Q-T interval and sudden death. *Am. Heart J.* 1957; **54**: 59–68.

175. Wang, Q., Curran, M.E., Splawski, I. *et al.* Positional cloning of a novel potassium channel gene: KVLQT1 mutations cause cardiac arrhythmias. *Nat. Genet.* 1996; **12**: 17–23.

176. Trudeau, M.C., Warmke, J.W., Ganetzky, B., & Robertson, G.A. HERG, a human inward rectifier in the voltage-gated potassium channel family. *Science* 1995; **269**: 92–95.

177. Sanguinetti, M.C., Jiang, C., Curran, M.E., & Keating, M.T. A mechanistic link between an inherited and an acquired cardiac arrhythmia: HERG encodes the IKr potassium channel. *Cell* 1995; **81**: 299–307.

178. Jiang, C., Atkinson, D., Towbin, J.A. *et al.* Two long QT syndrome loci map to chromosomes 3 and 7 with evidence for further heterogeneity. *Nat. Genet.* 1994; **8**: 141–147.

179. Duggal, P., Vesely, M.R., Wattanasirichaigoon, D., Villafane, J., Kaushik, V., & Beggs, A.H. Mutation of the gene for IsK associated with both Jervell and Lange–Nielsen and Romano–Ward forms of Long-QT syndrome. *Circulation* 1998; **97**: 142–146.

180. Splawski, I., Tristani-Firouzi, M., Lehmann, M.H., Sanguinetti, M.C., & Keating, M.T. Mutations in the hminK gene cause long QT syndrome and suppress IKs function. *Nat. Genet.* 1997; **17**: 338–340.

181. Bellocq, C., van Ginneken, A.C., Bezzina, C.R. *et al.* Mutation in the KCNQ1 gene leading to the short QT-interval syndrome. *Circulation* 2004; **109**: 2394–2397.

182. Priori, S.G., Pandit, S.V., Rivolta, I. *et al.* A novel form of short QT syndrome (SQT3) is caused by a mutation in the KCNJ2 gene. *Circ. Res.* 2005; **96**: 800–807.

183. Brugada, R., Hong, K., Dumaine, R. *et al.* Sudden death associated with short-QT syndrome linked to mutations in HERG. *Circulation* 2004; **109**: 30–35.

184. Priori, S.G., Napolitano, C., Tiso, N. *et al.* Mutations in the cardiac ryanodine receptor gene (hRyR2) underlie catecholaminergic polymorphic ventricular tachycardia. *Circulation* 2001; **103**: 196–200.

185. Laitinen, P.J., Brown, K.M., Piippo, K. *et al.* Mutations of the cardiac ryanodine receptor (RyR2) gene in familial polymorphic ventricular tachycardia. *Circulation* 2001; **103**: 485–490.

186. Postma, A.V., Denjoy, I., Hoorntje, T.M. *et al.* Absence of calsequestrin 2 causes severe forms of catecholaminergic polymorphic ventricular tachycardia. *Circ. Res.* 2002; **91**: e21–e26.

187. Lahat, H., Pras, E., Olender, T. *et al.* A missense mutation in a highly conserved region of CASQ2 is associated with autosomal recessive catecholamine-induced polymorphic ventricular tachycardia in Bedouin families from Israel. *Am. J. Hum. Genet.* 2001; **69**: 1378–1384.

188. Chen, Q., Kirsch, G.E., Zhang, D. *et al.* Genetic basis and molecular mechanism for idiopathic ventricular fibrillation. *Nature* 1998; **392**: 293–296.

189. Antzelevitch, C. The Brugada syndrome: ionic basis and arrhythmia mechanisms. *J. Cardiovasc. Electrophysiol.* 2001; **12**: 268–272.

190. Julian, D.G., Valentine, P.A., & Miller, G.G. Disturbances of rate, rhythm and conduction in acute myocardial Infarction: a prospective study of 100 consecutive unselected patients with the aid of electrocardiographic monitoring. *Am. J. Med.* 1964; **37**: 915–927.

191. MacMahon, S., Collins, R., Peto, R., Koster, R.W., & Yusuf, S. Effects of prophylactic lidocaine in suspected acute myocardial infarction. An overview of results from the randomized, controlled trials. *J. Am. Med. Assoc.* 1988; **260**: 1910–1916.

192. Hine, L.K., Laird, N.M., Hewitt, P., & Chalmers, T.C. Meta-analysis of empirical long-term antiarrhythmic therapy

after myocardial infarction. *J. Am. Med. Assoc.* 1989; **262**: 3037–3040.

193. Antman, E.M., & Berlin, J.A. Declining incidence of ventricular fibrillation in myocardial infarction. Implications for the prophylactic use of lidocaine. *Circulation* 1992; **86**: 764–773.

194. Norris, R.M., Barnaby, P.F., Brown, M.A. *et al.* Prevention of ventricular fibrillation during acute myocardial infarction by intravenous propranolol. *Lancet* 1984; **2**: 883–886.

195. Bigger, J.T., Jr., Fleiss, J.L., Kleiger, R., Miller, J.P., & Rolnitzky, L.M. The relationships among ventricular arrhythmias, left ventricular dysfunction, and mortality in the 2 years after myocardial infarction. *Circulation* 1984; **69**: 250–258.

196. Mukharji, J., Rude, R.E., Poole, W.K. *et al.* Risk factors for sudden death after acute myocardial infarction: two-year follow-up. *Am. J. Cardiol.* 1984; **54**: 31–36.

197. Denniss, A.R., Richards, D.A., Cody, D.V. *et al.* Correlation between signal-averaged electrocardiogram and programmed stimulation in patients with and without spontaneous ventricular tachyarrhythmias. *Am. J. Cardiol.* 1987; **59**: 586–590.

198. Gomes, J.A., Winters, S.L., Stewart, D., Horowitz, S., Milner, M., & Barreca, P. A new noninvasive index to predict sustained ventricular tachycardia and sudden death in the first year after myocardial infarction: based on signal-averaged electrocardiogram, radionuclide ejection fraction and Holter monitoring. *J. Am. Coll. Cardiol.* 1987; **10**: 349–357.

199. Kuchar, D.L., Thorburn, C.W., & Sammel, N.L. Prediction of serious arrhythmic events after myocardial infarction: signal-averaged electrocardiogram, Holter monitoring and radionuclide ventriculography. *J. Am. Coll. Cardiol.* 1987; **9**: 531–538.

200. Buxton, A.E., Marchlinski, F.E., Flores, B.T., Miller, J.M., Doherty, J.U., & Josephson, M.E. Nonsustained ventricular tachycardia in patients with coronary artery disease: role of electrophysiologic study. *Circulation* 1987; **75**: 1178–1185.

201. Denniss, A.R., Richards, D.A., Cody, D.V. *et al.* Prognostic significance of ventricular tachycardia and fibrillation induced at programmed stimulation and delayed potentials detected on the signal-averaged electrocardiograms of survivors of acute myocardial infarction. *Circulation* 1986; **74**: 731–745.

202. Mancini, D.M., Wong, K.L., & Simson M.B. Prognostic value of an abnormal signal-averaged electrocardiogram in patients with nonischemic congestive cardiomyopathy. *Circulation* 1993; **87**: 1083–1092.

203. Effect of prophylactic amiodarone on mortality after acute myocardial infarction and in congestive heart failure: meta-analysis of individual data from 6500 patients in randomised trials. Amiodarone Trials Meta-Analysis Investigators. *Lancet* 1997; **350**: 1417–1424.

204. Miller, D.D., Waters, D.D., Szlachcic, J., & Theroux, P. Clinical characteristics associated with sudden death in patients with variant angina. *Circulation* 1982; **66**: 588–592.

205. Cobb, L.A., Baum, R.S., Alvarez, H., 3rd, & Schaffer, W.A. Resuscitation from out-of-hospital ventricular fibrillation: 4 years follow-up. *Circulation* 1975; **52**: III223–III235.

206. Myerburg, R.J., Conde, C.A., Sung, R.J. *et al.* Clinical, electrophysiologic and hemodynamic profile of patients resuscitated from prehospital cardiac arrest. *Am. J. Med.* 1980; **68**: 568–576.

207. Wilber, D.J., Garan, H., Finkelstein, D. *et al.* Out-of-hospital cardiac arrest. Use of electrophysiologic testing in the prediction of long-term outcome. *N. Engl. J. Med.* 1988; **318**: 19–24.

208. Freedman, R.A., Swerdlow, C.D., Soderholm-Difatte, V., & Mason, J.W. Prognostic significance of arrhythmia inducibility or noninducibility at initial electrophysiologic study in survivors of cardiac arrest. *Am. J. Cardiol.* 1988; **61**: 578–582.

209. Swerdlow, C.D., Freedman, R.A., Peterson, J., & Clay, D. Determinants of prognosis in ventricular tachyarrhythmia patients without induced sustained arrhythmias. *Am. Heart J.* 1986; **111**: 433–438.

210. Morady, F., DiCarlo, L., Winston, S., Davis, J.C., & Scheinman, M.M. Clinical features and prognosis of patients with out of hospital cardiac arrest and a normal electrophysiologic study. *J. Am. Coll. Cardiol.* 1984; **4**: 39–44.

211. Kehoe, R., Tommaso, C., Zheutlin, T. *et al.* Factors determining programmed stimulation responses and long-term arrhythmic outcome in survivors of ventricular fibrillation with ischemic heart disease. *Am. Heart J.* 1988; **116**: 355–363.

212. Kelly, P., Ruskin, J.N., Vlahakes, G.J., Buckley, M.J., Jr., Freeman, C.S., & Garan, H. Surgical coronary revascularization in survivors of prehospital cardiac arrest: its effect on inducible ventricular arrhythmias and long-term survival. *J. Am. Coll. Cardiol.* 1990; **15**: 267–273.

213. Haissaguerre, M., Shah, D.C., Jais, P. *et al.* Role of Purkinje conducting system in triggering of idiopathic ventricular fibrillation. *Lancet* 2002; **359**: 677–678.

214. Haissaguerre, M., Shoda, M., Jais, P. *et al.* Mapping and ablation of idiopathic ventricular fibrillation. *Circulation* 2002; **106**: 962–967.

215. Haissaguerre, M., Extramiana, F., Hocini, M. *et al.* Mapping and ablation of ventricular fibrillation associated with long-QT and Brugada syndromes. *Circulation* 2003; **108**: 925–928.

216. Saliba, W., Abul Karim, A., Tchou, P., & Natale, A. Ventricular fibrillation: ablation of a trigger? *J. Cardiovasc. Electrophysiol.* 2002; **13**: 1296–1299.

217. Bansch, D., Oyang, F., Antz, M. *et al.* Successful catheter ablation of electrical storm after myocardial infarction. *Circulation* 2003; **108**: 3011–3016.

218. Li, Y.G., Gronefeld, G., Israel, C., & Hohnloser, S.H. Catheter ablation of frequently recurring ventricular fibrillation in a patient after aortic valve repair. *J. Cardiovasc. Electrophysiol.* 2004; 15: 90–93.

219. Zipes, D.P., Fischer, J., King, R.M., Nicoll, A.D., & Jolly, W.W. Termination of ventricular fibrillation in dogs by depolarizing a critical amount of myocardium. *Am. J. Cardiol.* 1975; **36**: 37–44.

220. Chen, P.S., Shibata, N., Dixon, E.G., Martin, R.O., & Ideker, R.E. Comparison of the defibrillation threshold and the upper limit of ventricular vulnerability. *Circulation* 1986; **73**: 1022–1028.

221. Efimov, I.R., Cheng, Y.N., Biermann, M., Van Wagoner, D.R., Mazgalev, T.N., & Tchou, P.J. Transmembrane voltage changes produced by real and virtual electrodes during monophasic defibrillation shock delivered by an implantable electrode. *J. Cardiovasc. Electrophysiol.* 1997; **8**: 1031–1045.

222. Efimov, I.R., Cheng, Y., Van Wagoner, D.R., Mazgalev, T., & Tchou, P.J. Virtual electrode-induced phase singularity: a basic mechanism of defibrillation failure. *Circ. Res.* 1998; **82**: 918–925.

223. Weaver, W.D., Copass, M.K., Bufi, D., Ray, R., Hallstrom, A.P., & Cobb, L.A. Improved neurologic recovery and survival after early defibrillation. *Circulation.* 1984; **69**: 943–948.

224. Weaver, W.D., Cobb, L.A., Dennis, D., Ray, R., Hallstrom, A.P., & Copass, M.K. Amplitude of ventricular fibrillation waveform and outcome after cardiac arrest. *Ann. Intern. Med.* 1985; **102**: 53–55.

225. Kerber, R.E., & Sarnat, W. Factors influencing the success of ventricular defibrillation in man. *Circulation* 1979; **60**: 226–230.

226. Gliner, B.E., Lyster, T.E., Dillion, S.M., & Bardy, G.H. Transthoracic defibrillation of swine with monophasic and biphasic waveforms. *Circulation.* 1995; **92**: 1634–1643.

227. Bardy, G.H., Ivey, T.D., Allen, M.D., Johnson, G., Mehra, R., & Greene, H.L. A prospective randomized evaluation of biphasic versus monophasic waveform pulses on defibrillation efficacy in humans. *J. Am. Coll. Cardiol.* 1989; **14**: 728–733.

228. Winkle, R.A., Mead, R.H., Ruder, M.A. *et al.* Improved low energy defibrillation efficacy in man with the use of a biphasic truncated exponential waveform. *Am. Heart J.* 1989; **117**: 122–127.

229. Tang, W., Weil, M.H., Sun, S. *et al.* The effects of biphasic and conventional monophasic defibrillation on postresuscitation myocardial function. *J. Am. Coll. Cardiol.* 1999; **34**: 815–822.

230. Leng, C.T., Paradis, N.A., Calkins, H. *et al.* Resuscitation after prolonged ventricular fibrillation with use of monophasic and biphasic waveform pulses for external defibrillation. *Circulation* 2000; **101**: 2968–2974.

231. Xie, J., Weil, M.H., Sun, S. *et al.* High-energy defibrillation increases the severity of postresuscitation myocardial dysfunction. *Circulation* 1997; **96**: 683–688.

232. Osswald, S., Trouton, T.G., O'Nunain, S.S., Holden, H.B., Ruskin, J.N., & Garan, H. Relation between shock-related myocardial injury and defibrillation efficacy of monophasic and biphasic shocks in a canine model. *Circulation* 1994; **90**: 2501–2509.

233. Schneider, T., Martens, P.R., Paschen, H. *et al.* Multicenter, randomized, controlled trial of 150-J biphasic shocks compared with 200- to 360-J monophasic shocks in the resuscitation of out-of-hospital cardiac arrest victims. Optimized response to cardiac arrest (ORCA) investigators. *Circulation* 2000; **102**: 1780–1787.

234. Valenzuela, T.D., Roe, D.J., Nichol, G., Clark, L.L., Spaite, D.W., & Hardman, R.G. Outcomes of rapid defibrillation by security officers after cardiac arrest in casinos. *N. Engl. J. Med.* 2000; **343**: 1206–1209.

235. Nichol, G., Valenzuela, T., Roe, D., Clark, L., Huszti, E., & Wells, G.A. Cost effectiveness of defibrillation by targeted responders in public settings. *Circulation* 2003; **108**: 697–703.

236. Ramaswamy, K., & Page, R.L. The automated external defibrillator: critical link in the chain of survival. *Annu. Rev. Med.* 2003; **54**: 235–243.

237. Page, R.L., Joglar, J.A., Kowal, R.C. *et al.* Use of automated external defibrillators by a U.S. airline. *N. Engl. J. Med.* 2000; **343**: 1210–1216.

238. Mirowski, M., Reid, P.R., Mower, M.M. *et al.* Termination of malignant ventricular arrhythmias with an implanted automatic defibrillator in human beings. *N. Engl. J. Med.* 1980; **303**: 322–324.

239. Echt, D.S., Barbey, J.T., & Black, J.N. Influence of ventricular fibrillation duration on defibrillation energy in dogs using bidirectional pulse discharges. *Pacing Clin. Electrophysiol.* 1988; **11**: 1315–1323.

240. Winkle, R.A., Mead, R.H., Ruder, M.A., Smith, N.A., Buch, W.S., & Gaudiani, V.A. Effect of duration of ventricular fibrillation on defibrillation efficacy in humans. *Circulation* 1990; **81**: 1477–1481.

241. Bardy, G.H., Ivey, T.D., Johnson, G., Stewart, R.B., & Greene, H.L. Prospective evaluation of initially ineffective defibrillation pulses on subsequent defibrillation success during ventricular fibrillation in survivors of cardiac arrest. *Am. J. Cardiol.* 1988; **62**: 718–722.

242. Platia, E., Waclawski, S.H., & Pluth, T.A. Automatic implantable defibrillator (AICD): Implication of delayed and subthreshold shocks. *Circulation* 1987; **76**(suppl IV): IV–311.

243. Guarnieri, T., Tomaselli, G., Griffith, L.S., & Brinker, J. The interaction of antiarrhythmic drugs and the energy for cardioversion of chronic atrial fibrillation. *Pacing Clin. Electrophysiol.* 1991; **14**: 1007–1012.

244. Hernandez, R., Mann, D.E., Breckinridge, S., Williams, G.R., & Reiter, M.J. Effects of flecainide on defibrillation thresholds in the anesthetized dog. *J. Am. Coll. Cardiol.* 1989; **14**: 777–781.

245. Fain, E.S., Dorian, P., Davy, J.M., Kates, R.E., & Winkle, R.A. Effects of encainide and its metabolites on energy requirements for defibrillation. *Circulation* 1986; **73**: 1334–1341.

246. Jung, W., Manz, M., Pizzulli, L., Pfeiffer, D., & Luderitz, B. Effects of chronic amiodarone therapy on defibrillation threshold. *Am. J. Cardiol.* 1992; **70**: 1023–1027.

247. Troup, P.J., Chapman P.D., Olinger GN, & Kleinman LH. The implanted defibrillator: relation of defibrillating lead configuration and clinical variables to defibrillation threshold. *J. Am. Coll. Cardiol.* 1985; **6**: 1315–1321.

248. Guarnieri, T., Levine, J.H., Veltri, E.P. *et al.* Success of chronic defibrillation and the role of antiarrhythmic drugs with the automatic implantable cardioverter/defibrillator. *Am. J. Cardiol.* 1987; **60**: 1061–1064.

249. Echt, D.S., Black, J.N., Barbey, J.T., Coxe, D.R., & Cato, E. Evaluation of antiarrhythmic drugs on defibrillation energy requirements in dogs. Sodium channel block and action potential prolongation. *Circulation* 1989; **79**: 1106–1117.

250. Fogoros, R.N. Amiodarone-induced refractoriness to cardioversion. *Ann. Intern. Med.* 1984; **100**: 699–700.

251. Marinchak, R.A., Friehling, T.D., Kline, R.A., Stohler, J., & Kowey, P.R. Effect of antiarrhythmic drugs on defibrillation threshold: case report of an adverse effect of mexiletine and review of the literature. *Pacing Clin. Electrophysiol.* 1988; **11**: 7–12.

252. Eisenberg, M.S., Copass, M.K., Hallstrom, A., Cobb, L.A., & Bergner, L. Management of out-of-hospital cardiac arrest. Failure of basic emergency medical technician services. *J. Am. Med. Assoc.* 1980; **243**: 1049–1051.

253. Weaver, W.D., Cobb, L.A., Hallstrom, A.P., Fahrenbruch, C., Copass, M.K., & Ray, R. Factors influencing survival after out-of-hospital cardiac arrest. *J. Am. Coll. Cardiol.* 1986; **7**: 752–757.

254. Weaver, W.D., Cobb, L.A., Hallstrom, A.P. *et al.* Considerations for improving survival from out-of-hospital cardiac arrest. *Ann. Emerg. Med.* 1986; **15**: 1181–1186.

255. Halperin, H.R., Tsitlik, J.E., Guerci, A.D. *et al.* Determinants of blood flow to vital organs during cardiopulmonary resuscitation in dogs. *Circulation* 1986; **73**: 539–550.

256. Sanders, A.B., Ewy, G.A., & Taft, T.V. Prognostic and therapeutic importance of the aortic diastolic pressure in resuscitation from cardiac arrest. *Crit. Care Med.* 1984; **12**: 871–873.

257. Niemann, J.T., Criley, J.M., Rosborough, J.P., Niskanen, R.A., & Alferness, C. Predictive indices of successful cardiac resuscitation after prolonged arrest and experimental cardiopulmonary resuscitation. *Ann. Emerg. Med.* 1985; **14**: 521–528.

258. Warner, L.L., Hoffman, J.R., & Baraff, L.J. Prognostic significance of field response in out-of-hospital ventricular fibrillation. *Chest* 1985; **87**: 22–28.

259. Hargarten, K.M., Stueven, H.A., Waite, E.M. *et al.* Prehospital experience with defibrillation of coarse ventricular fibrillation: a ten-year review. *Ann. Emerg. Med.* 1990; **19**: 157–162.

260. Martin, T.G., Hawkins, N.S., Weigel, J.A., Rider, D.E., & Buckingham, B.D. Initial treatment of ventricular fibrillation: defibrillation or drug therapy. *Am. J. Emerg Med.* 1988; **6**: 113–119.

261. Niemann, J.T., Cairns, C.B., Sharma, J., & Lewis, R.J. Treatment of prolonged ventricular fibrillation. Immediate countershock versus high-dose epinephrine and CPR preceding countershock. *Circulation* 1992; **85**: 281–287.

262. Weiss, J.N., Qu, Z., Chen, P.S. *et al.* The dynamics of cardiac fibrillation. *Circulation* 2005; **112**: 1232–1240.

263. Chen, P.S., Wu, T.J., Ting, C.T. *et al.* A tale of two fibrillations. *Circulation* 2003; **108**: 2298–2303.

The neuroendocrine response to global ischemia and reperfusion*

Martin W. Dünser, Stefan Jochberger, Karl-Heinz Stadlbauer, and Volker Wenzel

Department of Anesthesiology and Critical Care Medicine, Innsbruck Medical University, Innsbruck, Austria

The neuroendocrine system

Early during evolution, the *neuroendocrinium* developed as its own organ system. With its numerous intercellular and inter-organ mediators, the hormones, it fulfills important functions to synchronize and connect organs and tissues. Likewise, during stress, the neuroendocrine system, as a complex orchestra with not yet fully understood interactive mechanisms, plays one of the most important roles in the body's adaptation to harmful events, such as injury or disease.

Operational definitions (by Jacobo Wortsman, M.D.)

In general terms the endocrine system comprises hormone-producing organs (glands) that regulate the function of other organs. On functional activation, endocrine organs release their secretory products into the blood. Thus, activation can be assumed to occur when there is evidence of increased hormone concentrations in plasma.

Stress may be defined as any changes in the external or internal environment that elicit a highly organized and synchronized neuroendocrine response. Whereas changes in the internal environment can be quantified according to the degree of interference with homeostasis, changes in the external environment (psychologic stress) cannot be quantified in this manner. Thus, the description of stress must include both the nature of the stressful stimulus and the subsequent functional changes. Nevertheless, because of the universal and severe organ involvement during

cardiac arrest, it can be safely assumed that this condition *per se* represents a stress of maximal degree, without consideration of hormone levels.

The term neuroendocrine response, as used in the description of endocrine reactions to stress, emphasizes the regulatory control placed by the hypothalamus over the entire endocrine system. This control is exerted through the production of specific peptides that are translocated to the anterior lobe of the pituitary gland *via* a venous portal system. The hypothalamus has direct nerve connections with the posterior lobe of the pituitary gland, which stores and releases hormonal products. The peripheral endocrine glands (adrenal cortex, thyroid, and gonads), however, receive pituitary trophic stimulation *via* the general circulation. An important exception to this organizational pattern is the direct regulatory control of the adrenal medullae by the central nervous system.

Methodologic issues in studies of the neuroendocrine response to cardiac arrest (by Jacobo Wortsman, M.D.)

Studies on cardiac arrest in human subjects are fraught with interpretive errors because of the rapidity and intensity of physiologic changes, the use of strong therapeutic agents, and the unpredictability of outcome. For example, uncertainties about the exact time of the cardiac arrest and attendant variability in the interval between arrest and initiation of resuscitation procedures (downtime) make determination of the actual sequence of response events difficult. In general, when cardiac arrest occurs in an intensive care unit,

---

* revision of the chapter by Jacobo Wortsman, M.D. in the 1st edition.
Cardiac Arrest: The Science and Practice of Resuscitation Medicine. 2nd edn., ed. Norman Paradis, Henry Halperin, Karl Kern, Volker Wenzel, Douglas Chamberlain. Published by Cambridge University Press. © Cambridge University Press, 2007.

downtime is usually extremely short (seconds), whereas it is much longer (minutes) in out-of-hospital events. The interfering effect of drug therapy must also be considered since patients at risk for cardiac arrest are often receiving multiple drugs. Furthermore, cell death due to cardiac arrest could produce postmortem release of hormones unrelated to the stress reaction. Thus, if possible, biochemical analyses should be performed to identify hormonal products rigorously since substances appearing during global ischemia could differ from the normal circulating products. Of particular concern for studies in endocrine physiology is the abnormally low and irregular blood flow inherent to cardiac arrest and resuscitation maneuvers.[1, 2] The resulting altered hemodynamics could produce plasma compartmentalization; and, in such cases, samples of peripheral blood obtained during cardiopulmonary resuscitation (CPR) might not reflect the rates of hormone secretion and removal that prevail in the intact circulation.

Animal models provide extremely important tools for the study of cardiac arrest and resuscitation. Notably, however, the experimental approach carries the limitations imposed by the evolutionary gap when applied to the stress response of humans. It is reasonable to assume that the crucial role and involvement of higher centers in the central nervous system (as initiators or targets of the stress reaction) can only be determined in humans.

Neuroendocrine response in the immediate cardiac arrest period

Pathophysiologically, the period of acute cardiac arrest with cessation of systemic blood flow is inevitably associated with global ischemia. Depending on the type and function of the cells, cellular and organ dysfunction occurs, that is followed sooner or later by cell destruction, organ failure, and death. Clinically, the period of cardiac arrest represents a period of global ischemia including the downtime and later the period of cardiopulmonary resuscitation with mechanical, electrical, and pharmacological interventions. The immediate cardiac arrest period ends either when spontaneous circulation returns and reperfusion starts, or when resuscitative efforts are withdrawn.

Pituitary gland

The anterior lobe of the pituitary gland produces and releases peptides that control the function of the adrenal cortex (adrenocorticotropin), the thyroid gland (thyrotropin), and the gonads (gonadotropins). In addition, the anterior pituitary synthesizes other peptides such as growth

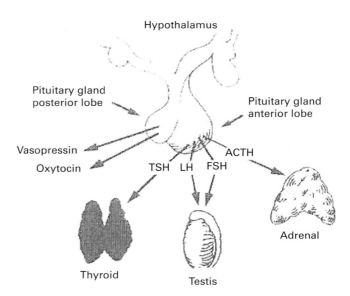

Fig. 7.1. The pituitary gland. Endocrine organs controlled by the anterior lobe of the pituitary gland. Not represented in the figure are pituitary hormones acting on non-endocrine targets, such as prolactin, growth hormone, and β-endorphin.

hormone (GH), prolactin, β-endorphin, and β-lipotropin which act on different neuroendocrine targets. Secretion of anterior pituitary hormones is regulated by specific hypothalamic releasing factors that are transported through the portal hypophyseal vascular system (Fig. 7.1).[3]

Anterior lobe

Pro-opiomelanocortin complex
The main product of the corticotrophic cells of the adenohypophysis is the pro-opiomelanocortin (POMC) complex which is a 266-amino acid molecule. During post-translational processing, prohormone convertase enzymes can cleave the POMC complex into different hormones. This generates adrenocorticotropin (ACTH) and β-lipoprotein (β-LPH). ACTH can be further processed to generate 7- or α-melanocyte stimulating hormone (7- or α-MSH), and corticotropin-like intermediate lobe peptide (CLIP), whereas β-LPH can be processed to generate β-LPH and β-endorphin.[4] Under physiologic conditions, POMC is mainly processed to the N-terminal glycopeptide, ACTH, and β-LPH; smaller amounts of the other peptides are also present.[5] Additional posttranslational modifications of the POMC complex have been described,[6, 7] but their biologic activities remain to be determined.

From those hormones that can be processed in the POMC complex, ACTH, 7- or α-MSH, and β-endorphin have been evaluated in the acute setting of cardiac arrest.

Table 7.1. Plasma hormone concentrations during cardiopulmonary resuscitation in resuscitated and non-resuscitated patients[20]

Hormone	Resuscitated patients (n=20)	Non-resuscitated patients (n=14)	p
Adrenocorticotropin (pg/ml) (25–50)	237 (29–572)	45 (1–794)	0.018
Cortisol (μg/dl) (5.0–25.0)	32.6 (5.9–74.7)	18.4 (9.6–70.1)	0.481
Arginine vasopressin (pg/ml) (1–3)	122 (20–469)	88 (5–156)	0.049
Renin (ng/l) (10–30)	46.5 (22–88)	11 (9–40)	0.017

Data are shown as median and range. The normal range of values is displayed after the name of the hormone in the left column.

ACTH

ACTH is the principal regulator of cortisol production in the *zona fasciculata* of the adrenal cortex, whereas it is of secondary significance in aldosterone and adrenal androgen production. The peripheral effects of ACTH are mediated *via* cyclic adenosine 3′, 5′-phosphate (cAMP)-coupled receptors on adrenal cell membranes. ACTH stimulates cortisol synthesis and secretion by affecting several steps in the steroidogenesis pathway. Although cortisol is not stored in the adrenal cortex, but is synthesized within minutes, the effects of ACTH on adrenal cortisol production can be readily measured after secretion of the hormone.

The synthesis of POMC and hence the secretion of ACTH is under the control of the corticotropin-releasing hormone (CRH) and to a lesser degree of arginine vasopressin. Both hormones are synthesized in the parvocellular cells of the paraventricular hypothalamic nucleus, and are under the negative control of circulating glucocorticoids. Vasopressin stimulates ACTH release only weakly by itself, but is strongly synergstic with the effects of CRH.[8] Other endocrinologic and non-endocrinologic factors have been shown to modulate ACTH release. While the vasoactive intestinal peptide (VIP),[9] catecholamines,[10] ghrelin,[11,12] as well as pro-inflammatory cytokines[13] stimulate ACTH release by indirect modulation of CRH secretion, angiotensin II was reported to stimulate ACTH release directly from pituitary cells.[14] Opiates and opioid peptides,[15] and probably also the atrial natriuretic peptide (ANP),[16, 17] decrease ACTH production.

During cardiac arrest and CPR in patients on the intensive care unit, ACTH levels were significantly higher when compared to those in other critically ill patients. This elevation was detectable within the first 10 minutes after cardiac arrest, when the plasma concentrations reached a mean value of 166 pg/ml (normal range <130 pg/ml), and remained elevated throughout the first hour.[18] In a study of a large population of patients with out-of-hospital cardiac arrest (n=205), it was found that the mean ACTH level (160 pg/ml) was similar to that observed in intensive care

unit cardiac arrest.[19] Further evaluation of patients with out-of-hospital cardiac arrest showed that initial plasma ACTH levels were lower in individuals in whom spontaneous circulation did not return (133 ± 227 pg/ml; n = 161) than in those who had return of spontaneous circulation (229 ± 260 pg/ml, n = 44, p<0.05).[19] Similar results were observed in two other studies, including 34 and 60 patients with out-of-hospital cardiac arrest (Table 7.1). In both studies, ACTH concentrations were higher in patients who had a return of spontaneous circulation compared to concentrations in the patients who could not be resuscitated.[20, 21] In 10 patients who underwent testing of "implanted cardioverter defibrillator" devices, a short period of cardiac arrest under light sedation slightly increased ACTH concentrations, but did not appear to stimulate catecholamine secretion.[22] In an animal experiment, serum ACTH concentrations were observed to be significantly higher in pigs resuscitated with vasopressin (0.4 IU/kg, n = 7) when compared to pigs receiving epinephrine (0.045 mg/kg, n = 7) (ACTH, p = 0.001; cortisol, p = 0.005).[23]

β-Endorphins

Endorphins play an important role as possible neuroregulators in pain transmission, analgesia, tolerance and dependence, as well as in behavior and endocrine pathways, mainly those related to the hypothalamo-pituitary axes.[24] β-Endorpin is known to be released during pain stimulation in the rat and during thermal injury or surgical procedures in humans.[4, 25, 26] β-Endorphin binds to opioid receptors and is thought to be an endogenous mediator for stress-induced analgesia.[5] Moreover, recent data suggest that endorphins act not only as neuroregulators, but also have direct effects on calcium channels of the cerebral vasculature.[6]

Only few studies so far have examined β-Endorphins during cardiac arrest. During cardiopulmonary resuscitation, β-Endorphins were found to be significantly elevated when compared to intensive care unit patients without cardiac arrest.[18] Such an increase in β-Endorphin levels was most pronounced in hypoxic cardiac arrest.[27] β-Endorphin concentrations remained high at least for 10 to 20 minutes after cardiac arrest.[18] The sudden increment of β-Endorphin in brain tissue and body fluids of dogs who were conscious at the moment of cardiac arrest led to the hypothesis that β-Endorphins could participate in the sensations narrated by subjects in the so-called near-death experience.[28]

Melanocyte stimulating hormones (MSH)

The general designation – γ-MSH refers to peptide fragments that are derived from the aminoterminal region of the POMC and have partial structural homology to the melanotropins.[29,30] Among the several amino acid sequences that have been postulated for – γ-MSH peptides, 73-MSH is the most extensively investigated.[31] Although γ_3-MSH exerts only weak melanotropic activity, it can enhance the adrenal-stimulating effect of ACTH.[32,33]

α-MSH is a tridecapeptide melanocortin structurally related to ACTH. It is found principally in the brain and the pituitary, although keratinocytes and blood monocytes can also release α-MSH. Moreover, α-MSH has potent anti-inflammatory actions in both the brain and in peripheral tissues.

Only one clinical study has investigated MSH levels in patients during cardiac arrest. In this analysis, γ_3-MSH immunoreactivity was found to be consistently elevated in patients with cardiac arrest when compared to intensive care unit controls (162 ± 20 vs. 35 ± 6 pg/ml; $p < 0.001$). γ_3-MSH seems to be an important component of the massive release of pituitary and adrenal glandular hormones during cardiac arrest.[18]

An interesting study in rats with prolonged global ischemia due to respiratory arrest demonstrated that if an intravenous injection of α-MSH was given at the start of mechanical ventilation there was an immediate (<1 minute) increase in cardiac output, heart rate, mean arterial pressure, and pulse pressure, with full recovery of electroencephalographic patterns and blood gas parameters after 30 to 45 minutes. All animals eventually recovered completely.[34] These results suggest that melanocortin peptides not only affect resuscitation during pre-terminal ischemia, but may also have potential therapeutic values in global and local ischemia.

Prolactin

Prolactin is a mammotrophic peptide that is unique among the pituitary hormones for being only under tonic inhibitory control by the hypothalamus. The hypothalamic factor that suppresses prolactin secretion is thought to be dopamine.[3] In addition to promoting mammary gland development and milk production, prolactin plays a pivotal role in the immune system. Physiologic studies have demonstrated the presence of prolactin receptors on human T- and B-lymphocytes,[35] and showed that T-lymphocytes depend on prolactin for maintaining immune competence.[36]

Cardiac arrest is associated with a marked elevation in serum prolactin concentrations (44 ± 10.2 ng/ml; frequency of abnormally high values 60%; $n = 15$). Prolactin levels increase within the first 10 minutes of cardiopulmonary resuscitation and remain elevated throughout resuscitation.[18] Another study of prolactin serum levels in patients with out-of-hospital cardiac arrest found that prolactin levels were significantly higher in patients who could be successfully resuscitated when compared to patients in whom cardiopulmonary resuscitative efforts remained ineffective (95.9 ± 13.6 vs. 23.9 ± 5.6 ng/ml; $p = 0.0001$). Decreased prolactin concentrations in non-resuscitated patients may have been a result of exhaustion of the neuroendocrine system, or due to differences in bioavailability at the site of blood sampling, on the basis of differences in hemodynamics.[37]

Prolactin release during cardiac arrest was speculated to be mediated by β-endorphin,[38] but the correlation between prolactin and β-endorphin concentrations was found to be small and non-significant ($r = -0.1$; $p > 0.1$; $n = 117$).[18] The correlation of prolactin with another marker of stress intensity, serum cortisol, was highly significant ($r = 0.44$; $p < 0.01$).[18]

Growth hormone (GH)

GH, or somatotropin, is released in a pulsatile fashion from somatotrophs of the pituitary gland. Two hypothalamic hormones control GH secretion: GH-releasing hormone, which stimulates the production and induces the release of GH; and somatostatin, which acts as an inhibitor.[3] GH affects body growth and metabolism directly and indirectly through stimulation of the liver to produce insulin-like growth factor-1 (IGF-1, also known as somatomedin C). Apart from its general effects causing growth, GH has multiple specific metabolic effects, including enhancement of total body protein, mobilization of fat stores, and conservation of carbohydrates.

Since the 1980s, a series of synthetic GH-releasing peptides and non-peptide analogs, together labeled GH secretagogues, have been developed with potent GH-releasing capacities acting through a specific G-protein-coupled receptor located in the hypothalamus and the pituitary.[39,40] The endogenous ligand for the GH receptor is known as ghrelin, a highly conserved 28-amino-acid peptide[41] originating in the stomach as well as in the hypothalamic arcuate nucleus, that has recently emerged as a key factor together with GH-releasing hormone and somatostatin, involved in the complex control of GH secretion. These regulatory factors act in concert to achieve a pulsatile secretion of GH.

To date, there are no studies on the GH response during global ischemia or cardiac arrest, although a significant release would be expected to maintain at least cerebral glucose supply.

Neurohypophysis (posterior lobe)

Vasopressin

Vasopressin is an endogenous nonapeptide hormone with antidiuretic, vasomotoric, hemostatic, and central nervous effects. The hormone is produced in the magnocellular nuclei of the hypothalamus and stored in neurosecretory vesicles of the neurohypophysis. It is secreted upon osmotic, hemodynamic, and endocrinologic stimuli. Most newly synthesized vasopressin is stored intracellularly; only 10%–20% of the total hormonal pool within the posterior pituitary can be readily released.

Important hemodynamic signals for secretion are reduced atrial filling, as well as decreased arterial blood pressure. Any reduction in blood volume or venous return stimulates vasopressin secretion via activation of stretch receptors located in the left atrium and pulmonary arteries (Gauer–Henry reflex). Activation of baroreceptors in the aortic and carotid sinus further augments vasopressin secretion *via* the glossopharyngeus and vagal nerves.[42] Baroreceptor-mediated vasopressin secretion, however, is the primary stimulation release in hypotensive states.[43]

In addition to osmolar and hemodynamic stimuli, endotoxin as well as pro-inflammatory cytokines can stimulate secretion of vasopressin independently of plasma osmolarity, blood pressure, or intravascular volume status.[44–46] Endocrinologically, angiotensin II and III, as well as endothelins (ET), norepinephrine, and epinephrine are physiologic secretagogues of vasopressin,[42, 47, 48] whereas ANP suppresses vasopressin secretion.[49, 50]

In plasma, vasopressin is bound to proteins; 10% at basal plasma concentrations and up to 40% at higher concentrations. Serum half-life varies between 8 and 15 minutes. Splanchnic and renal enzymatic degradation are primary pathways of inactivation. Renal clearance of vasopressin results from glomerular filtration, degradation, or reabsorption in the proximal nephron, and additional secretion into the distal nephron. Ten percent of vasopressin is excreted as active hormone. Renal clearance remains unaffected by changes in serum concentration over a broad range.[51] Splanchnic clearance of vasopressin is accomplished almost equally by the intestine and the liver.[52] Because the sum of splanchnic and renal elimination of vasopressin is less than estimates of its metabolic rate, there seems to be a pharmacologically significant clearance of vasopressin by other organs.[51]

Peripheral effects of vasopressin are mediated by three different G protein-coupled receptors. V1a-receptors have been found on vascular smooth muscle cells and induce vasoconstriction by an increase in cytoplasmic ionized calcium *via* the phosphatidyl-inositol-bisphosphonate cascade.[53] In contrast to catecholamine-mediated vasoconstriction, effects of vasopressin are also preserved during hypoxia and severe acidosis.[54] Vasopressin-mediated vascular effects differ substantially within particular vascular beds, however. Physiologically, most arterial beds exhibit vasoconstriction in response to vasopressin,[55, 56] with vasopressor effects being strongest in the splanchnic, muscular, and cutaneous vasculature.[57]

Paradoxical vasodilatation to vasopressin has been described in the pulmonary, coronary, vertebrobasilar, and gastrointestinal circulation.[58–60] The underlying mechanisms seem to be nitric oxide dependent.[58] Recently, there is increasing evidence of hemodynamically relevant V1a-receptors on cardiomyocytes. *In vitro* and animal experiments have demonstrated an increase in intracellular calcium concentration and inotropy after stimulation of myocardial V1a-receptors.[61,62] V1a-receptors are further expressed on thrombocytes. Upon stimulation, they induce an increase in intracellular calcium, thereby facilitating thrombocyte aggregation.[63] Vasopressin also increases expulsion of thrombocytes from the bone marrow.[64] Other hemostatic effects are mediated by V2-receptors. Prostacyclin generation is stimulated; tissue-type plasminogen activator activity, factor VIII-related antigen activity, factor VIII coagulant activity, and von Willebrand factor multimeres all increase upon V2-receptor stimulation.[65] Stimulation of V1a-receptors on hepatocytes increases glycolysis and glycogenolysis, gluconeogenesis, and esterification and oxidation of free fatty acids, as well as production of ketone bodies.[66]

V1b-receptors are found on the anterior hypophysis. Stimulation induces liberation of ACTH and consequently enhanced cortisol secretion from the adrenal glands.[67] Accordingly, Kornberger *et al.*[23] reported significantly higher serum ACTH and cortisol concentrations in animals resuscitated from cardiac arrest with vasopressin when compared to epinephrine. V1b-receptors are further expressed on pancreatic isle cells where they induce insulin secretion.[68] Nevertheless, stimulation of insulin secretion by vasopressin only seems to be relevant during moderate to severe hyperglycemia.[69]

In the kidney, V2-receptors are located on distal tubules and collecting ducts. Upon stimulation, they facilitate integration of aquaporines into the luminal cell membrane, leading to increased resorption of free water *via* an adenylate cyclase-dependent mechanism.[42] Despite this antidiuretic effect, a paradoxical increase of urine output has been reported during continuous vasopressin infusion in vasodilatory shock.[70–72] One explanation for this observation is the selective V1a-receptor-mediated vasodilatation of the afferent and vasoconstriction of efferent glomerular arterioles which results in a significantly increased glomerular filtration pressure.[70] V2-receptor-associated natriuretic and diuretic effects as well as release of the atrial natriuretic factor may also be involved.[72] Additional physiological effects of vasopressin on specific brain functions, temperature regulation, and myometrical contractions have been reported.[42, 73]

During cardiac arrest, serum vasopressin levels were found to increase significantly. A canine study of 10 minutes of fibrillatory cardiac arrest showed that AVP levels increased from 1.7 ± 1 pg/ml during spontaneous circulation to 29.9 ± 33.3 pg/ml during cardiac arrest and cardiopulmonary resuscitation ($p = 0.01$). In this model, there was a moderate positive correlation between aortic pressure and circulating endogenous vasopressin levels after the first dose of epinephrine ($r = 0.5$). Additionally, animals with return of spontaneous circulation showed a trend towards higher concentrations of vasopressin in serum ($p = 0.12$).[9] In a study including 34 patients with out-of-hospital cardiac arrest, vasopressin concentrations were significantly increased. Resuscitated patients had significantly higher vasopressin concentrations than did non-resuscitated patients (122 pg/ml vs. 88 pg/ml; $p = 0.049$).[20] In another study of 60 patients with out-of-hospital cardiac arrest, vasopressin serum levels before and after the first epinephrine dosage were significantly higher in patients with return of spontaneous circulation when compared with those in patients who could not be resuscitated (193 ± 28 vs. 70 ± 9 pg/ml, $p < 0.001$; 177 ± 27 vs. 58 ± 9 pg/ml, $p < 0.001$).[21] According to these data, it can be assumed that endogenous vasopressin release may have an important effect on patient outcome from cardiac arrest.

Thyroid gland

Thyroid hormones

The thyroid gland is composed of follicles filled with colloid. Colloid consists of the protein thyroglobulin, which serves as the matrix for synthesis of the thyroid hormones. On glandular stimulation by pituitary thyrotropin (TSH), thyroid hormones are released into the circulation, accompanied by small amounts of thyroglobulin.[16] The thyroid hormones triiod-thyronine with three iodine atoms *per* molecule (T3) and thyroxine with four iodine atoms (T4) have important effects on calorigenesis, somatic growth, and cardiovascular function.[16] T3 and T4 differ significantly in their metabolism.[16] Whereas T4 is synthesized exclusively in the thyroid, T3 is mainly produced in peripheral tissues by deiodination of T4. Reverse T3 is an alternate product of T4 deiodination that is biologically inactive.[16, 74]

Studies performed in 24 cardiac arrest patients in the intensive care unit showed low concentrations of total T4 (3.8 ± 0.6 µg/dl; normal range: 1.2–4.2 µg/dl) and T3 (48 ± 6 ng/dl; normal range: 80–200 ng/dl).[14] On the other hand, reverse T3 was increased to 53.5 ± 9.7 ng/dl (normal range: 8–26 ng/dl) and dialyzable T4 to $0.029 \pm 0.0003\%$ (normal range: 0.016–0.028%).[14] Although TSH was slightly higher in cardiac arrest than in non-cardiac arrest patients in intensive care units (6.2 ± 2 µg/ml vs. 3.6 ± 3.3 µg/ml), the difference was not statistically significant.[14] Serum thyroglobulin levels remained unchanged throughout resuscitation.[14] A similar hormonal profile of decreased T4, free T4, T3, and free T3, as well as increased reverse T3 was noted in dogs after cardiac arrest periods of 30 seconds to 9 minutes.[75] Analysis of 473 patients with out-of-hospital cardiac arrest found that patients exhibiting total T4, T3, and reverse T3 closer to the normal range and TSH levels that were higher, were significantly more likely to survive than were patients with low thyroid hormone levels.[76]

It appears that the thyroid profile of cardiac arrest is most compatible with peripheral hypothyroidism, and the relatively higher TSH concentrations in these patients suggest an appropriate response to a state of hypothyroidism. Taken together, the current data provide strong evidence against active participation of thyroid hormones in cardiac arrest.

Calcitonin

Calcitonin is a peptide hormone that is synthesized in and secreted from the parafollicular cells, also known as C cells, of the thyroid gland. The primary stimulus for calcitonin secretion is increased plasma calcium concentration. Whereas in young subjects calcitonin rapidly decreases blood calcium by reducing the function and formation of osteoclasts, calcitonin has only weak effects on plasma calcium levels in adults.[77]

Although there are no clinical or experimental studies that examine the course of calcitonin concentrations during cardiac arrest, calcitonin was measured in acutely traumatized patients ($n = 11$). Ninety-one percent of these patients had increased serum calcitonin concentrations on admission to the emergency department. Median calcitonin concentrations in acutely traumatized patients were higher throughout the study period than in elective surgery patients ($P<0.05$). Interestingly, despite these increased calcitonin concentrations and hypocalcemia in most patients, loss of urinary calcium was within the normal range.[78]

Parathyroid glands

The parathyroid consists of four small glands that are variably located behind the four poles of the thyroid gland. The parathyroid glands are the body's main location of parathyroid hormone production. The parathyroid hormone is a classical peptide hormone whose secretion is almost completely dependent on plasma calcium concentrations. Once released into the circulation, parathyroid hormone increases plasma calcium and reduces phosphate concentrations. While the parathyroid hormone-induced fall in phosphate concentration occurs rapidly, the rise in calcium can be divided into a rapid and a slow phase. The rapid effect is mostly due to parathyroid hormone-induced inhibition of renal calcium excretion. Calcium and phosphate absorption from the bone by stimulation of osteoclasts is responsible for the slow effects of parathyroid hormone on plasma calcium concentrations.[77]

No data currently exist on parathryoid hormone concentrations in patients with cardiac arrest. One clinical study, however, analyzed parathyroid hormone levels during global ischemia in acutely ill patients admitted to the emergency department. Elevated parathyroid hormone concentrations (>55 pg/ml) were observed in 16% of patients, most frequently in patients with myocardial infarction (28%) and congestive heart failure (42%). Parathyroid hormone levels significantly correlated with the APACHE II score ($P<0.0001$) and also with the length of hospital stay ($P<0.002$). Moreover, in that study, parathyroid hormone concentrations were identified as a strong predictor of patient outcome, with significantly higher serum concentrations observed in patients who subsequently died than in patients who eventually survived ($P<0.03$).[79]

Adrenal glands

The adrenal glands comprise two embryologically different tissues, the adrenal cortex and medulla. Although anatomically and histologically distinct, there is no strict separation in localization of the two tissues. Recent studies have proven that chromaffin cells, once thought to be located exclusively in the medulla, can also be found in all cortical zones, and that cortical cells are found in the adrenal medulla as well.[79, 80] This close co-localization is assumed to be a prerequisite for paracrine interactions.[81]

The adrenal medulla takes a special position within the endocrinologic system since it is not integrated into specific endocrinologic axes, but is directly innervated by terminal nerves of the sympathic trunk. Although the adrenal cortex is largely under the control of the hypothalamus and the adenohypophysis, a direct influence of autonomic nerve terminals on adrenocortical cells has been suggested.[82] The detection of chemo- and baroreceptors in the adrenal cortex further suggests efferent innervation as well.[83,84]

Adrenal medulla

In addition to the terminal sympathetic nerve endings, the adrenal medulla is the main source of plasma norepinephrine. For epinephrine, the adrenal glands are the only plasma source. Thus, plasma concentrations of epinephrine do not only represent activation of the adrenal medulla, but are also considered the most sensitive marker for activation of the neuroendocrine response to stress.[85]

Catecholamines

Epinephrine levels in cardiac arrest are markedly elevated to the highest concentrations ever reported.[86] Whereas the normal resting values of epinephrine are 0.034 ± 0.002 ng/ml, peak levels may reach 10.3 ± 2.9 ng/ml during cardiac arrest ($p<0.01$)[86] and the highest recorded spontaneous plasma epinephrine concentration during cardiac arrest was 35.6 ng/ml.[86] Extraordinarily elevated epinephrine levels have also been observed in porcine and canine models of cardiac arrest.[87, 88] Activation of the adrenal medulla is probably initiated by the cessation of blood flow, which produces maximal stimulation of vascular receptors in the cardiocirculatory system and results in massive discharge of epinephrine.[89, 90] Extensive manipulations associated with cardiopulmonary resuscitation do not appear to contribute to this elevation in epinephrine plasma levels, because peak concentrations are similar in dogs during cardiopulmonary resuscitation, or assisted with cardiopulmonary bypass (Fig. 7.2).[91]

Plasma norepinephrine levels also markedly increased during resuscitation, from normal resting levels of 0.52 ± 0.06 ng/ml up to 7.37 ± 1.8 ng/ml.[85] In addition, the correlation between simultaneous increases in plasma concentrations of epinephrine and norepinephrine during cardiac arrest is highly significant.[86, 92] Since experimental adrenalectomy before cardiac arrest produces almost total (about 80%) suppression of the rise in plasma epinephrine and norepinephrine,[88, 93] it appears that the two plasma

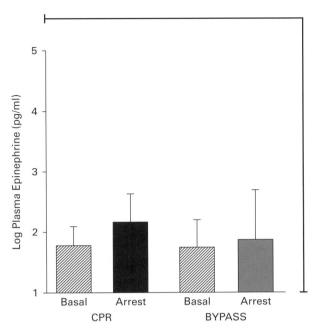

Fig. 7.2. Plasma epinephrine levels during experimental cardiac arrest in dogs.[91] Left, animals resuscitated with standard CPR; right, animals resuscitated with cardiopulmonary bypass. There are no differences in basal or peak epinephrine levels between the two groups.

catecholamines share a common adrenomedullary source in cardiac arrest. Recent evidence suggests, however, that the release of epinephrine precedes that of norepinephrine. The marked rise in plasma epinephrine precipitated by the administration of epinephrine at therapeutic dosages in cardiac arrest is followed by proportional increases in plasma norepinephrine levels.[94] Therefore, stimulation by epinephrine is likely to be the mechanism for the previously unexplained observation of higher plasma norepinephrine levels among cardiac arrest patients treated with epinephrine.[86] Taken together, the data suggest that plasma epinephrine itself may be the primary and perhaps most important stimulus driving the rise of plasma norepinephrine during cardiac arrest. Whether norepinephrine released during cardiac arrest is primarily derived from adrenal or extra-adrenal compartments (neurogenic or non-neurogenic) is not yet clear.

The effects of epinephrine administration in cardiac arrest have been the subject of numerous studies performed in the clinical or experimental setting. It has been concluded that administration of epinephrine may improve the outcome of cardiac arrest.[95–99] Thus epinephrine has become an important component in the therapy of cardiac arrest.

Adrenal cortex

The adrenal cortex is the main steroid hormone-producing organ of the body. More than 30 steroid hormones have been isolated from the adrenal cortex, but only two are of exceptional importance to the normal endocrine function: aldosterone and cortisol. According to functional and histological grading, the adrenal cortex can be divided into three different zones.

- The outer *zona glomerulosa* represents the site of mineralocorticoid production with its physiologically most important representative, aldosterone. The function of the *zona glomerulosa* is mainly modulated by the extracellular fluid content of angiotensin II, potassium, but also to a lesser degree by ACTH.
- The central *zona fasciculata* constitutes about 75% of the adrenal cortex and is the main site for synthesis of glucocorticoids. Apart from ACTH, numerous cytokines and other intercellular mediators influence the biosynthesis of glucocorticoids, of which cortisol is the most important and 95% of the glucocorticoid activity of the *zona fasciculata* is provided by cortisol.
- The inner *zona reticularis* is the site of adrenal androgen production. The *zona reticularis* does not only synthesize dehydroepiandrostenedione and androstenedione, however, but also synthesizes small amounts of estrogen and some glucocorticoids. ACTH regulates secretion of these hormones, although other factors such as cortical androgen-stimulating hormone, released from the pituitary, may be involved as well.

Cortisol

Cortisol is the predominant corticosteroid produced in the human body. In a healthy, unstressed person, cortisol is secreted according to a diurnal pattern. Circulating cortisol is bound to corticosteroid-binding globulin (CBG), with less than 10% in the free, bioavailable form. Its effects are mainly mediated by stimulation of nuclear receptors and modulation of genetic transcription. During recent years, however, studies show that there may be increasing numbers of cortisol effects that are not mediated by nuclear, but by cytosolic or membrane receptors.

As one of the most important physiologic stress hormones, cortisol has catabolic, anti-inflammatory, and vasoactive properties on the peripheral vasculature. Thus, cortisol also contributes to the peripheral vascular tone by facilitating adrenergic vasoconstriction and exerting permissive effects on the synthesis of catecholamines and other vasoactive peptides.[100, 101] Furthermore, cortisol has inotropic effects and can modulate free water distribution within the vascular compartment.[102] Another effect that may be of relevance during and after cardiac arrest, is the possible involvement of cortisol in the modulation of neuronal death during ischemia. An animal study shows that adrenalectomy and administration of a glucocorticoid receptor blocker reduced neuronal cell death after transient global ischemia, suggesting adverse effects of cortisol on neuronal cell survival from ischemia.[103]

Cardiac arrest in intensive care unit patients was associated with a significant elevation of serum cortisol concentrations (48.3 ± 7.6 μg/dl).[18] Overall, high serum cortisol concentrations were found in 86% of intensive care patients during cardiac arrest. Levels of CBG, on the other hand, were significantly decreased when compared with non-cardiac arrest patients in the intensive care unit.[18] Such a decrease in CBG results in a significant increase of its free serum portion and bioavailability during cardiac arrest. In 10 patients undergoing testing of implanted cardioverter defibrillator devices, serum cortisol concentrations increased significantly from 367 ± 62 to 539 ± 64 nmol/l ($p < 0.001$) during induced ventricular fibrillation.[22]

A study of serum cortisol profiles in patients with out-of-hospital cardiac arrest[19] presented results similar to those observed in patients with cardiac arrest in the intensive care unit. Initial serum cortisol levels in these patients were increased to 32 ± 33.1 μg/dl ($n = 205$) with the free fraction being equally elevated to 25% of the total cortisol level. Another trial including 60 patients with out-of-hospital cardiac arrest observed lower, but still supranormal cortisol levels (18 ± 3 and 15 ± 2 μg/dl in survivors and non-survivors, respectively).[21]

Initial serum cortisol concentrations at the time of cardiac arrest may therefore be an ancillary predictor of survival. Indeed, subjects with serum cortisol levels below 30 μg/dl at the time of cardiac arrest had a 96% mortality at 6 hours and a 100% mortality at 24 hours.[19,104] A recent trial found a significant difference in serum cortisol concentrations shortly after cardiac arrest between survivors (34.1 ± 11.2 μg/ml) and non-survivors (19 ± 2.8 μg/ml; $p = 0.0034$). Interestingly, there was no correlation between serum ACTH concentrations and patient outcome.[105] The possible biological significance of cortisol release during cardiac arrest is difficult to interpret and has not yet been studied. Therefore, it remains to be established whether cortisol plays a direct role in the maintenance of cellular functions during global ischemia or is simply a prognostic marker.

Renin–angiotensin–aldosterone system

Angiotensin II is one of the most potent endogenous vasoconstrictive peptides. It is cleaved from angiotensin I by the angiotensin-converting-enzyme whose major site of production is the lung epithelium.[106] Strong vasoconstrictive effects can partly be explained by angiotensin II-induced release of ET[33] and central activation of the sympathetic nervous system.[8] Another major effect of angiotensin II is the stimulation of aldosterone production and release from the adrenal glands.

In addition to the adrenal cortex, aldosterone is also locally produced in the heart and the vessel wall.[107–110] Since neither the aldosterone synthase nor 11-beta-hydroxylase has so far been detected in the myocardium or the vascular smooth muscle cells, it is hypothesized that aldosterone is extracted from the circulation by yet unknown mechanisms. Secretion of aldosterone from the adrenal cortex, the heart, and the vessels is mainly stimulated by angiotensin II and III. ET and serotonin are less potent stimulators, while potassium, the natriuretic peptides, and dopamine inhibit aldosterone secretion.[110]

Once released into the circulation, aldosterone exerts its effects by stimulation of cytoplasmic and transmembrane mineralocorticoid receptors, inducing both genomic and non-genomic effects. Such aldosterone receptors have been observed on endothelial cells, vascular smooth muscle cells, renal tubules, the colon, salivary glands, heart, and brain. Aldosterone plays a key role in the maintenance of sodium and water balance by regulation of epithelial tubular sodium absorption and transcription of sodium-potassium ATPase. By activation of central sympathetic neural pathways, aldosterone can also increase blood pressure. Non-epithelial effects of aldosterone are mediated through a second messenger system that involves activation of the sodium/hydrogen antiporter.[111]

Whereas aldosterone levels have not yet been examined in cardiac arrest, there are data on its precursors, renin and the angiotensins. Patients with out-of-hospital cardiac arrest presented with significantly increased renin concentrations when compared with a normal population (4.6 ng/dl; normal range: 1–3 ng/dl).[20] Elevation of plasma renin activity, however, appeared to be restricted to those who subsequently achieved return of spontaneous circulation, whereas renin elevation was not observed in non-resuscitated patients (1.1 ng/dl; $p < 0.2$ vs. resuscitated patients).[20] Also angiotensin II levels were found to be significantly elevated in canine cardiac arrest, where angiotensin II concentrations increased from 14.7 ± 12.9 pg/ml during spontaneous circulation to 151 ± 105 pg/ml during cardiac arrest and cardiopulmonary resuscitation ($p < 0.05$).[9]

Because of its potent vasoconstrictive effects, administration of angiotensin II has also been studied as a resuscitation drug during cardiac arrest. Infusion of 0.05 mg/kg of angiotensin II resulted in a significant improvement of both myocardial blood flow and short-term survival in a pig model of cardiac arrest.[112] Similar effects of angiotensin

II injection on diastolic aortic pressure as well as myocardial and cerebral blood flow were observed in another animal model of cardiac arrest.[113,114] The hemodynamic effects of angiotensin II during cardiac arrest apparently are not caused exclusively by direct arteriolar vasoconstriction *via* angiotensin II receptors, but are also mediated by a massive catecholamine release with adrenergic peripheral vasoconstriction.[115]

Unconventional endocrine organs

Endothelium

Endothelin (ET) was first isolated by Yanagisawa *et al.* in 1998. They identified the endothelium-derived contracting factor as a 21-amino acid peptide from porcine aortic endothelium cells. The peptide possessed strong vasoconstrictive properties and was at least ten times as potent as those of angiotensin II. This peptide was named ET-1 and together with ET-2 and ET-3 belongs to the ET isopeptide family.[116] ET-1 synthesis is not limited to the endothelium, but it is also produced in a broad variety of other cells, including vascular smooth muscle cells,[117] mucosal epithelium,[118] macrophages,[119] mast cells,[120] cardiomyocytes,[121] neurons,[122] tracheal epithelium,[123] renal medulla,[123] hepatic sinusoids, and Kupffer cells.[124]

Factors known to stimulate the endothelium to release ET-1 include low vascular shear stress,[125] hypoxia,[126] endotoxin,[127] transforming growth factor β,[128] adrenalin,[129] thrombin and angiotensin II.[130] Inhibition of ET-1 release occurs in response to prostacyclin,[131] nitric oxide,[132] ANP,[133] and heparin.[133]

Under physiologic conditions, ET-1 is considered to act as a paracrine mediator, and effects are mediated by at least two types of G-protein-coupled receptors, the ET_A and the ET_B receptors.[134,135] In addition to its highly potent vasoconstrictive effects, *in vitro* and animal studies have shown that ET is a particularly strong constrictor of renal mesangial and coronary vessels. ET receptor stimulation has further been associated with bronchoconstriction, endocrine regulation, and stimulation of monocytes to produce interleukins (interleukin-1, 6, 8), prostaglandin E_2, and substances that trigger formation of superoxide radicals.

During cardiac arrest, ET serum concentrations were found to be slightly increased over those under normal conditions. There was no significant difference in serum ET levels during cardiac arrest between patients who were successfully resuscitated and who were not (4.3 ± 0.9 vs. 5.5 ± 0.4 pg/ml).[21]

Because of its strong vasoconstrictive effects, ET-1 injection (50–300 μg) was studied during cardiac arrest soon after its physiologic identification. First studies underlined the potent vasopressor activities of ET-1 and reported significantly increased cerebral perfusion pressures, diastolic aortic pressure, as well as vital organ blood flow after ET-1 injection.[136–139] Nonetheless, ET-1 administration did not elevate myocardial blood flow because of sustained coronary vasoconstriction.[137] During cardiopulmonary resuscitation, ET-1 administration resulted in a lower endtidal carbon dioxide partial pressure presumably due to decreased cardiac output. After return of spontaneous circulation, the continued ET-1-mediated intense vasoconstriction led to higher aortic diastolic pressure and very narrow pulse pressure. Of greater importance, postresuscitation mortality was significantly higher in the ET-1 group (6 of 8 vs. 0 of 8 with epinephrine-treated animals, $p < 0.01$).[140,141]

Heart

The myocardium is known to produce and secrete natriuretic peptides which lower blood pressure by vascular relaxation and stimulate renal sodium excretion. Currently, the ANP and the brain natriuretic peptide (BNP) have been extensively examined. Both hormones are released into the blood in response to atrial distension.[142–145] They play a complex role in promoting natriuresis and diuresis, inhibiting the renin-angiotensin-aldosterone axis, and acting as a direct vasodilator.[146,147] Natriuretic peptides have been shown to reduce myocardial pre- and afterload, improve left ventricular function, dilate coronary arteries, and ameliorate exercise-induced myocardial ischemia.[148–151] BNP has a half-life of about 3 minutes as it is removed from circulation by binding to natriuretic peptide clearance receptors (c-type receptors), which are located on endothelial cells, and it is inactivated through cleavage by neutral endopeptidases.[152]

In dogs, the ANP response to cardiopulmonary resuscitation consists of an elevation from baseline values of 55 ± 46 pg/ml during spontaneous circulation to 293 ± 73 pg/ml during cardiac arrest.[9] ANP was measured in plasma of patients with out-of-hospital cardiac arrest ($n = 14$) by an assay with a detectability limit of 50 pg/ml.[153] The peptide was detectable in 3 of 29 healthy controls and in 8 of 14 cardiac arrest patients, where ANP serum levels were also significantly higher ($p < 0.01$ vs. controls).[152] Furthermore, the distribution of ANP levels in cardiac arrest correlated significantly with the presence of a pressor response to adrenalin.[153] Thus, a significant pressor response (> 3 mmHg) was observed among cardiac arrest patients who had low (undetectable) rather than measurable ANP levels.[153] As a result, the actual concentration of ANP had a strong predictive power for development of an adrenalin pressure response during cardiopulmonary resuscitation.[153]

Kidney

In addition to its important physiologic functions in controlling water, electrolyte, and acid base homeostasis, the kidney is also an endocrinologic organ. While the kidneys control the production of calcitriol, a hormone essential to regulation of calcium homeostasis, renin and erythropoietin are the most important hormones in the body's response to global ischemia and reperfusion.

Renin

The juxtaglomerular complex consists of macula densa cells in the initial portion of the distal tubule and juxtaglomerular cells in the walls of the afferent and efferent arterioles. Experimental studies suggest that volume depletion and low blood pressure decrease glomerular filtration and may thus slow the flow rate in the loop of Henle. This increases reabsorption of sodium and chloride cells in the ascending tubule and reduces the concentration of sodium chloride in the macula densa cells. Such a decrease in sodium chloride concentration, in turn, initiates a signal by the macula densa to stimulate renin secretion from the juxtaglomerular cells of the afferent and efferent arterioles, which are the major storage sites for renin. Plasma renin functions as an enzyme to increase the formation of angiotensin I, which is converted to angiotensin II. Finally, angiotensin II constricts the efferent arterioles, thereby increasing glomerular hydrostatic pressure and contributing to normalization of the glomerular filtration rate.[154]

Patients with out-of-hospital cardiac arrest presented with significantly increased renin concentrations when compared with a normal population (4.6 ng/dl; normal range: 1–3 ng/dl) (17 am), but elevation of plasma renin activity appeared to be restricted to those who subsequently achieved return of spontaneous circulation. In contrast, renin elevation was not observed in non-resuscitated patients (1.1 ng/dl; $p < 0.2$ vs. resuscitated patients).[20]

Erythropoietin

Erythropoietin is a glycoprotein hormone that is secreted from the kidney. Currently, it is not known exactly where erythropoietin is formed in the kidney, but production in the renal tubular epithelial cells seems to be likely. Whereas the kidneys produce approximately 90% of the circulating erythropoietin, the remaining portion of the hormone is synthesized in the liver. Anemia, global ischemia, and hypoxia are the major stimuli for production and secretion of erythropoietin. Interestingly also, local hypoxia in other parts of the body, but not in the kidneys, also stimulates secretion of renal erythropoietin, which suggests that there might be some non-renal sensor sending additional signals to the kidneys. Moreover, norepinephrine, epinephrine, and several prostaglandins can stimulate release of erythropoietin. Erythropoietin not only stimulates production of proerythroblasts from the hemopoietic stem cells in the bone marrow, but also increases the rate at which these cells pass through the different erythroblastic stages.[155]

Although no clinical or experimental data yet exist on erythropoietin in the immediate cardiac arrest period, it can be assumed that global ischemia induces a significant increase of erythropoietin secretion. In healthy individuals, increased plasma erythropoietin concentrations are observed within 2 hours of exposure to acute hypoxic or anemic conditions.[156, 157]

Gastrointestinal tract

Insulin

Insulin is synthesized as a prehormone in the β-cells of the islets of Langerhans in the pancreas. After posttranslational processing, insulin secretion is mainly regulated by plasma glucose levels. Elevated serum glucose concentrations cause increased glucose uptake in the pancreatic islet cells and led to an increase in cellular metabolism, causing an elevation of the ATP/ADP ratio. This leads to inhibition of the ATP-sensitive potassium channels, that again results in depolarization of the cell, leading to calcium influx and insulin secretion. Once released into the circulation, first into the hepatic circulation, insulin exerts its profound metabolic effects principally by stimulation of membranous insulin receptors. While in the liver, insulin increases the storage of glucose together with a decrease in hepatic glucose release, and in most nonhepatic tissues, insulin increases the glucose uptake by increasing the number of different plasma membrane glucose transporters (GLUT 1–4).

In addition to its central role in regulating glucose metabolism, insulin stimulates lipogenesis, diminishes lipolysis, and increases amino acid transport into cells. Moreover, insulin is known to alter the cellular content of numerous messenger RNAs and thus may control protein synthesis.

Despite marked hyperglycemia, plasma insulin levels progressively decrease during cardiac arrest.[158, 159] Although the hypoinsulinemia of cardiac arrest can be explained by decreased pancreatic blood flow, the absence of a decrease in pancreatic polypeptide (PP) levels does not support such an interpretation.[160] Moreover, hypoinsulinemia and hyperglycemia persist long after the return of spontaneous circulation.[158, 159] It is possible that the low splanchnic blood flow associated with CPR[1] masks systemic PP and/or insulin release. Washout increases failed to develop after return of spontaneous circulation, however.[61] These experimental results suggest that the endocrine digestive system products are not actively released by the neuroendocrine response to the stress of cardiac arrest.

Intestinal hormones

A number of substances found in abundance in the enteric and pancreatic nervous system affect gastrointestinal motility and the composition of digestive secretions.[162] Among the factors with functional activity are the peptides pancreatic polypeptide (PP), neurotensin, substance P, and VIP. These peptides are also produced in the central nervous system and are secreted in response to both food and neural stimulation.[161] Immunohistochemical studies of nervous tissue have shown that these generically called gastrointestinal neuropeptides are localized to specific nerve endings. Thus, they are thought to have important roles as neurotransmitters.[161] However, synthesis of neuropeptides occurs not only in enteric nerves and central nerves, but also in immune cells of lymphoid tissues in the gut. Lymphocytes express receptors for most of these neuropeptides, but other immune cells, such as macrophages and mast cells, are capable of responding to the intestinal hormones. The neuropeptides differ in their ability to generate lymphoproliferative responses, cytokine production, and immunoglobulin synthesis. Some neuropeptides, particularly cholecystokinin, gastrin-releasing peptide, and neurotensin, appear to play an important role in maintaining mucosal immunity in patients who cannot receive enteral feeding during critical illness or after intestinal resection.[162]

The blood levels of gastrointestinal neuropeptides have been determined in experimental cardiac arrest to evaluate a possible involvement of the gastrointestinal tract in the neuroendocrine response to stress.[160] This protocol examined the effects of ventricular fibrillation and return of spontaneous circulation in sham-operated and adrenalectomized dogs.[160] Measurement of PP, VIP, neurotensin, and substance P showed that only VIP was affected by experimental manipulations. VIP increased significantly after cardiac arrest, but only in the sham-operated group.[160] Of note, adrenalectomy *per se* appeared to affect some of the peptides, since both plasma PP and VIP levels were higher in adrenalectomized than in sham-operated animals.[160]

Neuroendocrine response in the postcardiac arrest period

Pathophysiologically, reperfusion after cardiac arrest begins with return of spontaneous circulation and renewed supply of oxygen to the cells. Clinically, the reperfusion phase reflects the postcardiac arrest period of critical illness in the emergency department and/or the intensive care unit. Although global ischemia is terminated in the reperfusion phase, formation of free oxygen radicals and systemic activation of the immune, coagulation, and neuroendocrine system contribute to ongoing cell dysfunction and death. Overwhelming systemic inflammation and multiple organ dysfunction are frequent complications during the reperfusion period after cardiac arrest, and have recently been summarized by the term "post-resuscitation disease."

Postresuscitation disease is associated with hemodynamic instability and multiple organ dysfunction that can contribute to adverse neurologic outcome.[163] The hemodynamic status of postresuscitation disease shares common features with septic shock and is typically associated with reversible myocardial dysfunction and vasodilation with low filling pressures requiring volume expansion, as well as inotropic and vasoactive drugs.[164] Moreover, the immunoinflammatory and coagulatory profile observed in patients after return of spontaneous circulation typically resembles that of patients with systemic inflammatory response syndrome or sepsis, thus characterizing a sepsis-like syndrome.[165, 166]

The distinct neuroendocrine response patterns in acute and prolonged critical illness

It was previously assumed that the stress response during the acute life-threatening event persisted throughout the course of critical illness, but this assumption has been disproved. During the initial response to an acute stress event, such as global ischemia and reperfusion, severe trauma, sepsis, or major surgery, the anterior pituitary actively releases its hormones into the circulation, while in the periphery, anabolic target organ hormones are inactivated. This response is thought to be beneficial and adaptive in order to overcome the acute disease. When critical illness becomes prolonged, however, pulsatile secretion of hormones becomes uniformly reduced and high stress hormone levels begin progressively to decrease to physiological or even subnormal values. In the pituitary gland, however, this is most probably due to several complex mechanisms, such as decreased (hypothalamic) stimulation, depletion of hormone stores, reduced activity of target tissues, and impaired anabolism.[167, 168]

Pituitary gland (anterior lobe)

ACTH

After the return of spontaneous circulation, plasma ACTH concentrations remain persistently elevated for at least 6 hours.[19] Indeed, in one study, ACTH did not decrease to a mean level of 65 pg/ml until 24 hours after cardiac arrest.[19]

Although high levels of ACTH and cortisol coexist in cardiac arrest,[18] a causative relationship between ACTH and cortisol has not yet been detected. Thus, comparison with healthy subjects showed that only 23% of postcardiac arrest intensive care unit samples had ACTH concentrations above the normal range, whereas serum cortisol was elevated in 86% of these samples.[18] Moreover, the overall correlation between cortisol and ACTH was low and did not even reach statistical significance ($r = 0.26$; $p > 0.2$).[18] The most important evidence against an ACTH-mediated stimulation of cortisol release is the response to a challenge with exogenous ACTH in out-of-hospital cardiac arrest. Testing of this population showed no serum cortisol response at either 6 or 24 hours after resuscitation, indicating that the adrenal was refractory to ACTH.[19] Therefore, it appears that adrenocortical ACTH release during and after cardiac arrest may be driven through a pathway other than ACTH, possibly including ET.[169] The reason for the low levels of ACTH during this phase of severe stress is unclear, although a role of ANP or substance P has been suggested.[169] It is interesting that additional evidence of perturbed ACTH secretion has been uncovered in critical illness, where ACTH levels are both not suppressed after administration of dexamethasone and also show an exaggerated response to its releasing factor (CRH).[170]

Therefore, global ischemia and in particular reperfusion is associated with dysregulated ACTH secretion and obvious loss of adrenal responsiveness to ACTH. The latter could represent specific adrenal dysfunction or just irregular adrenal perfusion. Regardless of the mechanism of the adrenal defect, the data indicate that plasma ACTH is biologically ineffective during cardiac arrest and the immediate postresuscitation phase. High levels of ACTH in the postresuscitation period can therefore only be taken as an indicator of the intensity of the neuroendocrine stress response.

β-Endorphins
No study so far has specifically evaluated β-endorphin concentrations in the post-resuscitation phase after cardiac arrest. Only Wortsman et al. have reported on elevated β-endorphin levels during the resuscitation phase after cardiac arrest.[18] Nonetheless, there are some reports on changes in β-endorphin concentrations during chronic and acute stress, such as shock or critical illness.[171] In an animal model of shock, β-endorphin was substantially increased during hemorrhage[172] and sepsis.[173] Similarly, Schmidt *et al.* observed significantly elevated β-endorphin levels that paralleled epinephrine and norepinephrine plasma concentrations during acute and chronic stress in

critically ill patients.[174] High levels of β-endorphin are assumed to modulate hemodynamic stability, neuroendocrine, and cytokine responses during stress, such as hemorrhagic shock.[175]

Of great interest with respect to cardiac arrest is an inhibitory effect of β-endorphin on plasma membrane calcium currents.[6] Recent studies have attributed such a possible neuroprotective effect of endogenous opioid peptides to the μ-receptor coupled to G(o)-type GTP-binding protein.[176, 177] β-Endorphin also acts as a direct vasodilator on the cerebral circulation and may thus have additional neuroprotective effects.[6] Nonetheless, administration of naloxone to dogs with cardiac arrest failed to have a beneficial effect on outcome.[7]

Melanocyte stimulating hormones
MSH concentrations have so far not been investigated in the postcardiac arrest period, although, several studies have reported a potential role of melanotropins in the treatment of global and local ischemia as well as reperfusion.

α-MSH and other ACTH fragments were reported to improve significantly blood pressure, pulse amplitude, and survival in otherwise fatal hemorrhagic shock in rats.[178] Similar effects of melanocortin peptides were observed in myocardial ischemia and reperfusion injury when MSH administration prevented free radical discharge, the development of severe ventricular arrhythmias, and an abrupt fall in systemic arterial resistance, with a consequent increase in survival.[179–181] The protective effects of melanocortins may be due to MC_3 receptor-mediated inhibition of oxygen free radical discharge and a reduced inflammatory response. Anti-inflammatory effects of MSH can be linked to stimulation of central melanocortin receptors,[182, 183] and to the inhibition of NF-κB activation.[184]

Based on the immune modulating effects of α-MSH, Delgado-Hernandez et al. have demonstrated that intrathecal injections of α-MSH can abrogate the inflammatory response in the peritoneum and lung after intraperitoneal administration of lipopolysaccharide, whereas intraperitoneal injections of similar dosages of α-MSH did not reduce this inflammatory response.[185]

Prolactin
Following the rapid increase in serum prolactin concentrations shortly after cardiac arrest, prolactin levels remain elevated throughout the postresuscitation period.[18] In one study, 5, 15, 30, and 60 minutes after restoration of spontaneous circulation, prolactin serum concentrations were significantly elevated (Fig. 7.3).[37] Cytokines again may play an important role. Although prolactin appears to have immunostimulatory properties in animal models as well

as in humans,[186–188] it remains unclear whether relative hyperprolactinemia during the initial phase of critical illness contributes to the activation of the inflammatory cascade.

In prolonged critical illness, serum prolactin levels are no longer elevated, and its secretory pattern is characterized by a reduction in the pulsatile fraction.[189, 190] It is not known whether the blunted prolactin secretion plays a role in the anergic immune dysfunction or the increased susceptibility of long-term critically ill patients to infections.[191, 192] In addition to endogenous suppressing factors, therapeutic interventions, such as dopamine infusion, may also reduce prolactin production and release. Thus, dopamine was shown to aggravate both T-lymphocyte dysfunction and impaired neutrophil chemotaxis.[188, 193, 194]

Growth hormone

Secretion of GH and its biologic activity have recently been studied in critically ill patients. In these subjects, circulating levels of GH were observed to be persistently elevated, whereas GH-binding activity in plasma was decreased.[8,195,196] These alterations of physiologic GH homeostasis have been interpreted as acquired peripheral resistance to GH.[195, 196]

During the initial phase of reperfusion and acute illness, serum levels of GH increase, and both peak and interpulse GH levels are elevated.[195, 197, 198] Although the physiologic mechanisms involved in the GH release in response to stress are yet to be elucidated, they may be similar to those observed in starvation, when an enhancement of circulating GH levels occurs in response to elevated levels of GH releasing hormone and absence of somatostatin.[199]

In the acute phase of critical illness, however, there is a reduction in circulating IGF-1 levels, despite elevated GH concentrations. Serum levels of IGF-binding proteins are concomitantly decreased.[196, 200] It has been hypothesized that these alterations in GH homeostasis during the initial phase of critical illness are mediated by inflammatory cytokines such as tumor necrosis factor α, and interleukin-1 and –6.[201] High concentrations of IGF-binding protein-1 in serum have been observed to correlate specifically with intensive care unit mortality in the chronic phase of critical illness, weeks before death.[202] The predictive value of a high serum IGF-binding protein-1 concentration was comparable to that of a high APACHE-II score.[203]

Although during prolonged critical illness, GH continues to be released in a high frequency pulsatile fashion, the amount of GH released with each pulse is significantly reduced.[189, 201, 204] Hence, mean GH serum levels during prolonged critical illness can reach values observed during health, but are substantially lower than are those during acute stress.[197] This relative deficiency of GH,

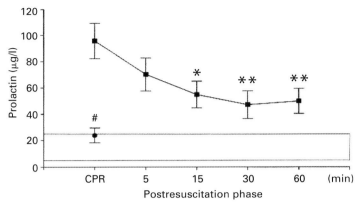

Fig. 7.3. Plasma prolactin concentrations during cardiopulmonary resuscitation (CPR) and within the first hour after restoration of spontaneous circulation.[37] Solid squares, values for resuscitated patients; solid circle, values for non-resuscitated patients; shaded rectangle, the normal range of prolactin. *P< 0.01 vs. CPR; **P< 0.001 vs. CPR; P< 0.0001 vs. values of resuscitated patients. Values are expressed as mean +/−SEM.

which is often observed in the chronic phase of critical illness, may help to explain the catabolic "wasting syndrome" which frequently occurs in long-term critically ill patients. Interestingly, a greater loss of pulsatility and regularity within the GH secretory pattern and lower IGF-1 serum concentrations have been observed in male compared with female patients.[168] Although the underlying disease process contributing to these alterations in the GH axis during prolonged critical illness are not completely understood, some authors suggested that a dysfunctional pituitary gland may fail to produce GH and thus contribute to low GH levels. Alternatively, reduced stimulation of somatotrophic cells by endogenous releasing factors, such as GH releasing hormone or ghrelin, as well as increased bioavailability of somatostatin, or endogenous or exogenous dopamine may decrease GH secretion.[201]

Clinical studies have shown that administration of GH improved negative nitrogen balance in patients with severe burns,[205] postsurgical patients,[206] patients in the early phase of sepsis,[207] and other critically ill patients.[208] Some small studies have even indicated that this improvement in nitrogen balance resulted in a shorter duration of mechanical ventilation, and a shorter stay in the intensive care unit or the hospital.[209–213] In an animal study of hemorrhagic shock after trauma and sepsis, however, administration of GH and IGF-1 resulted in more severe metabolic acidosis and impaired compensation of hemorrhage.[214] Similarly, a large multicenter study found that in patients with prolonged critical illness, high doses of GH were associated with increased morbidity and mortality ($p<0.001$; relative risk of death for patients receiving GH was 2.4). Among survivors, both the intensive care and hospital length of stay were prolonged in the GH group,[215] Exact reasons for increased morbidity and mortality associated with high GH levels in critically ill patients remain unclear, but direct and indirect modulation of immune function appears to play an important role.[215]

Gonadotropins

The pituitary gonadotropins, follicle-stimulating hormone (FSH) and luteinizing hormone (LH), act on the gonads (ovaries or testes) to determine sexual development and the reproductive potential. Secretion of gonadotropin is controlled by the hypothalamus and by a negative feedback mechanism triggered by testicular testosterone and ovarian estrogens.[3]

Although the gonadotropin hormonal response to cardiac arrest has not yet been studied, a significant amount of data has been collected on FSH and LH levels during critical illness. Patients in medical or surgical intensive care units usually present with a reversible impairment of gonadotropin secretion,[216] this effect is related to both the severity and duration of the underlying illness.[217] Studies in critically ill postmenopausal women, who normally have high FSH and LH levels, have shown suppressed gonadotropin concentrations.[218] In one study, levels somewhat below the expected concentrations of 30 IU/ml were found in 69% of patients, with concentrations frankly depressed (<5 IU/ml) in an additional 25%.[216] Since these patients did not respond to the hypothalamic peptide gonadotropin-releasing hormone, it was concluded that the gonadotropin secretory defect may involve predominantly the pituitary gland.[216] Studies in men with critical illness have shown comparable decreases in serum LH and FSH.[216, 219]

Endogenous dopamine or opiates may be involved in the pathogenesis of hypogonadotropic hypogonadism, while iatrogenic factors such as exogenous dopamine and opioids may further diminish blunted LH secretion.[219, 220] Animal data suggest that prolonged exposure of the brain to interleukin-1 may also contribute by suppressing synthesis of LH releasing hormone.[221]

Nevertheless, these abnormalities are reversible, and patients tested after recovery had normal gonadotropin concentrations.[217] In some types of less severe acute stress, such as minor surgical procedures or short-term fasting, gonadotropin levels were not found to be decreased.[222, 223] Therefore, it may be concluded that reproductive hormones are generally suppressed during chronic stress of high intensity, but not acute stress of minimal intensity.

The extent of the impairment of gonadotropin secretion has been reported to correlate with patient outcome. Patients presenting with hypogonadotropism during critical illness were more severely ill, had a longer duration of treatment in intensive care units and hospitalization as well as a higher incidence of parenteral hyperalimentation, lower serum albumin levels, and a higher mortality when compared with patients presenting with gonadotropin levels within the expected serum range (>30 IU/L).[216]

Neurohypophysis (posterior lobe)

Vasopressin

Thus far, vasopressin serum levels have not yet been examined during critical illness after cardiac arrest. However, several recent studies have focused on the evaluation of the role of endogenous vasopressin levels during septic shock.

As animal and human studies both showed, plasma vasopressin levels demonstrate a biphasic pattern during septic shock. In early septic shock, vasopressin concentrations significantly increase, while they begin to decline as early as 6 hours after the onset of septic shock. At 36 hours, vasopressin concentrations were found to be inappropriately low for the degree of hypotension in one-third of patients, and may thus represent a relative deficiency of vasopressin.[224] Similarly, Landry and coworkers have repeatedly observed inadequately low vasopressin concentrations in the course of septic shock,[225] vasodilatory shock after cardiac surgery[226] and cardiac transplantation,[227] late hemorrhagic shock,[228] as well as in hemodynamically unstable organ donors.[229]

Low vasopressin levels are most likely due to impaired vasopressin secretion, rather than increased metabolism as vasopressinase levels remain undetectable during established septic shock.[230, 231] A single study of three patients reported undetectable levels of vasopressinase in plasma, which were attributed to renal and hepatic dysfunction commonly seen in septic patients.[231] Hence, proposed mechanisms for decreased serum vasopressin levels in late septic shock include exhaustion of pituitary stores caused in response to baroreceptor-mediated release, autonomic dysfunction, inhibitory effects of increased concentrations of norepinephrine in serum, and increased release of nitric oxide in the posterior pituitary.[225, 230, 232] It is known that neurohypophyseal stores of vasopressin may easily be depleted after profound osmotic stimulation,[229, 233] and probably also after profound baroreflex stimulation. In support of this hypothesis, immunohistochemical analysis of the neurohypophysis in dogs revealed that vasopressin all but disappeared after 1 hour of severe hemorrhagic hypotension (Fig. 7.4).[230] Moreover, sepsis and a massive

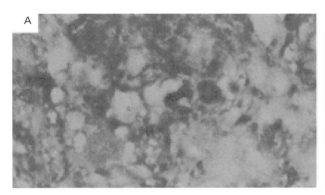 

Fig. 7.4. Vasopressin immunoreactivity in the neurohypophysis in dogs. [230] (a) section of the neurohypophysis from a normal dog. There is staining of the macrovesicles with antivasopressin serum, a reaction indicative of replete stores of vasopressin. (b) section of the neurohypophysis from a dog after severe hemorrhagic hypotension (mean arterial pressure, ≤ 40 mm Hg) for 1 hour. There is minimal staining with antivasopressin serum. For both panels, paraformaldehyde-fixed pituitary glands were sequentially incubated with a vasopressin monoclonal mouse antibody, a horse antimouse IgG conjugated to biotin, and avidin-conjugated horseradish peroxidase and stained with 3,3-diaminobenzidine in the presence of hydrogen peroxide (x 320).

surge of proinflammatory cytokines, as also occurs during postresuscitation disease, may lead to hypothalamic dysfunction and nitric oxide-mediated impairment of vasopressin synthesis, transport, storage, and release.[234]

Serum vasopressin concentrations 24 hours after admission to the intensive care unit were significantly higher in 239 mixed critically ill patients when compared with healthy controls (11.9 ± 20.6 vs. 0.92 ± 0.38 pg/ml, $p < 0.001$).[235] There was no detectable relationship between endogenous vasopressin levels and any specific hemodynamic index, indicating that endogenous AVP concentrations contribute only little to the maintenance of arterial blood pressure in critical illness. Whereas patients with hemodynamic dysfunction still had a detectable correlation between AVP serum concentration and the incidence of cardiovascular function ($p = 0.042$), however, patients in shock completely lost such a relationship ($p = 0.334$). This suggests that the physiologic association between hemodynamic parameters and AVP serum concentrations is substantially altered in critically ill patients with hemodynamic dysfunction, and completely lost in patients with shock. Additionally, during this early phase of critical illness, only 32/239 patients (13.4%) fulfilled the criteria for relative vasopressin deficiency. Absolute vasopressin deficiency, defined as serum vasopressin concentrations < 0.83 pg/ml, was detected in only four study patients (1.7%) and was not associated with diabetes insipidus, but with a low degree of organ dysfunction and beneficial patient outcome.

Leptin

Adipocytes are the body's main site of leptin production and secretion. Circulating leptin is known to correlate positively with fat mass and body weight in healthy volunteers, as well as in subjects with obesity and with conditions of chronic undernutrition.[236, 237] Adipocytes have been shown to release leptin in a pulsatile fashion, following a marked circadian rhythmicity with elevated nocturnal values.[238, 239] Factors known to influence leptin release from adipocytes in man are insulin, GH, IGF-1, thyroid hormones, glucocorticoids, cytokines, and β-adrenoreceptor agonists.[240–243]

Leptin is not only a central hormone in appetite control and regulation of energy expenditure,[244] but has recently emerged as an important regulator of T-cell-dependent immunity.[245, 246] Furthermore, as a cytokine, leptin affects thymic homeostasis and, similar to other pro-inflammatory mediators, it promotes cytokine production.[247] Leptin exerts its effects by stimulation of its receptors in hypothalamic neurons. Its peripheral effects are mainly mediated by melanocortins.[248]

Recent animal and human studies have suggested that leptin secretion is closely related to the function of the hypothalamic–pituitary–adrenal axis and the immune system, both of which crucially influence the course and outcome of critical illness. Mean leptin plasma concentrations were threefold higher (18.9 ± 4.5 ng/ml) in critically ill patients when compared to those in healthy controls (3.8 ± 1 ng/ml; $p < 0.05$). Patients surviving septic shock had significantly higher leptin plasma concentrations than did non-survivors (25.5 ± 6.2 vs. 8 ± 3.7 ng/ml; $p < 0.01$).[249] Another study demonstrated that leptin serum concentrations in critically ill patients with sepsis lost their correlation with body mass index, but correlated significantly with serum IGF-1 concentrations.[250] Similarly, Carlson *et al.* found no correlation between serum leptin concentrations and resting energy expenditure or insulin sensitivity in human sepsis.[251]

Thyroid gland

Thyroid hormones

Similar to the acute cardiac arrest period, thyroid hormone levels have been found to be low during reperfusion, indicative of a continuing hypothyroid state in the immediate post-cardiac arrest period. Twelve hours after a 9-minute cardiac arrest period in dogs, total and free T4 as well as T3 serum concentrations were found to be significantly decreased when compared to pre-arrest levels. Reverse T3 concentrations were elevated, indicating a peripheral metabolizing block of T4 during the first 24 hours after cardiac arrest.[75, 252]

During the later course of critical illness, peripheral hypothyroidism can advance to transient central hypothyroidism characterized by low total T4 and T3 levels, as well as low serum TSH concentrations.[253] In particular, this phenomenon has been observed in patients with sepsis and referred to as the "euthyroid sick syndrome,"[254] or "non-thyroidal illness syndrome."[253] Although the exact mechanisms of such a hypothyroid state in severe illness is not yet clear, several authors have proposed that decreased peripheral deiodination of T4 and reduced binding by plasma thyroid hormone binding proteins might explain the observed changes in thyroid hormone homeostasis.[255] Clinically, reduced plasma concentrations of T3 and T4 may cause ileus, insulin resistance, impaired triglyceride levels, reduced inotropy, and reduced protein synthesis and metabolism in muscle.[197]

Studies have repeatedly shown that hypothyroxinemia after cardiac arrest and during sepsis was a powerful predictor of mortality in critically ill patients (Fig. 7.5).[256] Notably, free T4 concentrations have been observed to be tightly associated with poor outcome.[257] Thus, T4 levels below 3 mg/dl after admission to the intensive care unit were reported to correlate with a 84% mortality rate. Mortality decreased with increasing T4 levels.[257]

In view of these results, several attempts have been made to substitute thyroid hormones and evaluate changes in patient outcome resulting from such an intervention. One randomized, double-blind study evaluating T3 substitution therapy in cardiac surgery patients demonstrated improved hemodynamic stability, as well as a decrease in postoperative ischemia in patients treated with T3.[258] Similarly, two studies performed in animals after 9 minutes of cardiac arrest reported improved cardiocirculatory and neurologic function after administration of L-T4.[252, 259]

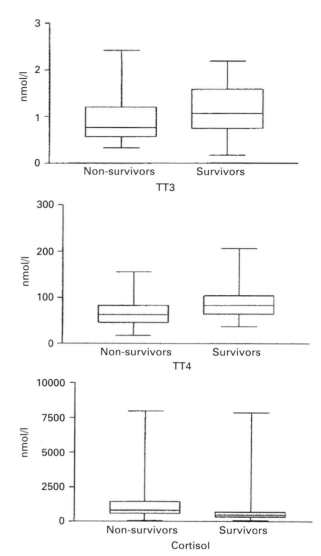

Fig. 7.5. Thyroid hormone concentrations measured on admission to ICU in survivors and non-survivors (range, 25th, 50th, and 75th percentiles).[256]

Administration of thyroid hormones was associated with a significant increase in systemic oxygen consumption.[260] Other studies found that neither hemodynamic variables nor morbidity or mortality were different between thyroid hormone-substituted and not substituted patients.[261, 262] Many authors, however, argue that administration of thyroid hormones to critically ill patients may inhibit TSH secretion and suppress an important mechanism for normalization of thyroid function during recovery.[263]

In conclusion, there is currently no scientific evidence to support subsitution of thyroid hormones in critically ill patients after cardiac arrest. At present, development of the so-called "euthyroid sick syndrome" can simply be interpreted as an indicator of the severity of disease.

Calcitonin

During the first 24 hours after admission to the intensive care unit, critically ill patients were found to have significantly increased calcitonin serum concentrations. In particular, patients suffering from sepsis had higher calcitonin levels than did non-septic patients ($p < 0.004$). Moreover, calcitonin levels were not only correlated with the APACHE II and the Multiple Organ Failure Score, but also demonstrated a positive correlation with length of stay in the intensive care unit. In the same study, survivors had significantly higher calcitonin concentrations than did non-survivors ($p < 0.03$). Interestingly, serum calcitonin concentrations were not related to the degree of total serum calcium concentrations.[264] In critically ill children, basal serum calcitonin levels were significantly increased and correlated with low concentrations of ionized calcium in blood.[265]

Parathyroid glands

In critically ill patients, both increased and decreased parathyroid hormone concentrations have been reported.[266–268] Carlsted *et al.* reported on significantly increased serum parathyroid hormone levels in a mixed critically ill patient population.[269] In this study, parathyroid hormone levels were related to the severity of disease and also to patient outcome. Similar to a more recent publication,[270] increased parathyroid hormone levels were particularly evident in two specific disease groups, patients with sepsis and patients undergoing major surgery (50–70% of healthy controls). Regardless of the nature of the critical illness, the elevation of parathyroid hormone serum concentrations during the early period of intensive care treatment was an unfavorable prognostic sign.[269]

In studies performed in healthy subjects, catecholamine infusion resulted in altered parathyroid hormone levels, most probably due to a decrease in circulating calcium levels.[270] Nonetheless, increased catecholamine serum concentrations, such as typically found in critically ill patients, could exert a direct action on parathyroid hormone secretion, as β-adrenergic receptors have been detected on parathyroid cells.[271–273] Furthermore, the systemic inflammatory response which inevitably occurs to a certain extent during sepsis or after major surgery, but also after resuscitation from cardiac arrest, seems to further influence homeostasis of parathyroid hormone. Tumor necrosis factor-α and interleukin-1 may impair the responsiveness to parathyroid hormone by downregulating parathyroid hormone receptors in osteoblast-like cells.[273] Interleukin-6

was shown to be a downstream effector of parathyroid hormone, which stimulates bone resorption.[274, 275]

Adrenal glands

Catecholamines

Plasma epinephrine, norepinephrine, and dopamine concentrations are markedly increased during the first 60 minutes after return of spontaneous circulation, even when exogenous epinephrine is not administered during resuscitation efforts. Peak levels of endogenous catecholamines are observed shortly after restoration of circulation and are probably due to "washout" of catecholamines released after arrest onset and during global ischemia.[276]

To date, only one other study evaluated the course of plasma catecholamine levels following conventional resuscitation that included the injection of epinephrine. Prengel and coworkers described the elimination kinetics of epinephrine in patients successfully resuscitated from out-of-hospital cardiac arrest. They failed to demonstrate a correlation between non-invasively determined hemodynamic variables, such as heart rate or mean arterial blood pressure, or glucose and lactate and measured serum epinephrine and norepinephrine concentrations, which consisted of endogenous and exogenous catecholamines.[277]

High plasma catecholamine concentrations persist for prolonged periods after the initial epinephrine and norepinephrine surge and appear to be driven by post-resuscitation hypotension. The adrenergic response not only leads to a compensatory increase in systemic vascular resistance, but also to detrimental effects on cardiac function during the postresuscitation period. Accordingly, Niemann *et al.* reported on a negative correlation between norepinephrine plasma concentrations and left ventricular stroke work.[276] This potentially detrimental effect of a presumed adrenergic compensatory response shares some close similarities with chronic congestive heart failure.[278, 279] As in patients with chronic heart failure, a recent investigation examining the effects of β-blockade during the early postresuscitation phase could prove to have a beneficial effect on myocardial function.[280]

After the immediate reperfusion period and postresuscitation phase, catecholamines remain significantly elevated in critically ill patients when compared to healthy controls.[281] Particularly high plasma epinephrine and norepinephrine concentrations have been reported during endoxemia and septic shock.[282] Boldt and colleagues reported significantly higher mortality rates in critically ill patients with high concentrations of plasma catecholamines. While epinephrine and norepinephrine plasma concentrations were elevated in non-survivors on the day of admission to the intensive care unit and were tremendously increased during the days following, plasma catecholamine concentrations significantly decreased in critically ill patients who survived.[283] Interestingly, in another study analyzing patients with septic shock, not only the absolute height of plasma catecholamine concentrations, but also the adrenal response to a head-up tilt was predictive of poor outcome. During a 60-degree head-up tilt, the increase in plasma norepinephrine levels was significantly higher in survivors than in non-survivors, suggesting an adequate response of the sympathetic nervous system including the adrenal medulla.[284]

Cortisol

A recent study examined the incidence and prognostic value of relative adrenal insufficiency after cardiac arrest. Out of 64 patients hospitalized in the intensive care unit after successful resuscitation of out-of-hospital cardiac arrest, 33 patients (52%) fulfilled the criteria for relative adrenal insufficiency defined as an incremental response of less than 9 μg/dl 60 minutes after administration of 250 μg of tetracosactide. Baseline cortisol concentrations were higher in patients with adrenal insufficiency than in patients without (41 vs. 22.8 μg/dl; $p = 0.001$). A long interval before initiation of cardiopulmonary resuscitation was associated with occurrence of relative adrenal insufficiency indicating a pathogenetic role of hypoxia. Presence of adrenal insufficiency after cardiac arrest was identified as a poor prognostic factor of shock-related mortality ($p = 0.02$).[285]

Adrenal function appears to be strongly dependent on age during critical illness. Adrenal insufficiency occurred 2.5 times more frequently in patients older than 55 years than in younger patients.[286] While patients older than 60 years had paradoxically higher serum cortisol concentrations than did patients younger than 30 years, their response to ACTH stimulation was significantly smaller on both low (1 μg) and standard dose (250 μg) tests.[287]

The mechanisms of adrenal insufficiency after cardiac arrest or major surgery as well as during severe sepsis and septic shock are complex and not yet fully understood. The systemic inflammatory response syndrome, which to a certain extent always accompanies the reperfusion period of global ischemia, results in the release of proinflammatory cytokines (TNF-α, IL-1, IL-6), which in vitro suppress the pituitary response to the hypothalamic corticotropin releasing hormone,[288, 289] and the release of cortisol from ACTH-stimulated adrenocortical cells.[290, 291] Nevertheless, although cortisol synthesis and secretion are impaired during critical illness, it appears that the function of the entire hypothalamic-pituitary–adrenal axis is also severely impaired.

Moreover, CBG, a liver-derived plasma protein that is the main carrier protein for cortisol (>90%), also appears to be another important regulator of the amount of biologically free cortisol during critical illness.[292] While during the initial phase of reperfusion in septic shock and multitrauma patients, CBG levels were found to be extremely low, reflecting higher levels of free cortisol, protracted critical illness is characterized by increasing and normalizing CGB levels, independent of clinical parameters.[293] Similar results have been observed in patients after major surgery.[294] Several mechanisms have been proposed to explain CBG depletion during reperfusion after shock: increased metabolic clearance, decreased synthesis in the liver, and capillary leakage.[295, 296] In view of the influence of hypoproteinemia on total cortisol concentrations, measurement of free cortisol levels or calculation of a correction factor, the free cortisol index (total cortisol/CBG concentration), has been suggested for assessment of adrenal function.[293, 294]

In the postresuscitation period, suppression of adrenal function can also be caused and aggravated by administration of drugs. For example, transient adrenal insufficiency has been reported after high-dose fluconazol therapy and more than one hypnotic dosage of etomidate.[297]

Renin–angiotensin–aldosterone system

Plasma aldosterone concentrations were reported to be increased in approximately two thirds of critically ill patients when compared to healthy controls. Secondary hyperaldosteronism in the early phase of critical illness, is hypothesized to be mainly due to the stimulatory effects of ACTH or ACTH-related peptides. Thereby, it is considered to be an epiphenomenon of the stress mechanisms of acute critical illness.[298]

Nonetheless, a significant portion of critically ill patients (up to 21% in one study) present with a dissociation of plasma renin activity and aldosterone production.[299] Hyper-reninemic hypoaldosteronism is characterized by normal metabolic clearance of aldosterone, normal production of angiotensin II, appropriate hypercortisolemia, and decreased levels of 18-hydroxycorticosterone, which is an aldosterone precursor. Clinically, this syndrome was reported to be frequently accompanied by hypotension and hemodynamic instability.[300] Such a dissociation is most probably not due to an impairment of angiotensin II production or changes in plasma ACTH or potassium. Pathophysiologically, tumor necrosis factor α and interleukin 1 as well as other cytokines (IGF-1, transforming growth factor β), which are known to stimulate renin activity, but inhibit aldosterone secretion, may contribute to this state of hyper-reninemic hypoaldosteronism.[301] Some authors have reported increased severity of the underlying disease and increased mortality associated with this syndrome.[299, 300, 302]

In light of evidence of decreased adrenal androgen secretion during severe illness, the dissociation of renin and aldosterone may represent another adrenal adaptation mechanism to promote cortisol production. Nonetheless, inappropriately low aldosterone levels were reported to be associated with high mortality during critical illness. Interestingly, a recent prospective study evaluating the effects of hydrocortisone substitution on patient outcome in patients with septic shock combined hydrocortisone with fludrocortisone substitution (50 μg) and reported a significant improvement in patient survival.[303]

Gonads

The neuroproductive axis is also significantly suppressed during critical illness. The degree of both central and peripheral suppression of the gonads in acute illness has been demonstrated to be related to the severity of the underlying disease. Such a suppression was not attributed to other factors, as age, drugs, head trauma, or hepatic failure, which are otherwise known to alter sexual hormone concentrations independently from critical illness.[217] Both men and women uniformly develop transient hypogonadotropic gonadal insufficiency during critical illness.[304]

Testes

Serum testosterone levels during critical illness fall to prepubertal levels secondary to decreased secretion of gonadotropins and a decreased Leydig cell response to LH. At the same time, serum estrogen concentrations rise as the result of an increased rate of peripheral aromatization.[305] The low testosterone concentrations are not due to reduced sex-hormone binding capacity.[304] Studies evaluating the therapeutic potential of androgen subistution in prolonged critical illness failed to demonstrate conclusive clinical benefit.[306]

Ovaries

Studies of serum levels of female gonadal hormones during critical illness in postmenopausal women showed increased levels of estrone and estradiol, whereas testosterone levels were decreased.[13] Since critical illness suppresses gonadotropin levels,[13, 216] it was suggested that the increase in gonadal hormones in this population reflects an adrenal rather than ovarian origin, presumably a consequence of excess ACTH.[13]

Non-conventional endocrine organs

Endothelium

Plasma immunoreactive endothelin (ET) concentrations in patients following cardiac arrest (5.4 ± 2.3 pg/ml) were not different from those in healthy subjects (5.1 ± 1.2 pg/ml). There was no significant difference in ET concentrations between survivors and non-survivors.[307] However, systemic ET were found to increase during hypoperfusion and all shock forms.[308–310] Particularly high ET serum levels have been reported during septic shock.[310,311] The possible involvement of the ET system in human septic shock is further supported by a clear positive correlation of ET plasma levels and morbidity and mortality in patients with sepsis.[312, 313]

Interestingly, critically ill patients with high ET levels did not have increased systemic vascular resistance. This was hypothesized to be due to prostaglandin E2-mediated vasodilation predominating over ET-mediated vasoconstriction.[308] Furthermore, activation of the ET system has been associated with several pathophysiological conditions complicating septic shock, such as acute respiratory distress syndrome, cardiac dysfunction, splanchnic hepatic and renal hypoperfusion, as well as disseminated intravascular coagulation.[116] Accordingly, high ET-1 levels during the initial phase of critical illness appeared to be a sensitive predictor of death from septic shock.[314]

Recent evidence suggests that persistently high ET serum concentrations in the first 24 hours after cardiac arrest were associated with increased cerebrovascular resistance and delayed cerebral hypoperfusion.[315] Supporting this hypothesis, application of the ET_A receptor antagonist BQ123 during the early reperfusion period after cardiac arrest in rats shortened postischemic cerebral hypoperfusion and accelerated the restoration of the cerebrovascular CO_2 reactivity and recovery of the electrophysiologic function (Fig. 7.6).[316] Furthermore, in the same model, blockage of the ET_A receptor 15 minutes after return of spontaneous circulation following a 12-minute period of cardiac arrest significantly improved neurologic outcome.[317]

Heart

In a study including 401 patients with out-of-hospital cardiac arrest, BNP concentrations on arrival at the emergency room correlated well with subsequent patient outcome. Increasing concentrations of BNP were predictive of an increased risk of death in hospital and unfavorable neurologic outcomes at the time of hospital discharge. A multiple logistic regression analysis revealed BNP to be a strong independent factor in survival to hospital discharge.

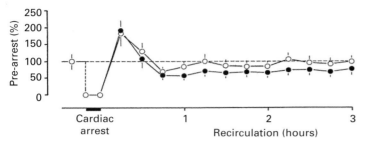

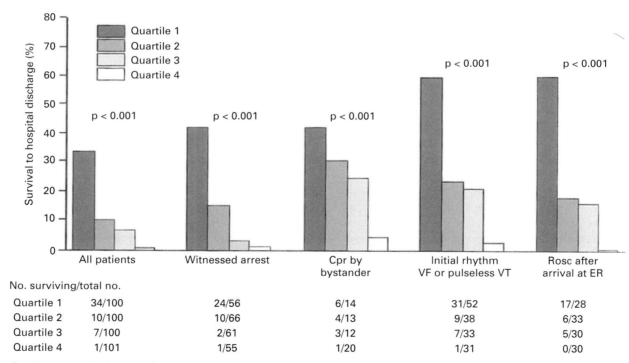

Fig. 7.6. Measurement of cerebral blood flow by laser-Doppler flowmetry during resuscitation from 12 min of cardiac arrest.[316] Comparison of untreated animals (*filled circles*) with animals treated with the selective endothelin type A antagonist BQ123 (*unfilled circles*) at 15 min after return of spontaneous circulation. Note initial hyperperfusion followed by delayed postischemic hypoperfusion in both groups but faster recovery from postischemic hypoperfusion in treated animals (mean ± sd, statistical significance between treated and untreated groups *$P < 0.05$, two-tailed analysis of variance for repeated measurements).

Serum concentrations of 100 pg/ml were determined to be the optimal cut-off point for BNP regarding survival to hospital discharge (Fig. 7.7).[318]

Similarly, patients with myocardial dysfunction due to sepsis or septic shock exhibited significantly higher serum BNP concentrations than did patients with adequate myocardial function. BNP levels were also significantly higher on days two and three in patients who died during their intensive care unit stay ($p < 0.05$).[319] In contrast, a study analyzing ANP and BNP plasma concentrations in 178 mixed critically ill patients reported increased plasma concentrations of both hormones compared with those in healthy controls (ANP, 14.3 ± 5.8 vs. 8.8 ± 3.2 pmol/l, $p < 0.05$; BNP, 26.2 ± 10.7 vs. 4.6 ± 2.8 pmol/l, $p < 0.0001$). The relative increases in ANP plasma levels were comparable in all diseases. BNP concentrations, by contrast, showed a wider variation, with largest concentrations in patients undergoing cardiac surgical procedures and with subarachnoid hemorrhage. In this study population, serum concentrations of ANP and BNP did not correlate with the severity of the disease and could not predict patient outcome.[320] Although another study in 78 mixed critically

No. surviving/total no.

	All patients	Witnessed arrest	Cpr by bystander	Initial rhythm VF or pulseless VT	Rosc after arrival at ER
Quartile 1	34/100	24/56	6/14	31/52	17/28
Quartile 2	10/100	10/66	4/13	9/38	6/33
Quartile 3	7/100	2/61	3/12	7/33	5/30
Quartile 4	1/101	1/55	1/20	1/31	0/30

Fig. 7.7. Association between the B-type natriuretic peptide level and the rate of survival to hospital discharge (primary end point) in all patients and in selected subgroups.[317] CPR, cardiopulmonary resuscitation; ER, emergency room; ROSC, return of spontaneous circulation; VF, ventricular fibrillation; VT, ventricular tachycardia. The range of B-type natriuretic peptide levels was as follows: 2.0–33.8 pg/ml (quartile 1), 33.9–152.0 pg/ml (quartile 2), 152.1–392.0 pg/ml (quartile 3), and 392.1–2620.0 pg/ml (quartile 4). *P* values are for the trend within each group.

ill patients indicated that BNP serum concentrations 24 hours after admission to the intensive care unit were significantly higher in patients with sepsis or septic shock ($p = 0.02$), in patients ≥ 65 years ($p = 0.04$), and in patients with raised serum creatinine concentrations ≥ 110 μmol/l ($p = 0.02$), BNP serum levels neither correlated with intensive care unit nor with hospital mortality.[321]

Kidney

Renin

During critical illness complicated by persistent hypotension, serum renin activities were found to be significantly elevated.[300] In 44 patients critically ill with septic shock, plasma renin activity on admission to the intensive care unit was significantly increased. Although in survivors, plasma renin activity significantly decreased following intensive care therapy, no change was observed in non-survivors.[322]

Erythropoietin

A recent clinical trial analyzed the acute phase response together with the course of erythropoietin plasma concentrations in 22 patients after cardiac arrest. During the intensive care unit stay after return of spontaneous circulation, plasma erythropoietin levels (mean values in healthy, non-anemic volunteers, 17.9 mU/ml; 95% CI, 11–31 mU/ml) increased from 23.5 after cardiac arrest to 26.5 (day 1), 25.5 (day 2), and 31 mU/ml (day 3), but this increase was not statistically significant ($p > 0.05$). At the same time, hemoglobin concentrations fell gradually from a median of 14 g/dl on admission to 12.8 (day 1), 11.6 (day 2), and 10.7 g/dl on day 3. Plasma erythropoietin concentrations in patients surviving with or without a neurologic deficit were not different, but in non-survivors erythropoeitin levels were significantly higher on the third day of intensive care therapy after cardiac arrest than in survivors.[323]

Similarly, in 44 patients with septic shock, non-survivors had significantly higher serum erythropoietin levels than did survivors on admission to the intensive care unit.[322] Abnormally high plasma erythropoeitin levels have been reported to be a negative prognostic indicator in patients suffering from septic shock in other studies.[324, 325] Analysis of receiver operating characteristic curves showed that a cutoff for serum erythropoeitin levels of 50 mU/ml on admission was optimal for predicting death. While in survivors from septic shock, plasma erythropoietin was negatively correlated with blood hemoglobin concentrations ($p < 0.001$), no such correlation was observed in non-survivors.[322]

Although initial plasma erythropoietin levels were significantly increased in a mixed medical and surgical patient population in an intensive care unit, erythropoietin concentrations rapidly decreased thereafter. In the period of prolonged critical illness, erythropoietin diminished to levels that were indistinguishable from those in patients with non-renal anemia.[326] Regardless of the underlying disease, the erythropoietin response to anemia in intensive care patients, particularly during protracted critical illness, seems to be severely blunted.[325, 327] Inadequate erythropoietin production is therefore likely to contribute to the development of anemia in long-term critically ill patients. This phenomenon is assumed to be particularly pronounced in patients with concomitant acute renal failure or sepsis.[327]

Gastrointestinal tract

Insulin

Critical illness, including the postresuscitation phase, is characterized by hyperglycemia and glucose intolerance associated with hyperinsulinemia and insulin resistance.[328] These metabolic alterations have been summarized under the rubric "diabetes of injury."[329,330] Pathophysiologically, the neuroendocrine stress response to global ischemia and/or reperfusion and the systemic activation of the immune system are held responsible for the "diabetes of injury."[330] While catecholamines, cortisol, glucagon, and GH were all shown to affect glucose and insulin metabolic pathways directly, pro-inflammatory cytokines influence glucose homeostasis indirectly, by altering insulin receptor signaling.[330–333]

Until recently, the "diabetes of injury" was widely accepted as a beneficial adaptive response to severe disease and, as such, to be important for survival. In particular, the overall increase in glucose turnover and the fact that hyperglycemia persists despite abundantly released insulin were considered arguments in favor of tolerating moderately elevated blood glucose levels during critical illness. Consequently, blood glucose concentrations of 160–200 mg/dl were recommended to maximize cellular glucose uptake while avoiding hyperosmolarity.[334]

In 2001, however, a large, prospective, randomized, single-center study impressively demonstrated that titration of insulin infusion during intensive care to strict normoglycemia (90–110 mg/dl) reduced the mortality of critically ill patients when compared with conventional insulin treatment aimed to prevent blood glucose levels >200 mg/dl (20.2% vs. 10.6%, $p = 0.005$) (Fig. 7.8).[335] The benefit of intensive insulin therapy in critically ill patients was particularly apparent among patients with prolonged critical illness that required intensive care for more than 5 days, with mortality reduced from 20.2% to 10.6%.

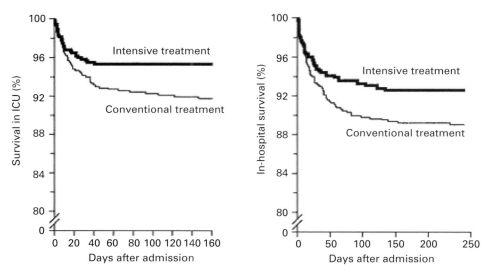

Fig. 7.8. Kaplan–Meier curves showing cumulative survival of patients who received intensive insulin treatment or conventional treatment in the intensive care unit (ICU).[334] Patients discharged alive from the ICU (a) and from the hospital (b) were considered to have survived. In both cases, the differences between the treatment groups were significant (survival in ICU, nominal $P = 0.005$ and adjusted $P < 0.04$; in-hospital survival, nominal $P = 0.01$). P values were determined with the use of the Mantel–Cox log-rank test.

Moreover, strict control of blood glucose levels reduced the incidence of complications, such as severe nosocomial infections, acute renal failure, liver dysfunction, critical illness, polyneuropathy, muscle weakness, and anemia and thus reduced the time that patients were dependent on intensive care. A recently published report confirmed the survival benefit of implementing tight blood glucose control with insulin in a mixed medical-surgical intensive care population.[336]

Intestinal hormones

Thus far, no study has examined plasma concentrations of intestinal hormones in the postresuscitation period after cardiac arrest. Since postresuscitation disease shares similarities with overwhelming systemic inflammation and sepsis, however, it was thought that observations made in animals and patients with sepsis might indicate comparable changes in the postcardiac arrest period.

During endotoxin-induced shock in animals, there are consistent data to show significantly increased plasma concentrations of cholecystokinin and VIP.[337–339] Since VIP is a potent vasodilator, it was postulated to contribute to vasodilatation and hypotension in septic shock. Although Broner *et al.* had established that infusion of VIP resulted in profound hypotension and lactic acidosis,[339] another animal study suggested that endogenous VIP levels may not be responsible for the vasodilatation during sepsis.[337]

In this study, during the first 24 hours of sepsis, VIP was released without a concomitant decrease in blood pressure, suggesting that during septic shock it was released by a direct mechanism rather than as a result of hypotension. Similarly, during peak VIP release, which occurred 2 to 4 hours after induction of sepsis, no decrease in systemic vascular resistance or mean arterial pressure was noted.[337] Zamir *et al.* showed that proinflammatory cytokines were involved in the release of intestinal peptides during sepsis and systemic inflammation. Whereas interleukin-1 did not affect plasma concentrations of gastrin, VIP, peptide YY, and secretin, tumor necrosis factor α induced a significant increase in peptide YY levels.[340]

In human sepsis, a similar increase in VIP serum concentrations was found in five patients with fulminant septic shock. Although none of these patients had VIP levels >2.5 pM before the septic episode, VIP increased >4 pM during the septic episode. Sequentially collected samples from three patients showed rapidly declining VIP levels after initiation of adequate antibiotic and fluid treatment.[341]

Summary

It appears that the differences between the neuroendocrine response to global ischemia/cardiac arrest and reperfusion/early phase of critical illness are more quantitative than qualitative. During both phases, all components of the neuroendocrine system are significantly altered to adapt to maximal stress. Whereas secretion of adrenomedullary hormones, cortisol, vasopressin, and the pituitary hormones prolactin, ACTH, β-endorphin, β-lipoprotein, and probably GH is significantly increased, thyroidal, gonadal, and endocrine gastrointestinal hormones are not released during the intense stress of cardiac arrest and global ischemia. Likewise, adrenal androgens and presumably mineralocorticoid secretions do not participate in the acute stress response, whereas secretion of pituitary gonadotropin may be actively impaired. Interestingly, during cardiac arrest, but not during critical illness, 73-MSH serum concentrations are elevated significantly. Cardiopulmonary resuscitation itself may be the mechanism for the release of ANP that may simply reflect atrial distension. Whereas most endocrinologic systems are activated during cardiac arrest and also in the early phase of critical illness, it appears that the neuroendocrine system is uncoupled from its stimulators during chronic stress. Thus, during prolonged critical illness, return of stress hormones to physiologic values often results in the occurrence of relative and absolute hormone deficiencies. Immune suppression, limited organ reserves, and severe catabolism may originate in part from these profound changes in the neuroendocrine response to global ischemia and reperfusion during prolonged critical illness.

When summarizing the results of most studies, an adequate neuroendocrine response to cardiac arrest and during the postresuscitation period appears to be tightly connected with beneficial patient outcome, whereas an inadequate stress response seems to be associated with high morbidity and poor outcome.

REFERENCES

1. Voorhees, W.D., Babbs, C.F., & Tacker, W.A., Jr. Regional blood flow during cardiopulmonary resuscitation in dogs. *Crit. Care Med.* 1980; **8**(3): 134–136.

2. Holmes, H.R., Babbs, C.F., Voorhees, W.D., Tacker, W.A., Jr., & de Garavilla, B. Influence of adrenergic drugs upon vital organ perfusion during CPR. *Crit. Care Med.* 1980; **8**(3): 137–140.

3. Thorner, M.O., Vance, M.L., Horvath, E., & Kovacs, K. The anterior pituitary. In Wilson, J.D., Foster, D.W., eds. *Williams Textbook of Endocrinology*. Philadelphia: W.B. Saunders, 1992: 221–310.

4. Dubois, M., Pickar, D., Cohen, M.R., Roth, Y.F., Macnamara, T., & Bunney, W.E., Jr. Surgical stress in humans is accompanied by an increase in plasma beta-endorphin immunoreactivity. *Life Sci.* 1981; **29**(12): 1249–1254.

5. Amit, Z., & Galina, Z.H. Stress-induced analgesia: adaptive pain suppression. *Physiol. Rev.* 1986; **66**(4): 1091–1120.

6. Dalayeun, J.F., Nores, J.M., & Bergal, S. Physiology of beta-endorphins. A close-up view and a review of the literature. *Biomed. Pharmacother.* 1993; **47**(8): 311–320.

7. Foley, P.J., Tacker, W.A., Voorhees, W.D., Ralston, S.H., & Elchisak, M.A. Effects of naloxone on the adrenomedullary response during and after cardiopulmonary resuscitation in dogs. *Am. J. Emerg. Med.* 1987; **5**(5): 357–361.

8. Ross, R.J., Miell, J.P., Holly, J.M. *et al.* Levels of GH binding activity, IGFBP-1, insulin, blood glucose and cortisol in intensive care patients. *Clin. Endocrinol. (Oxf.)* 1991; **35**(4): 361–367.

9. Paradis, N.A., Rose, M.I., & Garg, U. The effect of global ischemia and reperfusion on the plasma levels of vasoactive peptides. The neuroendocrine response to cardiac arrest and resuscitation. *Resuscitation* 1993; **26**(3): 261–269.

10. Zaloga, G.P., Chernow, B., Smallridge, R.C. *et al.* A longitudinal evaluation of thyroid function in critically ill surgical patients. *Ann. Surg.* 1985; **201**(4): 456–464.

11. Arem, R., Wiener, G.J., Kaplan, S.G., Kim, H.S., Reichlin, S., & Kaplan, M.M. Reduced tissue thyroid hormone levels in fatal illness. *Metabolism* 1993; **42**(9): 1102–1108.

12. Adriaanse, R., Romijn, J.A., Brabant, G., Endert, E., & Wiersinga W.M. Pulsatile thyrotropin secretion in nonthyroidal illness. *J. Clin. Endocrinol. Metab.* 1993; **77**(5): 1313–1317.

13. Spratt, D.I., Longcope, C., Cox, P.M., Bigos, S.T., & Wilbur-Welling, C. Differential changes in serum concentrations of androgens and estrogens (in relation with cortisol) in postmenopausal women with acute illness. *J. Clin. Endocrinol. Metab.* 1993; **76**(6): 1542–1547.

14. Wortsman, J., Premachandra, B.N., Chopra, I.J., & Murphy, J.E. Hypothyroxinemia in cardiac arrest. *Arch. Intern. Med.* 1987; **147**(2): 245–248.

15. Fisher, D.A. Thyroid function in the fetus and newborn. *Med. Clin. North. Am.* 1975; **59**(5): 1099–1107.

16. Larsen, P.R., Ingbar, S.H. The thyroid gland. In: Wilson, J.D., & Foster, D.W., eds. *Williams Textbook of Endocrinology*. Philadelphia: W.B. Saunders; 1992: 357–487.

17. Lindner, K.H., Brinkmann, A., Pfenninger, E.G., Lurie, K.G., Goertz, A., & Lindner, I.M. Effect of vasopressin on hemodynamic variables, organ blood flow, and acid-base status in a pig model of cardiopulmonary resuscitation. *Anesth. Analg.* 1993; **77**(3): 427–435.

18. Wortsman, J., Frank, S., Wehrenberg, W.B., Petra, P.H., & Murphy, J.E. Gamma 3-Melanocyte-stimulating hormone immunoreactivity is a component of the neuroendocrine response to maximal stress (cardiac arrest). *J. Clin. Endocrinol. Metab.* 1985; **61**(2): 355–360.

19. Schultz, C.H., Rivers, E.P., Feldkamp, C.S. *et al.* A characterization of hypothalamic–pituitary–adrenal axis function during and after human cardiac arrest. *Crit. Care Med.* 1993; **21**(9): 1339–1347.

20. Lindner, K.H., Strohmenger, H.U., Ensinger, H., Hetzel, W.D., Ahnefeld, F.W., & Georgieff, M. Stress hormone response during and after cardiopulmonary resuscitation. *Anesthesiology* 1992; **77**(4): 662–668.

21. Lindner, K.H., Haak, T., Keller, A., Bothner, U., & Lurie, K.G. Release of endogenous vasopressors during and after cardiopulmonary resuscitation. *Heart* 1996; **75**(2): 145–150.

22. O'Leary, M.J., Timmins, A.C., Appleby, J.N. *et al.* Dissociation of pituitary–adrenal and catecholamine activation after induced cardiac arrest and defibrillation. *Br. J. Anaesth.* 1999; **82**(2): 271–273.

23. Kornberger, E., Prengel, A.W., Krismer, A. *et al.* Vasopressin-mediated adrenocorticotropin release increases plasma cortisol concentrations during cardiopulmonary resuscitation. *Crit. Care Med.* 2000; **28**(10): 3517–3521.

24. Chretien, M., Seidah, N.G., & Scherrer, H. [Endorphins: structure, roles and biogenesis]. *Can. J. Physiol. Pharmacol.* 1981; **59**(5): 413–431.

25. Guillemin, R., Vargo, T., Rossier, J. *et al.* Beta-Endorphin and adrenocorticotropin are selected concomitantly by the pituitary gland. *Science* 1977; **197**(4311): 1367–1369.

26. Vescovi, P.P., Gerra, G., Pioli, G., Pedrazzoni, M., Maninetti, L., & Passeri, M. Circulating opioid peptides during thermal stress. *Horm. Metab. Res.* 1990; **22**(1): 44–46.

27. Tsunoda, K., Douge, K., Akiya, Y., & Watanabe, T. Beta-endorphin secretion at the time of sudden death due to cardiac or respiratory failure. *Nippon Hoigaku Zasshi* 1992; **46**(3): 182–188.

28. Sotelo, J., Perez, R., Guevara, P., & Fernandez, A. Changes in brain, plasma and cerebrospinal fluid contents of beta-endorphin in dogs at the moment of death. *Neurol. Res.* 1995; **17**(3): 223–225.

29. Smith, A.I., & Funder, J.W. Proopiomelanocortin processing in the pituitary, central nervous system, and peripheral tissues. *Endocr. Rev.* 1988; **9**(1): 159–179.

30. Slominski, A., Costantino, R., Wortsman, J., Paus, R., & Ling, N. Melanotropic activity of gamma MSH peptides in melanoma cells. *Life Sci.* 1992; **50**(15): 1103–1108.

31. Ling, N., Ying, S., Minick, S., & Guillemin, R. Synthesis and biological activity of four gamma-melanotropin peptides derived from the cryuptic region of the adrenocorticotropin/beta-lipotropin precursor. *Life Sci.* 1979; **25**(20): 1773–1779.

32. Pedersen, R.C., & Brownie, A.C. Adrenocortical response to corticotropin is potentiated by part of the amino-terminal region of pro-corticotropin/endorphin. *Proc. Natl Acad. Sci. USA* 1980; **77**(4): 2239–2243.

33. Seger, M.A., & Bennett, H.P. Structure and bioactivity of the amino-terminal fragment of pro-opiomelanocortin. *J. Steroid Biochem.* 1986; **25**(5B): 703–710.

34. Guarini, S., Bazzani, C., & Bertolini, A. Resuscitating effect of melanocortin peptides after prolonged respiratory arrest. *Br. J. Pharmacol.* 1997; **121**(7):1454–1460.

35. Russell, D.H. New aspects of prolactin and immunity: a lymphocyte-derived prolactin-like product and nuclear protein kinase C activation. *Trends Pharmacol. Sci.* 1989; **10**(1): 40–44.

36. Bernton, E.W., Meltzer, M.S., & Holaday, J.W. Suppression of macrophage activation and T-lymphocyte function in hypoprolactinemic mice. *Science* 1988; **239**(4838): 401–404.

37. Strohmenger, H.U., Lindner, K.H., Keller, A., Lindner, I.M., Bothner, U., & Georgieff, M. Concentrations of prolactin and prostaglandins during and after cardiopulmonary resuscitation. *Crit. Care Med.* 1995; **23**(8): 1347–1355.

38. Voigt, K.H., Frank, D., Duker, E., Martin, R., & Wuttke, W. Dopamine-inhibited release of prolactin and intermediate lobe-POMC-peptides: different modulation by opioids. *Life Sci.* 1983; **33** Suppl 1: 507–510.

39. Bowers, C.Y., Momany, F.A., Reynolds, G.A., & Hong, A. On the in vitro and in vivo activity of a new synthetic hexapeptide that acts on the pituitary to specifically release growth hormone. *Endocrinology* 1984; **114**(5): 1537–1545.

40. Howard, A.D., Feighner, S.D., Cully, D.F. *et al.* A receptor in pituitary and hypothalamus that functions in growth hormone release. *Science* 1996; **273**(5277): 974–977.

41. Kojima, M., Hosoda, H., Date, Y., Nakazato, M., Matsuo, H., & Kangawa, K. Ghrelin is a growth-hormone-releasing acylated peptide from stomach. *Nature* 1999; **402**(6762): 656–660.

42. Wutke, T. Endocrinology. In Schmidt, R.F., Thews, G., eds. *Human Physiology.* Berlin, Heidelberg, New York: Springer, 1993: 390–420.

43. Thrasher, T.N., & Keil, L.C. Systolic pressure predicts plasma vasopressin responses to hemorrhage and vena caval constriction in dogs. *Am. J. Physiol. Regul. Integr. Comp. Physiol.* 2000; **279**(3): R1035–R1042.

44. Chikanza, I.C., Petrou, P., & Chrousos, G. Perturbations of arginine vasopressin secretion during inflammatory stress. Pathophysiologic implications. *Ann. NY Acad. Sci.* 2000; **917**: 825–834.

45. Mastorakos, G., Weber, J.S., Magiakou, M.A., Gunn, H., & Chrousos, G.P. Hypothalamic-pituitary-adrenal axis activation and stimulation of systemic vasopressin secretion by recombinant interleukin-6 in humans: potential implications for the syndrome of inappropriate vasopressin secretion. *J. Clin. Endocrinol. Metab.* 1994; **79**(4): 934–939.

46. Zelazowski, P., Patchev, V.K., Zelazowska, E.B., Chrousos, G.P., Gold, P.W., & Sternberg, E.M. Release of hypothalamic corticotropin-releasing hormone and arginine-vasopressin by interleukin 1 beta and alpha MSH: studies in rats with different susceptibility to inflammatory disease. *Brain Res.* 1993; **631**(1): 22–26.

47. Yamamoto, T., Kimura, T., Ota, K. *et al.* Central effects of endothelin-1 on vasopressin and atrial natriuretic peptide release and cardiovascular and renal function in conscious rats. *J. Cardiovasc. Pharmacol.* 1991; **17** Suppl. **7**: S316–S318.

48. Shichiri, M., Hirata, Y., Kanno, K., Ohta, K., Emori, T., & Marumo, F. Effect of endothelin-1 on release of arginine-vasopressin from perifused rat hypothalamus. *Biochem. Biophys. Res. Commun.* 1989; **163**(3): 1332–1337.

49. Standaert, D.G., Cechetto, D.F., Needleman, P., & Saper, C.B. Inhibition of the firing of vasopressin neurons by atriopeptin. *Nature* 1987; **329**(6135): 151–153.

50. Obana, K., Naruse, M., Inagami, T. *et al.* Atrial natriuretic factor inhibits vasopressin secretion from rat posterior pituitary. *Biochem. Biophys. Res. Commun.* 1985; **132**(3): 1088–1094.

51. Share, L., Kimura, T., Matsui, K., Shade, R.E., & Crofton, J.T. Metabolism of vasopressin. *Fed. Proc.* 1985; **44**(1 Pt 1): 59–61.

52. Matsui, K., Share, L., Brooks, D.P., Crofton, J.T., & Rockhold, R.W. Splanchnic clearance of plasma vasopressin in the dog: evidence for prehepatic extraction. *Am. J. Physiol.* 1983; **245**(6): E611–E615.

53. Birnbaumer, M. Vasopressin receptors. *Trends Endocrinol. Metab.* 2000; **11**(10): 406–410.

54. Fox, A.W., May, R.E., & Mitch, W.E. Comparison of peptide and nonpeptide receptor-mediated responses in rat tail artery. *J. Cardiovasc. Pharmacol.* 1992; **20**(2): 282–289.

55. Garcia-Villalon, A.L., Garcia, J.L., Fernandez, N., Monge, L., Gomez, B., & Dieguez, G. Regional differences in the arterial response to vasopressin: role of endothelial nitric oxide. *Br. J. Pharmacol.* 1996; **118**(7): 1848–1854.

56. Moursi, M.M., van Wylen, D.G., & D'Alecy, L.G. Regional blood flow changes in response to mildly pressor doses of triglycyl desamino lysine and arginine vasopressin in the conscious dog. *J. Pharmacol. Exp. Ther.* 1985; **232**(2): 360–368.

57. Steckel, R.J., Kolin, A., MacAlpin, R.N. *et al.* Differential effects of Pitressin on blood flow and oxygen extraction in canine vascular beds. *Am. J. Roentgenol.* 1978; **130**(6): 1025–1032.

58. Wallace, A.W., Tunin, C.M., & Shoukas, A.A. Effects of vasopressin on pulmonary and systemic vascular mechanics. *Am. J. Physiol.* 1989; **257**(4 Pt 2): H1228–H1234.

59. Okamura, T., Ayajiki, K., Fujioka, H., & Toda, N. Mechanisms underlying arginine vasopressin-induced relaxation in monkey isolated coronary arteries. *J. Hypertens.* 1999; **17**(5): 673–678.

60. Suzuki, Y., Satoh, S., Oyama, H., Takayasu, M., Shibuya, M., & Sugita, K. Vasopressin mediated vasodilation of cerebral arteries. *J. Auton. Nerv. Syst.* 1994; **49** Suppl.: S129–S132.

61. Xu, Y.J., & Gopalakrishnan, V. Vasopressin increases cytosolic free [Ca^{2+}] in the neonatal rat cardiomyocyte. Evidence for V1 subtype receptors. *Circ. Res.* 1991; **69**(1): 239–245.

62. Fujisawa, S., & Iijima, T. On the inotropic actions of arginine vasopressin in ventricular muscle of the guinea pig heart. *Jpn. J. Pharmacol.* 1999; **81**(3): 309–312.

63. Filep, J., & Rosenkranz, B. Mechanism of vasopressin-induced platelet aggregation. *Thromb. Res.* 1987; **45**(1): 7–15.

64. Heck, M., & Fresenius, M. Coagulation. In: Heck, M., & Fresenius, M., eds. *Repetitorium Anaesthesiology (in German)*. Berlin, Heidelberg, New York: Springer, 1999: 881–918.

65. Mannucci, P.M., Canciani, M.T., Rota, L., & Donovan, B.S. Response of factor VIII/von Willebrand factor to DDAVP in healthy subjects and patients with haemophilia A and von Willebrand's disease. *Br. J. Haematol.* 1981; **47**(2): 283–293.

66. Matsuoka, T., & Wisner, D.H. Hemodynamic and metabolic effects of vasopressin blockade in endotoxin shock. *Surgery* 1997; **121**(2): 162–173.

67. Bilezikjian, L.M., & Vale, W.W. Regulation of ACTH secretion from corticotrophs: the interaction of vasopressin and CRF. *Ann. N Y Acad. Sci.* 1987; **512**: 85–96.

68. Lee, B., Yang, C., Chen, T.H., al-Azawi, N., & Hsu, W.H. Effect of AVP and oxytocin on insulin release: involvement of V1b receptors. *Am. J. Physiol.* 1995; **269**(6 Pt 1): E1095–E1100.

69. Richardson, S.B., Laya, T., & VanOoy, M. Vasopressin-stimulated insulin secretion and inositol phosphate production: interactions with glucose and phorbol esters. *J. Endocrinol.* 1995; **145**(2): 221–226.

70. Landry, D.W., Levin, H.R., Gallant, E.M. *et al.* Vasopressin pressor hypersensitivity in vasodilatory septic shock. *Crit. Care Med.* 1997; **25**(8): 1279–1282.

71. Tsuneyoshi, I., Yamada, H., Kakihana, Y., Nakamura, M., Nakano, Y., & Boyle, W.A., 3rd: Hemodynamic and metabolic effects of low-dose vasopressin infusions in vasodilatory septic shock. *Crit. Care Med.* 2001; **29**(3): 487–493.

72. Holmes, C.L., Walley, K.R., Chittock, D.R., Lehman, T., & Russell, J.A. The effects of vasopressin on hemodynamics and renal function in severe septic shock: a case series. *Intens. Care Med.* 2001; **27**(8): 1416–1421.

73. Pittman, Q.J., Chen, X., Mouihate, A., Hirasawa, M., & Martin, S. Arginine vasopressin, fever and temperature regulation. *Prog. Brain Res.* 1998; **119**: 383–392.

74. Engler, D. & Burger, A.G. The deiodination of the iodothyronines and of their derivatives in man. *Endocr. Rev.* 1984; **5**(2): 151–184.

75. Facktor, M.A., Mayor, G.H., Nachreiner, R.F. & D'Alecy, L.G. Thyroid hormone loss and replacement during resuscitation from cardiac arrest in dogs. *Resuscitation* 1993; **26**(2): 141–162.

76. Longstreth, W.T., Jr., Manowitz, N.R., DeGroot, L.J. *et al.* Plasma thyroid hormone profiles immediately following out-of-hospital cardiac arrest. *Thyroid* 1996; **6**(6): 649–653.

77. Guyton, A.C. & Hall, J.E. Parathyroid hormone, calcitonin, calcium and phosphate metabolism, vitamin, D., bone, and teeth. In Guyton, A.C., & Hall, J.E., eds. *Textbook of Medical Physiology.* 10th edn. Philadelphia: WB Saunders, 2000: 909.

78. Koch, S.M., Mehlhorn, U., Baggstrom, E., Donovan, D., & Allen, S.J. Hypercalcitoninemia and inappropriate calciuria in the acute trauma patient. *J. Crit. Care* 1996; **11**(3): 117–121.

79. Carlstedt, F., Lind, L., Wide, L. *et al.* Serum levels of parathyroid hormone are related to the mortality and severity of illness in patients in the emergency department. *Eur. J. Clin. Invest.* 1997; **27**(12): 977–981.

80. Bornstein, S.R., Ehrhart-Bornstein, M., Usadel, H., Bockmann, M., & Scherbaum, W.A. Morphological evidence for a close interaction of chromaffin cells with cortical cells within the adrenal gland. *Cell Tissue Res.* 1991; **265**(1): 1–9.

81. Bornstein, S.R., Gonzalez-Hernandez, J.A., Ehrhart-Bornstein, M., Adler, G., & Scherbaum, W.A. Intimate contact of chromaffin and cortical cells within the human adrenal gland forms the cellular basis for important intra-adrenal interactions. *J. Clin. Endocrinol. Metab.* 1994; **78**(1): 225–232.

82. Ehrhart-Bornstein, M., Hinson, J.P., Bornstein, S.R., Scherbaum, W.A., & Vinson, G.P. Intraadrenal interactions in the regulation of adrenocortical steroidogenesis. *Endocr. Rev.* 1998; **19**(2): 101–143.

83. Vinson, G.P., Hinson, J.P., & Toth, I.E. The neuroendocrinology of the adrenal cortex. *J Neuroendocrinol* 1994; **6**(3): 235–246.

84. Niijima, A., & Winter, D.L. Baroreceptors in the adrenal gland. *Science* 1968; **159**(813): 434–435.

85. Herd, J.A. Cardiovascular response to stress. *Physiol Rev.* 1991; **71**(1): 305–330.

86. Wortsman, J., Frank, S., & Cryer, P.E. Adrenomedullary response to maximal stress in humans. *Am. J. Med.* 1984; **77**(5): 779–784.

87. Schoffstall, J.M., Spivey, W.H., Davidheiser, S., Fuhs, L., & Kirkpatrick, R., Jr. Endogenous and exogenous plasma catecholamine levels in cardiac arrest in swine. *Resuscitation* 1990; **19**(3): 241–251.

88. Foley, P.J., Tacker, W.A., Wortsman, J., Frank, S., & Cryer, P.E. Plasma catecholamine and serum cortisol responses to experimental cardiac arrest in dogs. *Am. J. Physiol.* 1987; **253**(3 Pt 1): E283–289.

89. Mancia, G., Ferrari, A., Gregorini, L. *et al.* Plasma catecholamines do not invariably reflect sympathetically induced changes in blood pressure in man. *Clin. Sci. (Lond.)* 1983; **65**(3): 227–235.

90. Grassi, G., Gavazzi, C., Cesura, A.M., Picotti, G.B., & Mancia, G. Changes in plasma catecholamines in response to reflex modulation of sympathetic vasoconstrictor tone by cardiopulmonary receptors. *Clin. Sci. (Lond.)* 1985; **68**(5): 503–510.

91. Wortsman, J., Nowak, R.M., Martin, G.B., Paradis, N.A., & Cryer, P.E. Plasma epinephrine levels in resuscitation with cardiopulmonary bypass. *Crit. Care Med.* 1990; **18**(10): 1134–1137.

92. Little, R.A., Frayn, K.N., Randall, P.E. *et al.* Plasma catecholamines in patients with acute myocardial infarction and in cardiac arrest. *Q. J. Med.* 1985; **54**(214): 133–140.

93. Huyghens, L.P., Calle, P.A., Moerman, E.J., Buylaert, W.A., & Bogaert, M.G. Plasma norepinephrine concentrations during resuscitation in the dog. *Am. J. Emerg. Med.* 1991; **9**(5): 426–431.

94. Wortsman, J., Paradis, N.A., Martin, G.B. *et al.* Functional responses to extremely high plasma epinephrine concentrations in cardiac arrest. *Crit. Care Med.* 1993; **21**(5): 692–697.

95. Lindner, K.H., Ahnefeld, F.W., & Bowdler, I.M. Comparison of different doses of epinephrine on myocardial perfusion and resuscitation success during cardiopulmonary resuscitation in a pig model. *Am. J. Emerg. Med.* 1991; **9**(1): 27–31.

96. von Planta, I., Wagner, O., von Planta, M., & Ritz, R. Determinants of survival after rodent cardiac arrest: implications for therapy with adrenergic agents. *Int. J. Cardiol.* 1993; **38**(3): 235–245.

97. Brown, C.G., & Werman, H.A. Adrenergic agonists during cardiopulmonary resuscitation. *Resuscitation* 1990; **19**(1): 1–16.

98. Gonzalez, E.R., Ornato, J.P., Garnett, A.R., Levine, R.L., Young, D.S., & Racht, E.M. Dose-dependent vasopressor response to epinephrine during CPR in human beings. *Ann. Emerg. Med.* 1989; **18**(9): 920–926.

99. Paradis, N.A., & Koscove, E.M. Epinephrine in cardiac arrest: a critical review. *Ann. Emerg. Med.* 1990; **19**(11): 1288–1301.

100. Bernton, E.W., Long, J.B., & Holaday, J.W. Opioids and neuropeptides: mechanisms in circulatory shock. *Fed. Proc.* 1985; **44**(2): 290–299.

101. Svedmyr, N. Action of corticosteroids on beta-adrenergic receptors. Clinical aspects. *Am. Rev. Respir. Dis.* 1990; **141**(2 Pt 2): S31–S38.

102. Dorin, R.I., & Kearns, P.J. High output circulatory failure in acute adrenal insufficiency. *Crit. Care Med.* 1988; **16**(3): 296–297.

103. Antonawich, F.J., Miller, G., Rigsby, D.C., & Davis, J.N. Regulation of ischemic cell death by glucocorticoids and adrenocorticotropic hormone. *Neuroscience* 1999; **88**(1): 319–325.

104. Ito, T., Saitoh, D., Takasu, A., Kiyozumi, T., Sakamoto, T., & Okada, Y. Serum cortisol as a predictive marker of the outcome in patients resuscitated after cardiopulmonary arrest. *Resuscitation* 2004; **62**(1): 55–60.

105. Karnezis, I.A. Variations in serum angiotensin-converting enzyme activity following lung resection: a controlled study in a clinical setting. *Ann. Clin. Biochem.* 1999; **36** (Pt 2): 212–215.

106. Mizuno, Y., Yoshimura, M., Yasue, H. *et al.* Aldosterone production is activated in failing ventricle in humans. *Circulation* 2001; **103**(1): 72–77.

107. Rocha, R., & Stier, C.T., Jr. Pathophysiological effects of aldosterone in cardiovascular tissues. *Trends Endocrinol. Metab.* 2001; **12**(7): 308–314.

108. Weber, K.T. Aldosterone in congestive heart failure. *N. Engl. J. Med.* 2001; **345**(23): 1689–1697.

109. Gomez-Sanchez, C.E., & Gomez-Sanchez, E.P. Editorial: Cardiac steroidogenesis—new sites of synthesis, or much ado about nothing? *J. Clin. Endocrinol. Metab.* 2001; **86**(11): 5118–5120.

110. Orth, D.N., & Kovacs, W.J. The adrenal cortex. In Wilson, J.D., & Foster, D.W., eds. *Williams Textbook of Endocrinology.* Philadelphia: W.B. Saunders, 1998.

111. Rocha, R., & Williams, G.H. Rationale for the use of aldosterone antagonists in congestive heart failure. *Drugs* 2002; **62**(5): 723–731.

112. Lindner, K.H., Prengel, A.W., Pfenninger, E.G., & Lindner, I.M. Effect of angiotensin II on myocardial blood flow and acid-base status in a pig model of cardiopulmonary resuscitation. *Anesth. Analg.* 1993; **76**(3): 485–492.

113. Little, C.M., & Brown, C.G. Angiotensin II administration improves cerebral blood flow in cardiopulmonary arrest in swine. *Stroke* 1994; **25**(1): 183–188.

114. Little, C.M., Hobson, J.L., & Brown, C.G. Angiotensin II effects in a swine model of cardiac arrest. *Ann. Emerg. Med.* 1993; **22**(2): 244–247.

115. Lindner, K.H., Prengel, A.W., Pfenninger, E.G., & Lindner, I.M. Angiotensin II augments reflex activity of the sympathetic nervous system during cardiopulmonary resuscitation in pigs. *Circulation* 1995; **92**(4): 1020–1025.

116. Wanecek, M., Weitzberg, E., Rudehill, A., & Oldner, A. The endothelin system in septic and endotoxin shock. *Eur. J. Pharmacol.* 2000; **407**(1–2): 1–15.

117. Resink, T.J., Hahn, A.W., Scott-Burden, T., Powell, J., Weber, E., & Buhler, F.R. Inducible endothelin mRNA expression and peptide secretion in cultured human vascular smooth muscle cells. *Biochem. Biophys. Res. Commun.* 1990; **168**(3): 1303–1310.

118. Takahashi, K., Jones, P.M., Kanse, S.M. *et al.* Endothelin in the gastrointestinal tract. Presence of endothelinlike immunoreactivity, endothelin-1 messenger RNA, endothelin receptors, and pharmacological effect. *Gastroenterology* 1990; **99**(6): 1660–1667.

119. Ehrenreich, H., Anderson, R.W., Fox, C.H. *et al.* Endothelins, peptides with potent vasoactive properties, are produced by human macrophages. *J. Exp. Med.* 1990; **172**(6): 1741–1748.

120. Ehrenreich, H., Burd, P.R., Rottem, M. *et al.* Endothelins belong to the assortment of mast cell-derived and mast cell-bound cytokines. *New Biol.* 1992; **4**(2): 147–156.

121. Suzuki, T., Kumazaki, T., & Mitsui, Y. Endothelin-1 is produced and secreted by neonatal rat cardiac myocytes in vitro. *Biochem. Biophys. Res. Commun.* 1993; **191**(3): 823–830.

122. Giaid, A., Gibson, S.J., Ibrahim, B.N. *et al.* Endothelin 1, an endothelium-derived peptide, is expressed in neurons of the human spinal cord and dorsal root ganglia. *Proc. Natl Acad. Sci. USA* 1989; **86**(19): 7634–7638.

123. Endo, T., Uchida, Y., Matsumoto, H. *et al.* Regulation of endothelin-1 synthesis in cultured guinea pig airway epithelial cells by various cytokines. *Biochem. Biophys. Res. Commun.* 1992; **186**(3): 1594–1599.

124. Liu, B., Zhou, J., Chen, H. *et al.* Expression and cellular location of endothelin-1 mRNA in rat liver following endotoxemia. *Chin. Med. J. (Engl.)* 1997; **110**(12): 932–935.

125. Yoshizumi, M., Kurihara, H., Sugiyama, T. *et al.* Hemodynamic shear stress stimulates endothelin production by cultured endothelial cells. *Biochem. Biophys. Res. Commun.* 1989; **161**(2): 859–864.

126. Kourembanas, S., Marsden, P.A., McQuillan, L.P., & Faller, D.V. Hypoxia induces endothelin gene expression and secretion in cultured human endothelium. *J. Clin. Invest.* 1991; **88**(3): 1054–1057.

127. Maemura, K., Kurihara, H., Morita, T., Oh-hashi, Y., & Yazaki, Y. Production of endothelin-1 in vascular endothelial cells is regulated by factors associated with vascular injury. *Gerontology* 1992; **38** Suppl 1: 29–35.

128. Kurihara, H., Yoshizumi, M., Sugiyama, T. *et al.* Transforming growth factor-beta stimulates the expression of endothelin mRNA by vascular endothelial cells. *Biochem. Biophys. Res. Commun.* 1989; **159**(3): 1435–1440.

129. Yanagisawa, M., Kurihara, H., Kimura, S. *et al.* A novel potent vasoconstrictor peptide produced by vascular endothelial cells. *Nature* 1988; **332**(6163): 411–415.

130. Emori, T., Hirata, Y., Ohta, K., Shichiri, M., & Marumo, F. Secretory mechanism of immunoreactive endothelin in cultured bovine endothelial cells. *Biochem. Biophys. Res. Commun.* 1989; **160**(1): 93–100.

131. Razandi, M., Pedram, A., Rubin, T., & Levin, E.R. PGE2 and PGI2 inhibit ET-1 secretion from endothelial cells by stimulating particulate guanylate cyclase. *Am. J. Physiol.* 1996; **270**(4 Pt 2): H1342–H1349.

132. Boulanger, C., & Luscher, T.F. Release of endothelin from the porcine aorta. Inhibition by endothelium-derived nitric oxide. *J. Clin. Invest.* 1990; **85**(2): 587–590.

133. Hanehira, T., Kohno, M., & Yoshikawa, J. Endothelin production in cultured vascular smooth muscle cells – modulation by the atrial, brain, and C-type natriuretic peptide system. *Metabolism* 1997; **46**(5): 487–493.

134. Arai, H., Hori, S., Aramori, I., Ohkubo, H., & Nakanishi, S. Cloning and expression of a cDNA encoding an endothelin receptor. *Nature* 1990; **348**(6303): 730–732.

135. Sakurai, T., Yanagisawa, M., Takuwa, Y. *et al.* Cloning of a cDNA encoding a non-isopeptide-selective subtype of the endothelin receptor. *Nature* 1990; **348**(6303): 732–735.

136. DeBehnke, D.J., & Benson, L. Effects of endothelin-1 on resuscitation rate during cardiac arrest. *Resuscitation* 2000; **47**(2): 185–189.

137. DeBehnke, D. The effects of graded doses of endothelin-1 on coronary perfusion pressure and vital organ blood flow during cardiac arrest. *Acad. Emerg. Med.* 2000; **7**(3): 211–221.

138. DeBehnke, D.J., Spreng, D., Wickman, L.L., & Crowe, D.T. The effects of endothelin-1 on coronary perfusion pressure during cardiopulmonary resuscitation in a canine model. *Acad. Emerg. Med.* 1996; **3**(2): 137–141.

139. Holzer, M., Sterz, F., Behringer, W. *et al.* Endothelin-1 elevates regional cerebral perfusion during prolonged ventricular fibrillation cardiac arrest in pigs. *Resuscitation* 2002; **55**(3): 317–327.

140. Hilwig, R.W., Berg, R.A., Kern, K.B., & Ewy, G.A. Endothelin-1 vasoconstriction during swine cardiopulmonary resuscitation improves coronary perfusion pressures but worsens postresuscitation outcome. *Circulation* 2000; **101**(17): 2097–2102.

141. Wenzel, V., Ewy, G.A., & Lindner, K.H. Vasopressin and endothelin during cardiopulmonary resuscitation. *Crit. Care Med.* 2000; **28**(11 Suppl): N233–N235.

142. Pluta, R., Lossinsky, A.S., Wisniewski, H.M., & Mossakowski, M.J. Early blood-brain barrier changes in the rat following transient complete cerebral ischemia induced by cardiac arrest. *Brain Res.* 1994; **633**(1–2): 41–52.

143. Ferrari, R., & Agnoletti, G. Atrial natriuretic peptide: its mechanism of release from the atrium. *Int. J. Cardiol.* 1989; **25** Suppl 1: S3–S15.

144. Inagami, T. Atrial natriuretic factor. *J. Biol. Chem.* 1989; **264**(6): 3043–3046.

145. Woods, R.L., Oliver, J.R., & Korner, P.I. Direct and neurohumoral cardiovascular effects of atrial natriuretic peptide. *J. Cardiovasc. Pharmacol.* 1989; **13**(2): 177–185.

146. Levin, E.R., Gardner, D.G., & Samson, W.K. Natriuretic peptides. *N. Engl. J. Med.* 1998; **339**(5): 321–328.

147. de Denus, S., Pharand, C., & Williamson, D.R. Brain natriuretic peptide in the management of heart failure: the versatile neurohormone. *Chest* 2004; **125**(2): 652–668.

148. Naruse, M., Takeyama, Y., Tanabe, A. *et al.* Atrial and brain natriuretic peptides in cardiovascular diseases. *Hypertension* 1994; **23**(1 Suppl): I231–I234.

149. Morita, E., Yasue, H., Yoshimura, M. *et al.* Increased plasma levels of brain natriuretic peptide in patients with acute myocardial infarction. *Circulation* 1993; **88**(1): 82–91.

150. Yoshimura, M., Yasue, H., Morita, E. *et al.* Hemodynamic, renal, and hormonal responses to brain natriuretic peptide infusion in patients with congestive heart failure. *Circulation* 1991; **84**(4): 1581–1588.

151. Lai, C.P., Egashira, K., Tashiro, H. *et al.* Beneficial effects of atrial natriuretic peptide on exercise-induced myocardial ischemia in patients with stable effort angina pectoris. *Circulation* 1993; **87**(1): 144–151.

152. Stein, B.C., & Levin, R.I. Natriuretic peptides: physiology, therapeutic potential, and risk stratification in ischemic heart disease. *Am. Heart. J.* 1998; **135**(5 Pt 1): 914–923.

153. Gardner, D.G. Designer natriuretic peptides. *J. Clin. Invest.* 1993; **92**(4): 1606–1607.

154. Guyton, A.C., & Hall, J.E. eds. Urine formation by the kidneys: glomerular filtration, renal blood flow, and their control. In Guyton, A.C., & Hall, J.E. *Textbook of Medical Physiology.* 10th edn. Philadelphia: W.B. Saunders, 2000: 279–294.

155. Guyton, A.C., & Hall, J.E. eds. Red blood cells, anemia, and polycythemia. In *Textbook of Medical Physiology.* 10th edn. Philadelphia: W.B. Saunders, 2000: 381–391.

156. Eckardt, K.U., Boutellier, U., Kurtz, A., Schopen, M., Koller, E.A., & Bauer, C. Rate of erythropoietin formation in humans in response to acute hypobaric hypoxia. *J. Appl. Physiol.* 1989; **66**(4): 1785–1788.

157. Erslev, A.J., Caro, J., Miller, O., & Silver, R. Plasma erythropoietin in health and disease. *Ann. Clin. Lab. Sci.* 1980; **10**(3): 250–257.

158. Wortsman, J., Foley, P.J., Malarkey, W.B., O'Dorisio, T.M., Tacker, W.A., & Frank, S. Effect of adrenal function on gastrointestinal peptide release in experimental cardiac arrest. *J. Lab. Clin. Med.* 1988; **111**(1): 104–109.

159. Martin, G.B., O'Brien, J.F., Best, R., Goldman, J., Tomlanovich, M.C., & Nowak, R.M. Insulin and glucose levels during CPR in the canine model. *Ann. Emerg. Med.* 1985; **14**(4): 293–297.

160. Green, D.W., Gomez, G., & Greeley, G.H., Jr. Gastrointestinal peptides. *Gastroenterol Clin. North Am.* 1989; **18**(4): 695–733.

161. Levin, E.R. Natriuretic peptide C-receptor: more than a clearance receptor. *Am. J. Physiol.* 1993; **264**(4 Pt 1): E483–E489.

162. Genton, L., & Kudsk, K.A. Interactions between the enteric nervous system and the immune system: role of neuropeptides and nutrition. *Am. J. Surg.* 2003; **186**(3): 253–258.

163. Negovsky, V.A. Postresuscitation disease. *Crit. Care Med.* 1988; **16**(10): 942–946.

164. Laurent, I., Monchi, M., Chiche, J.D. *et al.* Reversible myocardial dysfunction in survivors of out-of-hospital cardiac arrest. *J. Am. Coll. Cardiol.* 2002; **40**(12): 2110–2116.

165. Adrie, C., Adib-Conquy, M., Laurent, I., *et al.* Successful cardiopulmonary resuscitation after cardiac arrest as a "sepsis-like" syndrome. *Circulation* 2002; **106**(5): 562–568.

166. Adrie, C., Laurent, I., Monchi, M., Cariou, A., Dhainaou, J.F., & Spaulding, C. Postresuscitation disease after cardiac arrest: a sepsis-like syndrome? *Curr. Opin. Crit. Care* 2004; **10**(3): 208–212.

167. Van den Berghe, G. Neuroendocrine pathobiology of chronic critical illness. *Crit. Care Clin.* 2002; **18**(3): 509–528.

168. Van den Berghe, G., Baxter, R.C., Weekers, F., Wouters, P., Bowers, C.Y., & Veldhuis, J.D. A paradoxical gender dissociation within the growth hormone/insulin-like growth factor I axis during protracted critical illness. *J. Clin. Endocrinol. Metab.* 2000; **85**(1): 183–192.

169. Vermes, I., Beishuizen, A., Hampsink, R.M., & Haanen, C. Dissociation of plasma adrenocorticotropin and cortisol levels in critically ill patients: possible role of endothelin and atrial natriuretic hormone. *J. Clin. Endocrinol. Metab.* 1995; **80**(4): 1238–1242.

170. Reincke, M., Allolio, B., Wurth, G., & Winkelmann, W. The hypothalamic-pituitary-adrenal axis in critical illness: response to dexamethasone and corticotropin-releasing hormone. *J. Clin. Endocrinol. Metab.* 1993; **77**(1): 151–156.

171. Lim, A.T., & Funder, J.W. Stress-induced changes in plasma, pituitary and hypothalamic immunoreactive beta-endorphin: effects of diurnal variation, adrenalectomy, corticosteroids, and opiate agonists and antagonists. *Neuroendocrinology* 1983; **36**(3): 225–234.

172. Rosolski, T., Gruska, S., & Konkel, J. [Opioid peptides in hemorrhagic shock]. *Anaesthesiol. Reanim.* 1991; **16**(4): 235–242.

173. Legakis, I., Saramantis, A., Voros, D., Chalevelakis, G., & Tolis, G. Dissociation of ACTH, beta-endorphin and cortisol in graded sepsis. *Horm. Metab. Res.* 1998; **30**(9): 570–574.

174. Schmidt, C., & Kraft, K. Beta-endorphin and catecholamine concentrations during chronic and acute stress in intensive care patients. *Eur. J. Med. Res.* 1996; **1**(11): 528–532.

175. Molina, P.E. Opiate modulation of hemodynamic, hormonal, and cytokine responses to hemorrhage. *Shock* 2001; **15**(6): 471–478.

176. Rusin, K.I., & Moises, H.C. Mu-Opioid receptor activation reduces multiple components of high-threshold calcium current in rat sensory neurons. *J. Neurosci.* 1995; **15**(6): 4315–4327.

177. Moises, H.C., Rusin, K.I., & Macdonald, R.L. Mu-Opioid receptor-mediated reduction of neuronal calcium current occurs via a G(o)-type GTP-binding protein. *J. Neurosci.* 1994; **14**(6): 3842–3851.

178. Bertolini, A., Guarini, S., Rompianesi, E., & Ferrari, W. Alpha-MSH and other ACTH fragments improve cardiovascular

function and survival in experimental hemorrhagic shock. *Eur. J. Pharmacol.* 1986; **130**(1–2): 19–26.

179. Bazzani, C., Guarini, S., Botticelli, A.R., *et al.* Protective effect of melanocortin peptides in rat myocardial ischemia. *J. Pharmacol. Exp. Ther.* 2001; **297**(3): 1082–1087.

180. Guarini, S., Schioth, H.B., Mioni, C. *et al.* MC(3) receptors are involved in the protective effect of melanocortins in myocardial ischemia/reperfusion-induced arrhythmias. *Naunyn Schmiedebergs Arch. Pharmacol.* 2002; **366**(2): 177–182.

181. Bazzani, C., Mioni, C., Ferrazza, G., Cainazzo, M.M., Bertolini, A., & Guarini, S. Involvement of the central nervous system in the protective effect of melanocortins in myocardial ischaemia/reperfusion injury. *Resuscitation* 2002; **52**(1): 109–115.

182. Catania, A., Delgado, R., Airaghi, L. *et al.* alpha-MSH in systemic inflammation. Central and peripheral actions. *Ann. NY Acad. Sci.* 1999; **885**: 183–187.

183. Catania, A., & Lipton, J.M. The neuropeptide alpha-melanocyte-stimulating hormone: a key component of neuroimmunomodulation. *Neuroimmunomodulation* 1994; **1**(2): 93–99.

184. Mioni, C., Giuliani, D., Cainazzo, M.M. *et al.* Further evidence that melanocortins prevent myocardial reperfusion injury by activating melanocortin MC3 receptors. *Eur. J. Pharmacol.* 2003; **477**(3): 227–234.

185. Delgado Hernandez, R., Demitri, M.T., Carlin, A. *et al.* Inhibition of systemic inflammation by central action of the neuropeptide alpha-melanocyte-stimulating hormone. *Neuroimmunomodulation* 1999; **6**(3): 187–192.

186. Reichlin, S. Neuroendocrine-immune interactions. *N. Engl. J. Med.* 1993; **329**(17): 1246–1253.

187. Carrier, M., Wild, J., Pelletier, L.C., & Copeland, J.G. Bromocriptine as an adjuvant to cyclosporine immunosuppression after heart transplantation. *Ann. Thorac. Surg.* 1990; **49**(1): 129–132.

188. Devins, S.S., Miller, A., Herndon, B.L., O'Toole, L., & Reisz, G. Effects of dopamine on T-lymphocyte proliferative responses and serum prolactin concentrations in critically ill patients. *Crit. Care Med.* 1992; **20**(12): 1644–1649.

189. Van den Berghe, G., de Zegher, F., Veldhuis, J.D. *et al.* Thyrotrophin and prolactin release in prolonged critical illness: dynamics of spontaneous secretion and effects of growth hormone-secretagogues. *Clin. Endocrinol. (Oxf.)* 1997; **47**(5): 599–612.

190. Van den Berghe, G., de Zegher, F., Baxter, R.C. *et al.* Neuroendocrinology of prolonged critical illness: effects of exogenous thyrotropin-releasing hormone and its combination with growth hormone secretagogues. *J. Clin. Endocrinol. Metab.* 1998; **83**(2): 309–319.

191. Goins, W.A., Reynolds, H.N., Nyanjom, D., & Dunham, C.M. Outcome following prolonged intensive care unit stay in multiple trauma patients. *Crit. Care Med.* 1991; **19**(3): 339–345.

192. Meakins, J.L., Pietsch, J.B., Bubenick, O. *et al.* Delayed hypersensitivity: indicator of acquired failure of host defenses in sepsis and trauma. *Ann. Surg.* 1977; **186**(3): 241–250.

193. Van den Berghe, G., de Zegher, F., Wouters, P. et al. Dehydroepiandrosterone sulphate in critical illness: effect of dopamine. *Clin. Endocrinol. (Oxf.)* 1995; **43**(4): 457–463.

194. Van den Berghe, G., de Zegher, F., & Lauwers, P. Dopamine and the sick euthyroid syndrome in critical illness. *Clin. Endocrinol. (Oxf.)* 1994; **41**(6): 731–737.

195. Ross, R., Miell, J., Freeman, E. *et al.* Critically ill patients have high basal growth hormone levels with attenuated oscillatory activity associated with low levels of insulin-like growth factor-I. *Clin. Endocrinol. (Oxf.)* 1991; **35**(1): 47–54.

196. Baxter, R.C., Hawker, F.H., To, C., Stewart, P.M., & Holman, S.R. Thirty-day monitoring of insulin-like growth factors and their binding proteins in intensive care unit patients. *Growth Horm IGF Res* 1998; **8**(6): 455–463.

197. Van den Berghe, G., de Zegher, F., & Bouillon, R. Clinical review 95: acute and prolonged critical illness as different neuroendocrine paradigms. *J. Clin. Endocrinol. Metab.* 1998; **83**(6): 1827–1834.

198. Voerman, H.J., Strack van Schijndel, R.J., de Boer, H., van der Veen, E.A., & Thijs, L.G. Growth hormone: secretion and administration in catabolic adult patients, with emphasis on the critically ill patient. *Neth. J. Med.* 1992; **41**(5–6): 229–244.

199. Hartman, M.L., Veldhuis, J.D., Johnson, M.L. *et al.* Augmented growth hormone (GH) secretory burst frequency and amplitude mediate enhanced GH secretion during a two-day fast in normal men. *J. Clin. Endocrinol. Metab.* 1992; **74**(4): 757–765.

200. Rodriguez-Arnao, J., Yarwood, G., Ferguson, C., Miell, J., Hinds, C.J., & Ross, R.J. Reduction in circulating IGF-I and hepatic IGF-I mRNA levels after caecal ligation and puncture are associated with differential regulation of hepatic IGF-binding protein-1, -2 and -3 mRNA levels. *J. Endocrinol.* 1996; **151**(2): 287–292.

201. Van den Berghe, G. Dynamic neuroendocrine responses to critical illness. *Front. Neuroendocrinol.* 2002; **23**(4): 370–391.

202. Van den Berghe, G., Wouters, P., Weekers, F. *et al.* Reactivation of pituitary hormone release and metabolic improvement by infusion of growth hormone-releasing peptide and thyrotropin-releasing hormone in patients with protracted critical illness. *J. Clin. Endocrinol. Metab.* 1999; **84**(4): 1311–1323.

203. Mesotten, D., Delhanty, P.J., Vanderhoydonc, F. *et al.* Regulation of insulin-like growth factor binding protein-1 during protracted critical illness. *J. Clin. Endocrinol. Metab.* 2002; **87**(12): 5516–5523.

204. Van den Berghe, G., de Zegher, F., Veldhuis, J.D. *et al.* The somatotropic axis in critical illness: effect of continuous growth hormone (GH)-releasing hormone and GH-releasing peptide-2 infusion. *J. Clin. Endocrinol. Metab.* 1997; **82**(2): 590–599.

205. Gore, D.C., Honeycutt, D., Jahoor, F., Wolfe, R.R., & Herndon, D.N. Effect of exogenous growth hormone on whole-body and isolated-limb protein kinetics in burned patients. *Arch. Surg.* 1991; **126**(1): 38–43.

206. Ponting, G.A., Halliday, D., Teale, J.D., & Sim, A.J. Postoperative positive nitrogen balance with intravenous hyponutrition and growth hormone. *Lancet* 1988; **1**(8583): 438–440.

207. Voerman, H.J., van Schijndel, R.J., Groeneveld, A.B. *et al.* Effects of recombinant human growth hormone in patients with severe sepsis. *Ann. Surg.* 1992; **216**(6): 648–655.

208. Voerman, B.J., Strack van Schijndel, R.J., Groeneveld, A.B., de Boer, H., Nauta, J.P., & Thijs, L.G. Effects of human growth hormone in critically ill nonseptic patients: results from a prospective, randomized, placebo-controlled trial. *Crit. Care Med.* 1995; **23**(4): 665–673.

209. Herndon, D.N., Barrow, R.E., Kunkel, K.R., Broemeling, L., & Rutan, R.L. Effects of recombinant human growth hormone on donor-site healing in severely burned children. *Ann. Surg.* 1990; **212**(4): 424–429; discussion 430–421.

210. Hammarqvist, F., Stromberg, C., von der Decken, A., Vinnars, E., & Wernerman, J. Biosynthetic human growth hormone preserves both muscle protein synthesis and the decrease in muscle-free glutamine, and improves whole-body nitrogen economy after operation. *Ann. Surg.* 1992; **216**(2): 184–191.

211. Jiang, Z.M., He, G.Z., Zhang, S.Y. *et al.* Low-dose growth hormone and hypocaloric nutrition attenuate the protein-catabolic response after major operation. *Ann. Surg.* 1989; **210**(4): 513–524; discussion 524–515.

212. Knox, J.B., Wilmore, D.W., Demling, R.H., Sarraf, P., & Santos, A.A. Use of growth hormone for postoperative respiratory failure. *Am. J. Surg.* 1996; **171**(6): 576–580.

213. Pape, G.S., Friedman, M., Underwood, L.E., & Clemmons, D.R. The effect of growth hormone on weight gain and pulmonary function in patients with chronic obstructive lung disease. *Chest* 1991; **99**(6): 1495–1500.

214. Unneberg, K., Balteskard, L., Mjaaland, M., & Revhaug, A. Growth hormone impaired compensation of hemorrhagic shock after trauma and sepsis in swine. *J. Trauma* 1996; **41**(5): 775–780.

215. Takala, J., Ruokonen, E., Webster, N.R. *et al.* Increased mortality associated with growth hormone treatment in critically ill adults. *N. Engl. J. Med.* 1999; **341**(11): 785–792.

216. Gebhart, S.S., Watts, N.B., Clark, R.V., Umpierrez, G., & Sgoutas, D. Reversible impairment of gonadotropin secretion in critical illness. Observations in postmenopausal women. *Arch. Intern. Med.* 1989; **149**(7): 1637–1641.

217. Spratt, D.I., Cox, P., Orav, J., Moloney, J., & Bigos, T. Reproductive axis suppression in acute illness is related to disease severity. *J. Clin. Endocrinol. Metab.* 1993; **76**(6): 1548–1554.

218. van Steenbergen, W., Naert, J., Lambrecht, S., Scheys, I., Lesaffre, E., & Pelemans, W. Suppression of gonadotropin secretion in the hospitalized postmenopausal female as an effect of acute critical illness. *Neuroendocrinology* 1994; **60**(2): 165–172.

219. Van den Berghe, G., de Zegher, F., Lauwers, P., & Veldhuis, J.D. Luteinizing hormone secretion and hypoandrogenaemia in critically ill men: effect of dopamine. *Clin. Endocrinol. (Oxf.)* 1994; **41**(5): 563–569.

220. Cicero, T.J., Bell, R.D., Wiest, W.G., Allison, J.H., Polakoski, K., & Robins, E. Function of the male sex organs in heroin and methadone users. *N. Engl. J. Med.* 1975; **292**(17): 882–887.

221. Rivier, C., & Vale, W. In the rat, interleukin-1 alpha acts at the level of the brain and the gonads to interfere with gonadotropin and sex steroid secretion. *Endocrinology* 1989; **124**(5): 2105–2109.

222. Adashi, E.Y., Rebar, R.W., Ehara, Y., Naftolin, F., & Yen, S.S. Impact of acute surgical stress on anterior pituitary function in female subjects. *Am. J. Obstet. Gynecol.* 1980; **138**(6): 609–614.

223. Beitins, I.Z., Barkan, A., Klibanski, A. *et al.* Hormonal responses to short term fasting in postmenopausal women. *J. Clin. Endocrinol. Metab.* 1985; **60**(6): 1120–1126.

224. Sharshar, T., Blanchard, A., Paillard, M., Raphael, J.C., Gajdos, P., & Annane, D. Circulating vasopressin levels in septic shock. *Crit. Care Med.* 2003; **31**(6): 1752–1758.

225. Landry, D.W., Levin, H.R., Gallant, E.M. *et al.* Vasopressin deficiency contributes to the vasodilation of septic shock. *Circulation* 1997; **95**(5): 1122–1125.

226. Argenziano, M., Chen, J.M., Choudhri, A.F. *et al.* Management of vasodilatory shock after cardiac surgery: identification of predisposing factors and use of a novel pressor agent. *J. Thorac. Cardiovasc. Surg.* 1998; **116**(6): 973–980.

227. Argenziano, M., Chen, J.M., Cullinane, S. *et al.* Arginine vasopressin in the management of vasodilatory hypotension after cardiac transplantation. *J Heart Lung Transpl.* 1999; **18**(8): 814–817.

228. Morales, D., Madigan, J., Cullinane, S. *et al.* Reversal by vasopressin of intractable hypotension in the late phase of hemorrhagic shock. *Circulation* 1999; **100**(3): 226–229.

229. Chen, J.M., Cullinane, S., Spanier, T.B. *et al.* Vasopressin deficiency and pressor hypersensitivity in hemodynamically unstable organ donors. *Circulation* 1999; **100**(19 Suppl): II244–246.

230. Landry, D.W., & Oliver, J.A. The pathogenesis of vasodilatory shock. *N. Engl. J. Med.* 2001; **345**(8): 588–595.

231. Sharshar, T., Carlier, R., Blanchard, A. *et al.* Depletion of neurohypophyseal content of vasopressin in septic shock. *Crit. Care Med.* 2002; **30**(3): 497–500.

232. Goldsmith, S.R. Vasopressin deficiency and vasodilation of septic shock. *Circulation* 1998; **97**(3): 292–293.

233. Cooke, C.R., Wall, B.M., Jones, G.V., Presley, D.N., & Share, L. Reversible vasopressin deficiency in severe hypernatremia. *Am. J. Kidney. Dis.* 1993; **22**(1): 44–52.

234. Rivier, C. Role of nitric oxide in regulating the rat hypothalamic-pituitary-adrenal axis response to endotoxemia. *Ann. N Y Acad. Sci.* 2003; **992**: 72–85.

235. Jochberger, S., Mayr, V.D., Luckner, G. *et al.* Serum vasopressin concentrations in critically Ill patients. *Crit. Care Med.* 2006; In press.

236. Considine, R.V., Sinha, M.K., Heiman, M.L. *et al.* Serum immunoreactive-leptin concentrations in normal-weight and obese humans. *N. Engl. J. Med.* 1996; **334**(5): 292–295.

237. Grinspoon, S., Gulick, T., Askari, H. *et al.* Serum leptin levels in women with anorexia nervosa. *J. Clin. Endocrinol. Metab.* 1996; **81**(11): 3861–3863.

238. Sinha, M.K., Ohannesian, J.P., Heiman, M.L. *et al.* Nocturnal rise of leptin in lean, obese, and non-insulin-dependent

diabetes mellitus subjects. *J. Clin. Invest.* 1996; **97**(5): 1344–1347.

239. Licinio, J., Mantzoros, C., Negrao, A.B. *et al.* Human leptin levels are pulsatile and inversely related to pituitary-adrenal function. *Nat. Med.* 1997; **3**(5): 575–579.

240. Kolaczynski, J.W., Nyce, M.R., Considine, R.V. *et al.* Acute and chronic effects of insulin on leptin production in humans: studies in vivo and in vitro. *Diabetes* 1996; **45**(5): 699–701.

241. Bianda, T.L., Glatz, Y., Boeni-Schnetzler, M., Froesch, E.R., & Schmid, C. Effects of growth hormone (GH) and insulin-like growth factor-I on serum leptin in GH-deficient adults. *Diabetologia* 1997; **40**(3): 363–364.

242. Berneis, K., Vosmeer, S., & Keller, U. Effects of glucocorticoids and of growth hormone on serum leptin concentrations in man. *Eur. J. Endocrinol.* 1996; **135**(6): 663–665.

243. Valcavi, R., Zini, M., Peino, R., Casanueva, F.F., & Dieguez, C. Influence of thyroid status on serum immunoreactive leptin levels. *J. Clin. Endocrinol. Metab.* 1997; **82**(5): 1632–1634.

244. Ahima, R.S., Prabakaran, D., Mantzoros, C. *et al.* Role of leptin in the neuroendocrine response to fasting. *Nature* 1996; **382**(6588): 250–252.

245. Peelman, F., Iserentant, H., Eyckerman, S., Zabeau, L., & Tavernier, J. Leptin, immune responses and autoimmune disease. Perspectives on the use of leptin antagonists. *Curr. Pharm. Des.* 2005; **11**(4): 539–548.

246. Batra, A., Zeitz, M., & Siegmund, B. [The role of leptin in the immune system—a linking of endocrinology and immunology]. *Dtsch Med. Wochenschr.* 2005; **130**(5): 226–229.

247. Matarese, G., Moschos, S., & Mantzoros, C.S. Leptin in immunology. *J. Immunol.* 2005; **174**(6): 3137–3142.

248. Pankov, Iu. A. [The role of leptin and its peptide mediators in neurophysiology]. *Vestn. Ross. Akad. Med. Nauk.* **2005**(2): 44–48.

249. Bornstein, S.R., Licinio, J., Tauchnitz, R. *et al.* Plasma leptin levels are increased in survivors of acute sepsis: associated loss of diurnal rhythm, in cortisol and leptin secretion. *J. Clin. Endocrinol. Metab.* 1998; **83**(1): 280–283.

250. Van den Berghe, G., Wouters, P., Carlsson, L., Baxter, R.C., Bouillon, R., & Bowers, C.Y. Leptin levels in protracted critical illness: effects of growth hormone-secretagogues and thyrotropin-releasing hormone. *J. Clin. Endocrinol. Metab.* 1998; **83**(9): 3062–3070.

251. Carlson, G.L., Saeed, M., Little, R.A., & Irving, M.H. Serum leptin concentrations and their relation to metabolic abnormalities in human sepsis. *Am. J. Physiol.* 1999; **276**(4 Pt 1): E658–E662.

252. D'Alecy, L.G. Thyroid hormone in neural rescue. *Thyroid* 1997; **7**(1): 115–124.

253. Chopra, I.J. Clinical review 86: euthyroid sick syndrome: is it a misnomer? *J. Clin. Endocrinol. Metab.* 1997; **82**(2): 329–334.

254. Brierre, S., Kumari, R., & Deboisblanc, B.P. The endocrine system during sepsis. *Am. J. Med. Sci.* 2004; **328**(4): 238–247.

255. Wiersinga, W.M. Nonthyroidal illness. In Braverman, L.E., & Utiger, R.D., eds. *The Thyroid: A Fundamental and Clinical Text.* Baltimore: Lippincott Williams & Wilkins, 2000: 121.

256. Ray, D.C., Macduff, A., Drummond, G.B., Wilkinson, E., Adams, B., & Beckett, G.J. Endocrine measurements in survivors and non-survivors from critical illness. *Intens. Care Med.* 2002; **28**(9): 1301–1308.

257. Slag, M.F., Morley, J.E., Elson, M.K., Crowson, T.W., Nuttall, F.Q., & Shafer, R.B. Hypothyroxinemia in critically ill patients as a predictor of high mortality. *J. Am. Med. Assoc.* 1981; **245**(1): 43–45.

258. Mullis-Jansson, S.L., Argenziano, M., Corwin, S. *et al.* A randomized double-blind study of the effect of triiodothyronine on cardiac function and morbidity after coronary bypass surgery. *J. Thorac. Cardiovasc. Surg.* 1999; **117**(6): 1128–1134.

259. Whitesall, S.E., Mayor, G.H., Nachreiner, R.F., Zwemer, C.F., & D'Alecy, L.G. Acute administration of T3 or rT3 failed to improve outcome following resuscitation from cardiac arrest in dogs. *Resuscitation* 1996; **33**(1): 53–62.

260. Zwemer, C.F., Whitesall, S.E., Nachreiner, R.F., Mayor, G.H., & D'Alecy, L.G. Acute thyroid hormone administration increases systemic oxygen delivery and consumption immediately following resuscitation from cardiac arrest without changes in thyroid-stimulating hormone. *Resuscitation* 1997; **33**(3): 271–280.

261. Klemperer, J.D., Klein, I., Gomez, M. *et al.* Thyroid hormone treatment after coronary-artery bypass surgery. *N. Engl. J. Med.* 1995; **333**(23): 1522–1527.

262. Bennett-Guerrero, E., Jimenez, J.L., White, W.D., D'Amico, E.B., Baldwin, B.I., & Schwinn, D.A. Cardiovascular effects of intravenous triiodothyronine in patients undergoing coronary artery bypass graft surgery. A randomized, double-blind, placebo-controlled trial. Duke T3 study group. *J. Am. Med. Assoc.* 1996; **275**(9): 687–692.

263. Brent, G.A., & Hershman, J.M. Thyroxine therapy in patients with severe nonthyroidal illnesses and low serum thyroxine concentration. *J. Clin. Endocrinol. Metab.* 1986; **63**(1): 1–8.

264. Lind, L., Bucht, E., & Ljunghall, S. Pronounced elevation in circulating calcitonin in critical care patients is related to the severity of illness and survival. *Intens. Care Med.* 1995; **21**(1): 63–66.

265. Sanchez, G.J., Venkataraman, P.S., Pryor, R.W., Parker, M.K., Fry, H.D., & Blick, K.E. Hypercalcitoninemia and hypocalcemia in acutely ill children: studies in serum calcium, blood ionized calcium, and calcium-regulating hormones. *J. Pediatr.* 1989; **114**(6): 952–956.

266. Burchard, K.W., Gann, D.S., Colliton, J., & Forster, J. Ionized calcium, parathormone, and mortality in critically ill surgical patients. *Ann. Surg.* 1990; **212**(4): 543–549; discussion 549–550.

267. McKay, C., Beastall, G.H., Imrie, C.W., & Baxter, J.N. Circulating intact parathyroid hormone levels in acute pancreatitis. *Br. J. Surg.* 1994; **81**(3): 357–360.

268. Brodrick, J.W., Largman, C., Ray, S.B., & Geokas, M.C. Proteolysis of parathyroid hormone in vitro by sera from acute pancreatitis patients. *Proc. Soc. Exp. Biol. Med.* 1981; **167**(4): 588–596.

269. Carlstedt, F., Lind, L., Rastad, J., Stjernstrom, H., Wide, L., & Ljunghall, S. Parathyroid hormone and ionized calcium levels

are related to the severity of illness and survival in critically ill patients. *Eur. J. Clin. Invest.* 1998; **28**(11): 898–903.

270. Lind, L., Carlstedt, F., Rastad, J. *et al.* Hypocalcemia and parathyroid hormone secretion in critically ill patients. *Crit. Care Med.* 2000; **28**(1): 93–99.

271. Joborn, H., Hjemdahl, P., Larsson, P.T. *et al.* Effects of prolonged adrenaline infusion and of mental stress on plasma minerals and parathyroid hormone. *Clin. Physiol.* 1990; **10**(1): 37–53.

272. Brown, E.M., Hurwitz, S., Woodard, C.J., & Aurbach, G.D. Direct identification of beta-adrenergic receptors on isolated bovine parathyroid cells. *Endocrinology* 1977; **100**(6): 1703–1709.

273. Katz, M.S., Gutierrez, G.E., Mundy, G.R., Hymer, T.K., Caulfield, M.P., & McKee, R.L. Tumor necrosis factor and interleukin 1 inhibit parathyroid hormone-responsive adenylate cyclase in clonal osteoblast-like cells by down-regulating parathyroid hormone receptors. *J. Cell Physiol.* 1992; **153**(1): 206–213.

274. Greenfield, E.M., Shaw, S.M., Gornik, S.A., & Banks, M.A. Adenyl cyclase and interleukin 6 are downstream effectors of parathyroid hormone resulting in stimulation of bone resorption. *J. Clin. Invest.* 1995; **96**(3): 1238–1244.

275. Weryha, G., & Leclere, J. Paracrine regulation of bone remodeling. *Horm. Res.* 1995; **43**(1–3): 69–75.

276. Niemann, J.T., & Garner, D. Post-resuscitation plasma catecholamines after prolonged arrest in a swine model. *Resuscitation* 2005; **65**(1): 97–101.

277. Prengel, A.W., Lindner, K.H., Ensinger, H., & Grunert, A. Plasma catecholamine concentrations after successful resuscitation in patients. *Crit. Care Med.* 1992; **20**(5): 609–614.

278. Pepper, G.S., & Lee, R.W. Sympathetic activation in heart failure and its treatment with beta-blockade. *Arch. Intern. Med.* 1999; **159**(3): 225–234.

279. Bristow, M.R. Beta-adrenergic receptor blockade in chronic heart failure. *Circulation* 2000; **101**(5): 558–569.

280. Ditchey, R.V., Rubio-Perez, A., & Slinker, B.K. Beta-adrenergic blockade reduces myocardial injury during experimental cardiopulmonary resuscitation. *J. Am. Coll. Cardiol.* 1994; **24**(3): 804–812.

281. Maddens, M., & Sowers, J. Catecholamines in critical care. *Crit. Care Clin.* 1987; **3**(4): 871–882.

282. Jones, S.B., & Romano, F.D. Dose- and time-dependent changes in plasma catecholamines in response to endotoxin in conscious rats. *Circ. Shock* 1989; **28**(1): 59–68.

283. Boldt, J., Menges, T., Kuhn, D., Diridis, C., & Hempelmann, G. Alterations in circulating vasoactive substances in the critically ill – a comparison between survivors and non-survivors. *Intens. Care Med.* 1995; **21**(3): 218–225.

284. Benedict, C.R., & Rose, J.A. Arterial norepinephrine changes in patients with septic shock. *Circ. Shock* 1992; **38**(3): 165–172.

285. Pene, F., Hyvernat, H., Mallet, V. *et al.* Prognostic value of relative adrenal insufficiency after out-of-hospital cardiac arrest. *Intens. Care Med.* 2005; **31**(5): 627–633.

286. Barquist, E., & Kirton, O. Adrenal insufficiency in the surgical intensive care unit patient. *J. Trauma* 1997; **42**(1): 27–31.

287. Beale, E., Zhu, J., & Belzberg, H. Changes in serum cortisol with age in critically ill patients. *Gerontology* 2002; **48**(2): 84–92.

288. Pinsky, M.R., Vincent, J.L., Deviere, J., Alegre, M., Kahn, R.J., & Dupont, E. Serum cytokine levels in human septic shock. Relation to multiple-system organ failure and mortality. *Chest* 1993; **103**(2): 565–575.

289. Gaillard, R.C., Turnill, D., Sappino, P., & Muller, A.F. Tumor necrosis factor alpha inhibits the hormonal response of the pituitary gland to hypothalamic releasing factors. *Endocrinology* 1990; **127**(1): 101–106.

290. Jaattela, M., Ilvesmaki, V., Voutilainen, R., Stenman, U.H., & Saksela, E. Tumor necrosis factor as a potent inhibitor of adrenocorticotropin-induced cortisol production and steroidogenic P450 enzyme gene expression in cultured human fetal adrenal cells. *Endocrinology* 1991; **128**(1): 623–629.

291. Spangelo, B.L., Judd, A.M., Call, G.B., Zumwalt, J., & Gorospe, W.C. Role of the cytokines in the hypothalamic–pituitary–adrenal and gonadal axes. *Neuroimmunomodulation* 1995; **2**(5): 299–312.

292. Ekins, R. Measurement of free hormones in blood. *Endocr. Rev.* 1990; **11**(1): 5–46.

293. Beishuizen, A., Thijs, L.G., & Vermes, I. Patterns of corticosteroid-binding globulin and the free cortisol index during septic shock and multitrauma. *Intens. Care Med.* 2001; **27**(10): 1584–1591.

294. Hamrahian, A.H., Oseni, T.S., & Arafah, B.M. Measurements of serum free cortisol in critically ill patients. *N. Engl. J. Med.* 2004; **350**(16): 1629–1638.

295. Rosner, W. The functions of corticosteroid-binding globulin and sex hormone-binding globulin: recent advances. *Endocr. Rev.* 1990; **11**(1): 80–91.

296. Pugeat, M., Bonneton, A., Perrot, D. *et al.* Decreased immunoreactivity and binding activity of corticosteroid-binding globulin in serum in septic shock. *Clin. Chem.* 1989; **35**(8): 1675–1679.

297. Absalom, A., Pledger, D., & Kong, A. Adrenocortical function in critically ill patients 24 h after a single dose of etomidate. *Anaesthesia* 1999; **54**(9): 861–867.

298. Jungmann, E., Schifferdecker, E., Rumelin, A., Althoff, P.H., & Schoffling, K. [Plasma renin activity and aldosterone behavior in critically ill patients]. *Klin. Wochenschr.* 1987; **65**(2): 87–91.

299. Findling, J.W., Waters, V.O., & Raff, H. The dissociation of renin and aldosterone during critical illness. *J. Clin. Endocrinol. Metab.* 1987; **64**(3): 592–595.

300. Zipser, R.D., Davenport, M.W., Martin, K.L. *et al.* Hyperreninemic hypoaldosteronism in the critically ill: a new entity. *J. Clin. Endocrinol. Metab.* 1981; **53**(4): 867–873.

301. Antonipillai, I., & Horton, R. Paracrine regulation of the renin-aldosterone system. *J Steroid Biochem. Mol. Biol.* 1993; **45**(1–3): 27–31.

302. Davenport, M.W., & Zipser, R.D. Association of hypotension with hyperreninemic hypoaldosteronism in the critically ill patient. *Arch. Intern. Med.* 1983; **143**(4): 735–737.

303. Annane, D., Sebille, V., Charpentier, C. *et al*. Effect of treatment with low doses of hydrocortisone and fludrocortisone on mortality in patients with septic shock. *J. Am. Med. Assoc.* 2002; **288**(7): 862–871.

304. Woolf, P.D., Hamill, R.W., McDonald, J.V., Lee, L.A., & Kelly, M. Transient hypogonadotropic hypogonadism caused by critical illness. *J. Clin. Endocrinol. Metab.* 1985; **60**(3): 444–450.

305. Spratt, D.I. Altered gonadal steroidogenesis in critical illness: is treatment with anabolic steroids indicated? *Best Pract. Res. Clin. Endocrinol. Metab.* 2001; **15**(4): 479–494.

306. Tweedle, D., Walton, C., & Johnston, I.D. The effect of an anabolic steroid on postoperative nitrogen balance. *Br. J. Clin. Pract.* 1973; **27**(4): 130–132.

307. Haynes, W.G., Hamer, D.W., Robertson, C.E., & Webb, D.J. Plasma endothelin following cardiac arrest: differences between survivors and non-survivors. *Resuscitation* 1994; **27**(2): 117–122.

308. Huribal, M., Cunningham, M.E., D'Aiuto, M.L., Pleban, W.E., & McMillen, M.A. Endothelin levels in patients with burns covering more than 20% body surface area. *J. Burn Care Rehabil.* 1995; **16**(1): 23–26.

309. Haak, T., Jungmann, E., Kasper-Dahm, G., Ehrlich, S., & Usadel, K.H. Elevated endothelin 1 levels in critical illness. *Clin. Investig.* 1994; **72**(3): 214.

310. Magder, S., & Cernacek, P. Role of endothelins in septic, cardiogenic, and hemorrhagic shock. *Can. J. Physiol. Pharmacol.* 2003; **81**(6): 635–643.

311. Battistini, B., Forget, M.A., & Laight, D. Potential roles for endothelins in systemic inflammatory response syndrome with a particular relationship to cytokines. *Shock* 1996; **5**(3): 167–183.

312. Weitzberg, E., Lundberg, J.M., & Rudehill, A. Elevated plasma levels of endothelin in patients with sepsis syndrome. *Circ. Shock* 1991; **33**(4): 222–227.

313. Pittet, J.F., Morel, D.R., Hemsen, A. *et al*. Elevated plasma endothelin-1 concentrations are associated with the severity of illness in patients with sepsis. *Ann. Surg.* 1991; **213**(3): 261–264.

314. Brauner, J.S., Rohde, L.E., & Clausell, N. Circulating endothelin-1 and tumor necrosis factor-alpha: early predictors of mortality in patients with septic shock. *Intensive Care Med.* 2000; **26**(3): 305–313.

315. Buunk, G., van der Hoeven, J.G., Frolich, M., & Meinders, A.E. Cerebral vasoconstriction in comatose patients resuscitated from a cardiac arrest? *Intens. Care Med.* 1996; **22**(11): 1191–1196.

316. Krep, H., Brinker, G., Schwindt, W., & Hossmann, K.A. Endothelin type A-antagonist improves long-term neurological recovery after cardiac arrest in rats. *Crit. Care Med.* 2000; **28**(8): 2873–2880.

317. Krep, H., Brinker, G., Pillekamp, F., & Hossmann, K.A. Treatment with an endothelin type A receptor-antagonist after cardiac arrest and resuscitation improves cerebral hemodynamic and functional recovery in rats. *Crit. Care Med.* 2000; **28**(8): 2866–2872.

318. Nagao, K., Hayashi, N., Kanmatsuse, K. *et al*. B-type natriuretic peptide as a marker of resuscitation in patients with cardiac arrest outside the hospital. *Circ. J.* 2004; **68**(5): 477–482.

319. Charpentier, J., Luyt, C.E., Fulla, Y. *et al*. Brain natriuretic peptide: A marker of myocardial dysfunction and prognosis during severe sepsis. *Crit. Care Med.* 2004; **32**(3): 660–665.

320. Berendes, E., Schmidt, C., Van Aken, H. *et al*. A-type and B-type natriuretic peptides in cardiac surgical procedures. *Anesth. Analg.* 2004; **98**(1): 11–19, table of contents.

321. Cuthbertson, B.H., Patel, R.R., Croal, B.L., Barclay, J., & Hillis, G.S. B-type natriuretic peptide and the prediction of outcome in patients admitted to intensive care. *Anaesthesia* 2005; **60**(1): 16–21.

322. Tamion, F., Le Cam-Duchez, V., Menard, J.F., Girault, C., Coquerel, A., & Bonmarchand, G. Erythropoietin and renin as biological markers in critically ill patients. *Crit. Care* 2004; **8**(5): R328–R335.

323. Oppert, M., Gleiter, C.H., Muller, C. *et al*. Kinetics and characteristics of an acute phase response following cardiac arrest. *Intens. Care Med.* 1999; **25**(12): 1386–1394.

324. Abel, J., Spannbrucker, N., Fandrey, J., & Jelkmann, W. Serum erythropoietin levels in patients with sepsis and septic shock. *Eur. J. Haematol.* 1996; **57**(5): 359–363.

325. Krafte-Jacobs, B., Levetown, M.L., Bray, G.L., Ruttimann, U.E., & Pollack, M.M. Erythropoietin response to critical illness. *Crit. Care Med.* 1994; **22**(5): 821–826.

326. Elliot, J.M., Virankabutra, T., Jones, S. *et al*. Erythropoietin mimics the acute phase response in critical illness. *Crit. Care* 2003; **7**(3): R35–R40.

327. Rogiers, P., Zhang, H., Leeman, M. *et al*. Erythropoietin response is blunted in critically ill patients. *Intens. Care Med.* 1997; **23**(2): 159–162.

328. Robinson, L.E., & van Soeren, M.H. Insulin resistance and hyperglycemia in critical illness: role of insulin in glycemic control. *AACN Clin. Issues* 2004; **15**(1): 45–62.

329. Thorell, A., Nygren, J., & Ljungqvist, O. Insulin resistance: a marker of surgical stress. *Curr. Opin. Clin. Nutr. Metab. Care* 1999; **2**(1): 69–78.

330. McCowen, K.C., Malhotra, A., & Bistrian, B.R. Stress-induced hyperglycemia. *Crit. Care Clin.* 2001; **17**(1): 107–124.

331. Van den Berghe, G. How does blood glucose control with insulin save lives in intensive care? *J. Clin. Invest.* 2004; **114**(9): 1187–1195.

332. Grimble, R.F. Inflammatory status and insulin resistance. *Curr. Opin. Clin. Nutr. Metab. Care* 2002; **5**(5): 551–559.

333. Marette, A. Mediators of cytokine-induced insulin resistance in obesity and other inflammatory settings. *Curr. Opin. Clin. Nutr. Metab. Care* 2002; **5**(4): 377–383.

334. Mizock, B.A. Alterations in carbohydrate metabolism during stress: a review of the literature. *Am. J. Med.* 1995; **98**(1): 75–84.

335. van den Berghe, G., Wouters, P., Weekers, F. *et al*. Intensive insulin therapy in the critically ill patients. *N. Engl. J. Med.* 2001; **345**(19): 1359–1367.

336. Krinsley, J.S. Effect of an intensive glucose management protocol on the mortality of critically ill adult patients. *Mayo Clin. Proc.* 2004; **79**(8): 992–1000.

337. Fuortes, M., Blank, M.A., Scalea, T.M., Pollock, T.W., & Jaffe, B.M. Release of vasoactive intestinal peptide during hyperdynamic sepsis in dogs. *Surgery* 1988; **104**(5): 894–898.

338. Riepl, R., Jenssen, T.G., Revhaug, A., Burhol, P.G., Gierchksky, K.E., & Lehnert, P. [Increase of plasma cholecystokinin by *Escherichia coli* endotoxin-induced shock in swine]. *Z. Gastroenterol.* 1986; **24**(11): 691–699.

339. Broner, C.W., O'Dorisio, M.S., Rosenberg, R.B., & O'Dorisio, T.M. Cyclic nucleotides and vasoactive intestinal peptide production in a rabbit model of Escherichia coli septicemia. *Am. J. Med. Sci* 1995; **309**(5): 267–277.

340. Zamir, O., Hasselgren, P.O., Higashiguchi, T., Frederick, J.A., & Fischer, J.E. Effect of sepsis or cytokine administration on release of gut peptides. *Am. J. Surg.* 1992; **163**(1): 181–184; discussion 184–185.

341. Brandtzaeg, P., Oktedalen, O., Kierulf, P., & Opstad, P.K. Elevated VIP and endotoxin plasma levels in human gram-negative septic shock. *Regul. Pept.* 1989; **24**(1): 37–44.

8

Inflammatory and immunologic responses to ischemia and reperfusion

Jason S. Haukoos[1], Ronald J. Korthuis[2], and James T. Niemann[3]

[1] Department of Emergency Medicine, Denver Health Medical Center, Department of Preventive Medicine and Biometrics, University of Colorado Health Sciences Center, Denver, CO, USA
[2] Department of Medical Pharmacology & Physiology and, The Dalton Cardiovascular Research Center, University of Missouri, Columbia, MO, USA
[3] Department of Emergency Medicine, Harbor-UCLA Medical Center, Torrance, CA, USA, David Geffen School of Medicine at UCLA, Los Angeles, CA, USA

Introduction

Despite advances in the treatment of cardiac arrest, the development of organ dysfunction following return of spontaneous circulation causes considerable morbidity and mortality. The complex pathophysiologic mechanisms underlying this postresuscitation syndrome likely result from global ischemia, reperfusion, and the triggering of a profound systemic inflammatory response syndrome.[1,2] To understand such mechanisms and to improve therapy for victims of cardiac arrest, it is essential to identify the principal mediators that contribute to this disease process, and to identify their roles in the development of organ dysfunction.[3] By understanding the roles of key inflammatory and immunologic mediators during the resuscitation and postresuscitation periods, it may be possible to improve understanding of the whole-body response to ischemia and reperfusion, and to develop effective therapeutic strategies for patients who suffer cardiac arrest and for those who achieve return of spontaneous circulation.

Systemic inflammatory response

The pathophysiology of cardiac arrest is complex and, like sepsis, induces a profound systemic inflammatory response syndrome.[4–12] Unlike sepsis, however, the systemic inflammatory response syndrome following cardiac arrest results from whole-body ischemia (i.e., low or no-flow) and reperfusion (i.e., restoration of flow following ischemia).[1,13] The development of a systemic inflammatory

response syndrome has been divided into three stages.[14] The first stage occurs in response to an insult, resulting in a local cytokine response primarily intended to evoke an inflammatory response to promote local cellular repair by recruiting cells from the reticuloendothelial and immune systems. The second stage involves release of small quantities of cytokines into the systemic circulation in order to enhance, or magnify, this local response. This acute-phase response is usually tightly controlled by endogenous proinflammatory antagonists, and cytokines and immunologic mediators are kept in check by specific downregulation and antagonism. This local process generally continues until the inciting focus is resolved. Occasionally, however, the third stage develops. This massive systemic reaction results in destruction rather than protection because of an imbalance of pro- and anti-inflammatory cytokines, the formation of oxygen-free radicals, and activation of leukocytes, and if left unchecked, commonly progresses to multiple organ failure and death (Fig. 8.1).

Cytokines and reperfusion injury

Proinflammatory and anti-inflammatory cytokine cascade

The systemic inflammatory response syndrome is characterized by a complex interplay of molecules and cells, resulting in increased concentrations of systemic inflammatory cytokines, activation of the clotting cascade, release of potent vasoactive substances and adhesion molecules, and activation of the immune system.[15,16] Cytokines are

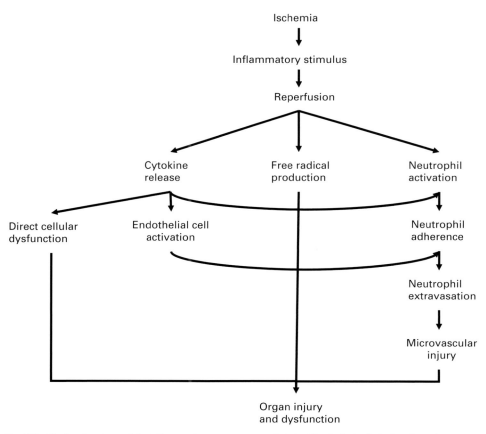

Fig. 8.1. Mechanism to explain inflammatory process associated with whole-body ischemia and reperfusion and the development of organ dysfunction following cardiac arrest.

soluble, cell-secreted, non-immunoglobulin proteins that, in minute quantities, modulate host cell function and include such diverse molecules as growth factors, interleukins, interferons, and colony-stimulating factors.[17] Altogether, there are at least 30 different cytokines that are generally divided into either pro-inflammatory or anti-inflammatory categories (Table 8.1). Of these, tumor necrosis factor (TNF)-α, interleukin (IL)-1, IL-6, IL-8, and IL-10 appear to play the most significant pathophysiologic roles during reperfusion following ischemia.[1,2,18] While the majority of basic science and clinical research has focused on the roles of cytokines in patients with sepsis, a growing body of literature has focused on their roles during ischemia and reperfusion.[19–23]

Two of the most widely studied proinflammatory cytokines include TNF-α and IL-1β. These two cytokines initiate elaboration and release of other downstream cytokines (e.g., IL-6, IL-8, IL-10, the Fas/Fas ligand system, and the CD40/CD40 ligand system), and stimulate an acute-phase response from the liver. This cascade results in widespread systemic inflammation resulting in direct physiologic alterations and tissue injury.

Tumor necrosis factor-α

Tumor necrosis factor-α was first described in 1975 for its oncolytic effects on solid tumors.[23] Since then, it has been found to have an abundance of physiologic effects, including but not limited to, triggering the development of fever, shock, myocardial depression, acute respiratory distress syndrome, edema, acute renal tubular necrosis, suppression of erythropoiesis, and disseminated intravascular coagulation.[24] Although several cell types can produce TNF-α, including the cardiac myocyte, it is primarily synthesized by macrophages as a 26-kD membrane protein from which a 17-kD extracellular peptide is cleaved by the enzyme TNF convertase. Three 17-kD peptides become non-covalently associated to form a homotrimeric complex that is biologically active.[25,26] TNF-α is released into the circulation after an insult within minutes and

Table 8.1. Sources and systemic effects of cytokines released during ischemia and reperfusion

Proinflammatory cytokines	Major sources	Systemic effects
TNF-α	Monocytes, macrophages, lymphocytes, neutrophils, endothelium, fibroblasts, and keratinocytes	Myocardial depression, hypotension, leukocyte and endothelial activation, promotion of hypercoagulability, and stimulation of IL-1, IL-6, and IL-8
IL-1β	Monocytes, macrophages, lymphocytes, neutrophils, endothelium, fibroblasts, and keratinocytes	Myocardial depression, hypotension, leukocyte and endothelial activation, promotion of hypercoagulability, and stimulation of TNF-α, IL-6, and IL-8
IL-8	Monocytes, macrophages, lymphocytes, endothelium, fibroblasts, and keratinocytes	Recruitment and activation of neutrophils
Anti-inflammatory cytokines		
IL-6	Monocytes, macrophages, T cells, endothelium, fibroblasts, and keratinocytes	Induction of hepatic acute-phase response, decreases IL-1β and TNF-α

reaches peak concentrations between 90 and 120 minutes, and the serum half-life is approximately 20 to 40 minutes.[27,28] TNF-α is removed from the serum by binding to TNF-receptors and soluble TNF-binding proteins (also known as soluble receptors) and by clearance of the protein complexes by the kidney and liver.[29]

TNF-α interacts with at least two distinct membrane-associated receptors called TNF-R1 and TNF-R2, both of which exhibit similar TNF-α binding affinities. Both receptors are ubiquitous, existing on essentially all cell type surfaces except red blood cells. The two receptors utilize distinct intracellular signaling pathways, however. Both receptors also exist in soluble forms produced by proteolytic cleavage of their extracellular domains. Whereas the mechanism underlying the specific cleavage is not well understood, it is thought that these soluble receptors function to antagonize the effects of TNF-α when concentrations are high. When TNF-α concentrations are lower, soluble receptors stabilize TNF-α in order to slow the spontaneous decay of its bioactivity.[29]

The role of TNF-α in ischemia and reperfusion injury is relatively well documented. Initial studies evaluated its role during re-implantation as well as in models of rat hepatic ischemia and reperfusion.[30] Plasma TNF-α concentrations significantly increased between 30 minutes and 3 hours after reperfusion in these models.

Interleukin-1

IL-1 was first described in the 1940s as a heat-labile protein that when injected into animals induced fever, and was further described as a 10- to 20-kD peptide in the 1970s.[31,32]

It exists in two forms, IL-1α and Il-1β, both of which possess a wide spectrum of inflammatory, metabolic, physiologic, hematopoietic, and immunologic properties. IL-1β, in the setting of endotoxemia, is rapidly transcribed and released extracellularly, with peak concentrations occurring in approximately 3 to 4 hours. Although both forms of IL-1 arise from distinct gene products, both recognize the same cell surface receptors and have overlapping biological effects. Several nucleated cell lineages have been shown to synthesize and release IL-1, including monocytes, macrophages, neutrophils, and endothelial cells.[33]

The physiologic effects of IL-1 are extensive and in many respects parallel those of TNF-α. These effects are not limited to, but include the development of fever, anorexia, and neutrophilia, and the systemic effects of high dose IL-1 after injection into animals include hypotension, depressed myocardial function, and decreased systemic vascular resistance.[24] Additionally, it has been shown that TNF-α potentiates the effects of IL-1, and their synergistic activities seem to be caused by second messenger molecules rather than upregulation of receptors.[33] In experimental settings in which a systemic inflammatory response syndrome was induced in volunteers, serum TNF-α concentrations reached peak levels between 60 and 90 minutes, whereas serum IL-1 concentrations reached peak levels in 3 to 4 hours.[34,35]

Other inflammatory cytokines

More downstream inflammatory cytokines include IL-6, IL-8, and IL-10. IL-6 is considered a weak inflammatory peptide that acts as an endogenous pyrogen and an inducer of acute-phase responses.[36] IL-8 functions to recruit and activate neutrophils in the development of inflammation and tissue damage. IL-10 is considered an anti-inflammatory cytokine and inhibits the production of TNF-α, IL-1β, IL-6, and IL-8, as well as expression of matrix metalloproteinases, and attenuates neutrophil infiltration at the site of injury.[20]

CD40 is a membrane glycoprotein belonging to the TNF receptor superfamily and is expressed on a relatively diverse line of cells, including lymphocytes, monocytes, macrophages, platelets, and endothelial cells.[37] CD40 ligand (CD40L), also known as CD154, is a cell surface glycoprotein that also belongs to the TNF family of cytokines, which also includes TNF-α and Fas ligand. CD40-CD40L interactions have been most extensively studied in the context of T- and B-lymphocyte interactions, but also more recently have been studied in settings of atherosclerosis and chronic inflammation, and ischemia and reperfusion.[38–40] Although it is unclear to what extent CD40-CD40L signaling plays a role in whole-body ischemia and reperfusion following cardiac arrest, it is known to play a key role in inflammation through the induction of cellular adhesion molecules, tissue factor in endothelial cells, enhancement of the production of proinflammatory cytokines, and activation of platelets.[41,42]

Soluble Fas-ligand (FasL) is cleaved by metalloproteinases from its membrane-bound form on T-lymphocytes and neutrophils, and serum FasL concentrations have been shown to increase dramatically following cardiac arrest.[43] Fas is a widely occurring apoptotic signal receptor molecule expressed by almost any type of cell, and the level of its soluble form has been shown to correlate with the degree of multiple organ dysfunction and survival in critically ill patients.[44]

Nitric oxide (NO) is a relatively stable free radical that has been proposed to contribute to reperfusion injury. NO is produced from L-arginine by the enzyme nitric oxide synthase (NOS), which is found predominantly in endothelial cells where NO has beneficial effects, including the promotion of vasodilation and preservation of endothelial activities. NO reacts with superoxide to produce peroxynitrite, a toxic, highly reactive compound capable of producing irreversible cellular injury. Inhibition of NOS in cardiac arrest models appears to decrease generation of free radicals generation by inhibiting the production of peroxynitrite and reduces the requirements for epinephrine and closed-chest compressions, but has not demonstrated survival benefit.[45–47]

Matrix metalloproteinases (MMPs) are a family of zinc-dependent endopeptidases involved in remodeling of the extracellular matrix during various physiologic and pathologic conditions, including wound healing and inflammation.[48] MMPs are synthesized in a latent, or pro-MMP, form and are activated by proteolytic cleavage or conformational change, and the expression of MMPs is transcriptionally regulated by growth factors, hormones, and cytokines.[48] Recent studies emphasize not only soluble factors but also cell-matrix and cell-cell interactions as key in gene expression of MMPs.[49,50] Inhibition of MMPs has been shown to improve postischemic left ventricular function in models of cardiac stunning after ischemia and reperfusion.[51]

Role of cytokines in the development of postischemic organ injury

Whole-body ischemia and reperfusion injury lead to the synthesis and widespread release of proinflammatory cytokines by macrophages, neutrophils, and endothelial cells. Cytokines play critically important roles by: (1) inducing the expression of cell surface adhesion receptors on a variety of cell types, thus serving to localize phagocytic cells to areas of inflammation; and (2) directly affecting parenchymal cell function (Fig. 8.1).

TNF-α, granulocyte/macrophage colony stimulating factor (GM-CSF), and IL-8 mobilize adhesion receptors on neutrophils, which facilitates adherence of these cells to sites of inflammatory injury.[52,53] Additionally, TNF-α and IL-1 induce the expression of adhesive glycoproteins on endothelial cell surfaces, which serve as receptors for activated neutrophils.[54] Cytokines also induce the expression of adhesion receptors on parenchymal cells. TNF-α, IL-1, and IL-6 induce expression of intercellular adhesion molecule (ICAM)-1 on cardiac myocytes, facilitating neutrophil adherence and activation.[55–57] Thus cytokines are able to induce the expression of adhesion receptors on a variety of cell types, which serves to localize neutrophils and other immunologic cells to areas of inflammation and injury.

Cytokines also directly affect several functions of parenchymal cells. The direct effect of TNF-α on endothelial cells results in suppression of NO production.[58] NO has been identified as an endothelial-derived relaxing factor that also demonstrates potent inhibitory actions on platelet and neutrophil function. Therefore, the cytokine-induced loss of endothelial-derived NO activity may contribute to both platelet and neutrophil adhesion during reperfusion.

It is also well known that patients who develop the systemic inflammatory response syndrome manifest cardiac dysfunction.[59] The hemodynamic effects of both TNF-α and IL-1 are characterized by decreased myocardial contractility and ejection fraction, hypotension, decreased systemic vascular resistance, and biventricular dilatation.[60–63] Two specific time-dependent phases have been described

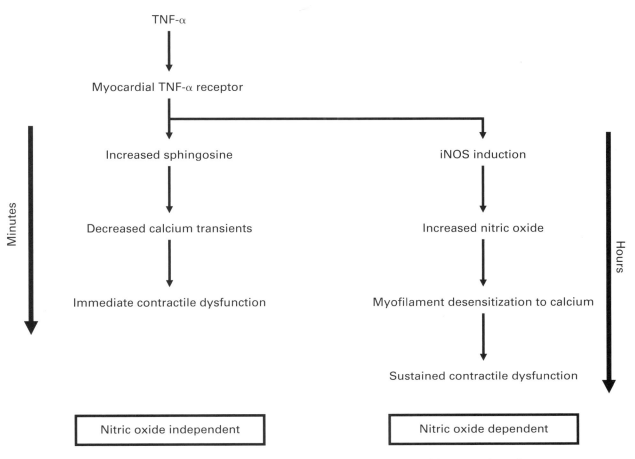

TNF-α

↓

Myocardial TNF-α receptor

Minutes →

Increased sphingosine

↓

Decreased calcium transients

↓

Immediate contractile dysfunction

iNOS induction

↓

Increased nitric oxide

↓

Myofilament desensitization to calcium

↓

Sustained contractile dysfunction

Hours →

Nitric oxide independent

Nitric oxide dependent

Fig. 8.2. Mechanism of tumor necrosis factor-alpha on myocardial contractility (iNOS = inducible nitric oxide synthase).

to characterize TNF-α-related myocardial dysfunction.[64,65] The immediate phase occurs minutes after TNF-α exposure, is nitric oxide (NO)-independent, and is mediated by sphingosine disruption of calcium-induced calcium release by the sarcoplasmic reticulum.[66,67] The late phase occurs over a period of hours after exposure to TNF-α, is temporally associated with inducible NO synthase induction, and is due to NO-induced myofilament desensitization to calcium (Fig. 8.2).[68–71] Additional research supports down-regulation of adrenergic receptors, an independent reduction in their responsiveness and their signal transduction pathways, the formation of free radicals, and apoptosis as contributors to the development of myocardial dysfunction when exposed to TNF-α and IL-1.[72–77] A recent investigation demonstrated an association between elevated serum TNF-α concentrations and myocardial dysfunction in a porcine cardiac arrest model.[78]

Other cytokines appear to exert protective effects on damaged cells. IL-8 prevents neutrophil migration and neutrophil-mediated damage to ischemic myocardium.[79] Also, IL-8 has been shown to inhibit neutrophil adhesion to endothelium and to preserve the ability of endothelium to relax after coronary artery occlusion and reperfusion.[80] Alternatively, transforming growth factor (TGF)-β prevents reperfusion-induced endothelial dysfunction after myocardial ischemia and reperfusion.[81] The protective effects of TGF-β may be related to its ability to decrease neutrophil-endothelial adhesion, suppress the release of TNF-α, or depress the formation of oxidants.[82,83]

In summary, cytokines produced by tissue macrophages, circulating or adherent neutrophils, or endothelial cells in response to ischemia may stimulate the production or mobilization of adhesion molecules on neutrophils, endothelial cells, and parenchymal cells that regulate the entrapment or sequestration of immunologic cells. Proinflammatory cytokines appear also to alter important endothelial functions directly and mediate negative inotropic effects at the level of the myocyte.

The immune system and reperfusion injury

The recruitment of leukocytes to sites of inflammation is critical in the response to tissue injury following ischemia and reperfusion, and the elucidation of molecules mediating the extravasation of leukocytes from the vascular space into the extravascular space is central to the understanding of the complex regulation of the host's response to inflammation. The recruitment of leukocytes from blood to the site of inflammation proceeds through an orderly process that includes: tethering or capture, rolling, activation and firm adhesion, and migration across the endothelium (also known as diapedesis).[84] Each of these steps is mediated by distinct adhesion molecule families that are expressed on the surface of both endothelial cells and adherent leukocytes.

Polymorphonuclear leukocytes and postischemic cellular dysfunction

It is widely accepted that neutrophils contribute to tissue damage following ischemia and reperfusion and several approaches have been used to examine the role of leukocytes in postischemic tissue injury. When blood supply is reduced (ischemia) and then subsequently reestablished (reperfusion), the ability of arterioles to regulate the distribution of blood flow is impaired, many capillaries fail to reperfuse (also known as capillary no-reflow), microvascular permeability is increased, and white blood cells become adherent to and emigrate across the walls of postcapillary venules. Once in the tissues, these inflammatory phagocytes attack parenchymal cells, thereby exacerbating injury induced by ischemia.

One approach to examining the role of leukocytes in postischemic tissue is to monitor the tissue entrapment of radiolabeled leukocytes or to measure granulocyte-specific enzymes, such as myeloperoxidase. Data derived from these techniques indicate that reperfusion of ischemic tissues is associated with massive leukocyte infiltration.[85,86]

Regulation of molecular determinants of leukocyte adherence

The observation that ischemia and reperfusion-induced tissue damage is attenuated by blocking neutrophil–endothelial adhesive interactions not only lends support to the concept that neutrophils directly mediate postischemic tissue dysfunction, but also emphasizes that the initial neutrophil–microvascular endothelial adhesion is the critical and rate-limiting step in later neutrophil–endothelial cell interactions. Adhesion molecules located

on both endothelial cells and circulating leukocytes are in large part responsible for guiding the process of leukocyte extravasation.[87] The egress of neutrophils from the vascular lumen to the extravascular compartment, where tissue damage occurs, requires several steps in which the neutrophil first intimately contacts endothelial cells and then becomes firmly adherent. The fact that this adhesive mechanism can be rapidly activated, that it may be rapidly reversed or sustained (depending on the inciting stimulus), and that it may be either site-specific or generalized implies that these adhesion molecules are under tight physiologic control. Research has shown that multiple, differentially expressed adhesion molecules on both the neutrophil and endothelial cell control the complex process of neutrophil adherence.[88]

The molecular events associated with establishing the adhesive interaction between neutrophils and microvascular endothelium appear to involve at least three families of adhesion molecules: (1) the leukocyte β_2-integrins (CD11$_a$/CD18, CD11$_b$/CD18, and CD11$_c$/CD18); (2) the immunoglobulin gene superfamily (intercellular adhesion molecule 1 [ICAM-1], vascular cell adhesion molecule 1 [VCAM-1], and platelet/endothelial cell adhesion molecule 1 [PECAM-1]); and (3) the glycoprotein adhesion molecule family of selectins (leukocyte (L)-selectin, endothelial (E)-selectin, and platelet (P)-selectin).[89–92] L-selectin is expressed on most leukocytes, including neutrophils and monocytes, whereas P- and E- selectins are expressed mainly on the surface of cytokine-activated endothelial cells.[91]

Endothelial activation

It was once thought that vascular endothelium functioned to prevent cellular adhesion and to compartmentalize the intravascular space. Substantial evidence exists to support an adhesive function, however, that is pivotal in modulating the localization of neutrophils to sites of inflammation. Adhesion molecules expressed on the surface of the microvascular endothelium modulate the neutrophil-endothelial interaction associated with inflammation after ischemia and reperfusion. Three of the best characterized endothelial cell adhesion molecules are P-selectin, E-selectin, and ICAM-1.[86,92–95]

P-selectin is normally found in secretory granules within platelets and can also be expressed by endothelial cells. After stimulation with complement, thrombin, or histamine, P-selectin is mobilized to the endothelial cell surface within minutes, remains there transiently, is associated with reversible PMN adhesion, and is rapidly removed by endocytosis.[96,97] In contrast, activation of endothelial cells by certain oxidants (e.g., hydrogen per-oxide) produced during reperfusion results in a sustained rather than transient expression of P-selectin.[98,99] Thus, the failure to reinternalize P-selectin may be caused by an impaired regulatory mechanism when microvascular endothelium is overwhelmed by oxidants produced by reperfusion. It is noteworthy, however, that protein synthesis-dependent P-selectin expression can occur within hours of exposure to appropriate stimuli, thereby providing another route for prolonged expression of this adhesive ligand.

E-selectin is not constitutively present on endothelium, but its expression, which requires new protein synthesis and reaches a maximum within 4 hours of stimulation, is induced by cytokines and by lipopolysaccharides.[91,100,101] The absence of E-selectin on unstimulated endothelium and the time course for its induced expression on activated endothelium suggests that it may target circulating PMNs to ischemic sites at later stages of reperfusion.[93]

ICAM-1 and VCAM-1 are also constitutively present on endothelium, but their expression can be upregulated in a protein synthesis-dependent manner, with maximal expression occurring within 4 to 8 hours after endothelial exposure to cytokines.[86,102,103] ICAM-1 persists on the cell surface for up to 24 hours and plays an important role in firm PMN-endothelial cell adherence.[104]

Leukocyte adhesion

The strength of adhesive interactions between adhesion molecules expressed on the surface of leukocytes and endothelial cells is important in determining whether a neutrophil adheres to the microvascular endothelium. The best characterized of the leukocyte adhesion molecules are L-selectin and the $CD11_{a,b,c}/CD18$ glycoprotein adherence complex.

L-selectin is expressed on the surface of unstimulated neutrophils where it appears to mediate the initial weak adhesion or rolling of neutrophils along cytokine-activated endothelium.[88,105] This form of neutrophil–endothelium interaction is fundamentally different from neutrophil margination as it occurs during inflammatory processes.

An interesting feature of L-selectin expression is the ability of soluble chemotactic substances (e.g., platelet activating factor [PAF] and endothelial IL-8) produced by activated endothelium to cause the rapid shedding (within minutes) or downregulation of the neutrophil L-selectin molecule.[94,106] Although the physiologic relevance of this downregulation is unclear, it may facilitate the transition of subsequent neutrophil-mediated tissue injury, and it is thought that it may help limit the sequestration of neutrophils at distant sites where injury has not occurred. Alternatively, this downregulation may facilitate the transition of neutrophils from adhesion to tissue extravasation.[107] This downregulation of L-selectin, however, occurs simultaneously with the upregulation of the next phase of neutrophil adhesion, namely, the $CD11_{a,b,c}/CD18$ glycoprotein complex.[94,106] The $CD11_{a,b,c}/CD18$ glycoprotein complex, located on the surface of neutrophils, has been shown to respond to chemotactic peptides (e.g., complement factor $C5_a$) and lipid mediators (e.g., leukotriene B_4 and PAF).[86,95,100] These glycoproteins regulate neutrophil extravasation, oxidant production, and degranulation, all of which have been implicated in neutrophil-mediated tissue dysfunction associated with ischemia and reperfusion.[108–110]

Selectins bind to a variety of glycans or mucins that possess the Sialyl Lewis[x] moiety, a carbohydrate known to play a vital role in cell–cell recognition.[111,112] For example, L-selectin binds to a group of mucins on the activated endothelial cells, including glycosylation-dependent cell adhesion molecule 1. The ligand for P-selectin, P-selectin glycoprotein ligand 1 (PSGL-1), which also contains Sialyl Lewis[x], is found on leukocytes and endothelial cells. PSGL-1, which is expressed constitutively on neutrophils and monocytes, serves as the dominant ligand for P- and E-selectin on endothelial cells.[113] Engagement of PSGL-1 enhances tether strength and stabilizes neutrophil and monocyte cell rolling on endothelial cells. In addition, engagement of PSGL-1 also may regulate gene expression in monocytes. Inhibition of PSGL-1/selectin interactions may be an effective tool to attenuate inflammation.

Coordination of leukocyte adhesion and extravasation

Neutrophils are localized to sites of inflammation by a highly coordinated and dynamic sequence of events in which each of the known adhesion molecules plays a distinct role.[93] The initial adhesive interaction between neutrophils and the endothelium involves upregulation of adhesion molecules (P-selectin, E-selectin, ICAM-1, and VCAM-1) on the surface of endothelial cells adjacent to sites of inflammation. L-selectin, located on the surface of neutrophils, appears to mediate the initial rolling and reversible adherence between non-activated neutrophils and activated endothelium. Weakly bound neutrophils are then activated by triggering substances (e.g., PAF and IL-8) produced by the activated endothelium itself, or by other circulating molecules, including cytokines and complement.[114,115] The $CD11_{a,b,c}/CD18$ glycoprotein complex interacts with ICAM-1, strengthening the neutrophil-endothelium interaction and promoting extravasation.

Table 8.2. Leukocyte adhesion stages and molecular determinants

Stage of migration	Phagocyte molecule	Endothelial cell molecule	Other
Capture or tethering	L-selectin PSGL-1	GlyCAM-1 E- and P-selectin	P-selectin is released by platelets and E-selectin is induced on endothelial cells by TNF-α and IFN-γ
Rolling	L-selectin PSGL-1	GlyCAM-1 E- and P-selectin	
Activation	Increased avidity of integrins		L-selectin shedding induced by chemokines (e.g., IL-8 and MCP-1)
Firm adhesion	CD11$_a$/CD18 CD11$_b$/CD18	ICAM-1 and ICAM-2	
Diapedesis	VE-cadherin PECAM-1	VE-cadherin PECAM-1	

Critical to diapedesis is the binding of vascular endothial (VE)-cadherin or platelet/endothelial cell adhesion molecule (PECAM)-1, both of which are present at the adherence junctions between the endothelial cells and on the leukocytes (Table 8.2). After neutrophil extravasation, oxidant production and degranulation occurs, resulting in tissue damage.

Mechanisms of neutrophil-mediated tissue injury

Activated neutrophils secrete an impressive number of antibacterial and antiseptic agents that are also cytotoxic to normal cells and that dissolve connective tissue.[116] These toxins can be conveniently divided into two groups based on their location with the cell: (1) plasma membrane-bound nicotinamide adenine dinucleotide phosphate (NADPH) oxidase; and (2) intracellular granules.

The NADPH oxidase system enables neutrophils to produce reactive oxygen species. The NADPH oxidase system utilizes NADPH to generate superoxide anion and hydrogen peroxide, both of which damage host tissue but are short-lived and rapidly consumed in other reactions.[117,118] The combination of NADPH oxidase-derived hydrogen peroxide and myeloperoxidase, a constituent of the neutrophil's intracellular granule system, however, produces hypochlorous acid, an oxidizing agent of immense destructive potential.

Activated neutrophils secrete myeloperoxidase, which catalyzes the conversion of hydrogen peroxide and chloride ions to hypochlorous acid. Hypochlorous acid destroys a wide variety of biological molecules, cellular contents, and plasma constituents, and also participates in the production of other chlorinated oxidants, which further impair the host's defense mechanisms against granular proteinases.[116]

Neutrophil proteinases (e.g., elastase, collagenase, and gelatinase) are target-specific enzymes that destroy extracellular matrix proteins, leading, in part, to increased vascular permeability. The simultaneous secretion of both oxidants and granular enzymes produces a synergistic reaction in which the destructive potential of neutrophils can be fully expressed. The cumulative effect of the cascade of cytotoxic reactions associated with neutrophil activation results in damage to structural, contractile, and transport proteins, enzymes, and membrane receptors and causes peroxidation of lipid membranes. As a consequence, normal cellular functions are impaired, membrane fluidity and integrity are lost, and extracellular matrix structure and repair processes are destroyed.

Neutrophils also may contribute to reperfusion abnormalities and tissue damage by occluding capillaries.[119,120] Neutrophils are large, stiff cells that when activated after exposure to hypoxic and acidotic conditions become larger and stiffer, making it more difficult for these cells to traverse capillary beds. Ischemia and reperfusion also reduces capillary diameters by inducing endothelial cell edema and interstitial edema. Such mechanisms create microcirculatory perfusion abnormalities (also known as no-reflow) that may persist despite restoration of normal blood flow. Both neutropenia and blockade of neutrophil adhesion molecules prevent the development of the no-reflow phenomenon.[121] Antibodies against endothelial cell determinants of neutrophil adhesion also effectively attenuate postischemic capillary no-reflow.[122]

Mechanisms of macrophage-mediated tissue injury

Neutrophils, monocytes, and macrophages combine to make up the mononuclear phagocytic system. This system includes promonocytes and their precursors in the bone

Table 8.3. Selected products generated by macrophages

Product	Function
Enzymes	
Plasminogen activators	Inflammatory; tissue repair
Collagenases	Inflammatory
Elastase	Inflammatory
Complement components	Antimicrobial; inflammatory
Coagulation factors	Tissue repair
Arginase	Immunoregulatory
Neutral proteinases	Inflammatory; tissue repair
Acid hydrolases	Inflammatory
Lysozymes	Antimicrobial
Enzyme inhibitors	
α_2 – macroglobulin	Regulation of plasma enzyme activities
Plasminogen activator inhibitor	Regulation of plasma enzyme activities
Cytokines	
IL-1	Inflammatory; tissue repair
TNF-α	Inflammatory; tissue repair
INF-α and β	Antiviral
Reactive oxygen metabolites	
Superoxide (O_2^-)	Microbicidal; inflammatory
Hydrogen peroxide (H_2O_2)	Microbicidal; inflammatory
Hydroxyl radical (OH^-)	Microbicidal; inflammatory
Arachidonic acid metabolites	
Prostaglandin E_1 and E_2	Inflammatory; immunomodulation
Thromboxane A_2	Inflammatory; immunomodulation
Leukotriene C	Inflammatory; immunomodulation

marrow, monocytes in the circulation, and macrophages in tissues. Monocytes remain in circulation for 1 to 3 days, whereas macrophages reside in tissues for up to 3 months.[123]

The mononuclear phagocytic system comprises a critical aspect of host defense against infection, and like neutrophils, macrophages play an important role in host tissue damage in non-infectious diseases, including after ischemia and reperfusion.[124,125] Macrophages secrete an impressive variety of enzymes, oxidants, cytokines, and chemotactic substances that are important for killing microbes, immunoregulation, and modulation of inflammation (Table 8.3).[126]

Monocytes and macrophages are important sources of IL-1, which has a potent effect on the inflammatory response.[33] IL-1 attracts neutrophils, lymphocytes, and monocytes to sites of injury and inflammation and enhances degranulation and adhesion to endothelium.

The ability of IL-1 to activate and thereby induce endothelium to express adhesion molecules may be a means by which distant organs are recruited into a whole-body inflammatory response after cardiac arrest.

TNF-α is another macrophage product responsible for many of the manifestations of inflammation. It has been implicated in the organ dysfunction and multiple organ failure in the setting of sepsis, and has also been associated with reperfusion injury following cardiac arrest.[24]

Therapeutic implications and future research

Resuscitation, postresuscitation, hemodynamic decompensation, multiple organ dysfunction, and survival

Cardiac arrest creates an immediate no-flow state, which produces an immediate systemic inflammatory response syndrome. Therefore, if perfusion is restored, an overwhelming inflammatory response ensues resulting in what many refer to as the metabolic phase of resuscitation.[3] The postresuscitation syndrome is characterized by increased levels of inflammatory cytokines, activation of the clotting cascade, release of potent vasoactive substances, and activation of leukocytes, all of which contributes to altered intracellular oxygen utilization and direct inflammatory injury, resulting in hemodynamic instability, organ dysfunction and failure, and subsequent death if left untreated.[1,2]

In light of the intricately coordinated molecular and cellular events that govern ischemia and reperfusion injury following cardiac arrest, it is not surprising that successful therapeutic efforts directed at the postresuscitation syndrome have been limited.[127] Nonetheless, the significant progress made in the understanding of the molecular and cellular events governing ischemia and reperfusion offers great promise for new therapeutic approaches. For example, ischemia and reperfusion injury following reperfusion after cardiac arrest may be significantly attenuated by inhibition of key inflammatory cytokines (e.g., TNF-α or IL-1) or by inhibition of leukocyte adhesion. Specific cytokines may exert anti-inflammatory effects following reperfusion and consequently offer new therapeutic avenues for those suffering from ischemia-reperfusion injury. The ability of some cytokines to exert protective cellular and tissue effects suggests their possible use as therapeutic agents in reperfusion injury. Alternatively, agents that interfere with the production of, or enhance the removal of, proinflammatory cytokines may provide other therapeutic avenues for treating such injury. A more broad approach to removing significant inflammatory mediators has recently been reported using high-volume hemofiltration during the postresuscitation period.[127]

One of the most important areas of continued and expanded research will be to identify major mediators released on reperfusion that trigger the sequelae of reperfusion injury. In particular, identification of the most upstream or influential mediators and their subsequent therapeutic attenuation might provide protection, by halting the amplification of the systemic inflammatory response, to individuals and their organ systems following cardiac arrest.[78]

The site specificity of neutrophil and macrophage adhesion at inflammatory sites implies that widespread expression of adhesion molecules by the endothelium occurs during ischemia and reperfusion. Familiarity with mediators of endothelial determinants of neutrophil adhesion suggests additional targets for therapeutic interventions. For example, immunologic intervention before the induction of P-selectin expression may prevent local and generalized organ system dysfunction, whereas later intervention may inhibit the continuous neutrophil recruitment and exacerbation of tissue injury.

Interference with substances released by activated endothelium may provide yet another opportunity to interrupt the cycle of neutrophil activation, adherence, migration, and subsequent tissue injury. In addition, inactivation, by using soluble receptors or antibodies, of systemic molecules (e.g., TNF-α or IL-1) may offer an opportunity to prevent the activation of endothelium or leukocytes, or may attenuate the direct effects of such molecules on organ systems, namely, the direct myocardial dysfunction induced by TNF-α.

A growing body of evidence indicates that the inflammatory sequelae to ischemia and reperfusion can be prevented by antecedent exposure to adenosine, nitric oxide, ethanol or short bouts of ischemia. Understanding the mechanisms whereby these preconditioning interventions induce the development of a preconditioned state, wherein the endothelium undergoes an adaptive transformation to an anti-inflammatory phenotype, may allow for prophylactic treatment of individuals at risk for cardiovascular disease.[128,129]

Conclusions

Although the overall survival rate of out-of-hospital cardiac arrest has remained low and relatively constant over the past four decades, understanding the molecular and cellular events of ischemia and reperfusion has increased substantially, and may, at some point in the future, have an impact on how clinicians treat patients following cardiac arrest. Translation of basic sciences research to clinical research will be the important next steps in determining how to invoke therapies that may improve resuscitation and survival rates for victims of cardiac arrest.

REFERENCES

1. Adrie, C., Laurent, I., Monchi, M. *et al.* Postresuscitation disease after cardiac arrest: a sepsis-like syndrome? *Curr. Opin. Crit. Care* 2004; **10**: 208–212.

2. Adrie, C., Adib-Conquy, M., Laurent, I. *et al.* Successful cardiopulmonary resuscitation after cardiac arrest as a "sepsis-like" syndrome. *Circulation* 2002; **106**: 562–568.

3. Weisfeldt, M.L., & Becker, L.B. Resuscitation after cardiac arrest: a 3-phase time-sensitive model. *J. Am. Med. Assoc.* 2002; **288**: 3035–3038.

4. Ito, T., Saitoh, D., Fukuzuka, K. *et al.* Significance of elevated serum interleukin-8 in patients resuscitated after cardiopulmonary arrest. *Resuscitation* 2001; **51**: 47–53.

5. Gando, S., Nanzaki, S., Morimoto, Y. *et al.* Tissue factor and tissue factor pathway inhibitor levels during and after cardiopulmonary resuscitation.

6. Bottiger, B.W., Motsch, J., Braun, V. *et al.* Marked activation of complement and leukocytes and an increase in the concentrations of soluble endothelial adhesion molecules during cardiopulmonary resuscitation and early reperfusion after cardiac arrest in humans. *Crit. Care Med.* 2001; **30**: 2473–2480.

7. DeBehnke, D.J., & Benson, L. Effects of endothelin-1 on resuscitation rate during cardiac arrest. *Resuscitation* 2000; **47**: 185–189.

8. Gando, S., Nanzaki, S., Morimoto, Y. *et al.* Out-of-hospital cardiac arrest increases soluble vascular endothelin adhesion molecules and neutrophil elastase associated with endothelial injury. *Intens. Care Med.* 2000; **26**: 38–44.

9. Shyu, K.G., Chang, H., Lin, C.C. *et al.* Concentrations of serum interleukin-8 after successful cardiopulmonary resuscitation in patients with cardiopulmonary arrest. *Am. Heart J.* 1997; **134**: 551–556.

10. Gando, S., Nanzaki, S., Morimoto, Y. *et al.* Alterations of soluble L- and P-selectins during cardiac arrest and CPR. *Intens. Care Med.* 1999; **25**: 588–593.

11. Geppert, A., Zorn, G., Karth, G.D. *et al.* Soluble selectins and the systemic inflammatory response syndrome after successful cardiopulmonary resuscitation. *Crit. Care Med.* 2000; **28**: 2360–2365.

12. Oppert, M., Gleiter, C.H., Muller, C. *et al.* Kinetics and characteristics of an acute phase response following cardiac arrest. *Intens. Care Med.* 1999; **25**: 1386–1394.

13. Bone, R.C. Toward a theory regarding the pathogenesis of the systemic inflammatory response syndrome: what we do and

do not know about cytokine regulation. *Crit. Care Med.* 1996; **24**: 163–172.

14. Davies, M.G., & Haagen, P.O. Systemic inflammatory response syndrome. *Br. J. Surg.* 1997; **84**: 920–935.

15. Kim, P.K., & Deutschman, C.S. Inflammatory responses and mediators. *Surg. Clin. N. Am.* 2000; **80**: 885–894.

16. Nystrom, P.O. The systemic inflammatory response syndrome: definitions and aetiology. *J. Antimicrob. Chemo.* 1998; **41**: A1–A7.

17. Nathan, C., & Sporn, M. Cytokines in context. *J. Cell Biol.* 1991; **113**: 981–986.

18. Cairns, C.B., Panacek, E.A., Harken, A.H. *et al.* Bench to bedside: tumor necrosis factor-alpha: from inflammation to resuscitation. *Acad. Emerg. Med.* 2000; **7**: 930–941.

19. Krishnadasan, B., Naidu, B.V., Byrne, K. *et al.* The role of proinflammatory cytokines in lung ischemia-reperfusion injury. *J. Thorac. Cardiovasc. Surg.* 2003; **125**: 261–272.

20. Welborn, M.B., Moldawer, L.L., Seeger, J.M. *et al.* Role of endogenous interleukin-10 in local and distant organ injury after visceral ischemia-reperfusion. *Shock* 2003; **20**: 35–40.

21. Welborn, M.B., Douglass, W.B., Abouhamze, Z. *et al.* Visceral ischemia-reperfusion injury promotes tumor necrosis factor (TNF) and interleukin-1 (IL-1) dependent organ injury in the mouse. *Shock* 1996; **6**: 171–176.

22. Gaines, G.C., Welborn, M.B., Moldawer, L.L. *et al.* Attenuation of skeletal muscle ischemia/reperfusion injury by inhibition of tumor necrosis factor. *J. Vasc. Surg.* 1999; **29**: 370–376.

23. Carswell, E.A., Old, L.J., Kassel, F.L. *et al.* An endotoxin-induced serum factor that causes necrosis of tumors. *Proc. Natl. Acad. Sci. USA* 1975; **72**: 3666–3671.

24. Strieter, R.M., Kunkel, S.L., & Bone, R.C. Role of tumor necrosis factor-alpha in disease states and inflammation. *Crit. Care Med.* 1993; **21**: S447–S463.

25. Kalra, D.K., Zhu, X., Ramchandani, M.K. *et al.* Increased myocardial gene expression of tumor necrosis factor-alpha and nitric oxide synthase-2: a potential mechanism for depressed myocardial function in hibernating myocardium in humans. *Circulation* 2002; **105**: 1537–1540.

26. Smith, R.A., & Baglioni, C. The active form of tumor necrosis factor is a trimer. *J. Biol. Chem.* 1987; **262**: 6951–6954.

27. Beutler, B.A., Milsark, I.W., & Cerami, A. Cachectin/tumor necrosis factor: production, distribution, and metabolic fate in vivo. *J. Immunol.* 1985; **135**: 3972–3977.

28. Waage, A. Production and clearance of tumor necrosis factor in rats exposed to endotoxin and dexamethasone. *Clin. Immunol. Immunopathol.* 1987; **45**: 348–355.

29. Pfizenmaier, K., Himmler, A., Schutze, S. *et al.* TNF receptors and TNF signal transduction. In: Beutler, B. (ed). *Tumor necrosis factors: the molecules and their emerging role in medicine.* New York, Raven Press 1993: 439–472.

30. Colletti, L.M., Remick, D.G., Burtch, G.D. *et al.* Role of tumor necrosis factor-alpha in the pathophysiologic alterations after hepatic ischemia/reperfusion injury in the rat. *J. Clin. Invest.* 1990; **85**: 1936–1943.

31. Atkins, E. Pathogenesis of fever. *Physiol. Rev.* 1960; **40**: 580–646.

32. Dinarello, C.A., Renfer, L., & Wolff, S.M. Human leukocytic pyrogen: purification and development of a radioimmunoassay. *Proc. Natl. Acad. Sci. USA* 1977; **74**: 4624–4627.

33. Dinarello, C.A. Interleukin-1 and interleukin-1 antagonism. *Blood* 1991; **77**: 1627–1652.

34. Cannon, J.G., Tompkins, R.G., Gelfand, J.A. *et al.* Circulating interleukin-1 and tumor necrosis factor in septic shock and experimental endotoxin fever. *J. Inf. Dis.* 1990; **161**: 79–84.

35. Michie, H.R., Manogue, K.R., Spriggs, D.R. *et al.* Detection of circulating tumor necrosis factor after endotoxin administration. *N. Engl. J. Med.* 1988; **318**: 1481–1486.

36. Jones, S.A., Richards, P.J., Scheller, J. *et al.* IL-6 transsignaling: the in vivo consequences. *J. Interferon Cytokine Res.* 2005; **25**: 241–253.

37. Tan, J., Town, T., Mori, T. *et al.* CD40 is expressed and functional on neuronal cells. *EMBO J.* 2002; **21**: 643–652.

38. Mach, F., Schonbeck, U., & Libby, P. CD40 signaling in vascular cells: a key role in atherosclerosis? *Atherosclerosis* 1998; **137**: S89–S95.

39. Ishikawa, M., Vowinkel, T., Stokes, K.Y. *et al.* CD40/CD40 ligand signaling in mouse cerebral microvasculature after focal ischemia/reperfusion. *Stroke* 2005; **111**: 1690–1696.

40. Phipps, R.P., Loumas, L., Leung, E. *et al.* The CD40–CD40 ligand system: a potential therapeutic target in atherosclerosis. *Curr. Opin. Investig. Drugs* 2001; **2**: 773–777.

41. Monaco, C., Andreakos, E., Young, S. *et al.* Cell mediated signaling to vascular endothelium: induction of cytokines, chemokines, and tissue factor. *J. Leukoc. Biol.* 2002; **71**: 659–668.

42. Henn, V., Slupsky, J.R., Grafe, M. *et al.* CD40 ligand on activated platelets triggers an inflammatory reaction of endothelial cells. *Nature* 1998; **391**: 591–594.

43. Iwama, H., Tohma, J., & Nakamura, N. High serum soluble Fas-ligand in cardiopulmonary arrest patients. *Am. J. Emerg. Med.* 2000; **18**: 348.

44. Papathanassoglou, E.D., Moynihan, J.A., Vermillion, D.L. *et al.* Soluble fat levels correlate with multiple organ dysfunction severity, survival and nitrate levels, but not with cellular apoptotic markers in critically ill patients. *Shock* 2000; **14**: 107–112.

45. Krismer, A.C., Linder, K.H., Wenzel, V. *et al.* Inhibition of nitric oxide improves coronary perfusion pressure and return of spontaneous circulation in a porcine cardiopulmonary resuscitation model. *Crit. Care Med.* 2001; **29**: 482–486.

46. Clark, C.B., Zhang, Y., Martin, S.M. *et al.* The nitric oxide synthase inhibitor N(G)-nitro-L-arginine decreases defibrillation-induced free radical generation. *Resuscitation* 2004; **60**: 351–357.

47. Zhang, Y., Boddicker, K.A., Rhee, B.J. *et al.* Effect of nitric oxide synthase modulation on resuscitation success in a swine ventricular fibrillation cardiac arrest model. *Resuscitation* 2005; [electronic publication ahead of print version].

48. Nagase, H., & Woessner, J.F. Matrix metalloproteinases. *J. Biol. Chem.* 1999; **274**: 21491–21494.

49. Spiegel, S., Foster, D., & Kolesnick, R. Signal transduction through lipid second messengers. *Curr. Opin. Cell. Biol.* 1996; **8**: 159–167.

50. Malik, N., Greenfield, B.W., Wahl, A.F. *et al.* Activation of human monocytes through CD40 induces matrix metallo-proteinases. *J. Immunol.* 1996; **156**: 3952–3960.

51. Klawitter, P.F., & Gregory, M. Inhibition of matrix metallopro-teinases during ischemia and reperfusion in the perfused rat heart attenuates infarction size. *Acad. Emerg. Med.* 2005; **12**: S154–S155.

52. Griffin, J.D., Sperrini, O., Ernst, T.J. *et al.* Granulocyte-macrophage colony-stimulating factor and other cytokines regulate surface expression of the leukocyte adhesion mole-cule-J on human neutrophils, monocytes, and their precur-sors. *J. Immunol.* 1990; **145**: S76–S84.

53. Lo, S.K., Detmers, P.A., Levin, S.M. *et al.* Transient adhesion of neutrophils to endothelium. *J. Exp. Med.* 1989; **169**: 1779–1794.

54. Bevilaqua, M.P., Strengelin, S., Gimbrone, M.A. *et al.* Endothelial leukocyte adhesion molecule **1**: an inducible receptor for neutrophils related to complement regulatory proteins and lectins. *Science* 1989; **243**: 1160–1165.

55. Smith, C.W., Entman, M.L., Lane, C.L. *et al.* Adherence of neu-trophils to canine cardiac myocytes in vitro is dependent on intercellular adhesion molecule-1. *J. Clin. Invest.* 1991; **88**: 1216–1223.

56. Frangogiannis, N.G., Youker, K.A., Rossen, R.D. *et al.* Cytokines and the microcirculation in ischemia and reperfu-sion. *J. Mol. Cell. Cardiol.* 1998; **30**: 2567–2576.

57. Colletti, L.M., Cortis, A., Lukacs, N. *et al.* Tumor necrosis factor up-regulates intercellular adhesion molecule 1, which is important in the neutrophil-dependent lung and liver injury associated with hepatic ischemia and reperfusion in the rat. *Shock* 1998; **10**: 182–191.

58. Lefer, A.M., & Aoki, N. Leukocyte-dependent and leukocyte-independent mechanisms of impairment of endothelium-mediated vasodilation. *Blood Vessels* 1990; **27**: 162–168.

59. Snell, R.J., & Parrillo, J.E. Cardiovascular dysfunction in septic shock. *Chest* 1991; **99**: 1000–1009.

60. Ellrodt, A.G., Riedinger, M.S., Kimchi, A. *et al.* Left ventricular performance in septic shock: reversible segmental and global abnormalities. *Am. Heart J.* 1985; **110**: 402–409.

61. Parker, M.M., Shelhammer, J.H., Backarach, S.L. *et al.* Profound but reversible myocardial depression in patients with septic shock. *Ann. Intern. Med.* 1984; **100**: 483–490.

62. Parker, M.M., McCarthy, K.E., Ognibene, F.P. *et al.* Right ven-tricular dysfunction and dilation, similar to left ventricular changes, characterize the cardiac depression in septic shock in humans. *Chest* 1990; **97**: 126–131.

63. Schulz, R., Panas, D.L., Catena, R. *et al.* The role of nitric oxide in cardiac depression induced by interleukin-1β and tumor necrosis factor-α. *Br. J. Pharmacol.* 1995; **114**: 27–34.

64. Meldrum, D.R. Tumor necrosis factor in the heart. *Am. J. Physiol.* 1998; **274**: R577–R595.

65. Murray, D.R., & Freeman, G.L. Tumor necrosis factor-α induces a biphasic effect on myocardial contractility in con-scious dogs. *Circ. Res.* 1996; **78**: 154–160.

66. Oral, H., Dorn, G.W., & Mann, D.L. Sphingosine mediates the immediate negative inotropic effects of tumor necrosis factor-α in the adult mammalian cardiac myocyte. *J. Biol. Chem.* 1997; **272**: 4836–4842.

67. Yokoyama, T., Vaca, L., Rossen, R.D. *et al.* Cellular basis for the negative inotropic effects of tumor necrosis factor-α in the adult mammalian heart. *J. Clin. Invest.* 1993; **92**: 2303–2312.

68. Goldhaber, J.L., Kim, K.H., Natterson, P.D. *et al.* Effects of TNF-α on $[Ca^{2+}]_i$ and contractility in isolated adult rabbit ventricu-lar myocytes. *Am. J. Physiol.* 1996; **271**: H1449–H1455.

69. Sugishita, K., Kinugawa, K., Shimizu, T. *et al.* Cellular basis for the acute inhibitory effects of IL-6 and TNF-α on excita-tion-contraction coupling. *J. Mol. Cell. Cardiol.* 1999; **31**: 1457–1467.

70. Ferdinandy, P., Danial, H., Ambrus, I. *et al.* Peroxynitrite is a major contributor to cytokine-induced myocardial contrac-tile failure. *Circ. Res.* 2000; **87**: 241–247.

71. Finkel, M.S., Oddis, C.V., Jacob, T.D. *et al.* Negative inotropic effects of cytokines on the heart mediated by nitric oxide. *Science* 1992; **257**: 387–389.

72. Bucher, M., Kees, F., Taeger, K. *et al.* Cytokines down-regulate $α_1$-adrenergic receptor expression during endotoxemia. *Crit. Care Med.* 2003; **31**: 566–571.

73. Gulick, T., Chung, M.K., Pieper, S.J. *et al.* Interleukin 1 and tumor necrosis factor inhibit cardiac myocyte β-adrenergic responsiveness. *Proc. Natl Acad. Sci. USA* 1989; **86**: 6753–6757.

74. Kumar, A., Kosuri, R., Kandula, P. *et al.* Effects of epinephrine and amrinone on contractility and cyclic adenosine monophosphate generation of tumor necrosis factor-α-exposed cardiac myocytes. *Crit. Care Med.* 1999; **27**: 286–292.

75. Krown, K.A., Page, M.T., Nguyen, C. *et al.* Tumor necrosis factor alpha-induced apoptosis in cardiac myocytes: involve-ment of the sphingolipid signaling cascade in cardiac cell death. *J. Clin. Invest.* 1996; **98**: 2854–2865.

76. Cheng, X.S., Shimokawa, H., Momii, H. *et al.* Role of superox-ide anion in the pathogenesis of cytokine-induced myocardial dysfunction in dogs in vivo. *Cardio. Res.* 1999; **42**: 651–659.

77. Bkaily, G., & D'orleans-Juste, P. Cytokine-induced free radi-cals and their roles in myocardial dysfunction. *Cardio. Res.* 1999; **42**: 576–577.

78. Niemann, J.T., Garner, D., & Lewis, R.J. Tumor necrosis factor-alpha is associated with early postresuscitation myocardial dysfunction. *Crit. Care Med.* 2004; **32**: 1753–1758.

79. Lefer, A.M., Johnson, G., Ma, X.L. *et al.* Cardioprotective and endothelial protective effects of [Ala-IL8]77 in a rabbit model of myocardial ischemia and reperfusion. *Br. J. Pharmacol.* 1991; **103**: 1153–1159.

80. Grimbose, M.A., Obin, M.S., Brock, A.F. *et al.* Endothelial interleukin-8: a normal inhibitor of leukocyte-endothelial interactions. *Science* 1989; **246**: 1601–1603.

81. Lefer, A.M., & Ma, X.L. Cytokines and growth factors in endothelial dysfunction. *Crit. Care Med.* 1993; **21**: S9–S14.

82. Aoki, N., Siegfried, M., & Lefer, A.M. Anti-EDRF effect of tumor necrosis factor in isolated, perfused cat carotid arteries. *Am. J. Physiol.* 1989; **256**: H1509–H1512.

83. Lefer, A.M., Tsao, P.S., Aoki, N. *et al.* Mediation of cardioprotection by transforming growth factor-beta. *Science* 1990; **249**: 61–64.

84. Lui, H., & Pope, R.M. Phagocytes: mechanisms of inflammation and tissue destruction. *Rheum. Dis. Clin. N. Am.* 2004; **30**: 19–39.

85. Granger, D.N. Role of xanthine oxidase and granulocytes in ischemia-reperfusion injury. *Am. J. Physiol.* 1988; **255**: H1269–H1275.

86. Korthuis, R.J., & Granger, D.N. Pathogenesis of ischemia/reperfusion: role of neutrophil-endothelial cell adhesion. In Born, G.V.R., Guatrecasas, P., Herken, H., & Schwartz, A., eds. *Handbook of Experimental Pharmacology.* Berlin: Springer-Verlag, 1993.

87. Catalina, M.D., Estess, P., & Siegelman, M.H. Selective requirements for leukocyte adhesion molecules in models of acute and chronic cutaneous inflammation: participation of E- and P-but not L-selectins. *Blood* 1999; **93**: 580–589.

88. Albelda, S.M., Smith, C.W., & Ward, P.A. Adhesion molecules and inflammatory injury. *FASEB J.* 1994; **8**: 504–512.

89. Bevilacqua, M.P. Endothelial-leukocyte adhesion molecules. *Annu. Rev. Immunol.* 1993; **11**: 767–804.

90. Lorenzon, P., Vecile, E., Nardon, E. *et al.* Endothelial cell E- and P-selectin and vascular cell adhesion molecule-1 function as signaling receptors. *J. Cell. Biol.* 1998; **142**: 1381–1391.

91. McEver, R.P. Selectins: novel adhesion receptors that mediate leukocyte adhesion during inflammation. *Thromb. Haematol.* 1991; **65**: 223–229.

92. Smith, C.W. Molecular determinants of neutrophil-endothelial cell adherence reactions. *Am. J. Respir. Cell. Molec. Biol.* 1990; **2**: 223–229.

93. Kishimoto, T.K. A dynamic model for neutrophil localization to inflammatory sites. *J. NIH Res.* 1991; **3**: 75–77.

94. Kishimoto, T.K., Jutila, M.A., Berg, E.L. *et al.* Neutrophil Mac-1 and MEL-14 adhesion proteins are inversely regulated by chemotactic factors. *Science* 1989; **245**: 1238–1241.

95. Tonnesen, M.G. Neutrophil-endothelial cell interactions: mechanisms of neutrophil adherence to vascular endothelium. *J. Invest. Dermatol.* 1989; **93**: S53–S58.

96. Lorant, D.E., Patel, K.D., McIntyre, T.M. *et al.* Coexpression of GMP-140 and PAF by endothelium stimulated by histamine or thrombin: a juxtacrine system for adhesion and activation of neutrophils. *J. Cell. Biol.* 1991; **115**: 223–234.

97. Lorant, D.E., Topham, M.K., Whatley, R.E. *et al.* Inflammatory roles of P-selectin. *J. Clin. Invest.* 1993; **92**: 559–570.

98. Patel, K.D., Zimmerman, G.A., Prescott, S.M. *et al.* Oxygen radicals induce human endothelial cells to express GMP-140 and bind neutrophils. *J. Cell. Biol.* 1991; **112**: 749–759.

99. Lorant, D.E., McEver, R.P., McIntyre, T.M. *et al.* Activation of polymorphonuclear leukocytes reduces their adhesion to P-selectin and causes redistribution of ligands for P-selectin on their surfaces. *J. Clin. Invest.* 1995; **96**: 171–182.

100. Bevilacqua, M.P., Strengelin, S., Gimbrone, M.A., *et al.* Endothelial leukocyte adhesion molecule 1: an inducible receptor for neutrophils related to complement regulatory proteins and lectins. *Science* 1989; **243**: 1160–1165.

101. Bevilacqua, M.P., Corless, C., & Lo, S.K. Endothelial-leukocyte adhesion molecule 1 (ELAM-1): a vascular selectin that regulates inflammation. In Cochrane, C.G., Gimbrone, M.G., eds. *Cellular and Molecular Mechanisms of Inflammation. Vascular Adhesion Molecules.* San Diego: Academic Press, 1991; **2**: 1–14.

102. Granger, D.N., Russell, J.M., Arfors, K.E. *et al.* Role of CD18 and ICAM-1 in ischemia/reperfusion-induced leukocyte adherence and emigration in mesenteric venules. *FASEB J.* 1991; **5**: A1753.

103. Elices, M.J., Osborn, L., Takada, Y. *et al.* VCAM-1 on activated endothelium interacts with the leukocyte integrin VLA-4 at a site distinct from the VLA-4/fibronectin binding site. *Cell* 1990; **60**: 577–584.

104. Springer, T. Adhesion receptors of the immune system. *Nature* 1990; **346**: 425–434.

105. Alon, R., Chen, S., Puri, K.D. *et al.* The kinetics of L-selectin tethers and the mechanics of selectin-mediated rolling. *J. Cell. Biol.* 1997; **138**: 1169–1180.

106. Smith, C.W., Kishimoto, T.K., Abbass, O. *et al.* Chemotactic factors regulate lectin adhesion molecule 1 (LE CAM 1)-dependent neutrophil adhesion to cytokine-stimulated endothelial cells in vitro. *J. Clin. Invest.* 1991; **87**: 609–618.

107. Kishimoto, T.K., Larsen, R.S., Corbi, A.L. *et al.* Antibodies against human neutrophil LECAM-1 (DREG56/LAM-1/Leu-8 antigen) and endothelial cell ELAM-1 inhibit a common CD-18-independent adhesion pathway in vitro. *Blood* 1990; **78**: 805–811.

108. Duilio, C., Ambrosio, G., Kuppusamy, P. *et al.* Neutrophils are primary source of oxygen radicals during reperfusion after prolonged myocardial ischemia. *Am. J. Physiol. Heart Circ. Physiol.* 2001; **280**: H2649–H2657.

109. Hansen, P.R. Role of neutrophils in myocardial ischemia and reperfusion. *Circulation* 1995; **91**: 1872–1885.

110. Jordan, J.E., Zhao, Z.Q., & Vinten-Johansen, J. The role of neutrophils in myocardial ischemia-reperfusion injury. *Cardiovasc. Res.* 1989; **43**: 860–878.

111. Beauharnois, M.E., Lindquist, K.C., Marathe, D. *et al.* Affinity and kinetics of sialyl Lewis-X and core-2 based oligosaccharides binding to L- and P-selectin. *Biochemistry* 2005; **44**: 9507–9519.

112. Walcheck, B., Leppanen, A., Cummings, R.D. *et al.* The monoclonal antibody CHO-131 binds to a core 2 O-glycan terminated with sialyl-Lewis, x., which is a functional glycan ligand for P-selectin. *Blood* 2002; **99**: 4063–4069.

113. Hirose, M., Kawashima, H., & Miyasaka, M. A functional epitope on P-selectin that supports binding of P-selectin to P-selectin glycoprotein ligand-1 but not to sialyl Lewis X oligosaccharides. *Int. Immunol.* 1998; **10**: 639–649.

114. Wahle, M., Greulich, T., Baerwald, C.G. *et al.* Influence of catecholamines on cytokine production and expression

of adhesion molecules of human neutrophils in vitro. *Immunobiology* 2005; **210**: 43–52.

115. Shandelya, S.M., Kuppusamy, P., Weisfeldt, M.L. *et al.* Evaluation of the role of polymorphonuclear leukocytes on contractile function in myocardial reperfusion injury. Evidence for plasma-mediated leukocyte activation. *Circulation* 1993; **87**: 536–546.

116. Weiss, S.J. Tissue destruction by neutrophils. *N. Engl. J. Med.* 1989; **320**: 365–376.

117. Decoursey, T.E., & Ligeti, E. Regulation and termination of NADPH oxidase activity. *Cell. Mol. Life Sci.* 2005;[electronic publication ahead of print].

118. Halliwell, B., & Gutteridge, J.M.C. *Free Radicals in Biology and Medicine*. Oxford, UK: Clarendon Press, 1989.

119. Ritter, L.S., & McDonagh, P.F. Low-flow reperfusion after myocardial ischemia enhances leukocyte accumulation in coronary microcirculation. *Am. J. Physiol.* 1997; **273**: H1154–H1165.

120. Engler, R.L., Schmid-Schonbein, G.W., & Pavelec, R.S. Leukocyte capillary plugging in myocardial ischemia and reperfusion in dogs. *Am. J. Pathol.* 1983; **111**: 98–111.

121. Jerome, S.N., Smith, C.W., & Korthuis, R.J. CD18-dependent adherence reactions play an important role in the development of the no-reflow phenomenon. *Am. J. Physiol.* 1992; **263**: H1637–H1642.

122. Jerome, S.N., Dore, M., Paulson, J.C. *et al.* P-selectin and ICAM-1 dependent adherence reactions: role in the genesis of postischemic no-reflow. *Am. J. Physiol.* 1994; **266**: H1316–H1321.

123. Johnston, R.B. Monocytes and macrophages. *N. Engl. J. Med.* 1988; **318**: 747–751.

124. Formigli, L., Manneschi, L.I., Nediani, C. *et al.* Are macrophages involved in early myocardial reperfusion injury? *Ann. Thorac. Surg.* 2001; **71**: 1596–1602.

125. Fiser, S.M., Tribble, C.G., Long, S.M. *et al.* Pulmonary macrophages are involved in reperfusion injury after lung transplant. *Ann. Thorac. Surg.* 2001; **71**: 1134–1138.

126. Takemura, R., & Werb, Z. Secretory products of macrophages and their physiological functions. *Am. J. Physiol.* 1984; **246**: C1–C9.

127. Laurent, I., Adrie, C., Vinsonneau, C. *et al.* High-volume hemofiltration after out-of-hospital cardiac arrest: a randomized study. *J. Am. Coll. Cardiol.* 2005; **46**: 432–437.

128. Dayton, C., Yamaguchi, T., Warren, A. *et al.* Ischemic preconditioning prevents postischemic arteriolar, capillary and postcapillary venular dysfunction: signaling pathways mediating the adaptive metamorphosis to a protected phenotype in preconditioned endothelium. *Microcirculation* 2002; **9**: 73–89.

129. Korthuis, R.J., Yamaguchi, T., Dayton, C.B. *et al.* Ethanol induces the development of an anti-inflammatory phenotype. *Pathophysiology* 2004; **10**: 131–139.

Resuscitation research

9

Methodology of laboratory resuscitation research

Menekhem Zviman and Henry Halperin

Johns Hopkins University School of Medicine, Baltimore, MD, USA

Up to 1000 cardiac arrests occur every day in the United States alone.[1] The ultimate goal of cardiopulmonary resuscitation (CPR) research is to find ways of improving the survival and post-resuscitation quality of life of the cardiac arrest victim. New CPR techniques may improve survival by various mechanisms, but development of new techniques must be based on a comprehensive understanding of the process of CPR to ensure that the results have a sound basis. Many CPR studies are devoted to understanding the physiologic mechanisms taking place in the patient during CPR and the relationship among the physiologic mechanisms, the technique of resuscitation, and the actions performed by the rescuer.

The sequence of major events during cardiac arrest is shown in Fig. 9.1. Both the actions by the rescuer and the underlying physiology play important roles in the eventual outcome of the resuscitation effort. The patient's status during each intervention can be characterized by hemodynamic, neurologic, biochemical, electrophysiologic, and mechanical properties. Some of these properties, such as blood pressure or arterial blood gases, can be *measured (quantified)* under experimental and clinical conditions. Often, clinicians or researchers utilize *qualitative* properties, such as the size of the pupils or the pulse pressure, that are more easily evaluated but are less likely to provide accurate information. It is unfortunate that many important properties that directly influence the outcome, such as the force of compression and sternal displacement, often are not measured at all, even in animal studies. Measurements during CPR studies are difficult, especially in humans. Even in animal studies, blood flow, pleural pressure, compression force, and other physiologic determinants of flow are difficult to measure.

Measurement of blood flow, for example, requires surgical manipulation of the neck or chest to implant flow probes, which can significantly alter the underlying physiology, making the results potentially suspect. Placement of the transducer for measurement of compression force may interfere with mechanics of delivery of force during CPR. Significant limitations are placed on CPR studies by the necessity of minimizing the downtime and the short time of the CPR procedure itself. In humans, there are serious limitations because cardiac arrest is not a planned event, and it often occurs in places and at times of the day inconvenient for collecting data. In addition, ethical and patient safety considerations, as well as government regulations, limit the extent of measurements that can be made during CPR.

This chapter examines the methodology of measurements and evaluation of measurement errors. Issues pertinent to the specific conditions of measurements during CPR studies will also be discussed. To avoid obscuring the main concepts in complex mathematic equations, we have chosen to use only simple mathematic equations. Table 9.1 lists many of the measurements performed during clinical CPR, human research, or animal research. As representative examples, measurements of compression force, vascular pressures, and blood flow are addressed in detail.

Basics of theory of measurements

Definition of measurement and units of measurement

Measurement of "some property of a thing is an operation that yields as an end result a number that indicates how

Cardiac Arrest: The Science and Practice of Resuscitation Medicine. 2nd edn., ed. Norman Paradis, Henry Halperin, Karl Kern, Volker Wenzel, Douglas Chamberlain. Published by Cambridge University Press. © Cambridge University Press, 2007.

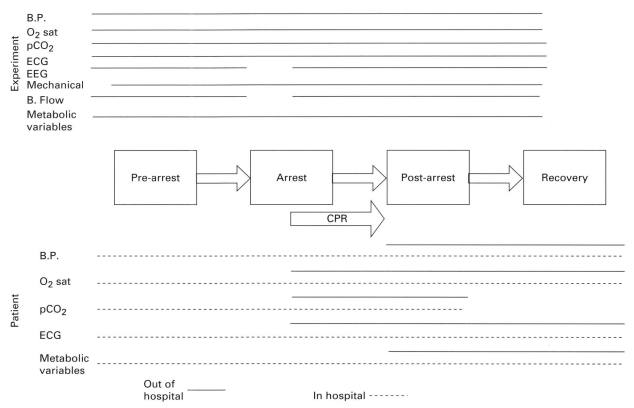

Fig. 9.1. Data available during the different phases of cardiac arrest.

much of the property the thing has".[2] In physics and engineering the measurements are performed on physical properties that can be expressed as multiples of some unit quantities. For example, blood pressure can be measured as a number of millimeters of mercury (mm Hg) or thousands of pascals (kPa). In clinical research, measurements are also used for such attributes as gender and mortality, as well as for such abstract constructs as coma score[3] or quality of life. This chapter addresses only measurement of physical properties.

Measurements require a system of measuring units. The current international standard is the modern metric system termed the *International System of Units (SI from its French name – Système International d'Unités)*. It is based on seven *base units* (Table 9.2)[4,5] and two *supplementary units* (Table 9.2) that are defined. Units for other physical properties are derived from the combination of basic, supplementary, and other derived units (Table 9.3 contains the most commonly used derived units). To extend the units, SI uses decimal multipliers denoted by prefixes (Table 9.4). In United States medical practice, the SI units are used for most measurements, but some old units, such as mm Hg for pressure, still prevail.

True value, errors of measurement and accuracy

In any measuring process, the true value of the property of interest is sought. The discrepancy between the result of measurement (x) and the true value (τ) is the *error of measurement*:[2]

$$\varepsilon = x - \tau \tag{9.1}$$

The error, or closeness of the measured value to the true value, determines the *accuracy* of the measurement.

The "real" true value is unknown and unknowable[2] since all measurements contain some errors. The value measured by a method accepted by experts as exemplary for the measured property is accepted as the true value.[2,6] For example, in calibrating a measuring instrument, the values measured by the standard instrument are accepted as true values for the tested unit.

Figure 9.2 shows inputs acting on a subject and measurement arrangements. The objects of measurements may be the properties of the treatment or environmental inputs to the subject, the treatment outputs, and/or the subject's physiologic properties. Sources of the measurement errors are (*a*) the variability of the property measured, (*b*) the

Table 9.1. Measurements performed during clinical and research CPR[a]

Properties	Clinical CPR	Human research CPR	Animal research CPR
Mechanical properties			
Sternal compression force	M	Y	Y
Sternal displacement	N	Y	Y
Abdominal movement	N	M	M
Blood pressures			
Heart chamber pressures	M	Y	Y
Aortic pressure	Y	Y	Y
Central venous pressure	M	Y	Y
Peripheral arterial pressure	Y	Y	Y
Peripheral venous pressure	Y	Y	Y
Blood flow			
Aorta blood flow by flow meter	N	N	Y
Peripheral artery blood flow	N	N	Y
Coronary blood flow	N	N	Y
Average organ perfusion flow (microspheres)	N	N	Y
Cardiac output			
By microspheres	N	N	Y
By measuring left ventricular dimensions (ultrasound imaging)	N	E	E
By measuring left ventricular dimensions (ultrasound crystals)	N	N	E
Intracranial pressure	M	M	Y
Pleural pressure	N	N	M
Esophageal pressure	Y	Y	Y
Arterial and venous blood gases			
Blood pH	Y	Y	Y
Blood Po_2	Y	Y	Y
Blood Pco_2	Y	Y	Y
Respiratory parameters			
Airway pressure	M	Y	Y
Respiratory flow	M	Y	Y
End-respiratory CO_2	Y	Y	Y

[a] Y, measurement is or can be performed with reasonable ease; M, measurement may be performed but requires special setup; E, measurement has been performed, but it is error prone; N, measurement cannot be performed.

Table 9.2. International system of units: base and supplementary units

Parameter	Unit	Abbreviation
Base units		
Length	meter	m
Mass	kilogram	kg
Time	second	s
Electric current	ampere	A
Thermodynamic temperature	Kelvin	K
Luminous intensity	candela	cd
Amount of substance	mole	mol
Supplementary units		
Plane angle	radian	rad
Solid angle	steradian	sr

interaction of the sensor and subject, and (c) the measuring instrument. One example of the sensor–subject interaction might be measurement of pleural pressure by a fluid-filled catheter. The thickness of the pleural space is 10 to 50 μm, whereas any catheter inserted into the pleural space has a diameter that is on the order of millimeters. Therefore the catheter distorts the pleural space drastically. In addition, propagation of the pressure from the limited volume of the pleural liquid in the pleural space to the liquid in the catheter is questionable. The error introduced by the measuring instrument depends on such factors as the quality and characteristics of the measuring instrument used the performance of the measuring technique by the operator, and the conditions under which the measurement is made.

Table 9.3. International system of units: derived units

Parameter	Unit	Abbreviation	Equivalent
Frequency	hertz	Hz	1/s
Force	newton	N	kg-m/s^2
Pressure	pascal	Pa	N/m^2
Work or energy	joule	J	N·m
Power	watt	W	J/s
Electric potential	volt	V	W/A
Electric resistance	ohm	$$	V/A
Conductance	siemens	S	A/V
Quantity of charge	coulomb	C	A·s
Electric capacitance	farad	F	C/V
Magnetic flux	weber	Wb	V·s
Magnetic flux density	tesla	T	Wb/m^2
Inductance	henry	H	Wb/A
Celsius temperature	degree	ºC	K

Table 9.4. International system of units: prefixes

Multiplication factor	Prefix	Symbol
10^{18}	exa	E
10^{15}	peta	p
10^{12}	tera	T
10^{9}	giga	G
10^{6}	mega	M
10^{3}	kilo	k
10^{2}	hecto	h
10^{1}	deka	da
10^{-1}	deci	d
10^{-2}	centi	c
10^{-3}	milli	m
10^{-6}	micro	μ
10^{-9}	nano	n
10^{-12}	pico	p
10^{-15}	femto	f

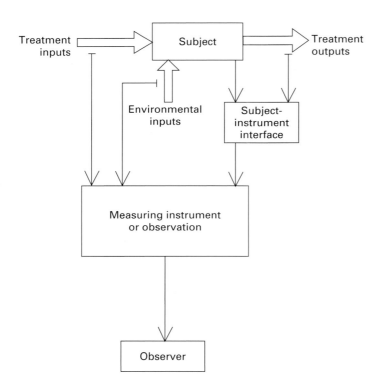

Fig. 9.2. Block diagram of measurement arrangements.

Depending on the nature of errors, they can be divided into *systematic errors* and *random errors*. A systematic error, or *bias*, is the same for all measurements of the same value by a particular instrument, whereas a random error may differ for every reading. The errors may be further subdivided into *static* and *dynamic errors*. The static error occurs when the measuring signal is constant or changes slowly in time; the dynamic error occurs when the measured value changes quickly.

The error expressed in units of measurement (Eq 9.1) is an *absolute error*. However, it is often more informative to report the error as a *relative error*, that is, as a fraction of the measured value (*reading*).

The relative error ε_r is usually expressed in percents of reading:

$$\varepsilon_r = \frac{\varepsilon}{\tau} 100\% \qquad (9.2)$$

Instrument manufacturers routinely quote the allowable maximum error, or the uncertainty (see below) of their instrument as a *percentage of the full-scale reading*. The type of error (systematic or random) is usually not specified. For example, the pressure monitor has the full scale of 300 mm Hg and a quoted uncertainty of ±1%; that means that the error for any measurement will not exceed 3 mm Hg if the instrument is properly used. It is important to emphasize that at the upper end of the scale the relative error of the instrument is close to the full-scale error, whereas at the lower end, the relative error becomes very large. Indeed, when the measurement is 30 mm Hg the error is (3/30)100%, or 10%. A lower, more sensitive scale of 50 mm Hg may have a slightly higher full-scale uncertainty of 2%; that is, the absolute error is not higher than 1 mm Hg. Thus measurement of 30 mm Hg pressure on this scale will have an error of not more than (1/30)100%, or 3.3%. For this reason, many modern measuring devices, such as pressure monitors, have switches that allow alternate full-scale measurements. The scales for extremely low or extremely high limits may have a slightly higher full-scale uncertainty.

Characteristics of measurement instruments and errors of measurement

Measuring instruments are designed to provide *functional relationships* between the value of the input signal and the output signal displayed by the instrument. The ideal characteristic of an element of the measuring instrument is a straight line relating the input (x_{inp}) and the output (y_{out}) variables (Fig. 9.3(a)):

$$Y_{out} = S \cdot x_{inp} \tag{9.3}$$

where S is a coefficient. The same characteristic is also applicable to a measuring instrument in which the input and output variables have different units. When input and output units are the same, the ideal characteristic is a line of identity ($S = 1$). (Fig. 9.3(b)). In an ideal instrument the output would be exactly equal to the measured value. Any discrepancy of the result of measurements from the straight line characteristics is the error of measurements (Fig. 9.3).

The values of properties measured by the instrument are limited by the minimal value (most often zero value) and the full-scale value. Most medical instruments have alternate switchable full scales. The transducer and other elements are limited by the range where their characteristics are linear. When the input signals change very slowly, the characteristics of any instrument can be described by its *static characteristics* and can be expressed using only simple algebraic equations. In contrast, the response of the instrument and its associated elements to fast-changing input signals is described by its *dynamic characteristics* and can only be represented using differential equations. For common measuring instruments the final functional characteristics of the instrument are defined by the superimposition of both its static and dynamic characteristics.[6]

Static characteristics and static errors of measurement

The static characteristic of a unit (an instrument or an element) describes the reaction of this unit to constant or slow-changing input signals.[6–8] As described above, the ideal characteristic is a straight line (Eqn 3, Fig. 9.3). The major parameter of the static characteristics is its sensitivity. *Sensitivity* of either the transducer or the measuring instrument is the slope of the characteristic:

$$S = \frac{\Delta y_{out}}{\Delta x_{inp}} \tag{9.4}$$

For the instrument with input and output values having the same units, sensitivity is equal to one. Sensitivity of the transducer to the primary signal should be many times larger than the sensitivities to interfering and modifying signals.

The smallest incremental quantity that can be measured or can be discriminated is termed *resolution*. An instrument has high resolution when this discriminated value is small. For an instrument to have high accuracy and

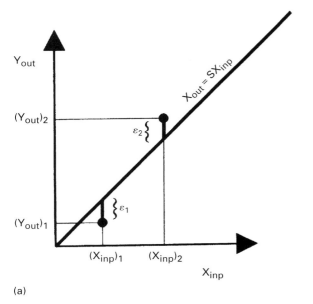

(a)

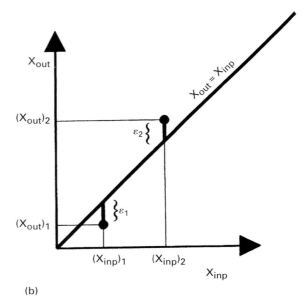

(b)

Fig. 9.3. Characteristics of a measurement instrument or an element of the measuring instrument. (a) Characteristic of a measuring instrument or an element with different input and output units. (b) Characteristic of a measuring instrument with the same input and output units. ε, error.

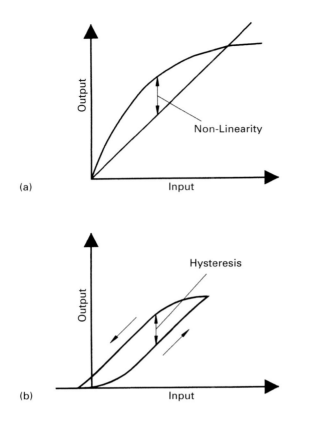

(a)

(b)

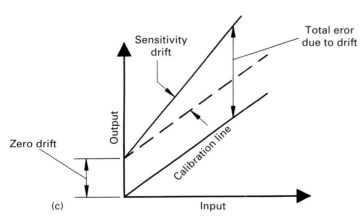

(c)

Fig. 9.4. Sources of systematic errors. (a) Non-linearity. (b) Hysteresis. (c) Zero and sensitivity drift.

precision (the term *precision* is defined in the section on random errors), it must have high resolution. Obviously this condition is necessary but not sufficient, since all errors of a high-accuracy instrument must be small.

Deviation of the real characteristic of an instrument, or an element, from a straight line is termed *linearity* (a more correct term would be non-linearity) (Fig. 9.4(*a*)).

In blood pressure transducers, non-linearity is the result of non-linear deformability of the membrane material when pressure is applied. If the measured value is first increased monotonically from zero to a maximum value and then decreased back to zero, the output signal at some particular value of the input value may be different (Fig. 9.4(*b*)). This difference defines *hysteresis* of the instrument or the element. In a pressure transducer, hysteresis is caused by internal friction in the membrane material during deformation.

Stability and *repeatability* define how accurately the device or sensor repeats the output signal when the input signal is repeated after cycles of input and temperature changes. Repeatability is a short-term specification; stability is a long-term specification.[7]

The characteristics of elements and the instrument change (*drift*) (Fig. 9.4(*c*)) with temperature. Changes can be in the slope of characteristics (*sensitivity drift*) and in zero offset (*zero drift*). To limit the changes in the working range of temperatures, transducers are often temperature compensated.

Sources of systematic errors are non-linearity, stability, and changes of characteristic with temperature, whereas repeatability and hysteresis are the sources of random error. Non-linearity and temperature changes can be measured during calibration. If the instrument contains a microprocessor and a temperature sensor, the characteristics may be stored in the memory and these systematic errors may then be compensated for during measurements. Currently, industry manufactures *smart transducers*, which contain microprocessors and provide such compensation.[7]

Dynamic characteristics

Many properties that are measured during CPR change rapidly. Examples of such properties are sternal compression force, blood pressure, and blood flow. The response of the measuring system to fast-changing input is characterized by a dynamic characteristic of the system that can be represented by differential equations. It is beyond the scope of this book to give detailed mathematic analysis of these equations, which are available elsewhere.[6,8,9]

Many real measurement systems, such as those measuring pressure or force, can be characterized by two parameters, *resonant frequency* and *damping coefficient*. Resonance occurs when the frequency of energy impacting on a system is close to the natural frequency of vibration of this system, resulting in storing of energy and amplification of oscillations. In damping, the system dissipates impacting energy, which results in much lower oscillations. For example, automobile shock absorbers are designed to dampen (attenuate) the vibrations of the car wheels and to provide a smooth ride, even on bumpy roads. Depending on the combination of the resonant frequency and damping coefficient, the measuring system may amplify the input signals of frequencies close to resonant frequency, and therefore the output magnitude will be larger than the input magnitude. Quite often, the signal will be attenuated, with the output magnitude smaller than the input magnitude.

Periodic signals such as aortic blood pressure can be represented as a sum of sinusoids.[10] In many practical measuring systems the components of different frequencies are amplified or damped to a different degree. As a result, the shape of the signal is distorted. In addition, the pulse pressure swing – the difference between the diastolic and systolic pressure – can be either amplified or damped. When the measuring system is strongly damped, the measured pulse pressure oscillations decrease and the measurement gets closer to showing just mean pressure. Thus the error of measurements of systolic, diastolic, and pulse pressure could be very large, whereas the error of the mean pressure measurement may be small.

To ensure a small dynamic measurement error, the dynamic characteristic of the measuring system should be close to ideal in the frequency range of the input signal components; in technical terms this is defined as a *flat dynamic characteristic* in the necessary frequency range. It is also referred to as a *high-fidelity* characteristic.

The contribution to limitations of quality of a dynamic characteristic can come from any element in the measuring arrangement. It can come from subject-instrument interface, from elements transmitting the signal, from a transducer, from electronics, or from a combination of some of the elements. For example, dynamic limitation of the pleural pressure measurement usually comes from subject–instrument interaction, whereas limitation of the aortic blood pressure measurements comes from the fluid-filled catheter and the fluid-filled transducer dome.

To choose a measuring system that provides sufficiently accurate measurements, the researcher has first to determine the dynamic parameters of the measured property, and second, to choose or design a measuring system with a dynamic characteristic close to ideal in the appropriate frequency range. Determination of the dynamic parameters of the measured property can be based on (*a*) previous experience (including a literature search), (*b*) analysis of the physical nature of the parameter and subject-transducer interaction, and (*c*) measurement of the property by means of a calibrated transducer known to have a dynamic characteristic of sufficient quality in the appropriate frequency range. Dynamic characteristics of the measuring system can be found from analysis of the equipment manufacturer's data and analysis of the complete measuring system, and by dynamic calibration of the measuring systems, that is, by measuring the dynamic characteristics of the system.

Random errors

Multiple measurements of the same true value produce dissimilar results because of random errors of measurement. (Extensive treatment of random errors can be found in refs)[2,4,6,11] An example of multiple measurements could be a set of independently performed measurements of a patient's temperature made over a short period of time with the same electronic thermometer. Although the patient's temperature was constant during this brief measurement period, the measurements made during this period can differ from one another by a few tenths of a degree Celsius. These variations represent random errors in measurement around the true temperature value. If the thermometer also were improperly calibrated, however, the measurements will be offset by a certain amount (i.e., the thermometer will have a systematic error).

If the number of measurements performed was very large, the measurements would comprise a *population* of measurements. A limited number of measurements constitute a *sample* of the population. The measurements (x_i) of the sample are concentrated around the *sample mean* or *average value*:

$$\bar{x} = \frac{\sum_{i=1}^{N} x_i}{N} \tag{9.5}$$

For a particular measurement, the value $\delta_i = x_i - \bar{x}$ (9.6)

is defined as *deviation* (or *residual*).

The magnitude of the random error for multiple measurements of a single value is characterized by the *sample variance*:

$$s^2 = \frac{\sum_{i=1}^{N} (x_i - \bar{x})^2}{N-1} \tag{9.7}$$

and the *standard deviation of the sample (SDS)* is defined as follows:

$$s = \sqrt{s^2} \tag{9.8}$$

As the number of measurements increases, the values of the sample mean ($\bar{x}$) and the sample standard deviation (SDS) (s) approach their limits, the population or limiting mean (μ) and the population standard deviation (σ). Therefore $\bar{x}$ and s are the estimates of parameters μ and σ respectively.[2] The error of estimating the population mean

(μ) by the sample mean ($\bar{x}$) decreases with the number of independent measurements. It is characterized by the *standard error of estimation of the mean (SEEM)*:

$$\sigma_{\bar{x}} = \frac{\sigma}{\sqrt{n}} \tag{9.9}$$

Here, σ is the standard deviation as above, which in fact is the standard deviation of a single measurement $(x_i)^2$.

The difference between the mean value (μ) and the true value (τ) is a systematic error of measurements, or bias:

$$\varepsilon_b = \mu - \tau \tag{9.10}$$

The estimate of bias, or the systematic error, is as follows:

$$b = \bar{x} - \tau \tag{9.11}$$

The total error for a measurement therefore is as follows:

$$\varepsilon_i = b + \delta_i \tag{9.12}$$

Many studies of random errors demonstrated that smaller random errors occur more often than large errors.[12] Therefore during multiple measurements most of the measurements are close to the mean value. The closeness of the measurements to the mean value is characterized by the standard deviation. Multiple measurements can decrease error in estimation of the mean value. The systematic error or bias can be found only by calibration of the measurement instrument, that is, by measurement of the same value by an instrument with higher accuracy.

As stated above, the true value is unknown, and therefore, the magnitude of error of a particular measurement is uncertain. Nevertheless, by knowing the distribution of errors it is possible to state with a predetermined probability (*confidence level*) that a true value of a property is located within the defined *confidence interval*[2,4,6,11] from a measured value.

Accuracy, precision, bias, and uncertainty

The closeness of the measured value to the true value defines the *accuracy* of the instrument. The total error of measurements, containing both the systematic and random errors, determines the accuracy of the measurements: the smaller the error of measurement, the smaller the inaccuracy of the measurement and therefore the higher the accuracy of the instrument used. Requirements of accuracy depend on the intended use of the instrument.[2] Of note, the price of the instrument increases with increased accuracy (decreased inaccuracy) of that instrument.

The error of estimation of the true value by the limiting mean is a systematic error, or bias.[2] The systematic error is the result of an imperfection in the instrument.[4] Multiple measurements can improve estimation of the limiting mean; however, the systematic error cannot be corrected by multiple measurements. It can only be determined by calibration of a measuring instrument.

The standard variance and hence standard deviation are measures of the *precision*, or more appropriately imprecision, of the measurement process. Imprecision characterizes a disagreement between repeated measurements of the same true value.[2]

Reports of measurements should contain both the estimation of systematic error and the random error. *Metrology* (science of measuring) recommends reporting not the error but the *measurement uncertainty*.[4,11] The term itself emphasizes the uncertainty of knowing the true value based on the measured value. The measurement uncertainty defines the range of values, usually centered on the measured value, which contains the true value with defined confidence. The uncertainty of a measuring instrument is usually determined by the *instrument calibration*.[4]

Static calibration

Calibration is performed for two reasons: (*a*) to verify the performance of the instrument being tested and (*b*) to adjust the response of the instrument being tested.[4,6] The quality of calibration is ensured by the fact that the standard reference, or the known instrument to which the calibrated instrument is compared, has been previously calibrated against better instruments. This chain of calibration guarantees traceability of the calibration of any device to the national standards. In the United States it means traceability to the National Institute of Standards and Technology (NIST) (previously the National Bureau of Standards) in Rockville, Maryland.

Calibration assures the clinician or investigator of the quality of his or her measurements. Moreover, the law and regulations require calibration of measuring instruments used for the acquisition of data that will be used by regulatory agencies to approve new drugs or medical devices.

Calibration of a measuring instrument or system is a measuring process performed when input values (true values being measured) are known. The input values are varied over some range of values while all other properties are held constant. During static calibration the input signal is changed in stepwise fashion, and time is given for the output to stabilize. The input signal is often changed in increasing and decreasing directions. The input signal is either provided by standards (serving as reference) or measured by standard instruments (test equipment).

Calibration should be performed with standards or instruments that are much more accurate than the instrument being calibrated. An instrument cannot be calibrated to accuracy better than that of the test equipment. An accepted practice in metrology is that the *ratio of total uncertainties (TUR)* of the unit under test and the standard should be not less than 4:1.[4]

Dynamic calibration

Dynamic errors of the measuring system depend on both the dynamic parameters of the property measured and the dynamic characteristics of the systems. In many cases the measured property can be presented as a sum of harmonics of different frequencies and magnitudes. Knowing the frequency content of the signal allows development of requirements to the measuring system and the choice of a method for its calibration.

If the measuring system is known to have a flat dynamic characteristic in the frequencies exceeding the frequency components of the measuring system, the system can be calibrated statically, and the result can be used for dynamic signal. For example, it is well established that the pressure transducers with the silicon piezoresistive sensors at the catheter tip have flat characteristics far beyond any blood pressure harmonics. As long as the electronics to which the transducer is connected do not distort the pressure signal, it is sufficient to calibrate this system statically.

The methods of dynamic calibration of the particular measuring devices should be chosen according to the physical principles of the property measured. The calibration of the system for measuring vascular pressures and the chest compression force is addressed below.

Notably, however, the measurements of the dynamic properties of the measuring system are usually conducted in somewhat idealized conditions. The system used for real measurement quite often has a lower resonant frequency and higher damping.

Thoracic compression

Sternal compression force measurement

Resuscitation is performed by applying a compression force to the sternum of the patient (Fig. 9.5(*a*)). The compression force is the major determinant of CPR effectiveness; however, in most studies this force is neither measiured nor controlled.

Examples of recordings of compression forces during mechanical and manual resuscitation in a dog are shown in Fig. 9.6(*a*),[13] which also presents the corresponding aortic and right atrial pressures. Figure 9.6(*b*) illustrates the force[14] generated by the mechanical resuscitator Thumper

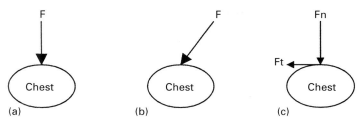

Fig. 9.5. Direction of application of chest compression force. (a) Compression force (*F*) perpendicular to sternum. (b) Compression force (*F*) applied to sternum at an angle different from normal. (c) Components of compression force are normal (F_n) and tangential (F_t).

(Michigan Instrument Inc., Grand Rapids, Michigan), which is used in the practice of CPR.

In measuring the compression force, three issues must be addressed: (*a*) direction of the application of the compression force; (*b*) dynamic properties of the force values; and (*c*) the shape of the force-time curve. The device for measuring force should not interfere with the delivery of CPR, nor should it alter the area and place where force is applied during CPR without the device.

Direction of compression force

Quite often, the rescuer applies the compression force not perpendicular to the sternum, but at some angle (Fig. 9.5(*b*)), in which case the total force can be represented by two components: normal to the sternum and tangential to the sternum (Fig. 9.5(*c*)). Sternal compression is brought about by the perpendicular force. Although tangential force does not directly affect the sternal displacement, this force contributes to changes in the shape of the thorax (what some call chest conditioning), especially in dogs, thereby affecting the mechanical properties of the chest and the effectiveness of the sternal compression.

An ideal assembly for measuring compression force would measure both force components separately, but there are no known devices capable of measuring both components. Devices currently in use measure the main component of the force, the normal component (e.g., a device in reference).[15]

Frequency characteristic of compression force

The analysis of frequency characteristics of the compression signals in Fig. 9.6 showed that for faithful reproduction of compression force, it is sufficient if the measuring system measures the signal of frequency up to 20 Hz without distortion. Some force application, however,

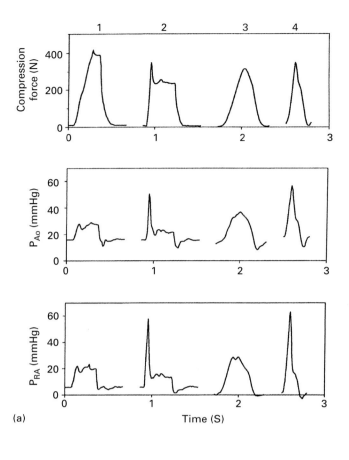

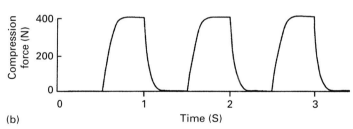

Fig. 9.6. (a) A Recording of compression forces (*upper panel*), corresponding aortic pressures (*middle panel*), and right atrial pressures (*lower panel*). *Vertical columns 1* and *2*, compressions with specially designed mechanical resuscitator; *vertical columns 3* and *4*, manual compressions. (b) Compressions with mechanical resuscitator Thumper (Michigan Instruments, Inc., Grand Rapids, Michigan). (a) From ref. 13. (b) From ref. 14.

as with the ACD (active compression–decompression) devices being promoted by AMBU, should require much higher frequency response. Indeed, in the ACD device, the central part is lifted from the chest and then brought into contact with the chest with high speed; in other words, this device provides an impulse load on the sternum.

Additional studies are required to measure the frequency characteristics of such loading.

Compression force–time course

The force-time curves of compression forces (i.e., the *time course of the compression force*) can differ (Fig. 9.6). Figure 9.6(*a*) also shows that the time course of compression force significantly influences the time course of the aortic and right atrial pressures. The characterization of CPR results and the comparison of the results of different compression sequences and different studies thus require characterization of the compression forces applied during resuscitation. Here we introduce the compression force–time course classification and the nomenclature of parameters describing most of the usually seen patterns of force–time curves.

Most of the observed time courses of the compression force can be divided into the following classes.

Class I: Semisinusoidal course

The force rises monotonically until it reaches the maximum force and then decreases monotonically to the minimum force (see curves 3 and 4 in Fig. 9.6(*a*)). The pattern of the force–time curve is similar to a distorted half-sinusoid.

Class II: Time course with plateau

For at least 20 milliseconds the force maintains a constant value; that is, the force–time curve contains a plateau. Class 2 can be subdivided into two subclasses.

Class 2A: Time course
The force reaches a plateau asymptotically without exceeding its value (see curve in Fig. 9.6(*b*)).

Class 2B: Time course
The force reaches the maximum value, then decreases to a plateau level, and then decreases to the minimum force (see curves 1 and 2 in Fig. 9.6(*a*)).

Some suggested definitions for use in describing the sternal compression force are given below. An example is shown in Fig. 9.7, which is the class 2B force–time course (curve 2 in Fig. 9.6(*a*)).

1. *Compression period (T)* (measured in seconds) is the time interval between the moments in two consecutive cycles when the rising compression force reaches the value of 50 N (Fig. 9A.7(*a*)).
2. *Compression rate* of CPR (*CR*) is the frequency of the compressions expressed as number of compressions per minute:

$$CR = \tfrac{1}{T}\, 60 \; Compressions/min \qquad (9.13)$$

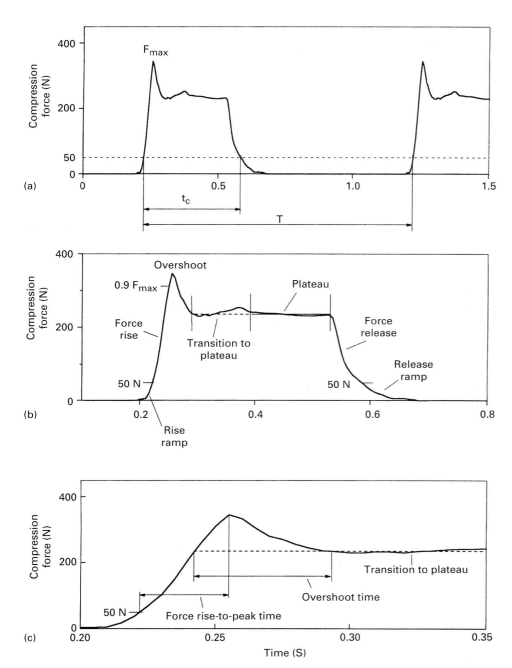

Fig. 9.7. Nomenclature of time course of compression force. (a) Complete cycle. (b) and (c) Time expansions of compression time course in (a).

3. *Compression duration (t_c)* (measured in seconds) is the time interval from the moment when the rising force reaches 50 N to the moment when the decreasing force returns to 50 N (Fig. 9.7(*a*)).

4. *Duty cycle (D.C.)* expresses what part of the compression period is spent in compression:

$$D.C. = \frac{T_c}{T}100\%$$

(9.14)

5. *Maximum force* (F_{max}) (measured in newtons) is the maximum value of force for class 1 compressions or the maximum value of overshoot for class 2B compressions (Fig. 9.7(*a*)).

6. *Plateau* is a part of the compression duration where the force is larger than 50 N, and the rate of change in compression force is less than 0.5 kN/s for at least 20 milliseconds (Fig. 9A.7(b)).
7. *Plateau force* (F_{pl}) is the average force during the plateau time interval.
8. *Force rise time* (t_r) is the time required for the force to change from the level of 50 N to 90% of peak force for class 1 and 2B compressions or to 90% of plateau force for class 2A compressions.
9. *Force peak time* (t_p) is the time required for the force to change from the level of 50 N to the maximum force–time for class 1 and 2B compressions (Fig. 9.7(c)).
10. *Overshoot time* (t_{OS}) is the time interval from the moment when the rising force reaches the level of F_{pl} to the moment when the force decreases to that level (Fig. 9.7(c)). This is applicable to class 2B compressions.
11. *Force relaxation time* (t_{Rel}) is the time required for the force to change from the maximum force to 50 N for class 1 compressions or from the plateau force to 50 N for classes 2A and 2B compressions (Fig. 9.7(b)).

This nomenclature, although somewhat arbitrary, is based on analysis of many records of compression forces and corresponding vascular pressures. It does not preclude introduction of other parameters that would appear necessary from other studies.

Devices for measuring chest compression force

The compression force can be measured accurately only by placing the appropriate transducer between the compressing element (e.g., rescuer's hands, mechanical piston, or circumferential vest or band) and the place of force application. Both the area of contact between the transducer and the patient's chest and the mechanical properties of the material in contact with the chest can affect the delivery of CPR. The goal of the researcher is to minimize these effects.

All force-measuring devices use mechanical elastic elements that produce mechanical deflection proportional to the applied force. In traditional mechanical devices, this deflection is calibrated in units of force. The modern force-measuring devices, the *load cells*, use flexible elements that focus the effect of a load into an isolated uniform field of small deformations (strain field).[16] The resistance strain-gages attached (bonded) to the flexing surface produce an electric signal proportional to these deformations. Problems may arise in choosing a load cell for measuring the compression force. Many of the industrial cells are designed to be used in such applications when the force is applied perpendicular to their loading surface. Presence of the tangential force causes unpredictable errors in their output. Cells that measure the component along the load cell axis but reject bending and side loads are also available. These cells use elastic devices with parallel linkages.[15–17] Gruben *et al.*[15] reported on an assembly that was specially designed to measure accurately the force component normal to the sternum (Fig. 9.8(a)). The assembly uses a coin-shaped force cell placed inside thick wall housing. The cell is isolated from bending moments and side forces by two parallel diaphragms. The industrial unidirectional force cells use

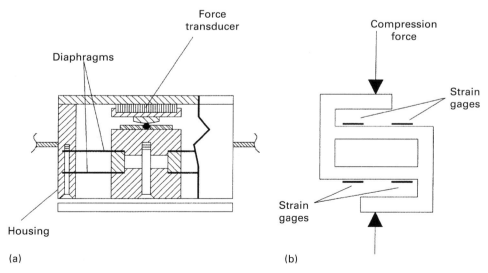

(a)   (b)

Fig. 9.8. (a) Force measuring assembly that selectively measures perpendicular component of manually applied compression force. (b) Coupled dual–beam spring element of a load cell. (a) From ref. 15. (b) Courtesy of Measurements Group, Inc., Raleigh, North Carolina.

a sensing element (Fig. 9.8(b)) that contains two beams joined by relatively massive sections at both sides.[16] With this configuration, tangential forces are counteracted by axial forces in these beams.

The commercial load cells have natural resonance frequency on the order of hundreds and even thousands of hertz and can provide an adequate measurement of dynamic CPR compression forces. Incorporation of additional masses can decrease the natural frequency of the assembly. Thus the device by Gruben *et al.*[15] had a peak error of 14 N at oscillating loading with the force not exceeding 400 N with the frequency of 2.8 Hz.

Attention should be paid to amplifiers used in conjunction with the load cells. Many commercial amplifiers allow their frequency responses to be defined by the settings on the amplifiers. These amplifiers should be set for a range from DC to not less than 50 Hz.

Calibration of force measurement devices

The static calibration of the force-measuring devices can be performed with calibrated weights. Because the forces applied during CPR should not exceed 500 N, calibration for a maximum mass of 60 kg is sufficient, and a load cell of an uncertainty of 5 N is acceptable. Since the standards should be at least more accurate than the device that is being calibrated (recommended TUR = 4:1) the uncertainty of calibrating mass should be less than 0.13 kg. The NIST class F weights have tolerance of 0.01%: for the 60-kg mass, the uncertainty is 6 g.

Static calibration of the force-measuring assembly should be performed before and after every study. The effect of non-perpendicular loading and the dynamic properties of the force-measuring assembly should be tested at least once at the beginning of each series of experiments. Gruben *et al.*[15] describe a simple method for testing the force assembly on an inclined surface and for an off-center loading. Tests of dynamic properties of the cells and the assemblies can be performed on vibration stands.

Deformation measurement

Thoracic compression deforms the thorax resulting in intrathoracic pressure that moves the blood (see Chapter . . .). It is therefore useful to measure both the deformation and the intrathoracic pressure.

Intrathoracic pressure

Pressure in the thorax can be measured using a manometer attached to a fluid-filled catheter. The catheter is terminated with a small fluid-filled balloon (Fig. 9.9). Such a

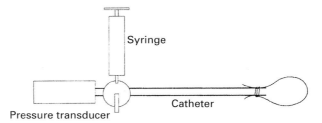

Fig. 9.9. Fluid-filled catheter for measurement of intrathoracic pressure. A small balloon (latex) is secured to the end of the catheter. By using the syringe, the catheter is filled with saline. Care is taken to insure that no air remains in the catheter.

catheter is then inserted to a cavity in the thorax that does not have direct communication with the blood pool and does not have a route to release the pressure. For example, the esophagus has been used.[18]

MRI

Compression force and sternal displacement measurements do not reveal the complete details of thorax deformation. This is particularly pertinent to circumferential compression. While force and displacement of the anterior surface of the chest might be good measures of manual CPR quality, a fuller assessment of deformation is required to understand the underlying mechanisms that propel blood during CPR. Figure 9.10 illustrates measurements feasible by MRI of the thorax during CPR. Images were acquired using fast gradient echo with and without motion tagging. The acquisition was synchronized to the CPR device and images could be acquired at a temporal resolution of 30 ms during the compression-release cycle. Multiple slices can be scanned such that the whole thorax is imaged. Thus a sequence of volumes can be generated covering the complete compression-release cycle. External measurement of the displacement of the chest during compression yields a one-dimensional measure of chest deformation. Panels (a) and (b) of Fig. 9.10 illustrate the additional measurements provided by MRI. In addition to the anterior-posterior distance (light blue line) volumes of the heart chambers (red, LV) and the thoracic cavity (green) can be calculated. It is also apparent that the simple sternal displacement is not a sufficient parameter to estimate the sternal to spine distance (blue arrow).

The use of motion tagging allows the creation of 4D volumes where strain is mapped during the compression-release cycle. Panels (c) and (d) of Figure 9.10 depict such tags. Tags in a form of a grid are created before compression starts and can be imaged throughout the

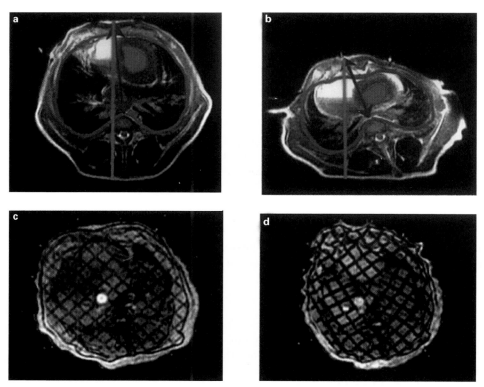

Fig. 9.10. Axial MRI images of pig thorax during CPR. Left panels (a and c) are images during relaxed phase. Right panels (b and d) are at peak compression. Panels a and b illustrate the type of measurements that can be performed. The light blue line demonstrates the anterior-posterior distance of the sternum. Areas of the sections through the left ventricle (red) and the intrathoracic cavity (green) can be readily calculated. The image in panel a was taken before compression and panel b at the peak compression (20% AP distance). Deformation of the chest wall, the heart and other organs is clearly visible. Also visible is that the direction of compression was not through the sternum-spine axis (blue arrow), thus shortening at this axis can not be calculated simply from the AP distance. Panels c and d illustrate the use of tagging. MRI images are acquired during multiple phases of the compression-release cycle. Recording the movement of the tagged grid produces a strain map. The complex features of deformations during the circumferentially compressed phase are clear (panel d). (See Plate 9.10.)

compression-release cycle. Following the displacement of the tags results in a strain map. Figure 9.10 (panels (c) and (d)) show an axial slice of an animal chest before and at the peak of circumferential compression.

Blood pressure measurement

The most commonly measured blood pressures in CPR studies are the aortic and the central venous (or the right atrial) pressures. Figure 9.6(*a*) shows examples of recordings of these pressures. The largest difference between the pressures at CPR and the normal pressures of the beating heart is that the right atrial pressure has the same magnitude as the aortic. Sometimes the peak right atrial

pressure is even larger than the peak arterial. Since the pressure generating the blood flow to the myocardium (coronary perfusion pressure) is the difference between the arterial and right atrial pressures, even small errors in measurement of the latter pressures can produce relatively large errors in the estimation in the perfusion pressure. In addition, change of resuscitation techniques may produce large changes in absolute values in the aortic and the right atrial pressures while producing small changes in the heart perfusion pressure. Therefore requirements for accuracy of measurement of blood pressures during CPR are high. The pressure-time curves may have a complex shape with short spikes. Consequently, faithful reproduction of these shapes requires pressure

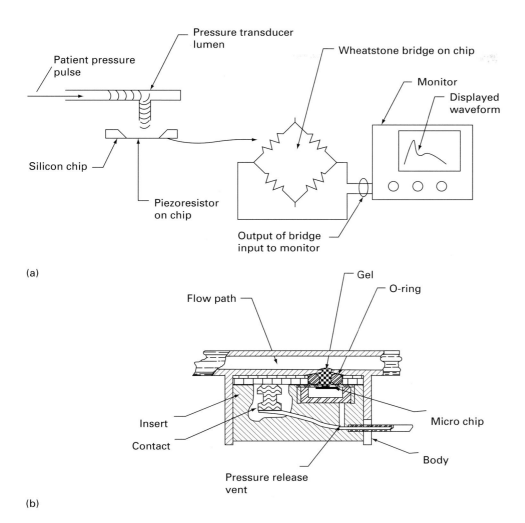

Fig. 9.11. (a) Transducing a pressure pulse to extravascular pressure transducer with displaying output signaling on a monitor. (b) Extravascular pressure transducer (ARGON CDX) with piezoresistors on microchip. (Used with permission of ARGON, a division of MAXXIM Medical.)

transducers that measure signals of frequency up to 20 Hz without distortion.

Methods of measuring blood pressure

The non-invasive indirect measurement of blood pressure that is common in clinical practice uses an inflatable cuff placed around the upper arm. Systolic and diastolic pressures are determined during deflation of the cuff either by listening to Korotkoff sounds or by utilizing the oscillatory method.[8,19,20] Due to the low peripheral blood pressure during CPR, these methods have limited applicability. Invasive techniques for measuring blood pressure place catheters inside a blood vessel. Measuring arrangements

are of two types: either a fluid-filled catheter is connected to the tubing outside the body, which in turn is connected to an *extravascular pressure transducer* (Fig. 9.11),[9–21] or a catheter with a transducer at its tip is placed so that an *intravascular pressure transducer* contacts the blood directly (Fig. 9.12).

Similar to force transducers, a pressure transducer contains a mechanical elastic element (membrane or diaphragm) (Fig. 9.11(*b*) and 9.12). One side of the membrane is exposed to measured pressure, and the other is vented to atmospheric pressure. The deflection of the membrane is converted into an electrical signal by the strain gages. In nearly all modern pressure transducers,

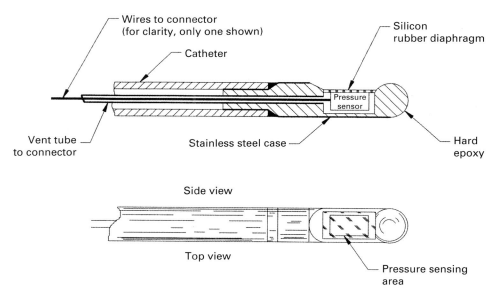

Fig. 9.12. Intravascular pressure transducer. (Courtesy of Millar Instruments, Inc., Houston, Texas.)

the strain gages (sometimes called piezoresistors) are produced on one silicon chip.

Choice of pressure transducers for CPR studies

Blood pressure transducers with direct coupling, the Mikro-Tip Catheter Pressure Transducers (Millar Instruments, Inc., Houston) (Fig. 9.12), have a natural frequency of 50 kHz and provide non-distorted measurements of the blood pressure during CPR.

The transducers used in measurement of blood pressure with fluid coupling by itself have high dynamic quality. The CDX Transducer (ARGON, a division of MAXXIM Medical, Athens, Texas) (Fig. 9.11(b)), for example, has a dynamic response in excess of 100 Hz. The combination of mass of liquid in the connecting fluid-filled catheter, the elasticity of the catheter, and the hydraulic resistance of the catheter contributes to resonance within the hydraulic system. The resonance selectively amplifies different frequency components of the blood pressure signal, significantly distorting the signal. Extensive evaluation of the dynamic properties of the system for measuring blood pressure with fluid coupling can be found in References 8, 19–21.

Simultaneous recordings of the same aortic pressure with both types of transducers are shown in Figure 9.13(a) with direct coupling by intravascular Mikro-Tip Catheter Pressure Transducers SPC-470 (Millar, Inc., Houston); and in Fig. 9.13(b)) with fluid coupling by extravascular transducer P23 ID (Statham-Gould, Oxnard, California) and 7 Fr fluid-filled catheter. The Mikro-Tip transducer gives a correct recording of the pressure wave. The resonance of the fluid-coupling system on rising and decreasing fronts of the pressure signal distorts the signal and overestimates pulse pressure. Both measuring systems give similar mean pressure for compression and release intervals. Optimization of the dynamic characteristics of the fluid-coupling system may reduce the resonance but cannot eliminate it.

If the objective of the study is to record the correct vascular pressures, then the application of a pressure measuring system with direct coupling is essential. Because intravascular transducers cost significantly more than extravascular pressure transducers and are much more fragile, intravascular transducers are not readily available and are not a part of routine monitoring in hospitals. Thus these transducers are not already in patients at the beginning of an in-hospital arrest. Placing catheters with transducers during CPR is a difficult task, but it can be done in prolonged resuscitation.[22] In animal studies, however, the use of intravascular transducers should be routine for recording intravascular pressures.

Accuracy of blood pressure measurement

Accuracy of 1 to 2 mm Hg is easily achievable. Blood pressure transducers should be calibrated before each study, if possible, and calibration should be verified after each study. Usually, calibration is performed with mercury manometers, which are readily available in hospitals.

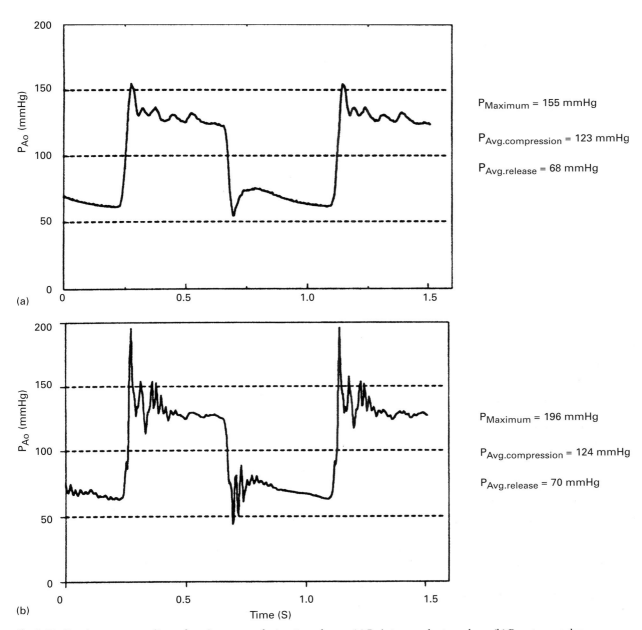

Fig. 9.13. Simultaneous recordings of aortic pressures by two transducers. (a) By intravascular transducer (b) By extravascular transducer. Note ringing at pressure upstrokes and down strokes, which distorts pressure waveforms as compared to waveforms measured with high-fidelity transducer in (a).

With appropriate care, pressure can be established with an accuracy of 0.2 to 0.3 mm Hg. Calibration with electrical means on the monitors or on connecting boxes (for Mikro-Tip Transducers) may add 1 to 2 mm Hg of calibration error.

The biggest challenge in blood pressure measurement is establishing the zero pressure level. External transducers have a port that can be exposed to ambient pressure for establishing zero pressure level, which is generally placed at the level of the right atrium. The same zero level can be established for different extravascular pressure transducers independent of the position of the ends of the attached fluid-filled catheters. The output signal for zero input pressure for intravascular transducers should be established before insertion of the transducer into the vessel and checked after the experiment. Since the zero level pressure in these transducers depends on the position of the tip of the catheter in the body, this discrepancy can reach 1 to 2 mm Hg. Therefore the post-experiment zero level should be checked in vivo (if the experiment allows).

Blood flow measurement in cardiopulmonary resuscitation

Blood flow is a critical determinant of survival. Blood flow is quantified as the volume of fluid passing through a cross-section of a blood vessel per unit time. If a small volume of blood (δV) has passed through the cross-section in a short time (δt) then the flow is as follows:

$$F = \frac{\delta V}{\delta t} \tag{9.15}$$

The flow can also be related to velocity of liquid in the cross-section. If the velocity is the same across the cross-section, then the volume of liquid that will pass the section in the time interval δt is as follows:

$$\delta V = uA\delta t \tag{9.16}$$

Here, u is a velocity of liquid in the cross-section, and A is the area of the cross-section. From Eqns 15 and 16, it follows that, when velocity is the same across the cross-section, the flow is as follows:

$$F = uA \tag{9.17}$$

When the velocity is not constant across the vessel cross-section, it should be substituted in Eqn 17 by an average across the cross section value of the velocity $\bar{u}\,(A)$:

$$F = \bar{u}(A) \cdot A \tag{9.18}$$

From Eqn (9.15), it follows that if flow is constant, the volume that passes the cross section in time interval Δt from t_1, to t_2 (i.e., $\Delta t = t_2 - t_1$) is as follows:

$$V = F(t_2 - t_1) \tag{9.19}$$

If the flow is changing in time, then constant flow (F) in Eqn (9.19) has to be substituted for mean (average in time) flow ($\bar{F}$):

$$V = \bar{F}(t_2 - t_1) \tag{9.20}$$

Flow is characterized by both magnitude and direction. *Antegrade blood flow* is usually assigned a positive value, whereas *retrograde flow* (e.g., the valve regurgitation flow) is assigned a negative value. During CPR the blood flow in vessels usually changes direction from antegrade to retrograde during one chest compression cycle. The resulting

mean flow defines the blood supply to the organs. The measurement of the *regional tissue blood flows*, or *organ per-fusion*, during CPR provides information on distribution of cardiac output to different organs. Success of CPR depends on sufficient blood supply to the heart and brain.

Methods of measuring blood flow

Both non-invasive and invasive techniques are used for measuring blood flow. An example of a non-invasive technique is the transcutaneous or the intraesophageal ultrasound echo Doppler technique.[23] Some invasive techniques require placement of catheters into blood vessels by transcutaneous or surgical cutdown access; examples are cardiac output measurements by the Fick principle or by thermo dilution.[19,24–27] Other invasive techniques require surgical procedures to access the external surface of the blood vessels to place a flow probe.[19,25,26,28] Measurement of regional blood flow by labeled microspheres requires sacrifice of an animal for acquiring tissue samples.[29,30]

Methods of blood flow measurements can be classified as follows: (*a*) use of tracers of various sorts (e.g., thermodilution or labeled microspheres);[25,26,29] (*b*) utilizing electromagnetic flow probes;[25,26,28] (*c*) methods utilizing transit-time ultrasonic flow probes,[31,32] (*d*) ultrasound echo Doppler technique,[23] and laser–Doppler flow methods.[33–35]

Distinctive features of blood flow measurement

Compression on the chest produces extensive mechanical movement and vibration of the chest, organs, and vasculature inside the chest and abdomen; consequently techniques such as transcutaneous or intraesophageal ultrasound echo Doppler, which require steady positioning of the transducer relative to the blood vessels, cannot be used during CPR.

During cardiac arrest, arterial pressure drops to the level of the mean systemic pressure (7 to 10 mm Hg), causing a significant decrease in aortic and arterial radii. During resuscitation the aortic and arterial pressures increase but still can be much lower than before arrest. Therefore, the arteries will be smaller than before arrest. Such arterial shrinkage will cause changes in mechanical coupling of the flow probes to the aorta and arteries.

During CPR, blood flow is usually substantially lower than in the intact circulation. In addition, during CPR, blood flow in most vessels alternates between antegrade and retrograde directions (Fig. 9.14). While the magnitude of the antegrade *instantaneous flow* (the flow at a particular time moment) can be large, subsequent retrograde flow negates some of it. Consequently, the mean flow for a

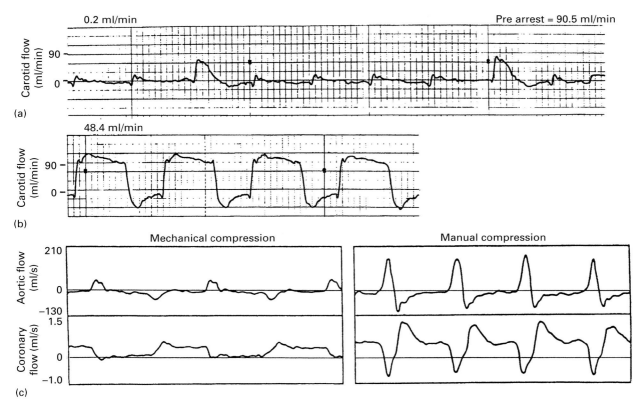

Fig. 9.14. Recording of blood flow during resuscitation by electromagnetic flow meters. (a) Carotid flow during conventional resuscitation. (b) Carotid flow during simultaneous compression and ventilation resuscitation. (c) Aortic and coronary flow during fast rise time-short duration resuscitation. (a) and (b) From ref. 51. (c) From ref. 50.

whole compression cycle could be rather small. Therefore it is of paramount importance to verify the output signal of the flowmeter when the flow rate is equal to zero.

This section will evaluate current methods of blood flow measurement by microsphere injection and with flow probes.

Measurement of blood flow with microspheres

Measurements of blood flow by known concentrations of tracers in the blood have been used for more than a century. In 1870 Fick introduced measurements of cardiac output by measurements of oxygen or carbon dioxide concentrations in arterial and venous blood and the uptake of oxygen or release of carbon dioxide by lungs. The tracers can be introduced into the bloodstream continuously or as a single bolus injection. Although single-bolus injection is utilized in the clinically popular measurement of cardiac output by thermodilution, this technique is not applicable during CPR because of low blood flow and extensive movement of the body.

Measurement of organ perfusion by injection of radionuclide-labeled microspheres in animal CPR studies was extensively studied by Koehler *et al.*[29] in the 1980s and is now widely accepted. In general, a known amount of tracer (Q) is injected into the bloodstream as a bolus (Fig. 9.15(a)) during a short time interval. Arterial blood is sampled by withdrawal by a syringe with a calibrated rate. To ensure accuracy of blood flow measurement, the tracer should be uniformly mixed with blood (i.e., the concentration [c] of the tracer in any cross-section in a vessel after the mixing chamber is constant); in addition, tracer particles should move with the same velocity as the flow particles.[27] After the bolus injection the concentration of the tracer in the blood distal to the mixing chamber changes with time, as shown in Fig. 9.15(*b*).

It can be shown[25,26] that if the amount of the tracer is known, the flow can be calculated as follows:

$$F = \frac{Q}{\int c \cdot dt} \qquad (9.21)$$

Here the denominator of Eqn 21 ($\int c \cdot dt$) is the area under the tracer concentration curve in Fig. 9.15(*b*). Thus, if the

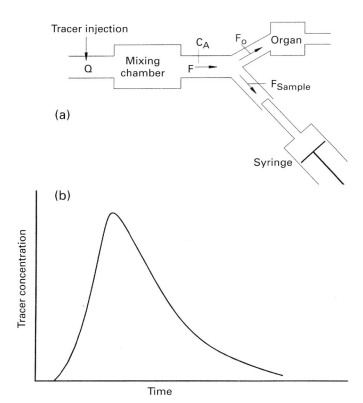

Fig. 9.15. (a) Principle of measuring organ perfusion by microsphere injection. (b) Concentration-time curve after fast injection of microspheres.

total amount of the tracer injected into the bloodstream is known, and the concentration of tracer in the blood after the mixing chamber can be measured, then the blood flow can be calculated. This method is used in cardiac output measurements with thermo dilution. During resuscitation, organ flow is measured with 15-μm diameter microspheres. These microspheres are nearly completely trapped in the capillaries, and therefore the rate at which the tracer leaves the organ is negligible. To avoid measurements of concentration of the spheres in the bloodstream, the reference sample of blood is withdrawn from an artery with a constant known flow (F_{sample}) (Fig. 9.15(a)). The syringe that withdraws the arterial blood can be looked on as another organ with known blood flow to it (F_{sample}). Since only the amount of microspheres in the sample is important, withdrawal starts before the microsphere injection and continues until the blood is cleared of spheres. It can be shown that the blood flow to an organ is as follows:

$$F_o = F_{sample} \frac{Q_o}{Q_{sample}} \qquad (9.22)$$

In CPR research the amount of microspheres in an organ is measured as the amount trapped in 1 g of tissue. Substituting Q_{100} in Eqn (9.22) for Q_o we get for the blood flow to 100 g of tissue:

$$F\left(\frac{ml}{min \cdot g}\right) = F_{sample} \frac{Q}{Q_{sample} \cdot w} \qquad (9.23)$$

where w is the assayed tissue weight in grams.

The number of spheres is measured as the amount of radioactivity or concentration of dye, depending on the type of microspheres that were used.[29,33,35–40] Multiple injections could be performed with microspheres labeled with different radioactive nuclides, different colors or different isotopes. The numbers of each different microsphere in one sample are then determined by differential spectroscopy,[29,30,38] or colorimetry.[36,37,39,40]

Practical considerations

While measuring organ blood flow with radionuclide-labeled microspheres, the spheres are injected into the left ventricle via a catheter. The number of spheres injected should be about 1 to 3 times 10^6. Additional fast flushing of the catheter with 10 ml of saline ensures that no spheres are left in the catheter and improves mixing of the spheres with blood in the left ventricle. The amount of injected microspheres depends on the minimal amount that is required for reliable assay. The estimate of the injection amount can be calculated as follows:

$$n = \frac{n_{min}}{F \cdot S \cdot CO_f} \qquad (9.24)$$

where $F \equiv \dfrac{F_{reduced}}{F_{normal}}$; $S \equiv \dfrac{\text{tissue sample weight}}{\text{Organ weight}}$;

$CO_f \equiv \dfrac{\text{normal flow to organ}}{\text{normal cardiac output}}$; n_{min} is the minimal amount required for reliable assay and n is the injected amount.

The reference samples are taken from at least two arteries lying on both sides. Closeness of counts in the two arteries ensures that spheres have been well mixed in the blood. The reference sample withdrawal time should be at least 2 minutes.[29] Instability of blood flow for such a long time would introduce significant errors in estimations of blood flow. Spheres with lower energy emissions (e.g., ^{113}Sn) should be injected when the flow is greatest; before arrest.

For radioactive microspheres, the numbers of microspheres in blood and tissues are counted on gamma spectrometers. The overlap of counts in tissue from high-energy isotopes into windows of lower-energy emission is subtracted to obtain a corrected count value for each isotope by differential spectroscopy.[30]

The following factors can cause error.

1. Instability of blood flow during blood sampling time, which should extend for at least 2 minutes.[29]
2. Any interruption of CPR during sampling time.
3. Poor mixing of microspheres in the left ventricle and sedimentation of spheres.
4. Any problems with the pump that withdraws the reference blood sample and discrepancy between counts in two samples (Koehler *et al.*[29] reported a discrepancy on the order of 1.5%).
5. Microsphere shunting across the venous bed and recirculation of spheres (Koehler *et al.*[29] found that shunting across the cerebral bed was $4.1 \pm 2.3\%$ during CPR).
6. Small numbers of spheres in some tissue samples.
7. Pulsatility of blood flow.[24]

Currently, we do not have realistic measurements of accuracy of regional blood flow during CPR by radionuclide-labeled microspheres. We can only estimate that the uncertainty of these measurements is at least 10% of the measurement. If the technique of the investigator is not perfect, the uncertainty can be 20% to 50% of measurement or even much higher.

Non-radioactive microspheres

Non-radioactive microspheres with affixed fluorescent non-leaching labels or neutron-activated isotopes have been added to regional blood flow measurements for four major reasons: (*a*) the cost of disposal of radioactive waste is becoming prohibitively expensive; (*b*) there is a danger to the health of laboratory personnel, however small; (*c*) animals injected with radioactive material are difficult and expensive to maintain; and (*d*) new technology of tissue processing and color analysis is improving in quality and is less costly.

Color

Fluorescent microspheres alleviate the problems associated with using radioactive material in animals. The use of fluorescent and radioactive microspheres is similar. Instead of detecting the amount of microspheres trapped in tissue sample by nuclear spectroscopy, fluorescent microsphere amounts are detected by fluorometry. In order to assay the fluorescence of the microspheres in tissue samples, the tissue has to be processed. Van Oosterhout *et al.*[37] describe a method for extracting the microspheres from the blood and tissue and than extracting the dye from the microspheres so it can be assayed using a luminescence spectrophotometer. It was later shown that fluorescent microspheres were superior to their radioactive counterparts when blood flow was

measured in chronic experiments.[36] Detailed technical discussion of the use of fluorescent microspheres can be found in the manufacturers' documentation.[39,40]

Neutron-activated

The latest microsphere technology is neutron-activated microspheres.[38] Like the fluorescent microspheres, it is not hampered by the use of radioactive material. At the same time, like the radioactive microspheres, it does not require digestion of the tissue. The microspheres are loaded with non-radioactive isotopes. Once tissue is harvested it is rinsed and dried in the investigator laboratory and sent to the manufacturer for assay. The assay procedure involves activation of the isotopes by neutron bombardment and measurements of the decay of the different isotopes in the sample. Currently, 12 different isotopes are available.

Blood flow measurement with flow meters

Blood flow meters contain at least two major parts: a flow probe producing a signal functionally related to the flow (usually proportional) and an electronic unit supplying energy to the flow probe, processing the output signal of the flow probe, and presenting the result to the observer. Blood flow measurement with flow meters requires placing a flow probe in the circulation. The degree of surgical intervention depends on the vessel in which the blood flow is measured and on the design of the flow probes. Independent of the physical principles on which flow measuring is based, we can distinguish three major types of flow probe design: perivascular, cannulating, and intravascular.

The perivascular probe is placed around the vessel. The required tightness of fit of the perivascular probe to the vessel depends on the physical principles of the flow measurement.

The cannulating flow probe is composed of a short tube with a sensor in the middle part. The vessel is transected and the flow probe interposed between the cut ends. Thus the entire volume of blood flowing through the vessel goes through the flow probe. The advantage of the cannulating flow probe is the fixed geometry, which guarantees the fixed velocity profile inside the probe, whereas the major disadvantage is that the anatomy of the vessel is altered, which might alter the hemodynamics.

The intravascular flow probe measures the velocity in the vicinity of the probe rather than the flow. Hence, such flow probes are often termed *velocity meters*. Measurements of the flow by these probes rely on knowing the vessel cross section and the velocity profile in this section and on stability of the cross section and the profile during measurement. Because these conditions are uncertain during CPR, intravascular flow probes have very limited use during CPR research.

Electromagnetic flow meters

The principle of electromagnetic flow meters is based on Faraday's law; namely, the electromotive force is generated when the conducting medium (blood) moves across the magnetic field (Fig. 9.16). The electromagnet produces the magnetic field with the magnetic flux density (*B*), across the vessel. Blood moves across the field with velocity (*u*), and as a result electromotive force (*E*) is generated in the blood. This voltage is picked up by the electrodes positioned on the walls. In a cannulating flow probe, the tube is made from an isolating material and the electrodes are placed inside the tube so that they are in contact with the flowing blood. In a perivascular flow probe the body of the probe is placed tightly around the blood vessel so that

the electrodes on the internal surface of the probe do not lose contact with the blood vessel.

It has been shown[28] that, under ideal conditions, distribution of the voltages and currents in the flow probes produces the voltage *E* on the electrodes that is proportional to the average across the cross-section flow velocity

$$\overline{u}(A) : E = dB\overline{u}(A) \tag{9.25}$$

where *d* is the diameter of the blood vessel and *B* is the magnetic inductance. Thus it follows from Eqns 18 and 25 that the electromagnetic flow meter generates a signal proportional to the flow. The signal of the flow probe is on the order of microvolts so that the flow meter requires high-quality, powerful amplification. The flow probe produces voltage proportional to flow, as long as flow is axially symmetric. The cannulating flow probe provides the proper flow profile, since it has a tube of sufficient length. The perivascular flow probe measures flow accurately in

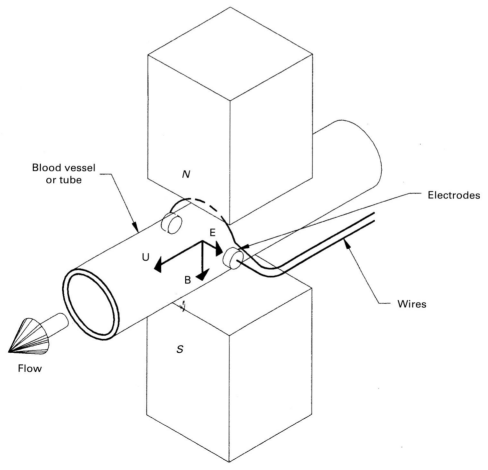

Fig. 9.16. Principle of electromagnetic flow meter, *B*, density of magnetic flux; *u*, velocity of blood; *E*, flow-induced electromotive force.

most arteries but not in the aorta, where the profile is non-symmetric.[9] When the perivascular flow probe is implanted and has become attached to the vessel by connective tissue, the shape of the vessel may be distorted, which can cause a non-symmetric flow profile.

Polarization of the electrodes in contact with blood or vessel produces voltages of higher magnitude than that of the flow signal. To exclude the polarization effect, the magnetic fields of the flow probes are produced by alternating electric current.

Some of the flow meters utilize a sinusoidal current of 400 to 700 Hz. In addition to the signal proportional to the flow, these flow probes also generate what is called a *transformer voltage*, which is not flow-related. This voltage is generated because of interaction of the winding of the probe, which produces the magnetic field, with a circuit comprising the electrodes, the blood between them, and the wires leading to the electrodes. The probe winding and this circuit function as primary and secondary windings for an unintentional de facto transformer. It is fortunate that the transformer voltage has a 90-degree phase shift in reference to the flow signal. The flow probe manufacturers reduce the transformer voltage by proper alignment of the wires leading to the electrodes. Nevertheless, complete compensation of the transformer voltage cannot be achieved. The flow meter electronics utilize different schemes of gating to overcome this voltage. Some of the flow meters have a gate knob that can be properly set. The appropriate gate number for the particular flow probe can be either supplied by the manufacturer or measured according to the flow meter manual.

The square-wave flow meters utilize power supplies that deliver constant current into a flow probe for a very short time interval, switching the direction of the current. The transformer voltage in these flow probes has the form of short spikes, which are gated out by the flow meter electronics. These spikes do, however, have the unwanted effect of producing eddy currents in the blood.

The biggest problem encountered with the use of electromagnetic flow meters is a zero flow variation. In sinusoidal flow meters the zero shift is caused by uncompensated transformer voltage and by currents leaking into the electrode circuitry. In square-wave flow meters, the major zero instability is caused by presence of the eddy currents during the field switching. The most reliable zero flow checking is by complete occlusion of the vessel while the flow meter is on. We estimate the uncertainty of flow measurement with electromagnetic flow meters to be 5 to 10% of full scale range.

Transit-time ultrasonic flow meters

A transit-time ultrasonic flow probe manufactured by Transonic Systems Inc. (Ithaca, New York) consists of a probe body, which houses two ultrasonic transducers, and a fixed acoustic reflector (Fig. 9.17). The transducers are positioned on one side of the vessel under study, and the reflector is positioned midway between two transducers on the opposite side.

An electrical excitation causes the downstream transducer to emit a wide plane wave of ultrasound, illuminating the vessel's full width. This ultrasonic wave intersects the vessel in the upstream direction, then bounces off the acoustic reflector, again intersects the vessel, and is received by the upstream transducer, where it is converted into an

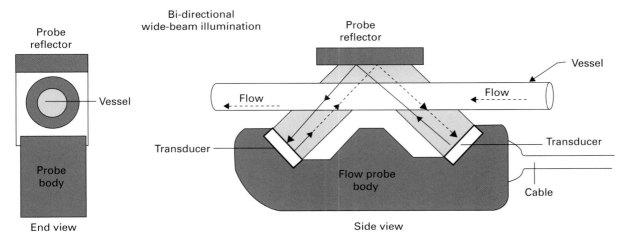

Fig. 9.17. Schematic view of perivascular ultrasonic volume flow meter. By means of wide beam illumination, two transducers pass ultrasonic signal back and forth, alternately intersecting flowing blood in upstream and downstream direction. (Courtesy of Transonic Systems Inc., Ithaca, New York.)

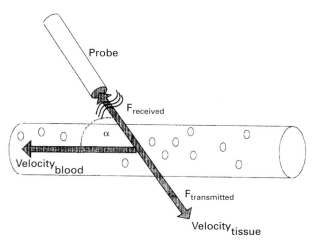

Fig. 9.18. Schematic view of ultrasound Doppler echo frequency determination.

electrical signal. From these signals the flow meter derives an accurate measure of the *transit time* taken for the wave of ultrasound to travel from one transducer to the other.

The same transit-receive sequence of the upstream cycle is repeated but with the transmitting and receiving functions of the transducers reversed so that the blood flow is bisected by an ultrasonic wave in the downstream direction. Again, the flow meter derives and records an accurate measure of transit time from this transmit-receive sequence.

During the upstream cycle the sound wave travels against flow, and total transit time is increased by a flow-dependent amount. During the downstream cycle the sound wave travels with flow, and total transit time is decreased by the same flow-dependent amount. The flow meter subtracts the downstream transit time from the upstream transit time and calculates the average velocity of the liquid along the path of the beam.[31] The beam illuminates the vessel's entire cross section, and the flow meter yields volume flow: average velocity multiplied by the vessel's cross-sectional area. Since the transit time is sampled at all points across the vessel, volume flow measurement is independent of the flow velocity profile. An electronic zero-flow reference signal is generated by subtracting two consecutive upstream measurements instead of using an upstream and a downstream measurement. This eliminates the need for clamping the vessel to establish the zero flow baseline.[32]

Transonic Systems Inc. manufactures both perivascular and in-line (cannulating) flow probes. Perivascular probes are non-constricting and allow some misalignment of the flow probe with the vessel. The free space in the probe should be filled with jelly, which serves as an acoustic couplant. The company guarantees high accuracy of the flow probes: for a perivascular probe appropriate for a 4-mm

vessel, the maximum uncertainty of zero offset is 4 ml/min, and the maximum uncertainty of the calibration slope is 10%; for a cannulating flow probe with 3.2-mm internal diameter (maximum flow range, 150 ml/min), the maximum uncertainty of zero offset is 2 ml/min, and the calibration slope is 7%. The zero flow uncertainty is usually smaller for most of the probes, and the slope uncertainty can be reduced by *in situ* calibration.

Ultrasound Doppler flow meters

Ultrasound Doppler flow meters[41] also known as color Doppler sonography have not been commonly used to quantify blood flow during CPR Experiments. Figure 9.18. depicts the principle of the velocity measurements using Doppler effect. The received frequency ($f_{received}$) is:

$$f_{received} = f_{transmitted}\left(1 + 2\frac{V_{blood}}{V_{tissue}}\cos\alpha\right) \qquad (9.26)$$

where V_{tissue} is the velocity of sound in the tissue, V_{blood} is the velocity of the blood, and α is the Doppler angle of incident ultrasound beam.[42] Newer Amplitude-coded Doppler solves problems of aliasing and angle dependence.[42] Unlike older continuous wave monitors, pulsed ultrasound is location-specific. This technology has been widely used in postresuscitation assessment of blood flow and cardiac output.[43,44]

Trans-esophageal echo (TEE) has been used in animals[45] and humans[46] during resuscitation to measure cardiac output. While extravascular probes are difficult to use during resuscitation because the motion caused by compressions, newer intravascular probes might facilitate the use of ultrasound Doppler[47,48] during experiments.

Laser Doppler flow meters

Tissue blood flow can be measured using Laser Doppler flow meter. The principles of operation of laser Doppler are similar to ultrasound Doppler flow meter. Here to the transmitted beam is reflected, or more accurately scattered, by the cells in the blood. The shift in the frequency of the light is than used to calculate velocity. Small probes can be implanted close to an area of interest to monitor blood flow. Nordmark and Rubertsson[34] implanted a probe (Periflux, Perimed) directly over the frontal cortex of piglets via a burr hole to monitor blood flow continuously during CPR.

MRI

Magnetic resonance imaging can be used to measure blood flow by using established clinical protocols. Krep *et al.*[49] report additional use of MRI and NMR to assess perfusion and the metabolic state of the brain during CPR. Diffusion-weighted imaging was used to monitor brain perfusion by calculating water diffusion coefficient which is sensitive to intracellular water and cell volume. Proton spectroscopy (^{1}H-NMR) was used to monitor brain lactate as an indicator of metabolic state.

Application of flow meters in CPR research

The specific features of cardiac arrest and the CPR procedure present significant challenges to the use of flow probes. As noted above, the resuscitation process produces significant motion and vibrations in the subject's body. As a result, the acutely placed perivascular probes may move around the vessel, changing their placement position and angle. In addition, the aorta and arteries are smaller during cardiac arrest and resuscitation than they are before arrest. This decrease in the vessel's size exaggerates the flow probe movement. In electromagnetic probes, arterial shrinkage will cause partial or even complete loss of contact of electrodes with the vessel. In ultrasound flow probes, the reduction in vessel size will cause disruption of sound coupling. The vibration can also cause leakage of the acoustic coupling jelly.

The implanted perivascular electromagnetic flow probes have been used by Wolfe *et al.*[50] for aortic and coronary flow measurements (Fig. 9.12(*c*)). Scarring of the flow probe prevents the implanted flow probe from losing contact with the vessel. Vibrations of the subject cause vibrations of the probe in relation to the vessel, however, which may influence the flow measurements. Another concern is that the scarring prevents the vessel from the shrinkage that is natural during CPR (see above). This modification of the vessel anatomy by the flow probe may influence the flow. Of note also, the implanted flow probes should be calibrated *in vivo*.[25,26] Chandra *et al.*[51] used cannulating flow probes to measure carotid flow (Fig. 9.14). Although cannulating probes present significant difficulties in their placement, they guarantee the best accuracy.

As already noted, blood flow during CPR alternates directions in the vessels (Fig. 9.12(a)). High magnitude of the positive and negative flow values requires the use of large full scale ranges. At the same time the mean flow value could be small, on the order of the error of measurement for the chosen scale. Thus measurements of phasic blood flow by flow meters during CPR require continuous development. It is conceivable that transit-time ultrasonic flow meters may provide, in the future, the necessary accuracy.

Air flow

It is of interest to measure the air flow during CPR. Air flow can be measured using a pneumotach. Most pneumotach transducers are low differential pressure transducers. Air is made to flow through some small resistance such as a number of thin glass tubes. At slow flow rates, the difference between the pressure before and after the resistance is proportional to the flow. The pneumotach is calibrated by blowing a known volume of air through it while recording the transducer response. The relationship between the voltage and flow can be calculate as: $V = \int_{t_s}^{t_e} v(t)\,dt$ where V is the volume, $v(t)$ is the transducer voltage, t_s and t_e are the starting and ending times. A pneumotach system that provided heating if the resistive elements is preferred. Heating prevents condensation in the resistive elements and thus prevents changes in the resistance.

Regulatory aspects of calibration in CPR research

In the United States, requirements for proper calibration are clearly spelled out for manufacture of medical equipment[52] and for non-clinical laboratory studies,[53] which are performed to provide the data in support of applications for investigational device exemption[54,55] or marketing permits for medical equipment.[56]

The regulations entitled *Good Laboratory Practice for Nonclinical Laboratory Studies*[53] state that "equipment used for generation, measurement, or assessment of data shall be adequately tested, calibrated and/or standardized," that "written standard operating procedures [are] required," and that "written records shall be maintained of all inspections, maintenance, testing, calibrating and/or standardizing operations." Therefore, any experimental data submitted to the US Food and Drug Administration for approval of a drug or device must have been acquired by use of instruments that meet these criteria.

CPR research uses many measurements performed in clinical laboratories. The quality of measurements in these laboratories is strictly regulated. In the United States, clinical laboratories have to be certified by federal and local governments.[57] To acquire certification, the laboratories must have written procedure manuals for performance of all analytic methods used by the laboratory. Procedure manuals must include, when applicable to the test procedure, calibration and calibration verification procedures. Extensive work for developing calibration procedures for clinical laboratories has been performed by the National Committee for Clinical Laboratory Standards, which has produced many publications on this topic.[58] Both the scientific community in CPR research and the manufacturers of equipment for CPR should devote more attention to developing standardized methods of static and dynamic calibration of measuring devices used in CPR research.

REFERENCES

1. Clinical perspective: defibrillation: ensuring success. In *Health Devices*; 1990; **19**: 32.

2. Eisenhart, C. Realistic evaluation of the precision and accuracy of instrument calibration systems. In Ku, H., ed. *Precision Measurement and Calibration. Selected NBS papers on statistical concepts and procedures.*: NBS Special Publication 300; 1969: 21–47.

3. Teasdale, G. & Jennet, B. Assessment of coma and impaired consciousness: a practical scale. *Lancet* 1974; **2**(7872): 81–84.

4. *Calibration: Philosophy in Practice*. 2 edn. Everett, Washington: Fluke Corporation, 1994.

5. E380–91. Standard practice for use of the International System of Units (SI) (The Modernized Metric System). In. Philadelphia: American Society for Testing and Materials (ASTM); 1991.

6. Doebelin, E. *Measurement System: Application and Design*. 4th edn. New York: McGraw-Hill, 1990.

7. Tandeske, D. *Pressure Sensors: Selection and Application*. New York: Marcel Dekker, 1991.

8. Webster, J., ed. *Medical Instrumentation: Application and Design*. Dallas: Houghton Mifflin, 1992.

9. Ogata, K. *Modern Control Engineering*. 2nd edn. Englewood Cliffs: Prentice-Hall, 1990.

10. Milnor, W. *Hemodynamics*. 2nd edn. Baltimore: Williams & Wilkins, 1989.

11. Eisenhart, C. Expressions of the uncertainties of final results. In Ku, H., ed. *Precision Measurement and Calibration. Selected NBS papers on statistical concepts and procedures.*: NBS Special Publication 300; 1969: 69–72.

12. Youden, W. *Experimentation and Measurement. NIST Special Publication 672.*: NIST; 1991.

13. Gruben, K. Mechanics of pressure generation during cardiopulmonary resuscitation. PhD dissertation. Baltimore: The Johns Hopkins University, 1993.

14. Tsitlik, J., Weisfeldt, M., Chandra, N., Effron, M., Halperin, H. & Levin, H. Elastic properties of the human chest during cardiopulmonary resuscitation. *Crit Care Med* 1983; **11**: 685–692.

15. Gruben, K., Romlein, J., Halperin, H. & Tsitlik, J. System for mechanical measurements during cardiopulmonary resuscitation. *IEEE Trans Biomed Eng* 1990; **37**: 204–209.

16. *Strain Gauge Based Transducers*. Raleigh, North Carolina: Measurement Group, Inc; 1988.

17. Bray, A., Barbato, G. & Levi, R. *Theory and Practice of Force Measurement*. London: Academic Press, 1990.

18. Halperin, H.R., Paradis, N., Ornato, J.P. *et al.* Cardiopulmonary resuscitation with a novel chest compression device in a porcine model of cardiac arrest: Improved hemodynamics and mechanisms. *J. Am. Coll. Cardiol.* 2004; **44**: 2214–2220.

19. Geddes, L. *Cardiovascular Devices and Their Applications*. New York: John Wiley & Sons, 1984.

20. Geddes, L. & Baker, L. *Principles of Applied Biomedical Instrumentation*. 3rd edn. New York: Wiley-Interscience Publication, 1989.

21. AAMI TIR No. 9–1992. Evaluation of clinical systems for invasive blood pressure monitoring. In. Arlington, Virginia: Association for Advancement of Medical Instrumentation (AAMI); 1993.

22. Halperin, H., Tsitlik, J. & Gelfand, M. A preliminary study of cardiopulmonary resuscitation by circumferential compression of the chest with the use of a pneumatic vest. *N. Engl. J. Med.* 1993; **329**: 762–768.

23. Goldberg, S., Allen, H., Marx, G. & Donnerstein, R. *Doppler Echocardiography*. 2nd edn. Philadelphia: Lea & Febiger, 1988.

24. Cropp, G. & Burton, A. Theoretical consideration and model experiments on the validity of indicator dilution methods for measurements of variable flow. *Circ. Res.* 1966; **18**: 26–48.

25. Mathie, R., ed. *Blood Flow Measurement in Man*. Kent: Castle House Publications Ltd, 1982.

26. Woodcock, J. *Theory and Practice of Blood Flow Measurement*. London: Butterworth & Co Ltd, 1975.

27. Meier, P. & Zierler, K. On the theory of the indicator-dilution method for measurement of blood flow and volume. *J. Appl. Physiol.* 1954; **6**: 731–744.

28. Shercliff, J. *The Theory of Electromagnetic Flow Measurement*. Cambridge: The University Press, 1962.

29. Koehler, R., Chandra, N., Guerci, A. *et al.* Augmentation of cerebral perfusion by simultaneous chest compression and lung inflation with abdominal binding after cardiac arrest in dogs. *Circulation* 1983; **67**: 266–275.

30. Heyman, M., Payne, B., Hoffman, J. & Rudolph, A. Blood flow measurement with radionuclide-labeled particles. *Prog. Cardiovasc. Dis.* 1977; **20**: 55.

31. Drost, C. Vessel diameter-independent volume flow measurements using ultrasound. *Proc San-Diego Biomed. Symp.*; 1978: 299–302.

32. Burton, R. & Gorewit, R. Ultrasonic flowmeter uses wide-beam transit-time technique. *Med. Electron.* 1984; **15**: 68–73.

33. Wadhwani, K. & Rapoport, S. Blood flow on the central and peripheral nervous systes. In Shepherd, A. & Oberg, P., eds. *Laser-Doppler Flowmetry*. Boston: Kluwer Academic Publishers, 1990: 265–288.

34. Nordmark, J. & Rubertsson, S. Induction of mild hypothermia with infusion of cold (4°C) fluid during ongoing experimental CPR. *Resuscitation* 2005; **66**: 357–365.

35. Tabrizchi, R. & Pugsley, M.K. Methods of blood flow measurement in the arterial circulatory system. *J. Pharmacol. Toxicol. Methods* 2000; **44**: 375–384.

36. Van Oosterhout, M.F.M., Prinzen, F.W., Sakurada, S., Glenny, R.W. & Hales, J.R.S. Fluorescent microspheres are superior to radioactive microspheres in chronic blood flow measurements *Am. J. Physiol. Heart Circ. Physiol.* 1998; **275**: H110–H115.

37. Van Oosterhout, M.F., Willigers, H.M., Reneman, R.S. & Prinzen, F.W. Fluorescent microspheres to measure organ

perfusion: validation of a simplified sample processing technique *Am. J. Physiol. Heart Circ. Physiol.* 1995; **269**: H725–H733.

38. Reinhardt, C.P., Dalhberg, S., Tries, M.A., Marcel, R. & Leppo, J.A. Stable labeled microspheres to measure perfusion: validation of a neutron activation assay technique *Am. J. Physiol. Heart Circ. Physiol.* 2001; **280**: H108–H116.

39. E-Z TRAC® Colored Ultraspheres® For measuring regional blood flow. In *Interactive Medical Technology*, 2006.

40. FluoSpheres Fluorescent Microspheres for Blood Flow Determination. In *Molecular Probes*, 2002.

41. Wells, P.N.T. Doppler studies of the vascular system. *Eur. J. Ultrasound.* 1998; **7**: 3–8.

42. Kollmann, C., Turetschek, K. & Mostbeck, G. Amplitude-coded colour Doppler sonography: physical principles and technique. *Eur. Radiol.* 1998; **8**: 649–656.

43. Nava, G., Adams, J.A., Bassuk, J., Wu, D., Kurlansky, P. & Lamas, G.A. Echocardiographic comparison of cardiopulmonary resuscitation (CPR) using periodic acceleration (pGz) versus chest compression. *Resuscitation* 2005; **66**: 91–97.

44. Sundgreen, C., Larsen, F.S., Herzog, T.M., Knudsen, G.M., Boesgaard, S. & Aldershvile, J. Autoregulation of cerebral blood flow in patients resuscitated from cardiac arrest. *Stroke* 2001; **32**: 128–132.

45. Lichtenberger, M., DeBehnke, D., Crowe, D.T. & Rudloff, E. Comparison of esophageal Doppler monitor generated minute distance and cardiac output in a porcine model of ventricular fibrillation. *Resuscitation* 1999; **41**: 269–276.

46. Hwang, S.O., Lee, K.H., Cho, J.H., Yoon, J. & Choe, K.H. Changes of aortic dimensions as evidence of cardiac pump mechanism during cardiopulmonary resuscitation in humans. *Resuscitation* 2001; **50**: 87–93.

47. Schumacher, M., Yin, L., Swaid, S., Oldenburger, J., Gilsbach, J.M. & Hetzel, A. Intravascular ultrasound Doppler measurement of blood flow velocity. *J. Neuroimaging* 2001; **11**: 248–252.

48. Vesely, T., Gherardini, D. & Krivitski, N. Preliminary experiences using intravascular blood flow Monitor. *J. Am. Soc. Nephrol.* 1999; **10**: 221A.

49. Krep, H., Bottiger, B.W., Bock, C. *et al.* Time course of circulatory and metabolic recovery of cat brain after cardiac arrest assessed by perfusion- and diffusion-weighted imaging and MR-spectroscopy. *Resuscitation* 2003; **58**: 337–348.

50. Wolfe, A., Maier, G. & Newton, J. Physiologic determinants of coronary blood flow during cardiac massage. *J. Thorac. Cardiovasc. Surg.* 1988; **95**: 523–532.

51. Chandra, N., Weisfeldt, M., Tsitlik, J. *et al.* Augmentation of carotid flow during cardiopulmonary resuscitation by ventilation at high airway pressure simultaneous with chest compression. *Am. J. Cardiol.* 1981; **48**: 1053–1063.

52. Lurie, K., Voelckel, W., Iskos, D. *et al.* Combination drug therapy with vasopressin, adrenaline (epinephrine) and nitroglycerin improves vital organ blood flow in a porcine model of ventricular fibrillation. *Resuscitation* 2002; **54**: 187.

53. Iwao, Y., Kawashima, Y., Seo, N. *et al.* [Perioperative mortality and morbidity for the year 2000 in 532 Japanese Society of Anesthesiologists certified training hospitals: with a special reference to surgical sites – report of the Japan Society of Anesthesiologists Committee on Operating Room Safety]. *Masui* 2002; **51**: 791–800.

54. Larzon, T., Jansson, H., Holmstrom, B. *et al.* A Salvage of an acutely ruptured thoracic aortic aneurysm during CPR. *J. Endovasc. Ther.* 2002; **9** Suppl 2: II67–II71.

55. Investigational device exemptions manual. In *HHS Publication FDA 92–4159*. Washington, DC: US Department of Health and Human Services, Food and Drug Administration.; 1992.

56. Bessho, R. & Chambers, D.J. Myocardial protection with oxygenated esmolol cardioplegia during prolonged normothermic ischemia in the rat. *J. Thorac. Cardiovasc. Surg.* 2002; **124**: 340–351.

57. Korn, P., Kroner, A., Schirnhofer, J. *et al.* Quinaprilat during cardioplegic arrest in the rabbit to prevent ischemia-reperfusion injury. *J. Thorac. Cardiovasc. Surg.* 2002; **124**: 352–360.

58. NCCLS Publication EP6-P. Evaluation of the linearity of quantitative analytical methods; proposed guideline. Villanova, Pennsylvania: National Committee for Clinical Laboratory Standards (NCCLS); 1986.

10

The methodology of clinical resuscitation research

Johan Herlitz[1], Anouk van Alem[2], Volker Wenzel[3], Karl Wegscheider[4]

[1] Department of Cardiology, Sahlgrenska University Hospital, SE-413 45 Göteborg, Sweden
[2] Department of Cardiology, Academic Medical Center, Room B2-238, Meibergdreef 9 1105 AZ, Amsterdam, The Netherlands
[3] Department of Anesthesiology and Critical Care Medicine, Innsbruck Medical University, Anichstrasse 35, 6020 Innsbruck, Austria
[4] Institute for Statistics and Econometry, University of Hamburg, Von-Melle-Park 5, 20146 Hamburg, Germany

This chapter is designed to provide a comprehensive, systematic account of the methods of conducting clinical research in resuscitation, in particular, how to set up and carry out a comprehensive and meaningful clinical trial. We will follow the natural conduct of a study, from designing the protocol through data collection to evaluation and interpretation. As an example of some of the difficulties and also the satisfactions of a job well done, in the Appendix we present Professor Wenzel's personal description of the trials and tribulations of determining the role of vasopressin in treatment for cardiac arrest.

Study design

Study objectives

Clinical research in cardiac arrest has developed slowly during the last few decades as compared with other disciplines. The objectives of completed, scheduled, or planned studies can roughly be divided into three categories: (1) epidemiology, i.e., collection of information on prevalence, chance and risks of clinical conditions that require resuscitation attempts; for example, anecdote in the Appendix, elevated endogenous vasopressin levels in survivors of cardiac arrest were found in previous epidemiological studies; (2) evaluation of established treatments and algorithms for resuscitation that are practiced with or without proof of efficacy; for example, in the anecdote, historical data on CPR with vasopressin were available; (3) randomized clinical trials performed to collect evidence on the efficacy and safety of established or new interventions or therapeutic strategies following cardiac arrest; for example, the anecdote describes a randomized clinical trial performed to gain evidence on the efficacy of vasopressin as compared to the established epinephrine injections during out-of-hospital CPR.

Study protocol

For all clinical trials and indeed other experimental studies, a comprehensive protocol is required that summarizes in detail the study objectives and procedures before the study starts. This protocol is the foundation for all decisions of sponsors, ethics committees, review boards, insurance companies or regulators, for conduct, evaluation, and publication. It provides detailed guidelines for study participants (researchers and patients), on how the study must be carried out (for example, recruitment and inclusion and exclusion criteria), and how to deal with potential conflicts. Although time-consuming, a well-designed and well-written protocol will prove invaluable during the course of the study.

Fundamental decisions in study design

When planning a clinical study in resuscitation or in other medical subjects, there are a few basic options that require fundamental decisions. The best choices will depend on the study objectives and on the practical restrictions of the researcher.

External vs. internal validity

Two potentially conflicting goals have to be in accord in a study: (1) Any conclusion from a study is based on some comparison. Usually, these comparisons involve a

Cardiac Arrest: The Science and Practice of Resuscitation Medicine. 2nd edn., ed. Norman Paradis, Henry Halperin, Karl Kern, Volker Wenzel, Douglas Chamberlain. Published by Cambridge University Press. © Cambridge University Press, 2007.

reference group or control group that does not exhibit the characteristic or experience the intervention under study. If the study allows a fair comparison to the reference group, the differences between the study groups can be ascribed to the characteristics or interventions under study only; such studies are called **internally valid**. In general, the best method to attain internal validity is by randomization. (2) Usually, the conclusions that apply to a general population or target population are of interest. For this purpose, the study population should be representative of the target population. If representiveness is guaranteed to a sufficient degree, the study is called **externally valid**. Ideally, external validity is accomplished by random selection from the target population. This can be accomplished by a broad selection of study centers in different countries, which may or may not represent all providers of resuscitation.

It is almost impossible to achieve perfect internal and external validity in a single study. For example, registers are usually selections from a target population that are complete for a defined period of time and thus ideally represent that period, but lack internal validity because of several confounding influences. On the other hand, randomized trials allow optimal internal comparisons, but, in order to permit randomization and attain a study of high quality, special centers and patients have to be selected that agree to randomization and fulfill restrictive inclusion and exclusion criteria, resulting in a lack of generalizability of the conclusions to routine health care. Thus, a decision must be made with respect to which goal is more important in the particular study. In epidemiology, external validity is usually considered to be more important in order to receive information from 'the real world' and thus, epidemiologic studies should include at best all patients suffering from cardiac arrest and considered for CPR from a well-defined area. On the other hand, proof of efficacy of a therapy requires high internal validity and would be better targeted in randomized controlled trials. Studies on health care usually try to give equal weight to both aspects.

Observational vs. interventional approach

A decision closely linked to the competing goals of external and internal validity is the choice between observational[7] and interventional[8–11] study approaches. In an observational study, once the study population is selected, patients are simply observed in the natural course of the disease with the therapies that they would receive anyway, regardless of whether they are in a study or not. By contrast, in an interventional study, the treatments under investigation will be allocated to the patients according to some allocation scheme that is designated in the study protocol.

Interventional studies obviously raise serious questions on ethical and practical issues. Physicians or patients may find it difficult to accept that the treatment a patient receives is determined by some arbitrary or random allocation scheme that is not derived from an individual clinical judgment. The justification for interventional studies is methodological. In observational studies, the treatments under study are always allocated in some way according to the characteristics of a patient or his/her disease; thus, it is never known, whether differences between groups are due to the treatment or to the different characteristics confounded with the treatment effect. For example, when comparing patients who receive bystander CPR with those who do not, the former group might be favored by being younger, with fewer co-morbid diseases, and thus bystander CPR might look more favorable in a study than it does in the real world. The differences may be measured and statistically corrected by adjustment, but there will always be some differences between groups in characteristics that cannot be or were not measured, introducing a hidden bias. In principle, this possibility limits the conclusions from observational studies. This problem can be overcome by artificial (optimally random) allocation of the patients to the treatments, so that all treatment groups under comparison have the same chances of success if treatments are equally effective. This argument alone renders randomized controlled trials sufficient and necessary to collect strong evidence on the efficacy of a treatment, despite ethical and practical concerns.

Interventional studies cannot be avoided if a high standard of internal validity is required. On the other hand, a high standard of external validity and reflection of 'real world' performance of a therapy can be accomplished more easily by observational studies. Nonetheless, the choice between the two approaches is determined by the practicability of the study (e.g., recruitment, timing of procedures), the potential participants, conclusions to be drawn, final acceptance in the scientific community and opportunities for publication. It is difficult or seem to be impossible to randomize resuscitation trials, in particular when early defibrillation,[12,13] bystander CRP,[14,15] or early call for ambulance is studied; on the other hand, the published observational studies raise concerns about confounding factors that may have biased the results.

Confirmatory vs. exploratory analysis

At the end of the study, the groups are usually compared for a wide variety of results in order to receive a complete picture of all clinical aspects. While this approach reflects the desire of a physician not to miss anything of relevance, it has the risk of overinterpretation of chance findings. Thus, the thorough search for differences is "frowned upon" by methodologists as "fishing expeditions." In contrast, to control random effects and error probabilities in a scientific study, the pre-specification of what is called 'primary analysis' is required, consisting of the exact definition of a primary endpoint, statistical hypotheses on the differences between groups, establishing a method of statistical evaluation, and a sample size calculation. The hypothesis to be tested is derived from a therapeutic model and from previous experience. The model is obtained by integrating the assumed mechanism of action of the intervention to the pathophysiology of the disease. Past experience is published from relevant studies of any kind before the start of the new trial. In principle, it is possible to have more than one primary endpoint in a trial, but this requires a larger sample size or a prior ordering of hypotheses that may be wrong, so the restriction to one endpoint is usually recommended.

In general, an analysis as described, with pre-specified hypotheses and evaluation schemes, is called 'confirmatory' since it is performed to confirm a pre-specified assumption. This approach is the only generally accepted way to attain a high level of evidence for a presumption. All other comparisons between study groups are called 'exploratory' since they can only generate new possibilities, but not prove them. Further studies are required to confirm these new hypotheses.

It is of utmost importance when dealing with study results to distinguish those that are confirmatory from those that are exploratory of, for example, a randomized trial. The results of analyses that were not specified before the trial cannot be taken for granted even if they stem from a randomized study.

In the Appendix, a randomized controlled study was performed. It was pre-specified that vasopressin treatment should be compared to epinephrine treatment with respect to survival to hospital admission. No significant difference was found between treatment groups. Surprisingly, better performance was found in patients who received epinephrine after unsuccessful use of vasopressin. Since this comparison was neither pre-specified, nor randomized, however, a new hypothesis that possibly vasopressin and epinephrine should be given in combination was generated, but not proven. This would require a new randomized controlled trial.

Once the objectives of the study are defined and the fundamental decisions are made, study type, study population, endpoints, and sample sizes have to be settled in the study protocol. These partly technical points are discussed below.

Study types

Responses, factors, and covariates

In general, clinical studies are designed to evaluate the influence of certain characteristics, exposures, or treatments (called 'factors' if discrete and 'covariates' if continuous, by statisticians) on clinically relevant endpoints (called 'responses' by statisticians).

The number of variables to be studied in cardiac arrest epidemiology research is substantial. The endpoints mostly deal with aspects of survival, e.g., immediate survival (i.e., return of spontaneous circulation), admitted alive to hospital, alive after 24 hours, alive at hospital discharge, alive at 1 month after cardiac arrest, and alive at 6 months after cardiac arrest, cerebral function, and quality of life. Few studies in the past have been adequately powered to address whether an intervention can increase survival to discharge from hospital. But in the future, more studies should be powered to address this issue and also to address whether it is possible to increase the proportion of patients who survive to hospital discharge with good cerebral function.

Factors and covariates include (a) demographics, (age, sex and co-morbidity), (b) circumstances around the cardiac arrest (witnessed status, place, etiology, presenting rhythm, time of day, week and year), and (c) aspects on treatment (including delay to start of treatment, use of medication, intubation, and so on).

Prospective, cross-sectional, and retrospective sampling

There are three sampling schemes that permit the associations of endpoints and factors to be studied. In cross-sectional studies, a target population is examined for the coincidence of factors and responses. In prospective studies, patients are sampled according to the exposure or treatment of interest, and the subsequent responses are observed. In retrospective sampling, cases (patients with critical outcome) are matched with similar controls without critical outcome, and exposure or treatment is collected from records. Each of the sampling schemes has advantages and disadvantages. Statistical analysis should be oriented according to the sampling scheme.

Observational studies: register, cohort studies, case-control studies

Medical registers document specific health care situations. Thus, external validity is of highest priority. Registers are observational by nature. Complete documentation of all cases or cross-sectional sampling (preferably random sampling) are natural approaches. The limitation of registers is the lack of internal validity because of significant confounding. Hence, registers are sometimes not valued by scientists who are only interested in first-class evidence for cause–effect relations. Recent experiences with safety problems in licensed drugs, however, have raised awareness that registers are indispensable for pharmacovigilance and optimization of use of principally effective treatments in daily life. In particular, in resuscitation medicine, there is an urgent need for registers, since routine data are collected according to local customs and cannot easily be compared or combined.

While medical registers are well suited to give an overall picture of the epidemiology and practice of resuscitation medicine (objective 1), they may be suboptimal for addressing specific research questions on certain accustomed or newly introduced interventions (objective 2). If suspicion is raised that there is a problem requiring a quick answer, or if study funds are severely limited, case-control studies that apply retrospective sampling, as described above, are good choices. Today, these studies can frequently be performed by selection from existing databases, possibly after linkage of different sources of information. Two limitations of case-control studies cannot be overcome, however: (1) missing data can usually not be retrieved retrospectively; and (2) criteria for choice of controls are usually neither unique nor exhaustive; different choices of controls may affect the result of the study, leaving researchers unable to assess which analysis they should trust.

Within the observational approach, both limitations can be overcome by a prospective study design. The collection of data can be monitored, and there is a natural control group: the unexposed or not treated patients. Two types of prospective studies are common: studies with historical controls, and cohort studies.

If a new treatment is introduced and data are collected, the observed successes can be compared with the previous successes in the same unit before the new treatment was introduced. Such a control group of patients is called 'historical'. For example, the hypothesis that early chest compression prior to defibrillation improves survival stems from a historical control study.[16] In this study a new routine (early chest compression) was introduced and outcome after ventricular fibrillation was compared before and after introduction of this new routine. The limitations of this approach are obvious: other aspects might have changed as well, including the study population, the skilfulness of the ambulance crew, and other treatment regimens. In studies with historical controls, the general medical progress is attributed to the new treatment and takes it piggy-back. Thus, a subsequent randomized confirmation trial will frequently end in disappointment. In consequence, a study with historical controls alone cannot be relied upon if a new treatment is considered for routine application.

In cohort studies, groups are prospectively and simultaneously sampled according to the treatments under study and are subsequently observed by identical procedures. The disadvantage of this study type is that it may be prolonged until a sufficient number of endpoints is reached, and the study may be expensive. On the other hand, this study type produces the most reliable results of all observational studies. Cohort differences in observed baseline variables can be controlled by statistical model building. The resulting adjusted effect estimates should be the primary endpoints. Hidden biases may occur, however, and thus spurious results cannot be excluded even if the cohort study meets high quality standards. Only interventional studies can overcome this limitation.

Interventional studies: randomized controlled trials, superiority, non-inferiority and equivalence trials, cluster-randomized trials

Randomization results in an equal distribution of chances between treatment groups. Thus, effects can be analyzed relying on the laws of probability. Observed group differences that are unlikely in case of no effect can thus be ascribed to the intervention with controlled error probabilities.

While randomization balances the baseline chances, however, a random treatment allocation does not exclude every sort of bias that can occur during the follow-up. For example, it is possible that after randomization the patients in the intervention group are consciously or unconsciously better treated or more thoroughly observed by physicians than are patients in the control group. To avoid such biases, the optimal approach is to keep patient and physician blinded as to the group in which the patient is enrolled. This can easily be accomplished if, for example, the study intervention consists of a drug to be infused, and a saline infusion that looks identical can be given to a control patient. If the intervention consists of the application of a mechanical device or a change in the order of treatments, however, blinding may be impossible. In this case, at least the evaluation of treatment successes should be done by a person blinded to the treatment allocation ('blinded reading').

In planning a randomized controlled trial, the appropriate choice of the control treatment is important.[17] The control may be inactive (e.g., placebo) or active (e.g., traditional intervention). It is particularly important to include three factors: (i) what doctors or other health care providers usually accomplish in their practice; (ii) what is recommended by guidelines; and (iii) the available evidence. If the available evidence does not demonstrate that an already known treatment is efficient, the appropriate choice is inactive. Therefore it can be argued that, for example, vaso-pressin in a number of studies has been compared with adrenaline (a treatment without scientific documentation in cardiac arrest) instead of placebo. Naturally, adrenaline has been used because it is recommended in guidelines.

In so-called superiority trials, the intervention must be shown to be better than the control. This is usually the case if the control is inactive or the intervention is supposed to improve the therapeutic efficacy. In some cases, however, the new treatment is not required to be more effective, but only easier to be applied, more tolerable, or safer than is a standard therapy. In this case, only non-inferiority or equivalence with respect to survival is required. Contrary to what would be expected, non-inferiority trials are harder to perform since the new therapy must prove to be not worse than the old one, but it also requires that the trial would have been able to demonstrate a clinically relevant difference, i.e., had a sufficient sample size and quality. Thus, non-inferiority trials require previous knowledge of the effect size of the standard therapy and huge sample sizes, which may explain why non-inferiority trials so far have been rare in resuscitation medicine.

Usually, individual patients are randomized. Some-times, however, interventions cannot be fitted to an indi-vidual patient, but require that a center be reorganized, and the intervention has then to be performed in every patient included in that specific center. In this situation, centers or time periods can be randomized instead of patients. Such trials are called cluster-randomized. They have to be analyzed differently from individually random-ized trials since patients of the same cluster will be more similar than patients from different clusters, compromis-ing the usual independence assumption of classical statis-tics. The statistical quality of such trials is governed by the number of clusters rather than by the total number of patients. A minimum of 30 clusters to be randomized per group is usually postulated. Cluster-randomized trials are thus not very efficient, but frequently this approach is the only way to study complex interventions in the hospital or ICU.

Technically, the best way to randomize is by telephone, which cannot be manipulated in case of local irregularities. Nevertheless, this kind of randomization is expensive and not always practicable. Out-of-hospital studies are some-times better performed by using randomization envelopes or coded study drugs. Irrespective of the method, however, randomization is crucial in such studies and this must be explained in detail to physicians and patients or their rela-tives to be accepted. Moreover, it has to be taken into account that some people will wish to crack the codes just because it is forbidden.

Summaries: systematic reviews, meta-analysis, metaregression, pooled analyses

An essential part of clinical research is the regular summary of evidence from studies. This can be done quali-tatively as a systematic review, by using formal methods of meta-analyses or meta-regression, or by pooling the indi-vidual data of the patients. The last mentioned is the most informative, but also the most elaborate and time-consuming. Quantitative methods rely heavily on advanced statistics and should be performed with great care.

Study population

Criteria for including patients in randomized clinical trials

Study populations can be defined as restrictive, to achieve homogeneity, or liberal, to achieve generalizability. If internal validity is found to be most desirable, homogene-ity is advantageous since sample sizes can be reduced and trials will be shorter, but external validity may be com-promised. Liberal inclusion criteria allow better general-ization but are more expensive. In drug development, restrictive inclusion criteria are applied in phase II, if proof of principle is sought. Liberal inclusion criteria are mandatory in phase III trials to confirm broad clinical effi-cacy. In principle, similar considerations should apply to resuscitation trials.

Most cardiac arrest trials tend to include cases with a presumed cardiac etiology in order to make the patient groups more homogeneous. Nevertheless, patients with other etiologies, including cerebral hemorrhage, will occa-sionally be included as well. It will be extremely difficult to evaluate the effects of interventions on subsets of cardiac arrest patients other than those with a presumed cardiac etiology, because these subsets are likely to be very small. Thus, it may be argued that all cardiac arrests should be included regardless of etiology, if there is no reason to assume that the intervention is particularly advantageous for patients whose arrest had a cardiac cause.

When evaluating the impact of a new intervention in cardiac arrest, patients with a prolonged delay between collapse and start of the intervention have not been included. Such a decision is based on the assumption that the chance of resuscitating a patient with a prolonged delay is extremely low, and therefore the inclusion of such patients will only weaken the chance of proving the effi-cacy of the intervention. Consequently, patients with a non-witnessed cardiac arrest and those with a delay above a certain time limit from either collapse or call for ambu-lance until start of the intervention are often excluded from participation. Although this might be a wise decision, it is important not to make the upper time limit too short, as this would limit the proportion of "available" patients to be included and if the intervention turns out to be positive, there will always be problems how eventually to extrapolate the data from the trial to clinical practice.

Similarly, previous interventions often have specifically addressed patients with a variety of rhythms admitted by the ambulance crew. For example, when evaluating the impact of an anti-arrhythmic agent on outcome, it would be logical to study patients in ventricular fibrillation. It has sometimes been argued that patients in asystole are found so late in their course, that the chance for rescue is minimal, even with the best of interventions. Perhaps it is wise to include patients with all types of rhythms in intervention trials, except for those on antiarrhythmic agents, and clearly state in the protocol that a secondary hypothesis will be to analyse separately the results of the intervention in the three major rhythm groups: ventricular fibrillation, asystole, and pulseless electrical activity.

Sample sizes

The requirement of representativeness and the desire to identify prognostically relevant factors or to collect evidence on treatment effects influence sample size requirements of clinical studies on resuscitation, both observational studies and clinical trials. To provide a representative cardiac arrest population, the sample size generally needs to be substantial, owing to the heterogeneity of patient populations. This is particularly true when subset analyses are to be performed, such as a description of men versus women, or patients with a shockable versus a non-shockable rhythm. Nevertheless, clinically relevant treatment effects can be small in a statistical sense and thus require big trials, particularly for survival endpoints in cardiac arrest because of the low survival rates.

If a confirmatory analysis is prespecified, e.g., in randomized controlled trials, a formal power calculation for determination of sample sizes is possible and desirable. The power of a trial is its ability to provide evidence to support the existence of the postulated treatment effect. Therefore, it should not only have sufficient statistical power but also pharmacodynamic power (i.e., optimal dose for a medication, or regimen for a mechanical device) and design power (optimal design). The power of a trial usually refers to statistical power, which indicates the chance that the expected difference could be detected at a pre-specified level of statistical significance. Sample size calculation is implemented so as to have a high chance of detecting a worthwhile effect, if it exists, and concomitantly to be reasonably sure that no such benefit exists if

it is not found in the trial. Obviously, the greater the power of the study, the more convincing the trial, but a greater power requires a larger sample. The vast majority of clinical trials aiming at evaluating the impact of various interventions in cardiac arrest have been underpowered, and thus have been too small to detect an improvement in long-term survival, such as discharge alive from hospital. Unless the true treatment effect is large, small trials can yield a - statistically significant result only if, by chance, the observed difference in the sample is much larger than the real difference.

Whereas it is evident that a formal sample size calculation is advantageous before start of a trial, the precision of a formal sample size calculation should not be overestimated. Formulae produce exact counts that look (pseudo) precise. But the input to the formulae consists of rough estimates of effect sizes and variances. Clearly, the calculated sample sizes cannot be more precise than the input, that is, previous knowledge from earlier studies. The risk of missing adequate power is always substantial and must be accepted, as inevitable, by the study participants. There is no silver bullet for trial success. Sample size calculations should thus be understood as an instrument to give a rough idea of the required efforts and the risks of a study. Nevertheless, once the sample size is fixed in the protocol, every change has to be justified to avoid the suspicion of manipulation of the results.

Data collection

Data exchange

The classical instrument for data exchange between centers and data management is the Case Record Form (CRF). The development of a CRF is not easy: it must be explicit, unequivocal, unambiguous, and complete; the order must be accurate, clear, concise, and easy to complete. Any mistake in the CRF will subsequently require considerable corrective work, and may result in misunderstanding, data losses, and errors. Frequently, CRFs are produced under pressure since everybody is anxious to begin the study. Nonetheless, we recommend testing the final CRF with a few pilot patients and, if necessary, to improve it.

Today, electronic CRFs, data exchange, and even data entry via the internet are used more frequently. Although electronic media simplify the process and allow immediate plausibility checks, the technical standard at each site must be of high quality to be successful. Data safety and security must be guaranteed. While CRFs are documents that can be used for source verification and reconstruction of data at any time, files can (and will) accidentally be lost, overwritten, exchanged, or deleted. In particular, in out-of-hospital resuscitation medicine, documentation should be easy to handle independent of the location and time, so classical (non-electronic) CRFs may be preferable in some studies.

Monitoring and auditing, plausibility checks

Data quality is absolutely essential in clinical trials, or medical registers. Thus, monitoring (concomitant assistance in data collection, for example, by study nurses/monitors) and auditing (systematic checks and source validation by an independent institution) are valuable instruments, even if expensive, to guarantee the required level of data quality. Alternatively, peer auditing among centers is possible as described in the anecdotal report, (Appendix) but may be less perfect.

The central database should perform prompt plausibility checks soon after the data are submitted and immediately ask for corrections or completion of missing data. 'Clean file' should be declared before any statistical evaluation starts, unless interim analyses are required for the trial to be continued.

Interim analyses

Interim examination of the data may be performed for safety reasons or for efficacy. Both aspects cannot always easily be separated. For example, mortality differences between study groups should be considered for safety reasons, but may at the same time be the primary efficacy endpoint of the study. These issues are discussed below.

Safety interim analyses

Safety aspects should be considered regularly (e.g., for every 50 patients included) to protect the study participants from harm. They are usually done informally. To avoid early stopping due to chance clusters of adverse events in one of the study groups, however, it is advisable to calculate p values, adjusted for the multiplicity of inspections.

Efficacy interim analyses

At study start, the required sample size is estimated based on limited knowledge. One method to deal with this problem is to define milestones (numbers of patients recruited, intervals in calendar time) when the sample size or even the study design may be recalibrated, taking into regard the last interim results and the growing body of scientific knowledge from other studies. Actions after interim examination of the data may compromise the intended study goals, however. As an extreme example, consider a researcher who examines the new data daily and calculates the primary endpoint. If he stops the trial once the endpoint has crossed the significance border, he will end up with a positive study with a probability far above the significance level, even if there is no treatment effect. This phenomenon is called 'alpha-explosion.' To avoid such pitfalls, such interim analyses of efficacy should be pre-specified and complex calculations of the error probabilities performed in advance. The result will be a group sequential plan or an adaptive design. Sequential or adaptive designs allow early stopping of the trial because of success or futility, as well as prolongation as a result of new power calculations, but only according to the pre-specified rules.

Efficacy interim analyses can only be useful if changes to the study design or conduct are still possible. If recruitment phase and treatment duration are short compared to the follow-up interval, interim analyses are useless. In resuscitation research, however, the recruitment phase is usually long and the follow-up to the primary endpoint is short, and thus efficacy interim analyses are frequently mandatory to avoid longer studies than necessary.

Data and Safety Monitoring Board

The interim monitoring, analyses, and recommendations should be performed by an independent Data and Safety Monitoring Board (DSMB) comprising scientists not otherwise involved in the study, in order to avoid conflicts of interest. Ideally, a committee should consist of an uneven number of members (three or five) for clear decisions, and at least one of them should have statistical expertise.

Evaluation and interpretation

Analysis populations

The choice of the analysis populations will depend on the objectives of the study. In medical registers or observational studies, usually the maximal available dataset will be applied that will be representative of the study population. In randomized controlled trials, a valid superiority conclusion requires an endpoint comparison between the random groups according to the intention-to-treat principle, regardless of the actual treatment, in order to avoid masking of bad outcomes in one of the random groups by treatment switch. In contrast, in non-inferiority trials, the actual treatment groups should be compared, but only with patients who were treated strictly according to protocol. Safety evaluations should be performed with all patients who received one of the study treatments at least once.

Unfortunately, so far, most of the cardiac arrest databases suffer from considerable missing information. A major reasons is that a cardiac arrest is one of the most chaotic events in medicine. Thus, missing data will continue to be a serious challenge during the statistical analysis of the study. Missing values may compromise conclusions even from the primary analysis, in particular if the missing data differ between study groups.[18] Unless the percentage of missing values is so small that it can have absolutely no impact on results, there should be some means of handling the missing data. Neither ignoring them nor excluding patients with missing data will suffice. Instead, the application of different methods of imputation and the report on the results in terms of a sensitivity analysis is recommended. Classical imputation methods like mean replacement or LOCF (last observation carried forward) in follow-up-studies are unsatisfactory. Maximum-likelihood imputation or multiple imputation are methods of choice.

For evaluation of response systems and cardiac arrest programs, accurate time registration is important. Often reconstruction of the time of collapse is necessary. Estimation of time intervals is hard in these circumstances,[19] but an observer who can concentrate on the different time sources and correct them with a standard clock. is most likely to be successful.

Choice of statistical method

In randomized trials with two groups, simple two-sample comparisons will be sufficient. Adjustment for baseline differences may slightly improve the power, but it is not required.[20] Subgroup analyses have to be pre-specified and should be evaluated using so-called interaction tests with p-value adjustment for multiplicity.[21] The statistical analysis plan should be finalized before unblinding the study.

In contrast, in observational studies, adjustments for factors and covariates are mandatory for confounder control. Thus, statistical models have to be applied, particularly for longitudinal analyses/analyses of follow-up data with complicated dependence structure that requires a deeper understanding of modern statistical model-building tools.

Interpretation

Interpretation of study results is a major task, even if there is agreement on the statistical evaluation. It requires the close cooperation of physicians and biometricians since neither group can overlook all the consequences and pitfalls alone. Various plotting techniques are helpful for

communication. Effects should be presented with confidence limits to give an account of other possible outcomes that would only differ by chance from the observed one. Conflicting views are frequent and may remain even after a thorough and honest discussion. Convergence of opinions is neither guaranteed nor required (not even in randomized trials) and should be reported in the final publication. In many cases, the result of a study is not what the authors had expected when they started, and thus some may be disappointed in the results. But the impact of a clinical study depends on both confirmation of the expected and/or detection of the unexpected, although the latter will need confirmation in further studies. In this manner, any study, either positive or negative, will contribute to a deeper understanding of the disease or treatment under study and will be reviewed and subjected to meta-analyses. In this sense, a well-performed study is always successful.

Future aspects

Survival in cardiac arrest has remained relatively unchanged during the last decades. One of the main reasons is that clinical research has not contributed much information on the documentation of effects of new interventions. The only hopeful major step forward so far, is research on hypothermia.[22,23]

The solution to this dilemma lies in large randomized clinical trials. If they were introduced it might be possible to forecast a more marked improvement in outcome during subsequent decades.

We need proper interventions to test, however, and most important such trials must be interpreted adequately. This means that the implementation of a new treatment must be based on the results of these trials. Not before all these requirements are fulfilled can we expect to see a more marked improvement in outcome after cardiac arrest.

REFERENCES

1. Lindner, K.H., Strohmenger, H.U., Ensinger, H., Hetzel, W.D., Ahnefeld, F.W. & Georgieff, M. Stress hormone response during and after cardiopulmonary resuscitation. *Anesthesiology* 1992; **77**: 662–668.
2. Lindner, K.H., Prengel, A.W., Pfenninger, E.G. *et al.* Vasopressin improves vital organ blood flow during closed-chest cardiopulmonary resuscitation in pigs. *Circulation* 1995; **91**: 215–221.
3. Wenzel, V., Lindner, K.H., Krismer, A.C., Miller, E.A., Voelckel, W.G. & Lingnau, W. Repeated administration of vasopressin but not epinephrine maintains coronary perfusion pressure

after early and late administration during prolonged cardiopulmonary resuscitation in pigs. *Circulation* 1999; **99**: 1379–1384.

4. Wenzel, V., Lindner, K.H., Krismer, A.C. *et al.* Survival with full neurologic recovery and no cerebral pathology after prolonged cardiopulmonary resuscitation with vasopressin in pigs. *J. Am. Coll. Cardiol.* 2000; **35**: 527–533.

5. Wenzel, V., Krismer, A.C., Arntz, H.R., Sitter, H., Stadlbauer, K.H. & Lindner, K.H. A comparison of vasopressin and epinephrine for out-of-hospital cardiopulmonary resuscitation. *N. Engl. J. Med.* 2004; **350**: 105–113.

6. McIntyre, K.M. Vasopressin in asystolic cardiac arrest. *N. Engl. J. Med.* 2004; **350**: 179–181.

7. Rosenbaum, P.R. *Observational Studies.* New York, Berlin, Heidelberg: Springer, 2002.

8. Meinert, C.L. *Clinical Trials: Design, Conduct, and Analysis.* Oxford: Oxford University Press, 1986.

9. Pocock, S.J. *Clinical Trials: A Practical Approach.* New York: Wiley, 1996.

10. ICH-E8: Note for guidance on general considerations for clinical trials (CPMP/ICH/291/95 – adopted Sept. 97), http://www.emea.eu.int/htms/human/ich/efficacy/ichfin.htm.

11. ICH-E9: Note for guidance on statistical principles for clinical trials (CPMP/ICH/363/96 – adopted Mar. 98), http://www.emea.eu.int/htms/human/ich/efficacy/ichfin.htm.

12. Weaver, W.D. Considerations for improving survival from out-of-hospital cardiac arrest. *Ann. Emerg. Med.* 1986; **15**: 1181–1186.

13. Holmberg, M., Holmberg, S. & Herlitz, J. Incidence, duration and survival of ventricular fibrillation in out-of-hospital cardiac arrest patients in Sweden. *Resuscitation* 2000; **44**: 7–17.

14. Gallagher, E.J., Lombardi, G. & Gennis, P. Effectiveness of bystander cardiopulmonary resuscitation and survival following out-of-hospital cardiac arrest. *J. Am. Med. Assoc.* 1995; **274**: 1922–1925.

15. Holmberg, M., Holmberg, S. & Herlitz, J. Factors modifying the effect of bystander – CPR on survival in out-of-hospital cardiac arrest patients in Sweden. *Eur. Heart J.* 2001; **22**: 511–519.

16. Cobb, L.A., Fahrenbruch, C.E., Walsh, T.R. *et al.* Influence of cardiopulmonary resuscitation prior to defibrillation in patients with out-of-hospital ventricular fibrillation. *J. Am. Med. Assoc.* 1999; **281**(13): 1182–1188.

17. ICH-E10: Note for guidance on choice of control group for clinical trials (CPMP/ICH/364/96 – adopted July 2000), http://www.emea.eu.int/htms/human/ich/efficacy/ichfin.htm.

18. Points to consider on missing data (CPMP/EWP/1776/99 – adopted November 2001), http://ultra.eudra.org/search/query/search.jsp?usearch.p_mode=Basic.

19. Cordell, W.H., Olinger, M.L., Kozak, P.A. & Nyhuis, A.W. Does anybody know what time it is? Does anybody really care? *Ann. Emerg. Med.* 1994; **23**: 1032–1036.

20. Points to consider on adjustment for baseline covariates (CPMP/EWP/2863/99 – adopted May 2003), http://ultra.eudra.org/search/query/search.jsp?usearch.p_mode=Basic.

21. Points to consider on multiplicity issues in clinical trials. (CPMP/EWP/908/99 – adopted September 2002), http://ultra.eudra.org/search/query/search.jsp?usearch.p_mode=Basic.

22. The Hypothermia after Cardiac Arrest Study Group. Mild therapeutic hypothermia to improve the neurologic outcome after cardiac arrest. *N. Engl. J. Med.* 2002; **346**: 549–556.

23. Bernard, S.A., Gray, T.W., Buist, M.D. *et al.* Treatment of comatose survivors of out-of-hospital cardiac arrest with induced hypthermia. *N. Engl. J. Med.* 2002; **346**: 557–563.

Appendix: Experience with a large randomized clinical trial in cardiac arrest

It started in the early 1990s, when it was found that survivors of prehospital cardiac arrest had significantly higher endogenous vasopressin levels than did non-survivors.[1] Multiple experiments in the laboratory followed, which confirmed that vasopressin resulted in superior effects compared with epinephrine during CPR;[2–3] further, neurological recovery was excellent even in pigs undergoing prolonged CPR;[2] results from in-hospital- and out-of-hospital CPR with vasopressin were promising as well;[4] therefore, we decided to organize a randomized controlled clinical trial in Europe to determine effects of vasopressin vs. epinephrine during out-of-hospital CPR. First, a team had to be assembled in both Innsbruck, Austria to do the routine work and organize the trial, and abroad to monitor and control efforts. Colleagues from the European Resuscitation Council offered help. The next step was to provide the study protocol, which obviously required important decisions with respect to inclusion/exclusion criteria, sample size (N=1500), randomizing centers (German-speaking countries Germany, Austria and Switzerland proved to be the most appropriate since everybody involved spoke the same language), and study endpoints (hospital admission and hospital discharge). The importance of the protocol should not be underestimated; bad decisions preclude any subsequent success – multiple face-to-face meetings were beneficial in assessing advantages vs. disadvantages of the protocol.

One continuous threat to the study was lack of funding, which was in large part due to the expired patent of arginine vasopressin. Although we were able to organize funds for the study itself, we were never able to pay anybody for personal efforts. One major expense was travel costs; another big expense was the drug we studied. At first, we had to buy hundreds of arginine vasopressin ampoules; we later convinced the manufacturer to donate arginine vasopressin to us; however, even the manufacturer himself had several unanticipated delivery problems. The study drugs were prepared by a pharmacist in Belgium in a clean-room laboratory in his spare time at night and weekends without pay – he was only reimbursed for expenses for supplies, and a large box of chocolate which he donated to his technicians. From Belgium, the study drugs were shipped to Innsbruck, and sent to the participating centers. During one particularly tense situation with several centers on the brink of running out of study drugs, we had a courier drive the 900 km from Antwerp, Belgium to Innsbruck with the drugs arriving on Christmas Day – they were shipped out to participating centers immediately. The third large expense (~100 Euro/patient) was the patient's insurance to be covered should severe unanticipated complications occur; this was first paid by us, and then sponsored by Pfizer Inc.

Organizing the study itself was the next, exhausting step-two dozen institutional review boards in three countries had to be convinced that the study was worthwhile. Interestingly, many institutional review boards were pragmatic and accepted each other's decision; however, some wanted to have the protocol changed during the study, and one institutional review board did not understand our intention to randomize between treatment arms. Almost all institutional review boards required adaptations of the informed consent form. With the institutional review board's approval, we traveled thousand of kilometers in central Europe to meet and convince colleagues responsible for emergency medical services to randomize patients for the study. This was generally no problem, but it had to be done personally- and many friendships developed.

With the start of the study, the case record form had to be entirely self-explanatory to ensure that the protocol was followed in detail. The study drug kit was self-made, and our medical students were frequent visitors to the local post office hauling material for the study. The study was very well received, and many people supported us who did not benefit from it at all – for example, we first considered black film boxes as containers for the study drugs, and received 1000 of them free one day after a single phone call. Once the study started, grant applications had to be written again: while many applications were rejected, in some cases money surfaced from areas we did not expect; total cost without any salary support was ~250, 000 Euro/US-Dollars.

During the study, we sent to the 44 randomizing emergency medical services in 33 cities packets with coffee with a sticker on each pack entitled "We are unable to pay you for your efforts, but may we invite you for a cup of coffee?" A regular newsletter about any new development ensured continuous updating. Despite all efforts, money was running out in Spring 2002, and we had to stop the study; however, 1219 patients had been randomized. We ensured data quality by doing several cross-checks in the data base (example: did the code of a study drug being sent to Hamburg, Germany, return from Hamburg, Germany?); also, two separate blinded investigators verified that original data were adequately entered into the database. Data analysis should not be underestimated; it is complicated and must be absolutely correct. The database had to be ready to be handed to, for example, Government authorities, who may cross-check any analysis.

These enormous efforts ended up with results indicating no overall difference between vasopressin and adrenaline in terms of survival after out of hospital cardiac arrest. Nevertheless, the study generated several interesting hypotheses: (1) compared with adrenaline vasopressin might improve survival among patients found in asystole; (2) among patients with a more complicated cardiac arrest the combination of vasopressin and epinephrine might be more advantageous than either drug alone;[5,6.] These two hypotheses need to be tested in further prospective clinical trials. Such trials are already being planned (P.Y. Gueugniaud, personal communication).

11

The special problem of consent for resuscitation research

Henry B. Halperin[1] and Douglas Chamberlain[2]

[1] Johns Hopkins University School of Medicine, Baltimore, MD, USA
[2] Prehospital Research Unit, School of Medicine, Cardiff University, UK

Introduction

Over 300 000 Americans die each year from catastrophic medical and surgical emergencies.[1,2] New interventions, based on sound research, could save lives. These research studies must be done in an ethical framework that traditionally includes obtaining prospective informed consent from the research subject. The ethical framework for the conduct of Human Research began with the development of the Nuremberg Code[3,4] in 1949. This code states that (1) informed consent of volunteers must be obtained without coercion of any form, (2) human experiments should be based on prior animal experiments, (3) the anticipated scientific results should justify the experiment, (4) only qualified scientists should conduct medical research, (5) physical and mental suffering should be avoided, and (6) no death or disabling injury should be expected from the research study.

The Declaration of Helsinki[5] was issued in 1964 and defines rules for clinical research. It repeats the ethical concerns stated in the Nuremberg Code, but also gives a provision for enrolling certain patients in clinical research without their consent, by using either proxy consent, or waiver of consent in minimal risk studies.

The subsequent Belmont Report,[6] which was published in 1979, is the cornerstone of ethical principles upon which current federal regulations for the protection of subjects are based. The Report conveys the three major premises of ethical conduct of studies: respect for persons, beneficence, and justice. The Report also provides elements used by Institutional Review Boards for evaluating the ethical standards for individual research proposals. The ethical principles presented in both the Belmont Report and the Declaration of Helsinki have been expanded and clarified in the most recent guidelines published by the Council for International Organizations of Medical Sciences (CIOMS),[7] especially for providing guidelines for applying ethical standards in local circumstances.

A dilemma arises in research studies of interventions for life-threatening emergencies, such as cardiac arrest, catastrophic neurological emergencies, and some instances of major trauma. In these circumstances, a victim may be eligible for a research study, but be unable to give prospective consent because of unconsciousness, or severe alteration in cognition, caused by the life-threatening emergency. Often with such research protocols, the subject must be enrolled immediately so that the potential physiological effects of the experimental intervention can be maximized before the onset of irreversible organ damage.[8,9]

The FDA defines the "therapeutic window" as "the time period, based on available scientific evidence, during which administration of the test article might reasonably produce a demonstrable clinical effect."[10] It is this therapeutic window that is limited or non-existent for research studies of life-threatening emergencies. There generally is not time to seek out a legally authorized patient representative for disclosure and consent. In addition, consent under such emergency circumstances may not meet the standards of informed consent, since there is little time for the investigator to explain the study, and little time for the patient representative to assess the various treatment options available.[11] In addition, the emotional state of the patient representative may eliminate the possibility of reflecting objectively on the situation. Obtaining informed consent is especially difficult in pediatric populations where it has been shown that "the emotional trauma of the

Cardiac Arrest: The Science and Practice of Resuscitation Medicine. 2nd edn., ed. Norman Paradis, Henry Halperin, Karl Kern, Volker Wenzel, Douglas Chamberlain. Published by Cambridge University Press. © Cambridge University Press, 2007.

diagnosis decreases a mother's ability to absorb and understand vital information, and the emergent nature of the children's condition and the urgency to begin treatment further compromise informed consent."[12]

Clinical trials involving research on emergency patients who were unable to give prospective informed consent were traditionally carried out in the United States by either receiving a waiver of informed consent from the local IRB, or by deferred consent.[13,14] In 1993, however, the Office for Protection from Research Risks (OPRR) at the National Institutes of Health and the FDA questioned the legality of the deferred consent practice (45 CFR 46.102(i)).[15] Because of problems with obtaining consent in studies of life-threatening emergencies,[16,17] and its impact on performing such studies, a Coalition Conference of Acute Resuscitation and Critical Care Researchers was held in October 1994. Representatives from over 20 organizations participated in discussions that explored informed consent in emergency research and produced consensus recommendations.[18] In 1996, the FDA and the Department of Health and Human Services published regulations (21 CFR 50.24)[19] for the ethically and legally acceptable conduct of emergency research. Emergency research must operate under exemption from consent, either because of no or minimal risk, or through community exception of consent regulations as outlined by the Office for Human Research Protections (OHRP) and the FDA. These guidelines aim to protect patients from participation in a study they would not consent to if they had decisional capacity. For research that is subject to FDA regulation (i.e., conducted under an Investigational Device Exemption (IDE) or Investigational New Drug (IND) permit), exception from consent can be applied to emergency research if explicit criteria are met (Table 11.1): (a) an IDE or IND is in effect; (b) the research involves human subjects who cannot consent because of their emerging life-threatening medical condition for which available treatments are unproven or unsatisfactory; (c) the intervention must be administered before informed consent from the patient's legally authorized representative is feasible; (d) the sponsor has prior written permission from the FDA; (e) an independent data monitoring committee exists; and (f) the relevant IRB has documented that these conditions were met. In addition, the ethical framework for performing such studies mandates that there is an independent assessment of the risks and benefits of the protocol.

For all research that is supported by federal funding (e.g., NIH), even if the study does not use a drug or device regulated by the FDA, similar criteria are required to determine whether exception to informed consent is warranted for an emergency research study. Further, for research that is not supported by federal funding or subject to FDA regulation

(e.g., a trial of a novel method of manual cardiopulmonary resuscitation), IRBs generally apply similar criteria to determine whether exception from consent is warranted for an emergency research study.

Prior to the initiation of the study, **Community Consultation** and **Public Disclosure** must be provided for each emergency research protocol for which an exception from informed consent is requested.[19] In March 2000, the FDA issued "Draft Guidance" to help clarify the concepts of community consultation and public disclosure.[10] This report stated: "[C]ommunity consultation means providing the opportunity for discussions with, and soliciting opinions from the community(ies) in which the study will take place and from which study subjects will be drawn." The three primary goals of the community consultation process are: (1) to explain the nature of the research, with its attendant risks and benefits; (2) to state that informed consent will not be obtained from individual subjects prior to study participation; and (3) to explain the process by which potential subjects can refuse to participate in research studies.[10] The FDA guidance defines public disclosure as ". . .dissemination of information about the emergency research sufficient to allow a reasonable assumption that communities are aware that the study will be conducted, and later, that the communities and scientific researchers are aware of the study results."[10]

The regulations indicate that each IRB is to exercise its own discretion in determining appropriate community consultation activities and public disclosure, allowing considerations specific to the local community(ies) to be taken into account. The regulations do not explicitly state the amount or types of community consultation and public disclosure that are required to achieve compliance, although the FDA Guidance document does give some general considerations.[10] These requirements for community consultation and public disclosure, although reasonable, sometimes lead to delays in obtaining approval for research studies that use the emergency exception process. Each IRB may lack experience in determining what types of consultation and disclosure are necessary. In addition, there is ambiguity in the regulations as to how individual IRBs should implement such community consultation and public disclosure. In a study in 2003, Shah and Sugarman examined emergency research protocols at 36 centers and reported that to satisfy the public disclosure requirement the majority of these centers used a one-way disclosure method (press releases, institutional and local newsletters, radio and television announcements). A minority of the centers reported using two-way disclosures with the community, including public forums, telephone polls, and written communications.[20]

Table 11.1. Summary of the exception from informed consent requirements for emergency research (21CFR50.24)

Justifications

(1) The research involves a medical condition or situation in which:
   (a) Human subjects are in a life-threatening situation.
   (b) Available treatments are unproven or unsatisfactory.
   (c) Evidence is necessary to determine the safety and effectiveness of particular interventions.
(2) Obtaining informed consent is not feasible because:
   (a) The subject is not able to give consent due to his or her medical condition;
   (b) The intervention must be administered before obtaining consent from legal representative is feasible.
   (c) There is no reasonable way to identify eligible subjects prospectively.
(3) Participation holds out the prospect of direct benefit to the subjects because:
   (a) Subjects face a life-threatening situation which requires intervention.
   (b) Preliminary investigations, including animal studies, and related evidence suggest that this intervention may provide a direct benefit to the individual subject.
   (c) The risks are reasonable.
(4) The clinical investigation could not practically be carried out without the waiver.

Obligations of the investigator

(5) The proposed study protocol defines the length of the potential therapeutic window, and the investigator:
   (a) Commits to attempt to contact and, if feasible, to obtain consent from a legally authorized representative for each subject within that window of time; and
   (b) If a legal representative is not available, commits to attempt to contact within that window some other family member and ask if that family member objects to the subject's inclusion; and
   (c) Will summarize the efforts made to contact legal representatives and family members and make this information available to the IRB at the time of continuing review.
(6) Consultation with representatives of the communities in which the research will be conducted.
(7) Public disclosure to the communities where the research is conducted:
   (a) Prior to initiation of the trial regarding the study plans, risks and benefits;
   (b) After completion, of the results and subject demographics.
(8) Perform the study under a separate investigational new drug application (IND) or investigational device exemption (IDE) from the Food and Drug Administration, even if an IND or IDE already exists.

Obligations of the IRB

(9) The IRB has reviewed and approved procedures and documents for:
   (a) Use in situations when obtaining informed consent is feasible;
   (b) Use when providing an opportunity for a family member to object is feasible.
(10) The IRB is responsible for assuring that procedures are in place to:
   (a) Inform each subject, or a legally authorized representative or family member (if the subject is incapacitated) of his or her inclusion in the study and details of the study;
   (b) Inform each subject or representative that he or she may discontinue participation in the trial;
   (c) Inform subjects who become competent after initial notification to representatives of incompetent subjects;
   (d) Inform a legally authorized representative or family member of subjects who die prior to notification about the trial.
(11) If an IRB determines that it cannot approve a proposed study because it does not meet the criteria for justifying the need for a waiver or for other ethical concerns, the IRB must provide these findings promptly to the investigator and sponsor in writing.
(12) The IRB must retain the determinations and documentation required by the above regulations for three years after completion of the investigation.

Obligation of the sponsor

(13) Develop the protocol in collaboration with appropriate investigators.
(14) Establishment of an independent data monitoring committee to exercise oversight of the clinical investigation.
(15) If an IRB denies approval of a protocol per item 12, the sponsor of the investigation must promptly disclose this information to the FDA, the clinical investigators and other IRBs that have been or are asked to review the same or a substantially equivalent trial. The sponsor must track all information disclosed and assure that disclosed information in placed on the FDA's public docket.

Effect of 21 CFR 50.24 on study approvals

Standardization of community consultation and public disclosure are necessary because there has been inconsistent interpretation of current procedures for implementing research with the exception of informed consent process. There are significant variations in local IRB's interpretation of what is necessary for fulfilling the FDA requirements for community consultation as well as what constitutes the proper venue for the community to provide feedback. These variations make it difficult for the investigator to "guess" what will be necessary for IRB approval in this section of the regulations and this often significantly prolongs the approval process. IRB membership and experience change over time so that the investigator is faced with an ongoing and evolving set of criteria that needs to be met for initial, as well as, continuing approval. Local IRBs place very different demands on different investigators, sometimes making it so onerous to perform Exception of Informed Consent research in certain circumstances that the research is simply not performed, or is moved outside the USA,[21–23] resulting in a lack of availability of potentially life-saving therapies to the entire population.

In addition, the process of community consultation and feedback can be extremely costly and time-consuming. Current processes vary substantially from institution to institution. Financial implications, therefore, vary widely from investigator to investigator. It is very difficult for investigators to know how much money to include for consultation costs, because the costs vary greatly from one IRB to another.

In one large multicenter trial of 24 sites studying defibrillation approaches, it took up to 404 days (median 108), up to 7 submissions (median 2), and cost up to $13,000 (median $1300) to obtain IRB approval.[24] The types and numbers of activities undertaken at each site to fulfill the community consultation and public disclosure requirements were quite diverse. There were public meetings, press releases, letters, brochures, newsletters, e-mails, radio, television or print advertisements, notices, feature stories, and radio and television appearances. Of over 1000 comments received, 96% were reported as "positive," and only 1% were reported as negative".[24] No IRB rejected the project for approval on the basis of negative comments. The experience from this trial in performing community consultation and public disclosure under Exception to Informed Consent demonstrates that despite numerous, costly, time-consuming, and different methods, there was minimal community input in this multi-center study, and that what negative input was expressed did not prohibit the conduct of the trial.

Effect of 21 CFR 50.24 on the number of research studies performed

A number of groups have completed statistics on the number of research studies performed before and after 21 CFR 50.24 was implemented. One group conducted a MEDLINE search using the strategy: "Heart Arrest" or "Cardiac Arrest" and "Human" not including Case Reports.[25] The results were hand-searched by two reviewers for US cardiac arrest articles that met criteria for Exception from Informed Consent. The group compared the fraction of all publications on research in the US during the 4 years since the promulgation of 21 CFR 50.24 to the 4 years before the moratorium.

Between 1990 and 1993 MEDLINE listed 1 090 395 clinical publications, of which 46 were US cardiac arrest studies meeting exception criteria; between 1997 and 2000 there were 1 288 460 clinical publications, of which 13 met cri-teria ($P < 0.001$).[25] Despite this dramatic drop in the number of studies published, it was noted by the group that publication delay may shift the effect time of these events such that a study performed before the moratorium appeared in the literature after the New Rule took effect. This decrease may also represent a lack of familiarity with the new Rule rather than an intrinsic negative effect of the Rule on emergency research. They concluded, however, that there has been a significant decrease in the number of published US emergency human cardiac arrest clinical trials under the new FDA Rule.

Effect of 21 CFR 50.24 on commercial entities

The effects of delays in obtaining study approvals can be extreme for commercial entities, where each month of delay incurs substantial cost to the commercial entity because of ongoing requirements for operating expenses. Companies that ceased commercial operations, and which were attempting to perform studies to determine the safety and efficacy of unapproved devices include Cardiologic Systems, Inc,[26] and Theracardia, Inc.[23] It is unlikely that the delays in study approval were the sole reason for the demise of those companies, but they may have contributed substantially. Other commercial entities have opted to perform emergency medicine studies in other countries, where approvals can proceed expeditiously. Industry's decision to move many trials on potentially life-saving therapies for diseases where conventional therapies are woefully inadequate to countries with less stringent and ambiguous regulations may deprive the United States population of the possible benefit of these interventions.

Studies with non-approved drugs or devices

IRB approval can be even more difficult if the drug or device to be studied has not been approved for sale by the FDA. The issue for the IRB is that they are asked to approve a research study where a drug or device that has not been approved by the FDA is used on test subjects without their consent, there is likely to be a fatal outcome because of the inherent disease state, and the next of kin will be notified of these details. In many emergency situations, such as cardiac arrest, mortality may exceed 90%. This is obviously why the research is critical. Because of the large numbers of victims of these conditions, even small increases in survival could save many lives. Even if the experimental drug of device would only reduce mortality from 90 to 80% – that would translate into a potential saving of more than 20 000 lives per year for that one therapy. Some IRBs have expressed great reluctance to approve such studies because of fear of liability. They believe that they can be successfully sued for enrolling research subjects into research studies without the subject's consent, even if appropriate federal guidelines have been followed. In general, companies sponsoring studies under an IND or IDE of drugs or devices are required by the study sites (universities, and others) to provide indemnification (insurance). This is a "cost of doing business." Large companies expect this. Small companies are often surprised, and the need for expensive liability insurance can be a substantial barrier to performing studies dealing with emergency research.

Community consultation and public disclosure template

The American Heart Association has published recommendations for implementation of Community Consultation and Public Disclosure.[27] A template is presented that (1) provides for quantification of the minimum requirements that an IRB might adopt, (2) gives examples to help IRBs quickly become familiar with the process of implementing and reviewing studies proposed with Exception to Informed Consent, and (3) proposes that trials of interventions approved by the FDA for the indication being studied should require levels of community consultation and public disclosure different from studies of unapproved interventions. The template gives a common interpretation of the requirements, and provides a list of actions acceptable for the implementation of community consultation and public disclosure.

Ethics

The guiding ethical principle for the template is that there is a range of actions that are acceptable to protect subjects' autonomy, depending on the risk of the study. The risk referred to here is the incremental risk of participation in the proposed study, over and above the risks of having sustained a life-threatening emergency and being treated with standard interventions. The higher the risk of the study, the more stringent are the actions that are required to protect subjects' autonomy. Since there is a range of risk associated with different study interventions, different levels of community consultation and public disclosure can be used to balance subjects' autonomy appropriately with the public good.

A trial of an approved therapy should not require the same level of community notification and consultation as one where non-approved or not-generally-accepted interventions are being introduced for the first time. For interventions that were not approved by the FDA, the risk of the therapy could be incrementally higher, and the level of community consultation and public disclosure for the study should similarly be higher.

It was, therefore, proposed that it is ethically acceptable to stratify the intensity of community consultation and public disclosure based upon the anticipated incremental risks to subjects participating in a research study. It was acknowledged that any research study may have unanticipated risks, but the argument for stratifying community consultation and public disclosure was based on the reasonable and prudent prediction of subject risk.

The proposal regarding stratifying community consultation is analogous to how IRBs currently review research protocols and informed consent documents. For example, IRB review of a protocol that studies unlinked serum samples will not require the same considerations as a project involving the use of a novel immunosuppressive agent in kidney transplantation. The study of unlinked serum samples may be considered to have minimal risk and therefore be eligible for expedited review, while the transplantation study requires standard IRB review. Similarly, the informed consent document may be shorter and simpler for the serum sample study than for the transplantation study. Indeed, for the transplantation study, the IRB may suggest in addition to an extensive consent protocol, the use of supplemental educational material or the involvement of a patient advocate to ensure that subjects fully understand the risks, benefits, and alternatives to participation. The point is that while all emergency research that is not minimal risk requires some level of public disclosure and community consultation, emergency research studies that have less incremental risk, and are not politically and culturally controversial, may be performed ethically with lesser degrees of community consultation and public disclosure than would be needed for high risk or controversial studies.

Stratification of risk

The template breaks studies into categories of minimal, low, intermediate, and high incremental risk. Any sudden, catastrophic, life-threatening condition places patients at high risk for substantial morbidity and mortality. Instead of paying heed only to the inherent risk of the underlying disease, which is present whether the patient is enrolled in the study or not, we recommend evaluating the incremental risk from participating in the proposed study. That evaluation can then be used to determine the degree of community consultation and public disclosure appropriate for the proposed study.

Certain studies are justifiable without documented consent under minimal risk criteria. Consider the study of a therapy approved by the FDA for the indications being studied being compared to another therapy that was approved or did not need approval (e.g., manual CPR). The study likely would carry a risk that was minimally above the risk of being treated with either approved therapy. In the absence of a research protocol, physicians could ethically and legally choose to treat patients with a life-threatening condition with either of these interventions. The only additional factors introduced by a research study of these interventions are (1) that the patients are being randomized to one of the approved interventions, and (2) the loss of privacy and confidentiality during review of the clinical record after the intervention has been applied. Therefore, if the randomization procedure does not introduce any significant delay in applying the approved therapies, such a study is justifiable without documented consent under minimal risk criteria. The rationale for not having an informed consent document is described in the preamble to the final rule for 21 CFR 50:

The agency thinks that it may not always be possible to develop a meaningful informed consent document for continued participation in the research, because the relevant information may vary significantly depending upon when it becomes feasible to provide the information to the subject or legally authorized representative. The agency is, therefore, not requiring that such a form be developed. The agency notes however that Sec. 50.24 (a)(6) places the responsibility on the IRB to review and approve

"informed consent procedures and an informed consent document" for use with subjects or their legal representatives, and procedures and information to be used in consultations with family members, in situations where use of such procedures is feasible. [Page 51520]

During the comment period for these regulations, the agency received feedback that the subject should be able to choose to continue to participate fully in a study, to continue the intervention but not have their data included in the research database or results, or to discontinue the intervention and use of the subject's data. This was rejected on the following grounds:

FDA regulations . . . require investigators to prepare and maintain adequate case histories recording all observations and other data pertinent to the investigation on each individual treated with the drug or exposed to the device. The agency needs all such data in order to be able to determine the safety and effectiveness of the device. The fact of having been in an investigation cannot be taken back. Also, if a subject were able to control the use (inclusion and exclusion) of his or her data, and particularly if the clinical investigation were not blinded, the bias potential would be immense. (Page 51520)

The factors that can help decide the degree of incremental risk added by a particular study are shown in Table 11.2. It was proposed that IRBs use the following criteria to determine incremental risk: (1) FDA labeling status of the investigational therapeutic drug or device, for studies of interventions; (2) an evaluation of whether the study introduces any additional risk of harm over that of simply using the investigational therapeutic drug or device (such as any delays in applying therapy that may be introduced by the randomization process); (3) the degree of invasiveness and need for real-time clinical decisions, for studies of diagnostics; and (4) the potential sensitive nature of the study from the community(ies)' perspective, including political cultural and religious considerations. For a therapeutic intervention, therefore, the study would have minimal, low, intermediate, or high incremental risk based on the FDA labeling status of the therapy and the assessment of whether there was minimal risk of being in the study (Table 11.2, "Intervention" row), unless it were placed in a higher risk category based on the community(ies)' sensitivity (Table 11.2, bottom row). The same would be true for the study of a diagnostic, where the type of diagnostic would place it in minimal, intermediate, or high risk categories on the basis of the degree of invasiveness, the need for real-time decision-making, and whether the diagnostic is FDA-approved (Table 2, "Diagnostic" row), unless it were placed in a higher risk category by the perceived community(ies)' sensitivity (Table 11.2, bottom row).

Table 11.2. Assessment of incremental risk of research studies

Study Type	Potential incremental risk added by study			
	Minimal	Low	Intermediate	High
Intervention (Device/drug)	(1) FDA-approved for proposed study indication (2) and/or already in clinical use for study indication (3) and have minimal risk of harm from being in the study. (e.g., Approved mechanical CPR devices standard CPR; amiodarone vs lidocaine)	(1) FDA-approved for proposed study indication (2) and/or already in clinical use for study indication (3) and have higher than minimal risk of harm from being in the study	(1) FDA-approved for clinical use, (2) but not for the study indication.	Not FDA-approved for any indication yet.
Diagnostic (Test/device/ feature)	(1) Non-invasive, (2) and not used for real-time clinical decisions. (e.g.: non-invasive monitor, low volume blood drawing)		(1) Minimally invasive, (2) and not used for real-time clinical decisions. (e.g., transconjunctival oxygen saturation)	(1) More than minimally invasive, (2) or used for real-time clinical decisions, (3) or not FDA approved. (e.g., intracranial pressure monitor)
Community's potential sensitivity (Political, cultural, religious)	Very unlikely to have community sensitivity	Very unlikely to have community sensitivity	Possibly to have community sensitivity	Likely to have community sensitivity

For a therapy, the study would have minimal, low, intermediate, or high incremental risk based on the FDA labeling status of the therapy, and the assessment of whether there was minimal risk from being in the study ("Intervention" row), unless it were placed in a higher risk category based on the community(ies)' sensitivity (bottom row). For a diagnostic: the study would have minimal, intermediate, or high risk categories based on the degree of invasiveness and the need for real-time decision making ("Diagnostic" row), unless it were placed in a higher risk category by the perceived community(ies)' sensitivity (bottom row).

Levels of community consultation and public disclosure

Once the degree of incremental risk is determined, it was proposed that the amount and types of community consultation and public disclosure be guided by Table 11.3. For minimal risk studies, no community consultation or public disclosure is required, although minimal community consultation should be considered. For low incremental risk studies, minimal community consultation would be needed. For example, review and feedback from an appropriate group, committee, panel, or organization representative of the study community could allow appropriate community consultation without excessive time being needed to wait for public comment from a published advertisement. Alternatively, there could be solicitation through a website or public notices (such as through a mass media piece), with a call-in number and/or web address provided for feedback. For a high incremental risk study, however, more community consultation would be required, including an appropriate number of mass media solicitations, community meetings, and contact with prominent community organizations. Specific examples of community consultations and public disclosures are available at: www.americanheart.org/emergencyexception. It was emphasized that the recommendations of Table 11.3 are simply guidelines. Individual IRBs will set their own standards based on their individual considerations. It was also emphasized that involvement of the community

Table 11.3. Levels of community consultation and public disclosure suggested at different degrees of incremental risk

	Potential incremental risk added by study		
	Low	Intermediate	High
Community Consultation Options	Review and feedback from an appropriate group, committee, panel or organization representative of the study community. Alternatively, consider solicitation through website or public notices (such as through a mass media piece), with a call-in number and/or web address provided for feedback	(1) As in Low (2) Plus consider solicitation through website or public notices (such as through a few mass media pieces). (3) Call-in number and/or web address provided for feedback	(1) Review and feedback from at least one group, committee, panel, or organization representative of the study community, (2) Public forum(s) or presentation at municipal government meeting(s) in the study community. (3) Solicitation via a number of mass media pieces. (4) Call-in number and/or web address provided for feedback
Public Disclosure Options	Single targeted effort deemed most likely to reach study community: This could be through a mass media piece or distribution of information in more focused manner to likely subjects. (e.g., targeted: poster, brochure, or newsletter article in senior citizen center where study will be conducted.)	At least one targeted effort and a mass media piece. Consider website.	Multiple efforts, including both targeted efforts and mass media pieces, as deemed necessary to reach the community adequately. Website recommended.
Patient / family notification of participation	Reasonable attempts required for written communication regardless of patient survival status (e.g., letter, including invitation to meet with investigator or study coordinator to discuss)		

For minimal risk, no community consultation or public disclosure is needed, although a single announcement could be considered. A mass media piece refers to a newspaper article or advertisement, or a radio announcement, or a television spot.

should include attempts to consult with targeted, at-risk, or interested populations.

Definition of Community for Pediatric Studies

There is a unique problem in the definition of what constitutes a "Community" for pediatric studies. For many pediatric populations, the "Community" could be defined to include a group of patients with a specific disease, their families, as well as the appropriate health care providers (especially in the in-hospital environment). In these types of situations, rather than a particular geographic based community, consultation with the "Community at risk"

may be most appropriate. This process should be differentiated, however, from prospective informed consent of all patients at risk, as the latter process may not be feasible because of the potentially large numbers of patients involved.

Definition of Community for Hospital-based Studies

Also there is a unique problem in the definition of what constitutes a "community" for hospital-based studies. For many hospital populations, the "community" could be defined to include a group of patients who present to the ambulatory, emergency, and wards of the hospital, their families, visitors, as well as the appropriate health care providers. In these types of situations, where it is not feasible to consent every individual who enters the grounds of the hospital, consultation with the "community at risk" may be most appropriate. This process should be differentiated, however, from prospective informed consent of all patients at risk, as the latter process may not be feasible owinge to the potentially large numbers of patients involved.

The situation in Europe

Difficulties in the United States have been mirrored in Europe – at least within the European Union (EU) – although the major problems came later. Differences exist among Member States despite an intention for a uniform approach.

Until relatively recently, emergency research in Europe was conducted in accordance with the terms of the revised Declaration of Helsinki[5] that permitted research involving mentally incompetent subjects subject to appropriate safeguards. The situation changed, however, with a Clinical Trials Directive from the EU in 2001[28] that had to be implemented by all EU countries by May 2004. This Directive reiterated the general principle that research involving medicinal products required the written informed consent from participating subjects, but it did make reference in its Article 5 to the inclusion of incapacitated adults who had neither given nor refused informed consent before the onset of their incapacity. Nine conditions were set out; whilst some of them were unexceptionable, others have put major obstacles in the way of research in emergency situations.

Without the ability to obtain consent from the subject, the Directive stated that informed consent must be obtained from a legal representative, either the next of kin or a suitable person independent of the research team. Considerable uncertainty exists in some parts of the EU about the definition of a legal representative which was intended to be determined by national law. But in any case the stipulation for prior written consent is impractical for emergency research where interventions have to be made either immediately or at least within minutes. These include resuscitation from sudden cardiac arrest, but also treatment of acute heart attacks, stroke, serious head injury, and many forms of shock. Some member states have waived the requirement to seek prior written consent from a legal representative if treatment must be started urgently. Whilst this is outside the strict wording of the Directive, no objections seem to have been raised to this liberal interpretation. The alternative approach has generally been to seek consent later from any subject who regains mental competence, or otherwise from a legal representative who is preferably a close family member. With this arrangement, ongoing treatment would certainly be halted if consent were refused, but the position is less clear for cases in which it had already been completed: is it then permissible to retain the data for analysis? If not, the possibility of bias is clear. A person whose condition has improved may be more likely to consent to inclusion of data than family members whose relative has not recovered. On the other hand, in some types of study a survivor may be unwilling to continue with treatment, whereas non-survivors would not be in a position to withdraw from participation.

The Directive also stipulates that research without individual consent can be considered only to validate data obtained from persons able to give consent or from other research methods: this does have reasonable flexibility since treatments would hardly be considered unless some previous clinical or experimental evidence is available. An additional clause is, however, more problematic: it states that the research must relate *directly* to the condition from which the subject suffers. Interpreted narrowly this prevents research that involves the general care of incapacitated patients. A relevant example might be research into the rate or volume of ventilatory support in those being treated during or after cardiac arrest, the importance of which was highlighted in recent observational and experimental studies.[29] Such research would not relate directly to the condition causing the cardiac arrest but rather to supportive therapy, and therefore would be unacceptable according to a strict acceptance of this provision from the Directive.

An even greater problem with the European Directive springs from a paragraph that requires an *expectation* that administration of experimental medicinal treatment will produce a benefit outweighing any risk or produce no risk at all. Almost any intervention carries some risk, however small. Moreover, the notion that a treatment under investigation must be more likely than not to offer benefit undermines the whole principle of equipoise that should be an ethical basis for randomized controlled trials!

The Directive has not been implemented in a uniform way by Member States. Variations are not restricted to the interpretation of the term "legal representative" mentioned above. Some Member States have have sought to widen the provisions of the Directive to include not only medicinal products but all research, whereas the legal framework in others is loose enough to impose little restriction on research that most ethicists would accept as legitimate. The variations within Europe have been reviewed by Lemaire and colleagues.[30] Within the United

Kingdom a review has been undertaken of the regulations that implemented the Directive. These were acknowledged by the Government to have been unduly restrictive as they were closely based on the Directive. The anticipated changes in the implementing legislation will thus permit a resumption of emergency research that is currently impossible to conduct lawfully. Curtailment of important studies has existed from the time of the publication of the Directive, 3 years before it became mandatory, because of fears that any on-going studies that remained incomplete by May 2004 may have to be terminated prematurely. The danger to emergency research was foreseen by many active in the field[31] but by then the terms of the Directive could not be changed.

The hope now is that Member States that have interpreted the Directive strictly in their implementing legislation may be prepared to introduce modifications in line with the perceived intention of the Directive to permit some flexibility. The initiative within the United Kingdom may encourage others to follow suit. To give guidance to this approach, a working group assembled in Vienna in May 2005 under the auspices of the Department for Ethics in Medical Research of the Vienna Medical University, in cooperation with other relevant groups, and recommendations have been published.[32]

Conclusions

In conclusion, obtaining informed consent from patients or surrogates is difficult in the setting of serious emergency conditions. Current regulations do allow studies to be performed with Exception to Informed Consent, but ambiguities in implementing studies under current regulations can be onerous for IRBs and investigators, and may discourage research to evaluate promising interventions. The proposed template to help guide IRBs to comply with the Federal Regulations may help with striking an appropriate balance between protecting eligible patients, and preserving the public good in the United States. For the moment, however, a serious barrier to the development of evidence-based treatments for many emergency conditions exists in Europe as in the United States.

REFERENCES

1. Zheng, Z.J., Croft, J.B., Giles, W.H. & Mensah, G.A. Sudden cardiac death in the United States, 1989 to 1998. *Circulation* 2001; **104**: 2158–2163.
2. *MMWR Morb Mortal Wkly Rep.* 2002; **51**: 126.
3. Trials of war criminals before the Nuremberg military tribunals under Control Council Law. *US Government Printing Office.* 1949; **2**: 181–182.
4. Katz, J. The Nuremberg Code and the Nuremberg Trial. A reappraisal. *J. Am. Med. Assoc.* 1996; **276**: 1662–1666.
5. Rickham, P.P. Human Experimentation. Code of Ethics of the World Medical Association. Declaration of Helsinki. *Br. Med. J.* 1964; **5402**: 177.
6. Protection of human subjects: Belmont Report – ethical principles and guidelines for the protection of human subjects of research. *Federal Register* 1979; **44**: 23192–23197.
7. International Ethical Guidelines for Biomedical Research Involving Human Subjects. Geneva: Council for International Organizations of Medical Sciences (CIOMS) in collaboration with the World Health Organization (WHO); 2002.
8. Weaver, W.D., Cobb, L.A., Hallstrom, A.P., Fahrenbruch, C., Copass, M.K. & Ray, R. Factors influencing survival after out-of-hospital cardiac arrest. *J. Am. Coll. Cardiol.* 1986; **7**: 752–757.
9. Eisenberg, M.S., Bergner, L. & Hallstrom, A. Out-of-hospital cardiac arrest: improved survival with paramedic services. *Lancet* 1980; **1**: 812–815.
10. Guidance for Institutional Review Boards, Clinical Investigators, and Sponsors: Exception from Informed Consent Requirements for Emergency Research. In: FDA; http://www.fda.gov/ora/compliance_ref/bimo/err_guide.htm; 2000.
11. Williams, B.F., French, J.K. & White, H.D. Informed consent during the clinical emergency of acute myocardial infarction (HERO-2 consent substudy): a prospective observational study. *Lancet* 2003; **361**: 918–922.
12. Stevens, P.E. & Pletsch, P.K. Ethical issues of informed consent: mothers' experiences enrolling their children in bone marrow transplantation research. *Cancer Nurs* 2002; **25**: 81–87.
13. Frost, N. & Robertson, J. Deferring consent with incompetent patients in an intensive care unit. *IRB: A Review of Human Subjects Research* 1980; **2**: 5–6.
14. Abramson, N.S., Meisel, A. & Safar, P. Deferred consent. A new approach for resuscitation research on comatose patients. *J. Am. Med. Assoc.* 1986; **255**: 2466–2471.
15. Protection of human subjects. *45 CFR46.102(i).* 1993.
16. Lurie, K.G., Shultz, J.J., Callaham, M.L. *et al.* Evaluation of active compression–decompression CPR in victims of out-of-hospital cardiac arrest. *J. Am. Med. Assoc.* 1994; **271**: 1405–1411.
17. Biros, M.H. Research without consent: current status, 2003. *Ann. Emerg. Med.* 2003; **42**: 550–564.
18. Biros, M.H. Development of the multiorganizational document regarding emergency research consent. *Acad. Emerg. Med.* 1996; **3**: 101–105.
19. US Department of Health and Human Services; Protection of Human Subjects: Informed Consent and Waiver of Informed Consent Requirements in Certain Emergency Research. Final Rules. Codified at 21 CFR, Part 50, and 45 CFR, Part 46. *Federal Register.* 1996; **61**: 51500–51533.
20. Shah, A.N. & Sugarman, J. Protecting research subjects under the waiver of informed consent for emergency

research: experiences with efforts to inform the community. *Ann. Emerg. Med.* 2003; **41**: 72–78.

21. Plaisance, P., Lurie, K.G., Vicaut, E. *et al.* A comparison of standard cardiopulmonary resuscitation and active compression–decompression resuscitation for out-of-hospital cardiac arrest. French Active Compression–Decompression Cardiopulmonary Resuscitation Study Group. *N. Engl. J. Med.* 1999; **341**: 569–575.

22. Weston, C., de Laorre, F., Dick, W., Chamberlain, D. & Bossaert, L. Vest CPR system: results of a multicenter randomized pilot study. *J. Am. Coll. Cardiol.* 1998; **4**: S910.

23. Rozenberg, A., Incagnoli, P., Delpech, P. *et al.* Prehospital use of minimally invasive direct cardiac massage (MID-CM): a pilot study. *Resuscitation* 2001; **50**: 257–262.

24. Mosesso, V.N., Jr., Brown, L.H., Greene, H.L. *et al.* Conducting research using the emergency exception from informed consent: the Public Access Defibrillation (PAD) Trial experience. *Resuscitation* 2004; **61**: 29–36.

25. Paradis, N., Tashkin, J., Heard, K. & Halperin, H. Effect of the FDAs final rule on informed consent and waiver of informed consent in emergency research circumstances on human cardiac arrest research in the United States. *Circulation* 2002; **106**: II-367.

26. Kremers, M.S., Whisnant, D.R., Lowder, L.S. & Gregg, L. Initial experience using the Food and Drug administration guidelines for emergency research without consent. *Ann. Emerg. Med.* 1999; **33**: 224–229.

27. Halperin, H., Paradis, N., Mosesso, V. *et al.* Recommendations for Implementation of Community Consultation and Public Disclosure under the FDA "Exception from Informed Consent Requirements for Emergency Research" An American Heart Association Scientific Statement from the Emergency Cardiovascular Care Committee. *Circulation.*

28. Directive 2001/20/EC on the approximation of the laws, regulations and administrative provisions of the Member States relating to the implementation of good clinical practice in the conduct of clinical trials on medical products for human use. 2001.

29. Aufderheide, T.P., Sigurdsson, G., Pirrallo, R.G. *et al.* Hyperventilation-induced hypotension during cardiopulmonary resuscitation. *Circulation* 2004; **109**: 1960–1965.

30. Lemaire, F., Bion, J., Blanco, J. *et al.* The European Union Directive on Clinical Research: present status of implementation in EU member states' legislations with regard to the incompetent patient. *Intens. Care Med.* 2005; **31**: 476–479.

31. Sterz, F., E.A.S., Bottiger, B., Chamberlain, D., Baskett, P., Bossaert, L. & Steen, P. A serious threat to evidence based resuscitation within the European Union. *Resuscitation* 2002; **53**: 237–238.

32. Liddell, K., Chamberlain, D., Menon, D.K. *et al.* The European Clinical Trials Directive Revisited: the VISEAR recommendations. *Resuscitation*, 2006.

Part III

The pathophysiology of global ischemia and reperfusion

12

The etiology of sudden death

Sunil K. Sinha, Arthur J. Moss[1], and Hugh G. Calkins

Johns Hopkins Hospital, Baltimore, MD, USA
[1] and University of Rochester Medical Center, Rochester, NY, USA

Definition

Sudden death is natural death, heralded by loss of consciousness within 1 hour of the onset of acute symptoms. The time and mode of death are unexpected. This definition is meant to satisfy medical and scientific considerations as well legal and social concerns.[1] Included within this construct are four temporal elements: (a) prodromes, (b) onset of terminal event, (c) cardiac arrest, and (d) progression to biological death. Prodromes, if any, are new or worsening symptoms that begin during an arbitrarily defined period of up to 24 hours before the onset of cardiac arrest. The 1-hour time period described in the definition refers to the duration of the terminal event leading to cardiac arrest. Following cardiac arrest – the clinician's synonym for *sudden death*, biological death may ensue within minutes, or alternatively, due to community-based interventions and life support systems, may be delayed for a long period of time and even aborted altogether. Nonetheless, for legal, forensic, and certain social considerations, *biological death* is used as the absolute definition of death.

Epidemiology and Causation

A large prospective cohort study – the Framingham study – observed that over a 26-year period, 13% of all deaths were sudden in nature as defined by death within 1 hour of the onset of symptoms.[2,3] In the Western hemisphere, cardiac causes currently predominate in sudden deaths among adults. One large retrospective analysis of death certificates in the United States reported that 88% of sudden deaths were due to cardiac causes.[4] Hence, an estimated 300 000 sudden cardiac deaths occur annually in the United States, accounting for about 50% of all deaths due to cardiovascular disease.[5,6] Accordingly, the general incidence of sudden cardiac death in the unselected United States population > 35 years of age is 1 – 2/1000 (0.1%–0.2%) per year.

A number of diseases are associated with cardiac and non-cardiac sudden death in adults (Table 12.1). Several subgroups at high risk for sudden cardiac death have been accurately identified. These include those individuals who have already survived a cardiac arrest, those with coronary artery disease (especially prior myocardial infarction), and those with left ventricular hypertrophy or systolic dysfunction.[7] Conventional, modifiable atherosclerosis risk factors such as cigarette smoking, hypertension, diabetes mellitus, dyslipidemia, and obesity serve as readily identifiable markers of increased risk, although their primary significance lies in their link to coronary artery disease, the predominant disease predisposing to sudden cardiac death.[8,9] The clinical dilemma that remains is that *the majority of sudden cardiac deaths occur in people who are not currently recognized as being at high risk* (Fig. 12.1(a), (b)).

Neurological causes, such as large acute ischemic or hemorrhagic stroke and seizures, constitute a distant second leading cause of sudden death. Respiratory compromise leading to hypoxia, catecholamine excess, metabolic acidosis, and asphyxia from a variety of causes may result in a fatal event. Likewise, significant metabolic and electrolyte derangements may cause sudden death. Acute infections may lead to sudden unexpected death due to meningitis, myocarditis, and endocarditis. A variety of toxins, including prescription and non-prescription drugs,

Cardiac Arrest: The Science and Practice of Resuscitation Medicine. 2nd edn., ed. Norman Paradis, Henry Halperin, Karl Kern, Volker Wenzel, Douglas Chamberlain. Published by Cambridge University Press. © Cambridge University Press, 2007.

Table 12.1. Acute and subacute causes of sudden death in adults

I.   Coronary atherosclerosis (acute ischemia, prior infarction)
II. Congestive heart failure
     a. Chronic
     b. Acute
III. Valvular heart disease (e.g., critical aortic stenosis)
IV. Ventricular hypertrophy
     a. Acquired (hypertensive heart disease)
     b. Congenital (hypertrophic cardiomyopathy)
     c. Cor pulmonale
V.   Aortic dissection
V.   Congenital heart disease
     a. Coronary artery anomalies
     b. Complex congenital defects (especially if complicated by Eisenmenger's physiology)
     c. Surgically corrected defects (e.g., Tetralogy of Fallot repair)
     d. Hypertrophic cardiomyopathy
     e. Arrhythmogenic right ventricular dysplasia
     f. Cardiac ion channelopathies
     g. Wolff–Parkinson–White syndrome
     h. Idiopathic ventricular tachycardia
     i. Idiopathic ventricular fibrillation
     j. Congenital heart block
VI. Acquired conduction abnormalities
     a. Lenegre's disease
     b. Lev's disease
VII. Infiltrative cardiomyopathy
     a. Sarcoidosis
     b. Chagas disease
     c. Amyloidosis
     d. Hemachromatosis
VIII. Pericardial disease (pericardial effusion causing cardiac tamponade)
IX. Cardiac tumors (e.g., atrial myxoma with acute valvular obstruction)
X.   Neurological
     a. Cerebrovascular accident (ischemic or hemorrhagic)
     b. Seizures
XI. Infectious
     a. Septic shock
     b. Meningitis
     c. Myocarditis
     d. Endocarditis
XII. Respiratory
     a. Severe bronchospasm
     b. Massive pulmonary embolism
     c. Acute pneumonitis
     d. Aspiration
     e. Sleep apnea (central or obstructive)
XIII. Immunological
     a. Anaphylactic shock
     b. Angioedema (causing asphyxiation)

Table 12.1. (continued)

XIV. Rheumatological
      a. Myocarditis
      b. Coronary arteritis
      c. Endocarditis (Libman–Sacks disease)
      d. Cerebritis
XV.   Toxic agents
      a. Recreational drugs (such as cocaine, heroin, alcohol)
      b. Pharmaceutical drugs (such as drug-induced long QT syndrome)
XVI. Electrolyte and metabolic disturbances
      a. Hyperglycemia (diabetic ketoacidosis, hyperosmolar non-ketotic acidosis) or hypoglycemia
      b. Hyperkalemia or hypokalemia
      c. Hypocalcemia
      d. Metabolic acidosis
XVII. Trauma
      a. Hemorrhagic shock
      b. Spinal shock
      c. Pneumothorax
      d. Blunt cardiac trauma (commotio cordis)
      e. Myocardial or aortic rupture

illegal narcotics, and alcohol may yield fatal consequences especially when used in excess. Sudden death due to trauma may ensue from a direct cardiac insult such as blunt cardiac trauma (*commotio cordis*) (Chapter 65), myocardial or aortic rupture, and acute cardiac tamponade, or indirectly from massive exsanguination or the triggering of one or more of the other causal processes mentioned above.

Sudden death in the pediatric and young adult population contains several unique features. In particular, *sudden infant death syndrome* is most likely to strike between birth and 6 months of age and has an incidence of 0.1%–0.3% of live births.[10] Established risk factors for sudden infant death include male sex, premature birth, maternal smoking, bed sharing, gastroesophageal reflux, and prone position.[11–13] This syndrome likely consists of a variety of causes both cardiac (such as cardiac ion channelopathies, high risk atrioventricular accessory pathways) and noncardiac (central nervous system respiratory dysfunction).[14–18] In contrast to adults, studies indicate that only 19% of sudden deaths in children between 1–13 years of age and 30% of sudden deaths in those 14–21 years of age are of cardiac origin.[19] Among the general population of adolescents and young adults < 30 years of age, the overall risk of sudden cardiac death is estimated to be 1/100 000 (0.001%) per year.[20,21] A significant element of sudden cardiac deaths in this population consists of either familial or spontaneous genetic mutations expressed as hypertrophic cardiomyopathy, arrhythmogenic right ventricular

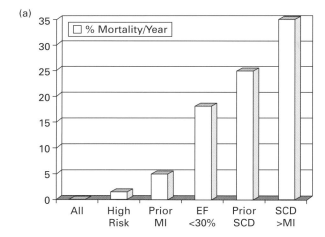

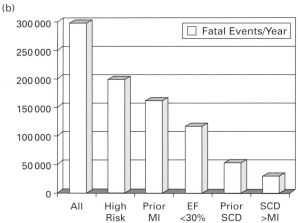

Fig. 12.1(a). Estimates of incidence (percent/year) of sudden death are shown for the overall adult population (**ALL**) and increasingly higher risk subgroups in the United States[5] (**HIGH RISK,** multiple coronary risk factors; **Prior MI,** prior myocardial infarction; **EF < 30%,** left ventricular ejection fraction < 30%; **Prior SCD,** prior resuscitated or aborted sudden cardiac death; **SCD > MI,** resuscitated or aborted VT/VF postacute myocardial infarction).

(**b**) Estimates of the total annual number (events/year) of sudden deaths are shown for the overall adult population and increasingly higher risk subgroups in the United States (abbreviated group labels as per Fig. 12.1(a)). The progressively smaller denomination of increasingly higher risk subgroups results in an inverse relationship between the total number of fatal events and the actual incidence of sudden death[5] (as displayed in Fig. 12.1(a)).

dysplasia, cardiac ion channelopathies, and congenital heart disease. Neurological catastrophe, usually seizures, is also an important contributor to sudden death in the young. An analysis of sudden death between 1 and 21 years of age noted that epilepsy accounted for 15% of deaths.[19]

Sudden cardiac death in athletes

Sudden cardiac death in athletes is rare but usually strikes individuals with previously unrecognized cardiac disease.[22,23] In athletes < 35 years of age, hypertrophic cardiomyopathy, with or without left ventricular outflow tract obstruction, represents the most common cause of sudden cardiac death.[24] The second most common cause is due to congenital coronary artery anomalies.[25] In particular, anomalous origin of the left main coronary artery from the right (anterior) sinus of Valsalva, predisposing to kinking at the origin of the coronary artery or compression of the artery between the aorta and pulmonary artery trunk during exercise, engenders a significant risk of sudden cardiac death in athletes.[26] Arrhythmogenic right ventricular dysplasia may present with syncope or sudden cardiac death – often exercise related.[27] Indeed, in Italy, where comprehensive clinical and electrocardiographic screening has effectively excluded most athletes with hypertrophic cardiomyopathy from competition, arrhythmogenic right ventricular dysplasia is the most common cause of sport-related sudden cardiac death.[28] Acute myocarditis, even in the absence of severe left ventricular dysfunction, is another potentially fatal cause.[29] In a report of 19 sudden cardiac deaths among previously screened United States Air Force recruits, eight had evidence of myocarditis at postmortem examination – the majority of whom had their cardiac arrest during strenuous exertion.[30] Other less common causes include premature coronary atherosclerosis, commotio cordis, severe aortic stenosis, dilated cardiomyopathy, deep myocardial bridging of intramural coronary arteries, long QT syndrome – particularly LQTS1, and idiopathic ventricular fibrillation.[31–36] On the other hand, athletes > 35 years of age are most likely to die suddenly from coronary artery disease.[23,37]

Pathophysiology

Pathological studies of victims of sudden cardiac death correspond well with the established epidemiological preponderance of coronary artery disease.[8,38] Autopsy studies have consistently revealed that > 80% of cases demonstrate significant stenosis (> 75%) in at least one major epicardial coronary artery.[39,40] However, < 40% exhibit evidence of recent plaque fissuring, platelet aggregation, and coronary thrombosis.[41,42] Coronary artery spasm as a cause of sudden death is recognizable postmortem in rare cases.[43] The incidence of acute myocardial infarction on necropsy averages 20%–30% and healed myocardial infarction is noted in about 40%–70%.[8,39,44] Additionally, left ventricular hypertrophy confers an acute mortality risk seemingly independent of hypertension, left ventricular dysfunction, or coronary artery disease.[45]

Clinically, malignant cardiac arrhythmias represent the final step of a complex pathophysiological process usually facilitated by established *structural heart disease* modulated by *functional variations*.[46] In this biological model of sudden cardiac death, structural abnormalities may include chronic coronary atherosclerosis, acute or healed myocardial infarction, ventricular hypertrophy or myopathy, or a congenital ion channelopathy. Functional alterations of abnormal anatomic substrate may result from interactions with dynamic influences, such as acute myocardial ischemia and reperfusion (coronary plaque

rupture, thrombosis, or spasm), hypoxia, acidosis, electrolyte imbalance, catecholamine excess, autonomic dysfunction, toxins, and proarrhythmic drugs. The final pathway is the triggering of a fatal arrhythmia – usually ventricular tachyarrhythmias (80%–90%), or less commonly bradyarrhythmias, asystole, or pulseless electrical activity.[47] For example, in athletes with premature coronary atherosclerosis, increased myocardial oxygen demand with a fixed supply may provide a mechanism for exercise-induced ventricular tachyarrhythmia during intense physical activity.[48]

At the level of the cardiac myocyte, ischemia results in an efflux of potassium, influx of calcium, intracellular acidosis, reduction of transmembrane resting potentials, and

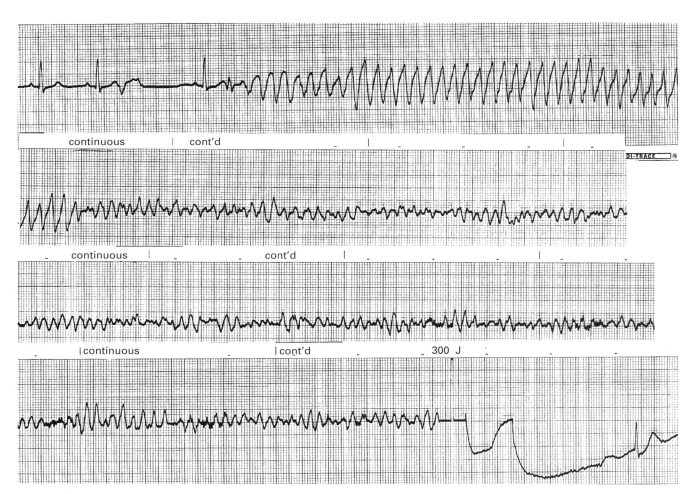

Fig. 12.2. Cardiac telemetry strips recorded from a patient 2 days postmyocardial infarction. Initially, the patient is in sinus rhythm at 70 beats per minute (bpm) with the first premature ventricular contraction (PVC) falling upon the T wave resulting in a compensatory ventricular pause. The second PVC upon the latter aspect of the T wave results in ventricular tachycardia, however, which soon progresses to ventricular flutter at 300 bpm (top strip), which in turn devolves in to coarse ventricular fibrillation (second strip from top) until an external 300 joule monophasic shock restores sinus rhythm (bottom strip).

an often heterogeneous enhancement of automaticity. Additionally, formation of superoxide radicals, fatty acid metabolites, adrenergic stimulation, and alterations in autonomic tone may contribute to electrical instability.[49,50] The resultant susceptible myocardium is prone to slow conduction and unidirectional block and, in the setting of premature impulses (premature ventricular contractions), can manifest a *re-entrant* ventricular tachyarrhythmia leading to ventricular fibrillation (Fig. 12.2). Furthermore, heterogeneously *enhanced automaticity* may trigger rapid bursts of depolarization and uncoordinated conduction leading to ventricular fibrillation.

Failure of normal sinus node and atrioventricular node function with concomitant failure of subordinate automatic activity to assume pacemaking function is the basis of the electrophysiological mechanism of bradyarrhythmias and asystole. At the cellular level, increased extracellular potassium concentration, anoxia, acidosis, shock, and hypothermia may result in partial depolarization of pacemaker cells in the His-Purkinje system, decreasing the slope of spontaneous phase 4 depolarization with loss of automaticity.[51] This phenomenon is likely to be more common in hearts with pre-existing His-Purkinje system conduction abnormalities due to *Lenegre's disease* (primary fibrosis) or *Lev's disease* (secondary mechanical injury).[52,53]

Pulseless electrical activity represents electrical depolarization of myocardium in the absence of effective mechanical myocardial contraction. Secondary pulseless electrical activity (pseudo-electromechanical dissociation) is caused by near or complete cessation of cardiac venous return due to large pulmonary embolism, cardiac tamponade, and massive exsanguination. Primary pulseless electrical activity results from a *failure of electromechanical coupling*.[54] The cellular mechanism for failure of electromechanical coupling probably includes abnormal metabolism of intracellular calcium, intracellular acidosis, and depletion of adenosine triphosphate. This usually occurs in the setting of end-stage heart disease, acute ischemia, or electrical resuscitation from a prolonged cardiac arrest.

Conclusions

Death is inevitable. Nevertheless, a thorough understanding of its multifaceted etiology holds the key for designing successful community- and patient-based strategies to delay its grim arrival. Familial clusterings of sudden cardiac death may provide us with the key to success by allowing us to delineate accurately specific genetic abnormalities that predispose to sudden cardiac death and target therapies accordingly.[55–58]

REFERENCES

1. Myerburg, R.J. & Castellanos, A. Chapter 26: Cardiac arrest and sudden cardiac death. In *Heart Disease: A Textbook of Cardiovascular Medicine*, 6th edn, W.B. Saunders, 2001: 890–909.

2. Schatzkin, A., Cupples, L.A., Heeren, T., *et al.* The epidemiology of sudden unexpected death: Risk factors for men and women in the Framingham Heart Study. *Am. Heart J.* 1984; **107**: 1300–1306.

3. Schatzkin, A., Cupples, L.A., Heeren, T., *et al.* Sudden death in the Framingham Heart Study: differences in incidence and risk factors by sex and coronary disease status. *Am. J. Epidemiol.* 1984; **120**: 888–899.

4. Kuller, L.H. Sudden death: definition and epidemiologic considerations. *Progr. Cardiovasc. Dis.* 1980; **23**: 1–12.

5. Myerburg, R.J., Kessler, K.M. & Castellanos, A. Sudden cardiac death: Structure, function, and time-dependence of risk. *Circulation* 1992; **85** (Suppl. 1): I2–I10.

6. Yusuf, S., Venkatesh, G. & Teo, K.K. Critical review of the approaches to the prevention of sudden death. *Am. J. Cardiol.* 1993; **72**: 51F–58F.

7. Sinha, S.K., Mehta, D. & Gomes, A.J. Prevention of sudden cardiac death: the role of the implantable cardioverter-defibrillator. *Mount Sinai J. Med.* 2005; **72**: 1–9.

8. Myerburg, R.J., Interian, A., Mitrani, R.M., *et al.* Frequency of sudden cardiac death and profiles of risk. *Am. J. Cardiol.* 1997; **80**: 10F–19F.

9. Sinha, S.K., Winslow, R. & Mehta, D. Prevention of sudden cardiac death and diabetes mellitus. *Curr. Diabetes Rep.* 2004; **4**: 155–157.

10. Burch, G.E. & DePasquale, N.P. Sudden, unexpected, natural death. *Am. J. Med. Sci.* 1965; **249**: 86–97.

11. Scragg, R., Mitchell, E.A., Taylor, B.J. *et al.* Bed sharing, smoking, and alcohol in the sudden infant death syndrome: New Zealand Cot Death Study Group. *Br. Med. J.* 1993; **307**: 1312–1318.

12. Byard, R.W. & Moore, L. Gastroesophageal reflux and sudden infant death syndrome. *Pediatr. Pathol.* 1993; **13**: 53–57.

13. Ponsonby, A.L., Dwyer, T. Gibbons, L.E., Cochrane, J.A. & Wang, Y.G. Factors potentiating the risk of sudden infant death syndrome associated with the prone position. *N. Engl. J. Med.* 1993; **329**: 377–382.

14. Spitzer, A.R. Current controversies in the pathophysiology and prevention of sudden infant death syndrome. *Curr. Opin. Pediatr.* 2005; **17**(2): 181–185.

15. Antzelevitch, C., Brugada, P., Borggrefe, M. *et al.* Brugada syndrome: report of the second consensus conference. *Heart Rhythm* 2005; **2**(4): 429–440.

16. Moss, A.J., Long QT syndrome. *J. Am. Med. Assoc.* 2003; **289**(16): 2041–2044.

17. Brugada, R., Hong, K., Cordeiro, J.M. & Dumaine, R. Short QT syndrome. *Can. Med. Assoc. J.* 2005; **173**(11): 1349–1354.

18. Southall, D.P., Richard, J.M., de Swiet, M. *et al.* Identification of infants destined to die unexpectedly during infancy.

Evaluation of predictive importance of prolonged apnea and disorders of cardiac rhythm or conduction. *Br. Med. J.* 1983; **286**: 1092–1099.

19. Neuspiel, D.R. & Kuller, L.H. Sudden and unexpected natural death in childhood and adolescence. *J. Am. Med. Assoc.* 1985; **254**: 1321–1325.

20. Kuisma, M., Souminen, P. & Korpela, R. Pediatric out-of-hospital cardiac arrests: Epidemiology and outcome. *Resuscitation* 1995; **30**: 141–150.

21. Steinberger, J., Lucas, R.V., Edwards, J.E. & Titus, J.L. Causes of sudden, unexpected cardiac death in the first two decades of life. *Am. J. Cardiol.* 1996; **77**: 992–995.

22. Maron, B.J. Sudden death in young athletes – lessons from the Hank Gathers affair. *N. Engl. J. Med.* 1993; **329**: 55–57.

23. Maron, B.J., Epstein, S.E. & Roberts, W.C. Causes of sudden death in competitive athletes. *J. Am. Coll. Cardiol.* 1986; **7**: 204–214.

24. Maron, B.J., Epstein, S.E. & Roberts, W.C. Hypertrophic cardiomyopathy: A common cause of sudden death in the young competitive athlete. *Eur. Heart J.* 1983; **4**(Suppl. F): 135–144.

25. Maron, B.J., Shirani, J., Poliac, L.C. *et al.* Sudden death in young competitive athletes: clinical, demographic, and pathological profiles. *J. Am. Med. Assoc.* 1996; **276**: 199–204.

26. Taylor, A.J., Rogan, K.M. & Virmani, R. Sudden cardiac death associated with isolated congenital coronary artery anomalies. *J. Am. Coll. Cardiol.* 1992; **20**: 640–647.

27. Thiene, G., Nava, A., Corrado, D. *et al.* Right ventricular cardiomyopathy and sudden death in young people. *N. Engl. J. Med.* 1988; **318**: 129–133.

28. Furlanello, F., Bertoldi, A., Dallago, M. *et al.* Cardiac arrest and sudden death in competitive athletes with arrhythmogenic right ventricular dysplasia. *Pacing Clin. Electrophysiol.* 1998; **21**: 331–335.

29. Topaz, O. & Edwards, J.E. Pathologic features of sudden death in children, adolescents, and young adults. *Chest* 1985; **87**: 476–482.

30. Phillips, M., Rabinowitz, M., Higgins, J.R. *et al.* Sudden cardiac death in air force recruits. *J. Am. Med. Assoc.* 1986; **256**: 2696–2699.

31. Roberts, W.C. & Maron, B.J. Sudden death while playing professional football. *Am. Heart J.* 1981; **102**: 1061–1063.

32. Maron, B.J., Poliac, L.C., Kaplan, J.A., *et al.* Blunt impact to the chest leading to sudden death from cardiac arrest during sports activities. *N. Engl. J. Med.* 1995; **33**: 337–342.

33. Geddes, L.A. & Roeder, R.A. Evolution of our knowledge of sudden death due to commotio cordis. *Am. J. Emerg. Med.* 2005; **23**(1): 67–75.

34. Morales, A.R., Romanelli, R. & Boucek, R.J. The mural left anterior descending coronary artery, strenuous exercise, and sudden death. *Circulation* 1980; **62**: 230–237.

35. Moss, A.J. & Kass, R.S. Long QT syndrome: from channels to cardiac arrhythmias. *J. Clin. Investigation.* 2005; **115**(8): 2018–2024.

36. Joint Steering Commitees of the Unexplained Cardiac Arrest Registry of Europe and of the Idiopathic Ventricular Fibrillation Registry of the United States. Survivors of out-of-hospital cardiac arrest with apparently normal heart. *Circulation* 1997; **95**: 265–272.

37. Waller, B.F. Exercise-related sudden death in young and old conditioned subjects. *Exercise and the Heart* Philadelphia: F.A. Davis, 1985; 9–73.

38. Myerburg, R.J., Conde, C.A., Sung, R.J. *et al.* Clinical, electrophysiologic, and hemodynamic profile of patients resuscitated from prehospital cardiac arrest. *Am. J. Med.* 1980; **68**: 568–576.

39. Liberthson, R.R., Nagel, E.L., Hirschman, J.C. *et al.* Pathophysiologic observations in prehospital ventricular fibrillation and sudden cardiac death. *Circulation* 1974; **49**: 790–798.

40. Perper, J.A., Kuller, J.H. & Cooper, M. Arteriosclerosis of coronary arteries in sudden, unexpected deaths. *Circulation* 1975; **52** (Suppl. 3): 27–33.

41. Davies, M.J. & Thomas, A. Thrombosis and acute coronary artery lesions in sudden cardiac ischemic death. *N. Engl. J. Med.* 1984; **310**: 1137–1140.

42. Farb, A., Burke, A.P., Tang, A.L. *et al.* Coronary plaque erosion without rupture into a lipid core: a frequent cause of coronary thrombosis in sudden cardiac death. *Circulation* 1996; **93**: 1354–1363.

43. Roberts, W.C., Currey, R.C., Isner, J.M. *et al.* Sudden death in Prinzmetal's angina with coronary spasm documented by angiography. *Am. J. Cardiol.* 1982; **50**: 203–210.

44. Newman, W.P., Tracy, R.E., Strong, J.P., *et al.* Pathology of sudden cardiac death. *Ann. NY Acad. Sci.* 1982; **382**: 39–49.

45. Cooper, R.S., Simmons, B.E., Castaner, A. *et al.* Left ventricular hypertrophy is associated with worse survival independent of ventricular function and number of coronary arteries severely narrowed. *Am. J. Cardiol.* 1990; **65**: 441–445.

46. Myerburg, R.J., Kessler, K.M., Bassett, A.L. & Castellanos, A. A biological approach to sudden cardiac death: Structure, function, and cause. *Am. J. Cardiol.* 1989; **63**: 1512–1516.

47. Bayes de Luna, A., Coumel, P. & Leclercq, J.F. Ambulatory sudden cardiac death: mechanisms of production of fatal arrhythmia on the basis of data from 157 cases. *Am. Heart J.* 1989; **117**: 151–159.

48. Cobb, L.A. & Weaver, W.D. Exercise: a risk for sudden death in patients with coronary heart disease. *J. Am. Coll. Cardiol.* 1986; **7**: 215–219.

49. Surawicz, B. Ventricular fibrillation. *J. Am. Coll. Cardiol.* 1985; **5** (Suppl. 6): 43B–54B.

50. Opie, L.H. Products of myocardial ischemia and electrical instability of the heart. *J. Am. Coll. Cardiol.* 1985; **5** (Suppl. 6): 162B–165B.

51. Vassalle, M. On the mechanisms underlying cardiac standstill: Factors determining success or failure of escape pacemakers in the heart. *J. Am. Coll. Cardiol.* 1985; **5** (Suppl. 6): 35B–42B.

52. Lenegre, J. Etiology and pathology of bilateral bundle branch block in relation to complete heart block. *Progr. Cardiovasc. Dis.* 1964; **6**: 409–444.

53. Lev, M. Anatomic basis for atrioventricular block. *Am. J. Med.* 1964; **37**: 742–748.

54. Fozzard, H.A. Electromechanical disassociation and its possible role in sudden cardiac death. *J. Am. Coll. Cardiol.* 1985; **5** (Suppl. 6): 31B–34B.

55. Friedlander, Y., Siscovick, D.S., Weinmann, S. *et al.* Family history as a risk factor for primary cardiac arrest. *Circulation* 1998; **97**: 155–160.

56. Marban, E. Cardiac channelopathies. *Nature* 2002; **415**: 213–218.

57. Priori, S.G., Barhanin, J., Hauer, R.N.W., *et al.* Genetic and molecular basis of cardiac arrhythmias: Impact on clinical management. *Circulation* 1999; **99**: 518–528.

58. Rubart, M. & Zipes, D.P. Mechanisms of sudden death. *J. Clin. Invest.* 2005; **115**(9): 2305–2315.

13

Global brain ischemia and reperfusion

Brian J. O'Neil[1], Raymond C. Koehler[2], Robert W. Neumar[3], Uwe Ebmeyer[4], and Gary S. Krause[5]

[1] Department of Emergency Medicine, William Beaumont Hospital, Royal Oak, MI, USA
[2] Department of Anesthesiology, Johns Hopkins University, Baltimore, MD, USA
[3] Department of Emergency Medicine, University of Pennsylvania School of Medicine, Philadelphia, PA, USA
[4] Klinik für Anaesthesiologie und Intensivtherapie, Otto-von-Guericke Universität, Magdeburg, Germany
[5] Department of Emergency Medicine, Wayne State University, Detroit, MI, USA

Introduction

Sudden, unexpected death claims nearly 1000 lives each day in the United States and is the fifth leading cause of all deaths in the western world.[1,2] Cardiac arrest occurs over 300 000 times per year both in the United States and Europe with the risk for persons 35 years and older estimated at 1 per 1000. In those patients resuscitated from cardiac arrest, nearly 60% die from a neurological cause. Despite every effort, only 3%–10% of all resuscitated patients are able to resume their former lifestyles.[3]

To date, there are no clinically effective pharmacologic tools for amelioration of brain damage by ischemia and reperfusion. Clinical trials conducted more than a decade ago utilizing postresuscitation treatment with barbiturates[4] or calcium antagonists[5] were disappointing. More recently, clinical treatment of stroke with a radical scavenger (trilazad),[6] intercellular adhesion molecule-1 antagonist (Enlimomab),[7] glutamate receptor antagonist (Aptiganel, gavestinel),[8,9] glutamate release inhibitor (Lubeluzole),[10] ganglioside administration (GM1),[11] calcium channel blockade,[12] or upregulation of the GABA receptor (Clomethiazole)[13] were all found ineffective. This suggests that our understanding of the mechanisms involved in damage and repair in neurons remains incomplete and further therapeutic progress will require the delineation of the primary mechanisms involved in neuronal injury and repair.

Although the picture is still incomplete, a few things are clear.

1. The majority of damage occurs not during ischemia but during reperfusion. Nevertheless, the two processes work sequentially to increase neuronal damage (i.e., lipolysis during ischemia potentiates the radical-mediated peroxidation of polyunsaturated fatty acids (PUFAs) during reperfusion).

2. Since in practice the initial ischemic damage has already occurred, suppression of further damage and promotion of acute repair is the key to minimizing permanent neurological injury.

3. Regulation of calcium influx or its intracellular release plays a sequential role in neuronal pathology.

4. Postischemic competence for protein synthesis is crucial to the neuron's ability both to limit and to repair damage during early reperfusion.

5. Competence for both antioxidant defense and membrane synthesis and repair in terminally differentiated brain neurons is regulated at a fundamental level by selected growth factors and proto-oncogenes.

Experimental models of global cerebral ischemia

Because the brain is particularly vulnerable to even short periods of ischemia, rapid defibrillation of the heart and restoration of spontaneous circulation are extremely critical. With each passing minute of cardiac arrest, the magnitude of neuronal injury progressively increases. For example, experimental studies in dogs have shown that increasing ischemic duration beyond 8 minutes results in progressively worse neurologic deficits.[14,15,16] Examination of brain histology, however, reveals that certain neuronal populations are injured after periods of ischemia as short as 5 minutes, whereas others can survive 30 or more minutes of ischemia.[17–23] Indeed, partial recovery of metabolism and electrophysiologic function is possible

Cardiac Arrest: The Science and Practice of Resuscitation Medicine. 2nd edn., ed. Norman Paradis, Henry Halperin, Karl Kern, Volker Wenzel, Douglas Chamberlain. Published by Cambridge University Press. © Cambridge University Press, 2007.

after 1 hour of ischemia.[24,25] In addition, selective neuronal populations do not die immediately, raising the possibility of a temporal therapeutic window. Considerable effort has been directed at understanding the mechanism of delayed neuronal death that typically occurs 1 to 3 days after the insult. The mechanisms by which ischemia causes neuronal death are multifactorial and vary by brain region and by connectivity of specific neuronal populations.

When evaluating the large body of literature concerning cerebral ischemia, it is critical to consider the severity, duration, and distribution of reduced blood flow in the particular experimental model used in each study. Although ventricular fibrillation produces zero blood flow throughout the body, cardiac arrest is not used in many experimental models of cerebral ischemia because of the difficulty of cardiac resuscitation after prolonged arrest and the need for intensive care in animals with impaired brain-stem and thalamic function. Models of complete cerebral ischemia (zero blood flow) include ventricular fibrillation,[26,27] aortic occlusion with preserved coronary blood flow,[28,29] brachiocephalic and subclavian arterial occlusion plus arterial hypotension (to reduce inflow from spinal accessory arteries),[25,30] neck cuff inflation,[31,32] and compression models in which intracranial pressure is elevated above arterial pressure by ventricular fluid infusion.[33,34] Models of nearly complete global forebrain ischemia have been developed in which blood flow to cortex, striatum, and hippocampus is reduced to extremely low levels (0–5 ml/min per 100 g), whereas blood flow to caudal structures is adequate for preserving respiratory and cardiovascular stability. Global forebrain ischemia models include the four-vessel occlusion model, in which vertebral arteries are permanently occluded and carotid arteries are reversibly occluded,[35] and the carotid occlusion plus arterial hypotension model.[36] These two models of global forebrain ischemia have been the most widely used because they are relatively easy to prepare, particularly in the rat, and require less postoperative care than do cardiac arrest models. In addition, gerbils are sometimes used because the Circle of Willis is incomplete and carotid occlusion without hypotension produces near-complete forebrain ischemia. The nature and topography of injury in global models of cerebral ischemia, in which the duration of cerebral ischemia is typically less than 20 minutes, differs from focal ischemia models of stroke, in which a spatial gradient of blood flow reduction is produced for durations typically greater than 1 hour, and in which an inflammatory response occurs that leads to infarction. Therapies that are effective in experimental stroke may not necessarily be effective after cardiac arrest.

Cardiac arrest as well as other neuronal injury-triggering processes can lead to selective and delayed neuronal death.[37] Postischemic recovery depends on the type and the duration of the ischemic insult, which correlates with the level of cellular damage during reperfusion.[38] Cell death after global cerebral ischemia can be due to apoptosis or necrosis, depending on the duration of the insult and the quality of postischemic reperfusion.[39,40] If cardiac arrest times are exceedingly long or return of spontaneous circulation (ROSC) is not robust, then primary brain necrosis results. Resuscitation and cerebral reperfusion with shorter time periods may lead to cellular restitution or a delayed type of cellular death (apoptosis). The term *apoptosis* was promulgated by Kerr and Wylli to describe a cell death process without necrosis.[41,42] Specific morphological and biochemical features distinguish apoptosis from necrosis.[43] Necrotic cell death begins with a swelling of the cell body and the mitochondrial elements. Soon thereafter cell membranes disintegrate. The release of cytoplasmic contents triggers inflammatory reactions in the surrounding tissue. In contrast, apoptosis is a well-regulated process. Apoptotic cells take an active part in their own "shut down," packing, and dismantling process.[44] The highly regulated physiological "programmed cell death" process is characterized by specific morphological features such as changes in the plasma membrane, condensation of cytoplasm and nucleolus, and internucleosomal cleavage of DNA. Intracellular processes degrade the cells without rupture of the plasma membrane. At the end of the apoptotic process, shrunken cells become fragmented into "apoptotic bodies."[45] Finally phagocytic cells eliminate these cell fragments without significant inflammatory damage to the surrounding cells. The newest research results indicate that postischemic neuronal death most likely involves a combination of both apoptosis and necrosis even at the level of individual neurons.[46] Furthermore, both forms of cell demise seem to represent the extremes of a continuum.[37,47]

Energy metabolism, ion fluxes, tissue pH, and cerebral circulation

Energy metabolism and ionic fluxes during ischemia

High-energy phosphates in mature brain are derived primarily from oxidative metabolism of glucose. With sudden cardiac arrest, high-energy phosphates are depleted more rapidly in brain than in most other organs. Both the tissue freeze-clamp technique and the phosphorus magnetic resonance spectroscopy (MRS) technique demonstrate

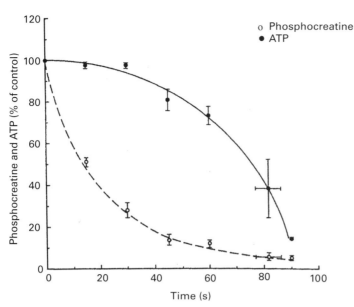

Fig. 13.1. Percent changes in phosphocreatine and ATP concentrations obtained from neocortex frozen at different times after cardiac arrest in rats. Note the rapid decrease in phosphocreatine, followed shortly by a decrease in ATP. The time of anoxic depolarization corresponded to an ATP concentration of 30–40% of control. (From ref. 59.)

that phosphocreatine is largely depleted within 1 minute and ATP is almost completely depleted within 2 to 3 minutes of the onset of complete cerebral ischemia.[34,48–50] Consciousness is lost within 10 seconds, and electroencephalographic (EEG) activity becomes isoelectric within 20 seconds.[51,52] As shown in Fig. 13.1, the decline in ATP over time is not linear because: (1) phosphocreatine initially acts to buffer the decrease in ATP[49,50] (2) EEG silence reduces ATP demand and the rate of decline in tissue PO_2, whereas subsequent cell depolarization increases ATP demand[53,48] and (3) anaerobic metabolism of tissue stores of glucose and glycogen produces small amounts of ATP for several minutes.

Recordings from ion-sensitive microelectrodes in brain interstitial space reveal two phases in the temporal ionic response.[54,55] During the initial phase after cardiac arrest, interstitial K^+ concentration gradually increases from 3 to approximately 10 mM. Moderate increases in intracellular Ca^{2+} also occur during this early phase of anoxia.[56,57] Magnetic resonance measurements of Na^+ and water diffusion constant also suggest an early influx of Na^+ and water.[48–59] Spontaneous electrical activity is lost during this phase (Fig. 13.2), although evoked responses can still be generated. Within 2 minutes of cardiac arrest, interstitial

K^+ activity begins to increase at a progressively faster rate, resulting in cell membrane depolarization of neurons and glia (anoxic depolarization), increases in ion conductance, and further increases in interstitial K^+ activity to 60–100 mM. The onset of this second phase is associated with rapid decreases in interstitial Na^+, Cl^-, and Ca^{2+} activity and shrinkage of the interstitial space as these ions and water move intracellularly.[59,60] At this time, tissue ATP levels are reduced to approximately 30% of normal and are inadequate to maintain Na^+–K^+ ATPase at maximum activity.[48] The large influx of Ca^{2+} leads to activation of proteolytic enzymes and phospholipase A_2 and to a consequent rise in free fatty acid levels in tissue.[49]

Therefore, complete cessation of cerebral blood flow

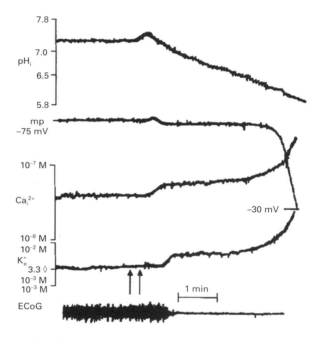

Fig. 13.2. Recordings of intracellular pH (pH_i), membrane potential (mp), and intracellular calcium activity (Ca_i^{2+}) from a triple-barreled microelectrode inserted into a cell in CA1 region of hippocampus. Extracellular potassium activity (K_e^+) was recorded from a microelectrode in the contralateral hippocampus, and electrocorticogram (ECoG) activity was recorded from frontal cortex. Global forebrain ischemia was produced in the rat (at the first arrow) and PO_2 in separately recorded tissue fell to zero (at the second arrow). After a transient alkaline shift, pH_i progressively decreases due in part to ATP hydrolysis. ECoG is rapidly lost. At about this time, small increases in Ca_i^{2+} and K_e^+ occur. After an approximately 2-minute delay, large increases in Ca_i^{2+} and K_e^+ occur and the membrane depolarizes. Thus, changes in Ca_i^{2+} are detectable before membrane depolarization. (From ref. 64.)

results in a very rapid sequence of physiologic and metabolic events, involving: (1) loss of consciousness, (2) loss of EEG activity, (3) small increases in interstitial K^+ and intracellular Ca^{2+} activity, (4) membrane depolarization when ATP is approximately 30% of normal, and (5) a large influx of Ca^{2+}, Na^+, Cl^-, and water and an efflux of K^+. This sequence of events can be delayed to a small extent by increasing tissue glucose stores with preischemic hyperglycemia[63] or by decreasing the rate of ATP utilization with barbiturates,[61] and to a greater extent with preischemic hypothermia.[62]

Energy metabolism during early reperfusion

When cerebral perfusion is fully reinstituted after 3 to 12 minutes of global ischemia, transcellular ionic gradients for K^+, Na^+ and Ca^{2+} are largely restored within several minutes.[48,55,57,63–65] Tissue levels of ATP also recover rapidly.[66] Recovery of Na^+ and K^+ gradients, however, precedes full recovery of ATP,[48,63] presumably because the affinity constant of Na^+–K^+ ATPase for ATP is lower than when ATP levels are normal. Hence, much of the ATP initially produced during reperfusion is utilized for restoration of ionic gradients and high ATPase activity delays recovery of ATP concentration.

When ischemia is prolonged beyond 15 minutes, recovery of ionic gradients and ATP becomes progressively slower.[67–70] Furthermore, steady-state recovery of ATP is 20%–40% below normal.[71,72] Slower ATP recovery may be the result of depressed mitochondrial function[73,74] secondary to acidosis,[75,76] formation of oxygen radicals,[77] degradation of mitochondrial phospholipids,[78] increased Ca^{2+} load, and opening of mitochondrial permeability transition pores.[79] Recovery of oxidative metabolism after prolonged ischemia might also be limited by loss of adenosine base through the adenosine deaminase pathway,[80,81] by defective production of NADH,[82] by heterogeneous patches of poor reflow and oxygenation,[33,83,84] and by sustained ionic membrane leaks that cause wasteful utilization of a limited ATP supply for ionic pump activity. In addition, initial recovery of ATP after prolonged ischemia might be followed by a secondary decline in ATP, as loss of adenosine, loss of NADH, and microcirculatory stasis worsening over a period of several hours.[85]

With short periods of ischemia, full restoration of transcellular ionic gradients and high-energy phosphates in tissue should not be taken as evidence that metabolism is completely restored throughout the cell. Critical abnormalities may persist in dendritic processes far removed from the cell body, particularly at synaptic sites. Postsynaptic microregions deluged by neurotransmitters are expected to show an imbalance in second messenger systems, with effects that will persist into reperfusion. Astrocyte processes responsible for ATP-dependent uptake and metabolism of neurotransmitters, such as glutamate, require restoration of their Na^+ gradient for inward glutamate transport. Presynaptic neuronal processes depleted of neurotransmitters during anoxic depolarization might also be active in reuptake and synthesis of neurotransmitters and synaptic vesicles.[86] Consequently, defects in neurotransmission can persist. Appearance of spontaneous EEG activity can be considerably delayed after restoration of ionic gradients and ATP, and if the duration of ischemia is prolonged, the EEG may remain abnormal.[27,51,87] Furthermore, the amplitude of evoked potentials may remain depressed even after brief ischemia. Thus, functional neurotransmission can remain impaired despite recovery of global oxidative metabolism and ionic gradients.

Cerebral acidosis during ischemia and reperfusion

Because acidosis has traditionally been assumed to play an important role in ischemic injury, it is useful to understand the factors that influence cerebral pH during ischemia. Normal intracellular pH in brain is approximately 7.1, and normal extracellular pH is approximately 7.3.[88,89] This transcellular pH gradient is the net result of intracellular production of acids, proton and bicarbonate antiporters, and membrane voltage.[88] With the onset of complete cerebral ischemia, intracellular pH falls rapidly to approximately 6.1–6.2 within 6–10 minutes.[48,90,91] Extracellular pH decreases in parallel with the decrease in intracellular pH, but appears to remain more alkaline than intracellular pH.[92,93]

One major source of protons during complete ischemia is the hydrolysis of ATP and other nucleoside triphosphates.[94,95] The net hydrolysis of ATP stores (0.3 mmol/kg) in brain is expected to produce approximately 2–4 mmol/kg of protons, depending on Mg^{2+} concentration and pH.[95] Another source of protons is anaerobic glycolysis, whereby 1 mole of glucose forms 2 moles of ATP and 2 moles of lactate anions. When these 2 moles of ATP are eventually hydrolyzed, approximately 2 moles of protons are produced. During complete ischemia, the amount of protons produced depends on glucose and glycogen stores in the tissue, which to a large extent, depend on the history of plasma glucose concentration before the onset of ischemia.[96] During incomplete ischemia, proton production also depends on continued delivery of glucose to the brain and, hence, on arterial glucose concentration.[97]

Ordinarily, changes in intracellular pH are passively buffered by proteins, particularly those with abundant histidine groups (p*k*a 6.9), and by inorganic phosphate (p*k*a 6.7) and bicarbonate ions (p*k*a 6.1). Because extracellular protein concentration is low in brain, extracellular pH is buffered primarily by bicarbonate ions. In addition, active regulation of intracellular pH that accompanies changes in acid loads is mediated by various proton and bicarbonate antiporters.[88,98] During complete ischemia, CO_2 is not cleared and bicarbonate ions become an ineffective buffer. Marked changes in Na^+ and Cl^- gradients during ischemia render extrusion of acid equivalents by antiporters unfavorable. Upon full reperfusion, CO_2 is cleared within a few minutes and tissue pH increases by approximately 0.3–0.4 unit.[55,91,92] Full recovery of tissue pH requires from 15 to 60 minutes, however[31,48,67,99,100] depends on the duration of ischemia, and lags behind recovery of calcium,[101] sodium,[48] and ATP. The delay in pH recovery might be due to (1) persistent anaerobic glycolysis and production of metabolic acids from other sources during early reperfusion, (2) the need for re-establishment of Na^+ and Cl^- gradients for appropriate function of proton and bicarbonate transporters, and (3) the magnitude of the buffered and unbuffered proton load that must be extruded out of the brain.

Influence of acidosis on ischemic injury

Major evidence that acidosis contributes to ischemic injury is largely derived from studies in which tissue pH is manipulated by varying blood glucose levels to influence the magnitude of anaerobic glycolysis during ischemia.[102,103] Induction of hyperglycemia before global ischemia augments histopathologic damage.[104,105] The most severe damage with hyperglycemia has been reported in models of incomplete global ischemia, in which blood flow is reduced by at least 75% and the duration of ischemia is extended to at least 30 minutes.[106,107] In this case, intracellular pH falls to values in the 5–6 range[97] and is not restored during reperfusion. Additional consequences of these events include: temporary recovery of energy metabolism,[102,108,109] glial and endothelial swelling during early reperfusion,[107,110] patchy, heterogeneous reperfusion,[111] and large areas of necrosis.[104] Conversion of the histopathologic injury from one of selective necrosis of individual neurons typically seen after normoglycemic ischemia to one of microregions of overt necrosis after hyperglycemic ischemia, probably depends on the presence of critically low levels of tissue pH. An alternative mechanism of injury that involves elevated corticosterone during hyperglycemia has been proposed.[112]

In addition to the importance of severity of intraischemic pH, acidosis during reoxygenation might promote from damage oxygen radicals. Postischemic hyperglycemia can delay pH recovery[113] and worsen neurologic deficit.[114] Furthermore, imposing carbonic acidosis during early reperfusion depresses electrophysiologic recovery,[91] whereas antioxidant treatment accelerates pH recovery and improves electrophysiologic recovery.[115]

The mechanism whereby acidosis augments ischemic injury remains unclear. It is generally assumed that, by altering protein charge, acidosis affects functions of a wide array of enzymes, receptors, ion channels, and intracellular messenger systems. Acidosis in the absence of ischemia does not produce neuronal and glial injury, unless it is severe (pH $<$ 6) and prolonged.[98,116–121] Therefore, if acidosis contributes to normoglycemic ischemic injury, it presumably interacts synergistically with other mechanisms that come into play after the loss of oxygenation and depletion of energy.

One way by which acidosis might augment ischemic injury is by augmenting increases in free intracellular Ca^{2+}.[122] This might occur via indirect effects on endoplasmic reticulum and mitochondrial Ca^{2+} sequestration sites, rather than on effects of acidosis on N-methyl-D-aspartate (NMDA) channels. Extracellular acidosis inhibits Ca^{2+} influx through NMDA channels in vitro,[123] and induction of metabolic alkalemia by infusion of carbicarb before incomplete cerebral ischemia depressed the recovery of energy metabolism through an NMDA channel-sensitive mechanism.[124] Acid-sensitive ion channels permit influx of cations, including Ca^{2+}, and blocking these channels protects the brain from focal cerebral ischemia.[125] The role of these acid-sensitive channels in brain injury from cardiac arrest remains to be elucidated.

Another mechanism by which acidosis might augment ischemic injury is through interactions with oxygen radical mechanisms. Iron-dependent lipid peroxidation is promoted by metabolic acidosis,[126] but not by carbonic acidosis.[127] This difference raised the possibility that lactic acid attacks iron that is bound to protein by carbonate bridges, such as occurs on transferrin, whereas carbonic acidosis acts to stabilize these carbonate bridges.[127] Mobilized iron, found in the brain after cardiac arrest,[128,129] will enhance the formation of reactive oxygen species during reoxygenation. The percent of iron bound to low-molecular-weight species after ischemia can be augmented in cerebral cortex by increasing acidosis with hyperglycemia.[130] Moreover, superoxide formed during reperfusion might mobilize additional iron from ferritin[131] and enhance lipid peroxidation.[132] Once abundant free iron is present, free radical production may proceed at a rapid rate and deplete endogenous antioxidants. Because tissue pH during reperfusion usually remains acidotic for 15 to 60 minutes, persistent acidosis during reperfusion might continue to augment this adverse process. An interaction of metabolic acidosis with oxygen radical damage is supported by evidence that shows that the depressed metabolic recovery associated with enhanced lactic acidosis during hyperglycemic ischemia[97] is ameliorated by treatment with an iron chelator[133,134] or an antioxidant,[135] whereas enhancing carbonic acidosis during ischemia does not depress metabolic recovery despite intra-ischemic pH falling to 5.7.[136] The importance of this mechanism in normoglycemic cardiac arrest is unclear, however because both carbonic acidosis and metabolic acidosis contribute to the drop in tissue pH when there is no blood flow to clear CO_2.

Intra-ischemic acidosis augmented by hyperglycemia affects protein kinases and protein phosphorylation during recovery in a manner different from acidosis augmented by hypercapnia and from normoglycemic ischemia.[137] Other potential mechanisms of acidotic damage include changes in gene expression and protein synthesis and activation of endonucleases, leading to DNA damage.[138] Therefore, the precise mechanism of interactions between acidosis and other mechanisms of ischemic injury remains uncertain and appears to depend on the nature of the acid load (metabolic acid vs. CO_2), the range of pH during ischemia, the range of pH during reperfusion, and the severity and duration of the ischemic insult.

Bioenergetics during chest compression CPR

In most experimental studies of global cerebral ischemia, reperfusion is initiated by rapidly restoring cerebral perfusion pressure to normal levels and producing a hyperemic response in the vasodilated vascular bed. In the typical clinical setting of cardiac arrest, however, a variable period of chest compression CPR, which generates subnormal levels of arterial blood pressure, occurs before the return of spontaneous circulation. Because the increase in intrathoracic pressure during each chest compression increases intracranial pressure,[139,140] cerebral perfusion pressure during CPR is considerably lower than arterial blood pressure. For example, cerebral perfusion pressures in the range of 15–30 mmHg averaged over a chest compression cycle have been measured in standard CPR.[141] At these low levels of cerebral perfusion pressure, cerebral blood flow is expected to be less than 50% of the normal value, which is insufficient to restore cerebral ATP and pH.[142] On the other hand, a low level of reperfusion achieved with experimental CPR does not worsen intracellular pH (Fig. 13.3), which might be of concern if the low level of blood flow restored glucose delivery without concurrently providing sufficient oxygen for aerobic energy

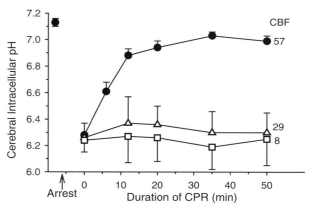

Fig, 13.3. Recovery of cerebral intracellular pH measured by phosphorus MRS during prolonged CPR started at 6 minutes of ventricular fibrillation in dogs. When cerebral perfusion pressure (arterial minus sagittal sinus pressure) was regulated at 80 mmHg during vest CPR and cerebral blood flow (CBF) was near normal (57 ml/min/100g), intracellular pH recovered to near prearrest levels. When cerebral perfusion pressure was regulated at 30 mmHg by adjusting the inflation pressure of a pneumatic thoracic vest, intracellular pH did not recover in a group with a CBF of 29 ml/min/100 g, despite partial recovery of ATP. In a group with poor CBF (8 ml/min/100 g at 12 minutes and lower flow thereafter), intracellular pH did not decrease further during CPR. Recovery of intracellular pH requires normal levels of CBF, but trickle flow does not worsen tissue acidosis. (Curves drawn from refs. 121 and 192.)

metabolism. With advanced CPR techniques that permit higher levels of cerebral blood flow (50%–100% of normal) to be generated, cerebral ATP partially recovers, but energy supply is insufficient to restore cerebral pH (Fig. 13.3) unless blood flow is near the normal level.[90,142] Most importantly, brief delays in the onset of CPR after cardiac arrest have a major effect on the level of cerebral blood flow that can be generated (Fig. 13.4). As the delay in the onset of CPR is increased from 0 minutes to 12 minutes, the relationship of blood flow to perfusion pressure progressively shifts to higher perfusion pressures.[143,144] Consequently, the ability to regenerate ATP becomes markedly impaired (Fig. 13.4). The increase in the zero-flow intercept on the pressure axis might be related to progressive swelling of astrocyte processes that surround capillaries, limiting flow at low perfusion pressures. Aquaporin-4 water channels are preferentially localized on astrocyte foot processes near blood vessels and appear to contribute to ischemia-induced swelling.[145,146] Additional delivery of water into the microcirculation that accompanies low perfusion might lead to additional astrocyte swelling and further shifts in the pressure–flow relationship.

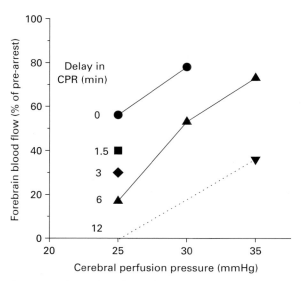
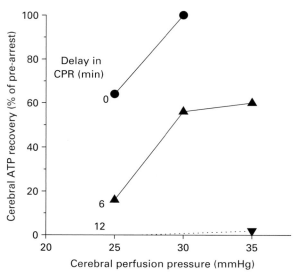

Fig. 13.4. Left. Forebrain blood flow generated during CPR vs. cerebral perfusion pressure (arterial minus sagittal sinus pressure) when CPR was started at different times after cardiac arrest in dogs. Cerebral perfusion pressure was regulated by adjusting inflation pressure of a pneumatic thoracic vest during a continuous epinephrine infusion. Note the progressive decrease in blood flow at a particular perfusion pressure when the CPR is delayed from 0 minutes to 1.5, 3, 6, and 12 minutes. Right. Percent recovery of cerebral ATP becomes progressively lower when CPR is delayed from 0 minutes to 6 and 12 minutes at a particular level of perfusion pressure. (Curves drawn from refs. 192 and 195.)

Therefore, intermediate levels of blood flow during reperfusion generate intermediate levels of ATP recovery, but recovery of tissue pH appears to require near normal levels of blood flow and near normal levels of ATP recovery. Consequently, it can be speculated that clinical CPR provides partial recovery of energy metabolism, at least after relatively short arrest times (6 minutes), but that cerebral acidosis persists until return of spontaneous circulation. After longer arrest times, however, metabolic recovery is likely to be poorer. These observations emphasize the importance of early defibrillation.

Cerebral circulation after return of spontaneous circulation

With return of spontaneous circulation and normal cerebral perfusion pressure after complete ischemia, cerebral blood flow initially increases to above normal levels and then decreases to below normal levels. The mechanism of initial vasodilatation is multifactorial and includes elevated extracellular concentrations of potassium,[147] adenosine,[148] and nitric oxide,[149,150] decreases in extracellular pH and calcium, and possibly trigeminal sensory afferent activation.[151] The magnitude of the flow changes might also depend on estrogen.[152] Studies with iodoantipyrine in rats[33] and with stable xenon in dogs[153] indicate that

initial hyperemia is relatively heterogeneous among brain regions. The microvascular pressure required to start reflow of a non-Newtonian fluid in individual capillaries might be greater than the pressure required to maintain flow, particularly if swollen astrocytes reduce capillary diameter sufficiently to impede the flow of red cells and the less deformable white cells.[154] Thus, reperfusion at subnormal perfusion pressure is expected to result in poor reflow capillaries. Reperfusion accompanied by hypertension and hemodilution for several hours has been used to promote reflow and has been found to improve neurologic recovery in animals.[26,155] The existence of brain capillaries with true zero blood flow at a time when perfusion pressure is normal after resuscitation remains uncertain, however, because the spatial resolution of most blood flow techniques employed after ischemia[33,153] does not resolve individual capillary red cell flux.

Postischemic hyperemia typically lasts 5 to 40 minutes and depends on the duration of ischemia.[34] This hyperemic phase is followed by a period during which cerebral blood flow falls to subnormal levels and is termed "delayed hypoperfusion." The transition from hyperperfusion to hypoperfusion has been assumed to depend on the gradual clearance of vasoactive metabolites, although some evidence suggests that the transition can occur abruptly.[156] Delayed hypoperfusion does not appear to be the result of neurogenic vasoconstriction[157] or loss of neurogenic vasodilatation.[30] Both cerebral blood flow and oxygen consumption are reduced in comatose cardiac arrest victims during the first 6 hours after resuscitation[158] and can remain depressed in those with persistent coma.[159] Postischemic reductions in oxygen consumption are also observed in most experimental models of complete ischemia.[34,91,160] Therefore, reduced metabolic demand may contribute to hypoperfusion. Nevertheless, increases in oxygen extraction observed by some investigators[153] suggest that postischemic reductions in metabolic rate do not fully account for postischemic reductions in blood flow.

Delayed hypoperfusion generally lasts 2 to 6 hours. In a 1989 study, patients who regained consciousness after cardiac arrest had normal cerebral blood flow before regaining consciousness, whereas those who died without regaining consciousness surprisingly exhibited increased cerebral blood flow by 24 hours after resuscitation.[161] The pathologic significance of delayed hypoperfusion remains uncertain because its severity does not necessarily correlate with the neurologic outcome in animals,[162] and treatment with nimodipine to reduce delayed hypoperfusion did not improve outcome in patients[163] or animals.[164,165]

On the other hand, perfusion defects in individual capillaries have been observed[84] and could result in neuronal damage. Leukocytes, which are much less deformable than red cells and can be a major source of oxygen radicals, may contribute to hypoperfusion by plugging compressed capillaries.[166] Endothelium-dependent vasodilatation is impaired in pial arterioles[167] by an oxygen radical-dependent mechanism,[168] and this impairment in female animals is augmented by the loss of estrogen.[169,170] Furthermore, cerebral blood flow responses to CO_2 are largely impaired, whereas flow responses to hypoxia and changes in blood pressure are only modestly affected.[28,171–173] Oxygen radicals appear to be involved in loss of CO_2 reactivity.[168,174] Delayed hypoperfusion is attenuated by antioxidant treatment after cardiac arrest,[175,176] but not by osmotic or thrombolytic therapy.[177] Therefore, selective abnormalities in vascular regulation occur during the delayed hypoperfusion period at both the macrocirculatory and microcirculatory levels. The consequence of hypoperfusion on neuronal injury, however, remains unclear.

Mechanisms implicated in selective vulnerability

The selectively vulnerable areas of the brain are the hippocampus CA1 region, the cerebral cortical layers 3–5, and the cerebellar Purkinje cells. The phenomenon of selective neuronal vulnerability can be explained by two main hypotheses: the excitotoxic neurotransmitter hypothesis, based largely upon events during ischemia, and the free radical hypothesis, primarily due to events during reperfusion. The excitotoxic neurotransmitter theory suggests that the selectively vulnerable cell bodies and dendrites receive afferent projections that release large amounts of amino acid neurotransmitters (i.e. glutamate) during ischemia-induced depolarization.[178] There are two classes of glutamate receptors, one being the inotropic receptors, which are the ligand-gated ion channels, and second the metabotropic glutamate receptors (mGluR), which are coupled to cellular effectors via GTP-binding proteins. On the vulnerable neurons glutamate may bind to the two inotropic receptors that are distinctively activated by either N-methyl-D-aspartate (NMDA) or α-amino-3-hydroxy-5-methyl-4-isoxazole propionic acid (AMPA). NMDA receptor activation opens a Ca^{2+} channel, allowing Ca^{2+} influx, and AMPA receptor activation opens a Na^+ channel, allowing Na^+ influx. The increased intracellular Na^+ concentration (Na^+_i) is thought to induce reversal of normal Ca^{2+} extrusion through a $3\,Na^+/Ca^{2+}$ antiporter, thereby also resulting in increased intracellular Ca^{2+}_i. Studies with brain slices and cell cultures suggest that the mGluRs are coupled to several second messenger systems in situ, including those involved in activation of phospho-inositide hydrolysis, regulation of cAMP formation, and ion (calcium and potassium) channel modulation. The mGluR agonists have two unusual effects. First, they reduce transmission of excitatory amino acid (glutamate) and reduces inhibitory postsynaptic potentials (probably via decreased GABA release). Second, in the hippocampal CA1 region mGluR agonists induce long-term synaptic potentiation (thought to be how memory is formed), probably mediated by protein kinase C-induced escalation in NMDA receptor currents.[179] Intraocular injection of the metabotropic receptor agonists protects against retinal damage induced by NMDA, but intra-hippocampal injections of mGluR agonists caused massive hippocampal damage in some rat strains.[180,181]

There is convincing evidence for glutamate release during complete global ischemia.[178] The resultant calcium influx stimulates even more glutamate release from presynaptic vesicles.[182] In addition reuptake of glutamate is inhibited by arachidonic acid[183] and other products of lipid peroxidation.[184] Magnesium, which inhibits synaptic transmitter release and, as a natural calcium antagonist also inhibits cell death in vitro.[185,186] Nevertheless, NMDA receptor antagonists have generally failed definitively to salvage neurons after complete global ischemia. There is little evidence for sustained exposure to elevated glutamate during reperfusion, calling into question whether glutamate plays a role in the progressive neuronal reperfusion injury. Further, the hydrogen ions that accumulate intra- and extracellularly during ischemia have been shown to inhibit the NMDA receptor.[187] There is however more promising evidence that AMPA receptor blockade is neuroprotective following complete global ischemia.[188] Excitotoxic mechanisms mediated at this receptor may play a larger role in complete global ischemia and reperfusion injury than that mediated by the NMDA receptor. In total this evidence reinforces the role of ischemia-induced Ca^{2+} overload as a principal mechanism in neuronal death.

The free radical hypothesis of selective vulnerability asserts that neurons are more susceptible to radical-induced damage (specifically lipid peroxidation) during reperfusion because (1) they are deficient in glutathione peroxidase,[189] and (2) they are surrounded by oligodendrocytes that have iron stores which are released during ischemic reperfusion and catalyze formation of free radicals.[190,191] Indeed, White *et al.* reported direct histochemical evidence that during the first 90 minutes of reperfusion following a 10 minute cardiac arrest in rats, lipid peroxidation was concentrated in the selectively vulnerable zones.[192] In particular the lipid peroxidation products localized to the area of the Golgi apparatus, an important site of membrane recycling, and in the apical dendrite, an area rich in mitochondria.[193,194]

Since the two theories primarily involve different phases in an injury continuum (*i.e.*, ischemia then reperfusion), the glutamate and free radical hypotheses are by no means mutually exclusive. Furthermore substantial evidence exists for membrane damage caused by both calcium activation of phospholipases and generation of free radicals during reperfusion. Later in the chapter we will explore the idea that damage to membrane lipids plays a central role in postischemic brain injury. In the next section we will explore the loss of calcium homeostasis as mediated by both energy depletion and glutamate receptor activation during ischemia.

Calcium flux and calcium activated proteases

Disruption of neuronal Ca^{2+} homeostasis during global brain ischemia and reperfusion

In vivo microelectrode measurements of hippocampal CA1 pyramidal neurons indicate that cytosolic $[Ca^{2+}]$ increases from a baseline of 60–90 nM to 20–200 μM within 8 minutes of transient forebrain ischemia.[195,196] If reperfusion occurs after brief to moderate durations of ischemia, cytosolic $[Ca^{2+}]$ returns to baseline within 20 minutes.[65,21,22] A

secondary increase in cytosolic Ca^{2+}, however, is detected as early as 4–6 hours after reperfusion.[197] Unfortunately, no direct measurements of cytosolic Ca^{2+} beyond 6 hours have been reported. Less quantitative histochemical techniques have demonstrated a transient increase in mitochondrial Ca^{2+} by 10 minutes of reperfusion that returns to baseline within 1–2 hours.[198–200] Secondary increases in mitochondrial Ca^{2+} appear 24 hours after reperfusion in the hippocampal CA1 sector prior to evidence of ATP depletion or the morphologic appearance of cell death.[201] In contrast to the cytosol and mitochondria, endoplasmic reticulum Ca^{2+} is persistently depleted in postischemic CA1 pyramidal neurons.[202] Ultimately, total tissue Ca^{2+} in the CA1 hippocampus begins to increase 48 hours after reperfusion and reaches a peak at 72 hours corresponding to histopathological evidence of neuronal death.[203,204]

Overall, these measurements show that cytosolic and mitochondrial Ca^{2+} overload observed during ischemia and early reperfusion is reversible, but sustained ER Ca^{2+} depletion and delayed secondary cytosolic and mitochondrial Ca^{2+} overload occur in neurons that eventually die. Understanding the mechanism of delayed secondary disruption of Ca^{2+} homeostasis is essential to discovering the cause of delayed postischemic neuronal death. Dysfunction of a number of Ca^{2+} regulatory proteins has been implicated, including plasma membrane Ca^{2+}-ATPase, the L-type voltage-gated Ca^{2+} channel, NMDA receptor, AMPA receptor and transient receptor potential melastatin (TRPM7)[205–212] and endoplasmic reticulum proteins including endoplasmic reticulum Ca^{2+} ATPase, the IP_3 receptor and the ryanodine receptor.[32,213]

The calpain/calpastatin system

Calpains (EC 3.4.22.17) are a family of non-lysosomal neutral cysteine proteases. Their activity is absolutely dependent on Ca^{2+} and is regulated by a specific endogenous inhibitor calpastatin.[214,215] The two ubiquitous calpain isoforms are μ-calpain (calpain I) and m-calpain (calpain II). Immunohistochemical studies have demonstrated that μ-calpain is concentrated in neurons, while m-calpain appears to be relatively more abundant in glia, and calpastatin is evenly distributed between the two cell types.[216–219] μ-Calpain and m-calpain are heterodimeric proteins that have nearly identical substrate specificity, but require different Ca^{2+} concentration ($[Ca^{2+}]$) for activity.[41] The $[Ca^{2+}]$ required for in vitro proteolytic activity of μ-calpain is 3–50 μM and for m-calpain is 200–1000 μM.[220] The two isoforms have unique 80-kDa catalytic subunits with only 50% sequence homology, but share a common 30-kDa regulatory subunit. The catalytic subunits of μ calpain and m-calpain undergo N-terminal autoproteolysis at a $[Ca^{2+}]$ slightly greater than that required for substrate proteolysis. The result of autoproteolysis is a decreased Ca^{2+} requirement for subsequent proteolytic activity (0.6–0.8 μM for μ-calpain and 50–150 μM for m-calpain).[221–223] This reduced Ca^{2+} requirement of autolyzed calpains may be a mechanism of potentiated proteolytic activity in response to recurrent intracellular Ca^{2+} overload such as occurs in postischemic neurons.

In vivo calpain activity is measured by demonstrating autoproteolysis and/or substrate degradation. Autoproteolysis of calpain I reduces the mass of the 80-kDa subunit first to 78-kDa and then to 76-kDa, and these forms can be resolved by SDS-PAGE and detected by Western blotting.[224] Autoproteolysis of the 80-kDa calpain II subunit reduces the mass to 78-kDa, but this usually cannot be resolved by SDS-PAGE. Calpain substrate degradation is detected by the loss of intact protein or the appearance of calpain-specific degradation fragments, the latter of which is much more sensitive. For the cytoskeletal protein α-spectrin, antibodies have been generated that bind specifically to the α-spectrin fragment uniquely generated by calpain proteolysis.[225,226] This method appears to be the most sensitive way for detecting in vivo calpain activity in rodent models of brain ischemia.

Calpains are physiologically involved in regulation of the cell cycle, mitosis, motility, signal transduction, gene expression, long-term potentiation, and synaptic remodeling.[41,42,227,228] Functional knockout of both ubiquitous isoforms is achieved by knockout of the common regulatory subunit and is embryonically lethal.[229,230] Knockout of m-calpain is also embryonically lethal,[42] whereas μ-calpain knockout mice survive and are fertile.[231] Honda et al.[232] recently reported that RNAi-mediated knockdown of m-calpain but not μ-calpain caused aberrant mitosis and abnormal chromosome alignment. Taken together these results strongly suggest that the two isoforms have unique physiologic roles despite their common substrate profile. Under physiologic conditions, calpain activity is likely to be stimulated by transient localized increases in cytosolic Ca^{2+} and to be tightly regulated by the presence of calpastatin. In contrast, the massive unlocalized increase in cytosolic Ca^{2+} that occurs during brain ischemia is likely to overwhelm endogenous regulatory systems and thus result in pathologic calpain activity.

Neuronal calpain activity during global brain ischemia and reperfusion

The initial increase in cytosolic Ca^{2+} during severe brain ischemia is clearly adequate to cause increased μ-calpain

activity and autoproteolysis based on in vitro kinetic data. We have demonstrated μ-calpain autoproteolysis and calpain substrate degradation within 10–20 minutes of cardiac arrest in rabbits.[233,234] Yamashima et al.[235] used immunohistochemistry with an antibody specific to the 76-kDa autolyzed form of calpain I to demonstrate the appearance of autolyzed μ-calpain in the cytosol of CA1 and cortical pyramidal neurons after 20 minutes of global brain ischemia in monkeys. In our rat model of transient forebrain ischemia, a transient increase in calpain-mediated α-spectrin cleavage product is detected in the CA1 hippocampus 1 hour after reperfusion followed by a ten-fold greater rise beginning between 24 and 48 hours after reperfusion.[236] This result is consistent with that published by several other investigators using different models or species.[52,53,237]

Studies with calpain inhibitors provide evidence that neuronal death following both global and focal brain ischemia may be caused by increased calpain activity.[238–244] However, these studies must be interpreted with caution, because all synthetic calpain inhibitors effective in vivo have significant activity against other proteases[245,246] including cathepsins, which have also been mechanistically implicated in postischemic neuronal necrosis acting downstream of calpains.[247,248] Furthermore, studies of calpain inhibitor cannot elucidate the relative role of μ-calpain and m-calpain because all known calpain inhibitors are effective against both isoforms. Bendarski et al.,[249] reported, however, that anti-sense-induced translation suppression of μ-calpain in cultured neurons decreased spectrin proteolysis and improved recovery of evoked synaptic responses after NMDA-induced injury. This observation supports the hypothesis that μ-calpain is primarily responsible for pathologic calpain activity in postischemic neurons.

Nitric oxide

Nitric oxide (NO) is a free radical generated from the conversion of arginine to citrulline by the three isoforms of the enzyme nitric oxide synthase (NOS). Constitutive isoforms are regulated by calcium and calmodulin and are located in endothelium, periarterial nerves,[250] and in approximately 2% of parenchymal neurons,[251,252] whereas a calcium-independent isoform can be induced in microglia, macrophages, and astrocytes. Parenchymal NOS neurons are highly arborized,[253] permitting NO to diffuse to many neighboring neurons, where it can stimulate soluble guanyl cyclase.[254] The activity of neuronal NOS, anchored by postsynaptic density proteins, is coordinated by calcium entry through NMDA receptors.[255,256] In addition, activation of AMPA, kainate, and metabotropic glutamate receptors can result in stimulation of NOS activity.[257–261] Overstimulation of these glutamate receptors during and after ischemia is thought to lead to an overproduction of NO in neurons.[262,263]

Nitric oxide can form reactive peroxynitrite anions, nitrosonium cations and nitroxyl anions, and alterations of metalloprotein redox state.[264,265] Most important, ischemia and reperfusion increase superoxide production which, in the presence of increased NO availability, rapidly generates excess peroxynitrite anion.[266] In the presence of carbon dioxide, peroxynitrite forms the nitrogen dioxide intermediate, which leads to nitration of tyrosine residues and altered protein function, nitrosylation of sulfhydryl groups on proteins, and hypochlorous acid.[264,267] Peroxynitrite can form hydroxyl radicals without a requirement for iron, leading to DNA damage[268,269] and lipid peroxidation.[270] Reduced NMDA toxicity and reduced ischemic damage by both Cu,Zn-superoxide dysmutase overexpression and NOS inhibitors are consistent with a peroxynitrite-mediated mechanism.[253,271] Damage to DNA causes activation of the nuclear repair enzyme poly(ADP-ribose) polymerase (PARP). Overactivation of PARP, however, causes caspase-independent cell death by stimulating translocation of apoptosis-inducing factor from the mitochondria to the nucleus[272] and possibly by depleting NAD$^+$.[273,274] Inhibitors of PARP reduce toxicity from NMDA and from NO donors in neuronal culture.[269] Translocation of apoptosis-inducing factor into the nucleus has been described in hippocampal neurons after global ischemia.[275]

The role of neuronally derived NO in ischemic damage is largely supported by evidence from focal ischemia in male animals, in which administration of NOS or PARP inhibitors or gene deletion of neuronal NOS or the PARP-1 isoform reduce infarct size.[276–279] Unexpectedly, this mechanism appears to differ in female animals that are subjected to focal ischemia.[280] In contrast to focal ischemia, the role of NO in global ischemia in vivo is less convincing. Studies in gerbil,[281,282] rat,[283] and cat[284] with NOS inhibitors failed to detect an improvement in histopathology, although some reports have described a positive effect.[285] Moreover, endothelial NOS exerts protective effects in focal ischemia by promoting blood flow and limiting platelet aggregation and inflammation. The use of inhibitors that act on both neuronal and endothelial NOS could result in offsetting effects. In contrast to the pharmacologic strategy, neuronal NOS-deficient mice were found to have reduced hippocampal neuronal cell loss in the CA1 region after global cerebral ischemia.[286] Moreover, the PARP-1 isoform appears to be important in neuronal injury from global ischemia, because PARP-1-deficient mice had improved neuronal viability in striatum and hippocampus after cardiac arrest and resuscitation.[287] Therefore, genetically altered mice support a link among neuronally derived NO, PARP activation, and hippocampal injury after global ischemia, but more robust biochemical and molecular evidence will be required to substantiate that the observed effects are not related to developmental effects of gene deletion. Furthermore, additional work is required to elucidate how these mechanisms may differ in the female, where injury in the hippocampus, but not striatum, after cardiac arrest appears to be linked to gender and where overexpression of superoxide dismutase has no additional protective effect.[288]

Because the inducible isoform of NOS (iNOS) is calcium independent, it can produce a large amount of NO continuously if substrate is available. Induction of iNOS has been studied in experimental focal ischemia, where induction in microglia and astrocytes in the peri-infarct region increases over a 48-hour period.[289] The iNOS inhibitor aminoguanidine given as late as 24 hours after focal ischemia can attenuate the progression of the infarction.[290] A role for iNOS in the infarction process is also supported by the reduced infarct size seen in iNOS null mice.[291] But the role of iNOS in neuronal injury that arises from global cerebral ischemia in which infarction does not occur has not been well studied. In one study of four-vessel occlusion in the rat, aminoguanidine was shown to reduce the nitrite and nitrate metabolites of NO at 24 hours of reperfusion in hippocampus, restore long-term potentiation in the hippocampus, and improve performance on a short-term memory task.[292] In another study, aminoguanidine was found to increase the number of viable pyramidal neurons in the hippocampus and reduce the number of NADPH-diaphorase-positive cells (presumed to represent iNOS in activated microglia and macrophages) over 14 days of reperfusion.[293] Therefore, increased activity of iNOS over many days of reperfusion may contribute to the delayed neuronal loss in the hippocampus after global ischemia.

Membrane Damage by Brain Ischemia and Reperfusion

Enzymatic lipolysis during brain ischemia and reperfusion

ATP stores in the brain are depleted within 4 minutes of complete ischemia. This depletion is associated with loss of the normal transmembrane gradient of Ca^{2+} the resultant increase in Ca^{2+}_i catalyzes lipolysis during ischemia. (The subsequent free fatty acid (FFA) release metabolism generates superoxide radicals ($\cdot O_2^-$) during reperfusion.) Initially, phospholipases are activated during early ischemia.[294–296] The phospholipases are a ubiquitous family of enzymes, found in the cytosol, plasmalemma, and mitochondrial membrane, that hydrolyze functional groups from phospholipids.[297,298] Of particular interest is phospholipase A_2, which has an absolute requirement for calcium[299,300] and cleaves fatty acyl chains from the β-position of phospholipids. Arachidonic acid in mammalian cells is esterified almost exclusively at the β-position. Thus, lipolysis during ischemia results in accumulation of free fatty acids, especially arachidonic acid, whose metabolism during reperfusion produces $\cdot O_2^-$. Cyclooxygenase catalyzes the addition of two molecules of O_2 to an unsaturated fatty acid, like arachidonic acid, and produces prostaglandin PGG, which is rapidly peroxidized to PGH with concomitant release of $\cdot O_2^-$[182] There is evidence that the rate of lipolysis in the selectively vulnerable zones is significantly greater than it is in other areas of the brain.[296]

The release of FFA appears to continue during reperfusion.[301] Enzymatic lipolysis and lipid peroxidation may act synergistically in membrane destruction during reperfusion, as erythrocytes damaged by lipid peroxidation are lyzed more rapidly by phospholipase than are normal membranes.[302,303] Thus, fatty acids that have been peroxidized are better substrate for phospholipase and some products of lipid peroxidation stimulate phospholipase.[304,305] In addition to the lipid peroxidation, there is evidence of substantial inhibition of the lipid repair enzymes, lysophosphatidylcholine acyltransferase and fatty acyl CoA synthetase during reperfusion.[306] Lipid hydroperoxides, a product of lipid peroxidation, also interfere with the reacylation (salvage pathway) of neuronal phospholipids.[307]

Lipid peroxidation during brain reperfusion

The morphological progression of injury during reperfusion led to the hypothesis[308] that accelerated structural damage is a consequence of excessive generation of oxygen radicals followed by lipid peroxidation. The resultant changes in the conformation or configuration of the fatty acids alters the permeability and fluidity of the membrane leading to compromised receptors and ion channels.

Lipid peroxidation comprises a set of radical-mediated chemical chain reactions whereby the double bonds in the unsaturated fatty acid side chains are rearranged.[309] The cell membrane contains a large number of unsaturated fatty acids in a monolayer and is a favorable environment for a lipid peroxidation chain reaction.[310] The divinyl hydrogens in the PUFA side chains of membrane lipids are particularly susceptible to attack by oxidizing chemical species.[311] After initial abstraction of the divinyl hydrogen and rearrangement of double bonds in the PUFA to form a conjugated diene, the consequent lipid alkyl radical reacts with O_2 to form the lipid peroxyl radical, which then abstracts a divinyl hydrogen from a second PUFA, yielding a lipid hydroperoxide and another lipid alkyl radical. In the presence of a transition metal, the lipid hydroperoxide can be converted to a lipid alkoxyl radical, which is electrophilic enough to initiate further lipid peroxidation.[312] This allows geometric expansion of the chain reactions. PUFA hydroperoxides and alcohols undergo a number of subsequent catabolic reactions that generate several aldehydic products, including malondialdehyde.[313]

The identity of the initiating oxidizer remains unclear despite intense investigation,[309,314] although it is well established that the presence of a transition metal is required as a catalyst. Iron is undoubtedly the biologically relevant transition metal catalyst. The brain glia have abundant stores of oxidized (ferric) iron,[315] mostly in ferritin and transferrin[316] which is unable to act as a catalyst for oxygen radical reactions. Nonetheless, $\cdot O_2^-$ promotes reduction of ferric and release of ferrous iron from ferritin,[132] a reaction possible only during reperfusion. Iron delocalization into low-molecular weight species is seen in the brain during postischemic reperfusion.[129] Kinetic modeling has shown that membrane lipid peroxidation can be initiated in the presence of 1 μM iron by reduction via $\cdot O_2^-$[317]

Membrane lipids are extensively peroxidized by iron-dependent radical reactions during reperfusion.[318–323] Sakamoto *et al.* demonstrated increased in vitro formation of N-tert-butyl-a-phenyl-nitrone (PBN – a radical spin trap) spin adducts during reperfusion following 10 to 20 minutes of carotid occlusion in rats, and interpreted this as representing a burst of free radical production.[322] They found that the PBN adduct reached a peak at 5 minutes of reperfusion, and this peak increased with longer ischemic time. Furthermore, they noted products of lipid peroxidation were increased as early as 30 minutes after 10 minutes of ischemia, and the degree of lipid peroxidation also increased with longer ischemic time. Bromont *et al.* found brain lipid peroxide levels were selectively increased in the hippocampus, striatum, and cortex between 8 and 72 hours of reperfusion after 30 minutes of 4-vessel occlusion in the rat.[321] In our work, by 8 hours of reperfusion, there was loss of 30% of the lipid double bond content and ultrastructural evidence of large gaps in the neuron plasmalemma.[324] At this point, the neurons were no longer able to maintain ionic homeostasis. The biochemical effects we observed were significantly inhibited by treatment with deferoxamine during the first 15 minutes of reperfusion.[325]

We have utilized a rat model of 10-minute cardiac arrest and resuscitation[326] to study cellular localization of reperfusion-induced lipid peroxidation. By 90 minutes postresuscitation, reperfusion-induced fluorescent products of the reaction between thiobarbituric acid and lipid aldehydes formed by lipid peroxidation are found in the pyramidal neurons in the infragranular layers of the cerebral cortex, including layers 5 and upper layer 6, and in the pyramidal layer of Ammon's horn in the hippocampus. Our observations are consistent with the chemical data on lipid peroxidation during reperfusion and verify the study of Bromont *et al.* showing that the selectively vulnerable neurons are damaged specifically by lipid peroxidation during early reperfusion.

These reactions also appear to be involved in the genesis of the postischemic hypoperfusion phenomenon, which is inhibited by superoxide dismutase and deferoxamine[327] or U74006F,[328] a lipid peroxidation chain terminator.[329] Thus, there is now evidence implicating membrane damage by reperfusion-induced lipid peroxidation in both histological damage to neurons and in the genesis of the postischemic hypoperfusion syndrome.

Protein synthesis and brain ischemia and reperfusion

At the onset of reperfusion following global ischemia, protein synthesis is inhibited in neurons throughout the entire brain,[330] but it recovers over a 6–24-hour period in neurons more resistant to ischemic damage. In the brain region most vulnerable to transient ischemia, the CA1 of the hippocampus, normal levels of protein synthesis never recover during reperfusion even after relatively brief durations of ischemia.[331] Indeed, a number of investigators have suggested that persistent suppression of protein is a marker for neurons destined to die in the reperfused brain. Because proteins have such fundamental roles in the cell, including enzymatic reactions governing intermediary metabolism, transport, and storage, as well as intracellular signaling and cellular structure, significant changes in the ability of neurons to produce and maintain proteins would be expected to have considerable effects on the capacity of the cells to survive. The brain has a substantial requirement for protein synthesis just to maintain homeostasis. It expresses the largest percentage of its DNA of any organ, and its protein turnover is approximately equal to 100% of its protein content every 48 hours. Additionally, as a result of ischemia and reperfusion, there is a significant need for replacement of proteins damaged by calpain-mediated proteolysis and membrane lipid peroxidation (neuronal

membranes are ~50% protein). We will first review the regional and temporal pattern of protein suppression occurring as a consequence of brain ischemia and reperfusion and then review the pathophysiological mechanisms responsible.

Patterns of protein suppression in reperfused brain

Postischemic suppression of protein synthesis was first reported in 1971 by Kleihues and Hossman.[332] When cats were given ^{14}C-labeled amino acids intravenously during reperfusion and the protein was extracted from brain homogenates 30 minutes later, a 30% decrease in label incorporation was observed after 4 hours of reperfusion following 30 minutes of ischemia. Evidence now indicates that in the selectively vulnerable neurons the post-ischemic suppression of brain protein synthesis is severe and prolonged. Cooper *et al.* measured [^{14}C]phenylalanine incorporation by in vitro translation utilizing the postmitochondrial supernatant from rat brain homogenates.[333] Incorporation was normal in the homogenates derived from rats after 15 minutes of ischemia, but had fallen 80% after 15 minutes of reperfusion. They concluded that the reduction of protein synthesis was a consequence of reperfusion. Nowak *et al.* found that in vitro amino acid incorporation by the postmitochondrial fraction prepared from gerbil brain homogenates was normal after 30 minutes of ischemia without reperfusion.[334] After 10 minutes of recirculation, however, protein synthesis had decreased 90% and slowly recovered to 60% of baseline by six hours of reperfusion. Moreover, these studies show that as little as 3 minutes of ischemia triggers suppression of protein synthesis during reperfusion. The degree of suppression was dependent on the duration of the ischemia for ischemic periods of less than 5 minutes; longer ischemic times did not result in any additional suppression. Recovery of protein synthesis was not affected by the duration of ischemia in this model. In contrast, Dienel *et al.* found that increasing the duration of ischemia delays the recovery of in situ protein synthesis in the surviving areas.[335]

Translational competence in the brain after ischemia/reperfusion is not regionally homogeneous; the cortex, hippocampus, and caudate show severe and prolonged suppression of protein synthesis, while the brainstem and midbrain structures are relatively unaffected.[336] Araki *et al.*, using a bilateral carotid occlusion model in the gerbil, demonstrated regional differences in L-[methyl-^{14}C]methionine incorporation and corroborated the existence of an ischemic threshold for suppression of protein synthesis.[331] They found that 1 minute of ischemia did not suppress protein synthesis during reperfusion. After 2 minutes of ischemia, however, there was a severe, but reversible suppression, and 3 minutes of ischemia produced a severe loss of protein synthesis in the neocortex, striatum, the whole hippocampus, and the thalamus that slowly recovered during the following 5–24 hours; the CA1 region of the hippocampus never recovered its ability to incorporate label. These areas are also the ones most susceptible to delayed neuronal death following ischemia, indicating that a prolonged deficit in postischemic protein synthesis correlates with the selective vulnerability of these areas to ischemia and reperfusion.

Mechanisms of protein suppression in reperfused brain

Although the patterns of postischemic suppression of protein synthesis in the brain are well described, the mechanisms that cause it are still under investigation. Protein synthesis is a complex process requiring (1) high energy phosphates, (2) intact DNA, (3) intact transcription machinery, (4) processing and transport of mRNA from the site of transcription to the site of translation, and (5) intact translation machinery. Each of these steps is a potential site of disruption following ischemia and reperfusion.

Energy supply

Because protein synthesis requires energy, depletion of ATP/GTP stores is responsible for its cessation during ischemia. Nowak *et al.* showed that the postmitochondrial supernatant fraction isolated from ischemic brain would incorporate amino acids into polypeptides if a source of high-energy phosphates was added.[337] High-energy phosphate depletion cannot account for the prolonged suppression of protein synthesis seen during reperfusion, however, ATP, phosphocreatine, and GTP, all essentially zero after 5 minutes of ischemia, are normal by 15 minutes of recirculation.[334]

DNA stability and transcription

When a particular protein is to be made, the nucleotide sequence from the appropriate section of the chromosomal DNA is first transcribed into an RNA molecule. These transcripts are then subjected to a series of processing steps that includes capping on the 5′ end, removal of intron sequences by splicing, and polyadenylation on the 3′ end before the messenger RNA is permitted to exit from the nucleus and be translated into protein.

Brain DNA does not accrue any significant damage by either endonucleolytic or free radical mechanisms during cardiac arrest or during early reperfusion. We developed sensitive assays able to detect low levels of damage (1 radical-mediated single-strand nick in 200 000 base pairs), but found no evidence of radical-mediated base damage nor of strand scission in brain genomic or mitochondrial DNA after a 20 minute cardiac arrest followed by up to 8 hours of reperfusion.[338,339] Furthermore, neither thymine glycols nor thymine dimers, formed by free radical mechanisms and known to cause premature termination of transcription, were seen in the same model. Hours later, however, apoptosis can be triggered in neurons, and as a part of that response, Ca^{2+}/Mg^{2+}-dependent endonucleases are activated that cleave DNA into the characteristic 200-base pair pieces.

mRNA processing

Following synthesis by RNA polymerase II, the 5′ terminus of the nascent transcript is modified by the addition of a 7-methylguanosine (m^7G) cap; this cap helps the RNA to be properly processed, exported, and attached to a ribosome for translation. After capping, the pre-mRNA enters the splicing pathway where the introns (sequences of bases interspersed between coding sequences) are removed and the transcript is brought to its mature sequence. In animals, all mRNAs, except histone mRNAs, are terminated on the 3′ end by a polyadenylate tail [poly(A)$^+$], 100 to 200 nucleotides in length, which increases the stability of the message and appears to act as a signal for transport to the cytoplasm.

Intron-containing mRNAs are tightly bound to the nuclear matrix, most likely by the splicing system, which appears to be an integral part of matrix structure. Transit through the splicing pathway seems to be a prerequisite for transport of at least some transcripts out of the nucleus. Nuclear placement of a single cDNA coding for the 16S mRNA of SV40 results in normal transcription, processing, and cytoplasmic transport of the message only if there is at least one intron contained in the gene.

There is some evidence that splicing, and presumably the resulting proteins, are altered in neurons following a transient ischemic event.[340] Splice-site selection depends on the relative concentration of splicing regulatory proteins. When C57BL/6 mice were subjected to transient focal cerebral ischemia for 1 hour and various recirculation times, splicing regulatory proteins tra2-β1 and SAM68 changed their intracellular localization from the nucleus to the cytoplasm in neurons. This relocalization was an active process and not the result of a non-specific breakdown of the nuclear envelope; the splicing factor rSLM-2 and ribosomal RNA complexes remained in the nucleus, and there was no evidence of apoptosis. These effects seem to be specific, because the splicing patterns of *Bax*, *Bcl*, and *SERCA2* genes were not affected. The changes in pre-mRNA splicing pathways caused by the relocalization of proteins that regulate splice-site selection were due to a change in the calcium concentration associated with ischemia.[341] Alternative splicing has also been shown to be a regional phenomenon. Neurexin IIIα mRNA is up-regulated in postischemic CA3 and contained the insert corresponding to the fourth splicing site, whereas the transcripts in postischemic CA1 neurons and control CA3 neurons lacked the insert.

The effects of alternative splicing are unknown, but may be profound. The transcripts of most genes that encode apoptotic regulators are subject to alternative splicing, which can result in the production of anti- or pro-apoptotic protein isoforms. Daoud *et al.* studied the *ICH-1* gene that can generate two isoforms: ICH-1L, which promotes apoptosis, and ICH-1S, which prevents apoptosis.[342] In C57BL/6 mice subjected to transient focal cerebral ischemia, the ischemic episode stimulated inclusion of an alternative exon and the formation of the ICH-1S form. Conversely, a study of Bax κ, a splice variant of Bax, found that expression of Bax κ mRNA and protein was up-regulated in the hippocampus after cerebral ischemic injury. The increased Bax κ mRNA was distributed mainly in selectively vulnerable hippocampal CA1 neurons that are destined to die after global ischemia. In vitro, overexpression of Bax κ protein in HN33 mouse hippocampal neuronal cells induces cell death.

Non-intron-containing transcripts are not affected because they do not require splicing, but there is some evidence suggesting that translation of these transcripts depends upon the sequence of the 5′ leader.

Nucleocytoplasmic transport of mRNA

To reach the cytoplasm, the mRNA must transit through a nuclear pore complex (NPC), which spans the nuclear envelope and serves as a gateway of communication between the nucleus and cytoplasm.[343] The pore is a huge structure with 50 individual nuclear pore proteins that allows proteins of less than 5-kDa to pass unimpeded, but large molecules must be actively transported. Correctly processed mRNAs interact with the NPC in the form of large ribonucleoprotein complexes (mRNPs) rather than the naked mRNA molecule. mRNP complexes contain nuclear mRNAs, the cap binding proteins CBP20 and CBP80, general RNA binding proteins, splicing factors (for those mRNAs derived from spliced precursors), and other factors involved in pre-mRNA processing. In general mRNA export does not depend on a specific nucleotide motif.

A group of evolutionarily conserved proteins known as nuclear export factors (NXFs) is responsible for exporting the majority of cellular mRNAs to the cytoplasm. Recruitment of export factors to nascent mRNA starts cotranscriptionally and involves elaborate systems of quality control. NXFs mediate the interaction between the mRNA export cargo and components of the NPC required for translocation. Presumably, export factors can load onto mRNA in both a relatively non-specific way as well as via splicing-coupled mechanisms.

Release of mature mRNA from the nuclear matrix requires ATP and DNA topoisomerase II and is the rate limiting step in mRNA nuclear translocation. Mechanical disruption of the nuclear membrane does not increase mRNA efflux; as immature (intron-containing) mRNA remains matrix-bound. Transport of poly(A)$^+$ mRNA requires hydrolysis of ATP or GTP, and is mediated by a nucleoside-triphosphatase (NTPase) that is associated with the inner nuclear membrane and the nuclear lamina. The NTPase is stimulated in situ by poly(A)$^+$ mRNA, but not by poly(A)$^-$ mRNA; an effect that is mediated by a pore-associated poly(A)$^+$ binding protein.[344]

There are some observations suggesting that newly synthesized mRNA does not efficiently reach the cytoplasm following ischemia and reperfusion. Autoradiograms of pulse-labeled RNA in gerbils reperfused after 5 minute forebrain ischemia showed accumulation of newly synthesized RNA in the nucleus with little appearing in the cytoplasm.[345] Moreover, there are normal levels of newly synthesized mRNA in the nucleus and mitochondria during reperfusion but decreased new mRNA in the microsomal and ribosomal fractions. Similarly, there is apparent retention of RNA in the nucleus during reperfusion by using acridine orange staining. Together, this indicates a reduction in mRNA transport from nucleus to cytoplasm has occurred, and an increased population of messages is being retained in the nucleus.

To study poly(A)$^+$ mRNA transport and NTPase activity, we prepared nuclear envelopes (NEVs) from dog brain cortices after a 15-minute cardiac arrest followed by up to 6 hours of reperfusion.[346] The rate of ATP-dependent poly(A)$^+$ mRNA export from NEVs was examined after ^{3}-H-uridine-labeled poly(A)$^+$ mRNA was incorporated in NEVs during their preparation. The kinetic constants for ATP hydrolysis by the brain NEVs were not significantly affected by ischemia and reperfusion. Furthermore, appropriate poly(A) stimulation of the rate of ATP hydrolysis occurred without significant differences between animal treatment groups. In vitro exposure of the NEVs to hydroxyl radical completely abolished NTPase activity. Similarly, the rate of poly(A)$^+$ mRNA egress was stimulated by ATP in all samples, and the ATP-stimulated egress rates were unaffected by ischemia and reperfusion. Thus, brain ischemia and reperfusion do not induce direct inhibition of nucleo-cytoplasmic transport of poly(A)$^+$ mRNA, although micromolar quantities of hydroxyl radical completely inhibit the NTPase. Therefore postischemic inhibition of protein synthesis and reduced brain nuclear mRNA egress is not caused by direct damage to the poly(A)$^+$ transport system of the nuclear membrane. Similarly, we found that the nucleocytoplasmic translocation system for the poly(A)$^-$ hsp-70 mRNA at the nuclear membrane is intact during postischemic brain reperfusion.

mRNA following ischemia and reperfusion

Although total RNA synthesis is normal during reperfusion,[347] several studies have used gene arrays to show that there is considerable variation in individual mRNA expression after both focal[348] and global brain ischemia.[349] Nonetheless, caution is required in extrapolating changes in mRNA expression to changes in protein levels. In a meta-analysis of studies comparing mRNA expression levels and protein levels for 2044 molecules, Greenbaum *et al.* reported a poor correlation ($r^2 = 0.43$).[350] In yeast, Gygi *et al.* found that that similar mRNA expression levels could be accompanied by up to 20-fold difference in protein levels, and in some instances similar protein levels were accompanied by a 30-fold difference in mRNA levels.[351] Given this lack of correlation between mRNA and protein levels, it is not possible to predict protein expression levels from quantitative mRNA data. For example, during reperfusion, cells of the CA1 sector of the hippocampus express massively increased amounts of hsp-70 mRNA with little or no accumulation of HSP-70 protein. Eukaryotic mRNA has a half-life estimated at several hours and there is no evidence of a generalized increase in mRNA degradation during ischemia and reperfusion nor in other processes characterized by disaggregation of polyribosomes. Thus, taken together the data suggest a dissociation of transcription and translation that does not involve either failed transcription or an acceleration of mRNA degradation. We will now turn our attention to translation.

Translation

Translation of mRNA into protein requires the presence of functional ribosomal subunits, translation factors, aminoacyl-tRNAs, amino acids, an energy supply, and an appropriate ionic environment. Ischemia and reperfusion appears to alter significantly some but not all of these components. For example, ischemia does not alter the intracellular levels of amino acids.[352] Levels of aminoacyl-tRNAs, required for chain elongation, fall to no less than 64% of control values during reperfusion, and the energy supplies normalize upon circulatory return. Ribosomes can tolerate prolonged periods of ischemia without apparent functional impairment. Nowak *et al.* demonstrated stable in vitro incorporation of amino acids by brain polysomes after 1 hour of decapitation ischemia.[337] Marotta *et al.* reported that human brain ribosomes obtained 2–6 hours postmortem could synthesize proteins in vitro.[353] Dienel *et al.* found that polysomes isolated from rat brains subjected to 30 minutes of ischemia and 3 hours of reperfusion qualitatively produced the same protein patterns, with the addition of heat shock proteins, on 2D-PAGE gels as polysomes isolated from non-ischemic rat brains.[354] Our own work demonstrated that the rate of in vitro translation by purified ribosomes was not inhibited after 20 minutes of cardiac arrest or by 2 or 8 hours of reperfusion,[355] a time when protein synthesis is suppressed both in vivo and by in vitro translation systems utilizing an unfractionated postmitochondrial supernatant. The above evidence argues against any significant damage to the ribosomes themselves.

Several lines of evidence are consistent with the hypothesis that protein synthesis may be suppressed at initiation during early reperfusion, thereby deranging the "assembly line" involved in transport of mRNA. Ribosomal sedimentation profiles obtained from reperfused brains show a preponderance of monomeric ribosomal subunits suggesting a block in the formation of the initiation complex. In the study by Cooper *et al.* using an in vitro translation system, the addition of a chain initiation inhibitor (polyinosinic acid) decreased protein synthesis 63% in control animals as expected.[333] Polyinosinic acid had no effect on in vitro translation with the postmitochondrial supernatant obtained after 15 minutes of reperfusion, however, indicating that translation initiation was already maximally inhibited.

Formation of the translation initiation complex

The rate limiting step in translation is initiation.[356] This step entails the formation of the initiation complex (Fig. 13.5) which involves over 140 proteins and requires the coordinated assembly of the 40S and 60S ribosomal subunits, the mRNA to be translated, and the charged amino-acyl tRNA coding for the first amino acid (always methionine in eukaryotic cells). The process is orchestrated by a family of proteins collectively known as eukaryotic initiation factors (eIFs), and several eIFs are altered as a consequence of brain ischemia and reperfusion.

The initiation complex begins with free 40S ribosomal subunits; however, under normal physiologic conditions,

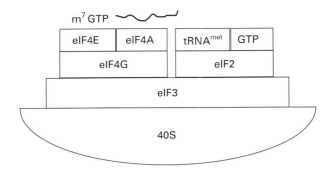

Fig. 13.5. Translation Initiation Complex

formation of inactive 80S ribosomes is favored. Binding of eIF6 to the 60S subunit and of eIF3 plus eIF4C to the 40S subunit act to keep the subunits disassociated. Next, eIF2 joins GTP and the initiator tRNA into a ternary complex (eIF2/GTP/Met-tRNA$_i$) which binds via eIF3 to the 40S subunit. The mRNA to be translated binds to eIF4E, which recognizes the m^{7}G cap at the 5′ end of the mRNA. eIF4A, eIF4E, and eIF4G form a complex which, together with eIF4B, unwinds the mRNA near the cap structure and binds it via eIF3 to the 40S subunit. At this point, the combined complexes migrate along the mRNA in the 5′ to 3′ direction to locate the AUG start codon. Once the appropriate match is made, eIF5 triggers the hydrolysis of the bound GTP molecule and the release of eIF2/GDP. A conformational change occurs such that the 60S subunit joins the 40S subunit to complete the 80S initiation complex.

Initiation is primarily regulated by modulating the degree of phosphorylation of the initiation factors required for the formation of the ternary complex (eIF2) and the recognition of mRNAs (eIF4E and eIF4G).

Cells determine which mRNAs bind to the ribosome by modulating phosphorylation of the mRNA cap binding protein, eIF4E. Cellular mRNAs vary greatly in their binding efficiency to eIF-4E, and increasing the activity or availability of the limited amount of eIF4E in cells appears to favor translation of those mRNAs that compete poorly for the mRNA-specific initiation factors. eIF4E is found in the nucleus as well as the cytoplasm and may play a role in post-transcriptional processing as well as translation initiation. Brain ischemia has been variably reported to induce transient dephosphorylation of eIF4E that normalizes rapidly with reperfusion.[357,358]

eIF4G is phosphorylated at multiple sites, which is thought to correspond with increased binding of eIF4E and enhanced protein synthesis. We found that µ-calpain (a calcium-activated protease) is activated during brain ischemia and proteolyzed eIF4G;[359] eIF4G is also a target of caspase-3, which cleaves it at multiple sites, but leaves a stable 76-kDa "middle fragment." In our model, multiple fragments of eIF4G persist in the forebrain at 90 minutes of reperfusion following a 10-minute cardiac arrest.[357] Martin de la Vega *et al.* confirmed proteolysis of eIF4G during ischemia and showed reduced eIF4G levels (~ 65% of control) in the vulnerable CA1 region at 4 hours of reperfusion.[360]

Nonetheless, we[357] and others[334] have found little or no inhibition of the overall rate of in vitro translation in brain homogenates after up to 30 minutes of complete global ischemia without reperfusion despite eIF4G degradation during ischemia. The surprisingly limited effect of eIF4G degradation on in vitro protein synthesis by brain homogenates obtained after ischemia without reperfusion suggests that either the residual amount of eIF4G is adequate to support translation initiation or that proteolytic fragments of eIF4G may be active in supporting initiation of translation. In either case, the proteolytic degradation of eIF4G may have major implications for message selection.[361] Fragmented eIF4G causes failure of the docking of eIF4E-bound m^{7}G-capped mRNAs to the small ribosomal subunit during initiation of translation and favors translation of messages that contain "Internal ribosome entry sites" (IRES).

Cells downregulate the overall rate of global protein synthesis primarily by decreasing the initiation rate via phosphorylating serine 51 on the α subunit of eIF2. Phosphorylated eIF2α [eIF2α (P)] is a competitive inhibitor of eIF2B, the factor that exchanges GTP for GDP once the eIF2/GDP complex is released after the start codon has been located. Because the ratio of eIF2 to eIF2B is approximately 5:1 in the brain, initiation translation will be nearly completely inhibited when ~20% of eIF2 contains a phosphorylated α-subunit.

Postischemic brain reperfusion induces a very rapid and large increase in eIF2α (P)[362] that is seen in highly vulnerable as well as less vulnerable neurons throughout the entire brain. After 10 minutes of reperfusion following a 10-minute cardiac arrest, phosphorylated eIF2α in brain homogenates has increased ~20-fold and represents ~23% of the total eIF2α. This extent of eIF2α phosphorylation will inhibit almost all protein synthesis. This level of eIF2α (P) remains relatively stable throughout the first 4 hours reperfusion. We used immunohistology to study the regional and cellular distribution of eIF2α (P) in normal, ischemic, and reperfused rat brains.[362] The small amount of eIF2α (P) in normal brains is predominantly localized to astrocytes, which lose their eIF2α (P) during ischemia, presumably due to unopposed action of phosphatases. In the early minutes of reperfusion, heavy eIF2α (P) immunostaining appears in the cytosol of neurons, and is most pronounced in the vulnerable neurons in cortical layers 3 and 5 and in the hilus and CA1 of the hippocampus; eIF2α (P) also appears in ischemia-resistant neurons of the dentate gyrus during early reperfusion. By 1 hour of reperfusion eIF2α (P) is largely undetected in ischemia-resistant neurons but remains prominent in vulnerable neurons, which also now display intense nuclear eIF2α (P) staining. By 4 hours of reperfusion, the pattern of nuclear eIF2α (P) immunostaining in vulnerable neurons suggests nuclear condensation consistent with the early stages of apoptosis. In addition, although eIF2α (P) is initially localized exclusively in neuronal cytoplasm, we found that by 1 hour of reperfusion, there is a substantial amount of eIF2α (P) only in the nuclei of vulnerable neurons; phosphorylated eIF2α was never found within the nuclei of neurons in the ischemia-resistant areas of the brain. These observations raise questions whether eIF2α is phosphorylated in the cytoplasm and migrates to the nucleus or is also phosphorylated in the nucleus itself. This could reflect a conformational change in eIF2α (P) that exposes the RRRIR nuclear localization signal adjacent to the Ser-51 phosphorylation site, and suggests the possibility that the nuclear localization of eIF2α (P) in vulnerable neurons by 1-hour reperfusion has important consequences for transcription.

Insulin and insulin-like growth factors administered during post-ischemic brain reperfusion substantially reduce both neuronal death and the final extent of neurologic disability independent of any hypoglycemia.[363] Insulin has several effects on the translation initiation system that, in general, increase protein synthesis; in particular, insulin rapidly decreases eIF2α phosphorylation, increases eIF2B activity and the association of eIF4E with eIF4G. We investigated the effect of insulin on protein synthesis during reperfusion utilizing immunostaining for eIF2α (P) and autoradiography of in situ [35] S amino acid incorporation.[364] After resuscitation from 10 minutes of cardiac arrest, rats were given 0, 2, 10 or 20 U/kg of intravenous insulin and reperfused for 90 minutes. Controls had abundant protein synthesis and no eIF2α (P) in neurons of the hippocampal CA1 and hilus. Untreated reperfused brains had intense staining for eIF2α (P) and little protein synthesis in these neurons, and animals receiving 2 or 10 U/kg of insulin, however, demonstrated little improvement. All animals treated with 20 U/kg of insulin, however, had complete clearing of eIF2α (P) and extensive label incorporation in vulnerable neurons. Interestingly, insulin did not block phosphorylation of eIF2α of the neurons after a 5-minute reperfusion. This is a direct demonstration that it is possible to reverse the phosphorylation of eIF2α (P) and the loss of protein synthesis in vulnerable neurons during early reperfusion.

Role of eIF2α (P) in message selection

The modifications to eIF2α induced by brain ischemia/reperfusion last for at least several hours and affect not only the rate of protein synthesis, but also the repertoire of peptides actually synthesized from the available mRNAs. High levels of eIF2α (P) cause a generalized decrease in global rate of translation, whereas lower levels of eIF2α (P) play a role in message selection. Because eIF2α (P) competitively inhibits the reaction needed to recycle eIF2, translation does not completely cease, and there is always some capacity for residual translation. There are at least two alternative translation initiation pathways, bypass scanning and IRES-mediated initiation, that exist and either of these can have profound influences on message selection.

Bypass scanning is a form of residual translation that occurs when the 5' untranslated region of an mRNA contains upstream open reading frames (uORF).[365] In situations where there are high levels of eIF2 α (P), there is inefficient delivery of the initial methionine tRNA to the ribosome. Thus the ORF that is translated under normal conditions may be bypassed because of the lack of an initiator tRNA at the time when the scanning ribosome reaches the start codon. If an initiator tRNA becomes available at a later point as the ribosome scans the remainder of the mRNA, translation can be initiated on a downstream, normally untranslated, ORF. Upstream open reading frames are important control elements of growth and differentiation of cells. Although less than 10% of vertebrate mRNAs contain an uORF, about two thirds of mRNAs encoding vertebrate growth-regulatory proteins have uORFs. This paradoxical eIF2α (P)-induced enhancement of translation has been shown to occur for the pro-apoptotic proteins CHOP and ATF4, and may contribute to directing reperfused neurons down a cell death pathway.

Initiation of translation from the vast majority of cellular mRNAs occurs via scanning; the 40 S ribosomal subunit binds to the m^7G-cap and then moves along the mRNA until an initiation codon is encountered. Nevertheless, the 5' untranslated region of some mRNAs contain regions, called internal ribosomal entry sites (IRES), and cellular stress can stimulate translation from some cellular IRESs via a mechanism that requires the phosphorylation of eIF2α.[366] It is thought that some mammalian mRNAs use IRES-mediated translation to provide cells with proteins essential for survival when the nutrient supply is limited.[367] Although cellular stress can stimulate translation from some cellular IRESs via a mechanism that requires the phosphorylation of eIF2α, there are distinct regulatory patterns for different cellular mRNAs that contain IRESs within their 5′-untranslated regions. Thus it will be crucial to determine if, for example, APAF-1 (Apoptosis-Activating Factor-1), which is produced only by an IRES-mediated mechanism and serves to maintain sufficient levels of APAF-1 even when cap-dependent translation initiation mechanisms are compromised, is being synthesized after brain ischemia/reperfusion.

The combination of bypass scanning and IRES-mediated translation initiation means it is not possible to predict precisely which peptides are being made from examining changes in mRNA in the reperfused brain. An elevation in capped mRNAs does not mean that they will get translated under conditions of IRES-mediated translation initiation. Furthermore, even in the subset of IRES-containing mRNAs, it will be impossible to determine which ORF is being used from study of the available mRNAs by bypass scanning.

Mechanisms to hyperphosphorylate eIF2a following transient global brain ischemia

Protein synthesis is downregulated by phosphorylating eIF2α in response to a wide variety of cellular stresses, including transient brain ischemia.[362] It appears that specific eIF2α kinases have evolved that directly sense specific cellular stresses and respond by regulating translation. There are four known eIF2α kinases, GCN2, HRI, PKR, and PERK that, either individually or in combination, could mediate eIF2α phosphorylation in the reperfused brain. Because many of the stimuli that signal for inhibition of protein synthesis occur as a consequence of transient brain ischemia, it remained to be determined which eIF2α kinase(s) was activated under these stresses; in one in vitro system, at least three of the eIF2α kinases were activated simultaneously in response to a single chemical insult.

Although all four kinases share homology in the kinase catalytic domain, their regulatory mechanisms are quite different. GCN2 (general control non-derepressible-2), which is expressed in mammalian brain, is activated in response to amino acid starvation in mammalian cells. During ischemia, lowered ATP levels in neurons make it possible that uncharged tRNAs accumulate thereby activating GCN2. However, Munoz *et al.* were unable to demonstrate GCN2 activity in PC12 neurons following in vitro ischemia.[368] HRI (heme-regulated inhibitor) coordinates globin synthesis with heme availability in erythroid cells, but it can be activated by transition metals and reactive oxygen species both of which are characteristic of post-ischemic brain reperfusion. Little, if any, HRI is present in brain, however.[369] PKR (double-stranded RNA-activated protein kinase) can be activated in neuronal cell

culture by calcium overload induced by the calcium ionophore A23187. In addition, PKR can be activated upon its cleavage in vitro by recombinant caspase-3, caspase-7, and caspase-8. Calcium overload and caspase activation are well-known events in reperfused brain, and Burda *et al.* have suggested that PKR was responsible for increased eIF2α (P) during reperfusion.[358] Although PKR can be activated by calcium overload, it is not required for increased eIF2α phosphorylation or inhibition of protein synthesis in response to amino acid deprivation or endoplasmic reticulum stress. PERK (also known as PEK) is an endoplasmic reticulum transmembrane protein that couples protein folding in the endoplasmic reticulum to translation initiation rates in the cytoplasm.[370] Hypoxia can induce PERK activation and subsequent phosphorylation of eIF2 in fibroblasts.[371] Previously, we have shown that PERK is present in the brain and is activated early in reperfusion following transient ischemia.[372]

The development of knockout mice has allowed us to address the question of which kinase is responsible for the dramatic increase in eIF2α (P) during reperfusion. Previously, we have shown that mice with homozygous functional knockouts for the gene encoding either GCN2, HRI, or PKR had large increases in brain eIF2α (P) following ischemia and reperfusion similar to wild type mice;[372,373] this argues against one of these kinases being solely responsible. Nevertheless, in a transgenic mouse line with targeted disruption of the *Perk* gene, we found that phosphorylated eIF2α is absent in the non-ischemic mice.[374] This implies that PERK is the kinase chiefly responsible for modulating the basal level of eIF2α (P). More important, there was only a minimal change in phosphorylated eIF2α levels and there was a substantial rescue of protein translation in the reperfused transgenic mice compared to the wild type. Together, these data demonstrate that PERK is responsible for the large increase in phosphorylated eIF2α early in reperfusion that suppresses protein synthesis following transient global brain ischemia.

It is possible that increased phosphorylation of eIF2α could also result from a loss of an eIF2α (P) phosphatase activity, but we found no reduction in eIF2α (P) phosphatase activity in reperfused brain homogenates.[373]

An alternative mechanism was suggested by a series of studies by Gupta and colleagues which identified a 67-kDa glycoprotein (p67) that binds to the γ-subunit of eIF2 and protects its α-subunit from phosphorylation.[375] Depletion of p67, either by preincubation of brain homogenates with antibody against p67 or by antisense-mediated reduction of p67 in KRC-7 cells results in greatly increased eIF2α phosphorylation. In p67-depleted KRC-7 cells, eIF2α (P) approached 100% of eIF2α and was associated with a three-fold reduction in protein synthesis, and induction of apoptosis. The binding of p67 to eIF2 is regulated by glycosylation of p67; when deglycosylated, p67 is unable to prevent phosphorylation of eIF2α.

Because glycosylated p67 is present in rat brain, these findings suggested at least two testable hypotheses might explain the large and prolonged increase in eIF2α (P) in vulnerable neurons during reperfusion. First, activation of the p67 deglycosylase and subsequent deglycosylation of brain p67 might occur during ischemia and/or early reperfusion and be more extensive in vulnerable neurons. Second, the vulnerable neurons, such as those in the CA1, could normally express smaller amounts of p67 than more resistant neurons, such as those in the CA2. We found no reperfusion-induced loss of total or glycosylated p67 by Western blots or by immunohistochemical staining in vulnerable neurons, however.[376] Thus the mechanism by which eIF2α is phosphorylated during reperfusion is due solely to the activation of PERK.

Role of PERK in the UPR

PERK is activated only by the ER stress signaling system termed the unfolded protein response (UPR).[377] Thus, inhibition of protein synthesis following brain reperfusion is likely to be part of a more comprehensive cellular response that contributes to the ultimate fate of reperfused neurons.

The UPR is activated to overcome ER stress by temporarily slowing accumulation of new proteins in the ER lumen, while simultaneously upregulating transcription of genes for ER-resident chaperones and enzymes that abate the effects of ER stress.[377] In higher eukaryotes, prolonged activation of the UPR can also activate pro-apoptotic mechanisms. PERK contributes to a pro-survival response by attenuating accumulation of new protein in the ER through phosphorylation of eIF2α leading to a generalized decrease of protein synthesis. Several studies have presented evidence of ER dysfunction following ischemia and reperfusion.[372,378] Thus, we have hypothesized that regional differences in expression of the UPR in brain may contribute to selective vulnerability following ischemia and reperfusion.[379]

The primary effectors of the UPR in mammalian brain are three ER-transmembrane proteins: PERK, IRE1α, and ATF6, and it is thought that activation of all three is required for a full response to ER stress.[379] In transient focal cerebral ischemia, Paschen et al. found a marked increase in processed xbp1 mRNA levels during reperfusion, indicating activation of IRE1α, that was most pronounced after a 1-hour occlusion of the right middle cerebral artery.[380] The rise in processed xbp1 mRNA was not paralleled by a

similar increase in its cognate protein levels, however, because transient ischemia induces severe suppression of translation. In contrast, our data indicates that there is dysfunction in the UPR during global brain ischemia and reperfusion.[381] In rats subjected to 10 minutes of global brain ischemia, PERK was maximally activated at 10 minutes of reperfusion, which correlated with maximal eIF2α phosphorylation and protein synthesis inhibition. Neither ATF6 nor IRE1α show evidence of activation, however. IRE1α's substrate, xbp1 mRNA, had not been processed nor was there expression of the UPR effector proteins XBP1 (55-kDa), CHOP or ATF4. In other systems, failure to mount the UPR results in increased cell death.

Translation in late reperfusion

Finally, during the later reperfusion period, other mechanisms may be responsible for continued inhibition of translation. Apoptosis can inhibit protein synthesis via the caspase-dependent cleavage of initiation factors eIF4G, eIF4B, eIF2α and the p35 subunit of eIF3.[382,383] Substantial shifts in potassium, magnesium, and calcium occur that could affect translation. Ribosome activity is very sensitive to concentrations of potassium and magnesium, both of which are important for assembly of the ribosomal subunits. Decreased Mg^{2+} concentrations result in disaggregation of polysomes, increased missense errors, and decreased protein elongation. Normal pH and tissue concentrations of Na^+, K^+ and Ca^{2+} are recovered early in reperfusion. However, a secondary loss of ionic homeostasis is seen by 8 hours of reperfusion following a 15-minute cardiac arrest in dogs with concomitant loss of 30% of the lipid double bond content and ultrastructural evidence of large gaps in the neuron plasmalemma.[324] Finally Liu et al. have shown evidence of irreversible aggregation of translational components after prolonged ischemic times.[384]

Thus, the evidence we have reviewed suggests that postischemic suppression of protein synthesis in the brain has different etiologies depending on the time examined. During ischemia, suppression of protein synthesis is due to the lack of high energy phosphates needed to support the energy-requiring synthetic process. Although the high energy phosphate level quickly returns to normal during early reperfusion, there is inhibition of formation of the translation initiation complex secondary to the phosphorylation of eIF2α by PERK. Nuclear retention of newly synthesized mRNA probably reflects a "backup" of mRNA traffic. Later in the reperfusion period, lipid peroxidation eventually destroys the integrity of the plasmalemma for ionic partitioning, and after this time protein synthesis will be halted because the cell can no longer maintain the requisite ionic milieu.

Surprisingly, it is not clear that restoring protein synthesis in the reperfused brain is beneficial. There is contradictory evidence from studies with mutant variations of eIF2α and PERK as to whether activation of PERK, phosphorylation of eIF2α, and inhibition of translation are protective,[385] pro-apoptotic,[386] or neutral.[387] While the conflicting conclusions in the above studies could be ascribed to different insults administered to different cell lines, we theorize that there may be some time points following an insult where translation is protective, while at other times it may induce death. During early reperfusion, eIF2α(P)-mediated inhibition of translation may well be a protective response to cope with ischemia-induced ER stress. It is clear, however, that at some stage protein synthesis must be restored to ensure survival.[388] The contribution of postischemic inhibition of cerebral protein synthesis inhibition to neuronal death is a crucial issue that has yet to be resolved.[389,390,391]

Mitochondria: membrane potential, cytochrome

As previously stated, since the contribution of apoptosis to postischemic neuronal death appears to have enormous therapeutic relevance, the following reflections will focus on apoptosis. Two apoptotic pathways have been identified: the extrinsic, death receptor protein-mediated pathway, and the intrinsic, mitochondria-mediated, pathway.[392] In neuronal ischemia both pathways may be activated. Apoptosis is an energy-dependent, programmed form of cell death.[41,45] Mitochondria have long been considered as subcellular targets of ischemia. Disturbed mitochondrial function appears to be a key player in the pathogenesis of post ischemic neurodegeneration and a critical factor in the cellular "life-or-death" decision.[393–396] Mitochondrial dysfunction is a trigger for development of necrotic as well as apoptotic neuronal death.[397] In general, relatively mild mitochondrial injury results primarily in apoptotic cell death, whereas more extensive injury leads more toward necrosis. Thereby, alterations in mitochondrial oxidative phosphorylation, Ca^{2+} transport, free radical generation, and release of apoptotic factors[394,398,399] are major events in the damaging process. Two of the earliest events that can tip the balance toward neurodegeneration following transient ischemia are the accumulation of Ca^{2+} and generation of ROS by mitochondria. It is generally accepted that the mitochondrial membrane potential ($\Delta\Psi_m$) is an important factor in the maintenance of mitochondrial homeostasis:

both the influx of Ca^{2+} and production of ROS are attenuated following a decrease in $\Delta\Psi_m$.[394,395,399] Under normal conditions, more than 90% of the available cellular oxygen is consumed by the mitochondria during oxidative phosphorylation.[400,401] Which is driven by the electron donors NADH and FADH. These electron carriers enter the mitochondrial electron transport chain via complex I (NADH) and complex II (FADH). Electrons are transferred to oxygen via cytochrome c oxidase and other components of the electron transport chain.

Cytochrome oxidase, located in the inner mitochondrial membrane, is composed of 13 subunits. To function properly this complex requires intact catalytic, regulatory and structural subunits as well as maintenance of the inner mitochondrial membrane environment.[402]

Cytochrome c is a vital component of the mitochondrial electron transport chain. It is a water-soluble protein whose primary function is to transport electrons between coenzyme Q and cytochrome c oxidase. Cytochrome c resides in the mitochondrial interspace where it interacts with the redox partners of complexes III and IV. The entire process generates an electrochemical proton gradient across the mitochondrial membrane driving ATP synthesis by complex V.[403] Electron transport along the electron transport chain and ATP synthesis are closely related, in this case respiration is functionally "coupled."

The disturbance of energy dependent processes during early ROSC is thought to have a major influence on the development of temporary and permanent neurological deficits. As previously noted, ischemia results in rapid loss of high-energy phosphate stores. The amount of available ATP becomes insufficient to sustain normal function of active transport systems and to maintain proper ionic gradients.[404–406] Inadequate oxygen supply but also insufficient amounts of available electrons (donated from NADH or FADH) influence the cellular redox state and lead to mitochondrial damage.[403,407] The ability to produce ATP via oxidative phosphorylation is impaired in the integrated cellular substrate pathway (NADH, complex I).[408,46] Initially, brief periods of ischemia damage complex I in the proximal electron transport chain followed by damage to complex III.[402] Disturbances of the electron transport chain may cause a reduced cellular redox state even under normal oxygen concentrations.[408–410] Electron transport and ATP synthesis become "decoupled." Decoupled mitochondria reduce cell viability,[411] may result in further disturbances of electron transport,[46,412,413] produce reactive oxygen and nitrogen species,[414,415] and can lead to free radical damage.[46] Initially these changes are reversible, but the release of cytochrome c and the opening of the mitochondrial permeability transition pore pave the way to irreversible damages and finally to cell death. Opening of the mitochondrial permeability transition pores causes depolarization of the mitochondrial membrane potential ($\Delta\Psi_m$) and transforms mitochondria from ATP producers to ATP consumers by reversing ATP synthesis in an attempt to maintain $\Delta\Psi_m$.[416] In addition, prolonged membrane dysfunction can lead to excessive water influx, matrix swelling and outer mitochondrial membrane rupture. The release of proapoptotic molecules, including cytochrome c and Apaf-1, triggers cell death via caspase-dependent as well as caspase-independent mechanisms.[416] Therefore, increased mitochondrial permeability and reduction of $\Delta\Psi_m$ are key factors in triggering apoptosis in a variety of cell types.[417]

Mitochondria under normal conditions generate small amounts of cytotoxic reactive oxygen species (ROS), like hydroxyl radicals ($^\bullet OH$), superoxide anions ($O_2^{\bullet-}$), hydrogen peroxide (H_2O_2), nitric oxide (NO), peroxynitrite ($ONOO^-$) and other radical substances.[402,418] ROS production is essentially a toxic by-product mainly generated by complex III of the mitochondrial electron transport chain. As reactive oxygen species may damage cellular components, cells have developed various strategies to dissipate free radicals and remove their oxidation products.[40] Superoxide dismutase (SOD), glutathione peroxidase (GSHPx), and catalase constantly scavenge physiological amounts of free radicals.[419] SOD specifically processes O_2^- into H_2O_2. Catalase and GSHPx deactivate H_2O_2 into H_2O and O_2, which is especially important as hydroxyl radicals may be generated from H_2O_2 through the Fenton reaction.[400] Unfortunately, during oxidative stress, cytochrome c oxidase generates greater amounts of ROS.[400] Under these conditions, up to 2% of the consumed oxygen can be converted to free radicals.[397] The degree of ROS production depends on the type of the cell, the available substrate and the polarization of the mitochondrial membrane. The resulting overload of free radicals may cause cerebral damage during ischemia as well as reperfusion.[418,419,420] Permeabilization of the mitochondrial membrane caused by these reactive oxygen species is one of the basic underlying mechanisms of active cell death.[421] Mitochondrial membrane permeabilization can lead to an increased translocation of Bax from cytosol to the mitochondria,[422,423] and a release of cytochrome c and apoptosis inducing factor (AIF). Translocation of mitochondrial cytochrome c to the cytoplasm has been reported to be a key step in the initiation and/or amplification of the intrinsic pathway of apoptosis.[392,424,425] Release of cytochrome c into the cytosol leads to the formation of a complex comprising apoptotic-protease-activating factor-1 (Apaf-1), procaspase-9, and ATP. This complex ultimately cleaves and activates pro-caspase-9, activating the intrinsic pathway for the induction of apoptosis.[426–429] Additionally, cerebral ischemia

causes and activates the neuronal form of nitric oxide synthase (nNOS) and triggers the expression of the inducible iNOS in glia cells, both of which result in the production of an excessive amount of nitric oxide (NO).[430] Nitric oxide is a diffusable free radical that may prevent or promote cell death depending on cell type and NO concentration. NO interacts directly and indirectly with mitochondria. Binding of NO to cytochrome c oxidase causes respiratory inhibition.[431] As a result, NO may trigger apoptosis by one of the following mechanisms: decreased mitochondrial membrane potential, release of cytochrome c from mitochondria, direct activation of several caspases, degradation of caspase-activated DNAse inhibitors, and activation of caspase-activated DNAse.[430] Several homozygous e/i/nNOS knockout mice mutants have been developed to investigate the role of NO in intra- and postischemic pathophysiology.[418] By using these knockout models, a substantial reduction in lesion size after focal ischemia was noted in nNOS knockouts[432–434] as well as the influence on the blood flow-dependent development of cerebral lesions noted in eNOS knockouts.[435] Other studies indicate that NO produced by iNOS in non-neuronal cells may contribute to cerebral ischemic damage.[436]

Cell signaling: Bcl-2, .. caspases

Release of cytochrome c, apoptotic protease activating factor 1 (Apaf-1), and caspase-9 from mitochondria are central mechanisms for triggering the caspase cascade and therefore for inducing apoptosis. Cysteine-requiring aspartate directed proteases (caspases or cell death proteases) and Bcl-2 family proteins represent core components of the apoptotic process.[45] Recently, it has been suggested that "caspase-mediated-cell death" might be a more accurate description than "apoptosis" for the ischemia triggered programmed cell death.[45] Fourteen distinct caspases have been identified thus far, although two of them (caspase-11 and caspase-12) have no identified human counterparts.[45] Under normal conditions caspases are expressed as zymogens composed of an N-terminal prodomain, a large subunit and a small subunit, which undergo proteolytic processes upon apoptotic stimuli.[437] The subunits within some or the procaspases are separated by small linker peptides. Activation results from proteolytic cleavage of the procaspase into its three component parts, usually by other activated caspases.[438] Caspases can be subdivided into two broad groups: those of the interleukin-1 converting enzyme family (caspases-1, -4, -5, -11, -12, and -14) that are involved in the maturation of cytokines and the induction of inflammation and those caspases directly involved in apoptosis (caspase-2, -3, -6, -7, -8, -9, and -10).[439,440] By using functional aspects, the latter caspase proteins can be classified into upstream "initiators" (caspase-2, -8, -9, and -10) that act as signal transducers and downstream "effectors" (caspase-3, -6, and -7).[442] The initiator caspases have long prodomains that interact with the death domains of other transmembrane and intracellular proteins involved in initiating apoptosis and thus translate a range of pro-apoptotic stimuli into proteolytic activity. In contrast, the effector caspases have short prodomains and are directly responsible for the cleavage of cellular substrates that are in turn responsible for most of the morphological and biochemical features of apoptosis.[45,441] There are two main pathways of caspase activation: death receptor-mediated and mitochondria mediated. The extrinsic pathway is triggered by Fas and TNF-1 and leads via the formation of a "death-inducing signaling complex" to the activation of the

initiator caspases-8 and -10.[391,441] Binding of death receptors by their cognate ligands causes trimerization of the receptors and interaction between cytoplasmic death domains in these receptors and intracellular adapter proteins.[439] The mitochondrial pathway of caspase activation can be initiated by several proteins. Central to this pathway are proteins in the Bcl-2 family. The Bcl-2 family proteins are central modulators of intracellular apoptotic processes by regulating the cytochrome c-dependent pathways of caspase activation. Bcl-2 family proteins are either members of the anti-apoptotic (Bcl-2, Bcl-X_L, Bcl-w) or the pro-apoptotic (Bax, Bak, Bad, Bid) faction.[441] Post-translational modification can change anti-apoptotic members to pro-apoptotic forms.[442] The degree of formation of homo- and heterodimers of these proteins coincides with either cell death or survival. Unfavorable alterations in the ratio of anti- and pro-apoptotic caspases accelerate programmed cell death.[443] Anti-apoptotic members of the Bcl-2 family, including Bcl-2 and Bcl-X_L, are associated with the mitochondrial outer membrane and can inhibit the release of cytochrome c.[444] In contrast the pro-apoptotic protein Bax promotes apoptosis by forming oligomers onto the mitochondrial outer membrane and creating a channel for the release of cytochrome c and other apoptotic substances.[417] Another pro-apoptotic protein Bad binds to Bcl-2 and Bcl-X_L and inhibits their anti-apoptotic functions.[444] Some of the Bcl-2 family proteins are regulated directly by caspases. Therefore the caspase-mediated effects on Bcl-2 family proteins provide a link between the death receptor and mitochondrial pathways for apoptosis.

It was suggested that, after dephosphorylation, interactions of Bad with Bcl-2 and Bcl-X_L on mitochondria may initiate the opening of mitochondrial permeability transition pores and the consequent release of cytochrome c.[444] Cytochrome c together with Apaf-1 and dATP can activate the initiator caspase-9 by activating pro-caspase-9446.[392] Cytochrome c, Apaf-1, and caspase-9 are responsible for the formation of the apoptosome. The apoptosome cleaves and activates procaspase-3 the key effector of caspase-mediated cell death. The critical nature of caspase-3 activation to apoptosis is demonstrated nicely by the decreased neuronal damage in caspase-3 knock-out mice.[437,445] Following these two steps of apoptotic activation other caspases such as caspase-2, -6, and -7 are activated. Activation of the caspase cascade results in cell death through disassembly of the nuclear envelope, degradation of DNA repair enzymes, inactivation of the inhibitor of caspase-activated DNase (ICAD), and the release of caspase-activated DNase (CAD) leading to the apoptotic fragmentation of nuclear DNA.[44,446] The mechanisms of apoptosis is summarized in Fig. 13.6

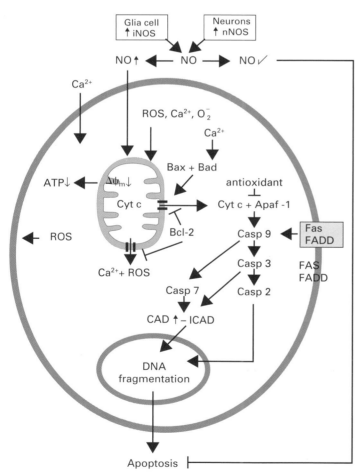

Fig. 13.6. Mechanisms of cerebral ischemia-induced neuronal apoptosis; modified from refs. 9,10,52.

Competence of neurons for antioxidant defense and repair of membrane damage

Regulatory control of the cell cycle may affect the capacity for endogenous defense and repair and may be critical in surviving ischemia and reperfusion. Terminally differentiated, therefore non-replicating cells, such as those in the glomeruli, the myocardium, and the central nervous system, are quite sensitive to damage by ischemia and reperfusion. Traditionally, it was postulated that non-replicating cells without stem cell support were irreplaceable. Nevertheless, there are data suggesting that non-replicating status is associated with chronic downregulation of (1) the transcription promoter binding complex called activator-protein-1 (AP-1), known to act at promoter regions of a family of antioxidant enzymes, and (2) lipid synthesis that would be important for efficient membrane repair.

Cell replication status and membrane synthesis

The theory that DNA replication and membrane synthesis were linked would be easily explained since both are required for cell replication. This idea is supported by evidence from both prokaryotic and eukaryotic systems, including cultured human cell lines. In prokaryotes experimental manipulations that specifically inhibit lipid synthesis block DNA replication,[447] and blocked DNA replication is associated with down-regulation of phospholipid synthesis.[448] Fewer studies have addressed such questions in eukaryotic cells; however, in a human promyelocytic cell line, sterol and phospholipid synthesis are markedly decreased following induction of myeloid differentiation. Although lipid synthesis before and after neuronal differentiation has not been studied in detail, it is known that there is a 90% decrease in cholesterol synthesis in neurons after completion of differentiation in fetal rats. There is also important evidence that the degree of differentiation is directly related to susceptibility to radical oxidant-induced death in many cell culture lines.[449] Tumor cells, in which replication machinery is fully switched on, are not easily killed by lipid peroxidation.[450] It appears that terminal differentiation is associated with a substantial reduction in the capacity for lipid neogenesis and membrane synthesis.

This theoretical approach predicts that terminal differentiation of neuroblasts to neurons should be associated with a significant increase in susceptibility to cell death induced by membrane damaging mechanisms such as free radical induced lipid peroxidation. We have observed substantial enhancement of radical-induced death in neuroblastoma B104 (NB104) cells after neuronal differentiation,[451] induced by dibutyryl cyclic AMP and theophylline. Electron microspic examination of the differentiated cells after radical damage confirms significantly increased ultrastructural injury. Of note, the altered Golgi morphology was nearly identical to that observed in vulnerable neurons of reperfused brains.[452]

Fundamental cellular regulatory systems in neuronal ischemia and reperfusion

Cell growth, proliferation, and differentiation are regulated, in part, by growth factors.[453] The brain has receptors for several growth factors, including insulin,[454,455] fibroblast growth factor (FGF),[456] and nerve growth factor (NGF),[457] all of which have been found in the selectively vulnerable hippocampal and cerebral cortical neurons. Similarly, transforming growth factor beta (TGF-),[458] insulin-like growth factor-1 (IGF-1),[459] and epidermal growth factor (EGF)[460] have been found in the brain and elsewhere in the central nervous system. Receptor proteins for all these growth factors characteristically include a ligand-activated tyrosine kinase at the inner surface of the plasmalemma.

The mechanisms by which these growth factors influence cellular growth and differentiation are not completely understood, particularly with respect to control of synthesis of membrane components. The general consensus, however, is that the effects are mediated through receptor kinase-induced "phosphorylation cascades" leading to transcription of the immediate-early genes,[461] which include the proto-oncogenes c-*fos* and c-*jun*. Proteins of the cFOS family form heterodimers with proteins of the cJUN family to constitute the AP-1 complex that binds with high affinity and specificity to DNA transcription factor binding sequences upstream of target genes.[462]

Brain ischemia and reperfusion elicit the production of both growth factors and proto-oncogene products in at least some neuronal populations. Examples of growth factor responses following ischemia are an increase in basic FGF in the rat hippocampus, caudate, putamen, and cortex;[463] increased production of mRNAs for brain-derived neurotrophic factor and NGF in rat dentate gyrus and in the rat hippocampus CA_1 and CA_2 regions;[464] and increased levels of IGF-1 in the lateral cortex, hippocampus, striatum, thalamus, and pyriform cortex.[465]

With regard to proto-oncogene products, c-*fos* and c-*jun* transcripts are elevated in brain homogenates within 30 minutes of postischemic reperfusion both in rats[466] and gerbils.[467] In situ cytochemistry has shown, however, that within 1 hour after cortical ischemia, the cFOS protein found in rat cerebral cortex is higher in layers II and VI than in the selectively vulnerable layers III-V.[468] Delayed c-*fos* transcription[469] and translation[470] were also observed in the selectively vulnerable CA$_1$ layer of the rat hippocampus, with transcripts appearing at 24 hours reaching peak at 72 hours of reperfusion. Examination of various cell types during early reperfusion showed that c-*fos* mRNA is transcribed in large amounts in the damage-resistant dentate granule cells, whereas only modest expression was found in CA$_1$ and CA$_3$ pyramidal layers of the hippocampus.[471] Wessel *et al*, using in situ hybridization, studied c-*fos* and c-*jun* transcripts in the rat brain following 20 minutes of transient ischemia.[472] There was strong expression of both genes within 30 minutes of reperfusion in the dentate gyrus; however, expression in the CA$_1$ region of the hippocampus was delayed 1–2 hours and showed a biphasic response. The initial moderate peak had returned to baseline by 6 hours, followed by a weaker response at 24 hours of reperfusion.

There are important links between induction of c-*fos* and the translation of important stress proteins.[473] Heat shock proteins (HSPs),[477] can be induced by a wide variety of insults and are highly conserved from prokaryotes to humans. HSPs appear to facilitate correct folding of proteins[474] and rRNA,[475] dissociate clathrin baskets in the presence of ATP (which is a presumed requirement for cell membrane recycling),[476] interact with cellular tumor suppressor p53,[476] have a calmodulin binding site,[478] are proposed to be involved in membrane synthesis[479] appear to protect cultured neurons from glutamate toxicity,[480] and are induced by insulin in a human tumor cell line.[481] Heat shock messages[482] and proteins[483] are expressed in the brain during reperfusion. After an ischemic insult, the selectively vulnerable neurons in the hippocampus and cortex transcribe large quantities of *hsp-70* mRNA, but translation of *hsp*-70 is considerably decreased when compared to surviving areas of the hippocampus (i.e., the dentate gyrus).[482] The c-*fos*/c-*jun*/*hsp* system is directly activated by ionizing radiation,[484] presumably by hydroxyl radical-mediated events. Also, there is evidence that the HSP response is induced in the presence of free radicals,[485] but not by increased intracellular calcium alone.[486] Clearly, an interesting case can be made that the heat shock response is primarily a free radical defense.[487] The selectively vulnerable brain neurons that display delayed expression of c-*fos* correspond to those with poor translation of *hsp*-70 transcripts. These results suggest the important association of early transcription and translation of c-*fos*, c-*jun*, and *hsp-70* with neuronal survival.

The activator protein library: defense against neuronal damage

The evidence for brain reperfusion-induced transcription of *fos* and *jun* led us to conduct a comprehensive literature search for proteins known to have in their genes' promoters or enhancers sequences responsive to transcriptional regulation by the AP-1 heterodimer.

General observations

On its DNA promoter sequence, the AP-1 complex binds the protein that recognizes the "TATA box" and thus facilitates initiation of transcription.[488] AP-1 DNA binding is modulated by a few known mechanisms, which include regulatory phosphorylation and antagonism by the glucocorticoid receptor. Inhibitory protein-1 (IP-1) inhibits AP-1 binding to DNA, and this inhibition is blocked when IP-1 is phosphorylated by protein kinase C (PKC).[489] Protein phosphatase A$_2$ (a serine-threonine phosphatase) activates AP-1 DNA binding by a dephosphorylation reaction with Jun,[490] but tyrosine phosphatases decrease AP-1 activation of transcription.[491] Both ligand-activated glucocorticoid receptors and retinoic acid-receptors block the DNA binding activity of AP-1.[492,493] In particular the glucocorticoid receptor and AP-1 appear antagonistic for DNA binding; for example, in the promoter region of the genes for α-fetoprotein[494] and insulin-like binding protein 1[495] there are overlapping and mutually exclusive sequences for the glucocorticoid receptor and AP-1. This antagonism could explain the general failure of glucocorticoids and the 21-aminosteroids ("lazaroids") to protect neuronal soma.

Activator protein library

Our search identified 42 proteins with AP-1 sites and 31 with AP-2 sites in the promoter regions of the genes. Most of these genes fall into groups related to (1) antioxidants, (2) growth factors and their receptors, (3) cytokines and their receptors, (4) lipid management, (5) structural proteins, (6) neurotransmitter management, (7) phosphorylation regulation, (8) protease regulation, and (9) electrolyte and water management (Table 13.1).

Theoretical speculation about what the *fos-jun* reperfusion response means

This list of AP-regulated genes makes it difficult to believe that the reperfusion-induced *fos-jun* response is not intended for cell salvage. In particular, the AP-1 and AP-2 systems stimulate production of a family of enzymes that one investigator group has characterized as belonging to an "electrophile counterattack." For AP-1 these include glutathione transferase, NAD(P)H quinone reductase, epoxide

Table 13.1.

AP-1	AP-2
Antioxidants	
Glutathione transferase	Glutathione peroxidase
NAD(P)H quinone reductase epoxide hydrolase	S-adenosylmethionine decarboxylase
UDP glucuronsyltransferase heme oxygenase I	
S-adenosylmethionine decarboxylase	
Growth factors and receptors	
Insulin-like GF-2	Fibroblast GF receptor
Insulin-like GF-1	IGF-1 receptor
IGF binding protein 5	Insulin receptor
Nerve GF	TGF β 2 and 3
IGF binding protein 1	Vascular endothelial growth factor
Fibroblast GF receptor	IGF binding protein 5
TGF β1	
Vascular endothelial GF	
Cytokines and receptors	
Interleukin 2	TNF α 1
Interleukin 6	IL7 receptor
TNF α	
IL7 receptor	
Nuclear Factor-Kappa B	
Interleukin 1 type 1 receptor	
Lipid management	
Apolipoprotein CIII	5-Lipoxygenase activating protein
	Acetyl CoA carboxylase
	Branched chain α-ketoacid dehydrogenase-E1α
	BCαKAD E2 dihydrolipoyl transacylase
Structural proteins	
α-Actin	Elastin
vimentin	Neurofilament light protein
lysosomal membrane glycoprotein 2	Calreticulin
N-Cell Adhesion Molecule	Nidogen
I-CAM	
Cytoactin	
Neurotransmitter management	
NO synthetase	Glutamate dehydrogenase
Tyrosine hydroxylase	NO synthetase
Glutamate dehydrogenase	Aromatic amino acid decarboxylase
Cholecystokinin	Phenylalanine hydroxylase
Phosphorylation regulation	
Protein kinase C	Germ cell alkaline phosphatase
	Protein tyrosine kinase (SRC homolog)
	cAMP-dependent kinase
Protease regulation	
HSP 47 (serine protease inhibitor)	Cathepsins H and L (cysteine proteases)
Stromolysin 1 (metalloproteinase) 92 kDa collagenase	Cathepsin D
Electrolyte and water management	
Atrial natruiretic protein	
Na/H exchanger	
Miscellaneous	
c-jun and c-fos	ADP ribosylation Factor II
α-fetoprotein	α -subunit mitochondrial ATP synthase
Histone H 3.2	
α-subunit pyruvate dehydrogenase amyloid precursor protein	

hydrolase, and UDP glucuronyl transferase, and transcripts for these enzymes are induced by a large number of electrophiles. Glutathione peroxidase and S-adenosylmethionine decarboxylase have AP-2 binding sites in the 5′ promoter region. A search for the SOD and catalase promoters reveals that both of these classic radical scavenging enzymes are regulated by SP1[496] (housekeeping) promoter sequences and have neither AP-1 nor AP-2 promoter sequences.

This suggests that, since the activator proteins are significantly involved at the level of the cell cycle, there are a group of important antioxidant enzymes that are upregulated during DNA replication. The potential evolutionary rationale could be that relaxed repair of electrophilic DNA damage is acceptable during non-division states, but DNA damage during replication could lead to nonsense copies. Upregulated DNA synthesis and growth factor stimulation of the activator proteins suggests that neurons may respond to ischemia and reperfusion with a augmented transcription of both antioxidant and membrane repair competence. This would potentially explain the resistance to free radical damage conferred by growth factors in primary neuron cultures. Because it has long been known that pretreatment with barbiturates induces substantial resistance to brain damage by ischemia and reperfusion, it is interesting that phenobarbital induces transcription of glutathione transferase and NAD(P)H reductase[497] through a radical-mediated mechanism (quite possibly related to cytochrome p450 metabolism of barbiturates).

The second theory is derived from reports[498] of interactions between cytokines and growth factors inducing phosphorylation of a 91-kDa constitutive protein (STAT-91) that marks it for nuclear localization, DNA binding [to the SIE sequence-*fos* promoter][499], and transcription initiation. Further the AP library has multiple positive feedback loops between promotion of cytokines, growth factors, and growth factor receptors. This system may represent a coordinated mechanism for stimulating growth factors, receptors, regulatory tyrosine phosphorylation, transcription machinery, and the "electrophile counterattack." It may be possible to manipulate these activities by administration of growth factors.

Growth Factors

Since growth factors are involved in cellular reproduction, including transcription of the AP-1 components and most probably membrane synthesis and repair, it is not surprising that the administration of growth factors has improved post-ischemic neuronal survival.[500] Fibroblast growth factor substantially inhibits glutamate receptor-mediated neuronal damage.[501] Nerve growth factor administered either before or after 5 minutes of carotid occlusion in Mongolian gerbils significantly reduced the loss of hippocampal CA_1 neurons.[502] Treatment with IGF-1 2 hours after an ischemia–hypoxia insult in rats reduced cortical neuronal loss.[465] Treatment with insulin, either pre- or postischemia in the rat, reduced cortical and striatal neuronal necrosis and reduced infarction in the cerebral cortex, thalamus, and substantia nigra pars reticularis.[503,504]

Insulin

The observed role of insulin in prevention of postischemic brain injury is particularly interesting. The improvement in neurologic outcome seen with postischemic administration of insulin is independent of any hypoglycemic effect,[503] a predictable outcome as glucose transport to the brain is insulin-independent. The poorer neurologic outcome observed with hyperglycemia prior to brain ischemia was commonly attributed to increased lactic acidosis.[106] However, the involvement of acidosis in tissue injury appears unlikely, however, because generation of the same low tissue pH by hypercarbia did not cause any evident damage. The effects previously ascribed to hyperglycemia are equally plausible as alternative interpretations involving insulin; that is, hyperglycemic experimental animals (typically fasted rats made ischemic and hyperglycemic) do not do well, potentially due to either fasting-induced insulin deficiency or downregulation of insulin receptors.

Insulin effects are complex and affect fundamental cell regulatory functions well beyond the management of glucose. For example, insulin receptor-mediated protein phosphorylation cascades have many actions: they stimulate transcription of c-*fos*/c-*jun*, increase mRNA efflux from the nucleus, induce enzymatic systems for *de novo* lipogenesis, activate the mitochondrial pyruvate dehydrogenase complex, modify the phosphatidylinositol transcytoplasmic signaling system, and stimulate the heat shock response.[389]

The actions of insulin are mediated by a membrane receptor tyrosine kinase that shares homology with other growth factor receptors. The initial effect of insulin receptor activation is tyrosine autophosphorylation and activation of the intrinsic tyrosine kinase. Secondarily, other proteins are phosphorylated by activated kinases or dephosphorylated by activated phosphatases. It is the modulation of the phosphate content of specific proteins that appears to direct cellular regulation. A germane example involves the Ca^{2+}-calmodulin complex, which activates phospholipases; calmodulin is phosphorylated by the insulin receptor,[505] thereby reducing its ability to bind calcium, a reaction that potentially modulates insulin's antilipolytic effects.

Selectively vulnerable neurons, including specifically the cortical pyramidal ones and those in the CA$_1$ hippocampus, show marked elevation of the level of both insulin receptors and phosphotyrosine-containing proteins, which co-map extensively.[506] Furthermore, phosphotyrosine-containing proteins show the highest concentrations in the nuclei of these selectively vulnerable neurons,[506] consistent with a transcriptional regulatory function.

This evidence suggests that the postischemic neuroprotective effects of insulin are modulated during reperfusion by kinases, phosphatases, and prompt transcriptional regulation mediated by protein tyrosine–phosphorylation. Indeed, we have reported a reperfusion-specific insulin-induced ~10-fold increase in tyrosine phosphorylation on a 90-kDa brain nuclear protein and Sullivan et al. have shown a significant decrease in eIF2α phosphorylation with supranormal recovery of protein synthesis with insulin administration at ROSC.[507] The insulin-induced neuro-protective responses are likely specifically to include (1) activation of appropriate early transcription for the components of AP-1 in the vulnerable zones with subsequent upregulation of antioxidant defenses; (2) inhibition of calcium-calmodulin-activated lipolysis; (3) stimulation of the lipid synthesis systems vital to membrane repair; and (4) insulin-dependent promotion of the heat shock response.

The data regarding the involvement of insulin in neuronal salvage raise may explain in part the observed increase in ROSC, but no improvement in neuronal recovery.[508] Catecholamines, such as epinephrine, cause prompt and prolonged inhibition of insulin secretion by the pancreas[509] and reduce the tyrosine kinase activity of the insulin receptor by cAMP-induced phosphorylation of serine and threonine residues on the receptor.[510] These difficulties may be further aggravated by epinephrine-induced glucocorticoid secretion with consequent ligand activation of glucocorticoid receptors and interference with transcriptional activation by AP-1. Moreover, catecholamines, including dopamine, norepinephrine, and epinephrine, promote iron-mediated lipid peroxidation[511] and neuronal death[512] in vitro. We have carried out a preliminary examination of the interrelationships of insulin and epinephrine levels during the first 3 hours postresuscitation in cardiac arrest patients.[513] We have observed, as have others, very high endogenous levels of catecholamines in patients during cardiac arrest. In resuscitated patients we have observed two distinct subgroups; in one, insulin and C-peptide were initially high and then significantly decreased over time, and in the other, insulin and C-peptide were initially normal with a trend for C-peptide levels to increase with time. An obvious trend is noted for epinephrine levels to be higher at all times (~10-fold higher at ROSC) in the group with falling insulin levels. These results suggest that very high epinephrine levels are associated with a progressive decrease in insulin and C-peptide levels during reperfusion. Further the stroke and critical care literature provide data that bolsters this theory. The Capes et al meta-analysis reveals that an elevated initial glucose predicts an increase in mortality by 3-fold in non-diabetic cerebro vascular accident (CVA) patients.[514] The TOAST study reports initial hyperglycemia predicts poor outcome from CVA. Further, Parsons et al. proved by MRI and MR spectroscopy a mechanistic link between acute hyperglycemia and increased infarct volume and lactate production,[515] and that persistent hyperglycemia is an independent predictor of increased stroke volume and poor neurologic outcome.[516] Insulin use in diabetics with acute myocardial infarct (AMI) decrease morbidity and mortality,[517] and strict glucose control with insulin decreases ICU mortality from 8% to 4.6%.[518]

Summary

We have tried diligently to summarize the existing evidence related to brain injury by global ischemia and reperfusion (Fig. 13.7). Ischemia results in rapid loss of high energy phosphate compounds and generalized depolarization. Selectively vulnerable neurons are characterized by their dendritic fields receiving large amounts of glutamate released by the general depolarization during ischemia. Under these circumstances, both voltage-dependent calcium channels and glutamate-regulated calcium channels allow a massive increase in intracellular calcium to occur. This takes place in concert with initiation of lipolysis, a process that occurs more intensely in the selectively vulnerable neurons. Early during reperfusion, there is a burst of excess oxygen radical production and iron release from storage proteins. The availability of this transition metal allows initiation of lipid peroxidation. This process preferentially occurs in the selectively vulnerable neurons. The vulnerable neurons respond with transcription products for heat shock proteins and immediate-early genes, a response that appears directed toward enhancing antioxidant and membrane repair competence. Unfortunately, translation initiation is significantly depressed and thus the transcriptional response does not lead to translation of the appropriate protein products. Under these circumstances, the processes of membrane damage during reperfusion proceed unchecked, leading to loss of integrity in partitioning ions and cell death. Growth factors represent a physiologically based intervention strategy to enhance

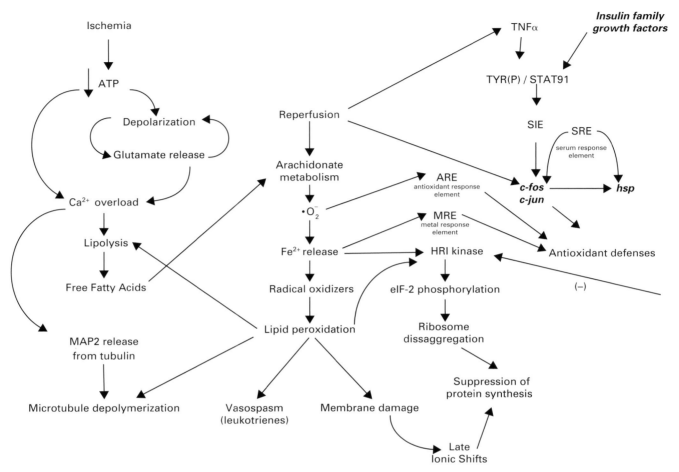

Fig. 13.7. Schematic of the major mechanisms involved in neuronal ischemia and reperfusion.

appropriate transcriptional responses and translation competence. Antioxidant drugs reduce the rate of membrane damage, but do not alter the ultimate outcome in the absence of an effective physiological response by the neurons. The role of high levels of adrenergic agonists in this process is not yet completely worked out, but it appears likely that these compounds may act to enhance the damage and impede the appropriate physiologic response. We believe that based on appreciation of these fundamental principles, it will be possible to design effective clinical strategies to improve neurologic outcome significantly following cardiac arrest and resuscitation.

REFERENCES

1. CDC. Mortality from coronary heart disease and acute myocardial infarction: United States, 1998. *MMWR Morb Mortal Wkly Rep.* 2001; **50**: 90–93.

2. De Vreede-Swagemakers, J.J., Gorgels, A.P., Dubois-Arbouw, W.J. *et al.* Out-of-hospital cardiac arrest in the 1990's: a population based study in the Maastricht area on incidence, characteristics and survival. *J. Am. Coll. Cardiol.* 1997; **30**: 1500–1505.

3. Krause, G.S., Kumar, K., White, B.C., Aust, S.D., & Wiegenstein, J.G. Ischemia, resuscitation, and reperfusion: mechanisms of tissue injury and prospects for protection. *Am. Heart J.* 1986; **111**: 768–780.

4. Brain Resuscitation Clinical Trial I Study Group: Study of thiopental loading in comatose survivors of cardiac arrest. *N. Engl. J. Med.* 1986; **314**: 397–401.

5. Brain Resuscitation Clinical Trial II Study Group: A randomized clinical study of a calcium-entry blocker (lidoflazine) in the treatment of comatose survivors of cardiac arrest. *N. Engl. J. Med.* 1991; **324**: 1225–1231.

6. RANITAS investigators: a randomized trial of trilazad mesylate in patients with acute stroke. *Stroke* 1996; **27**: 1453–1458.

7. Enlimomab acute stroke trial investigators. Use of anti-ICAM-1 therapy in ischemic stroke: results of the Enlimomab acute stroke trial. *Neurology* 2001; **23**: 1428–1434.

8. Albers, G.W., Goldstein, L.B., Hall, D., & Lesko, L.M. Aptiganel hydrochloride in acute ischemic stroke. *J. Am. Med. Assoc.* 2001; **286**: 2673–2682.

9. Sacco, R.L., DeRosa, J.T., Haley, E.C. Jr. *et al.* Glycine antagonist in neuroprotection for patients with acute stroke: GAIN Americas: a randomized controlled trial. *J. Am. Med. Assoc.* 2001; **285**: 1719–1728.

10. Gandolfo, C., Sandercock, P., & Conti, M. Lubeluzole for acute ischaemic stroke (Cochrane Review). *Cochrane Database Syst. Rev.* 2002; (1): CD001924.

11. Ganglioside GM1 in acute ischemic stroke. The SASS trial. *Stroke* 1994; **25**: 1141–1148.

12. Horn, J., & Limburg, M. Calcium antagonists for ischemic stroke: a systematic review. *Stroke* 2001; **32**: 570–576.

13. Lyden, P., Shuaib, A., Ng, K. *et al.* The CLASS-I/H/T Investigators. Clomethiazole Acute Stroke Study in ischemic stroke (CLASS-I): final results. *Stroke* 2002; **33**: 122–128.

14. Brockman, S., & Jude, J.R. The tolerance of the dog brain to total arrest of circulation. *Bull. Johns Hopkins Hosp.* 1960; **106**: 74–80.

15. Radovsky, A., Safar, P., Sterz, F., Leonov, Y., Reich, H., & Kuboyama, K. Regional prevalence and distribution of ischemic neurons in dog brains 96 hours after cardiac arrest of 0 to 20 minutes. *Stroke* 1995; **26**: 2127–2133.

16. Sanders, A.B., Kern, K.B., Bragg, S., & Ewy, G.A. Neurologic benefits from the use of early cardiopulmonary resuscitation. *Ann. Emerg. Med.* 1987; **16**: 142–146.

17. Arsenio-Nunes, M.L., Hossmann, K.A., & Frakas-Bargeton, E. Ultrastructural and histochemical investigation of the cerebral cortex of cat during and after complete ischemia. *Acta Neuropathol.* 1973; **26**: 329–344.

18. de la Torre, J.C., Saunders, J., Fortin, T., Butler, K., & Richard, M. Return of ATP/PCr and EEG after 75 min of global brain ischemia. *Brain Res.* 1991; **542**: 71–76.

19. Ginsberg, M.D., Graham, D.I., Welsh, F.A., & Budd, W.W. Diffuse cerebral ischemia in the cat: III. Neuropathological sequelae of severe ischemia. *Ann. Neurol.* 1979; **5**: 350–358.

20. Hatakeyama, T., Matsumoto, M., Brengman, J.M., & Yanagihara, T. Immunohistochemical investigation of ischemic and postischemic damage after bilateral carotid occlusion in gerbils. *Stroke* 1988; **19**: 1526–1534.

21. Helfaer, M.A., Ichord, R.N., Martin, L.J., Hurn, P.D., Castro, A., & Traystman, R.J. Treatment with the competitive NMDA antagonist GPI 3000 does not improve outcome after cardiac arrest in dogs. *Stroke* 1998; **29**: 824–829.

22. Jenkins, L.W., Povlishock, J.T., Lewelt, W., Miller, J.D., & Becker, D.P. The role of postischemic recirculation in the development of ischemic neuronal injury following complete cerebral ischemia. *Acta Neuropathol. (Berl.)* 1981; **55**: 205–220.

23. Myers, R.E., & Yamaguchi, S. Nervous system effects of cardiac arrest in monkeys. Preservation of vision. *Arch. Neurol.* 1977; **34**: 65–74.

24. Kleihues, P., Hossmann, K.A., Pegg, A.E., Kobayashi, K., & Zimmermann, V. Resuscitation of the monkey brain after one hour complete ischemia. III. Indications of metabolic recovery. *Brain Res.* 1975; **95**: 61–73.

25. Schmidt Kastner, R., Hossmann, K.A., & Grosse Ophoff, B. Relationship between metabolic recovery and the EEG prolonged ischemia of cat brain. *Stroke* 1986; **17**: 1164–1169.

26. Safar, P., Stezoski, W., & Nemoto, E.M. Amelioration of brain damage after 12 minutes' cardiac arrest in dogs. *Arch. Neurol.* 1976; **33**: 91–95.

27. Todd, M.M., Dunlop, B.J., Shapiro, H.M., Chadwick, H.C., & Powell, H.C. Ventricular fibrillation in the cat: a model for global cerebral ischemia. *Stroke* 1981; **12**: 808–815.

28. Koch, K.A., Jackson, D.L., Schmiedl, M., & Rosenblatt, J.I. Total cerebral ischemia: effect of alterations in arterial PCO2 on cerebral microcirculation. *J. Cereb. Blood Flow Metab.* 1984; **4**: 343–349.

29. Miller, C.L., Lampard, D.G., Alexander, K., & Brown, W.A. Local cerebral blood flow following transient cerebral ischemia. I Onset of impaired reperfusion within the first hour following global ischemia. *Stroke* 1980; **11**: 534–541.

30. Macfarlane, R., Tasdemiroglu, E., Moskowitz, M.A., Uemura, Y., Wei, E.P., & Kontos, H.A. Chronic trigeminal ganglionectomy or topical capsaicin application to pial vessels attenuates postocclusive cortical hyperemia but does not influence postischemic hypoperfusion. *J. Cereb. Blood Flow Metab.* 1991; **11**: 261–271.

31. Chopp, M., Frinak, S., Walton, D.R., Smith, M.B., & Welch, K.M. Intracellular acidosis during and after cerebral ischemia: in vivo nuclear magnetic resonance study of hyperglycemia in cats. *Stroke* 1987; **18**: 919–923.

32. Steen, P.A., Gisvold, S.E., Milde, J.H. *et al.* Nimodipine improves outcome when given after complete cerebral ischemia in primates. *Anesthesiology* 1985; **62**: 406–414.

33. Kagstrom, E., Smith, M.L., & Siesjo, B.K. Local cerebral blood flow in the recovery period following complete cerebral ischemia in the rat. *J. Cereb. Blood Flow Metab.* 1983; **3**: 170–182.

34. Nishijima, M.K., Koehler, R.C., Hurn, P.D. *et al.* Postischemic recovery rate of cerebral ATP, phosphocreatine, pH, and evoked potentials. *Am. J. Physiol. Heart Circ. Physiol.* 1989; **257**: H1860–H1870.

35. Pulsinelli, W.A., & Duffy, T.E. Regional energy balance in rat brain after transient forebrain ischemia. *J. Neurochem.* 1983; **40**: 1500–1503.

36. Kagstrom, E., Smith, M.L., & Siesjo, B.K. Recirculation in the rat brain following incomplete ischemia. *J. Cereb. Blood Flow Metab.* 1983; **3**: 183–192.

37. Krajewska, M., Rosenthal, R.E., Mikolajczyk, J. *et al.* Early processing of Bid and caspase -6, -8, -10, -14 in the canine brain during cardiac arrest and resuscitation. *Exp. Neurol.* 2004; **189**(2): 261–279.

38. Safar, P., & Bircher, N. *Cardiopulmonary–Cerebral Resuscitation*. 3 edn. London: W. B. Saunders Co., 1994.

39. Hossmann, K.A. Neuronal survival and revival during and after cerebral ischemia. *Am. J. Emerg. Med.* 1983; **1**(2): 191–197.

40. Hossmann, K.A., Oschlies, U., Schwindt, W., & Krep, H. Electron microscopic investigation of rat brain after brief cardiac arrest. *Acta Neuropathol. (Berl.)* 2001; **101**(2): 101–113.

41. Kerr, J.F., Wyllie, A.H., & Currie, A.R. Apoptosis: a basic biological phenomenon with wide-ranging implications in tissue kinetics. *Br. J. Cancer* 1972; **26**(4): 239–257.

42. Wyllie, A.H. Apoptosis: cell death under homeostatic control. *Arch. Toxicol Suppl.* 1987; **11**: 3–10.

43. Waldmeier, P.C. Prospects for antiapoptotic drug therapy of neurodegenerative diseases. *Prog. Neuro-Psychopharmacol. Biol. Psychiatry* 2003; **27**(2): 303–321.

44. Rami, A. Ischemic neuronal death in the rat hippocampus: the calpain-calpastatin-caspase hypothesis. *Neurobiol. Dis.* 2003; **13**(2): 75–88.

45. Love, S. Apoptosis and brain ischaemia. *Prog. Neuropsychopharmacol. Biol. Psychiatry* 2003; **27**(2): 267–282.

46. Cairns, C.B., Moore, F.A., Haenel, J.B. *et al.* Evidence for early supply independent mitochondrial dysfunction in patients developing multiple organ failure after trauma. *J. Trauma* 1997; **42**(3): 532–536.

47. Nicotera, P., Leist, M., & Manzo, L. Neuronal cell death: a demise with different shapes. *Trends Pharmacol. Sci.* 1999; **20**(2): 46–51.

48. Eleff, S.M., Maruki, Y., Monsein, L.H., Traystman, R.J., Bryan, R.N., & Koehler, R.C. Sodium, ATP, and intracellular pH transients during reversible complete ischemia of dog cerebrum. *Stroke* 1991; **22**: 233–241.

49. Katsura, K., Rodriguez de Turco, E.B., Folbergrova, J., Bazan, N.G., & Siesjo, B.K. Coupling among energy failure, loss of ion homeostasis, and phospholipase A2 and C activation during ischemia. *J. Neurochem.* 1993; **61**: 1677–1684.

50. Ljunggren, B., Schutz, H., & Siesjo, B.K. Changes in energy state and acid-base parameters of the rat brain during complete compression ischemia. *Brain Res.* 1974; **73**: 277–289.

51. Hossmann, K.A., & Grosse Ophoff, B. Recovery of monkey brain after prolonged ischemia. I Electrophysiology and brain electrolytes. *J. Cereb. Blood Flow Metab.* 1986; **6**: 15–21.

52. Rossen, R., Kabat, H., & Anderson, J.P. Acute arrest of cerebral circulation in man. *Arch. Neurol. Psychiatry* 1943; **50**: 510–528.

53. Raffin, C.N., Harrison, M., Sick, T.J., & Rosenthal, M. EEG suppression and anoxic depolarization: influences on cerebral oxygenation during ischemia. *J. Cereb. Blood Flow Metab.* 1991; **11**: 407–415.

54. Hansen, A.J. Effect of anoxia on ion distribution in the brain. *Physiol. Rev.* 1985; **65**: 101–148.

55. Silver, I.A., & Erecinska, M. Intracellular and extracellular changes of $[Ca^{2+}]$ in hypoxia and ischemia in rat brain in vivo. *J. Gen. Physiol.* 1990; **95**: 837–866.

56. Folbergrova, J., Minamisawa, H., Ekholm, A., & Siesjo, B.K. Phosphorylase alpha and labile metabolites during anoxia: correlation to membrane fluxes of K^+ and Ca^{2+}. *J. Neurochem.* 1990; **55**: 1690–1696.

57. Uematsu, D., Greenberg, J.H., Reivich, M., Kobayashi, S., & Karp, A. In vivo fluorometric measurement of changes in cytosolic free calcium from the cat cortex during anoxia. *J. Cereb. Blood Flow Metab.* 1988; **8**: 367–374.

58. Eleff, S.M., Mclennan, I.J., Hart, G.K., Maruki, Y., Traystman, R.J., & Koehler, R.C. Shift reagent enhanced concurrent ^{23}Na and ^{1}H magnetic resonance spectroscopic studies of transcellular sodium distribution in the dog brain in vivo. *Magn. Reson. Med.* 1993; **30**: 11–17.

59. Decanniere, C., Eleff, S., Davis, D., & van Zijl, P.C. Correlation of rapid changes in the average water diffusion constant and the concentrations of lactate and ATP breakdown products during global ischemia in cat brain. *Magn. Reson. Med.* 1995; **34**: 343–352.

60. Hansen, A.J., & Olsen, C.E. Brain extracellular space during spreading depression and ischemia. *Acta Physiol. Scand.* 1980; **108**: 355–365.

61. Mrsulja, B.B., Ueki, Y., Wheaton, A., Passonneau, J.V., & Lust, W.D. Release of pentobarbital-induced depression of metabolic rate during bilateral ischemia in the gerbil brain. *Brain Res.* 1984; **309**: 152–155.

62. Sutton, L.N., Clark, B.J., Norwood, C.R., Woodford, E.J., & Welsh, F.A. Global cerebral ischemia in piglets under conditions of mild and deep hypothermia. *Stroke* 1991; **22**: 1567–1573.

63. Ekholm, A., Katsura, K., Kristian, T., Liu, M., Folbergrova, J., & Siesjo, B.K. Coupling of cellular energy state and ion homeostasis during recovery following brain ischemia. *Brain Res.* 1993; **604**: 185–191.

64. Hansen, A.J., Gjedde, A., & Siemkowicz, E. Extracellular potassium and blood flow in the post-ischemic rat brain. *Pflugers Arch.* 1980; **389**: 1–7.

65. Siemkowicz, E., & Hansen, A.J. Brain extracellular ion composition and EEG activity following 10 minutes ischemia in normo- and hyperglycemic rats. *Stroke* 1981; **12**: 236–240.

66. Ljunggren, B., Ratcheson, R.A., & Siesjo, B.K. Cerebral metabolic state following complete compression ischemia. *Brain Res.* 1974; **73**: 291–307.

67. Behar, K.L., Rothman, D.L., & Hossmann, K.A. NMR spectroscopic investigation of the recovery of energy and acid–base homeostasis in the cat brain after prolonged ischemia. *J. Cereb. Blood Flow Metab.* 1989; **9**: 655–665.

68. Hossmann, K.A., Sakaki, S., & Zimmerman, V. Cation activities in reversible ischemia of the cat brain. *Stroke* 1977; **8**: 77–81.

69. Kobayashi, M., Lust, W.D., & Passonneau, J.V. Concentrations of energy metabolites and cyclic nucleotides during and after bilateral ischemia in the gerbil cerebral cortex. *J. Neurochem.* 1977; **29**: 53–59.

70. Mayevsky, A., Friedli, C.M., & Reivich, M. Metabolic, ionic, and electrical responses of gerbil brain to ischemia. *Am. J. Physiol. Regul. Integr. Comp. Physiol.* 1985; **248**: R99–107.

71. Kleihues, P., Kobayashi, K., & Hossmann, K.A. Purine nucleotide metabolism in the cat brain after one hour of complete ischemia. *J. Neurochem.* 1974; **23**: 417–425.

72. Nordstrom, C.H., Rehncrona, S., & Siesjo, B.K. Restitution of cerebral energy state, as well as of glycolytic metabolites, citric acid cycle intermediates and associated amino acids

after 30 minutes of complete ischemia in rats anaesthetized with nitrous oxide or phenobarbital. *J. Neurochem.* 1978; **30**: 479–486.

73. Rehncrona, S., Mela, L., & Siesjo, B.K. Recovery of brain mitochondrial function in the rat after complete and incomplete cerebral ischemia. *Stroke* 1979; **10**: 437–446.

74. Sims, N.R. Selective impairment of respiration in mitochondria isolated from brain subregions following transient forebrain ischemia in the rat. *J. Neurochem.* 1991; **56**: 1836–1844.

75. Hillered, L., Siesjo, B.K., & Arfors, K.E. Mitochondrial response to transient forebrain ischemia and recirculation in the rat. *J. Cereb. Blood Flow Metab.* 1984; **4**: 438–446.

76. Hillered, L., Smith, M.L., & Siesjo, B.K. Lactic acidosis and recovery of mitochondrial function following forebrain ischemia in the rat. *J. Cereb. Blood Flow Metab.* 1985; **5**: 259–266.

77. Hillered, L., & Ernster, L. Respiratory activity of isolated rat brain mitochondria following in vitro exposure to oxygen radicals. *J. Cereb. Blood Flow Metab.* 1983; **3**: 207–214.

78. Nakahara, I., Kikuchi, H., Taki, W. *et al.* Degradation of mitochondrial phospholipids during experimental cerebral ischemia in rats. *J. Neurochem.* 1991; **57**: 839–844.

79. Abe, T., Takagi, N., Nakano, M., & Takeo, S. The effects of monobromobimane on neuronal cell death in the hippocampus after transient global cerebral ischemia in rats. *Neurosci. Lett.* 2004; **357**: 227–231.

80. Phillis, J.W., Walter, G.A., & Simpson, R.E. Brain adenosine and transmitter amino acid release from the ischemic rat cerebral cortex: effects of the adenosine deaminase inhibitor deoxycoformycin. *J. Neurochem.* 1991; **56**: 644–650.

81. Sciotti, V.M., & Van Wylen, D.G. Increases in interstitial adenosine and cerebral blood flow with inhibition of adenosine kinase and adenosine deaminase. *J. Cereb. Blood Flow Metab.* 1993; **13**: 201–207.

82. Welsh, F.A., O'Connor, M.J., Marcy, V.R., Spatacco, A.J., & Johns, R.L. Factors limiting regeneration of ATP following temporary ischemia in cat brain. *Stroke* 1982; **13**: 234–242.

83. Lin, S.R., & Kormano, M. Cerebral circulation after cardiac arrest. Microangiographic and protein tracer studies. *Stroke* 1977; **8**: 182–188.

84. Theilen, H., Schrock, H., & Kuschinsky, W. Capillary perfusion during incomplete forebrain ischemia and reperfusion in rat brain. *Am. J. Physiol. Heart Circ. Physiol.* 1993; **265**: H642–H648.

85. Phillis, J.W., O'Regan, M.H., Estevez, A.Y., Song, D., & VanderHeide, S.J. Cerebral energy metabolism during severe ischemia of varying duration and following reperfusion. *J. Neurochem.* 1996; **67**: 1525–1531.

86. Dagani, F., & Erecinska, M. Relationships among ATP synthesis, K⁺ gradients, and neurotransmitter amino acid levels in isolated rat brain synaptosomes. *J. Neurochem.* 1987; **49**: 1229–1240.

87. Lin, S.R., O'Connor, M.J., King, A., Harnish, P., & Fischer, H.W. Effect of dextran on cerebral function and blood after cardiac arrest. An experimental study on the dog. *Stroke* 1979; **10**: 13–20.

88. Chesler, M. Regulation and modulation of pH in the brain. *Physiol. Rev.* 2003; **83**: 1183–1221.

89. Petroff, O.A., Prichard, J.W., Behar, K.L., Alger, J.R., den Hollander, J.A., & Shulman, R.G. Cerebral intracellular pH by ^{31}P nuclear magnetic resonance spectroscopy. *Neurology* 1985; **35**: 781–788.

90. Eleff, S.M., Schleien, C.L., Koehler, R.C. *et al.* Brain bioenergetics during cardiopulmonary resuscitation in dogs. *Anesthesiology* 1992; **76**: 77–84.

91. Maruki, Y., Koehler, R.C., Eleff, S.M., & Traystman, R.J. Intracellular pH during reperfusion influences evoked potential recovery after complete cerebral ischemia. *Stroke* 1993; **24**: 697–703.

92. von Hanwehr, R., Smith, M.L., & Siesjo, B.K. Extra- and intracellular pH during near-complete forebrain ischemia in the rat. *J. Neurochem.* 1986; **46**: 331–339.

93. Kraig, R.P., & Chesler, M. Astrocytic acidosis in hyperglycemic and complete ischemia. *J. Cereb. Blood Flow Metab.* 1990; **10**: 104–114.

94. Erecinska, M., & Silver, I.A. ATP and brain function. *J. Cereb. Blood Flow Metab.* 1989; **9**: 2–19.

95. Siesjo, B.K., Katsura, K., Mellergard, P., Ekholm, A., Lundgren, J., & Smith, M.L. Acidosis-related brain damage. *Prog. Brain Res.* 1993; **96**: 23–48.

96. Kraig, R.P., Pulsinelli, W.A., & Plum, F. Carbonic acid buffer changes during complete brain ischemia. *Am. J. Physiol. Regul. Integ. Comp. Physiol.* 1986; **250**: R348–R357.

97. Hurn, P.D., Koehler, R.C., Norris, S.E., Blizzard, K.K., & Traystman, R.J. Dependence of cerebral energy phosphate and evoked potential recovery on end-ischemic pH. *Am. J. Physiol. Heart Circ. Physiol.* 1991; **260**: H532–H541.

98. Chesler, M. Failure and function of intracellular pH regulation in acute hypoxic-ischemic injury of astrocytes. *Glia* 2005; **50**: 398–406.

99. Martin, G.B., Nowak, R.M., Paradis, N. *et al.* Characterization of cerebral energetics and brain pH by 31P spectroscopy after graded canine cardiac arrest and bypass reperfusion. *J. Cereb. Blood Flow Metab.* 1990; **10**: 221–226.

100. Smith, M.L., von Hanwehr, R., & Siesjo, B.K. Changes in extra- and intracellular pH in the brain during and following ischemia in hyperglycemic and in moderately hypoglycemic rats. *J. Cereb. Blood Flow Metab.* 1986; **6**: 574–583.

101. Silver, I.A., & Erecinska, M. Ion homeostasis in rat brain in vivo: intra- and extracellular [Ca²⁺] and [H⁺] in the hippocampus during recovery from short-term, transient ischemia. *J. Cereb. Blood Flow Metab.* 1992; **12**: 759–772.

102. Rehncrona, S., Rosen, I., & Siesjo, B.K. Brain lactic acidosis and ischemic cell damage: 1. Biochemistry and neurophysiology. *J. Cereb. Blood Flow Metab.* 1981; **1**: 297–311.

103. Welsh, F.A., Ginsberg, M.D., Rieder, W., & Budd, W.W. Deleterious effect of glucose pretreatment on recovery from diffuse cerebral ischemia in the cat. II. Regional metabolite levels. *Stroke* 1980; **11**: 355–363.

104. Pulsinelli, W.A., Waldman, S., Rawlinson, D., & Plum, F. Moderate hyperglycemia augments ischemic brain damage:

a neuropathologic study in the rat. *Neurology* 1982; **32**: 1239–1246.

105. Warner, D.S., Gionet, T.X., Todd, M.M., & McAllister, A.M. Insulin-induced normoglycemia improves ischemic outcome in hyperglycemic rats. *Stroke* 1992; **23**: 1775–1780.

106. Kalimo, H., Rehncrona, S., Soderfeldt, B., Olsson, Y., & Siesjo, B.K. Brain lactic acidosis and ischemic cell damage: 2. Histopathology. *J. Cereb. Blood Flow Metab.* 1981; **1**: 313–327.

107. Paljarvi, L. Brain lactic acidosis and ischemic cell damage: a topographic study with high-resolution light microscopy of early recovery in a rat model of severe incomplete ischemia. *Acta Neuropathol. (Berl.)* 1984; **64**: 89–98.

108. Wagner, K.R., Kleinholz, M., & Myers, R.E. Delayed neurologic deterioration following anoxia: brain mitochondrial and metabolic correlates. *J. Neurochem.* 1989; **52**: 1407–1417.

109. Wagner, K.R., Kleinholz, M., & Myers, R.E. Delayed onset of neurologic deterioration following anoxia/ischemia coincides with appearance of impaired brain mitochondrial respiration and decreased cytochrome oxidase activity. *J. Cereb. Blood Flow Metab.* 1990; **10**: 417–423.

110. Paljarvi, L., Rehncrona, S., Soderfeldt, B., Olsson, Y., & Kalimo, H. Brain lactic acidosis and ischemic cell damage: quantitative ultrastructural changes in capillaries of rat cerebral cortex. *Acta Neuropathol.* 1983; **60**: 232–240.

111. Ginsberg, M.D., Welsh, F.A., & Budd, W.W. Deleterious effect of glucose pretreatment on recovery from diffuse cerebral ischemia in the cat. I. Local cerebral blood flow and glucose utilization. *Stroke* 1980; **11**: 347–354.

112. Payne, R.S., Tseng, M.T., & Schurr, A. The glucose paradox of cerebral ischemia: evidence for corticosterone involvement. *Brain Res.* 2003; **971**: 9–17.

113. Tyson, R., Peeling, J., & Sutherland, G. Metabolic changes associated with altering blood glucose levels in short duration forebrain ischemia. *Brain Res.* 1993; **608**: 288–298.

114. Siemkowicz, E. Hyperglycemia in the reperfusion period hampers recovery from cerebral ischemia. *Acta Neurol. Scand.* 1981; **64**: 207–216.

115. Maruki, Y., Koehler, R.C., Kirsch, J.R., Blizzard, K.K., & Traystman, R.J. Effect of the 21-aminosteroid tirilazad on cerebral pH and somatosensory evoked potentials after incomplete ischemia. *Stroke* 1993; **24**: 724–730.

116. Cohen, Y., Chang, L.H., Litt, L. *et al.* Stability of brain intracellular lactate and 31P-metabolite levels at reduced intracellular pH during prolonged hypercapnia in rats. *J. Cereb. Blood Flow Metab.* 1990; **10**: 277–284.

117. Kraig, R.P., Petito, C.K., Plum, F., & Pulsinelli, W.A. Hydrogen ions kill brain at concentrations reached in ischemia. *J. Cereb. Blood Flow Metab.* 1987; **7**: 379–386.

118. Nedergaard, M., Goldman, S.A., Desai, S., & Pulsinelli, W.A. Acid-induced death in neurons and glia. *J. Neurosci.* 1991; **11**: 2489–2497.

119. Petito, C.K., Kraig, R.P., & Pulsinelli, W.A. Light and electron microscopic evaluation of hydrogen ion- induced brain necrosis. *J. Cereb. Blood Flow Metab.* 1987; **7**: 625–632.

120. Staub, F., Baethmann, A., Peters, J., Weigt, H., & Kempski, O. Effects of lactacidosis on glial cell volume and viability. *J. Cereb. Blood Flow Metab.* 1990; **10**: 866–876.

121. Xu, Y., Cohen, Y., Litt, L., Chang, L.H., & James, T.L. Tolerance of low cerebral intracellular pH in rats during hyperbaric hypercapnia. *Stroke* 1991; **22**: 1303–1308.

122. O'Donnell, B.R., & Bickler, P.E. Influence of pH on calcium influx during hypoxia in rat cortical brain slices. *Stroke* 1994; **25**: 171–177.

123. Giffard, R.G., Monyer, H., Christine, C.W., & Choi, D.W. Acidosis reduces NMDA receptor activation, glutamate neurotoxicity, and oxygen-glucose deprivation neuronal injury in cortical cultures. *Brain Res.* 1990; **506**: 339–342.

124. Hurn, P.D., Koehler, R.C., & Traystman, R.J. Alkalemia reduces recovery from global cerebral ischemia by NMDA receptor-mediated mechanism. *Am. J. Physiol. Heart Circ. Physiol.* 1997; **272**: H2557–H2562.

125. Xiong, Z.G., Zhu, X.M., Chu, X.P. *et al.* Neuroprotection in ischemia: blocking calcium-permeable acid-sensing ion channels. *Cell* 2004; **118**: 687–698.

126. Siesjo, B.K., Bendek, G., Koide, T., Westerberg, E., & Wieloch, T. Influence of acidosis on lipid peroxidation in brain tissues in vitro. *J. Cereb. Blood Flow Metab.* 1985; **5**: 253–258.

127. Rehncrona, S., Hauge, H.N., & Siesjo, B.K. Enhancement of iron-catalyzed free radical formation by acidosis in brain homogenates: differences in effect by lactic acid and CO_2. *J. Cereb. Blood Flow Metab.* 1989; **9**: 65–70.

128. Komara, J.S., Nayini, N.R., Bialick, H.A. *et al.* Brain iron delocalization and lipid peroxidation following cardiac arrest. *Ann. Emerg. Med.* 1986; **15**: 384–389.

129. Krause, G.S., Nayini, N.R., White, B.C. *et al.* Natural course of iron delocalization and lipid peroxidation during the first eight hours following a 15-minute cardiac arrest in dogs. *Ann. Emerg. Med.* 1987; **16**: 1200–1205.

130. Lipscomb, D.C., Gorman, L.G., Traystman, R.J., & Hurn, P.D. Low molecular weight iron in cerebral ischemic acidosis in vivo. *Stroke* 1998; **29**: 487–492.

131. Biemond, P., van Eijk, H.G., Swaak, A.J., & Koster, J.F. Iron mobilization from ferritin by superoxide derived from stimulated polymorphonuclear leukocytes. Possible mechanism in inflammation diseases. *J. Clin. Invest.* 1984; **73**: 1576–1579.

132. Thomas, C.E., Morehouse, L.A., & Aust, S.D. Ferritin and superoxide-dependent lipid peroxidation. *J. Biol. Chem.* 1985; **260**: 3275–3280.

133. Davis, S., Helfaer, M.A., Traystman, R.J., & Hurn, P.D. Parallel antioxidant and antiexcitotoxic therapy improves outcome after incomplete global cerebral ischemia in dogs. *Stroke* 1997; **28**: 198–204.

134. Hurn, P.D., Koehler, R.C., Blizzard, K.K., & Traystman, R.J. Deferoxamine reduces early metabolic failure associated with severe cerebral ischemic acidosis in dogs. *Stroke* 1995; **26**: 688–694.

135. Maruki, Y., Koehler, R.C., Kirsch, J.R., Blizzard, K.K., & Traystman, R.J. Tirilazad pretreatment improves early

cerebral metabolic and blood flow recovery from hyperglycemic ischemia. *J. Cereb. Blood Flow Metab.* 1995; **15**: 88–96.

136. Hurn, P.D., Koehler, R.C., Norris, S.E., Schwentker, A.E., & Traystman, R.J. Bicarbonate conservation during incomplete cerebral ischemia with superimposed hypercapnia. *Am. J. Physiol. Heart Circ. Physiol.* 1991; **261**: H853–H859.

137. Kurihara, J., Katsura, K., Siesjo, B.K., & Wieloch, T. Hyperglycemia and hypercapnia differently affect postischemic changes in protein kinases and protein phosphorylation in the rat cingulate cortex. *Brain Res.* 2004; **995**: 218–225.

138. Siesjo, B.K., Katsura, K.I., Kristian, T., Li, P.A., & Siesjo, P. Molecular mechanisms of acidosis-mediated damage. *Acta Neurochir.* Suppl 1996; **66**: 8–14.

139. Guerci, A.D., Shi, A.Y., Levin, H., Tsitlik, J., Weisfeldt, M.L., & Chandra, N. Transmission of intrathoracic pressure to the intracranial space during cardiopulmonary resuscitation in dogs. *Circ. Res.* 1985; **56**: 20–30.

140. Koehler, R.C., Chandra, N., Guerci, A.D. *et al.* Augmentation of cerebral perfusion by simultaneous chest compression and lung inflation with abdominal binding after cardiac arrest in dogs. *Circulation* 1983; **67**: 266–275.

141. Paradis, N.A., Martin, G.B., Goetting, M.G. *et al.* Simultaneous aortic, jugular bulb, and right atrial pressures during cardiopulmonary resuscitation in humans. Insights into mechanisms. *Circulation* 1989; **80**: 361–368.

142. Eleff, S.M., Kim, H., Shaffner, D.H., Traystman, R.J., & Koehler, R.C. Effect of cerebral blood flow generated during cardiopulmonary resuscitation in dogs on maintenance versus recovery of ATP and pH. *Stroke* 1993; **24**: 2066–2073.

143. Shaffner, D.H., Eleff, S.M., Brambrink, A.M. *et al.* Effect of arrest time and cerebral perfusion pressure during cardiopulmonary resuscitation on cerebral blood flow, metabolism, adenosine triphosphate recovery, and pH in dogs. *Crit. Care Med.* 1999; **27**: 1335–1342.

144. Shaffner, D.H., Eleff, S.M., Koehler, R.C., & Traystman, R.J. Effect of the no-flow interval and hypothermia on cerebral blood flow and metabolism during cardiopulmonary resuscitation in dogs. *Stroke* 1998; **29**: 2607–2615.

145. Amiry-Moghaddam, M., Otsuka, T., Hurn, P.D. *et al.* An alpha-syntrophin-dependent pool of AQP4 in astroglial end-feet confers bidirectional water flow between blood and brain. *Proc. Natl Acad. Sci. USA* 2003; **100**: 2106–2111.

146. Manley, G.T., Fujimura, M., Ma, T. *et al.* Aquaporin-4 deletion in mice reduces brain edema after acute water intoxication and ischemic stroke. *Nat. Med.* 2000; **6**: 159–163.

147. Kirshner, H.S., Blank, W.F., Jr., & Myers, R.E. Brain extracellular potassium activity during hypoxia in the cat. *Neurology* 1975; **25**: 1001–1005.

148. Phillis, J.W., DeLong, R.E., & Towner, J.K. Adenosine deaminase inhibitors enhance cerebral anoxic hyperemia in the rat. *J. Cereb. Blood Flow Metab.* 1985; **5**: 295–299.

149. Greenberg, R.S., Helfaer, M.A., Kirsch, J.R., & Traystman, R.J. Effect of nitric oxide synthase inhibition on post-ischemic cerebral hyperemia. *Am. J. Physiol. Heart Circ. Physiol.* 1995; **239**: H341–H347.

150. Schleien, C.L., Kuluz, J.W., & Gelman, B. Hemodynamic effects of nitric oxide synthase inhibition before and after cardiac arrest in infant piglets. *Am. J. Physiol. Heart Circ. Physiol.* 1998; **274**: H1378–H1385.

151. Moskowitz, M.A., Sakas, D.E., Wei, E.P. *et al.* Postocclusive cerebral hyperemia is markedly attenuated by chronic trigeminal ganglionectomy. *Am. J. Physiol. Heart Circ. Physiol.* 1989; **257**: H1736–H1739.

152. Hurn, P.D., Littleton-Kearney, M.T., Kirsch, J.R., Dharmarajan, A.M., & Traystman, R.J. Postischemic cerebral blood flow recovery in the female: effect of 17 beta-estradiol. *J. Cereb. Blood Flow Metab.* 1995; **15**: 666–672.

153. Leonov, Y., Sterz, F., Safar, P., Johnson, D.W., Tisherman, S.A., & Oku, K. Hypertension with hemodilution prevents multifocal cerebral hypoperfusion after cardiac arrest in dogs. *Stroke* 1992; **23**: 45–53.

154. Fischer, E.G., Ames, A., III, Hedley-Whyte, E.T., & O'Gorman, S. Reassessment of cerebral capillary changes in acute global ischemia and their relationship to the "no-reflow phenomenon." *Stroke* 1977; **8**: 36–39.

155. Sterz, F., Leonov, Y., Safar, P., Radovsky, A., Tisherman, S.A., & Oku, K. Hypertension with or without hemodilution after cardiac arrest in dogs. *Stroke* 1990; **21**: 1178–1184.

156. Frerichs, K.U., Siren, A.L., Feuerstein, G.Z., & Hallenbeck, J.M. The onset of postischemic hypoperfusion in rats is precipitous and may be controlled by local neurons. *Stroke* 1992; **23**: 399–406.

157. Blomqvist, P., Lindvall, O., & Wieloch, T. Delayed postischemic hypoperfusion: evidence against involvement of the noradrenergic locus ceruleus system. *J. Cereb. Blood Flow Metab.* 1984; **4**: 425–429.

158. Beckstead, J.E., Tweed, W.A., Lee, J., & MacKeen, W.L. Cerebral blood flow and metabolism in man following cardiac arrest. *Stroke* 1978; **9**: 569–573.

159. Edgren, E., Enblad, P., Grenvik, A. *et al.* Cerebral blood flow and metabolism after cardiopulmonary resuscitation. A pathophysiologic and prognostic positron emission tomography pilot study. *Resuscitation* 2003; **57**: 161–170.

160. Michenfelder, J.D., & Milde, J.H. Postischemic canine cerebral blood flow appears to be determined by cerebral metabolic needs. *J. Cereb. Blood Flow Metab.* 1990; **10**: 71–76.

161. Cohan, S.L., Mun, S.K., Petite, J., Correia, J., Tavelra Da Silva, A.T., & Waldhorn, R.E. Cerebral blood flow in humans following resuscitation from cardiac arrest. *Stroke* 1989; **20**: 761–765.

162. LaManna, J.C., Crumrine, R.C., & Jackson, D.L. No correlation between cerebral blood flow and neurologic recovery after reversible total cerebral ischemia in the dog. *Exp. Neurol.* 1988; **101**: 234–247.

163. Forsman, M., Aarseth, H.P., Nordby, H.K., Skulberg, A., & Steen, P.A. Effects of nimodipine on cerebral blood flow and cerebrospinal fluid pressure after cardiac arrest: correlation with neurologic outcome. *Anesth. Analg.* 1989; **68**: 436–443.

164. Milde, L.N., Milde, J.H., & Michenfelder, J.D. Delayed treatment with nimodipine improves cerebral blood flow after complete cerebral ischemia in the dog. *J. Cereb. Blood Flow Metab.* 1986; **6**: 332–337.

165. Steen, P.A., Newberg, L.A., Milde, J.H., & Michenfelder, J.D. Cerebral blood flow and neurologic outcome when nimodipine is given after complete cerebral ischemia in the dog. *J. Cereb. Blood Flow Metab.* 1984; **4**: 82–87.

166. Grogaard, B., Schurer, L., Gerdin, B., & Arfors, K.E. Delayed hypoperfusion after incomplete forebrain ischemia in the rat. The role of polymorphonuclear leukocytes. *J. Cereb. Blood Flow Metab.* 1989; **9**: 500–505.

167. Mayhan, W.G., Amundsen, S.M., Faraci, F.M., & Heistad, D.D. Responses of cerebral arteries after ischemia and reperfusion in cats. *Am. J. Physiol. Heart Circ. Physiol.* 1988; **255**: H879–H884.

168. Nelson, C.W., Wei, E.P., Povlishock, J.T., Kontos, H.A., & Moskowitz, M.A. Oxygen radicals in cerebral ischemia. *Am. J. Physiol. Heart Circ. Physiol.* 1992; **263**: H1356–H1362.

169. Watanabe, Y., Littleton-Kearney, M.T., Traystman, R.J., & Hurn, P.D. Estrogen restores postischemic pial microvascular dilation. *Am. J. Physiol. Heart Circ. Physiol.* 2001; **281**: H155–H160.

170. Qin, X., Hurn, P.D., & Littleton-Kearney, M.T. Estrogen restores postischemic sensitivity to the thromboxane mimetic U46619 in rat pial artery. *J. Cereb. Blood Flow Metab.* 2005; (Article in Press).

171. Christopherson, T.J., Milde, J.H., & Michenfelder, J.D. Cerebral vascular autoregulation and CO_2 reactivity following onset of the delayed postischemic hypoperfusion state in dogs. *J. Cereb. Blood Flow Metab.* 1993; **13**: 260–268.

172. Kagstrom, E., Smith, M.L., & Siesjo, B.K. Cerebral circulatory responses to hypercapnia and hypoxia in the recovery period following complete and incomplete cerebral ischemia in the rat. *Acta Physiol. Scand.* 1983; **118**: 281–291.

173. Nemoto, E.M., Snyder, J.V., Carroll, R.G., & Morita, H. Global ischemia in dogs: cerebrovascular CO2 reactivity and autoregulation. *Stroke* 1975; **6**: 425–431.

174. Kirsch, J.R., Helfaer, M.A., Haun, S.E., Koehler, R.C., & Traystman, R.J. Polyethylene glycol-conjugated superoxide dismutase improves recovery of postischemic hypercapnic cerebral blood flow in piglets. *Pediatr. Res.* 1993; **34**: 530–537.

175. Cerchiari, E.L., Hoel, T.M., Safar, P., & Sclabassi, R.J. Protective effects of combined superoxide dismutase and deferoxamine on recovery of cerebral blood flow and function after cardiac arrest in dogs. *Stroke* 1987; **18**: 869–878.

176. Liu, X.L., Wiklund, L., Nozari, A., Rubertsson, S., & Basu, S. Differences in cerebral reperfusion and oxidative injury after cardiac arrest in pigs. *Acta Anaesthesiol. Scand.* 2003; **47**: 958–967.

177. Krep, H., Bottiger, B.W., Bock, C. *et al.* Time course of circulatory and metabolic recovery of cat brain after cardiac arrest assessed by perfusion- and diffusion-weighted imaging and MR-spectroscopy. *Resuscitation* 2003; **58**: 337–348.

178. Siesjö, B.K. Pathophysiology and treatment of focal cerebral ischemia. I. Pathophysiology. *J Neurosurg* 1992; **77**: 169–184.

179. Schoepp, D.D., & Conn, P.J. Metabotropic glutamate receptors in brain function and pathology. *TiPS* 1993; **14**: 13–20

180. Siliprandi, R., Lipartiti, M., Fadda, E. *et al.* Activation of glutamate metaboprobiic receptor protects retina against N-methyl-D-aspartate toxicity. *Eur. J. Pharmacol.* 1992; **219**(1): 173–174.

181. Lipartiti, M., Fadda, E., Savioni, G. *et al.* In rats, the metaboprobic receptor-triggered hippocampal neuronal damage is strain-dependant. *Life Sci.* 1993; **52**:PL85–PL90.

182. Krause, G.S., White, B.C., Aust, S.D., & Nayini, N.R. Brain cell death following ischemia and reperfusion: a proposed biochemical sequence. *Crit. Care Med.* 1988; **16**: 714–726.

183. Chan, P.H., Kerlan, R., & Fishman, R.A. Reductions of gama-aminobutyric acid and glutamate and $(Na^+ + K^+)$-ATPase activity in brain slices and synaptosomes by arachidonic acid. *J. Neurochem.* 1983; **40**: 309–315.

184. Braughler, J.M.: Lipid peroxidation-induced inhibition of gama-aminobutyric acid uptake in rat brain synaptosomes. Protection by glucocorticoids. *J. Neurochem.* 1985; **44**: 1282–1286.

185. Ames, A. III. Earliest irreversible changes during ischemia. *Am. J. Emerg. Med.* 1983; **2**: 139–143.

186. Drejer, J., Benveniste, H., Diemer, N.Y. *et al.* Cellular origin of ischemic-induced glutamate release from brain tissue *in vivo* and *in vitro*. *J. Neurochem.* 1985; **45**: 145–150.

187. Traynelis, S.F., & Cull-Candy, S.G. Proton inhibition of N-methyl-D-Aspartate receptors in cerebellar neurons. *Nature* 1990; **345**: 347–350.

188. Nellgård, B., & Wieloch, T. Postischemic blockade of AMPA but not NMDA receptors mitigates neuronal damage in the rat brain following severe cerebral ischemia. *J. Cereb. Blood Flow Metab.* 1992; **12**: 2–11.

189. Ushijima, K., Miyazaki, H., & Morioka, T. Immunohistochemical localization of glutathione peroxidase in the brain of the rat. *Resuscitation* 1986; **13**: 97–105.

190. Tiffany, B.R., White, B.C., & Krause, G.S. Nuclear-envelope nucleoside triphosphatase kinetics and mRNA transport following brain ischemia and reperfusion. *J. Neurochem.*, submitted March 1994.

191. Zaleska, M.M., & Floyd, R.A. Regional lipid peroxidation in rat brain *in vitro*: Possible role of endogenous iron. *Neurochem. Res.* 1985; **10**: 397–410.

192. White, B.C., Rafols, J.A., DeGracia, D.J., Skjaerlund, J.M., & Krause, G.S. Fluorescent histochemical localization of lipid peroxidation during brain reperfusion. *Acta Neuropathol. (Berl.)* 1993; **86**: 1–9.

193. Farquhar, M.G. Traffic of products and membranes through the Golgi complex. In Silverstein, KSC (ed.), *Transport of Macromolecules in Cellular Systems*. Berlin: Dahlem Konferenzen, 1978: 341–362.

194. Voelker, D.R. Lipid transport pathways in mammalian cells. *Experientia* 1990; **46**: 569–579.

195. Silver, I.A., & Erecinska, M. Intracellular and extracellular changes of $[Ca^{2+}]$ in hypoxia and ischemia in rat brain in vivo. *J. Gen. Physiol.* 1990; **95**: 837–866.

196. Erecinska, M., & Silver, I.A. Relationships between ions and energy metabolism: Cerebral calcium movements during ischaemia and subsequent recovery. *Can. J. Physiol. Pharmacol.* 1992; **70**: S190–S193.

197. Silver, I.A., & Erecinska, M. Ion homeostasis in rat brain in vivo: intra- and extracellular Ca2+ and H+ in the hippocampus during recovery from short-term, transient ischemia. *J. Cereb. Blood Flow Metab.* 1992; **12**: 759–772.

198. Borgers, M., Thone, F., & Van Neuten, J.M. Subcellular distribution of calcium and the effects of calcium-antagonists as evaluated with combined oxalate-pyroantimonate technique. *Acta Histochem.* 1981; **24** (Suppl): 327–332.

199. Simon, R.P., Griffiths, T., Evans, M.C., Swan, J.H., & Meldrum, B.S. Calcium overload in selectively vulnerable neurons of the hippocampus during and after ischemia: an electron microscopy study in the rat. *J. Cereb. Blood Flow Metab.* 1984; **4**: 350–361.

200. Zaidan, E., & Simms, N.R. The calcium content of mitochondria from brain subregions following short-term forebrain ischemia and recirculation in the rate. *J. Neurochem.* 1994; **63**: 1912–1919.

201. Dux, E., Mies, G., Hossmann K.-A., & Siklos, L. Calcium in the mitochondria following brief ischemia of the gerbil brain. *Neurosci. Lett.* 1987; **78**: 295–300.

202. Kohno, K., Higuchi, T., Ohta, S., Kohno, K., Kumon, Y., & Sakaki, S. neuroprotective nitric oxide synthase inhibitor reduces intracellular calcium accumulation following transient global ischemia in the gerbil. *Neurosci. Lett.* 1997; **224**: 17–20.

203. Deshpande, J.K., Siesjo, B.K., & Wieloch, T. Calcium accumulation and neuronal damage in the rat hippocampus following cerebral ischemia. *J. Cereb. Blood Flow Metab.* 1987; **7**: 89–95.

204. Martins, E., Inamura, K., Themner, K., Malmqvist, K.G., & Siesjo, B.K. Accumulation of calcium and loss of potassium in the hippocampus following transient cerebral ischemia: a proton microprobe study. *J. Cereb. Blood Flow Metab.* 1988; **8**: 531–538.

205. Parsons, J.T., Churn, S.B., & DeLorenzo, R.J. Global ischemia-induced inhibition of the coupling ratio of calcium uptake and ATP hydrolysis by rat whole brain microsomal Mg^{2+}/Ca^{2+}-ATPase. *Brain Res.* 1999; **834**: 32–41.

206. Oguro, K., Nakamura, M., & Masuzawa, T. Histochemical study of Ca2+-ATPase activity in ischemic CA1 pyramidal neurons in the gerbil hippocampus. *Acta Neuropathol.* 1995; **90**: 448–453.

207. Pellegrini-Giampietro, D.E., Zukin, R.S., Bennett, M.V.L., Cho, S., & Pulsinellini, W.A. Switch in glutamate receptor subunit gene expression in CA1 subfield of hippocampus following global ischemia in rats. *Proc. Natl Acad. Sci. USA* 1992; **89**: 10499–10503.

208. Hu, P., Diemer, N.H., Bruhn, T., & Johansen, F.F. Effects of the AMPA-receptor antagonist, NBQX, on neuron loss in dentate hilus of the hippocampal formation after 8, 10, or 12 min of cerebral ischemia in the rat. *J. Cereb. Blood Flow Metab.* 1997; **17**: 147–152.

209. Gorter, J.A., Petrozzino, J.J., Aronica, E.M. *et al.* Global ischemia induces downregulation of GluR2 mRNA and increases AMPA receptor-mediated Ca^{2+} influx in hippocampal CA neurons of gerbil. *J. Neurosci.* 1997; **17**: 6179–6188.

210. Kawasaki-Yatsugi, S., Yatsugi, S., Koshiya, K., & Shimizu-Sasamata, M. Neuroprotective effect of YM90K, an AMPA-receptor antagonist, against delayed neuronal death induced by transient global cerebral ischemia in gerbils and rats. *Jpn J. Pharmacol.* 1997; **74**: 253–260.

211. Aronica, E.M., Gorter, J.A., Grooms, S. *et al.* Aurintricarboxylic acid (ATA) prevents GLUR2 mRNA down-regulation and delayed neurodegeneration in hippocampal CA1 neurons of gerbil after global ischemia. *Proc. Natl Acad. Sci. USA* 1998; **95**: 7115–7120.

212. Aarts, M., Iihara, K., Wei, W.L. *et al.* A key role for TRPM7 channels in anoxic neuronal death. *Cell* 2003; **115**: 863–877.

213. Panfoli, I., Rosina, F., Musante, L., Morelli, A., Cugnoli, C., & Pepe, I.M. Endoplasmic reticulum Ca^{2+}-ATPase in microsomal vesicles isolated from bovine retinae. *Ital. J. Biochem.* 1995; **44**: 247–257.

214. Croall, D.E., & DeMartino, G.N. Calcium-activated neutral protease (Calpain) system: Structure, function, and regulation. *Physiol. Rev.* 1991; **3**: 813–847.

215. Goll, D.E., Thompson, V.F., Li, H., Wei, W., & Cong, J. The calpain system. *Physiol. Rev.* 2003 **83**: 731–801.

216. Siman, R., Gall, C., Perlmutter, L., Christian, C., Baudry, M., & Lynch, G. Distribution of calpain, I., an enzyme associated with degenerative activity in rat brain. *Brain Res.* 1985; **347**: 399–403.

217. Hamakubo, T.R., Kannagi, R., Murachi, T., & Matus, A. Distribution of calpains I and II in rat brain. *J. Neurosci.* 1986; **6**: 3103–3111.

218. Fukuda, T., Adachi, E., Kawashamia, S., Yoshiya, I., & Hashimoto, P.H. Immunohistochemical distribution of calcium-activated neutral proteinases and endogenous CANP inhibitor in the rabbit hippocampus. *J. Comp. Neurol.* 1990; **302**: 100–109.

219. Kamakura, K., Ishiura, S., Imajoh, S., Nagata, N., & Sugita, H. Distribution of calcium-activated neutral protease inhibitor in the central nervous system of the rat. *J. Neurosci. Res.* 1992; **31**: 543–548.

220. Cong, J., Goll, D.E., Peterson, A.M., & Kapprell, H.P. The role of autolysis in activity of the Ca2+-dependent proteinases (mucalpain and m-calpain). *J. Biol. Chem.* 1989; **264**: 10096–10103.

221. Goll, D.E., Thompson, V.F., Taylor, R.G., & Zalewska, T. Is calpain activity regulated by membranes and autolysis or by calcium and calpastatin? *BioEssays* 1992; **14**: 549–556.

222. Suzuki, K., Saido, T., & Hirai, S. Modulation of cellular signals by calpain. *Ann. N Y Acad. Sci.* 1992; **674**: 218–227.

223. Croall, D.E., & DeMartino, G.N. Regulation of calcium-dependent protease activity in vitro: Clues for determining their physiological functions. In Mellgren, R.L., Murachi T. eds. *Intracellular Calcium-Dependent Proteolysis.* Boca Raton: CRC Press Inc., 1990: 103–114.

224. Hayashi, M., Inomata, M., Saito, Y., Ito, H., & Kawashima, S. Activation of intracellular calcium-activated neutral proteinase in erythrocytes and its inhibition by exogenously added inhibitors. *Biochim. Biophys. Acta* 1991; **1094**: 249–256.

225. Saido, T.C., Yokota, M., Nagao, S. *et al.* Spatial resolution of fodrin proteolysis in post-ischemic brain. *J. Biol. Chem.* 1993; **268**: 25239–25243.

226. Roberts-Lewis, J.M., Savage, M.J., Marcy, V.R., Pinsler, L.R., & Siman, R. Immunolocalization of calpain I-mediated spectrin degradation to vulnerable neurons in the ischemic gerbil brain. *J. Neurosci.* 1994; **14**: 3934–3944.

227. Seubert, P., & Lynch, G. Plasticity and pathology: brain calpains as modifiers of synaptic structure. In Mellgren, R.L., Murachi, T. eds. *Intracellular Calcium-Dependent Proteolysis*. Boca Raton: CRC Press, Inc., 1990: 251–264.

228. Song, D.K., Malmstrom, T., Kater, S.B., & Mykles, D.L. Calpain inhibitors block Ca2+-induced suppression of neurite outgrowth in isolated hippocampal pyramidal neurons. *J. Neurosci. Res.* 1994; **39**: 474–481.

229. Arthur, J.S.C., Elce, J.S., Hegadorn, C., Williams, K., & Greer, P.A. Disruption of the murine calpain SC subunit gene, Capn4: calpain is essential for embryonic development but not for cell growth and division. *Mol. Cell. Biol.* 2000; **20**: 4474–4481.

230. Zimmerman, U.J., Boring, L., Pak, J.H., Mukerjee, N., & Wang, K.K. The calpain small subunit gene is essential: its inactivation results in embryonic lethality. *IUBMB Life* 2000; **50**: 63–68.

231. Azam, M., Andrabi, S.S., Sahr, K.E., Kamath, L., Kuliopulos, A., & Chishti, A.H. Disruption of the mouse mu-calpain gene reveals an essential role in platelet function. *Mol. Cell. Biol.* 2001; **21**: 2213–2220.

232. Honda, S., Marumoto, T., Hirota, T. *et al.* Activation of m-calpain is required for chromosome alignment on the metaphase plate during mitosis. *J. Biol. Chem.* 2004; **279**: 10615–10623.

233. Neumar, R.W., Hagle, S.M., DeGracia, D.J., Krause, G.S., & White, B.C. Brain m-calpain autolysis during global cerebral ischemia. *J. Neurochem.* 1996; **66**: 421–424.

234. Zhang, C., Siman, R., Xu, Y.A., Mills, A.M., & Neumar, R.W. Comparison of calpain and caspase activities in the adult rat brain following transient forebrain ischemia. *Neurobiol. Dis.* 2002; **10**: 289–305.

235. Yamashima, T., Saido, T.C., Takita, M. *et al.* Transient brain ischaemia provokes Ca^{2+}, PIP2, and calpain responses prior to delayed neuronal death in monkeys. *Eur. J. Neurosci.* 1996; **8**: 1932–1944.

236. Neumar, R.W., Meng, F.H., Mills, A.M. *et al.* Calpain activity in the rat brain after transient forebrain ischemia. *Exp. Neurol.* 2001; **170**: 27–35.

237. Bartus, R.T., Dean, R.L., Mennerick, S., Eveleth, D., & Lynch, G. Temporal ordering of pathogenic events following transient global ischemia. *Brain Res.* 1998; **790**: 1–13.

238. Hong, S.C., Goto, Y., Lanzino, G., Soleau, S., Kassell, N.F., & Lee, K.S. Neuroprotection with a calpain-inhibitor in a model of focal cerebral ischemia. *Stroke* 1994; **25**: 663–669.

239. Hong, S.C., Lanzino, G., Goto, Y. *et al.* Calcium-activated proteolysis in rat neocortex induced by transient focal ischemia. *Brain Res.* 1994; **661**: 43–50.

240. Lee, K.S., Frank, S., Vanderklish, P., Arai, A., & Lynch, G. Inhibition of proteolysis protects hippocampal neurons from ischemia. *Proc. Natl Acad. Sci. USA* 1991; **88**: 7233–7237.

241. Rami, A., & Krieglstein, J. Protective effects of calpain inhibitors against neuronal damage caused by cytotoxic hypoxia in vitro and ischemia in vivo. *Brain Res.* 1993; **609**: 67–70.

242. Markgraf, C.G., Velayo, N.L., Johnson, M.P. *et al.* Six-hour window of opportunity for calpain inhibition in focal cerebral ischemia in rats. *Stroke* 1998; **29**: 152–158.

243. Li, P.A., Howlett, W., He, Q.P., Miyashita, H., Siddiqui, M., & Shuaib, A. Postischemic treatment with calpain inhibitor MDL-28170 ameliorates brain damage in a gerbil model of global ischemia. *Neurosci. Lett.* 1998; **247**: 17–20.

244. Yokota, M., Tani, E., Tsubuki, S. *et al.* Calpain inhibitor entrapped in liposomes rescues ischemic neuroanl damage. *Brain Res.* 1999; **819**: 8–14.

245. Donkor, I.O. A survey of calpain inhibitors. *Curr. Med. Chem.* 2000; **7**: 1171–1188.

246. Wang, K.K., & Yuen, P.W. Development and therapeutic potential of calpain inhibitors. *Adv. Pharmacol.* 1997; **37**: 117–152.

247. Yamashima, T. Implication of cysteine proteases calpain, cathepsin and caspase in ischemic neuronal death of primates. *Prog. Neurobiol.* 2000; **62**: 273–295.

248. Syntichaki, P., Xu, K., Driscoll, M., & Tavernarakis, N. Specific aspartyl and calpain proteases are required for neurodegeneration in *C. elegans*. *Nature* 2002; **419**: 939–944

249. Bednarski, E., Vanderklish, P., Gall, C., Saido, T.C., Bahr, B.A., & Lynch, G. Translational suppression of calpain I reduces NMDA-induced spectrin proteolysis and pathophysiology in cultured hippocampal slices. *Brain Res.* 1995; **694**: 147–157.

250. Nozaki, K., Moskowitz, M.A., Maynard, K.I. *et al.* Possible origins and distribution of immunoreactive nitric oxide synthase-containing nerve fibers in cerebral arteries. *J. Cereb. Blood Flow Metab.* 1993; **13**: 70–79.

251. Bredt, D.S., Glatt, C.E., Hwang, P.M., Fotuhi, M., Dawson, T.M., & Snyder, S.H. Nitric oxide synthase protein and mRNA are discretely localized in neuronal populations of the mammalian CNS together with NADPH diaphorase. *Neuron* 1991; **7**: 615–624.

252. Valtschanoff, J.G., Weinberg, R.J., Kharazia, V.N., Nakane, M., & Schmidt, H.H. Neurons in rat hippocampus that synthesize nitric oxide. *J. Comp. Neurol.* 1993; **331**: 111–121.

253. Dawson, V.L., Dawson, T.M., Bartley, D.A., Uhl, G.R., & Snyder, S.H. Mechanisms of nitric oxide-mediated neurotoxicity in primary brain cultures. *J. Neurosci.* 1993; **13**: 2651–2661.

254. Bredt, D.S., & Snyder, S.H. Nitric oxide mediates glutamate-linked enhancement of cGMP levels in the cerebellum. *Proc. Natl Acad. Sci. USA* 1989; **86**: 9030–9033.

255. Christopherson, K.S., Hillier, B.J., Lim, W.A., & Bredt, D.S. PSD-95 assembles a ternary complex with the N-methyl-D-aspartic acid receptor and a bivalent neuronal NO synthase PDZ domain. *J. Biol. Chem.* 1999; **274**: 27467–27473.

256. Sattler, R., Xiong, Z., Lu, W.Y., Hafner, M., MacDonald, J.F., & Tymianski, M. Specific coupling of NMDA receptor activation to nitric oxide neurotoxicity by PSD-95 protein. *Science* 1999; **284**: 1845–1848.

257. Bhardwaj, A., Northington, F.J., Ichord, R.N., Hanley, D.F., Traystman, R.J., & Koehler, R.C. Characterization of ionotropic glutamate receptor-mediated nitric oxide production in vivo in rats. *Stroke* 1997; **28**: 850–857.

258. Bhardwaj, A., Northington, F.J., Martin, L.J., Hanley, D.F., Traystman, R.J., & Koehler, R.C. Characterization of metabotropic glutamate receptor-mediated nitric oxide production in vivo. *J. Cereb. Blood Flow Metab.* 1997; **17**: 153–160.

259. Garthwaite, J., Southam, E., & Anderton, M. A kainate receptor linked to nitric oxide synthesis from arginine. *J. Neurochem.* 1989; **53**: 1952–1954.

260. Southam, E., East, S.J., & Garthwaite, J. Excitatory amino acid receptors coupled to the nitric oxide/cyclic GMP pathway in rat cerebellum during development. *J. Neurochem.* 1991; **56**: 2072–2081.

261. Okada, D. Two pathways of cyclic GMP production through glutamate receptor-mediated nitric oxide synthesis. *J. Neurochem.* 1992; **59**: 1203–1210.

262. Goyagi, T., Goto, S., Bhardwaj, A., Dawson, V.L., Hurn, P.D., & Kirsch, J.R. Neuroprotective effect of σ-receptor ligand 4-phenyl-1-(4-phenylbutyl) piperidine (PPBP) is linked to reduced neuronal nitric oxide production. *Stroke* 2001; **32**: 1613–1620.

263. Tomonaga, T., Sato, S., Ohnishi, T., & Ohnishi, S.T. Electron paramagnetic resonance (EPR) detection of nitric oxide during forebrain ischemia of the rat. *J. Cereb. Blood Flow Metab.* 1994; **14**: 715–722.

264. Ischiropoulos, H., & Beckman, J.S. Oxidative stress and nitration in neurodegeneration: cause, effect, or association? *J. Clin. Invest.* 2003; **111**: 163–169.

265. Stamler, J.S., Singel, D.J., & Loscalzo, J. Biochemistry of nitric oxide and its redox-activated forms. *Science* 1992; **258**: 1898–1902.

266. Beckman, J.S., Beckman, T.W., Chen, J., Marshall, P.A., & Freeman, B.A. Apparent hydroxyl radical production by peroxynitrite: implications for endothelial injury from nitric oxide and superoxide. *Proc. Natl Acad. Sci. USA* 1990; **87**: 1620–1624.

267. Radi, R., Beckman, J.S., Bush, K.M., & Freeman, B.A. Peroxynitrite oxidation of sulfhydryls. The cytotoxic potential of superoxide and nitric oxide. *J. Biol. Chem.* 1991; **266**: 4244–4250.

268. Wink, D.A., Kasprzak, K.S., Maragos, C.M. *et al.* DNA deaminating ability and genotoxicity of nitric oxide and its progenitors. *Science* 1994; **254**: 1001–1003.

269. Zhang, J., Dawson, V.L., Dawson, T.M., & Snyder, S.H. Nitric oxide activation of poly(ADP-ribose) synthetase in neurotoxicity. *Science* 1994; **263**: 687–689.

270. Radi, R., Beckman, J.S., Bush, K.M., & Freeman, B.A. Peroxynitrite-induced membrane lipid peroxidation: the cytotoxic potential of superoxide and nitric oxide. *Arch. Biochem. Biophys.* 1991; **288**: 481–487.

271. Sampei, K., Mandir, A.S., Asano, Y. *et al.* Stroke outcome in double-mutant antioxidant transgenic mice. *Stroke* 2000; **31**: 2685–2691.

272. Yu, S.W., Wang, H., Poitras, M.F. *et al.* Mediation of poly(ADP-ribose) polymerase-1-dependent cell death by apoptosis-inducing factor. *Science* 2002; **297**: 259–263.

273. Alano, C.C., Ying, W., & Swanson, R.A. Poly(ADP-ribose) polymerase-1-mediated cell death in astrocytes requires NAD+ depletion and mitochondrial permeability transition. *J. Biol. Chem.* 2004; **279**: 18895–18902.

274. Ying, W., Alano, C.C., Garnier, P., & Swanson, R.A. NAD+ as a metabolic link between DNA damage and cell death. *J. Neurosci. Res.* 2005; **79**: 216–223.

275. Cao, G., Clark, R.S., Pei, W. *et al.* Translocation of apoptosis-inducing factor in vulnerable neurons after transient cerebral ischemia and in neuronal cultures after oxygen-glucose deprivation. *J. Cereb. Blood Flow Metab.* 2003; **23**: 1137–1150.

276. Eliasson, M.J., Huang, Z., Ferrante, R.J. *et al.* Neuronal nitric oxide synthase activation and peroxynitrite formation in ischemic stroke linked to neural damage. *J. Neurosci.* 1999; **19**: 5910–5918.

277. Huang, Z., Huang, P.L., Panahian, N., Dalkara, T., Fishman, M.C., & Moskowitz, M.A. Effects of cerebral ischemia in mice deficient in neuronal nitric oxide synthase. *Science* 1994; **265**: 1883–1885.

278. Eliasson, M.J.L., Sampei, K., Mandir, A.S. *et al.* Poly(ADP-ribose) polymerase gene disruption renders mice resistant to cerebral ischemia. *Nat. Med.* 1997; **3**: 1089–1095.

279. Goto, S., Xue, R., Sugo, N. *et al.* Poly (ADP-ribose) polymerase (PARP-1) impairs early and long-term experimental stroke therapy. *Stroke* 2002; **33**: 1101–1106.

280. McCullough, L.D., Zeng, Z., Blizzard, K.K., Debchoudhury, I., & Hurn, P.D. Ischemic nitric oxide and poly (ADP-ribose) polymerase-1 in cerebral ischemia: male toxicity, female protection. *J. Cereb. Blood Flow Metab.* 2005; **25**: 502–512.

281. Sancesario, G., Iannone, M., Morello, M., Nistico, G., & Bernardi, G. Nitric oxide inhibition aggravates ischemic damage of hippocampal but not of NADPH neurons in gerbils. *Stroke* 1994; **25**: 436–443.

282. Shapira, S., Kadar, T., & Weissman, B.A. Dose-dependent effect of nitric oxide synthase inhibition following transient forebrain ischemia in gerbils. *Brain Res.* 1994; **668**: 80–84.

283. Buchan, A.M., Gertler, S.Z., Huang, Z.G., Li, H., Chaundy, K.E., & Xue, D. Failure to prevent selective CA1 neuronal death and reduce cortical infarction following cerebral ischemia with inhibition of nitric oxide synthase. *Neuroscience* 1994; **61**: 1–11.

284. Kirsch, J.R., Bhardwaj, A., Martin, L.J., Hanley, D.F., & Traystman, R.J. Neither L-arginine nor L-NAME affects neurological outcome after global ischemia in cats. *Stroke* 1997; **28**: 2259–2264.

285. Caldwell, M., O'Neill, M., Earley, B., & Leonard, B. Nω-Nitro-L-arginine protects against ischaemia-induced increases in nitric oxide and hippocampal neuro-degeneration in the gerbil. *Eur. J. Pharmacol.* 1994; **260**: 191–200.

286. Panahian, N., Yoshida, T., Huang, P.L. *et al.* Attenuated hippocampal damage after global cerebral ischemia in mice mutant in neuronal nitric oxide synthase. *Neuroscience* 1996; **72**: 343–354.

287. Kofler, J., Sawada, M., Hattori, K., Dawson, V.L., Hurn, P.D., & Traystman, R.J. Brain injury after cardiac arrest and cardiopulmonary resuscitation (CPR). In Krieglstein, J., ed. *Pharmacology of Cerebral Ischemia 2002.* Stuttgart, Germany: Medpharm Scientific Publishers; 2003: 397–403.

288. Kofler, J., Hurn, P.D., & Traystman, R.J. SOD1 overexpression and female sex exhibit region-specific neuroprotection after global cerebral ischemia due to cardiac arrest. *J. Cereb. Blood Flow Metab.* 2005; (in Press).

289. Iadecola, C., Zhang, F., Xu, S., Casey, R., & Ross, M.E. Inducible nitric oxide synthase gene expression in brain following cerebral ischemia. *J. Cereb. Blood Flow Metab.* 1995; **15**: 378–384.

290. Nagayama, M., Zhang, F., & Iadecola, C. Delayed treatment with aminoguanidine decreases focal cerebral ischemic damage and enhances neurologic recovery in rats. *J. Cereb. Blood Flow Metab.* 1998; **18**: 1107–1113.

291. Iadecola, C., Zhang, F., Casey, R., Nagayama, M., & Ross, M.E. Delayed reduction of ischemic brain injury and neurological deficits in mice lacking the inducible nitric oxide synthase gene. *J. Neurosci.* 1997; **17**: 9157–9164.

292. Mori, K., Togashi, H., Ueno, K.I., Matsumoto, M., & Yoshioka, M. Aminoguanidine prevented the impairment of learning behavior and hippocampal long-term potentiation following transient cerebral ischemia. *Behav. Brain. Res.* 2001; **120**: 159–168.

293. Danielisova, V., Nemethova, M., & Burda, J. The protective effect of aminoguanidine on cerebral ischemic damage in the rat brain. *Physiol. Res.* 2004; **53**: 533–540.

294. Yoshida, S., Inoh, S., Asano, T. *et al.* Effect of transient ischemia on free fatty acids and phospholipids in the gerbil brain. *J. Neurosurg.* 1980; **53**: 323–331.

295. Yasuda, H., Kishiro, K., Izumi, N., & Nakanishi, M. Biphasic liberation of arachidonic and stearic acids during cerebral ischemia. *J. Neurochem.* 1985; **45**: 168–172.

296. Umemura, A. Regional difference in free fatty acids release and the action of phospholipase during ischemia in rat brain. *No To Shinkei* 1990; **42**: 979–986.

297. Irvine, R.F. How is the level of free arachidonic acid controlled in mammalian cells? *Biochem. J.* 1982; **204**: 3–16.

298. Van Den Bosch, H. Intracellular phospholipases A. *Biochim. Biophys. Acta* 1980; **604**: 191–246.

299. Drenth, J., Enzing, C.M., Kalk, K.H., & Vessies, J.C. Structure of porcine pancreatic phospholipase A2. *Nature* 1976; **264**: 373–377.

300. Moskowitz, N., Schook, W., & Puskin, S. Regulation of endogenous calcium-dependent synaptic membrane phospholipase A2. *Brain Res.* 1984; **290**: 273–280.

301. Rosenthal, R.E., & Fiskum, G. Phospholipid deterioration and free fatty acid release in the cerebral cortex following cardiac arrest and resuscitation. Abstract, *Ann. Emerg. Med.* 1991; **20**: 478.

302. Barker, M.O., & Brin, M. Mechanisms of lipid peroxidation in erythrocytes of vitamin E deficient rats and in phospholipid model systems. *Arch Biochem Biophys* 1975; **166**: 32–40.

303. Sevanian, A., Muakkassah-Kelly, S.F., & Montestruque, S. The influence of phospholipase A2 and glutathione peroxidase on the elimination of membrane lipid peroxides. *Arch. Biochem. Biophys.* 1983; **223**: 441–452.

304. Au, A.M., Chan, P.H., & Fishman, R.A. Stimulation of phospholipase A2 activity by oxygen-derived free radicals in isolated brain capillaries. *J. Cell. Biochem.* 1985; **27**: 449–453.

305. Chan, P.H., Yurko, M., & Fishman, R.A. Phospholipid degradation and cellular edema induced by free radicals in brain cortical slices. *J. Neurochem.* 1982; **38**: 525–531.

306. Das, D.K., Engelman, R.M., Rousou, J.A., Breyer, R.H., Otani, H., & Lemeshow, S. Role of membrane phospholipids in myocardial injury induced by ischemia and reperfusion. *J. Physiol.* 1986; **251**: H71–H79.

307. Zaleska, M.M., & Wilson, D.F. Lipid hydroperoxides inhibit reacylation of phospholipids in neuronal membranes. *J. Neurochem.* 1989; **52**: 255–260.

308. Demopoulos, H.B., Flamm, E.S., Pietronigro, D.D., & Seligman, M.L. The free radical pathology and the microcirculation in the major central nervous system disorders. *Acta Physiol. Scand.* 1980; **492** (suppl.): 91–119.

309. Halliwell, B., & Gutteridge, J. Oxygen toxicity, oxygen radicals, transition metals, and disease. *Biochem. J.* 1984; **19**: 1–14.

310. Mead, J.F. Free radical mechanisms of lipid damage and consequences for cellular membranes. In Pryor, W.A. (ed). *Free Radicals in Biology* Vol 1. New York: Academic Press, 1976: 51–68.

311. Freeman, B.A., & Crapo, J.D. Free radicals and tissue injury. *Lab. Invest.* 1982; **47**: 412–426.

312. Aust, S.D., Morehouse, L.A., & Thomas, C.E. Role of metals in oxygen radical reactions. *J. Free Radi. Biol. Med.* 1985; **1**: 3–25.

313. Janero, D.R. Malondialdehyde and thiobarbituric acid reactivity as diagnostic indices of lipid peroxidation and peroxidative tissue injury. *Free Radi. Biol. Med.* 1990; **9**: 515–540.

314. Mead, J.F. Free radical mechanisms of lipid damage and consequences for cellular membranes. In Pryor, W.A. (ed). *Free Radicals in Biology* Vol 1. New York: Academic Press, 1976: 51–68.

315. Harrison, W.W., Netsky, M.G., & Brown, M.D. Trace elements in the human brain: Copper, iron, and magnesium. *Clin. Chim. Acta* 1968; **21**: 55–60.

316. Crichton, R.R. Interactions between iron metabolism and oxygen activation. In *Oxygen Free Radicals and Tissue Damage.* Ciba Foundation Symposium 65, New York: Excerpta Medica, 1979: 57–66.

317. Babbs, C.F., & Steiner, M.G. Simulation of free radical reactions in biology and medicine: A new two-compartment

kinetic model of intracellular lipid peroxidation. *Free Radi. Biol. Med.* 1990; **8**: 471–485.

318. Zaleska, M.M., & Floyd, R.A. Regional lipid peroxidation in rat brain *in vitro*: Possible role of endogenous iron. *Neurochem. Res.* 1985; **10**: 397–410.

319. Kogure, K., Watson, B.D., Busto, R., & Abe, K. Potentiation of lipid peroxides by ischemia in rat brain. *Neurochem. Res.* 1982; **7**: 437–454.

320. Watson, B.D., Busto, R., Goldberg, W.J., Santiso, M., Yoshida, S., & Ginsberg, M.D. Lipid peroxidation *in vivo* induced by reversible global ischemia in rat brain. *J. Neurochem.* 1984; **42**: 268–274.

321. Bromont, C., Marie, C., & Bralet, J. Increased lipid peroxidation in vulnerable brain regions after transient forebrain ischemia in rats. *Stroke* 1989; **20**: 918–924.

322. Sakamoto, A., Ohnishi, S.T., Ohnishi, T., & Ogawa, R. Relationship between free radical production and lipid peroxidation during ischemia-reperfusion injury in rat brain. *Brain Res.* 1991; **554**: 186–192.

323. Rosenthal, R.E., Chanderbhan, R., Marshall, G., & Fiskum, G. Prevention of post-ischemic brain lipid conjugated diene production and neurological injury by hydroxyethyl starch-conjugated deferoxamine. *Free Rad. Biol. Med.* 1992; **12**: 29–33.

324. Kumar, K., Goosmann, M., Krause, G. *et al.* Ultrastructural and ionic studies in global ischemic dog brain. *Acta Neuropathol. (Berl.)* 1987; **73**: 393–399.

325. White, B.C., Nayini, N.R., Krause, G.S. *et al.* Effect on biochemical markers of brain injury of therapy with deferoxamine or superoxide dismutase following cardiac arrest. *Am. J. Emerg. Med.* 1988; **6**: 569–576.

326. Skjaerlund, J.M., Krause, G.S., O'Neil, B.J., & White, B.C. The effect of EMHP on post-cardiac arrest survival of rats. *Resuscitation* 1991; **22**: 139–149.

327. Cerchiari, E.L., Hoel, T.M., Safar, P., & Sclabassi, R.J. Protective effects of combined superoxide dismutase and deferoxamine on recovery of cerebral blood flow and function after cardiac arrest in dogs. *Stroke* 1987; **18**: 869–878.

328. Hall, E.D., & Yonkers, P.A. Attenuation of post-ischemic cerebral hypoperfusion by the 21-aminosteroid U74006F. *Stroke* 1988; **10**: 340–344.

329. Braughler, J.M., Pregenzer, J.F., Chase, R.L., Duncan, L.A., Jacobsen, E.J., & McCall, J.M. Novel 21-amino steroids as potent inhibitors of iron-dependent lipid peroxidation. *J. Biol. Chem.* 1987; **262**: 10438–10440.

330. Krause, G.S., & Tiffany, B.R. Suppression of protein synthesis in the reperfused brain. *Stroke* 1993; **24**: 747–755.

331. Araki, T., Kato, H., Inoue, T., & Kogure, K. Regional impairment of protein synthesis following brief cerebral ischemia in the gerbil. *Acta Neuropathol. (Berl.)* 1990; **79**: 501–505.

332. Kleihues, P., & Hossmann, K.A. Protein synthesis in the cat brain after prolonged cerebral ischemia. *Brain Res.* 1971; **35**: 409–418.

333. Cooper, H.K., Zalewska, T., Kawakami, S., & Hossman, K.A. The effect of ischemia and recirculation on protein synthesis in the rat brain. *J. Neurochem.* 1977; **28**: 929–934.

334. Nowak, T.S. Jr, Fried, R.L., Lust, D., & Passonneau, J.V. Changes in brain energy metabolism and protein synthesis following transient bilateral ischemia in the gerbil. *J. Neurochem.* 1985; **44**: 487–494.

335. Dienel, G., Pulsinelli, W., & Duffy, T. Regional protein synthesis in rat brain following acute hemispheric ischemia. *J. Neurochem.* 1980; **35**: 1216–1226.

336. Bodsch, W., Takahashi, K., Barbier, A., Grosse Ophoff, B., & Hossmann, K.A. Cerebral protein synthesis and ischemia. *Prog. Brain Res.* 1985; **63**: 197–210.

337. Nowak, T.S. Jr, Carty, E.R., Lust, W.D., & Passonneau, J.V. An *in vitro* amino acid incorporation method for assessing the status of *in vivo* protein synthesis. *Anal. Biochem.* 1984; **136**: 285–292.

338. White, B.C., DeGracia, D.J., Krause, G.S. *et al.* Brain DNA survives cardiac arrest and reperfusion. *Free Rad. Bilo. Med.* 1991; **10**: 125–135.

339. White, B.C., Tribhuwan, R.C., Vander Lann, D.J., DeGracia, D.J., Krause, G.S., & Grossman, L.I. Brain mitochondrial DNA is not damaged by prolonged cardiac arrest or reperfusion. *J. Neurochem.* 1992; **58**: 1716–1722.

340. Pichiule, P., Chavez, J.C., Xu, K., & LaManna, J.C. Vascular endothelial growth factor upregulation in transient global ischemia induced by cardiac arrest and resuscitation in rat brain. *Brain Res. Mol. Brain Res.* 1999; **74**: 83–90.

341. Daoud, R., Mies, G., Smialowska, A., Olah, L., Hossmann, K.A., & Stamm, S. Ischemia induces a translocation of the splicing factor tra2-beta 1 and changes alternative splicing patterns in the brain. *J. Neurosci.* 2002; **22**: 5889–5899.

342. Wang, L., Miura, M., Bergeron, L., Zhu, H., & Yuan, J. Ich-1, an Ice/ced-3-related gene, encodes both positive and negative regulators of programmed cell death. *Cell* 1994; **78**: 739–750.

343. Erkmann, J.A., & Kutay, U. Nuclear export of mRNA: from the site of transcription to the cytoplasm. *Exp. Cell. Res.* 2004; **296**: 12–20.

344. Schroder, H.C., Bachmann, M., Diehl-Seifert, B., & Muller W.E.G. Transport of mRNA from nucleus to cytoplasm. *Prog. Nucl. Acid Res. Mol. Biol.* 1987; **34**: 89–142.

345. Sakaguchi, T., Yamada, K., Hayakawa, T. *et al.* Malfunction of gene expression as a possible cause of delayed neuronal death. *No To Shinkei Brain Nerve* 1988; **40**: 629–635.

346. Tiffany, B.R., White, B.C., & Krause, G.S. Nuclear-envelope nucleoside triphosphatase kinetics and mRNA transport following brain ischemia and reperfusion. *Ann. Emerg. Med.* 1995; **25**: 809–817.

347. Matsumoto, K., Yamada, K., Hayakawa, T., Sakaguchi, T., & Mogami, H. RNA synthesis and processing in the gerbil brain after transient hindbrain ischaemia. *Neurol. Res.* 1990; **12**: 45–48.

348. Lu, A., Tang, Y., Ran, R., Clark, J.F., Aronow, B.J., & Sharp, F.R. Genomics of the periinfarction cortex after focal cerebral ischemia. *J. Cereb. Blood Flow Metab.* 2003; **23**: 786–810.

349. Jin, K., Mao, X.O., Eshoo, M.W., Nagayama, T., Minami, M., Simon, R.P., & Greenberg, D.A. Microarray analysis of hippocampal gene expression in global cerebral ischemia. *Ann Neurol.* 2001; **50**: 93–103.

350. Greenbaum, D., Colangelo, C., Williams, K., & Gerstein, M. Comparing protein abundance and mRNA expression levels on a genomic scale. *Genome Biol.* 2003; **4**: 117.

351. Gygi, S.P., Rochon, Y., Franza, B.R., & Aebersold, R. Correlation between protein and mRNA abundance in yeast. *Mol. Cell. Biol.* 1999: **19**: 1720–1730.

352. Raley-Susman, K.M. & Lipton, P. *In vitro* ischemia and protein synthesis in the rat hippocampal slice: The role of calcium and NMDA receptor activation. *Brain Res.* 1990; **515**: 27–38.

353. Marotta, C.A., Brown, B.A., Strocchi, P., Bird, E.D., & Gilbert, J.M. *In vitro* synthesis of human brain proteins including tubulin and actin by purified post mortem polysomes. *J. Neurochem.* 1981; **36**: 966–975.

354. Dienel, G., Kiessling, M., Jacewicz, M., & Pulsinelli, W.A. Synthesis of heat shock proteins in rat brain cortex after transient ischemia. *J. Cereb. Blood Flow Metab.* 1986; **6**: 505–510.

355. DeGracia, D.J., O'Neil, B.J., Frisch, C. *et al.* Studies of the protein synthesis system in the brain cortex during global ischemia and reperfusion. *Resuscitation* 1993; **21**: 161–170.

356. Pain, V.M. Initiation of protein synthesis in eukaryotic cells. *Eur. J. Biochem.* 1996; **236**: 747–771.

357. DeGracia, D.J., Neumar, R.W., White, B.C., & Krause, G.S. Global brain ischemia and reperfusion: Modifications in eukaryotic initiation factors are associated with inhibition of translation initiation. J. *Neurochem.* 1996; **67**; 2005–2012.

358. Burda, J., Martin, M.E., Gottlieb, M. *et al.* The intraischemic and early reperfusion changes of protein synthesis in the rat brain. eIF-2 alpha kinase activity and role of initiation factors eIF-2 alpha and eIF-4E. *J. Cereb. Blood Flow Metab.* 1998; **18**: 59–66.

359. Neumar, R.W., DeGracia, D.J., Konkoly, L.L., Khoury, J.I., White, B.C., & Krause, G.S. Calpain mediates eukaryotic initiation factor 4G degradation during global brain ischemia. *J Cereb Blood Flow Metab.* 1998; **18**: 876–881.

360. Martin de la Vega, C., Burda, J., Nemethova, M. *et al.* Possible mechanisms involved in the down-regulation of translation during transient global ischemia in the rat brain. *Biochem J.* 2001; **357**: 819–826.

361. Johannes, G., Carter, M.S., Eisen, M.B., Brown, P.O., & Sarnow, P. Identification of eukaryotic mRNAs that are translated at reduced cap binding complex eIF4F concentrations using a cDNA microarray. *Proc. Natl Acad. Sci. USA* 1999; **96**: 13118–13123.

362. DeGracia, D.J., Sullivan, J.M., Neumar, R.W. *et al.* Effect of brain ischemia and reperfusion on the localization of phosphorylated eukaryotic initiation factor 2α. *J. Cereb. Blood Flow Metab.* 1997; **17**: 1291–1302.

363. Voll, C.L., & Auer, R.N. Insulin attenuates ischemic brain damage independent of its hypoglycemic effect. *J. Cereb. Blood Flow Metab.* 1991; **11**: 1006–1014.

364. Sullivan, J.M., Alousi, S.S., Hikade, K.R., Rafols, J.A., Krause, G.S., & White, B.C. Insulin induces dephosphorylation of eIF2α and restores protein synthesis in vulnerable hippocampal neurons following transient brain ischemia. *J. Cereb. Blood Flow Metab.* 1999; **19**: 1010–1019.

365. Meijer, H.A., & Thomas, A.A.M. Control of eukaryotic protein synthesis by upstream open reading frames in the 5′-untranslated region of an mRNA. *Biochem J.* 2002; **367**: 1–11.

366. Gerlitz, G., Jagus, R., & Elroy-Stein, O. Phosphorylation of initiation factor-2 alpha is required for activation of internal translation initiation during cell differentiation. *Eur. J. Biochem.* 2002; **269**: 2810–2819.

367. Fernandez, J., Yaman, I., Merrick, W.C. *et al.* Regulation of internal ribosome entry site-mediated translation by eukaryotic initiation factor-2α phosphorylation and translation of a small upstream open reading frame. *J. Biol. Chem.* 2002; **277**: 2050–2058.

368. Munoz, F., Martin, M.E., Manso-Tomico, J., Berlanga, J., Salinas, M., & Fando, J.L. Ischemia-induced phosphorylation of initiation factor 2 in differentiated PC12 cells: role for initiation factor 2 phosphatase. *J. Neurochem.* 2000; **75**: 2335–2345.

369. Pal, J.K., Chen, J.J., & London, I.M. Tissue distribution of heme-regulated eIF-2α kinase determined by monoclonal antibodies. *Biochemistry* 1991; **30**: 2555–2562.

370. Harding, H.P., Zhang, Y., & Ron, D. Protein translation and folding are coupled by an endoplasmic-reticulum-resident kinase. *Nature* 1999; **397**: 271–274.

371. Koumenis, C., Naczki, C., Koritzinsky, M. *et al.* Regulation of protein synthesis by hypoxia via activation of the endoplasmic reticulum kinase PERK and phosphorylation of the translation initiation factor eIF2α. *Mol. Cell. Biol.* 2002; **22**: 7405–7416.

372. Kumar, R., Azam, S., Sullivan, J.M. *et al.* Brain ischemia and reperfusion activates the eukaryotic initiation factor 2α kinase, PERK. *J. Neurochem.* 2001; **77**: 1418–1421.

373. DeGracia, D.J., Adamczyk, S., Folbe, A.J. *et al.* Eukaryotic initiation factor 2α kinase and phosphatase activity during post-ischemic brain reperfusion. *Exp. Neurol.* 1999; **155**: 221–227.

374. Owen, C.R., Kumar, R., Zhang, P., McGrath, B.C., Cavener, D.R., & Krause, G.S. PERK is responsible for the increased phosphorylation of eIFα and the severe inhibition of protein synthesis after transient global brain ischemia. *J. Neurochem.* 2005; **94**: 1235–1242.

375. Ray, M.K., Datta, B., Chakraborty, A., Chattopadhyay, A., Meza-Keuthen, S., & Gupta, N.K. The eukaryotic initiation factor 2-associated 67-kDa polypeptide (p67) plays a critical role in regulation of protein synthesis initiation in animal cells. *Proc. Natl Acad. Sci. USA* 1992; **89**: 539–543.

376. Owen, C., Lipinski, C., Page, A. *et al.* Characterization of the eIF2-associated protein p67 during brain ischemia and reperfusion. In Bazan, N. G., Ito, U., Marcheselli, V. L., Kuroiwa, T., & Klatzo, I. (eds). *Maturation Phenomenon in Cerebral Ischemia, IV.* Springer-Verlag, Berlin Heidelberg, 2001: 19–24.

377. Ron, D., & Harding, H.P. PERK and translational control by stress in the endoplasmic reticulum. In Sonenberg, N., Hershey, J.W.B., Mathews, M.B., eds, *Translational Control of Gene Expression* New York: Cold Spring Harbor Laboratory Press, 2000: 547–560.

378. Hu, B.R., Martone, M.E., Jones, Y.Z., & Liu, C.L. Protein aggregation after transient cerebral ischemia. *J. Neurosci.* 2000; **20**: 3191–3199.

379. DeGracia, D.J., Kumar, R., Owen, C.R., Krause, G.S., & White, B.C. Molecular pathways of protein synthesis inhibition during brain reperfusion: Implications for neuronal survival or death. *J. Cereb. Blood Flow Metab.* 2002; **22**: 127–141.

380. Paschen, W., Aufenberg, C., Hotop, S., & Mengesdorf, T. Transient cerebral ischemia activates processing of xbp1 messenger RNA indicative of endoplasmic reticulum stress. *J. Cereb. Blood Flow Metab.* 2003; **23**: 449–461.

381. Kumar, R., Krause, G.S., Yoshida, H., Mori, K., & DeGracia, D.J. Dysfunction of the unfolded protein response during global brain ischemia and reperfusion. *J. Cereb. Blood Flow Metab.* 2003; **23**: 462–471.

382. Bushell, M., Wood, W., Clemens, M.J., & Morley, S.J. Changes in integrity and association of eukaryotic protein synthesis initiation factors during apoptosis. *Eur. J. Biochem.* 2000; **267**: 1083–1091.

383. Clemens, M.J., Bushell, M., Jeffrey, I.W., Pain, V.M., & Morley, S.J. Translation initiation factor modifications and the regulation of protein synthesis in apoptotic cells. *Cell Death Differ.* 2000; **7**: 603–615.

384. Liu, C.L., Ge, P., Zhang, F., & Hu, B.R. Co-translational protein aggregation after transient cerebral ischemia. *Neuroscience* 2005; **134**: 1273–1284.

385. Harding, H.P., Zhang, Y., Bertolotti, A., Zeng, H., & Ron, D. Perk is essential for translational regulation and cell survival during the unfolded protein response. *Mol. Cell.* 2000; **5**: 897–904.

386. Srivastava, S.P., Kumar, K.U., & Kaufman, R.J. Phosphorylation of eukaryotic translation initiation factor 2 mediates apoptosis in response to activation of the double-stranded RNA-dependent protein kinase. *J. Biol. Chem.* 1998; **273**: 2416–2423.

387. Murtha-Riel, P., Davies, M.V., Scherer, B.J., Choi, S.Y., Hershey, J.W., & Kaufman, R.J. Expression of a phosphorylation-resistant eukaryotic initiation factor 2α-subunit mitigates heat shock inhibition of protein synthesis. *J. Biol. Chem.* 1993; **268**: 12946–12951.

388. Novoa, I., Zhang, Y., Zeng, H., Jungreis, R., Harding, H.P., & Ron, D. Stress-induced gene expression requires programmed recovery from translational repression. *EMBO J.* 2003; **22**: 1180–1187.

389. Lipton, P. Ischemic cell death in brain neurons. *Physiol. Rev.* 1999; **79**: 1431–1568.

390. White, B.C., Sullivan, J.M., DeGracia, D.J. *et al.* Brain ischemia and reperfusion: Molecular mechanisms of neuronal injury. *J. Neurol. Sci.* 2000; **179**: 1–33.

391. Paschen, W. Shutdown of translation: lethal or protective? Unfolded protein response versus apoptosis. *J. Cereb. Blood Flow Metab.* 2003; **23**: 773–779.

392. Yin, X.M., Luo, Y., Cao, G. *et al.* Bid-mediated mitochondrial pathway is critical to ischemic neuronal apoptosis and focal cerebral ischemia. *J. Biol. Chem.* 2002; **277**(44): 42074–42081.

393. Dluzniewska, J., Beresewicz, M., Wojewodzka, U., Gajkowska, B., & Zablocka, B. Transient cerebral ischemia induces delayed proapoptotic Bad translocation to mitochondria in CA1 sector of hippocampus. *Brain Res. Mol. Brain Res.* 2005; **133**(2): 274–280.

394. Fiskum, G. Mechanisms of neuronal death and neuroprotection. *J. Neurosurg. Anesthesiol.* 2004; **16**(1): 108–110.

395. Korde, A.S., Pettigrew, L.C., Craddock, S.D., & Maragos, W.F. The mitochondrial uncoupler 2,4-dinitrophenol attenuates tissue damage and improves mitochondrial homeostasis following transient focal cerebral ischemia. *J. Neurochem.* 2005; **94**(6): 1676–1684.

396. Friberg, H., Connern, C., Halestrap, A.P., & Wieloch, T. Differences in the activation of the mitochondrial permeability transition among brain regions in the rat correlate with selective vulnerability. *J. Neurochem.* 1999; **72**(6): 2488–2497.

397. Schild, L., & Reiser, G. Oxidative stress is involved in the permeabilization of the inner membrane of brain mitochondria exposed to hypoxia/reoxygenation and low micromolar Ca^{2+}. *FEBS J.* 2005; **272**(14): 3593–3601.

398. Bogaert, Y.E., Sheu, K.F., Hof, P.R. *et al.* Neuronal subclass-selective loss of pyruvate dehydrogenase immunoreactivity following canine cardiac arrest and resuscitation. *Exp. Neurol.* 2000; **161**(1): 115–126.

399. Starkov, A.A., Chinopoulos, C., & Fiskum, G. Mitochondrial calcium and oxidative stress as mediators of ischemic brain injury. *Cell Calcium* 2004; **36**(3–4): 257–264.

400. Cairns, C.B. Rude unhinging of the machinery of life: metabolic approaches to hemorrhagic shock. *Curr. Opin. Crit. Care* 2001; **7**(6): 437–443.

401. Jobsis, F.F. Noninvasive, infrared monitoring of cerebral and myocardial oxygen sufficiency and circulatory parameters. *Science* 1977; **198**(4323): 1264–1267.

402. Lesnefsky, E.J., Chen, Q., Moghaddas, S., Hassan, M.O., Tandler, B., & Hoppel, C.L. Blockade of electron transport during ischemia protects cardiac mitochondria. *J. Biol. Chem.* 2004; **279**(46): 47961–47967.

403. Ouyang, Y.B., & Giffard, R.G. Cellular neuroprotective mechanisms in cerebral ischemia: Bcl-2 family proteins and protection of mitochondrial function. *Cell Calcium* 2004; **36**(3–4): 303–311.

404. Sulkowski, G., Waskiewicz, J., Walski, M., Januszewski, S., & Rafalowska, U. Synaptosomal susceptibility on global ischaemia caused by cardiac arrest correlated with early and late times after recirculation in rats. *Resuscitation* 2002; **52**(2): 203–213.

405. Siesjo, B.K., & Siesjo, P. Mechanisms of secondary brain injury. *Eur. J. Anaesthesiol.* 1996; **13**(3): 247–268.

406. Siesjo, B.K. *Brain Energy Metabolism*. New York: John Wiley & Sons, 1978.

407. Siesjo, B.K., Elmer, E., Janelidze, S. *et al.* Role and mechanisms of secondary mitochondrial failure. *Acta Neurochir. Suppl (Wien)* 1999; **73**: 7–13.

408. Cairns, C.B., Moore, F.A., Haenel, J.B. *et al.* Evidence for early supply independent mitochondrial dysfunction in patients developing multiple organ failure after trauma. *J. Trauma* 1997; **42**(3): 532–536.

409. Gattinoni, L., Brazzi, L., Pelosi, P. *et al.* A trial of goal-oriented hemodynamic therapy in critically ill patients. SvO2 Collaborative Group. *N. Engl. J. Med.* 1995; **333**(16): 1025–1032.

410. Alberts, B. Energy conversion. In Alberts, B., ed. *Mol. Biol. Cell.* New York: Garland Publishing, 1994: 676.

411. Fosslien, E. Mitochondrial medicine–molecular pathology of defective oxidative phosphorylation. *Ann. Clin. Lab. Sci.* 2001; **31**(1): 25–67.

412. Shoemaker, W.C., Appel, P.L., Kram, H.B., Waxman, K., & Lee, T.S. Prospective trial of supranormal values of survivors as therapeutic goals in high-risk surgical patients. *Chest* 1988; **94**(6): 1176–1186.

413. Shoemaker, W.C., Appel, P.L., & Kram, H.B. Role of oxygen debt in the development of organ failure sepsis, and death in high-risk surgical patients. *Chest* 1992; **102**(1): 208–215.

414. Proctor, H.J., Sylvia, A.L., & Jobsis, F. Failure of brain cytochrome alpha, alpha 3 redox recovery after hypoxic hypotension as determined by in vivo reflectance spectrophotometry. *Stroke* 1982; **13**(1): 89–92.

415. Zhang, J., & Piantadosi, C.A. Mitochondrial oxidative stress after carbon monoxide hypoxia in the rat brain. *J. Clin. Invest.* 1992; **90**(4): 1193–1199.

416. Honda, H.M., Korge Paav, & Weiss, J.N. Mitochondria and Ischemia/Reperfusion Injury. *Ann. NY Acad Sci.* 2005; **1047**(1): 248–258.

417. Lin, C.H., Lu, Y.Z., Cheng, F.C., Chu, L.F., & Hsueh, C.M. Bax-regulated mitochondria-mediated apoptosis is responsible for the in vitro ischemia induced neuronal cell death of Sprague Dawley rat. *Neurosci. Lett.* 2005; **387**(1): 22–27.

418. Sugawara, T., & Chan, P.H. Reactive oxygen radicals and pathogenesis of neuronal death after cerebral ischemia. *Antioxid. Redox. Signal* 2003; **5**(5): 597–607.

419. Chan, P.H. Reactive oxygen radicals in signaling and damage in the ischemic brain. *J. Cerebr. Blood Flow Metab.* **21**(1), 2–14. 2001.

420. Patt, A., Harken, A.H., Burton, L.K. *et al.* Xanthine oxidase-derived hydrogen peroxide contributes to ischemia reperfusion-induced edema in gerbil brains. *J. Clin. Invest.* 1988; **81**(5): 1556–1562.

421. Anderson, T., & Vanden Hoek, T.L. Preconditioning and the oxidants of sudden death. *Curr. Opin. Crit. Care* 2003; **9**(3): 194–198.

422. Andrabi, S.A., Spina, M.G., Lorenz, P., Ebmeyer, U., Wolf, G., & Horn, T.F. Oxyresveratrol (trans-2,3′,4,5′-tetrahydroxystilbene) is neuroprotective and inhibits the apoptotic cell death in transient cerebral ischemia. *Brain Res.* 2004; **1017**(1–2): 98–107.

423. Antonsson, B. Bax and other pro-apoptotic Bcl-2 family "killer-proteins" and their victim the mitochondrion. *Cell Tissue Res.* 2001; **306**(3): 347–361.

424. Fujimura, M., Morita-Fujimura, Y., Murakami, K., Kawase, M., & Chan, P.H. Cytosolic redistribution of cytochrome c after transient focal cerebral ischemia in rats. *J. Cereb. Blood Flow Metab.* 1998; **18**(11): 1239–1247.

425. Fujimura, M., Morita-Fujimura, Y., Kawase, M. *et al.* Manganese superoxide dismutase mediates the early release of mitochondrial cytochrome C and subsequent DNA fragmentation after permanent focal cerebral ischemia in mice. *J. Neurosci.* 1999; **19**(9): 3414–3422.

426. Yin, R., Reddihough, D.S., Ditchfield, M.R., & Collins, K.J. Magnetic resonance imaging findings in cerebral palsy. *J. Paediatr. Child Health* 2000; **36**(2): 139–144.

427. Ashkenazi, A., & Dixit, V.M. Death receptors: signaling and modulation. *Science* 1998; **281**(5381): 1305–1308.

428. Green, D.R., & Reed, J.C. Mitochondria and apoptosis. *Science* 1998; **281**(5381): 1309–1312.

429. Gross, A., McDonnell, J.M., & Korsmeyer, S.J. BCL-2 family members and the mitochondria in apoptosis. *Genes Dev.* 1999; **13**(15): 1899–1911.

430. Nomura, Y. Neuronal apoptosis and protection: effects of nitric oxide and endoplasmic reticulum-related proteins. *Biol. Pharm. Bull.* 2004; **27**(7): 961–963.

431. Kim, J.S., Ohshima, S., Pediaditakis, P., & Lemasters, J.J. Nitric oxide: a signaling molecule against mitochondrial permeability transition- and pH-dependent cell death after reperfusion. *Free Radi. Biol. Med.* 2004; **37**(12): 1943–1950.

432. Huang, Z., Huang, P.L., Panahian, N., Dalkara, T., Fishman, M.C., & Moskowitz, M.A. Effects of cerebral ischemia in mice deficient in neuronal nitric oxide synthase. *Science* 1994; **265**(5180): 1883–1885.

433. O'Dell, T.J., Huang, P.L., Dawson, T.M. *et al.* Endothelial NOS and the blockade of LTP by NOS inhibitors in mice lacking neuronal NOS. *Science* 1994; **265**(5171): 542–546.

434. Zaharchuk, G., Hara, H., Huang, P.L. *et al.* Neuronal nitric oxide synthase mutant mice show smaller infarcts and attenuated apparent diffusion coefficient changes in the peri-infarct zone during focal cerebral ischemia. *Magn. Reson. Med.* 1997; **37**(2): 170–175.

435. Huang, Z., Huang, P.L., Ma, J. *et al.* Enlarged infarcts in endothelial nitric oxide synthase knockout mice are attenuated by nitro-L-arginine. *J. Cereb. Blood Flow Metab.* 1996; **16**(5): 981–987.

436. Iadecola, C. Bright and dark sides of nitric oxide in ischemic brain injury. *Trends Neurosci.* 1997; **20**(3): 132–139.

437. Cho, S., Liu, D., Gonzales, C., Zaleska, M.M., & Wood, A. Temporal assessment of caspase activation in experimental models of focal and global ischemia. *Brain Res.* 2003; **982**(2): 146–155.

438. White, B.C., & Sullivan, J.M. Apoptosis. *Acad. Emerg. Med.* 1998; **5**(10): 1019–1029.

439. Strasser, A., O'Connor, L., & Dixit, V.M. Apoptosis signaling. *Annu. Rev. Biochem.* 2000; **69**: 217–245.

440. Earnshaw, W.C., Martins, L.M., & Kaufmann, S.H. Mammalian caspases: structure, activation, substrates, and functions during apoptosis. *Annu. Rev. Biochem.* 1999; **68**: 383–424.

441. Krajewska, M., Rosenthal, R.E., Mikolajczyk, J. *et al.* Early processing of Bid and caspase-6, -8, -10, -14 in the canine brain during cardiac arrest and resuscitation. *Exp. Neurol.* 2004; **189**(2): 261–279.

442. Basanez, G., Zhang, J., Chau, B.N. *et al.* Pro-apoptotic cleavage products of Bcl-xL form cytochrome c-conducting pores in pure lipid membranes. *J. Biol. Chem.* 2001; **276**(33): 31083–31091.

443. Antonawich, F.J. Translocation of cytochrome c following transient global ischemia in the gerbil. *Neurosci. Lett.* 1999; **274**(2): 123–126.

444. Abe, T., Takagi, N., Nakano, M., Furuya, M., & Takeo, S. Altered bad localization and interaction between Bad and Bcl-xL in the hippocampus after transient global ischemia. *Brain Res.* 2004; **1009**(1–2): 159–168.

445. Le, D.A., Wu, Y., Huang, Z. *et al.* Caspase activation and neuroprotection in caspase-3- deficient mice after in vivo cerebral ischemia and in vitro oxygen glucose deprivation. *Proc. Natl Acad. Sci. USA* 2002; **99**(23): 15188–15193.

446. Lundberg, K.C., & Szweda, L.I. Initiation of mitochondrial-mediated apoptosis during cardiac reperfusion. *Arch. Biochem. Biophys.* 2004; **432**(1): 50–57.

447. Loewy, B., Marczynski, G.T., Dingwall, A., & Shapiro, L. Regulatory interactions between phospholipid synthesis and DNA replication in *Caulobacter crescentus. J. Bacteriol.* 1990; **172**: 5523–5530.

448. Contreras, I.R., Bender, R.A., Mansour, J., Henry, S., & Shapiro, L. *Caulobacter cresentus* mutant defective in membrane phospholipid synthesis. *J. Bacteriol.* 1979; **140**: 612–619.

449. Dianzani, M.U. Lipid peroxidation and cancer: A critical reconsideration. *Tumori* 1989; **75**: 351–357.

450. Benedetti, A., Malvaldi, G., Fulceri, R., & Comporti, M. Loss of lipid peroxidation as a histochemical marker for preneoplastic hepatocellular foci of rats. *Cancer Res.* 1984; **44**: 5712–5717.

451. O'Neil, B.J., Chapman, S., & White, B.C. Increased radical-induced cell death after neuronal differentiation. *Ann. Emerg. Med.* 1993; **22**: 928.

452. O'Neil, B.J., White, B.C., & Rafols, J.A: Neuronal Golgi apparatus ultrastructure: brain reperfusion and radicals. For Presentation at the International Symposia on Pharmacology of Cerebral Ischemia, Marburg, Germany, July 1994. Abstract to be published in J Cereb Blood Flow Metab, 1994.

453. Cattaneo, E., & McKay, R. Proliferation and differentiation of neuronal stem cells regulated by nerve growth factor. *Nature* 1990; **347**: 762–765.

454. Havarankova, J., & Roth, J. Insulin receptors are widely distributed in the central nervous system of the rat. *Nature* 1978; **272**: 827–829.

455. Werther, G.A., Hogg, A., Oldfield, B.J. *et al.* Localization and characterization of insulin receptors in rat brain and pituitary gland using *in vitro* autoradiography and computerized densitometry. *Endocrinology* 1987; **121**: 1562–1570.

456. Wanaka, A., Johnson, E.M. Jr, & Milbrandt, J. Localization of FGF receptor mRNA in the adult rat central nervous system by *in situ* hybridization. *Neuron* 1990; **5**: 267–281.

457. Taniuchi, M., Schweitzer, J.B., & Johnson, E.M. Nerve growth factor receptor molecules in rat brain. *Proc. Natl. Acad Sci. USA* 1986; **83**: 1950–1954.

458. Unsicker, K., Flanders, K.C., Cissel, D.S., Lafyatis, R., & Sporn, M.B. Transforming growth factor beta isoforms in the adult rat central and peripheral nervous system. *Neuroscience* 1991; **44**: 613–625.

459. Marks, J.L., King, M.G., & Baskin, D.G. Localization of insulin and type 1 IGF receptors in rat brain by *in vitro* autoradiography and *in situ* hybridization. *Adv. Exp. Med. Biol.* 1991; **293**: 459–470.

460. Plata-Salaman, C.R. Epidermal growth factor and the nervous system. *Peptides* 1991; **12**: 653–663.

461. Larsson, L.G., Gray, H.E., Totterman, T., Pettersson, U., & Nilsson, K. Drastically increased expression of *myc* and *fos* proto-oncogenes during *in vitro* differentiation of chronic lymphocytic cells. *Proc. Natl Acad. Sci. USA* 1987; **84**: 223–227.

462. Angel, P., & Karin, M. The role of Jun, Fos and the AP-1 complex in cell-proliferation and transformation. *Biochim. Biophys. Acta* 1991; **1072**: 129–157.

463. Kiyota, Y., Takami, K., Iwane, M. *et al.* Increase in basic fibroblast growth factor-like immunoreactivity in rat brain after forebrain ischemia. *Brain Res.* 1991; **545**: 322–328.

464. Lindvall, O., Ernfors, P., Bengzon, J. *et al.* Differential regulation of mRNAs for nerve growth factor, brain-derived neurotrophic factor, and neurotrophin 3 in the adult rat brain following cerebral ischemia and hypoglycemic coma. *Proc. Natl Acad. Sci. USA* 1992; **89**: 648–652.

465. Gluckman, P., Klempt, N., Guan, J. *et al.* A role for IGF-1 in the rescue of CNS neurons following hypoxic-ischemic injury. *Biochem. Biophys. Res. Commun.* 1992; **182**: 593–599.

466. Onodera, H., Kogure, K., Ono, Y., Igarashi, K., Kiyota, Y., & Nagaoka, A. Proto-oncogene c-*fos* transiently induced in the rat cerebral cortex after forebrain ischemia. *Neurosci. Lett.* 1989; **98**: 101–104.

467. Kindy, M.S., Carney, J.P., Dempsey, R.J., & Carney, J.M. Ischemic induction of protooncogene expression in gerbil brain. *J. Mol. Neurosci.* 1991; **2**: 217–228.

468. Uemura, Y., Kowall, N.W., & Moskowitz, M.A. Focal ischemia in rats causes time-dependent expressin of c-Fos immunoreactivity in widespread regions of ipsilateral cortex. *Brain Res.* 1991; **552**: 99–105.

469. Jorgensen, M.B., Deckert, J., Wright, D.C., & Gehlert, D.R. Delayed c-*fos* proto-oncogene expression in the rat hippocampus induced by transient global ischemia: An *in situ* hybridization study. *Brain Res.* 1989; **484**: 393–398.

470. Jorgensen, M.B., Johansen, F.F., & Diemer, N.H. Post-ischemic and kanic acid-induced c-Fos protein expression in the rat hippocampus. *Acta Neurol. Scand.* 1991; **84**: 352–356.

471. Nowak, T.S. Jr, Ikeda, J., & Nakajima, T. 70 kDa heat shock protein and c-*fos* gene expression after transient ischemia. *Stroke* 1990; **21**(Suppl III): 107–111.

472. Wessel, T.C., Joh, T.H., & Volpe, B.T. *In situ* hybridization analysis of c-*fos* and c-*jun* expression in the rat brain following transient forebrain ischemia. *Brain Res.* 1991; **567**: 231–240.

473. Schiaffonati, L., Rappocciolo, E., Tacchini, L., Cairo, G., & Bernelli-Zazzera, A. Reprogramming of gene expression in

post-ischemic rat liver: Induction of proto-oncogenes and *hsp-70* gene family. *J. Cell. Physiol.* 1990; **143**: 79–87.

474. Beckmann, R.P., Mizzen, L.A., & Welch, W.J. Interaction of HSP-70 with newly synthesized proteins: Implications for protein folding and assembly. *Science* 1990; **248**: 850–854.

475. Welch, W.J., & Feramisco, J.R. Nuclear and nucleolar localization of the 72,000-dalton heat shock protein in heat-shocked mammalian cells. *J. Biol. Chem.* 1984; **259**: 4501–4513.

476. Schlesinger, M.J. Heat shock proteins: The search for funtions. *J. Cell Bio.* 1986; **103**: 321–325.

477. Burdon, R.H. Heat shock and heat shock proeins. *J. Biochem.* 1986; **240**: 313–324.

478. Stevenson, M.A., & Calderwood, S.K. Members of the 70-kilodalton heat shock family contain a highly conserved calmodulin-binding domain. *Mol. Cell. Biol.* 1990; **10**: 1234–1238.

479. Hightower, L.E. Heat shock, stress proteins, chaperones, and proteotoxicity. *Cell* 1991; **66**: 191–197.

480. Rordorf, G., Koroshetz, W.J., & Bonventre, J.V. Heat shock protects cultureed neurons from glutamate toxicity. *Neuron* 1991; **7**: 1043–1051.

481. Ting, L.P., Tu, C.L., & Chou, C.K. Insulin-induced expression of human heat shock protein gene *hsp-70*. *J. Biol. Chem.* 1989; **264**(6): 3404–3408.

482. Nowak, T.S. Jr. Localization of 70 kDa stress protein mRNA induction in gerbil brain after ischemia. *J. Cereb. Blood Flow Metab.* 1991; **11**: 432–439.

483. Nowak, T.S. Jr. Synthesis of a stress protein following transient ischemia in the gerbil. *J. Neurochem.* 1985; **45**: 1635–1641.

484. Higo, H., Lee, J.Y., Satow, Y., & Higo, K. Elevated expression of proto-oncogenes accompany enhanced induction of heat-shock genes after exposure of rat embryos *in utero* to ionizing radiation. *Teratogenesis, Carcinogenesis, Mutagenesis* 1989; **9**: 191–198.

485. Privalle, C.T., & Fridovich, I. Induction of superoxide dismutase in *E coli* by heat shock. *Proc. Natl Acad. Sci. USA* 1987; **84**: 2723–2726.

486. Drummond, I.A., McClure, S.A., Poenie, M., Tsien, R.Y., & Steinhardt, R.A. Large changes in intracellular pH and calcium observed during heat shock are not responsible for the induction of heat shock proteins in *Drosophila melanogaster*. *Mol. Cell. Biol.* 1986; **6**: 1767–1775.

487. Loven, DP: A role for reduced oxygen species in heat-induced cell killing and the induction of thermotolerance. *Med. Hypotheses* 1988; **26**: 39–50.

488. Ransone, L.J., Kerr, L.D., Schmitt, M.J., Wamsley, P., & Verma, I.M. The bZIP domains of Fos and Jun mediate a physical association with the TATA box-binding protein. *GeneExpr* 1993; **3**: 37–48.

489. Auwerx, J., & Sassone-Corsi, P. AP-1 (Fos-Jun) regulation by IP-1: effect of signal transduction pathways and cell growth. *Oncogene* 1992; **7**: 2271–2280.

490. Alberts, A.S., Deng, T., Lin, A. *et al.* Protein phosphatase 2A potentiates activity of promoters containing AP-1-binding elements. *Mol. Cell. Biol.* 1993; **13**: 2104–2112.

491. Champion-Arnaud, P., Gesnel, M.C., Foulkes, N., Ronsin, C., Sassone-Corsi, P., & Breathnach, R: Activation of transcription via AP-1 or CREB regulatory sites is blocked by protein tyrosine phosphatases. *Oncogene* 1991; **6**: 1203–1209.

492. Schule, R., Rangarajan, P., Yang, N. *et al.* Retinoic acid is a negative regulator of AP-1-responsive genes. *Proc. Natl Acad. Sci. USA* 1991; **88**: 6092–6096.

493. Kerppola, T.K., Luk, D., & Curran, T. Fos is a preferential target of glucocorticoid receptor inhibition of AP-1 activity *in vitro*. *Mol. Cell. Biol.* 1993; **13**: 3782–3791.

494. Zhang, X.K., Dong, J.M., & Chiu, J.F. Regulation of alpha-feto-protein gene expression by antagonism between AP-1 and the glucocorticoid receptor at their overlapping binding site. *J. Biol. Chem.* 1991; **266**: 8248–8254.

495. Unterman, T.G., Lacson, R.G., McGary, E., Whalen, C., Purple, C., & Goswami, R.G. Cloning of the rat insulin-like growth factor binding protein-1 gene and analysis of its 5′ promoter region. *Biochem. Biophys. Res. Commun.* 1992; **185**: 993–999.

496. Levanon, D., Lieman-Hurwitz, J., Dafni, N. *et al.* Architecture and anatomy of the chromosomal locus in human chromosome 21 encoding the Cu/Zn superoxide dismutase. *EMBO J.* 1985; **4**: 77–84.

497. Pinkus, R., Bergelson, S., & Daniel, V. Phenobarbital induction of AP-1 binding activity mediates activation of glutathione S-transferase and quinone reductase gene expression. *Biochem J.* 1993; **290**: 637–640.

498. Montminy, M. Trying on a new pair of SH2s. *Science* 1993; **261**: 1694–1695.

499. Ruff-Jamison, S., Chen, K., & Cohen, S. Induction by EGF and Interferon-γ of tyrosine phosphorylated DNA binding proteins in mouse liver nuclei. *Science* 1993; **261**: 1733–1735.

500. Varon, S., Hagg, T., & Manthorpe, M. Nerve growth factor in CNS repair and regeneration. *Adv. Exp. Med. Biol.* 1991; **296**: 267–276.

501. Mattson, M.P., Murrain, M., Guthrie, P.B., & Kater, S.B. Fibroblast growth factor and glutamate: Opposing roles in the generation and degeneration of hippocampal neuroarchitecture. *J. Neurosci.* 1989; **9**: 3728–3740.

502. Shigeno, T., Mima, T., Takakura, K. *et al.* Amelioration of delayed neuronal death in the hippocampus by nerve growth factor. *J. Neurosci.* 1991; **11**: 2914–2919.

503. Voll, C.L., & Auer, R.N. Insulin attenuates ischemic brain damage independent of its hypoglycemic effect. *J. Cereb. Blood Flow Metab.* 1991; **11**: 1006–1014.

504. LeMay, D.R., Gehua, L., Zelenock, G.B., & D'Alecy, G. Insulin administration protects neurological function in cerebral ischemia in rats. *Stroke* 1988; **19**: 1411–1419.

505. Laurino, J.P., Colca, J.R., Pearson, J.D., DeWald, D.B., & McDonald, J.M. The *in vitro* phosphorylation of calmodulin by the insulin receptor tyrosine kinase. *Arch. Biochem. Biophys.* 1988; **265**: 8–21.

506. Moss, A.M., Unger, J.W., Moxley, R.T., & Livingston, J.N. Location of phosphotyrosine-containing proteins by immunocytochemistry in the rat forebrain corresponds to

the distribution of the insulin receptor. *Proc. Natl Acad. Sci. USA* 1990; **87**: 4453–4457.

507. DeGracia, D.J., O'Neil, B.J., White, B.C. *et al.* Insulin treatment during post-ischemic brain reperfusion induces tyrosine phosphorylation of a 90 kDa protein. *Exp. Neurol.* 1993; **124**: 351–356.

508. Callaham, M., Madsen, C.D., Barton, C.W., Saunders, C.E., Daley, M., & Pointer, J. A randomized clinical trial of high-dose epinephrine and norepinephrine versus standard-dose epinephrine in prehospital cardiac arrest. Abstract, *Ann. Emerg. Med.* 1992; **21**: 606, presented at the meeting of the Society for Academic Emergency Medicine, Toronto, May, 1992.

509. Drews, G., Debuyser, A., Nenquin, M., & Henquin, J.C. Galanin and epinephrine act on distinct receptors to inhibit insulin release by the same mechanisms, including an increase in K+ permeability of the β-cell membrane. *Endocrinology* 1990; **126**: 1646–1653.

510. Yu, K.T., Pessin, J.E., & Czech, M.P. Regulation of insulin receptor kinase by multisite phosphorylation. *Biochime* 1985; **67**: 1081–1090.

511. Sotomatsu, A., Nakano, M., & Hirai, S. Phospholipid peroxidation induced by the catechol-Fe3+ (Cu2+) complex: a possible mechanism of nigrostriatal cell damage. *Arch. Biochem. Biophys.* 1990; **283**: 334–341.

512. Tanaka, M., Sotomatsu, A., Kanai, H., & Hirai, S. Dopa and dopamine cause cultured neuronal death in the presence of iron. *J. Neurol. Sci.* 1991; **101**: 198–203.

513. O'Neil, B.J., Loewe, C., White, S., Harris, M., & Benson, D: Preliminary study of insulin, c-peptide, and catecholamines after resuscitation from cardiac arrest. *Acad. Emerg. Med.* (abstract) 1994; **1**: A86–A87.

514. Capes, S.E., Hunt, D., Malmberg, K., Pathak, P., & Gerstein, H.C. Stress hyperglycemia and prognosis of stroke in nondiabetic and diabetic patients: a systematic overview. *Stroke* 2001; **32**(10): 2426–2432.

515. Parsons, M.W., Barber, P.A., Desmond, P.M. *et al.* Acute hyperglycemia adversely affects stroke outcome: a magnetic resonance imaging and spectroscopy study. *Ann. Neurol.* 2002; **52**(1): 20–28.

516. Baird, T.A., Parsons, M.W., Phanh, T. *et al.* Persistent poststroke hyperglycemia is independently associated with infarct expansion and worse clinical outcome. *Stroke* 2003; **34**(9): 2208–2214. Epub 2003 Jul 31.

517. Malmberg, K. Prospective randomised study of intensive insulin treatment on long term survival after acute myocardial infarction in patients with diabetes mellitus: DIGAMI (Diabetes Mellitus, Insulin Glucose Infusion in Acute Myocardial Infarction) Study Group. *BMJ* 1997; **314**: 1512–1515.

518. Van den Berghe, G., Wouters, P., Weekers, F. *et al.* Intensive insulin therapy in critically ill patients. *N. Engl. J. Med.* 2001; **345**: 1359–1367.

14

Reperfusion injury in cardiac arrest and cardiopulmonary resuscitation

Thomas Aversano

Johns Hopkins Hospital, Baltimore, MD, USA

Except for a single group of papers written in the mid-1980s[1–3] and a more recent preliminary report,[4] there are no studies and no literature on myocardial reperfusion injury in the setting of cardiac arrest and cardiopulmonary resuscitation (CPR). From this perspective, the following discussion may be, as Iago claims Cassio's soldiership to be in Shakespeare's *Othello*, "mere prattle without practice." It is to be hoped, however, that this discussion will serve to identify cardiac arrest and CPR as a setting in which reperfusion injury may occur; that it will point out where reperfusion injury may be relevant mechanistically and therapeutically in this particular clinical circumstance; and, ultimately, that it will encourage basic and clinical research in an area that remains largely unexplored.

Reperfusion injury

The primary therapy for myocardial ischemia is reestablishment of normal blood flow. Yet despite the proven benefit of reperfusion in ischemic syndromes such as acute myocardial infarction,[5–7] evidence shows that some of this benefit may be lessened by injury caused by reperfusion itself.[8]

The term *reperfusion injury* includes a number of potentially deleterious effects of reperfusion after a period of ischemia, including myocardial stunning, reperfusion arrhythmia, and reperfusion-related myonecrosis.[9] Depending on the particular setting in which ischemia and reperfusion occur, these several types of reperfusion injury may be present alone or in combination.

Clinical settings in which reperfusion injury is thought to be important include postcardiopulmonary bypass, heart transplantation, and acute myocardial infarction treated with either thrombolytic therapy or immediate angioplasty.[10] Although generally not recognized as such, cardiac arrest with CPR is clearly an instance, albeit a very complex one, of ischemia and reperfusion; and, as argued in what follows, reperfusion injury may very well play an important role in determining its course and outcome.

Cardiac arrest and cardiopulmonary resuscitation: a setting for reperfusion injury

Cardiac arrest results in myocardial ischemia. Initiation of CPR may result in reperfusion if coronary perfusion pressure is sufficient to provide normal or near-normal coronary blood flow. However, CPR may not provide an adequate coronary driving pressure, either because the developed aortic–right atrial pressure gradient is inadequate or because of coronary artery stenoses. Even minimal coronary stenoses may lead to marked reduction of coronary flow during CPR, particularly in the endocardium.[11] Further, the heart is often fibrillating during CPR, so that levels of coronary flow that might be adequate in the diastolically arrested heart may be insufficient to meet the higher oxygen demands of the fibrillating heart. Thus how long ischemia (defined as the mismatch between myocardial oxygen supply and demand) lasts during cardiac arrest and CPR is often unclear and depends on the time delay between the onset of cardiac arrest and the initiation of CPR and on the adequacy of CPR in restoring a level of coronary blood flow sufficient to meet metabolic demand. As a result, reperfusion may occur once CPR is instituted, once spontaneous circulation is established, or perhaps only after sufficient pharmacologic or mechanical

Cardiac Arrest: The Science and Practice of Resuscitation Medicine. 2nd edn., ed. Norman Paradis, Henry Halperin, Karl Kern, Volker Wenzel, Douglas Chamberlain. Published by Cambridge University Press. © Cambridge University Press, 2007.

hemodynamic support allows for development of adequate coronary perfusion pressure. To make matters more complex, the setting of cardiac arrest and CPR often involves multiple, recurring episodes of ischemia and reperfusion and obviously requires administration of a number of pharmacologic agents, which may influence coronary flow and myocardial oxygen consumption.

These considerations make it likely that the full spectrum of reperfusion injury may be seen in the setting of cardiac arrest and CPR. It is important to reiterate that, except for the three studies mentioned above, no studies have been performed to date specifically addressing the question of reperfusion injury in this setting.

The potential importance of defining the extent of reversible or preventable dysfunction or injury caused by reperfusion in this very special setting cannot be overstated. Therapies aimed at *preventing* reperfusion injury may preserve cardiac function and muscle mass and minimize recurrent arrhythmias, critical determinants of survival in the early and late postresuscitation period. Further, *treatment* of reperfusion injury with effective therapeutic modalities utilized for the proper duration can mean the difference between long-term survival and death.

This chapter will review what is known about myocardial reperfusion injury and attempt to relate information gleaned from these studies to the setting of cardiac arrest and CPR, keeping in mind that most of what is known comes from studies meant to examine experimental or clinical circumstances *other than* cardiac arrest and CPR.

Myocardial stunning

Definition

As first reported by Heyndrickx *et al.* in 1975,[12] myocardial stunning refers to the prolonged but reversible ventricular dysfunction that follows a relatively brief, non-lethal ischemic period. The key features of stunning are that myocardial dysfunction occurs despite normal blood flow, that this dysfunction is reversible, and that it occurs in the absence of significant myonecrosis.

Recognition of stunning after cardiac arrest and CPR is important since the associated dysfunction is reversible. Failure to recognize this possibility may adversely and wrongly affect the physician's assessment of the patient's prognosis in the immediate postresuscitation period. Further, as potential treatments for stunning are developed, particularly those directed at its prevention, they may be applied to this clinical situation.

Stunned myocardium in animal models

The original description of stunning involved regional ischemia and reperfusion[12] in the dog. Since then, many studies have shown that the degree and duration of postischemic dysfunction depend on the duration of ischemia (Fig. 14.1(a).[12–15] Five minutes of ischemia may be followed by 3 hours of reduced systolic wall thickening, and 15 minutes of ischemia may be followed by 24 hours of reduced function.[14] In one of the few studies that directly relates to CPR, Cerchiari *et al.*[15] studied the effect of cardiac arrest of 7.5-, 10-, and 12.5-minute duration on ability to resuscitate, mortality, neurologic deficit scores, and cardiac function. There was no difference in any category except that cardiac output was depressed for more than 12 hours after CPR and more severe arrhythmias occurred in the animals with cardiac arrest of 12.5-minute duration (Fig. 14.1(b)).[15] The prolonged depression of cardiac output with a gradual return toward normal probably represents myocardial stunning, the extent and duration of which are functions of the duration of the ischemic episode. Moreover, the degree of postreperfusion dysfunction is directly related to the reduction of blood flow reduction during the ischemic period[16] and consequently can be influenced by collateral flow.

Repeated brief episodes of ischemia followed by reperfusion periods can also lead to stunning.[17,18] Deterioration of systolic function is greatest after the first occlusion-reperfusion period and reaches its nadir after the third repetition.[17,18] The reason functional deterioration does not continue is unclear, but it appears to be related to a "preconditioning" effect of a first, brief period of ischemia that protects the myocardium from further functional deterioration and adenosine triphosphate (ATP) loss[19] and minimizes myonecrosis[20] in subsequent ischemic periods.

Stunning has also been observed in the isolated heart after brief periods of global ischemia followed by reperfusion in a number of species.[21] Although global ischemia might be considered a better model of cardiac arrest and CPR than regional ischemia models, many such models fail to document a full return of function since the preparation most often used, the isolated heart, deteriorates significantly over time.[21]

In addition to systolic dysfunction, it has been appreciated more recently that diastolic dysfunction can also occur in stunned myocardium. In previously ischemic regions, the rate and degree of diastolic wall thinning were reduced for several hours after a 15-minute coronary occlusion in the conscious dog.[22]

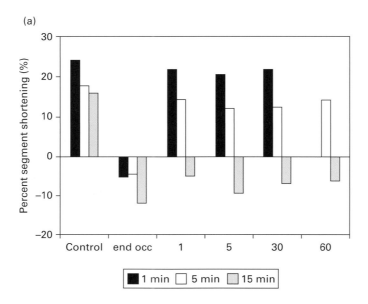

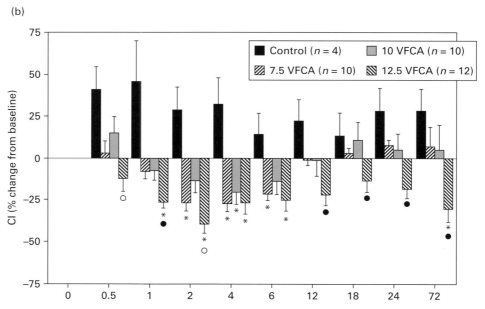

Fig. 14.1. (a) Effect of ischemic duration on regional myocardial function after reperfusion in dogs. (b) Effect of time to initiation of CPR in dogs. *VFCA*, minutes in ventricular fibrillation circulatory arrest before CPR initiated. In both cases, the longer the ischemic duration the longer and more profound the dysfunction in the reperfusion period. (a) Adapted from ref. 14.) (b) Adapted from ref. 15.)

Interestingly, cessation of coronary blood flow is not necessary to produce stunning: transient dysfunction has been noted after exercise-induced ischemia. For example, Homans *et al.*[23] have shown progressive deterioration in wall thickening in dogs with critical coronary stenoses made to exercise for 10 minutes with 60-minute rest periods between. Thus it is ischemia *per se* (i.e., the mismatch between myocardial oxygen supply and demand), not how it is produced, that when followed by reperfusion results in myocardial stunning.

Finally, factors other than ischemia may produce stunning. Particularly important to the setting of cardiac arrest

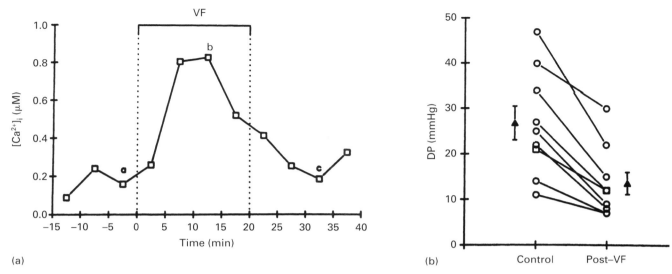

Fig. 14.2. Ventricular fibrillation (*VF*) is associated with, (a) a transient rise in intracellular Ca^{2+} and (b) a postfibrillation reduction in cardiac function (stunning) recorded as a reduction in developed pressure (*DP*). (From ref. 24.)

and CPR, ventricular fibrillation alone, in the absence of ischemia, may produce prolonged ventricular dysfunction after its cessation (Fig. 14.2).[24]

Stunned myocardium in humans

Clinical settings in which stunning may occur include reperfusion therapy for acute myocardial infarction (whether pharmacologic or mechanical), following cardiopulmonary bypass, cardiac transplantation, and even after ischemia-producing exercise in patients with coronary artery disease.[9]

Ellis *et al.*[25] have shown that with prolonged ischemia sufficient to produce subendocardial infarction, followed by reperfusion, non-necrotic myocardium surrounding infarcted myocardium is probably stunned and function in this region returns gradually over a 2-week period. By analogy, after thrombolytic therapy for acute myocardial infarction, several studies have shown a gradual return of function over days to weeks.[26] Whereas some functional recovery may be due to infarct healing and the effect of drugs and other factors, recovery of stunned myocardium is a likely additional factor.

Perhaps the best clinical example of stunning is the transient myocardial dysfunction that follows cardiopulmonary bypass (Fig. 14.3). Although a number of factors may play a role in postbypass dysfunction, including the prolonged metabolic effects of hypothermia and effects caused by handling of the heart during surgery, it is likely that much is due to reperfusion injury.[27] Systolic

dysfunction[28,29] and diastolic dysfunction[30] have been reported in the early hours after bypass, with complete recovery within hours, days, or, in some instances, weeks.[31]

As in animal models, it is ischemia *per se*, the mismatch between coronary flow and myocardial oxygen demand, rather than cessation of coronary flow, that results in stunning. Exercise-induced stunning has been demonstrated in studies that reveal transient regional dysfunction after an exercise period that provoked ischemia in patients with coronary artery disease.[32]

Mechanisms of stunned myocardium

A number of mechanisms have been proposed for stunned myocardium, including a decline in myocyte ATP levels, alterations of Ca^{2+} metabolism, change in subcellular organelles, and production of free radicals.

Stunned myocardium is characterized by a persistent reduction in ATP level and in the total purine nucleotide pool[33] for a variable time following reperfusion. In stunned myocardium, less ATP synthesis can occur via the salvage pathway because of loss of the requisite precursors during ischemia. Therefore *de novo* purine precursor resynthesis is required to replenish ATP, a process that may require several days.[33] The parallel reduction in myocardial function and ATP levels and their gradual, parallel return toward normal levels in stunned myocardium strongly suggest a causal relationship between the two. A number of studies have shown, however, that myocardial function and the level of ATP can be dissociated in stunned

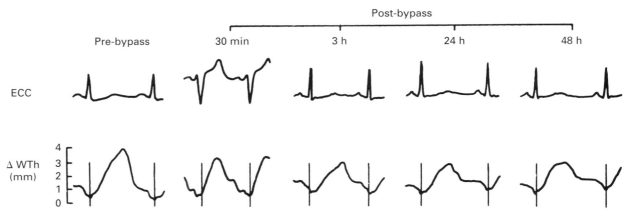

Fig. 14.3. Evidence for prolonged dysfunction following cardiopulmonary bypass in a patient for more than 48 hours after being taken off bypass. Δ *Wth*, change in wall thickening. (From ref. 29.)

myocardium. For example, function can be increased and sustained at normal or supranormal levels with catecholamines or postextrasystolic potentiation in stunned myocardium[18] without changing ATP levels. Conversely, ATP levels can be increased to near normal levels in stunned myocardium by administration of requisite precursors without reversing dysfunction.[34] Thus the prolonged but reversible dysfunction that characterizes stunned myocardium is not related to myocyte ATP levels.

Strong evidence suggests that at least part of the prolonged dysfunction after reperfusion in stunned myocardium is mediated by abnormalities of calcium homeostasis. Intracellular calcium levels rise during ischemia and during early reperfusion.[35] The mechanism for the increase in cytosolic Ca^{2+} appears to be a metabolic inhibition of the sarcolemmal Na–K ATPase with a consequent rise in intracellular Na^+. At reperfusion the Na–Ca exchange mechanism, which usually pumps Ca^{2+} out of the cell in exchange for Na^+, reverses direction in response to relative intracellular Na^+-loading, now extruding Na^+ in exchange for Ca^{2+}.

That the transient rise in intracellular Ca^{2+} is causally related to stunning is supported by several lines of evidence. Reducing the rise in intracellular calcium with acidosis[36] or perfusion with low calcium[37] minimizes stunning. In addition, other non-ischemic maneuvers that result in intracellular calcium loading such as perfusion with high calcium concentration perfusate[38] or following a period of ventricular fibrillation[24] mimic ischemia-mediated stunning functionally and histologically.

How this transient rise in intracellular Ca^{2+} leads to depressed function is unclear. Nevertheless, systolic dysfunction in stunned myocardium is associated with a decline in maximal calcium-activated force production

and a decrease in the sensitivity of the myofilaments to calcium.[39,40] Similarly, the mechanism of postfibrillation dysfunction has been related to intracellular Ca^{2+} overload and a resulting decline in the sensitivity of myocyte contractile elements to Ca^{2+}.[24] It is possible that increased intracellular Ca^{2+} may activate protein kinases, which may then phosphorylate and therefore alter the function of contractile proteins.[41] Finally, reduced uptake of calcium by sarcoplasmic reticulum has been observed in stunned myocardium[42] and may be related to both impaired systolic and diastolic function. Impaired diastolic relaxation may also be caused by abnormal myofilament relaxation, perhaps secondary to changes in intracellular inorganic phosphate.[43]

Paradoxically, despite a decline in ATP levels and a parallel reduction in function, myocardial oxygen consumption is increased in stunned myocardium.[44,45] This mismatch between oxygen consumption and function is related neither to uncoupling of oxidative phosphorylation nor to a rise in basal (non-contractile-related) myocyte oxygen requirements.[46] Instead, it appears to be caused by a reduction in the calcium sensitivity of myofilaments in the postischemic period,[47,48] noted above.

Evidence also exists that oxygen-based radicals are important mediators of stunned myocardium. Within 1 minute of reperfusion there is a marked production of free radical species including O_2, H_2O_2, and OH,[49] which, while declining rapidly, is sustained for several hours after reperfusion.[49] Treatment with superoxide dismutase (SOD) (which prevents production of O_2) and catalase (which prevents production of H_2O_2 and OH) minimizes free radical production[49] and minimizes the degree of postischemic dysfunction as well.[50] The relationship between degree of dysfunction in the reperfusion period and the degree of blood flow reduction during the ischemic period noted above may reflect the close association between the degree of ischemia and the level of oxygen radicals subsequently produced during reperfusion.[51] The only literature that actually specifically addresses reperfusion injury in the setting of cardiac arrest and CPR involved administration of the iron chelator deferoxamine to inhibit generation of oxygen radicals by inhibiting the Haber–Weiss reaction.[1–3] Interestingly, deferoxamine was given 5 minutes *after* return of spontaneous circulation and therefore after reperfusion[2,3] and after the expected early, large burst of free radical generation; yet inhibition of free radical generation at this relatively late time still appeared to have a marked beneficial effect as measured by *late survival*: in the deferoxamine-treated group, late neurologically intact survival was twice that of controls.[2,3]

It is likely that the pathogenesis of stunning involves both free radical–mediated injury and calcium-mediated injury; the two mechanisms are not mutually exclusive.[41,52] Although a number of ways the two mechanisms may work together to effect myocardial stunning have been suggested,[41,52] their complex interrelations remain to be elucidated.

Clinical issues relevant to cardiac arrest and cardiopulmonary resuscitation

The critical aspect of stunning important to the setting of cardiac arrest and CPR is that stunning may lead to profound, prolonged, but *reversible*, myocardial dysfunction despite restoration of normal coronary blood flow and preservation of cerebral function. The clinician must be aware that stunned myocardium *will* recover if given sufficient time and that support of the stunned heart, often for protracted periods of time, may be required. Better methods to identify viable but dysfunctional myocardium could be of obvious value in the postarrest setting.

Minimization of arrest time before initiation of CPR and restoration of adequate coronary blood flow would be important since the degree of stunning is directly related to the duration of ischemia. Clinical studies have repeatedly demonstrated a direct relationship between early and late survival and minimization of the time between cardiac arrest and institution of CPR.[53,54] Clearly, while rapid institution of CPR may minimize myocardial stunning, other beneficial effects are probably as, or even more, important.

During CPR, maintenance of the highest perfusion pressure possible is of clear importance since stunning depends in part on the degree of ischemia. The requisite pressure can be significantly higher than that required for cerebral perfusion, because the elevated oxygen consumption of the fibrillating heart and the presence of coronary artery stenoses increase the aortic pressure required to maintain adequate coronary blood flow. Since stunning depends on an imbalance between oxygen supply and demand, improvement of this balance in the course of CPR might minimize stunning. Epinephrine, which is often used in high doses to improve coronary perfusion pressure during CPR, can also increase myocardial oxygen demand. If the improvement in flow fails to match the increase in demand, then the setting exists for myocardial stunning. In a recent animal study the combination of phenylephrine and propranolol resulted in lower myocardial lactate levels and higher myocardial ATP levels than either high-dose epinephrine or phenylephrine alone.[55] Presumably, phenylephrine allowed for an increase in aortic pressure during CPR, while propranolol reduced myocardial oxygen consumption, suggesting that use of this combination of drugs during CPR may minimize subsequent stunning. Whether this will translate into a useful therapeutic strategy remains to be seen.

Following restoration of spontaneous circulation, the postarrest heart may be stunned and require support, either mechanical[31] or pharmacologic.[18] Left ventricular assist devices[31] and peripheral bypass are both potential forms of therapy. Stunned myocardium can be made to develop normal contractile performance pharmacologically by use of inotropic drugs, such as catecholamines.[18] The duration of support can be quite extraordinary (Fig. 14.4): one patient undergoing coronary artery bypass surgery was reported to have an ejection fraction of 6% postoperatively (50% preoperatively).[31] After more than

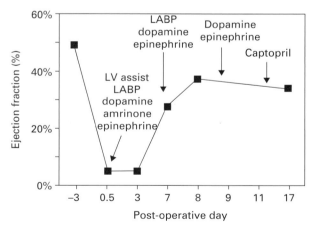

Fig. 14.4. Dysfunction caused by stunned myocardium may be profound and prolonged, requiring pharmacologic and mechanical support for a protracted period of time. *IABP*, intraaortic balloon pump. (Adapted from ref. 31.)

2 weeks of mechanical and pharmacologic (inotropic) support, cardiac function recovered and the (unsupported) ejection fraction was 38%.[31] The clinician caring for the postarrest patient must recognize the potential for stunned myocardium to recover over such protracted periods of time.

In the future, further study of the mechanisms of stunning in cardiac arrest and CPR may lead to other ways of preventing its occurrence. Thus inhibition of free radical formation with SOD and catalase administered during CPR may prevent or minimize postarrest myocardial dysfunction. Inhibition of the transient postischemic rise in intracellular Ca^{2+} or reversal of its longer lasting effects on target proteins or subcellular structures could also be a future preventive strategy.

Reperfusion arrhythmias

At one time, arrhythmias, including ventricular tachycardia and fibrillation, were thought to herald successful reperfusion after thrombolytic therapy for acute myocardial infarction. Closer study of large numbers of patients, however, revealed that reperfusion arrhythmias are insensitive and non-specific markers of reperfusion in this setting.[56,57] Nevertheless, reperfusion arrhythmias have been repeatedly demonstrated in animal models of ischemia and reperfusion. It is interesting that reperfusion after brief (5 to 20 minutes) ischemic periods may be associated with more frequent and more severe ventricular arrhythmias than more prolonged periods (hours).[9] A discussion of reperfusion arrhythmias is warranted for at least two reasons. First, as will be discussed below, reperfusion arrhythmias can be the proximate cause of cardiac arrest. Second, since the ischemic period associated with cardiac arrest and CPR is usually relatively brief (minutes not hours), the reperfusion that attends restoration of adequate coronary flow either from CPR itself or from the return of spontaneous circulation may create the electrophysiological milieu associated with reperfusion arrhythmias.

Animal models of reperfusion arrhythmias

Reperfusion arrhythmias have been documented in several species, and in general their frequency and severity depend on the duration of ischemia.[58] This relationship is not linear, however. Very brief episodes of ischemia lead to no or infrequent reperfusion arrhythmias; longer periods of ischemia that end before the onset of significant irreversible injury are associated with the highest frequency and most severe ventricular arrhythmias; and very long ischemic periods (long enough to lead to irreversible myonecrosis) again lead to less frequent and less severe ventricular arrhythmias.[58] The exact timing of these events depends on the species and the model (intact or isolated heart) examined. In the isolated rat heart, for example, reperfusion ventricular fibrillation occurs infrequently after less than 5 or more than 30 minutes of ischemia but occurs in virtually all animals after 15 minutes of ischemia.[58] In the intact dog, ischemic durations less than 5 to 10 minutes or greater than 60 to 90 minutes infrequently lead to reperfusion fibrillation, whereas more than 50% of animals fibrillate on reperfusion after 20 to 30 minutes of ischemia.[58] In addition to the duration of ischemia, development of serious ventricular arrhythmias appears to be related to the level of collateral flow and high-energy phosphates: the higher the collateral flow during the ischemic period, the less likely arrhythmias follow reperfusion.[59]

Reperfusion arrhythmias in humans

As noted above, prolonged ischemia followed by reperfusion, as occurs in acute myocardial infarction treated with thrombolytic therapy, is sometimes but not usually associated with ventricular arrhythmias. One large study of 500 patients with acute myocardial infarction, some treated with and others without thrombolytic therapy, showed no increase in ventricular arrhythmias in patients treated with reperfusion therapy,[60] suggesting that these arrhythmias, when they occur, are not necessarily related to reperfusion.

In other clinical settings, brief periods of ischemia followed by reperfusion have been shown to be associated with development of serious ventricular arrhythmias. For example, Previtali et al.[61] studied a group of patients with Prinzmetal's variant angina. Continuous Holter monitoring identified a subgroup of these patients who had ventricular arrhythmias either during ST segment elevation (during ischemia) or after resolution of ST elevation (reperfusion). Of the group who developed ventricular arrhythmias, the arrhythmia was associated with reperfusion in one-third (10 out of 27).[61] Similarly, Myerburg et al.[62] described a small group of patients with transient, silent ST segment elevation associated with life-threatening ventricular arrhythmias, 40% (two out of five) of whom developed the arrhythmia during resolution of the preceding ST segment elevation (i.e., during reperfusion).

From these observations it is clear that reperfusion arrhythmias occur in humans, particularly after brief episodes of ischemia. It is also clear that reperfusion arrhythmias can be the initiating event in cardiac arrest.

Mechanisms of reperfusion arrhythmias

Re-entry, increased automaticity, and triggered activity have all been suggested as potential mechanisms of reperfusion arrhythmias.

The ionic and electrophysiologic consequences of ischemia and reperfusion are complex and incompletely understood; the nature and degree of these alterations depend on the duration of ischemia and on the model used for study. Since reperfusion ventricular arrhythmias seem to occur most often after relatively brief durations of ischemia (15 to 30 minutes in most species), this discussion will center around changes that occur in that time frame.

Ischemia rapidly leads to an increase in extracellular K^+ and a rise in intracellular Na^+, in part a result of metabolic inhibition of the sarcolemmal Na–K ATPase pump. The myocyte transmembrane potential becomes depolarized, and action potential duration is shortened. On reperfusion, there is a rise in intracellular Ca^{2+} mediated, in part, by the Na–Ca exchanger mentioned above. Extracellular K^+ is washed out and returns toward normal or subnormal levels, and action potential duration returns to normal or becomes prolonged.

Restoration of coronary blood flow returns the electrophysiologic properties of ischemic myocardium toward normal. However, since coronary blood flow is restored in a non-homogeneous manner, with islands of high and low flow, restoration of the normal ionic and electrophysiologic milieu is also not homogeneous. Hariman et al.[63] showed that in the dog, reperfusion after 20 minutes of ischemia was associated with a marked spatial heterogeneity of regional blood flow, extracellular K^+ concentration, and electrogram duration within the reperfused zone in the first minutes of reperfusion. Similarly, Coronel et al.[64] demonstrated marked heterogeneity of extracellular K^+ and action potential duration between reperfused and normal myocardium in early reperfusion after 10 minutes of coronary occlusion in the isolated pig heart.

This heterogeneity leads to a dispersion of refractoriness, which forms the ideal substrate for re-entry. Although various studies differ on the precise nature of the electrophysiologic changes involved, most support the notion that reperfusion is marked by a dispersion of refractory periods either within the previously ischemic region or between the reperfused and normal regions. For example, Levites et al. demonstrated a marked dispersion of refractoriness in dog hearts subjected to 15 to 30 minutes of coronary occlusion followed by reperfusion.[65] After shortening during the ischemic period, the refractory period was prolonged in the previously ischemic region within 3 minutes of flow restoration.[65] They concluded that the dispersion of refractoriness and its temporal relation to the onset of ventricular arrhythmias suggested re-entry was an important mechanism of reperfusion arrhythmia.[65] Naimi et al. also demonstrated a dispersion of effective refractory periods in ischemic and reperfused dog hearts following either 5 or 15 minutes of regional ischemia.[66] In this study the effective refractory period was actually shortened in the first minute of reperfusion; the increased dispersion of refractory periods between normal and reperfused myocardium led to a large electrical gradient between the two regions.[66]

Although re-entry constitutes a common, if not the most common, mechanism for production of reperfusion arrhythmias, other mechanisms are also likely to be operative. For example, reperfusion arrhythmias have been attributed to triggered arrhythmias: early and delayed afterdepolarizations.

Priori et al. demonstrated, in an in vivo cat model of 10 minutes of coronary occlusion followed by reperfusion, that early afterdepolarization occurs in early reperfusion and can be an important mechanism of reperfusion arrhythmias.[67] Rozanski and Witt[68,69] showed that in isolated cardiac Purkinje fibers recovering from ischemia like conditions (hypoxia, high external K^+, and acidosis), action potential duration is prolonged, setting the stage for early afterdepolarizations (Fig. 14.5). Further, generation of such depolarizations was critically dependent on intracellular acidosis.[68] The ionic basis for early afterdepolarizations is not completely clear but may involve an inward current carried by Ca^{2+} through sarcolemmal voltage-gated Ca^{2+} channels,[70] which, in part because of prolongation of action potential duration, have time to recover from their inactive state and reopen at or near the plateau potential. Alternatively, the ionic current could be carried by Na^+ through Na^+ channels or may be caused by a reduction or delay in outward, repolarizing current.[68] The requirement for a preceding intracellular acidosis suggests that Ca^{2+} may be important in creating the conditions necessary for early afterdepolarizations. That is, the rise in intracellular Ca^{2+} after reperfusion may depend on an increase in intracellular Na^+; and the rise in intracellular Na^+ may depend not only on metabolic inhibition of the Na–K ATPase pump but also on Na–H exchange. The rise in intracellular Ca^{2+} occurs on reperfusion when the Na–Ca exchanger pumps out Na^+ and takes in Ca^{2+}. These reperfusion-associated changes in intracellular Ca^{2+}, although transient, may lead to longer-lasting alterations in membrane electrophysiologic properties,[68] just as they lead to longer-lasting changes in function in the case of myocardial stunning.

Delayed afterdepolarizations have also been suggested as a cause of reperfusion arrhythmias. Delayed

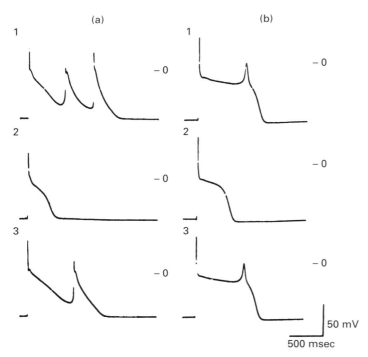

Fig. 14.5. Early afterdepolarizations and triggered activity in a model of ischemia and reperfusion. Inhibition by lidocaine. (From ref. 68.)

afterdepolarizations are related to spontaneous oscillations in intracellular Ca^{2+} caused by release from the sarcoplasmic reticulum.[70] Increases in such release, as may be seen with the relative calcium overload that occurs with ischemia and reperfusion, can be associated with such depolarizations. In a model consisting of isolated, superfused canine papillary muscle–Purkinje fiber preparations, Ferrier *et al.* demonstrated that "reperfusion" following ischemia-like conditions (hypoxia, acidosis) resulted in a stereotyped sequence of events: first hyperpolarization, then progressive depolarization, and then a return to control membrane potential.[71] During the depolarization phase, delayed afterdepolarizations could initiate extrasystoles,[71] but whether or not they actually can initiate repetitive ventricular activity in the setting of in vivo ischemia and reperfusion is unclear.

Similar to altered cardiac function following ischemia and reperfusion, changes in the electrophysiologic properties of reperfused myocardium have been attributed to alterations in Ca^{2+} homeostasis and changes caused by free radical damage. Relevant changes in Ca^{2+} homeostasis were outlined above.

The extent to which electrophysiologic changes are the result of free radical injury is more difficult to determine,

and the relationship between free radical–induced injury and reperfusion arrhythmias remains unclear. Some studies suggest that the time course of changes in electrophysiologic properties such as action potential duration is too slow to be associated with reperfusion arrhythmias,[72] whereas other studies suggest changes can occur within 1 minute of exposure to free radical–generating systems.[73] And although some studies have shown a reduction in ventricular arrhythmias associated with reperfusion after treatment with free radical scavengers such as SOD and catalase,[74,75] others have failed to show such a benefit.[73,76] Thus, although free radicals are generated in the first moments of reperfusion, their relationship to arrhythmias in this period remains uncertain.

Other potential mechanisms involved in reperfusion arrhythmias include α-adrenergic activation[77] and angiotensin II production.[78] Blockade of α-adrenergic activation with phentolamine[77] and angiotensin converting enzyme (ACE) inhibition[78] has been reported to reduce the frequency and severity of ventricular reperfusion arrhythmias in animal models.

Influence of comorbid conditions and common drugs on reperfusion arrhythmias

Comorbid conditions that affect cardiac arrest victims, such as hypertension and diabetes, may influence reperfusion arrhythmias. Isolated hearts from hypertensive rats subjected to 10 minutes of regional ischemia followed by reperfusion have a higher incidence of ventricular fibrillation than do normal hearts.[79] On the other hand, diabetic rats (streptozotocin-induced) appear to have a somewhat lower incidence of sustained ventricular fibrillation after 10 minutes of regional ischemia followed by reperfusion,[80] perhaps because these hearts have a higher content of free radical–scavenging enzymes, prolonged action potential duration, and reduced activity of Na^+–H^+ and Na^+–Ca^{2+} exchange.[80]

Concomitant drug administration can also influence reperfusion arrhythmias. The incidence and duration of ventricular fibrillation are increased in isolated rat hearts made globally ischemic for 25 minutes and reperfused after administration of ouabain,[81] probably because of ouabain-induced augmentation of Ca^{2+} overload. Other drugs may have a beneficial effect. For example, ACE inhibitors have also been shown to reduce the incidence, severity, and duration of reperfusion arrhythmias.[82] Still other drugs have a mixed action. Glibenclamide, an oral hypoglycemic, has been shown to increase the frequency of delayed afterdepolarizations and triggered activity in eperfused myocardium;[83] yet it also appears to reduce re-entrant ventricular tachycardia and fibrillation in the same setting.[83,84]

Clinical relevance of reperfusion arrhythmias to cardiac arrest and cardiopulmonary resuscitation

Reperfusion arrhythmias may initiate cardiac arrest, as noted above, and may be an important cause of sudden death. In addition, reestablishment of coronary flow by CPR, either by creating an adequate coronary driving pressure or restoration of spontaneous circulation, results in reperfusion, which may in turn lead to reperfusion arrhythmias either during CPR or in the early postresuscitation period.

The approach to these arrhythmias is standardized and directed for the most part at treating re-entry, the mechanism that is probably most common and for which there is strongest evidence. Thus lidocaine, bretyllium, and magnesium sulfate, in that order, are used for serious ventricular arrhythmias in the setting of CPR. In addition, lidocaine has been reported to be effective in suppressing both early[85] and delayed[86] afterdepolarizations, making it a drug of first choice in this setting. At present, no specific therapies can be aimed at *preventing* these arrhythmias.

It is clear that the ability to identify mechanisms of reperfusion-related arrhythmias beside re-entry at the bedside may be important in the future when specific therapies for these arrhythmic mechanisms are available. In addition, methods of modifying the effects of increased intracellular Ca^{2+} or minimizing the ionic and metabolic disturbances that lead to Ca^{2+} overload and its lingering aftereffects may be available in the future and used for prevention. Finally, to the extent that free radicals mediate reperfusion arrhythmias, treatment with free radical scavengers during CPR may minimize postresuscitation arrhythmias.

Myonecrosis and vascular injury

Definition

Reperfusion-related myonecrosis occurs after more prolonged ischemic periods. Ischemia alone obviously can produce irreversible injury, but this reperfusion-related myonecrosis extends this injury and produces additional cell death.

Whereas myocardial stunning and reperfusion arrhythmias are important to both therapy and a fundamental understanding of cardiac arrest and CPR, whether the myonecrosis caused by reperfusion after more prolonged ischemic periods is relevant in this setting is much less clear. Indeed, whether this type of reperfusion injury occurs at all in any setting remains unresolved. Further, since a more prolonged ischemic insult is required to produce lethal myocyte injury, the relevance to the setting of cardiac arrest and CPR is less clear: an arrest time greater than a few minutes is incompatible with meaningful neurologic recovery.

Nevertheless, it is possible to imagine a circumstance in which CPR was begun soon after cardiac arrest and produced an adequate coronary perfusion pressure. However, if one or more coronary arteries had critical stenoses, then the regional ischemic period could be relatively long if CPR is continued for a prolonged period; this could be sufficient to produce irreversible injury. On return of spontaneous circulation and better coronary perfusion pressure and flow, reperfusion injury could occur and result in additional myonecrosis.

Reperfusion-related myonecrosis in animals

The most direct evidence for reperfusion injury comes from a study of Becker *et al.*[87] Dogs were subjected to 90 minutes of coronary occlusion followed by variable periods of reperfusion. Electron microscopic evidence for irreversible injury was assessed in biopsies taken from ischemic regions reperfused for 0, 5, 90, or 180 minutes. Nearly all biopsies from ischemic regions with very low flow ($<0.05\,ml/g$ per min) showed irreversible injury independent of the reperfusion period. In biopsies from ischemic regions with less severe flow reduction ($>0.05\,ml/g$ per min), however, irreversible injury increased as a function of reperfusion period, with more samples showing irreversible injury as reperfusion time increased. These results are consistent with reperfusion injury. Whether this injury was inevitable and would have occurred whether or not reperfusion had occurred cannot be gleaned from this study.

Rather than demonstrating reperfusion injury directly, most studies attempt to demonstrate reperfusion-related myonecrosis by trying to minimize it. Such studies rely on using some agent or maneuver to reduce reperfusion injury compared to a control condition. Infarct size (mass) is the most common outcome variable measured: if the agent reduces reperfusion injury, infarct size will be smaller in the treated than in the control group. A critical conceptual issue in such studies is that most interventions designed to reduce reperfusion injury may minimize infarct size in other ways as well and therefore are not absolutely specific.

Review of the numerous agents used in such studies is beyond the scope of this chapter. Agents that appear to reduce infarct size by minimizing reperfusion-related myonecrosis include (a) those that interfere with neutrophil sequestration in the reperfused region or neutrophil function,[88–90] (b) agents that interfere with free radical formation,[1,3,91,92] and (c) other agents that work through various or uncertain mechanisms.[93–95] All such studies demonstrate, at best, an association between a reduction in infarct size and the agent's use but do not prove that the mechanism has any connection with limitation of reperfusion injury. Further, for each of these approaches, studies that fail to show benefit exist as well. For this reason the issue of reperfusion-related myonecrosis remains controversial and unresolved.

Evidence for reperfusion-related myonecrosis in humans

No direct or indirect evidence exists of reperfusion-related myonecrosis in humans. Two agents that have been shown to reduce infarct size in animal models of ischemia and reperfusion (presumably by limiting reperfusion injury), SOD and the perfluorochemical Fluosol, had no beneficial effect when administered just before reperfusion in recent trials of patients undergoing thrombolysis or angioplasty for acute myocardial infarction.[96,97]

Mechanisms of reperfusion-related myonecrosis

The potential elements involved in reperfusion-related myonecrosis are numerous, complex, interrelated, and incompletely understood. The leukocyte, endothelial cell, platelet, cytokines, free radicals, Ca^{2+}, and other factors all may be involved in a complex and interconnected way.

The polymorphonuclear leukocyte (PMN) is sequestered in the reperfused region shortly after reestablishment of flow by the action of specific adhesion molecules that allow for adherence of the PMN to the endothelial cell and subsequent diapedesis into the interstitial space.[98] Deleterious effects of these PMNs include release of lysosomal enzymes and free radicals, which cause both myocyte and endothelial cell damage, and direct plugging of the microvasculature.

Free radical production occurs from sequestered PMNs and also from endothelial cells on reperfusion,[99] resulting in both muscle and microvascular injury.[87] Experiments demonstrating that inhibition of free radical formation limits infarct size support this as a potential mechanism but do not identify the source of radical formation directly.

Clinical relevance of reperfusion-related myonecrosis in cardiopulmonary resuscitation

Since the existence of reperfusion-related myonecrosis is itself controversial, its relevance to cardiac arrest and CPR is tenuous indeed. Nevertheless, to the extent that reperfusion-related myonecrosis may be important, therapeutic strategies that are currently being designed and tested in animal models may be appropriate potential therapies in the setting of prolonged CPR. These include antineutrophil therapies designed to interfere with neutrophil sequestration in reperfused myocardium and inhibition of free radical formation.

Summary

Cardiac arrest and CPR provide a setting in which reperfusion injury can occur (Fig. 14.6). Relatively brief episodes of ischemia lasting less than 10 to 20 minutes followed by reperfusion are probably relatively common and may be regional or global, depending on the time between circulatory collapse and initiation of CPR, the adequacy of CPR in restoring coronary blood flow, the presence of coronary stenoses, the time to recovery of spontaneous circulation and normal hemodynamics, and the pharmacologic agents administered.

Durations of ischemia in this range can be followed by two types of reperfusion injury, myocardial stunning and

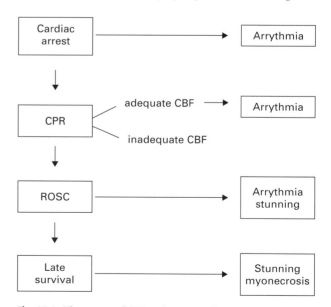

Fig. 14.6. The course of CPR and associated events potentially associated with reperfusion injury. *CBF,* coronary blood flow; ROSC, re turn of spontaneous circulation.

reperfusion arrhythmias. One common mechanism underlying the functional and electrophysiologic derangements in these two types of reperfusion injury is altered Ca^{2+} homeostasis. The transient Ca^{2+} overload that characterizes ischemia and reperfusion is related to the rise in intracellular Na^+ that occurs secondary to inhibition of the sarcolemmal Na–K ATPase pump and to intracellular acidosis with subsequent Na–H exchange that occurs during ischemia. On reperfusion the rise in intracellular Na^+ results in a rise in intracellular Ca^+ as Na^+ is extruded in exchange for Ca^+ via the Na–Ca exchanger. This transient rise in intracellular Ca^{2+} leads to longer-lasting derangements in the functional and electrophysiologic properties of the cardiac myocytes by as yet undermined mechanisms, perhaps involving alteration of myofilament or membrane proteins through activation of protein kinases. As a result, reperfusion after brief ischemic periods can result in prolonged cardiac dysfunction and a dispersion of refractoriness, which lead to myocardial stunning and re-entrant reperfusion arrhythmias.

Other mechanisms of stunning and reperfusion arrhythmias may exist, such as free radical injury. Although experimental support for the importance of free radical–mediated injury in animal models of stunning is strong, the relationship of free radical generation to reperfusion arrhythmias is less clear.

Whether more prolonged ischemia can lead to reperfusion-related myonecrosis and whether this is really applicable to the setting of cardiac arrest and CPR are more difficult to assess.

Current therapeutic considerations center around recognition and treatment of the potentially prolonged dysfunction that may occur in stunned myocardium and the important discrimination of stunned from irreversibly injured heart. Pharmacologic and mechanical support of the postresuscitation stunned heart can be protracted but ultimately can be rewarded with improved functional survival. Re-entry is probably the most common mechanism for reperfusion arrhythmias, which appear to be appropriately treated with currently recommended agents.

Future therapies will attempt to prevent or minimize reperfusion injury. Altered Ca^{2+} homeostasis may be prevented by limiting the entry of intracellular Na^+ during ischemia or reversing the effects of intracellular Ca^{2+} accumulation on target proteins and subcellular structures once these are identified. Restriction of the effects of such agents to injured tissue may be the biggest challenge to their development. Free radical generation could be limited by treatment with free radical scavengers during CPR and for some time after return of spontaneous circulation to prevent the functional and electrophysiologic consequences of their formation.

Conclusions

Cardiac arrest and CPR constitute a setting in which reperfusion injury in its various forms may occur. Almost nothing is directly known about myocardial reperfusion injury in this circumstance, because studies to date have been designed to model other clinical settings, such as cardiopulmonary bypass or myocardial infarction treated with thrombolytics. Nevertheless, knowledge gained from these models can be applied to cardiac arrest and CPR to speculate on how reperfusion injury might occur in this setting. Recognition of the potentially critical role that reperfusion injury may play in the course and outcome of cardiac arrest and CPR will, it is hoped, stimulate research in an area that has remained largely unexplored. Until then our speculations, although perhaps at a level just above "mere prattle," remain "without practice."

REFERENCES

1. Babbs, C.F. Role of iron ions in the genesis of reperfusion injury following successful cardiopulmonary resuscitation: preliminary data and a biochemical hypothesis. *Ann. Emerg. Med.* 1985; **14**: 777–783.

2. Badylak, S.F. & Babbs, C.F. The effect of carbon dioxide, lidoflazine and deferoxamine upon long term survival following cardiorespiratory arrest in rats. *Resuscitation* 1986; **13**(3): 165–173.

3. Zweier, J.L., Kuppusamy, P. & Lutty, G.A. Measurement of endothelial cell free radical generation: evidence for a central mechanism of free radical injury in postischemic tissues. *Proc. Natl Acad. Sci. USA* 1988; **85**: 4046–4050.

4. Kern, K.B., Rhee, K.H., Raya, T.E. *et al.* Global myocardial stunning following successful resuscitation from cardiac arrest [Abstract]. *Circulation* 1994; **90**: 1–5.

5. Gruppo Italiano per lo Studio della Streptochinasi nell'Infarto Miocardico (GISSI). Effectiveness of intravenous thrombolytic treatment in acute myocardial infarction. *Lancet* 1986; **1**(8478): 397–402.

6. Guerci, A.D., Gerstenblith, G., Brinker, J.A. *et al.* A randomized trial of intravenous tissue plasminogen activator for acute myocardial infarction with subsequent randomization to elective coronary angioplasty. *N. Engl. J. Med.* 1987; **317**(26): 1613–1618.

7. Kennedy, J.W., Ritchie, J.L., Davis, K.B. & Fritz, J.K. Western Washington randomized trial of intracoronary streptokinase in acute myocardial infarction. *N. Engl. J. Med.* 1983; **309**(24): 1477–1482.

8. Braunwald, E. & Kloner, R.A. Myocardial reperfusion: a double-edged sword? *J. Clin. Invest.* 1985; **76**: 1713–1719.

9. Kloner, R.A. Does reperfusion injury exist in humans? *J. Am. Coll. Cardiol.* 1993; **21**: 537–545.

10. Braunwald, E. Is myocardial stunning important from a clinical standpoint? In Kloner, R.A., Przyklenk, K., eds. *Stunned Myocardium.* New York: Marcel Dekker, Inc, 1993; 441–452.

11. Kern, K.B. & Ewy, G.A. Minimal coronary stenoses and left ventricular blood flow during CPR. *Ann. Emerg. Med.* 1992; **21**: 1066–1072.

12. Heyndrickx, G.R., Millard, R.W., McRitchie, R.J., Maroko, P.R. & Vatner, S.F. Regional myocardial functional and electrophysiological alterations after brief coronary artery occlusion in conscious dogs. *J. Clin. Invest.* 1975; **56**: 978–985.

13. Heyndrickx, G.R., Baig, H., Nellens, P., Leusen, I., Fishbein, M.C. & Vatner, S.F. Depression of regional blood flow and wall thickening after brief coronary occlusions. *Am. J. Physiol.* 1978; **234**: H653–H659.

14. Kloner, R.A., Ellis, S.G., Lange, L. & Braunwald, E. Studies of experimental coronary artery reperfusion: effects on infarct size, myocardial function, biochemistry, ultrastructure, and microvascular damage. *Circulation* 1983; **68**(Suppl 1): 1–8.

15. Cerchiari, E.L., Safar, P., Klein, E., Cantadore, R. & Pinsky, M. Cardiovascular function and neurologic outcome after cardiac arrest in dogs: the cardiovascular post-resuscitation syndrome. *Resuscitation* 1993; **25**: 9–33.

16. Bolli, R., Zhu, W.X., Thornby, J.I., O'Neill, P.G. & Roberts, R. Time course and determinants of recovery of function after reversible ischemia in conscious dogs. *Am. J. Physiol.* 1988; **254**: H102–H114.

17. Nicklas, J.M., Becker, L.C. & Healy-Bulkley, B. Effects of repeated brief coronary occlusion on regional left ventricular function and dimension in dogs. *Am. J. Cardiol.* 1985; **56**: 473.

18. Becker, L.C., Levine, J.H., DiPaula, A.F., Guarnieri, T. & Aversano, T. Reversal of dysfunction in postischemic stunned myocardium by epinephrine and postextrasystolic potentiation. *J. Am. Coll. Cardiol.* 1986; **7**: 580–589.

19. Murry, C.E., Jennings, R.B. & Reimer, K.A. Preconditioning with ischemia: a delay of lethal cell injury in ischemic myocardium. *Circulation* 1986; **74**: 1124–1136.

20. Murry, C.E., Richard, V.J., Reimer, K.A. & Jennings, R.B. Ischemic preconditioning slows energy metabolism and delays ultrastructural damage during a sustained ischemic episode. *Circ. Res.* 1990; **66**: 913–931.

21. Przyklenk, K. & Apstein, C.S. Stunned myocardium in the isolated perfused heart preparation. In Kloner, R.A., Przyklenk, K., eds. *Stunned Myocardium.* New York: Marcel Dekker, Inc, 1993; 109–134.

22. Charlat, J.L., O'Neill, R.G., Hartly, C.J., Roberts, R. & Bolli, R. Prolonged abnormalities of left ventricular diastolic wall thinning in the "stunned" myocardium in conscious dogs: time course and relation to systolic function. *J. Am. Coll. Cardiol.* 1989; **13**: 185–194.

23. Homans, D.C., Laxson, D.D., Sublett, E., Lindstrom, P. & Bache, R.J. Cumulative deterioration of myocardial function after repeated episodes of exercise-induced ischemia. *Am. J. Physiol.* 1989; **89**: H1462–H1471.

24. Koretsune, Y. & Marban, E. Cell calcium in the pathophysiology of ventricular fibrillation and in the pathogenesis of post-arrhythmic contractile dysfunction. *Circulation* 1989; **80**: 369–379.

25. Ellis, S.G., Henschke, C.I., Sandor, T., Wynne, J., Braunwald, E. & Kloner, R.A. Time course of functional and biochemical recovery of myocardium salvaged by reperfusion. *J. Am. Coll. Cardiol.* 1983; **1**: 1047.

26. Pfisterer, M., Zuber, M., Wenzel, R. & Burkart, F. Prolonged myocardial stunning after thrombolysis: can left ventricular function be assessed definitely at hospital discharge? *Eur. Heart J.* 1991; **12**: 214–217.

27. Wilson, I.C. & Gardner, T.J. Stunned myocardium in cardiac surgery. In Kloner, R.A., Przyklenk, K., eds. *Stunned Myocardium.* New York: Marcel Dekker, Inc, 1993; 379–399.

28. Roberts, A.J., Spies, S.M., Sanders, J.H. *et al.* Serial assessment of left ventricular performance following coronary artery bypass grafting: early post-operative results with myocardial protection afforded by multidose hypothermic potassium crystalloid cardioplegia. *J. Thorac. Cardiovasc. Surg.* 1981; **81**: 69–84.

29. Bolli, R., Hartley, C.J., Chelly, J.E. *et al.* An accurate non-traumatic ultrasonic method to monitor myocardial wall thickening in patients undergoing cardiac surgery. *J. Am. Coll. Cardiol.* 1990; **15**: 1055–1065.

30. Fremes, S.E., Weisel, R.D., Mickle, D.A. *et al.* Myocardial metabolism and ventricular function following cold potassium cardioplegia. *J. Thorac. Cardiovasc. Surg.* 1985; **89**: 531–546.

31. Ballantyne, C.M., Verani, M.S., Short, H.D., Hyatt, C. & Noon, G.P. Delayed recovery of severely "stunned" myocardium with the support of a left ventricular assist device after coronary artery bypass graft surgery. *J. Am. Coll. Cardiol.* 1987; **10**: 710–712.

32. Schneider, R.M. Rate of left ventricular functional recovery by radionuclide angiography after exercise in coronary artery disease. *Am. J. Cardiol.* 1986; **57**: 927–932.

33. Reimer, K.A., Hill, M.L. & Jennings, R.B. Prolonged depletion of ATP and of the adenine nucleotide pool due to delayed resynthesis of adenine nucleotides following reversible myocardial ischemia in dogs. *J. Mol. Cell. Cardiol.* 1981; **13**: 229–239.

34. Ambrosio, G., Jacobus, W.E., Mitchell, M.C., Litt, M.R. & Becker, L.C. Effects of ATP precursors on ATP and free ADP content and functional recovery of postischemic hearts. *Am. J. Physiol.* 1989; **256**: H560–H566.

35. Marban, E., Kitakaze, M., Koretsune, Y., Yue, D.T., Chacko, V.P. & Pike, M.M. Quantification of $[Ca^{2+}]_i$ in perfused hearts: critical evaluation of the 5F-BAPTA/NMR method as applied to the study of ischemia and reperfusion. *Circ. Res.* 1990; **66**: 1255–1267.

36. Kitakaze, M., Weisfeldt, M.L. & Marban, E. Acidosis during early reperfusion prevents myocardial stunning in perfused hearts. *J. Clin. Invest.* 1988; **82**: 920–927.

37. Kuroda, H., Ishiguro, S. & Mori, T. Optimal calcium concentration in the initial reperfusate for post-ischemic myocardial performance (calcium concentration during reperfusion). *J. Mol. Cell. Cardiol.* 1986; **18**: 625–633.

38. Kitakaze, M., Weisman, H.F. & Marban, E. Contractile dysfunction and ATP depletion after transient calcium overload in perfused ferret hearts. *Circulation* 1988; **77**: 685–695.

39. Kusuoka, H., Porterfield, J.K., Weisman, H.F., Weisfeldt, M.L. & Marban, E. Pathophysiology and pathogenesis of stunned myocardium: depressed Ca^{2+} activation of contraction as a consequence of reperfusion-induced cellular calcium overload in ferret hearts. *J. Clin. Invest.* 1987; **79**: 950–961.

40. Kusuoka, H., Koretsune, Y., Chacko, V.P., Weisfeldt, M.L. & Marban, E. Excitation contraction coupling in postischemic myocardium: does failure of activator Ca^{2+} transients underlie "stunning"? *Circ. Res.* 1990; **66**: 1268–1276.

41. Kusuoka, H. & Marban, E. Role of altered calcium homeostasis in stunned myocardium. In Kloner, R.A., Przyklenk, K., eds. *Stunned Myocardium.* New York: Marcel Dekker, Inc, 1993; 197–213.

42. Krause, S.M., Jacobus, W.E. & Becker, L.C. Alterations in cardiac sarcoplasmic reticulum calcium transport in the postischemic "stunned" myocardium. Circ Reïrations in oxidative function and respiratory regulation in the post-ischemic myocardium. *J. Biol. Chem.* 1989; **264**: 12402–12530.

43. Bertoni, A.G., Adrian, S., Mankad, S. & Silverman, H.S. Impaired post-hypoxic relaxation in single cardiac myocytes: role of intracellular pH and inorganic phosphate. *Cardiovasc. Res.* 1993; **27**: 1983–1990.

44. Stahl, L.D., Weiss, H.R. & Becker, L.C. Myocardial oxygen consumption, oxygen supply/demand heterogeneity, and microvascular patency in regionally stunned myocardium. *Circulation* 1988; **77**: 865–872.

45. Zimmer, S.D., Ugurbill, K., Michurski, S.P., Mohanakrishnan, P., Ulstad, V.K. & Foker, J.E., From AHL. Alterations in oxidative function and respiratory regulation in the postischemic myocardium. *J. Biol. Chem.* 1989; **264**: 12402–12411.

46. Zimmer, S.D. & Bache, R.J. Metabolic correlates of reversibly injured myocardium. In Kloner, R.A., Przyklenk, K., eds. *Stunned Myocardium.* New York: Marcel Dekker, Inc, 1993; 41–70.

47. Hofmann, P.A., Miller, W.P. & Moss, R.L. Altered calcium sensitivity of isometric tension in myocyte-sized preparations of porcine postischemic stunned myocardium. *Circ. Res.* 1993; **72**: 50–56.

48. Kusuoka, H., Koretsune, Y., Chacko, V.P., Weisfeldt, M.L. & Marban, E. Excitation-contraction coupling in postischemic myocardium: Does failure of activator Ca^{2+} transients underlie stunning? *Circ. Res.* 1990; **66**: 1268–1276.

49. Bolli, R., Jeroudi, M.O., Patel, B.S., DuBose, C.M., Lai, E.K., Roberts, R. & McCay, P.B. Direct evidence that oxygen-derived free radicals contribute to postischemic myocardial dysfunction in the intact dog. *Proc. Natl Acad. Sci. USA* 1989; **86**: 4695–4699.

50. Triana, J.F., Li, X.Y., Jamaluddin, U., Thornby, J.I. & Bolli, R. Post-ischemic myocardial "stunning": identification of major

differences between the open-chest and conscious dog and evluation of the oxy-radical hypothesis in the latter model. *Circ. Res.* 1991; **69**: 731–747.

51. Bolli, R., Patel, B.S., Jeroudi, M.O., Lai, E.K. & McCay, P.B. Demonstration of free radical gneration in "stunned" myocardium of intact dogs with the use of the spin trap α-phenyl N-tert-butyl nitrone. *J. Clin. Invest.* 1988; **82**: 476–485.

52. Bolli, R. Role of oxygen radical in myocardial stunning. In Kloner, R.A., Przyklenk, K., eds. *Stunned Myocardium.* New York: Marcel Dekker, Inc, 1993; 155–195.

53. Martens, P.R., Mullie, A., Calle, P. & van Hoeyweghen, T. Influence on outcome after cardiac arrest of time elapsed between call for help and start of bystander basic CPR: the Belgian Cerebral Resuscitation Study Group. *Resuscitation* 1993; **25**(3): 227–234.

54. Wilcox-Gok, V.L. Survival from out-of-hospital cardiac arrest. a multivariate analysis. *Med. Care* 1991; **29**(2): 104–114.

55. Ditchey, R.V. & Slinker, B.K. Phenylephrine plus propranolol improves the balance between myocardial oxygen supply and demand during experiments in cardiopulmonary resuscitation. *Am. Heart J.* 1994; **127**(2): 324–330.

56. Kircher, B.J., Topol, E.J., O'Neill, W.W. & Pitt, B. Prediction of infarct coronary artery recanalization after intravenous thrombolytic therapy. *Am. J. Cardiol.* 1987; **59**: 513–515.

57. Calif, R.M., O'Neil, W., Stack, R.S. *et al.* and the TAMI Study Group. Failure of simple clinical measurements to predict perfusion status after intravenous thrombolysis. *Ann. Intern. Med.* 1988; **108**: 658–662.

58. Manning, A.S. & Hearse, D.J. Reperfusion-induced arrhythmias: mechanisms and prevention. *J. Mol. Cell. Cardiol.* 1984; **16**: 497–518.

59. Hale, S.L., Lange, R., Alker, K.J. & Kloner, R.A. Correlates of reperfusion ventricular fibrillation in dogs. *Am. J. Cardiol.* 1984; **53**: 1397–1400.

60. Burney, R.E., Walsh, D., Kaplan, L.R., Fraser, S., Tung, B. & Overmyer, J. Reperfusion arrhythmia: myth or reality. *Ann. Emerg. Med.* 1989; **18**: 240–243.

61. Previtali, M., Klersy, C., Salerno, J.A. *et al.* Ventricular tachyarrhythmias in Prinzmetal's variant angina: clinical significance and relation to the degree and time course of S-T segment elevation. *Am. J. Cardiol.* 1983; **52**: 19–25.

62. Myerburg, R.J., Kessler, K.M., Mallon, S.M., Cox, M.M., deMarchena, E., Interin, A. & Castellanos, A. Life-threatening ventricular arrhythmias in patients with silent myocardial ischemia due to coronary artery spasm. *N. Engl. J. Med.* 1992; **326**: 1451–1455.

63. Hariman, R.J., Louie, E.K., Krahmer, R.L. *et al.* Regional changes in blood flow, extracellular potassium and conduction during myocardial ischemia and reperfusion. *J. Am. Coll. Cardiol.* 1993; **21**: 798–808.

64. Coronel, R., Wilms-Schopman, F.J., Opthof, T., Cinca, J., Fiolet, J.W. & Janse, M.J. Reperfusion arrhythmias in isolated perfused pig hearts: inhomogeneities in extracellular potassium, ST and TQ potentials, and transmembrane action potentials. *Circ. Res.* 1992; **71**: 1131–1142.

65. Levites, R., Banka, V.S. & Helfant, R.H. Electrophysiologic effects of coronary occlusion and reperfusion: observations of dispersion of refractoriness and ventricular automaticity. *Circulation* 1975; **52**(5): 760–765.

66. Naimi, S., Avitall, B., Mieszala, J. & Levine, H.J. Dispersion of effective refractory period during abrupt reperfusion of ischemic myocardium in dogs. *Am. J. Cardiol.* 1977; **39**(3): 407–412.

67. Priori, S.G., Mantica, M., Napolitano, C. & Schwartz, P.J. Early afterdepolarizations induced in vivo by reperfusion of ischemic myocardium: a possible mechanism for reperfusion arrhthmias. *Circulation* 1990; **81**(6): 1911–1920.

68. Rozanski, G.J. & Witt, R.C. Early afterdepolarizations and triggered activity in rabbit cardiac Purkinje fibers recovering from ischemic-like conditions: role of acidosis. *Circulation* 1991; **83**: 1352–1360.

69. Rozanski, G.J. & Witt, R.C. Alterations in repolarization of cardiac Purkinje fibers recovering from ischemic-like conditions: genesis of early afterdepolarizations. *J. Cardiovasc Electrophysiol* 1993; **4**: 134–143.

70. Marban, E., Robinson, S.W. & Wier, W.G. Mechanisms of arrhythmiogenic delayed and early afterdepolarizations in ferret ventricular muscle. *J. Clin. Invest.* 1986; **78**(5): 1185–1192.

71. Ferrier, G.R., Moffat, M.P. & Lukas, A. Possible mechanisms of ventricular arrhythmias elicited by ischemia followed by reperfusion: studies on isolated canine ventricular tissues. *Circ. Res.* 1985; **56**(2): 184–194.

72. Cerbai, E., Ambrosio, G., Porciatti, F., Chiariello, M., Giotti, A. & Mugelli, A. Cellular electrophysiological basis for oxygen radical-induced arrhythmias: a patch-clamp study in guinea pig ventricular myocytes. *Circulation* 1991; **84**(4): 1773–1782.

73. Coetzee, W.A., Owen, P., Dennis, S.C., Saman, S. & Opie, L.H. Reperfusion damage: free radicals mediate delayed membrane changes rather than early ventricular arrhythmias. *Cardivasc. Res.* 1990; **24**(2): 156–164.

74. Tosaki, A., Droy-Lefaix, M.T., Pali, T. & Das, D.K. Effects of SOD, catalase, and a novel antiarrhythmic drug, EGB 761, on reperfusion-induced arrhythmias in isolated rat hearts. *Free Radic. Biol. Med.* 1993; **14**(4): 361–370.

75. Hagar, J.M., Hald, S.L., Ilvento, J.P. & Kloner, R.A. Lack of significant effects of superoxide dismutase and catalase on development of reperfusion arrhythmias. *Basic Res. Cardiol.* 1991; **86**(2): 127–135.

76. Minezaki, K.K., Nakazawa, H., Shinozaki, Y., Ichimori, K. & Okino, H. The failure of radical scavengers to attenuate the incidence of reperfusion arrhythmias despite improvement of cardiac function. *Heart Vessels* 1992; **7**(1): 31–36.

77. Heusch, G. Alpha-adrenergic mechanisms in myocardial ischemia. *Circulation* 1990; **81**(1): 1–13.

78. Linz, W., Wiemer, G. & Scholkens, B.A. ACE-inhibition induces NO-formation in cultured bovine endothelial cells and protects isolated ischemic rat hearts. *J. Mol. Cell. Cardiol.* 1992; **24**(8): 909–919.

79. Baxter, G.F. & Yellon, D.M. Attenuation of reperfusion-induced ventricular fibrillation in the rat isolated hypertrophied heart by preischemic diltiazem treatment. *Cardiovasc. Drug Ther.* 1993; **7**: 225–231.

80. Kusama, Y., Hearse, D.J. & Avkiran, M. Diabetes and susceptibility to reperfusion-induced ventricular arrhythmias. *J. Mol. Cell. Cardiol.* 1992; **24**: 411–421.

81. Tani, M. & Neely, J.R. Deleterious effects of digitalis on reperfusion-induced arrhythmias and myocardial injury in ischemic rat hearts: possible involvements of myocardial Na$^+$ and Ca^{2+} imbalance. *Basic Res. Cardiol.* 1991; **86**: 340–354.

82. McKenna, W.J. & Haywood, G.A. The role of ACE inhibitors in the treatment of arrhythmias. *Clin. Cardiol.* 1990; 13(6; Suppl 7):VII49–VII52.

83. Pasnani, J.S. & Ferrier, G.R. Differential effects of glyburide on premature beats and ventricular tachycardia in an isolated tissue model of ischemia and reperfusion. *J. Pharmacol. Exp. Ther.* 1992; **262**(3): 1076–1084.

84. Tosaki, A., Szerdahelyi, P., Engelman, R.M. & Das, D.K. Potassium channel openers and blockers: do they possess proarrhythmic or antiarrhythmic activity in ischemic and reperfused rat hearts? *J. Pharmacol. Exp. Ther.* 1993; **267**(3): 1355–1362.

85. Arnsdorf, M.F. The effect of antiarrhythmic drugs on triggered sustained rhythmic activity in cardiac Purkinje fibers. *J. Pharmacol. Exp. Ther.* 1977; **201**: 689–700.

86. Rosen, M.R. & Danilo, P. Effects of tetrodo-toxin, lidocaine, verapamil and AHR-2666 on oubain-induced delayed afterdepolarizations in canine Purkinje fibers. *Circ. Res.* 1980; **46**: 117–124.

87. Becker, L.C., Schaper, J., Jeremy, R. & Schaper, W. Severity of ischemia determines the occurrence of myocardial reperfusion injury. *Circulation* 1991; **84**:(Suppl II):II–254.

88. Litt, M.R., Jeremey, R.W., Weisman, H.F., Winkelstein, J.A. & Becker, L.C. Neutrophil depletion limited to reperfusion reduces myocardial infarct size after 90 minutes of ischemia: evidence for neutrophil-mediated reperfusion injury. *Circulation* 1989; **80**: 1816–1827.

89. Aversano, T., Zhou, W., Nedelman, M., Nakada, M. & Weisman, H. A chimerid IgG4 monoclonal antibody directed against CD18 reduces infarct size in a primate model of myocardial ischemia and reperfusion. *J. Am. Coll. Cardiol.* 1995; **25**: 781–788.

90. Forman, M.B., Puett, D.W., Wilson, B.H. *et al.* Beneficial long-term effect of intracoronary perfluorochemical on infarct size and ventricular function in a canine reperfusion model. *J. Am. Coll. Cardiol.* 1987; **9**: 1082–1090.

91. Jolly, S.R., Kane, W.J., Bailie, M.B., Abrams, G.D. & Lucchesi, B.R. Canine myocardial reperfusion injury: its reduction by the combined administration of superoxide dismutase and catalase. *Circ. Res.* 1984; **54**: 277–285.

92. Kompala, S.D., Babbs, C.F. & Blaho, K.E. Effect of deferoxamine on late deaths following CPR in rats. *Ann. Emerg. Med.* 1986; **15**(4): 405–407.

93. Kloner, R.A. & Przyklenk, K. Experimental infarct size reduction with calcium channel blockers. *J. Am. Coll. Cardiol.* 1991; **18**: 876–878.

94. Olfson, B., Forman, M.B., Puett, D.W. *et al.* Reduction of reperfusion injury in the canine preparation by intracoronary adenosine: importance of the endothelium and the no-reflow phenomenon. *Circulation* 1987; **76**: 1135–1145.

95. DeGraeff, P.A., van Gilst, W.H., Bel, K., de Langen CDF, Kingma, J.H. & Wesseling, H. Concentration-dependent protection by captopril against myocardial damage during ischemia and reperfusion in a closed chest pig model. *J. Cardiovacs. Pharmacol.* 1987; **9**(Suppl 2): 537–542.

96. Flaherty, J.T., Pitt, B., Gruber, J.W. *et al.* Recombinant human superoxide dismutase (h-SOD) fails to improve recovery of ventricular function in patients undergoing coronary angioplasty for acute myocardial infarction. *Circulation* 1994; **89**: 1982–1991.

97. Wall, T.C., Califf, R.M., Blankenship, J. *et al.* Intravenous fluosol in treatment of acute myocardial infarction: results of the thrombolysis and angioplasty in myocardial infarction 9 trial. *Circulation* 1994; **90**: 114–120.

98. Bevilacqua, M.P. Endothelial-leukocyte adhesion molecules. *Ann. Rev. Immunol.* 1991; **11**: 767–804.

99. Przykleuk, K. & Kloner, R.A. "Reperfusion injury" by oxygen-derived free radicals? Effect of superoxide dismutase plus catalase, given at the time of reperfusion, on myocardial infarct size, contractile function, coronary microvasculature, and regional blood flow. *Circ. Res.* 1989; **64**: 86–96.

ADDITIONAL READINGS

1. Bolli, R., Jeroudi, M.O., Patel, B.S. *et al.* Marked reduction of free radical generation and contractile dysfunction by antioxidant therapy begun at the time of reperfusion: evidence that myocardial "stunning" is a manifestation of reperfusion injury. *Circ. Res.* 1989; **65**: 607–622.

2. Coronar, R., Wilms-Schopman, F.J., Opthof, T., Cinca, J., Fiolet, J.W. & Janse, M.J. Reperfusion arrhythmias in isolated perfused pig heart: inhomogeneities in extracellular potassium, ST and TQ potentials, and transmembrane action potentials. *Circ. Res.* 1992; **71**: 1131–1142.

3. Hariman, R.J., Louie, E.K., Krahmer, R.L. *et al.* Regional changes in blood flow, extracellular potassium and conduction during myocardial ischemia and reperfusion. *J. Am. Coll. Cardiol.* 1993; **21**: 798–808.

4. Whittaker, P., Boughner, D.R., Kloner, R.A. & Przyklenk, K. Stunned myocardium and myocardial collagen damage: differential effects of single and repeated occlusion. *Am. Heart J.* 1991; **131**: 434.

5. Zhao, M.J., Zhang, H., Robinson, T.F., Factor, S.M., Sonnenblick, E.H. & Eng, C. Profound structural alterations in the extracellular collagen matrix in postischemic dysfunctional ("stunned") but viable myocardium. *J. Am. Coll. Cardiol.* 1987; **6**: 1322–1334.

Visceral organ ischemia and reperfusion in cardiac arrest

Kevin R. Ward and Andreas W. Prengel

Department of Emergency Medicine Virginia Commonwealth University and Virginia Commonwealth University Reanimation Engineering Shock Center
Department of Anesthesiology, Critical Care Medicine and Pain Therapy, Ruhr University Hospital, Bochum, Germany

During CPR, therapy focuses primarily on restarting the arrested heart and ensuring cerebral perfusion. For the splanchnic and renal circulation, the period of CPR represents a time of very low perfusion. When vasopressors are given during CPR in order to increase vital organ perfusion, splanchnic and renal blood flow may come close to zero.[1,2]

Negovsky[3] and Safar[4] have long maintained that self-intoxication from visceral organ ischemia as a result of cardiac arrest delays or prevents full neurologic recovery and may be a secondary cause of neuronal injury. Nevertheless, the effects of visceral organ ischemia and reperfusion (I/R) on the postresuscitation syndrome, which is characterized by a systemic inflammatory response similar to that observed in other systemic inflammatory conditions such as sepsis,[5] are not fully understood.

In the non-cardiac arrest setting, the two major directions of research on visceral organ ischemia are the contribution of individual visceral organs to development of secondary organ dysfunction and multiple organ failure; and studies of visceral organ injury, surgery, or transplant-ation resulting in or requiring ischemia. This chapter reviews the mechanisms of ischemia and reperfusion injury of the visceral organs; puts them in the context of cardiac arrest, the period of resuscitation (CPR), and the postresuscitation period; and considers how visceral organ ischemia may contribute to the postresuscitation syndrome.

Splanchnic circulation

Splanchnic circulation refers to the vasculature that brings blood to and from the major abdominal organs including the liver, spleen, stomach, pancreas, and small and large intestine. The splanchnic vascular system is regarded as the major blood reservoir containing 20% to 40% of total blood volume, and making the splanchnic circulation the primary source for mobilizing blood during critical situations. While transient reduction of splanchnic perfusion may be life-saving under certain circumstances, splanchnic hypoperfusion may contribute to the pathogenesis of systemic inflammation and multiple organ dysfunction via several mechanisms, including I/R injury, increased mucosal permeability for endotoxins and bacteria, and activation of inflammatory mediators.[6]

Regardless of the organ studied, all organs share a similar complex response to oxygen deprivation from I/R. The relative contribution of ischemia versus reperfusion to the final injury is an area of great debate and is probably related to the period of initial ischemia.[7] If the ischemic insult is not severe enough to cause massive cell death resulting in organ failure, several mechanisms of injury are postulated to exist during the period of reperfusion that contribute to further damage.[8–11]. These involve complex molecular, neural, hormonal, and immunologic responses that cause secondary ischemic damage not only to the involved organ itself, but also to other organ systems (Fig. 15.1). The degree of contribution of each of these mechanisms is unknown and likely varies among organs.

Intestines

The mesenteric circulation receives 10% to 15% of the body's normal cardiac output, which provides a resting intestinal blood flow ranging between 50 and 70 ml/min/ 100 g of tissue.[12] The mucosal and submucosal layers receive about

Cardiac Arrest: The Science and Practice of Resuscitation Medicine. 2nd edn., ed. Norman Paradis, Henry Halperin, Karl Kern, Volker Wenzel, Douglas Chamberlain. Published by Cambridge University Press. © Cambridge University Press, 2007.

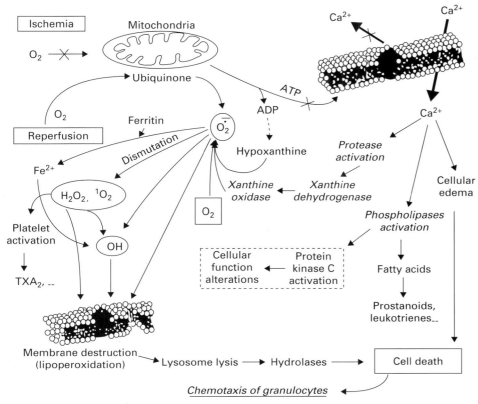

Fig. 15.1. General scheme of biochemical events responsible for I/R cellular damage. Extent to which each of the mechanisms is responsible for damage is unknown. Complex interaction of cytokines not shown. (From Pincemail J- Biochemical alterations in ischemia and reperfusion, In Vincent, J.L., ed. Yearbook of intensive care and emergency medicine. Berlin: Springer-Verlag, 1992:104. Copyright Springer-Verlag; Gmbh & Co, KG.)

70% of this flow, and the muscularis and submucosal layers receive the rest.[12] Regulation of mesenteric flow is complex: beside metabolic and myogenic control, intricate neural and hormonal factors affect flow.[13] Activation of both neural and systemic circulating humoral vasoconstrictors results in disproportionate vasoconstriction of the splanchnic vascular bed, which, although helping to redistribute blood to the heart, brain, and kidneys, causes selective splanchnic ischemia itself.[14,15] Table 15.1 lists a number of these agents.

Of particular interest are the vasoactive peptides vasopressin and angiotensin II. Vasopressin primarily affects the splanchnic resistance vasculature, with the response being disproportionately greater than that of the systemic vasculature.[14,15] Receptors for the potent vasoconstrictor angiotensin II exist on splanchnic vascular smooth muscle. The splanchnic circulation is hypersensitive to non-pharmacologic levels of angiotensin II compared to the rest of the circulation,[12,13] as demonstrated by studies of shock.[14,15]

The main findings from studies of intestinal ischemia are more easily interpreted if the severity and duration of the insult to the intestine are known. Studies have revealed that oxygen extraction is maintained when flow is kept above a critical level (about 25 ml/min/per 100 g tissue).[16,17] Because of compensatory mechanisms, even 2-hour reductions in flow result in little or no detectable injury as long as O_2 consumption is maintained above 50% of normal.[17] When ischemic damage occurs, it begins at the villous layer of the mucosa. For any given reduction in blood flow, mucosal hypoxia is amplified because of the countercurrent exchange of oxygen at the base of the villus. This mechanism results in the villous base remaining oxygenated at the expense of the tip of the villus.[16,18]

Few studies have examined the response of high-energy phosphates to levels of I/R and correlated them with degree of histologic damage. One study with phosphorus 31 (^{31}P) magnetic resonance spectroscopy reported complete loss of phosphocreatine and adenosine triphosphate

Table 15.1. Effects of vasoconstrictor agents on splanchnic circulation

Agent	Dose	Action*	Significance
Autonomic nervous system			
Sympathomimetics			Mediates non-selective arteriolar vasoconstriction
Norepinephrine	0.01-1.0 μg/kg/min	1	Mediates ambient arteriolar tone
Epinephrine	0.1-1.0 μg	1	(does not mediate selective vasoconstriction)
Dopamine	5-20 μg/kg/min	1	Mediates postcapillary venous vasconstriction
Sympatholytics (propranolol)	0.1 μg/kg bolus	2	Blocks ambient β-vasodilator tone
Parasympatholytics (atropine)	50 μg/kg bolus	2	Blocks ambient cholinergic vasodilator tone
Parasympathomimetics			
Physostigmine	0.15-0.9 μg/kg/min	2	Blood flow reduction 2% to muscular contraction
Vasoconstrictor peptides			
Vasopressin	0.7-50 mU/kg	1	Potent, selective, important to shock
Angiotensin II	0.01-0.05 μg/kg/min	1	Very potent, highly selective, primary mediator of selective splanchnic vasoconstriction
Gastrointestinal polypeptides			
Vasoactive intestinal peptide	1.75-175 ng/min	?2	Many act via renin release
Glucagon	50 μg/kg/hr	?	Usually a dilator; may act as a constrictor
Miscellaneous peptides			
Prolactin	0.6 μg/hr	?	Unknown
Thyrotropin releasing hormone	2 mg/kg	?	Unknown
Arachidonic acid metabolites			
Prostaglandin F_{2a}	12.5-50 μg/min	1	Potent, selective
Prostaglandin B_2	12.5-50 μg/min	1	Selective
Prostaglandin D_2	0.1-0.3 μg bolus	1	Selective
Thromboxane (U46619)	0.01-0.1 μg bolus, i.a.	?	Selective
Leukotrienes C_4 and D_4	0.3-3.0 μg bolus, i.a.	?	Selective
Indomethacin	8 mg/kg bolus	2	Blocks ambient vasodilator tone
Aspirin	100 mg/kg bolus	2	Effect caused by prostaglandins
Meclofenamate	2$$		
Digitalis glycosides			
Ouabain	5 μg/min	1	Potent, selective
Digoxin	50 μg/kg bolus	1	Role in non-occlusive mesenteric ischemia
Serotinin	30-100 μg/kg/min	?1	Unknown

From Reilly, P.M., Bulkley, G.B. Vasoactive mediators and splanchnic perfusion. *Crit. Care Med.* 1993; **21**(2): S60.
* 1, primary; 2, secondary.

(ATP) after 20 minutes of ischemia, with significant recovery after 60 minutes of reperfusion.[19] In contrast, direct biopsies revealed that complete ischemia reduced ATP levels to 40% of baseline after 30 minutes, with no further depletion even after 120 minutes.[20] The reasons for these discrepancies are unclear. The exact role of high-energy phosphate depletion in the final amount of tissue damage remains to be elucidated. Since studies show histologic damage within 10 minutes of ischemia and that damage is reversible after 60 minutes of complete ischemia, this suggests that high-energy phosphate loss is only one of many factors contributing to I/R injury.[16]

As with other organs, it is likely that further damage to the intestine is caused after return of blood flow and that this injury is affected, at least in part, by generation of oxygen free radicals. Nevertheless, the functional importance of the injury that occurs during reperfusion is unclear. If ischemia times are 1 hour or more, injury from the initial insult may be so severe that no further exacerbation can occur.[18] There appears to be a window of time during which reperfusion contributes to total organ damage (Fig. 15.2).

Much attention has been given to the role of xanthine oxidase in I/R injury of the intestine. The intestinal mucosa is one of the richest sources of its precursor, xanthine dehydrogenase.[9] There is no doubt that the oxidase can produce toxic free radical species, but it is unclear if these species directly harm the cell. Rather, the enzyme and the free radicals it produces may act mainly as chemotoxins in recruiting polymorphonuclear white blood cells (PMNs) that promote the major portion of free radical damage (Fig.15.3).[9] Studies reveal that intestinal xanthine dehydrogenase is converted to the oxidase between 1 and 120 minutes of intestinal ischemia.[9, 21] Administration of allopurinol prevents reperfusion injury when given before ischemia or when reperfusion is initiated.[9,10] It was assumed that allopurinol acts by competitively inhibiting xanthine oxidase. Nevertheless, some studies indicate that allopurinol may reduce damage by acting as a free radical scavenger itself or by stabilizing mitochondrial membranes.[22]

Although lipid peroxidation by free radicals is implicated as a cause of intestinal I/R injury, it is unclear if its inhibition will prevent injury to the intestinal mucosa. In rats treated with U74389F no decrease in mucosal damage was detected.[9, 22, 23]

The role of the PMN is currently under investigation as a cause not only of injury to the intestine itself during I/R, but also of subsequent injury to distant organs.[24] PMNs are capable of producing free radicals as well as proteolytic enzymes, such as elastase, in the intestine in response to I/R. What triggers this response of PMNs already in the intestine and subsequent sequestration of additional PMNs from the systemic circulation is unclear. Free radicals produced by xanthine oxidase and lipid peroxidation as

well as substances produced by phospholipase A_2 may act as potent chemoattractants and chemoactivators of PMNs.[9,25] This influx of PMNs and release of their toxins increase microvascular permeability and dysfunction of the mucosal barrier of the intestine.[11,25, 26] The mechanisms underlying PMN adhesion in the intestine are unknown but may involve complement and the selectin family of glycoproteins. Antagonism of PMN elastase with secretory leukocyte protease inhibitor (SLPI) and inhibition of activation and adhesion with IL-1ra and tumor necrosis factor (TNF) binding protein do not prevent local intestinal injury after 60 minutes of ischemia and 4 hours of reperfusion.[25]

Activation of phospholipase A_2 in the ischemic intestine may also cause reperfusion injury.[9] When inhibitors of this enzyme, such as quinacrine and hydrocortisone, are used, some studies showed decreased damage and others showed no change.[23]

The role of nitric oxide (NO) in I/R injury of the intestine is also unclear. Exogenous sources of NO, such as nitroprusside and L-arginine, are found to reduce I/R-induced intestinal permeability. This occurs even though NO does not increase intestinal blood flow. NO may counter superoxide and reduce PMN-mediated injury.[27]

Toxic factors in the lumen are also implicated in causing intestinal injury during ischemia.[28] Hydrochloric acid, bile salts, proteases, and lipases normally secreted during digestion are likely to induce further injury to the mucosa. Studies in which the pancreatic duct is ligated or protease

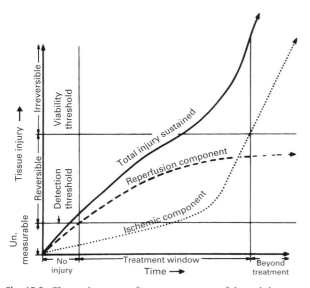

Fig. 15.2. Theoretic curves of two components of tissue injury (ischemia and reperfusion). Therapy directed at free radical–mediated reperfusion injury will not be effective at a certain point of ischemia. (From Hoshmo, T., Maley, W.R., Bulkley, G.B., Williams, G.M. Ablation of free radical–mediated reperfusion injury for the salvage of kidneys from non-heartbeating donors–Transplantation 1988;45:288.)

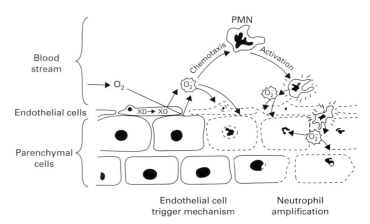

Fig. 15.3. Both parenchyma and endothelial cells produce free radicals via xanthine oxidase that attract neutrophils. Neutrophils in turn amplify injury by producing various free radicals and enzymes. (From Bulkey GB: Mediators of splanchmic organ injury: overview and perspective. In: Marston, A., Bulkey, G.B., Fiddian-Green, R.G., Hagland, U.H., eds. Splanchnic ischemia and multiple organ failure. Copyright 1989 by Adrian Marston, Gregory, B. Bulkey, Richard, G., Fidden-Green, Ulf H. Hagland Reproduced by permission of Hodder & Stoughton Ltd., London.)

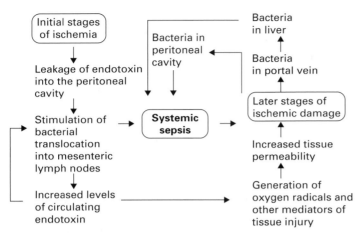

Fig. 15.4. Hypothesis outlining relationship among mild and acute mesenteric ischemia, bacterial translocation, and systemic sepsis. (From Wells, C.L., Maddans, M.A., Simmons, R.L., Bacterial translocation. In: Marston, A., Bulkley, G.B., Fiddian-Green, R.G., Haglund, U.H., eds., Splanchnic ischemia and multiple organ failure. (Copyright @ 1989 by Adrian Marston, Gregory, B., Bulkley, Richard, G., Fiddian-Green, Ulf H., Haglund. Reproduced by permission of Hodder & Stoughton Ltd., London.)

inhibitors are administered intraluminally showed reduced injury to the intestine during ischemia.[28]

Bacterial overgrowth is commonly observed in states of ischemia. Under normal conditions several mechanisms keep more than 500 species of bacteria in the intestinal tract and not in the systemic circulation.[29] These mechanisms include the resident mesenteric lymph nodes and PMNs in the intestine, as well as the Kupffer cell system of the liver and the alveolar macrophage system of the lungs.[29,30] The mechanisms operate in series, and thus there are several opportunities to remove intestinal toxins before they reach the systemic circulation. Both aerobic and anaerobic species are capable of producing various toxins, with the majority of gastrointestinal infections caused by aerobic organisms. *Enterobacteriaceae* organisms release the endotoxin lipopolysaccharide, which can produce profound local and systemic effects. Despite normal defenses, intestinal ischemia is known to promote translocation of bacteria and endotoxin from the intestine to the systemic circulation.[29,31] Endotoxin can also be recovered in the peritoneal cavity, suggesting an additional mechanism of translocation. It is thought that in the early stages of ischemia, intestinal permeability increases, which allows molecules such as endotoxin (but not bacteria) to leak into the peritoneal cavity. Such endotoxins potentiate translocation of intestinal bacteria into mesenteric lymph nodes, which results in increasing levels of circulating endotoxin. These levels further raise the rate of

bacterial translocation into mesenteric lymph nodes, because they are potent activators of inflammation, which increases permeability. Endotoxin also stimulates macrophage-released cytokines. This activates PMNs to adhere to endothelium and by diapedesis and phagocytosis to detroy bacteria by lysosomal production of free radicals and non-oxidative enzymes.

The exact role of endotoxin in PMN priming is not known; indeed, it may not be needed.[32] Free radical production is usually counteracted by the scavenger superoxide dismutase (SOD) also produced by the PMN. Although this usually occurs only intracellularly at the infection site, when massive and persistent endotoxemia persists, free radical production overcomes SOD protection.[30] This in turn leads to an out of control inflammatory response in multiple organs and finally to tissue destruction and dysfunction. In the intestines, increased destruction of the mucosal barrier evolves,[29–31] which facilitates escape of bacteria directly through the damaged mucosa and through the portal vein into the liver. Injury caused by toxins, bacteria, and proteases may well depend on the extent and duration of the ischemic period. This general theory is outlined in Fig. 15.4.

Although the effects of intestinal ischemia of sufficient duration will obviously be most prominent in the intestine itself, extraintestinal consequences of such ischemia are now recognized. Ischemia insufficient to cause transmural intestinal infarction can nevertheless be devastating to other organ systems. Once the mucosal barrier is compromised, portal and systemic absorption of bacteria, endotoxins, digestive enzymes, and inflammatory mediators may take place, which is thought to be a major inciting factor leading to the systemic inflammatory response syndrome and multiple organ system dysfunction and failure. The intestines are now thought to serve as the "motor" for multiorgan dysfunction and failure in many forms of shock.[33]

Hepatic injury following intestinal I/R is characterized by acute increases in serum hepatocellular enzymes, reduction of bile flow, and PMN sequestration. After 120 minutes of intestinal ischemia followed by 60 minutes of reperfusion, hepatocytes are exposed to oxidant stress as demonstrated by increased levels of oxidized glutathione.[34] Nevertheless, lipid peroxidation products do not increase significantly despite increases in the number of PMNs, suggesting that hepatocellular injury is reversible in this setting. Moreover, sufficient intestinal I/R induces TNF and IL-1 production by the hepatic Kupffer system, which in turn activates various other mediators and PMNs.[25] Hepatocellular injury can be ameliorated by administering various free radical scavengers such as SOD and catalase. Rendering animals neutropenic or administering agents that inhibit activation and adhesion of PMNs as well as secretion of PMN elastase also decreases intestinal I/R-produced hepatocellular damage. I/R of the intestine also impairs Kupffer cell function, which enhances the toxicity of translocated endotoxin and bacteria.[35]

Intestinal I/R also appears to be very damaging to the pulmonary system by similar mechanisms. Circulating xanthine oxidase from the ischemic intestine has been shown to mediate sequestration of PMNs in the lung after intestinal I/R. Treatment with allopurinol decreases the level of circulating enzyme and results in decreases in pulmonary PMNs.[36,37] In addition, elevated levels of cytokines, eicosanoids, and other inflammatory mediators act as potent chemoattractants for PMNs. Neutropenia before intestinal I/R and treatment with SOD, catalase (CAT), SLPI, IL-1ra, and TNFbp reduce pulmonary capillary leak.[11,25,38] With the exception of TNFbp these treatments also reduce the level of PMN sequestration in the lungs. ATP levels in pulmonary endothelium were reduced when cells were incubated with plasma from reperfused ischemic intestine, but the mechanism is currently unknown. The time of peak ATP depletion correlates with the known time sequence of peak procoagulant activity, cytokine synthesis and release, and expression of the adhesion molecules.[39] The role of endotoxin in lung injury is unclear, but the effect may be indirect.[40]

Cardiac contractile dysfunction has also been demonstrated after periods of intestinal ischemia for only 20 minutes and reperfusion for 2 hours.[41,42] Left ventricular pressure is decreased, together with a right-ward shift in the left ventricular function curve and decreased responsiveness to Ca^{2+} perfusate. Allopurinol given before I/R prevents this dysfunction, providing evidence that free radicals played some role.[43] Prior treatment with pentoxifylline, which decreases PMN adhesion, also prevents dysfunction.[43]

Different end points have been used as a measure of intestinal ischemia, ranging from morphologic changes to functional changes in mucosal and capillary permeability. One hour of local hypotension (30 to 40 mm Hg) with blood flows of 5 to 15 ml/min/100 g tissue followed by 1 hour of reperfusion results in increases in capillary perfusion but no histologic damage even in the superficial mucosa.[10,16,44] With complete ischemia for 1 to 4 hours and 30 minutes of reperfusion, the degree of mucosal permeability and villous damage is proportional to the time of ischemia. Free radical scavengers given before treatment apparently fail to prevent the injury, which suggests that under these conditions the majority of injuries are not caused by reperfusion. Prolonged hypoperfusion with perfusion pressures of 25 to 35 mm Hg without reperfusion, however, causes villous tip necrosis, which is exacerbated by reperfusion at normal flows and can be prevented to a large degree by free radical scavengers.[45] In an in vivo perfusion model, Chiu et al. demonstrated that although complete vascular occlusion for 1 hour produced total destruction of villi, it took 4 hours of perfusion at 5 ml/min/kg to produce the same findings. Perfusion at 15 ml/min per kg for 4 hours produced no demonstrable histologic changes.[44] Rats subjected to intestinal strangulation showed transmucosal necrosis after 4 hours. The viability of the muscularis was largely preserved with antibiotics and fluids. This integrity of the bowel wall was largely maintained, and the mucosa eventually regenerated.[46,47]

In summary, the degree of injury appears to be related in large part to the duration and completeness of the initial ischemic insult. Complete occlusion produces the most rapid injury, from increased permeability at 30 minutes to complete loss of villi at 60 minutes to transmucosal necrosis and infarction at 4 hours. After complete ischemia of 1 hour, administration of free radical scavengers is not effective, indicating a window of therapeutic effectiveness.[47]

The recovery of intestinal mucosa after an ischemic injury is remarkable. After 45 to 60 minutes of complete ischemia, variable mucosal repair occurs within 3 hours of reperfusion, with only rare defects remaining at 24 hours. At 90 minutes of ischemia, mucosal repair at 18 hours is complete. No visual histologic difference from controls exists. Mucosal reconstitution takes place by migration of nearby mucosal cells to cover mucosal defects.[16,44,46,47]

Liver

Blood flow to the liver is supplied by the hepatic arteries and portal vein. The liver is probably susceptible to ischemic injury in part because 70% of its blood is supplied by venous effluent from the gut via the portal system. The liver contains 25 to 30 ml of blood per 100 g of tissue and, therefore, 14% of the total blood volume.[35] In shock, parallel drops in both arterial and venous portal flow occur, which probably reflect selective vasoconstriction of both the hepatic and mesenteric arterial vasculature mediated largely by an increase in sensitivity to angiotensin II.

Damage to the liver parenchyma is a combination of ischemic hypoxia, free radicals, lipid peroxidation, and inflammatory mediated injury if reperfusion is restored within certain time limits. The effects of these events on such responses as production of heat shock protein and programmed cell death are being vigorously studied.[11]

During complete ischemia, ATP levels drop to 25% of normal within the first 10 minutes. After 60 minutes of ischemia, ATP levels are decreased to 5% of control with no further decrease to 120 minutes, at which time the total adenine pool has decreased to 22% of control, and lactate levels reach 20 times control values. After 15 minutes of ischemia, followed by 120 minutes of reperfusion, ATP and lactate levels return to normal. After 60 minutes of ischemia, lactate levels are normalized after 120 minutes of reperfusion, but ATP levels are not completely restored. After 120 minutes of ischemia and 120 minutes of reperfusion, lactate levels decrease but do not normalize, and ATP levels only increase to 17% of control values.[48, 49]

The role of Ca^{2+} in I/R hepatic injury has been clearly demonstrated by marked reductions in hepatic I/R damage after administration of various Ca^{2+} channel blockers such as verapamil and diltiazem during warm I/R.[50] The exact mechanisms for this are unknown but probably involve a combination of blocking of Ca^{2+} channels that leads to a reduction in protease activation and free radical production, and to vasodilatory effects that improve reperfusion flow.

Large contributions to liver I/R injury are thought to be made by free radicals produced within the liver itself from hepatocytes, Kupffer cells, neutrophils, and the endothelium. Regardless of the source, evidence that free radicals cause damage is in part based on observations that glutathione (GSH), which is particularly abundant in the liver, is reduced during I/R. If GSH is experimentally depleted before I/R, hepatic damage is greatly exacerbated and products of lipid peroxidation are increased.[51]

In common with other organs, the molecular source of these free radicals has been debated. With loss of ATP during ischemia, these free radicals are thought to be produced from the activity of xanthine oxidase, although the rate of xanthine dehydrogenase conversion to the oxidase varies. In one study, up to 60 minutes of ischemia was necessary for conversion of 50% of the dehydrogenase to the oxidase.[52] Other investigators have found even smaller rates of conversion, raising the question of the importance of xanthine oxidase as a cause of hepatic cellular injury.[53] If indeed xanthine oxidase is produced in the liver and released, it might cause system injury by contributing to local PMN-induced injury and injury to distant organs.[9,10,36] Regardless of the source, administration of various free radical scavengers such as SOD and α-tocopherol decreases I/R hepatic damage, giving additional evidence that these reactive oxygen species are responsible in part for some of the hepatic damage and dysfunction caused by I/R.[54]

Lipid peroxidation occurs in the liver in response to I/R, as demonstrated by increases in products of lipid peroxidation.[55] These changes are ameliorated by administration of substances known to reduce lipid peroxidation such as α-tocopherol.[55] The total contribution of lipid peroxidation to the final damage is unknown.

PMNs, Kupffer cells, and the inflammatory mediator eicosanoids, peptide cytokines, platelet activating factor (PAF), and complement all appear to play a major role in hepatic I/R injury and are intricately related.[56,57] It is unclear whether they cause injury to the hepatocyte directly or via microcirculatory damage. It appears that I/R primes Kupffer cell-induced oxidant stress and also primes Kupffer cells and PMNs for increased production of oxygen free radicals by activation of the complement system.[57] PMN infiltration and adhesion in the liver also are apparently mediated by the complement system rather than the CD-18 mechanism since blockade of CD-18 receptor does not result in decreased neutrophil adhesion.[58] Complement depletion results in significantly fewer hepatic PMNs during I/R.[57] Superoxide radicals produced during I/R have also been shown to be responsible for PMN accumulation.[56] The damage done by PMNs in the liver is likely due to a combination of free radical and protease production and plugging of the microvasculature.[59]

PAF produced by Kupffer cells during I/R appears to be responsible for much of the late-phase hepatocellular damage by its ability to attract and activate PMNs. Endotoxin from intestinal I/R is thought to have a similar effect.[60]

Peptide cytokines, probably produced by I/R-activated Kupffer cells, are also likely to play a role in hepatic I/R injury. After 60 minutes of ischemia followed by reperfusion, TNF was produced and reached peak levels after 30 minutes. IL-6 was also detected, independent of TNF. Administration of TNF antiserum decreased hepatic damage from I/R.[61] TNF is known to cause production of PAF by Kupffer cells. The presence of endotoxin is not necessary for production of liver TNF.[61]

Irrespective of the degree of damage imposed by the above mechanisms, all affect the microcirculation. Whereas 60 minutes of flow-controlled reperfusion significantly reduces hepatocellular damage, pressure-controlled reperfusion causes massive cell death. By microscopic visualization, fewer sinusoids conducted flow during the pressure-controlled method, which depends entirely on intrahepatic vascular resistance. Thus reperfusion injury may simply represent more ongoing ischemia.[59]

The function of the reticular endothelium system is also greatly affected by ischemic injury; in the liver, hypoxia and acidosis can reduce clearance by this system by 20% to 25%.[35] This is important because the liver clears the portal vein, which drains the intestines. Since velocity of blood flow and tissue perfusion are inversely related to reticular endothelial system function, some injury other than hypoperfusion is at least partially responsible for its dysfunction. Depression of the reticular endothelial system in hepatic ischemia is probably multifactorial. Epinephrine, norepinephrine, angiotensin II, vasopressin, and cholinergic and histamine antagonists all decrease the phagocytic function of the system. Hepatic ischemia itself, depletion of opsonic glycoprotein fibronectin, and release of a reticular endothelial system depressant factor from other splanchnic sites have also been implicated.[35]

I/R injury to the liver is also thought to effect injury to distant organs, including the lung and heart. Several models have demonstrated that I/R of the liver itself of 60 minutes' duration can produce cardiac dysfunction,[60] possibly by mechanisms similar to those of the intestine. The lungs are also damaged by hepatic I/R injury, and this damage is likely to be mediated through PMN activation by a variety of mechanisms, such as production of TNF and PAF.[62,63]

The exact limits of hepatic ischemia are unknown and probably depend on whether other organ systems are concomitantly injured. In isolated hepatic ischemia of 30 minutes followed by reperfusion, no hepatic cell necrosis is detected at 24 hours. If ischemia is extended to 60 and 90 minutes, focal necrosis is seen, but the majority of the hepatocytes are intact. After 2 to 3 hours of complete ischemia, more than two-thirds of the liver is necrotic at 24 hours.[35,59] Hepatic parenchymal cells can regenerate via mitosis if not severely damaged.[35]

Pancreas

The mechanism of pancreatic I/R is much less clear than that of the intestines, liver, and kidney. As an exocrine and endocrine organ, even the structure of its microcirculation is controversial. The pancreas comprises about 98% acini by weight, which receive up to 90% of blood flow, whereas the remaining 10% of flow is directed to the islet system. The magnitude of total pancreatic flow (40 to 120 ml/min per 100 g tissue) is similar to that of the other splanchnic organs.[35,63] Blood flow and oxygen consumption of the pancreas are under complex neurohormonal control: blood flow can be severely reduced with vasoactive agents such as epinephrine, norepinephrine, dopamine, vasopressin, and angiotensin II.[13]

In models of hemorrhagic and endotoxic shock, the pancreas becomes disproportionately hypoperfused compared to other splanchnic organs, but it appears to be quite resistant to isolated ischemia per se for up to 1 hour. Hypoperfusion to 20% of control values appears to be tolerated,[63] probably because the pancreas can increase oxygen extraction by metabolic and myogenic autoregulation.[35] States of hypoperfusion that affect multiple organ systems

appear to place the pancreas at greater risk for ischemia, possibly by activation of the renin-angiotensin system.[13] Nevertheless, ischemic pancreatitis is not usually included in the picture of multiorgan failure.

The exact mechanisms whereby ischemia produces pancreatic injury and the part played by reperfusion injury are unclear. Among multiple etiologies suggested as causing ischemic pancreatitis are trauma, hypovolemia, splanchnic vasoconstriction, and hypercalcemia.[35] Intracellular release of lysosomal enzymes and zymogen hydrolases may speed up necrosis. Perfusion of the isolated pancreas with a perfusate high in amylase after a period of ischemia exacerbates damage.[35,63] Some involvement of free radicals in the I/R process is suggested by studies showing a decrease in I/R damage by administration of allopurinol.[35] Pancreatic proteases are known to be capable of converting xanthine dehydrogenase to its oxidase form. Protease inhibitors such as α_1-antitrypsin are probably overwhelmed during periods of ischemia when significant leakage from damaged cell membranes occurs. Other factors, such as TNF, may increase pancreatic edema.[35]

There appears to be little doubt that, regardless of the mechanisms, the microcirculation is adversely affected. Studies reveal better pancreatic function and less damage by optimizing the rheologic properties of the blood by hemodilution with agents such as dextran 62, thereby enhancing oxygen delivery to the pancreas.[64]

I/R damage to the pancreas likely affects distant organ systems such as the heart and lung in a manner similar to other visceral organs. Of particular interest is the release of a myocardial depressant factor that is thought to be produced from a compartmentalized protein by cathepsins. Zymogen granules and lysosomes are thought to release trypsin and cathepsins in response to hypoxia; in turn, trypsin activity promotes phospholipase A, causing further release of cathepsins. This myocardial depressant factor appears to compromise cardiac output, which further jeopardizes subsequent perfusion to the visceral organs.[35,65]

Kidney

Partial or complete I/R can disrupt the homeostatic and excretory function of the kidney. Much debate exists on the extent to which components of vascular changes, tubular obstruction, and tubular cell death and necrosis itself cause ischemic renal failure.[48]

As renal perfusion is decreased, blood flow shifts from the outer cortical nephrons to the medullary nephrons. The renal cortex depends primarily on aerobic metabolism with ketones, lactate, fatty acids, and glutamine as its primary fuel. The renal medulla, however, has a small amount of O_2-independent glycolysis,[48] as illustrated by the finding that renal cortical ATP levels fall by 65% to 75% within several minutes, whereas medullary ATP levels fall by 19% to 33% in the same period. Lactate increases up to 3.7-fold in the cortex, whereas it increases by up to 8.3% in the medulla, demonstrating the greater capacity of the medulla for anaerobic glycolysis.[48] Overall, during complete renal ischemia, ATP levels decrease to between 20% and 50% of control after 10 minutes but decline more slowly thereafter to between 13% and 30% of control after 40 minutes.

Review of the transplant literature indicates that the kidney may function normally after 60 minutes of warm ischemia followed by an additional 72 hours of cold ischemia. On final reperfusion, ATP levels are regenerated to various degrees, but these levels do not correlate closely with the total ischemic time. Consequently ATP content or adenylate charge itself at the end of the ischemic period has not been found to correlate with ultimate recovery of renal function. The ability to use ATP in critical functions after the ischemic period may be a more important indicator of post-I/R function.[66]

Mitochondrial swelling occurs at rates correlating with durations of ischemia up to 120 minutes and is attributable to increases in permeability of the inner mitochondrial membrane to electrolytes. It is reversible if ATP is added. After 2 to 4 hours of warm ischemia, however, swelling is not reversible, possibly because alterations in the phospholipid membrane increase the level of free fatty acids in mitochondria and inhibit electron transport.[48]

With loss of volume regulation by ongoing ATP depletion of the ischemic cell, free cytosolic Ca^{2+} is elevated from both extracellular and intracellular sources such as the mitochondria, and increased Ca^{2+} activates phospholipases and proteases that are involved in free radical production. Many models have shown improved renal tolerance and function to ischemia when calcium channel blockers are added before the ischemic insult or on reperfusion.[48]

With several exceptions, many studies have indicated that after 30 minutes of ischemia, xanthine dehydrogenase is converted to the oxidase in the kidney and during reperfusion as a result of sulfhydryl oxidation and Ca^{2+}-induced proteolysis and that the oxidase is an important source of the superoxide free radical.[67] The proximal tubular cells, as well as the endothelial cells, are a major source of oxidase-derived free radicals.[68] Administration of allopurinol confers protection presumably by inhibiting xanthine oxidase activity, although this has not been conclusively proven since allopurinol itself is a free radical scavenger.[69] Further, allopurinol is relatively insoluble at physiologic pH, raising doubts whether it has access to the xanthine oxidase in cells.[69]

On the basis of observations that inhibition by catalase and glutathione peroxidase causes larger increases in hydrogen peroxide production and reduced function in I/R of renal cells, it is thought that other radicals such as the hydroxyl radical also promote reperfusion injury.[68,70] Further, iron chelators such as deferoxamine have been shown to be protective, presumably by preventing hydroxyl radical formation by the Harber–Weiss reaction[68,70] The amount of damage caused by free radical–induced lipid peroxidation is unclear, but damage is decreased and function improved by administration of the 21-aminosteroid U74006F during reperfusion after 45 minutes of ischemia.[71]

The role of the PMN in renal I/R damage is less clear than that in the intestine and liver. PMNs can perturb the microcirculation by their adherence to endothelial cells and accumulation in the ascending vasa recta in the outer and inner medullas.[68,72] The addition of PMNs during perfusion of an isolated kidney after ischemia worsens functional and histologic injury. It appears, however, that these PMNs may require "priming" by such substances as lipopolysaccharide, phorbol myristate acetate, PAF, TNF, and interleukins. These primed PMNs may then be fully activated in the ischemic kidney by release of chemotactic phospholipid or other products of phospholipases, including leukotrienes or prostaglandins, that are released by the injured renal cell. Once activated, PMNs then may release free radicals, elastases, and other harmful substances that have been shown to cause significant degradation of the glomerular basement membrane. Nevertheless, some activation of unprimed PMNs within the renal parenchyma is likely to occur. These mechanisms may account in part for the high incidence of renal failure in the setting of relatively mild renal hypoperfusion.[72]

Phospholipase A_2 activity has been studied in the setting of renal I/R. Mitochondrial and microsomal phospholipase A_2 activity increases during ischemia, but cytosolic phospholipase A_2 does not. With reperfusion, phospholipase A_2 activity increases in all fractions. Since mitochondrial membranes are composed of 65% unsaturated fatty acids, they are good targets for phospholipase A_2.[73]

How all of these mechanisms affect glomerular hemodynamics is controversial. Production of eicosanoids by free radicals likely plays a role. PGE_2, $PGF_{2\alpha}$, 6-keto-$PGF_{1\alpha}$, and TXB_2 are produced by renal cells in response to exposure to free radicals and phospholipase A_2 activity resulting from Ca^{2+} influx.[74] In addition, a newly reported non-cyclooxygenase–produced prostaglandin, 8-epi-PGF$_{2\alpha}$, has been detected after I/R in the kidney.[74] These substances may increase arteriolar resistance, with resulting decreases in glomerular ultrafiltration. Although PGI$_2$ has hemodynamic effects opposite to TXB$_2$, increases in PGI$_2$ and PGE$_2$ may cause increases in cyclic adenosine monophosphate (cAMP) within the cells of the glomeruli.[75] This in turn may stimulate renin synthesis, with local formation of angiotensin and resultant extended renal hypoperfusion, long after the initial insult. Of interest, administration of atrial natriuretic factor (ANF) may increase PGI$_2$, thus altering the TXB$_2$:PGI$_2$ ratio to favor vasodilation rather than constriction.[76]

The role of NO in renal I/R is unclear. Whereas some authors have shown that it contributes to sustained ischemic renal failure and increases PAF, others think that it may have a protective effect by reducing vasoconstriction.[68]

Although evidence for reperfusion injury appears to be overwhelming, one model has demonstrated that ischemia with intermittent reperfusion actually reduces renal functional and morphologic damage.[77]

The role of the cytokines TNF and IL-1 that are increased after I/R of the kidneys is not fully understood, but they are likely to worsen function by augmenting both production of cyclooxygenase-mediated products and PAF and PMN adhesion. They seem to have a greater effect when renal I/R is accompanied by additional concurrent organ I/R. Administration of the immunosuppressant FK 506 before I/R reduces TNF and renal damage by an as yet unknown mechanism.[78] It is likely that a combination of humoral-mediated vasoconstriction, mechanical obstruction by vascular congestion (erythrocytes and PMNs), and endothelial and tubule cell swelling (by Ca^{2+} and free radical damage) is responsible for the observed low or no-flow phenomena in the kidney after I/R.[79]

Adrenal glands

Virtually no work has been performed on the mechanisms of adrenal I/R. Adrenal dysfunction can lead to cardiovascular collapse refractory to conventional treatments and also to electrolyte imbalances.[80,81] Cortisol and catecholamines act synergistically to augment vascular tone and myocardial contractility.[80,81] The majority of shock states produce increased levels of circulating cortisol, thus demonstrating an intact hypothalamic–pituitary–adrenal axis.[82] Circulating catecholamines are also increased, which likely represents an outpouring from the adrenal gland.[82] Apparently adrenal failure caused by various forms of shock is rare, possibly because the adrenal gland can preserve flow to itself secondary to the local action of adrenergic receptors and endogenous catecholamines on its vasculature.[83] When I/R damage occurs, it probably shares previously discussed mechanisms of damage.

Visceral organ ischemia in the context of cardiac arrest

Under the conditions of low systemic perfusion, blood flow to vital organs is maintained at the expense of the perfusion of visceral organs.[84–89] Despite a large capacity to increase oxygen extraction,[90] prolonged splanchnic ischemia results in increased mucosal permeability[91] and finally in tissue damage and necrosis. Increased mucosal permeability allows endotoxin and other bacterial products to pass through the gut wall into lymphatic and systemic circulation[92–94] and to cause injury to distant organs.[95] Multiple organ failure and death have been associated with such changes.[96, 97] Thus, long term survival after cardiac arrest is determined not only by the duration of circulatory arrest, but also by the ability to ensure adequate organ perfusion during CPR as well as during the postresuscitation phase.

While individual visceral organs can tolerate complete ischemia of 1 hour, in CPR models, the time from actual arrest to the time of beginning CPR ranges from beginning resuscitation immediately after arrest up to waiting 20 minutes thereafter.[98] Typical downtimes for models of pre-hospital cardiac arrest range from 7 to 13 minutes. The actual time of resuscitation to the point of return of spontaneous circulation (ROSC) also varies with the particular model, but the maximum time of no flow (downtime) and low flow (CPR) rarely exceeds 20 minutes before ROSC. Most models of CPR are studied within this time period in order to assess (*a*) the effects of a particular drug or CPR technique on cerebral and myocardial perfusion pressures and blood flow, (*b*) the rates of ROSC from a particular drug or CPR technique, and (*c*) the neurologic or cardiovascular function after ROSC in response to a drug or CPR technique or post-ROSC modality.

With regard to visceral organs, important factors in the context of cardiac arrest and CPR are the amount of blood flow during CPR, the impact of drug therapy during CPR on the splanchnic circulation, and possible development of systemic inflammatory response syndrome and multiorgan dysfunction similar to those of other shock states due to I/R. The most important question in this context is whether visceral organ I/R injury of cardiac arrest does affect outcome.

Visceral organ blood flow during cardiopulmonary resuscitation

Only a few cardiac arrest studies have been performed for specifically examining blood flow to visceral organs during or after CPR. Visceral organ blood flow is generally measured using radiolabeled microspheres. The technique is problematic during low flow for several reasons, the most pertinent of which is microsphere quantification. As flows get lower, the accuracy of quantifying microspheres also decreases. A minimum of 400 spheres per tissue sample is needed to achieve 95% accuracy with repetitive measurements.[99,100] This becomes a problem for visceral organs since their flow is particularly low during CPR. Dramatically increasing the number of injected spheres to achieve adequate microsphere deposition and accuracy to compensate for the low flow would increase expense and create problems in disposing of the animals after experiments because of radiation concerns.

In the few cardiac arrest studies in canine and swine models reporting intestinal blood flow, the durations of no flow before CPR ranged from 0 to 10 minutes.[100,101] Baseline blood flows have been between 20 and 60 ml/min per 100 g tissue; flows during standard external CPR without intervention were between 0 and 10 ml/min/100 g tissue. In efforts to enhance flow, use of interposed abdominal compression (IAC)-CPR did not increase blood flow compared to standard CPR;[102] with simultaneous compression ventilation (SCV)-CPR, however, intestinal blood flow was significantly increased when the abdomen was bound and no epinephrine was given, but it decreased to standard CPR levels over time. With SCV-CPR without abdominal binding but with standard dose epinephrine no significant increase in intestinal blood flow occurs.[103]. When SCV-CPR is combined with abdominal binding and epinephrine, no increase in intestinal flow over standard CPR is seen,[101] nor is flow increased with combined standard CPR and abdominal binding.[104]

Regardless of technique, blood flow decreases over time.[104] Administration of various vasoconstrictors such as epinephrine, phenylephrine, angiotensin II, and vasopressin not only failed to increase intestinal blood flow during CPR but, depending on the study and dose, further decreased intestinal blood flow compared to CPR alone.[103,105,106]

Perhaps the most compelling evidence of the limited improvement in intestinal blood flow during CPR is provided by studies by Linder *et al.* on the effects of vasopressin on organ blood flow during CPR.[105] In a 4-minute swine model of ventricular fibrillation cardiac arrest, open chest CPR only produced intestinal blood flows between 2 and 26 ml/min per 100 g tissue. Administration of epinephrine, 0.045 mg/kg, with continued internal massage did not increase blood flow. Administration of vasopressin, which increased blood flow to brain, heart, and kidney, resulted in significantly decreased blood flow to almost non-detectable levels in the small intestine.

In a closed chest cardiac arrest model in swine, after 3 minutes of CPR, blood flow to the small intestine was approximately 10 ml/min per 100 g during CPR before drug administration, and did not change after administration of epinephrine 0. 2 mg/kg. After administration of different doses of vasopressin (0.2, 0.4, or 0. 8 U/kg), intestinal blood flow was below 1 ml/min per 100 g tissue.[107]

The level of intestinal blood flow in the postresuscitation period has been investigated in only a small number of studies. Among factors likely to affect blood flow are pre-existing intestinal disease, length of arrest, amount and type of vasopressors used during CPR, and the state of the cardiovascular status on ROSC. In one study designed specifically to examine splanchnic and renal blood flow after CPR with epinephrine and vasopressin in pigs, blood flow to the small intestines was measured with radiolabeled microspheres and was not significantly impaired after 30, 90, and 240 minutes after CPR in comparison to pre-arrest control values.[108] In another study in pigs, blood flow through the superior mesenteric artery was measured with an ultrasound flow probe. After CPR, including the administration of either epinephrine 0.045 mg/kg, or vasopressin 0. 4 U/kg, superior mesenteric artery blood flow was significantly lower after vasopressin compared with epinephrine at 5 minutes after ROSC (332 vs. 1087 ml/min), and at 15 minutes after ROSC (450 vs. 1130 ml/min).[109]

Only a few measurements of liver blood flow during CPR have been reported.[101,103,104,108,110]. Baseline flows in these studies range between 40 and 50 ml/min per 100 g tissue, compared with between 0.1 and 10 ml/min per 100 g tissue during CPR. SVC-CPR with or without abdominal binding and epinephrine failed to increase hepatic artery blood flow compared to standard CPR.[101,103] Standard CPR with abdominal binding also did not increase hepatic blood flow.[103]

Postresuscitation hepatic blood flows after a 5-minute arrest without epinephrine were not depressed from baseline, whereas with longer periods of arrest, hepatic flows were significantly lower than prearrest baseline.[111] When hepatic blood flow was measured by means of a constant infusion of indocyanine green[108] or with a hepatic artery ultrasound flow probe[109] after 4 minutes of cardiac arrest, postresuscitation blood flow was not significantly different in animals that received epinephrine 0.045 mg/kg or vasopressin 0. 4 U/kg.

Pancreatic blood flow during CPR, including IAC- or SVC-CPR, has been measured to be, for all practical purposes, zero.[101–103,112]. Postresuscitation flows are significantly decreased from prearrest baselines after only 5 minutes of arrest without epinephrine administration.[110,111] With administration of vasopressors during CPR, pancreatic blood flow at 30 minutes after CPR is reduced by 50% with epinephrine, and by 70% with vasopressin, respectively.[108] It is not known whether postresuscitation blood flow is sufficient to meet the organ's demand.

In contrast to the other visceral organs studied, where blood flow is further reduced by administration of vasopressors during CPR, blood flow to the adrenal glands is increased. Adrenal blood flows during normal sinus rhythm have been measured to be between 140 and 500 ml/min/per100 g tissue,[83,102,108] and during CPR, flow decreased to between 5 and 128 ml/min per 100 g tissue. In a swine model of cardiac arrest, however, administration of epinephrine or angiotensin during CPR increased blood flow to normal sinus rhythm baseline;[83] administration of both agents decreased CPR blood flow to 50 ml/min per 100 g tissue. Simultaneously measured renal blood flows were very low during CPR and were further reduced after administration of epinephrine or angiotensin II or both agents. In a pig model of CPR, both vasopressin and epinephrine produced significantly higher medullary and cortical adrenal gland perfusion during CPR than did a saline placebo, but vasopressin resulted in significantly higher medullary adrenal gland blood flow when compared with epinephrine.[113] On ROSC, adrenal blood flow was substantially higher than in baseline controls despite lower than normal renal flows.[108] Thus, adrenal blood flow seems to be preserved during CPR with and without use of vasopressor drugs.

Renal blood flow during closed chest CPR of various durations without any vasopressors is between zero and 75 ml/min per 100 g of tissue as determined in both dogs and swine,[99,103,104,106,112,114–116] compared with baseline flows between 50 and 500 ml/min per 100 g of tissue. In all studies the flows produced by CPR are far below that required to meet the oxygen requirements of the kidney. IAC-CPR, vest CPR, and standard CPR with abdominal binding also failed to increase renal blood flow significantly compared to baseline CPR.[101–104,117] SVC-CPR performed with abdominal binding and without epinephrine administration[103] did show some increase in flow, but after 20 minutes flow returned to levels equivalent to standard CPR. Active compression-decompression CPR has been shown to increase renal blood flow over standard CPR, but downtimes in this study were very short. It is unclear

how long these increases can be sustained and whether these levels will prevent damage.[118]

Studies with various doses of vasopressors including epinephrine, angiotensin II, and vasopressin revealed that renal blood flow is significantly decreased or unchanged compared to CPR alone.[2, 106, 114–116, 119, 120] Linder *et al.* examined blood flows in a swine model of open chest CPR in the presence of angiotensin II and vasopressin.[105, 120] Baseline renal blood flow was 190 ± 77 ml/min per 100 g of tissue. With open chest CPR after 4 minutes of cardiac arrest, renal flows were reduced to between 17 and 25 ml/min per 100 g of tissue. When angiotensin was administered, renal blood flow decreased to 4. 6 ml/min per 100 g of tissue after 90 seconds and further decreased to 1.1 ml/min per 100 g of tissue after 5 minutes. When standard dose epinephrine was given, renal blood flow decreased from 17 ml/min/ 100 g of tissue to 14 ml/min per 100 g of tissue 90 seconds after drug administration and further decreased to 8 ml/min per 100 g of tissue. With vasopressin, blood flow decreased from 24 ml/min/per 100 g of tissue to between 14 and 19 ml/min/per 100 g of tissue 90 seconds after drug administration but increased to 34 to 40 ml/min/per 100 g of tissue 5 minutes after administration. Of note, these measurements were made during open chest CPR, which is a superior mode of reperfusion.

Few data exist on the postresuscitation renal blood flows after cardiac arrest. With prearrest baselines of 170 to 265 ml/min per 100 g of tissue and arrest times of 10 minutes, postresuscitation blood flows measured at 5 and 15 minutes after ROSC ranged from 17 to 90 ml/min per 100 g of tissue.[83, 100, 119] With arrest times of 4 minutes and administration of epinephrine 0.045 mg/kg, or vasopressin 0.4 U/kg, renal blood flow in pigs ranged from 450 ml/min per 100 g of tissue in control animals to 370 ml/min per 100 g (vasopressin), and 300 ml/min per 100 g (epinephrine) at 30 minutes after ROSC.[108] With arrest times of 5 minutes without vasopressors, post-ROSC renal flow is not depressed.[111]

On the basis of the available data, it does not appear that blood flow to the intestines, liver, pancreas, and kidney can be sufficiently increased by current CPR techniques and vasopressors. Current efforts to improve myocardial and cerebral blood flow with high doses of vasopressor agents will likely further reduce flow to these organs during CPR. Even open chest CPR appears to produce blood flows below those needed to reverse ischemia, especially if the descending aorta is cross-clamped.[2,120] Since with isolated visceral organ ischemia, most organs are tolerant for up to 60 minutes of warm ischemia, it does not appear that increasing visceral organ blood flow during CPR would be advantageous. It is probably more valuable to use techniques that shorten the duration of ischemia before ROSC, thus restoring visceral organ blood flow as soon as possible, even if these techniques further reduce visceral organ blood flow during CPR. The exception to this may be the use of pharmacologic agents that increase cerebral and myocardial blood flow at the expense of visceral flow after ROSC.

To summarize, the period of arrest before institution of CPR represents a time of complete ischemia. The period of CPR with or without administration of vasopressors represents a time of extremely low perfusion. Flows to the visceral organs during CPR, especially the intestines, liver, and pancreas, are likely to be close to zero for the most part, especially if vasopressors are needed. The ability to increase oxygen extraction in such extreme conditions is likely to be unhelpful during arrest and CPR since oxygen delivery to these organs is close to zero. The period of CPR should probably be considered additional complete ischemia time for the visceral organs.

In models of isolated visceral organ ischemia, organs experience periods of reduced flow on reperfusion for various reasons, but which may be largely the result of reperfusion injury. The time course for this decrease in flow during reperfusion has not been clearly delineated for each organ. In the limited reports of arrest times of 10 minutes, it appears that post-ROSC blood flow to all visceral organs except the adrenal glands is reduced. Whether there are periods of heterogeneous no-flow or very low flow in areas within the individual visceral organs on reperfusion after ROSC is not known.[121,122] The need for post-ROSC vasopressors and the body's natural response to shunt blood from the visceral organs to preserve flow to the heart and brain, however, may account for most of the decreases in post-ROSC blood flow to the visceral organs, rather than actual reperfusion injury in each individual visceral organ tissue bed. Recent clinical studies on global body oxygen delivery and consumption measured using lactate levels and mixed venous blood gas indicate that blood flow is not sufficient.[123,124]

It has been well documented in animals and humans that endogenous levels of epinephrine, norepinephrine, angiotensin, and vasopressin are all elevated during CPR and in the post-ROSC period.[125–127] Although these levels may not correlate with post-ROSC blood pressure or heart rate, the visceral organ vasculature is hypersensitive to these elevated endogenous levels, which may exacerbate microvasculature failure and increase I/R damage by jeopardizing oxygen delivery (DO_2) and oxygen consumption (VO_2). Further visceral organ I/R might be expected with the addition of exogenous vasopressors to maintain blood pressure.

Visceral organ damage from cardiac arrest

Organ dysfunction may cause considerable mortality and morbidity after restoration of spontaneous circulation. It was not until Cerchiari *et al.* examined the effects of visceral organ damage from cardiac arrest and CPR on neurologic outcome that there was any systematic attempt to examine visceral organ function after cardiac arrest.[128] This study was performed on dogs placed in arrest for periods of 7.5, 10, and 12.5 minutes. After resuscitation, all animals received standard postresuscitation intensive care and had various visceral organ functions as well as neurologic measures assessed up to 72 hours. Transient visceral organ dysfunctions were found in all groups, with most functions returning to normal over time. Although trends were noted, no correlations existed among arrest times, visceral dysfunction, and neurologic outcome.

Intestines

When systematically examined in the canine model of cardiac arrest with complete ischemia times of 7.5, 10.0, and 12.5 minutes devised by Cerchiari *et al.*, no alteration in cerebral outcome could be attributed to intestinal ischemia.[128] Each group contained 13 dogs. Despite negative blood cultures before arrest, all but five dogs at 6 hours after ROSC and all but two dogs at 24 hours after resuscitation had positive blood cultures. At 6 hours after ROSC, cultures were generally positive for a single organism whereas multiple organisms were found at 72 hours. Most organisms were enteric aerobic gram-negative bacilli, of which *Enterobacter* was the most common. When poor neurologic outcomes did occur in these animals, sepsis caused by bacteremia was not present. Histopathology of these animals 72 hours after ROSC revealed diffuse petechial hemorrhages in the mesentery and intestinal serosa in only one of nine animals arrested for 7.5 minutes and three of nine animals arrested for 12.5 minutes.

Although ulceration, intractable acidosis of intestinal origin, bloody diarrhea, and sepsis have been reported in the post-ROSC period, this does not appear to be a uniform problem.[124,129] Only one human study has specifically examined the incidence of intestinal dysfunction and failure as exemplified by bacteremia and diarrhea after cardiac arrest.[130] In this study, of 39 patients resuscitated from out-of-hospital arrest, 12 had fetid diarrhea several hours after admission and subsequently developed bacteremia with positive blood cultures for enteric organisms, including streptoccocus D, *Escherichia coli*, *Pseudomonas aeruginosa*, *Acinetobacter*, and *Enterobacter*, which were also recovered from the stool. Interestingly, the average dose of epinephrine given during the resuscitation did not differ between bacteremic and non-bacteremic groups (mean dose range, 9 to 13 mg). Both groups had similar CPR times of 6 minutes, but no estimate of downtimes before CPR was given. Although all patients who developed diarrhea died, none of these patients was thought to have died from sepsis. The results clearly provided evidence of ischemia-induced bacterial translocation. No comment was made, however, about the hemodynamic course and use of vasopressors in both groups after ROSC; therefore, it is difficult to know why some but not all patients developed diarrhea and bacteremia. In another study, gastrointestinal hemorrhage after in-hospital cardiac arrest was reported:[129] of 63 patients 25 developed some type of upper or lower gastrointestinal hemorrhage. These complications were not associated with increased mortality.

Liver

In the same canine ventricular fibrillation cardiac arrest model of Cerchiari et al., no permanent liver damage was detected histopathologically 72 hours after cardiac arrest.[128] Hepatocyte swelling and occasional centrilobular necrosis were seen, but this was not severe enough to impair liver function. Serum bilirubin and glutamyl-transpeptidase (GTP) levels were normal throughout the postresuscitation period in all three groups. Aspartate aminotransferase (AST) was significantly elevated up to 72 hours after arrest, whereas alanine aminotransferase (ALT) was significantly elevated in all three groups only up to 24 hours after arrest, but since these enzymes are not specific for liver damage, the elevations may have been due to myocardial injury. Ammonia levels were significantly elevated at 24 hours in the 10-minute arrest group but not at 72 hours; in contrast, the 12.5-minute arrest group demonstrated significantly elevated ammonia levels only at 72 hours. Animals that regained consciousness had significantly lower ammonia levels than those that did not, although the standard deviation was high. However, there were no significant differences in neurologic outcome between arrest time groups.

Interesting patterns in the amino acid profiles were noted in this model. The branched chain amino acids were significantly increased in dogs with poor outcome but were unchanged in those with good outcome. Although the aromatic amino acids increased in both groups, they were significantly higher in those animals with poor neurologic outcome. The branched chain:aromatic amino acid ratio was worse in animals with poor outcome. None of these

patterns, however, was significantly correlated with arrest times. In addition, the authors of this study point out that liver dysfunction cannot account for all of this imbalance since the elevated levels of aromatic amino acids (metabolized by the liver) were not accompanied by decreased levels of branched chain amino acids, which are utilized by skeletal muscle. These patterns of ammonia and amino acids were not reflected by worse neurohistopathology.

Only one clinical study examined hepatic function after in-hospital cardiac arrest.[129] In this study, 18 of 63 patients had some elevation of liver function tests. However, eight of these patients were in congestive heart failure before arrest and had some elevation of liver function tests at that time. An additional smaller number were found to have passive liver congestion on autopsy. It is therefore difficult to ascribe the abnormal liver function in this study to hepatic ischemia and necrosis from the ischemic time of the cardiac arrest itself. Since animal and clinical studies suggest that livers can be successfully harvested and transplanted from donors after cardiac arrest that involved warm ischemia times from 30 to 60 minutes, complete ischemia of moderate duration cardiac arrest apparently does not impose insurmountable injury.[131]

Pancreas

No formal animal or human studies have examined pancreatic function after cardiac arrest. Clinical pancreatitis has not been reported as a common postresuscitation complication. Up to 39% of pancreatic donors who have undergone some period of ischemia have hyperamylasemia.[132] Pancreatitis secondary to ischemia is, however, extremely difficult to diagnose.

An interesting finding that may have bearing on neuronal salvaging is that insulin production by the pancreas appears to be blunted in the early postresuscitation period. Whether this is secondary to the ischemia of cardiac arrest itself or to the exogenously administered epinephrine given during CPR is not known.[133]

Kidneys

When systematically studied in the canine animal model of Cerchiari et al., renal function is found to recover promptly after only transient periods of anuria and oliguria.[128] Histopathologic examination 72 hours after cardiac arrest in this model revealed scattered renal infarcts that were more consistent with iatrogenic emboli from indwelling catheters than ischemic insults. Blood urea nitrogen

(BUN), creatinine, serum osmolality levels, and serum electrolytes were all reported to be normal at 6 hours after resuscitation.

After CPR including the administration of vasopressors, in the postresuscitation phase neither urinary output nor calculated renal function indices differed significantly between animals after having received epinephrine or vasopressin.[109] Calculated glomerular filtration showed no difference between groups and calculated fractional excretion of sodium was elevated in both groups at 60 minutes after ROSC, with an ongoing elevation in the vasopressin group for 2 hours after ROSC. Relationship of osmolarity between urine and plasma was not impaired at any time point during the postresuscitation phase. In summary, with respect to renal blood flow and renal function after ROSC, there was no significant difference between either vasopressor given during CPR.

Only one study to date has specifically examined the prevalence of acute renal failure in humans following CPR;[134] 30% of patients who were resuscitated from in-hospital cardiac arrest developed acute renal failure. Analysis revealed that the group developing acute renal failure had a significantly longer duration of actual CPR (12 minutes vs. 7 minutes), although the estimated downtime before institution of CPR was not reported. It was also found that the group developing acute renal failure received larger doses of epinephrine (1.8 mg vs. 0.9 mg) and the frequency of preexisting congestive heart failure, coronary artery disease, and compromised renal function was significantly higher in this group. As expected, the group with acute renal failure had significantly worse long-term survival compared to the group without such failure (6.3% vs. 47.5%). More patients who recovered renal function had cardiac arrest secondary to ventricular fibrillation than did those who developed renal failure. The report does not mention which patients required post-ROSC vasopressor blood pressure support or what measures were taken to avoid postarrest renal failure. No study has reported post-ROSC electrolyte disturbances that could be attributed to renal I/R.

In contrast to the intestines and liver, preexisting renal insufficiency is common in cardiac arrest patients and thus is likely to affect renal outcome after arrest. Volume status and renal function are normal in virtually all current animal models of cardiac arrest, thus making these factors, which are common in the clinical setting, difficult to study experimentally unless altered by design.

Many examples exist in which kidneys have been successfully harvested and transplanted from non-resuscitated donors after cardiac arrest times approaching 60 minutes.[135] It appears therefore that complete ischemia from cardiac arrest of moderate duration does not impose an insurmountable insult to the kidneys if they were not significantly impaired before arrest

Adrenal gland

Adrenal function during cardiac arrest has recently been evaluated in both the laboratory and clinical settings. One study found that cortisol concentrations in human victims of cardiac arrest were lower than those reported in other stress states.[82] In this study there was an apparent association between cortisol levels and at least short-term survival from cardiac arrest. Increases in cortisol levels were observed by 6 hours after ROSC but not at 24 hours. Adrenocorticotropic hormone (ACTH) levels were increased, but they decreased 6 hours after ROSC. There was no significant response to cosyntropin stimulation at 6 and 24 hours, suggesting that low levels of cortisol may represent primary adrenal dysfunction, the etiology of which is unclear. Interestingly, increased levels of cortisol have been found in dying intensive care unit (ICU) patients and in patients who suffered cardiac arrest in the ICU and underwent immediate CPR.[136] In cases of sudden cardiac death, it is unlikely that cortisol levels would be increased before arrest. Even if the adrenal gland were capable of responding during CPR it is possible that the volume of distribution of the cortisol is too low, secondary to the low flow of CPR, and thus any advantage it would impose on the catecholamine response, for example, would be lost. Nevertheless, secondary causes of cardiac arrest may be preceded with stress states, such as cardiogenic shock or sepsis, in which the adrenal gland increases cortisol production and flow is sufficient to distribute it. In the study by Schultz et al., patients achieving ROSC tended to have higher cortisol levels,[82] as well as shorter arrest times, and more presented in pulseless electrical activity. Therefore the underlying etiology of the arrest may affect adrenal function and vice versa. Despite ROSC, many individuals did not achieve cortisol levels greater than 30 µg/dl in this stressful state, thus indicating some ongoing adrenal dysfunction after ROSC, possibly secondary to I/R damage caused by the prolonged downtimes and resuscitation times. Again no significant response to cosyntropin stimulation at 6 or 24 hours indicated some primary adrenal dysfunction, possibly in the form of a "stunned" adrenal cortex.

In a pig model of cardiac arrest including the administration of epinephrine 0.045 mg/kg or vasopressin 0.4 U/kg during CPR, ACTH and cortisol plasma concentrations were measured before arrest, during CPR before drug administration, and at 90 seconds and 5 minutes after drug administration.[137] ACTH and cortisol concentrations remained unchanged in epinephrine-treated animals, but increased significantly after administration of vasopressin and were significantly higher (12.5 μg/dl) than in epinephrine-treated animals 5 minutes after drug administration (5.5 μg/dl). Vasopressin is a potent stimulus for ACTH secretion during CPR. The increased plasma cortisol concentrations caused by the enhanced ACTH release after vasopressin may be one factor contributing to the improved outcome repeatedly observed with vasopressin in animal models of CPR.

Future models of cardiac arrest examining visceral organ I/R may require modifications to mimic the clinical setting more closely, such as longer downtimes and resuscitation times, larger epinephrine doses, and predetermined pauses between ROSC and institution of postresuscitation intensive care.

Relationship among visceral organ I/R of cardiac arrest, systemic inflammatory response syndrome, and multisystem organ dysfunction or failure

Although no exact numbers exist, some resuscitated patients will develop multiorgan dysfunction syndrome and failure, leading to death. This has been termed the postresuscitation syndrome.

The mechanism underlying this postresuscitation disease involves a whole-body-ischemia and reperfusion syndrome, and shares many features with systemic inflammatory response syndrome (SIRS) and sepsis, including plasma cytokine elevation with dysregulated cytokine production, the presence of endotoxin in plasma, coagulation abnormalities, and adrenal dysfunction.

The SIRS and resulting organ dysfunction represent a response to injury; four general events can incite this response: infection, perfusion deficits, inflammation, and dead or injured tissue. These inciting events may overlap. Free radicals, inflammatory mediators, immunologic factors, and neurohormonal factors all play a role in SIRS and its progression to MODS. These mediators are probably produced from the visceral organs as a result of the inciting events. The SIRS response generally reaches a peak in 3 to 4 days and abates in 7 to 10 days, and the patient recovers. If SIRS continues, however, MODS develops and may eventually lead to death.[11]

Drastic increases in mortality from 40% to as much as 100% may occur after the transition of SIRS to MODS. The postresuscitation response of an organ or organism after

any insult is based on multiple factors, including the severity of the initial injury, the patient's organ reserve, the time interval from insult to resuscitation, and the adequacy of resuscitation. Failure to control infection or correct perfusion deficits, for example, will convert a stable SIRS patient to one with MODS progressing to failure and death.[11]

Recently, TNF has been detected 6 hours after ROSC in patients resuscitated from cardiac arrest, indicating an inflammatory response and possible SIRS. TNF was not found in patients surviving less than 4 hours.[138] Patients surviving longer than 20 days in this study had no TNF detectable at 6 hours, although TNF did eventually appear. Patients surviving for more than 12 hours, but who died within 72 hours, had the highest levels.

In other models of shock and I/R, TNF has been found to reach a peak between 30 and 180 minutes after reperfusion.[139] The different time lags for detection of TNF between these states and the cardiac arrest study discussed above suggest that the stimulus for TNF may not be the initial ischemia time of cardiac arrest and CPR, but rather the postresuscitation course that follows ROSC. There is good evidence that derangements of oxygen delivery and consumption exist long after ROSC, and these may underlie the majority of visceral organ injuries that occur in the postresuscitation state.[123,124]

Cytokines and soluble receptors increase in the circulation as early as 3 hours after cardiac arrest. Plasma concentrations of interleukin-6 (IL-6) show greater elevations in non-survivors than in survivors and were higher in patients requiring vasopressor therapy. IL-6 and soluble TNF receptor II are closely correlated with plasma lactate concentrations, suggesting a relation among ischemia, reperfusion injury, and inflammatory responses. Elevated levels of plasma endotoxin within 2 days after successful resuscitation may be explained by translocation of endotoxin through sites of gut-wall ischemia. Increased soluble intercellular adhesion molecule-1, soluble vascular-cell adhesion molecule-1, and P and E selectins were found after successful CPR, suggesting neutrophil activation and subsequent endothelial injury in patients with SIRS, including patients after recovery from cardiac arrest, however, hyporesponsiveness of circulating leucocytes has been observed, and may allow protection against overwhelming dysregulation of the inflammatory process, but may also induce immune paralysis with an increased risk of subsequent infection.

The relationship between the SIRS progression to MODS of other shock states and that of cardiac arrest may depend on the etiology of arrest as well as postarrest events. Cardiac arrest from trauma or sepsis would likely have been preceded by some degree of SIRS. In addition, lung or liver trauma caused by CPR, infectious foci occurring secondarily, such as catheter-related infections or sepsis, and aspiration pneumonitis might induce SIRS not due to the primary ischemia. Because of these complex relationships, it remains questionable whether the primary ischemia of cardiac arrest itself, or cofactors in the context of CPR may induce a sepsis-like syndrome after successful resuscitation from cardiac arrest.

The oxygen debt incurred during the cardiac arrest itself is not likely to represent a lethal insult in producing postresuscitation mortality and the development of multisystem organ failure. Studies of critically ill surgical patients demonstrate little or no mortality from development of multisystem organ failure when oxygen debt is less than $4100\,ml/m^2$. Mortality increases to 50% and 95% when cumulative oxygen debt is $4900\,ml/m^2$ and $5800\,ml/m^2$, respectively.[140] In contrast, for a 70-kg individual with a baseline oxygen consumption of $120\,ml/min/m^2$, a 30-minute cardiac arrest would create an oxygen debt of $3600\,ml/m^2$. Postresuscitation hemodynamic derangements may cause further accumulation of oxygen debt to more lethal ranges.

The preponderance of evidence indicates that ischemia of cardiac arrest per se may not promote a systemic inflammatory response leading to the multiorgan dysfunction syndrome of the postresuscitation syndrome unless ischemia times are extremely prolonged. Rather, it seems more likely that protracted hemodynamic derangements, many of which may be iatrogenic in nature (often from neglect), in the post-ROSC period are mainly responsible.

Treatment

Little work has been performed specifically to prevent postresuscitation visceral organ damage. Therapies should probably be aimed at reducing injury at reperfusion and at preventing further I/R injury in the postresuscitation state, keeping in mind that the majority of visceral organ injury may occur in the post-ROSC phase. Several strategies aimed at stabilizing cells, inhibiting molecularly mediated damage, correcting derangements of oxygen transport, and reducing complications of visceral organ injury will be examined.

Prevention of free radical and inflammatory mediator injury

Since primary ischemia from most cardiac arrests is less than 1 hour, there is likely to be a window of opportunity for inhibition of various molecularly mediated causes of I/R injury. Many agents have been studied with the hope of limiting damage not only to the individual visceral organ itself, but also to distant organ systems.

Many potential antioxidant therapies have been proposed because they were used to demonstrate that a particular oxidant was responsible for the injury. In numerous instances, however, this required that the antioxidant be given before the ischemic insult or at the start of reperfusion. Consequently, although the antioxidant may have proved beneficial in these cases, extrapolation to the clinical setting of cardiac arrest has numerous problems. This again relates to the concept of a window of opportunity for these therapies to be effective (Fig. 15.2). No agent has been shown to make a clinically significant difference in outcome and is in routine use. Table 15.2 lists the exogenous antioxidant agents that may be useful in limiting visceral organ I/R damage. If the postresuscitation phase of cardiac arrest is considered a period of ongoing ischemia, administration of these agents may be helpful.

If antioxidant therapy becomes a clinical reality, its use in the cardiac arrest patient will require examination of dose-response curves and timing of administration. Administration during CPR would offer no advantage before ROSC, because of the short half-lives of many of these agents and because their distribution would be limited by the low blood flow to the visceral organs. On the other hand, sufficient concentrations of antioxidants in the circulation would permit their rapid delivery to the visceral organs after ROSC. Administration of these agents to patients who are immediately at risk for sudden cardiac death, such as those who present with an evolving myocardial infarction, might be of greater benefit. If the patient arrests and is resuscitated, antioxidant therapy will then be available for maximal effect. Even if these individuals do not arrest, many will develop a protracted and difficult course of cardiogenic shock, which will produce varied degrees of visceral organ I/R injury.

Other therapies with great potential include suppressing or blocking molecular mediators of the inflammatory response that lead to organ dysfunction, for example by altering the PMN-endothelial interaction, the arachidonic acid and eicosanoid response, the peptide cytokines, PAF, complement, and NO. The role of molecular mediators as inhibitors of visceral organ ischemia from cardiac arrest is purely speculative at this time. Figure 15.5 illustrates the points of action of many of the free radical scavenging agents.

In experimental models of sepsis and ischemia-reperfusion injury, isovolemic high-volume hemofiltration by using a synthetic high-cutoff membrane removes

Table 15.2. Exogenous antioxidants and antineutrophil agents with potential to decrease visceral organ I/R

Enzyme inhibitor	Species affected
Xanthine oxidase inhibitors	
Allopurinol	Xanthine oxidase
Oxypurinol	
Folic acid	
Pterin aldehyde	
Tungsten	
Other inhibitor	
Soybean trypsin inhibitor	Xanthine dehydrogenase
NADPH oxidase inhibitors	
Adenosine	NADPH oxidase
Local anesthetics, calcium-channel blockers	
NSAIDs	
Cetiedil	
CHIP	
Monoclonal abs to NADPH oxidase	
Superoxide dismutase	
Native SOD	O_2
IgA hinge-linked SOD	
PEG-SOD	
Liposome-encapsulated SOD	
SOD Mimics	
Cu^{2+} chelates	O_2
Desferal Mn	
Cyclic nitroxides	
Catalase	
Native catalase	H_2O_2
PEG-catalase	
Liposome-encapsulated catalase	
Other non-enzymatic free radical scavengers	
Mannitol	OH^-
Albumin	LOOH, HOCl
DMSO	OH^-
DMTU	OH^-, H_2O_2
Lazaroids	$LOOH_1$ O_2
Inhibitors of iron redox cycling	
Deferoxamine	Fe^{3+}
Ceruloplasmin	
Augmentation of endogenous antioxidant activity	
Oltipraz	
Ebselen	
Glutathione	
N-Acetylysteine	
Antineutrophil agents	
Antineutrophil serum	Neutrophil

Table 15.2. (continued)

Antiadhesion agents	Adhesion molecules
Monoclonal Abs to CD11/CD 18	
Soluble GMP 140	
Platelet-activating factor	PAF-dependent
Antagonists	adhesion molecules
BN 52021	
WEB 2086	

From Schiller, H.J., Reilly, P.M., Bulkley, G.B., Antioxidant therapy. *Crit. Care Med.* 1993; **21** (2) S97.

medium molecular-weight molecules responsible for ischemia-reperfusion injury. The potential effects of high-volume hemofiltration have been evaluated by randomizing 61 patients with out-of-hospital cardiac arrest into three groups: control patients and those with high-volume hemofiltration with or without hypothermia.[141] The 6-month survival curves of the three groups were significantly different, with better survival in the hemofiltration group and in the hemofiltration-hypothermia group. The authors of this study stated that definitive conclusions should await clinical trials in a larger cohort of survivors of cardiac arrest.

Oxygen delivery and consumption

Resuscitation of the cardiac arrest victim does not end on ROSC. It is clear from many studies examining other forms of shock that patients may remain underresuscitated for days after the initial insult. This is likely to occur for the victim of cardiac arrest in whom aggressive treatment was delayed because of concerns for neurologic viability. Measures such as heart rate, blood pressure, and urine output have clearly been shown to be poor indicators of the adequacy of resuscitation.[123,124] As discussed earlier, microcirculatory failure is likely to be protracted, making it a major factor in ongoing injury, and ultimately additional oxygen deprivation of the tissues results. Since for practical purposes, flow to the visceral organs during CPR is likely to be zero, the main factors affecting oxygen debt will be time elapsed between arrest and ROSC and post-ROSC blood flows below the level of critical oxygen delivery. The requirement of exogenous vasopressors to maintain myocardial and cerebral perfusion pressure may pose a problem since ongoing visceral I/R mediated by these vasopressors is possible.

VO_2 values vary widely in critically ill patients. Certain shock states show decreases in oxygen consumption,

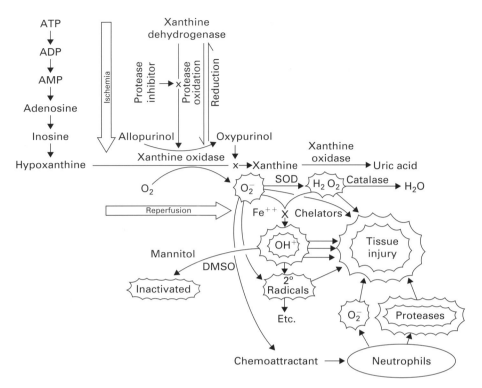

Fig. 15.5. Points of action (indicated by x) in free radical cascade where various scavenging agents may be effective (From Bulkley, G.B.: Mediators of splanchnic organ injury: overview and perspective. In: Marston, A., Bulkley, G.B. Fiddian-Green, R.G., Haglund, U.H., eds Splanchnic ischemia and multiple organ failure. Copyright @ 1989 by Adrian Marston, Gregory B. Bulkley, Richard, G. Fiddian-Green,Ulf H. Haglund. Reproduced by permission of Hodder & Stoughton Ltd., London.)

whereas others show higher levels. Studies reveal that survival is associated with increased levels of VO_2. It has been suggested that increasing DO_2 to levels above 600 ml/min per m² [140,142-144] would be helpful to overcome VO_2 defects, even though proper extraction and utilization of O_2 are not guaranteed. The exact role of this type of therapy in the postresuscitation phase of cardiac arrest is not entirely clear. In sudden cardiac death, cardiogenic shock probably predominates; however, even in this setting, postarrest cardiogenic shock is likely to be quite different from primary cardiogenic shock. Rivers *et al.* have demonstrated severe derangements in DO_2, VO_2, and oxygen extraction ratios in the postarrest state up to 6 hours after ROSC.[123] Patients receiving more than 14 mg of epinephrine showed further impairment of systemic oxygen utilization after ROSC.

Both endogenous and exogenous catecholamines, as well as the endogenous vasoactive peptides angiotensin II and vasopressin, are likely to mediate much of the VO_2 impairment that is occurring in the visceral organ

microcirculation. Studies quantifying plasma epinephrine levels during cardiac arrest have shown resting levels of 160 pmol/l, which can reach levels as high as 2 144 994 pmol/l before administration of exogenous epinephrine.[108,127] Norepinephrine levels have been found to be increased up to 90-fold after administration of epinephrine.[145] On the basis of the sensitivity of the visceral organ vasculature along with plugging of the microvasculature mediated by reperfusion, the visceral organs are at tremendous risk for VO_2 defects. VO_2 may thus be limited by constraints of diffusion, which, combined with the difficulties in increasing DO_2, put these organs at further risk.

DO_2 in the setting of postarrest cardiogenic shock is difficult to optimize. The use of catecholamines requires a delicate balance. With respect to sudden cardiac death from coronary vascular occlusion, serious consideration should be given to very early coronary angiography and angioplasty, since cardiac reserve will limit the usefulness of catecholamines in increasing cardiac index while still exerting negative effects in the visceral organs.

Intraluminal oxygenation

Part of the pathophysiology and anatomy of intestinal I/R involves injury that begins at the villous surface because of the countercurrent exchange mechanism of oxygen. This results in an early breach of the intestinal barrier to bacteria and other intestinal toxins. Since systemic perfusion to the intestine is likely to be compromised, an alternate route of O_2 via the intraluminal surface is being studied. Supplying O_2 to the intestinal lumen either by providing gaseous oxygen to the mucosa or by perfusing the lumen with oxygenated fluids has been shown in animals to prevent, in part, the development of mucosal injury.[18] Intestinal I/R-produced falls in blood pressure are significantly smaller, possibly secondary to decreased amounts of cardiotoxic substances formed and released in the intestine. In animal studies mortality has been reduced with this technique. Intraluminal oxygenation also results in increased Po_2 of the intestinal venous effluent and reduced endotoxin translocation.[18] Its ability to improve intestinal function and overall organ system function from the I/R of cardiac arrest is unclear.

Hyperbaric oxygen therapy

Theoretically the use of hyperbaric oxygen should help repay oxygen debt and reverse ongoing ischemia secondary to decreased DO_2 and VO_2. Inspiration of 100% oxygen at 3.0 atmospheres can raise PaO_2 levels to 1800 mm Hg;[146] this level dissolved in the plasma can meet the metabolic demands of the body. Areas where blood flow is intact but compromised and at risk for ischemia are supplied with O_2 because of large diffusion gradients created by nearby well-perfused areas with their high PaO_2.[146] In addition, hyperbaric oxygen has been shown to increase the deformability of red blood cells and decrease platelet aggregation, thus making their transit through debris-filled vessels easier. The end result is increased DO_2 to all areas not subject to complete vascular occlusion.

There is also evidence that hyperbaric oxygen can ameliorate reperfusion injury. In several models of I/R, hyperbaric oxygen has been shown to decrease neutrophil adherence to the endothelium, decrease lipid peroxidation, and cause increased activity of superoxide dismutase.[145,146] In addition, hyperbaric oxygen increases the ability of PMNs to kill bacteria. In theory, hyperbaric oxygen could prevent or reverse ongoing ischemia of the visceral organs, especially in the hemodynamically unstable postarrest patient who depends on vasopressors and is likely to be at risk for ongoing visceral I/R.

Intraaortic balloon pumping

Another potentially promising technique that has not been well studied is intraaortic balloon pumping. Although not proven, early use of this technique in the postresuscitation phase may reduce the requirement for vasopressors and thus decrease the incidence of vasopressor-induced visceral organ ischemia. Intraaortic balloon pumping may increase blood flow to the visceral organs as shown in one model of hemorrhagic shock.[149] Its use to decrease visceral organ I/R requires further study.

Hypothermia

Hypothermia is another potential treatment for reducing the effects of ischemia in the visceral organs. Creation of postresuscitation hypothermia has been vigorously investigated as a neuronal salvaging tactic.[150] In visceral organ ischemia, hypothermia has been studied during harvesting of organs for transplantation. Rapidly induced hypothermia in donors with recent cessation of circulation appears to extend the viability of several organs for transplantation, including the liver and kidney.[151,152] The exact mechanism by which hypothermia salvages or prevents further ischemic damage is unknown, but it may be related to slowing certain reactions that cause secondary damage at the molecular level, as well as decreasing the metabolic rate of the organ.[66,153]

Hemodilution

If disturbances in the microcirculation exist after ROSC, improving the rheologic properties of blood flow may enhance flow to ischemic organs. There appears to be little advantage in keeping hemoglobin levels above 10 g/dl.[64] Endogenous visceral organ ischemia is ongoing, taking place in the postresuscitation phase in the face of relatively normal central hemodynamics. Yano and Takori found that even after only 5 minutes of cardiac arrest without administration of vasopressors, flow to some visceral organs is decreased up to 90 minutes after arrest and that this could be prevented by hemodilution with dextran.[111] If flow to these organs can be improved by hemodilution without jeopardizing myocardial and cerebral O_2 delivery and consumption, the visceral organs may benefit. Lenov and colleagues attempted a similar hemodilution strategy to decrease postresuscitation hypoperfusion of the brain.[122] Although their attempt was successful, the hematocrit of 20 to 25% decreased oxygen content to the point that overall DO_2 was not increased. Hemodilution may have its greatest benefit when coupled with other postresuscitation maneuvers such as hyperbaric oxygen therapy, whereby oxygen content can be supplemented.

Alteration of neural-humoral and hormonal response

Since the splanchnic vasculature is exquisitely sensitive to vasopressor agents, especially endogenous agents such as angiotensin II and vasopressin, temporary ablation of this response might prove beneficial.[13] In states of shock where these agents are endogenously produced at greater rates, it has been shown that the response of the splanchnic vasculature is disproportionately greater than is that of the rest of the vascular system. In models of cardiogenic shock, decreases in splanchnic blood flow occur for prolonged periods, even when the underlying cause is reversed.[154–156]

Manipulation of atrial natriuretic factor might also be beneficial. Atrial natriuretic factor is increased during cardiac arrest, possibly caused by atrial distension. Higher levels of this factor appear to blunt the pressor response to exogenously given vasopressors. Blocking the effect of the factor to increase the vasopressor response during cardiac arrest has been considered.[157] Again this must be weighed against the potentially detrimental effects on I/R damage to the visceral organs that might be incurred in the postresuscitation phase.

As previously discussed, cortisol levels may be depressed in the postresuscitation period. Supplementation of cortisol may reduce the need for potent exogenous vasopressors. One animal study demonstrated a trend toward earlier resuscitation and requirements for less epinephrine when cortisol was administered during resuscitation.[158]

Other treatments

Gut decontamination

Since ischemia may cause a breach of the intestinal barrier, selective decontamination of the gastrointestinal tract with non-absorbable antibiotics such as polymyxin, amphotericin, and tobramycin has been shown to reduce the content of gut organisms and to lower concentrations of endotoxins and cytokines.[159] It appears to lower the rate of endotoxemia and its associated complications as well as possibly reducing the incidence of nosocomial pneumonia.[160] The antibiotics work by a combination of binding lipopolysaccharide and keeping gram-negative organism concentrations in check. Other maneuvers that may aid decontamination include gut lavage with whole gut irrigation as well as early institution of enteral nutrition.[159]

Extracorporeal therapy

Several forms of extracorporeal therapy have been proposed to reduce visceral organ ischemia and its complications. Major techniques include use of activated carbon hemoperfusion and early renal dialysis. Activated carbon or charcoal hemabsorption has been proposed as an adjunct to aid in the recovery of the severely damaged ischemic liver.[161] Acute ischemic liver damage leading to hepatic failure is associated with a host of complications, including cerebral dysfunction. Charcoal can adsorb a wide range of water- and lipid-soluble molecules of size range 113 to 40 000 Da, which are both beneficial and toxic.[162] These toxic substances include, but are not limited to mercaptans, gamma-aminobutyric acid (GABA), aromatic amino acids, phenols, and other false transmitters.[161] Hemoperfusion is also capable of removing and reducing certain bacterial species such as *E. coli* and *P. aeruginosa*, as well as endotoxins.[163] The liver is responsible for removing many toxins in addition to breaking down and maintaining plasma amino acid levels within a physiologic range and clearing bacteria and endotoxin. Since many of these functions are compromised after an ischemic insult, methods to reduce the work load of the liver may be helpful.

To date, only two studies have examined the value of charcoal hemoperfusion after cardiac arrest: one showed no improvement, and the other was only minimally helpful.[162,164] Both models used cardiac arrest times between 10 and 15 minutes. In the most recent of the two studies, dogs were in arrest between 12.5 and 15 minutes.[162] Despite significant decreases in the concentrations of aromatic amino acids, the overall neurologic outcome of animals receiving charcoal hemoperfusion was no better than in controls. Aromatic amino acids increased after treatment was stopped. Blood cultures in both groups were positive. The authors suggest that a more prolonged trial of charcoal hemabsorption should be performed.

Indications for the use of renal hemodialysis in the postresuscitation phase of cardiac arrest are unclear. Early dialysis in some shock states apparently decreases the incidence of prolonged renal failure and its associated complications. The true incidence of postresuscitation renal failure is unknown, but it appears to be higher in patients than in animal models.[128,134]

Monitoring

Monitoring for visceral organ I/R would be helpful, but what should be monitored and when remain unclear. Obviously, aggressive resuscitation must continue immediately on ROSC, and monitoring of heart rate and blood pressure as guides to treatment response is insufficient. Monitoring of isolated organs will be difficult.

Pulmonary artery catheter monitoring

Since a large oxygen debt accumulates during cardiac arrest, the ability to repay this debt may be a major determinant of survival or progression to the postresuscitation syndrome and death. Rivers *et al.* indicate that derangements in oxygen utilization exist and are likely due to a combination of reperfusion-mediated events and catecholamine use during and after resuscitation.[123,124] In short, utilization defects are probably best recognized and corrected by invasive monitoring. Since the utilization defects are due to a combination of problems with DO_2 and VO_2, monitoring with an oximetric pulmonary artery catheter would provide the clinician with the most useful information allowing flow-dependent VO_2 to be better recognized.

Lactate

Normal arterial lactate level is considered to be less than 1.8 mEq/l. Levels greater than 2 mEq/l have been associated with increased mortality. Lactate accumulation may occur not only from increased production in ischemic tissue beds, but also from decreased hepatic oxidation. Liver failure only modestly increases the clearance time for lactate.[165]

Washout of lactate from ischemic tissue beds is usually short-lived and does not significantly affect lactate clearance. Following CPR, arterial lactate levels have been found to decrease by one-half over a period of 60 to 90 minutes if adequate perfusion is restored.[166] During circulatory shock, lactic acid clearance is significantly delayed and may require hours to normalize, which likely reflects the times involved for full reversal of the underlying cause of the tissue hypoperfusion. Unless arterial-venous lactate measurements are made across specific tissue beds, they cannot predictably pinpoint ischemia to a particular organ system.

Other peripheral measures of perfusion

Additional techniques that measure peripheral perfusion have been advocated as a means to recognize inadequate resuscitation and to guide treatment (see Chapter 38): these include measurement of transcutaneous oxygen and carbon dioxide, transconjunctival oxygen, subcutaneous oxygen, and temperature gradients between the great toe and ambient air.[167] None has been specifically correlated with visceral organ blood flow. An ideal situation would be to measure indicators of ischemia for each organ.

Local measures

Recently, D(-)-lactate stemming from bacterial overgrowth has been shown in animal models to be specific for intestinal ischemia. D(-)-Lactate is produced by bacteria indigenous to the gastrointestinal tract, including *Klebsiella, E. coli, Lactobacillus*, and *Bacteroides* species. Overproduction of D(-)-lactate coupled with breaches in the integrity of the mucosal barrier likely contributes to elevation of this product in the serum.[168] Although not tested in humans, this will probably become a valuable marker of intestinal ischemia.

Another endogenous marker potentially specific for ischemia to an individual visceral organ is the arterial:ketone body ratio. This is a measure of the ability of liver mitochondria to maintain a critical level of energy production via oxidation–reduction pathways, and it has been used to assess postperfusion function of liver grafts.[169] Recently, urine oxygen tension has been used to predict postoperative renal function in patients undergoing cardiac surgery.[170] More study is needed to validate these markers. A new and exciting measure of visceral organ ischemia now in use is the monitoring of gastrointestinal intramucosal pH (pHi) by gastric tonometry.[142] It is thought to reflect visceral organ blood flow as a whole because of the similar responses of all visceral organs to shock. Titration of therapy to maintain a normal pHi may be associated with improved outcomes in some forms of shock.[171] The pHi is calculated by using the Henderson-Hasselbalch equation from the PCO_2 content obtained from a nasogastrically placed tonometer and the bicarbonate concentration of an arterial blood gas.[171] The validity of this measure relies on the observation that the PCO_2 of a fluid placed in the lumen of a hollow viscus will rapidly equilibrate with the PCO_2 in the wall of the viscus and that arterial and gastric cell bicarbonate levels are the same. Although tonometrically and directly measured pHi levels generally show good correlation in states of ischemia from septic shock, they may be somewhat less reliable in states of low flow where arterial bicarbonate is not likely to provide a true reflection of intestinal bicarbonate. The use of gastric tonometry in the postresuscitation phase of cardiac arrest has not been studied.

Magnetic resonance spectroscopy (MRS) is capable of non-invasive and repetitive measurements of the relative concentrations of different metabolites in many organs, including the brain, heart, skeletal muscle, liver, kidney, and intestine.[172,173] With different MRS techniques these metabolites include intracellular high-energy phosphates and lactate. In addition, intracellular pH, free magnesium, and intermediary metabolism can be studied. Regional blood flow measurements with MRS are also being developed. Phosphorous MRS has been used for diagnosing intestinal ischemia.[174] This technique appears promising for other visceral organs.

Summary

Damage produced to the visceral organs is complex. With regard to visceral organ I/R in the setting of cardiac arrest, the majority of the damage may take place in the postresuscitation phase because of ongoing occult ischemia. Although the postresuscitation syndrome of cardiac arrest and the MODS of other shock states are similar, it is unclear whether a state of SIRS precedes it. Better resuscitation and postresuscitation therapies guided by appropriate monitoring aimed at reducing use of vasopressors and improving postresuscitation oxygen transport may be key factors in avoiding visceral organ damage leading to the postresuscitation visceral organ syndrome. Therapies that also blunt the inflammatory mediator response need exploring. To understand these issues, animal models should be developed without regard to neurologic outcome since once effective neuronal salvaging agents are found, MODS will not overshadow their effectiveness.

REFERENCES

1. Michael, J.R., Guerci, A., Koehler, R.C. *et al.* Mechanisms by which epinephrine augments cerebral and myocardial perfusion during cardiopulmonary resuscitation in dogs. *Circulation* 1984; **69**: 822–835.
2. Linder, K.H., Brinkmann, A., Pfenninger, E.G., Lurie, K.G., Goertz, A., & Lindner, I.M. Effect of vasopressin on hemodynamic variables, organ blood flow, and acid-base status in a pig model of cardiopulmonary resuscitation. *Anesth. Analg.* 1993; **77**: 427–435.
3. Negovsky, V.A. Postresuscitation disease. *Crit. Care Med.* 1988; **16**: 942–946.
4. Safar, P. Effects of the postresuscitation syndrome on cerebral recovery from cardiac arrest. *Crit. Care Med.* 1985; **13**: 932–935.
5. Adrie, C., Laurent, I., Monchi, M., Cariou, A., Dhainaou, & Spaulding, C. Postresuscitation disease after cardiac arrest: a sepsis-like syndrome? *Curr. Opin. Crit. Care* 2004; **10**; 208–212.
6. Jakob, S.M. Splanchnic blood flow in low-flow states. *Anesth. Analg.* 2003; **96**: 1129–1138.
7. Hoshino, T., Maley, W.R., Bulkley, G.B., & Williams, G.M. Ablation of free radical-mediated reperfusion injury for the salvage of kidneys from non-heartbeating donors. *Transplantation* 1988; **45**: 284–289.
8. Siesjo, B.K. Mechanisms of ischemic brain damage. *Crit. Care Med.* 1988; **16**: 954–963.
9. Schoenberg, M.H., & Berger, H.G. Reperfusion injury after intestinal ischemia. *Crit. Care Med.* 1993; **21**: 1376–1386.
10. Schiller, H.J., Reilly, P.M., & Bulkley, G.B. Antioxidant therapy. *Crit. Care Med.* 1993; **21**: S92–S102.
11. Cipolle, M.D., Pasquale, M.D., & Cerra, F.B. Secondary organ dysfunction. *Crit. Care Clin.* 1993; **9**: 261–298.
12. Lundgren, O. Physiology of the intestinal circulation. In Marston, A., Bulkley, G.B., Fiddian-Green, R.G., & Haglund, U.H., eds. *Splanchnic Ischemia and Multiple Organ Failure*. St. Louis: Mosby, 1989: 29–40.
13. Reilly, P.M., & Bulkley, G.B. Vasoactive mediators and splanchnic perfusion. *Crit. Care Med.* 1993; **21**: S55–S68.
14. McNeill, J.R., Stark, R.D., & Greenway, C.V. Intestinal vasoconstriction after hemorrhage: roles of vasopressin and angiotensin. *Am. J. Physiol.* 1970; **219**: 1342–1347.
15. Adar, R., Franklin, A., Spark, R.F., Rosoff, C.B., & Salzman, E.W. Effect of dehydration and cardiac tamponade on superior mesenteric artery flow: role of vasoactive substances. *Surgery* 1976; **79**: 534–543.
16. Haglund, U., Bulkley, G.B., & Granger, D.N. Of the pathophysiology of intestinal ischemic injury. *Acta Chir. Scand.* 1987; **153**: 321–324.
17. Bulkley, G.B., Kvietys, P.R., Parks, D.A., Perry, M.A., & Granger, D.N. Relationship of blood flow and oxygen consumption to ischemic injury in the canine small intestine. *Gastroenterology* 1986; **89**: 852–857.
18. Haglund, U. Therapeutic potential of intraluminal oxygenation. *Crit. Care Med.* 1993; **21**: S69–S71.
19. Blum, H., Barlow, C., & Chance, B. Acute intestinal ischemia studies by phosphorus nuclear magnetic resonance spectroscopy. *Ann. Surg.* 1986; **204**: 83–88.
20. Cighetti, G., Del Puppo, M., Paroni, R., & Kienlee, M.G. Lack of conversion of xanthine dehydrogenase to xanthine oxidase during warm renal ischemia. *FEBS Lett.* 1990; **274**: 82–84.
21. Parks, D.A., Williams, T.K., & Bechman, J.S. Conversion of xanthine dehydrogenase to oxidase in ischemic rat intestine: a reevaluation. *Am. J. Physiol.* 1988; **254**: G768–G774.
22. Moorehouse, P.C., Grootveld, M., Halliwell, B.J. *et al.* Allopurinol and oxypurinol are hydroxyl scavengers. *FEBS Lett* 1987; **213**: 23–28.

23. Boros, M., Karacsony, G., Kasszaki, J., & Nagy, S. Reperfusion mucosal damage after complete intestinal ischemia in the dog: the effects of antioxidant and phospholipase A_2 inhibitor therapy. *Surgery* 1993; **113**: 184–191.

24. Poggetti, R.S., Moore, F.A., Moore, E.E., Bensard, D.D., Anderson, B.O., & Banerjee, A. Liver injury is a reversible neutrophil-mediated event following gut ischemia. *Arch. Surg.* 1992; **127**: 175–179.

25. Simpson, R., Alon, R., Kobzik, L., Valen, C.R., Shepro, D., & Hechtman, H.B. Neutrophil and nonneutrophil-mediated injury in intestinal ischemia-reperfusion. *Ann. Surg.* 1993; **218**: 444–454.

26. Brown, M.F., Ross, A.J., Dasher, J., Turley, D.L., Ziegler, M.M., & O'Neill, J.A. The role of leukocytes in mediating mucosal injury of intestinal ischemia/reperfusion. *J. Pediatr. Surg.* 1990; **25**: 214–217.

27. Payne, D. & Kubes, P. Nitric oxide donors reduce the rise in reperfusion-induced intestinal mucosal permeability. *Am. J. Physiol.* 1993; **265**: G189–G195.

28. Borgstrom, A., & Haglund, U.H. Proteases: role in mucosal injury. In Marston, A., Bulkley, G.B., Fiddian-Green, R.G., & Haglund, U.H., eds. *Splanchnic Ischemia and Multiple Organ Failure*. St. Louis: Mosby, 1989: 159–166.

29. Kibbler, C.C. Enteric bacterial toxins. In Marston, A., Bulkley, G.B., Fiddian-Green, R.G., & Haglund, U.H., eds. *Splanchnic Ischemia and Multiple Organ Failure*. St. Louis: Mosby, 1989: 167–181.

30. Wells, C.L., Maddaus, M.A., & Simmons, R.L. Bacterial translocation. In Marston, A., Bulkley, G.B., Fiddian-Green, R.G., & Haglund, U.H., eds. *Splanchnic Ischemia and Multiple Organ Failure*. St. Louis: Mosby, 1989: 195–204.

31. Ledingham, I. & Ramsay, G. Endotoxins. In Marston, A., Bulkley, G.B., Fiddian-Green, R.G., & Haglund, U.H., eds. *Splanchnic Ischemia and Multiple Organ Failure*. St. Louis: Mosby, 1989: 205–211.

32. Read, R., Moore, E.E., Moore, F.A., & Carl, V. Lipopolysaccharide-induced CD11B-mediated neutrophil-endothelial adhesion is not required for polymorphonuclear cell priming. *J. Trauma* 1994; **37**: 13–17.

33. Meakins, J.L., & Marshall, J.C. The gut as the motor of multiple system organ failure. In Marston, A., Bulkley, G.B., Fiddian-Green, R.G. & Haglund, U.H., eds. *Splanchnic Ischemia and Multiple Organ Failure*. St. Louis: Mosby, 1989: 229–236.

34. Turnage, R.H., Bagnasco, J., Berger, J., Guice, K.S., Oldham, K.T., & Hinshaw, D.B. Hepato-cellular-oxidant stress following intestinal ischemia–reperfusion injury. *J. Surg. Res.* 1991; **51**: 467–471.

35. Grull, N.J. Ischemia of the liver and pancreas. In Marston, A., Bulkley, G.B., Fiddian-Green, R.G., & Haglund, U.H., eds. *Splanchnic Ischemia and Multiple Organ Failure*. St. Louis: Mosby, 1989: 107–120.

36. Poggetti, R.S., Moore, F.A., Moore, E.E., Koeike, K., & Banerjee, A. Simultaneous liver and lung injury following gut ischemia is mediated by xanthine oxidase. *J. Trauma* 1992; **32**: 723–728.

37. Terada, L.S., Dormish, J.J., Shanley, P.F., Leff, J.A., Anderson, B.O., & Repine, J.E. Circulating xanthine oxidase mediates lung neutrophil sequestration after intestinal ischemia–reperfusion. *Am. J. Physiol.* 1992; **263**: L394–L401.

38. Caty, M.G., Guice, K.S., Kunkel, S.I. *et al.* Evidence for tumor necrosis factor-induced pulmonary microvascular injury after intestinal ischemia-reperfusion injury. *Ann. Surg.* 1990; **212**: 694–699.

39. Gerkin, T.M., Oldham, K.T., Guice, K.S., Hinshaw, D.B., & Ryan, U.S. Intestinal ischemia-reperfusion injury causes pulmonary endothelial cell ATP depletion. *Ann. Surg* 1993; **217**: 46–48.

40. Koike, K., Moore, E.E., Moore, F., Read, R., Carl, V., & Banerjee, A. Gut ischemia/reperfusion produces lung injury independent of endotoxin. *Crit. Care Med.* 1994; **22**: 1438–1444.

41. Horton, J.W., & White, D.J. Cardiac contractile injury after intestinal ischemia–reperfusion. *Am. J. Physiol.* 1991; **261**: H164–H170.

42. Horton, J.W., & White, D.J. Lipid peroxidation contributes to cardiac deficits after ischemia and reperfusion of the small bowel. *Am. J. Physiol.* 1993; **264**: H1686–H1692.

43. Horton, J.W., & White, D.J. Free radical scavengers prevent intestinal ischemia–reperfusion-mediated cardiac dysfunction. *J. Surg. Res.* 1993; **55**: 282–289.

44. Chiu, C.J., McArdle, A.H., Brown, R., Scott, H.J., & Gurd, F.N. Intestinal mucosal lesion in low-flow states. *Arch. Surg.* 1970; **101**: 478–483.

45. Schoenberg, M.H., Grogard, B., Sellin, D. *et al.* Posthypotensive generation of superoxide free radicals – possible role in the pathogenesis of the intestinal mucosal damage. *Acta Chir. Scand.* 1984; **150**: 301–309.

46. Park, P.O. Haglund, U., Bulkley, G.B., & Falt, K. The sequence of development of intestinal tissue injury after strangulation ischemia and reperfusion. *Surgery* 1990; **107**: 574–580.

47. Park, P.O., & Haglund, U. Regeneration of small bowel mucosa after intestinal ischemia. *Crit. Care Med.* 1992; **20**: 135–139.

48. Humes, H.D. & Weinberg, J.M. Cellular energetics in acute renal failure. In Brenner, B.M. & Lazarus, J.M., eds. *Acute Renal Failure*. Philadelphia: Saunders, 1983: 47–98.

49. Kito, K., Arai, T., Mori, K., Morikawa, S., & Inubushi, T. Hepatic blood flow and energy metabolism during hypotension induced by prostaglandin E_1 nicardipine in rabbits: an in vivo magnetic resonance spectroscopic study. *Anesth. Analg.* 1993; **77**: 606–612.

50. Hisanaga, M., Nakajima, Y., Wada, T. *et al.* Protective effect of the calcium channel blocker diltiazem on hepatic function following warm ischemia. *J. Surg. Res.* 1993; **55**: 404–410.

51. Stein, H.J., Oosthuizen, M.M.J., Hinder, R.A., & Lamprechts, H. Oxygen free radicals and glutathione in hepatic ischemia/reperfusion injury. *J. Surg. Res.* 1991; **50**: 398–402.

52. Yoshifumi, Y., Beckman, J.S., Beckman, T.K. *et al.* Circulating xanthine oxidase: potential mediator of ischemic injury. *Am. J. Physiol.* 1990; **258**: G564–G570.

53. Marubayashi, S., Dohi, K., Yamada, K., & Kawasaki, T. Role of conversion of xanthine dehydrogenase to oxidase in ischemic rat liver cell injury. *Surgery* 1991; **110**: 537–543.

54. Marubayashi, S., Dohi, K., Ochi, K., & Kawasaki, T. Role of free radicals in ischemic rat liver cell injury: prevention of damage by α-tocopherol administration. *Surgery* 1986; **99**: 184–192.

55. Lee, S.M., & Clemens, M.G. Effect of α-toco-pherol on hepatic mixed function oxidase in hepatic ischemia/reperfusion. *Hepatology* 1992; **15**: 276–281.

56. Schlag, G., Red, L., & Hallstrom, S. The cell in shock: the origin of multiple organ failure. *Resuscitation* 1991; **21**: 137–180.

57. Jaeschke, H., Farhood, A., Bautissta, A.P., Spolarics, Z., & Spitzer, J.J. Complement activates Kupffer cells and neutrophils during reperfusion after hepatic ischemia. *Am. J. Physiol.* 1993; **264**: G801–G809.

58. Langdale, L.A., Flaherty, L.C., Liggitt, H.D., Harlan, J.M., Rice, C.L., & Winn, R.K. Neutrophils contribute to hepatic ischemia-reperfusion injury by a CD18-independent mechanism. *J. Leuko. Biol.* 1993; **53**: 511–517.

59. Chun, K., Zhang, J., Biewer, J., Ferguson, D., & Clemens, M.G. Microcirculatory failure determines lethal hepatocyte injury in ischemic/reperfused rat livers. *Shock* 1994; **1**: 3–9.

60. Zhou, W., McCollum, M.O., Levine, B.A., & Olson, M.S. Inflammation and platelet-activating factor production during hepatic ischemia/reperfusion. *Hepatology* 1992; **16**: 1236–1240.

61. McCurry, K.R., Campbell, D.A., Scales, W.E., Warren, J.S., & Remick, D.G. Tumor necrosis factor, interleukin 6, and the acute phase response following hepatic ischemia/reperfusion. *J. Surg. Res.* 1993; **55**: 49–54.

62. Pretto, E.A. Cardiac function after hepatic ischemia-anoxia and reperfusion injury: a new experimental model. *Crit. Care Med.* 1991; **19**: 1188–1194.

63. Clemens, J.A., Bulkley, G., & Cameron, J.L. Ischemia pancreatitis. In Marston, A., Bulkley, G.B., Fiddian-Green, R.G., & Haglund, U.H., eds. *Splanchnic Ischemia and Multiple Organ Failure*. St. Louis: Mosby, 1989: 273–277.

64. Klar, E., Foitzik, T., Buhr, H., Messmer, K., & Herfarth, C. Isovolemic hemodilution with dextran 60 as treatment of pancreatic ischemia in acute pancreatitis: clinical practicability of an experimental concept. *Ann. Surg.* 1993; **217**: 369–374.

65. Haglund, U.H. Myocardial depressant factors. In Marston, A., Bulkley, G.B., Fiddian-Green, R.G., & Haglund, U.H., eds. *Splanchnic Ischemia and Multiple Organ Failure*. St. Louis: Mosby, 1989: 229–236.

66. Southard, J.H., Lindell, S.L., & Belzer, F.O. Energy metabolism and renal ischemia. *Renal Failure* 1992; **14**: 251–255.

67. Neumayer, H.H., Gellert, J., & Luft, F.C. Calcium antagonist and renal protection. *Renal Failure* 1993; **15**: 353–358.

68. Baud, L., & Ardaillou, R. Involvement of reactive oxygen species in kidney damage. *Br. Med. Bull.* 1993; **49**: 621–629.

69. Linas, S.L., Whittenburg, D., & Repine, J.E. Role of xanthine oxidase in ischemia/reperfusion injury. *Am. J. Physiol.* 1990; **2588**: F711–F716.

70. Greene, E.L., & Paller, M.S. Oxygen free radical in acute renal failure. *Miner. Electrolyte Metab.* 1991; **17**: 124–132.

71. Stanley, J.J., Goldblum, J.R., Frank, T.S., Zelenock, G.B., & D'Alecy, L.G. Attenuation of renal reperfusion injury in rats by the 21-aminosteroid U74006F. *J. Vasc. Surg.* 1993; **17**: 685–689.

72. Linas, S.L., Whittenburg, D., Parsons, P.E., & Repine, J.E. Mild renal ischemia activates primed neutrophils to cause acute renal failure. *Kidney Int.* 1992; **42**: 610–616.

73. Nakamura, H., Nemenoff, R.A., Gronich, J.H., & Bonventre, J.V. Subcellular characteristics of phospholipase A_2 activity in the rat kidney. *J. Clin. Invest.* 1991; **87**: 1810–1818.

74. Takahashi, K., Nammour, T.M., Fukunaga, M. *et al.* Glomerular actions of a free radical-generated novel prostaglandin, 8-epi-prostaglandin $F_{2\alpha}$, in the rat. *J. Clin. Invest.* 1992; **90**: 136–141.

75. Paller, M.S., Manivel, J.C., Patten, M., & Barry, M. Prostaglandins protect kidneys against ischemic and toxic injury by cellular effect. *Kidney Int.* 1992; **42**: 1345–1354.

76. Gianello, P., Besse, T., Gustin, T. *et al.* Atrial natriuretic factor, arachidonic acid metabolites and acute renal ischemia: experimental protocol in the rat. *Eur. Surg. Res.* 1990; **22**: 57–62.

77. Frank, R.S., Frank, T.S., Zelenock, G.B., & D'Alecy, L.G. Ischemia with intermittent reperfusion reduces functional and morphologic damage following renal ischemia in the rat. *Ann. Vasc. Surg.* 1993; **7**: 150–155.

78. Sakr, M., Zetti, G., McClain, C. *et al.* The protective effect of FK506 pretreatment against renal ischemia/reperfusion injury in rats. *Transplantation* 1992; **53**: 987–991.

79. Lennon, G.M., Ryan, P.C., Gaffney, E.F., & Fitzpatrick J.M. Changes in regional renal perfusion following ischemia/reperfusion injury to the rat kidney. *Urol. Res.* 1991; **19**: 259–264.

80. Dorin, R.I. & Kearns, P.J. High output circulatory failure in acute adrenal insufficiency. *Crit. Care Med.* 1988; **16**: 296–297.

81. Hubay, C.A., Weckesser, E.C., & Levy, R.P. Occult adrenal insufficiency in surgical patients. *Ann. Surg.* 1975; **181**: 325–332.

82. Schultz, C., Rivers, E.P., Feldkamp, C. *et al.* A characterization of hypothalamic–pituitary–adrenal axis function during and after human cardiac arrest. *Crit. Care Med.* 1993; **21**: 1339–1347.

83. Little, C.M., Angelos, M.G., & Brown, C.G. Adrenal perfusion in CPR is preserved despite vasopressor drugs [Abstract]. *Ann. Emerg. Med.* 1994; **23**: 608.

84. Bulkley, G.B., Kvietys, P.R., Perry, M.A., & Granger, D.N. Effects of cardiac tamponade on colonic hemodynamics and oxygen uptake. *Am. J. Physiol.* 1983; **244**: G604–G612.

85. Sapirstein, L.A., Sapirstein, E.H., & Bredemeyer, A.S. Effect of hemorrhage on the cardiac output and its distribution in the rat. *Circ. Res.* 1960; **8**: 130–139.

86. Vatner, S.F. Effects of hemorrhage on regional blood flow distribution in dogs and primates. *J. Clin. Invest.* 1974; **54**: 225–235.

87. Bailey, R.W., Bregman, M.L., Fuh K.C. *et al.* Hemodynamic pathogenesis of ischemic hepatic injury following cardiogenic shock/resuscitation. *Shock* 2000; **14**: 451–459.

88. Reilly, P.M., Wilkins, K.B., & Fuh, K.C. The mesenteric hemodynamic response to circulatory shock: an overview. *Shock* 2001; **15**: 329–342.

89. Toung, T., Reilly, P.M., Fuh, K.C. *et al.* Mesenteric vasoconstriction in response to hemorrhagic shock. *Shock* 2000; **13**: 267–273.

90. Rowell, L.B., Blackmon, J.R., Kenny, M.A., & Escourrou, P. Splanchnic vasomotor and metabolic adjustments to hypoxia and exercise in humans. *Am. J. Physiol.* 1984; **247**: H251–H258.

91. Khanna, A., Rossman, J.E., Fung, H.L., & Caty, M.G. Intestinal and hemodynamic impairment following mesenteric ischemia/reperfusion. *J. Surg. Res.* 2001; **99**: 114–119.

92. Grotz, M.R., Ding, J., Guo, W. *et al.* Comparison of plasma cytokine levels in rats subjected to superior mesenteric artery occlusion in hemorrhagic shock. *Shock* 1995; **3**: 362–368.

93. Ljungdahl, M., Lundholm, M., Katouli, M. *et al.* Bacterial translocation in experimental shock is dependent on the strains in the intestinal flora. *Scand. J. Gastroenterol.* 2000; **35**: 389–397.

94. Bone, R.C. Towards an epidemiology and natural history of SIRS. *J. Am. Med. Assoc.* 1992; **268**: 3452–3455.

95. Aranow, J.S. & Fink, M.P. Determinants of intestinal barrier failure in critical illness. *Br. J. Anaesth.* 1996; **77**: 71–81.

96. Kirton, O.C., Windsor, J., Wedderburn, R. *et al.* Failure of splanchnic resuscitation in the acutely injured trauma patient correlates with muliple organ system failure and length of stay in the ICU. *Chest* 1998; **113**: 1064–1069.

97. Doglio, G.R., Pusajo, J.F., Egurrola, M.R. *et al.* Gastric mucosal pH as a prognostic index of mortality in critically ill patients. *Crit. Care Med.* 1991; **19**: 1037–1040.

98. Idris, A., Becker, L., Wenzel, V., Fuerst, R., & Gravenstein, M. Lack of uniform definitions and reporting in laboratory models of cardiac arrest: a review of the literature and a proposal for guidelines. *Ann. Emerg. Med.* 1994; **23**: 9–16.

99. Taylor, R.B., Brown, C.G., Bridges, T., Werman, H.A., Ashton, J., & Hamlin, R.L. A model for regional blood flow measurements during cardiopulmonary resuscitation in a swine model. *Resuscitation* 1988; **16**: 107–118.

100. Marcus, M.L., Heistad, D.D., Ehrhardt, J.C. *et al.* Total and regional cerebral blood flow measurement with 7–10, 15, 25, and 50 µm microspheres. *J. Appl. Physiol.* 1975; **40**: 501–507.

101. Koehler, R.C., Chandra, N., Guerci, A.D. *et al.* Augmentation of cerebral perfusion by simultaneous chest compression and lung inflation with abdominal binding after cardiac arrest in dogs. *Circulation* 1983; **67**: 266–275.

102. Voorhees, W.D., Ralston, S.H., & Babbs, C.F. Regional blood flow during cardiopulmonary resuscitation with abdominal counterpulsation in dogs. *Am. J. Emerg. Med.* 1983; **2**: 123–128.

103. Michael, J.R., Guerci, A., Koehler, R.C. *et al.* Mechanisms by which epinephrine augments cerebral and myocardial perfusion during cardiopulmonary resuscitation in dogs. *Circulation* 1984; **69**: 822–835.

104. Sharff, J.A., & Pantley, G. Effect of time on regional organ perfusion during two methods of cardiopulmonary resuscitation. *Ann. Emerg. Med.* 1984; **13**: 649–656.

105. Linder, K.H., Brinkman, A., Pfenninger, E.G., Goertz, A., & Lindner, I.M. Effect of vasopressin on hemodynamic variables, organ blood flow, and acid–base status in a pig model of cardiopulmonary resuscitation. *Anesth. Analg.* 1993; **77**: 427–435.

106. Berkowitz, I.D., Gervais, H., Schleien, C.L., Koehler, R.C., Dean, J.M., & Traystman, R.J. Epinephrine dosage effects on cerebral and myocardial blood flow in an infant swine model of cardiopulmonary resuscitation. *Anesthesiology* 1991; **75**: 1041–1050.

107. Lindner, K.H., Prengel, A.W., Pfenninger, E.G. *et al.* Vasopressin improves vital organ blood flow during closed-chest cardiopulmonary resuscitation in pigs. *Circulation* 1995; **91**: 215–221,

108. Prengel, A.W., Lindner, K.H., Wenzel, V., Tugtekin, I., & Anhäupl, T. Splanchnic and renal blood flow after cardiopulmonary resuscitation with epinephrine and vasopressin in pigs. *Resuscitation* 1998; **38**: 19–24.

109. Voelckel, W.G., Lindner, K.H., & Wenzel, V. Effects of vasopressin and epinephrine on splanchnic blood flow and renal function during and after cardiopulmonary resuscitation in pigs. *Crit. Care Med.* 2000; **28**: 1083–1088.

110. Angelos, M.G., Ward, K.R., Hobson, J., & Beckley, P.D. Organ blood flow following cardiac arrest in a swine low-flow cardiopulmonary bypass model. *Resuscitation* 1994; **27**: 245–254.

111. Yano, H., & Takaori, M. Effect of hemodilution on capillary and arteriolovenous shunt flow in organs after cardiac arrest in dogs. *Crit. Care Med.* 1990; **18**: 1146–1151.

112. Voorhees, W.D., Babbs, C.F., & Tacker, W.A. Regional blood flow during cardiopulmonary resuscitation in dogs. *Crit. Care Med.* 1980; **8**: 134–136.

113. Krismer, A.C., Wenzel, V., & Voelckel, W.G. Effects of vasopressin on adrenal gland regional perfusion during experimental cardiopulmonary resuscitation. *Resuscitation* 2003; **56**: 223–228.

114. Lindner, K.H., Ahnefeld, F.W., & Bowdler, I.M. Comparison of different doses of epinephrine on myocardial perfusion and resuscitation success during cardiopulmonary resuscitation in a pig model. *Am. J. Emerg. Med.* 1991; **9**: 27–31.

115. Brown, C.G., Werman, H.A., Davis, E.A., Hobson, J., & Hamlin, R.L. The effects of graded doses of epinephrine on regional myocardial blood flow during cardiopulmonary resuscitation in swine. *Circulation* 1987; **75**: 491–497.

116. Holmes, H.R., Babbs, C.F., Voorhees, W.D., Tacker, W.A., & De Garavilla, B. Influence of adrenergic drugs upon vital organ perfusion during CPR. *Crit. Care Med.* 1980; **8**: 137–140.

117. Halperin, H.R., Guerci, A.D., Chandra, N. *et al.* Vest inflation without simultaneous ventilation during cardiac arrest in dogs; improved survival from prolonged cardiopulmonary resuscitation. *Circulation* 1986; **74**: 1407–1415.

118. Chang, M.W., Coffeen, P., Lurie, K.G. *et al.* Tissue perfusion during standard vs. active compression decompression CPR in the dog [Abstract]. *Circulation* 1992; **86**: 1–233.

119. Little, C.M., & Brown, C.G. Angiotensin II improves myocardial blood flow in cardiac arrest. *Resuscitation* 1993; **26**: 203–210.

120. Linder, K.H., Prengel, A.W., Pfenninger, E.G., & Lindner, I.M. Effect of Angiotensin II on myocardial blood flow and acid–base status in a pig model of cardiopulmonary resuscitation. *Anesth. Analg.* 1993; **76**: 485–492.

121. Ames, A. III, Wright, R.L., Kowanda, M., Thurston, J.M., & Majino, G. Cerebral ischemia. II. The no-reflow phenomenon. *Am. J. Pathol.* 1968; **152**: 437–453.

122. Lenov, Y., Sterz, F., Safar, P., Johnson, D., Tisherman, S.A., & Oku, K. Hypertension with hemodilution prevents multifocal cerebral hypoperfusion after cardiac arrest in dogs. *Stroke* 1992; **23**: 45–53.

123. Rivers, E.P., Rady, M.Y., Martin, G.B. *et al.* Venous hyperoxia after cardiac arrest: characterization of a defect in systemic oxygen utilization. *Chest* 1992; **102**: 1787–1793.

124. Rivers, E.P., Wortsman, J., Rady, M.Y. *et al.* The effect of the total cumulative epinephrine dose administered during human CPR on hemodynamic oxygen transport and utilization variables in the post-resuscitation period. *Chest* 1994; **106**: 1499–1507.

125. Prengel, A., Linder, K., Ensinger, H., & Grunert, A. Plasma catecholamine concentrations after successful resuscitation in patients. *Crit. Care Med.* 1992; **20**: 609–614.

126. Paradis, N.A., Rose, M.I., & Garg, U. The effect of global ischemia and reperfusion on the plasma levels of vasoactive peptides: the neuroendocrine response to cardiac arrest and resuscitation. *Resuscitation* 1993; **26**: 261–269.

127. Wortsman, J., Paradis, N.A., Martin, G.B. *et al.* Functional responses to extremely high plasma epinephrine concentrations in cardiac arrest. *Crit. Care Med.* 1993; **21**: 692–697.

128. Cerchiari, E.L., Safar, P., Klein, E., & Diven, W. Visceral and bacteriologic changes and neurologic outcome after cardiac arrest in dogs: the visceral postresuscitation syndrome. *Resuscitation* 1993; **25**: 119–136.

129. Bjork, R.J., Snyder, B.D., Campion, B.C., & Lowenson, R.B. Medical complications of cardiopulmonary arrest. *Arch. Intern. Med.* 1982; **142**: 500–503.

130. Gaussorgues, P., Gueugniaud, P.Y., Vedrine, J.M., Salord, F., Mercatteello, A., & Robert, D. Bacteremia following cardiac arrest and cardiopulmonary resuscitation. *Intens. Care Med.* 1988; **14**: 575–577.

131. Schon, M.R., Hunt, C.J., Peff, D.E., & Wight, D.G. The possibility of resuscitating livers after warm ischemic injury. *Transplantation* 1993; **56**: 24–31.

132. Hess, A.D.J., Najarian, J.J.S., & Sutherland, D.E.R. Amylase activity and pancreas transplants. *Lancet* 1985; **2**: 726.

133. White, B.C., Grossman, L.I., & Krause, G.S. Brain injury by global ischemia and reperfusion: a theoretical perspective on membrane damage and repair. *Neurology* 1993; **43**: 1656–1665.

134. Mattana, J., & Singhala, P.C. Prevalence and determinants of acute renal failure following cardiopulmonary resuscitation. *Arch. Intern. Med.* 1993; **153**: 235–239.

135. Koffman, C.G., Bewick, M., Chang, R.W.S., & Compton, F. Comparative study of the use of systolic and asystolic kidney donors between 1988 and 1991. *Transpl. Proc.* 1993; **25**: 1527–1529.

136. Wortsman, J., Frank, S., Wehrenberg, W.B. *et al.* Melanocyte-stimulating hormone immunoreactivity is a component of the neuroendocrine response to maximal stress (cardiac arrest). *J. Clin. Endocrinol. Metab.* 1985; **61**: 355–360.

137. Kornberger, E., Prengel, A.W., Krismer, A. *et al.* Vasopressin-mediated adrenocorticotropin release increases plasma cortisol concentrations during cardiopulmonary resuscitation. *Crit. Care Med.* 2000; **28**: 3517–3521.

138. Basha, M.A., Meyere, G.S., Kunkel, S.L. Strieter, R.M., Rivers, E.P. & Popovich, J. Presence of tumor necrosis factor in humans undergoing cardiopulmonary resuscitation with return of spontaneous circulation. *Crit. Care.* 1991; **6**: 185–189.

139. Tracy, K.J. & Cerami, A. Tumor necrosis factor: an updated review of its biology. *Crit. Care Med.* 1993; **21**: S415–S422.

140. Shoemaker, W.C., Appel, P.L., & Kram, H.B. Tissue oxygen debt as a determinant of lethal and nonlethal postoperative organ failure. *Crit. Care Med.* 1988; **16**: 1117–1121.

141. Laurent, I., Adrie, C., Vinsonneau, C. *et al.* High-volume hemofiltration after out-of-hospital cardiac arrest. *J. Am. Coll. Cardiol.* 2005; **46**: 432–437.

142. Leach, R.M.M. & Treacher, D.F. The relationship between oxygen delivery and consumption. *Dis. Month.* 1994; **XL**: 301–368.

143. Moore, F.A., Haenel, J.B., Moore, E.E., & Whitehill, T.A. Incommensurate oxygen consumption in response to maximal oxygen availability predicts postinjury multiple organ failure. *J. Trauma* 1992; **33**: 58–67.

144. Shoemaker, W.C., Appel, P.L., Kram, H.B., Waxman, K., & Lee, T.S. Prospective trial of supranormal values of survival as therapeutic goals in the high risk surgical patient. *Chest* 1988; **94**: 1176–1186.

145. Wortsman, J., Frank, S., & Cryer, P.E. Adreno-medullary response to maximal stress in humans. *Am. J. Med.* 1984; **77**: 779–784.

146. Grim, P.S., Gottileb, L.J., Boddie, A., & Baston, E. Hyperbaric oxygen therapy. *J. Am. Med. Assoc.* 1990; **263**: 2216–2220.

147. Hammarlund, C. The physiologic effects of hyperbaric oxygen. In Kindwall, E.P., ed. *Hyperbaric Medicine Practice*. Flagstaff, Arizona: Best, 1994: 17–32.

148. Zamboni, W.A., Roth, A.C., Russell, R.C., Graham, B., Suchy, H., & Kucan, J.O. Morphologic analysis of the microcirculation during reperfusion of ischemic skeletal muscle and the effect of hyperbaric oxygen. *Plast. Reconstr. Surg.* 1993; **91**: 1110–1123.

149. Landreneau, R.J.J., Horton, J.W., & Cochran, R.P. Splanchnic blood flow response to intraaortic balloon pump assist of hemorrhagic shock. *J. Surg. Res.* 1991; **51**: 281–287.

150. Safar, P. Cerebral resuscitation after cardiac arrest: research initiatives and future directions. *Ann. Emerg. Med.* 1993; **22**: 324–349.

151. Gomez, M., Alvarez, J., Arias, J. *et al.* Cardiopulmonary bypass and profound hypothermia as a means for obtaining kidney grafts from irreversible cardiac arrest donors: cooling techniques. *Transpl. Proc.* 1993; **25**: 1501–1502.

152. Moriyama, Y.Y., Morishita, R., Shimokawa, S., & Taira, A. Multiple organ procurement for transplantation: the effect of peritoneal cooling. *Transpl. Proc.* 1991; **23**: 2324–2325.

153. Pelky, T.J., Frank, R.S., Stanley, J.J. *et al.* Minimal physiologic temperature variations during renal ischemia alter functional and morphologic outcome. *J. Vasc. Surg.* 1992; **15**: 619–625.

154. Bailey, R.W., Bulkley, G.B., Hamilton, S.R., Morris, J.B.B., & Haglund, U.H. Protection of the small intestine from nonocclusive mesenteric ischemia injury due to cardiogenic shock. *Am. J. Surg.* 1987; **205**: 597–612.

155. McNeil, J.R., Stark, R.D., & Greenway, C.V. Intestinal vasoconstriction after hemorrhage: roles of vasopressin and angiotensin. *Am. J. Physiol.* 1970; **219**: 1342–1347.

156. Bulkley, G.B., Oshima, A., & Bailey, R.W. Pathophysiology of hepatic ischemia in cagiogenic shock. *Am. J. Surg.* 1986; **151**: 87–97.

157. Paradis, N.A., Wortsman, J., Malarkey, W.B. *et al.* High atrial natriuretic peptide concentrations blunt the pressor response during cardiopulmonary resuscitation in humans. *Crit. Care Med.* 1994; **22**: 213–218.

158. Smithline, H., Rivers, E., Appleton, T., & Nowak, R. Corticosteroid supplementation during cardiac arrest in rats. *Resuscitation* 1993; **25**: 257–264.

159. Fink, M.P., & Fiddian-Green, R.G. Care of the gut in the critically ill. In Marston, A., Bulkley, G.B., Fiddian-Green, R.G., & Haglund, U.H., eds. *Splanchnic Ischemia and Multiple Organ Failure*. St. Louis: Mosby, 1989; 349–363.

160. Tetteroo, G., Wagenvoort, J., Mulder, P.G., Ince, C., & Bruining, H. Decrease mortality rate and length of hospital stay in surgical intensive care unit patients with successful selective decontamination of the gut. *Crit. Care Med.* 1994; **21**: 1692–1698.

161. O'Grady, J., Gimson, E.S., O'Brien, C.J., Pucknell, A., Hughes, R.D., & Williams, R. Controlled trials of charcoal hemoperfusion and prognostic factors in fulminant hepatic failure. *Gastroenterology* 1988; **94**: 1186–1192.

162. Sterz, F., Safar, P., Diven, W., Leonov, Y., Radovsky, A., & Odu, K. Detoxification with hemabsorption after cardiac arrest does not improve neurologic recovery: review and outcome study in dogs. *Resuscitation* 1993; **25**: 137–160.

163. Bende, S., & Bertok, L. Elimination of endotoxin from the blood by extracorporeal activated charcoal hemoperfusion in experimental canine endotoxin shock. *Circ. Shock* 1986; **18**: 239–244.

164. Negovsky, V.A., Saks, I.O., & Shapiro, V.M. Experimental extracorporeal hemabsorption in the post-resuscitation period in dogs. *Resuscitation* 1979; **77**: 145–149.

165. Almenoff, P.P., Leavy, J., Weil, M.H. *et al.* Prolongation of the half-life of lactate after maximal exercise in patients with hepatic dysfunction. *Crit. Care Med.* 1989; **17**: 870–873.

166. Leavy, J., Weil, M.H., & Rackow, E. Lactate washout following circulatory arrest. *J. Am. Med. Assoc.* 1988; **260**: 622–664.

167. Astiz, M.E. & Rackow, E.C. Assessing perfusion failure during circulatory shock. *Crit. Care Clin.* 1993; **9**: 299–312.

168. Murray, M.J., Barbose, J.J. & Cobb, C.F. Serum D(-)-lactate levels as a predictor of acute intestinal ischemia in a rat model. *J. Surg. Res.* 1993; **54**: 507–509.

169. Egawa, H., Shaked, A., Konishi, Y. *et al.* Arterial ketone body ratio in pediatric liver transplantation. *Transplantation* 1993; **55**: 522–526.

170. Kainuma, M., Kimura, N., Yamashit, N., & Marukawa, T. Intraoperative urine oxygen tension predicts postoperative renal function [Abstract]. *Anesthesiology* 1993; **79**: A545.

171. Gutierrez, G., Palizas, F., Poglia, G. *et al.* Gastric intramucosal pH as a therapeutic index of tissue oxygenation in critically ill patients. *Lancet* 1992; **339**: 195–199.

172. Bottomley, P.A. Human in vivo NMR spectroscopy in diagnostic medicine: clinical tool or research probe? *Radiology* 1989; **170**: 1–15.

173. Matson, G.G.B., Twieg, D.B., Karczmar, G.S. *et al.* Application of image-guided surface coil P-31 MR spectroscopy to human liver, heart, and kidney. *Radiology* 1988; **169**: 541–547.

174. Temes, R.T., Kauten, R., & Schwartz, M.Z. Nuclear magnetic resonance as a noninvasive method of diagnosing intestinal ischemia: technique and preliminary results. *J. Pediatr. Surg.* 1991; **26**: 775–779.

16

Mechanisms of forward flow during external chest compression

Henry R. Halperin

Johns Hopkins University School of Medicine, Baltimore, MD, USA

There are more than 300 000 victims of cardiac arrest each year, and attempts to resuscitate them are usually unsuccessful.[1,2] Laboratory and clinical studies have shown that restoration of cardiac function after cardiac arrest is related to the level of coronary perfusion generated during resuscitation.[3-6] It has also been shown that adequate cerebral perfusion is necessary for preservation of brain function.[7,8] There is therefore a critical need for determining methods to augment blood flow generated during resuscitation. A key factor in enhancing flow is understanding the mechanisms of blood flow operative during chest compression, since it may be possible to optimize flow by exploiting those mechanisms.

Fluid movement in any hydraulic system results from the interaction of a pump, or driving force for fluid movement, and a load. In the intact cardiovascular system, the pump is obviously the heart, and the load is the vascular resistance and compliance. During resuscitation, however, the pump and load are less well defined. Continuing controversy exists over the nature of the pump operative during chest compression.[9-23] Pumps that have been proposed include direct cardiac compression,[19,22,24] intrathoracic pressure rises,[16,18,25] and a combination of both.[15,26,27] It is important to determine the nature of the pump, since the method of chest compression for optimizing flow may be different depending on which pump is operative.[4,15,28]

For optimizing flow, it may also be important to understand the effects of a number of techniques that have been investigated which may modify the pump. These techniques include: (*a*) abdominal compression,[29-32] (*b*) airway manipulation,[29,33-41] (*c*) circumferential chest compression,[4,28,42-45] and (*d*) sternal force applied during chest relaxation (active decompression).[39,46-52] A detailed understanding of how these techniques modify the pump to affect blood flow may facilitate development of methods that harness the optimal features of each technique.

In addition, the vascular load during resuscitation may have profound effects on coronary and cerebral blood flow.[4,53-56] Increases in peripheral resistance may preferentially shunt flow to the heart and brain,[4,53] whereas low peripheral resistance states may lead to vascular collapse with reduction of flow.[53,57] Changes in the distribution of arterial compliance may also affect flow.[58,59] Vasoconstrictor drugs are used routinely during resuscitation to increase peripheral resistance and improve coronary flow.[2] Other drugs used during resuscitation for other indications, however, may have profound effects on the vascular load, some of which may decrease flow. For example, calcium and some analgesics may cause vasodilation, which reduces peripheral resistance. Non-pharmacologic means, such as abdominal binding, may also change the vascular load.[60] Consequently, understanding how the vascular load affects blood flow and how the vascular load can be altered may be useful in determining means for optimizing flow.

This chapter deals with mechanisms of blood flow operative during external chest compression cardiopulmonary resuscitation (CPR), since external chest compression is not only a part of standard CPR, but also a part of the newer forms of CPR that may replace or supplement standard CPR.[4,28,49,61-63] The mechanisms discussed include the pump, techniques that can modify the pump, and the vascular load.

Cardiac Arrest: The Science and Practice of Resuscitation Medicine. 2nd edn., ed. Norman Paradis, Henry Halperin, Karl Kern, Volker Wenzel, Douglas Chamberlain. Published by Cambridge University Press. © Cambridge University Press, 2007.

Basic science

The pump

With the *cardiac compression pump*, it is postulated that chest compression does not cause intrathoracic pressure to rise. Instead, the heart (and possibly some vascular structures) is compressed between the sternum and vertebral column (Fig. 16.1).[22] It is presumed that blood is squeezed from the heart into the arterial circulation during chest compression, with the cardiac valves preventing retrograde blood flow. With release of chest compression, the heart would expand and fill with blood. Coronary flow and cerebral flow are presumed to occur in a way similar to that in the intact circulation.

With the *intrathoracic pressure pump*, it is postulated that chest compression causes a rise in intrathoracic pressure, which is transmitted to the intrathoracic vasculature (Fig. 16.1).[16,18] Intrathoracic arterial pressure is transmitted fully to extrathoracic arteries. Intrathoracic venous pressure is not, however, transmitted to the extrathoracic veins because of the large extrathoracic venous compliance and because of closure of venous valves (Fig. 16.2).[18,26,64] This differential transmission of intrathoracic pressure to the extrathoracic vasculature produces extrathoracic arterial-venous pressure gradients, which cause blood to flow out of the thorax. With release of chest compression, intrathoracic pressure would fall and venous blood would return from the periphery into the thoracic venous system. Coronary flow, which is entirely inside the thorax, appears

Cardiac compression pump

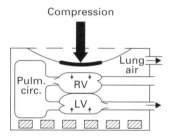

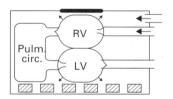

Intrathoracic pressure pump

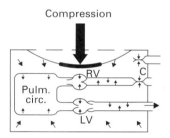

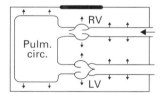

Fig. 16.1. Schematic representation of cardiac compression pump (*left panel*) and intrathoracic pressure pump (*right panel*). With cardiac compression pump, it is postulated that chest compression causes left ventricle (*LV*) and possibly right ventricle (*RV*) of heart to be compressed between sternum and vertebral column. It is presumed that blood is squeezed from heart into arterial circulation during chest compression, with cardiac valves preventing retrograde blood flow. It is also presumed that air moves freely out of the lungs, so that intrathoracic pressure does not rise and pulmonary circulation (*pulm. circ.*) is not affected by chest compression. With chest relaxation, heart would expand and fill with blood, and air would passively return to lungs. With intrathoracic pressure pump, it is postulated that chest compression causes a rise in intrathoracic pressure (*large arrows*), which is transmitted to intrathoracic vasculature. It is presumed that intrathoracic pressure can rise because of collapse of airways (above the C) which reduces movement of air out of lungs. All intrathoracic structures are reduced in size but not necessarily equally. There is also collapse of venous structures at thoracic inlet (below the C), which helps prevent retrograde venous blood flow. With chest relaxation, intrathoracic pressure would fall, with return of venous blood from periphery into thoracic venous system.

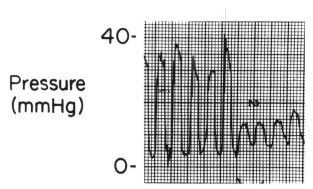

Fig. 16.2. Pressure tracing during catheter pullback in patient undergoing chest compression. Pressure catheter was placed in internal jugular vein and advanced into thorax. Each oscillation is pressure recorded during each chest compression. As catheter tip crossed thoracic inlet during pullback, amplitude of pressure oscillations decreased substantially, indicating site of collapse. (Reproduced with permission from ref. 18. Copyright 1980 American Heart Association.)

to depend on the extrathoracic arteries (Fig. 16.3).[59] As intrathoracic pressure rises during chest compression, blood moves from intrathoracic arteries to extrathoracic arteries. As intrathoracic pressure falls during chest relaxation, it appears that some blood from the extrathoracic arteries flows retrograde into the intrathoracic arteries to perfuse the coronary arteries.[15,59,65]

History

Nearly lost in the medical literature are observations by Crile and Dolley[25] in 1906 and Eisenmenger[66] in the 1930s, who demonstrated, in experimental animals with cardiac arrest and to some extent in humans, that circulation of blood could be achieved through fluctuations of intrathoracic pressure. In 1960 the era of modern CPR was begun by Kouwenhoven, Jude, and Knickerbocker.[22] From anatomic considerations it was suggested that chest compression resulted in direct compression of the heart between the sternum and the vertebral column. Later in the 1960s, a series of investigations was performed that demonstrated, however, that no intrathoracic arterial-venous pressure gradient was present during external chest compression in the dog.[67,68] In addition, very high right atrial pressures were present during external chest compression in humans.[68] If direct cardiac compression were responsible for movement of blood, an arterial-venous pressure gradient across the heart would be expected. Arterial pressure should exceed venous pressure to provide the necessary peripheral and coronary perfusion pressures.

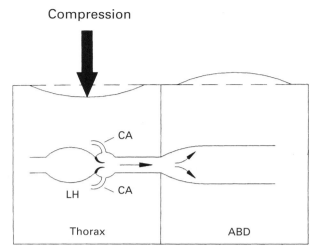

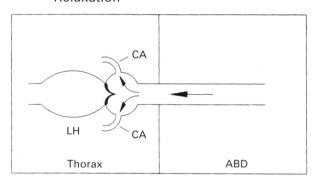

Fig. 16.3. Schematic of mechanism for generation of coronary blood flow by rises in intrathoracic pressure. As intrathoracic pressure rises during chest compression, blood moves from intrathoracic arteries to extrathoracic arteries. Blood does not flow into coronary arteries (*CA*) during chest compression because of high intrathoracic venous pressure. As intrathoracic pressure falls during chest relaxation, it appears that aortic valve closes and some blood from extrathoracic arteries flows retrograde into intrathoracic arteries to perfuse coronary arteries. *ABD*, abdomen; *LH*, left heart.

In 1976 Criley and associates observed that as long as a patient with cardiac arrest began to cough before unconsciousness occurred, the patient would not lose consciousness provided that coughing at a rate of 40 to 60 times per minute was continued.[9] It was suggested that blood flow resulted from direct compression of the heart by thoracic structures during the cough maneuver. Later, Niemann *et al.* performed a series of elegant cine-angiographic and hemodynamic studies in dogs which demonstrated that movement of blood during the cough was most likely a reflection of a rise and fall in intrathoracic pressure.[10] The cough was shown to be extremely efficient at producing cyclic fluctuations in intrathoracic and vascular pressures. [9,10,69]

In 1980 Rudikoff *et al.* suggested that blood movement during external chest compression CPR can be accounted for by a general rise in intrathoracic pressure.[18] This suggestion was based on several observations made in patients. First, they noted that in two patients who had traumatically flail sternums and subsequently suffered cardiac arrest, no measurable arterial blood pressure fluctuations or forward carotid blood flow velocity could be generated by external chest compression. If the chest wall was bound to prevent the paradoxic expansion of the rest of the chest, however, a measurable arterial blood pressure fluctuation with each compression did occur. They reasoned that a patient with a flail sternum should be ideally suited for direct cardiac compression but that binding the chest during sternal displacement would allow intrathoracic pressure to rise. Second, they observed that the compression cycle after ventilation was the cycle that produced the greatest pressure elevation and the highest velocity of carotid blood flow. If cardiac compression were the driving force for blood movement, they reasoned that generated pressures should be lower on the cycle after ventilation, since the sternum would be further from the heart at the beginning of the cycle.

Thus by 1980 controversy existed as to whether the pump operative during external chest compression was direct cardiac compression or induced rises in intrathoracic pressure. The controversy has continued, and, more recently, investigators have suggested that both mechanisms may be operative.[26,27,65] The following discussion describes a number of approaches that have been used in attempts to determine more definitively the nature of the pump.

Determining the pump

Intrathoracic pressure

It seems the most straightforward way of gaining insight into whether blood moves because of intrathoracic pressure changes or through direct cardiac compression or both would be to measure simultaneously the generated vascular pressures and regional intrathoracic pressure. If vascular pressures were significantly higher than intrathoracic pressure, then rises in intrathoracic pressure could not account for the generated vascular pressures. There have been a number of attempts to make such simultaneous measurements.[17,19,21,29] Some investigators have reported that there is a very close correlation between the *change* in intrathoracic vascular pressures and estimates of the change in intrathoracic pressure.[17]

Those investigators presume that changes in pressure, rather than generated peak pressures, are important. They reason that pressures in the various vascular compartments may be different at the beginning of chest compression, and a rise in intrathoracic pressure would *add* to the existing pressure. Other investigators have reported, however, that changes in vascular pressures are much larger than changes in intrathoracic pressure, suggesting that intrathoracic pressure fluctuations are not primarily responsible for generating vascular pressures.[19] The following problems, however, make these studies difficult to interpret: (*a*) use of sensors for measuring intrathoracic pressure that had limited frequency response; (*b*) sensors that required entry of pleural liquid where the pleural liquid may not be present in sufficient volume; (*c*) surgical manipulation of the chest, where a pneumothorax, or alteration of anatomic relations, might be present; and (*d*) no consensus as to what method or methods give valid measurement of pleural pressures.

Venting intrathoracic pressure, while measuring vascular pressures before and after venting, has also been attempted as a method for providing insight into the driving force for blood movement. If the pressures before and after venting were essentially the same, it could be reasoned that manipulation of intrathoracic pressure had little to do with generation of vascular pressure. Based on this reasoning, some studies were done with thoracic venting attempted via bilateral chest tubes.[21] The major problem with these studies was that intrathoracic pressure was incompletely vented because of sealing of the chest tubes by the pleura,[70] so that the results are questionable.

Aortic and cardiac dimensions

Another way to gain insight into the nature of the pump operative during chest compression is to visualize changes in aortic and cardiac dimensions. Angiograms have shown that aortic size decreases during chest compression, rather than increasing as would be expected if blood flow occurred as a result of direct heart compression.[14] Direct heart compression should drive blood from the left ventricle into the aorta, leading to distension, not collapse, of the proximal aorta. Intrathoracic pressure changes, however, would tend to reduce the size of all intrathoracic vascular structures. One limitation of this study is that direct compression of the aorta could have occurred, which could decrease the anteroposterior dimension of the aorta.

Cardiac dimensional changes have been studied with chronically implanted ultrasonic crystals in dogs,[19] and with echocardiography in humans.[27,71–73] In dogs, certain left ventricular dimensions were reported to decrease during chest compression, suggesting that there is direct left ventricular compression leading to forward blood flow.[19] Other left ventricular dimensions, however, increased, and total left ventricular volume was not measured. It is unclear therefore whether there was a change in total left ventricular volume. Similar limitations in determination of left ventricular volume were present in the echocardiographic studies of humans, also making the results of those studies inconclusive.

Mitral valve motion

A third way that has been explored for determining the driving force for blood movement during external chest compression CPR has been through investigation of mitral valve motion. It was previously shown in some preparations that the mitral and aortic valves were open during chest compression, with the heart acting as a passive conduit for flow.[72,73] It was presumed therefore that if the mitral valve closed during chest compression, then cardiac compression (without rises in intrathoracic pressure) was operative. The reasoning was that if during chest compression the left ventricular volume decreased and there were pressure gradients from the left ventricle to the left atrium,

closing of the mitral valve during chest compression established that direct compression of the heart was the cause. The conclusions of those studies are problematic, however, since (*a*) there is sufficient motion of the heart that different portions of the heart may be used for volume determinations made during chest compression and relaxation and (*b*) intrathoracic pressure was not measured. In addition, left ventricular to left atrial pressure gradients can be caused by "pure" rises in intrathoracic pressure.[23]

The ability of "pure" rises in intrathoracic pressure to close the mitral valve was demonstrated by using large-bore chest tubes placed into the thorax of dogs. The chest tubes were used to cyclically inflate the thorax, while left ventricular and left atrial pressures were measured and echocardiograms were recorded. With the trachea open to atmosphere during thoracic inflation, air moved out of the lungs, and the mitral valve leaflets approximated (Fig. 16.4, *upper panels*). With thoracic deflation, however, the mitral leaflets separated widely (Fig. 16.4, *lower panels*). During most of the high-pressure portion of the cycle, left ventricular pressure was higher than left atrial pressure[23] (Fig. 16.5a). With lung ventilation alone, however, the

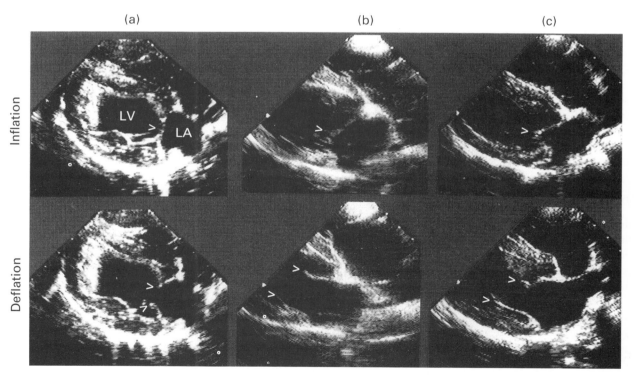

(a)   (b)   (c)

Fig. 16.4. Parasternal long-axis echocardiographic views of hearts of three dogs (*a*), (*b*), (*c*) from right chest wall during inflation and deflation of thorax through large-bore port. Port had a baffle that directed airflow away from heart. During inflation (*upper panels*), mitral valve leaflets close (*arrow*). During deflation (*lower panels*), mitral valve leaflets open (*arrows*). *LV*, left ventricle; *LA*, left atrium. (Reproduced with permission from ref. 23. Copyright 1988 American Heart Association.)

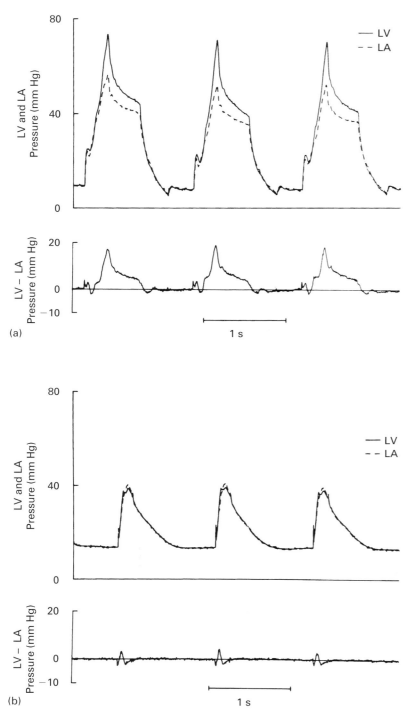

Fig. 16.5. (a) Plot of intracardiac pressures during thoracic inflation and deflation in one dog. Left ventricular (*LV*) pressure is higher than left atrial (*LA*) pressure during most of the high-pressure phase, and the difference in those pressures (*LV – LA*) is shown separately. (b) Plot of intracardiac pressures during lung ventilation in one dog. Left ventricular (*LV*) pressure is nearly identical to left atrial (*LA*) pressure during entire cycle, and difference in those pressures (*LV – LA*) is shown separately. (Reproduced with permission from ref. 23. Copyright 1988 American Heart Association.)

mitral valve leaflets remained separated during both inspiration and expiration, and no left ventricular to left atrial pressure gradient was present[23] (Fig. 16.5b). These thoracic inflation and lung ventilation studies demonstrate therefore that mitral valve motion can depend on how intrathoracic pressure is generated.

Some echocardiographic studies of CPR in humans have shown that the mitral valve can be open during chest compression.[72,73] Since those studies tended to be late in the course of cardiac arrest, decreases in peripheral resistance may have strongly affected forward flow and resulting valve motion.[74] In addition, low compression rates and increased intravascular volume are associated with more antegrade flow through the heart during compression, whereas higher rates and decreased intravascular volume are associated with elimination of antegrade flow during compression.[74] In those echocardiographic studies of CPR in humans, therefore, it is not known (a) whether the level of intrathoracic pressure generated was insufficient to produce significant intracardiac pressure gradients, (b) whether the heart was simply a passive conduit for flow produced by intrathoracic pressure changes, (c) whether the degree of cardiac compression was insufficient to produce mitral valve closure, (d) how the duration of cardiac arrest affected the observed findings, (e) what the effects of the rate of compression were, or (f) what the effect of the intravascular volume status was. Other echocardiographic studies in humans have shown variable relationships between chest compression and mitral valve motion,[27] suggesting either that mitral valve motion gives no insight into mechanisms or that the mechanisms change during the course of chest compression.

Thus, rises in intrathoracic pressure with accompanying lung deflation can produce higher pressures in the left ventricle than in the left atrium and cause the mitral valve to close. Cardiac compression can also cause the mitral valve to close. Mitral valve closure during chest compression, therefore, does not distinguish whether blood moves because of direct cardiac compression or because of intrathoracic pressure rises.

Effects of changes in rate and duration of compression

A fourth way that has been explored for determining the driving force for blood movement during external chest compression CPR has been to examine the hemodynamic consequences of changes in applied compression rate (cycles per minute) and compression duration (percentage of cycle in compression). These indirect studies avoid the problems with pleural pressure measurements and surgical manipulation of the chest but depend on models. A mathematical model was developed that predicts that blood flow caused by intrathoracic pressure fluctuations should be insensitive to compression rate over a wide range but should depend on the applied force and compression duration.[59] With intrathoracic pressure rises, increasing the applied force should increase generated intrathoracic pressure. Blood flow should continue as the duration of compression is prolonged, as long as the venous capacitance bed is not filled with blood. If direct compression of the heart plays a major role, however, the model predicts that flow should depend on compression rate and force but, above a threshold, should be insensitive to compression duration. With cardiac compression, stroke volume should be a function of chest compression force, and an increased rate would cause more stroke volumes per unit time to be pumped into the arterial bed. Prolonging compression beyond that necessary for maximum sternal displacement would have no effect, however, because the entire stroke volume would be ejected as soon as maximum cardiac compression occurred.

The model was validated for direct cardiac compression by studying the hemodynamics of cyclic cardiac deformation following thoracotomy in dogs. As predicted by the model, no change in myocardial or cerebral perfusion pressures occurred when the duration of compression was increased from 15 to 45% of the cycle at a constant rate of 60 compressions/min. There was, however, a significant increase in perfusion pressures when the rate was increased from 60 to 150 compressions/min at a constant duration of 45%. The model was validated for intrathoracic pressure changes by studying the hemodynamics produced by a circumferential thoracic vest (vest CPR). The vest contained a bladder that was inflated and deflated. Vest CPR changed intrathoracic pressure without direct cardiac compression, since sternal displacement was less than 0.8 cm and was usually away from the heart. As predicted by the model, and opposite to direct cardiac compression, there was no change in perfusion pressures when the rate was increased from 60 to 150 compressions/min at a constant duration of 45% of the cycle.

The hemodynamic effects of changes in applied sternal force, compression rate, and compression duration were then studied during manual CPR in dogs (Fig. 16.6). In these studies there was no surgical manipulation of the chest. Myocardial and cerebral blood flows were determined with radioactive microspheres and behaved as predicted from the model of intrathoracic pressure – flow was significantly increased when the duration of compression was increased from short (13 to 19% of the cycle) to long (40 to 47%), at a rate of 60 compressions/min, but flow was unchanged for an increase in rate from 60 to 150 compressions/min at constant compression duration.[16]

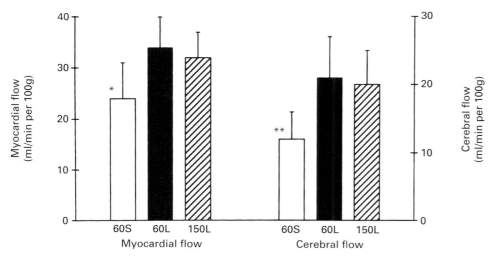

Fig. 16.6. Microsphere-determined myocardial and cerebral blood flows at different rates and compression durations (percent of cycle in compression) during manual CPR in dogs ($n = 8$). Both myocardial and cerebral flows are less when manual CPR is performed at 60 compressions/min with short (15%) duration (*60S*) than when it is performed at 60 compressions/min with long (45%) duration (*60L*) or at 150 compressions/min with long duration (*150L*). There is no increase in flow when rate is increased from 60 to 150 compressions/min at same duration of compression. * = $P < 0.05$; ** = $P < 0.02$.

Similar results were found in patients. Taylor and associates demonstrated in humans that higher mean arterial pressure and Doppler-estimated carotid artery blood flow velocity were achieved by longer (50 to 60% of the cycle) rather than shorter (30% of the cycle) chest compression duration at constant maximum chest compression force and compression rate.[75] In that study a mechanical chest compression device was used to control these variables precisely. The increased compression duration itself, rather than an increase in sternal displacement with prolonged compression duration, explained the increased flow. Later studies in humans confirmed that no significant increase occurred in sternal displacement when the compression duration was increased at a constant chest compression force.[76] In contrast to the increase in pressures and flows with prolonged compression duration, very little difference in mean pressure or estimated flow occurred with changes in rate between 40 and 80 cycles/min.

In studies of chronically instrumented dogs, faster compression rates have been reported to increase blood flow,[19] suggesting that cardiac compression was the driving force for blood movement. This conclusion, however, is questionable when compression duration is also considered. In these latter studies, rate may have been important since compression duration and perhaps force were not controlled. The time of compression at each rate appears nearly constant, so that at higher rates, compression occurred for

an increased percentage of the cycle. Optimal cardiac output occurred at a rate of 120 compressions/minute, where it appears that compression was approximately 50% of the cycle.[19] Since compression force was not measured, it is possible that some of the increase in flow reflects an increase related to greater compression force at faster rates.

In summary, the above data suggest that generated changes in intrathoracic pressure can move blood during external chest compression CPR. Intrathoracic pressure rises probably are responsible for the bulk of blood movement during external chest compression. Direct cardiac compression can, however, contribute to a variable extent.

Modifiers of the pump

Abdominal pressure

Abdominal pressure influences the intrathoracic pressure pump directly, since manipulation of abdominal pressure can affect the level of generated intrathoracic pressure.[34,53,60,77] The effect of abdominal pressure on the cardiac compression pump is, however, less clear. Manipulation of abdominal pressure has been studied during both chest compression,[43,53,60] and chest relaxation.[63,78]

Increases in abdominal pressure during chest compression have generally been accomplished by applying a circumferential binder to the abdomen.[53,60] The binder restricts movement of the thoracic contents into the abdomen during chest compression. As thoracic volume is reduced by chest compression, the thoracic contents are restricted from moving away from the compression force, and intrathoracic pressure is augmented. Right atrial pressure, however, appears to be raised excessively, which reduces the pressure gradient from the aorta to the right atrium.[53] Since the resulting decrease in coronary blood flow can reduce the likelihood of restoring the heartbeat,[4,53,79] abdominal binding is generally not considered a useful adjunct to chest compression.

Application of force to the abdomen during chest relaxation has generally been done manually and sometimes with a pressure measuring device.[63,80] This approach has been termed interposed abdominal compression (or abdominal counterpulsation) CPR.[63,80,81] In addition to an increase in intrathoracic pressure, it is presumed that abdominal compression between chest compressions can compress the aorta and produce greater retrograde aortic flow into the chest.[65] As with intraaortic balloon pumping, the resulting increase in aortic pressure would augment coronary flow. Animal studies of interposed abdominal compression have shown variable results,[32,82–84] but abdominal mechanics in humans and animals may be quite different. In humans, direct compression of the aorta by abdominal compression might be more effective than in dogs. Increasing intrathoracic pressure during chest relaxation may prolong the duration of intrathoracic pressure, which could augment coronary flow.[16,75] Alternatively, right atrial pressure may be raised relative to aortic pressure, which could decrease coronary flow. Since hemodynamic data in humans are not available, this approach requires further investigation.

Airway mechanics

For the cardiac compression pump, it would be assumed that airway mechanics are not important, since the driving force for blood movement is thought to be determined simply by the amount of cardiac deformation. For the intrathoracic pressure pump, however, airway mechanics are probably critical, since the trachea is generally not obstructed during chest compression.

It has been shown that increasing the duration of sternal compression maintains intrathoracic and vascular pressures while augmenting flow.[58,75] It has also been shown that arterial pressure is generally higher on the first compression after ventilation than on subsequent compressions.[18] In addition, high levels of intrathoracic pressure and improved survival can be produced by circumferential thoracic compressions from a pneumatic vest,[4,28] and by anterior-posterior chest compressions from a load distributing band,[85,86] despite an unobstructed trachea. If the airways were open during chest compression, then intrathoracic pressure would rise with the initial compression of the thoracic contents. Intrathoracic pressure would subsequently fall as the lungs emptied, despite sustained chest compression. If, however, the airways closed during chest compression, then the lungs would not empty, and intrathoracic pressure would remain elevated during the period of chest compression.

It has been demonstrated that airway collapse with air trapping does occur during chest compression, which explains how intrathoracic pressure can be generated and maintained despite an unobstructed airway.[85,87] Air trapping appears to result from vigorous chest compression, which alters the properties of the airways, leading to their collapse. This air trapping probably reduces the deformation of the chest wall needed to raise intrathoracic pressure and increases the transmission of pressure to the thoracic structures. In addition, air trapping is probably greater when chest compressions begin at higher lung volumes, since chest compressions after ventilation result in larger increases in intrathoracic pressure than chest compressions without prior ventilation.[18,87]

Three phenomena have been noted in dogs that show that airway collapse and air trapping occur. First, with ventilation just before chest compression, only a portion of the inspired tidal volume moved out of the lungs during chest compression (Fig. 16.7). After chest relaxation, however, more air moved out of the lungs, indicating that a portion of the inspired tidal volume was trapped during chest compression. The trapped air was passively discharged by the elastic recoil of the respiratory system. During cycles without prior ventilation, the amount of air expired by chest compression can decrease, paradoxically, at higher levels of chest compression, indicating that air was trapped at the higher levels. Second, with a micro-manometer advanced 5 to 8 cm distal to the carina, a zone of high pressure was noted, indicating a zone of airway collapse distal to the carina. Withdrawal of the catheter only a few centimeters caused a marked decrease in the recorded phasic pressure changes, again indicating that there was a locus of constriction or collapse approximately 4 to 6 cm distal to the carina, in small or medium airways. Finally, the site of collapse was directly visualized with cineradiography during chest compression, by instillation of contrast into the airway (Fig. 16.8). The collapse site was found to be coincident with the site in the airway where the large phasic changes in airway pressure were noted.

Airway manipulation

Positive airway pressure administered simultaneously with chest compression has been used to augment intrathoracic

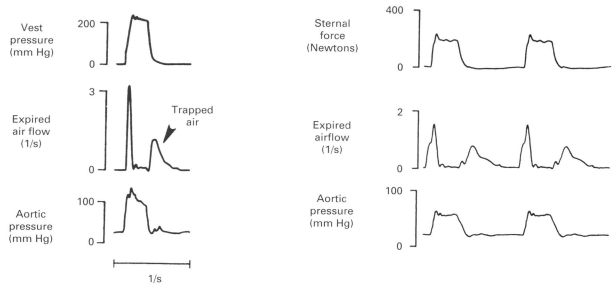

Fig. 16.7. Original recording during vest inflation (*left*) and during sternal displacement from a pneumatic piston (*right*). Inspiration with 500 ml occurred just before each vest inflation or piston actuation. Only expired airflow is shown. Inspired airflow is not shown since it did not go through airflow sensor. During vest inflation, note that a portion of inspired tidal volume was trapped (trapped air), since more air moved out of thorax after vest deflation. Note similar finding with piston compression. (Reproduced with permission from ref. 87. Copyright 1989 American Heart Association.)

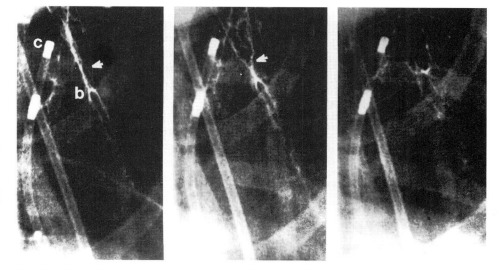

Fig. 16.8. Cineradiograms of airways during vest deflation. *Left frame* was taken just as vest deflation started. Airway collapse is noted by *arrow*. Airway bifurcates (*b*) distal to collapse site. *Center frame* was taken 17 milliseconds later and shows airway partially open (*arrow*). *Right frame* was taken another 17 milliseconds later and shows airway fully open. Bipolar electrode catheter (c) is in right ventricle and is approximately 2 mm in diameter. (Reproduced with permission from ref. 87. Copyright 1989 American Heart Association.)

pressure directly and has been termed simultaneous compression-ventilation CPR.[29,34,53,77] As with airway collapse, the mechanism for augmentation of intrathoracic pressure is the elimination of expiratory airflow during chest compression. The requirement of endotracheal intubation and a device to administer simultaneous compression and high-pressure ventilation, however, has limited use of this technique.

Obstruction of the airway with a valve has also been used to augment intrathoracic pressure.[88] The valve is generally closed during chest compression, and the mechanism of action appears to be similar to that of airway collapse. The contribution of this airway obstruction over that of intrinsic airway collapse is unknown.

Negative airway pressure has been administered during chest relaxation to produce negative intrathoracic pressure.[29,38,40,89] It was suggested that negative intrathoracic pressure, between chest compressions, would augment venous return and thereby augment forward flow.

Circumferential chest compression

Circumferential chest compression has been studied as a more effective way of generating intrathoracic pressure fluctuations[4,65] and is generally accomplished with a pneumatic vest.[28,90] The vest contains a bladder that is cyclically inflated and deflated. The increased intrathoracic pressure fluctuations appear to be mediated through increased reduction of thoracic volume and through increased air trapping.[87] In addition, chest compression force is substantially higher than that used with standard manual CPR, since the force is distributed around the thorax.[28] The increased chest compression force would raise intrathoracic pressure in relation to the reduction in thoracic volume, assuming air trapping occurred. By reducing expiratory airflow, air trapping could also increase the efficiency with which vest pressure is transmitted to the intrathoracic space. Any decrease in expiratory airflow would reduce the amount of chest deformation at any level of vest pressure. At the reduced amount of chest deformation, less of the force applied to the chest would be needed to compress the elastic structures of the thorax, resulting in greater transmission of vest pressure to the intrathoracic space.

Load distributing band

The load distributing band is an evolution of the circumferential vest compression concept.[85,91] With the load distributing band system, an electromechanical band is placed around the chest and the band is tightened and loosened by a rotating motor that is contained in a backboard assembly. The band system produces anterior-posterior chest compressions, but distributes the chest compression force over the entire anterior chest.[85,91] Similar airway collapse has been noted with the band system as with the circumferential chest compression system.[85,87]

Active chest decompression

Active, rather than passive, decompression of the chest has been reported to augment vascular pressures[48,92], and return of spontaneous circulation.[46,93] The technique has been termed active compression–decompression CPR and utilizes a suction-cup device to pull up on the chest during chest relaxation (see Chapter 31). The mechanisms operative during active decompressions have not been determined, but such active decompressions could result in greater chest expansion and filling with air between compressions. The amount of air trapped in the lungs could thereby be increased, which could augment the generated intrathoracic pressure.[87] In addition, active decompressions could induce negative intrathoracic pressure between compressions, which could augment venous return. Increased venous return could enhance the forward flow produced by cardiac compression or by intrathoracic pressure fluctuations. Few data sources are available, however, on the level of chest compression force used with this technique, so it is not known if the reported benefit for active decompression CPR results simply from an increased *total force* (peak compression to peak decompression force) applied to the chest. For example, if a 400-newton compression force and a 100-newton decompression force were applied to the chest, is it equivalent to simply applying 500-newtons of compression force, or does the decompression force have unique physiologic effects that improve blood flow? Results of studies to date have not resolved these issues.

The device used to apply the active compressions and decompressions[36] may also give the rescuer a mechanical advantage in performing chest compression, which could result in substantially higher sternal forces being applied than with standard manual CPR. These increased forces could augment the generated intrathoracic pressure or enhance cardiac compression, which could increase short-term survival. Trauma, however, could reduce long-term survival.

Impedance threshold device

This device is placed in the airway circuit and is used to impede the flow of air into the chest during chest decompression, thereby producing a particular level of negative intrathoracic pressure. This device has allowed the use of negative intrathoracic pressure between chest compressions to come into clinical use,[36,38,40,89,94] and improvements in hemodynamics and short-term survival have been reported with this device.[39,41]

The load

As with the intact circulation, the vascular load during external chest compression is probably the arterial resistance and compliance. Their values during CPR may, however, differ substantially from those of the intact circulation because of changes in neural-humoral conditions, ischemia, administered drugs, and mechanical maneuvers such as applying pressure to the abdomen.

Arterial resistance

The arterial (peripheral) resistance appears to be the most critical loading factor that influences coronary and cerebral flow. Numerous studies have shown that administering drugs that increase peripheral resistance increases coronary perfusion pressure, cerebral and coronary blood flow (Fig. 16.9), and return of spontaneous circulation.[4,53,54,56,95–100] These improvements were present regardless of the type of CPR performed. Because of the difficulty in making direct measurements in humans, both electrical and mathematic models have been developed to study the hemodynamic effects of changes in peripheral resistance.[58,59,101] These models predict increases in cerebral and myocardial flows similar to those that have been measured experimentally. One extensively validated model[59] predicts that increased peripheral resistance improves myocardial and cerebral blood flow because of an increase in the mean aortic pressure during chest compression. The increased peripheral resistance probably decreases the runoff of blood into the periphery during chest compression, maintaining higher levels of aortic pressure, regardless of the nature of the pump.

Increasing peripheral resistance may not, however, have equivalent effects on the coronary flow produced by different CPR techniques. One study in pigs showed that active decompression CPR produced more coronary blood flow than standard CPR when vasoconstrictors were not used[48] but showed no difference in coronary flow when vasoconstrictors were used. The vasoconstrictors increased the coronary flow produced by standard CPR more than that produced by active decompression CPR, so that both flows became similar.[48] The mechanisms causing these differences are unknown, since it is assumed that peripheral resistance was increased an equivalent amount by the vasoconstrictors with each technique.

In contrast to the increase in cerebral and myocardial flow with increased peripheral resistance, there appears to be a paradoxical fall in cardiac output.[102] This fall in cardiac output is most consistent with the intrathoracic pressure pump as the driving force for blood movement. With a fixed level of intrathoracic pressure determining vascular pressure, cardiac output would be inversely related to peripheral resistance, because the mean pressure across the vascular bed would be equal to the mean flow through the bed times the resistance of the bed.[103] It would be expected therefore that with use of vasoconstrictors, cardiac output would fall as peripheral resistance rises, since the driving pressure would not change. Because myocardial blood flow during CPR is a major determinant of survival from cardiac arrest,[3,4] it is possible that with the periodic use of epinephrine, changes in

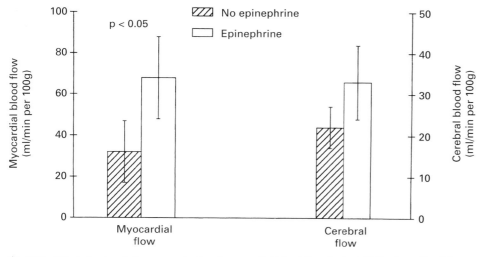

Fig. 16.9. Effect of epinephrine on cerebral and myocardial blood flow during CPR in dogs. Blood flows were measured with radioactive microspheres.

cardiac output may be uncoupled with changes in coronary blood flow, so that cardiac output would have no correlation with survival. Consequently, indicators of cardiac output, such as end-tidal CO_2 measurements, may be very limited in their utility as indicators of the efficacy of CPR.

Arterial compliance

The distribution of arterial compliance (intrathoracic versus extrathoracic) also appears to be an important determinant of myocardial blood flow.[58,59] This effect was predicted by at least two cardiovascular models[58,59] and is consistent with the intrathoracic pressure pump as the driving force for blood movement. With the intrathoracic pressure pump, intrathoracic pressure appears to be transmitted to the intrathoracic arteries collectively, so that all of the intrathoracic arteries can be represented by a single compliance. The extrathoracic arteries can also be represented by a single compliance. On the basis of using these two compliances, the models predict that coronary blood flow will be maximized when the intrathoracic arterial compliance is minimized (Fig. 16.10). The mechanisms appear to be related to bidirectional arterial flow (Fig. 16.3). During chest compression, blood will move from intrathoracic arteries to extrathoracic arteries. During

chest relaxation, however, some blood will move retrograde from the extrathoracic arteries back into the intrathoracic arteries to perfuse the coronary arteries. The less compliant are the intrathoracic arteries, the higher will be the aortic relaxation-phase pressure. If the intrathoracic arteries were very compliant, however, a greater volume of blood would be needed to fill these arteries immediately after release of chest compression, to maintain aortic relaxation-phase pressure – the intrathoracic arteries would have collapsed more during compression. Thus, if intrathoracic arterial compliance is small, blood returning to the thoracic arteries during chest relaxation quickly fills the arterial bed and improves myocardial blood flow. For the cardiac compression pump mechanism, however, the distribution of arterial compliance is probably less important.

Despite the possible importance of the distribution of arterial compliance (intrathoracic versus extrathoracic) in determining blood flow, this compliance distribution cannot be measured directly in intact animal preparations or in humans. Therefore, computer models have been used to show that the ratio of mean aortic relaxation-phase pressure to mean aortic compression-phase pressure (pressure ratio) can be used as an index of the distribution of arterial compliance between the extrathoracic and intrathoracic compartments.[59] There is an excellent correlation (r = .99) between this ratio and the ratio of extrathoracic to total arterial compliance. This pressure ratio was found to be a potent predictor of coronary blood flow in a canine model of cardiac arrest.[59]

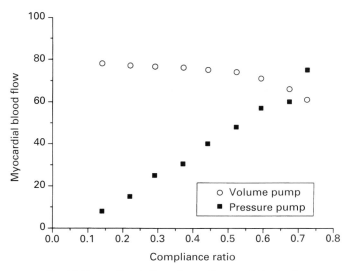

Fig. 16.10. Predicted effect of compliance ratio (ratio of extrathoracic to total arterial compliance) on myocardial blood flow for two different models of blood movement in CPR. For volume pump (cardiac compression), there is little effect of compliance ratio on myocardial blood flow. For pressure pump (intrathoracic pressure), however, there is a linear increase in myocardial flow with increasing compliance ratio. These data are predictions from a mathematic model of CPR (see text).

Abdominal pressure

In addition to the effect of abdominal pressure on the level of generated vascular pressure, abdominal pressure appears also to be a factor in changing the vascular load. Abdominal binding, which reduces coronary blood flow,[53] increases abdominal pressure during chest compression.[34,53] The cardiovascular model[59] confirms that as the level of abdominal pressure increases, the generated myocardial flow decreases (r = .99) (Fig. 16.11). The mechanism of reduction of coronary blood flow with increased abdominal pressure appears to be through a reduction in the effective extrathoracic arterial compliance. The reduced extrathoracic arterial compliance would limit the amount of blood stored in extrathoracic arteries during chest compression, so that less blood could flow retrograde during chest relaxation to perfuse the coronary arteries. In addition, increased abdominal pressure could alter the distribution of intravascular volume or resistance.

Therapy

The goal of external chest compression CPR, after defibrillation fails or is not indicated, is to maximize the generated coronary and cerebral blood flow. Restoration of native cardiac activity and preservation of brain function are directly related to these flows. Cerebral and coronary flows should be maximized by optimizing the driving force for blood movement and the loading conditions.

Optimizing the pump

For intrathoracic pressure fluctuations, the amount of thoracic volume reduction produced by chest compression appears to be critical. By Boyle's law, the more the chest volume is reduced, the more the intrathoracic pressure will rise. In current clinical practice, chest volume is reduced by the standard anteroposterior sternal displacement technique (see Chapter 30), although other techniques are being studied that may prove to be more effective.[28,40,61,85] For maximizing cardiac compression, however, the amount of thoracic volume reduction is probably not important. The major determinant of cardiac compression is probably the amount of anteroposterior chest displacement, although the exact determinants of cardiac compression are unknown. *Whether the driving force for blood movement is intrathoracic pressure fluctuations or direct cardiac compression, the amount of chest compression is a critical determinant of flow (Fig. 16.12), and the quality of chest compression will probably be a major factor in the effectiveness of CPR.*

The ability of even properly performed chest compressions to generate adequate levels of intrathoracic pressure or cardiac compression is probably marginal, since only about 15% of cardiac arrest victims survive. Nevertheless, external chest compression is the only technique for CPR that is widely available, and many lives are saved each year by standard CPR. Proper chest compression requires that the arms are locked relatively straight (see Chapter 30) and that the whole body is used in the compressions. Often, just the arms are used for chest compression, which is extremely tiring and probably will not generate sufficient compression force.

Although the amount of chest compression force or displacement appears to be a major determinant of the level of generated vascular pressure,[16] chest compression has to be applied at the optimal rate and compression duration (Fig. 16.6). Blood flow from intrathoracic pressure fluctuations should be insensitive to rate over a wide range but dependent on the compression duration.[16,59,75] If direct compression of the heart plays a major role, however, flow

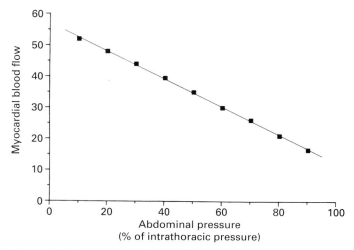

Fig. 16.11. Predicted effect of abdominal pressure on myocardial blood flow for pressure pump model of CPR. Abdominal pressure is expressed as a percentage of intrathoracic pressure. Predictions are from mathematic model.

should depend on rate but, above a threshold, should be insensitive to compression duration. The current recommendation of a rate of 80 to 100 compressions/minute probably maximizes blood flow from either pump. At that rate, the compression duration tends to be around 50%,[19] which is optimal for blood movement by intrathoracic pressure fluctuations,[59] and the rate of 80 to 100 compressions/minute is near the maximum that can be administered for any length of time by a rescuer, and would maximize the number of stroke volumes delivered to the circulation by a cardiac compression pump.[59]

The level of generated vascular pressures is likely to be affected by techniques that modify the pump, including abdominal compression,[63,80] airway manipulations,[34,40,43] circumferential chest compression,[4,28] load distributing band chest compression,[85,91] and active decompression.[50,51] The efficacy of abdominal compression, circumferential chest compression, load distributing band chest compression, and active chest decompression has not been definitively determined, so that their use in routine practice should be considered only when personnel are available who have been adequately trained in their use. Airway inflation between chest compressions should, however, be considered for routine use at this time. This airway inflation is used for ventilation, but it can also augment vascular pressures generated by the intrathoracic pressure pump. Lung inflation before chest compression can increase the amount of air trapped in the lungs during chest compression,[87] thereby augmenting the generated intrathoracic and vascular pressures and improving the efficacy of CPR.

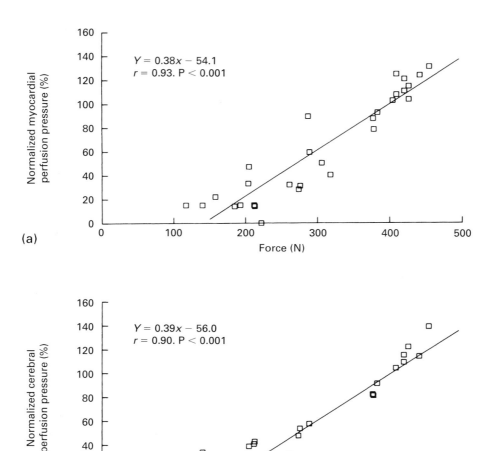

Fig. 16.12. (a) Correlation between normalized myocardial perfusion pressure and applied sternal force for manual CPR at 60 compressions/min with prolonged duration in dogs. Perfusion pressures for each dog are expressed as a percentage of perfusion pressure obtained at a sternal force of 400 newtons for that dog. (b) Correlation between normalized cerebral perfusion pressure and applied sternal force for manual CPR at 60 compressions/min with prolonged duration in dogs. Perfusion pressures for each dog are expressed as above. (Reproduced with permission from ref. 16. Copyright 1986 American Heart Association.)

Optimizing the vascular load

The peripheral resistance is probably the component of the vascular load that has the largest effect on blood flow. Numerous studies have shown that vascular pressures are augmented and produce increased flow to the heart muscle and brain when vasoconstrictors are used.[3,4,48,54,56,100,102] This increased flow appears to be mediated through a-adrenergic agonism,[96–98] which increases peripheral resistance and decreases runoff of blood to the periphery. Decreased runoff

slows decay of arterial pressure during the release phase of chest compression, thereby raising aortic pressure, myocardial perfusion pressure (aortic minus right atrial mean release phase pressure), and cerebral perfusion pressure (carotid minus intracranial mean pressure).

The vasoconstrictor most commonly used today is epinephrine, which has both α- and β-agonist effects. It is clear that the α-agonist effects are responsible for improvement in vital organ flows (Fig. 16.9). The utility of the β-agonist effects, however, is controversial. Some investigators believe that β-agonism is detrimental because of increased myocardial work,[96,100] whereas others believe that β-agonism is beneficial by increasing inotropy.[96] The efficacy of epinephrine compared with other vasoconstrictors remains to be determined. Higher doses of epinephrine have, however, been found to be toxic[104] and are no longer recommended.

In contrast to increasing blood flow to the myocardium and brain, increased peripheral resistance can reduce total cardiac output. Cardiac output is reduced because the increases in peripheral resistance are greater than the increases in generated vascular pressures that are secondary to the increases in peripheral resistance.[102] This decreased cardiac output can explain the observation that end-tidal CO_2 can decrease with increased doses of epinephrine.[102] End-tidal CO_2 has been studied as a non-invasive method of determining the adequacy of resuscitation, since it appears to correlate with cardiac output and resuscitation success in some circumstances.[105]

In addition to the effects of vascular resistance and compliance on blood flow during CPR, it appears that the volume status contributes independently. If excessive volume is present in the vascular spaces during CPR, the venous pressures tend to be elevated during the release phase of chest compression, which can reduce the coronary perfusion pressure.[106] This finding strongly suggests that excessive volume should not be infused during resuscitation. If insufficient volume is present, however, forward flow appears to be compromised by inducing arterial collapse. Selective arterial infusion does appear to be of potential value in reversing this arterial collapse.[107]

In summary with what is currently known, the factors that appear to have the most influence on generating blood flow by external chest compression are (a) maximizing the amount of chest compression and (b) using the proper doses of vasoconstrictors. Maximization of chest compression force includes using the proper sternal force, as well as minimizing interruptions in the application of force. With standard external chest compression, the type of pump operative probably is not important, since standard external chest compression does not allow selection of a particular mechanism over that which occurs naturally.

The future

Determining the pump

Controversy continues about the nature of the pump operative during external chest compression. Future studies could potentially help resolve this controversy, but it now

seems that the driving force for blood flow produced by standard external chest compression is some combination of intrathoracic pressure fluctuations and direct cardiac compression. Although standard external chest compression does not appear to allow selective utilization of intrathoracic pressure or cardiac compression, it is likely that more clever ways of applying force to the patient will be developed in the future, based on exploiting specific mechanisms.

By its more directed application of force, cardiac compression is probably more potent than intrathoracic pressure fluctuations in moving blood for a given amount of pressure rise. It remains to be determined, however, whether external CPR can compress the heart the large amount necessary to generate adequate vascular pressures.[16] It is also unclear how cardiac compression can specifically be augmented during non-invasive CPR, since the determinants of cardiac compression have not been defined. These issues could potentially be clarified with further research.

Improving standard chest compression

One simple way of potentially increasing blood flow would be to increase the amount of chest compression force and displacement. There is clearly a minimum amount of chest compression force that has to be applied to generate blood flow[16] (Fig. 16.12). It is very likely, therefore, that ineffective CPR occurs because inadequate chest compression force is applied. In routine clinical practice, there is no objective way for a rescuer to determine if adequate chest compression is applied. The American Heart Association recommends that there should be 1.5 to 2 inches of chest displacement during chest compression,[2] but it is not known whether that amount of chest compression is applied routinely or whether that amount of compression is optimal. More emphasis should be placed on ensuring that adequate chest compression is performed. This could consist of more training. Retention of trained skills is limited, however, and even well-trained rescuers have no objective way of judging whether they are performing chest compressions adequately. The widespread use of gauges or other measuring aids may increase the likelihood that chest compression is performed properly. Although it is probably true that "any CPR" (i.e., any blood flow) is better than no CPR, the available data suggest very strongly that better CPR (i.e., CPR that generates more blood flow) will improve survival.[3,4,16,53] There is little chance that ischemia will be relieved, or that drugs will be delivered adequately, if blood flow is insufficient. Increasing the level of chest compression beyond that normally used may improve blood flow and survival. It has not been determined, however, whether increased sternal force would have a greater effect on improving blood flow and enhancing survival or on increasing trauma and limiting survival. External chest compression could also be modified by altering the point or points of force application and the rate of the force rise. Studies should be performed to investigate the influence of changes in chest compression force on blood flow and survival.

Alternative compression techniques

Understanding the mechanisms of blood flow during external chest compression is probably most important for development of improved compression techniques, since they can be aimed at exploiting specific mechanisms.

Circumferential chest compressions (vest CPR)[28] may be a more efficient way of generating vascular pressures and flow, because the amount of reduction in thoracic volume is critical for generation of intrathoracic pressure rises. There is a geometric advantage in reducing thoracic volume by a circumferential, rather than a point, compression, since the volume will decrease roughly as the square of the decrease in radius. The circumferential compression may also allow increased force to be used because the force is distributed over a much larger area than it is with standard external chest compression. Since only preliminary data are available, however, the role of vest CPR in treating cardiac arrest remains to be determined.

Chest compressions with the Load Distributing Band system[85,91] may be a more practical way of improving chest compression than the Vest CPR System. The Load Distributing Band system is much more compact than the Vest CPR system and applies forces to the entire anterior chest. Hemodynamic results with the Load Distributing Band system seem to be similar to those with the Vest CPR System.[28,85,91]

Intrathoracic pressure changes could also be enhanced through increased air trapping, which could be achieved by ventilation before each chest compression or through active chest decompressions.[46,51] The active decompressions could result in greater chest expansion and filling with air between compressions, so that the next compression results in a greater rise in intrathoracic pressure and increased flow. In addition, the impedance threshold device can be used to enhance negative intrathoracic pressure changes in between chest compressions,[41] that may augment venous return and aid either the intrathoracic pressure or cardiac compression pumps.

Last, application of force to the abdomen during chest relaxation may augment vascular pressure.[63,80] Animal studies of such abdominal compression have shown variable results, and few objective hemodynamic data are available in humans. Further studies of these techniques are therefore needed.

Improved adjuncts

The efficacy of CPR may be improved by using drugs or mechanical techniques to modify the pump or the load. Such interventions could potentially increase peripheral resistance to levels higher than currently achieved, favorably alter the distribution of arterial compliance (intrathoracic versus extrathoracic), increase air trapping, and augment venous return.

It is possible that peripheral resistance could be increased to higher levels by using increased doses of epinephrine or by using other vasoconstrictor drugs. Clearly the α-agonist effects of epinephrine increase peripheral resistance.[97,98] There is controversy, however, about the utility of the β-agonist effects. Some investigators believe that β-agonism is detrimental because of increased myocardial work,[100,108] whereas others believe that β-agonism is beneficial by increasing inotropy.[96] Increased doses of epinephrine likely have direct toxic effects on tissues, may exacerbate ischemic damage to other tissues by shunting blood away from them, and are no longer recommended for general clinical use.[104] The roles of other vasoconstrictor drugs, however, have not been resolved.

REFERENCES

1. Zheng, Z.J., Croft, J.B., Giles, W.H., & Mensah, G.A. Sudden cardiac death in the United States, 1989 to 1998. *Circulation* 2001; **104**: 2158–2163.
2. 2005 American Heart Association Guidelines for Cardiopulmonary Resuscitation and Emergency Cardiovascular Care. *Circulation* 2005; **112**: IV1–203.
3. Ralston, S.H., Voorhees, W.D., & Babbs, C.F. Intrapulmonary epinephrine during prolonged cardiopulmonary resuscitation: improved regional blood flow and resuscitation in dogs. *Ann. Emerg. Med.* 1984; **13**: 79–86.
4. Halperin, H.R., Guerci, A.D., Chandra, N. *et al.* Vest inflation without simultaneous ventilation during cardiac arrest in dogs: improved survival from prolonged cardiopulmonary resuscitation. *Circulation* 1986; **74**: 1407–1415.
5. Pearson, J.W., & Redding, J.S. Peripheral vascular tone on cardiac resuscitation. *Anesth. Analg.* 1965; **44**: 746–752.
6. Paradis, N.A., Martin, G.B., Rivers, E.P. *et al.* Coronary perfusion pressure and the return of spontaneous circulation in human cardiopulmonary resuscitation. *J. Am. Med. Assoc.* 1990; **263**: 1106–1113.
7. Eleff, S.M., Kim, H., Shaffner, D.H., Traystman, R.J., & Koehler, R.C. Effect of cerebral blood flow generated during

cardiopulmonary resuscitation in dogs on maintenance versus recovery of ATP and, pH. *Stroke* 1993; **24**: 2066–2073.

8. Eleff, S.M., Schleien, C.L., Koehler, R.C. *et al.* Brain bioenergetics during cardiopulmonary resuscitation in dogs. *Anesthesiology* 1992; **76**: 77–84.

9. Criley, J.M., Blaufuss, A.H., & Kissel, G.L. Cough-induced cardiac compression. Self-administered from of cardiopulmonary resuscitation. *J. Am. Med. Assoc.* 1976; **236**: 1246–1250.

10. Niemann, J.T., Rosborough, J.P., Hausknecht, M., Garner, D., & Criley, J.M. Pressure-synchronized cineangiography during experimental cardiopulmonary resuscitation. *Circulation* 1981; **64**: 985–991.

11. Criley, J.M. The thoracic pump provides a mechanism for coronary perfusion. *Arch. Intern. Med.* 1995; **155**: 1236.

12. Criley, J.M., Niemann, J.T., Rosborough, J.P., Ung, S., & Suzuki, J. The heart is a conduit in CPR. *Crit. Care Med.* 1981; **9**: 373–374.

13. Niemann, J.T., Rosborough, J., Hausknecht, M., Ung, S., & Criley, J.M. Blood flow without cardiac compression during closed chest CPR. *Crit. Care Med.* 1981; **9**: 380–381.

14. Guerci, A.D., Halperin, H.R., Beyar, R. *et al.* Aortic diameter and pressure-flow sequence identify mechanism of blood flow during external chest compression in dogs. *J. Am. Coll. Cardiol.* 1989; **14**: 790–798.

15. Weisfeldt, M.L., & Halperin, H.R. Cardiopulmonary resuscitation: beyond cardiac massage. *Circulation* 1986; **74**: 443–448.

16. Halperin, H.R., Tsitlik, J.E., Guerci, A.D. *et al.* Determinants of blood flow to vital organs during cardiopulmonary resuscitation in dogs. *Circulation* 1986; **73**: 539–550.

17. Chandra, N., Guerci, A., Weisfeldt, M.L., Tsitlik, J., & Lepor, N. Contrasts between intrathoracic pressures during external chest compression and cardiac massage. *Crit. Care Med.* 1981; **9**: 789–792.

18. Rudikoff, M.T., Maughan, W.L., Effron, M., Freund, P., & Weisfeldt, M.L. Mechanisms of blood flow during cardiopulmonary resuscitation. *Circulation* 1980; **61**: 345–352.

19. Maier, G.W., Tyson, G.S., Jr., Olsen, C.O. *et al.* The physiology of external cardiac massage: high-impulse cardiopulmonary resuscitation. *Circulation* 1984; **70**: 86–101.

20. Feneley, M.P., Maier, G.W., Gaynor, J.W. *et al.* Sequence of mitral valve motion and transmitral blood flow during manual cardiopulmonary resuscitation in dogs. *Circulation* 1987; **76**: 363–375.

21. Babbs, C.F., Bircher, N., Burkett, D.E., Frissora, H.A., Hodgkin, B.C., & Safar, P. Effect of thoracic venting on arterial pressure, and flow during external cardiopulmonary resuscitation in animals. *Crit. Care Med.* 1981; **9**: 785–788.

22. Kouwenhoven, W.B., Jude, J.R., & Knickerbocker, G.G. Closed chest cardiac massage. *J. Am. Med. Assoc.* 1960; **173**: 1064–1067.

23. Halperin, H.R., Weiss, J.L., Guerci, A.D. *et al.* Cyclic elevation of intrathoracic pressure can close the mitral valve during cardiac arrest in dogs. *Circulation* 1988; **78**: 754–760.

24. Deshmukh, H.G., Weil, M.H., Gudipati, C.V., Trevino, R.P., Bisera, J., & Rackow, E.C. Mechanism of blood flow generated by precordial compression during CPR. I. Studies on closed chest precordial compression. *Chest* 1989; **95**: 1092–1099.

25. Crile, G., & Dolley, D.H. An experimental research into the resuscitation of dogs killed by anesthetics and asphyxia. *J. Exp. Med.* 1906; **8**: 713.

26. Paradis, N.A., Martin, G.B., Goetting, M.G. *et al.* Simultaneous aortic, jugular bulb, and right atrial pressures during cardiopulmonary resuscitation in humans. Insights into mechanisms. *Circulation* 1989; **80**: 361–368.

27. Porter, T.R., Ornato, J.P., Guard, C.S., Roy, V.G., Burns, C.A., & Nixon, J.V. Transesophageal echocardiography to assess mitral valve function and flow during cardiopulmonary resuscitation. *Am. J. Cardiol.* 1992; **70**: 1056–1060.

28. Halperin, H.R., Tsitlik, J.E., Gelfand, M. *et al.* A preliminary study of cardiopulmonary resuscitation by circumferential compression of the chest with use of a pneumatic vest. *N. Engl. J. Med.* 1993; **329**: 762–768.

29. Chandra, N., Weisfeldt, M.L., Tsitlik, J. *et al.* Augmentation of carotid flow during cardiopulmonary resuscitation by ventilation at high airway pressure simultaneous with chest compression. *Am. J. Cardiol.* 1981; **48**: 1053–1063.

30. Krischer, J.P., Fine, E.G., Weisfeldt, M.L., Guerci, A.D., Nagel, E., & Chandra, N. Comparison of prehospital conventional and simultaneous compression-ventilation cardiopulmonary resuscitation. *Crit. Care Med.* 1989; **17**: 1263–1269.

31. Babbs, C.F., Sack, J.B., & Kern, K.B. Interposed abdominal compression as an adjunct to cardiopulmonary resuscitation. *Am. Heart J.* 1994; **127**: 412–421.

32. Babbs, C.F. Interposed abdominal compression CPR: a comprehensive evidence based review. *Resuscitation* 2003; **59**: 71–82.

33. Melker, R.J. Asynchronous and other alternative methods of ventilation during CPR. *Ann. Emerg. Med.* 1984; **13**: 758–761.

34. Chandra, N., Rudikoff, M., & Weisfeldt, M.L. Simultaneous chest compression and ventilation at high airway pressure during cardiopulmonary resuscitation. *Lancet* 1980; **1**: 175–178.

35. Babbs, C.F., Tacker, W.A., Paris, R.L., Murphy, R.J., & Davis, R.W. CPR with simultaneous compression and ventilation at high airway pressure in 4 animal models. *Crit. Care Med.* 1982; **10**: 501–504.

36. Lurie, K.G., Coffeen, P., Shultz, J., McKnite, S., Detloff, B., & Mulligan, K. Improving active compression–decompression cardiopulmonary resuscitation with an inspiratory impedance valve. *Circulation* 1995; **91**: 1629–1632.

37. Lurie, K.G., Mulligan, K.A., McKnite, S., Detloff, B., Lindstrom, P., & Lindner, K.H. Optimizing standard cardiopulmonary resuscitation with an inspiratory impedance threshold valve. *Chest* 1998; **113**: 1084–1090.

38. Lurie, K., Voelckel, W., Plaisance, P. *et al.* Use of an inspiratory impedance threshold valve during cardiopulmonary resuscitation: a progress report. *Resuscitation* 2000; **44**: 219–230.

39. Plaisance, P., Lurie, K.G., & Payen, D. Inspiratory impedance during active compression–decompression cardiopulmonary

resuscitation: a randomized evaluation in patients in cardiac arrest. *Circulation* 2000; **101**: 989–994.

40. Lurie, K.G., Zielinski, T., McKnite, S., Aufderheide, T., & Voelckel, W. Use of an inspiratory impedance valve improves neurologically intact survival in a porcine model of ventricular fibrillation. *Circulation* 2002; **105**: 124–129.

41. Pirrallo, R.G., Aufderheide, T.P., Provo, T.A., & Lurie, K.G. Effect of an inspiratory impedance threshold device on hemodynamics during conventional manual cardiopulmonary resuscitation. *Resuscitation* 2005; **66**: 13–20.

42. Luce, J.M., Ross, B.K., O'Quin, R.J. *et al.* Regional blood flow during cardiopulmonary resuscitation in dogs using simultaneous and nonsimultaneous compression and ventilation. *Circulation* 1983; **67**: 258–265.

43. Niemann, J.T., Rosborough, J.P., Niskanen, R.A., Alferness, C., & Criley, J.M. Mechanical "cough" cardiopulmonary resuscitation during cardiac arrest in dogs. *Am. J. Cardiol.* 1985; **55**: 199–204.

44. Swenson, R.D., Weaver, W.D., Niskanen, R.A., Martin, J., & Dahlberg, S. Hemodynamics in humans during conventional and experimental methods of cardiopulmonary resuscitation. *Circulation* 1988; **78**: 630–639.

45. Beyar, R., Kishon, Y., Dinnar, U., & Neufeld, H.N. Cardiopulmonary resuscitation by intrathoracic pressure variations – in vivo studies and computer simulation. *Angiology* 1984; **35**: 71–78.

46. Cohen, T.J., Tucker, K.J., Redberg, R.F. *et al.* Active compression–decompression resuscitation: a novel method of cardiopulmonary resuscitation. *Am. Heart J.* 1992; **124**: 1145–1150.

47. Shultz, J.J., Coffeen, P., Sweeney, M. *et al.* Evaluation of standard and active compression–decompression CPR in an acute human model of ventricular fibrillation. *Circulation* 1994; **89**: 684–693.

48. Lindner, K.H., Pfenninger, E.G., Lurie, K.G., Schurmann, W., Lindner, I.M., & Ahnefeld, F.W. Effects of active compression–decompression resuscitation on myocardial and cerebral blood flow in pigs. *Circulation* 1993; **88**: 1254–1263.

49. Lurie, K.G., Lindo, C., & Chin, J. CPR: the P stands for plumber's helper. *J. Am. Med. Assoc.* 1990; **264**: 1661.

50. Mauer, D.K., Nolan, J., Plaisance, P. *et al.* Effect of active compression–decompression resuscitation (ACD-CPR) on survival: a combined analysis using individual patient data. *Resuscitation* 1999; **41**: 249–256.

51. Plaisance, P., Lurie, K.G., Vicaut, E. *et al.* A comparison of standard cardiopulmonary resuscitation and active compression–decompression resuscitation for out-of-hospital cardiac arrest. French Active Compression–Decompression Cardiopulmonary Resuscitation Study Group. *N. Engl. J. Med.* 1999; **341**: 569–575.

52. Voelckel, W.G., Lurie, K.G., Sweeney, M. *et al.* Effects of active compression–decompression cardiopulmonary resuscitation with the inspiratory threshold valve in a young porcine model of cardiac arrest. *Pediatr. Res.* 2002; **51**: 523–527.

53. Michael, J.R., Guerci, A.D., Koehler, R.C. *et al.* Mechanisms by which epinephrine augments cerebral and myocardial perfusion during cardiopulmonary resuscitation in dogs. *Circulation* 1984; **69**: 822–835.

54. Gonzalez, E.R., & Ornato, J.P. The dose of epinephrine during cardiopulmonary resuscitation in humans: what should it be? *DICP* 1991; **25**: 773–777.

55. Gervais, H.W., Schleien, C.L., Koehler, R.C., Berkowitz, I.D., Shaffner, D.H., & Traystman, R.J. Effect of adrenergic drugs on cerebral blood flow, metabolism, and evoked potentials after delayed cardiopulmonary resuscitation in dogs. *Stroke* 1991; **22**: 1554–1561.

56. Berkowitz, I.D., Gervais, H., Schleien, C.L., Koehler, R.C., Dean, J.M., & Traystman, R.J. Epinephrine dosage effects on cerebral and myocardial blood flow in an infant swine model of cardiopulmonary resuscitation. *Anesthesiology* 1991; **75**: 1041–1050.

57. Yin, F.C., Cohen, J.M., Tsitlik, J., Zola, B., & Weisfeldt, M.L. Role of carotid artery resistance to collapse during high-intrathoracic-pressure CPR. *Am. J. Physiol.* 1982; **243**: H259–H267.

58. Babbs, C.F., Ralston, S.H., & Geddes, L.A. Theoretical advantages of abdominal counterpulsation in CPR as demonstrated in a simple electrical model of the circulation. *Ann. Emerg. Med.* 1984; **13**: 660–671.

59. Halperin, H.R., Tsitlik, J.E., Beyar, R., Chandra, N., & Guerci, A.D. Intrathoracic pressure fluctuations move blood during CPR: comparison of hemodynamic data with predictions from a mathematical model. *Ann. Biomed. Eng.* 1987; **15**: 385–403.

60. Chandra, N., Snyder, L.D., & Weisfeldt, M.L. Abdominal binding during cardiopulmonary resuscitation in man. *J. Am. Med. Assoc.* 1981; **246**: 351–353.

61. Lurie, K.G. Active compression–decompression CPR: a progress report. *Resuscitation* 1994; **28**: 115–122.

62. Babbs, C.F. Preclinical studies of abdominal counterpulsation in CPR. *Ann. Emerg. Med.* 1984; **13**: 761–763.

63. Sack, J.B., Kesselbrenner, M.B., & Jarrad, A. Interposed abdominal compression-cardiopulmonary resuscitation and resuscitation outcome during asystole and electromechanical dissociation. *Circulation* 1992; **86**: 1692–1700.

64. Fisher, J., Vaghaiwalla, F., Tsitlik, J. *et al.* Determinants and clinical significance of jugular venous valve competence. *Circulation* 1982; **65**: 188–196.

65. Halperin, H.R., & Weisfeldt, M.L. New approaches to CPR. Four hands, a plunger, or a vest. *J. Am. Med. Assoc.* 1992; **267**: 2940–2941.

66. Eisenmenger, R. Suction and air pressure over the abdomen, its application and effects [in German]. *Med. Wochenschr.* 1939; **89**: 807.

67. Weale, F.E., & Rothwell-Jackson, R.L. The efficiency of cardiac massage. *Lancet* 1962; **1**: 990–992.

68. Mackenzie, G.J., Taylor, S.H., McDonald, A.H., & Donald, K.W. Haemodynamic effects of external cardiac compression. *Lancet* 1964; **18**: 1342–1345.

69. Niemann, J.T., Rosborough, J., Hausknecht, M., Brown, D., & Criley, J.M. Cough–CPR: documentation of systemic perfusion in man and in an experimental model: a "window" to the mechanism of blood flow in external CPR. *Crit. Care Med.* 1980; **8**: 141–146.

70. Weisfeldt, M.L., Chandra, N., & Tsitlik, J. Increased intrathoracic pressure – not direct heart compression – causes the rise in intrathoracic vascular pressures during CPR in dogs and pigs. *Crit. Care Med.* 1981; **9**: 377–378.

71. Tucker, K.J., Redberg, R.F., Schiller, N.B., & Cohen, T.J. Active compression–decompression resuscitation: analysis of transmitral flow and left ventricular volume by transesophageal echocardiography in humans. Cardiopulmonary Resuscitation Working Group. *J. Am. Coll. Cardiol.* 1993; **22**: 1485–1493.

72. Werner, J.A., Greene, H.L., Janko, C.L., & Cobb, L.A. Visualization of cardiac valve motion in man during external chest compression using two-dimensional echocardiography. Implications regarding the mechanism of blood flow. *Circulation* 1981; **63**: 1417–1421.

73. Rich, S., Wix, H.L., & Shapiro, E.P. Clinical assessment of heart chamber size and valve motion during cardiopulmonary resuscitation by two-dimensional echocardiography. *Am. Heart J.* 1981; **102**: 368–373.

74. Beattie, C., Guerci, A.D., Hall, T. *et al.* Mechanisms of blood flow during pneumatic vest cardiopulmonary resuscitation. *J. Appl. Physiol.* 1991; **70**: 454–465.

75. Taylor, G.J., Tucker, W.M., Greene, H.L., Rudikoff, M.T., & Weisfeldt, M.L. Importance of prolonged compression during cardiopulmonary resuscitation in man. *N. Engl. J. Med.* 1977; **296**: 1515–1517.

76. Tsitlik, J.E., Weisfeldt, M.L., Chandra, N., Effron, M.B., Halperin, H.R., & Levin, H.R. Elastic properties of the human chest during cardiopulmonary resuscitation. *Crit. Care Med.* 1983; **11**: 685–692.

77. Koehler, R.C., Chandra, N., Guerci, A.D. *et al.* Augmentation of cerebral perfusion by simultaneous chest compression and lung inflation with abdominal binding after cardiac arrest in dogs. *Circulation* 1983; **67**: 266–275.

78. Babbs, C.F. Abdominal counterpulsation in cardiopulmonary resuscitation: animal models and theoretical considerations. *Am. J. Emerg. Med.* 1985; **3**: 165–170.

79. Ralston, S.H., Babbs, C.F., & Niebauer, M.J. Cardiopulmonary resuscitation with interposed abdominal compression in dogs. *Anesth. Analg.* 1982; **61**: 645–651.

80. Babbs, C.F. Relative effectiveness of interposed abdominal compression CPR: sensitivity analysis and recommended compression rates. *Resuscitation* 2005; **66**: 347–355.

81. Bircher, N.G., & Abramson, N.S. Interposed abdominal compression CPR (IAC-CPR): a glimmer of hope. *Am. J. Emerg. Med.* 1984; **2**: 177–178.

82. Niemann, J.T., Rosborough, J.P., & Criley, J.M. Continuous external counterpressure during closed-chest resuscitation: a critical appraisal of the military antishock trouser garment and abdominal binder. *Circulation* 1986; **74**: IV102–107.

83. Mateer, J.R., Stueven, H.A., Thompson, B.M., Aprahamian, C., & Darin, J.C. Interposed abdominal compression CPR versus standard CPR in prehospital cardiopulmonary arrest: preliminary results. *Ann. Emerg. Med.* 1984; **13**: 764–766.

84. McDonald, J.L. Effect of interposed abdominal compression during CPR on central arterial and venous pressures. *Am. J. Emerg. Med.* 1985; **3**: 156–159.

85. Halperin, H.R., Paradis, N., Ornato, J.P. *et al.* Cardiopulmonary resuscitation with a novel chest compression device in a porcine model of cardiac arrest: improved hemodynamics and mechanisms. *J. Am. Coll. Cardiol.* 2004; **44**: 2214–2220.

86. Ikeno, F., Kaneda, H., Hongo, Y. *et al.* Augmentation of tissue perfusion by a novel compression device increases neurologically intact survival in a porcine model of prolonged cardiac arrest. *Resuscitation* 2006; **68**: 109–118.

87. Halperin, H.R., Brower, R., Weisfeldt, M.L. *et al.* Air trapping in the lungs during cardiopulmonary resuscitation in dogs. A mechanism for generating changes in intrathoracic pressure. *Circ. Res.* 1989; **65**: 946–954.

88. Kimmel, E., Beyar, R., Dinnar, U., Sideman, S., & Kishon, Y. Augmentation of cardiac output and carotid blood flow by chest and abdomen phased compression cardiopulmonary resuscitation. *Cardiovasc. Res.* 1986; **20**: 574–580.

89. Lurie, K.G., Voelckel, W.G., Zielinski, T. *et al.* Improving standard cardiopulmonary resuscitation with an inspiratory impedance threshold valve in a porcine model of cardiac arrest. *Anesth. Analg.* 2001; **93**: 649–655.

90. Luce, J.M., Rizk, N.A., & Niskanen, R.A. Regional blood flow during cardiopulmonary resuscitation in dogs. *Crit. Care Med.* 1984; **12**: 874–878.

91. Timerman, S., Cardoso, L.F., Ramires, J.A., & Halperin, H. Improved hemodynamic performance with a novel chest compression device during treatment of in-hospital cardiac arrest. *Resuscitation* 2004; **61**: 273–280.

92. Cohen, T.J., Tucker, K.J., Lurie, K.G. *et al.* Active compression–decompression. A new method of cardiopulmonary resuscitation. Cardiopulmonary Resuscitation Working Group. *J. Am. Med. Assoc.* 1992; **267**: 2916–2923.

93. Tucker, K.J., Khan, J.H., & Savitt, M.A. Active compression–decompression resuscitation: effects on pulmonary ventilation. *Resuscitation* 1993; **26**: 125–131.

94. Lurie, K., Zielinski, T., McKnite, S., & Sukhum, P. Improving the efficiency of cardiopulmonary resuscitation with an inspiratory impedance threshold valve. *Crit. Care Med.* 2000; **28**: N207–N209.

95. Lindner, K.H. Adrenergic agonist drug administration during cardiopulmonary resuscitation. *Crit. Care Med.* 1993; **21**: S324–325.

96. Halperin, H.R., & Guerci, A.D. Vasoconstrictors during CPR. Are they used optimally? *Chest* 1990; **98**: 787–789.

97. Redding, J.S., & Pearson, J.W. Evaluation of drugs for cardiac resuscitation. *Anesthesiology* 1963; **24**: 203–207.

98. Yakaitis, R.W., Otto, C.W., & Blitt, C.D. Relative importance of alpha and beta adrenergic receptors during resuscitation. *Crit. Care Med.* 1979; **7**: 293–296.

99. Ralston, S.H., Babbs, C.F., & Joseph, S. Redding's contributions to cardiac resuscitation. *Am. J. Emerg. Med.* 1985; **3**: 247–251.

100. Ditchey, R.V., & Slinker, B.K. Phenylephrine plus propranolol improves the balance between myocardial oxygen supply and demand during experimental cardiopulmonary resuscitation. *Am. Heart J.* 1994; **127**: 324–330.

101. Beyar, R., Kishon, Y., Kimmel, E., Neufeld, H., & Dinnar, U. Intrathoracic and abdominal pressure variations as an efficient method for cardiopulmonary resuscitation: studies in dogs compared with computer model results. *Cardiovasc. Res.* 1985; **19**: 335–342.

102. von Planta, I., Wagner, O., von Planta, M., & Scheidegger, D. Coronary perfusion pressure, end-tidal CO_2 and adrenergic agents in haemodynamic stable rats. *Resuscitation* 1993; **25**: 203–217.

103. Milnor, W. *Hemodynamics.* Baltimore: Williams and Wilkins, 1982.

104. Brown, C.G., Werman, H.A., Davis, E.A., Katz, S., & Hamlin, R.L. The effect of high-dose phenylephrine versus epinephrine on regional cerebral blood flow during CPR. *Ann. Emerg. Med.* 1987; **16**: 743–748.

105. Falk, J.L., Rackow, E.C., & Weil, M.H. End-tidal carbon dioxide concentration during cardiopulmonary resuscitation. *N. Engl. J. Med.* 1988; **318**: 607–611.

106. Ditchey, R.V., & Lindenfeld, J. Potential adverse effects of volume loading on perfusion of vital organs during closed-chest resuscitation. *Circulation* 1984; **69**: 181–189.

107. Paradis, N.A., Rose, M.I., & Gawryl, M.S. Selective aortic perfusion and oxygenation: an effective adjunct to external chest compression-based cardiopulmonary resuscitation. *J. Am. Coll. Cardiol.* 1994; **23**: 497–504.

108. Ditchey, R.V., & Lindenfeld, J. Failure of epinephrine to improve the balance between myocardial oxygen supply and demand during closed-chest resuscitation in dogs. *Circulation* 1988; **78**: 382–389.

17

Hemodynamics of cardiac arrest

Michael. P. Frenneaux and Stig Steen

Department of Cardiovascular Medicine, University of Birmingham, UK
Department of Cardiothoracic Surgery, University Hospital of Lund, Sweden

Stroke volume and cardiac output

Each ventricle normally ejects approximately 70–75 ml with each heart beat (the stroke volume) at a rate of approximately 70 beats per minute, resulting in a cardiac output of approximately 5 litres per minute.

Stroke volume is determined by:

1. the intrinsic contractile properties of the heart (which are modified by the effects of ischemia, by circulating hormones, and by autonomic stimulation);
2. the degree of stretch of the left ventricle during diastole, i.e., its "preload" (the Frank–Starling phenomenon). This in turn is dependent on:
   (a) total blood volume,
   (b) venous tone, which determines the distribution of blood volume between the venous and central compartments
   (c) left ventricular compliance – determined by intrinsic left ventricular myocardial compliance, and in some circumstances by external constraint from the right ventricle, pericardium, and mediastinal structures (see later)
3. The "Afterload" against which the heart contracts. When the heart contracts against a high afterload, stroke volume tends to fall.

Arterial physiology and hemodynamics

Small arteries and arterioles

Mean arterial blood pressure (⅔ diastolic BP + ⅓ systolic BP) is the product of cardiac output and systemic vascular resistance. Systemic vascular resistance is a static resistance, principally determined by the tone of arterioles. This tone is controlled by humoral and neural factors (particularly sympathetic tone)[1] and by paracrine factors (including nitric oxide, prostaglandins, endothelium-derived hyperpolarizing factor, and endothelin).[2] Systemic vascular resistance represents the global resistance produced by small artery and arteriolar tone. At a local level, changes in resistance vessel tone modulate tissue perfusion.

Large arteries

The large arteries are more than simply passive conduits. The fixed and dynamic properties of the large arteries profoundly affect blood pressure and left ventricular performance. In healthy young subjects the large arteries (such as the aorta, and iliac vessels) are very compliant and exert a damping effect on pulsatile left ventricular outflow, resulting in a relatively lower systolic pressure and a higher diastolic pressure. Aging of the large arteries renders them less compliant, impairing this damping function and resulting in relatively higher systolic and lower diastolic blood pressures for any given mean blood pressure. Furthermore, in the elderly, central aortic pressure is augmented by pressure wave reflection from the periphery. Following left ventricular ejection there is a forward travelling pressure wave which is then reflected back from branch sites (where there is impedance mismatch). In healthy young arteries the pressure wave travels relatively slowly and returns to the aorta in diastole, where it helps to maintain diastolic pressure and flow, whereas in stiffer elderly arteries it travels more rapidly, returning to the central aorta in systole, augmenting the systolic pressure.[3]

In summary, whereas the arterioles modulate static resistance, the properties of the large arteries determine dynamic impedance, which is analogous to resistance but relates to pulsatile rather than to steady flow.

Venous capacitance

The capacitance vessels serve a reservoir function. Over 70% of total blood volume is located in the venous compartment. Of this, the vast majority is in the small veins and venules, with the minority in the medium sized and large veins. Because of the large volume of blood within the venous compartment, relatively small changes in venous tone markedly alter the distribution of blood volume. An increase in venous tone shifts blood from the venous compartment to the heart, increasing intracardiac pressures, whereas a reduction in venous tone has the opposite effect. In patients with heart failure, for example, diuretic treatment may reduce total blood volume yet central blood volume (and jugular venous pressure) may remain high because of venoconstriction. Unlike the arteries, the venous system exerts only a modest resistance to blood flow.

Coronary blood flow

Whereas flow in most organs occurs predominantly in systole, flow in the coronary arteries occurs mainly during diastole.[4] The high pressures generated in the left ventricle during systole impede flow through the intramural microvessels (i.e., coronary vascular resistance rises markedly during systole) by generating a backward travelling compression wave, and forward flow in the coronary arteries during the latter part of isovolumic relaxation is mainly a "suction" phenomenon due to rapid relaxation of the left ventricle, with an associated rapid reduction in the pressure within the intramural coronary microvessels.[5]

Compared with other tissues, the perfusion gradient across the heart is smaller. Because flow occurs in diastole, the upstream pressure is aortic diastolic rather than mean pressure. Furthermore, although the coronary sinus drains into the right atrium, coronary microvascular pressure is markedly influenced by left ventricular diastolic pressure, which is usually substantially higher than right atrial pressure. The perfusion of the heart may be compromised by a reduction in aortic diastolic pressure, the presence of stenoses in the epicardial coronary arteries, an increase in coronary microvascular resistance, or an increase in left ventricular end diastolic pressure.

Hemodynamic changes occurring following cardiac arrest

Most of the experimental studies published have examined the hemodynamic changes occurring after the onset of ventricular fibrillation (VF). VF results in totally incoordinate ventricular activity, with effective cessation of ventricular contraction. Interestingly, as first described by William Harvey,[6] atrial contractions may continue for a considerable period after the onset of cardiac arrest. The effects of these atrial contractions may be evident in the aortic pressure tracing (Fig. 17.1).

At the instant of cardiac arrest, a large pressure gradient exists between the central aorta (mean arterial pressure) and the right side of the heart. Despite cessation of ventricular contraction, this pressure gradient drives antegrade blood flow which will continue until the pressure gradient has been completely dissipated. Direct visual inspection and cardiac MRI studies have shown a rapid increase in right ventricular volume following cardiac arrest, as blood is translocated from the systemic circulation to the right side of the heart along its pressure gradient (Fig. 17.2).[7,8] There is also a pressure gradient between pulmonary artery and left atrium, and flow therefore continues through the pulmonary circulation to dissipate this gradient. When these pressures equalise, this flow ceases and the pulmonary vasculature including the extrapericardial component of the pulmonary veins is distended with blood (Fig. 17.3). The theoretical pressure at which the pressures converge throughout the circulation was termed "Statischer Fullungsdruck" by Weber in 1851,[9] or "Static Blood Pressure" by Starr in 1940.[10] Guyton proposed that arterial and systemic venous pressure would almost reach equilibrium (at a pressure he called "Mean Circulatory Filling Pressure") 30–50 seconds after the heart stopped beating.[11] This equilibrium pressure is determined by total blood volume and by total vascular "capacitance" (of which venous capacitance provides the largest contribution). Consequently, this concept has been used by physiologists to assess the effects of interventions on venous capacitance in animal models. Mean circulatory filling pressure is estimated during brief induced ventricular fibrillation. As blood pressure falls however, baroreflex inactivation may be expected to increase sympathetic outflow, increasing venous tone and leading to an equilibrium pressure which overestimates the venous tone that existed prior to cardiac arrest. Consequently, some groups have calculated a theoretical equilibrium pressure on the basis of the pressure changes in the arteries and veins occurring during the first few seconds after onset of VF.[12] Postmortem studies have

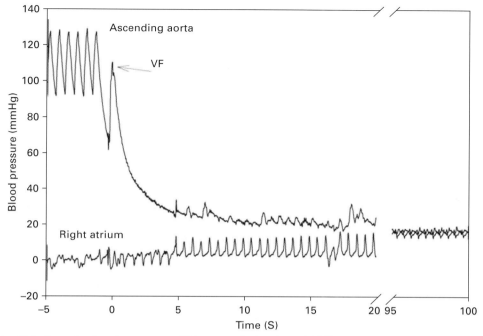

Fig. 17.1. Example of aortic pressure and RA pressure in the pig model following the onset of VF cardiac arrest. Phasic changes in both pressures are seen due to continuing atrial contraction. (Figure provided by S. Steen.)

shown an equilibrium pressure in human corpses (well after death) of approximately 6 mmHg.[10]

Studies in animals and in man have shown that the decay in arterial pressure and the increase in venous pressure does not conform to a single mono-exponential function.[8,13] Schipke and colleagues recently studied patients with heart failure who had undergone implantation of an automatic implantable cardioverter defibrillator (AICD).[13] Ventricular fibrillation was induced in order to assess the defibrillation threshold. Haemodynamic changes were assessed during an average of 13 seconds of VF. In a subgroup, the duration of VF was over 20 seconds. The averaged data for this subgroup is shown in Fig. 17.4. As expected, LV and aortic pressure were almost identical, and both decayed rapidly. Right atrial pressure increased rapidly. Nevertheless, even at 20 seconds an arteriovenous pressure gradient of almost 10 mmHg persisted. It is clear from the data that Guyton's prediction that an equilibrium pressure would exist throughout the circulation in 30–50 seconds is not correct. This study showed that the decay in arterial pressure and the increase in right arterial pressures both conformed best to exponential curves. Exponential curves should approach an equilibrium at five times the time constant of the curve. During the first few seconds the time constant of the arterial pressure decay was

2.9 seconds – which would have predicted a plateau at approximately 14.5 seconds, yet this was not seen. The reason is that the time constant of the exponential decay progressively lengthened. Why might this be so? First, hypotension-induced baroreflex withdrawal would be expected to increase sympathetic outflow, and indeed a marked increase in sympathetic circulating catecholamines of adrenal, and to a lesser extent neural, origin has been reported after cardiac arrest.[14–16] This would be expected to increase arteriolar tone and also to increase venous tone. Secondly, it may be due to "waterfall" phenomena. As arterial pressure falls, some microvascular beds may close down, resulting in a net increase in vascular resistance. In anesthetised dogs a "waterfall" has also been demonstrated in the inferior vena cava at the level of the diaphragm.[17] However, no significant inferior vena cava waterfall was demonstrated at the level of the diaphragm before or during VF in humans.[12]

Steen and colleagues studied the hemodynamic changes occurring in anesthetised pigs during much longer periods of VF.[8] A typical example of the changes in arterial and right atrial pressures occurring after the onset of VF in non-ventilated pigs is shown in Fig. 17.5. The first 20 seconds of this recording are very similar to the human data reported by Schipke *et al.*[13] There is an early progressive reduction of

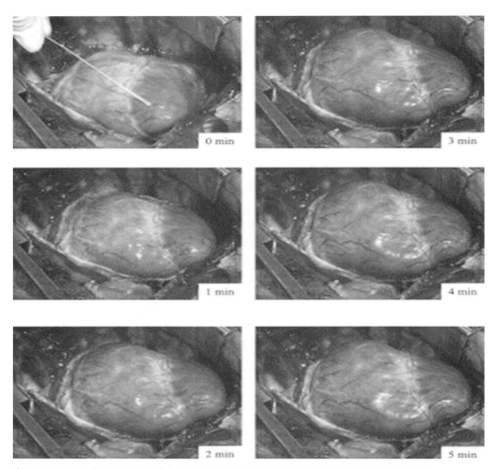

Fig. 17.2. External appearance of the heart following VF Cardiac Arrest in Pig Model. The right ventricular volume rapidly increases as blood flows from the aorta to the right heart. (Reproduced with permission from *Resuscitation*.[8])

aortic pressure, reaching a minimum of 20 mmHg after about 30 seconds. Aortic pressure then increases slightly to about 25 mmHg at 2 minutes, thereafter gradually decreasing over the next 5 minutes to approximately 10 mmHg. Right atrial pressure increases gradually after induction of VF, reaching a peak of about 18 mmHg after 2 min, decreasing thereafter to approximate aortic pressure by about 7 min. Mean circulatory filling pressure at this point is approximately 9 mmHg.

These findings cannot be explained purely by a "waterfall" effect. The increase in arterial pressure between 30 seconds and 2 minutes is probably related to transient sympathetically mediated vascular constriction. As the brainstem becomes more ischemic this sympathetic outflow is presumably reduced again, resulting in a fall in both arteriolar resistance and venous tone and a decline in both aortic and right atrial pressures.

Carotid blood flow changes following VF cardiac arrest

Figure 17.6 shows the changes in carotid blood flow following VF cardiac arrest in the anesthetised non-ventilated pig. Carotid blood flow declines exponentially after the onset of VF, but measurable carotid blood flow continues for approximately 4 minutes.

Coronary blood flow changes following VF cardiac arrest

The gradient between aorta and right atrium is often referred to as the "coronary perfusion pressure," i.e., the gradient during coronary blood flow during cardiac arrest. A "coronary perfusion pressure" of less than 15 mmHg

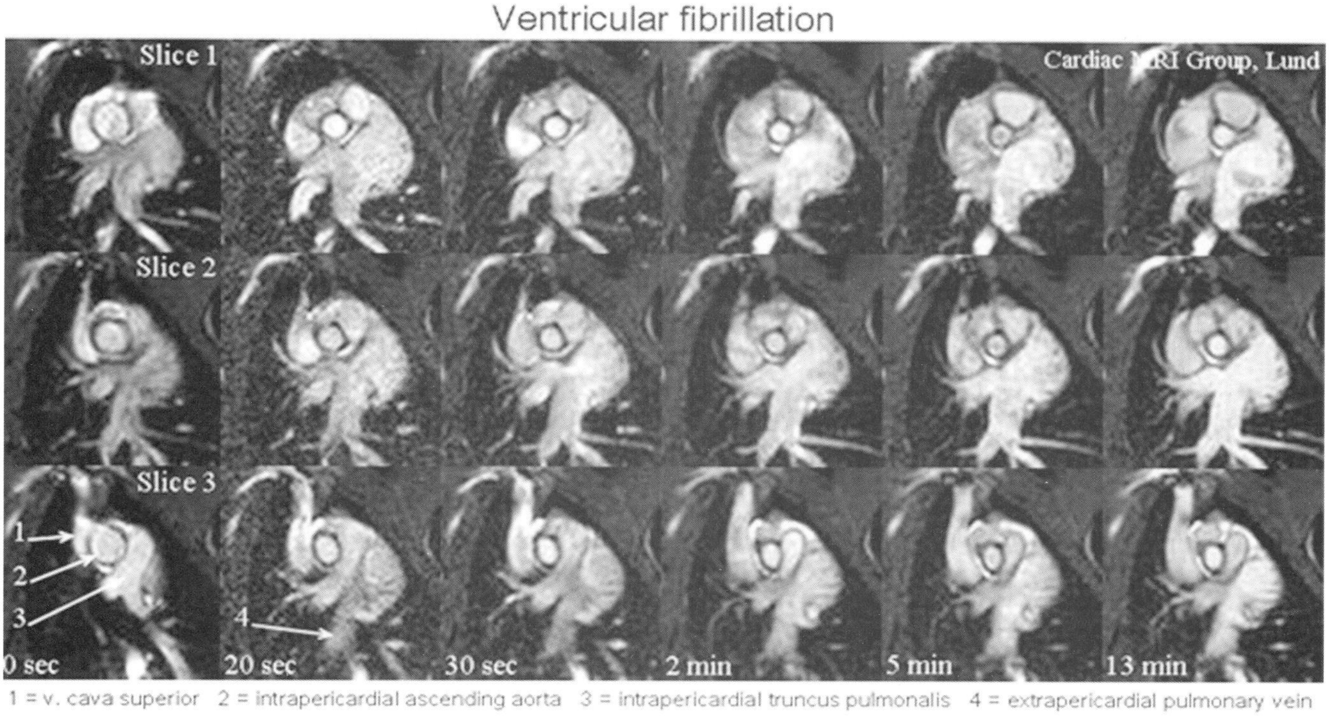

Ventricular fibrillation

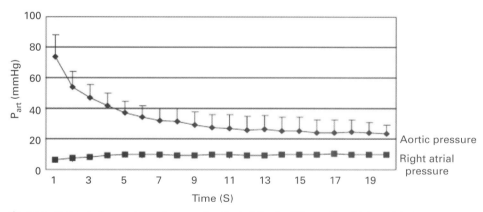

Fig. 17.3. MRI of pig heart following VF cardiac arrest. The extrapericardial component of the pulmonary vein becomes distended. (S. Steen – unpublished data.)

Fig. 17.4. Pressure changes in a subgroup of patients following VF arrest in which ventricular fibrillation lasted at least 20 s ($n=14$). There is progressive decrease in arterial pressure and an increase in right atrial pressure. These changes do not conform to single monoexponential functions. Note that, at 20 seconds, a significant arterio-venous pressure gradient (9.6 mmHg) persists. (Reproduced with permission from the *American Journal of Physiology*[11].)

during the release phase of CPR has been shown to be a good predictor that recovery of spontaneous circulation (ROSC) is unlikely in both humans and in animal models.[18,19] It has been assumed in the past that this was because, below this "coronary perfusion pressure," myocardial perfusion was totally inadequate to support

recovery of myocardial function after restoration of electrical activity.

In fact, the changes in coronary blood flow and of carotid blood flow following VF cardiac arrest without CPR do not parallel each other in the anesthetised non-ventilated pig model. As shown in Fig. 17.7, coronary blood flow rapidly

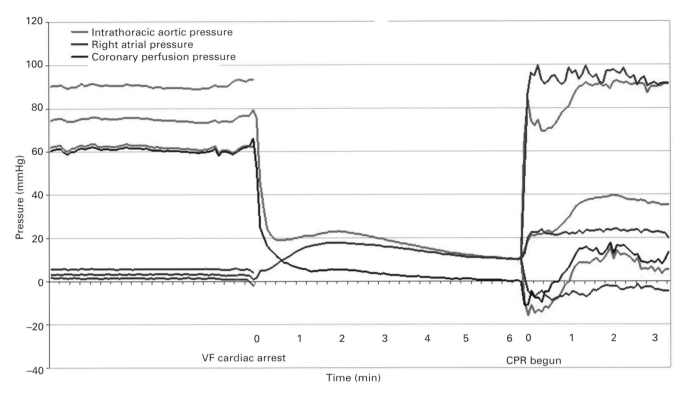

Fig. 17.5. Changes in aortic pressure, right atrial pressure and calculated coronary perfusion pressure in the pig model following VF cardiac arrest. (Reproduced with permission from *Resuscitation*.[8])

declines to zero by 1 minute. For the next 2 minutes, coronary blood flow is retrograde before declining again to zero.

These observations, suggest that the term "coronary perfusion pressure" may be misleading, because "coronary perfusion pressure" is positive during this period when coronary flow is retrograde. Although the coronary sinus drains into the right atrium and therefore the aortic minus right atrial pressure gradient might be expected to determine coronary blood flow, the intramural coronary microvascular pressure is also profoundly influenced by the left ventricular intracavity pressure. The conventional "coronary perfusion pressure" therefore provides an overestimate of the actual pressure gradient driving coronary blood flow – explaining the observations above.

Hemodynamics during cardiopulmonary resuscitation

How does CPR eject blood into the aorta?

Closed chest CPR results in phasic blood flow. There has been considerable controversy regarding the mechanisms responsible for this forward blood flow. According to the "cardiac compression theory," direct compression of the left and right ventricles between the sternum and vertebral column creates a pressure gradient between the ventricle and the aorta (or pulmonary artery in the case of the right ventricle). This pressure gradient closes the mitral (and tricuspid) valve and ejects blood forward out of the ventricle. According to this paradigm, the ventricle then refills during the decompression phase. The theory was proposed by Kouwenhoven and colleagues.[20] This view was essentially unchallenged until the 1970s. In 1976, Criley and colleagues described the phenomenon of "cough cardiopulmonary resuscitation" and ascribed the forward flow generated by coughing to the increased intrathoracic pressure generated during coughing.[21] In the 1980s, studies in dogs[22] and in man[23] led to the proposal of the "thoracic pump" theory for antegrade flow during CPR. According to the thoracic pump theory, external chest decompression increases intrathoracic pressure, forcing blood to flow from the thoracic to the systemic circulation. Retrograde flow from the right side of the heart to the systemic veins is prevented by the venous valves. According to this paradigm, the heart acts merely as a passive conduit without having a pump function.

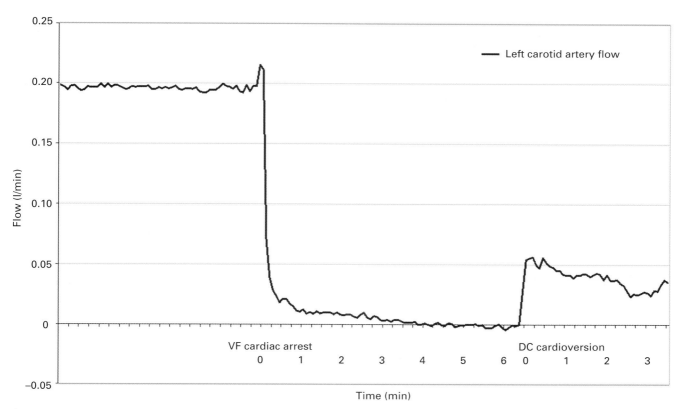

Fig. 17.6. Changes in carotid artery flow in the pig model following VF cardiac arrest. (Modified from Steen *et al. Resuscitation* 2003; **58**: 249–258. Reproduced with permission from *Resuscitation*.[8])

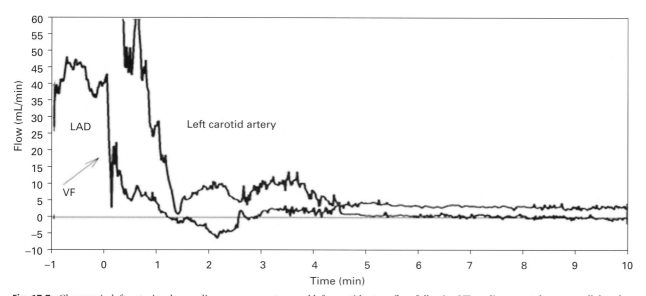

Fig. 17.7. Changes in left anterior descending coronary artery and left carotid artery flow following VF cardiac arrest do not parallel each other. (With permission from Professor S. Steen, University of Lund.)

This theory requires the AV valves to be open during the compression phase of CPR. Two transthoracic echocardiographic studies reported in the early 1980s during CPR in man supported the thoracic pump theory.[24,25] Guerci and colleagues also concluded, on the basis of observations of the aortic pressure-flow relation during CPR in dogs, that aortic flow was due to fluctuations in intrathoracic pressure.[26] Other studies performed in dogs and in pigs, however, supported the cardiac pump hypothesis.[27–29]

The availability of transesophageal echocardiography has provided the opportunity to study the mechanisms involved during CPR in man in much greater detail. Transesophageal echocardiography can be performed without interrupting cardiac massage and the quality and stability of the imaging is generally superior to transthoracic echocardiography. Several studies concluded that the mechanism of antegrade flow during CPR was consistent with the cardiac pump theory.[30,31] This conclusion was based on the observations that the mitral valve closed during the compression phase and opened during the decompression phase, and that the size of both left and right ventricular cavities fell during the compression phase. In contrast, another study performed in 17 patients undergoing CPR suggests that the physiological mechanisms responsible for antegrade flow may differ from patient to patient.[32] In this study both pulmonary venous and trans-mitral flow were assessed. In 5 of the 17 patients the mitral valve closed during the compression phase of CPR, with associated mitral regurgitation and forward aortic

flow, consistent with the cardiac pump theory. In the remaining 12 patients the mitral valve remained open during both the compression and decompression phases of CPR, and peak forward mitral flow also occurred during the compression phase in this group. In 8 of these 12 patients, forward mitral flow during the compression phase was accompanied by forward pulmonary vein flow, consistent with the classic "thoracic pump" mechanism. In the remaining 4 patients, forward mitral flow during the compression phase was accompanied by backwards pulmonary vein flow, which the authors suggested implied a "left atrial pump" mechanism, in which the left atrium rather than the left ventricle was the major target of chest compression. Downtime was much shorter in the 5 patients in whom the cardiac pump mechanism was thought to be operating than in the remaining 12 patients.

These three mechanisms are summarized schematically in Fig. 17.8. Whatever the mechanism, it is clear that antegrade flow occurs in both the thoracic aorta and the pulmonary artery during the compression phase of CPR and retrograde flow occurs in these vessels during the release or decompression phases.

Changes in aortic and pulmonary artery pressures during CPR

Steen and colleagues reported the hemodynamic effects of CPR using the LUCAS (Lund University Cardiac Arrest

Blood flow during chest compression

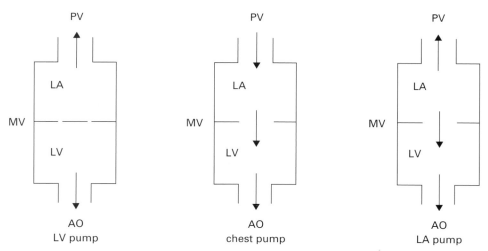

Fig. 17.8. Schematic representation of the three mechanisms by which CPR ejects blood into the aorta. LA – left atrium, LV – left ventricle, PV – pulmonary vein, Ao – aorta, MV – mitral valve. (Reproduced with permission from *Circulation*.[32])

System) device in anesthetised pigs.[33] The LUCAS device provides automatic mechanical chest compression; active "physiological" decompression.[33] CPR was instituted for 3–5 minutes after 6.5 minutes of VF (when the "coronary perfusion pressure" has reached zero). The hemodynamic effects in a typical animal are shown on the right of Fig. 17.5. Here, the compression phase is akin to "systole" and the decompression phase is akin to "diastole." During the entire 3½ minutes of CPR the compression pressure in the right atrium (top pressure trace) exceeded the pressure in the intrathoracic aorta (the second highest pressure trace). This reveals a negative "coronary perfusion pressure" during the compression phase. There was also a negative "coronary perfusion pressure" during the decompression phase for 1 minute after instituting CPR, but the "coronary perfusion pressure" during decompression then became positive, reaching a peak of 18 mmHg at 1½ minutes before declining slightly. Intrathoracic aortic pressure reached approximately 40 mmHg during CPR. Observations in man during CPR have shown peak systolic arterial pressures of between 60 and 80 mmHg.[34–36]

A study in pigs has shown that during closed chest CPR, compression phase pulmonary artery pressure was approximately 80–90 mmHg, mean pulmonary artery pressure was approximately 40 mmHg, and mean left atrial pressure approximately 3–4 mmHg lower than this.[37]

Cardiac output during CPR

Studies in dogs and in pigs have suggested that during optimal CPR, cardiac output is between 25% and 40% of pre-arrest values.[27,37–39]

Carotid and cerebral blood flow during CPR

In the pig model, Steen and colleagues showed that appreciable common carotid blood flow is apparent within seconds of initiating compression/decompression CPR using the LUCAS device. Values of approximately 300 ml/min were obtained when CPR was sustained, but even brief interruptions of CPR dramatically reduced carotid blood flow Fig. 17.9.[33] Cerebral blood flow is determined by the gradient between carotid artery and intracranial pressure. Assuming an ischemic threshold level of cerebral tissue oxygen content of 8 mmHg, a recent report suggested that, during standard CPR in

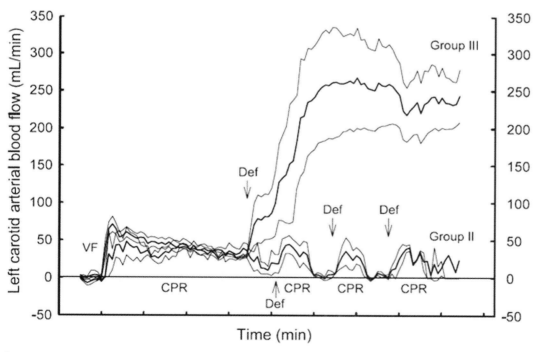

Fig. 17.9. The blood flow in the left internal carotid artery during 3.5 minutes of mechanical compressions followed by defibrillation attempts with (II) and (III) interrupting the chest compressions. Mean value ± S.E.M., $n=5$ in each group. (Reproduced with permission from *Resuscitation*.[8])

man, cerebral tissue oxygen content may be lower than this value much of the time. However, optimally performed CPR that maintained coronary perfusion pressure at least 25 mmHg was associated with cerebral tissue oxygen content greater than 8 mmHg.[40] A study in dogs demonstrated that if CPR is started immediately and "coronary perfusion pressures" are maintained above 25 mmHg, cerebral blood flow (measured by using microspheres) and cerebral ATP were both maintained at approximately 60% of pre-cardiac arrest values. In contrast, when CPR was delayed for 6 minutes after cardiac arrest, a coronary perfusion pressure of 35 mmHg was required to produce similar cerebral blood flow and cerebral ATP content. Furthermore, when CPR was delayed for 12 minutes, even this level of coronary perfusion pressure failed to restore cerebral blood flow.[41] Lindner and colleagues demonstrated that active compression–decompression CPR produced greater cerebral perfusion pressures and greater cerebral oxygen delivery than did standard CPR in a pig model.[42]

Coronary blood flow during CPR

Studies in animal models have shown that coronary flow is retrograde during the compression phase of CPR and antegrade during the release or decompression phase.[37,43,44] The retrograde flow during the compression phase continued even when the "coronary perfusion pressure" was raised throughout the CPR cycle by more effective CPR.[44] This presumably is related to the importance of left ventricular intra-cavity pressure in determining coronary blood flow. In the pig model, assessing CPR by using a mechanical device, even at 2.5-inch thumper strokes, coronary blood flow was less than 50% of pre-arrest values, and with thumper strokes of 1.5 inches, coronary flow was approximately 15% of baseline pre-arrest values.[43] Changes in coronary blood flow during CPR in dogs were related to changes in "coronary perfusion pressure."[45] Wolfe and colleagues observed that in dogs coronary blood flow fell at very high compression rates because of a reduction in "diastolic perfusion time" (i.e., the time spent in the relaxation phase during which antegrade coronary flow occurs). Optimal coronary flow occurred at a compression rate of 120/min.[46]

Effects of interruption of CPR on hemodynamics

Interrupting CPR for rescue breathing adversely affects hemodynamics. Berg and colleagues compared the effects of CPR at 100 compressions per minute with a brief rest period every minute for the rescuer to take 2 deep breaths vs. a protocol involving cycles of 15 compressions at 100 per minute each interrupted by 2 rescue breaths. The integrated coronary perfusion pressure over each cycle was substantially reduced in the rescue breathing group because of a reduction in aortic pressure during the rescue breathing phase, and because the number of chest compressions was also lower in this group.[47] Furthermore, Steen and colleagues showed in the pig model that periods of 30 seconds of CPR between defibrillation attempts were insufficient to generate an adequate "coronary perfusion pressure" (i.e., at least 15 mmHg) and, on the basis of these observations, the authors recommended at least 90 seconds of CPR between each defibrillation attempt.[8]

Coronary perfusion pressure and recovery of spontaneous circulation (ROSC)

In 1940, Wiggers noted that 3 to 5 minutes after the onset of VF (appreciably earlier than the "irretrievable failure of the central nervous system"), the heart enters an "atonic phase" in which "anoxia causes depression of contractile force and slows conduction."[48]

The impact of "coronary perfusion pressure" on the likelihood of ROSC has been described in animals and in man.[18,19,49,50] The probability of ROSC is low when coronary perfusion gradient is < 15–20 mmHg. **Fig. 17.10** shows human data relating likelihood of ROSC to coronary perfusion pressure during CPR.[19]

There are two potential reasons why this might be so.

1. At lower coronary perfusion pressures, profound myocardial ischemia may prevent ROSC. Ralston and colleagues have shown in a dog model that a mean myocardial blood flow less than 0.13 ml/min per g tissue was associated with no survival, whereas a flow of > 0.16 ml/min per g tissue was associated with survival.[51] Although this is likely to be a contributory factor, cardiac contractile function recovers after even relatively long periods of total ischemia. In the isolated perfused dog heart, postischemic contractile function was markedly depressed after 25 and 30 minutes of normothermic global ischemia, but the reduction in left ventricular contractile function after 15 to 20 minutes of global ischemia was only mild.[52] This threshold of 20 minutes is consistent with observations in other species.[53–55] In the swine model, even at 20 minutes of VF (without CPR), 89% of animals had myocardial ATP levels > 20% of control and adenylate charge ratio > 0.60 – values known to be associated with reversibility of myocyte injury.[56]

2. "Coronary perfusion pressure" is defined as the pressure difference between aorta and right atrium during the decompression phase. During VF aortic pressure is almost identical to LV pressure and right atrial pressure is almost

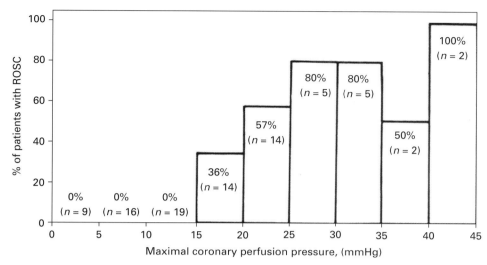

Fig. 17.10. Percentage of patients with return of spontaneous circulation (ROSC) as a function of the maximal coronary perfusion pressure.

identical to RV pressure. Accordingly, coronary perfusion pressure provides a measure of the pressure gradient across the interventricular septum during cardiac arrest. This is a measure of the true "preload" acting on the left ventricle. As discussed below, this may be an important determinant of ROSC, because it determines the degree of myocyte stretch and therefore, according to the Frank–Starling mechanism, the force of myocyte contraction when it is activated by electrical depolarization.

The concept of left ventricular preload and the Effect of Constraint from the Pericardium and Right Ventricle

Frank57 first described the importance of the degree of cardiac muscle stretch during diastole (preload) in determining its subsequent force of contraction. The mechanism of this observation is related predominantly to the nature of the actin-myosin interaction in the sarcomere. The force generated by a single sarcomere is proportional to the number of actin-myosin bonds and the available energy from ATP hydrolysis. Generation of optimal force is achieved when the sarcomere length is approximately 2.2 to 2.3 microns, which corresponds to the maximum number of actin–myosin interactions. At sarcomere lengths less than approximately 1.5 microns, there are no actin–myosin interactions and force generation is more or less eliminated. In addition to the actin–myosin interaction, the giant filamentous protein Titin which

spans the sarcomere, acts like a molecular "spring," storing potential energy when it is stretched and it may also play a role in development of stretch-dependent passive tension.58 As a result of the length dependency of the actin–myosin interaction and of titin tension development, below a certain "slack length," myocytes do not generate tension. Patterson and Starling observed that the output of the left ventricle was related to changes in the venous pressure.59 In clinical practice it has been assumed that changes in left atrial pressure (or LV end diastole pressure or pulmonary capillary wedge pressure) parallel those of LV diastole stretch ("preload") and that changes in pressure can be used as a surrogate for changes in stretch. Indeed, the literature commonly refers to the Frank-Starling relationship, as if Frank and Starling had described the same phenomenon. Within the physiological range, the use of change in LVEDP to predict changes in preload is generally valid, but in certain pathophysiological states it is not. The effective distending pressure acting on the left ventricle at end diastole is the left ventricular end diastolic pressure minus external pressures acting on the left ventricle from the pericardium, and from the right ventricle via the interventricular septum. In health, both RV end diastolic pressure and pericardial pressure are close to zero; therefore, changes in LVEDP generally parallel those of LV end diastolic volume. As the pericardium is stretched, however, there is an exponential increase in pericardial pressure (Fig. 17.11).60 In most situations, RVEDP and pericardial pressure are almost identical, because the RV is thin walled and therefore maintains only

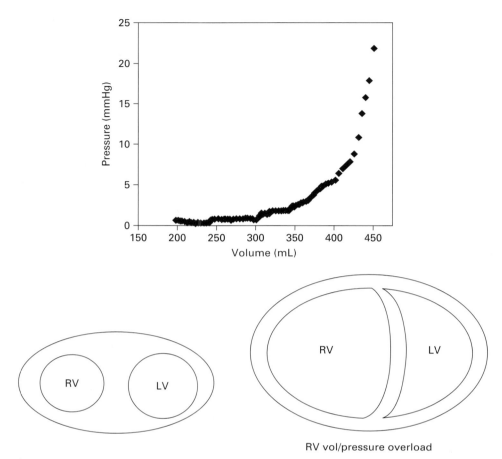

Fig. 17.11. The pericardium has a J-shaped stress–strain relation. When it is stretched (e.g., by right ventricular volume overload) pericardial pressure and RV end-diastolic pressure become elevated. The filling of the LV is then impeded by external constraint from the pericardium and RV, despite a high LVEDP. The interventricular septum is shifted to the left. From Frenneaux, M. Cardiopulmonary resuscitation: some physiological considerations. *Resuscitation* 2003; **58**: 259–265. Reproduced with permission from *Resuscitation*.

a small pressure gradient across it.[61] In experimental situations in which the pericardium is stretched by acute enlargement of the right ventricle (e.g., experimental pulmonary embolism), the pericardial and right ventricular end diastolic pressures may be substantially more than zero. In this situation the filling of the left ventricle is impeded by the external constraint from the pericardium (pericardial constraint) and from the right ventricle (diastolic ventricular interaction). The measured intracavity LVEDP overestimates the true LV preload. The interventricular septum, normally convex to the right at end diastole, becomes flattened, and the position of the septum at end diastole has been shown to be very closely related to the trans-septal pressure gradient, i.e., it reflects the degree of ventricular interaction.[62]

Pericardial constraint and diastolic ventricular interac-

tion have been well described in animal experimental models of acute right ventricular pressure and volume overload.[63] Important diastolic ventricular interaction is also seen in many patients with chronic heart failure.[64,65] Reducing central blood volume in these patients (using a lower body "suction" device) resulted in a fall in RV volume, and of right atrial and pulmonary capillary wedge pressures, but despite this, left ventricular diastolic volume increased (Fig. 17.12). The explanation was confirmed in a canine rapid pacing heart failure model. While central blood volume unloading reduced LV end diastolic pressure, it reduced pericardial pressure and RV end diastolic pressure even more; therefore, the effective distending pressure increased, resulting in an increase in LV diastolic volume and stroke volume.[66] These observations are shown in **Fig. 17.13**.

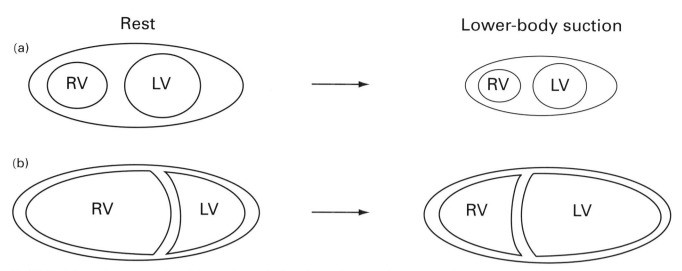

Fig. 17.12. Schematic representation of changes in ventricular volumes that occur during acute volume unloading such as that produced by application of lower body suction. (a) – Normal individuals, (b) – direct diastolic ventricular interaction in heart failure patients with pericardial constraint, RV – right ventricle, LV – left ventricle. (Reproduced with permission from *The Lancet*.[64])

Steen's observations in the pig model suggest that important pericardially mediated ventricular interaction may occur following cardiac arrest.[8] As noted previously, Steen and colleagues observed that as blood flowed along its pressure gradient from the aorta to the right side of the heart, the right ventricle became markedly distended. Furthermore, there was a progressive increase in right atrial pressure (and, by implication right ventricular pressure) during the first 2 minutes or so after cardiac arrest, before this slowly declined again. Pericardial pressure also rose progressively during the first 2 minutes after cardiac arrest before gradually declining. As expected, right atrial pressure and pericardial pressure changes paralleled each other almost exactly, with pericardial pressure marginally lower than right atrial pressure. These changes are shown in Fig. 17.14. These observations, performed in open chest pigs, clearly show that the pericardium was stretched sufficiently to raise pericardial pressure substantially. In the closed chest situation, this effect would be expected to be greater. Right ventricular volume fell slightly when right atrial and pericardial pressures started to decline. As discussed earlier, this decline in right atrial and pericardial pressures and right ventricular volume after about 3–4 minutes presumably reflects the withdrawal of sympathetic tone, as the brainstem vasomotor centers become profoundly ischemic.

As noted previously, there is also a temporary increase in aortic pressure between approximately 1 and 3 minutes after the onset of VF (Fig. 17.5), presumably due to the combined effects of increased sympathetic outflow and

"waterfall" phenomena, then aortic pressure starts to decline again, presumably because of a reduction in sympathetic outflow.

If we make the reasonable assumptions that intrathoracic aortic pressure approximates the left ventricular pressure and that right atrial pressure approximates the right ventricular pressure during cardiac arrest, then we can calculate the serial changes in left ventricular transmural pressure gradient (LV minus pericardial pressure) and trans-septal pressure gradient (left ventricular minus right ventricular pressure gradient). Changes in septal position and left ventricular volume would be expected to parallel changes in these gradients, which are in effect the distending pressures acting on the left ventricle. We have applied these calculations to a typical recording of aortic, RA, and pericardial pressures reported by Steen and colleagues.[8] A rapid initial fall in trans-septal and transmural gradients is followed by a slight increase, until approximately 4 minutes (corresponding to the period during which aortic pressures increase), followed by a subsequent decline to about zero. Berg and colleagues recently reported the changes in left and right ventricular volume after VF arrest in the pig.[7] Typical short axis MRI appearances are shown in Fig. 17.15. During the first 30 seconds after cardiac arrest there is a dramatic increase in right ventricular volume, with a shift of the interventricular septum to the left and a marked reduction in left ventricular volume. Between approximately 1 and 5 minutes, left ventricular volume increases modestly (but not back to baseline), although the interventricular septum remains

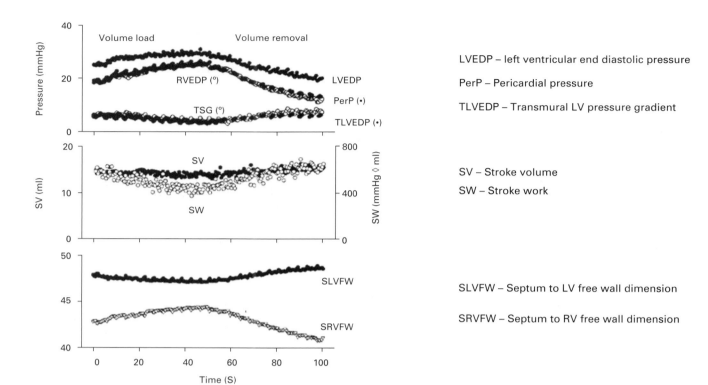

Fig. 17.13. Example of a study in the canine rapid pacing heart failure model. Volume unloading reduced pericardial pressure more than it reduced LV diastolic pressure, therefore true filling pressure increased and stroke volume increased. (Reproduced with permission from the *American Journal of Physiology*.[66])

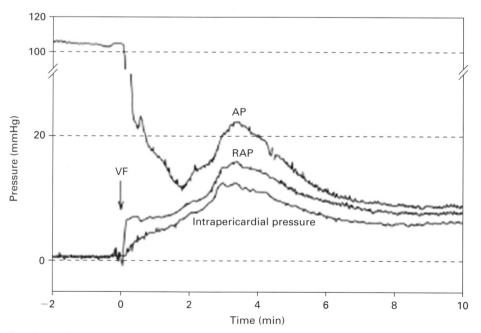

Fig. 17.14. Changes in aortic pressure (AP), right atrial pressure (RAP) and pericardial pressure following VF cardiac arrest in the pig Model. (Reproduced with permission from *Resuscitation*.[8])

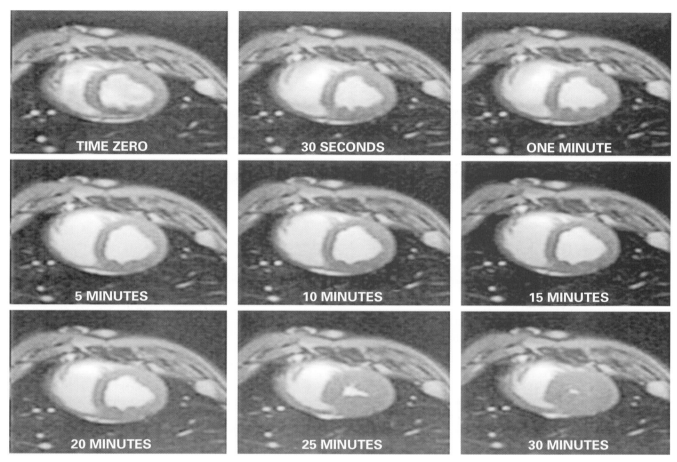

Fig. 17.15. Short-axis views of RV and LV through same mid-ventricular slice in 1 animal during 30 minutes of untreated VF. Time 0 refers to time VF was induced, and next 8 views were at respectively labeled duration of untreated VF. (Reproduced with permission from *Circulation*.[7])

dramatically flattened. Subsequently, left ventricular volume starts to decline again. These changes imply the rapid development of very marked ventricular interaction with some amelioration of this interaction between 1 and 5 minutes, and are entirely to be anticipated on the basis of the changes in the pressure gradient calculated form the data of Steen *et al.* In Fig. 17.16, the right and left ventricular volume changes reported by Berg and colleagues are plotted above the calculated changes in transmural gradient in the data reported by Steen and colleagues. As expected, the left ventricular volume changes closely mirror the changes in the transmural and trans-septal pressure gradients. Because, during cardiac arrest, aortic pressure is approximately LV pressure and since RA pressure is approximately RV pressure, AO-RA pressure is a close approximation to the pressure gradient between LV and RV (the "trans-septal" gradient).

This may have important implications for our understanding of the mechanism of ROSC. When ventricular interaction is marked, the degree of myocyte stretch may be so small that return of electrical activity generates only a minimal force of contraction, especially if the myocytes are also profoundly ischemic.

Effects of ventilation on hemodynamics during cardiac arrest

It is common practice to ventilate patients during cardiac arrest, on the assumption that this will improve oxygen delivery to the tissues, particularly the brain. Recent observations have called into question the validity of this assumption. Jellinek *et al.* reported the hemodynamic effects of positive airways pressure in patients undergoing

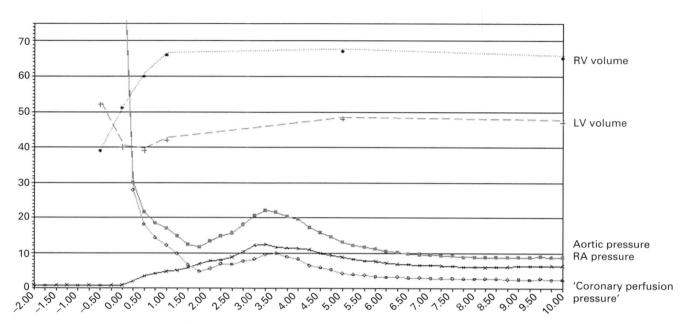

Fig. 17.16. The MRI calculated LV and RV volumes reported in the swine model by Berg *et al.*[63] are plotted against the changes in aortic, RA and coronary perfusion pressures reported by Steen *et al.*[8] There are no MRI data points between 1 and 5 minutes, but the changes in LV volume are predictable on the basis of changes in "coronary perfusion pressure."

AICD threshold testing. Before VF occurred, positive airway pressure increased right atrial pressure and reduced aortic pressure and left ventricular stroke volume. During VF arrest, positive airway pressure modestly reduced the coronary perfusion pressure. There was no evidence of collapse of the inferior vena cava, but in some patients there was a marked reduction in the diameter of the superior vena cava.[12] In the dog, positive airway pressure has been shown to cause collapse of the inferior vena cava resulting in a "waterfall effect."[17]

In addition to the direct effect of positive airways pressure on coronary perfusion pressure, ventilation is associated with substantial interruptions in compressions, and, as discussed above, this may cause substantial and prolonged reductions in coronary perfusion pressure. Woollard and colleagues reported on a randomized trial comparing compression-only vs. standard telephone CPR instructions in simulated cardiac arrest. Two and a half times more compressions were delivered during a standard ambulance response time in compression-only CPR in the compression-only group.[67] Furthermore, in pigs, CPR with rescue breathing was shown by Berg and colleagues to be associated with substantially lower "integrated coronary perfusion pressure" and left ventricular blood flow than compression-only CPR.[7]

An alternative approach to ventilation is the use of the so-called "inspiratory impedance threshold Device" (ITV). During the inflow phase, this provides a respiratory resistance which increases the negative intrathoracic pressure, analogous to the Müller maneuver. The hemodynamic effects of adding the device to the respiratory circuit in pigs was assessed during VF cardiac arrest. There was a non-significant increase in the coronary perfusion pressure (from $12.5. \pm 1.5$ to 14.8 ± 1.3 mmHg averaged during 28 minutes of CPR) associated with significant increases in left ventricular and cerebral blood flows.[68] Pilot studies in humans suggest that use of the ITV during CPR is associated with improved short term survival.[69,70]

The combination of positive end expiratory pressure ventilation (PEEP) with the inspiratory threshold device was reported to have particularly beneficial hemodynamic effects during active compression-decompression CPR in the pig. The addition of PEEP did not alter diastolic coronary perfusion pressure, but may nevertheless increase myocardial perfusion because the gradient of the diastolic aorta to left ventricular pressure was augmented, probably because PEEP reduces alveolar collapse, leading to an increase in indirect myocardial compression.[71]

Hemodynamic effects of spontaneous gasping during cardiac arrest

Gasping was first described by Legallois in 1812, in a variety of animal species including man.[72] It is very common in the human newborn and is also frequently observed after cardiac arrest. In this setting it appears to be triggered by ischemia of the brainstem and persists until the respiratory center in the caudal medulla is completely disabled. In the pig model it is typically observed between the first and second minute after the onset of cardiac arrest if no CPR is given. It begins weakly, increasing to a maximum, and then disappears typically by about 5 minutes, but sometimes longer. If effective cardiac compressions are given to gasping pigs they continue to gasp as long as the chest compressions create a minimum blood flow to the brainstem. Gasping produces gas exchange, and a sharp increase in arterial oxygen saturation, and a fall in arterial carbon dioxide tension typically follows the gasp.[73,74] As shown in **Fig. 17.17**, during the expiratory phase of a gasp there is

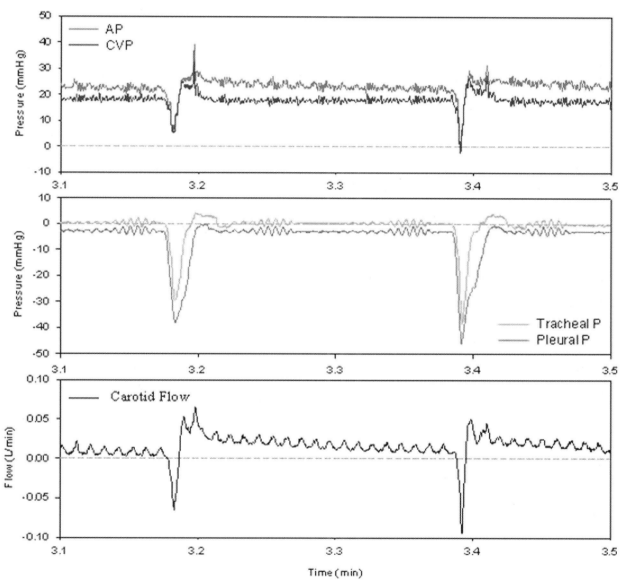

Fig. 17.17. The effects of a gasp on aortic pressure, central venous pressure, tracheal and pleural pressures and carotid flow in the swine VF model are shown. Note the effects of persistent atrial contractions following VF arrest. During the expiratory phase of the gasp there is an increase in carotid flow. (S. Steen, unpublished observations.)

an increase in aortic pressure and in carotid blood flow. The breath occurs against a partially closed airway and generates a negative intrapleural pressure of approximately 40 mmHg. This negative intrapleural pressure markedly reduces right atrial and pericardial pressures and increases the pressure gradient between aorta and RA. Xie and colleagues showed in the pig that during the inspiratory phase of the gasp, left ventricular area substantially increased and then returned to its "pre-gasp" value during the expiratory phase. This generated a stroke volume of approximately 60% of that seen in the spontaneously beating heart. The expiratory phase of the gasp was also associated with a substantial increase in end-tidal carbon dioxide.[75]

The appearance of gasping in a patient with cardiac arrest should not therefore be considered as a sign of recovery that discourages continued resuscitative measures, but implies that the brainstem is ischemic but still viable. The frequency of gasping has been reported to be predictive of the success of resuscitation.[76,77]

REFERENCES

1. Opie, L.H. Control of the circulation. In *Heart Physiology: From Cell to Circulation*. Philadelphia: Lippincott, Williams & Wilkins, 2004: 16–41.

2. Schiffrin, E.L. The endothelium and control of blood vessel function in health and disease. *Clin. Invest. Med.* 1994; **17**: 602–620.

3. Benetos, A., Waeber, B., Izzo, J. *et al.* Influence of age, risk factors, and cardiovascular and renal disease on arterial stiffness: clinical applications. *Am. J. Hypertens.* 2002; **15**: 1101–1108.

4. Downey, J.M. & Kirk, E.S. Inhibition of coronary blood flow by a vascular waterfall mechanism. *Circ. Res.* 1975; **36**: 753–763.

5. Sun, Y.H., Anderson, T.J., Parker, K.H. *et al.* Wave-intensity analysis: a new approach to coronary hemodynamics. *J. Appl. Physiol.* 2000; **89**: 1636–1644.

6. Harvey, W. *Excercitatio Anatomica de Motu Cordis et Sanguinis in Animalibus.* Frankfurt: 1628.

7. Berg, R.A., Sorrell, V.L., Kern, K.B. *et al.* Magnetic resonance imaging during untreated ventricular fibrillation reveals prompt right ventricular overdistention without left ventricular volume loss. *Circulation* 2005; **111**: 1136–1140.

8. Steen, S., Liao, Q., Pierre, L. *et al.* The critical importance of minimal delay between chest compressions and subsequent defibrillation: a haemodynamic explanation. *Resuscitation* 2003; **58**: 249–258.

9. Weber, E.H. *Uber die Anwendung der Wellenlehre auf die Lehre von Kreislauf des Blutes und insbesondere auf die Pulslehre.* 18th edn. 1851.

10. Starr, I. The role of the static blood pressure in abnormal increments in venous pressure, especially in heart failure. Part II. clin-

11. Guyton, A.C., Polizo, D. & Armstrong, G.G. Mean circulatory filling pressure measured immediately after cessation of heart pumping. *Am. J. Physiol.* 1954; **179**: 261–267.

12. Jellinek, H., Krenn, H., Oczenski, W. *et al.* Influence of positive airway pressure on the pressure gradient for venous return in humans. *J. Appl. Physiol.* 2000; **88**: 926–932.

13. Schipke, J.D., Heusch, G., Sanii, A.P. *et al.* Static filling pressure in patients during induced ventricular fibrillation. *Am. J. Physiol. Heart Circ. Physiol.* 2003; **285**: H2510–H2515.

14. Foley, P.J., Tacker, W.A., Wortsman, J. *et al.* Plasma catecholamine and serum cortisol responses to experimental cardiac arrest in dogs. *Am. J. Physiol.* 1987; **253**: E283–E289.

15. Lindner, K.H., Haak, T., Keller, A. *et al.* Release of endogenous vasopressors during and after cardiopulmonary resuscitation. *Heart* 1996; **75**: 145–150.

16. Kern, K.B., Elchisak, M.A., Sanders, A.B. *et al.* Plasma catecholamines and resuscitation from prolonged cardiac arrest. *Crit. Care Med.* 1989; **17**: 786–791.

17. Jungmann, E. Der transdiaphragmale Venendruckgradient und seine Abhangigkeit von Korperdrehung und Blutvolumen bei narkotisierten Hunden. Institut fur Experimentelle Anaesthesiologie der Heniriche-Heine-Universitat Dusseldorf, 1993.

18. Kern, K.B., Ewy, G.A., Voorhees, W.D. *et al.* Myocardial perfusion pressure: a predictor of 24-hour survival during prolonged cardiac arrest in dogs. *Resuscitation* 1988; **16**: 241–250.

19. Paradis, N.A., Martin, G.B., Rivers, E.P. *et al.* Coronary perfusion pressure and the return of spontaneous circulation in human cardiopulmonary resuscitation. *J. Am. Med. Assoc.* 1990; **263**: 1106–1113.

20. Moss, A.J., Kouwenhoven, W.B., Jude, J.R. & Knickerbocker, G.G. Closed-chest cardiac massage. *J. Am. Med. Assoc.* 1960; **173**: 1064–1067.

21. Criley, J.M., Blaufuss, A.H. & Kissel, G.L. Cough-induced cardiac compression. Self-administered from of cardiopulmonary resuscitation. *J. Am. Med. Assoc.* 1976; **236**: 1246–1250.

22. Rudikoff, M.T., Maughan, W.L., Effron, M. *et al.* Mechanisms of blood flow during cardiopulmonary resuscitation. *Circulation* 1980; **61**: 345–352.

23. Chandra, N., Rudikoff, M. & Weisfeldt, M.L. Simultaneous chest compression and ventilation at high airway pressure during cardiopulmonary resuscitation. *Lancet* 1980; **1**: 175–178.

24. Werner, J.A., Greene, H.L., Janko, C.L. *et al.* Visualization of cardiac valve motion in man during external chest compression using two-dimensional echocardiography. Implications regarding the mechanism of blood flow. *Circulation* 1981; **63**: 1417–1421.

25. Rich, S., Wix, H.L. & Shapiro, E.P. Clinical assessment of heart chamber size and valve motion during cardiopulmonary resuscitation by two-dimensional echocardiography. *Am. Heart J.* 1981; **102**: 368–373.

26. Guerci, A.D., Halperin, H.R., Beyar, R. *et al.* Aortic diameter and pressure-flow sequence identify mechanism of blood flow

during external chest compression in dogs. *J. Am. Coll. Cardiol.* 1989; **14**: 790–798.

27. Maier, G.W., Tyson, G.S., Jr., Olsen, C.O. *et al.* The physiology of external cardiac massage: high-impulse cardiopulmonary resuscitation. *Circulation* 1984; **70**: 86–101.

28. Feneley, M.P., Maier, G.W., Gaynor, J.W. *et al.* Sequence of mitral valve motion and transmitral blood flow during manual cardiopulmonary resuscitation in dogs. *Circulation* 1987; **76**: 363–375.

29. Hackl, W., Simon, P., Mauritz, W. *et al.* Echocardiographic assessment of mitral valve function during mechanical cardiopulmonary resuscitation in pigs. *Anesth. Analg.* 1990; **70**: 350–356.

30. Pell, A.C., Pringle, S.D., Guly, U.M. *et al.* Assessment of the active compression–decompression device (ACD) in cardiopulmonary resuscitation using transoesophageal echocardiography. *Resuscitation* 1994; **27**: 137–140.

31. Redberg, R.F., Tucker, K.J., Cohen, T.J. *et al.* Physiology of blood flow during cardiopulmonary resuscitation. A transesophageal echocardiographic study. *Circulation* 1993; **88**: 534–542.

32. Ma, M.H., Hwang, J.J., Lai, L.P. *et al.* Transesophageal echocardiographic assessment of mitral valve position and pulmonary venous flow during cardiopulmonary resuscitation in humans. *Circulation* 1995; **92**: 854–861.

33. Steen, S., Liao, Q., Pierre, L. *et al.* Evaluation of LUCAS, a new device for automatic mechanical compression and active decompression resuscitation. *Resuscitation* 2002; **55**: 285–299.

34. Chandra, N.C., Tsitlik, J.E., Halperin, H.R. *et al.* Observations of hemodynamics during human cardiopulmonary resuscitation. *Crit. Care Med.* 1990; **18**: 929–934.

35. Swenson, R.D., Weaver, W.D., Niskanen, R.A. *et al.* Hemodynamics in humans during conventional and experimental methods of cardiopulmonary resuscitation. *Circulation* 1988; **78**: 630–639.

36. Martin, G.B., Carden, D.L., Nowak, R.M. *et al.* Aortic and right atrial pressures during standard and simultaneous compression and ventilation CPR in human beings. *Ann. Emerg. Med.* 1986; **15**: 125–130.

37. Rubertsson, S., Grenvik, A. & Wiklund, L. Blood flow and perfusion pressure during open-chest versus closed-chest cardiopulmonary resuscitation in pigs. *Crit. Care Med.* 1995; **23**: 715–725.

38. Voorhees, W.D., Babbs, C.F. & Tacker, W.A., Jr. Regional blood flow during cardiopulmonary resuscitation in dogs. *Crit. Care Med.* 1980; **8**: 134–136.

39. Weil, M.H., Bisera, J., Trevino, R.P. *et al.* Cardiac output and end-tidal carbon dioxide. *Crit. Care Med.* 1985; **13**: 907–909.

40. Imberti, R., Bellinzona, G., Riccardi, F. *et al.* Cerebral perfusion pressure and cerebral tissue oxygen tension in a patient during cardiopulmonary resuscitation. *Intens. Care Med.* 2003; **29**: 1016–1019.

41. Shaffner, D.H., Eleff, S.M., Brambrink, A.M. *et al.* Effect of arrest time and cerebral perfusion pressure during cardiopulmonary resuscitation on cerebral blood flow, metabolism, adenosine triphosphate recovery, and pH in dogs. *Crit. Care Med.* 1999; **27**: 1335–1342.

42. Lindner, K.H., Pfenninger, E.G., Lurie, K.G. *et al.* Effects of active compression-decompression resuscitation on myocardial and cerebral blood flow in pigs. *Circulation* 1993; **88**: 1254–1263.

43. Bellamy, R.F., DeGuzman, L.R. & Pedersen, D.C. Coronary blood flow during cardiopulmonary resuscitation in swine. *Circulation* 1984; **69**(1): 174–180.

44. Kern, K.B., Hilwig, R. & Ewy, G.A. Retrograde coronary blood flow during cardiopulmonary resuscitation in swine: intracoronary Doppler evaluation. *Am. Heart J.* 1994; **128**: 490–499.

45. Halperin, H.R., Tsitlik, J.E., Guerci, A.D. *et al.* Determinants of blood flow to vital organs during cardiopulmonary resuscitation in dogs. *Circulation* 1986; **73**: 539–550.

46. Wolfe, J.A., Maier, G.W., Newton, J.R., Jr. *et al.* Physiologic determinants of coronary blood flow during external cardiac massage. *J. Thorac. Cardiovasc. Surg.* 1988; **95**: 523–532.

47. Berg, R.A., Sanders, A.B., Kern, K.B. *et al.* Adverse hemodynamic effects of interrupting chest compressions for rescue breathing during cardiopulmonary resuscitation for ventricular fibrillation cardiac arrest. *Circulation* 2001; **104**: 2465–2470.

48. Wiggers, C.J. The physiological basis for cardiac resuscitation from ventricular fibrillation: method for serial defibrillation. *Am. Heart J.* 1940; **20**: 413–422.

49. Michael, J.R., Guerci, A.D., Koehler, R.C. *et al.* Mechanisms by which epinephrine augments cerebral and myocardial perfusion during cardiopulmonary resuscitation in dogs. *Circulation* 1984; **69**: 822–835.

50. von, P.I., Weil, M.H., von Planta, M. *et al.* Cardiopulmonary resuscitation in the rat. *J. Appl. Physiol.* 1988; **65**: 2641–2647.

51. Ralston, S.H., Voorhees, W.D. & Babbs, C.F. Intrapulmonary epinephrine during prolonged cardiopulmonary resuscitation: improved regional blood flow and resuscitation in dogs. *Ann. Emerg. Med.* 1984; **13**: 79–86.

52. Palmer, B.S., Hadziahmetovic, M., Veci, T. *et al.* Global ischemic duration and reperfusion function in the isolated perfused rat heart. *Resuscitation* 2004; **62**: 97–106.

53. Bolli, R. & Marban, E. Molecular and cellular mechanisms of myocardial stunning. *Physiol. Rev.* 1999; **79**: 609–634.

54. Jennings, R.B., Murry, C.E., Steenbergen, C., Jr. *et al.* Development of cell injury in sustained acute ischemia. *Circulation* 1990; **82**: II2–II12.

55. Kloner, R.A., Ganote, C.E., Whalen, D.A., Jr. *et al.* Effect of a transient period of ischemia on myocardial cells. II. Fine structure during the first few minutes of reflow. *Am. J. Pathol.* 1974; **74**: 399–422.

56. Neumar, R.W., Brown, C.G., Van Ligten, P. *et al.* Estimation of myocardial ischemic injury during ventricular fibrillation with total circulatory arrest using high-energy phosphates and lactate as metabolic markers. *Ann. Emerg. Med.* 1991; **20**: 222–229.

57. Frank, O. Zur Dynamik der Hermuskels. *Z. Biol.* 1895; **32**: 3703.

58. Fukuda, N., Sasaki, D., Ishiwata, S. *et al.* Length dependence of tension generation in rat skinned cardiac muscle: role of titin in the Frank–Starling mechanism of the heart. *Circulation* 2001; **104**: 1639–1645.

59. Patterson, S.W. & Starling, S.E. On the mechanical factors which determine the output of the ventricles. *J. Physiol. (Lond.)* 2005; **48**: 348–356.

60. Lee, M.C., LeWinter, M.M., Freeman, G. *et al.* Biaxial mechanical properties of the pericardium in normal and volume overload dogs. *Am. J. Physiol.* 1985; **249**: H222–H230.

61. Tyberg, J.V., Taichman, G.C., Smith, E.R. *et al.* The relationship between pericardial pressure and right atrial pressure: an intraoperative study. *Circulation* 1986; **73**: 428–432.

62. Kingma, I., Tyberg, J.V. & Smith, E.R. Effects of diastolic transseptal pressure gradient on ventricular septal position and motion. *Circulation* 1983; **68**: 1304–1314.

63. Belenkie, I., Dani, R., Smith, E.R. *et al.* Effects of volume loading during experimental acute pulmonary embolism. *Circulation* 1989; **80**: 178–188.

64. Atherton, J.J., Moore, T.D., Lele, S.S. *et al.* Diastolic ventricular interaction in chronic heart failure. *Lancet* 1997; **349**: 1720–1724.

65. Dauterman, K., Pak, P.H., Maughan, W.L. *et al.* Contribution of external forces to left ventricular diastolic pressure. Implications for the clinical use of the Starling law. *Ann. Intern. Med.* 1995; **122**: 737–742.

66. Moore, T.D., Frenneaux, M.P., Sas, R. *et al.* Ventricular interaction and external constraint account for decreased stroke work during volume loading in CHF. *Am. J. Physiol. Heart Circ. Physiol.* 2001; **281**: H2385–H2391.

67. Woollard, M., Smith, A., Whitfield, R. *et al.* To blow or not to blow: a randomised controlled trial of compression-only and standard telephone CPR instructions in simulated cardiac arrest. *Resuscitation* 2003; **59**: 123–131.

68. Lurie, K.G., Mulligan, K.A., McKnite, S. *et al.* Optimizing standard cardiopulmonary resuscitation with an inspiratory impedance threshold valve. *Chest* 1998; **113**: 1084–1090.

69. Plaisance, P., Lurie, K.G., Vicaut, E. *et al.* Evaluation of an impedance threshold device in patients receiving active compression-decompression cardiopulmonary resuscitation for out of hospital cardiac arrest. *Resuscitation* 2004; **61**: 265–271.

70. Wolcke, B.B., Mauer, D.K., Schoefmann, M.F. *et al.* Comparison of standard cardiopulmonary resuscitation versus the combination of active compression–decompression cardiopulmonary resuscitation and an inspiratory impedance threshold device for out-of-hospital cardiac arrest. *Circulation* 2003; **108**: 2201–2205.

71. Voelckel, W.G., Lurie, K.G., Zielinski, T. *et al.* The effects of positive end-expiratory pressure during active compression decompression cardiopulmonary resuscitation with the inspiratory threshold valve. *Anesth. Analg.* 2001; **92**: 967–974.

72. Legallois, J.J.C. *Experimences sur le principe de la vie.* Paris: D. Hautel, 1812.

73. Guntheroth, W.G., & Kawabori, I. Hypoxic apnea and gasping. *J. Clin. Invest.* 1975; **56**: 1371–1377.

74. Noc, M., Weil, M.H., Sun, S. *et al.* Spontaneous gasping during cardiopulmonary resuscitation without mechanical ventilation. *Am. J. Respir. Crit. Care Med.* 1994; **150**: 861–864.

75. Xie, J., Weil, M.H., Sun, S. *et al.* Spontaneous gasping generates cardiac output during cardiac arrest. *Crit. Care Med.* 2004; **32**: 238–240.

76. Yang, L., Weil, M.H., Noc, M. *et al.* Spontaneous gasping increases the ability to resuscitate during experimental cardiopulmonary resuscitation. *Crit. Care Med.* 1994; **22**: 879–883.

77. Tang, W., Weil, M.H., Sun, S. *et al.* Cardiopulmonary resuscitation by precordial compression but without mechanical ventilation. *Am. J. Respir. Crit. Care Med.* 1994; **150**: 1709–1713.

Perfusion pressures

18

Coronary perfusion pressure during cardiopulmonary resuscitation

Karl B. Kern, James T. Niemann, and Stig Steen

University of Arizona Sarver Heart Center, Tucson, AZ, USA
Department of Emergency Medicine, Harbor-UCLA Medical Center, Torrance CA, USA
Department of Cardiothoracic Surgery, University Hospital of Lund, Sweden

Introduction

The resurgence of resuscitation research in the 1970s and 1980s initially focused on the physiological mechanisms for systemic blood flow during closed chest resuscitation for cardiac arrest.[1,2] At the same time, the importance of both myocardial and cerebral blood flow during cardiopulmonary resuscitation (CPR) became evident. Using contemporary, state-of-art techniques, investigators found that regional perfusion of vital organs occurs with closed chest compression CPR, but at substantially lower rates than that measured during normal sinus rhythm.[3–5] Such studies have shown that standard anteroposterior chest compressions can, at best, provide 30% to 40% of normal cerebral blood flow levels. Myocardial blood flow achieved with external chest compressions is often even lower, typically between 10% and 30% of normal. Peripheral perfusion is almost non-existent during CPR. Nevertheless, good CPR efforts can temporarily provide at least some perfusion to the myocardium and cerebrum until more definitive treatment (i.e., defibrillation) can be accomplished.

Myocardial perfusion during cardiac arrest can be estimated by measuring "coronary perfusion pressure" during the resuscitation effort. This perfusion pressure gradient correlates well with resultant myocardial blood flow generated with CPR and with the subsequent possibility of successful defibrillation.[3,4] The critical importance of coronary perfusion pressure during CPR has been confirmed in both laboratory and clinical studies of resuscitation. This part of the chapter focuses on coronary perfusion pressure during CPR: its generation and impact.

Determinants of coronary perfusion pressure during cardiopulmonary resuscitation

AoD pressure during CPR

The importance of an adequate perfusion pressure for resuscitation from cardiac arrest was first noted by Crile and Dolley in 1906.[6] While studying means of reversing cardiorespiratory arrest in dogs and cats asphyxiated with chloroform or ether (popular anesthetics of that time), they noted that "the basic problem, then, in resuscitations seems to us to be that of securing some means of some infusion – a coronary pressure, approximately amounting to 30 to 40 mm Hg." This concept was later reinforced by the work of Redding and Pearson.[7–10] These investigators showed that, when aortic diastolic pressure was raised above 40 mm Hg, usually with α-adrenergic drugs or other special maneuvers, experimental animals could be successfully resuscitated from cardiac arrest. When this diastolic pressure was not achieved, however, the animals could not be resuscitated. From this early work they deduced the mechanism of action for epinephrine and other α-adrenergic agonists during cardiac arrest. They postulated that such agents caused peripheral vasoconstriction, which raised the aortic diastolic pressure and increased coronary perfusion. Otto and coworkers confirmed this postulate in the late 1970s and early 1980s. By using selective blockade, they elucidated the relative importance of α- and β-adrenergic receptors during resuscitation. Animals that were α-blocked had difficulty in responding to epinephrine, i.e., diastolic aortic pressure did not increase and they were not resuscitated. In contrast, those that were β-blocked were successfully resuscitated and exhibited

Cardiac Arrest: The Science and Practice of Resuscitation Medicine. 2nd edn., ed. Norman Paradis, Henry Halperin, Karl Kern, Volker Wenzel, Douglas Chamberlain. Published by Cambridge University Press. © Cambridge University Press, 2007.

peripheral vasoconstriction with elevated aortic diastolic pressures in response to adrenergic agonists.[11–13]

AoD-RAD pressure during CPR

During the early 1980s, investigators not only confirmed the importance of a perfusion pressure (i.e., the aortic diastolic pressure) but also of a defined perfusion pressure gradient, which included a "downstream" pressure from the myocardial venous system acting as an impedance to forward flow. Voorhees *et al.*, measuring regional blood flow to the brain, heart, and other peripheral tissues, noted that the arteriovenous gradient was important during the compression phase of CPR for cerebral blood flow and postulated that the same arteriovenous gradient during the relaxation component of CPR was important for myocardial blood flow.[14] Both Niemann *et al.*[15] and Ditchey *et al.*[16] suggested that coronary perfusion pressure results from the difference in pressure between the aortic and the right atrium. Ditchey *et al.* found that coronary blood flow during CPR was a linear function of the mean pressure difference generated across the coronary circulation and that the ascending aortic and right atrial pressure difference and coronary flow were highest during the relaxation phase of each chest compression cycle (Fig. 18.1).

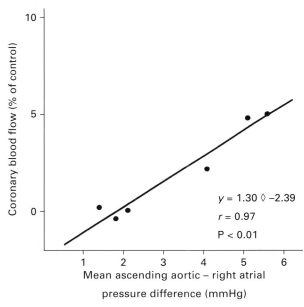

Fig. 18.1. Relationship as percent of control between coronary blood flow and coronary perfusion pressure defined as mean ascending aortic pressure minus mean right atrial pressure difference generated during CPR. (From ref. 16.)

Alternatives for calculating CPP

In spite of these insights on coronary perfusion pressure and its importance for generating myocardial blood flow and facilitating resuscitation, the best method for measuring coronary perfusion pressure during CPR has not been standardized. Some investigators suggested that subtracting the middiastolic right atrial pressure from simultaneously obtained middiastolic aortic pressure was sufficient,[3,17] whereas others suggested that coronary perfusion pressure be obtained by measuring the peak positive diastolic pressure gradient between the aorta and the right atrium.[18] Another approach has been to calculate the coronary perfusion pressure gradient by subtracting the mean right atrial diastolic pressure from the mean diastolic aortic pressure.[4,5] To address this uncertainty, the Utstein-style guidelines for reporting laboratory CPR research specify that the point just before compression be used as the reference point for measurement of coronary perfusion pressure. This point was selected because it is easily identified and more likely to be consistent among investigators.[19]

An alternative method for calculating coronary perfusion pressure is to measure the integrated area under the aortic diastolic pressure minus the right atrial diastolic pressure curves during each minute of cardiopulmonary resuscitation.[20] Since chest compression/relaxation cycles (i.e., the relaxation phase specifically) are responsible for generation of blood flow to the heart, a decrease in delivered chest compression cycles can markedly decrease the total amount of myocardial perfusion generated with the resuscitation effort. Calculating coronary perfusion pressure in the usual fashion (end-diastolic aortic minus right atrial pressures) does not account for periods when chest compression is interrupted. A more accurate method is to use the integrated area (iCPP) over each minute. The effect of chest compression pauses on coronary perfusion pressure becomes readily apparent, typically resulting in a 40% decrease in cumulative coronary perfusion (Fig. 18.2).

Interruption of chest compression/relaxation has direct effects on the amount of coronary perfusion pressure generated during the period of 15 compression cycles. We found that, at the beginning of each cycle of 15, the first 5–10 compressions/relaxations are "building-up" the coronary perfusion gradient and that it is not optimal until at least one-third of the series is completed.[21] Then, with cessation of chest compressions/relaxations, this diastolic gradient falls off rapidly, often returning to near zero within 5–10 seconds. Often the coronary perfusion pressure gradient falls even sooner to below the "critical closing pressure" predicting no forward flow after just a few seconds interruption of chest compression/relaxation. When chest compressions do resume, the coronary perfusion gradient must be rebuilt, usually starting from zero (Fig. 18.3).

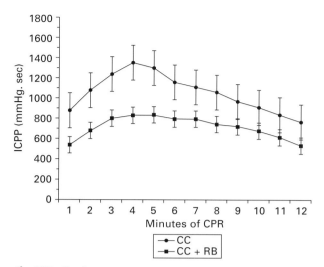

Fig. 18.2. Caption to come

AoS-RaS: no antegrade flow to myocardium

Several investigators have explored the possibility of whether coronary flow could occur during the compression phase of CPR.[15,16,22] Data from Schleien *et al.* suggested that forward coronary flow may occur during the compression phase of CPR, when epinephrine infusions are used, because a positive aortic to right atrial pressure gradient was observed during the compression phase. They concluded that the diastolic gradient as an index of coronary blood flow during CPR may be incomplete.[22] Subsequent work has shown that many methods of CPR routinely generate some degree of aortic to right atrial pressure difference during the compression phase, either positive or negative; hence, the potential for antegrade or even retrograde coronary blood flow exists during chest compression or CPR systole.[23]

Figure 18.4 shows a positive "gradient" during the compression phase of CPR. Total "net" flow during CPR may require consideration of the entire cardiac cycle (the compression phase and the relaxation phase). This hypothesis has been tested by using an intracoronary Doppler flow catheter to determine the relationship among (*a*) systolic or compression phase coronary perfusion pressure, (*b*) diastolic or relaxation-phase coronary perfusion, and (*c*) direction of coronary blood flow in the proximal left anterior coronary artery.[24] Retrograde coronary artery blood flow (from the coronary back into the ascending aorta) occurred routinely during the compression phase of manual CPR, regardless of the measured aortic to right atrial pressure gradient. Even in circumstances where the aortic pressure exceeded right atrial pressure during compressions, no antegrade coronary flow occurred. Rather, such antegrade coronary blood flow occurred exclusively during the relaxation phase of chest compression and correlated with a positive "diastolic" or relaxation-phase perfusion pressure gradient between the aorta and the right atrium. The greater the gradient, the larger the velocity of the antegrade coronary blood flow. Positive systolic coronary perfusion gradients occurring during the compression phase do not significantly improve

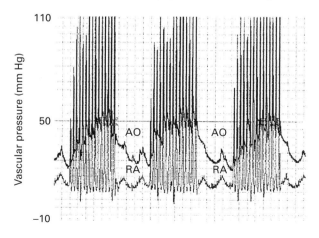

Fig. 18.3. Caption to come

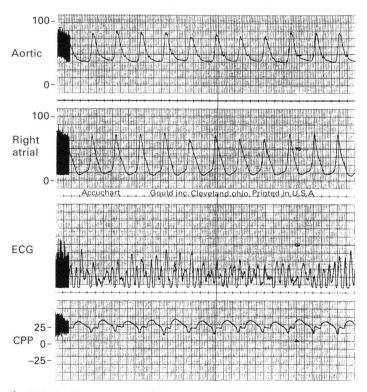

Fig. 18.4. Positive coronary perfusion pressure (*CPP*) gradient during compression phase of CPR where aortic systolic pressure minus right atrial systolic pressure remains positive.

antegrade blood flow and, indeed, can be associated with significant amounts of retrograde coronary flow. Hence, diastolic perfusion pressure gradients do account for the vast majority of cases of myocardial perfusion.

Under normal physiologic conditions, coronary perfusion pressure is conventionally defined as the difference in transmural myocardial pressure between the aortic and the left ventricular diastolic pressures. In subjects with normal ventricular filling pressures, the coronary driving pressure may be approximated by either the mean aortic pressure or the aortic diastolic pressure. When ventricular filling pressures are elevated, however, one of two corrections is typically used. First, the right atrial pressure could be subtracted since the coronary sinus drains into the right atrium, leaving the perfusion pressure then equal to the aortic pressure minus right atrial pressure.[25] Nevertheless, even the use of right atrial pressure tends to overestimate the perfusion pressure gradient when left ventricular diastolic pressure is increased. Second, the aortic pressure minus the left ventricular diastolic pressure could be used. CPR investigators have typically chosen the former formula and have used the right atrial pressure. Kern and coworkers (unpublished data) have assessed the relationship between transmural myocardial blood flow, measured with microspheres, and coronary perfusion pressure, which was defined as either aortic diastolic pressure minus right atrial diastolic pressure or, alternatively, aortic diastolic pressure minus left ventricular end-diastolic pressure. These investigators found that coronary perfusion pressure defined as aortic diastolic pressure minus right atrial diastolic pressure had a correlation coefficient of 0.58 with myocardial blood flow, whereas perfusion pressure defined as aortic diastolic pressure minus left ventricular end-diastolic pressure had a correlation coefficient of 0.47 during CPR.

Myocardial blood flow and coronary perfusion pressure during cardiopulmonary resuscitation

Regional perfusion or organ blood flow under nearly all physiologic conditions is determined by the pressure gradient across the vascular bed of interest divided by vascular resistance (flow equals arterial pressure minus venous pressure divided by vascular resistance or $Q = P_1 - P_2 / R$). During normal sinus rhythm in the heart in vivo, coronary vascular resistance depends on at least three physiologically distinct components termed R_1, R_2, and R_3.[26] R_1 is the resistance of the epicardial coronary conductive vessel. In the absence of vascular spasm or fixed coronary stenoses, R_1 contributes only a small percentage of the total coronary resistance. R_2, the autoregulatory resistance factor, is the major component of coronary resistance during normal

sinus physiology. R_2 results primarily from the smooth muscle tone of the arteriolar bed. The compressive resistance factor, R_3, results from intramyocardial pressure during systole compressing the intramural coronary vessels. It is the chief factor accounting for the observation that myocardial blood flow during normal sinus rhythm occurs primarily in the diastolic phase of the cardiac cycle. Other factors influencing R_3 include left ventricular diastolic pressure and transmural differences in vascular density.

During cardiac arrest, coronary vascular resistance is dramatically different. Intrinsic coronary tone (R_2) is minimal because of local, metabolically mediated coronary vasodilatation. Potential mediators of coronary vasodilatation include extracellular acidosis, endogenous adenosine release, and vasoactive compounds of endothelial origin, such as nitric oxide and endothelin. These ischemically induced vasodilatory substances are thought to induce maximal coronary vasodilatation relatively quickly during cardiac arrest, perhaps within the first 15 to 20 seconds. As a consequence, myocardial blood flow during cardiac arrest and artificial circulatory support by any method or technique will be largely determined by the driving force or "pressure head" across the coronary circulation, namely, the arterial pressure minus the venous pressure and the coronary vascular resistance. In the setting of ventricular fibrillation and CPR, coronary vascular resistance consists mainly of an R_1 component from epicardial coronary compression and R_3 from the intramyocardial pressure generated by the fibrillating myocardium and chest compression. In contrast to the resistance seen during normal sinus physiology, coronary vascular resistance during CPR is minimal during the relaxation phase of chest compression.

Careful study of the data illustrating the relationship between CPP and myocardial blood flow during CPR shows that no myocardial blood flow occurs until a minimum coronary perfusion pressure of approximately 5–10 mmHg is achieved. This corresponds to the "critical closing pressure" for coronary perfusion pressure, below which flow stops secondary to intrinsic smooth muscle tone in the arteriole wall literally causing physical closure of the arteriolar vessels.[27] Under normal physiologic conditions it is estimated that this critical closing pressure is about 30–40 mmHg, and that during intense vasodilatation it decreases to approximately 10–12 mmHg.[27] Data gathered during actual cardiac arrest suggest that during maximal vasodilatation this closing pressure may fall as low as 5–10 mmHg, but does not become zero, as some have previously postulated.[28] This "closing pressure," below which no flow seems to occur is a key concept in understanding the importance of limiting interruptions to chest compressions/relaxations during which the coronary perfusion pressure inevitably falls.

Correlation between CPP and MBF

Aortic and right atrial pressures can easily be measured in the laboratory and also, but with some effort, in the clinical setting. During the relaxation phase of chest compressions, aortic pressure largely depends upon intrinsic arterial tone. Right atrial pressure during the relaxation phase of CPR is largely determined by central venous return and venous capacitance. An excellent correlation has been established between the coronary perfusion pressure and simultaneously measured myocardial blood flow during CPR.[3–5,29] Data from three different laboratories demonstrate correlation coefficients in the range between 0.82 and 0.89. Ralston *et al.* found a correlation coefficient of 0.89 in dogs where no epinephrine was used and of 0.85 when epinephrine was used (Fig. 18.5).[3] Using epinephrine, Michael *et al.* found a

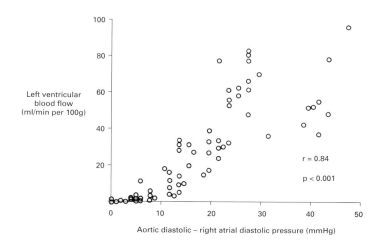

Fig. 18.6. Relationship between left ventricular blood flow and aortic diastolic pressure minus right atrial diastolic pressure during several forms of external CPR with and without use of epinephrine (From ref. 4.)

correlation coefficient of 0.84 (Fig. 18.6) and Halperin *et al.*, from the same laboratory at Johns Hopkins, found a correlation coefficient with multiple forms of CPR of 0.88 (Fig. 18.7).[4,5] Kern and coworkers reported a correlation coefficient of 0.82 between the coronary perfusion pressure achieved and the resultant myocardial blood flow to the anterior left ventricular wall.[29]

Many have noted, by general observation, that the typically low coronary perfusion pressures generated with standard CPR (10 to 20 mm Hg) produced only small

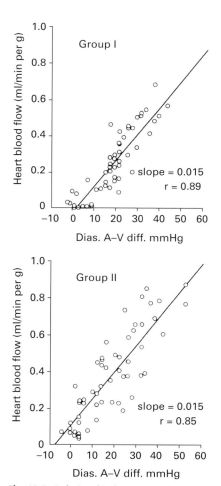

Fig. 18.5. Relationship between arterial minus venous diastolic pressure difference and heart blood flow during CPR in animals without epinephrine (group I) and those treated with epinephrine (group II). (From ref. 3.)

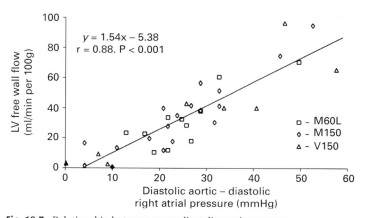

Fig. 18.7. Relationship between mean diastolic aortic pressure minus mean diastolic right atrial pressure and left ventricular free wall blood flow. Data include manual chest compressions at 60 compressions/min with prolonged duty cycle (M60L), manual compressions at 150 compressions/minute with prolonged duty cycle (M150), and vest CPR at 150 compressions/min with prolonged duration (V150). (From ref. 5.)

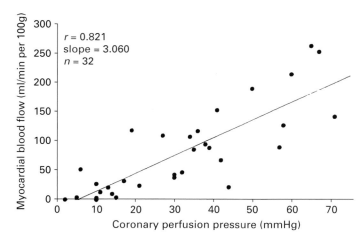

Fig. 18.8. Transmural anterior left ventricular myocardial blood flow resulting during CPR as function of coronary perfusion pressure. Note increase in myocardial blood flow with increasing coronary perfusion pressure generated during CPR. (From ref. 29.)

amounts of myocardial blood flow, usually no more than 20% of that observed during sinus rhythm. With a coronary perfusion pressure of 10 to 20 mm Hg, Ralston *et al.* found left ventricular flows of 15 to 20 ml/min/100 g.[3] Michael *et al.* found flows of 5 to 40 ml/min/100 g;[4] Halperin *et al.* found flows of 5 to 25 ml/min/100 g;[5] and Taylor *et al.* found flows of 10 to 15 ml/min/100 g.[30] These studies also demonstrated, however, that, if perfusion pressures are in the range of 40 to 60 mm Hg, excellent myocardial blood flow levels will result. Under these circumstances the following flows were found (all in milliliters per minute per 100 g): Ralston *et al.*, 60 to 90; Michael *et al.*, 40 to 100; Halperin *et al.*, 40 to 100; and Kern *et al.*, 50 to 200 (Fig. 18.8).[29]

In addition to obstructive epicardial coronary lesions that will affect the R_1 component of coronary resistance (discussed below), other interventions that increase one or more components of coronary resistance may alter the relationship between coronary perfusion pressure, and myocardial blood flow. One example of this is administration of endothelin-1. Early work with endothelin-1 as a pharmacologic adjunct for resuscitation demonstrated dramatic increases in coronary perfusion pressure, prompting initial enthusiasm for a promising new intervention.[31] Subsequent work demonstrated not only that coronary flow did not increase, but also that endothelin-1 adversely impacted affected survival 1 hour after resuscitation because sustained arterial vasoconstriction and increased cardiac work led to perfusion failure and refractory ventricular arrhythmias.[32,33]

Effect of coronary lesions on coronary flow

All of the previously described work correlating myocardial blood flow and coronary perfusion pressure was performed on experimental animals with normal coronary arteries and normal left ventricular function. The relationship between coronary perfusion pressure and myocardial blood flow during CPR has been helpful in understanding the physiology of blood flow production under these conditions. The established relationship, however, is derived from experiments in normal animals and may be limited in its applicability to humans, where the majority of sudden cardiac death victims have coronary artery disease.[34] To examine the effect of coronary artery lesions on the relationship between coronary perfusion pressure and myocardial blood flow during CPR, investigators at the University of Arizona evaluated a closed chest porcine model of fixed artificial coronary artery stenoses.[29] In this model with minimal collateral circulation, coronary artery lesions were found to have major effects on regional myocardial blood flow measured during CPR. With use of this closed chest model, chest compressions could be performed without compromising the integrity of the thoracic cage. Coronary stenoses greatly decrease the amount of distal coronary blood flow for any given coronary perfusion pressure produced. Complete coronary occlusion results in negligible distal myocardial perfusion, regardless of the coronary perfusion pressure. Myocardial blood flow measured during CPR continued to show a high correlation with coronary perfusion pressure, albeit with less myocardial blood flow for every increment in coronary perfusion pressure. With coronary perfusion pressures of 30 to 60 mm Hg, coronary stenosis resulted in an approximate 50% reduction in distal blood flow (Fig. 18.9). The data demonstrate that coronary lesions have an important effect on myocardial blood flow during CPR in that there was a substantial change in the relationship between coronary perfusion pressure and resultant myocardial blood flow. For any given coronary perfusion pressure generated with CPR, a 50% reduction in myocardial blood flow distal to the stenosis was seen (Fig. 18.10). This reduction occurred over a wide range of coronary perfusion pressures generated with external chest compressions. Previously determined levels of adequate perfusion pressure during CPR in models without coronary artery lesions may not be applicable to patients with coronary artery disease. Figure 18.11(a) and 18.11(b) shows the left anterior coronary artery before and after the creation of a 33% stenosis. Figure 18.12 shows left ventricular anterior endocardial blood flow proximal and

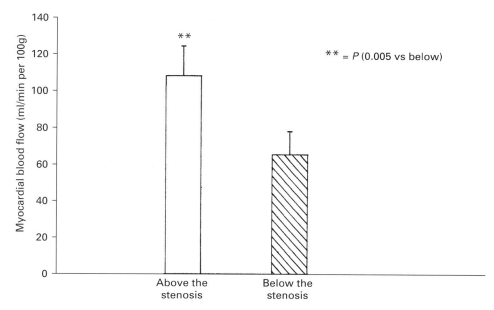

Fig. 18.9. Midleft anterior descending coronary artery stenosis results in significant reduction in distal myocardial blood flow over clinically realistic range of CPR-produced coronary perfusion pressures from 30 to 60 mm Hg. (From ref. 29.)

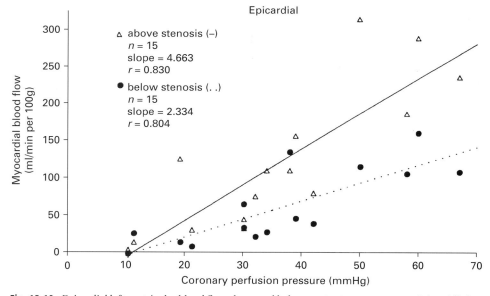

Fig. 18.10. Epicardial left ventricular blood flow above and below a patent coronary stenosis in midleft anterior descending coronary artery. Note decreased slope for myocardial blood flow as function of coronary perfusion pressure below stenosis when compared to that above stenosis. (From ref. 29.)

distal to the 33% diameter stenosis at 3 and 8 minutes of CPR. There was a significant difference between proximal and distal blood flow to the endocardium at 8 minutes of CPR. Therefore, even minimal or previously considered "insignificant" coronary lesions may have a profound effect on distal myocardial blood flow during the performance of CPR.[35]

The importance of coronary artery disease in victims of cardiac arrest had not been routinely considered in previous CPR research. Intuitive thinking would indicate that

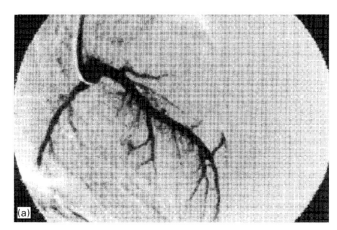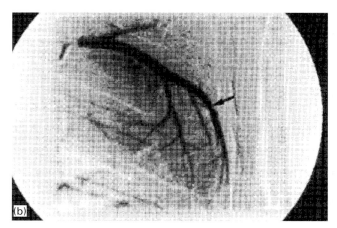

Fig. 18.11. (a) Digital cineangiography of porcine left anterior descending coronary artery before placement of Teflon cylinder creating midvessel stenosis. (b) Digital cineangiography of same porcine left anterior descending coronary artery after placement of Teflon cylinder creating 33% diameter stenosis (*arrow*). (From ref. 35.)

any coronary lesion that compromises myocardial blood flow under normal basal physiologic conditions will also be a potential problem during the extreme circumstances of CPR, but these findings of decreased blood flow below "clinically insignificant" lesions are noteworthy.

Effect of "resuscitation time" on CPP

Coronary perfusion pressure does not remain constant during the period of circulatory arrest and CPR. The highest pressure gradients and the greatest myocardial

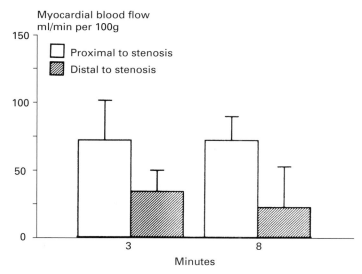

Fig. 18.12. Left ventricular anterior endocardial blood flow proximal and distal to 33% diameter stenosis at 3 and 8 minutes of CPR. (From ref. 35.)

perfusion occur during the first minutes of resuscitation. Prolonged resuscitation is characterized by a gradual decline in regional perfusion, most notably to the heart and brain.[36] This is due to the gradual decline in arterial tone and gradual increase in right heart pressures. Maintenance of minimal perfusion pressures generally requires the use of vasoactive drugs.[4]

The effect of "downtime" on subsequent coronary perfusion pressure generated during CPR was studied by Duggal *et al.*[37] They found no compromise in coronary perfusion pressure after extending the downtime from 9 minutes to 15 minutes of untreated ventricular fibrillation. They did note, however, that the previously established threshold levels of coronary perfusion pressure for resuscitability were not valid after the longer downtimes.

Coronary perfusion pressure, resuscitation, and survival

Correlation between CPP and resuscitation outcome

Coronary perfusion pressure is a determinant of myocardial blood flow during CPR and it has also been shown to be predictive of successful resuscitation, i.e., restoration of spontaneous circulation (ROSC), short-term outcome, and long-term survival. Both Ralston *et al.*[3] and Michael *et al.*[4] showed that increased coronary perfusion pressure translated into increased myocardial blood flow and better rates of successful resuscitation (Figs. 18.13 and 18.14). Other experimental studies have confirmed the predictive value of the myocardial perfusion gradient and longer-term survival rates, from 1- to 24-hour survival,[18,38–46] to 7-day survival rates.[47]

The ability of coronary perfusion pressure to serve as a direct monitoring adjunct during resuscitation efforts makes it attractive for use in clinical cardiac arrest. Over the last two decades, there have been reports of more than 200 patients who had coronary perfusion pressure measured during the performance of CPR.[48–57] A number of import-ant lessons have been learned. First, it is feasible to measure coronary perfusion pressure in victims of clinical cardiac arrest. The necessary instrumentation, including cannulation of the ascending aorta and right atrium, can be accomplished even during resuscitation efforts, and experience suggests that this can be done safely. It is unfortunate that, by the time the catheters are in place, the patient is often relatively late in the course of cardiac arrest, which may limit the utility of measuring coronary perfusion pressure in victims of unexpected cardiac arrest. In these cases the information is obtained so late in the course of cardiac arrest that it is not helpful. Occasionally, cardiac arrest occurs in patients who already have a pulmonary artery catheter or an arterial line. Such patients can easily be monitored for coronary perfusion pressure during CPR by the appropriate use of these pressure tracings.

The vast majority of measurements obtained in humans show poor coronary perfusion pressures. The mean coronary perfusion pressure reported in human series ranges from 0[43] to 15 mm Hg.[57] Consistent with these low values, most humans monitored for coronary perfusion pressure during CPR have not survived. Occasionally, however, survivors are reported. McDonald.[49] reported that 1 out of 12 patients survived and that patient had the highest coronary perfusion pressure from his series (16 mm Hg). Paradis *et al.*[55] reported on 100 patients, of whom 24 had return of spontaneous circulation. When coronary perfusion pressures between survivors and non-survivors were compared, there was a statistically significant difference in initial coronary perfusion pressure measured: those without return of spontaneous circulation had a mean coronary perfusion pressure of 2 mm Hg; those in whom spontaneous circulation returned had mean perfusion pressures of 13 mm Hg. Likewise, maximal coronary perfusion pressure was significantly different between the two groups: 8 mm Hg vs. 26 mm Hg. This series, in particular, substantiates the experimental data from animal models showing that coronary perfusion pressure can be a predictor of the return of spontaneous circulation. Paradis and colleagues noted that, in patients with prolonged cardiac arrest, coronary perfusion pressure was a better predictor of resuscitation outcome than was aortic pressure alone. A coronary perfusion pressure of 15 mm Hg

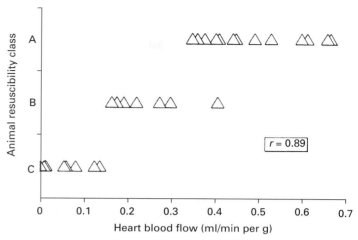

Fig. 18.13. Relationship between ease of resuscitation and heart blood flow produced during CPR. Class A animals were easy to resuscitate, class B were difficult, and class C could not be resuscitated. (From ref. 3.)

seemed to be necessary for the return of spontaneous circulation and may represent a reasonable goal.

CPR quality and coronary perfusion pressure

An effective myocardial perfusion gradient is dependent upon properly performed chest compressions during resuscitation efforts. Babbs and colleagues at Purdue Unversity showed that there is an effective compression threshold for generating both blood pressure and cardiac output with external chest compressions.[58] A number of studies support the contention that standard manual CPR must be properly performed to be of survival benefit. One study supporting this statement was performed in the United States and involved 2071 out-of-hospital resuscitations evaluated over a 6-month period in New York City.[59] The investigators attempted to determine whether the quality of bystander CPR affected eventual survival. CPR quality was determined to be effective or ineffective by emergency medical services (EMS) personnel in those instances in which bystander CPR was in progress at the time of their arrival on scene. CPR was judged to be effective if EMS personnel observed ventilations producing chest rise and chest compressions associated with palpable pulses in the carotid or femoral arteries in accordance with the American Heart Association guidelines. These guidelines specify 1.5 to 2 inches of sternal displacement. CPR was characterized as ineffective if effective compressions were accompanied by ineffective ventilations and vice versa, or if both compressions and ventilations were ineffective. Survival was defined as discharge from the

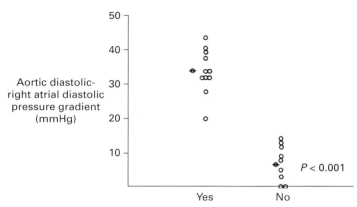

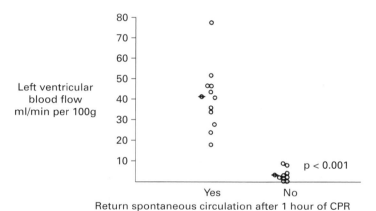

Fig. 18.14. Return of spontaneous circulation after 1 hour of cardiac arrest as function of coronary perfusion pressure generated during CPR. Animals with coronary perfusion pressures less than 20 in this experiment could not be resuscitated. (From ref. 4.)

assume that inadequate myocardial perfusion accompanying inadequately performed CPR was responsible for the failure to restore spontaneous circulation.

Number of chest compressions/min, coronary perfusion pressure, and ROSC

Several experimental studies indicate that interruptions in chest compressions during CPR lessen the likelihood of successful cardiac resuscitation. During pauses for artificial ventilation, aortic diastolic pressure begins to fall spontaneously toward the resting pressure which is determined by vascular tone. The initial compressions following a pause for ventilation generate a lower coronary perfusion pressure than those which precede a ventilation.[21] (Fig. 18.3) These changes in perfusion pressure result in lower myocardial perfusion than when chest compressions are performed in an uninterrupted fashion.[63] In addition, frequent interruptions for ventilation can also adversely effect neurological recovery in an animal model.[64] Additional reasons for stopping chest compressions frequently punctuate conventional resuscitation efforts. Such reasons would include rhythm interpretation, pulse checks, and defibrillator charging and discharging, all of which may alter hemodynamics and outcome.[65,66]

Recent observational clinical investigations of the quality CPR performed by paramedics, nurses, or physicians indicate that inappropriately slow chest compression rates, inappropriately high ventilation rates, inadequate depth of sternal depression, and frequent interruptions of compressions are common.[67,68] These latter studies did not evaluate the impact of poor CPR performance on outcome.

Improving outcome and coronary perfusion pressure

Since coronary perfusion pressure correlates with myocardial blood flow and myocardial blood flow correlates with resuscitation success, it follows that the greater the coronary perfusion pressure, the more likely is a successful outcome. However, achieving such benefit can rarely be accomplished by standard chest compressions alone. As seen in Fig. 18.15, the production of high levels of coronary perfusion pressure is not without problems. In an effort to maximize perfusion pressure, the use of excessive force in chest compressions may result in severe and even life-threatening injury. In an animal model (without coronary lesions) of cardiac arrest, a myocardial perfusion pressure of 30 mm Hg appears to be ideal for ensuring long-term

hospital to home. Non-survivors were patients who died or who discharged to a facility rather than home. For the 662 patients entered in the study, the overall survival was 2.9% for those who received CPR (effective or ineffective) and 0.8% for those who received no bystander CPR. For those receiving effective CPR, 4.5% survived, compared to 0%–2% for those judged to have received ineffective CPR. After adjustments or corrections for time from collapse to initiation of bystander CPR, time from collapse to advanced cardiac life support (ACLS), and the initial rhythm, effective CPR yielded an adjusted odds ratio of 3.9 for survival. These findings were similar to the results of studies conducted in Europe and New Zealand which demonstrated that good CPR was associated with a 16%–23% survival compared to the 1%–7% survival with bad bystander CPR.[60–62] Although coronary perfusion pressure was not measured in these studies, it is logical to

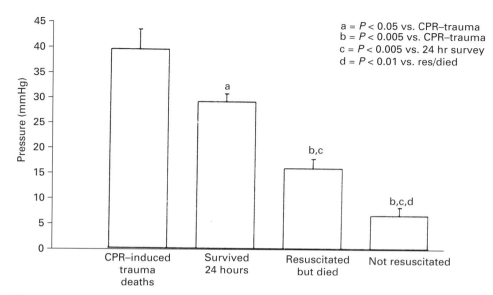

a = $P < 0.05$ vs. CPR–trauma
b = $P < 0.005$ vs. CPR–trauma
c = $P < 0.005$ vs. 24 hr survey
d = $P < 0.01$ vs. res/died

Fig. 18.15. Mean myocardial perfusion pressures between 10 and 15 minutes of CPR among animals that suffered CPR-induced trauma deaths, 24-hour survivors, animals that were resuscitated but died non-traumatic deaths before 24 hours, and animals that were never resuscitated. (From ref. 45.)

survival without a high degree of CPR injury. Efforts with external chest compressions to increase perfusion pressure above 30 mm Hg do not seem justified because of the resultant CPR-induced trauma and reduced rate of 24-hour survival.[45] In this series, animals that died from CPR-induced injury had a mean perfusion pressure of 39 mm Hg, whereas those that survived 24 hours had a mean perfusion pressure of 29 mm Hg. These results suggest that coronary perfusion pressure measured during CPR can also be used as a guide to avoid unnecessary injury when optimal levels have been achieved.

Although effective or good CPR is associated with a better outcome, the ability to perform effective or good CPR appears to be time-dependent, i.e., the longer CPR is performed, the less likely that compressions remain effective in terms of sternal displacement or rate per minute. This phenomenon has been demonstrated in a number of studies in which instrumented or "recording" manikins were used to record the chest compression rate and chest compression depth during uninterrupted, extended CPR (typically 5 minutes duration).[69–72] The study by Ochoa and colleagues perhaps demonstrates this time effect most dramatically.[70] In that investigation, the authors sought to evaluate the influence of rescuer fatigue on the quality of chest compressions and the influence of gender, age, weight, and height on the reduction of quality CPR. Thirty-eight healthcare professionals performed chest compressions on a recording manikin for five consecutive minutes. The manikin recorded the number of compressions per minute, the depth of sternal depression, and the location of the site of each compression (hand position). A marked decline in depth of sternal displacement was observed as early as the second minute of the trial and the mean time to fatigue, as verbalized by the participants, was 186 seconds. Although some compressions were effective, the majority were not.

A renewed interest in newer CPR methods and the development and use of automated devices for CPR[73,74] has been driven, in part, by the limitations of manual chest compressions, namely, decline in effectiveness over time and inherent interruptions. A number of alternative methods of CPR have been tested, for both CPP generation and outcome, and include, but are not limited to, the following.

Manual techniques

IAC-CPR

Interposed abdominal compression CPR (IAC-CPR) is a method of manual basic life support that has been proposed as a technique to improve coronary perfusion pressure during resuscitation. With this method, abdominal pressure is applied over the mid abdomen with two hands during the relaxation phase of chest compressions. Investigators at Purdue University rediscovered the hemodynamic advantages of intermittent abdominal compression during CPR.[75] Follow-up studies at Purdue University verified improvement in coronary perfusion pressure with the use of interposed abdominal compression CPR.[76] Two other reports examined the use of this form of CPR in experimental models, one of which found no improvement[42] and one of which did.[77] Three reports have been published concerning the use of interposed abdominal compression CPR in human subjects where coronary perfusion was measured. One patient reportedly had an increase in coronary perfusion pressure.[78] In a separate series, six patients had no significant increase,[49] and, in the largest series of 14 patients, interposed abdominal compression had inconsistent effects on the coronary perfusion pressure.[51] Despite these inconsistencies, four clinical trials comparing IAC-CPR and standard CPR demonstrated greater rates of initial successful resuscitation and a trend toward an increased survival rate to hospital discharge in the IAC-CPR group.[79]

ACD-CPR

Another new form or method of CPR is active compression-decompression CPR (ACD-CPR). Using a chest "suction cup" apparatus applied to the sternum, ACD-CPR pulls the anterior chest outward during the relaxation or release phase of chest compressions performed with the same device. In contrast, standard CPR allows passive thoracic recoil between compressions. The active "diastolic" component of ACD-CPR generates a negative intrathoracic pressure resulting in a lower diastolic right atrial pressure and a greater coronary perfusion pressure.[80] Several reports in experimental models have shown improved diastolic or relaxation-phase coronary perfusion pressure with the use of active compression-decompression CPR when compared to standard.[73] A number of clinical trials with this device have also been completed with conflicting results regarding benefit compared to standard CPR. However, a combined analysis, using chi-square trend analysis, of the nearly 3000 patients enrolled in these trials has demonstrated an increased overall survival rate.[81]

Mechanical techniques

Circumferential compression of the thorax with an inflatable vest-like garment was described in the 1980s and tested in small, selected clinical populations in the late 1980s and early 1990s.[52,56] The design of this device was based upon the concept of a "thoracic pump" as the driving force for blood flow during chest compression. Studies demonstrated that "Vest CPR" increased coronary perfusion pressure in experimental cardiac arrest models and in patients. However, the device was logistically difficult to incorporate into clinical resuscitation. Based upon the thoracic pump theory and success with a circumferential garment, redesign and experimentation led to substantial

revisions and re-introduction of a thoracic compression device (AutoPulse™, Revivant Inc., Sunnyvale, CA). This device incorporates a band applied over the anterior chest that is rhythmically tightened and released, resulting in a decrease in thoracic dimension or size of about 20%. Ongoing experimental animal and clinical studies indicate that the device produces greater coronary perfusion pressures than those measured during chest compression performed with a mechanical, pneumatic piston device.[57,82] An early clinical trial has demonstrated a greater rate of return of spontaneous circulation treated with the device when compared to a historical control group who received conventional, manual CPR.[83]

Another mechanical device, LUCAS, is also currently being evaluated. This device incorporates a gas-driven piston combined with active decompression. LUCAS CPR produces greater perfusion pressures and resuscitation rates in experimental animals than a standard, commercially available pneumatic piston device.[84]

Neither of these mechanical devices nor others in development have undergone extensive clinical testing.

Open chest CPR

Open chest cardiac massage or invasive CPR has probably been the most studied and the most impressive in its ability to improve coronary perfusion pressure.[85] Numerous studies by resuscitation research groups at the University of Pittsburgh and the University of Arizona have shown improvement in hemodynamics, specifically coronary perfusion pressure, with the institution of open chest cardiac massage.[39,40,44,47,86,87] Figure 18.16 is an excellent example of coronary perfusion pressure increasing with open chest cardiac massage.

A particularly clinically relevant investigation of open-chest resuscitation was undertaken by Sanders and colleagues. This study dramatically demonstrated the importance of the duration of inadequate coronary perfusion pressure on subsequent improvements in perfusion and ultimate resuscitation from cardiac arrest.[40] Invasive forms of resuscitation often have dramatic effects on coronary perfusion pressure but, because of morbidity associated with an invasive approach, these treatment options are often instituted late in the course of resuscitation. In an experimental model with closed chest CPR efforts for periods between 15 and 25 minutes, Sanders *et al.* found that aggressive intervention, such as open chest cardiac massage, could improve coronary perfusion pressure substantially above that achieved with continued closed chest compressions, but resuscitation would not result if such therapy was instituted beyond 15 minutes of cardiac

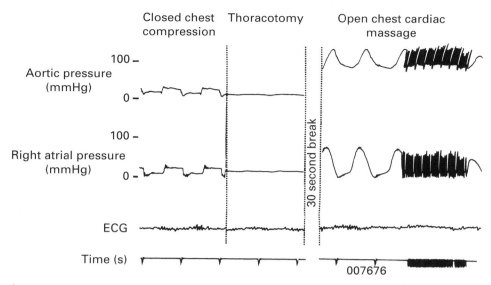

Fig. 18.16. Hemodynamic and electrocardiographic record from animal receiving closed chest compression CPR for 12 minutes after 3 minutes untreated cardiac arrest and then an emergent thorocotomy and 2 minutes of open chest cardiac message. (From ref. 47.)

arrest. Such data imply that improvements in coronary perfusion pressure may not translate into improved survival if they come too late in the course of resuscitation therapy.

In another series of experimental animals undergoing open chest cardiac massage after a period of ineffective closed chest compressions, tremendous improvements in mean coronary perfusion pressure were seen compared to continued closed chest efforts (65 mm Hg vs. 19 mm Hg). The animals that had improved coronary perfusion pressure during CPR not only were resuscitated more easily and survived 24 hours, but also had a better 7-day survival rate.[47] Thus it appears that even during a relatively short period of CPR, coronary perfusion pressure can be used to predict long-term 7-day survival.

CPR adjuncts

An inspiratory impedance valve has been developed and tested during several resuscitation methods or techniques. The valve is inserted into the ventilation circuit, typically between an endotracheal tube and self-inflating bag. During chest compression, the valve opens and allows passive expiration. During the relaxation phase, the valve blocks the circuit and negative intrathoracic pressure is increased. A lower intrathoracic pressure is transmitted to the right heart, resulting in a lower right atrial pressure and greater venous return.[80] Coronary perfusion pressure is increased as a result of the lower right atrial pressure. This valve has been tested during standard, conventional CPR as well as during ACD-CPR. Coronary perfusion pressure and systemic perfusion have been shown to be significantly better with the valve than without it.[88,89]

Pharmacologic interventions

One of the main avenues to improve coronary perfusion pressure has been the use of α-adrenergic agonists. As understanding of the importance of coronary perfusion pressure has increased, so has knowledge that certain α-adrenergic agonists improved coronary perfusion pressure by raising aortic diastolic pressure above increases in the right atrial diastolic pressure.[6–13] Epinephrine was one of the first agents shown to be effective in this regard.[6] Numerous investigators have clearly pointed out the advantageous increases in coronary perfusion pressure in response to epinephrine administration during CPR.[3–5,90–96]

Although adrenergic agonists increase coronary perfusion pressure, their effect on myocardial oxygen consumption is more controversial. Ditchey and Lindenfield were the first to describe the effect of epinephrine, not only on coronary perfusion pressure, but also on myocardial oxygen supply and demand.[97] They found that, in contrast to a placebo, epinephrine increased myocardial lactate concentration and decreased myocardial adenosine triphosphate (ATP) concentration after CPR. They suggested that large doses of epinephrine failed to improve the balance between myocardial oxygen supply and demand during CPR, even when such agents result in increased coronary blood flow. However, Brown *et al.* found that epinephrine improved the oxygen extraction ratio, which is defined as oxygen utilization divided by oxygen delivery, during CPR. They suggested that high-dose epinephrine improved not only myocardial blood flow, but also oxygen extraction ratios during CPR when compared with drugs having greater α-agonism, namely, phenylephrine in two different doses (0.1 mg/kg and 1.0 mg/kg).[92] Lindner *et al.* found that, although epinephrine effectively increased both perfusion pressure and myocardial blood flow, it also increased myocardial oxygen consumption.[96] Epinephrine led to greater increases in myocardial oxygen consumption than did norepinephrine, and any advantage in the slight increase in myocardial blood flow seen with epinephrine was negated. These authors concluded that norepinephrine improved the balance between myocardial oxygen delivery and myocardial oxygen consumption in contrast to epinephrine and thereby facilitated the restoration of spontaneous circulation.

Numerous animal studies have shown that epinephrine in doses of 0.2 mg/kg, so-called high-dose epinephrine, produces substantially higher coronary perfusion pressure and greater myocardial blood flow than does "standard"-dose epinephrine (0.02 mg/kg).[90,91,98] Figure 18.17

represents the graded response to different doses of epinephrine for both coronary perfusion pressure and myocardial blood flow. Clinical reports on the optimal dose for generation of coronary perfusion pressure during CPR are difficult to find. Gonzalez reported increases in radial artery systolic and diastolic pressures with stepwise increases in the dose of epinephrine administered to cardiac arrest patients.[99] Paradis and coworkers did study 32 patients whose cardiac arrests were refractory to advanced cardiac life support, measuring simultaneous aortic and right atrial pressures to calculate coronary perfusion pressure.[100] They found an increase in mean coronary perfusion pressure of 4 mm Hg after a standard dose of epinephrine, with a further increase of 11 mm Hg after high-dose epinephrine. They concluded that high-dose epinephrine seemed more likely to raise coronary perfusion pressure above the previously demonstrated critical value of 15 mm Hg in patients during cardiac arrest. Despite the preponderance of data supporting the benefit of high dose epinephrine in animal models, randomized trials of high-dose vs. standard-dose epinephrine in clinical cardiac arrest have failed to show an improved survival rate.[101,102] However, these studies do demonstrate some improvement in restoration of spontaneous circulation, i.e., successful cardiac resuscitation, with high dose epinephrine which would support improved myocardial perfusion during resuscitative efforts. Of note, data from

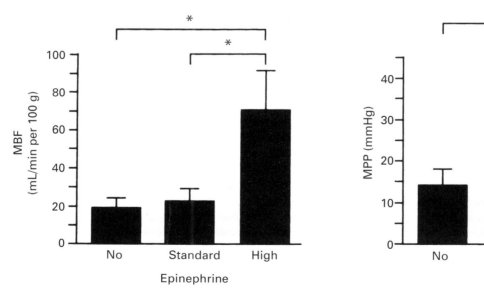

Fig. 18.17. Graded doses of epinephrine, including no epinephrine, standard-dose epinephrine (O.O2 mg/kg), and high-dose epinephrine (O.O2 mg/kg), and resultant myocardial perfusion pressures (*MPP*) and myocardial blood flows (*MBF*). High-dose epinephrine produced significantly more myocardial perfusion pressure and resultant myocardial blood flow than did either no adrenalin or standard-dose epinephrine. (From ref. 98.)

other studies suggest that epinephrine, even when administered frequently in standard doses, impairs postresuscitation circulatory dynamics and may worsen neurological outcome.[103,104]

The best adrenergic agonist for raising coronary perfusion pressures is likewise controversial. Brown *et al.* reported two studies: one compared epinephrine and phenylephrine for their effects on coronary perfusion pressure in an experimental model, and the other compared epinephrine vs. methoxamine. They found that epinephrine produced greater coronary perfusion pressures than did either of two doses of phenylephrine[92] and that epinephrine-treated animals had significantly higher coronary perfusion pressures than did methoxamine-treated animals.[105] Other authors compared the effects of epinephrine and either methoxamine or norepinephrine on aortic diastolic pressure and mean aortic pressure. Roberts *et al.* found that methoxamine produced greater diastolic aortic pressures than either high-dose or low-dose epinephrine.[106] Lindner *et al.* found epinephrine and norepinephrine to have equally potent effects on improving coronary perfusion pressure during CPR.[96] A growing body of recent literature demonstrates that vasopressin offers benefit in the resuscitation setting. Activation of vasopressin receptors in the peripheral circulation increases arterial tone and the coronary perfusion gradient. No consensus yet exists concerning the best adrenergic agonist for raising coronary perfusion pressure during resuscitation. A combination of vasopressin and epinephrine may be most beneficial.

Non-invasive alternatives to measuring coronary perfusion pressure during cardiopulmonary resuscitation

Because of its correlation with myocardial blood flow produced during CPR and with successful resuscitation outcome, coronary perfusion pressure is an ideal way to gauge effectiveness of CPR during the ongoing resuscitation effort. It is unfortunate that this measure of the effectiveness of ongoing CPR is limited in the clinical setting because these pressures are difficult to obtain and require intravascular catheters in the aorta and right atrium. Some clinical studies have accomplished such catheter placements and coronary perfusion pressure has been measured, but typically this takes 15 to 30 minutes after arrival at the hospital, and, although feasible in some patients, in many patients this is well beyond the usual time that resuscitation can be expected to be successful. There is a critical need for a simple, rapid, and preferably non-invasive measure of the effectiveness of CPR that can be used early in the resuscitation effort. Monitoring of end-tidal CO_2 exhaled during CPR is one such possibility. A second is monitoring characteristics of the VF waveform which may reflect myocardial perfusion during CPR and predict defibrillation outcome. Carbon dioxide is byproduct of tissue metabolism and is transported to the lung and eliminated during ventilation. Carbon dioxide delivery to the lung is dependent upon venous return which is equal to cardiac output. If ventilation is held constant, expired carbon dioxide is a measure of pulmonary perfusion and cardiac output. During cardiac arrest, the fall in cardiac output is accompanied by a decrease in carbon dioxide transport from the tissues to the pulmonary circulation and a reduction in carbon dioxide elimination from the lungs. With initiation of CPR and restoration of cardiac output, pulmonary perfusion is restored, to some degree, and carbon dioxide elimination returns.

Expired carbon dioxide can be measured by interposing a capnometer between the endotracheal tube and the ventilation source during CPR. Laboratory studies have shown excellent correlations between end-tidal CO_2 and coronary perfusion pressure,[107] as well as return of spontaneous circulation.[108–110] In one study the pattern of changes in end-tidal CO_2 during resuscitation proved to be more significant than any single reading. Over a 15-minute period of resuscitation, animals that were eventually resuscitated had constant and steady levels of end-tidal CO_2; animals that failed to be resuscitated exhibited a steady decline in such levels.[109] Other studies have shown minimal levels of end-tidal CO_2 below which no animals were resuscitated.[110] End-tidal CO_2 monitoring has also been used in humans to assess ongoing resuscitation efforts.[111–114] None of these studies measured coronary perfusion pressure, but several found minimal levels of end-tidal CO_2 that appeared to be required for successful resuscitation.[113,114] Although end-tidal CO_2 monitoring has the advantage of being non-invasive and easy to use, there has been some concern recently that administration of epinephrine during CPR may adversely affect the ability of end-tidal CO_2 monitoring to predict coronary perfusion pressure, as well as resuscitation outcome.[115–117] Nevertheless, a study in humans showed that although end-tidal CO_2 may decrease temporarily after epinephrine use, the predictive value of this measurement was not eliminated.[117] The electrocardiogram is closely monitored during resuscitation efforts and cardiac rhythms detected during such efforts dictate most resuscitative interventions. Recent data suggest that computer based analysis of the VF waveform may be useful in estimating "downtime," determining the effect of interventions, including CPR, and predicting the outcome of countershock. Such analyses typically include some component of the amplitude or frequency or both components of the recorded VF signal and include the mean frequency by Fourier transformation, both amplitude and frequency resulting in an amplitude spectrum analysis (AMSA), or fractal geometric analysis resulting in a scaling exponent.[118] Each of these methods has been shown to be predictive of countershock outcome in animal models of prolonged cardiac arrest due to VF. Two have been evaluated in the clinical population. Salutary changes in VF amplitude and frequency have been described following the initiation of CPR and are likely to reflect the adequacy of myocardial perfusion and the magnitude of the coronary perfusion gradient.

Summary

Coronary perfusion pressure obtained during CPR is a useful measurement. The aortic and right atrial pressure gradient during the relaxation phase of chest compressions defines coronary perfusion pressure during CPR. This gradient has correlated well with measured myocardial blood flow during CPR and with resuscitation outcome. Efforts to improve coronary perfusion pressure and success of resuscitation have centered around the use of adrenergic agonists and new methods of chest compression or resuscitation techniques, such as open chest cardiac massage, rapid manual CPR, interposed abdominal compression CPR, active compression–decompression CPR, and a number of new and investigational mechanical CPR methods. Measuring end-tidal CO_2 or the VF waveform may be reasonable non-invasive "surrogates" of coronary perfusion pressure in guiding resuscitation efforts.

REFERENCES

1. Chandra, N.C. Mechanisms of blood flow during CPR. *Ann. Emerg. Med.* 1993; **22**(part2): 281–288.
2. Gazmuri, R.J. & Becker, J. Cardiac resuscitation. The search for hemodynamically more effective methods. *Chest* 1997; **111**: 712–723.
3. Ralston, S.H., Voorhees, W.D., & Babbs, C.F. Intrapulmonary epinephrine during prolonged cardiopulmonary resuscitation: improved regional blood flow and resuscitation in dogs. *Ann. Emerg. Med.* 1984; **13**: 79–86.
4. Michael, J.R., Guerci, A.D., Koehler, R.C. *et al.* Mechanism by which epinephrine augments cerebral and myocardial perfusion during cardiopulmonary resuscitation in dogs. *Circulation* 1984; **69**: 822–835.
5. Halperin, H.R., Tsitlik, J.E., Guerci, A.D. *et al.* Determinants of blood flow to vital organs during cardiopulmonary resuscitation in dogs. *Circulation* 1986; **73**: 539–550.
6. Crile, G. & Dolley, D.H. Experimental research into resuscitation of dogs killed by anesthetics and asphyxia. *J. Exp. Med.* 1906; **8**: 713–738.
7. Redding, J.S. & Pearson, J.W. Evaluation of drugs for cardiac resuscitation. *Anesthesiology* 1963; **24**: 203–207.
8. Pearson, J.W. & Redding, J.S. Influence of peripheral vascular tone on cardiac resuscitation. *Anesth. Analg.* 1976; **44**: 746–752.
9. Redding, J.S., & Pearson, J.W. Resuscitation from ventricular fibrillation. *J. Am. Med. Assoc.* 1968; **203**: 255–260.
10. Redding, J.S. Abdominal compression in cardiopulmonary resuscitation. *Anesth. Analg.* 1971; **50**: 668–675.
11. Yakaitis, R.W., Otto, C.W., & Blitt, C.D. Relative importance of alpha and beta adrenergic receptors during resuscitation. *Crit. Care Med.* 1979; **7**: 293–296.
12. Otto, C.W., Yakaitis, R.W., & Blitt, C.D. Mechanism of action of epinephrine and resuscitation from asphyxia arrest. *Crit. Care Med.* 1981; **9**: 364–366.
13. Otto, C.W., Yakaitis, R.W., Redding, J.S., & Blitt, C.D. Comparison of dopamine, dobutamine, and epinephrine in CPR. *Crit. Care Med.* 1981; **9**: 366.
14. Voorhees, W.D., Babbs, C.F., & Tacker, W.A. Regional blood flow during cardiopulmonary resuscitation in dogs. *Crit. Care Med.* 1980; **8**: 134–136.
15. Niemann, J.T., Rosborough, J.P., Ung, S., & Criley, J.M. Coronary perfusion pressure during experimental cardiopulmonary resuscitation. *Ann. Emerg. Med.* 1982; **11**: 127–131.
16. Ditchey, R.V., Winkler, J.V., & Rhodes, C.A. Relative lack of coronary blood flow during closed-chest resuscitation in dogs. *Circulation* 1982; **66**: 297–302.
17. Sanders, A.B., Ewy, G.A., Alverness, C., Taft, T., & Zimmerman, M. Failure of a simultaneous chest compression, ventilation and abdominal binding technique of cardiopulmonary resuscitation. *Crit. Care Med.* 1982; **10**: 509–513.
18. Niemann, J.T., Rosborough, J.P., Niskanen, R.A., Alferness, C., & Criley, J.M. Mechanical "cough" cardiopulmonary resuscitation during cardiac arrest in dogs. *Am. J. Cardiol.* 1985; **55**: 199–204.
19. Idris, A.H., Becker, L.B., Ornato, J.P. *et al.* Utstein-style guidelines for uniform reporting of laboratory CPR research. *Circulation* 1996; **94**: 2324–2336.
20. Berg, R.A., Sanders, A.B., Kern, K.B. *et al.* Adverse hemodynamic effects of interrupting chest compressions for rescue breathing during cardiopulmonary resuscitation for ventricular fibrillation cardiac arrest. *Circulation* 2001; **104**: 2465–2470.
21. Kern, K.B., Hilwig, R.W., Berg, R.A. *et al.* Efficacy of chest compression-only BLS CPR in the presence of an occluded airway. *Resuscitation* 1998; **39**: 179–188.
22. Schleien, C.L., Dean, J.M., Koehler, R.C. *et al.* Effect of epinephrine on cerebral and myocardial perfusion in an infant

animal preparation of cardiopulmonary resuscitation. *Circulation* 1986; **73**: 809–817.

23. Raessler, K.L., Kern, K.B., Sanders, A.B., Tacker, W.A., & Ewy, G.A. Aortic and right atrial systolic pressures during cardiopulmonary resuscitation: a potential indicator of the mechanism of blood flow. *Am. Heart J.* 1988; **115**: 1021–1029.

24. Kern, K.B., Hilwig, R., & Ewy, G.A. Retrograde coronary blood flow during cardiopulmonary resuscitation in swine: Intracoronary doppler evaluation. *Am. Heart J.* 1994; **128**: 490–499.

25. Sakka, S.G., Wallbridge, D.R., & Heusch, G. Glossary: methods for the measurement of coronary blood flow and myocardial perfusion. *Basic Res. Cardiol.* 1996; **91**: 155–178.

26. Jones, C.J.H., Kuo, L., Davis, M.J., & Chilian, W.M. Regulation of coronary blood flow: coordination of heterogenous control mechanisms in vascular microdomains. *Cardiovasc. Res.* 1995; **29**: 585–596.

27. Marcus, M.L. Autoregulation in the coronary circulation. In *The Coronary Circulation in Health and Disease.* 1st edn, New York: McGraw-Hill, 1983, 93–112.

28. Alexander, R.S. Critical closure reexamined. *Circulation Research* 1977; **40**: 531.

29. Kern, K.B., Lancaster, L., Goldman, S., & Ewy, G.A. The effect of coronary artery lesions on the relationship between coronary perfusion pressure and myocardial flow during cardiopulmonary resuscitation in pigs. *Am. Heart J.* 1990; **120**: 324–333.

30. Taylor, R.B., Brown, C.G., Bridges, T., Werman, H.A., Ashton, J. & Hamlin, R.L. A model for regional blood flow measurements during cardiopulmonary resuscitation in a swine model. *Resuscitation* 1988; **16**: 107–118.

31. DeBehnke, D.J., Spreng, D., Wickman, L.L., & Crowe, D.T. The effects of endothelin-1 on coronary perfusion pressure during cardiopulmonary resuscitation in a canine model. *Acad. Emerg. Med.* 1996; **3**: 137–141.

32. DeBehnke, D. The effects of graded doses of endothelin-1 on coronary perfusion pressure and vital organ blood flow during cardiac arrest. *Acad. Emerg. Med.* 2000; **7**: 211–221.

33. Hilwig, R.W., Berg, R.A., Kern, K.B., & Ewy, G.A. Endothelin-1 vasoconstriction during swine cardiopulmonary resuscitation improves coronary perfusion pressures but worsens postresuscitation outcome. *Circulation* 2000; **101**: 2097–2102.

34. American Heart Association. *Heart and Stroke Statistical. Update.* Dallas, TX: American Heart Association, 2004, www. americanheart.org.

35. Kern, K.B. & Ewy, G.A. Minimal coronary stenoses and left ventricular blood flow during CPR. *Ann. Emerg. Med.* 1992; **21**: 1066–1072.

36. Sharff, J.A., Pantley, G., & Noel, E. Effect of time on regional organ perfusion during two methods of cardiopulmonary resuscitation. *Ann. Emerg. Med.* 1984; **13**: 649–656.

37. Duggal, C., Weil, M.H., Tang, W., Gazmuri, R.J., & Sun, S. Effect of arrest time on the hemodynamic efficacy of precordial compression. *Crit. Care Med.* 1995; **23**: 1233–1236.

38. Halperin, H.R., Guerci, A.D., Chandra, N. *et al.* Vest inflation without simultaneous ventilation during cardiac arrest in dogs: improved survival from prolonged cardiopulmonary resuscitation. *Circulation* 1986; **74**: 1407–1415.

39. Sanders, A.B., Kern, K.B., Ewy, G.A., Atlas, M., & Bailey, L. Improved resuscitation from cardiac arrest with open-chest massage. *Ann. Emerg. Med.* 1984; **13**: 672–675.

40. Sanders, A.B., Kern, K.B., Atlas, M., Bragg, S., & Ewy, G.A. Importance of the duration of inadequate coronary perfusion pressure on resuscitation from cardiac arrest. *J. Am. Coll. Cardiol.* 1985; **6**: 113–118.

41. Kern, K.B., Carter, A.B., Showen, R.L. *et al.* Manual versus mechanical cardiopulmonary resuscitation in an experimental canine model. *Crit. Care Med.* 1985; **13**: 899–903.

42. Kern, K.B., Carter, A.B., Showen, R.L. *et al.* Twenty-four hour survival in canine model of cardiac arrest comparing three methods of manual cardiopulmonary resuscitation. *J. Am. Coll. Cardiol.* 1986; **7**: 859–867.

43. Kern, K.B., Carter, A.B., Showen, R.L. *et al.* Comparison of manual techniques of cardiopulmonary resuscitation: survival and neurologic outcome in dogs. *Am. J. Emerg. Med.* 1987; **5**: 190–195.

44. Bircher, N. & Safar, P. Cerebral perfusion during cardiopulmonary resuscitation. *Crit. Care Med.* 1985; **13**: 185–190.

45. Kern, K.B., Ewy, G.A., Voorhees, W.D., Babbs, C.F., & Tacker, W.A. Myocardial perfusion pressure: a predictor of 24-hour survival during prolonged cardiac arrest in dogs. *Resuscitation* 1988; **16**: 241–250.

46. Feneley, M.P., Maier, G.W., Kern, K.B. *et al.* Influence of compression rate on initial success of resuscitation and 24-hour survival after prolonged manual and cardiopulmonary resuscitation in dogs. *Circulation* 1988; **77**: 240–250.

47. Kern, K.B., Sanders, A.B., Badylak, S.F. *et al.* Long term survival with open-chest cardiac massage after ineffective closed-chest compression in a canine model. *Circulation* 1987; **75**: 498–503.

48. Sanders, A.B., Ogle, M., & Ewy, G.A. Coronary perfusion pressure during cardiopulmonary resuscitation. *Am. J. Emerg. Med.* 1985; **3**: 11–14.

49. McDonald, J.L. Effect of interposed abdominal compression during CPR on central arterial and venous pressures. *Am. J. Emerg. Med.* 1985; **3**: 156–159.

50. Martin, G.B., Garden, D.L., Nowak, R.M., Lewinter, J.R., Johnston, W., & Tomlanovich, M.C. Aortic and right atrial pressures during standard and simultaneous compression and ventilation CPR in human beings. *Ann. Emerg. Med.* 1986; **15**: 125–130.

51. Howard, M., Carrubba, C., Foss, F., Janiak, B., Hogan, B., & Guinness, M. Interposed abdominal compressions CPR: its effects on parameters of coronary perfusion in human subjects. *Ann. Emerg. Med.* 1987; **16**: 253–259.

52. Swenson, R.D., Weaver, W.D., Niskanen, R.A., Martin, J., & Dahlberg, S. Hemodynamics in humans during conventional and experimental methods of cardiopulmonary resuscitation. *Circulation* 1988; **78**: 630–639.

53. Lewinter, J.R., Carden, D.L., Nowak, R.M., Enriquez, E., & Martin, G.B. CPR dependent consciousness: evidence for cardiac compression causing forward flow. *Ann. Emerg. Med.* 1989; **18**: 1111–1115.

54. Paradis, N.A., Martin, G.B., Goetting, M.G. *et al.* Simultaneous aortic, jugular bulb, and right atrial pressures during cardiopulmonary resuscitation in humans. *Circulation* 1989; **80**: 361–368.

55. Paradis, N.A., Martin, G.B., Rivers, E.P. *et al.* Coronary perfusion pressure and return of spontaneous circulation in human cardiopulmonary resuscitation. *J. Am. Med. Assoc.* 1990; **263**: 1106–1113.

56. Halperin, H.R., Tsitlik, J.E., Gelfand, M. *et al.* A preliminary study of cardiopulmonary resuscitation by circumferential compression of the chest with use of a pneumatic vest. *N. Engl. J. Med.* 1993; **329**: 762–768.

57. Timerman, S., Cardoso, L.F., Ramires J.A.F., & Halperin, H. Improved hemodynamic performance with a novel chest compression device during treatment of in-hospital cardiac arrest. *Resuscitation* 2004; 273–280.

58. Babbs, C.F., Voorhees, W.D., Fitzgerald, K.R., Holmes, H.R., & Geddes, L.A. Relationship of blood pressure and flow during CPR to chest compression amplitude: evidence for an effective compression threshold. *Ann. Emerg. Med.* 1983; **12**: 527–532.

59. Gallagher, E.J., Lombardi, G., & Gennis, P. Effectiveness of bystander cardiopulmonary resuscitation and survival following out-of-hospital cardiac arrest. *J. Am. Med. Assoc.* 1995; **274**: 1922–1925.

60. Wik, L., Steen, P.A., & Bircher, N.G. Quality of bystander cardiopulmonary resuscitation influences outcome after-prehospital cardiac arrest. *Resuscitation* 1994; **28**: 195–203.

61. Van Hoeyweghen, R.J., Bossaert, L.L., Mullie, A. *et al.* Quality and efficiency of bystander CPR. Belgian Cerebral Resuscitation Study Group. *Resuscitation* 1993; **26**: 47–52.

62. Crone, P.D. Auckland Ambulance Service cardiac arrest data 1991–1993. *N Z Med. J.* 1995; **108**: 297–299.

63. Berg, R.A., Sanders, A.B., Kern, K.B. *et al.* Adverse hemodynamic effects of interrupting chest compressions for rescue breathing during cardiopulmonary resuscitation for ventricular fibrillation cardiac arrest. *Circulation* 2001; **104**: 2465–2470.

64. Kern, K.B., Hilwig, R.W., Berg, R.A., Sanders, A.B., & Ewy, G.A. Importance of continuous chest compressions during cardiopulmonary resuscitation. Improved outcome during stimulated single lay-rescuer scenario. *Circulation* 2002; **105**: 645–649.

65. Yu, T., Weil, M.H., Tang, W. *et al.* Adverse outcomes of interrupted precordial compression during automated defibrillation. *Circulation* 2002; **106**: 368–372.

66. Valenzuela, T.D., Kern, K.B., Clark, L.L. *et al.* Interruptions of chest compressions during emergency medical systems resuscitation. *Circulation* 2005; **112**: 1259–1265.

67. Wik, L., Kramer-Johansen, J., Myklebust, H. *et al.* Quality of cardiopulmonary resuscitation during out-of-hospital cardiac arrest. *J. Am. Med. Assoc.* 2005; **293**: 299–304.

68. Abella, B.S., Alvarado, J.P., Myklebust, H. *et al.* Quality of cardiopulmonary resuscitation during in-hospital cardiac arrest. *J. Am. Med. Assoc.* 2005; **293**: 305–310.

69. Hightower, D., Thomas, S.H., Stone, C.K., Dunn, K., & March, J.A. Decay in quality of closed-chest compressions over time. *Ann. Emerg. Med.* 1995; **26**: 300–303.

70. Ochoa, F.J., Ramalle-Gomara, E., Lisa, V., & Saralegui, I. The effect of rescuer fatigue on the quality of chest compressions. *Resuscitation* 1998; **37**: 149–152.

71. Ashton, A., McClusky, A., Gwinnutt, C.L., & Keenan, A.M. Effect of rescuer fatigue on performance of continuous external chest compressions over 3 min. *Resuscitation* 2002; **55**: 151–155.

72. Baubin, M., Schirmer, M. Nogler, M. *et al.* Rescuer's work capacity and duration of cardiopulmonary resuscitation. *Resuscitation* 1996; **33**: 135–139.

73. Mauer, D., Wolcke, B., & Dick, W. Alternative methods of mechanical cardiopulmonary resuscitation. *Resuscitation* 2000; **44**: 81–85.

74. Babb, C.F. Circulatory adjuncts. Newer methods of cardiopulmonary resuscitation. *Cardiol. Clin.* 2002; **20**: 37–59.

75. Ralston, S.H., Babbs, C.F., & Niebauer, M.J. Cardiopulmonary resuscitation with interposed abdominal compression in dogs. *Anesth. Analg.* 1982; **61**: 645–651.

76. Voorhees, W.D., Niebauer, M.J., & Babbs, C.F. Improved oxygen delivery during cardiopulmonary resuscitation with interposed abdominal compressions. *Ann. Emerg. Med.* 1983; **12**: 128–135.

77. Lindner, K.H., Ahnefeld, F.W., & Bowdler, I.M. Cardiopulmonary resuscitation with interposed abdominal compression after asphyxia or fibrillatory cardiac arrest in pigs. *Anesthesiology* 1990; **72**: 675–681.

78. Berryman, C.R., & Phillips, G.M. Interposed abdominal compression CPR in human subjects. *Ann. Emerg. Med.* 1984; **13**: 226–229.

79. Babbs, C.F. Interposed abdominal compression CPR: a comprehensive evidence based review. *Resuscitation* 2003; **59**: 71–82.

80. Lurie, K. Mechanical devices for cardiopulmonary resuscitation. An update. *Emerg. Med. Clin. N. Am.* 2002; **20**: 771–784.

81. Mauer, D.K., Nolan, J., Plaisance, P. *et al.* Effect of active compression-decompression resuscitation (ACD-CPR) on survival: a combined analysis using individual patient data. *Resuscitation* 1999; **41**: 249–256.

82. Halperin, H.R., Paradis, N., Ornato, J.P. *et al.* Cardiopulmonary resuscitation with a novel chest compression device in a porcine model of cardiac arrest. *J. Am. Coll. Cardiol.* 2004; **44**: 2214–2220.

83. Casner, M., Andersen, D., & Isaacs, M. The impact of a new CPR assist device on rate of return of spontaneous circulation in out-of-hospital cardiac arrest. *Prehosp. Emerg. Care* 2005; **9**: 61–67.

84. Steen, S., Liao, Q., Pierre, L., Paskevicius, A., & Sjoberg, T. Evaluation of LUCAS, a new device for automatic mechanical

compression and active decompression resuscitation. *Resuscitation* 2002; **55**: 285–299.

85. Alzaga-Fernandez, A.G. & Varon, J. Open-chest cardiopulmonary resuscitation: past, present and future. *Resuscitation* 2005; **64**: 149–156.

86. Bircher, N., Safar, P., & Stewart, R. A comparison of standard, "MAST"-augmented and open-chest CPR in dogs. *Crit. Care Med.* 1980; **8**: 147–152.

87. Bircher, N. & Safar, P. Manual open-chest cardiopulmonary resuscitation. *Ann. Emerg. Med.* 1984; **13**: 770–773.

88. Wolcke, B.B., Mauer, D.K., Schoefmann, M.F. *et al.* Comparison of standard cardiopulmonary resuscitation versus the combination of active compression-decompression cardiopulmonary resuscitation and an inspiratory impedance threshold device of out-of-hospital cardiac arrest. *Circulation* 2003; **108**: 2201–2205.

89. Pirrallo, R.G., Aufderheide, T.P., Provo, T.A., & Lurie, K.G. Effect of an inspiratory threshold device on hemodynamics during conventional manual cardiopulmonary resuscitation. *Resuscitation* 2005; **66**: 13–20.

90. Brown, C.G., Werman, H.A., Davis, E.A., Hobson, J., & Hamlin, R.L. The effects of greater doses of epinephrine on regional myocardial blood flow during cardiopulmonary resuscitation in swine. *Circulation* 1987; **75**: 491–497.

91. Lindner, K.H., Ahnefeld, F.W., & Bowdler, I.M. Comparison of different doses of epinephrine on myocardial perfusion and resuscitation success during cardiopulmonary resuscitation in a pig model. *Am. J. Emerg. Med.* 1991; **9**: 27–31.

92. Brown, C.G., Taylor, R.B., Werman, H.A., Luu, T., Ashton, J., & Hamlin, R.L. Myocardial oxygen delivery/consumption during cardiopulmonary resuscitation: a comparison of epinephrine and phenylephrine. *Ann. Emerg. Med.* 1988; **17**: 302–308.

93. Lindner, K.H., Strohmenger, H.U., Prengel, A.W., Ensinger, H., Goertz, A., & Weichel, T. Hemodynamic and metabolic effect of epinephrine during cardiopulmonary resuscitation in a pig model. *Crit. Care Med.* 1992; **20**: 1020–1026.

94. Brown, C.G., Werman, H.A., Davis, E.A., Katz, S., & Hamlin, R.L. The effect of high dose phenylephrine versus epinephrine on regional cerebral blood flow during CPR. *Ann. Emerg. Med.* 1987; **16**: 743–748.

95. Lindner, K.H., Ahnefeld, F.W., & Bowdler, I.M. Comparison of epinephrine and dobutamine during cardiopulmonary resuscitation. *Intens. Care Med.* 1989; **15**: 432–438.

96. Lindner, K.H., Ahnefeld, F.W., Schuermann, W., & Bowdler, I.M. Epinephrine and norepinephrine in cardiopulmonary resuscitation. *Chest* 1990; **97**: 1458–1462.

97. Ditchey, R.V. & Lindenfeld, J. Failure of epinephrine to improve the balance between myocardial oxygen supply and demand during closed-chest resuscitation in dogs. *Circulation* 1988; **78**: 382–389.

98. Chase, P.B., Kern, K.B., Sanders, A.B., Otto, C.W., & Ewy, G.A. Effects of greater doses of epinephrine on both non-invasive and invasive measures of myocardial perfusion in blood flow during cardiopulmonary resuscitation. *Crit. Care Med.* 1993; **21**: 413–419.

99. Gonzalez, E.R., Ornato, J.P., Garnett, A.R., Levine, R.L., Young, D.S. & Racht, E.M. Dose-dependent vasopressors responses to epinephrine in human beings. *Ann. Emerg. Med.* 1989; **18**: 920–926.

100. Paradis, N.A., Martin, G.B., Rosenberg, J. *et al.* The effect of standard and high dose epinephrine on coronary perfusion pressure during prolonged cardiopulmonary resuscitation. *J. Am. Med. Assoc.* 1991; **265**: 1139–1144.

101. Vandycke, C. & Martens, P. High dose versus standard dose epinephrine in cardiac arrest-a meta-analysis. *Resuscitation* 2000; **45**: 161–166.

102. Perondi, M.B.M., Reis, A.G., Paiva, E.F., Nadkarni, V.M., & Berg, R.A. A comparison of high-dose and standard-dose epinephrine in children with cardiac arrest. *N. Engl. J. Med.* 2004; **350**: 1722–1730.

103. Rivers, E.P., Wortsman, J., Rady, M.Y., Blake, H.C., McGeorge, F.T. & Buderer, N.M. The effect of the total cumulative epinephrine dose administered during human CPR on hemodynamic, oxygen transport, and utilization variables in the postresuscitation period. *Chest* 1994; **106**: 1499–1507.

104. Behringer, W., Kittler, H., Sterz, F. *et al.* Cumulative epinephrine dose during cardiopulmonary resuscitation and neurologic outcome. *Ann. Intern. Med.* 1998; **129**: 450–456.

105. Brown, C.G., Katz, S.E., Werman, H.A., Luu, T., Davis, E.A., & Hamlin, R.L. The effect of epinephrine versus methoxamine on regional myocardial blood flow and defibrillation rates following a prolonged cardiorespiratory arrest in a swine model. *Am. J. Emerg. Med.* 1987; **5**: 362–369.

106. Roberts, D., Landolfo, K., Dobson, K., & Light, R.B. The effects of methoxamine and epinephrine on survival and regional distribution of cardiac output in dogs with prolonged ventricular fibrillation. *Chest* 1990; **98**: 999–1005.

107. Sanders, A.B., Atlas, M., Ewy, G.A., Kern, K.B., & Bragg, S. Expired PCO_2 as an index of coronary perfusion pressure. *Am. J. Emerg. Med.* 1985; **3**: 147–149.

108. Sanders, A.B., Ewy, G.A., Bragg, S., Atlas, M., & Kern, K.B. Expired PCO_2 as a prognostic indicator of successful resuscitation from cardiac arrest. *Ann. Emerg. Med.* 1985; **14**: 948–952.

109. Kern, K.B., Sanders, A.B., Voorhees, W.D., Babbs, C.F., Tacker, W.A. & Ewy, G.A. Changes in expired end-tidal carbon dioxide during cardiopulmonary resuscitation in dogs: a prognostic guide for resuscitation efforts. *J. Am. Coll. Cardiol.* 1989; **13**: 1184–1189.

110. Von Planta, M., Von Planta, I., Weil, M.H., Bruno, S., Bisera, J., & Rackow, E.C. End-tidal carbon dioxide as a hemodynamic determinate of cardiopulmonary resuscitation in the rat. *Cardiovasc. Res.* 1989; **23**: 364–368.

111. Garnett, A.R., Ornato, J.P., Gonzalez, E.R., & Johnson, E.D. End-tidal carbon dioxide monitoring during cardiopulmonary resuscitation. *J. Am. Med. Assoc.* 1987; **257**: 512–515.

112. Falk, J.L., Rackow, E.G., & Weil, M.H. End-tidal carbon dioxide concentration during cardiopulmonary resuscitation. *N. Engl. J. Med.* 1988; **318**: 607–611.

113. Sanders, A.B., Kern, K.B., Otto, C.W., Milander, M.M., & Ewy, G.A. End-tidal carbon dioxide monitoring during cardiopulmonary resuscitation. *J. Am. Med. Assoc.* 1989; **262**: 1347–1351.

114. Callaham, M. & Barton, C. Prediction of outcome of cardiopulmonary resuscitation from end-tidal carbon dioxide concentration. *Crit. Care Med.* 1990; **18**: 358–362.

115. Martin, G.B., Gentile, N.T., Paradis, N.A., Moeggenberg, J., Appleton, T.J., & Nowak, R.M. Effective epinephrine on end-tidal carbon dioxide monitoring during CPR. *Ann. Emerg. Med.* 1990; **19**: 396–398.

116. Tang, W., Weil, M.H., Gazmuri, R.J., Sun, S., Duggal, C., & Bisera, J. Pulmonary ventilation/perfusion defects induced by epinephrine during cardiopulmonary resuscitation. *Circulation* 1991; **84**: 2101–2107.

117. Callaham, M., Barton, C. & Matthay, M. Effect of epinephrine on the ability of end-tidal carbon dioxide readings to predict initial resuscitation from cardiac arrest. *Crit. Care Med.* 1992; **20**: 337–343.

118. Hayes, M.M., Berg, R.A. & Otto, C.W. Monitoring during cardiac arrest: are we there yet? *Curr. Opin. Crit. Care* 2003; **9**: 211–217.

19

Methods to improve cerebral blood flow and neurological outcome after cardiac arrest

Uwe Ebmeyer[1], Laurence M. Katz[2], and Alan D. Guerci[3]

[1] Klinik fur Anaesthesiologie und Intensivtherapie, Otto-von-Guericke University, Magdeburg, Germany
[2] Department of Emergency Medicine, University of North Carolina School of Medicine, Chapel Hill, NC, USA
[3] Klinik fur Anaesthesiologie und Intensivtherapie, Otto-von-Guericke University, Magdeburg, Germany

Ischemic neurological injury accounts for much of the mortality and most of the morbidity among persons who are initially resuscitated from cardiac arrest.[1,2] This chapter summarizes what is known about the determinants of cerebral blood flow during cardiopulmonary resuscitation (CPR) and the relationship of cerebral blood flow to neurological outcome.

Cerebral perfusion in the intact circulation has been characterized as a classical vascular waterfall. Arterial pressure is the upstream pressure, and cerebrospinal fluid pressure is the downstream pressure. Pressure in the venous sinuses is below the downstream pressure; that is, animal studies demonstrate a significant pressure gradient between the cortical veins and the sagittal sinus.[3–5]

Determinants of cerebral blood flow

Halperin *et al.* reported a close correlation ($r = 0.89$) between cerebral blood flow and the difference between carotid arterial pressure and pressure in the lateral ventricle during CPR in dogs.[6] Accordingly, the determinants of carotid arterial pressure and intracranial cerebrospinal fluid pressure will be reviewed.

At the outset of CPR in laboratory animals, carotid artery pressure is usually equal to thoracic aortic pressure. As time goes by, however, carotid arterial pressure tends to fall, and cerebral blood flow declines in parallel.[7] This phenomenon, termed carotid collapse, appears to be mediated by loss of vascular tone and physical collapse of the carotid artery at the thoracic inlet.[7,8] α-Adrenergic agents and pressor doses of adrenalin reverse carotid collapse, in part by increasing the rigidity of the carotid artery and in part by raising peripheral resistance, thus limiting the runoff of blood to non-essential vascular beds.[7] In animal studies, if CPR is begun immediately after the onset of cardiac arrest, carotid pressure remains as high as thoracic aortic pressure over periods of 1 hour or more as long as peripheral resistance is maximized.

Under conditions of intense α-adrenergic stimulation, carotid arterial pressure appears to be maximized by the same maneuvers that maximize thoracic aortic pressure. For the most part, this means applying the maximal amount of compression force that the sternum can withstand. Maintenance of compression for 40% to 60% of each compression-release cycle is important in dogs and probably in humans.[9] Binding the abdomen also increases thoracic aortic and carotid artery pressure, but, for the reasons cited below, abdominal binding may not maximize cerebral perfusion.

Intracranial cerebrospinal fluid pressure, the downstream pressure for cerebral blood flow, fluctuates synchronously with intrathoracic pressure during CPR. About one-third of the fluctuation in intrathoracic pressure is transmitted to the intracranial space in dogs with normal intracranial pressure. This pressure transmission takes place via non-valved veins (e.g., the paravertebral venous plexus) and cerebrospinal fluid. Evidence supporting this statement is summarized in the following paragraphs.

Intracranial pressure during CPR is unrelated to either carotid arterial or jugular venous pressure, as evidenced by the facts that balloon occlusion of the proximal aorta, which abolishes carotid flow and pressure, and interruption of the jugular venous valve at the thoracic inlet, which raises jugular pressure to the same level as intrathoracic pressure, have no effect on intracranial pressure changes

Cardiac Arrest: The Science and Practice of Resuscitation Medicine. 2nd edn., ed. Norman Paradis, Henry Halperin, Karl Kern, Volker Wenzel, Douglas Chamberlain. Published by Cambridge University Press. © Cambridge University Press, 2007.

during chest compression.[10] This lack of effect of jugular pressure on intracranial pressure is explained by more cephalad valves in the jugular system.

Ligation of the cervical spinal cord reduces fluctuations in intracranial pressure by about one-third. The remaining pressure transmission occurs along vascular channels, as indicated by exsanguination of dogs during CPR, a maneuver that abolishes changes in intracranial pressure. Ligation of the paraspinal veins substantially reduces the intracranial pressure changes, indicating that the paravertebral venous plexus and perhaps other non-valved veins in the posterior cerebral circulation are responsible for the bulk of transmission of intrathoracic pressure to the intracranial space.[10]

Intracranial capacitance

The magnitude of transmission of intracranial pressure to the intracranial space is increased under conditions of elevated intrathoracic pressure and by abdominal binding.[10] These observations are explained by the abrupt limits of intracranial capacitance. The translocation of any given amount of venous blood and cerebrospinal fluid from the thorax to the intracranial space will produce larger pressure fluctuations in a closed space that is already on the lower compliance part of its volume pressure curve (elevated intracranial pressure). Alternatively, maneuvers such as abdominal binding, which simultaneously increases intrathoracic pressure during chest compression and impedes the flow of blood and cerebrospinal fluid from the thorax into the abdomen, result in the translocation of more fluid into the intracranial space.

Relationship of cerebral perfusion pressure and blood flow to cerebral metabolism and neurologic outcome

In pentobarbital-treated dogs in which CPR is initiated immediately on induction of ventricular fibrillation, cerebral blood flow of approximately 30 ml/min per 100 g is sufficient to maintain cerebral oxygen consumption and adenosine triphosphate (ATP) at prearrest levels for almost 1 hour.[11] This level of cerebral perfusion can be achieved with a cerebral perfusion pressure of about 30 mmHg.[6,11] Under conditions of normal intracranial pressure, and in the absence of abdominal binding, this level of cerebral perfusion pressure occurs when mean aortic pressure is 55 to 60 mm Hg. Animals so treated wake up and appear normal after as much as 60 minutes of CPR. Despite

maintenance of constant cerebral perfusion pressure, cerebral blood flow may deteriorate over time when the initiation of CPR is delayed.[11] This phenomenon is thought to be mediated by a multitude of factors, including increased blood viscosity, intravascular coagulation, constriction of blood vessels, vascular/perivascular edema.[12]

Clinical implications

Abundant evidence exists that the human brain cannot tolerate more than 4 or 5 minutes of complete cessation of blood flow,[2] and there is some research in humans suggesting that CPR can generate cerebral perfusion pressures greater than 25 mmHg and potential normal oxygen tension if CPR is started immediately after cardiac arrest.[13] If CPR is delayed for even a few minutes after cardiac arrest, however, it is unlikely that standard CPR can generate sufficient cerebral blood flow to preserve normal cerebral viability until cardiac function is restored.[11] This observation may explain in part why cardiac arrest has such high neurological morbidity and mortality. Therefore, new methods are needed to improve cerebral blood flow and subsequent neurological outcome from cardiac arrest. Methods to improve cerebral blood flow and neurological outcome from cardiopulmonary resuscitation have included the following:
(1) medications (vasopressin and epinephrine, HBOC)
(2) CPR techniques and devices
    open chest CPR
    minimally invasive CPR
    AutoPulse Vest CPR
    active compression–decompression CPR
    intermittent threshold valve (ITV)
    intraaortic balloon
    cardiopulmonary bypass (CPB)
(3) hypothermia
(4) combination therapy
Vasopressin is a peptide of neuronal origin produced in the hypothalamus.[14] Vasopressin was recognized to have a role in cardiac arrest as early as the 1960s, but research into its use for treatment of cardiac arrest did not begin until the 1990s. The discovery that higher levels of this peptide were present in patients resuscitated from cardiac arrest motivated investigators to develop vasopressin as a therapy for cardiac arrest.[15] Laboratory studies have shown that vasopressin given during cardiac arrest increases cerebral blood flow via cerebral vasodilatation and by increasing central aortic and carotid systolic pressure, while producing return of spontaneous circulation similar to that of adrenalin.[16] In addition, when vasopressin was added to adrenalin therapy during cardiac arrest in laboratory animals, neurological

outcome improved. The result of vasopressin in clinical trials is less clear. A preliminary human study comparing epinephrine to vasopressin for the treatment of cardiac arrest showed an improved survival rate in the vasopressin group, but there was no difference in neurological outcome in survivors of either group.[17] A larger clinical trial showed no difference between epinephrine and vasopressin on survival or neurological outcome in cardiac arrest patients unless the cardiac arrest was prolonged. A subgroup analysis of these patients suggested that those patients with asystole may have improved survival if epinephrine was followed by vasopressin for resuscitation.[18] Nonetheless, a review of all clinical trials comparing vasopressin to epinephrine does not show a clear advantage of vasopressin over epinephrine in improving survival or neurological outcome from cardiac arrest.[19] Regardless, the International Liaison Committee on Resuscitation (ILCOR) and the American Heart Association's (AHA) 2001 guidelines state that "vasopressin can be used once as an alternative to epinephrine for the treatment of shock-refractory ventricular fibrillation."[20]

Hemoglobin-based oxygen-carrying (HBOC) agents have been extensively studied for use in the treatment of hemorrhagic shock.[21] In addition to their ability to deliver oxygen to tissues, HBOCs have significant vasopressor effects.[22] These properties of HBOC agents may explain why its intravenous administration during CPR in laboratory animals improved cerebral perfusion pressure and oxygen delivery to tissues when compared with normal saline.[23] HBOC agents also improve resuscitation rates in laboratory animals, but no studies on neurological outcome were performed. There are also no studies of use of HBOC agents in humans during cardiac arrest.

Experiments in laboratory animals have shown that open chest CPR is superior to closed chest CPR in generating blood flow to the brain during cardiac arrest and increasing resuscitation rates[24]. The neurological outcome is also significantly improved with open chest CPR.[25,26] These results were so impressive that open chest CPR was recommended for use in humans after failure of standard closed chest CPR.[27] However, the simplicity of closed chest CPR and the social, fear of infection, and financial and legal concerns about open chest cardiac massage have limited its use since the arrival of closed chest CPR in the 1960s.[28] Minimally invasive direct cardiac massage (MIDCM) was developed as an alternative to thoracotomy for performing direct cardiac massage during CPR and does increase resuscitation rates and blood flow to vital organs compared with closed chest CPR.[29] No clinical trials are currently available, however, to evaluate the efficacy of this method of resuscitation.

A multitude of mechanical methods have been developed to improve upon standard closed chest CPR. The methods have been developed to increase cerebral blood flow during cardiac arrest and improve resuscitation rates in the hope that these characteristics of the modified CPR will improve neurological outcome and survival as outlined above. A review of these devices was conducted by Smith in 2002.[30] A few of some of these methods with respect to cerebral blood flow and human application are provided below.

AutoPulse (Revivant, California) CPR is performed with a band that wraps around and compresses the chest with an automated device.[31] The device increased cerebral blood flow during cardiac arrest in swine when the resuscitation was initiated 1 minute after the onset of ventricular fibrillation.[31] The device has been applied to a group of terminally ill patients and hemodynamic monitoring demonstrated that the coronary perfusion pressure was increased from 15 mmHg (standard CPR) to 20 mmHg (AutoPulse). Several before and after cohort studies have reported improved short-term outcome; however, the ASPIRE trial (a randomized, prospective trial) reported no difference in 4-hour survival and a decrease in survival to hospital discharge rate with AutoPulse.

Active compression-decompression (ACD) CPR was discovered when a layperson used a plumber's plunger to resuscitate a family member.[32] ACD CPR is unique in that a suction device, instead of passive recoil of the chest during standard CPR, is used to re-expand the chest after a chest compression. ACD CPR in pigs increases cerebral blood flow and coronary blood flow when compared to standard CPR if the resuscitation is started 30 seconds after the onset of ventricular fibrillation.[33] An impedance threshold device (ITD) is a one-way valve that creates a negative pressure in the thorax during chest decompression and increases venous return to the heart and cerebral blood flow by 20% compared to standard CPR during cardiac arrest in pigs.[34] In a 3-year study that analyzed 210 victims of out of hospital cardiac arrest, ACD CPR in combination with the intermittent threshold device (ITD) significantly improved 24-hour survival.[35] In a subgroup analysis of patients with a greater than 10-minute delay in initiation of resuscitation by EMS, the 24-hour survival of the ACD with ITD group (44%) was even greater when compared with the standard CPR group (14%). Although the rate of hospital discharge for patients with witnessed arrest was 23% for the ACD with ITD group compared with 15% in the standard CPR group (15%), it did not reach statistical significance.[35] The percentage of patients with normal neurological outcome was higher in the ACD with ITD group (15%) compared with standard CPR (5%), but also did not reach statistical significance. To appreciate the potential benefit of ITD with ACD CPR, when 400 patients with prehospital cardiac arrest all had ACD performed and ITD was used only in the treatment group, the ITD group had a 40% 24-hour survival versus 29% in controls ($P<0.03$).[36] Six out of ten survivors in the ACD plus ITD group had normal neurological outcome, while one of eight survivors in the ACD non-ITD group had good neurological outcome, but again the results did not reach statistical significance ($P<0.10$).

Transfemoral balloon-catheter aortic occlusion during cardiac arrest in a canine model of open chest CPR increased coronary and cerebral perfusion pressure 100% when compared with controls.[37] In contrast, transfemoral catheter balloon occlusion of the aorta alone during CPR in a canine model of closed chest CPR did not improve coronary perfusion pressures or resuscitation rates when resuscitation efforts and balloon inflation were initiated 20 minutes after the onset of ventricular fibrillation.[38] In two separate studies, intraaortic balloon catheter occlusion did increase coronary and cerebral perfusion pressure [39] as well as return of spontaneous circulation [40] in a pig model, provided that the balloon and resuscitative efforts were initiated 8 minutes after the onset of ventricular fibrillation. When epinephrine was administered proximal to the occluded aorta via the aortic catheter during CPR, it increased coronary perfusion pressure as shown in earlier studies,[41] but provided no further increase in cerebral blood flow.[42] Administration of vasopressin through an intraaortic catheter proximal to the occluding aortic balloon increased cerebral blood flow more than the aortic occlusion alone during cardiac arrest when CPR was performed.[43] In addition, cerebral blood flow remained elevated during reperfusion even though the balloon was deflated, suggesting that vasopressin was better than the aortic balloon in maintaining elevated cerebral blood flow during reperfusion because of its vasodilatatory properties.[43] The intraaortic balloon catheter has also been used for selective perfusion of the aortic arch during CPR.[38,41] Perfusion with an oxygen-carrying solution increases resuscitation rates and the speed of resuscitation, but its combined effects on cerebral blood flow and neurological outcome are unknown.[44]

Cardiopulmonary bypass (CPB) increases resuscitation rates, cerebral blood flow, survival, and neurological recovery in laboratory experiments of cardiac arrest.[45,46] A feasibility study showed that CPB could be initiated in the emergency department and all cardiac arrest patients had a return of spontaneous circulation.[47] Nevertheless, CPB was not initiated until an average of 30 minutes after the onset of cardiac arrest and there were no long term survivors. A review of multiple human studies of CPB during cardiac arrest suggests that CPB may have a role in the future care of cardiac arrest victims.[48]

Mild hypothermia induced during cardiac arrest is the only therapy shown to improve survival and neurological outcome in victims of out of hospital cardiac arrests.[49–51] In addition to reducing brain injury caused by reperfusion disease, mild hypothermia attenuates the decrease in blood flow that occurs with delays in initiating CPR,[12] although a brief period of hypothermia after resuscitation from cardiac arrest did not alter regional blood flow when compared with normothermic controls.[52]

There currently is no single therapy that dramatically increases resuscitation rates from cardiac arrest and produces consistent normal neurological outcome. Therefore, it is likely that the combination of the above therapies in addition to development of new techniques and drug cocktails will be needed to achieve the breakthrough effect being sought to treat victims of cardiac arrest.

REFERENCES

1. Levy, D.E., Bates, D., Caronna, J.J. *et al.* Prognosis in nontraumatic coma. *Ann. Intern. Med.* 1981; **94**(3): 293–301.
2. Longstreth, W.T., Jr., Inui, T.S., Cobb, L.A. & Copass, M.K. Neurologic recovery after out-of-hospital cardiac arrest. *Ann. Intern. Med.* 1983; **98**(5 Pt 1): 588–592.
3. Luce, J.M., Huseby, J.S., Kirk, W. & Butler, J. A. Starling resistor regulates cerebral venous outflow in dogs. *J. Appl. Physiol.* 1982; **53**(6): 1496–1503.
4. Nakagawa, Y., Tsuru, M. & Yada, K. Site and mechanism for compression of the venous system during experimental intracranial hypertension. *J. Neurosurg.* 1974; **41**(4): 427–434.
5. Shulman, K. Small artery and vein pressures in the subarachnoid space of the dog. *J. Surg. Res.* 1965; **45**: 56–61.
6. Halperin, H.R., Tsitlik, J.E., Guerci, A.D. *et al.* Determinants of blood flow to vital organs during cardiopulmonary resuscitation in dogs. *Circulation* 1986; **73**(3): 539–550.
7. Michael, J.R., Guerci, A.D., Koehler, R.C. *et al.* Mechanisms by which epinephrine augments cerebral and myocardial perfusion during cardiopulmonary resuscitation in dogs. *Circulation* 1984; **69**(4): 822–835.
8. Yin, F.C., Cohen, J.M., Tsitlik, J., Zola, B. & Weisfeldt, M.L. Role of carotid artery resistance to collapse during high-intrathoracic-pressure CPR. *Am. J. Physiol.* 1982; **243**(2): H259–H267.
9. Taylor, G.J., Tucker, W.M., Greene, H.L., Rudikoff, M.T. & Weisfeldt, M.L. Importance of prolonged compression during cardiopulmonary resuscitation in man. *N. Engl. J. Med.* 1977; **296**(26): 1515–1517.
10. Guerci, A.D., Shi, A.Y., Levin, H., Tsitlik, J., Weisfeldt, M.L. & Chandra, N. Transmission of intrathoracic pressure to the

intracranial space during cardiopulmonary resuscitation in dogs. *Circ. Res.* 1985; **56**(1): 20–30.

11. Eleff, S.M., Kim, H., Shaffner, D.H., Traystman, R.J. & Koehler, R.C. Effect of cerebral blood flow generated during cardiopulmonary resuscitation in dogs on maintenance versus recovery of ATP and pH. *Stroke* 1993; **24**(12): 2066–2073.

12. Shaffner, D.H., Eleff, S.M., Koehler, R.C. & Traystman, R.J. Effect of the no-flow interval and hypothermia on cerebral blood flow and metabolism during cardiopulmonary resuscitation in dogs. *Stroke* 1998; **29**(12): 2607–2615.

13. Imberti, R., Bellinzona, G., Riccardi, F., Pagani, M. & Langer, M. Cerebral perfusion pressure and cerebral tissue oxygen tension in a patient during cardiopulmonary resuscitation. *Intens. Care Med.* 2003; **29**(6): 1016–1019.

14. Gainer, H., Loh, Y.P. & Russell, J.T. Biosynthesis of neuronal peptides: implications for neurobiology. *Prog. Biochem. Pharmacol.* 1980; **16**: 60–68.

15. Lindner, K.H., Strohmenger, H.U., Ensinger, H., Hetzel, W.D., Ahnefeld, F.W. & Georgieff, M. Stress hormone response during and after cardiopulmonary resuscitation. *Anesthesiology* 1992; **77**(4): 662–668.

16. Lindner, K.H., Prengel, A.W., Pfenninger, E.G. *et al.* Vasopressin improves vital organ blood flow during closed-chest cardiopulmonary resuscitation in pigs. *Circulation* 1995; **91**(1): 215–221.

17. Lindner, K.H., Dirks, B., Strohmenger, H.U., Prengel, A.W., Lindner, I.M. & Lurie, K.G. Randomised comparison of epinephrine and vasopressin in patients with out-of-hospital ventricular fibrillation. *Lancet* 1997; **349**(9051): 535–537.

18. Wenzel, V., Krismer, A.C., Arntz, H.R., Sitter, H., Stadlbauer, K.H. & Lindner, K.H. A comparison of vasopressin and epinephrine for out-of-hospital cardiopulmonary resuscitation. *N. Engl. J. Med.* 2004; **350**(2): 105–113.

19. Aung, K. & Htay, T. Vasopressin for cardiac arrest: a systematic review and meta-analysis. *Arch. Intern. Med.* 2005; **165**(1): 17–24.

20. Kern, K.B., Halperin, H.R., & Field, J. New guidelines for cardiopulmonary resuscitation and emergency cardiac care: changes in the management of cardiac arrest. *J. Am. Med. Assoc.* 2001; **285**(10): 1267–1269.

21. Arnoldo, B.D. & Minei, J.P. Potential of hemoglobin-based oxygen carriers in trauma patients. *Curr. Opin. Crit. Care* 2001; **7**(6): 431–436.

22. Reah, G., Bodenham, A.R., Mallick, A., Daily, E.K. & Przybelski, R.J. Initial evaluation of diaspirin cross-linked hemoglobin (DCLHb) as a vasopressor in critically ill patients. *Crit. Care Med.* 1997; **25**(9): 1480–1488.

23. Chow, M.S., Fan, C., Tran, H., Zhao, H. & Zhou, L. Effects of diaspirin cross-linked hemoglobin (DCLHb) during and post-CPR in swine. *J. Pharmacol. Exp. Ther.* 2001; **297**(1): 224–229.

24. Bircher, N. & Safar, P. Comparison of standard and "new" closed-chest CPR and open-chest CPR in dogs. *Crit. Care Med.* 1981; **9**(5): 384–385.

25. Bircher, N. & Safar, P. Cerebral preservation during cardiopulmonary resuscitation. *Crit. Care Med.* 1985; **13**(3): 185–190.

26. Kern, K.B., Sanders, A.B., Badylak, S.F. *et al.* Long-term survival with open-chest cardiac massage after ineffective closed-chest compression in a canine preparation. *Circulation* 1987; **75**(2): 498–503.

27. Del Guercio, L.R.M. Open chest cardiac massage: an overview. *Resuscitation* 1987; **15**: 9–11.

28. Kouwenhoven, W.B., Jude, J.R. & Knickerbocker, G.G. Closed-chest cardiac massage. *J. Am. Med. Assoc.* 1960; **173**: 1064–1067.

29. Paiva, E.F., Kern, K.B., Hilwig, R.W., Scalabrini, A. & Ewy, G.A. Minimally invasive direct cardiac massage versus closed-chest cardiopulmonary resuscitation in a porcine model of prolonged ventricular fibrillation cardiac arrest. *Resuscitation* 2000; **47**(3): 287–299.

30. Smith T. Alternative cardiopulmonary resuscitation devices. *Curr. Opin. Crit. Care* 2002; **8**(3): 219–223.

31. Halperin, H.R., Paradis, N., Ornato, J.P. *et al.* Cardiopulmonary resuscitation with a novel chest compression device in a porcine model of cardiac arrest: improved hemodynamics and mechanisms. *J. Am. Coll. Cardiol.* 2004; **44**(11): 2214–2220.

32. Lurie, K.G., Lindo, C. & Chin, J. CPR: the P stands for plumber's helper. *J. Am. Med. Assoc.* 1990; **264**(13): 1661.

33. Lindner, K.H., Pfenninger, E.G., Lurie, K.G., Schurmann, W., Lindner, I.M. & Ahnefeld, F.W. Effects of active compression-decompression resuscitation on myocardial and cerebral blood flow in pigs. *Circulation* 1993; **88**(3): 1254–1263.

34. Lurie, K.G., Mulligan, K.A., McKnite, S., Detloff, B., Lindstrom, P. & Lindner, K.H. Optimizing standard cardiopulmonary resuscitation with an inspiratory impedance threshold valve. *Chest* 1998; **113**(4): 1084–1090.

35. Wolcke, B.B., Mauer, D.K., Schoefmann, M.F. *et al.* Comparison of standard cardiopulmonary resuscitation versus the combination of active compression-decompression cardiopulmonary resuscitation and an inspiratory impedance threshold device for out-of-hospital cardiac arrest. *Circulation* 2003; **108**(18): 2201–2205.

36. Plaisance, P., Lurie, K.G., Vicaut, E. *et al.* Evaluation of an impedance threshold device in patients receiving active compression-decompression cardiopulmonary resuscitation for out of hospital cardiac arrest. *Resuscitation* 2004; **61**(3): 265–271.

37. Wesley, R.C., Jr. & Morgan, D.B. Effect of continuous intra-aortic balloon inflation in canine open chest cardiopulmonary resuscitation. *Crit. Care Med.* 1990; **18**(6): 630–633.

38. Paradis, N.A., Rose, M.I. & Gawryl, M.S. Selective aortic perfusion and oxygenation: an effective adjunct to external chest compression-based cardiopulmonary resuscitation. *J. Am. Coll. Cardiol.* 1994; **23**(2): 497–504.

39. Sesma, J., Labandeira, J., Sara, M.J., Espila, J.L., Arteche, A. & Saez, M.J. Effect of intra-aortic occlusion balloon in external thoracic compressions during CPR in pigs. *Am. J. Emerg. Med.* 2002; **20**(5): 453–462.

40. Gedeborg, R., Rubertsson, S. & Wiklund, L. Improved haemodynamics and restoration of spontaneous circulation with constant aortic occlusion during experimental cardiopulmonary resuscitation. *Resuscitation* 1999; **40**(3): 171–180.

41. Manning, J.E., Murphy, C.A., Jr., Hertz, C.M., Perretta, S.G., Mueller, R.A. & Norfleet, E.A. Selective aortic arch perfusion during cardiac arrest: a new resuscitation technique. *Ann. Emerg. Med.* 1992; **21**(9): 1058–1065.

42. Nozari, A., Rubertsson, S. & Wiklund, L. Intra-aortic administration of epinephrine above an aortic balloon occlusion during experimental CPR does not further improve cerebral blood flow and oxygenation. *Resuscitation* 2000; **44**(2): 119–127.

43. Nozari, A., Rubertsson, S. & Wiklund, L. Improved cerebral blood supply and oxygenation by aortic balloon occlusion combined with intra-aortic vasopressin administration during experimental cardiopulmonary resuscitation. *Acta. Anaesthesiol. Scand.* 2000; **44**(10): 1209–1219.

44. Manning, J.E., Batson, D.N., Payne, F.B. *et al.* Selective aortic arch perfusion during cardiac arrest: enhanced resuscitation using oxygenated perflubron emulsion, with and without aortic arch epinephrine. *Ann. Emerg. Med.* 1997; **29**(5): 580–587.

45. Safar, P., Abramson, N.S., Angelos, M. *et al.* Emergency cardiopulmonary bypass for resuscitation from prolonged cardiac arrest. *Am. J. Emerg. Med.* 1990; **8**(1): 55–67.

46. Sterz, F., Leonov, Y., Safar, P. *et al.* Multifocal cerebral blood flow by Xe-CT and global cerebral metabolism after prolonged cardiac arrest in dogs. Reperfusion with open-chest CPR or cardiopulmonary bypass. *Resuscitation* 1992; **24**(1): 27–47.

47. Martin, G.B., Rivers, E.P., Paradis, N.A., Goetting, M.G., Morris, D.C. & Nowak, R.M. Emergency department cardiopulmonary bypass in the treatment of human cardiac arrest. *Chest* 1998; **113**(3): 743–751.

48. Dunning, J. & Levine, A. Best evidence topic report. Cardiopulmonary bypass and the survival of patients in cardiac arrest. *Emerg. Med. J.* 2004; **21**(4): 499–501.

49. Mild therapeutic hypothermia to improve the neurologic outcome after cardiac arrest. *N. Engl. J. Med.* 2002; **346**(8): 549–556.

50. Bernard, S.A., Gray, T.W., Buist, M.D. *et al.* Treatment of comatose survivors of out-of-hospital cardiac arrest with induced hypothermia. *N. Engl. J. Med.* 2002; **346**(8): 557–563.

51. Holzer, M., Bernard, S.A., Hachimi-Idrissi, S., Roine, R.O., Sterz, F. & Mullner, M. Hypothermia for neuroprotection after cardiac arrest: systematic review and individual patient data meta-analysis. *Crit. Care Med.* 2005; **33**(2): 414–418.

52. Oku, K., Sterz, F., Safar, P. *et al.* Mild hypothermia after cardiac arrest in dogs does not affect postarrest multifocal cerebral hypoperfusion. *Stroke* 1993; **24**(10): 1590–1597.

20

Pharmacology of cardiac arrest and reperfusion

Tommaso Pellis, Jasmeet Soar, Gavin Perkins, and Raùl J. Gazmuri

The University Laboratory of Physiology, Oxford, UK,
Clinical and Medical Affairs, Biosite Incorporated, San Diego, CA, USA

Introduction

The pharmacology of resuscitation is largely based on anecdotal evidence and descriptive research rather than on objective scientific experimentation. Our understanding of the pharmacokinetics (PK) and pharmacodynamics (PD) of drugs used to resuscitate victims of cardiac arrest is also limited by ethical and experimental constraints.

Animal models of cardiac arrest and cardiopulmonary resuscitation (CPR), jointly with clinical studies, have considerably increased our understanding of the pathophysiology of cardiac arrest and significantly improved our ability to resuscitate victims of cardiac arrest.[1–7] The great majority of such studies, however, were designed to address interventions to improve resuscitation rather than to investigate the pharmacological profile of drugs used in settings of cardiac arrest and reperfusion.[8–10] Even less evidence is available on the PK of administration of multiple drugs, a more complex but realistic scenario. During resuscitative efforts, i.e., low flow reperfusion, significant shunting of blood to vital organs occurs.[11–13] The use of vasopressors in this setting further modifies the patterns of blood flow distribution, in all likelihood affecting the PK of concomitantly administered drugs.[11,14–18]

The time from onset of cardiopulmonary arrest until restoration of an effective spontaneous circulation is the single most important determinant of long-term survival and neurological outcome. Prompt initiation of CPR and defibrillation of ventricular fibrillation (VF) or pulseless ventricular tachycardia (VT) are more likely to alter patient outcome than is pharmacologic management.[19,20] Nevertheless, treatment with pharmacologic agents is frequently required in patients with VF or VT that is refractory to electrical shocks and in patients with asystole or pulseless electrical activity (PEA).[21,22]

The use of pharmacological agents during CPR has been associated with a poor clinical outcome, despite initial restoration of spontaneous circulation, ultimately leading to skepticism on the effectiveness of drug therapy during CPR.[8,19,20,23] Several factors may hamper the effectiveness of pharmacological interventions during CPR. Pharmacological agents are used during resuscitation efforts with scant, if any, knowledge of the patient history, underlying medical conditions, or current medical therapy. As for other interventions in settings of cardiac arrest, time appears to be a critical factor.[23] Therapeutic agents may well be administered too late or under suboptimal conditions throughout resuscitation efforts to have a significant impact on survival, with average delays in clinical trials as long as 20–25 minutes.[21,24] In settings of VF/VT, current guidelines advocate the use of vasopressors and antiarrhythmic agents only when such rhythms are recurrent or refractory to multiple shocks, thereby resulting in a considerable delay.[25,26] Airway management and vascular access may further delay drug administration and ultimately compromise delivery to end organ targets because of the poor blood flow generated during prolonged closed chest compression.[3,27,28] Moreover, the time interval that precedes the initiation of resuscitation efforts may be extremely variable or not known with precision. With the progression of ischemia, factors such as acidosis, hypoxemia, downregulation of receptors, target end organ damage, and impaired metabolism and excretion may all interfere with the PD properties of pharmacologic agents, thereby hindering drug effectiveness.[29] Despite our progress in understanding the derangements that follow

Cardiac Arrest: The Science and Practice of Resuscitation Medicine. 2nd edn., ed. Norman Paradis, Henry Halperin, Karl Kern, Volker Wenzel, Douglas Chamberlain. Published by Cambridge University Press. © Cambridge University Press, 2007.

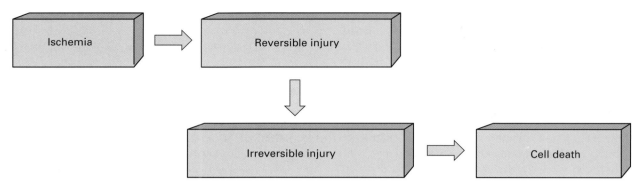

Fig. 20.1. Reversible and irreversible injury: ischemia initiates a sequence of events that, unless interrupted by early reperfusion, leads to cell death. (Modified from ref. 36.)

global myocardial ischemia, little is known about the PK and PD profiles of drugs in this setting.[13,30–35]

The present chapter provides an overview of the pathophysiology of cardiac arrest and reperfusion, reviews basic pharmacological concepts, their (increasingly studied) underlying genetic variability, and the clinical pharmacology pertinent to the drugs used in settings of cardiac arrest and reperfusion.

Pathophysiologic considerations during cardiac arrest and reperfusion

The pathophysiology of cardiac arrest is characterized by the abrupt cessation of forward blood flow. Within seconds, global myocardial ischemia initiates a continuum of progressive intracellular derangements (Fig. 20.1). These changes, which become progressively more severe with time, are initially reversible; eventually, however, with increasing duration of ischemia, irreversible injury occurs.[36] Both the heart and the brain have high metabolic demands despite a relatively small mass, thus tolerating only a very limited period of global ischemia.

This is particularly true during VF/VT when the myocardium consumption of high energy substrate increases dramatically.[37–39] Ischemic contracture soon develops as a manifestation of severe ischemia. It becomes manifest when ATP levels are less than 10% of normal[40] and is characterized by progressive thickening of the left ventricular wall leading to a ventricular cavity size.[3,28] As a result, ventricular preload is compromised, and the amount of blood ejected by chest compression is reduced,[41] partly explaining the characteristic time-dependent decreases in the hemodynamic efficacy of closed-chest resuscitation.[42]

Under normal conditions the brain receives approximately 15% of the body's cardiac output. Consciousness is lost within 15 seconds of cardiac arrest, and brain stem function ceases within 1 minute. Although neurons have been shown to maintain some electrical activity for up to 60 minutes of complete ischemia, the maintenance of adequate cerebral perfusion during CPR is essential for survival.[43–45] Brain adenosine triphosphate (ATP) is depleted after 4–6 minutes of no-flow and it returns nearly to normal within 6 minutes of starting CPR. Animal models suggest that good neurologic outcome may be possible for 10- to 15 minute periods of normothermic cardiac arrest, pending on prompt restoration of cerebral perfusion by artificial means.[46]

Intracellular metabolic derangements

Reductions in oxygen delivery and metabolic waste removal during cardiac arrest alter cellular function and homeostasis. Myocytes have three pathways of energy production: glycolysis, glucose oxidation, and fatty acid oxidation. In contrast, neurons are unable to metabolize fatty acids. Reduced oxygen delivery requires both neurons and myocytes to switch to the only anaerobic metabolism: glycolysis. Out of 1 molecule of glucose, this inefficient anaerobic process generates 2 molecules of ATP and lactate, as compared to the 38 molecules of ATP produced via the aerobic pathway. Glycolysis, which normally accounts of 1– 5% of energy production, under anaerobic conditions becomes the most important source of energy production at the expense of glucose and of free fatty acid oxidation.[47] The result is not only an increased production of lactate – responsible for intracellular acidosis – but also of free fatty acids, which are potent cytotoxic agents.[48]

The shift of global ischemic injury from reversibility to irreversibility is related to a critical decrease in concentrations of high-energy phosphate compounds and/or in free energy change of ATP hydrolysis.[49, 50] The decrease in high-energy phosphate levels inhibits the Na^+ pump, which results in Ca^{2+} overload. At this stage, reperfusion does not result in recovery, but instead it may actually aggravate the situation by activating positive feedback mechanisms.

Restoration of spontaneous circulation

The aim of CPR is to promote a low-flow state sufficient to maintain both brain and heart viablility. Hence, CPR therapy is directed at sustaining vital organ function until natural cardiac function is restored.

Available data suggest that a myocardial blood flow of at least 16 ml min^{-1} per 100 g, and a cerebral blood flow of at least 10 ml min^{-1} per 100 g, are required to meet these metabolic demands during VF.[51–57] Myocardial and cerebral blood flow in animal models of cardiac arrest, and coronary perfusion pressure (CPP) in humans, are usually below these minimal levels during standard external CPR, especially after prolonged CPR and without the use of vasopressor agents.[53,56,58,59] During cardiac arrest, pulmonary blood flow produced by conventional closed-chest CPR is less than 20% of normal, and transalveolar drug absorption is likely to be minimal.[16–18]

Vasopressor agents administered during CPR increase aortic diastolic pressure, but not right atrium diastolic pressure, hence increasing CPP (i.e., the difference between aortic diastolic pressure and right atrial diastolic pressure).[60] The rationale for administration of vasopressor agents during CPR is to restore threshold levels of CPP and, therefore, myocardial blood flow. Restoration of threshold levels of coronary perfusion is the single overriding determinant of the success of the resuscitation effort, especially when the duration of untreated cardiac arrest exceeds 4 minutes.[11,53,57,61–67]

Reperfusion

Restoration of coronary flow increases the release of oxygen free radicals, cytokines, and other pro-inflammatory mediators that activate both neutrophils and the coronary vascular endothelium. The end result of this cascade reaction is reperfusion injury with endothelial dysfunction, microvascular collapse and blood flow defects, and additional cell necrosis and apoptosis.[68]

Upon reperfusion, cells often swell owing to increased osmotic pressure generated during ischemia.[69] The resulting increase in extravascular resistance eventually occludes the nutritive vessels. The importance of this phenomenon has been demonstrated by observing improved recovery of electrical and biochemical functions when the osmotic

pressure of the reperfusing solution is increased to levels above normal to avoid cell swelling.[69]

Dangers secondary to reperfusion of ischemic tissue may also result from altered Ca^{2+} homeostasis. During ischemia the concentration of free Ca^{2+} may increase secondary to release of Ca^{2+} from the sarcoplasmic reticulum and mitochondria. Upon reperfusion the pH is rapidly restored, leading to considerable pH gradients. The sarcolemmal Na^+–H^+ exchanger restores intracellular pH after ischemia, leading to further increases in intracellular Na^+ levels. Increased sarcolemmal Na^+ influx with subsequent intracellular Na^+ overload resulting from the inability of the Na^+–K^+ pump to extrude Na^+ during myocardial ischemia has been recognized as an important pathogenic mechanism of cell injury during ischemia and reperfusion.[70–72] Na^+ becomes a "substrate" for reperfusion injury[73] and intensifies processes detrimental to cell function. The principal routes for Na^+ entry are Na^+–H^+ exchanger isoform 1 (NHE-1), the Na^+–HCO_3^- cotransporter, and Na^+ channels. Under conditions of ischemia and reperfusion, however, NHE-1 seems to be the predominant route. Na^+ overload can have detrimental effects on energy metabolism by intensifying ATP use for sodium extrusion by the Na^+–K^+ pump.[74] Sodium-induced sarcolemmal Ca^{2+} entry through the Ca^{2+}–Na^+ exchanger acting in its reverse mode appears to be the main mechanism of cell injury.[75] Experimental evidence suggests that the Ca^{2+}–Na^+ exchanger contributes to ischemia-reperfusion injury in settings of global and local myocardial ischemia. This process results in severe depletion of ATP and the development of ischemic contracture (stone heart).[3,28,40] Studies in a porcine model of cardiac arrest have demonstrated that ischemic contracture develops only after the beginning of closed-chest resuscitation, suggesting that reperfusion may be key to the development of ischemic contracture.[3] In humans, ischemic contracture has been reported during open-chest resuscitation after failure of closed-chest resuscitation as myocardial "firmness" and has been demonstrated to compromise resuscitability.[42] Sodium–hydrogen exchanger isoform 1 inhibition markedly ameliorates the aforementioned myocardial abnormalities that develop during cardiac arrest and reperfusion[76,77] and prevents increases in left ventricular wall thickness.[3]

Basic pharmacological concepts

Two major processes describe the events that occur between drug administration and its effects determined by the interaction with the target organ (Fig. 20.2).

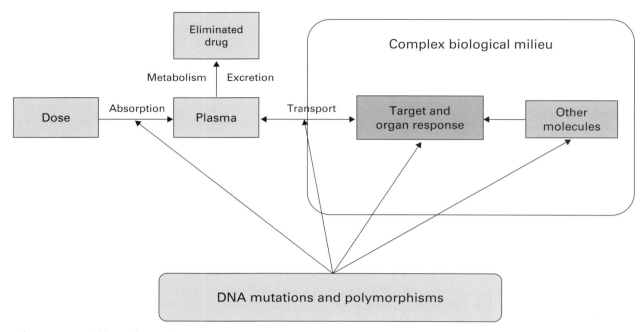

Fig. 20.2. A model for understanding variability in drug action. When a dose of a drug is administered, the processes of absorption, metabolism, excretion, and transport determine its access to specific molecular targets that mediate beneficial and toxic effects. The interaction between a drug and its molecular target then produces changes in molecular, cellular, whole organ, and ultimately whole patient physiology. This molecular interaction occurs in a complex biologic milieu modulated by multiple factors (some of which are disturbed to cause disease). DNA variants in the genes responsible for the processes of drug disposition, the molecular target, or the molecules determining the biological context in which the drug–target interaction occurs can all contribute to variability in drug action. (Modified from ref. 79.)

First, the drug must enter the systemic circulation and access its molecular site of action. The magnitude of the effect at the target is determined by the concentration of drug, and in some cases its metabolites, achieved in the plasma compartment. This process, named *pharmacokinetics*, describes drug delivery to and removal from the target molecule, and includes the processes of absorption, distribution, metabolism, and elimination (Fig. 20.3).

The second process that determines drug action has been termed *pharmacodynamics* and describes how the interaction between a drug and its specific molecular target generates effects at molecular, cellular, whole organ, and whole patient levels. Considerable intersubject variability in drug effects may arise from PD mechanisms because of the specifics of the target molecule and the complex biological milieu in which the interaction between drug and target occurs. Most frequently the biological context is altered by the same pathological processes for which that specific drug is administered.

It is only recently that the molecular basis of PK and PD has received increasing recognition, and that we have identified and characterized the genes that encode and regulate the expression of such individual molecules. At the same time it is apparent that there is extreme interindividual genetic variability, on the order of tens of millions of DNA variants. Some, termed *mutations*, are rare and result in specific diseases such as long-QT syndrome. Other more common variants, named *polymorphisms*, may or may not interfere with the function of the encoded protein, depending on whether the polymorphism results in a variation in the original amino acid sequence, or the amount of mRNA transcribed from the gene and, as a consequence, of the amount of protein produced. The most common type of variation is confined to a single nucleotide and thus is termed *single nucleotide polymorphism*.

The way multiple DNA variants within the genome modulate drug responses is called *pharmacogenomics*.[80–82] An accepted hypothesis considers polymorphisms as physiologically "silent" until superimposed stressors, such as acute myocardial ischemia or drug administration, alter the biological milieu. Only then, in the context of such pathophysiological conditions, may DNA polymorphisms promote highly individual responses.[83,84]

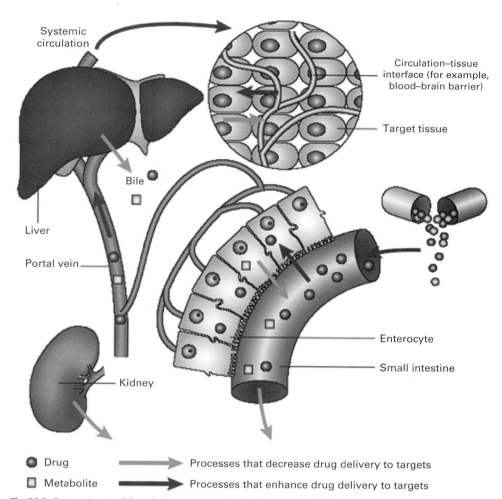

Fig. 20.3 Determinants of drug delivery to target sites. The processes of absorption, distribution into tissues, metabolism, and elimination determine the amount of drug and metabolites that are delivered to target sites. In this figure, black arrows indicate processes that enhance drug delivery, whereas gray ones show processes that decrease it. Although some of the processes shown here might occur passively, much of this drug handling is mediated by specific drug-uptake or drug-efflux transporters, as well as by drug-metabolizing enzyme complexes. An ingested drug enters enterocytes, where it can undergo metabolism, then efflux into the portal circulation, or efflux back into the gut lumen. Similarly, a drug delivered to hepatocytes can be metabolized and excreted into the bile, or returned to the systemic circulation, from where it can also be excreted, generally through biliary or renal routes. If the molecular target is not located within the circulation, further obstacles to a drug accessing its molecular targets might be encountered at plasma-tissue barriers, which could limit drug access to certain cell populations, such as the brain or testes. Some drugs must access intracellular molecular targets, in which case uptake into, and efflux out of, the target cell might be key determinants of drug delivery and hence of drug action. (From ref. 80.)

Pharmacokinetics

Administration of an intravenous drug bolus results in maximal drug concentrations at the end of the bolus and then a decline in plasma drug concentration over time (Fig. 20.4). Most frequently, however, drugs are administered by non-intravenous routes such as oral, sublingual, transcutaneous, or intramuscular. During CPR, when difficulties in venous access arise, the intratracheal or intraosseous routes of administration can be used. The intrasseous route has been shown to be effective for

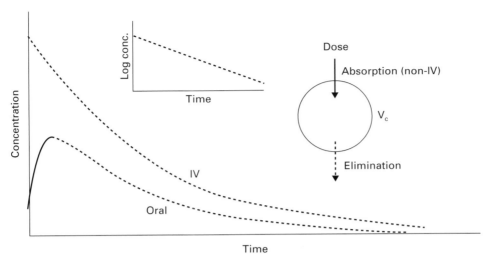

Fig. 20.4. Models of plasma concentrations as a function of time after a single dose of a drug. The simplest situation is one in which a drug is administered as a very rapid intravenous bolus into a volume (Vc) into which it is instantaneously and uniformly distributed. Elimination then takes place from this volume. In this case, drug elimination is monoexponential; that is, a plot of the logarithm of concentration versus time is linear, as shown in the inset. When the same dose of drug is administered orally, a distinct absorption phase is required prior to drug entry into Vc. Most absorption (shown here as a solid line) is completed prior to elimination (broken line), although the processes overlap. In this example, the amount of drug delivered by the oral route is less than that delivered by the intravenous route, assessed by the total areas under the two curves, indicating reduced bioavailability.(From ref. 79.)

administration of drugs and fluids in both children and adults, as well as laboratory analysis.[85–92] Evidence suggests that intraosseous infusion is much more reliable than tracheal administration of drugs during cardiac arrest. Two major differences distinguish the tracheal route of administration from the intravenous route. First, plasma concentrations are characterized by a rising phase as drugs slowly access the plasma compartment. Second, not all the drug administered may access the systemic circulation; thus, the plasma concentration may be less than that achieved by the intravenous route (Figs. 20.3 and 20.4). The amount of drug entering the systemic circulation by any route, compared to the same dose administered intravenously, is referred to as *bioavailability*. Bioavailability may be reduced because the drug is simply not absorbed from the site of administration or because the drug undergoes metabolism prior to entering the circulation – i.e., presystemic metabolism.

The simplest situation to describe is when a single dose of drug, administered as a rapid intravenous bolus, is eliminated in a monoexponential fashion (Fig. 20.4). The time in which 50% of the drug elimination occurs – *half-life* ($t_{1/2}$) – is a useful measure to describe its decline. After two half-lives, 75 % of the drug has been eliminated, after three half-lives 87.5 %, and after four 93.7% has been eliminated.

For practical purposes, elimination is complete after four to five elimination half-lives.

In other instances, the decline of drug concentration following administration of an intravenous bolus dose is multiexponential. The drug is not only eliminated but also undergoes more rapid distribution to peripheral tissues. Thus, the exponential term with the shorter half-life is generally associated with distribution and the longer one with elimination. Just as elimination may be usefully described by half-life, distribution half-life can also be derived from curves such as those shown in Fig. 20.5.

Rapid distribution can alter the way in which drug therapy should be initiated. When lidocaine is administered intravenously, it displays a prominent and rapid distribution phase ($t^{1/2} = 8$ min) prior to slower elimination ($t^{1/2} = 120$ min). As a consequence, an antiarrhythmic effect of lidocaine may be transiently achieved but very rapidly lost following a single bolus, due not to elimination, but to redistribution.[78] Administration of higher doses to circumvent this problem results in a greater likelihood of developing dose-related toxicity, often seizures. Hence, administration of a lidocaine loading dose of 3 to 4 mg kg^{-1} should occur over 10 to 20 minutes, a series of intravenous boluses (e.g., 50–100 mg every 5–10 minutes)

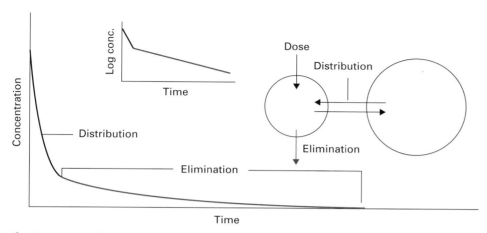

Fig. 20.5. Drug is delivered to the central volume, from which it is not only eliminated but also undergoes distribution to the peripheral sites. This distribution process is more rapid than elimination, resulting in a distinct biexponential disappearance curve. (From ref. 79.)

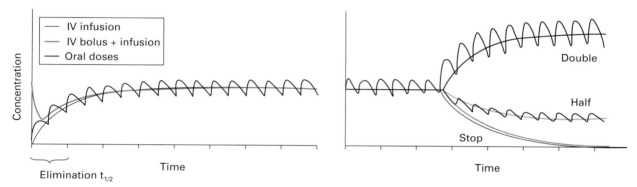

Fig. 20.6. Time course of drug concentrations when treatment is started or dose is changed. **Left.** The hash lines on the abscissa indicate one elimination half-life($t^{1/2}$). With a constant rate of intravenous infusion, plasma concentrations accumulate to steady state in four to five elimination half-lives. When a loading bolus is administered with the maintenance infusion, plasma concentrations are transiently higher but may dip, as shown here, prior to achieving the same steady state. When the same drug is administered by the oral route, the time course of drug accumulation is identical; in this case, the drug was administered at intervals of 50% of a $t^{1/2}$. Steady-state plasma concentrations during oral therapy fluctuate around the mean determined by intravenous therapy. **Right.** This plot shows that dosages are doubled or halved, or the drug is stopped during steady-state administration, and the time required to achieve the new steady state, four or five half-lives, is independent of the route of administration, (From ref. 79.)

or an intravenous infusion (e.g., 20 mg min^{-1} over 10–20 minutes).

With repeated doses or continuous infusions, drug levels accumulate to a *steady state*, the condition under which the rate of drug administration is equal to the rate of drug elimination in any given period of time. The elimination half-life describes not only the disappearance of a drug, but also the time course by which a drug accumulates to steady state. Whenever drug therapy is started, the drug dosage is changed, or the drug therapy is stopped, the time required to achieve a new steady-state plasma concentration is four

to five elimination half-lives (Fig. 20.6). It is important to distinguish between steady-state plasma concentrations, achieved in four to five elimination half-lives, and steady state drug effects, which may take longer to achieve. For some drugs, clinical effects develop immediately upon access to the molecular target: adrenergic agents to increase blood pressure, nitrates for angina, and nitroprusside to lower blood pressure, are all examples. In contrast, when an active metabolite must be generated first, drug effects follow plasma concentrations, but with a lag. Time may also be required for translation of the drug effect at the molecular site to a physiologic end point. Penetration of a drug into intracellular or other tissue sites of action may be required prior to development of drug effect; this is widely cited to explain the lag time between administration of amiodarone dosages and development of its chronic effects, although the exact mechanism underlying its effect remains poorly understood.

The mechanisms underlying drug elimination from the body are metabolism and excretion. Drug metabolism often occurs in the liver, although extrahepatic metabolism is increasingly well defined, i.e., in the circulation, lungs, intestine, and kidneys. In the liver, "phase I" drug metabolism generally involves oxidation of the drug by specific drug-oxidizing enzymes, a process that renders the drug more polar, hence more likely to undergo renal excretion.[94,95] Additionally, drugs or their metabolites often undergo conjugation with specific chemical groups to increase their water solubility; these conjugation reactions are also catalyzed by specific transferases and are designated "phase II" enzymes.[95, 96]

Some drugs undergo such extensive presystemic metabolism that the amount of drug required to achieve a therapeutic effect is much greater than that required for the same drug administered intravenously. Thus, small doses of intravenous propranolol (5 mg) may achieve slowing of heart rate equivalent to that observed with much larger oral doses (80–120 mg). Propranolol is actually well absorbed, but it undergoes extensive metabolism in the intestine and the liver prior to entering the systemic circulation. Another example is amiodarone, a highly lipophilic drug consequently with very limited water solubility, which has a bioavailability of only 30% to 50% when it is administered orally. Thus, an intravenous infusion of 0.5 mg min^{-1} (720 mg day^{-1}) is equivalent to 1.5 to 2 g day^{-1} orally.

Clearance is the most useful way of quantifying drug elimination. Clearance can be viewed as a volume of plasma that is "cleared" of drug in any given period of time, or as organ-specific (e.g., renal clearance, hepatic clearance), or whole body clearance. Reduction in clearance, by disease, drug interaction, or genetic factors, will increase drug concentrations and hence drug effects. An exception are drugs whose effects are mediated by generation of active metabolites. In this case, inhibition of drug metabolism may lead to accumulation of the parent drug, but loss of therapeutic efficacy.

Pharmacodynamics

Drugs can exert variable effects, even in the absence of PK variability. As depicted in Fig. 20.2, these disturbances can be secondary to alterations in the molecular targets with which drugs interact, as well as variability in the biologic milieu that hosts the drug-target interaction. This is a frequent mechanism of variability in drug effects, e.g., the effect of lytic therapy in a patient with no clot is evidently different from that in a patient with acute coronary thrombosis; the arrhythmogenic effects of digitalis depend on K^+ serum concentrations; the vasodilating effects of nitrates, although beneficial in patients with limited coronary flow, can be catastrophic in patients with aortic stenosis.

When aiming at rapidly correcting disturbances in physiology, a drug should be administered intravenously in doses designed to achieve a rapid therapeutic effect. Steady state is not synonymous with stable plasma concentration. Under the same conditions, a near steady-state drug concentration can be achieved rapidly by use of a loading dose (Fig. 20.6). Nevertheless, a potential disadvant-age is that a loading dose may induce drug-related side effects, especially with large loading doses. Accordingly, this approach is best justified when benefits clearly outweigh risks. Unless therapeutic and plasma concentrations are required urgently, such as when suppressing life-threatening arrhythmias, large intravenous drug boluses carry with them a disproportionate risk of enhancing drug-related toxicity, making this approach rarely appropriate. An exception is adenosine, which must be administered as a rapid bolus because it undergoes extensive and rapid elimination from plasma by uptake into virtually all cells; as a consequence, a slow bolus or infusion rarely achieves sufficiently high concentrations at the desired site of action – the coronary arteries – to terminate arrhythmias or to prevent the "no-reflow" phenomenon.[97]

The time required to achieve steady-state plasma concentrations is determined by elimination half-life, as discussed earlier. The main determinant of loading dose is the volume of distribution i.e., the theoretical volume of plasma into which the drug distributes. Loading dose = volume distribution × desired plasma concentration. The clearance and elimination half-life will determine the need and time at which to repeat doses.

It is unusual for a patient to receive chronic drug therapy with a single agent. Rather, the rule is multiple chronic drug regimens in patients with coexisting organ dysfunctions of varying degrees. Physicians should recognize the risk of unanticipated drug effects, particularly drug toxicity, in these settings. Moreover, a number of disturbances of drug elimination and drug sensitivity may alter either the therapeutic dose or tilt the balance between risks and benefits of therapy. Some ß-blockers (e.g., propranolol and metoprolol) and cimetidine reduce hepatic blood flow and the intrinsic clearance of lidocaine, respectively.[98–100] Patients with left ventricular hypertrophy often have baseline QT prolongation, and thus the risk of arrhythmias may increase; most guidelines suggest avoiding QT-prolonging antiarrhythmics in such patients.[78] In cases of heart failure, hepatic congestion can lead to decreased clearance and thus an increased toxicity with unadjusted doses of certain drugs, including lidocaine, ß-blockers, and some sedatives. In addition, patients with heart failure may have reduced renal perfusion and require dose adjustments on this basis. Heart failure is also characterized by a redistribution of regional blood flow that can lead to reduced volume of distribution and enhanced risk for drug toxicity. Lidocaine loading doses, for example, should be reduced in patients with heart failure because of altered distribution, whereas maintenance doses should be reduced in cases of both heart failure and liver disease because of altered clearance.

Drug interaction may also occur through PD mechanisms. Drugs may interact at the same effector site; the marked increase in isoproterenol dosage needed to increase heart rate in the presence of a ß-blocker is an example of a competitive agonist and antagonist interacting with the same target molecule, i.e., the β_1-adrenergic receptor. Drugs may also interact at the same time to produce synergistic effects, as in the case of two different antiarrhythmic Na^+ channel blockers with different dissociation characteristics, or drugs may allow additive pharmacologic effects while minimizing the risk of non-cardiac adverse effects present with high doses of a single drug.

More commonly, however, drugs interact by acting on different molecular targets, both of which modulate the end organ drug response. For example, low extracellular K^+ concentrations increase the potency of the rapidly activating component of delayed rectifier K^+ current (I_{Kr}) blockers;[101] thus, K^+-wasting diuretics act synergistically with I_{Kr} blockers to prolong the QT interval (same site). In addition, some diuretics also block the *slow* component of delayed rectifier K^+ current (I_{Ks}) to prolong the QT interval further.[102]

Pharmacogenetics

The variability of drug effects is increasingly recognized as dependent on DNA variants in genes that encode the drug targets and in key genes that control the biological milieu hosting the drug-receptor interaction.

A single nucleotide change can alter gene product function, and thus produce dramatic changes in physiology: the long QT syndromes or inherited errors in drug-biotransforming pathways are examples. Indeed, exogenous substrates, such as drugs, once aberrantly metabolized, produce unusual actions in affected patients.[79] Hence, these patients are phenotypically normal until an exogenous stressor – the drug – is added. These examples share the common mechanism of a DNA variant, a mutation, that severely disrupts protein function. Individuals and families with defects in genes encoding specific drug-metabolizing enzymes have been recognized. Individuals with defective CYP2D6, for example, exhibit markedly enhanced ß-blocking action (including bronchospasm and bradyarrhythmias) during propafenone therapy because of accumulation of the parent drug.[94,103]

In contrast to mutations, DNA polymorphisms are more common: one of the definitions of such polymorphisms is "a variant that occurs in more than 1% of a given study population." The distinction between *rare polymorphisms* and *mutations* however, can sometimes be blurred. Considerable effort is currently being devoted to identifying polymorphisms in the human genome, characterizing the way in which they alter protein function, and relating changes in polymorphism frequency to specific genotypes[80,81,104,105]

The mechanisms by which both mutations and polymorphisms can affect drug response are: (1) changes in PK; (2) changes in the target molecules; and (3) changes in the biologic context in which drug-target molecule interaction occurs (Fig. 20.7).

Specific drug-transport molecules, whose levels of expression and genetic variation are only now being explored, play a role not only in drug absorption and distribution but also excretion, generally into the urine or bile. Pharmacokinetic changes may derive from functionally important polymorphisms in the coding region of genes[107] or from variations in the mechanisms that regulate the amount of an individual messenger RNA generated by transcription of a single gene, that is, polymorphisms in the promoter,[107] including binding of multiple transcription factors to regulatory sequences of DNA. Thus, DNA variants may not only change the amino acid sequence of an encoded protein, but they may also change the amount of normally functioning protein generated by transcriptional control.[107,108]

Functionally important polymorphisms may also affect target molecules. Polymorphisms in the β_1 and β_2 receptor genes have been associated with variability in heart rate and blood pressure effects with ß-blockers and ß-agonists[110-112]. Torsades de pointes during QT-prolonging antiarrhythmic therapy have been linked to polymorphisms in ion channel genes. This adverse effect sometimes arises in patients with clinically latent congenitally long QT syndrome, emphasizing the strict relation among disease, genetic background, and drug therapy.[112,113]

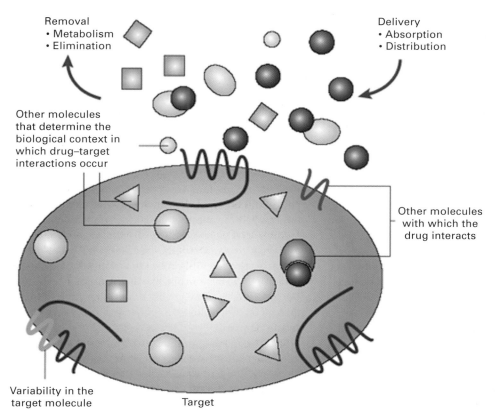

Fig. 20.7. Determinants of drug action at the target site. The drug is indicated as black circles, and the metabolite as gray squares. Delivery of drug and metabolite to, and removal from, target sites on the cell surface or within the cell are controlled by processes with activities that might be genetically determined. Variability in drug action can also arise through the pharmacodynamic mechanisms illustrated here: the drug might interact with several other targets, there might be variability in the function or expression level of the drug target, or other molecules might modulate the biological context within which the drug–target interaction takes place. DNA variants in elements that control each of these processes can lead to variable drug actions. (From ref. 80.)

Correlation between polymorphisms and variability of the biologic context in which drugs act has been exemplified by studies on the mechanisms of torsades de pointes. Virtually all drugs that cause torsades de pointes are I_{Kr} blockers.[114,115] The biologic milieu in which I_{Kr} blockers act includes other mechanisms that control the action potential as well as the normal autonomic function and serum K^+. Thus, variants in any of the genes modulating these processes in theory could modulate the extent to which I_{Kr} blockers prolong the QT interval and generate torsades de pointes. For an example, administration of a drug with I_{Kr} blocking properties does not ordinarily perturb cardiac repolarization excessively, probably because of the presence of other repolarizing currents, notably the slow component termed I_{Ks}; however, individuals with subclinical loss-of-function mutations in genes encoding I_{Ks}, who

have normal cardiac repolarization at baseline, have been shown to develop marked repolarization abnormalities and arrhythmias when challenged with an I_{Kr}-blocking drug.[116–118] Consistent with this reasoning, families have been described in which patients with mutations responsible for long QT syndromes are asymptomatic until exposed to a QT-prolonging drug.[112,116]

Drug transport is an active process that is also gene-regulated, making it an appealing target of genetic therapy. Indeed, drug entry into and efflux from cellular sites often reflects normal function and expression of specific energy-dependent drug transporters.[119,120] The most studied drug transporter is P-glycoprotein, the product of expression of the *MDR1* gene. P-glycoprotein is an efflux pump extensively expressed on the apical lumen of the enterocytes, the biliary aspect of hepatocytes, and the capillary endothelium of the brain.[121] In the latter, p-glycoprotein serves to limit access of drug to the central nervous system and thus forms an important component of the blood–brain barrier, representing at the same time a promising target for future therapeutic genetic interventions. Specific drug uptake and efflux transporters have not been identified in cardiac myocytes, and the mechanisms by which the drug accesses intracellular sites of action (relevant to virtually all antiarrhythmic drugs) is yet unknown.

Pharmacology of cardiac arrest

General considerations

Pharmacological therapies are used in cardiopulmonary resuscitation to supplement the key interventions of effective chest compression/ventilation and defibrillation. In contrast to other interventions (such as defibrillation), scientific evidence to support the use of drugs in cardiac arrest is limited. In the large Ontario Prehospital Advanced Life Support (OPALS) study, the addition of drug administration and intubation skills to the repertoire of skills of existing pre-hospital responders (trained in CPR and rapid defibrillation) had no effect on survival.[19] Despite the limited evidence to support its use, however, pharmacological therapy remains a central part of resuscitation protocols. Drugs used during cardiopulmonary resuscitation will be considered under the headings of vasopressors, antiarrhythmics, thrombolytics, and other drugs.

Specific considerations

Vasopressors

Vasopressors have been used as an adjunct to cardiopulmonary resuscitation for the last 40 years. Vasopressors are used in cardiac arrest in the belief that they will improve coronary and cerebral blood flow during CPR and thereby increase the chances of achieving a return of spontaneous circulation and neurologically intact survival. Despite their widespread inclusion in resuscitation guidelines, to date no randomized placebo-controlled clinical trials in humans have demonstrated improved survival to discharge with any of the vasopressor drugs.[25]

Several vasopressors have been studied in the context of cardiopulmonary resuscitation. Epinephrine has been the standard first-line drug for cardiac arrest for many decades. Vasopressin has been studied extensively in animal models and human clinical trials. Despite initially

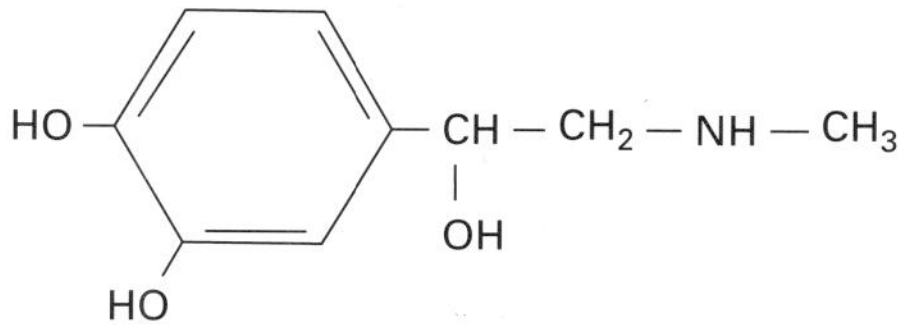

Fig. 20.8 Molecular structure of epinephrine.

promising results, a recent meta-analysis of five clinical trials failed to demonstrate that it was superior to epinephrine for improving the rate of return of spontaneous circulation, or of 24-hour or discharge survival.[122] The specific pharmacological actions and efficacy of epinephrine and vasopressin are considered below. The alternative vasopressors alpha-methyl norepinephrine and endothelin-1 have been investigated in laboratory models of cardiac arrest, but to date no clinical studies have been conducted.[25] These agents are not considered further in this chapter.

Epinephrine

Epinephrine is a naturally occurring hormone synthesized from L-tyrosine in the adrenal medulla and secreted in response to activation of the sympathetic nervous system (Fig. 20.8). It is a mixed adrenergic agonist, acting on both α- and β-adrenergic receptors. The adrenergic receptors are coupled to G-protein secondary messenger systems including cyclic adenosine monophosphate (β and α_2) (Fig. 20.9) and phospholipase C (α_1 receptor) (Fig. 20.10).

The beneficial effects of epinephrine in cardiac arrest are mostly mediated by activation of the α-adrenergic receptors. Activation of α-adrenergic receptors causes vascular smooth muscle contraction, leading to systemic arteriolar vasoconstriction, which maintains peripheral vascular tone and prevents arteriolar collapse. This has the effect of increasing aortic diastolic pressure, which increases coronary perfusion and cerebral perfusion pressures.

Stimulation of β-receptors by epinephrine has both inotropic and chronotropic effects on the beating heart that increase coronary and cerebral blood flow, but at the same time increase oxygen consumption, increase ventricular ectopic activity, and reduce subendocardial perfusion. Within the lung, stimulation of β_2 receptors by epinephrine can increase arteriovenous mismatching leading to transient hypoxemia.

Epinephrine is available in a variety of formulations and is usually given intravenously during cardiac arrest. It is metabolized by catechol-o-methyltransferase and monoamine oxidase, predominantly in the liver, to inactive metabolites, which are excreted in the urine. Intravenous administration has a rapid onset of action and half-life of

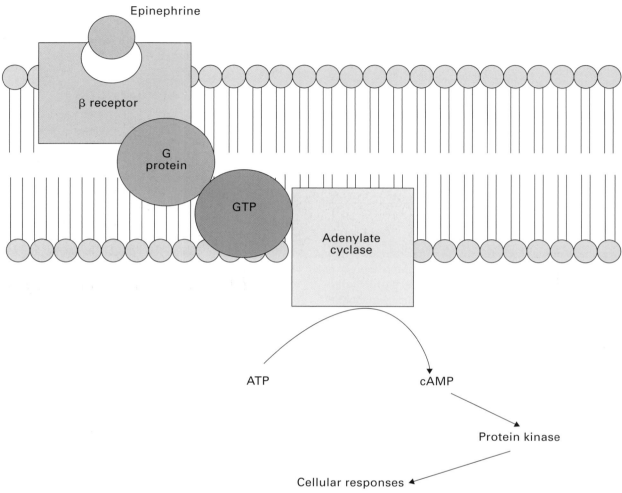

Fig. 20.9 β- and α_2-adrenergic receptors are coupled via G-proteins to the adenylate cyclase, leading, after drug-receptor interaction, to the production of the second messenger cyclic adenosine monophosphate (CAMP).

approximately 5–10 minutes. Absorption from subcutaneous and intramuscular injection of epinephrine is slow and erratic in cardiac arrest and should be avoided. Endotracheal epinephrine is recommended in resuscitation guidelines when intravenous access cannot be established.[25] Recent animal data suggest that tracheal administration can be associated with hypotension, mediated through pulmonary β_2 receptors.[123] This complication was avoided with endobronchial administration.[124]

Vasopressin

Arginine vasopressin (Fig. 20.11) is a naturally occurring hormone (antidiuretic hormone) synthesized and released by the posterior pituitary in response to changes in plasma osmolality and circulating volume. Physiological concentrations of vasopressin in humans range from 2–20 pg ml.[125]

Vasopressin receptors are membrane-bound receptors coupled to G-protein-activated intracellular signaling pathways. Three different subtypes have been described: V1 receptors (previously known as $V1_a$ receptors) are the most widespread type of vasopressin receptor and are found on vascular smooth muscle cells (where they regulate vasomotor tone), the kidney, myometrium, bladder, hepatocytes, platelets, adipocytes, and spleen. V2 receptors are located in the distal tubule and collecting ducts of the kidney and control urine volume through regulating the density of aquaporin channels on the cell surface. V3 receptors (previously known as $V1_b$) are found in the pituitary gland and stimulate adrenocorticotropic hormone (ACTH) secretion and regulate memory, blood pressure, temperature, and pituitary hormone release.[125]

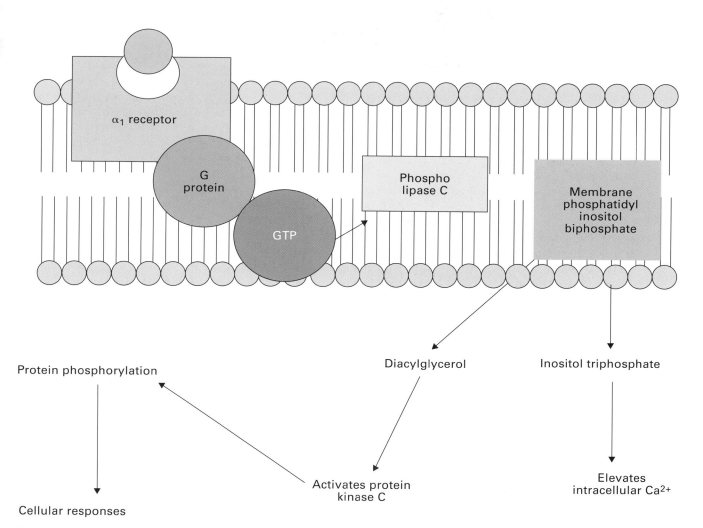

Fig. 20.10. The interaction of epinephrine with the α_1 adrenergic receptor determines the G-protein-mediated activation of the second messenger system via phospholipase C.

At physiological concentrations, vasopressin contributes to osmoregulation and maintenance of normovolemia. It also plays a role in hemostasis, temperature regulation, memory, and sleep. Synthetic vasopressin is available as an aqueous solution for intravenous, intramuscular or subcutaneous use. The intravenous route has been used exclusively in clinical trials in cardiac arrest patients. Animal data suggest that the intraosseous,[126] endotracheal, and intravenous routes[127,128] are equally effective. Vasopressin is not protein-bound and has a volume of distribution of 140 ml kg^{-1} and plasma half-life

Cys-Tyr-Phe-Gln-Asn-Cys-Pro-Arg-GlyNH$_2$

Fig. 20.11. Molecular structure of vasopressin.

of 24 minutes. Its is cleared by renal elimination (65%) and metabolism (35%) by tissue peptidases.[125]

Endogenous vasopressin concentrations increase rapidly within the first few minutes of cardiac arrest. Average vasopressin concentrations are significantly higher in patients who are successfully resuscitated from cardiopulmonary arrest than in non-survivors (177 pg ml^{-1} and 58 pg ml^{-1}, $P < 0.001$).[128]

The efficacy of vasopressin in animal cardiac arrest models has been studied extensively. In porcine models of ventricular fibrillation, compared to maximal dose epinephrine (200 µg kg^{-1}), vasopressin (0.8 µg kg^{-1}) produced superior coronary and cerebral perfusion and improved cerebral oxygen delivery and ventricular fibrillation mean frequency.[129] A meta-analysis of 33 randomized controlled animal studies (n=669) showed that vasopressin was associated with a higher rate of return of spontaneous circulation than was placebo (93% vs. 19%, P<0.001) or epinephrine (84% vs. 59%, P<0.001). Sub-group analysis demonstrated that vasopressin was superior to placebo in both VF and non-VF models.[130]

One of the first clinical studies to investigate vasopressin involved 8 patients in refractory cardiac arrest despite standard therapy with chest compression, epinephrine, and defibrillation; vasopressin administration (40 units) resulted in a prompt return of spontaneous circulation in all 8 cases. Of these, three subsequently survived and were discharged from hospital neurologically intact.[131] The first randomized controlled trial in humans to investigate vasopressin in cardiac arrest compared 40 U of IV vasopressin to 1 mg of epinephrine as the initial pharmacological treatment in 40 out-of-hospital subjects with shock-refractory VF. A significantly higher proportion of patients in the vasopressin group were successfully resuscitated and survived 24 hours compared to those treated with epinephrine.[132]

A prospective randomized controlled trial in 200 hospitalized cardiac arrest patients compared vasopressin (40 U) to epinephrine (1 mg) as the initial pharmacological treatment. This study failed to demonstrate any difference in the primary outcome measure of 1-hour survival (39% vasopressin vs. 35% epinephrine) or 30-day survival (vasopressin 13% vs. epinephrine 14%). The time to drug administration in these studies differed substantially (prehospital study 7.8–8.6 minutes compared to 1.1–1.3 minutes in the in-hospital study) and it was postulated at the time that vasopressin and epinephrine may be equipotent if administered early after the onset of cardiac arrest.[133]

The largest clinical trial to study the effect of vasopressin in cardiac arrest was conducted by the European Resuscitation Council Vasopressor during Cardiopulmonary Resuscitation Study Group. This study compared up to two injections of vasopressin 40 U or 1 mg of epinephrine, followed by additional treatment with epinephrine if required, during out-of-hospital cardiac arrest in Vienna, Germany, and Switzerland. The primary end point was survival to hospital admission and the secondary endpoint was survival to hospital discharge.[22]

A total of 1186 patients were randomized, of whom 589 received vasopressin and 597 epinephrine. The two treatment groups had similar characteristics at baseline. There was a trend toward improved rates of hospital admission in the vasopressin group compared to the epinephrine groups (36.3 vs. 31.2%, P = 0.06), but no difference in hospital discharge rates (9.9% both groups). A secondary post-hoc subgroup analysis found that patients in asystolic

cardiac arrest treated with vasopressin were more likely to survive to hospital admission (29% vs. 20.3%, P = 0.02) and subsequent discharge (4.7% vs. 1.5%, P = 0.04) than if they received epinephrine. This observation was not true for the VF or PEA groups. A second subgroup comprised 732 patients with prolonged cardiac arrest who received both the initial doses of vasopressin and then received epinephrine showed significantly better survival compared to those who received epinephrine alone (discharge survival 6.2% vs. 1.7%, P = 0.002). Nonetheless, half (10/20) the survivors in this subset of vasopressin patients were discharged comatose or with severe cerebral disability compared with 20% (1/5) in the epinephrine group.

A systematic review and meta-analysis of five clinical trials (1519 patients) comparing epinephrine and vasopressin (which included the data from the European Resuscitation Council Vasopressin study) found no difference in return of spontaneous circulation, admission or discharge survival, or the number of neurologically intact survivors. Subgroup analysis based on initial cardiac rhythm showed no statistically significant difference between drugs.[122]

In conclusion, despite promising laboratory studies, clinical studies have failed to demonstrate a consistent survival advantage for humans in cardiac arrest. The precise indications and timing of administration for vasopressin in the management of cardiac arrest therefore remains to be defined in future clinical trials.

Antiarrhythmics

There is no evidence that administration of any antiarrhythmic drug routinely during human cardiac arrest increases survival to hospital discharge. Amiodarone improves the short-term outcome of survival to hospital admission in shock-refractory VF when compared to lidocaine or placebo. Bretylium is no longer part of international guidelines for resuscitation. Amiodarone, lidocaine, and magnesium are considered below.

Amiodarone

Amiodarone was originally developed as an antianginal agent.[134] It has complex ion channel-blocking activities.[135,136] Acute intravenous administration decreases heart rate and blood pressure with minimal changes in QRS duration or QT interval. Chronic use may lead to bradycardia and increases in action potential duration in atrioventricular (AV) nodal and ventricular tissue, with increased QRS duration and QT interval.

Amiodarone is lipophilic and is taken up by many tissues (volume distribution approximately 60 liters kg^{-1}) with large interindividual variation and complex PK.[137–139] The short initial, context-sensitive half-life after intravenous administration represents drug redistribution. The actual elimination half-life is 40 to 60 days.

Amiodarone produces all four electrophysiological effects according to the Vaughan Williams classification. It has use-dependent class I activity, inhibition of inward Na^+ currents, and class II activity.[136] The antiadrenergic effect of amiodarone is non-competitive and additive to the effect of beta blockers. Amiodarone depresses sinoatrial node automaticity, slows the heart rate and conduction, and increases refractoriness of the AV node, properties useful in the management of supraventricular arrhythmia. Class III activity increases atrial and ventricular refractoriness and prolongs the QTc interval. Chronic amiodarone administration may increase the defibrillation threshold, although this is not observed after acute administration. Administration of amiodarone in a dog model of VF (12 dogs received acute IV amiodarone 10 mg kg^{-1} or placebo; 12 dogs were pretreated with chronic amiodarone 20 mg $kg^{-1} day^{-1}$ for 30 days or placebo before induction of VF) increased the organization of VF by several measures without lengthening the refractory period and without changing the defibrillation threshold.[141] Amiodarone has a long list of side effects. The most important is pulmonary toxicity, which may affect up to 1% of recipients.[141]

The ARREST – Amiodarone in the Resuscitation of Refractory Sustained Ventricular Tachyarrhythmias – study was a randomized, prospective, double blind, placebo-controlled trial of 504 patients with out-of-hospital cardiac arrest in VF/VT who failed to respond to $\geq$ 3 shocks. They received either placebo or amiodarone 300 mg IV. Treatment with amiodarone was an independent predictor of admission alive to hospital (44% vs. 34%, odds ratio 1.6; 95% confidence interval 1.1 – 2.4).[24]

In the randomized, controlled, double blind ALIVE – Amiodarone versus Lidocaine in Prehospital Ventricular Fibrillation Evaluation – study, amiodarone ($n = 180$) was compared to lidocaine ($n = 167$) in out-of-hospital VF/VT resistant to three shocks: 22.8% of amiodarone-treated patients survived to hospital admission compared to 12.0% of lidocaine-treated patients. Neither the ARREST nor ALIVE studies had a sufficient sample size to show any difference in survival to hospital discharge. One possible reason for the superiority of amiodarone may be that it is effective in severe acidosis; a laboratory study shows that amiodarone remains effective despite extracellular acidosis.[142]

Amiodarone caused a significantly lower CPP compared with epinephrine alone or the combination of epinephrine and amiodarone in a dog model of VF arrest.[143] Recent human data support this,[144] suggesting that it may actually

be the combination of amiodarone and a vasopressor that is beneficial in cardiac arrest.

A new aqueous formulation of amiodarone (Amio-Aqueous) does not contain the solvents of the standard formulation (polysorbate 80 and benzyl alcohol) that are used to keep amiodarone in solution. These solvents may be responsible for the hypotensive effects of the standard amiodarone formulation. Amio-Aqueous is also more effective than lidocaine in terminating shock-resistant VT.[145] A meta-analysis of four prospective clinical trials of patients with VT shows that Amio-Aqueous is as safe as lidocaine with respect to hypotensive side effects.[146]

Finally, animal studies suggest that amiodarone may not be effective in hypothermia.[147, 148]

Lidocaine

Lidocaine, a class 1B antiarrhythmic blocks a specific site on the Na^+ channel. It decreases automaticity by decreasing the slope of phase 4 depolarization and does not affect the PR interval, QRS complex, or QT interval.

It is no longer the drug of choice in shock-refractory VF or VT (see amiodarone above). Plasma lidocaine levels above 6 μg ml^{-1} are needed for an antifibrillatory effect. Levels above 8–10 μg ml^{-1} are associated with toxicity, which includes seizures and decreased cardiac output. Patients with significant conduction system abnormalities or hemodynamic compromise can develop toxicity at very low lidocaine concentrations. Active metabolites can also contribute to toxicity even with modest concentrations of lidocaine in plasma. Lidocaine is metabolized in the liver and excreted by the kidneys. The half-life of intravenous lidocaine is about 100 minutes, but because it is metabolized in the liver (which depends on liver flow), dosage should be reduced in patients with low cardiac output. In cardiogenic shock, the half-life may exceed 10 hours.

Magnesium

Magnesium sulfate has electrophysiological properties that might make it a useful antiarrhythmic agent. Specifically, its role as a coenzyme for the Na^+–K^+ ion exchange pump (the Na^+–K^+ ATPase) and its effects on K^+ channels and intracellular Ca^{2+} accumulation all contribute to decrease automaticity. Clinically, it has been found that AV nodal conduction is prolonged in patients treated with infusions of magnesium sulfate. It also has a high therapeutic ratio and is relatively devoid of negative inotropic effects. Magnesium use during resuscitation has been of interest since normomagnesemia appeared to be related to successful resuscitation.[149, 150]

Studies have failed to show any benefit of giving magnesium in cardiac arrest.[151–152] The only real indications for magnesium therapy seem to be hypomagnesemia and torsades de pointes. Magnesium sulfate 2 g (8 mmol) IV has also been tested as a neuroprotective agent after successful resuscitation from cardiac arrest. It did not improve neurological outcome compared to placebo when given immediately following ROSC after out-of-hospital cardiac arrest, either alone or in combination with diazepam.[156]

In summary, evidence from human studies does not favor routine use of magnesium during CPR. Recent animal data[160] point to a possible cardioprotective role of magnesium with respect to reducing oxygen free radical-induced damage and to preserving postdefibrillation left ventricular contractile function, but this requires further investigation.

Thrombolytics

Thrombolytics may be useful after initial failure of standard CPR techniques, particularly if arrest is caused by acute pulmonary embolism or other cardiac causes.[161–168] One large clinical trial[169] showed no benefit for thrombolytics in out-of-hospital patients with PEA cardiac arrest unresponsive to initial interventions. Several studies[161–164] and case series[165–168] show that there is no increase in bleeding complications with thrombolysis during CPR in non-traumatic cardiac arrest. Animal studies[170, 171] also show improved cerebral infusion with thrombolysis during CPR.

There is an argument for a more general positive effect of thrombolytic agents (even if administered prearrest or postarrest in those achieving ROSC) in preventing or diminishing no-reflow and microvascular thrombosis and organ dysfunction after cardiac arrest.[171] Several authors have suggested that this mechanism may improve neurological outcome in survivors of cardiac arrest.[164, 171, 172]

A large, prospective, randomized clinical trial – Thrombolysis In Cardiac Arrest ("TROICA") – is ongoing in Europe to study the potential value of prehospital fibrinolysis in adult, non-traumatic cardiac arrest patients who do not respond promptly to conventional therapy.

Tenecteplase can be given as a rapid intravenous bolus and hence is currently the agent of choice if thrombolysis is considered during cardiac arrest. Tenecteplase is a triple combination mutant variant of alteplase with high fibrin specificity and resistance to plasminogen activator inhibitor-1. The reduced rate of systemic clearance (fourfold slower) of the drug relative to alteplase allows tenecteplase to be given by rapid bolus injection. In patients with myocardial infarction tenecteplase has an initial plasma half-life of 20–24 minutes.

Atropine

Atropine should be considered in asystole and slow PEA. Several studies in adults[19, 23, 173–176] show that treatment with atropine is not associated with any consistent benefits after in-hospital or out-of-hospital cardiac arrests. There is, however, a physiological rationale for use of a vagolytic, as asystole can be precipitated by excessive vagal tone. Asystole is usually fatal and atropine is unlikely to have side effects in this setting.

Atropine has similar antagonist activity for all five muscarinic receptor subtypes. Thus far, the postsynaptic muscarinic receptors supposed to transduce parasympathetic impulses to the heart have been assigned to the M2 subtype, because mRNA for M1 or M3 receptors could not be found in heart muscle cells in experimental studies in adult animals. The direct effect of activation of M2 receptors in the heart is to decrease myocardial activity; that is, negative chronotropic, dromotropic, and inotropic effects occur. M2 receptors inhibit adenylate cyclase activity and enhance K^+ currents, both of which lead to decreased activation of myocardial cells. In pacemaker cells, this slows the rate of spontaneous depolarization. A negative inotropic effect decreases myocardial oxygen demand. These cardiodepressant effects are a predictable consequence of mimicking the parasympathetic nervous system and are consistent with energy conservation.

In asystolic patients 14% who received atropine survived to admission to the emergency department as opposed to 0 % who did not receive atropine.[177] In patients with severe bradycardia or asystole following administration of succinylcholine most cases resolve with atropine.[178]

Literature to refute the use of atropine is sparse and of limited quality. In a small prospective, controlled, nonrandomized study of out-of-hospital cardiac arrest patients, investigators found no difference in rhythm change, ROSC, or survival when patients were given 1–2 mg of atropine as their initial resuscitation medication versus control.[179] In a prospective, controlled, blinded canine asphyxial PEA model, no differences in ROSC or survival rates were noted between standard dose atropine and placebo groups.[180] In a prospective, controlled, nonblinded canine asphyxial PEA model, methoxamine was compared to atropine and calcium chloride. Fifty percent of the animals who received atropine had ROSC vs. 20% of the control group, but this did not reach statistical significance. Additionally, a prompt response to atropine, signifying pharmacologic effect, was not noted. Subtherapeutic doses of atropine in some of the animals and lack of epinephrine use may be significant.

Bernheim *et al.*[181] investigated 25 clinically stable heart transplant patients. After endomyocardial biopsy, a temporary pacemaker was introduced and patients were monitored. Atropine was given in increasing doses (0.004 mg kg^{-1} body weight initially, total cumulative dose

0.035 mg kg^{-1} body weight). In 20% of the patients (5/25), a paradoxical response to atropine was observed. Four patients exhibited third degree AV block, one of whom also demonstrated sinus arrest; a fifth patient showed sinus arrest only. Atropine may paradoxically cause high degree AV block in patients after cardiac transplantation. It should be used with caution and appropriate monitoring in these patients.

Atropine is a naturally occurring alkaloid of "Atropa belladonna" Atropine disappears rapidly from the blood and is distributed throughout the body. It is destroyed by enzymatic hydrolysis, particularly in the liver; from 13 to 50% is excreted unchanged in the urine. Its plasma half-life is approximately 2–4 hours.

REFERENCES

1. von Planta, M., von Planta, I., Wagner, O. *et al.* Adenosine during cardiac arrest and cardiopulmonary resuscitation: a placebo-controlled, randomized trial. *Crit. Care Med.* 1992; **20**(5): 645–649.

2. Tang, W., Weil, M.H., Sun, S. *et al.* K(ATP) channel activation reduces the severity of postresuscitation myocardial dysfunction. *Am. J. Physiol. Heart Circ. Physiol.* 2000; **279**(4): H1609–H1615.

3. Ayoub, I.M., Kolarova, J., Yi, Z. *et al.* Sodium-hydrogen exchange inhibition during ventricular fibrillation: beneficial effects on ischemic contracture, action potential duration, reperfusion arrhythmias, myocardial function, and resuscitability. *Circulation* 2003; **107**(13): 1804–1809.

4. Kaye, W., Mancini, M.E., & Rallis, S.F. Can better basic and advanced cardiac life support improve outcome from cardiac arrest? *Crit. Care Med.* 1985; **13**(11): 916–920.

5. Gazmuri, R.J., Ayoub, I.M., & Kolarova, J. Myocardial protection during resuscitation from cardiac arrest. *Curr. Opin. Crit. Care.* 2003; **9**(3): 199–204.

6. Bunch, T.J., White, R.D., Gersh, B.J. *et al.* Long-term outcomes of out-of-hospital cardiac arrest after successful early defibrillation. *N. Engl. J. of Med.* 2003; **348**(26): 2626–2633.

7. Hypothermia after Cardiac Arrest Study Group. Mild therapeutic hypothermia to improve the neurologic outcome after cardiac arrest. *N. Engl. J. Med.* 2002; **346**(8): 549–556.

8. Gonzalez, E.R. Pharmacologic controversies in CPR. *Ann. Emerg. Med.* 1993; **22**(2): 317–323.

9. Paret, G., Mazkereth, R., Sella, R. *et al.* Atropine pharmacokinetics and pharmacodynamics following endotracheal versus endobronchial administration in dogs. *Resuscitation* 1999; **41**(1): 57–62.

10. Grillo, J.A., Venitz, J., & Ornato, J.P. Prediction of lidocaine tissue concentrations following different dose regimes during cardiac arrest using a physiologically based pharmacokinetic model. *Resuscitation* 2001; **50**(3): 331–340.

11. Michael, J.R., Guerci, A.D., Koehler, R.C. *et al.* Mechanisms by which epinephrine augments cerebral and myocardial perfusion during cardiopulmonary resuscitation in dogs. *Circulation* 1984; **69**(4): 822–835.

12. Duggal, C., Weil, M.H., Gazmuri, R.J. *et al.* Regional blood flow during closed-chest cardiac resuscitation in rats. *J. Appl. Physiol.* 1993; **74**(1): 147–152.

13. Voorhees, W.D., Babbs, C.F., & Tacker, W.A., Jr. Regional blood flow during cardiopulmonary resuscitation in dogs. *Crit. Care Med.* 1980; **8**(3): 134–136.

14. Thrush, D.N., Downs, J.B., & Smith, R.A. Is epinephrine contraindicated during cardiopulmonary resuscitation? *Circulation* 1997; **96**(8): 2709–2714.

15. Wenzel, V., Lindner, K.H., Prengel, A.W. *et al.* Vasopressin improves vital organ blood flow after prolonged cardiac arrest with postcountershock pulseless electrical activity in pigs. *Crit. Care Med.* 1999; **27**(3): 486–492.

16. Gudipati, C.V., Weil, M.H., Bisera, J. *et al.* Expired carbon dioxide: a noninvasive monitor of cardiopulmonary resuscitation. *Circulation* 1988; **77**(1): 234–239.

17. Rubertsson, S., & Wiklund, L. Hemodynamic effects of epinephrine in combination with different alkaline buffers during experimental, open-chest, cardiopulmonary resuscitation. *Crit. Care Med.* 1993; **21**(7): 1051–1057.

18. Hornchen, U., Schuttler, J., & Stoeckel, H. Influence of the pulmonary circulation on adrenaline pharmacokinetics during cardiopulmonary resuscitation. *Eur. J. Anaesthesiol.* 1992; **9**(1): 85–91.

19. Stiell, I.G., Wells, G.A., Field, B. *et al.* Advanced cardiac life support in out-of-hospital cardiac arrest. *N. Engl. J. Med.* 2004; **351**(7): 647–656.

20. Holmberg, M., Holmberg, S., & Herlitz, J. Low chance of survival among patients requiring adrenaline (epinephrine) or intubation after out-of-hospital cardiac arrest in Sweden. *Resuscitation* 2002; **54**(1): 37–45.

21. Dorian, P., Cass, D., Schwartz, B. *et al.* Amiodarone as compared with lidocaine for shock-resistant ventricular fibrillation. *N. Engl. J. Med.* 2002; **346**(12): 884–890.

22. Wenzel, V., Krismer, A.C., Arntz, H.R. *et al.* A comparison of vasopressin and epinephrine for out-of-hospital cardiopulmonary resuscitation. *N. Engl. J. Med.* 2004; **350**(2): 105–113.

23. Stiell, I.G., Wells, G.A., Hebert, P.C. *et al.* Association of drug therapy with survival in cardiac arrest: limited role of advanced cardiac life support drugs. *Acad. Emerg. Med.* 1995; **2**(4): 264–273.

24. Kudenchuk, P.J., Cobb, L.A., Copass, M.K. *et al.* Amiodarone for resuscitation after out-of-hospital cardiac arrest due to ventricular fibrillation. *N. Engl. J. Med.* 1999; **341**(12): 871–878.

25. Nolan, J.P., Deakin, C.D., Soar, J. *et al.* European Resuscitation Council guidelines for resuscitation 2005. Section 4. Adult advanced life support. *Resuscitation* 2005; **67** Suppl 1: S39–S86.

26. 2005 American Heart Association Guidelines for Cardiopulmonary Resuscitation and Emergency Cardiovascular Care. *Circulation* 2005; **112**(24 Suppl): IV1–IV203.

27. Sharff, J.A., Pantley, G., & Noel, E. Effect of time on regional organ perfusion during two methods of cardiopulmonary resuscitation. *Ann. Emerg. Med.* 1984; **13**(9 Pt 1): 649–656.

28. Klouche, K., Weil, M.H., Sun, S. *et al.* Evolution of the stone heart after prolonged cardiac arrest. *Chest.* 2002; **122**(3): 1006–1011.

29. Apfelbaum, J.L., Gross, J.B., & Schaw, L.M. Changes in lidocaine protein binding may explain its increased CNS toxicity at elevated CO_2 tensions. *Anesthesiology.* 1984; **61**(3A): Abstract 213.

30. Pentel, P., & Benowitz, N. Pharmacokinetic and pharmacodynamic considerations in drug therapy of cardiac emergencies. *Clin. Pharmacokinet.* 1984; **9**(4): 273–308.

31. Doan, L.A. Peripheral versus central venous delivery of medications during CPR. *Ann. Emerg. Med.* 1984; **13**(9 Pt 2): 784–786.

32. Barsan, W.G., Levy, R.C., & Weir, H. Lidocaine levels during CPR: differences after peripheral venous, central venous, and intracardiac injections. *Ann. Emerg. Med.* 1981; **10**(2): 73–78.

33. Kuhn, G.J., White, B.C., Swetnam, R.E. *et al.* Peripheral vs central circulation times during CPR: a pilot study. *Ann. Emerg. Med.* 1981; **10**(8): 417–419.

34. Hedges, J.R., Barsan, W.B., Doan, L.A. *et al.* Central versus peripheral intravenous routes in cardiopulmonary resuscitation. *Am. J. Emerg. Med.* 1984; **2**(5): 385–390.

35. Redding, J.S., Asuncion, J.S., & Pearson, J.W. Effective routes of drug administration during cardiac arrest. *Anesth Analg.* 1967; **46**(2): 253–258.

36. Hearse, D.J. Myocardial protection during ischemia and reperfusion. *Mol. Cell. Biochem.* 1998; **186**: 177–184.

37. Redding, J.S., & Pearson, J.W. Evaluation of drugs for cardiac resuscitation. *Anesthesiology* 1963; **24**: 203–207.

38. Ditchey, R., & Lindenfeld, J. Failure of epinephrine to improve the balance between myocardial oxygen supply and demand during closed-chest resuscitation in dogs. *Circulation* 1988; **78**: 382–389.

39. Pellis, T., Weil, M.H., Tang, W. *et al.* Evidence favoring the use of an [alpha]2-selective vasopressor agent for cardiopulmonary resuscitation. *Circulation* 2003; **108**(21): 2716–2721.

40. Koretsune, Y., & Marban, E. Mechanism of ischemic contracture in ferret hearts: relative roles of $[Ca^{2+}]i$ elevation and ATP depletion. *Am. J. Physiol.* 1990; **258**(1 Pt 2): H9–H16.

41. Klouche, K., Weil, M.H., Sun, S. *et al.* Stroke volumes generated by precordial compression during cardiac resuscitation. *Crit. Care Med.* 2002; **30**(12): 2626–2631.

42. Takino, M., & Okada, Y. Firm myocardium in cardiopulmonary resuscitation. *Resuscitation* 1996; **33**(2): 101–106.

43. Hossmann, K.A., & Zimmermann, V. Resuscitation of the monkey brain after 1 h complete ischemia, I: physiological and morphological observations. *Brain Res.* 1974; **81**(1): 59–74.

44. Kleihues, P., Hossmann, K.A., Pegg, A.E. *et al.* Resuscitation of the monkey brain after one hour complete ischemia, III: indications of metabolic recovery. *Brain Res.* 1975; **95**(1): 61–73.

45. Kirsch, J.R., Dean, J.M., & Rogers, M.C. Current concepts in brain resuscitation. *Arch. Intern. Med.* 1986; **146**(7): 1413–1419.

46. Angelos, M., Safar, P., & Reich, H. A comparison of cardiopulmonary resuscitation with cardiopulmonary bypass after prolonged cardiac arrest in dogs: reperfusion pressures and neurologic recovery. *Resuscitation* 1991; **21**(2–3): 121–135.

47. Opie, L.H. Effects of regional ischemia on metabolism of glucose and fatty acids. Relative rates of aerobic and anaerobic energy production during myocardial infarction and comparison with effects of anoxia. *Circ. Res.* 1976; **38**(5 Suppl 1): I52–174.

48. Theroux, P. Protection of the myocardial cell during ischemia. *Am. J. Cardiol.* 1999; **83**(10A): 3G–9G.

49. Hearse, D.J. Oxygen deprivation and early myocardial contractile failure: a reassessment of the possible role of adenosine triphosphate. *Am. J. Cardiol.* 1979; **44**(6): 1115–1121.

50. Reimer, K.A., Hill, M.L., & Jennings, R.B. Prolonged depletion of ATP and of the adenine nucleotide pool due to delayed resynthesis of adenine nucleotides following reversible myocardial ischemic injury in dogs. *J. Mol. Cell. Cardiol.* 1981; **13**(2): 229–239.

51. Monroe, R.G., & French, G. Ventricular pressure-volume relationships and oxygen consumption in fibrillation and arrest. *Circ. Res.* 1960; **8**: 260–266.

52. Hashimoto, K., Shigei, T., Imai, S. *et al.* Oxygen consumption and coronary vascular tone in the isolated fibrillating dog heart. *Am. J. Physiol.* 1960; **198**: 965–970.

53. Paradis, N.A., Martin, G.B., Rivers, E.P. *et al.* Coronary perfusion pressure and the return of spontaneous circulation in human cardiopulmonary resuscitation. *J. Am. Med. Assoc.* 1990; **263**(8): 1106–1113.

54. Sundt, T.M., Jr., Sharbrough, F.W., Piepgras, D.G. *et al.* Correlation of cerebral blood flow and electroencephalographic changes during carotid endarterectomy: with results of surgery and hemodynamics of cerebral ischemia. *Mayo Clin. Proc.* 1981; **56**(9): 533–543.

55. Branston, N.M., Strong, A.J., & Symon, L. Extracellular potassium activity, evoked potential and tissue blood flow. Relationships during progressive ischaemia in baboon cerebral cortex. *J. Neurol. Sci.* 1977; **32**(3): 305–321.

56. Niemann, J.T. Differences in cerebral and myocardial perfusion during closed-chest resuscitation. *Ann. Emerg. Med.* 1984; **13**(9 Pt 2): 849–853.

57. Ralston, S.H., Voorhees, W.D., & Babbs, C.F. Intrapulmonary epinephrine during prolonged cardiopulmonary resuscitation: improved regional blood flow and resuscitation in dogs. *Ann. Emerg. Med.* 1984; **13**(2): 79–86.

58. Ditchey, R.V., Winkler, J.V., & Rhodes, C.A. Relative lack of coronary blood flow during closed-chest resuscitation in dogs. *Circulation* 1982; **66**(2): 297–302.

59. Lee, S.K., Vaagenes, P., Safar, P. *et al.* Effect of cardiac arrest time on cortical cerebral blood flow during subsequent standard external cardiopulmonary resuscitation in rabbits. *Resuscitation* 1989; **17**(2): 105–117.

60. Klocke, F.J., & Ellis, A.K. Control of coronary blood flow. *Annu. Rev. Med.* 1980; **31**: 489–508.

61. Cobb, L.A., Fahrenbruch, C.E., Walsh, T.R. *et al.* Influence of cardiopulmonary resuscitation prior to defibrillation in patients with out-of-hospital ventricular fibrillation. *J. Am. Med. Assoc.* 1999; **281**(13): 1182–1188.

62. Pearson, J.W., & Redding, J.S. Peripheral vascular tone on cardiac resuscitation. *Anesth. Analg.* 1965; **44**(6): 746–752.

63. Pearson, J.W., & Redding, J.S. The role of epinephrine in cardiac resuscitation. *Anesth. Analg.* 1963; **42**: 599–606.

64. Pearson, J.W., & Redding, J.S. Epinephrine in cardiac resuscitation. *Am. Heart J.* 1963; **66**: 210–214.

65. Kern, K.B., Ewy, G.A., Voorhees, W.D. *et al.* Myocardial perfusion pressure: a predictor of 24-hour survival during prolonged cardiac arrest in dogs. *Resuscitation* 1988; **16**: 241–250.

66. Sanders, A.B., Ewy, G.A., & Taft, T.V. Prognostic and therapeutic importance of the aortic diastolic pressure in resuscitation from cardiac arrest. *Crit. Care Med.* 1984; **12**(10): 871–873.

67. Sanders, A.B., Ogle, M., & Ewy, G.A. Coronary perfusion pressure during cardiopulmonary resuscitation. *Am. J. Emerg. Med.* 1985; **3**(1): 11–14.

68. Jordan, J.E., Zhao, Z.Q., & Vinten-Johansen, J. The role of neutrophils in myocardial ischemia-reperfusion injury. *Cardiovasc Res.* 1999; **43**(4): 860–878.

69. Tranum-Jensen, J., Janse, M.J., Fiolet, W.T. *et al.* Tissue osmolality, cell swelling, and reperfusion in acute regional myocardial ischemia in the isolated porcine heart. *Circ. Res.* 1981; **49**(2): 364–381.

70. Karmazyn, M. Amiloride enhances postischemic ventricular recovery: possible role of Na^+-H^+ exchange. *Am. J. Physiol.* 1988; **255**(3 Pt 2): H608–H615.

71. Lazdunski, M., Frelin, C., & Vigne, P. The sodium/hydrogen exchange system in cardiac cells: its biochemical and pharmacological properties and its role in regulating internal concentrations of sodium and internal pH. *J. Mol. Cell. Cardiol.* 1985; **17**(11): 1029–1042.

72. Avkiran, M. Rational basis for use of sodium-hydrogen exchange inhibitors in myocardial ischemia. *Am. J. Cardiol.* 1999; **83**(10A): 10G–17G; discussion 17G–18G.

73. Imahashi, K., Kusuoka, H., Hashimoto, K. *et al.* Intracellular sodium accumulation during ischemia as the substrate for reperfusion injury. *Circ Res.* 1999; **84**(12): 1401–1406.

74. Mosca, S.M., & Cingolani, H.E. Comparison of the protective effects of ischemic preconditioning and the Na^+/H^+ exchanger blockade. *Naunyn Schmiedebergs Arch. Pharmacol.* 2000; **362**(1): 7–13.

75. Mosca, S.M., & Cingolani, H.E. [The Na^+/Ca^{2+} exchanger as responsible for myocardial stunning]. *Medicina (B Aires).* 2001; **61**(2): 167–173.

76. Gazmuri, R.J., Ayoub, I.M., Hoffner, E. *et al.* Successful ventricular defibrillation by the selective sodium-hydrogen exchanger isoform-1 inhibitor cariporide. *Circulation* 2001; **104**(2): 234–239.

77. Gazmuri, R.J., Hoffner, E., Kalcheim, J. *et al.* Myocardial protection during ventricular fibrillation by reduction of proton-driven sarcolemmal sodium influx. *J. Lab. Clin. Med.* 2001; **137**(1): 43–55.

78. Roden, D.M. The principles of drug therapy. In Zipes, D.P., Libby, P., Bonow, R.O. *et al.*, eds. *Heart Disease.* 7th edn. Philadephia: Elsevier Saunders; 2005: 43–52.

79. Roden, D.M., & George, A.L., Jr. The genetic basis of variability in drug responses. *Nat. Rev. Drug Discov.* 2002; **1**(1): 37–44.

80. Evans, W.E., & Relling, M.V. Pharmacogenomics: translating functional genomics into rational therapeutics. *Science* 1999; **286**(5439): 487–491.

81. Roses, A.D. Pharmacogenetics and the practice of medicine. *Nature* 2000; **405**(6788): 857–865.

82. Meyer, U.A. Pharmacogenetics and adverse drug reactions. *Lancet* 2000; **356**: 1667–1671.

83. Collins, F.S., & Jegalian, K.G. Deciphering the code of life. *Sci. Am.* 1999; **281**(6): 86–91.

84. Collins, F.S. Shattuck lecture–medical and societal consequences of the Human Genome Project. *N. Engl. J. Med.* 1999; **341**(1): 28–37.

85. Banerjee, S., Singhi, S.C., Singh, S. *et al.* The intraosseous route is a suitable alternative to intravenous route for fluid resuscitation in severely dehydrated children. *Ind. Pediatr.* 1994; **31**(12): 1511–1520.

86. Brickman, K.R., Krupp, K., Rega, P. *et al.* Typing and screening of blood from intraosseous access. *Ann. Emerg. Med.* 1992; **21**(4): 414–417.

87. Fiser, R.T., Walker, W.M., Seibert, J.J. *et al.* Tibial length following intraosseous infusion: a prospective, radiographic analysis. *Pediatr Emerg Care.* 1997; **13**(3): 186–188.

88. Ummenhofer, W., Frei, F.J., Urwyler, A. *et al.* Are laboratory values in bone marrow aspirate predictable for venous blood in paediatric patients? *Resuscitation* 1994; **27**(2): 123–128.

89. Glaeser, P.W., Hellmich, T.R., Szewczuga, D. *et al.* Five-year experience in prehospital intraosseous infusions in children and adults. *Ann. Emerg. Med.* 1993; **22**(7): 1119–1124.

90. Guy, J., Haley, K., & Zuspan, S.J. Use of intraosseous infusion in the pediatric trauma patient. *J. Pediatr. Surg.* 1993; **28**(2): 158–161.

91. Macnab, A., Christenson, J., Findlay, J. *et al.* A new system for sternal intraosseous infusion in adults. *Prehosp. Emerg. Care.* 2000; **4**(2): 173–177.

92. Ellemunter, H., Simma, B., Trawoger, R. *et al.* Intraosseous lines in preterm and full term neonates. *Arch. Dis. Child. Fetal Neonatal Ed.* 1999; **80**(1): F74–F75.

93. Guengerich, F.P. Cytochrome P-450 3A4: regulation and role in drug metabolism. *Annu. Rev. Pharmacol. Toxicol.* 1999; **39**: 1–17.

94. Meyer, U.A., & Zanger, U.M. Molecular mechanisms of genetic polymorphisms of drug metabolism. *Annu. Rev. Pharmacol. Toxicol.* 1997; **37**: 269–296.

95. Weinshilboum, R.M., Otterness, D.M., & Szumlanski, C.L. Methylation pharmacogenetics: catechol O-methyltransferase, thiopurine methyltransferase, and histamine N-methyltransferase. *Annu. Rev. Pharmacol. Toxicol.* 1999; **39**: 19–52.

96. Innocenti, F., Iyer, L., & Ratain, M.J. Pharmacogenetics: a tool for individualizing antineoplastic therapy. *Clin. Pharmacokinet.* 2000; **39**(5): 315–325.

97. Quintana, M., Kahan, T., & Hjemdahl, P. Pharmacological prevention of reperfusion injury in acute myocardial infarction. A potential role for adenosine as a therapeutic agent. *Am. J. Cardiovasc. Drugs.* 2004; **4**(3): 159–167.

98. Conrad, K.A., Byers, J.M., 3rd, Finley, P.R. *et al.* Lidocaine elimination: effects of metoprolol and of propranolol. *Clin. Pharmacol. Ther.* 1983; **33**(2): 133–138.

99. Ochs, H.R., Carstens, G., & Greenblatt, D.J. Reduction in lidocaine clearance during continuous infusion and by coadministration of propranolol. *N. Engl. J. Med.* 1980; **303**(7): 373–377.

100. Wing, L.M., Miners, J.O., Birkett, D.J. *et al.* Lidocaine disposition – sex differences and effects of cimetidine. *Clin. Pharmacol. Ther.* 1984; **35**(5): 695–701.

101. Yang, T., & Roden, D.M. Extracellular potassium modulation of drug block of IKr. Implications for torsade de pointes and reverse use-dependence. *Circulation* 1996; **93**(3): 407–411.

102. Fiset, C., Drolet, B., Hamelin, B.A. *et al.* Block of IKs by the diuretic agent indapamide modulates cardiac electrophysiological effects of the class III antiarrhythmic drug dl-sotalol. *J. Pharmacol. Exp. Ther.* 1997; **283**(1): 148–156.

103. Lee, J.T., Kroemer, H.K., Silberstein, D.J. *et al.* The role of genetically determined polymorphic drug metabolism in the beta-blockade produced by propafenone. *N. Engl. J. Med.* 1990; **322**(25): 1764–1768.

104. Kalow, W. Pharmacogenetics, pharmacogenomics, and pharmacobiology. *Clin Pharmacol Ther.* 2001; **70**(1): 1–4.

105. McLeod, H.L., & Evans, W.E. Pharmacogenomics: unlocking the human genome for better drug therapy. *Annu. Rev. Pharmacol. Toxicol.* 2001; **41**: 101–121.

106. Kuehl, P., Zhang, J., Lin, Y. *et al.* Sequence diversity in CYP3A promoters and characterization of the genetic basis of polymorphic CYP3A5 expression. *Nat. Genet.* 2001; **27**(4): 383–391.

107. Wandel, C., Witte, J.S., Hall, J.M. *et al.* CYP3A activity in African American and European American men: population differences and functional effect of the CYP3A4*1B5'-promoter region polymorphism. *Clin. Pharmacol. Ther.* 2000; **68**(1): 82–91.

108. Schuetz, E.G., Strom, S., Yasuda, K. *et al.* Disrupted bile acid homeostasis reveals an unexpected interaction among nuclear hormone receptors, transporters, and cytochrome P450. *J. Biol. Chem.* 2001; **276**(42): 39411–39418.

109. Sofowora, G.G., Dishy, V., Muszkat, M. *et al.* A common beta1-adrenergic receptor polymorphism (Arg389Gly) affects blood pressure response to beta-blockade. *Clin. Pharmacol. Ther.* 2003; **73**(4): 366–371.

110. Dishy, V., Sofowora, G.G., Xie, H.G. *et al.* The effect of common polymorphisms of the beta2-adrenergic receptor on agonist-mediated vascular desensitization. *N. Engl. J. Med.* 2001; **345**(14): 1030–1035.

111. Johnson, J.A., & Terra, S.G. Beta-adrenergic receptor polymorphisms: cardiovascular disease associations and pharmacogenetics. *Pharm Res.* 2002; **19**(12): 1779–1787.

112. Yang, P., Kanki, H., Drolet, B. *et al.* Allelic variants in long-QT disease genes in patients with drug-associated torsades de pointes. *Circulation* 2002; **105**(16): 1943–1948.

113. Sesti, F., Abbott, G.W., Wei, J. *et al.* A common polymorphism associated with antibiotic-induced cardiac arrhythmia. *Proc. Natl. Acad. Sci. USA* 2000; **97**(19): 10613–10618.

114. Mitcheson, J.S., Chen, J., Lin, M. *et al.* A structural basis for drug-induced long QT syndrome. *Proc. Natl. Acad. Sci. USA* 2000; **97**(22): 12329–12333.

115. Roden, D.M. Taking the "idio" out of "idiosyncratic": predicting torsades de pointes. *Pacing Clin. Electrophysiol.* 1998; **21**(5): 1029–1034.

116. Donger, C., Denjoy, I., Berthet, M. *et al.* KVLQT1 C-terminal missense mutation causes a forme fruste long-QT syndrome. *Circulation* 1997; **96**(9): 2778–2781.

117. Napolitano, C., Schwartz, P.J., Brown, A.M. *et al.* Evidence for a cardiac ion channel mutation underlying drug-induced QT prolongation and life-threatening arrhythmias. *J. Cardiovasc. Electrophysiol.* 2000; **11**(6): 691–696.

118. Yang, P. Frequency of ion channel mutations and polymorphisms in a large population of patients with drug associated Long QT Syndrome. *Pacing Clin. Electrophys* 2001; **24**: 579.

119. Ambudkar, S.V., Dey, S., Hrycyna, C.A. *et al.* Biochemical, cellular, and pharmacological aspects of the multidrug transporter. *Annu. Rev. Pharmacol. Toxicol.* 1999; **39**: 361–398.

120. Zhang, L., Brett, C.M., & Giacomini, K.M. Role of organic cation transporters in drug absorption and elimination. *Annu. Rev. Pharmacol. Toxicol.* 1998; **38**: 431–460.

121. Mayer, U., Wagenaar, E., Dorobek, B. *et al.* Full blockade of intestinal P-glycoprotein and extensive inhibition of blood-brain barrier P-glycoprotein by oral treatment of mice with PSC833. *J. Clin. Invest.* 1997; **100**(10): 2430–2436.

122. Aung, K., & Htay, T. Vasopressin for cardiac arrest: a systematic review and meta-analysis. *Arch. Intern. Med.* 2005; **165**(1): 17–24.

123. Vaknin, Z., Manisterski, Y., Ben-Abraham, R. *et al.* Is endotracheal adrenaline deleterious because of the beta adrenergic effect? *Anesth Analg.* 2001; **92**(6): 1408–1412.

124. Efrati, O., Ben-Abraham, R., Barak, A. *et al.* Endobronchial adrenaline: should it be reconsidered? Dose response and haemodynamic effect in dogs. *Resuscitation* 2003; **59**(1): 117–122.

125. Kam, P.C., Williams, S., & Yoong, F.F. Vasopressin and terlipressin: pharmacology and its clinical relevance. *Anaesthesia* 2004; **59**(10): 993–1001.

126. Wenzel, V., Lindner, K.H., Augenstein, S. *et al.* Intraosseous vasopressin improves coronary perfusion pressure rapidly during cardiopulmonary resuscitation in pigs. *Crit. Care Med.* 1999; **27**(8): 1565–1569.

127. Efrati, O., Barak, A., Ben-Abraham, R. *et al.* Should vasopressin replace adrenaline for endotracheal drug administration? *Crit. Care Med.* 2003; **31**(2): 572–576.

128. Wenzel, V., Lindner, K.H., Prengel, A.W. *et al.* Endobronchial vasopressin improves survival during cardiopulmonary resuscitation in pigs. *Anesthesiology* 1997; **86**(6): 1375–1381.

129. Lindner, K.H., Prengel, A.W., Pfenninger, E.G. *et al.* Vasopressin improves vital organ blood flow during closed-chest cardiopulmonary resuscitation in pigs. *Circulation* 1995; **91**(1): 215–221.

130. Biondi-Zoccai, G.G., Abbate, A., Parisi, Q. *et al.* Is vasopressin superior to adrenaline or placebo in the management of cardiac arrest? A meta-analysis. *Resuscitation* 2003; **59**(2): 221–224.

131. Lindner, K.H., Prengel, A.W., Brinkmann, A. *et al.* Vasopressin administration in refractory cardiac arrest. *Ann. Intern. Med.* 1996; **124**(12): 1061–1064.

132. Lindner, K.H., Dirks, B., Strohmenger, H.U. *et al.* Randomised comparison of epinephrine and vasopressin in patients with out-of-hospital ventricular fibrillation. *Lancet* 1997; **349**(9051): 535–537.

133. Stiell, I.G., Hebert, P.C., Wells, G.A. *et al.* Vasopressin versus epinephrine for inhospital cardiac arrest: a randomised controlled trial. *Lancet* 2001; **358**(9276): 105–109.

134. Singh, B.N., & Vaughan Williams, E.M. The effect of amiodarone, a new antianginal drug, on cardiac muscle. *Br. J. Pharmacol.* 1970; **39**: 657.

135. Smith, W. Mechanisms of cardiac arrhythmias and conduction disturbances. In Hurst, J.W., ed. *The Heart, Arteries and Veins.* 7th edn. New York, NY: McGraw-Hill Health Professions Division; 1990: 473–488.

136. Pinter, A., & Dorian, P. Intravenous antiarrhythmic agents. *Curr. Opin. Cardiol.* 2001; **16**: 17.

137. Chow, M.S. Intravenous amiodarone: pharmacology, pharmacokinetics, and clinical use. *Ann Pharmacother.* 1996; **30**: 637.

138. Mitchell, L.B., Wyse, G., Gillis, A.M. *et al.* Electropharmacology of amiodarone therapy initiation. *Circulation* 1989; **80**: 34.

139. Holt, D.W., Tucker, G.T., Jackson, P.R. *et al.* Amiodarone pharmacokinetics. *Am. Heart J.* 1983; **106**(pt 2)(4): 840–847.

140. Huang, J., Skinner, J.L., Rogers, J.M. *et al.* The effects of acute and chronic amiodarone on activation patterns and defibrillation threshold during ventricular fibrillation in dogs. *J. Am. Coll. Cardiol.* 2002; **40**(2): 375–383.

141. Camus, P., Martin, W.J., & Rosenow, E.C. 3rd. Amiodarone pulmonary toxicity. *Clin. Chest Med.* 2004; **25**(1): 65–75.

142. Lin, C., Ke, X., Cvetanovic, I. *et al.* The influence of extracellular acidosis on the effect of IKr Blockers. *J. Cardiovasc. Pharmacol. Ther.* 2005; **10**(1): 67–76.

143. Paiva, E.F., Perondi, M.B., Kern, K.B. *et al.* Effect of amiodarone on haemodynamics during cardiopulmonary resuscitation in a canine model of resistant ventricular fibrillation. *Resuscitation* 2003; **58**(2): 203–208.

144. Skrifvars, M.B., Kuisma, M., Boyd, J. *et al.* The use of undiluted amiodarone in the management of out-of-hospital cardiac arrest. *Acta Anaesthesiol Scand.* 2004; **48**(5): 582–587.

145. Somberg, J.C., Bailin, S.J., Haffajee, C.I. *et al.* Intravenous lidocaine versus intravenous amiodarone (in a new aqueous formulation) for incessant ventricular tachycardia. *Am. J. Cardiol.* 2002; **90**(8): 853–859.

146. Somberg, J.C., Timar, S., Bailin, S.J. *et al.* Lack of a hypotensive effect with rapid administration of a new aqueous formulation of intravenous amiodarone. *Am. J. Cardiol.* 2004; **93**(5): 576–581.

147. Schwarz, B., Mair, P., Wagner-Berger, H. *et al.* Neither vasopressin nor amiodarone improve CPR outcome in an animal model of hypothermic cardiac arrest. *Acta. Anaesthesiol. Scand.* 2003; **47**(9): 1114–1118.

148. Stoner, J., Martin, G., O'Mara, K. *et al.* Amiodarone and bretylium in the treatment of hypothermic ventricular fibrillation in a canine model. *Acad. Emerg. Med.* 2003; **10**(3): 187–191.

149. Cannon, L.A., Heiselman, D.E., Dougherty, J.M. *et al.* Magnesium levels in cardiac arrest victims: relationship between magnesium levels and successful resuscitation. *Ann. Emerg. Med.* 1987; **16**(11): 1195–1199.

150. Tobey, R.C., Birnbaum, G.A., Allegra, J.R. *et al.* Successful resuscitation and neurologic recovery from refractory ventricular fibrillation after magnesium sulfate administration. *Ann. Emerg. Med.* 1992; **21**(1): 92–96.

151. Thel, M.C., Armstrong, A.L., McNulty, S.E. *et al.* Randomised trial of magnesium in in-hospital cardiac arrest. Duke Internal Medicine Housestaff. *Lancet* 1997; **350**(9087): 1272–1276.

152. Fatovich, D., Prentice, D., & Dobb, G. Magnesium in in-hospital cardiac arrest. *Lancet* 1998; **351**(9100): 446.

153. Allegra, J., Lavery, R., Cody, R. *et al.* Magnesium sulfate in the treatment of refractory ventricular fibrillation in the prehospital setting. *Resuscitation* 2001; **49**(3): 245–249.

154. Hassan, T.B., Jagger, C., & Barnett, D.B. A randomised trial to investigate the efficacy of magnesium sulphate for refractory ventricular fibrillation. *Emerg. Med. J.* 2002; **19**(1): 57–62.

155. Miller, B., Craddock, L., Hoffenberg, S. *et al.* Pilot study of intravenous magnesium sulfate in refractory cardiac arrest: safety data and recommendations for future studies. *Resuscitation* 1995; **30**(1): 3–14.

156. Longstreth, W.T., Jr., Fahrenbruch, C.E., Olsufka, M. *et al.* Randomized clinical trial of magnesium, diazepam, or both after out-of-hospital cardiac arrest. *Neurology* 2002; **59**(4): 506–514.

157. Brown, C.G., Griffith, R.F., Neely, D. *et al.* The effect of intravenous magnesium administration on aortic, right atrial and coronary perfusion pressures during CPR in swine. *Resuscitation* 1993; **26**(1): 3–12.

158. Siemkowicz, E. Magnesium sulfate solution dramatically improves immediate recovery of rats from hypoxia. *Resuscitation* 1997; **35**(1): 53–59.

159. Seaberg, D.C., Menegazzi, J.J., Check, B. *et al.* Use of a cardio-cerebral-protective drug cocktail prior to countershock in a porcine model of prolonged ventricular fibrillation. *Resuscitation* 2001; **51**(3): 301–308.

160. Zhang, Y., Davies, L.R., Martin, S.M. *et al.* Magnesium reduces free radical concentration and preserves left ventricular function after direct current shocks. *Resuscitation* 2003; **56**(2): 199–206.

161. Bottiger, B.W., Bode, C., Kern, S. *et al.* Efficacy and safety of thrombolytic therapy after initially unsuccessful cardiopulmonary resuscitation: a prospective clinical trial. *Lancet* 2001; **357**(9268): 1583–1585.

162. Lederer, W., Lichtenberger, C., Pechlaner, C. *et al.* Recombinant tissue plasminogen activator during cardiopulmonary resuscitation in 108 patients with out-of-hospital cardiac arrest. *Resuscitation* 2001; **50**(1): 71–76.

163. Janata, K., Holzer, M., Kurkciyan, I. *et al.* Major bleeding complications in cardiopulmonary resuscitation: the place of thrombolytic therapy in cardiac arrest due to massive pulmonary embolism. *Resuscitation* 2003; **57**(1): 49–55.

164. Lederer, W., Lichtenberger, C., Pechlaner, C. *et al.* Long-term survival and neurological outcome of patients who received recombinant tissue plasminogen activator during out-of-hospital cardiac arrest. *Resuscitation* 2004; **61**(2): 123–129.

165. Scholz, K.H., Hilmer, T., Schuster, S. *et al.* Thrombolysis in resuscitated patients with pulmonary embolism. *Dtsch. Med. Wochenschr.* 1990; **115**(24): 930–935.

166. Gramann, J., Lange-Braun, P., Bodemann, T. *et al.* Der Einsatz von Thrombolytika in der Reanimation als Ultima ratio zur Überwindung des Herztodes. *Intensiv.- und Notfallbehandlung.* 1991; **16**(3): 134–137.

167. Tiffany, P.A., Schultz, M., & Stueven, H. Bolus thrombolytic infusions during CPR for patients with refractory arrest rhythms: outcome of a case series. *Ann. Emerg. Med.* 1998; **31**(1): 124–126.

168. Ruiz-Bailen, M., Aguayo-de-Hoyos, E., Serrano-Corcoles, M.C. *et al.* Thrombolysis with recombinant tissue plasminogen activator during cardiopulmonary resuscitation in fulminant pulmonary embolism. A case series. *Resuscitation* 2001; **51**(1): 97–101.

169. Abu-Laban, R.B., Christenson, J.M., Innes, G.D. *et al.* Tissue plasminogen activator in cardiac arrest with pulseless electrical activity. *N. Engl. J. Med.* 2002; **346**(20): 1522–1528.

170. Lin, S.R., O'Connor, M.J., Fischer, H.W. *et al.* The effect of combined dextran and streptokinase on cerebral function and blood flow after cardiac arrest: and experimental study on the dog. *Invest Radiol.* 1978; **13**(6): 490–498.

171. Fischer, M., Böttiger, B.W., Popov-Cenic, S. *et al.* Thrombolysis using plasminogen activator and heparin reduces cerebral no-reflow after resuscitation from cardiac arrest: an experimental study in the cat. *Inten. Care Med.* 1996; **22**(11): 1214–1223.

172. Schreiber, W., Gabriel, D., Sterz, F. *et al.* Thrombolytic therapy after cardiac arrest and its effect on neurological outcome. *Resuscitation* 2002; **52**(1): 63–69.

173. Engdahl, J., Abrahamsson, P., Bang, A. *et al.* Is hospital care of major importance for outcome after out-of-hospital cardiac arrest? Experience acquired from patients with out-of-hospital cardiac arrest resuscitated by the same Emergency Medical Service and admitted to one of two hospitals over a 16-year period in the municipality of Goteborg. *Resuscitation* 2000; **43**(3): 201–211.

174. Dumot, J.A., Burval, D.J., Sprung, J. *et al.* Outcome of adult cardiopulmonary resuscitations at a tertiary referral center including results of "limited" resuscitations. *Arch. Intern. Med.* 2001; **161**(14): 1751–1758.

175. Engdahl, J., Bang, A., Lindqvist, J. *et al.* Factors affecting short- and long-term prognosis among 1069 patients with out-of-hospital cardiac arrest and pulseless electrical activity. *Resuscitation* 2001; **51**(1): 17–25.

176. Tortolani, A.J., Risucci, D.A., Powell, S.R. *et al.* In-hospital cardiopulmonary resuscitation during asystole. Therapeutic factors associated with 24-hour survival. *Chest* 1989; **96**(3): 622–626.

177. Stueven, H.A., Tonsfeldt, D.J., & Thompson, B.M. Atropine in asystole: Human studies. *Ann. of Emerg. Med.* 1984; **13**(9 II): 815–817.

178. Sorensen, M., Engbaek, J., Viby-Mogensen, J. *et al.* Bradycardia and cardiac asystole following a single injection of suxamethonium. *Acta. Anaesthesiol. Scand.* 1984; **28**(2): 232–235.

179. Coon, G.A., Clinton, J.E., & Ruiz, E. Use of atropine for brady-asystolic prehospital cardiac arrest. *Ann. Emerg. Med.* 1981; **10**(9): 462–467.

180. DeBehnke, D.J., Swart, G.L., Spreng, D. *et al.* Standard and higher doses of atropine in a canine model of pulseless electrical activity. *Acad. Emerg. Med.* 1995; **2**(12): 1034–1041.

181. Bernheim, A., Fatio, R., Kiowski, W. *et al.* Atropine often results in complete atrioventricular block or sinus arrest after cardiac transplantation: an unpredictable and dose-independent phenomenon. *Transplantation* 2004; **77**(8): 1181–1185.

21

Analysis and predictive value of the ventricular fibrillation waveform

Trygve Eftestøl, Hans-Ulrich Strohmenger and Colin Robertson

Department of Electrical and Computer Engineering, University of Stavanger, Norway
Department of Anaesthesiology and Critical Care Medicine, Medical University Innsbruck, 6020 Innsbruck, Austria, and
Department of Emergency Medicine, The Royal Infirmary of Edinburgh, UK

Introduction: Why analyze the waveform?

Ventricular fibrillation (VF) is the cardiac arrest rhythm most amenable to successful treatment, and the vast majority of survivors from human cardiac arrest have VF as their primary rhythm. Successful treatment in these patients almost invariably requires electrical defibrillation. While advances have been made in defibrillation therapy, particularly in the introduction of automatic and semi-automatic defibrillators (AED) with rhythm recognition and the use of novel defibrillatory waveforms, the primary determinant of successful defibrillation is the duration of the VF episode.[1] With the passage of time, the chances of successful defibrillation fall dramatically. Basic life support (BLS) procedures in general and myocardial perfusion due to closed-chest compression can only retard the metabolic deterioration of the myocardium. With prolonged duration of VF, an increasing likelihood of asystole, pulseless electrical activity, or persistent VF following countershock results.[2,3] Moreover, multiple countershocks that do not result in spontaneous circulation are probably harmful by causing thermal damage to the heart and increasing cumulative defibrillation energy decreases postresuscitation myocardial function and survival.[4,5]

For these reasons, researchers attempt to interrogate the VF waveform determined from the surface electrocardiogram (ECG) trace to ascertain knowledge of the myocardial state, to assess the probability of success of a defibrillating shock, and to investigate whether, by physical or pharmacological means, the situation can be changed to improve the likelihood of restoring a spontaneous perfusing rhythm.

Data acquisition and preprocessing

Logistic difficulties

Although the primary focus of analysis is the ECG-derived VF waveform itself, additional documentation such as patient demographics, electrical, pharmacological, and physical interventions, and outcome information is required to provide meaningful conclusions. In contrast to animal experiments, human studies need substantial time and effort to gather and store field information in a form suitable for detailed analysis.

To extract meaningful information, data are imported and integrated in a software environment that facilitates signal analysis.[6] Figure 21.1 illustrates some key information including the ECG time series, events from the defibrillation log, and rhythm annotations provided by medical experts. Human VF analysis involves considerable work to establish the databases, routines for storing and transferring electronic data from the emergency medical system (EMS) and linking it with information from the signal analysis.[7–9] Separate centers typically use different equipment so the coding format of electronic information for ECG, event logs, demographic information, and annotations vary. This lack of standardization makes research on this kind of data challenging.

Filtering techniques

Mechanical activity from chest compression and ventilation during CPR introduces artefact components in the ECG signal.[10–12] At present, it is necessary to stop CPR

Cardiac Arrest: The Science and Practice of Resuscitation Medicine. 2nd edn., ed. Norman Paradis, Henry Halperin, Karl Kern, Volker Wenzel, Douglas Chamberlain. Published by Cambridge University Press. © Cambridge University Press, 2007.

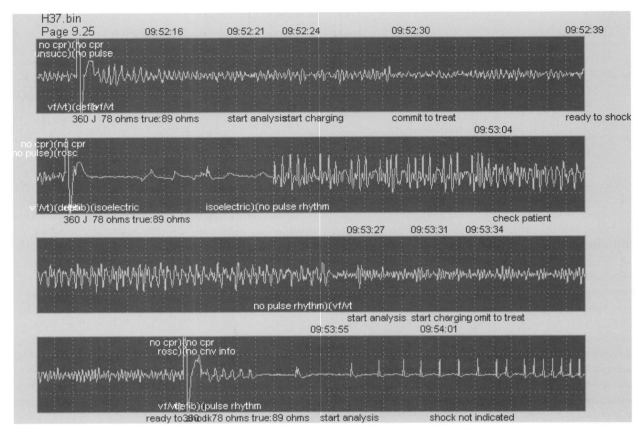

Fig. 21.1. ECG during resuscitation. ECG tracing illustrating VF, with artefacts from precordial chest compressions, hands-off intervals, countershocks and return of spontaneous circulation. Each line shows 30 seconds of ECG continuing from the previous line. The time stamps and defibrillator usage text above and below each line of tracing are read from the electronic defibrillator log file. The text within the tracing axes are the therapy, defibrillation outcome and rhythm annotations provided by the medical experts. (*After Eftestøl et al. Expert Rev. Cardiovasc. Ther. (2003)© Future Drugs 2003.*)

before analyzing (manually, or by AED) the artefact-free ECG rhythm. This intermittent cessation of CPR reduces the likelihood of successful defibrillation because, during these breaks, myocardial (and cerebral) perfusion does not occur.

Artefact removal has been successfully applied to animal ECGs by using high-pass digital filters with fixed coefficients.[13,14] In the human ECG, however, the frequency components of the artefacts overlap with dominant components in the human VF spectrum, and make separation by such filters unfeasible.

Adaptive filtering has been used to remove CPR artefacts in human out-of-hospital cardiac arrest ECG.[15] Reference signals that resemble different artefact types (e.g., compressions and ventilations) are recorded simultaneously with the ECG and "subtracted" from the ECG. CPR artefacts in the ECG can be reduced in this way, but not always well

enough for a shock/no-shock decision classifier. The time without blood flow from compressions can be reduced significantly by removing artefacts during CPR.[16]

Approaches to analysis

The search for one or more predictors of defibrillation outcome derived from the VF ECG waveform and for measuring the effects of therapy goes back 20 years.[2,7,10,17–21]

Time and frequency domain techniques

From a signal processing perspective, the main approaches to VF waveform analysis fall within the categories of time and frequency domain techniques. Typically, time domain approaches are applied to characterize specific events such as detection and description of P waves, QRS complexes, or T waves in the ECG of perfusing rhythms. Perfusing rhythms are, to some degree, deterministic: a term often used to describe biomedical signals of a quasiperiodic nature. The VF waveform signals, however, do not display clearly distinctive quasiperiodic events but are governed by processes that are described and analyzed statistically. These processes, related to cardiac arrest, change with time and therapy and the parameters describing these processes change accordingly. VF analysis seeks to identify parameters that can be used to distinguish features associated with a high probability of restoration of spontaneous circulation (ROSC) following countershock from those with a low countershock success rate.

Time domain techniques applied to VF involve characterization of the signal's amplitude behavior. These techniques attempt to describe the statistical properties of the amplitude or energy distribution of the signal-generating process. As an example, the expected amplitude value can be estimated by the signal's sample mean or the signal energy can be quantified as the dispersion of the squared amplitude about its mean.[22,23] In statistical terms, these are moments of the signal amplitude's first-order distribution or probability density function (PDF). Another important family of amplitude distributions is the second-order distributions, in which more amplitudes of one signal are involved. With these it is possible to analyze the relationship between amplitude variations of the same signal at different time instants. The autocorrelation function (ACF) estimated from the signal is an expression for this relationship. The VF signal typically does not exhibit one distinct periodic component, but rather a composite spectrum of several such components more naturally expressed in frequency rather than time units. Because of this, and because signals with such properties are commonly analyzed in the frequency domain, the power spectral density (PSD) function, which is the frequency domain equivalent of the VF ACF, has been widely used in the analysis of the signal's periodic behavior.

Chaos theory and non-linear dynamics

To the naked eye, the VF waveform appears entirely random or stochastic, but "random" phenomena can, on further investigation, show predictable features. Non-linear mathematical approaches, colloquially known as "chaos theory," have been used to search for underlying structure and predictability in VF. Such approaches are not simply "blue sky" in nature. A fundamental element of mathematically chaotic systems is that miniscule changes at an early stage can lead to subsequent dramatic perturbations – popularized as the "Butterfly effect."[24] If the VF waveform is chaotic then, instead of the 10–100s of joules required for conventional defibrillation, there is the possibility that a tiny electrical stimulus at a predetermined point could terminate the arrhythmia and restore a perfusing rhythm.

In some animal and computer models, spiral waves of electrical activity (vortices and rotors) travel through the myocardium, become fragmented and turbulent, and lead to persistence of VF.[25–27] The characterization of these initiating events, and of VF, as mathematically chaotic systems is a highly specialized area and differing analytical methods have made interpretation and extrapolation difficult. Nevertheless there is evidence that, at least in the early stages, VF does show specific phenomena of mathematical chaos with consistent exhibition of organized structure.[28–30]

Non-linear dynamic methods have been used to elucidate the fractal dimension of the VF signal and quantify its morphology and time course, independent of signal amplitude and spectral parameters. The practical difficulties of using these forms of analysis relate to the massive computer processing power needed and the necessity of using "clean," but unfiltered, signals. The ability to achieve this and provide real-time feedback will demand massive improvements before clinical therapy can be influenced.

Practically, the problem of prediction of defibrillation outcome is handled by extracting VF waveforms immediately before a defibrillation attempt with corresponding outcome information (ROSC or no-ROSC) from the available data. After this, signal analysis based on time domain, frequency domain, and/or non-linear dynamics techniques measures waveform characteristics (features) to be used in the shock outcome predictor.

Structuring the data in frequency and time-frequency representations

Characterization of the VF signal often involves a first stage in which the signal is restructured or transformed into a frequency domain representation or even combined time-frequency representations. These alternative representations are often a prelude to computing shock outcome predictors, but also offer alternative representations by which the hidden structures of VF have been revealed to the observer.

Fourier transforms

This technique involves splitting short segments of the VF waveform into small subunits and expressing each of these as the sum of multiple simpler sine/cosine waves of varying amplitude and frequency. These component waves can then provide an amplitude or power histogram by plotting the square of the amplitude against the frequency.[31,32] The Fourier transform gives this frequency domain information when applied to the time domain signal. The power spectral density (PSD) is theoretically defined as the Fourier transform of the ACF, and has been widely used in VF analysis.

A significant problem with Fourier transforms is that the PSD is strictly defined only for signals with stable, or stationary, statistical properties. VF is a non-stationary signal, and the short time PSD has to be determined for time-limited VF segments considered quasi-stationary. In practice the discrete Fourier transform (DFT) is used. This approach has disadvantages in that it assumes that the time limited VF segment under investigation repeats periodically ad infinitum. Further, the technique is limited when analyzing sharply changing signals (Gibbs phenomenon).

Wavelet transforms

Wavelet transforms use small wave-like functions that come in different shapes and sizes to transform the VF signal. Mathematically, the wavelet transform is a convolution of the wavelet function with the signal. If the wavelet matches the shape of the signal closely at a specific scale and location, then a large value of the transform results and vice versa. Changing the type of wavelet allows the investigator to concentrate on individual small scale high frequency components or to pick up larger scale low frequency components. An energy scalogram can be produced which plots the log of the band-pass center frequency against the time where darker areas represent a higher wavelet energy coefficient and lighter areas a lower wavelet energy coefficient (Fig. 21.2).[32]

The key advantage of the continuous wavelet transform technique is that it can elucidate local spectral and temporal information simultaneously within the VF waveform. Even if short time Fourier transform (STFT) is performed on small segments of the signal at a time and moved incrementally along, this spectrogram technique uses a window of fixed width and therefore averages short duration components "smearing" the information across the window and so might lose potentially valuable information.

Time-frequency analysis as offered by both short time Fourier and especially wavelet transform analysis has allowed the extraction of previously hidden information from the VF waveform, for example observations possibly related to coordinated independent atrial activity while the ventricles remain fibrillating.[12,34] In this case, the superior temporal resolution of the wavelet transform offers the possibility of detecting the instance of the pulse complexes.[34] In addition, in animal models, chest compression artefact is seen to be clearly distinct from other VF-related features (Fig. 21.3).[11,12]

Describing the data: extracting features

After the first stages of VF analysis, whether this involves filtering and/or frequency domain transforms or not, quantification of the signal characteristics follows. This is the feature extraction stage, to capture the signal characteristics distinguishing successful from unsuccessful defibrillations.

To evaluate the ability of a feature (alone or in combination) to discriminate between outcome categories, various approaches including receiver operating characteristics (ROC) analysis have been used to determine the sensitivities and specificities of outcome predictors. These thresholds are usually linear, but some pattern recognition methods based on Bayesian decision theory have been applied to define non-linear decision borders for feature combinations.[7,9,33,35,36] Figure 21.4 illustrates a set of two-dimensional feature combinations, each coordinate representing the features computed from VF preshock waveforms. The feature space is divided into decision regions separated by non-linear decision borders. The area under the curve (AUC) may be used to determine the discriminative power of features.

Approaches to analysis

Amplitude

The magnitude of the VF waveform voltage, or VF amplitude, can be described clinically: "Coarse" VF is high amplitude (> 0.2 mV) usually of recent onset and has a higher probability of ROSC following defibrillation. "Fine" VF is low amplitude (< 0.2 mV), results from prolonged global myocardial ischemia, and is less amenable to resuscitation.[2] The "natural history" of untreated VF is progressive reduction in VF amplitude from coarse to fine, but simple clinical interpretation of the VF waveform is poor and quantitative analysis is needed to guide therapy.[37]

VF amplitude analysis by measuring either the maximum[38] or the average[13] peak-to-trough ECG voltage for a predefined time window has become much easier with improvements in digital signal analysis and computa-

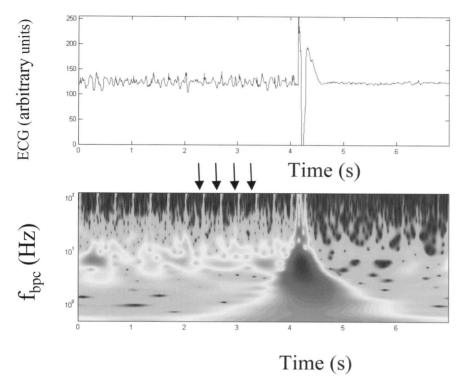

Fig. 21.2. Attempted defibrillation of human ventricular fibrillation. *Top:* 7 seconds of human ECG exhibiting VF containing a defibrillation shock event. *Bottom:* Scalogram corresponding to the ECG signal. Notice the high frequency spiking prior to the shock evident in the scalogram – indicated by arrows. (After Addison *et al., IEEE Eng. Med. Biol* (2002) © IEEE 2002.) (See Plate 21.2.)

tional technique. In animal models VF amplitude during CPR reflects myocardial perfusion and energy metabolism[39] and values immediately before defibrillation are significantly higher in succesfully resuscitated animals.[38,39] Human studies confirm that maximum VF amplitude before countershock can predict outcome of defibrillation,[38,40,41] but the predictive power and discriminative value of VF amplitude are limited because of interindividual variability resulting from the main fibrillatory vector direction, electrode placement, transthoracic impedance, and shape of the thorax.

Frequency/spectral analysis

The frequency domain features used in VF analysis have mostly been calculated from a PSD estimate derived by the periodogram method[42] or variations of this. The periodogram method for PSD estimation applies a Fourier transform to the squared signal samples for each extracted preshock VF segment. Examples of some of the

main features calculated from these include the peak power frequency, median frequency, energy, spectral flatness measure, amplitude spectrum analysis (AMSA), spectral edge frequency, fibrillation power or variations of these. These features capture discriminating characteristics from the PSD.

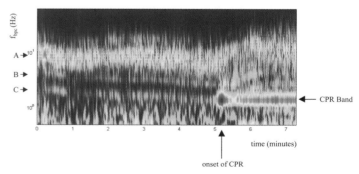

Fig. 21.3. The energy scalogram for the first seven minutes of porcine ventricular fibrillation. CPR is initiated at 5 minutes as indicated. (After Addison *et al.* (2000) © 2000 IEEE.) (See Plate 21.3.)

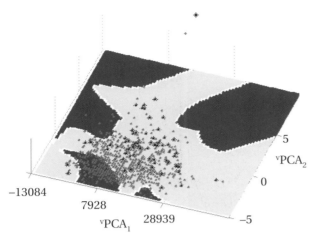

Fig. 21.4. Defibrillation outcome prediction. Decision regions corresponding to the ROSC/noROSC prediction problem. The classes are identified by the following color scheme: yellow = decision region for ROSC (restoration of spontaneous circulation), blue = decision region for noROSC. The coordinate corresponding to ROSC outcomes are shown as stars (*) and noROSC as points (.). To predict the outcome of an ECG tracing, the features vPCA1 and vPCA2 are computed from the tracing. If the coordinate point corresponding to (vPCA1,vPCA2) is mapped into the yellow decision area, an ROSC outcome is predicted. If it is found to be in the blue area, a no ROSC outcome is predicted. (After Eftestøl *et al. Resuscitation* (2005) © Elsevier 2005.) (See Plate 21.4.)

The peak power or dominant frequency is the frequency corresponding to the maximum amplitude frequency component in the PSD. The median frequency (sometimes termed mean or centroid frequency) is the frequency bisecting the PSD, corresponding to the point of mass in the spectrum.[42] Both this feature and the peak power frequency emphasize the low frequency content of VF.

Energy, which is closely related to amplitude features, expresses the "coarseness" of the waveform, and corresponds to the area under the PSD curve.

The spectral flatness measure characterizes the waveform complexity and is computed as the ratio of the geometric and arithmetic mean of the PSD.[7]

In retrospective human studies, areas under ROC curves for peak power and median frequency perform worse than in animal studies, with AUC ranging from 0.53 to 0.72.[8,19,41,43,44,8] Studies of combined features have demonstrated AUC at 0.80 in an independent test[9] of an outcome predictor developed earlier.[7]

Fibrillation power was originally defined as the (amplitude)[2] of frequency components in the VF power spectrum. Power has also been defined as the integral of the power spectrum between certain frequency limits, representing energy. In this sense, the PSD method was used to investi-

gate the distribution of fibrillation power with frequency and time before defibrillation. In a porcine model of cardiac arrest, VF power is a better predictor of countershock success than are features such as mean amplitude or mean fibrillation frequency.[44] Disappointingly, human studies did not confirm this high predictive value of fibrillation power (i.e., energy)[8,44] and did not reveal significant changes of energy during manual chest-compression. Nonetheless, the low correlation between power/energy and frequency or amplitude parameters[45] provided complementary information in feature combination for outcome prediction.[7]

AMSA is the sum of the frequency-weighted PSD amplitudes, and represents the area under the amplitude frequency relationship resulting from fast Fourier transform. The method emphasizes the high frequency content of the PSD.

AMSA has yielded promising results in animal experiments.[20,46] In a pig VF model, an AMSA value of 21 mV Hz predicted defibrillation success with negative and positive predictive values (95% and 78%) superior to those for coronary perfusion pressure, mean amplitude, or median frequency.[20]

An AMSA value of 13 mV Hz retrospectively applied to recordings of 108 out-of-hospital cardiac arrest episodes in 46 patients predicted defibrillation success with ROSC with a sensitivity of 91% and specificity of 94%.[47] Eftestøl found a sensitivity of 95% and specificity of 40% for the AMSA feature for outcome prediction, but showed that the parameter increased during ongoing chest compression.[8]

Wavelet time/frequency methods

Quantification of the time frequency characteristics extracted by wavelet methods from the VF signal has been used as a marker of shock outcome prediction, and principal component analysis has been used to improve system performance. The wavelet entropy marker, in particular, offers significant improvements in terms of sensitivity and specificity as compared to similar Fourier transform-based features derived from the same data set.[7,21] In a recent study, the continuous wavelet technique showed an improved performance when compared to median frequency, spectral energy, and AMSA methods.[33,35]

Non-linear dynamics methods

N(α) histogram analysis is a non-linear dynamic method that provides analysis independent of ECG-signal amplitudes or artefacts due to manual chest compression.[48] For every time interval, time-shifted ECG amplitudes are plotted in a three-dimensional coordinate system. The distribution of points found in spheres with a defined radius at specific points in space allows extraction of a local dimension α.

In a pig model the randomness of the VF ECG signal reflected by the width of $N(\alpha)$-histogram was a better predictor of countershock success than the median dimension. In addition, the more irregular the VF from the animal studied the more easily it could be defibrillated.[46] The principal disadvantage of this method, however, is the computation time requirement including sophisticated hardware and software.

The scaling exponent method has been used as a tool to quantify the self-similarity dimension of the VF waveform. The normal values of the scaling exponent D range from 1 – 2; low values indicate a high degree of organization of the VF signal and are associated with short downtime, and an increased probability of ROSC (PROSC) and hospital discharge rate.[19] Conversely, the scaling exponent increased with the duration of VF in animals and humans[19,49,50] and significantly higher values were found in patients with unfavorable outcomes.[19] Recently in a pig model of VF, scaling exponent D was used to guide the sequence of CPR interventions.[51] Although the predictive power of this single feature with respect to ROSC is low (reflected by an ROC curve area of 0.71), it may provide additional information to guide electrical therapy in human cardiac arrest.[19]

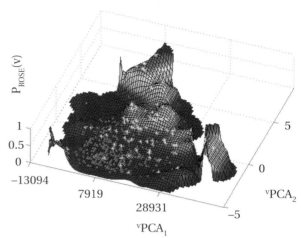

Fig. 21.5. The probability of ROSC. A functional relationship between the feature representations of all the VF waveforms extracts and corresponding ROSC/NO ROSC outcome with the feature representation coordinates from Figure 4 superimposed. This can be explained as a division of the feature space defined by vPCA1 and vPCA2 into equal-sized cells. In each cell the PROSC value is estimated as the number of ROSC coordinates divided by the total number of coordinates in the cell. To compute the probability of successful outcome of an ECG tracing, the features vPCA1 and vPCA2 are computed from the tracing. The coordinate point corresponding to (vPCA1,vPCA2) is mapped onto the PROSC function surface, where the probability value can be read directly. (After Eftestøl *et al. Expert Rev. Cardiovasc. Ther.* (2003) © Future Drugs 2003.) (See Plate 21.5.)

What to do with the results: Defibrillation success and PROSC

Whichever method of analysis is used, clinicians require guidance for the delivery of CPR and the timing of defibrillation. In its simplest form, this may be a YES/NO instruction based upon a predetermined probability of the technique used leading to ROSC (Fig. 21.5).[52]

Establishing these decision thresholds has its own difficulties. Using data from animal studies where all treatment groups divide clearly into ROSC/NoROSC gives a clear-cut problem that is simpler to analyze but less applicable to real-life clinical situations. Ideally, successful and unsuccessful outcomes should be mixed well in the treatment groups, although such studies have lower specificities.[53,54]

It is also important that when evaluating the performance of the parameter(s) chosen, the data set for training is separate from that used for testing. Several studies use variants of this approach, especially cross-validation tech-

niques, where the training and test sets are shifted among several data sets, providing several opportunities to give estimates of expected performance.[7,9,33,36] These methods attempt to provide an idea of how the predictor will perform on future data, but it is important to note that the test performances are considered in the design of the classifiers to choose the generalizing parameters. In a recent study, a final evaluation was performed on an independent data set not considered in the design process.[9]

PROSC values can also be used to monitor the efficacy of clinical interventions. In one study PROSC was used to evaluate the effect of interrupting precordial compressions and more recently to investigate the effects of giving precordial compressions. The studies demonstrated a negative change in PROSC when chest compressions were interrupted[55] and a positive change after prolonged sequences of compressions.[8]

The Future

The knowledge that, at least in its genesis and early stages, VF is not a random process and that the waveform contains elements of identifiable structure has been the first step in using the waveform for practical clinical purposes. The recognition that some of these elements can provide proxy information about the state of the underlying myocardial substrate leads to their potential to monitor and direct individual resuscitation efforts. The promise shown in animal studies has yet to be fully matched in humans and the mathematical tools used have limitations but, with continuing improvements in analytical techniques and computing power, it is inevitable that in the near future such techniques will be used clinically. The application of similar techniques to cerebrally generated waveforms holds the exciting prospect of performing and monitoring truly integrated cardiocerebral resuscitation.

REFERENCES

1. Yakaitis, R.W., Ewy, G.A., Otto, C.W., Taren, D.L. & Moon T.E. Influence of time and therapy on ventricular defibrillation in dogs. Crit. Care Med. 1980; **8**: 157–163.
2. Weaver, W.D., Cobb, L.A., Dennis, D., Ray, R., Hallstrom, A. & Copass, M.K. Amplitude of ventricular fibrillation waveform and outcome after cardiac arrest. *Ann. Intern. Med.* 1985; **102**: 53–55.
3. Martin, G., Cosin, J., Such, M., Hernandez, A. & Llamas, P. Relation between power spectrum time course during ventricular fibrillation and electromechanical dissociation. Effects of coronary perfusion and nifedipine. *Eur. Heart J.* 1986; **7**: 560–569.
4. Xie, J., Weil, M.H., Sun, S. *et al.* High-energy defibrillation increases the severity of postresuscitation myocardial dysfunction. *Circulation* 1997; **96**: 683–688.
5. Yamaguchi, H., Weil, M.H., Tang, W., Kamohara, T., Jin, X. & Bisera, J. Myocardial dysfunction after electrical defibrillation. *Resuscitation.* 2002; **54**: 289–296.
6. Värri, A., Kemp, B., Penzel, T. & Sclögl, A. Standards for biomedical signal databases. *IEEE Eng. Med. Biol. Mag.* 2001; **20**: 33–37.
7. Eftestol, T., Sunde, K., Aase, S.O., Husoy, J.H. & Steen, P.A. Predicting outcome of defibrillation by spectral characterization and nonparametric classification of ventricular fibrillation in patients with out-of-hospital cardiac arrest. *Circulation* 2000; **102**: 1523–1529.
8. Eftestol, T., Wik, L., Sunde, K. & Steen, P.A. Effects of cardiopulmonary resuscitation on predictors of ventricular fibrillation defibrillation success during out-of-hospital cardiac arrest. *Circulation* 2004; **110**: 10–15.
9. Eftestol, T., Losert, H., Kramer-Johansen, J., Wik, L., Sterz, F. & Steen, P.A. Independent evaluation of a defibrillation outcome predictor for out-of-hospital cardiac arrest patients. *Resuscitation* 2005; **67**: 55–60.
10. Strohmenger, H.U., Lindnder, K.H., Lindner, I.M., Pfenniger, E.G. & Bothner, U. Spectral analysis of ventricular fibrillation and closed-chest cardiopulmonary resuscitation. *Resuscitation* 1996; **33**: 155–161.
11. Watson, J., Addison, P.S., Clegg, G. *et al.* A novel wavelet transform based analysis reveals hidden structure inventricular fibrillation. *Resuscitation* 2000; **43**: 121–127.
12. Langhelle, A., Eftestøl, T., Myklebust, H. *et al.* Reducing CPR artefacts in ventricular fibrillation in vitro. *Resuscitation* 2001; **48**: 279–291.
13. Noc, M., Weill, M.H., Tang, W., Sun, S., Pernat, A. & Bisera, J. Electrocardiographic prediction of the success of cardiac resuscitation. *Crit. Care Med.* 1999; **27**: 708–714.
14. Strohmenger, H.U., Lindner, K.H., Keller, A., Lindner, I.M., Pfenninger, E.G. & Bothner, U. Effects of graded doses of vasopressin on median frequency in a porcine model of cardiopulmonary resuscitation: Results of a prospective, randomized, controlled trial. *Crit. Care Med.* 1996; **24**: 1360–1365.
15. Eilevstjønn, J., Eftestol, T., Aase, S.O., Myklebust, H., Husøy, J.H.H. & Steen, P.A. Feasability of shock advice analysis during CPR through removal of CPR artefacts from human ECG. *Resuscitation* 2004; **2**: 131–141.
16. Eilevstjønn, J. Removal of cardiopulmonary resuscitation artifacts in the human electrocardiogram. PhD thesis, Stavanger University College, Stavanger, Norway, September 2005.
17. Dalzell, G.W. & Adgey, A.A. Determinants of successful transthoracic defibrillation and outcome in ventricular fibrillation. *Br. Heart. J.* 1991; **65**: 311–316.
18. Brown, C.G., Griffith, R.F., Van Ligten, P. *et al.* Median frequency – a new parameter for predicting defibrillation success rate. *Ann. Emerg. Med.* 1991; **20**: 787–789.
19. Callaway, C.W., Sherman, L.D., Mosesso, V.N., Dietrich, T.J., Holt, E. & Clarkson, M.C. Scaling exponent predicts defibrillation success for out-of-hospital ventricular fibrillation cardiac arrest. *Circulation* 2001; **103**: 1656–1661.
20. Marn-Pernat, A., Weil, M.H., Tang, W., Pernat, A. & Bisera, J. Optimizing the timing of ventricular defibrillation. *Crit. Care Med.* 2001; **29**: 2360–2365.
21. Watson, J.N., Uchaipichat, N., Addison, P. *et al.* Improved prediction of defibrillation success for out-of-hospital VF cardiac arrest using wavelet transform methods. *Resuscitation* 2004; **63**: 269–275.
22. Rangayyan, R.M. Biomedical signal analysis: A case-study approach, IEEE press series on biomedical engineering, Piscataway, N.J., 2002.
23. van Bemmel, J.H. & Musen, M.A. (eds). *Handbook of Medical Informatics*, Houten, Bohn Stafleu Van Loghum, 1997.
24. Lorenz, E.N. Predictability: does the flap of as butterfly's wings in Brazil set off a tornado in texas? Title of december 1972 talk

to AAAS as quoted in *Chaos and Non Linear Dynamics* by R C Hilbourne OUP 1994.

25. Jalife, J. & Gray, R. Drifting vortices of electrical waves underlie ventricular fibrillation in the rabbit heart. *Acta. Physiol. Scand.* 1996; **157**: 123–131.

26. Witkowski, F.Y., Leon, L.J. & Penkoske, P.A. Spatiotemporal evolution of VF. *Nature* 1998; **392**: 78–82.

27. Panfilov, A.V. Spiral breakup as a model of ventricular fibrillation. *Chaos* 1998; **8**: 57–64.

28. Small, M., Yu, D.J., Harrison, R.J. *et al.* Characterising nonlinearity in ventricular fibrillation. *Computers Cardiol.* 1999; **26**: 17–20.

29. Small, M., Yu, D.J., Harrison, R.J. *et al.* Deterministic nonlinearity in ventricular fibrillation. *Chaos* 2000; **10**: 1–10.

30. Yu, D.J., Small, M., Harrison, R.J. *et al.* Measuring temporal complexity of ventricular fibrillation. *Phys. Lett. A* 2000; **265**: 68–75.

31. Cooley, J.W. & Tukey, J.W. An algorithm for the machine calculation of complex Fourier seies. In Rabiner, L.R. & Rader, C.M. *Digital Signal Processing* IEEE Press, 1972: 223–227.

32. Bergland, G.D.A. A guided tour of the Fast Fourier Transform. In Rabiner, L.R. & Rader, C.M. *Digital Signal Processing* IEEE Press 1972: 223–227.

33. Watson, J., Addison, P.S., Clegg, G. *et al.* Practical issues in the evaluation of methods for the prediction of shock outcome success in out of hospital cardiac arrest patients: COP, a case study. *Resuscitation* 2005a in press.

34. Addison, P., Watson, J.N., Clegg, G.R., Steen, P.A. & Robertson, C.E. Finding coordinated atrial activity during ventricular fibrillation using wavelet decomposition *IEEE Eng. Med. Biol.* 2002 Jan/Feb1–3.

35. Watson, J., Addison, P.S., Clegg, G. *et al.* Wavelet transfer-based prediction of the likelihood of successful defibrillation for patients exhibiting ventricular fibrillation. *Meas. Sci. Technol.* 2005; **616**: L1–L6.

36. Yang, Z., Yang, Z., Lu, W. *et al.* A probabilistic neural network as the predictive classifier of out-of-hospital defibrillation outcomes. *Resuscitation* 2005; **64**: 31–36.

37. Lightfoot, C.B., Sorensen, T.J., Garfinkel, M.D., Sherman, L.D., Callaway, C.W. & Menegazzi, J.J. Physician interpretation and quantitative measures of electrocardiographic ventricular fibrillation waveform. *Prehosp. Emerg. Care* 2001; **5**(2): 147–154.

38. Strohmenger, H.U., Lindner, K. & Brown, C.G. Analysis of ventricular fibrillation signal amplitude and frequency parameters as predictors of countershock success in humans. *Chest* 1997; **111**: 584–589.

39. Noc, M., Weil, M.H., Gazmuri, R.J., Bisera, J. & Tang, W. Ventricular fibrillation voltage as a monitor of the effectiveness of cardiopulmonary resuscitation. *J. Lab. Clin. Med.* 1994; **124**: 421–426.

40. Callaham, M., Braun, O., Valentine, W., Clark, D.M. & Zegans, D. Prehospital cardiac arrest treated by urban first responders: profile of patient response and prediction of outcome by ventricular fibrillation waveform. *Ann. Emerg. Med.* 1993; **22**: 1664–1677.

41. Strohmenger, H.U., Eftestol, T., Sunde, K. *et al.* The predictive value of ventricular fibrillation electrocardiogram signal frequency and amplitude variables in patients with out-of-hospital cardiac arrest. *Anesth. Analg.* 2001; **93**: 1428–1433.

42. Kay, Sm. *Modern Spectral Estimation: Theory and Application.* EnglewoodCliffs, NJ: Prentice Hall, 1988.

43. Brown, C. & Dzwonczyk, G.R. Signal analysis of the human electrocardiogram during ventricular fibrillation: frequency and amplitude parameters as predictors of successful countershock. *Ann. Emerg. Med.* 1996; **27**: 184–188.

44. Hamprecht, F.A., Achleitner, U., Krismer, A.C. *et al.* Fibrillation power, an alternative method of ECG spectral analysis for predition of countershock success in a porcine model of ventricular fibrillation. *Resuscitation* 2001; **50**: 287–296.

45. Hamprecht, F.A., Jost, D., Rüttimann, M., Calamai, F. & Kowaöski, J.J. Preliminary results on the prediction of countershock success with fibrillating power. *Resuscitation* 2001; **50**: 297–299.

46. Povoas, H.P., Weil, M.H., Tang, W. *et al.* Predicting the success of defibrillation by electrocardiographic analysis. *Resuscitation* 2002; **53**: 77–82.

47. Young, C., Bisera, J., Gehman, S., Snyder, D., Tang, W. & Weil, M.H. Amplitude spectrum area: measuring the probability of successful defibrillation as applied to human data. *Crit. Care Med.* 2004; **32**[Suppl]: S356–S358.

48. Amann, A., Achleitner, U., Antretter, H. *et al.* Analysing ventricular fibrillation ECG-signals and predicting defibrillation success during cardiopulmonary resuscitation employing N(alpha)-histograms. *Resuscitation* 2001; **50**: 77–85.

49. Callaway, C.W. & Menegazzi, J.J. Waveform analysis of ventricular fibrillation to predict defibrillation. *Curr. Opin. Crit. Care* 2005; **11**: 192–199.

50. Sherman, L.D., Callaway, C.W. & Menegazzi, J.J. Ventricular fibrillation exhibits dynamical properties and self-similarity. *Resuscitation* 2000; **47**: 163–173.

51. Menegazzi, J.J., Callaway, C.W., Sherman, L.D. *et al.* Ventricular fibrillation scaling exponent can guide timing of defibrillation and other therapies. *Circulation* 2004; **109**: 926–1031.

52. Eftestøl, T., Sunde, K., Aase, S.O. *et al.* "Probability of successful defibrillation" as a monitor during CPR in out-of-hospital cardiac arrested patients. *Resuscitation* 2001; **48**: 245–254.

53. Berg, R.A., Hilwig, R.W., Kern, K.B. *et al.* Precountershock cardiopulmonary resuscitation improves ventricular fibrillation median frequency and myocardial readiness for successful defibrillation from prolonged ventricular fibrillation: a randomized, controlled swine study *Ann. Emerg. Med.* 2002; **40**: 563–570.

54. Lightfoot, C.B., Nremt, P., Callaway, C.W. *et al.* Dynamic nature of electrocardiographic waveform predicts rescue shock outcome in porcine ventricular fibrillation. *Ann. Emerg. Med.* 2003; **42**: 230–241.

55. Eftestøl, T., Sunde, K. & Steen, P.A. The effects of interrupting precordial compressions on the calculated probability of defibrillation success during out-of-hospital cardiac arrest. *Circulation* 2002; **105**: 2270–2273.

22

Etiology, electrophysiology, and myocardial mechanics of pulseless electrical activity

Tom P. Aufderheide

Department of Emergency Medicine, Medical College of Wisconsin, Milwaukee, WI, USA

Pulseless electrical activity (PEA) is defined in this chapter based on its clinical presentation, the presence of organized electrical activity, and the absence of detectable pulses. This definition includes any pulseless organized rhythm irrespective of etiology, heart rate, or electrocardiogram (ECG) characteristics.

PEA may be viewed as a continuous mechanical and electrical phenomenon. Detectable pulses may be lacking because of the absence of synchronous myocardial fiber shortening. Detectable pulses may also be absent in the presence of weak myocardial contractions that produce measurable aortic pressures as evidenced by invasive monitoring. PEA can also be present with normotensive cardiac activity in patients with conditions such as cardiac tamponade, hypovolemic shock, or severe peripheral arteriovascular disease.

There is evidence to support the contention that the ECG characteristics in PEA reflect the degree of pathophysiologic derangement or time from onset of cardiac arrest.[1–3] Irrespective of PEA etiology, the more normal the ECG complex and the shorter the time from cardiac arrest, the higher is the likelihood of successful resuscitation or survival.[2] Conversely, the more abnormal the ECG complex, the longer time from cardiac arrest and the lower the likelihood of successful resuscitation or survival.[2] There probably has been no greater advance in understanding and managing PEA than the recent determination of a relationship between the integrity of the ECG complex and underlying mechanical activity.[1,2]

Pulseless electrical activity is classified by its clinical presentation into three groups: (a) normotensive PEA, (b) pseudo-PEA, and (c) true PEA. Normotensive PEA is defined as baseline cardiac contractions and myocardial fiber shortening in the absence of detectable pulses. Pseudo-PEA is the stage of pulseless electrical activity in which weak myocardial contractions produce detectable aortic pressure only measurable by invasive monitoring or echocardiography. True PEA is the stage of pulseless electrical activity in which myocardial contraction is absent.

PEA frequently results from a primary condition that profoundly decreases preload or afterload or causes severe inflow or outflow obstruction. The primary disorder results in hypoxia, acidosis, and increased vagal tone, which, if not rapidly reversed, affects the strength of myocardial contraction and eventually results in PEA. Causes for PEA include (a) mechanical, including tension pneumothorax, cardiac tamponade, and auto-PEEP (auto–positive end-expiratory pressure); (b) preload reduction, including hypovolemia, sepsis, and pulmonary embolism; (c) primary myocardial dysfunction, including acute myocardial infarction, congestive heart failure, drug ingestions, hyperkalemia, and hypothermia; and (d) pulmonary, including severe respiratory insufficiency or respiratory arrest (Fig. 22.1).

Another cause of pulseless electrical activity is termed *postdefibrillation PEA*; this refers to the variable electrical and mechanical cardiac activity that occurs following countershock from ventricular fibrillation. Prolonged ventricular fibrillation results in hypoxia, acidosis, and increased vagal tone, which produce a variable response to countershock, including baseline, decreased, or no cardiac contractions (Fig. 22.1).

The incidence of PEA depends on the patient population studied. The condition accounts for 16 to 22% of out-of-hospital cardiac arrests.[4,5] The frequency of PEA in-hospital cardiac arrests is higher. Raizes *et al.* found

Cardiac Arrest: The Science and Practice of Resuscitation Medicine. 2nd edn., ed. Norman Paradis, Henry Halperin, Karl Kern, Volker Wenzel, Douglas Chamberlain. Published by Cambridge University Press. © Cambridge University Press, 2007.

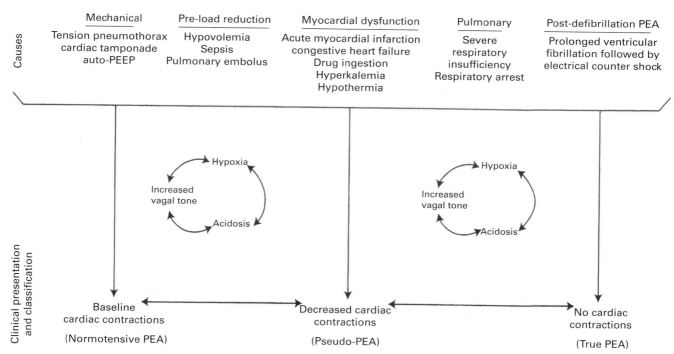

Fig. 22.1. Clinical spectrum of pulseless electrical activity

that PEA accounted for 68% of monitored in-hospital sudden deaths and 10% of all in-hospital deaths.[6] Vincent et al. reported PEA as the initial symptom in 66% of monitored in-hospital cardiac arrests.[7] Pirolo et al. reviewed the results of 50 autopsies of patients dying in PEA and found that 12 of 50 (24%) had primary PEA, 22 (44%) had secondary PEA, and in six (12%) the classification of PEA could not be determined.[8]

The average age of patients presenting in PEA is 70 years.[4] The incidence of PEA as a presenting cardiac arrest rhythm is higher in the elderly (15% vs. 3%).[9] When PEA and coarse ventricular fibrillation are compared with respect to demographics, patients who present in PEA are more likely to be female (43% versus 24%); they are also more likely to have no cardiac history (54% vs. 19%),[4] but a similar percentage of patients are likely to be on cardiac medication (43% vs. 42%).[4] It is possible that cardiac medications such as β-blockers or calcium antagonists may contribute to the presentation of PEA.[4]

The successful resuscitation and save rates in PEA patients are higher in prehospital compared with hospital patients. The largest clinical prehospital study of PEA patients reported 98 (19.5%) of 503 successful resuscitations and 22 (4.4%) of 503 discharged from the hospital alive.[2] Vincent et al. reviewed 50 hospitalized patients experiencing sudden onset of PEA in a hospital-based critical

care setting.[7] Only 3 of 50 (6%) were discharged alive from the critical care ward, and only 1 of 50 (2%) survived to hospital discharge.[7]

Basic science

Cellular basis of cardiac contraction

The myocardium consists of a syncytium of branching and anastomosing fibers that are divided into individual cells by modified, closely opposed cell membranes termed *intercalated* disks. This apposition provides a continuous "tight junction" with free passage of ions and action potentials from cell to cell throughout the syncytium. In contrast to skeletal muscle, the myocyte has a centrally located nucleus and is richly endowed with mitochondria, necessary for the generation of large amounts of adenosine triphosphate (ATP) required for cardiac contraction. The myocyte also has an abundant sarcoplasmic reticulum and an elaborate system of large T tubules. The T tubules provide a channel for ion fluxes, especially Ca^{2+} involved in cardiac contraction. The fibers within myocytes each contain multiple cross-banded myofibrils, which run the length of the fiber and are composed of a serially repeating structure, the sarcomere.

The sarcomere is the structural and functional unit of myocardial contraction and is delimited by two adjacent transverse Z lines. Sarcomeres are characterized by cross striations caused by prominent central dark A bands of a constant width of 1.5 μm. A bands are composed of thicker filaments, principally of the protein myosin. The A band is flanked by lighter I bands composed primarily of thinner filaments of actin. The thin actin filaments are attached at their outer ends to the Z lines and, at their inner ends, interdigitate partially between the myosin filaments. Thus the A band has partially overlapping myosin and actin filaments, whereas the I band contains only actin filaments. On electron-microscopic examination, bridges can be seen to extend between the thick and thin filaments within the A band (Fig. 22.2).[10,11]

The contractile process

Both the thick and thin filaments remain at a constant overall length, both at rest and during contraction, leading to a sliding model for myocardial contraction. During myocardial contraction, repetitive interactions occur at the bridges between the actin and myosin filaments, propelling the actin filaments further into the A band. During the contractile process, the A band remains at a constant width, whereas the I band narrows, and the Z lines move toward one another.

The myosin molecule is a complex fibrous protein with a molecular weight of approximately 500 000; it has a rodlike portion that is about 1500 Å in length with a globular portion at its end. This globular portion forms the bridges between myosin and actin and contains adenosine triphosphatase activity (ATPase). These bridges project outward so that they can interact with actin to generate force and shortening.

The thin filament actin is composed of a double helix of two chains of actin molecules wound around each other, has a molecular weight of 47 000, and is associated with two regulatory proteins, tropomyosin and troponin. Troponin can be separated into three components: troponins C, I, and T. Actin has no intrinsic enzymatic activity, but it has the ability to combine reversibly with myosin in the presence of ATP and Ca^{2+}, which activates the myosin ATPase. Tropomyosin inhibits this interaction in relaxed muscle. During activation, troponin C binds Ca^{2+}, resulting in a conformational change exposing the actin cross-bridge interaction sites. Physical changes in the cross bridges result in sliding of the actin along the myosin filaments causing muscle shortening or the development of tension. Cleavage of ATP into adenosine diphosphate (ADP) and inorganic phosphate dissociates the myosin cross bridge from actin. Linkages between actin and myosin filaments are made repeatedly as long as sufficient Ca^{2+} is present; linkages are broken when Ca^{2+} concentration decreases below a critical level. At this point the troponin-tropomyosin complex again prevents binding between myosin and actin filaments. Ionic calcium is the principal mediator of the inotropic state of the heart. Most positive inotropic drugs, including digitalis and catecholamines, act by increasing delivery of Ca^{2+} to the myofilament.

The abundant sarcoplasmic reticulum is a complex network of membrane-lined intracellular channels running longitudinally within the sarcomere in close proximity to the outside membrane but which have no direct continuity with the outside of the cell. Transverse or T tubules represent tubelike invaginations of the sarcolemma that are continuous with the extracellular space and traverse adjacent to the Z lines. This complex network of membrane channels assists ion fluxes during cardiac contraction (Fig. 22.3).[10,11]

Cardiac activation

The sarcomere at rest has an interior negative charge relative to the outside of the cell with a transmembrane potential of -80 to -100 mV. In the resting state the sarcolemma is largely impermeable to Na^+. The membrane has an Na^+ and a K^+ stimulated pump requiring ATP, which extrudes Na^+ from the cell and plays a critical role in establishing the resting potential of the membrane. The intracellular milieu is high in K^+ and low in Na^+, whereas the opposite is true extracellularly. In the resting state, at the same time, the extracellular concentration of Ca^{2+} greatly exceeds free intracellular Ca^{2+} concentration.[10,11]

During the plateau of the action potential in phase 2, there is a slow inward current reflecting primarily movement of Ca^{2+} within the cell. The absolute quantity of Ca^{2+} that crosses the surface membrane is relatively small. Nevertheless, the depolarizing current not only extends across the surface of the cell membrane but also penetrates deeply into the cell by the elaborate system of transverse tubules. Because of this transsarcolemmal movement of Ca^{2+}, much larger quantities of Ca^{2+} are released from the sarcoplasmic reticulum within the cell. This process is termed *regenerative release of* Ca^{2+}.[10,11]

The Ca^{2+} combines with troponin, and, by repressing the inhibitor of contraction, activates the myofilaments to produce contraction. The sarcoplasmic reticulum then reaccumulates Ca^{2+} by an ATP-dependent calcium pump, lowering intracellular Ca^{2+} concentration to a level that inhibits actin-myosin interaction and leading to muscle

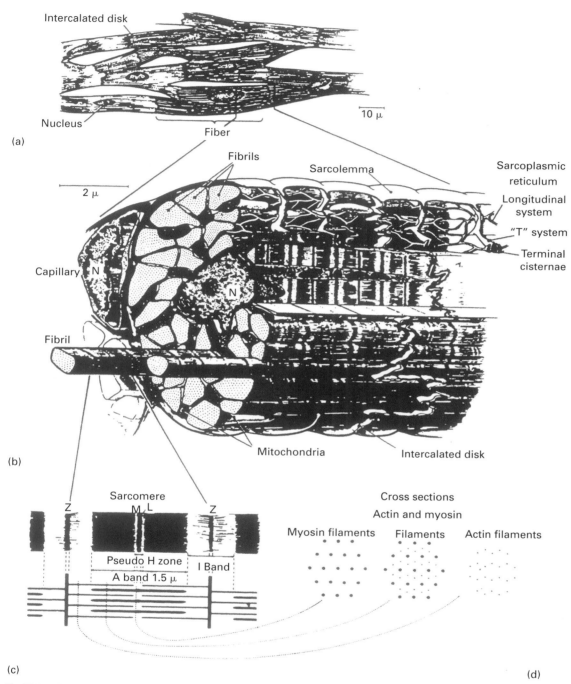

(a)

(b)

(c)

(d)

Fig. 22.2. Microscopic structure of heart muscle. (a) Myocardium as seen under light microscope. Branching of fibers is evident. Each fiber, or cell, contains centrally located nucleus. (b) Myocardial cell, reconstructed from electron micrographs. Each cell is composed of multiple parallel fibrils. Each fibril is composed of serially connected sarcomeres (N, nucleus). (c) Sarcomere from myofibril, with diagramatic representation of myofilaments. Thick filaments (1.5 μm long, composed of myosin) form A band, and thin filaments (1 μm long, composed primarily of actin) extend from Z line through I band into a band. Overlapping of thick and thin filaments is seen only in A band. (d) Cross-sections of sarcomere indicate specific lattice arrangements of myofilaments. In center of sarcomere only thick, or myosin, filaments arranged in a hexagonal array are seen. In distal portions of A band, both thick and thin, or actin, filaments are found, with each thick filament surrounded by six thin filaments. In I band only thin filaments are present. (Reproduced with permission from ref. 10.)

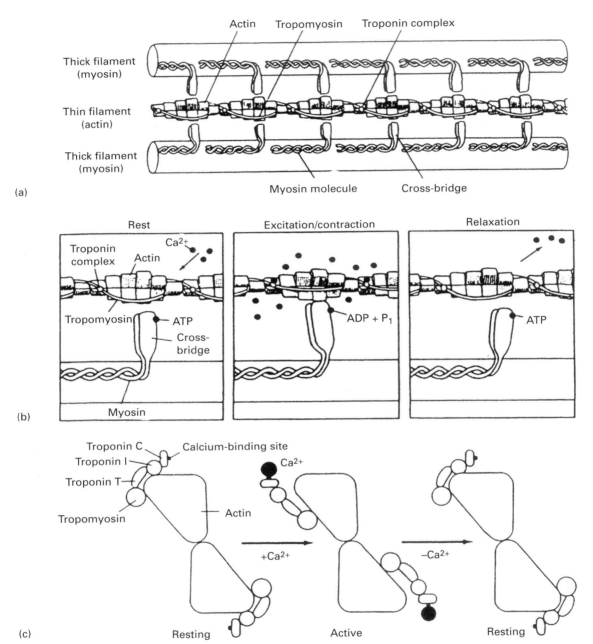

Fig. 22.3. Contractile protein interactions and role of calcium as activator messenger are shown schematically. (a) Contractile proteins (myosin and actin) and regulatory proteins (troponin complex and tropomyosin) shown in relative positions on myofilaments. (b) Contraction takes place when heads of myosin molecules, which form cross bridges of thick filament, bind to actin, followed by shift in orientation of cross bridge that pulls thin filament toward center of sarcomere. Activation requires calcium binding to troponin complex, reversing inhibition of interaction between myosin and actin. In cycle of chemical reactions underlying contraction, hydrolysis of ATP produces cross-bridge motion. Relaxation occurs when calcium becomes dissociated from troponin. (c) Molecular rearrangements at level of thin filament involve regulatory proteins (tropomyosin and troponins C, I, T) in allosteric effect. Calcium binding to troponin C loosens bond linking troponin I to actin; resulting dissociation of troponin T from actin backbone of thin filament displaces tropomyosin, exposing active sites for interaction with myosin. (From Katz AM, Smith VE. Myocardial relaxation abnormalities. Part I: mechanisms. Hosp Prac 1984; 19(1):69. Illustration by Bunji Tagawa.)

relaxation. In this way, the cell membrane, transverse tubules, and sarcoplasmic reticulum play a fundamental role in myocardial contraction and relaxation by their ability to transmit an action potential and to release and then reaccumulate Ca^{2+}.[10,11]

ATP is the principal source of energy for almost all of the mechanical work of myocardial contraction. The high-energy phosphate stores in ATP are in equilibrium with those present in creatine phosphate. The activity of the myosin ATPase determines the rate of forming and breaking the actin-myosin cross bridges and ultimately the velocity of muscle contraction (Fig. 22.4).[10,11]

Myocardial contraction

The mechanical activity of myocardial muscle can ultimately be explained by a combination of force and velocity of muscle contraction. The Frank–Starling relation (Starling's law of the heart) describes the relationship between the initial length of myocardial muscle fibers and the development of force. Within limits, the initial length of myocardial muscle (which is a function of left ventricular end-diastolic volume) is related to the force of ventricular contraction. It has been postulated that increasing the initial length of myocardial muscle to an optimum of 2.2 μm results in the most advantageous overlap of interdigitating contractile filaments within the sarcomere and also optimizes their sensitivity to Ca^{2+}.

Changes in the velocity of shortening the myocardial muscle may also occur, even at a constant muscle length. This type of shift in the force-velocity curve may be seen with administration of a positive inotropic agent such as digitalis or norepinephrine. It has also been postulated that increased velocity of myocardial contraction is ultimately related to either the concentration of Ca^{2+} in the vicinity of the myofilaments or their sensitivity to Ca^{2+} or both of these factors. Whatever the mechanism, velocity of myocardial contraction appears primarily related to increased availability of Ca^{2+} within the cell.

Ultimately, stroke volume is determined by three influences: (*a*) the length of the muscle at the onset of contraction (the preload), (*b*) the inotropic state of the heart, and (*c*) the tension that the myocardium must develop during contraction (the afterload).

Preload

Ventricular end-diastolic volume determines the length of the muscle fiber at the onset of contraction, affecting stroke volume. Depletion in total blood volume results in decreased ventricular end-diastolic volume, reflected in a reduction in ventricular performance. Ventricular enddiastolic volume can also be influenced by the distribution of blood between the intrathoracic and extrathoracic compartments. Gravitational forces tend to pool blood in dependent positions. Elevation of intrathoracic pressure, as occurs in tension pneumothorax or with positive end-expiratory pressure, impedes venous return to the heart, diminishes intrathoracic blood volume, and reduces ventricular end-diastolic volume. Elevated intrapericardial pressure, as with pericardial tamponade, interferes with ventricular filling, lowering stroke volume and ventricular work. Venoconstriction and the pumping action of skeletal muscle are active systems responsible for venous return to the heart. Their loss preceding and during cardiac arrest results in decreased intrathoracic blood volume.

Inotropic state

Many factors determine and influence the velocity of myocardial fiber shortening. Variations in sympathetic nerve activity modify the quantity of norepinephrine released to act on the β-adrenergic receptors of the myocardium. Sympathetic nerve activity is one of the most important mechanisms determining the position of the myocardium on the force-velocity and ventricular function curves under physiologic conditions. When stimulated by sympathetic nerve activity the adrenal medulla releases catecholamines, thus augmenting the inotropic state of the heart. Exogenously administered inotropic agents such as epinephrine, norepinephrine, isoproterenol, calcium, caffeine, and theophylline improve the myocardial force-velocity relation, increasing ventricular performance. Conversely, physiologic depressants, acting either singly or in combination, can exert a depressant effect on the myocardial force-velocity curve, lowering ventricular performance. Physiologic depressants include severe myocardial hypoxia, hypercapnia, ischemia, and acidosis. Pharmacologic depressants, including β-blockers, calcium channel blockers, barbiturates, local and general anesthetics, and many other drugs, likewise reduce ventricular work. Myocardial stunning or necrosis caused by ischemia may profoundly affect total ventricular performance.

Afterload

The force and velocity of myocardial muscle fiber shortening at any given diastolic fiber length and myocardial inotropic state are inversely related to the afterload imposed on the myocardium. Stroke volume is determined by myocardial fiber length and velocity of fiber shortening. In turn, stroke volume and heart rate produce cardiac output, which, with peripheral arterial resistance produce arterial pressure or afterload. As ventricular function becomes more impaired, left ventricular afterload becomes

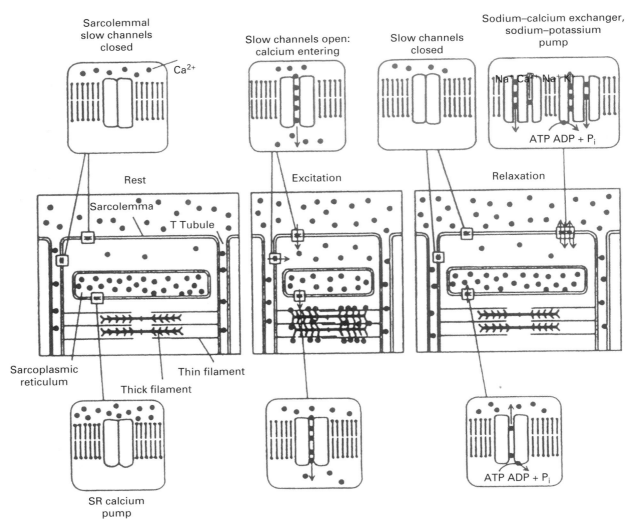

Fig. 22.4. Calcium fluxes that activate contraction are downhill, and those that cause relaxation are uphill. As depicted in heart muscle at rest, calcium channels in sarcolemmal membrane are closed, and intracellular calcium is stored in sarcoplasmic reticulum. With excitation and membrane depolarization, voltage-sensitive sodium channels (not shown) and calcium channels in sarcolemma open to allow rapid entry of extracellular sodium and calcium. Entry of calcium is now believed to cause release of calcium from sarcoplasmic reticulum that initiates contraction. Reuptake of calcium by sarcoplasmic reticulum by an ATP-dependent calcium pump is essential for heart to relax. Of importance, contraction is activated mainly by passive calcium fluxes from sarcoplasmic reticulum. By contrast, during diastole calcium must be pumped actively out of cytosol to accomplish relaxation. Energy also must be expended during diastole to restore sodium and calcium gradients across sarcolemma, which provide for depolarizing ionic currents that generate action potential. Sodium transport is accomplished by sarcolemmal sodium pump (Na^+-K^+ ATPase), which utilizes ATP to pump sodium out of the cell in exchange for potassium. Resultant sodium gradient is largely responsible for active transport of calcium out of cell during relaxation, via sodium-calcium exchange. (From Katz AM, Smith VE. Myocardial relaxation abnormalities. Part I: mechanisms. *Hosp.Prac.*1984; 19(1):69. Illustration by Bunji Tagawa.)

increasingly important in determining cardiac performance. Influences on the arterial bed of neural, humoral, or structural changes that increase afterload may further reduce cardiac output while myocardial oxygen requirements are increased.

Pulseless electrical activity feedback loop

Preceding the onset of PEA, as the force and velocity of myocardial contraction decrease, stroke volume is reduced. Although a transient compensatory increase in heart rate can be seen, eventually cardiac output and aortic pressure are decreased. Lowered aortic pressure decreases coronary artery perfusion, resulting in increased myocardial ischemia, hypoxemia, and reduced myocardial function. The force and velocity of myocardial fiber shortening are further reduced, exacerbating lowered stroke volume and further decreasing aortic pressure. This negative feedback loop characterizes the pathophysiology of PEA and represents the challenge for therapeutic intervention (Fig. 22.5).

Animal models of pulseless electrical activity

The various animal models for PEA provide insight into its pathophysiology and reflect its heterogeneous nature. PEA may be generated in the isolated perfused rat heart or intact dog by producing severe acidosis with a perfusion fluid of acetoacetate and glucose.[12] High concentrations of acetoacetate and lactic acid produced by cellular utilization of glucose via anaerobic glycolysis result in severe extracellular and intracellular acidosis that reliably inhibits ventricular contraction.[12] Perfusion of the heart in a calcium-free medium also produces PEA.[13] These animal models have been developed primarily to study techniques of open heart surgery and cardiopulmonary bypass.

The two animal models most commonly used to study resuscitation techniques in PEA are the asphyxia model and postdefibrillation model in dogs. In the asphyxia model, after anesthesia, intubation, and instrumentation, the endotracheal tube is occluded at the end of exhalation. This is followed by initial hypertension and tachycardia and then progressive hypotension and bradycardia until aortic pressure fluctuations cease approximately 10 minutes after airway obstruction. To simulate downtime in cardiac arrest, most experimental protocols continue airway obstruction without intervention for 5 to 10 minutes after the last systolic aortic pressure fluctuation. During this time period, the ECG of the dog shows normal or nearly normal sequences of P, QRS, and T waves, usually at a bradycardic rate unaccompanied by any fluctuation in aortic pressure. Following this predetermined downtime, the obstruction of the endotracheal tube is reversed, cardiopulmonary resuscitation (CPR) is started, and the experimental protocol is initiated.[14] Because ECG activity continues for prolonged periods after complete cessation of myocardial contraction, the asphyxia model can study the effects of interventions at either short or long downtimes.

Some investigators think that the asphyxia dog model for PEA more closely approximates the clinical presentation of patients with PEA who frequently have a respiratory cause for cardiac arrest and variable downtimes. This

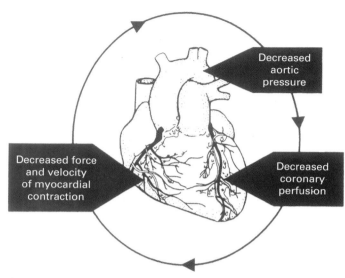

Fig. 22.5. PEA feedback loop.

model provides some evidence that following the onset and persistence of severe hypoxia in human patients, the presence of initial hypertension and tachycardia may indicate a grave sign of impending cardiac arrest.

In the postdefibrillation animal model, after anesthesia, intubation, and instrumentation, PEA is induced by passing an AC current through a bipolar electrode positioned at the right ventricle, initiating ventricular fibrillation. After a predetermined time (approximately 5 minutes) of ventricular fibrillation without artificial circulatory or ventilatory support, one or more transthoracic countershocks are administered until ventricular fibrillation is terminated. After this treatment responses can vary: there may be electrical activity with detectable pulses, electrical activity with absent pulses but measurable aortic pressures of 20 to 40 mm Hg, or electrical activity without detectable pulses and no measurable aortic pressures. With ventricular fibrillation times of 5 to 7 minutes, the most frequent response is spontaneous cardiac electrical activity accompanied by absent aortic pressure fluctuations. In such circumstances, CPR is begun and the experimental protocol initiated. The situation in the postdefibrillation animal model closely resembles the pulseless, spontaneous cardiac rhythm seen in up to 60% of resuscitation attempts following prehospital ventricular fibrillation.[15,16] The postdefibrillation animal model, however, has the disadvantage of a potentially variable response following defibrillation, which appears related to the time of ventricular fibrillation before the defibrillation attempt. This may be consistent with the clinical observation that postdefibrillation PEA may be more common after countershock of fine ventricular fibrillation in patients with longer downtimes.[17] Some investigators postulate that the development of PEA immediately following defibrillation represents a transitory recovery rhythm that in some cases improves spontaneously leading to the appearance of pulses, supraventricular activity, and stabilization of hemodynamic status.[18]

Another model, the acute cardiac tamponade model, is produced by making a small incision in the dog pericardium, inserting a polyethylene catheter into the pericardial sac, and fastening the cut pericardium around the catheter with a string suture. Tamponade is induced by injecting fixed volumes (60 ml/increment) of warmed saline (37 °C) into the pericardial cavity through the intrapericardial catheter until peak left ventricular pressure is depressed to 25 mm Hg. The intrapericardial volume is maintained until PEA occurs, as verified by the absence of left ventricular pressures corresponding with the QRS complex of the ECG. This acute cardiac tamponade model allows study of the role of the sympathetic and parasympathetic nervous systems in the initiation of PEA during acute cardiac tamponade and the response to therapeutic intervention.

Notably, the use of different models with different pathophysiologic processes and variable downtimes makes comparison between studies and application to the clinical setting difficult.

Normotensive, pseudo-, and true pulseless electrical activity

Pathophysiologic associations

Ischemia

Although the precise cause and pathogenesis of PEA remain poorly understood, much evidence points toward ischemia as the underlying cause of myocardial excitation contraction uncoupling.[19,20] Ischemia may occur locally or globally. Under experimental conditions, occlusion of a coronary vessel rapidly leads to disappearance of myocardial contraction in the area at risk, although electrical activity may be initially unchanged.[6,21,22] The clinical syndrome of PEA may arise when a large enough area of myocardium is rendered ischemic. Subsequent local ischemia may result in systolic or diastolic left ventricular dysfunction severe enough to produce hypotension that eventually leads to global ischemia (Fig. 22.5).

In studies of localized coronary artery occlusions of various durations in the anesthetized dog, the rate of improvement of myocardial function was shown to be inversely proportional to the duration of occlusion.[23–28] A period of coronary occlusion of less than 20 minutes may not be associated with the development of myocardial necrosis but may result in depressed myocardial contraction for several days.[29] Braunwald and Kloner postulated that ischemia may interfere with normal myocardial function, biochemical processes, and ultrastructure for prolonged periods, resulting in myocardial stunning.[29]

The development of PEA, however, is not thought to depend solely on local occlusion of a coronary artery. Global ischemia resulting in hypoxia, acidosis, and increased vagal tone from any source appears to make the myocardium vulnerable to global depolarization and the uncoupling of excitation and contraction.[8,22]

Calcium

With global ischemia there is neither washout of metabolites nor delivery of substrate; thus, after an initial rapid loss of myocardial function, further cellular damage is slowly progressive.[30] Some investigators have shown that it is reperfusion of ischemic tissues that actually causes the most significant damage.[31–33] The role of calcium in producing ultrastructural myocardial damage associated with ischemia and reperfusion was first examined by Shen and Jennings.[34,35] Forty minutes of ischemia followed by 10 minutes of arterial reperfusion in an animal model resulted in an 18-fold increase in calcium uptake in injured myocardial tissue.[30,34,35] Calcium uptake was accompanied by massive cellular swelling, mitochondrial and myofibrillar damage, and the appearance of contraction bands and intramitochondrial calcium phosphate deposits.

Calcium may be involved in the development of PEA by several mechanisms. Defects in excitatory Ca^{2+} release could occur because of the loss of the triggering Ca^{2+} current or because of a change in the sarcoplasmic reticular Ca^{2+} store.[19] The sensitivity of the contraction process to calcium may be reduced.[19] For example, the affinity of Ca^{2+} for troponin C necessary for excitation contraction coupling can be reduced by some metabolic factors, such as acidosis.[19]

Intracellular pH

Persistent ischemia or anoxia results in continued anaerobic glycolysis, lactic acid production, and acidosis. It has been proposed that intracellular acidosis changes the affinity of troponin C for Ca^{2+}, thus contributing to excitation contraction uncoupling. Whether acidosis initiates this process fast enough to entirely explain complete contractile failure in PEA remains unanswered. Measurements of intracellular pH changes by magnetic resonance provide values integrated over 3 to 4 minutes, and, as a result, the intracellular changes in the first few minutes of PEA are difficult to measure.[19,36] Further, magnetic resonance methodology uses the phase shift for inorganic phosphate to determine intracellular pH, which may be encountered by the contractile proteins.[19] Conversely, extracellular acidosis is known to occur quickly after the onset of ischemia. The decrease in affinity of troponin C for Ca^{2+} resulting from intracellular acidosis is probably partially responsible for excitation contraction coupling; however, there is insufficient evidence at this time to attribute contractile failure entirely to acidosis.

Adenosine triphosphate

Depletion of ATP may be a key factor in the development of PEA and in determining the potential reversibility of the process.[7,30,37,38] Some investigators have shown that intracellular ATP concentrations in ischemic myocardium fall to approximately 50% of normal after 15 minutes of ischemia.[29,39] Myocardial ATP levels in these studies also remained reduced for days following reperfusion.[29,39] Since recovery of myocardial function parallels the recovery of intracellular ATP concentrations, it is tempting to speculate that they are causally related.[29] It is possible that myocardial function remains depressed until ATP stores or at least the pool of ATP directly related to the contractile process has returned to normal. However, other factors including calcium flux also may be responsible.[29]

Other investigators have suggested that lowered but functional levels of ATP are maintained during ischemia and are present at the time of contractile failure.[40,41] ATP that is used during the early phases of development of ischemia is replaced by breakdown of phosphocreatine and, to a lesser degree, by anaerobic glycolysis. This process leads to substantial increases in inorganic phosphate and modest increases in ADP.[17] Increases in inorganic phosphates and ADP limit the free energy available from ATP, resulting in metabolic inefficiency.[19,22]

It has also been proposed that ischemia disrupts the modulatory function of ATP, possibly affecting calcium entry into cells, calcium efflux from the sarcoplasmic reticulum, or both.[20,22] Increased intracellular levels of inorganic phosphates may also contribute to the development of PEA by forming insoluble calcium phosphate precipitates, thus trapping calcium in the sarcoplasmic reticulum and mitochondria.[20,22]

Autonomic nervous system

Kostreva et al. studied the role of the autonomic nervous system in the initiation of PEA during acute cardiac tamponade in a dog model.[42] The onset of PEA in this model was significantly delayed by either surgical or pharmacologic sympathectomy, leading the authors to conclude that the sympathetic efferent component of the autonomic nervous system plays an important role in the initiation of PEA.[42] Cardiac sympathetic efferent stimulation increased the heart rate and double product (Heart rate × Peak left ventricular pressure ÷ 100), thereby increasing cardiac work and oxygen consumption and promoting the initiation of PEA. β-blockade with propranolol decreased the double product and heart rate, significantly delaying the onset of PEA. Although this PEA model did not show any apparent effect on initiation of PEA with bilateral vagotomy, other authors contend that the parasympathetic nervous system also plays an important role.

DeBehnke found that complete loss of vagal tone through surgical vagotomy significantly improved the rate of return of spontaneous circulation from experimental asphyxial PEA cardiac arrest in a dog model.[43] The greater incidence of inferior myocardial infarctions in patients with PEA also suggests a role of the autonomic nervous system.[6,22] Acute increases in parasympathetic activity or withdrawal of sympathetic activity may be partially responsible for initiating the condition. Precipitous decreases in heart rate and blood pressure attributed to the Bezold-Jarish reflex are frequently seen with inferior myocardial infarctions and the development of PEA.[44] The role of the autonomic nervous system in triggering the sequence of events leading to PEA is still undefined and remains a promising area for further research.

Other metabolic derangements

Hypoxia resulting in anaerobic glycolysis and severe lactic acidosis is thought to precipitate PEA in a significant proportion of patients. In an autopsy study, Pirolo et al. reported that approximately 20% of PEA patients had a respiratory cause of cardiac arrest.[8] In a prehospital study, Stueven et al. reported approximately 53% of successfully resuscitated prehospital PEA patients had a probable respiratory cause for their arrest.[4] After the onset of ischemia, cellular action potentials decrease and become sufficiently depolarized to become inexcitable. This depolarization is due almost entirely to an accumulation of extracellular potassium.[45,46]

There are predictable cardiovascular responses to hypothermia.[47] After an initial tachycardia, progressive bradycardia occurs, with a 50% decrease in the palpable pulse at 28 °C.[47] Because the conduction system is more sensitive to cold than is the myocardium, the cardiac cycle is prolonged.[48] The PR, QRS, and QT intervals are sequentially prolonged with reduction of core temperature.[48] Hypothermia decreases the mean arterial pressure and cardiac index. With core temperatures below 25 °C, ventricular fibrillation, PEA, or asystole can occur.[49] The

Table 22.1. Unsuccessful vs. successful resuscitations

Group [a]	Rate	Presence of P waves (%)	QT interval (SEC)	QRS interval (SEC)
Group I ($n=405$)	55 ± 27 } [b]	21.0 } [b]	0.56 ± 0.2 } [b]	0.12 ± 0.06 } [b]
Group II initial ($n=98$)	75 ± 45 }	42.9 }	0.46 ± 0.21 }	0.09 ± 0.04 }
Group II final ($n=98$)	114 ± 36 } [b]	60.0 } [c]	0.40 ± 0.11 } [c]	0.09 ± 0.03

[a] Group I, unsuccessful resuscitations; group II, successful resuscitations.
[b] $P\leq0.01$.
[c] $P\leq0.04$.

Table 22.2. Rate vs. outcome

		Group II			
		Initial		Final	
Rate (beats/min)	Group I(%)	Died (%)	Lived (%)	Died (%)	Lived (%)
Tachycardia (rate ≥100)	8.68	22.08	36.36	74.06	25.00
Normal rate (60–100)	28.68	35.06	27.27	18.54	68.75
Bradycardia (rate ≤60)	62.64	42.86	36.37	7.40	6.25

mechanism is poorly defined. Tissue hypoxia, acid-base disturbances, and autonomic dysfunction all have been implicated.[47]

A variety of medications reduce myocardial contractility and may result in PEA in drug overdoses. Tricyclic antidepressants, β-blockers, calcium channel blockers, and digitalis can produce PEA.[50]

Coronary perfusion pressure is well established as the most important predictor of return of spontaneous circulation in cardiac arrest patients.[51,52] With gradual loss of myocardial contractility that often occurs before the onset of PEA, myocardial hypoxia and acidosis are further intensified by the corresponding decrease in coronary perfusion pressure.

Effects of metabolic derangements on electrocardiographic characteristics

Aufderheide *et al.* studied the ECG characteristics in PEA in 503 prehospital adult cardiac arrest patients.[2] The initial and final ECG characteristics were compared for unsuccessfully (group I) and successfully (group II) resuscitated patients (Table 22.1). On initial prehospital presentation, patients with PEA who responded to therapy (group II) had significantly faster initial rates, a higher incidence of P waves, and average shorter QRS and QT intervals than did patients not responding to therapy (Group I). Successfully resuscitated patients were capable of increasing heart rates, shortening QT intervals, and developing the new

onset of P waves in response to treatment. Further, successfully resuscitated patients had an average initial and final QRS complex length within normal limits, and these remained unchanged with therapy (Table 22.1).

Successful resuscitations (Group II) were divided into those who lived and those who died. ECG parameters were not significantly different with respect to the presence of P waves or QT or QRS interval. Heart rate was significantly different in these two groups (Table 22.2). Patients who responded to therapy but eventually died increased their heart rate over baseline, and it remained significantly elevated when compared with patients who lived. In the group of patients who died, 74% presented to the emergency department with tachycardias. Conversely, those patients who were successfully resuscitated and lived had faster initial presenting heart rates and these tended to become normal with therapy; that is, bradycardias increased and tachycardias decreased. Nearly 69% of PEA saves (defined as discharged from the hospital alive) arrived at the emergency department with normal rates. Bradycardias were the predominant presenting rhythm in unsuccessful resuscitations (Table 22.2).

There appeared to be a relationship between the presence of sinoatrial activity and the rate of successful resuscitation and saves (Table 22.3). Successfully resuscitated patients had a significantly higher incidence of organized atrial activity on initial ECG than did non-responding patients. In addition, nearly 20% of successful resuscitations and 30% of

Table 22.3. Rhythm type vs. outcome

Rhythm type	Group I (%)	Group II			
		Initial		Final	
		Died (%)	Lived (%)	Died (%)	Lived (%)
Sinus activity related to QRS complex	12.40	32.47	45.46	53.69	75
Second- and third-degree atrioventricular block	7.93	7.79	0	0	0
Atrial fibrillation	0	2.60	4.55	3.70	0
Supraventricular tachycardia	0.99	0	0	12.96	0
Nodal	34.16	25.98	27.28	22.21	25
Wide complex rhythms without P waves	44.57	25.98	22.73	7.14	0

saves developed the new onset of organized atrial activity with treatment. No patient with an initial ECG rhythm of second- or third-degree atrioventricular (AV) block survived to hospital discharge. Similarly, supraventricular tachycardia appeared to be associated with a negative outcome. PEA saves were in those patients who presented to the emergency department following treatment and who had sinus activity related to the QRS complex (75%) or narrow complex nodal rhythms (25%).

The time from onset of cardiac arrest, as estimated by the paramedics, was significantly longer for unsuccessful resuscitations than for successful resuscitations.[2]

Earlier PEA ECG studies performed in animals and humans demonstrated a progression of ECG characteristics with time from onset of anoxia.[7,18,53–67] After the onset of anoxia, the vagi and the electrical cardiac conduction system respond to ever-worsening metabolic events, including lactic acidosis, hypoxia, electrolyte abnormalities, and depletion of intracellular metabolites including ATP and creatine phosphate.[19,25,28,29,39,68–70] These metabolic events worsen with time but are potentially reversible through pharmacologic and non-pharmacologic resuscitative intervention. It is tempting to speculate, therefore, that the observed ECG characteristics in PEA patients are a function of time from onset of anoxia and consequently provide a predictive indicator for successful resuscitation and survival.

Stueven *et al.* classified PEA patients into four groups based on initial ECG morphology and related this classification to patient outcome in 503 PEA patients treated in an emergency medical system.[3] Group 1 and group 2A classifications represented more normal ECG complexes. Thus PEA patients who were successfully resuscitated or saved had initial ECG complexes classified as group 1 or group 2A. Group 2B and group 3 represented more abnormal ECG complexes. Consequently, no PEA patient

Table 22.4. Duration of ECG components in patients with true PEA and pseudo-PEA[a]

	True PEA	Pseudo-PEA	P
QR	0.19 ± 0.13 (0.04–0.56)	0.07 ± 0.05 (0.02–0.20)	0.0004
RS	0.12 ± 0.08 (0.05–0.24)	0.09 ± 0.05 (0.04–0.24)	0.5
QRS	0.24 ± 0.12 (0.11–0.56)	0.12 ± 0.06 (0.04–0.26)	0.006

[a] Values are durations expressed in seconds, with range in parentheses.

classified in group 2B or group 3 was saved or successfully resuscitated. The authors of this study speculated that these four classifications represented progressive stages in the anoxic process, which accounted for their predictive value with respect to outcome or response to therapy (Fig. 22.6).[3]

Paradis *et al.* extended these findings by studying the relationship between the ECG and perfusion by measuring central aortic pressure in patients during PEA.[1] Ninety-four patients with PEA were classified as those with and those without aortic pulse pressures, and the ECG findings and rates of return of spontaneous circulation in the two groups were compared.[1]

Patients whose ECG showed regular, organized depolarizations but who lacked palpable carotid or femoral arterial pulses were designated to be in PEA: those without aortic pulse pressures were defined as being in true PEA ($n = 55$); those with regular aortic pulse pressures less than 60 mm Hg that were synchronous with ECG depolarizations were designated as having pseudo-PEA.

The QR and QRS durations of patients with true PEA and pseudo-PEA are compared in Table 22.4. Patients with pseudo-PEA had shorter QR and QRS durations than did patients with true PEA.

Group 1

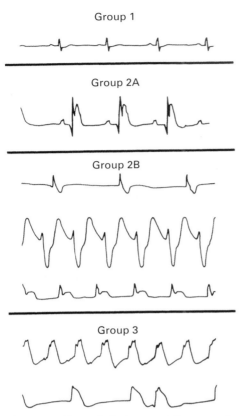

Group 2A

Group 2B

Group 3

Fig. 22.6. PEA morphologic presentation: group 1, normal QRS width, isoelectric ST waves and normal-appearing T waves; group 2A, atrial activity, widened QRS width ($\leq$ 0.12 msec) or abnormal ST or T waves (ST depression, elevation, slurring or T-wave inversion); group 2B, same as 2A but with no atrial activity; group 3, essentially monophasic, slurred RST complexes. These classifications may represent progressive stages in anoxic process of PEA. (From ref. 3.)

A concurrent study of the effect of high-dose epinephrine on CPR coronary perfusion pressure allowed assessment of the effects of standard- and high-dose epinephrine on each type of PEA (71). Eight (15%) of 55 patients in true PEA and 14 (36%) of 39 in pseudo-PEA responded to standard therapy, including epinephrine doses of 1 mg with return of spontaneous circulation ($P = .016$). Six (23%) of the 26 patients in true PEA who received high-dose epinephrine had return of spontaneous circulation. Of the 18 patients with pseudo-PEA who received high-dose epinephrine, 14 (78%) had return of spontaneous circulation. This was significantly greater than the proportion with return of spontaneous circulation after standard doses ($P = 0.003$) and was the best outcome among all combinations of PEA type and epinephrine dose ($P = 0.001$).

Table 22.5. Characteristics of patients with true PEA and pseudo-PEA

Characteristic	True PEA	Pseudo-PEA	P
Age (yr)	71 ± 15	65 ± 15	0.7
Total arrest time (min)	25 ± 11	21 ± 13	0.44
Witnessed arrests	22/55	26/39	0.01
PO_2 (mm Hg)	237 ± 168	310 ± 134	0.03
PCO_2 (mm Hg)	34 ± 23	24 ± 16	0.04
pH	7.23 ± .25	7.23 ± .25	0.7
Coronary perfusion pressure (mm Hg)	9.9 ± 11.5	19.2 ± 9.5	<0.0001

True and pseudo-pulseless electrical activity

These studies demonstrate that patients with a clinical diagnosis of PEA are in a spectrum of perfusion states that range from normotension to complete absence of perfusion. The fact that many patients clinically in PEA have mechanical cardiac activity should be considered when interpreting the results of cardiac arrest studies. Further, patients with pseudo-PEA appear to have a different short-term prognosis and response to therapy than do patients in true PEA. On the basis of the above preliminary data, administration of high-dose epinephrine may be considered in the treatment of narrow-complex PEA in the hope of improving patient outcome.[1]

Although the minimal perfusion present in patients with pseudo-PEA may be the reason for better short-term outcomes, it is also possible that pseudo-PEA is characterized by a less deranged pathophysiologic state and therefore is more amenable to resuscitation.[1,2] The characteristics of patients with true PEA and pseudo-PEA are shown in Table 22.5. The younger age and higher coronary perfusion pressures in patients with pseudo-PEA are consistent with this conclusion. The greater proportion of witnessed arrests in patients with pseudo-PEA suggests that arrest times are shorter.[1] Further, the estimated time from onset of cardiac arrest to arrival of paramedics has been found to be shorter in PEA patients responding to treatment.[2]

Rapid differentiation of true PEA and pseudo-PEA may be important because of the higher frequency of return of spontaneous circulation with standard and high doses of epinephrine previously mentioned. Consideration of the characteristics of patients with true PEA and pseudo-PEA (Table 22.5) may be helpful, as well as consideration of the ECG characteristics. Patients in PEA who are successfully resuscitated have average QRS intervals that are shorter (0.09 second ± 0.03 second) than those without return of spontaneous circulation (0.12 second ± 0.06 second).[2] The observation that patients in pseudo-PEA differ in their initial but not terminal QRS deflection indicates the importance of the initial QR deflection (Fig. 22.7).[2] Paradis *et al.* demonstrated that no patient with pseudo-PEA had a QRS interval or initial deflection in the QRS of more than 0.2 second.[1] A QRS duration of 0.12 second or less and especially a normal duration of the initial QR deflection occur most frequently in patients with pseudo-PEA. Nonetheless, there is significant overlap in the average ECG values acquired in PEA patient populations, and these values may not apply in specific cases.

Patients with baseline cardiac contractions (normotensive PEA) probably represent individuals in the first seconds to minutes after the onset of hypovolemia, tension pneumothorax, cardiac tamponade, or other sudden causes for severe preload or afterload reduction. No studies indicate that normotensive PEA represents a significant subset of PEA patients seen by practicing clinicians. It is included as a subset primarily for understanding the pathophysiology and clinical spectrum of PEA. Its detection, however, may assist the clinician in identifying a readily reversible cause for PEA.

Rapid and definitive differentiation among normotensive PEA, pseudo-PEA, and true PEA can be achieved by immediate emergency department echocardiography able to demonstrate myocardial wall motion in patients with clinical PEA. Placement of a Doppler probe over the femoral triangle may rapidly detect pulsatile blood flow. Establishing a peripheral (femoral or radial) arterial line may assist in the differentiation of pseudo-PEA.

Alternatively, placement of a central pressure monitoring catheter may alternatively demonstrate aortic pressures in patients without a clinically detectable pulse.

Causes of pulseless electrical activity

In many patients, PEA is not a primary cardiac arrest but rather a state of severe cardiogenic shock from another etiology. This severe hypotension may propagate the PEA feedback loop: hypotension causes decreased coronary perfusion, which impairs myocardial function, which results in greater hypotension (Fig. 22.5). Indeed, myocardial contractility is normal on initiation of PEA (normotensive PEA). As the process continues, decreased cardiac contractions occur (pseudo-PEA), eventually resulting in absent cardiac contractions (true PEA). The multiple causes of PEA play a central role in therapeutic intervention. Consequently, one major action that must be taken when PEA occurs is the rapid search for possible reversible causes.[50]

Pulmonary causes

The most common cause of PEA is probably severe and sustained respiratory insufficiency or respiratory arrest. Respiratory insufficiency has been implicated as the cause of PEA in 20 to 53% of cases.[4,8]

Preload reduction

Hypovolemia was reported as the cause of PEA in 4.4% of prehospital patients:[4] 3.3% had hemorrhage and 1.1%

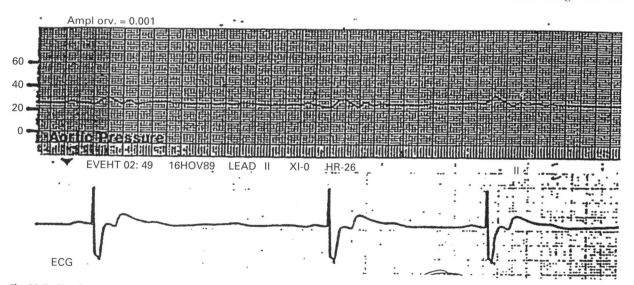

Fig. 22.7. Simultaneous aortic arch pressure (expressed in million meters of mercury) and lead II ECG from patient in pseudo-PEA. Total QRS duration of 0.12 msec or less and especially a normal duration of initial QR deflection are more frequently seen in patients with pseudo-PEA. (From ref. 1.)

had functional volume depletion as a result of sepsis.[4] *Pulmonary embolism* results in an increase in pulmonary vascular resistance resulting in an increase in pulmonary arterial pressure. If more than 50% of the pulmonary vascular tree is occluded, left ventricular enddiastolic volume is critically reduced and hemodynamic collapse occurs.

Mechanical causes

Mechanical causes of PEA are so classified because their etiology is related to anatomic structure and their resolution requires mechanical intervention. *Tension pneumothorax* compresses the affected lung, shifting the mediastinum toward the unaffected side and severely reducing cardiac output because of positive intrathoracic pressure decreasing venous return to the heart. *Cardiac tamponade* interferes with normal ventricular filling and results in critically low cardiac output.

Auto-PEEP is a recently described cause of PEA in patients with bronchospastic pulmonary disease during mechanical ventilation. When there is inadequate time for complete exhalation, dynamic forces such as increased respiratory frequency, airway collapse, tidal volume, percentage of inspiratory time (which reduces absolute expiratory time), or a combination of these factors results in air trapping or hyperinflation of the lungs.[72,73] An important consequence of dynamic hyperinflation is that alveolar pressure remains positive throughout expiration, leading to the development of "occult" PEEP. The hemodynamic consequences are identical to those caused by extrinsically applied PEEP that produce increasing intrathoracic pressure, increased pulmonary vascular resistance, and decreased venous return to the heart.[74–76]

Myocardial dysfunction

A direct myocardial dysfunction may cause PEA via a variety of conditions. *Acute myocardial infarction* may cause a critical loss of left ventricular contraction. *Myocardial ischemia* may interfere with normal myocardial function, biochemical processes, and ultrastructure for prolonged periods, resulting in "stunned" myocardium.[29] An autopsy study identified myocardial ischemia as the precipitating cause of PEA in 44% of cases.[8] Patients with end-stage *congestive heart failure* may develop hypotension that causes decreased coronary perfusion and results in myocardial ischemia that further impairs myocardial function. Drug overdoses with *tricyclic antidepressants*, β-*blockers, calcium channel blockers*, and *digitalis* can depress myocardial function and result in hemodynamic collapse. *Hyperkalemia* slows electrical cardiac conduction and depresses myocardial contractility.[77] *Hypothermia*

results in decreased spontaneous depolarization of pacemaker cells, bradydysrhythmias, decreased mean arterial pressure, and decreased cardiac index.[48,49]

Postdefibrillation pulseless electrical activity

Countershock of ventricular fibrillation may be followed by transient PEA in up to 60% of resuscitation attempts.[16] Hoffman and Stevenson reviewed 100 consecutive patients with prehospital ventricular fibrillation receiving countershock.[18] Thirteen (27%) of the forty-nine patients who developed immediate postdefibrillation PEA were admitted to the hospital, and four (8%) were discharged from the hospital alive.[18] These patients had statistically significantly better outcomes than the 25 patients who failed to achieve any organized rhythm in the field. As the initial cardiac arrest rhythm, postcountershock PEA may have a slightly better prognosis than does true PEA. Many patients immediately experiencing postcountershock PEA subsequently develop pulses. Although patients immediately developing supraventricular rhythms with pulses have a better survival rate, the development of postdefibrillation PEA has a prognosis that is neither better nor worse than before defibrillation and statistically better than the prognosis for patients in whom defibrillation fails to produce any organized rhythm. It is therefore postulated that the development of PEA immediately following defibrillation may represent a transient recovery rhythm that, in some cases, spontaneously improves, leading to the appearance of pulses, supraventricular activity, stabilization of hemodynamic status, and possible long-term survival.[18] The variability in return of spontaneous circulation following postcountershock PEA compared with PEA as the initial cardiac arrest rhythm should be considered when interpreting cardiac arrest studies.

Therapy

Therapy for PEA depends on correcting metabolic derangements, correcting anatomic structural derangements, and rapidly reversing underlying causes for PEA.

Correcting metabolic derangements

Because respiratory insufficiency is the cause of PEA in up to 53% of cases, reversal of hypoxia with immediate airway stabilization and hyperventilation with 100% oxygen is indicated in all patients. Maintaining adequate alveolar ventilation and restoration of tissue perfusion, first with chest compressions and then with rapid restoration of spontaneous circulation, should be the primary goal of acid-base therapy in cardiac arrest. Hyperventilation will partially correct respiratory acidosis by removing carbon dioxide.[78] Laboratory and clinical data fail to show conclusively that low blood pH adversely affects ability to restore spontaneous circulation or short-term survival.[79–81] The use of sodium bicarbonate for treatment of acidosis following return of spontaneous circulation after a long arrest interval is thought to increase cerebrospinal fluid acidosis, is thought to be insufficient to reverse myocardial acidosis, and indeed may be potentially harmful because of its reduction in coronary perfusion pressure.[82–86] The use of bicarbonate may be considered as a therapeutic option with the weight of evidence in favor of its usefulness and efficacy in patients with preexisting metabolic acidosis, hyperkalemia, or tricyclic or phenobarbital overdose.[50]

Treatment of the cardiotoxic effects of various drug overdoses can be effective in the shock state but has not been clearly demonstrated to be effective in cardiac arrest. The direct cardiotoxic effects of tricyclic antidepressant overdose can often be reversed by producing a systemic arterial pH above 7.5 by hyperventilation and the use of intravenous bicarbonate.[50] The cardiosuppressant effects of overdoses of β-blockers respond variably to intravenous glucagon, epinephrine, isoproterenol, and intravascular volume expansion. The cardiac suppressant effects of overdoses of calcium channel blockers can be reversed with intravenous calcium chloride or calcium gluconate. Massive digitalis overdose is treated with intravenous Digabind. The cardiotoxic effects of hyperkalemia are immediately reversed with intravenous calcium chloride or calcium gluconate, followed by intravenous bicarbonate, 10 units of regular insulin, and 1 ampule of intravenous D-50. Therapeutic options for reversing hypothermia include passive external rewarming or active external or core rewarming.[48,49]

Correcting severely reduced preload

Patients with hypotension caused by known hypovolemia should receive rapid intravenous volume expansion. Needle and tube thoracostomies may improve venous return to the heart in patients with tension pneumothorax. Subxiphoid pericardiocentesis may be lifesaving in patients with pericardial tamponade.

Reducing increased vagal tone

Atropine has been recommended by the American Heart Association in cases of bradycardic PEA (below 60 beats/min) or in patients with relative bradycardia.[50] Atropine may reduce increased vagal tone. It has been demonstrated that patients in PEA who respond to treatment with rate normalization have a higher resuscitation and save rate.[2] The atropine dose-response rate for human subjects in PEA has not been established.

Pharmacologically increasing coronary perfusion pressure

α-Adrenergic stimulation improves coronary perfusion pressure, which has been shown experimentally and clinically to predict return of spontaneous circulation.[51,87] Epinephrine has been the adrenergic agent of choice in cardiac arrest. Preliminary information suggests that patients with PEA have a higher rate of return of spontaneous circulation in response to high-dose rather than standard dose epinephrine.[88] Further, patients in pseudo-PEA may benefit from high-dose epinephrine (1). High-dose epinephrine may interrupt the feedback loop of hypotension that causes decreased coronary perfusion and further impairs myocardial function in such patients (Fig. 22.5).

Mechanically increasing coronary perfusion pressure

Maintaining adequate coronary perfusion pressure by utilizing closed chest CPR and intravenous adrenergic agents is the mainstay of therapy for PEA. Modifying existing CPR techniques may improve forward flow, thus increasing coronary perfusion pressure and possibly improving patient outcome. Interopposed abdominal compression CPR, circumferential compression of the chest with use of a pneumatic vest, and active compression-decompression CPR have been shown to improve coronary perfusion pressures and blood flow compared with standard CPR.[89–96]. Cardiopulmonary bypass implemented within 15 minutes after PEA arrest has improved return of spontaneous circulation rates compared with standard- and high-dose epinephrine in an animal postcountershock model.[97] Cardiopulmonary bypass may be a possible therapeutic option in appropriately staffed resuscitation institutions.

Assisting the cardiac electrical conduction system

Transvenous cardiac pacing was studied in a canine model of postcountershock PEA and was found to produce electrical capture but no cardiac contractions.[15] Until cardiac pacing in PEA is studied further, therapy should be aimed at increasing perfusion pressure with other interventions.

The future

PEA remains poorly understood at the biochemical, cellular, and clinical levels. Further investigation into the precise relationships between intracellular biochemical events and myocardial contraction is needed to define the pathologic biochemical cascade leading to uncoupling of excitation and contraction. Characterization of the mechanism for dysfunctional intracellular release and reaccumulation of

Ca^{2+} and the degree of change in affinity for Ca^{2+} during PEA are important areas for investigation. The presence and description of interfering structural changes between actin and myosin cross bridges, including tropomyosin and troponins T, I, and C, at the physiologic extremes seen in PEA may assist understanding of this pathologic process. Further characterization of the biochemical interactions of intracellular high-energy phosphate (ATP) might lead to interventions designed to minimize depletion and facilitate regeneration of myocardial ATP stores.

PEA clinically presents with a spectrum from normotensive to absent myocardial contraction, and there are numerous causes for this condition. Different etiologies may have significantly different pathophysiologic mechanisms and correspondingly different responses to treatment. Study of therapeutic options in PEA is currently limited to asphyxial, tamponade, and postdefibrillation animal models. There is a need to develop and study a much wider variety of animal models that reflect the types of PEA seen clinically, including tension pneumothorax, sepsis/hypovolemia, pulmonary embolus, and drug toxicity PEA animal models.

Perhaps the greatest recent advance in PEA has been the recognition of the important subset of pseudo-PEA patients and their apparent response to high-dose epinephrine therapy. Currently under development, portable and simplified echocardiographic technology may, in the near future, allow hospital and prehospital identification of such patients. Rapid and accurate identification of pseudo-PEA patients will allow clinicians to match PEA therapeutic intervention more accurately with underlying pathophysiology.

Acknowledgment

With appreciation to Ms. Dawn Kawa for her support of this project and superb manuscript preparation and revision.

REFERENCES

1. Paradis, N.A., Martin, G.B., Boetting, M.G., Rivers, E.P., Feingold, M., & Nowak, R.M. Aortic pressure during human cardiac arrest: identification of pseudo-electromechanical dissociation. *Chest* 1992; **101**(1): 123–128.
2. Aufderheide, T.P., Thakur, R.K., Stueven, H.A. *et al.* Electrocardiographic characteristics in EMD. *Resuscitation* 1989; **17**: 183–193.
3. Stueven, H.A., Aufderheide, T., Thakur, R.K., Hargarten, K., & Vanags, B. Defining electromechanical dissociation: morphologic presentation. *Resuscitation* 1989; **17**: 195–203.
4. Stueven, H.A., Aufderheide, T., Waite, E.M., & Mateer, J.R. Electromechanical dissociation: six years prehospital experience. *Resuscitation* 1989; **17**: 173–182.
5. Weaver, W.D., Copass, M.K., Hill, D.K. *et al.* Cardiac arrest treated with a new automatic external defibrillator by out-of-hospital first responders. *Am. J. Cardiol.* 1986; **57**: 1017–1021.
6. Raizes, G., Wagner, G.S., & Hacket, D.B. Instantaneous non-arrhythmic cardiac death in acute myocardial infarction. *Am. J. Cardiol.* 1973; **39**: 1–6.
7. Vincent, J.L., Thijs, L., Weil, M.H., Michaels, S., & Silverberg, R.A. Clinical and experimental studies on electromechanical dissociation. *Circulation* 1981; **64**: 18–67.
8. Pirolo, J.S., Hutchins, G.M., & Moore, G.W. Electromechanical dissociation: pathologic explanations in 50 patients. *Hum. Pathol.* 1985; **16**: 485–487.
9. Tresch, D.D., Thakur, R.K., Hoffman, R.G., Olson, D., & Brooks, H.L. Should the elderly be resuscitated following out-of-hospital cardiac arrest? *Am. J. Med.* 1989; **86**: 145–150.
10. Braunwald, E. Normal and abnormal myocardial function. In: Braunwald, E., Isselbacher, K.J., Petersdorf, R.G., Wilson, J.D., Martin, J.B., & Fauci, A.S., eds. *Harrison's Principles of Internal Medicine*, 11th edn. St Louis: McGraw-Hill, 1987: 896–905.
11. The heart. In: Cotran, R.S., Kumar, V., & Robbins, S.L., eds. *Robbins Pathologic Basis of Disease*, 4th ed. Philadelphia: WB Saunders, 1989: 597–656.
12. Zimmerman, A.N.E., Meijler, F.L., & Hulsmann, W.C. The inhibitory effect of acetoacetate on myocardial contraction [Letter]. *Lancet* 1962; Oct **13**: 757–758.
13. Zimmerman, A.N.E., Daems, W., Hulsmann, W.C., Snijder, J., Wisse, E., & Durrer, D. Morphological changes of heart muscle caused by successive perfusion with calcium-free and calcium-containing solutions (calcium paradox). *Cardiovasc. Res.* 1967; **1**: 201–209.
14. Redding, J.S., Haynes, R.R., & Thomas, J.D. Drug therapy in resuscitation from electromechanical dissociation. *Crit. Care Med.* 1983; **11**(9): 681–684.
15. Niemann, J.T., Haynes, K.S., Garner, D., Rennie, C.J., Jagels, G., & Stormo, O. Postcountershock pulseless rhythms: response to CPR, artificial cardiac pacing, and adrenergic agonists. *Ann. Emerg. Med.* 1986; **15**: 112–120.
16. Warner, L.L., Hoffman, J.R., & Baraff, L.J. Prognostic significance of field response in out-of-hospital ventricular fibrillation. *Chest* 1985; **87**: 22–28.
17. Weaver, W.D., Cobb, L.A., Dennis, D. *et al.* Amplitude of ventricular fibrillation waveform and outcome after cardiac arrest. *Ann. Intern. Med.* 1985; **102**: 53–55.
18. Hoffman, J.R., & Stevenson, L.W. Postdefibrillation idioventricular rhythm – a salvageable condition. *West J. Med.* 1987; **146**: 188–191.
19. Fozzard, H.A. Electromechanical dissociation and its possible role in sudden cardiac death. *J. Am. Coll. Cardiol.* 1985; **5**: 31B–34B.
20. Kubler, W., & Katz, A.M. Mechanism of early "pump" failure of the ischemic heart. *Am. J. Cardiol.* 1977; **40**: 467–471.

21. Tennant, R., & Wiggers, C.J. The effect of coronary occlusion on myocardial contraction. *Am. J. Physiol.* 1935; **112**: 351–361.

22. Charlap, S., Kahlam, S., Lichstein, E., & Frishman, W. Electro-mechanical dissociation: diagnosis, pathophysiology, and management. *Am. Heart J.* 1989; **118**(2): 355–360.

23. Heyndrickx, G.R., Baig, H., Nellers, P., Levsen, L., Fishbein, M.C., & Vatner, S.F. Depression of regional blood flow and wall thickening after brief coronary occlusions. *Am. J. Physiol.* 1978; **234**: H653.

24. Ellis, S.G., Henschke, C.I., Sandor, T., Wynne, J., Braunwald, E., & Kloner, R.A. Time course of functional and biochemical recovery of myocardium salvaged by reperfusion. *J. Am. Coll. Cardiol.* 1983; **1**(4):1047–1055.

25. Puri, P.S. Contractile and biochemical effects of coronary reperfusion after extended periods of coronary occlusion. *Am. J. Cardiol.* 1975; **36**: 244.

26. Weiner, J.M., Apstein, C.S., Arthur, J.H., Pirzada, F.A., & Hood, W.B. Persistence of myocardial injury following brief periods of coronary occlusion. *Cardiovasc. Res.* 1976; **10**: 678.

27. Wood, J.M., Hanley, H.G., Entman, M.L. *et al.* Biochemical ischemia in the dog. IV. Energy mechanisms during very early ischemia. *Circ. Res.* 1979; **44**: 52.

28. Hess, M.L., Barnhart, G.R., Crute, S., Komwatana, P., Krause, S., & Greenfield, L.J. Mechanical and biochemical effects of transient myocardial ischemia. *J. Surg. Res.* 1979; **26**: 175.

29. Braunwald, E., & Kloner, R.A. The stunned myocardium: prolonged, post-ischemic ventricular dysfunction. *Circulation* 1982; **66**(6): 1146–1149.

30. Martin, G.B. Use of calcium blockers in electromechanical dissociation. *Ann. Emerg. Med.* 1984; **13**(2): 846–848.

31. Nayler, W.G. The role of calcium in the ischemic myocardium. *Am. J. Pathol.* 1981; **102**: 267–270.

32. Weishaar, R.E., & Bing, R.J. The beneficial effect of a calcium channel blocker, diltiazem, on the ischemic-reperfused heart. *J. Mol. Cell. Cardiol.* 1980; **12**: 993–1009.

33. Ashraf, M., White, F., & Bloor, C.M. Ultrastructural influences of reperfusing dog myocardium with calcium-free blood after coronary artery occlusion. *Am. J. Pathol.* 1978; **90**: 423–428.

34. Shen, A.C., & Jennings, R.B. Kinetics of calcium accumulation in acute myocardial ischemic injury. *Am. J. Pathol.* 1972; **67**: 441–452.

35. Shen, A.C., & Jennings, R.B. Myocardial calcium and magnesium in acute ischemic injury. *Am. J. Pathol.* 1972; **67**: 417–440.

36. Allen, D.G., Morris, P.G., & Orchard, C.H. A transient alkalosis precedes acidosis during hypoxia in ferret heart. *J. Physiol. (Lond)* 1983; **343**: 58P–9.

37. Jennings, R.B., & Reimer, K.A. Lethal myocardial ischemic injury. *Am. J. Pathol.* 1981; **102**: 241–255.

38. Benson, E.S., Evans, G.T., Hallaway, B.E., Phibbs, C., & Frier, E.F. Myocardial creatine phosphate and nucleotides in anoxic cardiac arrest and recovery. *Am. J. Physiol.* 1961; **201**: 687–693.

39. DeBoer, L.W.V., Ingwall, J.S., Kloner, R.A., & Braunwald, E. Prolonged derangements of canine myocardial purine metabolism after a brief coronary artery occlusion not associated with anatomic evidence of necrosis. *Proc. Natl. Acad. Sci. USA* 1980; **77**(9): 5471–5475.

40. Katz, A.M. Effects of interrupted coronary flow upon myocardial metabolism and contractility. *Prog. Cardiovasc. Dis.* 1968; **10**: 450–465.

41. Kübler, W., & Katz, A.M. Mechanism of early "pump" failure of the ischemic heart. *Am. J. Cardiol.* 1977; **40**: 467–471.

42. Kostreva, D.R., Castaner, A., & Kampine, J.P. Role of autonomics in the initiation of electromechanical dissociation. *Am. J. Physiol.* 1981; **241**(*Regul. Integr. Comp. Physiol.* 10):R213–R221.

43. DeBehnke, D.J. Effects of vagal tone on resuscitation from experimental electro-mechanical dissociation. *Ann. Emerg. Med.* 1993; **22**: 1789–1794.

44. Frink, R.J., & James, T.N. Intracardiac route of the Bezold-Jarisch reflex. *Am. J. Physiol.* 1971; **221**: 1464–1469.

45. Hill, J.L., & Gettes, L.S. Effect of acute coronary artery occlusion on local myocardial extracellular K^+ activity in swine. *Circulation* 1980; **61**: 768–778.

46. Kléber, A.J. Resting membrane potential, extracellular potassium activity, and intracellular sodium activity during acute global ischemia in isolated perfused guinea pig hearts. *Circ. Res.* 1983; **52**: 442–450.

47. Danzl, D.F. Accidental hypothermia. In: Rosen, P., Barkin, R.M., eds. *Emergency Medicine: Concepts and Clinical Practice.* St Louis: Mosby-Year Book, 1992: 913–944.

48. Bashour, T.T., Gualberto, A., & Ryan, C. Atrioventricular block in accidental hypothermia – a case report. *Angiology* 1989; **40**: 63.

49. Harnett, R.M., Pruitt, J.R., & Sias, F.R. A review of the literature concerning resuscitation from hypothermia. II. Selected rewarming protocols. *Aviat. Space Environ. Med.* 1983; **54**: 487.

50. Emergency Cardiac Care Committee and Subcommittees, American Heart Association. Guidelines for cardiopulmonary resuscitation and emergency cardiac care. III. Adult advanced cardiac life support. *J. Am. Med. Assoc.* 1992; **268**: 2219.

51. Paradis, N.A., Martin, G.B., Rivers, E.P. *et al.* Coronary perfusion pressure and the return of spontaneous circulation in human cardiopulmonary resuscitation. *J. Am. Med. Assoc.* 1990; **263**(8):1106–1113.

52. Niemann, J.T., Garner, D., Pelikan, P.C.D., & Jagels, G. Predictive value of the ECG in determining cardiac resuscitation outcome in a canine model of postcountershock electro-mechanical dissociation after prolonged ventricular fibrillation. *Ann. Emerg. Med.* 1988; **17**: 567–571.

53. Rhomer. Ueber das elekrokardiogramm dies diphtherieherztodef. *Munchen Med. Wochenschr* 1911; **58**: 2358.

54. Robinson, G.C. A study with the electrocardiograph of the mode of death of the human heart. *J. Exp. Med.* 1912; **16**: 291–302.

55. Dieuaide, F.R., & Davidson, E.C. Terminal cardiac arrhythmias: report of three cases. *Arch. Int. Med.* 1921; **28**: 663–677.

56. Willius, F.A. Changes in the mechanism of the human heart preceding and during death. *Med. J. Rec.* 1924; **119**: 49.

57. Kahn, M.H., & Goldstein, I. The human dying heart. *Am. J. Med. Sci.* 1924; **168**: 388–412.

58. Turner, K.B. The mechanism of death of the human heart as recorded in the electrocardiogram. *Am. Heart J.* 1931; **6**: 743–757.

59. Hanson, J.F., Purks, W.K., & Anderson, R.G. Electrocardiographic studies of the dying human heart. *Arch. Int. Med.* 1933; **51**: 965–977.

60. Greene, C.W., & Gilbert, N.C. Studies on the responses of the circulation to low oxygen tension. III. Changes in the pacemaker and in conduction during extreme oxygen want as shown in the human electrocardiogram. *Arch. Int. Med.* 1921; **27**: 517–557.

61. Greene, C.W., & Gilbert, N.C. Studies in the responses of the circulation to low oxygen tension. IV. Sphygmographic study of the pulse during the rebreather test. *Arch. Int. Med.* 1921; **27**: 688–698.

62. Friedman, H.S., Gomes, J.A., Tardio, A.R., & Haft, J.I. The electrocardiographic features of acute cardiac tamponade. *Circulation* 1974; **50**: 260–265.

63. Sherrington, C.S. A mammalian spinal preparation. *J. Physiol.* 1909; **38**: 375–383.

64. Roaf, H.E., & Sherrington, C.S. Further remarks on the mammalian spinal preparation. *Q. J. Exp. Physiol.* 1910; **3**: 209–211.

65. Lewis, T., & Mathison, G.C. Auriculo-ventricular heart-block as a result of asphyxia. *Heart* 1910; **2**: 47–53.

66. Mathison, G.C. The cause of the heart-block occurring during asphyxia. *Heart* 1910; **2**: 54–73.

67. Kountz, W.B., & Gruber, C.M. The electrocardiographic changes in anoxemia. *Proc. Soc. Exp. Biol. Med.* 1929; **27**: 170–172.

68. Heyndrickx, G.R., Millard, R.W., McRitchie, R.J., Maroko, P.R., & Vatner, S.F. Regional myocardial functional and electrophysiological alterations after brief coronary artery occlusion in conscious dogs. *J. Clin. Invest.* 1975; **56**: 978–985.

69. Reimer, K.A., Hill, M.L., & Jennings, R.B. Prolonged depletion of ATP and of the adenine nucleotide pool due to delayed resynthesis of adenine nucleotides following reversible myocardial ischemic injury in dogs. *J. Mol. Cell. Cardiol.* 1981; **13**: 229–239.

70. Jennings, R.B., Hawkins, H.K., Lowe, J.E., Hill, M.L., Klotman, S., & Reimer, K.A. Relation between high energy phosphate and lethal injury in myocardial ischemia in the dog. *Am. J. Pathol.* 1978; **92**: 187–213.

71. Paradis, N.A., Martin, G.B., Ribers, E.P., Rosenberg, J., Appleton, T.J., & Nowak, R.M. The effect of standard- and high-dose epinephrine on coronary perfusion pressure during prolonged cardiopulmonary resuscitation. *J. Am. Med. Assoc.* 1991; **2650**: 1139–1144.

72. Rogers, P.L., Schlichtig, R., Miro, A., & Pinsky, M. Auto-PEEP during CPR: an "occult" cause of electromechanical dissociation? *Chest* 1991; **99**: 492–493.

73. Bergman, N.A. Intrapulmonary gas trapping during mechanical ventilation at rapid frequencies. *Anesthesiology* 1972; **37**: 626–633.

74. Pepe, P.E., & Marini, J.J. Occult positive end-expiratory pressure in mechanically ventilated patients with airflow obstruction: the auto-PEEP effect. *Am. Rev. Respir. Dis.* 1982; **126**: 166–170.

75. Whittenberger, J.L., McGregor, M., Berglund, E., & Borst, H.G. Influence of state of inflation of the lung on pulmonary vascular resistance. *J. Appl. Physiol.* 1960; **15**: 878–882.

76. Vincent, J.L., & Pinsky, M.R. Cough-induced syncope. *Intensive Care Med.* 1988; **14**: 591–594.

77. Fourman, P. Experimental observations on the tetany of potassium deficiency. *Lancet* 1954; **2**: 525.

78. Bishop, R.L., & Weisfeldt, M.L. Sodium bicarbonate administration during cardiac arrest: effect on arterial pH, PCO_2, and osmolality. *J. Am. Med. Assoc.* 1976; **235**: 506–509.

79. Kette, F., Weil, M.H., von Planta, M., Gazmuri, R.G., & Rackow, E.D. Buffer agents do not reverse intramyocardial acidosis during cardiac resuscitation. *Circulation* 1990; **81**: 1660–1666.

80. Kerber, R.E., Pandian, N.G., Hoyt, R. *et al.* Effect of ischemia, hypertrophy, hypoxia, acidosis, and alkalosis on canine defibrillation. *Am. J. Physiol.* 1983; **244**: H825–H831.

81. von Planta, M., Weil, M.H., Gazmuri, R.J., Bisera, J., & Rackow, E.C. Myocardial acidosis associated with CO_2 production during cardiac arrest and resuscitation. *Circulation* 1989; **80**: 684–692.

82. Weisfeldt, M.L., Bishop, R.L., & Greene, H.L. Effects of pH and PCO_2 on performance of ischemic myocardium. In *Recent Advances in Studies on Cardiac Structure and Metabolism.* Baltimore: University Park Press, 1975: vol 10.

83. Cingolani, H.E., Faulkner, S.L., Mattiazzi, A.R., Bender, H.W., & Graham Jr, T.P. Depression of human myocardial contractility with "respiratory" and "metabolic" acidosis. *Surgery* 1975; **77**: 427–432.

84. Cingolani, H.E., Mattiazzi, A.R., Blesa, E.S., & Gonzalez, N.C. Contractility in isolated mammalian heart muscle after acid-base changes. *Circ. Res.* 1970; **26**: 269–278.

85. Berenyi, K.J., Wolk, M., & Killip, T. Cerebrospinal fluid acidosis complicating therapy of experimental cardiopulmonary arrest. *Circulation* 1975; **52**: 319–324.

86. Khuri, S.F., Flaherty, J.T., O'Riordan, J.B. *et al.* Changes in intramyocardial ST segment voltage and gas tensions with regional myocardial ischemia in the dog. *Circ. Res.* 1975; **37**: 455–463.

87. Sanders, A.B., Ogle, M., & Ewy, G.A. Coronary perfusion pressure during cardiopulmonary resuscitation. *Am. J. Emerg. Med.* 1985; **3**: 11–14.

88. Brown, C.G., Martin, D.R., Pepe, P.E. *et al.* A comparison of standard-dose and high-dose epinephrine in cardiac arrest outside the hospital. *N. Engl. J. Med.* 1992; **327**: 1051–1055.

89. Lindner, K.H., Ahnefeld, F.W., & Bowdler, I.M. Cardiopulmonary resuscitation with interposed abdominal compression after asphyxial or fibrillatory cardiac arrest in pigs. *Anesthesiology* 1990; **72**: 675–681.

90. Ralston, S.H., Babbs, C.F., & Neibauer, M.J. Cardiopulmonary resuscitation with interposed abdominal compression in dogs. *Anesth Analg* 1982; **61**: 645–651.

91. Voorhees, W.D., Niebauer, M.J., & Babbs, C.F. Improved oxygen delivery during cardiopulmonary resuscitation with interposed abdominal compressions. *Ann. Emerg. Med.* 1983; **12**: 128–135.

92. Einagle, V., Bertrand, F., Wise, R.A., Roussos, C., & Magder, S. Interposed abdominal compressions and carotid blood flow during cardiopulmonary resuscitation: support for a thoracoabdominal unit. *Chest* 1988; **93**: 1206–1212.

93. Walker, J.W., Bruestle, J.C., White, B.C., Evans, A.T., Indreri, R., & Rialek, H. Perfusion of the cerebral cortex by use of abdominal counterpulsation during cardiopulmonary resuscitation. *Am. J. Emerg. Med.* 1984; **2**: 391–393.

94. Halperin, H.R., Guerci, A.D., Chandra, N. *et al.* Vest inflation without simultaneous ventilation during cardiac arrest in dogs: improved survival from prolonged cardiopulmonary resuscitation. *Circulation* 1986; **74**: 1407–1415.

95. Halperin, H.R., Tsitlik, J.E., Gelfand, M. *et al.* A preliminary study of cardiopulmonary resuscitation by circumferential compression of the chest with use of a pneumatic vest. *N. Engl. J. Med.* 1993; **329**: 762–768.

96. Lindner, K.H., Pfenninger, E.G., Lurie, K.G., Schürmann, W., Lindner, K.M., & Ahnefeld, F.W. Effects of active compression-decompression resuscitation on myocardial and cerebral blood flow in pigs. *Circulation* 1993; **88**: 1254–1263.

97. DeBehnke, D.J., Angelos, M.G., & Leasure, J.E. Use of cardiopulmonary bypass, high-dose epinephrine, and standard-dose epinephrine in resuscitation from post-countershock electromechanical dissociation. *Ann. Emerg. Med.* 1992; **21**: 1051–1057.

Addendum

Volker Wenzel

Innsbruck Medical University, Department of Anesthesiology and Critical Care Medicine, Austria

In a recent study of initial ECG rhythms in out-of-hospital cardiac arrest in Europe, ventricular fibrillation was observed in about 40%, asystole in about 45%, and pulseless electrical activity accounted for about 15%. In contrast, pulseless electrical activity was more likely during in-hospital CPR (children 24%, adults 32%). This is similar to a North American study, when pulseless electrical activity was the initial ECG rhythm in about 20%–40%.[2] Although exact CPR management was not analyzed according to the initial ECG rhythm in the in-hospital CPR study, survival of pulseless electrical activity patients to hospital discharge was relatively good (pediatrics 27%, adults 11%).[3] In a recent study comparing vasopressin vs. epinephrine during CPR (n=1219), pulseless electrical activity patients in Europe had a slightly better chance to be discharged from the hospital alive than did asystolic patients (about 6%–8% vs. 2%–5%), but the discharge rate was lower than that for ventricular fibrillation patients (about 18%–19%).[1] While this study was unable to determine an advantage of vasopressin over epinephrine, no pulseless electrical activity

patient receiving ≥3 mg of epinephrine during CPR (n=82) was discharged from the hospital alive, indicating that there may be a critical myocardial ischemia threshold in pulseless electrical activity patients for them to survive.[1] With use of a load-distributing band during out-of-hospital CPR, survival was not improved but differences in survival patterns between initial ECG rhythms (hospital discharge rate, ventricular fibrillation 14%–23%; pulseless electrical activity 3%–9%; asystole 1%–2%)[2] were similar to those in the vasopressin trial in Europe.

Comparable hospital discharge rates for pulseless electrical activity patients were found in Richmond, Virginia, where a load-distributing band was also employed, but survival was not improved over standard manual CPR.[4] When aminophylline vs. placebo was given to patients with bradyasystolic states during out-of-hospital CPR (n=971), it was difficult to evaluate effects in pulseless electrical activity patients (n=222), because asystolic patients (n=602), as well as ventricular fibrillation/tachycardia patients (n=147) were included as well. Nonetheless, overall hospital discharge rate in both groups was extremely low (5/971; 0.005%).[5] A different pharmacological strategy, fibrinolysis, was used in pulseless electrical activity victims in a prospective CPR study in Vancouver, Canada. Unfortunately, survival to hospital discharge was again very low (1/117 in the thrombolysis group, and none of 116 of patients receiving placebo), indicating that survival with pulseless electrical activity as initial ECG rhythm was extremely unlikely at least in this trial, and that any statement about treatment strategies was inconclusive.[6]

These clinical studies confirm that survival chances after cardiac arrest with pulseless electrical activity as the initial rhythm are significantly worse than after ventricular fibrillation, and may be only slightly better than survival chances after asystolic cardiac arrest. Moreover, the aforementioned clinical trials further confirm that there is no new promising therapy, such as a "hot track," for this cohort of patients that may be worth follow-up. As pathophysiology indicates, pulseless electrical activity reflects a myocardium that is virtually completely deprived of metabolic activity, and may therefore reflect a setting that is extremely difficult to convert to return of spontaneous circulation with subsequent long-term survival and full neurological recovery.

REFERENCES

1. Wenzel, V., Krismer, A.C., Arntz, H.R., Sitter, H., Stadlbauer, K.H. & Lindner, K.H. A comparison of vasopressin and epinephrine for out-of-hospital cardiopulmonary resuscitation. *N. Engl. J. Med.* 2004; **350**: 105–113.

2. Hallstrom, A., Rea, T.D., Sayre, M.R. *et al.* Manual chest compression vs use of an automated chest compression device during resuscitation following out-of-hospital cardiac arrest: a randomized trial. *J. Am. Med. Assoc.* 2006; **295**: 2620–2628.

3. Nadkarni, V.M., Larkin, G.L., Peberdy, M.A. *et al.* First documented rhythm and clinical outcome from in-hospital cardiac arrest among children and adults. *J. Am. Med. Assoc.* 2006; **295**: 50–57.

4. Ong, M.E., Ornato, J.P., Edwards, D.P. *et al.* Use of an automated, load-distributing band chest compression device for out-of-hospital cardiac arrest resuscitation. *J. Am. Med. Assoc.* 2006; **295**: 2629–2637.

5. Abu-Laban, R.B., McIntyre, C.M., Christenson, J.M. *et al.* Aminophylline in bradyasystolic cardiac arrest: a randomised placebo-controlled trial. *Lancet* 2006; **367**: 1577–1584.

6. Abu-Laban, R.B., Christenson, J.M., Innes, G.D. *et al.* Tissue plasminogen activator in cardiac arrest with pulseless electrical activity. *N. Engl. J. Med.* 2002; **346**: 1522–1528.

Part IV

Therapy of sudden death

23

Prevention of sudden cardiac death

Catherine Campbell, Ty J. Gluckman, Charles Henrikson, M. Dominique Ashen, and Roger S. Blumenthal

Johns Hopkins Ciccarone Preventive Cardiology Center, Baltimore, MD, USA

Sudden cardiac death (SCD) is defined as death from a cardiac cause that occurs suddenly (usually less than 1 hour) after the onset of symptoms. Most cases of sudden cardiac death are the result of ventricular arrhythmias, which may be the first manifestation of cardiac disease.[1] Chest pain, palpitations, dyspnea, and syncope are common but non-specific prodromal symptoms associated with SCD.

About 400 000–460 000 people in the United States die from SCD each year, accounting for over 60% of all cardiac deaths.[1] Despite the high age-adjusted incidence of SCD (206.5 per 100 000 men, 140.7 per 100 000 women, and 3.0 per 100 000 children and young adults aged ≤34 years[2]), it has been a difficult condition to study thus far. In this chapter we review the etiologies of SCD, the tools used to identify and stratify individuals at risk, and strategies for risk reduction.

Etiologies of sudden cardiac death

Coronary artery disease

Because most cases of SCD (approximately 70%) occur in individuals with at least moderate coronary artery disease (CAD), it remains the most common risk factor for this condition.[2] Individuals with a history of myocardial infarction (MI) have a 4- to 6-fold increased risk of SCD[3] due in large part to postinfarction ventricular remodeling.[4] Among patients with left ventricular dysfunction or heart failure, the risk of sudden death is highest (1.4% per month) in the first 30 days after an MI.[5] Coronary artery disease is a less significant risk factor for SCD in young

patients, as only about one fourth of young SCD victims have coronary artery disease.[6]

There are numerous conditions that increase an individual's risk for CAD (Table 23.1).[7] While many of these risk factors are causally linked with CAD, other predisposing and conditional factors are thought to play a role (Table 23.1). Identification of these risk factors is central to CAD risk reduction and, thus, a reduction in the incidence of SCD. The National Cholesterol Education Program Adult Treatment Panel III (ATP III) recommends calculation of the Framingham Risk Prediction Score to provide an estimate of risk for developing an MI or coronary heart disease (CHD) death over the course of 10 years.[8] Importantly, this score is utilized to determine the intensity of pharmacologic risk-reduction therapies. The ATP III also recognizes the impact of the metabolic syndrome on CAD risk, defined by the presence of at least three of the following: abdominal obesity (waist circumference >102 cm men, >88 cm women), hypertriglyceridemia (triglycerides ≥150 mg/dl), low high-density lipoprotein cholesterol (HDL <40 mg/dl men, <50 mg/dl women), elevated blood pressure (≥130/85 mmHg), and elevated fasting glucose (≥110 mg/dl).

Heart failure and left ventricular hypertrophy

The risk of SCD is increased 6- to 9-fold in individuals with congestive heart failure.[3] Ischemic cardiomyopathy is the most common cause of heart failure in developed countries; however, other cardiomyopathies may also cause heart failure and an increase in the risk of SCD. Structural and functional changes in the failing heart lead to action potential prolongation, abnormal calcium handling, and

Cardiac Arrest: The Science and Practice of Resuscitation Medicine. 2nd edn., ed. Norman Paradis, Henry Halperin, Karl Kern, Volker Wenzel, Douglas Chamberlain. Published by Cambridge University Press. © Cambridge University Press, 2007.

Table 23.1. Risk factors for coronary artery disease

Causal	Advancing age ($\geq$45 y men, $\geq$55 y women)
	Cigarette smoking
	Diabetes mellitus (fasting glucose $\geq$126 mg/dL; glucose $\geq$200 mg/dl post-glucose load)
	Elevated blood pressure (>120/80 mmHg)
	Elevated total ($\geq$200 mg/dL) and LDL ($\geq$130 mg/dL) cholesterol
	Low serum HDL cholesterol (<40 mg/dL)
Predisposing	Family history of premature coronary heart disease (first degree relative, <55 y men, <65 y women)
	Overweight and obese states (BMI >25 kg/m^2)
	Abdominal obesity (waist circumference >102 cm M, >88 cm F)
	Physical inactivity
	Ethnic characteristics
	Higher risk than whites:
	African-Americans, South Asians
	Lower risk than whites:
	Hispanics, Asians/Pacific Islanders
	Psychosocial factors (depression, phobias, chronic stressors)
Conditional	Elevated triglycerides ($\geq$150 mg/dL)
	High-sensitivity C-reactive protein ($\geq$2 mg/dL)
	Small LDL particles
	Other possible risk factors:
	• Homocysteine
	• Lipoprotein (a)
	• Lipoprotein-associated phospholipase A$_2$
	B-type natriuretic peptide

aberrant conduction, which are thought to underlie the increased risk of SCD.[9] The degree of functional impairment and left ventricular dysfunction are powerful predictors of the risk of death from an arrhythmic cause.[10–12]

Genetics

Evidence supporting a genetic predisposition for SCD comes from familial associations in population studies and rare genetic disease paradigms. Longitudinal population studies have demonstrated the importance of family history in determining risk for SCD. On the basis of work done in the Seattle[13] and Paris[14] population studies, the relative risk of SCD in an offspring of a parent with a history of SCD is more than 50% higher than the risk in an unaffected family. Of note, in the Paris population study, the relative risk of SCD in offspring with a history of SCD in both parents was 9 times that of the risk in an unaffected family.

Rare genetic disease paradigms also provide evidence for a familial predisposition to life-threatening arrhythmias. Many of these conditions result from mutations in genes that code for channel proteins, non-ion conduction proteins, structural proteins, and contractile proteins, as well as from mutations that alter the interaction of these proteins with regulatory proteins. Management options for these syndromes generally include an implantable cardioverter-defibrillator (ICD) for high-risk patients, and exercise restriction (Table 23.2). In many of these syndromes, β-blockers are also helpful (Table 23.2).

Long QT (LQT) syndrome is an inherited condition characterized by prolonged ventricular repolarization and episodic life-threatening arrhythmias. The autosomal dominant Romano Ward syndrome and the autosomal recessive Jervell and Lange–Nielsen syndromes were the first phenotypes identified.[15,16] It is now apparent that this syndrome is genetically heterogeneous, as more than 10 genes for cardiac ion channel subunits[17] and 1 gene for ankyrin B[18] (a structural protein) have been associated with this condition. Because many carriers of genes associated with long QT syndrome are asymptomatic, there is also variable penetrance.[19] Symptoms, when they do occur, are variable and can occur during sleep (i.e., LQT3), along with emotional stress (i.e., LQT2) and exercise (i.e., LQT1).[20]

The Brugada syndrome is an autosomal dominant disease characterized by right bundle branch block, ST segment elevation in leads V1 to V3, and ventricular tachyarrhythmias that may result in syncope or cardiac arrest.[21] Although an early study suggested that there was an

Table 23.2. Genetic syndromes associated with sudden cardiac death

Syndrome	Genetic mutations	Function Impaired	Management options
Long QT syndrome	Potassium channel: KCNQ1 (LQT1) HERG (LQT2) minK (LQT5) MiRP1 (LQT 6) Sodium channel: SCN5A (LQT3) Ankrin B: ANKB (LQT4)	Ion channel conduction Anchoring of ion channels to cellular membrane	• ICD • β-blockers • avoidance of medications that prolong QT interval • LQT1: avoidance of competitive sports, unsupervised swimming • LQT2: potassium supplementation; avoidance of alarm clocks, loud telephones • LQT3: mexiletene, pacemaker
Brugada syndrome	SCN5A (sodium channel)	Sodium channel conduction	• ICD
Catecholaminergic polymorphic ventricular tachycardia (CPVT)	RyR2 (ryanodine receptor) CASQ2 (calsequestrin)	Calcium signaling	• ICD • β-blockers • exercise restriction
Arrhythmogenic right ventricular dysplasia (ARVD)	RyR2 (ryanodine receptor) DSP (desmoplakin) JUP (junctional plakoglobin)	Calcium signaling	• ICD • β-blockers (sotalol) • exercise restriction
Hypertrophic cardiomyopathy (HCM)	Sarcomeric myofilament proteins	Muscle contraction, structural stability	• ICD • β-blockers • amiodarone • verapamil • septal ablation, myotomy, or myomectomy • exercise restriction

increased mortality rate (>30% over 3 years) among those not treated with an ICD,[22] more recent data suggest that asymptomatic patients have low mortality rates (0% over 3 years) and may not need an ICD.[23] Unfortunately, the pathogenesis of the Brugada syndrome is poorly understood. In fewer than 25% of cases, there is a mutation in SCN5A,[24] a gene that codes for a sodium channel protein associated with LQT3.

Catecholaminergic polymorphic ventricular tachycardia (CPVT) is an inherited disease characterized by stress- or exercise-induced ventricular arrhythmias and an increased risk of sudden cardiac death.[25,26] CPVT may be inherited by an autosomal dominant or autosomal recessive pattern. Genetic mutations in the ryanodine receptor gene (RyR2),[27,28] which encodes a cardiac sarcoplasmic reticulum calcium channel, and the calsequestrin gene (CASQ2),[29,30] which binds calcium and serves as a reservoir within the sarcoplasmic reticulum, are associated with CPVT.

Arrhythmogenic right ventricular dysplasia (ARVD) is a familial disease characterized by fatty-fibrous infiltrate of the right (and less frequently left) ventricular myocardium. The inheritance of ARVD is usually autosomal dominant, with its highest incidence among individuals in the Veneto region of northern Italy (12%–25% of SCD in young patients is associated with ARVD in this area).[31–33] Mutations in desmoplakin (DSP),[34] junctional plakoglobin (JUP),[35] and ryanodine receptor (RyR2)[36] are associated with ARVD. Desmoplakin and plakoglobin are key constituents of desmosomes, with mechanical forces applied to these cell–cell junctions activating calcium channels and calcium release from the ryanodine receptor.[34]

Hypertrophic cardiomyopathy (HCM) is an autosomal dominant genetic disorder characterized by idiopathic left ventricular hypertrophy and marked heterogeneity. The prevalence of HCM in young adults is about 2 per 1000.[37] About 60% of patients have mutations in sarcomeric protein genes, which function in cardiac muscle contraction and structural stability.[38] As most patients are asymptomatic, diagnosis often results from family screening. Sudden cardiac death in patients with HCM is usually due to ventricular arrrhythmias[38], with an annual risk of 1% in adults, compared with 2%–4% in children and adolescents.[38]

Medications

Further evidence for genetic predisposition to SCD comes from the interaction of drugs with specific genes. Many medications may prolong the QT interval and potentiate torsade de pointes through blockade of the potassium channel in cardiac myocytes.[39] Although antiarrhythmics are the most common offenders, many non-cardiac medications may also produce this effect (Table 23.3). Genetic polymorphisms that increase the risk of drug-induced long QT syndrome have also been identified.[40–42] These include polymorphisms in P450 metabolism pathways, which may lengthen the time that an individual is exposed to a medication that may prolong the QT interval.[41] This idea was first recognized in the early 1970s, when it was noted that certain families (which had a deficiency in the P450 cytokine, CYP2D6) were at higher risk of toxicity from warfarin and anti-seizure medications.[41]

Tools for risk stratification

Patients with a history of CAD, myocardial infarction, heart failure, or certain genetic syndromes should undergo some form of stratification to assess their risk of SCD. This is particularly important for those individuals who are being considered for an ICD.

Ejection fraction (EF) has been the primary SCD risk stratification tool used for inclusion in clinical trials.[43,44] For example, the Marburg Cardiomyopathy Study (MACAS) found that left ventricular EF was the only significant predictor of arrhythmia in patients with idiopathic dilated cardiomyopathy.[45] Despite this, 81% of individuals in the Maastricht prospective registry of cardiac arrest had an EF >30% prior to the event.[46]

Other methods used in SCD risk stratification include Holter monitoring, ECG analysis, and novel tools (Table 23.4).[47] Early studies suggested that ambient ventricular arrhythmias on 24-hour Holter monitoring were predictive of SCD in heart failure patients.[48] More recent studies, however, suggest that ambient ventricular arrhythmias on Holter monitoring are predictive of SCD in patients with HCM[49] but not in patients with heart failure.[50] Holter monitoring also offers the ability to measure reduced heart rate variability, which is associated with an increase in the risk of SCD.[51–55] Baroflex sensitivity, which measures the response to phenylephrine, may also be useful, as decreased sensitivity is associated with an increased risk of SCD.[54]

Table 23.3. Medications that may lead to torsade de pointes through QT prolongation.[39]

Cardiac medications	Non-cardiac medications
Amiodarone	**Anti-infective**
Bepridil	Clarithromycin
Disopyramide	Erythromycin
Dofetilide	Foscarnet
Flecainide	Gatifloxacin
Ibutilide	Halofantrine
Indapamide	Moxifloxacin
Isradipine	Pentamidine
Moexipril/HCTZ	Sparfloxacin
Nicardipine	**Anti-psychotic**
Procainamide	Chlorpromazine
Quinidine	Haloperidol
Sotalol	Mesoridazine
	Pimozide
	Quetiapine
	Risperidone
	Thioridazine
	Ziprasidone
	Anti-nausea
	Dolasetron
	Domperidone
	Droperidol
	Anti-convulsant
	Felbamate
	Fosphenytoin
	Pain control
	Levomethadyl
	Methadone
	GI stimulant
	Cisapride
	Asthma/COPD
	Salmeterol
	Anti-depressant
	Venlafaxine
	Acromegaly/Carcinoid diarrhea
	Octreotide
	Muscle relaxant
	Tizanidine

Finally, implantable loop recorders, which allow extended and continuous ECG monitoring in the evaluation of unexplained syncope[56] and detection of arrhythmias after myocardial infarction,[57] remain to be fully evaluated in identifying individuals at risk for SCD.

Standard ECG analysis, which includes analysis of the ST segment, QT interval, and QRS width and morphology, can be useful in providing clues to structural heart disease and genetic electrophysiologic syndromes. Using the standard

Table 23.4. Tools for risk stratification

	Risk measured	Predictive power
Traditional tools		
CAD risk factors	Underlying disease risk	Low positive predictive value to determine SCD risk in a particular individual
NYHA functional class/ Echocardiography Ejection fraction LVH	Structural disease	High predictive power for sudden cardiac death and overall cardiac death
Holter monitoring Ambient ventricular arrhythmias	SCD triggers	High predictive power in patients with hypertrophic cardiomyopathy; low predictive power in other patients unless combined with other factors
Heart rate variability/baroreflex sensitivity	Conditioning factors	Predictive power unknown
Implantable loop recorders ECG variables	SCD triggers	Predictive power unknown
Standard ECG QRS width QT dispersion	Electrical abnormalities	Low predictive power
Abnormalities suggestive of structural disease (e.g., LVH) or genetic syndromes (e.g., long QT)	Electrical abnormalities	High predictive power in identifying certain diseases
Novel tools		
High-resolution ECG		
T-wave alternans	Electrical abnormalities	High predictive power in high-risk patients, predictive power unknown for other patients
Late potentials	Electrical abnormalities	Predictive power highest in patients with ischemic cardiomyopathy. Low positive predictive value, high negative predictive value
EP testing: Inducibility of ventricular tachyarrhythmia	Arrhythmogenic substrate	Good positive predictive value in patients with ischemic cardiomyopathy; high rate of false negatives in high-risk patients
Imaging: MRI, MRS, MDCT	Scar tissue, coronary plaque	Predictive power unknown
Genotyping	Genetic predisposition	High predictive power for certain genetic syndromes; predictive power unknown for other patients

Abbreviations: CAD, Coronary artery disease; NYHA, New York Heart Association; LVH, left ventricular hypertrophy; ECG, electrocardiogram; EP, electrophysiologic; MRI, magnetic resonance imaging; MRS, magnetic resonance spectroscopy; MDCT, multi-detector computed tomography.

ECG, QT-interval dispersion has been proposed as a useful risk-stratifying tool. Although it measures the difference between minimal and maximal QT intervals in various ECG leads, it lacks accuracy and reliability.[58–60]

Usually, more information can be obtained with high-resolution signal-averaged electrocardiography (SAECG), by evaluating for T-wave alternans and late potentials. T-wave alternans, the beat-to-beat alteration in T-wave

Table 23.5. ABCs of cardiovascular disease risk management

A	Antiplatelet agents	
	Aspirin	• 75–325 mg daily in high-risk patients[81] • Controversial for low-risk patients: reduction in CVD risk seen in men,[82] but not in women[83]
	Clopidogrel	• High-risk patients resistant or intolerant to aspirin[84] • In addition to aspirin for at least 9–12 months following an acute coronary syndrome, particularly after percutaneous coronary intervention[85–87]
	Anticoagulant therapy: Warfarin	• Post-MI patients intolerant to aspirin[88] • Patients with left ventricular thrombus and/or atrial fibrillation
	Angiotensin-converting enzyme inhibitors (ACEIs)	• Patients with recent MI, heart failure, and/or left ventricular systolic dysfunction[89–91] • Patients with diabetes mellitus and/or CVD if systolic blood pressure is >120 mmHg[92–94]
	Angiotensin receptor blockers (ARBs)	• Patients with heart failure, diabetic nephropathy, or hypertension[95] • In patients with heart failure, primary therapy only in patients intolerant to ACEIs[96]
	Antianginals	• For patients with anginal symptoms: antianginals enable these patients to exercise
B	Blood pressure control	• Initiate blood pressure treatment in low-risk patients if blood pressure ≥140/90 mmHg.[97] • Initiate blood pressure treatment in patients with diabetes or chronic kidney disease if blood pressure ≥130/80 mmHg.[97] • First-line therapy: ACEIs, beta-blockers, thiazide diuretics • Second-line therapy: aldosterone antagonists, ARBs, calcium channel blockers
	β-Blockers	• Post-MI patients[98] • Heart failure patients[99] • Blood pressure control for CVD patients[97]
C	Cholesterol management	• Statins, ezetimibe, fibrates, nicotinic acid • LDL-C goal <100 mg/dL for high-risk patients, <130 mg/dL for intermediate-risk patients, <160 mg/dL for low-risk patients.[100] • Lowering LDL even further may reduce risk of CVD.[101–103] • Non-HDL-C goal is 30 mg/dL higher than LDL-C goal. Non-HDL-C goal <130 mg/dL for high-risk patients, <160 mg/dL for intermediate-risk patients, <190 mg/dL for low-risk patients. After LDL-C goal met, consider intensifying therapy with LDL-C lowering drug or adding nicotinic acid or fibrate to reach LDL-C goal.[100]
	Cigarette smoking cessation	• Counseling • Treatment with buproprion with or without nicotine patch more successful than placebo or nicotine patch alone.[104]
D	Diet and weight management	• ≥500 kcal/d caloric reduction • Patients with cardiovascular disease should be encouraged to follow a diet containing whole grains, vegetables, fruits, omega-3 fatty acids and nuts and low in refined grains, cholesterol and saturated fat.[105]
	Diabetes mellitus	• Patients with impaired fasting glucose (110–124 mg/dL) or impaired glucose tolerance (140–199 mg/dL) should be treated aggressively with lifestyle counseling and/or metformin to prevent diabetes.[106,107] • Goal hemoglobin A_{1c} <7%, lowest risk when hemoglobin A_{1c} <6%[108]

Table 23.5. (continued)

E	Exercise	• Aerobic, weight training
		• Exercise beneficial for primary[109] and secondary[110] prevention of CVD.
		• Cardiac rehabilitation programs should be considered for patients with left ventricular systolic dysfunction, recent coronary artery bypass surgery, recent MI, and/or chronic stable angina pectoris.[111]
	Ejection fraction	• ACEI and β-blocker for all patients with heart failure.[99]
		• Aldosterone inhibitors (spironolactone,[112] eplerenone[113]) indicated in post-MI patients with severe heart failure.
		• Digitalis can be used to treat symptoms of heart failure.[99]
		• Implantable cardioverter-defibrillator for high-risk patients[114,115]

amplitude, has been found to increase the risk of life-threatening arrhythmia in high-risk patients.[61–63] Late potentials or low-amplitude high-frequency potentials at the end of the QRS complex indicate delayed ventricular activation and have high negative predictive values. The value of late potentials appears to be highest in patients with ischemic cardiomyopathy.[64,65]

Electrophysiologic testing is used for risk stratification because it can assess the inducibility of ventricular tachyarrhythmias. While electrophysiologic testing is most useful in patients with an ischemic cardiomyopathy,[66,67] it is largely limited by a high false negative rate, particularly in high-risk patients.[68,69] In the Multicenter Unsustained Tachycardia Trial (MUSTT), the rate of cardiac arrest was highest in patients with an EF <30% and an inducible tachyarrhythmia. Patients with an EF <30% in whom tachyarrhythmia was not inducible had rates of cardiac arrest similar to those of patients with ejection fraction ≥30% and in whom tachyarrhythmia could be induced.[70]

Significant effort is being focused on novel methods to risk-stratify patients at risk for SCD. Methods include imaging techniques, such as magnetic resonance imaging and spectroscopy (MRI/MRS) and multi-detector computed tomography (MDCT). Genetic and proteomic biomarkers are also being evaluated, helped by the ability now to do large-scale unbiased screens of proteomic expression and genomic information. For example, the Oregon Sudden Unexpected Death Study[71] is collecting risk factor and genetic information for all sudden deaths in the Portland area over a 3-year period. In addition, the Johns Hopkins Donald W. Reynolds Project is utilizing novel technologies, such as whole genome association to identify the genetic determinants of SCD in groups such as the Oregon SUDS and patients with ICDs.

Strategies in the prevention of SCD

Only 1% to 5% of patients with out-of-hospital cardiac arrest survive.[72] Although widespread availability of automatic external defibrillators may increase survival rates,[73] the low survival rate from cardiac arrest requires a preventive focus.

Prevention of coronary artery disease

As patients with CAD are at high risk for SCD, it is imperative that efforts be undertaken to protect against the development of CAD through primary and secondary prevention. Recommended therapies for prevention of CAD are underutilized, with irregular practice patterns.[74–78] Furthermore, the trend towards earlier discharge after myocardial infarction has restricted the opportunity for counseling about modifications of lifestyle such as smoking cessation, diet, and exercise.[79]

A straightforward "ABC" approach to cardiovascular risk reduction may help to narrow the treatment gap in prevention of cardiovascular disease (Table 23.5).[80] This approach provides a checklist to encourage provider adherence to recommended practices. A simplified version of the approach facilitates patient–physician communication about the risk-reducing strategy. For patients at high risk of CHD events (>20% 10-year risk), aggressive risk-reduction therapies should be instituted. For patients at intermediate (10%–20% 10-year risk) or low risk (<10% 10-year risk) of CHD events, less aggressive risk-reduction therapies should be instituted. In addition to managing overall cardiovascular disease risk, lifestyle modifications, medications, and implantable devices can further reduce the risk of sudden cardiac death.

Lifestyle

Smoking is a major CAD risk factor and thus also increases risk for SCD. Smoking cessation should be encouraged in all patients, but particularly in those with CAD. It is also apparent that other lifestyle factors such as circadian variation, anxiety, exercise, and diet influence the risk of SCD. Indeed, SCD risk is increased in the morning[71] and in individuals with phobic anxiety.[116,117] In patients with certain genetic syndromes that increase SCD risk, exercise is generally discouraged as it may further increase risk of SCD (Table 23.2). In nearly all other patients, regular exercise should be encouraged, with participation in cardiac rehabilitation for those at highest risk.[111]

Regular exercise decreases the overall risk of SCD and CHD, but the relative risk of SCD during and shortly after vigorous exertion is greatly increased relative to other times.[118,119] Habitual exercise likely decreases SCD risk by increasing electrical stability through increased basal vagal tone and decreasing risk of plaque rupture through its beneficial effects on lipids and its tendency to decrease the hemodynamic stress experienced at a given workload.[119] The "exercise paradox" likely reflects the increased sympathetic tone of vigorous exertion that increases the risk of ventricular fibrillation and plaque rupture.[119]

Various dietary measures influence the risk of SCD (Table 23.5).[105] Fish consumption and increased levels of the omega-3 polyunsaturated fatty acids (PUFA) found in fish are associated with a reduced risk of SCD, likely because of membrane-stabilizing effects.[120–123] Because alpha-linolenic acid (ALA), an omega-3 fatty acid found in fatty fish and the precursor of eicosapentanoic acid (EPA) and docosahexaenoic acid (DHA), is associated with a reduced risk of SCD[124–126], the American Heart Association recommends regular consumption of fatty fish and other sources of ALA.[127,128] Fish oil capsules can be taken in lieu of fish consumption and may be a useful adjunct because of harm associated with increased mercury levels in fish.[129]

Potassium and magnesium intake and levels should be monitored in patients who are high risk, on diuretics, or are malnourished, because their deficiencies can increase the risk of SCD.[130] In addition, heavy drinking should be discouraged, as heavy alcohol consumption (>5 drinks per day) and, in particular, binge drinking is associated with an increased risk of CHD and SCD.[131,132] This likely results from alcohol's predilection to cause thrombosis and myocardial scarring and through a reduction in the threshold for ventricular arrhythmias.[133]

Medications

Angiotensin converting enzyme inhibitors (ACEIs), β-blockers, and lipid-lowering agents are staples of secondary prevention of CAD and thus SCD. In contrast, nearly all studies have shown a lack of benefit or an increase in mortality with the use of antiarrhythmic medications. The Cardiac Arrhythmia Suppression Trial (CAST) and the survival with d-sotalol (SWORD) trial are clear examples of antiarrhythmic failures. CAST evaluated the efficacy of three class I antiarrhythmic drugs (encainide, flecainide, and moricizine). CAST I was stopped early when encainide and flecainide were found to increase risk of sudden cardiac death relative to placebo.[134] CAST II evaluated moricizine versus placebo and was also stopped early because of a trend toward mortality in the moricizine group.[135] The SWORD trial evaluated the efficacy of the class II agent d-sotalol versus placebo in patients with ischemic cardiomyopathy.[136] The trial was stopped early because of increased mortality in the d-sotalol group. The paradoxical proarrhythmic tendencies of antiarrhythmic medications likely underlie their increased risk of SCD. Of all of the antiarrhythmic medications, only β-blockers and possibly amiodarone (in conjunction with a β-blocker) have shown any promise in reducing risk of SCD.[137,138] β-Blockers are also indicated for many genetic syndromes that predispose to SCD (Table 23.2). Because of the limitations of antiarrhythmics, much of the focus of SCD prevention has shifted to non-pharmacologic therapies.

Device-based therapy

Initial non-pharmacologic therapy involved surgical excision of scar tissue or intraoperative mapping of regions where ventricular tachycardia could be induced.[139,140] Since the development of ICDs, however, interest in these procedures has diminished considerably. ICDs reliably convert ventricular arrhythmias to sinus rhythm and substantially reduce mortality in patients at high risk for SCD. The initial trials, Antiarrhythmics vs. Implantable Defibrillators (AVID),[141] Canadian Implantable Defibrillator Study (CIDS),[142] and Cardiac Arrest Study Hamburg (CASH),[143] demonstrated the efficacy of ICDs in survivors of life-threatening arrhythmias. More recent trials have demonstrated efficacy in a broader group of patients.

The Multicenter Automatic Defibrillator Implantation Trial (MADIT) II included post-MI patients with EF<30% and demonstrated that ICDs reduce mortality by more than 30% when compared to "conventional medical therapy" (lipid-lowering medications, diuretics, beta-blockers, ACEIs).[43] Sudden Cardiac Death in Heart Failure Trial (SCD-HeFT) demonstrated a mortality benefit with ICDs of 23% in patients with New York Heart Association (NYHA) class II or III CHF and an ejection fraction less than 35%.[44] Of note, the Defibrillator in Acute Myocardial Infarction Trial (DINAMIT) found no mortality benefit with ICD implantation 6 to 40 days after MI in patients with EF less than 35%,[144] despite the high risk for sudden death in these patients.[5] Moreover, high-risk patients with genetic predisposition to sudden cardiac death may not be adequately managed with medication and may benefit from an ICD (Table 23.2). The broad categories of patients who may benefit from an ICD and the expense of the devices make risk stratification important. Furthermore, defibrillation is stressful, and many shocks may be inappropriate. Cardiac resynchronization may be less stressful for the patient, and recent trials have demonstrated the benefit of cardiac resynchronization in patients with heart failure and cardiac dyssynchrony.[114,115]

Future investigation

Because of the potential for cell-based therapy to allow for generation of new, functional myocardium, there is hope that this treatment may be useful in those at risk for SCD in years to come. At present, concurrent implantation of ICDs is mandatory as these cells may potentiate arrhythmogenicity by virtue of their limited ability to transmit current.

Conclusions

Sudden cardiac death is a frequent cause of death. CAD, heart failure, and genetic syndromes are the major risk factors for SCD. Assessing risk in these patients is crucial, given the cost implications of both pharmacologic therapies and ICDs. Treatment options include management of cardiovascular disease and heart failure, lifestyle modifications, and, in high-risk patients, implantable devices.

REFERENCES

1. Zheng, Z.J., Croft, J.B., Giles, W.H. & Mensah, G.A. Sudden cardiac death in the United States, 1989 to 1998. *Circulation* 2001; **104**: 2158–2163.
2. CDC. State-Specific Mortality from Sudden Cardiac Death – United States, 1999. *Morb. Mortal. Wkly Rep.* 2002; **51**: 123–126.
3. American Heart Association. Heart Disease and Stroke Statistics – 2005 Update. Dallas, TX: American Heart Association, 2004.
4. El-Sherif, N. & Turitto, G. Risk stratification and management of sudden cardiac death: A new paradigm. *J. Cardiovasc. Electr.* 2003; **14**: 1113–1119.
5. Solomon, S., Zelenkofske, S., McMurray, J. *et al.* Sudden death in patients with myocardial infarction and left ventricular dysfunction, heart failure, or both. *N. Engl. J. Med.* 2005; **352**: 2581–2588.
6. Liberthson, R.R. Current concepts – sudden death from cardiac causes in children and young adults. *N. Engl. J. Med.* 1996; **334**: 1039–1044.
7. Kannel, W., Dawber, T., Kagan, A., Revotskie, N. & Stokes, J. Factors of risk in the development of coronary heart disease – six year follow-up experience. The Framingham Study. *Ann. Intern. Med.* 1961; **55**: 33–50.
8. Cleeman, J.I., Grundy, S.M., Becker, D. *et al.* Executive summary of the Third Report of the National Cholesterol Education Program (NCEP) expert panel on detection, evaluation, and treatment of high blood cholesterol in adults (Adult Treatment Panel III). *J. Am. Med. Assoc.* 2001; **285**: 2486–2497.
9. Tomaselli, G.F. & Zipes, D.P. What causes sudden death in heart failure? *Circ. Res.* 2004; **95**: 754–763.
10. Moss, A.J. Risk stratification and survival after myocardial infarction. *N. Engl. J. Med.* 1983; **309**: 331–336.
11. Bigger, J.T., Fleiss, J.L., Kleiger, R., Miller, J.P. & Rolnitzky, L.M. The relationships among ventricular arrhythmias, left ventricular dysfunction, and mortality in the 2 years after myocardial infarction. *Circulation* 1984; **69**: 250–258.
12. Luu, M., Stevenson, W.G., Stevenson, L.W., Baron, K. & Walden, J. Diverse mechanisms of unexpected cardiac arrest in advanced heart failure. *Circulation* 1989; **80**: 1675–1680.
13. Friedlander, Y., Siscovick, D.S., Weinmann, S. *et al.* Family history as a risk factor for primary cardiac arrest. *Circulation* 1998; **97**: 155–160.
14. Jouven, X., Desnos, M., Guerot, C. & Ducimetiere, P. Predicting sudden death in the population – The Paris Prospective Study, I. *Circulation* 1999; **99**: 1978–1983.
15. Romano, C., Gemme, G. & Pongiglione, R. Rare cardiac arrythmias of the pediatric age. *Clin Pediatr.* 1963; **45**: 656–683.
16. Jervell, A. & Lange-Nielsen, F. Congenital deaf mutism, functional heart disease with prolongation of the QT interval, and sudden death. *Am. Heart J.* 1957; **54**: 59–68.
17. Keating, M.T. & Sanguinetti, M.C. Molecular and cellular mechanisms of cardiac arrhythmias. *Cell* 2001; **104**: 569–580.
18. Mohler, P.J., Schott, J.J., Gramolini, A.O. *et al.* Ankyrin-B mutation causes type 4 long-QT cardiac arrhythmia and sudden cardiac death. *Nature.* 2003; **421**: 634–639.
19. Vincent, G.M., Timothy, K.W., Leppert, M. & Keating, M. The spectrum of symptoms and QT intervals in carriers of the gene for the long QT syndrome. *N. Engl. J. Med.* 1992; **327**: 846–852.
20. Balaji, S. Medical therapy for sudden death. *Pediatr. Clin. N. Am.* 2004; **51**: 1379–1387.
21. Brugada, P. & Brugada, J. Right bundle branch block, persistent ST segment elevation and sudden cardiac death: a

distinct clinical and electrocardiographic syndrome. A multi-center rport. *J. Am. Coll. Cardiol.* 1992; **20**: 1391–1396.

22. Brugada, J., Brugada, R. & Brugada, P. Right bundle branch block and ST segment elevation in leads V-1 through V-3: a marker for sudden death in patients without demonstrable structural heart disease. *Circulation* 1998; **97**: 457–460.

23. Priori, S.G., Napolitano, C., Gasparini, M. *et al.* Clinical and genetic heterogeneity of right bundle branch block and ST-segment elevation syndrome: a prospective evaluation of 52 families. *Circulation* 2000; **102**: 2509–2515.

24. Priori, S.G., Napolitano, C., Gasparini, M. *et al.* Natural history of Brugada syndrome – insights for risk stratification and management. *Circulation* 2002; **105**: 1342–1347.

25. Leenhardt, A., Lucet, V., Denjoy, I., Grau, F., Dongoc, D. & Coumel, P. Catecholaminergic polymorphic ventricular tachycardia in children. A 7-year follow-up of 21 patients. *Circulation* 1995; **91**: 1512–1519.

26. Swan, H. & Laitinen, P. Familial polymorphic ventricular tachycardia—intracellular calcium channel disorder. *Cardiol Electrophysiol. Rev.* 2002; **6**: 81–87.

27. Priori, S.G., Napolitano, C., Tiso, N. *et al.* Mutations in the cardiac ryanodine receptor gene (hRyR2) underlie catecholaminergic polymorphic ventricular tachycardia. *Circulation* 2001; **103**: 196–200.

28. Laitinen, P.J., Brown, K.M., Piippo, K. *et al.* Mutations of the cardiac ryanodine receptor (RyR2) gene in familial polymorphic ventricular tachycardia. *Circulation* 2001; **103**: 485–490.

29. Lahat, H., Pras, E., Olender, T. *et al.* A missense mutation in a highly conserved region of CASQ2 is associated with autosomal recessive catecholamine-induced polymorphic ventricular tachycardia in Bedouin families from Israel. *Am. J. Hum. Genet.* 2001; **69**: 1378–1384.

30. Postma, A.V., Denjoy, I., Hoorntje, T.M. *et al.* Absence of calsequestrin 2 causes severe forms of catecholaminergic polymorphic ventricular tachycardia. *Circ. Res.* 2002; **91**: E21–E26.

31. Thiene, G., Nava, A., Corrado, D., Rossi, L. & Pennelli, N. Right ventricular cardiomyopathy and sudden death in young people. *N. Engl. J. Med.* 1988; **318**: 129–133.

32. Basso, C., Corrado, D. & Thiene, G. Cardiovascular causes of sudden death in young individuals including athletes. *Cardiol. Rev.* 1999; **7**: 127–135.

33. Corrado, D., Thiene, G., Nava, A., Rossi, L. & Pennelli, N. Sudden death in young competitive athletes: clinicopathological correlations in 22 cases. *Am. J. Med.* 1990; **89**: 588–596.

34. Rampazzo, A., Nava, A., Malacrida, S. *et al.* Mutation in human desmoplakin domain binding to plakoglobin causes a dominant form of arrhythmogenic right ventricular cardiomyopathy. *Am. J. Hum. Genet.* 2002; **71**: 1200–1206.

35. McKoy, G., Protonotarios, N., Crosby, A. *et al.* Identification of a deletion in plakoglobin in arrhythmogenic right ventricular cardiomyopathy with palmoplantar keratoderma and woolly hair (Naxos disease). *Lancet* 2000; **355**: 2119–2124.

36. Tiso, N., Stephan, D.A., Nava, A. *et al.* Identification of mutations in the cardiac ryanodine receptor gene in families

affected with arrhythmogenic right ventricular cardiomyopathy type 2 (ARVD2). *Hum. Mol. Genet.* 2001; **10**: 189–194.

37. Maron, B.J., Gardin, J.M., Flack, J.M., Gidding, S.S., Kurosaki, T.T. & Bild, D.E. Prevalence of hypertrophic cardiomyopathy in a general-population of young-adults – echocardiographic analysis of 4111 subjects in the CARDIA study. *Circulation* 1995; **92**: 785–789.

38. Elliott, P. & McKenna, W.J. Hypertrophic cardiomyopathy. *Lancet* 2004; **363**: 1881–1891.

39. Chiang, C. Congenital and acquired long QT syndrome: current concepts and management. *Cardiol. Rev.* 2004; **12**: 222–234.

40. Yang, P., Kanki, H., Drolet, B. *et al.* Allelic variants in long-QT disease genes in patients with drug-associated torsades de pointes. *Circulation* 2002; **105**: 1943–1948.

41. Roden, D.M. Pharmacogenetics and drug-induced arrhythmias. *Cardiovasc. Res.* 2001; **50**: 224–231.

42. Abbott, G.W., Sesti, F., Splawski, I. *et al.* MiRP1 forms I-Kr potassium channels with HERG and is associated with cardiac arrhythmia. *Cell* 1999; **97**: 175–187.

43. Moss, A.J., Zareba, W., Hall, W.J. *et al.* Prophylactic implantation of a defibrillator in patients with myocardial infarction and reduced ejection fraction. *N. Engl. J. Med.* 2002; **346**: 877–883.

44. Bardy, G.H., Lee, K.L., Mark, D.B. *et al.* Amiodarone or an implantable cardioverter-defibrillator for congestive heart failure. *N. Engl. J. Med.* 2005; **352**: 225–237.

45. Grimm, W., Christ, M., Bach, J., Muller, H.H. & Maisch, B. Noninvasive arrhythmia risk stratification in idiopathic dilated cardiomyopathy – results of the Marburg cardiomyopathy study. *Circulation* 2003; **108**: 2883–2891.

46. Gorgels, A.P.M., Gijsbers, C., de Vreede-Swagemakers, J., Lousberg, A. & Wellens, H.J.J. Out-of-hospital cardiac arrest – the relevance of heart failure. The Maastricht Circulatory Arrest Registry. *Eur. Heart. J.* 2003; **24**: 1204–1209.

47. Huikuri, H.V., Castellanos, A. & Myerburg, R.J. Medical progress: sudden death due to cardiac arrhythmias. *N. Engl. J. Med.* 2001; **345**: 1473–1482.

48. Doval, H.C., Nul, D.R., Grancelli, H.O. *et al.* Nonsustained ventricular tachycardia in severe heart failure: Independent marker of increased mortality due to sudden death. *Circulation* 1996; **94**: 3198–3203.

49. Monserrat, L., Elliott, P.M., Gimeno, J.R., Sharma, S., Penas-Lado, M. & McKenna, W.J. Non-sustained ventricular tachycardia in hypertrophic cardiomyopathy: an independent marker of sudden death risk in young patients. *J. Am. Coll. Cardiol.* 2003; **42**: 873–879.

50. Teerlink, J.R., Jalaluddin, M., Anderson, S. *et al.* Ambulatory ventricular arrhythmias in patients with heart failure do not specifically predict an increased risk of sudden death. *Circulation* 2000; **101**: 40–46.

51. Kleiger, R.E., Miller, J.P., Bigger, J.T. & Moss, A.J. Decreased heart-rate-variability and its association with increased mortality after acute myocardial-infarction. *Am. J. Cardiol.* 1987; **59**: 256–262.

52. Bigger, J.T., Fleiss, J.L., Steinman, R.C., Rolnitzky, L.M., Kleiger, R.E. & Rottman, J.N. Frequency-domain measures of heart period variability and mortality after myocardial-infarction. *Circulation* 1992; **85**: 164–171.

53. Nolan, J., Batin, P.D., Andrews, R. *et al.* Prospective study of heart rate variability and mortality in chronic heart failure – results of the United Kingdom heart failure evaluation and assessment of risk trial (UK-Heart). *Circulation* 1998; **98**: 1510–1516.

54. La Rovere, M.T., Pinna, G.D., Hohnloser, S.H. *et al.* Baroreflex sensitivity and heart rate variability in the identification of patients at risk for life-threatening arrhythmias – Implications for clinical trials. *Circulation* 2001; **103**: 2072–2077.

55. Huikuri, H.V., Makikallio, T.H., Peng, C.K. *et al.* Fractal correlation properties of R-R interval dynamics and mortality in patients with depressed left ventricular function after an acute myocardial infarction. *Circulation* 2000; **101**: 47–53.

56. Benditt, D.G., Ermis, C., Pham, S. *et al.* Implantable diagnostic monitoring devices for evaluation of syncope, and Tachy- and Brady-arrhythmias. *J. Interv. Card. Electr.* 2003; **9**: 137–144.

57. Huikuri, H.V., Mahaux, V., Bloch-Thomsen, P.E. & Inv, C. Cardiac arrhythmias and risk stratification after myocardial infarction: results of the CARISMA pilot study. *Pace* 2003; **26**: 416–419.

58. Kautzner, J., Yi, G., Camm, A.J. & Malik, M. Short-term and long-term reproducibility of Qt, Qtc, and Qt dispersion measurement in healthy subjects. *Pace* 1994; **17**: 928–937.

59. Zabel, M., Klingenheben, T., Franz, M.R. & Hohnloser, S.H. Assessment of QT dispersion for prediction of mortality or arrhythmic events after myocardial infarction – results of a prospective, long-term follow-up study. *Circulation* 1998; **97**: 2543–2550.

60. Okin, P.M., Devereux, R.B., Fabsitz, R.R., Lee, E.T., Galloway, J.M. & Howard, B.V. Principal component analysis of the T wave and prediction of cardiovascular mortality in American Indians – The Strong Heart Study. *Circulation* 2002; **105**: 714–719.

61. Klingenheben, T., Zabel, M., D'Agostino, R.B., Cohen, R.J. & Hohnloser, S.H. Predictive value of T-wave alternans for arrhythmic events in patients with congestive heart failure. *Lancet* 2000; **356**: 651–652.

62. Rosenbaum, D.S., Jackson, L.E., Smith, J.M., Garan, H., Ruskin, J.N. & Cohen, R.J. Electrical alternans and vulnerability to ventricular arrhythmias. *N. Engl. J. Med.* 1994; **330**: 235–241.

63. Gold, M.R., Bloomfield, D.M., Anderson, K.P. *et al.* A comparison of T-wave alternans, signal averaged electrocardiography and programmed ventricular stimulation for arrhythmia risk stratification. *J. Am. Coll. Cardiol.* 2000; **36**: 2247–2253.

64. Huikuri, H.V., Tapanainen, J.M., Lindgren, K. *et al.* Prediction of sudden cardiac death after myocardial infarction in the beta-blocking era. *J. Am. Coll. Cardiol.* 2003; **42**: 652–658.

65. Gomes, J.A., Cain, M.E., Buxton, A.E., Josephson, M.E., Lee, K.L. & Hafley, G.E. Prediction of long-term outcomes by signal-averaged electrocardiography in patients with unsustained ventricular tachycardia, coronary artery disease, and left ventricular dysfunction. *Circulation* 2001; **104**: 436–441.

66. Brugada, P., Green, M., Abdollah, H. & Wellens, H.J.J. Significance of ventricular arrhythmias initiated by programmed ventricular stimulation: the importance of the type of ventricular arrhythmia induced and the number of premature stimuli required. *Circulation* 1984; **69**: 87–92.

67. Prystowsky, E.N. Electrophysiologic–electropharmacologic testing in patients with ventricular arrhythmias. *Pace* 1988; **11**: 225–251.

68. Schmitt, H., Hurst, T., Coch, M., Killat, H., Wunn, B. & Waldecker, B. Nonsustained, asymptomatic ventricular tachycardia in patients with coronary artery disease: prognosis and incidence of sudden death of patients who are noninducible by electrophysiological testing. *Pace* 2000; **23**: 1220–1225.

69. Crandall, B.G., Morris, C.D., Cutler, J.E. *et al.* Implantable cardioverter-defibrillator therapy in survivors of out-of-hospital sudden cardiac death without inducible arrhythmias. *J. Am. Coll. Cardiol.* 1993; **21**: 1186–1192.

70. Buxton, A.E., Lee, K.L., Hafley, G.E. *et al.* Relation of ejection fraction and inducible ventricular tachycardia to mode of death in patients with coronary artery disease – an analysis of patients enrolled in the Multicenter Unsustained Tachycardia Trial. *Circulation* 2002; **106**: 2466–2472.

71. Chugh, S.S., Jui, J., Gunson, K. *et al.* Current burden of sudden cardiac death: multiple source surveillance versus retrospective death certificate-based review in a large US community. *J. Am. Coll. Cardiol.* 2004; **44**: 1268–1275.

72. Marenco, J.P., Wang, P.J., Link, M.S., Homoud, M.K. & Estes N.A.M. Improving survival from sudden cardiac arrest – the role of the automated external defibrillator. *J. Am. Med. Assoc.* 2001; **285**: 1193–1200.

73. Hallstrom, A.P., Ornato, J.P., Weisfeldt, M. *et al.* Public-access defibrillation and survival after out-of-hospital cardiac arrest. *N. Engl. J. Med.* 2004; **351**: 637–646.

74. Sueta, C.A., Chowdhury, M., Boccuzzi, S.J. *et al.* Analysis of the degree of undertreatment of hyperlipidemia and congestive heart failure secondary to coronary artery disease. *Am. J. Cardiol.* 1999; **83**: 1303–1307.

75. Frolkis, J.P., Zyzanski, S.J., Schwartz, J.M. & Suhan, P.S. Physician noncompliance with the 1993 National Cholesterol Education Program (NCEP–ATPII) guidelines. *Circulation* 1998; **98**: 851–855.

76. Pilote, L., Califf, R.M., Sapp, S. *et al.* Regional variation across the United-States in the management of acute myocardial infarction. *N. Engl. J. Med.* 1995; **333**: 565–572.

77. Stafford, R.S. & Radley, D.C. The underutilization of cardiac medications of proven benefit, 1990 to 2002. *J. Am. Coll. Cardiol.* 2003; **41**: 56–61.

78. Barnato, A., Lucas, F., Staiger, D., Wennberg, D. & Chandra, A. Hospital-level racial disparities in acute myocardial infarction treatment and outcomes. *Med. Care* 2005; **43**: 308–319.

79. Kaul, P., Newby, L.K., Fu, Y.L. *et al.* International differences in evolution of early discharge after acute myocardial infarction. *Lancet* 2004; **363**: 511–517.

80. Gluckman, T.J., Baranowski, B., Ashen, D. *et al.* A practical and evidence-based approach to cardiovascular disease risk reduction. *Arch. Intern. Med.* 2004; **164**: 1490–1500.

81. Hennekens, C.H., Dyken, M.L. & Fuster, V. Aspirin as a therapeutic agent in cardiovascular disease: a statement for healthcare professionals from the American Heart Association. *Circulation* 1997; **96**: 2751–2753.

82. Steering Committee of the Physicians' Health Study Research Group. Final report on the aspirin component of the ongoing Physicians Health Study. *N. Engl. J. Med.* 1989; **321**: 129–135.

83. Ridker, P.M., Cook, N.R., Lee, I.M. *et al.* A randomized trial of low-dose aspirin in the primary prevention of cardiovascular disease in women. *N. Engl. J. Med.* 2005; **352**: 1293–1304.

84. Pepine, C.J. Aspirin and newer orally active antiplatelet agents in the treatment of the post-myocardial infarction patient. *J. Am. Coll. Cardiol.* 1998; **32**: 1126–1128.

85. Yusuf, S., Fox K.A.A., Tognoni, G. *et al.* Effects of clopidogrel in addition to aspirin in patients with acute coronary syndromes without ST-segment elevation. *N. Engl. J. Med.* 2001; **345**: 494–502.

86. Mehta, S.R., Yusuf, S., Peters, R.J.G. *et al.* Effects of pretreatment with clopidogrel and aspirin followed by long-term therapy in patients undergoing percutaneous coronary intervention: the PCI-CURE study. *Lancet* 2001; **358**: 527–533.

87. Steinhubl, S.R., Berger, P.B., Mann, J.T. *et al.* Early and sustained dual oral antiplatelet therapy following percutaneous coronary intervention – a randomized controlled trial. *J. Am. Med. Assoc.* 2002; **288**: 2411–2420.

88. Hurlen, M., Abdelnoor, M., Smith, P., Erikssen, J. & Arnesen, H. Warfarin, aspirin, or both after myocardial infarction. *N. Engl. J. Med.* 2002; **347**: 969–974.

89. ISIS-4 (Fourth International Study of Infarct Survival) Collaborative Group. ISIS-4: a randomized factorial trial assessing early oral captopril, oral mononitrate, and intravenous magnesium sulfate in 58,050 patients with suspected acute myocardial infarction. *Lancet* 1995; **345**: 669–685.

90. Gruppo Italiano per lo Studio della Sopravvivenza nell'infarto Miocardico. GISSI-3: effects of lisinopril and transdermal glyceryl trinitrate singly and together on 6-week mortality and ventricular function after acute myocardial infarction. *Lancet* 1994; **343**: 1115–1122.

91. Ambrosioni, E., Borghi, C. & Magnani, B. The effect of the angiotensin-converting-enzyme inhibitor zofenopril on mortality and morbidity after anterior myocardial infarction. *N. Engl. J. Med.* 1995; **332**: 80–85.

92. Yusuf, S., Sleight, P., Pogue, J. *et al.* Effects of an angiotensin-converting-enzyme inhibitor, ramipril, on cardiovascular events in high-risk patients. *N. Engl. J. Med.* 2000; **342**: 145–153.

93. Fox, K.M., Bertrand, M., Ferrari, R. *et al.* Efficacy of perindopril in reduction of cardiovascular events among patients with stable coronary artery disease: randomised, double-blind, placebo-controlled, multicentre trial (the EUROPA study). *Lancet* 2003; **362**: 782–788.

94. Braunwald, E., Pfeffer, M.A., Domanski, M. *et al.* Angiotensin-converting-enzyme inhibition in stable coronary artery disease. *N. Engl. J. Med.* 2004; **351**: 2058–2068.

95. Kjeldsen, S.E., Dahlof, B., Devereux, R.B. *et al.* Effects of losartan on cardiovascular morbidity and mortality in patients with isolated systolic hypertension and left ventricular hypertrophy – a Losartan intervention for Endpoint reduction (LIFE) substudy. *J. Am. Med. Assoc.* 2002; **288**: 1491–1498.

96. Pourdjabbar, A., Lapointe, N. & Rouleau, J. Angiotensin receptor blockers: powerful evidence with cardiovascular outcomes? *Can. J. Cardiol.* 2002; **18**: 7A-14A.

97. Chobanian, A.V., Bakris, G.L., Black, H.R. *et al.* Seventh Report of the Joint National Committee on prevention, detection, evaluation, and treatment of high blood pressure. *Hypertension* 2003; **42**: 1206–1252.

98. Freemantle, N., Cleland, J., Young, P., Mason, J. & Harrison, J. beta Blockade after myocardial infarction: systematic review and meta regression analysis. *Br. Med. J.* 1999; **318**: 1730–1737.

99. Hunt, S.A., Baker, D.W., Chin, M.H. *et al.* Committee to revise the 1995 Guidelines for the evaluation and management of heart failure. ACC/AHA guidelines for the evaluation and management of chronic heart failure in the adult: executive summary: a report of the American College of Cardiology/American Heart Association Task Force on Practice Guidelines. *Circulation* 2001; **104**: 2996–3007.

100. Executive summary of the Third Report of the National Cholesterol Education Program (NCEP) expert panel on detection, evaluation, and treatment of high blood cholesterol in adults (Adult Treatment Panel III). *J. Am. Med. Assoc.* 2001; **285**: 2486–2497.

101. Nissen, S.E., Tuzcu, E.M., Schoenhagen, P. *et al.* Effect of intensive compared with moderate lipid-lowering therapy on progression of coronary atherosclerosis – a randomized controlled trial. *J. Am. Med. Assoc.* 2004; **291**: 1071–1080.

102. Cannon, C.P., Braunwald, E., McCabe, C.H. *et al.* Intensive versus moderate lipid lowering with statins after acute coronary syndromes. *N. Engl. J. Med.* 2004; **350**: 1495–1504.

103. LaRosa, J., Grundy, S., Waters, D. *et al.* Intensive lipid lowering with atorvastatin in patients with stable coronary disease. *N. Engl. J. Med.* 2005; **352**: 1425–1435.

104. Jorenby, D.E., Leischow, S.J., Nides, M.A. *et al.* A controlled trial of sustained-release bupropion, a nicotine patch, or both for smoking cessation. *N. Engl. J. Med.* 1999; **340**: 685–691.

105. Hu, F.B. & Willett, W.C. Optimal diets for prevention of coronary heart disease. *J. Am. Med. Assoc.* 2002; **288**: 2569–2578.

106. Tuomilehto, J., Lindstrom, J., Eriksson, J.G. *et al.* Prevention of type 2 diabetes mellitus by changes in lifestyle among subjects with impaired glucose tolerance. *N. Engl. J. Med.* 2001; **344**: 1343–1350.

107. Knowler, W.C., Barrett-Connor, E., Fowler, S.E. *et al.* Reduction in the incidence of type 2 diabetes with lifestyle intervention or metformin. *N. Engl. J. Med.* 2002; **346**: 393–403.

108. Stratton, I.M., Adler, A.I., Neil, H.A.W. *et al.* Association of gly-caemia with macrovascular and microvascular complications of type 2 diabetes (UKPDS 35): prospective observational study. *Br. Med. J.* 2000; **321**: 405–412.

109. Manson, J.E., Greenland, P., LaCroix, A.Z. *et al.* Walking compared with vigorous exercise for the prevention of cardiovascular events in women. *N. Engl. J. Med.* 2002; **347**: 716–725.

110. Wannamethee, S.G., Shaper, A.G. & Walker, M. Physical activity and mortality in older men with diagnosed coronary heart disease. *Circulation* 2000; **102**: 1358–1363.

111. Ades, P.A. Cardiac rehabilitation and secondary prevention of coronary heart disease. *N. Engl. J. Med.* 2001; **345**: 892–902.

112. Pitt, B., Zannad, F., Remme, W.J. *et al.* The effect of spirono-lactone on morbidity and mortality in patients with severe heart failure. *N. Engl. J. Med.* 1999; **341**: 709–717.

113. Pitt, B., Remme, W., Zannad, F. *et al.* Eplerenone, a selective aldosterone blocker, in patients with left ventricular dysfunction after myocardial infarction. *N. Engl. J. Med.* 2003; **348**: 1309–1321.

114. Cardiac Resynchronization-Heart Failure (CARE-HF) Study Investigators. The effect of cardiac resynchronization on morbidity and mortality in heart failure. *N. Engl. J. Med.* 2005; **352**: 1539–1549.

115. Bristow, M.R., Saxon, L.A., Boehmer, J. *et al.* Cardiac-resyn-chronization therapy with or without an implantable defib-rillator in advanced chronic heart failure. *N. Engl. J. Med.* 2004; **350**: 2140–2150.

116. Kawachi, I., Colditz, G.A., Ascherio, A. *et al.* Prospective study of phobic anxiety and risk of coronary heart disease in men. *Circulation* 1994; **89**: 1992–1997.

117. Albert, C.M., Chae, C.U., Rexrode, K.M., Manson, J.E. & Kawachi, I. Phobic anxiety and risk of coronary heart disease and sudden cardiac death among women. *Circulation* 2005; **111**: 480–487.

118. Siscovick, D.S., Weiss, N.S., Fletcher, R.H. & Lasky, T. The incidence of primary cardiac-arrest during vigorous exercise. *N. Engl. J. Med.* 1984; **311**: 874–877.

119. Albert, C.M., Mittleman, M.A., Chae, C.U., Lee, I.M., Hennekens, C.H. & Manson, J.E. Triggering of sudden death from cardiac causes by vigorous exertion. *N. Engl. J. Med.* 2000; **343**: 1355–1361.

120. Albert, C.M., Hennekens, C.H., O'Donnell, C.J. *et al.* Fish consumption and risk of sudden cardiac death. *J. Am. Med. Assoc.* 1998; **279**: 23–28.

121. Albert, C.M., Campos, H., Stampfer, M.J. *et al.* Blood levels of long-chain *n*-3 fatty acids and the risk of sudden death. *N. Engl. J. Med.* 2002; **346**: 1113–1118.

122. Valagussa, F., Franzosi, M.G., Geraci, E. *et al.* Dietary supple-mentation with *n*-3 polyunsaturated fatty acids and vitamin E after myocardial infarction: results of the GISSI-Prevenzione trial. *Lancet.* 1999; **354**: 447–455.

123. Marchioli, R., Barzi, F., Bomba, E. *et al.* Early protection against sudden death by *n*-3 polyunsaturated fatty acids after myocardial infarction – time-course analysis of the results of the Gruppo Italiano per lo Studio della Sopravvivenza nell'Infarto Miocardico (GISSI)-Prevenzione. *Circulation* 2002; **105**: 1897–1903.

124. de Lorgeril, M., Renaud, S., Mamelle, N. *et al.* Mediterranean alpha-linolenic acid-rich diet in secondary prevention of coronary heart disease. *Lancet* 1994; **343**: 1454–1459.

125. de Lorgeril, M., Salen, P., Martin, J.L., Monjaud, I., Delaye, J. & Mamelle, N. Mediterranean diet, traditional risk factors, and the rate of cardiovascular complications after myocardial infarction – Final report of the Lyon Diet Heart Study. *Circulation* 1999; **99**: 779–785.

126. Brouwer, I.A., Katan, M.B. & Zock, P.L. Dietary alpha-linolenic acid is associated with reduced risk of fatal coronary heart disease, but increased prostate cancer risk: a meta-analysis. *J. Nutr.* 2004; **134**: 919–922.

127. Krauss, R.M., Eckel, R.H., Howard, B. *et al.* AHA dietary guide-lines – Revision 2000: a statement for healthcare profession-als from the nutrition committee of the American Heart Association. *Circulation* 2000; **102**: 2284–2299.

128. Kris-Etherton, P.M., Harris, W.S., Appel, L.J. & Comm, N. Fish consumption, fish oil, omega-3 fatty acids, and cardiovascu-lar disease. *Circulation* 2002; **106**: 2747–2757.

129. Guallar, E., Sanz-Gallardo, M.I., van't Veer, P. *et al.* Mercury, fish oils, and the risk of myocardial infarction. *N. Engl. J. Med.* 2002; **347**: 1747–1754.

130. Macdonald, J.E. & Struthers, A.D. What is the optimal serum potassium level in cardiovascular patients? *J. Am. Coll. Cardiol.* 2004; **43**: 155–161.

131. Murray, R.P., Connett, J.E., Tyas, S.L. *et al.* Alcohol volume, drinking pattern, and cardiovascular disease morbidity and mortality: is there a U-shaped function? *Am. J. Epidemiol.* 2002; **155**: 242–248.

132. Britton, A. & McKee, M. The relation between alcohol and car-diovascular disease in Eastern Europe: explaining the paradox. *J. Epidemiol. Commun. Health* 2000; **54**: 328–332.

133. McKee, M. & Britton, A. The positive relationship between alcohol and heart disease in eastern Europe: potential physio-logical mechanisms. *J. Roy. Soc. Med.* 1998; **91**: 402–407.

134. Echt, D.S., Liebson, P.R., Mitchell, L.B. *et al.* Mortality and morbidity in patients receiving encainide, flecainide, or placebo – the cardiac-arrhythmia suppression trial. *N. Engl. J. Med.* 1991; **324**: 781–788.

135. Rogers, W.J., Epstein, A.E., Arciniegas, J.G. *et al.* Effect of the antiarrhythmic agent moricizine on survival after myocar-dial-infarction. *N. Engl. J. Med.* 1992; **327**: 227–233.

136. Waldo, A.L., Camm, A.J., deRuyter, H. *et al.* Effect of d-sotalol on mortality in patients with left ventricular dysfunction after recent and remote myocardial infarction. *Lancet* 1996; **348**: 7–12.

137. Kendall, M.J., Lynch, K.P., Hjalmarson, A. & Kjekshus, J. Beta-blockers and sudden cardiac death. *Ann. Intern. Med.* 1995; **123**: 358–367.

138. Boutitie, F., Boissel, J.P., Connolly, S.J. *et al.* Amiodarone inter-action with beta-blockers – Analysis of the merged EMIAT (European Myocardial Infarct Amiodarone Trial) and

CAMIAT (Canadian Amiodarone Myocardial Infarction Trial) databases. *Circulation* 1999; **99**: 2268–2275.

139. Guiraudon, G., Fontaine, G., Frank, R., Escande, G., Etievent, P. & Cabrol, C. Encircling endocardial ventriculotomy – new surgical treatment for life-threatening ventricular tachycardias resistant to medical treatment following myocardial infarction. *Ann. Thorac. Surg.* 1978; **26**: 438–444.

140. Josephson, M.E., Harken, A.H. & Horowitz, L.N. Endocardial excision – new surgical technique for the treatment of recurrent ventricular tachycardia. *Circulation* 1979; **60**: 1430–1439.

141. The Antiarrhythmics versus Implantable Defibrillators (AVID) Investigators. A comparison of antiarrhythmic-drug therapy with implantable defibrillators in patients resuscitated from near-fatal ventricular arrhythmias. *N. Engl. J. Med.* 1997; **337**: 1576–1583.

142. Connolly, S.J., Gent, M., Roberts, R.S. *et al.* Canadian implantable defibrillator study (CIDS): A randomized trial of the implantable cardioverter defibrillator against amiodarone. *Circulation* 2000; **101**: 1297–1302.

143. Kuck, K.H., Cappato, R., Siebels, J., Ruppel, R. & Investigators, C. Randomized comparison of antiarrhythmic drug therapy with implantable defibrillators in patients resuscitated from cardiac arrest : The Cardiac Arrest Study Hamburg (CASH). *Circulation* 2000; **102**: 748–754.

144. Hohnloser, S.H., Kuck, K.H., Dorian, P. *et al.* Prophylactic use of an implantable cardioverter-defibrillator after acute myocardial infarction. *N. Engl. J. Med.* 2004; **351**: 2481–2488.

24

Sequence of therapies during resuscitation: application of CPR

Leonard A. Cobb, M.D.

Harborview Medical Center University of Washington, Seattle, Washington, USA

Introduction

Intuitively, the order in which therapies are applied seems likely to be important for the treatment of many conditions. In the emerging field of cardiac resuscitation such ordering was initially established on the basis of empiricism and on interpretation of animal experiments. In this chapter, a reexamination of two long accepted therapies addresses the possibility that changes might be considered for the sequence of actions in carrying out basic CPR and in the delivery of precordial shocks for ventricular fibrillation.

The worldwide acceptance of the ABC sequence (airway, breathing, circulation) for CPR is impressive. Similarly the emphasis on rapid defibrillation would seem to be logical and has borne the test of time. On the other hand, there is scant evidence for the strict adherence to treatment guidelines in terms of what comes first.

An important reason for reexamining the sequence of steps is that the ground rules have changed over the course of some 40 plus years. CPR was initially developed for use by physicians, nurses, and specially qualified emergency rescue workers.[1] However, resuscitation is now commonly initiated outside the hospital, often by persons with minimal—or even no—formal training in the application of CPR. Notably, the widespread use of automated defibrillators (AEDs) has provided opportunities for new approaches. And clearly, the call for evidence-based medicine is increasingly heard.

The ABC sequence for basic CPR

Prior to 1960, attempts to alter the outcome of cardiac arrest entailed thoracotomy, direct cardiac compression, and internal defibrillation. Whereas open-chest resuscitation could be effective in controlled environments,[2] survivors of such an approach were uncommon. The inventions of effective external techniques to provide circulation, defibrillation, and rescue breathing markedly extended the possibilities for reversing cardiac arrest.[3] The initial steps in cardiac resuscitation were designated ABC shortly after their introduction. That acronym is noteworthy for its simplicity and ease of recall. But why ABC, and not CAB or ACB? The reasoning behind that choice is not clear but might well have been influenced by the possibility of encountering primary ventilatory failure or submersion injury.

Reasons to modify the ABC sequence

For the well-trained healthcare provider, there is probably little reason to modify the ABC sequence for initiating CPR. Thirty years of precedence suggest that immediate change is not mandatory and would likely not be met with enthusiasm. Nonetheless, in considering instruction for the general public, there is at least a practical basis for reexamining alternatives to ABC.

An important reason to replace the current ABC sequence in favor of CAB (or ACB) is to emphasize what is most often the principal goal of CPR: to restore tissue oxygenation as rapidly as possible. The vast majority of adults found in cardiac arrest do not have primary respiratory failure as the mechanism leading to collapse. Thus for most patients with cardiac arrest, efforts to afford oxygenation without circulation can be considered a waste of valuable moments. Furthermore, the difficulties in training persons to perform mouth-to-mouth ventilation correctly are considerable[4]

Cardiac Arrest: The Science and Practice of Resuscitation Medicine. 2nd edn., ed. Norman Paradis, Henry Halperin, Karl Kern, Volker Wenzel, Douglas Chamberlain. Published by Cambridge University Press. © Cambridge University Press, 2007.

and contrast with the relative simplicity of teaching and performing sternal chest compression.[5] Finally, at times there may be reluctance to initiate CPR because of perceived hygienic concerns about mouth-to-mouth ventilation.[6,7]

On the other hand, a case for the status quo, i.e., retaining ABC, can be made, particularly in treating infants and some children who are pulseless and unconscious because of primary respiratory failure. Similarly, adults with poisoning or primary ventilatory impairment may be more effectively managed with the ABC sequence.

An exception to the ABC sequence for the lay public was established in the Netherlands in the mid 1980s. CAB was chosen over ABC because of the possible advantage of circulating blood already oxygenated prior to sudden cardiac arrest.[8] It is noteworthy that the CAB sequence for lay public instruction in the Netherlands was recently abandoned in favor of ABC. As far as can be determined, that change was effected largely in an effort to achieve international conformity rather than demonstration of efficacy.[9]

Chest compressions alone

It has been suggested that the provision of chest compressions alone (without ventilation) during the initial minutes of resuscitation may be more efficacious than the ABC sequence, because interruptions of chest compression typically lead to reduced coronary perfusion pressure.[10] The value of chest compression alone has been demonstrated in animal models of cardiac arrest,[11,12] but its role in humans awaits clarification. The production of pulmonary gas exchange with chest compressions has also been demonstrated in experimental animals.[12]

It is relevant to note that EMS dispatchers, when giving transtelephonic instructions, were able to provide instruction more quickly and efficiently when offering instructions for chest compression only, compared to ABC instructions. Importantly, survival of patients in the former group tended to be greater than for those with ABC instruction (14.6% vs. 10.4%).[13]

Staged training for basic life support

Assar and colleagues in the UK have proposed an innovative, phased instructional approach for the training of the general public. Using the bronze, silver, and gold medal designations for the Olympic Games, three instructional programs have been proposed.[14] The bronze level offers instruction in chest compression and opening of the airway (without active ventilation). Silver adds on ventilation at a ratio of 50:5. The gold designation is for the full-course ABC sequence. This remarkably sensible approach was designed to encourage training of the public in the essentials of chest compression, at the same time making available instruction in the full ABCs whenever practical and desired. Such instructional innovation holds promise for enhancing the participation of the general public, thereby facilitating the primary goal of early intervention for sudden cardiac arrest.[15]

A solution

Whereas the CAB sequence seems to afford theoretical advantage over ABC, there is a likely downside, mainly a reluctance to change without evidence for efficacy. Furthermore, it appears unlikely that robust clinical evidence will soon be forthcoming. On the other hand, the goal of encouraging bystander intervention could be furthered quite simply by implementing the bronze, silver, gold format for training of the public. Ideally most of the public should be equipped and ready to carry out the ABC sequence; unfortunately that expectation has not been realized over the past 25 years.[16] If one considers the ease of teaching and the simplicity of application, widespread knowledge about the use of chest compression, with or without ventilation, appears to offer an opportunity for more of the general public to be prepared and willing to initiate resuscitative measures while awaiting arrival of EMS personnel. That approach to training of the public offers the potential advantage of making chest compressions nearly uniformly available because of the relative ease of training. Although the early implementation of training for the bronze stage was conducted over a course of 2 hours,[15] it is likely that the duration could be substantially reduced. Community-wide studies of staged training programs are highly desirable.

CPR before defibrillation?

For many years CPR guidelines have advocated the need for quick delivery of shocks for all patients discovered to be in cardiac arrest with ventricular fibrillation (or pulseless ventricular tachycardia).[17,18] A widely accepted judgment by many EMS experts was to "zap first."

Two observations, however, led some to question the wisdom of always shocking first:
1. Experiments in animals with induced VF showed that after several minutes of ventricular fibrillation, survival was significantly improved when shocks were delivered after a brief period of CPR (plus administration of epinephrine), compared to attempts at immediate defibrillation.[19,20]

2. In patients with out-of-hospital VF, survival was not improved when first responder AEDs were incorporated into mature tiered EMS systems. Contrary to expectations, exchanging immediate shock for CPR by first responders has not served to improve survival.[21,22] An additional consideration in questioning the wisdom of always directing primary attention to defibrillation was the simple observation that, for many patients found in cardiac arrest, VF is not the first identified rhythm; *most* patients found in cardiac arrest by EMS responders do not have VF when first examined.[23] In cases with pulseless electric activity or asystole the emphasis on application of an AED would appear to be counterproductive by delaying the institution of potentially useful therapy, i.e., CPR.

Notably, a policy of shocking all VF patients as soon as possible was actually a departure from the then accepted procedure of providing CPR prior to shock in order to coarsen VF and facilitate its conversion (unless a defibrillator was immediately available on the scene).

If countershock and spontaneous pulse do not occur within 60 seconds of collapse, CPR must be started . . . In unwitnessed arrest CPR Steps A-B-C are needed for about 2 minutes (to reoxygenate the myocardium) before an attempt to defibrillate has a chance to succeed. From Safar, P. and Bircher, N.G.[24]

In retrospect one might question the basis for modifying practice guidelines so as to shock first whenever VF was present. The development and widespread availability of AEDs was undoubtedly the principal stimulus for change. It is also likely that other considerations included the recognition that untreated VF is virtually always fatal, and it seemed to follow that the sooner it was removed, the greater the likelihood of survival. And indeed a number of studies had shown that survival was improved with more rapid response of defibrillator-equipped EMS vehicles.[25,26] Additionally, years of experience in hospital coronary care units convincingly demonstrated that recent onset VF in monitored patients was readily managed with the prompt delivery of shocks without need for CPR.[27] Whatever the explanation, most EMS systems adopted, as a number one priority, the deployment of AEDs as quickly as possible for virtually all patients found in cardiac arrest.

Clinical studies

The dictum to rely on the initial use of defibrillator shocks rather than CPR was challenged by the Seattle Medic One EMS providers.[21] In 1994 that group, prompted by the disappointing results after implementing the quick application of AEDs, modified their treatment protocol to provide

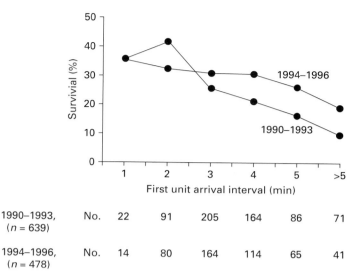

| 1990–1993, (n = 639) | No. | 22 | 91 | 205 | 164 | 86 | 71 |
| 1994–1996, (n = 478) | No. | 14 | 80 | 164 | 114 | 65 | 41 |

Fig. 24.1. Seattle report. Survival in the two study periods according to the response intervals of the first arriving unit. The CPR-first protocol was introduced in 1994. (Reproduced with permission from author and publisher.[21])

1.5 minutes of CPR by first responders prior to use of an AED. The Seattle experience was population-based and utilized a control period immediately before the change in treatment protocol.[21] A randomized trial comparing 3.0 minutes of CPR to immediate defibrillation was conducted in Oslo, Norway,[28] and another randomized trial of 1.5 minutes of CPR was recently performed in Perth, Australia.[29] The Seattle study, the largest to date, but limited by the use of historical controls, showed an overall survival benefit with a CPR-first strategy, restricted entirely to patients with initial response intervals 4 minutes or greater (Fig. 24.1). A qualitatively similar finding was observed in Oslo but without statistically significant benefit overall – only in those with longer initial response intervals (Fig. 24.2). In the Perth study there was no difference in survival rates between the two groups, but response intervals were prolonged to 9 minutes on average, and survival rates were considerably lower than in the other studies. The findings from these three reports are summarized in Table 24.1 below.

Limitations of the clinical studies

The Seattle experience,[21] although population-based, was less robust than a randomized clinical trial, and there is a possibility that the observed benefit could have been due to spontaneous variation in survival rates or that there were other unapparent reasons for increased survival rate. Nonetheless, the *a priori* hypothesis that improvement

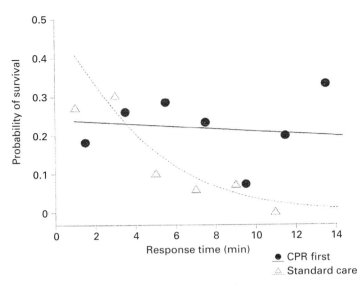

Fig. 24.2. Oslo study. Estimated probability of survival to hospital discharge plotted against response time. Average fraction of surviving patients for each 2-minute interval. Lines indicate logistic regression models with time as independent variable fitted separately for each of the two groups. (Reproduced with permission from author and publisher.[28])

would occur mainly in cases with longer response intervals proved to be the case.

The Oslo study[28] was likely underpowered in the number of patients, and the overall benefit of initial CPR did not achieve the generally accepted degree of significance. As in the Seattle study, however, survival benefit was demonstrated in those with longer initial response intervals.

The randomized trial in Perth[29] failed to show any benefit with the introduction of 1.5 minutes of CPR prior to shock. In that study, initial response intervals were lengthy, pharmacologic measures were not used, and tracheal intubation was infrequently employed. The low survival rates in that study raise the possibility that interventions done within those limitations might not be able to improve outcomes.

Thus, each of the three studies cited in Table 24.1 has limitations, and the advisability of extensive and immediate change is not certain. In two of the three reports, however, the findings are consistent with experimental studies in animals.

Three phases of resuscitation

Weisfeldt and Becker have developed an interesting conceptual framework relating to the treatment of VF; they proposed three phases with markedly differing therapeutic implications.[30]

1. *An electrical phase* persisting for a few minutes after onset of VF. The implication here is one of directing immediate attention to the management of the arrhythmia, i.e., prompt delivery of one or more shocks, without incurring delays for CPR or pharmacologic intervention. A relevant clinical scenario describes a patient who is observed to develop unexpected cardiac arrest and can be shocked for VF within 2 or 3 minutes. Prompt defibrillation in this situation has a high likelihood for successful resuscitation. The duration of the electrical phase may be only about 4 minutes.

2. *A proposed circulatory phase* immediately follows the electrical phase. During the circulatory phase the myocardium has become depleted of energy-rich substrates; tissue acidosis has developed; and cellular dysfunction is operative. In this phase, defibrillation attempts without attention to the state of the myocardium are much less effective than in the earlier period, and a shock is likely to result in asystole or to establishment of an organized cardiac rhythm without myocardial contraction. It is during the circulatory phase that oxygen delivery as well as removal of metabolic byproducts by CPR-generated blood flow prior to shock is likely to be of utility. Of note, most victims of out-of-hospital cardiac arrest, when first encountered by EMS, can be considered to be in the circulatory phase. The circulatory phase is estimated to persist for about 10 minutes if VF is not treated.

3. *A metabolic phase* is said to have developed after about 10 minutes of untreated cardiac arrest. In this stage, standard therapies become progressively ineffective, and survival rates are poor. The biochemical alterations leading to this state are not clearly defined, but are postulated to represent factors beyond those immediately due to ischemia or tissue reperfusion. Postresuscitation cooling has been shown to afford benefit;[31,32] other approaches are undergoing study.[33]

Estimating the duration of untreated VF

If the principles described above are accepted, including the position that in some patients it is advisable to provide CPR prior to delivery of shocks, how does one determine the appropriate intervention for the initial management of VF? A tentative estimate of "down time," based on the available clinical history, can sometimes be made on arrival at the scene of cardiac arrest, although the accuracy of that information is often unreliable. Additionally, if bystander

Table 24.1. Summary of three clinical studies: patients with VF on arrival of EMS

Design	Seattle[21] Population-based, historical controls	Oslo[28] Randomized clinical trial	Perth[29] Randomized clinical trial
No. patients			
CPR First	478	104	119
Shock ASAP	639	96	137
Overall survival to hosp.			
Discharge			
CPR First	30% } $p = 0.04$	22% } $p = 0.20$	4.2% } $p = 0.81$
Shock ASAP	24%	15%	5.1%
Avg. first response			
Interval (min)		6.5[c]	
CPR First	3.6[a]		9.3[b]
Shock ASAP	3.7[a]		9.0[b]
Bystander witnessed (%)			
CPR First	71%	91%	74%
Shock ASAP	73%	94%	80%
Bystander- initiated CPR		(0.40)	(0.13)
CPR First	58%	62%	54%
Shock ASAP	58%	56%	64%
Survival with longer response intervals			
Delay specified	$\geq 4\,min^a$	$>5\,min^a$	$> 5\,min^b$
Survival to hosp. discharge			
CPR first	27% (60/220) } $p < 0.01$	22% (14/64) } $p < 0.01$	4% (4/113)) } $p = 0.74$
Shock ASAP	17% (56/321)	4% (2/55)	5% (5/101))
Survival with shorter response intervals			
Response interval	$< 4\,min$	$\leq 5\,min$	$\leq 5\,min$
CPR First	32% (82/258)	23% (9/40)	12% (3/24)
Shock ASAP	31% (99/318)	29% (12/41)	0% (0/18)

[a] Measured from dispatch time.

[b] Measured from time call received.

[c] 6.5 min for all subjects (L. Wik, pers.commun., 9 October, 2005).

ASAP = as soon as possible.

CPR has been initiated, the qualitative aspects of that are usually not known. Thus, unfortunately, the arriving team has to rely to a certain extent on guesswork to untangle the situation.

Another approach is to examine the VF waveform, which declines in amplitude and frequency over the course of several minutes. To this end, several analytic approaches have been suggested as being helpful. These include measurements of signal amplitude[34,35] waveform frequency/spectral analyses,[35,36] application of chaos theory,[37] and combinations thereof. Such probes have an appeal in that they can be automated and the information transmitted to the EMS personnel, but the clinical utility of these measurements has yet to be established. The influence of time and of CPR on the VF waveform is shown in Fig. 24.3.

Summary

The ABC sequence for basic life support has withstood a test of time for health care professionals. On the other hand, a change in emphasis for the general public deserves consideration. The training requirements for mouth-to-mouth ventilation and the difficulty in its correct performance stand in sharp contrast to the relative ease in teaching and performing chest compressions. Furthermore, the provision of chest compressions appears to be the most vital element in the initial management of cardiac arrest Accordingly the use of staged training for the general public[14] (e.g., bronze, silver, gold) warrants further testing and application.

CPR prior to defibrillation is an attractive, but not fully evaluated, option in patients attended several minutes

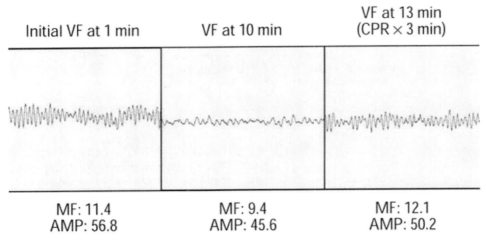

Fig. 24.3. From Berg, R.A. *et al.* Typical changes in VF waveform during untreated VF (after 1 and 10 min) and after 3 min. of CPR-first. MF, median frequency (in Hz); AMP, amplitude (in mV). (Reproduced with permission from author and publisher.[35])

after collapse. There are unanswered questions about when "several minutes" starts and how long CPR should continue before rhythm analysis and shock. The widespread acceptance of CPR prior to shock will require modifications in regard to the complete acceptance of the Chain of Survival as now promulgated, yet evidence to date does not support the practice of immediately shocking patients who are no longer in the electrical phase of ventricular fibrillation.[22,23,30,38]

REFERENCES

1. The closed-chest method of cardiopulmonary resuscitation. Benefits and hazards. Editorial. *Circulation* 1962; **26**: 324.

2. Beck, C.S., Pritchard, H. & Feil, S.H. Ventricular fibrillation of long duration abolished by electric shock. *J. Am. Med. Assoc.* 1947; **135**: 985–991.

3. Kouwenhoven, W.B., Jude, J.R. & Knickerbocker, G.G. Closed-chest cardiac massage. *J. Am. Med. Assoc.* 1960; **173**: 1064–1067.

4. Mandel, L.P. & Cobb, L.A. Initial and long term competency of citizens trained in CPR. *Emerg. Hlth. Serv. Quart.* 1982; **1**: 49–63.

5. Sanders, A.B. & Ewy, G.A. Cardiopulmonary resuscitation in the real world: When will the guidelines get the message? *J. Am. Med. Assoc.* 2005; **293**: 363–365.

6. Locke, C.J., Berg, R.A., Sanders, A.B. *et al.* Bystander cardiopulmonary resuscitation: concerns about mouth-to-mouth contact. *Arch. Intern. Med.* 1995; **155**: 938–943.

7. Ornato, J.P., Hallagan, L.F., McMahan, S.B., Peeples, E.H. & Rostafinski, A.G. Attitudes of BCLS instructors about mouth-to-mouth resuscitation during the AIDS epidemic. *Ann. Emerg. Med.* 1990; **19**: 151–156.

8. Meursing, B.T.J., Zimmerman, A.N.E. & van Heyst, A.N.P. Experimental evidence in favor of a reversed sequence in cardiopulmonary resuscitation. *J. Am. Coll. Cardiol.* 1983; **1**: 610. Abstract.

9. Meursing, B.T.J., Wulterkens, D.W., & van Kesteren, R.G. The ABC of resuscitation and the Dutch (re)treat. *Resuscitation* 2005; **64**: 279–286.

10. Steen, S., Liao, Q., Pierre, L., Paskevicius, A. & Sjöberg, T. The critical importance of minimal delay between chest compressions and subsequent defibrillation: a haemodynamic explanation. *Resuscitation* 2003; **58**: 249–258.

11. Kern, K.B., Hilwig, R.W., Berg, R.A. & Ewy, G.A. Efficacy of chest compression-only BLS CPR in the presence of an occluded airway. *Resuscitation* 1998; **39**: 179–188.

12. Kern, K.B., Hilwig, R.W., Berg, R.A., Sanders, A.B. & Ewy, G.A. Importance of continuous chest compression during cardiopulmonary resuscitation. Improved outcome during a simulated single lay-rescuer scenario. *Circulation* 2002; **105**: 645–649.

13. Hallstrom, A., Cobb, L., Johnson, E. & Copass, M. Cardiopulmonary resuscitation by chest compression alone or with mouth-to-mouth ventilation. *N. Engl. J. Med.* 2000; **342**: 1546–1553.

14. Assar, D., Chamberlain, D., Colquhoun, M. *et al.* A rationale for staged teaching of basic life support. *Resuscitation* 1998; **39**: 137–143.

15. Assar, D., Chamberlain, D., Colquhoun, M. *et al.* Randomized controlled trials of staged teaching for basic life support. I. Skill acquisition at bronze stage. *Resuscitation* 2000; **45**: 7–15.

16. Ewy, G.A. Cardiocerebral resuscitation. The new cardiopulmonary resuscitation. *Circulation* 2005; **111**: 2134–2142.

17. Chamberlain, D., Bossaert, L., Carli, P. *et al.* Guidelines for advanced life support: a statement by the Advanced Life Support Working Party of the European Research Council, 1992. *Resuscitation* 1992; **24**: 111–121.

18. Emergency Cardiac Care Committee and the Advanced Cardiac Life Support Subcommittee of the American Heart Association. Automated external defibrillators and ACLS: a new initiative from the American Heart Association. *Am. J. Emerg. Med.* 1991; **9**: 91–94.

19. Niemann, J.T., Cairns, C.B., Sharma, J. & Lewis, R.J. Treatment of prolonged ventricular fibrillation: immediate countershock versus high-dose epinephrine and CPR preceding counter-shock. *Circulation* 1992; **85**: 281–287.

20. Yakaitis, R.W., Ewy, G.A., Otto, C.W., Taren, D.L. & Moon, T.E. Influence of time and therapy on ventricular defibrillation in dogs. *Crit. Care Med.* 1980; **8**: 157–163.

21. Cobb, L.A., Fahrenbruch, C.E., Walsh, T.R. *et al.* Influence of cardiopulmonary resuscitation prior to defibrillation in patients with out-of-hospital ventricular fibrillation. *J. Am. Med. Assoc.* 1999; **281**: 1182–1188.

22. Sweeney, T., Runge, J., Gibbs, M. *et al.* EMT defibrillation does not increase survival from sudden cardiac death in a two-tiered urban-suburban EMS system. *Ann. Emerg. Med.* 1998; **31**: 234–240.

23. Cobb, L.A., Fahrenbruch, C.E., Olsufka, M. & Copass, M.K. Changing incidence of out-of-hospital ventricular fibrillation, 1980–2000. *J. Am. Med. Assoc.* 2002; **288**: 3008–3013.

24. Safar, P. & Bircher, N.G. *Cardiopulmonary Cerebral Resuscitation.* 3rd edn. Philadelphia: W.B. Saunders, 1988.

25. Weaver, W.D., Cobb, L.A., Hallstrom, A.P., Fahrenbruch, C., Copass, M.K. & Ray, R. Factors influencing survival after out-of-hospital cardiac arrest. *J. Am. Coll. Cardiol.* 1986; **7**: 752–757.

26. Larsen, M.P., Eisenberg, M.S., Cummins, R.O. & Hallstrom, A.P. Predicting survival from out-of-hospital cardiac arrest: a graphic model. *Ann. Emerg. Med.* 1993; **22**: 1652–1658.

27. Killip, T. & Kimball, J.T. Treatment of myocardial infarction in a coronary care unit: a two year experience with 250 patients. *Am. J. Cardiol.* 1967; **20**: 457–464.

28. Wik, L., Hansen, T.B., Fylling, F. *et al.* Delaying defibrillation to give basic cardiopulmonary resuscitation to patients with out-of-hospital ventricular fibrillation–a randomized trial. *J. Am. Med. Assoc.* 2003; **289**: 1389–1395.

29. Jacobs, I.G., Finn, J.C., Oxer, H.F. & Jelinek, G.A. CPR before defibrillation in out-of-hospital cardiac arrest; a randomized trial. *Emerg. Med. Austral.* 2005; **17**: 39–45.

30. Weisfeldt, M.L. & Becker, L.B. Resuscitation after cardiac arrest. A 3-phase time-sensitive model. *J. Am. Med. Assoc.* 2002; **288**: 3035–3038.

31. Bernard, S.A., Gray, T.W., Buist, M.D. *et al.* Treatment of comatose survivors of out-of-hospital cardiac arrest with induced hypothermia. *N. Engl. J. Med.* 2002; **346**: 557–563.

32. The Hypothermia After Cardiac Arrest Study Group. Mild therapeutic hypothermia to improve the neurologic outcome after cardiac arrest. *N. Engl. J. Med.* 2002; **346**: 549–556.

33. Anderson, T. & Vanden Hoek, T.L. Preconditioning and the oxidants of sudden death. *Curr. Opin. Crit. Care.* 2003; **3**: 194–198.

34. Weaver, W.D., Cobb, L.A., Dennis, D., Ray, R., Hallstrom, A.P. & Copass, M.K. Amplitude of ventricular fibrillation waveform and outcome after cardiac arrest. *Ann. Intern. Med.* 1985; **102**: 53–55.

35. Berg, R.A., Hilwig, R.W., Kern, K.B. & Ewy, G.A. Precountershock cardiopulmonary resuscitation improves ventricular fibrillation median frequency and myocardial readiness for successful defibrillation from prolonged ventricular fibrillation: a randomized, controlled swine study. *Ann. Emerg. Med.* 2002; **40**: 563–570.

36. Eftestøl, T., Wik, L.,Sunde, K. & Steen, P.A. Effects of cardiopulmonary resuscitation on predictors of ventricular fibrillation success during out-of-hospital cardiac arrest. *Circulation* 2004; **110**: 10–15.

37. Callaway, C.W., Sherman, L.D., Mosesso, V.N., Dietrich, T.J., Holt, E. & Clarkson, M.C. Scaling exponent predicts defibrillation success for out-of-hospital ventricular fibrillation cardiac arrest. *Circulation* 2001; **103**: 1656–1661.

38. Stotz, M., Albrecht, R., Zwicker, G., Drewe, J. & Ummenhofer, W. EMS defibrillation-first policy may not improve outcome in out-of-hospital cardiac arrest. *Resuscitation* 2003; **58**: 277–282.

25

Transthoracic defibrillation

Richard E. Kerber[1], Charles D. Deakin[2], and Willis A. Tacker[3] Jr.

[1] Department of Internal Medicine, University of Iowa, Iowa City, IA, USA
[2] Shackleton Department of Anesthesia, Southampton University Hospital NHS Trust, Southampton, UK
[3] Basic Medical Sciences, Purdue University, West Lafayette, IN, USA

Introduction and history of defibrillation

The passage of electrical current through the myocardium to terminate ventricular fibrillation (VF) or ventricular tachycardia is the definitive treatment and single most important factor in surviving cardiac arrest due to VF. This chapter will review the history and theory of defibrillation, current techniques, and future developments of this critically important therapy.

In 1775, the Danish veterinarian–physician Abildgaard demonstrated that chickens could be stunned and revived by electrical shocks administered to the head and to the heart.[1] Prevost and Batelli in 1899 showed that ventricular fibrillation in dogs could be terminated by electric shocks.[2] In the twentieth century, the Consolidated Edison Company of New York became concerned about the high rate of accidental electrocutions among maintenance workers, and funded research on the cardiac consequences of electrical shocks. Supported by this source, Hooker et al. published important studies on defibrillation in animals.[3] The first human defibrillation was performed in 1947 by Beck who administered shocks directly to the exposed epicardium in an operating room.[4] The first closed-chest human defibrillation was achieved by Zoll et al. in 1956.[5] Although alternating current was used originally, direct current quickly supplanted alternating current;[6] postshock atrial arrhythmias were found to be reduced by use of direct current.

An important consequence of the early canine studies of defibrillation was the observation that arterial pressure rose when electrodes were pressed against the animal chest. This recognition of the role of chest compression in blood circulation and arterial pressure maintenance ultimately resulted in the development of closed-chest massage by Kouwenhoven et al.[7] It is appropriate that the development of contemporary defibrillation techniques should have also resulted in the development of cardiopulmonary resuscitation (CPR), since these two techniques remain cornerstones of cardiac arrest therapy.

Basic science

Theory of defibrillation

Although defibrillation has been an effective cardiac tool for the termination of cardiac arrhythmias for over 45 years, the exact mechanism of defibrillation remains uncertain and controversial. For many years it was believed that a critical mass of myocardium was depolarized by the electrical current traversing the heart; those muscle cells that were not depolarized were thought to be inadequate to sustain the arrhythmia.[8] This hypothesis is supported by the difficulty of initiating and sustaining ventricular fibrillation in the hearts of small animals (e.g., rabbits). More recently, Ideker's group[9] has introduced the "upper limit of vulnerability" hypothesis. This hypothesis suggests that the most important factor in defibrillation is achieving a critical current density throughout the ventricular myocardium; if current density is inadequate, fibrillation may be transiently terminated but then reinitiated. Jones[10] has argued that to achieve defibrillation, shocks must extensively prolong refractoriness so that fibrillation wave fronts are not propagated and VF terminates. Neither Ideker's nor Jones' hypotheses necessarily repudiate the critical mass theory, since a critical mass effect may be important for their mechanisms also.

Cardiac Arrest: The Science and Practice of Resuscitation Medicine. 2nd edn., ed. Norman Paradis, Henry Halperin, Karl Kern, Volker Wenzel, Douglas Chamberlain. Published by Cambridge University Press. © Cambridge University Press, 2007.

The metabolic and biochemical environment in which defibrillation occurs is important. Myocardial levels of the so-called "high-energy phosphates" – adenosine triphosphate (ATP), adenosine diphosphate, adenosine monophosphate, and creatine phosphate–appear crucial.[11] These high-energy phosphates are essential for normal regulation of cell volume and maintenance of the normal ionic gradients via the Na^+/K^+ and $Ca^{2+}/ATPase$ pumps. When ventricular fibrillation occurs, myocardial perfusion ceases, myocytes become oxygen-deficient and are unable to continue normal aerobic metabolism, and contractile function stops.[12] Mitochondrial oxidative phosphorylation is inhibited, with uncoupling of high-energy phosphate production and utilization. The levels of the high-energy phosphates decline progressively as tissue lactate and hydrogen ion levels increase. Conversely, after the restoration of circulation, the regeneration of these compounds indicates a return to normal cellular activity and viability.

The depletion of myocardial high-energy phosphates correlates with the onset of myocardial cell injury. Ischemic myocardial contraction develops and ultrastructural studies show progressive evidence of injury such as disruption of the sarcolemma. ATP levels below 10% of normal strongly suggest irreversible myocardial injury.[13,14] Smaller degrees of depletion, such as may occur in the postischemic phase, are associated with myocardial dysfunction or stunning.

During ventricular fibrillation, the decline of ATP levels with time correlates closely with the success of attempted defibrillation. The levels may also predict poor contractile function and hemodynamic status following defibrillation of VF to a potentially perfusing electrocardiographic rhythm.[15,16]

The timing of defibrillation before or, if necessary, after a period of CPR has been debated. Although current guidelines advocate defibrillation as soon as possible, it has been suggested that a period of CPR before defibrillation may achieve better survival. This was first proposed by Cobb in 1999 who reported that the routine provision of approximately 90 seconds of CPR before use of AED was associated with increased survival when response intervals were 4 minutes or longer.[17] More recently, Wik has studied this in greater detail, reporting that CPR before defibrillation did not improve outcome for patients with ambulance response times shorter than 5 minutes, but for patients with ambulance response times longer than 5 minutes, better outcomes were achieved with 3 minutes of CPR before defibrillation.[18,19] It is known that cellular functioning and in particular active transmembrane ion channel functioning deteriorates rapidly during cardiac arrest. With depletion of high energy ATP reserves, successful defibrillation requires rapidly increasing energy levels. The results of these studies suggest that a period of external chest compression may improve cellular functioning to enable defibrillation to achieve a perfusing rhythm. External chest compression may also reverse distention of both ventricles, particularly the right, which occurs within the first few minutes of VF and subsequently impairs biventricular function after defibrillation.[20]

The ability to defibrillate and subsequent survival correlate with the "coarseness" (amplitude) and the frequency of the ventricular fibrillation waveform. Low-amplitude ventricular fibrillation waveforms are less likely to be associated with restoration of spontaneous circulation and discharge from hospital, and are more likely to convert to asystole following defibrillation.[21] Low-frequency ventricular fibrillation indicates a poor chance of successful resuscitation.[22] The median frequency of the VF waveform correlates with myocardial perfusion during CPR.[23] In an animal model a median frequency of 9.14 Hz or greater had 100% sensitivity in relation to defibrillation success.[23] This type of analysis could possibly be used to determine the most appropriate time to administer a defibrillating shock.[24–26]

Role of transthoracic impedance

Defibrillation involves the delivery of electrical energy across the thorax. Because present defibrillation guidelines specify the delivery of a fixed amount of energy, the magnitude of the transthoracic current (I_m) is determined by transthoracic impedance (TTI).

$$I_m \propto \sqrt{\frac{E}{Z}}$$

where:

I_m = peak discharge current (A)
Z = transthoracic impedance (Ω)
E = electrical energy (J)

The transthoracic impedance is an important determinant of the ensuing defibrillation waveform. The average transthoracic impedance to monophasic defibrillation shocks in adult humans is 70–80 ohms, with a range of 15–150 ohms.[27] Although the total amount of energy delivered is approximately the same, irrespective of the impedance, a low impedance results in a narrow waveform with high current, while high impedance results in a wide waveform with lower current. Excessively high current can cause morphological and physiological myocardial damage associated with postshock arrhythmias, whereas

Table 25.1. Factors that determine and alter human transthoracic impedance

Factor	Effect on impedance
Chest size or interelectrode distance (most important factor)	Larger chest results in higher impedance
Selected energy	Higher energy reduces impedance
Electrode size	Larger electrodes reduce impedance
Couplants between electrodes and chest wall	Failure to use a low resistivity couplant results in very high impedance and low current flow. Gels, electrodes, pastes, and saline-soaked gauze pads are all satisfactory
Multiple shocks	Multiple shocks reduce impedance
Phase of respiration	Inspiration increases impedance, expiration lowers impedance
Electrode-chest wall contact pressure	Firm pressure on hand-held paddles reduces impedance
Sternotomy	Sternotomy lowers impedance
Electrode placement on female breasts	Breast placement increases impedance
Specific arrhythmia (i.e., VF, VT, AFib, AF)*	No effect on impedance

* AFib, atrial fibrillation; AFL, atrial flutter; VF, ventricular fibrillation; VT, ventricular tachycardia.

low current may be inadequate to achieve defibrillation and the longer duration waveform may risk reinduction of ventricular fibrillation. Clinical studies with monophasic waveform defibrillators suggest that optimal success is achieved with a transthoracic current of 30–40 amperes.[27–34]

The challenge in delivering safe defibrillation across a range of impedance is to ensure optimal waveform and current across the entire range. Monophasic defibrillators are unable to adjust for transthoracic impedance and the resultant waveform varies considerably with impedance. Excessively high or low peak transthoracic current is associated with reduced effectiveness of monophasic waveform defibrillation. Minimizing transthoracic impedance will increase the chance of successful defibrillation. Factors affecting transthoracic impedance are listed in Table 25.1 and discussed in more detail below.

Paddle force

When using traditional hand-held defibrillation electrode "paddles," increasing paddle force improves electrical contact at the electrode–skin interface. Optimal paddle force in adults is approximately 8 kg;[35] in children 1–17 years the optimal paddle force is approximately 5 kg and in children <10 kg, approximately 3 kg.[36] Eight kg is a significant force and the physically strongest member of the resuscitation team should therefore be delegated to apply the electrode paddles.

Paddle orientation

Most external defibrillation pads and paddles are asymmetric. Placing the apical electrode in a craniocaudal direction minimizes transthoracic impedance.[37]

Couplant

A couplant is a high conductivity material that minimizes impedance at the electrode-skin interface. Pastes, creams, gels, saline-soaked gauze swabs, or preformed gel pads have all been used for this purpose. Although pastes, creams, and gels all provide good electrical contact, they are prone to be smeared across the chest, making external chest compression slippery and risking arcing between electrodes[38] with the production of a potentially dangerous spark. The low-impedance gel pathway also results in little current traversing the heart.[39] Preformed gel pads as a couplant for hand-held paddle electrodes are quick to apply, provide good electrical contact,[40] and minimize these risks. It is important not to use a high impedance gel (such as some ultrasound gels) since less current is conducted and also since arcing is more likely to occur with associated complications of skin burns or fire.

Shaving the chest

Chest hair increases transthoracic impedance through poor electrode contact and air trapping. Defibrillation across an unshaved chest is likely to result in more severe burns. Shaving the chest prior to defibrillation minimizes transthoracic impedance by improving electrical contact.[41,42] Shaving must not interfere with ongoing external chest compressions.

Lung volume

Lung volume is a major contributor to transthoracic impedance. Firm paddle force (8 kg) during defibrillation reduces overall thoracic volume and reduces transthoracic impedance by 16%.[43] Transthoracic impedance is also lower during the expiratory phase of respiration[31] and increases progressively with increasing positive end-expiratory pressure (PEEP).[44] Patients with acute asthma may have particularly high transthoracic impedance due to lung hyperinflation and auto-PEEP.

Hypothermia

In swine models of short duration (30 seconds) and long duration (8 minutes) VF, moderate (33.0 ºC) and severe (30.0 ºC) hypothermia was associated with a higher defibrillation success rate, despite an increase in transthoracic impedance. A higher resumption of spontaneous circulation was achieved. The improved shock success is thought to be due to a hypothermia-induced change in the mechanical or electrophysiological properties of the myocardium.[45,46]

Repeated shocks

Multiple monophasic shocks slightly reduce transthoracic impedance to subsequent shocks.[27,29] The reduced transthoracic impedance will result in a greater transmyocardial current with subsequent shocks even at the same energy. The mechanism for this reduction in impedance may be related to tissue hyperemia and edema in the current pathway.[47] The effect of repeated biphasic shocks on transthoracic impedance is unknown.

Impedance compensating waveforms

Biphasic waveforms are generated using discharge from a capacitor but electronic modification allows manipulation of the waveform. Instantaneous measurement of transthoracic impedance enables the waveform to be controlled by the defibrillator to provide both optimal current and waveform duration. Shock characteristics that may be altered in various commercially available biphasic defibrillators include the duration of the two pulses (individually and in total) and/or the leading-edge voltage of the pulses. This technology, not available on monophasic defibrillators, has resulted in more effective biphasic defibrillation across a wide range of transthoracic impedance, minimizing the effect of impedance on the success of defibrillation.[48]

Therapy

Electrodes

The optimal size of electrodes for adults is thought to be from 8.5 to 12 cm in diameter.[27,49,50] Although impedance can be reduced by using even larger electrodes, if the electrodes are too large, contact with the chest wall may be inadequate if rigid hand-held electrodes are used. Furthermore,

with very large electrodes a greater proportion of the current may traverse extracardiac pathways, thereby "missing" the heart.[51]

Traditionally, small electrodes have been used for infants and children, often labeled "pediatric" electrodes. This has primarily been based on the intuitive concept that smaller electrodes are more suitable for children. Very small electrodes may result in excessively high transthoracic impedance and inadequate current flow, however.[52] Larger "adult" electrodes are therefore more appropriate if the electrode paddles will fit completely on the child's thorax, which, for most children, is true at or above 1 year of age or 10 kg weight. Current flow is improved by using "adult" paddle electrodes in children.[53]

Electrodes should be placed so that the heart is located between them. The polarity of the paddles is unimportant.[54,55] It is now understood that current does not follow a straight line through the chest between electrodes, and a surprisingly low portion of the total current flow – only about 4% – actually traverses the myocardium during transthoracic defibrillation.[56] The most common electrode placement is apex-anterior: the anterior electrode is placed anteriorly to the right of the upper sternum below the clavicle, while the apical electrode is placed to the left of the nipple, just outside the position of the normal cardiac apex (V_{4-5} position)[57] (Fig. 25.1). The apical electrode must be placed sufficiently laterally to optimize transmyocardial current flow and prevent arcing of current across the chest wall.

It is important in female patients to avoid placing the defibrillator paddles or self-adhesive pads directly on the left breast. The breast should be elevated and the paddle or pad placed on the chest wall lateral to the breast in the expectation that this will reduce impedance and improve current flow.[34]

Other electrode positions have been used successfully: an anterior-posterior position where one electrode is placed anteriorly over the left precordium and the other posteriorly in the right or left infrascapular position or an apex-posterior position where the anterior paddle is placed over the cardiac apex with a posterior paddle in the right infrascapular location (Fig. 25.1). In any individual patient one position may be superior to others; in our experience, a shock will occasionally achieve defibrillation when electrode positions are altered and a new position is used, after several shocks have been administered unsuccessfully from a previously used position.

Putting the electrodes nearer the heart to increase the electrical field strength will increase success and may be achieved by a more invasive defibrillation route. Examples of this include epicardial or endocardial electrodes applied

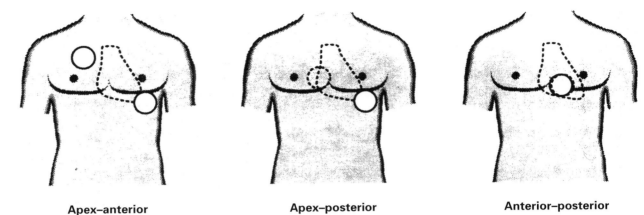

Apex–anterior   **Apex–posterior**   **Anterior–posterior**

Fig. 25.1. Recommended electrode placement for defibrillation. (From Tacker, W.A., ed., *Defibrillation of the Heart*. St. Louis, Mosby-Year Book, 1994:1630.)

either during open-chest resuscitation or by surgical implantation of automatic defibrillators. This also will lower impedance because the electrodes will be closer together. With invasive techniques, energy levels between 5 J and 25 J may be adequate.

Transesophageal electrode placement permits successful defibrillation of ventricular tachycardia and ventricular fibrillation at relatively low energy levels (100 J or less).[58] The technique, however, is unlikely to be applicable for routine resuscitation, and esophageal injury has been reported with higher energies.[59]

Defibrillation can also be performed by using disposable self-adhesive monitoring defibrillation pads that incorporate a conductive gel between the electrode and skin surface.[49,60,61] This is an attractive option: the pads enhance operator safety by physically separating the operator from the patient. In elective situations (electrophysiologic studies, cardiac catheterization laboratory, elective cardioversion) they can be preplaced, facilitating optimal placement without the extreme stress of an ongoing cardiac arrest. Transthoracic impedance is similar to that of standard hand-held electrodes.[49] Self-adhesive pads are routinely supplied with automatic external defibrillators, and are used to detect the surface electrocardiogram and permit its analysis and then to deliver the defibrillating shock.

Present recommendations for the size of pads used with these automatic external defibrillators are that the total area of the two electrodes be at least 150 cm^2.[50]

Defibrillation waveforms

The monophasic damped sinusoidal (MDS) waveform for defibrillation was introduced by Lown in 1962,[62] and remained the standard waveform for transthoracic defibrillation for 30 years. Monophasic truncated exponential waveform defibrillators were used less frequently,[63] and may be less effective.[64] More recently, biphasic truncated exponential waveforms have supplanted the damped sinusoidal monophasic waveform as the standard waveform for transthoracic defibrillation. Shocks given by using the BTE waveform have been shown to achieve higher rates of VF termination than MDS waveforms at equivalent energy levels.[65–67] Furthermore, there is experimental evidence that the BTE waveform is less damaging, as it is associated with less myocardial depression and fewer postshock arrhythmias.[68]

An available variant of the BTE waveform is characterized by a rectilinear (near-rectangular) first pulse followed after polarity reversal by a truncated exponential second pulse.[69]

Energy guidelines for defibrillation by use of monophasic waveform defibrillators have for many years emphasized a "stacked shocks" approach: 200 J, 200–300 J, 360 J. This was based on several studies which found that initial shocks of less than 200 J may generate inadequate current to defibrillate,[70] while higher energy initial shocks did not achieve higher initial success.[71] The newer biphasic truncated exponential waveforms, however, have been found to have much higher success rates (up to 98%) than monophasic waveforms at relatively low shock energies.[66,67,72,73] In view of this, a single-shock strategy might be preferable to three standard shocks, i.e., if the first shock fails to terminate VF, external chest compressions should be immediately resumed, rather than applying additional biphasic shocks which take time and are unlikely to be effective until a period of closed-chest compression has been administered.

Elapsed time during a cardiac arrest is a particularly important consideration when the new automated external defibrillators (AEDs) that analyze the ECG signal are used and, if an algorithm for VF detection is satisfied, the operator is advised to deliver a shock. No CPR can be performed while the analysis is in progress, because CPR produces artifacts in the ECG. The AED algorithms typically require 30 or more seconds for each analysis/charging cycle. Thus, requiring three failed stacked shocks before resuming CPR and administering agents such as epinephrine or vasopressin, could require as long as 1½–2 minutes during which no CPR was administered, thus reducing the chance of success of the resuscitation effort.

"Thumpversion" (precordial thump)

Ventricular tachycardia and, rarely, ventricular fibrillation can be terminated by striking the precordium with a closed fist – so-called "thumpversion" or precordial thump.[74–77] The success rate of this maneuver in terminating the arrhythmia is from 11 to 25% for ventricular tachycardia, and approximately 2% in ventricular fibrillation. However, such a thump can accelerate ventricular tachycardia or convert it to ventricular fibrillation, asystole, or electromechanical dissociation, thereby substantially worsening the patient's condition. "Thumpversion" should be considered in a witnessed cardiac arrest where the patient is pulseless and a defibrillator is not immediately available. If the patient has a pulse, the precordial thump should not be employed unless a defibrillator is immediately available.

Safety of defibrillation

Whereas the use of a defibrillator may be lifesaving for the patient, safety must not be compromised during defibrillation attempts. There are three significant areas of risk during defibrillation: risk to the patient, to the user, and to the equipment/environment. There is obviously some overlap between these.

Risk to the patient

Defibrillation of supraventricular arrhythmias should be synchronized to avoid delivering a shock on the "T" wave of the ECG, which may induce ventricular fibrillation. It is important to avoid inadvertent use of synchronization when shocking ventricular fibrillation in order to avoid delay in delivering a shock.

When paddles are used for monitoring, after one or more shocks an electrical voltage "offset" can result in the monitor incorrectly displaying an ECG trace mimicking asystole, even when the patient remains in VF.[78] This spurious appearance of asystole may last long enough to delay further shocks, because it may mislead rescuers who rely on monitoring through the paddles. Spurious asystole is more likely to occur after several successive shocks have been applied through gel pads and in the presence of high transthoracic impedance. This is probably due to the higher voltages applied with successive shocks. If asystole is seen following a shock while gel pads or paddles ("quick look paddles") are used, the rhythm must be confirmed immediately by attaching standard ECG electrodes.[78] They are less likely to have a prolonged voltage offset.

Increasing numbers of patients requiring defibrillation may have an implanted pacemaker or a cardioverter defibrillator. Both these devices may be damaged by the high current associated with defibrillation (this is one example of risk to equipment and to patient). Placing the electrodes 12–15 cm away from the device has been recommended to ensure both that the sensitive electrical components of the ICD are not damaged and that the defibrillation current does not stray down the low-impedance pathway of the internal pacing/defibrillation electrode.[79–81] This is not difficult to achieve in the majority of such patients, where the pacemaker generator is placed in a subcutaneous pocket in the left pectoral area. In these situations where a right pectoral location is present, anterior–posterior electrode placement can be used safely. All implanted cardioverter defibrillators and pacemakers should be checked promptly in patients after they have been defibrillated, because transient disturbances in sensing, capture, and pacing may occur.

Risk to the user

Accidental shock to the rescuer
The rate of accidental shocks during defibrillation by emergency medical technicians has been reported to be 1/1000 compared with 1/1700 for paramedics, fortunately without morbidity or mortality.[82] When defibrillation is carried out, it is important that no one is physically in direct contact with the patient. The operator must shout "stand clear" and check that all those present have done so before giving the shock. With automated systems, the team leader must ensure that voice commands from the machine are followed. Contact with intravenous infusions, wet clothing, and metallic contact with the patient (e.g., from a bed or trolley) must also be excluded. Electrode pastes can spread across the chest wall and/or onto the operator's hands, leading to arcing of the current and the potential for spark formation.

Risks to equipment and environment (also may carry risk to patient and user)

Oxygen   High oxygen concentrations may be present around patients during resuscitation attempts.[83] Sparks generated during defibrillation may ignite the oxygen and cause a fire and burns to the patient.[84,85] It is recommended that oxygen concentrations around the chest during defibrillation be minimized by avoiding disconnection of the ventilation circuit and ensuring that any free-flowing oxygen is moved away from the patient.

Transdermal drug patches   Nitroglycerine patches may explode if a defibrillating electrode is placed directly over the patch. The explosion is due to arcing and breakdown of the metal backing of the patch rather than explosion of the nitroglycerine itself.[86,87] Metal backing is present in other transdermal drug patches and therefore all should be removed before defibrillation.

Aircraft avionics   Defibrillation in aircraft is normally safe, provided that standard precautions are observed. Leakage currents of less than 1.5 mA have been recorded from standard battery-operated defibrillators and should cause no interference with avionic equipment.[88]

The future of defibrillation

Automated external defibrillators

The development of AEDs has revolutionized out-of-hospital resuscitation.

AEDs monitor the ECG via self-adhesive electrodes applied to the patient's chest. The rhythm is analyzed by a microprocessor in the defibrillator. If the algorithm for ventricular fibrillation is satisfied, semiautomatic versions of these devices sound an alarm and advise the operator to deliver a shock. In fully automatic systems, the defibrillation shock is applied without further input from the operator, but an audible warning is given for safety of any nearby personnel. An example of defibrillation accomplished by lay rescuers using an AED is shown in Fig. 25.2.

The algorithms used are accurate when tested against field-recorded electrocardiograms.[89,90] Specificity rates for diagnosing ventricular fibrillation approach 100%, i.e., that the machine will not shock non-VF rhythms. Sensitivity rates are somewhat lower, particularly with low-amplitude ventricular fibrillation waveforms.[91,92] AEDs may also fail to interpret the pacing "spike" of an implanted defibrillator pacemaker correctly, but instead recognize it incorrectly as

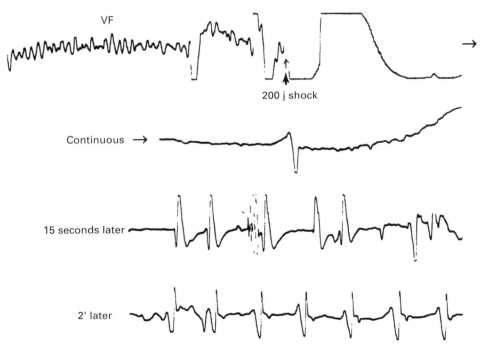

Fig. 25.2.   Defibrillation by a volunteer (lay) first responder emergency medical service using an automated external defibrillator. A single 200 J shock terminates ventricular fibrillation (VF); a brief period of asystole is followed by a perfusing rhythm. The patient survived.

a QRS complex.[93] Lower sensitivity rates can result in failure to shock ventricular fibrillation.

Emergency service personnel equipped with such automated defibrillators achieve higher resuscitation and survival rates than do those equipped with manual defibrillators or no defibrillators at all.[94] This is primarily due to the reduced time for delivery of the first shock when an AED is used. Also, AEDs have significant advantages over manual defibrillators in terms of reducing time and resources for initial training and periodic retraining.

The International Liaison Committee on Resuscitation (ILCOR), of which the American Heart Association is a member, has promulgated the concept of the "chain of survival" – early activation of the emergency medical service system, early CPR, early defibrillation, early advanced cardiac care – and strongly endorses and encourages the use of automated or manual defibrillators by all emergency personnel who may be called to diagnose and treat cardiac arrests: physicians, nurses, emergency medical technicians, and first responders, such as firefighters and police officers.[95]

Widespread availability of AEDs in the community, with selected lay personnel trained in the use of these devices, was shown to be practical and to offer a promising approach to improving survival from prehospital cardiac arrest.[95–97] In a subsequent large public access defibrillation (PAD) study, there were substantially more survivors to hospital discharge in scenarios where lay volunteers were trained in the use of AEDs plus CPR (23% survival), rather than CPR only (14%).[98]

Automatic implantable defibrillators

Fewer than half of the individuals who survive out-of-hospital resuscitation for sudden cardiac death have evidence of acute myocardial infarction. Ambulatory ECG recording indicates that ventricular fibrillation is often the terminal event, frequently preceded by ventricular tachycardia or multiple ventricular ectopic activities.[99,100] In an attempt to reduce the frequency of recurrent ventricular arrhythmias, antiarrhythmic drug therapy has been used, but these drugs are not always effective, have side effects, and can themselves be proarrhythmic (i.e., can cause life-threatening arrhythmias). Recent reports indicating an increase in mortality in patients taking drugs for arrhythmia control have highlighted this problem.[101]

A fully automatic implantable defibrillator (AID) was first described for use in treatment of sudden cardiac death in 1986.[102] These first devices were inserted by thoracotomy, but transvenous systems are now used for nearly all patients. They consist of a pulse generator that resembles a pacemaker and have electrodes for sensing the ECG and shocking the heart, with the electrodes located on leads that are usually positioned in the cardiac chambers and superior vena cava. Newer implantable devices have both pacing and defibrillation capability and are referred to as ICDs (implantable cardioverter defibrillators). The sensing electrodes detect occurrence of a dangerous arrhythmia and the device automatically applies pacing pulses (for ventricular tachycardia) or defibrillation shocks (for rapid ventricular tachycardia or ventricular fibrillation) to treat the disorder. Many patients are treated with both an ICD and antiarrhythmic drugs.

At the time of implantation, the patient's shock intensity required for defibrillation is determined by test shocks, because there is considerable patient-to-patient variability in shock intensity needed. Also, the ICDs allow for progressive increases with each shock in the event that the first shock(s) are unsuccessful. The intensity of shocks can be reprogrammed non-invasively at a later date if the patient's requirements change. If they are conscious, patients report that a shock feels like being hit or kicked in the chest.

Because many of these patients have extensive ischemic heart disease and poor ventricular function, mortality from heart failure remains high, but sudden death from arrhythmias is dramatically reduced and overall survival is improved after device implantation.[103]

Implantation of these devices has greatly increased as indications for use have increased and implantation has become easier. Three large trials have shown the effectiveness of ICDs to reduce mortality. The MADIT (multicenter automatic defibrillator implantation trial) and MUSTT (multicenter unsustained tachycardia trial) trials[104,105] showed that mortality decreased in patients who had ischemic heart disease, a reduced ejection fraction, non-sustained ventricular tachycardia and inducible sustained VT. The MADIT II study did not require non-sustained VT or electrophysiology testing, but did require a previous myocardial infarction and an ejection fraction <30%.[106] Notably, MADIT II showed that prophylactic ICD implantation, sometimes in combination with drug therapy, reduced patient mortality by 31%. This finding almost certainly will further increase the use of ICDs.

Home defibrillators

The great majority of prehospital sudden cardiac deaths occur in the home, not in public places.[107] AEDs are approved for use in a home setting. However, certain requirements for successful AED use must be present: the arrest must be witnessed (family members or spouses may be asleep or away) and the rescuer must be trained and able to locate the AED, apply the electrodes and operate the device correctly (a particular challenge for elderly or infirm spouses). The recent introduction of wearable defibrillators, which continuously monitor the ECG and which are fully automated, offers potential for overcoming some of these problems.[108] Possibly such devices could be provided to intermediate risk patients on a temporary lease basis to reduce costs – perhaps for several months after a myocardial infarction, or as a bridge before heart transplant in patients with severe dilated cardiomyopathy (such patients have high rates of sudden death while awaiting heart transplantation). Clearly, patients known to be a high risk for sudden cardiac death (previous cardiac arrests, malignant ventricular arrhythmias) should receive an implantable defibrillator.

Developing strategies for prompt diagnosis and treatment of VF occurring in the home remains a major challenge if we are to improve survival from cardiac arrest.

REFERENCES

1. Driscoll, T.E., Ratnoff, O.D. & Nygard, O.F. The remarkable Dr. Abildgaard and countershock. *Ann. Intern. Med.* 1975; **83**: 878–882.
2. Prevost, J.L. & Batelli, F. Sur quelques effets des descharges electriques sur le coueur des mammiferes. *C. R. Acad. Sci.* [III] 1899; **129**: 1267–1268.
3. Hooker, D.R., Kouwenhoven, W. & Langworthy, O. The effect of alternating electrical currents on the heart. *Am. J. Physiol.* 1933; **103**: 444–454.
4. Beck, C.S., Pritchard, W.H. & Feil, H.S. Ventricular fibrillation of long duration abolished by electric shock. *J. Am. Med. Assoc.* 1947; **135**: 985–986.
5. Zoll, P., Linenthal, A., Gibson, W., Paul, M. & Norman, L. Termination of ventricular fibrillation in man by externally applied electric countershock. *N. Engl. J. Med.* 1956; **254**: 727–732.
6. Lown, B., Neuman, J., Amarasingham, R. & Berkovits, B.V. Comparison of alternating current with direct electroshock across the closed chest. *Am. J. Cardiol.* 1962; **10**: 223–233.
7. Kouwenhoven, W.B., Jude, J.R. & Knickerbocker, G.G. Closed-chest cardiac massage. *J. Am. Med. Assoc.* 1960; **173**: 1064–1067.
8. Zipes, D.P., Fischer, J., King, R.M., Nicoll, A.D. & Jolly, W.W. Termination of ventricular fibrillation in dogs by depolarizing a critical amount of myocardium. *Am. J. Cardiol.* 1975; **36**: 37–44.
9. Shibata, N., Chen, P.S., Dixon, E.G. *et al.* Epicardial activation after unsuccessful defibrillation shocks in dogs. *Am. J. Physiol.* 1988; **255**: H902–H909.
10. Jones, J.L. Waveforms for implantable cardioverter defibrillators and transchest defibrillation. In Tacker, W.A. (ed.): Defibrillation of the heart. St. Louis: Mosby-Year Book, 1994: 46–81.
11. Neumar, R.W., Brown, C.G., Robitaille, P. & Altschuld, R.A. Myocardial high energy phosphate metabolism during ventricular fibrillation with total circulatory arrest. *Resuscitation* 1990; **19**: 199–226.
12. Kern, K.B., Garewal, H.S., Sanders, A.B. *et al.* Depletion of myocardial adenosine triphosphate during prolonged untreated ventricular fibrillation: effect on defibrillation success. *Resuscitation* 1990; **20**: 221–229.
13. Jennings, R.B., Reimar, K.A., Hill, M.L. & Mayer, S.E. Total ischemia in dog hearts, in vitro: comparison of high energy phosphate production, utilization and depletion and adenine nucleotide catabolism in total ischemia in vitro vs severe ischemia in vivo. *Circ. Res.* 1981; **49**: 892–900.
14. Schafer, J., Mulch, J., Winkler, B. & Schafer, W. Ultrastructural, functional and biochemical criteria for estimation of reversibility of ischemic injury. *J. Mol. Cell. Cardiol.* 1979; **11**: 521–541.
15. Kern, K.B., Garewal, H.S., Sanders, A.B. *et al.* Depletion of myocardial adenosine triphosphate during prolonged untreated ventricular fibrillation: effect on defibrillation success. *Resuscitation* 1990; **20**: 221–229.
16. Reibel, D.K. & Rovetto, M.J. Myocardial adenosine triphosphate synthesis and mechanical function following oxygen deficiency. *Am. J. Physiol.* **234**: H620–H624.
17. Cobb, L.A., Fahrenbruch, C.E., Walsh, T.R. *et al.* Influence of cardiopulmonary resuscitation prior to defibrillation in patients with out-of-hospital ventricular fibrillation. *J. Am. Med. Assoc.* 1999; **281**: 1182–1188.
18. Wik, L. Rediscovering the importance of chest compressions to improve outcome from cardiac arrest. *Resuscitation* 2003; **58**: 267–269.
19. Wik, L., Hansen, T.B., Fylling, F. *et al.* Delaying defibrillation to give basic cardiopulmonary resuscitation to patients with out-of-hospital ventricular fibrillation: a randomized trial. *J. Am. Med. Assoc.* 2003; **289**: 1389–1395.
20. Wik, L., Steen, P.A. & Bircher, N.G. Quality of bystander cardiopulmonary resuscitation influences outcome after prehospital cardiac arrest. *Resuscitation* 1994; **28**: 195–203.
21. Weaver, W.D., Cobb, L.A., Dennis, D. *et al.* Amplitude of ventricular fibrillation waveform and outcome after cardiac arrest. *Ann. Intern. Med.* 1985; **102**: 53–55.
22. Stewart, A.J., Allen, J.D. & Adgey, A.A.J. Frequency analysis of ventricular fibrillation and resuscitation success. *Q. J. Med.* 1992; **85**: 761–769.
23. Brown, C.G., Griffith, R.F., Van Ligten, P. *et al.* Median frequency – a new parameter for predicting defibrillation success rate. *Ann. Emerg. Med.* 1991; **20**: 787–789.
24. Callaway, C.W., Sherman, L.D., Mosesso, V.N., Jr. *et al.* Scaling exponent predicts defibrillation success for out-of-hospital ventricular fibrillation cardiac arrest. *Circulation* 2001; **103**: 1656–1661.
25. Eftestol, T., Sunde, K., Aase, S.O., Husoy, J.H. & Steen, P.A. Predicting outcome of defibrillation by spectral characterization and nonparametric classification of ventricular fibrillation in patients with out-of-hospital cardiac arrest. *Circulation* 2000; **102**: 1523–1529.

26. Eftestol, T., Wik, L., Sunde, K. & Steen, P.A. Effects of cardiopulmonary resuscitation on predictors of ventricular fibrillation defibrillation success during out-of-hospital cardiac arrest. *Circulation* 2004; **110**: 10–15.

27. Kerber, R.E., Grayzel, J., Hoyt, R., Marcus, M. & Kennedy, J. Transthoracic resistance in human defibrillation. Influence of body weight, chest size, serial shocks, paddle size and paddle contact pressure. *Circulation* 1981; **63**: 676–682.

28. Kerber, R.E., Kieso, R.A. & Kienzle, M.G. Current-based transthoracic defibrillation. *Am. J. Cardiol.* 1996; **78**: 1113–1118.

29. Geddes, L.A., Tacker, W.A., Cabler, P. *et al.* The decrease in transthoracic impedance during successive ventricular defibrillation trials. *Med. Instrum.* 1975; **9**: 179–180.

30. Dahl, C.F., Ewy, G.A., Ewy, M.D. & Thomas, E.D. Transthoracic impedance to direct current discharge: effect of repeated countershocks. *Med. Instrum.* 1976; **10**: 151–154.

31. Ewy, G.A., Hellman, D.A., McClung, S. & Taren, D. Influence of ventilation phase on transthoracic impedance and defibrillation effectiveness. *Crit. Care Med.* 1980; **8**: 164–166.

32. Sirna, S.J., Ferguson, D.W., Charbonnier, F. & Kerber, R.E. Factors affecting transthoracic impedance during electrical cardioversion. *Am. J. Cardiol.* 1988; **62**: 1048–1052.

33. Kerber, R.E., Vance, S., Schomer, S.J., Mariano, D.J. & Charbonnier, F. Transthoracic defibrillation: effect of sternotomy on chest impedance. *J. Am. Coll. Cardiol.* 1992; **20**: 94–97.

34. Pagan-Carlo, L.A., Spencer, K.T., Robertson, C.E. *et al.* Transthoracic defibrillation: importance of avoiding electrode placement directly on the female breast. *J. Am. Coll. Cardiol.* 1996; **27**: 449–452.

35. Deakin, C., Sado, D., Petley, G. & Clewlow, F. Determining the optimal paddle force for external defibrillation. *Am. J. Cardiol.* 2002; **90**: 812–813.

36. Deakin, C., Bennetts, S., Petley, G. & Clewlow, F. What is the optimal paddle force for paediatric defibrillation? *Resuscitation* 2002; **55**: 59.

37. Deakin, C.D., Sado, D.M., Petley, G.W. & Clewlow, F. Is the orientation of the apical defibrillation paddle of importance during manual external defibrillation? *Resuscitation* 2003; **56**: 15–18.

38. Hummel, R.S., 3rd, Ornato, J.P., Weinberg, S.M. & Clarke, A.M. Spark-generating properties of electrode gels used during defibrillation. A potential fire hazard. *J. Am. Med. Assoc.* 1988; **260**: 3021–3024.

39. Caterine, M.R., Yoerger, D.M., Spencer, K.T., Miller, S.G. & Kerber, R.E. Effect of electrode position and gel-application technique on predicted transcardiac current during transthoracic defibrillation. *Ann. Emerg. Med.* 1997; **29**: 588–595.

40. Deakin, C.D., Petley, G.W., Drury, N.E. & Clewlow, F. How often should defibrillation pads be changed?: the effect of evaporative drying. *Resuscitation* 2001; **48**: 157–162.

41. Bissing, J.W. & Kerber, R.E. Effect of shaving the chest of hirsute subjects on transthoracic impedance to self-adhesive defibrillation electrode pads. *Am. J. Cardiol.* 2000; **86**: 587–589.

42. Sado, D.M., Deakin, C.D., Petley, G.W. & Clewlow, F. Comparison of the effects of removal of chest hair with not doing so before external defibrillation on transthoracic impedance. *Am. J. Cardiol.* 2004; **93**: 98–100.

43. Deakin, C.D., Sado, D.M., Petley, G.W. & Clewlow, F. Differential contribution of skin impedance and thoracic volume to transthoracic impedance during external defibrillation. *Resuscitation* 2004; **60**: 171–174.

44. Deakin, C.D., McLaren, R.M., Petley, G.W., Clewlow, F. & Dalrymple-Hay, M.J. Effects of positive end-expiratory pressure on transthoracic impedance – implications for defibrillation. *Resuscitation* 1998; **37**: 9–12.

45. Rhee, B.J., Zhang, Y., Boddicker, K.A., Davies, L.R. & Kerber, R.E. Effect of hypothermia on transthoracic defibrillation in a swine model. *Resuscitation* 2005; **65**: 79–85.

46. Boddicker, K., Zhang, Y., Zimmerman, M.B., Davies, L.R. & Kerber, R.E. Hypothermia improves defibrillation success and resuscitation outcomes from ventricular fibrillation. *Circulation* 2005; **111**: 3195–3201.

47. Sirna, S.J., Kieso, R.A., Fox-Eastham, K.J. *et al.* Mechanisms responsible for decline in transthoracic impedance after DC shocks. *Am. J. Physiol.* 1989; **257**(2): H1180–H1183.

48. White, R.D. New concepts in transthoracic defibrillation. *Emerg. Med. Clin. North Am.* 2002; **20**: 785–807.

49. Kerber, R.E., Martins, J.B., Kelly, K.J. *et al.* Self-adhesive pre-applied electrode pads for defibrillation and cardioversion. *J. Am. Coll. Cardiol.* 1984; **3**: 815–820.

50. American National Standard: Automatic External Defibrillators and Remote Controlled Defibrillators (DF39). Arlington, Virginia: Association for the Advancement of Medical Instrumentation, 1993.

51. Hoyt, R., Grayzel, J. & Kerber, R.E. Determinants of intracardiac current in defibrillation. Experimental studies in dogs. *Circulation* 1981; **64**: 818–823.

52. Atkins, D.L., Sirna, S., Kieso, R., Charbonnier, F. & Kerber, R.E. Pediatric defibrillation: importance of paddle size in determining transthoracic impedance. *Pediatrics* 1988; **82**: 914–918.

53. Atkins, D.L. & Kerber, R.E. Pediatric defibrillation: current flow is improved by using "adult" electrode paddles. *Pediatrics* 1994; **94**: 90–93.

54. Bardy, G.H., Ivey, T.D., Allen, M.D., Johnson, G. & Greene, H.L. Evaluation of electrode polarity on defibrillation efficacy. *Am. J. Cardiol.* 1989; **63**: 433–437.

55. Schuder, J.C., Stoeckle, H., McDaniel, W.C. & Dbeis, M. Is the effectiveness of cardiac ventricular defibrillation dependent upon polarity? *Med. Instrum.* 1987; **21**: 262–265.

56. Lerman, B.B. & Deale, O.C. Relation between transcardiac and transthoracic current during defibrillation in humans. *Circ. Res.* 1990; **67**: 1420–1426.

57. Kerber, R.E. Electrical treatment of cardiac arrhythmias: defibrillation and cardioversion. *Ann. Emerg. Med.* 1993; **27**: 296–301.

58. McKeown, P., Khan, M.M., Croal, S. *et al.* Electrocardiographic recording, atrial pacing and defibrillation in the course of

electrophysiologic studies using the esophagus. *Coronary Artery Dis.* 1992; **3**: 383–391.

59. McKeown, P.P., Croal, S., Allen, J.D., Anderson, J. & Adgey, A.A.J. Transesophageal cardioversion. *Am. Heart J.* 1993; **125**: 396–404.

60. Tacker, W.A. & Paris, R. Transchest defibrillation effectiveness and electrical impedance using disposable conductive pads. *Heart Lung* 1983; **12**: 510–513.

61. Ewy, G.A., Horan, W.J. & Ewy, M.D. Disposable defibrillator electrodes. *Heart Lung* 1977; **6**: 127–130.

62. Lown, B., Neuman, J. & Amarasinghem, R. Comparison of alternating current with direct current electroshock across closed chest. *Am. J. Cardiol.* 1962; **10**: 223–227.

63. Anderson, G.J. & Suelzer, J. The efficacy of trapezoidal waveforms for ventricular defibrillation. *Chest* 1976; **70**: 298–300.

64. Behr, J.C., Hartley, L.L., York, D.K., Brown, D.D. & Kerber, R.E. Truncated exponential versus damped sinusoidal waveform shocks for transthoracic defibrillation. *Am. J. Cardiol.* 1996; **78**: 1242–1245.

65. Bardy, G.H., Marchlinski, F., Sharma, A. *et al.* Multicenter comparison of truncated biphasic shocks and standard damped sine wave monophasic shocks for transthoracic ventricular fibrillation. *Circulation* 1996; **94**: 2507–2514.

66. Schneider, T., Martens, P.R., Paschen, H. *et al.* Multicenter, randomized, controlled trial of 150-J biphasic shocks compared with 200- to 360-J monophasic shocks in the resuscitation of out-of-hospital cardiac arrest victims. *Circulation* 2000; **102**: 1780–1787.

67. van Alem, A.P., Chapman, F.W., Lank, P., Hart, A.A. & Koster, R.W. A prospective, randomised and blinded comparison of first shock success of monophasic and biphasic waveforms in out-of-hospital cardiac arrest. *Resuscitation* 2003; **58**: 17–24.

68. Tang, W., Weil, M.H., Sun, S. *et al.* The effects of biphasic and conventional monophasic defibrillation on postresuscitation myocardial function. *J. Am. Coll. Cardiol.* 1999; **34**: 815–822.

69. Mittal, S., Ayati, S., Stein, K.M. *et al.* Comparison of a novel rectilinear biphasic waveform with a damped sine wave monophasic waveform for transthoracic ventricular defibrillation. ZOLL Investigators. *J. Am. Coll. Cardiol.* 1999; **34**: 1595–1601.

70. Kerber, R.E., Martins, J.B., Kienzle, M.G. *et al.* Energy, current, and success in defibrillation and cardioversion: clinical studies using an automated impedance-based method of energy adjustment. *Circulation* 1988; **77**: 1038–1046.

71. Weaver, W.D., Cobb, L.A., Copass, M.K. & Hallstrom, A.P. Ventricular defibrillation: a comparative trial using 175-J and 320-J shocks. *N. Engl. J. Med.* 1982; **307**: 1101–1106.

72. Martens, P.R., Russell, J.K., Wolcke, B. *et al.* Optimal response to cardiac arrest study: defibrillation waveform effects. *Resuscitation* 2001; **49**: 233–243.

73. White, R.D., Blackwell, T.H., Russell, J.K., Snyder, D.E. & Jorgenson, D.B. Transthoracic impedance does not affect defibrillation, resuscitation or survival in patients with out-of-hospital cardiac arrest treated with a non-escalating

biphasic waveform defibrillator. *Resuscitation* 2005; **64**: 63–69.

74. Pennington, J.E., Taylor, J. & Lown, B. Chest thump for reverting ventricular tachycardia. *N. Engl. J. Med.* 1970; **283**: 1192–1195.

75. Robertson, C. The precordial thump and cough techniques in advanced life support. A statement for the Advanced Life Support Working Party of the European Resuscitation Council. *Resuscitation* 1992; **24**: 133–135.

76. Caldwell, G., Millar, G. & Quinn, E. Simple mechanical methods for cardioversion: Defence of the precordial thump and cough version. *Br. Med. J.* 1985; **291**: 627–630.

77. Miller, J., Tresch, D., Horwitz, L. *et al.* The precordial thump. *Ann. Emerg. Med.* 1984; **13**: 791–794.

78. Chamberlain, D. Gel pads should not be used for monitoring ECG after defibrillation. *Resuscitation* 2000; **43**: 159–160.

79. Waller, C., Callies, F. & Langenfeld, H. Adverse effects of direct current cardioversion on cardiac pacemakers and electrodes. Is external cardioversion contraindicated in patients with permanent pacing systems? *Europace* 2004; **6**: 165–168.

80. Altamura, G., Bianconi, L. & LoBianco, F. Transthoracic DC shock may represent a serious hazard in pacemaker dependent patients. *Pacing Clin. Electrophysiol.* 1995; **18**: 194–198.

81. Aylward, P., Blood, R. & Tonkin, A. Complications of defibrillation with permanent pacemaker in situ. *Pacing Clin. Electrophysiol.* 1979; **2**: 462–464.

82. Gibbs, W., Eisenberg, M. & Damon, S.K. Dangers of defibrillation: injuries to emergency personnel during patient resuscitation. *Am. J. Emerg. Med.* 1990; **8**: 101–104.

83. Robertshaw, H. & McAnulty, G. Ambient oxygen concentrations during simulated cardiopulmonary resuscitation. *Anaesthesia* 1998; **53**: 634–637.

84. Theodorou, A.A., Gutierrez, J.A. & Berg, R.A. Fire attributable to a defibrillation attempt in a neonate. *Pediatrics* 2003; **112**: 677–679.

85. Fires from defibrillation during oxygen administration. *Health Devices* 1994; **23**: 307–309.

86. Liddle, R. & Richmond, W. Investigation into voltage breakdown in glyceryl trinitrate patches. *Resuscitation* 1998; **37**: 145–148.

87. Wrenn, K. The hazards of defibrillation through nitroglycerin patches. *Ann. Emerg. Med.* 1990; **19**: 1327–1328.

88. Dedrick, D.K., Darga, A., Landis, D. & Burney, R.E. Defibrillation safety in emergency helicopter transport. *Ann. Emerg. Med.* 1989; **18**: 69–71.

89. Stults, K.R., Brown, D.D. & Kerber, R.E. Efficacy of an automated external defibrillator in the management of out-of-hospital cardiac arrest: validation of the diagnostic algorithm and initial clinical experience in a rural environment. *Circulation* 1986; **73**: 701–709.

90. Cummins, R.O., Stults, K.R., Haggar, B. *et al.* A new rhythm library for testing automatic external defibrillators: performance of three devices. *J. Am. Coll. Cardiol.* 1988; **11**: 597–602.

91. Dickey, W., Dalzell, G.W., Anderson, J.M. & Adgey, A.A. The accuracy of decision-making of a semi-automatic defibrillator during cardiac arrest. *Eur. Heart J.* 1992; **13**: 608–615.

92. Murray, A., Clayton, R.H. & Campbell, R.W. Comparative assessment of the ventricular fibrillation detection algorithms in five semi-automatic or advisory defibrillators. *Resuscitation* 1993; **26**: 163–172.

93. Singer, I., Guarnieri, T. & Kupersmith, J. Implanted automatic defibrillators: effects of drugs and pacemakers. *Pacing Clin. Electrophysiol.* 1988; **11**: 2250–2262.

94. Weaver, W.D., Hill, D., Fahrenbruch, C.E. *et al.* Use of the automatic external defibrillator in the management of out-of-hospital cardiac arrest. *N. Engl. J. Med.* 1988; **319**: 661–666.

95. Cummins, R.O., Ornato, J.P., Thies, W.H. & Pepe, P.E. Improving survival from sudden cardiac arrest: the "chain of survival" concept. A statement for health professionals from the Advanced Cardiac Life Support Subcommittee and the Emergency Cardiac Care Committee, American Heart Association. *Circulation* 1991; **83**: 1832–1847.

96. Cobb, L.A., Eliastam, M., Kerber, R.E. *et al.* Report of the American Heart Association Task Force on the Future of Cardiopulmonary Resuscitation. *Circulation* 1992; **85**: 2346–2355.

97. Walters, G., Glucksman, E. & Evans, T.R. Training St John Ambulance volunteers to use an automated external defibrillator. *Resuscitation* 1994; **27**: 39–45.

98. The Public Access Defibrillation Trial Investigators. Public-access defibrillation and survival after out-of-hospital cardiac arrest. *N. Engl. J. Med.* 2004; **351**: 637–646.

99. Cobb, L.A., Baum, R.S., Alvarez, H., 3rd & Schaffer, W.A. Resuscitation from out-of-hospital ventricular fibrillation: 4 years follow-up. *Circulation* 1975; **52**: III223–III235.

100. Kempf, F.C., Jr. & Josephson, M.E. Cardiac arrest recorded on ambulatory electrocardiograms. *Am. J. Cardiol.* 1984; **53**: 1577–1582.

101. Preliminary report: effect of encainide and flecainide on mortality in a randomized trial of arrhythmia suppression after myocardial infarction. The Cardiac Arrhythmia Suppression Trial (CAST) Investigators. *N. Engl. J. Med.* 1989; **321**: 406–412.

102. Mirowski, M., Reid, P.R., Mower, M.M. *et al.* Termination of malignant ventricular arrhythmias with an implanted automatic defibrillator in human beings. *N. Engl. J. Med.* 1980; **303**: 322–324.

103. Tchou, P.J., Kadri, N., Anderson, J. *et al.* Automatic implantable cardioverter defibrillators and survival of patients with left ventricular dysfunction and malignant ventricular arrhythmias. *Ann. Intern. Med.* 1988; **109**: 529–534.

104. Moss, A.J., Hall, W.J., Cannom, D.S. *et al.* Improved survival with an implanted defibrillator in patients with coronary disease at high risk for ventricular arrhythmia. Multicenter Automatic Defibrillator Implantation Trial Investigators. *N. Engl. J. Med.* 1996; **335**: 1933–1940.

105. Buxton, A.E., Lee, K.L., Fisher, J.D. *et al.* A randomized study of the prevention of sudden death in patients with coronary artery disease. Multicenter Unsustained Tachycardia Trial Investigators. *N. Engl. J. Med.* 1999; **341**: 1882–1890.

106. Moss, A.J., Zareba, W., Hall, W.J. *et al.* Prophylactic implantation of a defibrillator in patients with myocardial infarction and reduced ejection fraction. *N. Engl. J. Med.* 2002; **346**: 877–883.

107. Weaver, W.D. & Peberdy, M.A. Defibrillators in public places – one step closer to home. *N. Engl. J. Med.* 2002; **347**: 1223–1224.

108. Auricchio, A., Klein, H., Geller, C.J. *et al.* Clinical efficacy of the wearable cardioverter-defibrillator in acutely terminating episodes of ventricular fibrillation. *Am. J. Cardiol.* 1998; **81**: 1253–1256.

26

Automated external defibrillators

Rudolph W. Koster[1], Douglas Chamberlain[2], and Dianne L. Atkins[3]

[1] Department of Cardiology, Academic Medical Center, Amsterdam, The Netherlands
[2] School of Medicine, Cardiff University, Wales UK
[3] Division of Pediatric Cardiology, Children's Hospital of Iowa, Department of Pediatrics, Carver College of Medicine, University of Iowa, Iowa City, USA

History of AEDs

Automated external defibrillators (AEDs) as we now know them have had a rapid and interesting evolution. The first report of an "automatic cardiac resuscitator" was made by Diack *et al.* in 1979, who had developed the defibrillator, the Heart-Aid.[1] A first clinical report on successful ambulance use was published in 1982.[2] The design of this defibrillator was unusual for several reasons. First, it used a tongue electrode together with a chest electrode for defibrillation. Second, the tongue blade also contained a sensor for respiration, which prevented the defibrillator from delivering a shock as long as an air stream was detected over the tongue. Confidence in the algorithm to detect ventricular fibrillation (VF) by the ECG was not sufficient: a second independent sign of circulatory arrest was desired. Further automated analysis of the ECG and defibrillation in cardiac arrest was investigated first in defibrillators that were used by traditional responders such as Emergency Medical Technicians.[3,4] Then, when safety and efficacy were confirmed, the use was extended to fire fighters[5] who were already part of the Emergency Medical Services (EMS) and to police squads who had never been part of the EMS.[6] It became clear that the future of automated defibrillation was with lay rescuers with limited training, without the ability to interpret ECGs. Ease of use was paramount.

Therefore, new AEDs were designed with the lay rescuer in mind, with increasing simplicity and decreasing weight, volume, and cost. Also, these new AEDs offered assistance to the rescuer with voice prompts that could talk the rescuer through the still complicated process of applying defibrillation pads, defibrillation, checks for return of circulation, and resuming CPR when needed. The process could be repeated according to agreed protocols. These AEDs received rapid acceptance, especially when experiences were published with police[7,8] airline personnel,[9] casino attendants[10] airports[11] and the public domain.[12] Use of AEDs in pediatric cardiac arrest became better accepted when energy attenuators became available, limiting the energy delivered,[13] and the VF detection algorithm proved reliable in children.[14] Limitations in the delivering of the voice prompts became clear however,[15] they markedly curtailed the time during which CPR could be administered, thus decreasing the life-saving potential of AEDs. The 2005 AHA and ERC guidelines on resuscitation[16,17] suggest revision of voice prompts according to accumulated experience and new understanding of the prime importance of chest compressions.

Another trend is the addition of new tools to assist the rescuer in performing Basic Life Support, such as a metronome to enforce an optimal rate of chest compression and a displacement transducer that gives feedback on speed and depth of chest compressions.

AEDs have evolved into highly sophisticated, small, simple, and cheaper devices that are now applied in increasing numbers in out-of-hospital cardiac arrest.[18] The technological developments will clearly continue with new capabilities to optimize the chance of successful resuscitation.

The clinical application of AEDs

The principal applications of AEDs are for use by operators with modest training, although they have been used

Cardiac Arrest: The Science and Practice of Resuscitation Medicine. 2nd edn., ed. Norman Paradis, Henry Halperin, Karl Kern, Volker Wenzel, Douglas Chamberlain. Published by Cambridge University Press. © Cambridge University Press, 2007.

increasingly by healthcare professionals, including physicians and nurses, whose work does not bring them into frequent contact with cardiac emergencies so that they lack relevant experience for dealing with cardiac arrest.

AEDs are deployed in two strategies: "on-site," in which any use is expected to be close to where the device is kept; and "transported" in which the device is intended to be taken to an emergency remote from where it is kept.

On-site AEDs

The most obvious on-site use of AEDs is within the home, a concept that has been likened to keeping a fire extinguisher for an unlikely but grave emergency. But it is not an exact analogy. Even an AED requires both training and refresher training as well as battery maintenance. Moreover, the cost for *routine* home use would be prohibitive and many would find its presence intrusive. Thus the perceived risk of a family member developing a malignant arrhythmia must be great enough to justify its purchase for both reassurance and protection. Here, too, there is a caveat; if the risk is very great – as for example for an individual who has already suffered such an event – then an implantable defibrillator would be the usual strategy. Vest devices[19] also compete for favor if protection is required as a bridge whilst an implant is awaited. No consensus yet exists on the level of risk that might call for protection to be immediately available yet not merit implantation. One early small study showed no survival benefit.[20] Moreover, the psychological aspects cannot be assumed to be favorable. How many deemed at risk might fear to venture far from what may be perceived as a life-line? The strategy is currently being investigated comprehensively in the HAT (home external automatic defibrillator trial) trial that is expected to report in 2007.[21] Until more evidence is available, home applications should be regarded as of unproven value.

An extension of the home concept has been investigated as part of a larger trial that involved placement of units not only in public places, but also in blocks of dwellings. The need here was therefore based on a large number of individuals at relatively low risk rather than on single persons at high risk. The Public Access Defibrillation (PAD) trial[12] included 80 apartment complexes with volunteers trained to provide CPR for cardiac arrest and, for comparison, 77 others in which the volunteers also had the potential to deliver an AED within 3 minutes. Only a single individual survived in each group from a total of 70 definite cardiac arrests. The issues of ownership, training, and response times would inevitably have posed challenges that may have accounted for the poor result in the AED arm of the study. The declared target to have defibrillation available within 3 minutes would also be difficult to achieve in this situation, so that the strategy does not provide a typical example of "on-site" use.

The considerations are quite different in relation to the protection of individuals not known to be at high risk, but who are in areas remote from any chance of conventional rescue. Typical examples have been reported in relation to commercial aviation[9,22–25] but could apply equally well to ships, long distance trains, expeditions, and even remote settlements. Here, the problem of responsibility for using the device in an emergency can be settled readily because selected individuals will have a "duty to respond." The case for this strategy cannot generally be made on economic grounds unless, as was the situation aircraft, experience shows that expensive diversions can be avoided. Few AEDs would ever be used successfully to treat cardiac arrest during flight. A review of in-flight deaths reported to the International Air Transport Association suggested that cardiac arrest might occur once in every 3 million passenger flights.[26] The QANTAS experience[22] of one in a million passenger flights was higher; this may represent only statistical chance in small numbers, but under-reporting of events by airlines is also possible. The case for AEDs on aircraft, now adopted by almost all major carriers, was based in part on medicolegal considerations, because of the risk of liability arising from not having facilities available for defibrillation. More recently, in the United States the Federal Aviation Agency (FAA) has ruled that all commercial aircraft with at least one flight attendant must carry an AED: the law now adds an even more powerful motive.[27] The principle of equity might also be cited. All these reasons are valid and powerful: benefit cannot always be judged on clinical results alone.

The likelihood of need is clearly greatest where large numbers of sick patients are likely to be found. Whereas high dependency clinical areas are generally equipped with defibrillators with staff experienced in their use, most healthcare areas do not have resuscitation equipment available routinely – more than a decade after the first description of AEDs in hospital.[28] Many non-critical hospital wards, nursing homes, clinics, and physician or paramedical premises are also likely to have patients, either resident or visiting, who are at risk of sudden cardiac death. The use of automated defibrillation is ideal in such areas but has been unevenly exploited. All hospital areas with vulnerable patients should have defibrillation facilities immediately to hand, certainly sufficiently close to permit application within a couple of minutes in order to achieve defibrillation within the few minutes of the 'electrical phase' of cardiac arrest[29] while the prospects of success remain optimal. The notion that collapse in a ward area is a signal for summoning a remote cardiac arrest team is a recipe for unnecessary deaths! AEDs can provide a very desirable solution because all professional ward staff should then be able to provide immediate definitive treatment. Although observational studies attest to its value,[30,31] the strategy has not yet been widely implemented in some countries, nor fully in all. It should be seen as a priority. Primary care is another area where availability of defibrillation facilities has been disappointingly low. One can only regret that the excellent results obtained from the use of AEDs in the offices of general practitioners have not prompted a demand for the defibrillator being universally available.[32]

The concept of "on-site" defibrillators in public places is developed in Chapter 27 where Public Access Defibrillation is considered in greater detail. It has been a success story for the implementation of AEDs, with use in casinos,[10,33] airports, bus or ferry terminals, railway stations,[11,34] shopping malls,[12] and sports facilities.[35–39] Remarkable success for on-site defibrillation was also reported from a survey of rehabilitation programs even before devices were automated;[40] such equipment should now should be available routinely where cardiac rehabilitation is practiced. Authorities should consider carefully where else in the community they should be deployed. A survey in 1998 examined the annual incidence of cardiac arrest in public places.[41] A county jail came second only to an international airport; the needs of defibrillation facilities in detention centers can readily be overlooked! Data from emergency services should be used more frequently to guide community policies with regard to prompt defibrillation.

Vulnerability of any given population must be a key issue, but even the apparently fit merit consideration. At present we have no consensus on the numbers of healthy people gathered in one place that might constitute a recognized need for availability of defibrillation facilities. Numbers alone provide an insufficient guide, however, in assessing community risk. Average age of a population clearly has a bearing, but more important is the type of environment. In particular, environments that trigger high adrenergic drive have a disproportionately high incidence of cardiac arrest, but also an unusually high incidence of arrests with shockable rhythms, with fibrillation found in over 80% of cases in airports and railway stations[34] and over 90% of cases in a casino.[10] Moreover, where adrenergic drive is a major factor, a high proportion of arrests may occur in the absence of fresh infarction, so that resuscitation may have a greater chance of success. Although this is a reasonable hypothesis that is in keeping with observed data, it has not been studied formally.

Transported AEDs

Lay first-responder schemes are probably the most important area of development in which the use of AEDs could counter an important proportion of cases of sudden cardiac death. Although response times will generally be longer than for on-site defibrillation, they can still be appreciably shorter than those achieved by conventional emergency systems. This is hugely important when every minute of delay has been shown in a large database to reduce the average success rate in comparison with that of the previous minute by no less than 23%.[42] The strategy has not been adequately exploited for various reasons, but none of them is insuperable nor should any be seen as an overly daunting challenge in comparison with the size and nature of the problem that it could address. Complacency, lack of vision, and even ignorance within the medical community pose the greatest barriers.

The major barrier to reducing community mortality by first-responder defibrillation is perceived to be the site of most unexpected cardiac arrests. They do not occur in hospital, or even in public places. A large majority of persons die at home; in one epidemiological survey this was reported to be as high as 80%,[43] although it was appreciably lower at 61% in another study.[44] Not surprisingly, older people are more likely to suffer sudden cardiac arrest at home than are younger ones.[44,45] Most are witnessed by sight or by sound but the survival rate is poor, with prospects regarded as gloomy because of the belief that most patients with cardiac arrest outside hospital will never be in reach of publicly accessible defibrillators.[46]

The current situation is indeed unsatisfactory, particularly since most statistics for out-of-hospital cardiac arrest relate only to cases in which an attempt at resuscitation was made. In some areas this is close to zero, but even in areas with highly developed emergency services there is another problem. The proportion of victims found with shockable rhythms is usually reported to be about 40%.[47,48] Such unpromising figures are, however, due in large measure to slow response times that permitted the decay of fibrillation into asystole. Indeed, data from Gothenburg have suggested that the initial incidence of fibrillation is about 80%,[49] a percentage that has been exceeded in some studies of on-site AEDs as quoted above. The figure was derived by extrapolating backwards to zero time from the falling incidence found as delays increase. Although the proportion of cases with fibrillation has been noted to fall in recent years, defibrillation should be the appropriate option for far more victims than is currently observed: short response times are the key. An important concept must be accepted: *cardiac arrest in the community is a problem for the community and not primarily for ambulances*. It remains, however, a problem for the emergency services because it is the conventional emergency control systems that must activate responders in the shortest possible time. But if responders are activated only for cases believed to involve cardiac arrest, then at least half will be missed, and the responders will never develop the competence that comes from experience and confidence. Few data have yet been published to confirm that community responders can achieve greater success by attending all reported major emergencies. One study from Piacenza[50] in Italy, however, has attracted interest by showing that implementation of a scheme in which volunteers trained in AED use, but not CPR, tripled the community survival rate. Further detailed studies of well organized community schemes are urgently needed.

Far more extensively studied have been schemes in which non-healthcare professionals 'with a duty to respond' have been equipped with AEDs and given the remit of attending cardiac emergencies. These have largely been fire service and police personnel. In the United States and some other countries, the fire service is generally part of a unified emergency service but, where this is not the case, firemen could supplement ambulances and indeed can often reach victims sooner.[51] Fire services must be adequately staffed at all times for emergencies that are relatively infrequent. It therefore makes abundant sense to equip them with AEDs and use them as coresponders in order to achieve good response times at relatively modest cost. In some countries, however, the strategy has not been adopted or has been adopted imperfectly. Within the United Kingdom, union reservations from the professional fire service has held up progress. In other countries, interservice rivalry has lessened the beneficial impact.

Police forces offer another obvious method of rapid response to life-threatening emergencies. The highly successful experience by police in Rochester (Minnesota,[6,52] described in Chapter 27) shows how dramatically successful this can be. But even well-organized schemes[53,54] cannot match this success unless an effective system is in place to ensure that police are alerted as quickly as the regular ambulance service. When this is achieved, response times can be appreciably reduced.[55] Any shortcomings in this area may not be due to lack of cooperation. Apart from the complexities of linking control centers and the resultant delay, incidents of cardiac arrest cannot be identified accurately from public emergency calls, and few police services have the capacity or will to act as a routine

backup ambulance service. Moreover, one survey found that most law enforcement officers would not feel comfortable using an AED.[56] This area requires more research by those willing to follow the lead given by the 'goldstandard' Rochester co-responder scheme.

AEDs were not initially designed for healthcare professionals, but some of their most valuable contributions have been made by such personnel. Reference has already been made to their use by physicians and hospital staff with access to "on-site" units. Apart from general practitioner physicians who travel to emergencies equipped with their office AEDs,[32] they have found a role in the conventional or statutory ambulance services as well as independent private services and those provided by voluntary groups. The obvious benefit comes from the reduced training required compared with that for manual defibrillators, so that the use of ambulance defibrillation can be greatly extended. But there are other benefits. The algorithm decision plus screen interpretation of the waveform offers a double check that many believed would hasten decisions to shock. Some reports, however, showed that the adoption of AEDs in ambulances did not improve results overall[57] even when the previous option had been to provide CPR and await a second tier ambulance.[58] This is probably due to the considerable delays that have been required by AED algorithms before a shock can be given, comprising 'hands-off' analysis time, charge time, and human delay after the shock instruction is issued.[15] Experimental evidence now indicates that after cardiac arrest has been present for a very few minutes, any delay between compressions and shock greatly reduces the likelihood of a return of spontaneous circulation.[59] At present, this can reduce the efficacy of AEDs in comparison with manual defibrillation.[60] Improvements in design of the devices will shortly overcome this disadvantage. Once this has been achieved, we anticipate that AEDs will eventually displace manual units even for skilled professional use.

The inestimable value of AEDs has been shown in many different spheres of resuscitation. The role of automated and perhaps automatic (self-discharging) units is set to increase, both in terms of the numbers that a community will expect to have available and also for expanding indications for their use.

AED in children

As the advantages and availability of automated external defibrillators (AEDS) in both out-of-hospital and in-hospital sites increased, it became apparent that children were not eligible for this potential therapy. Since AEDs were not approved for use in young children, a child could receive only CPR and initial airway management by first responders. Rhythm analysis and defibrillation were delayed until the arrival of advanced paramedics with a variable dose manual defibrillator. The energy dose was substantially higher than recommended doses for children and the rhythm detection algorithms had been developed with adult rhythms only. Over the last 5 years, there has been an increasing effort to understand these risks and modify the AEDs to optimize use in children.

Cardiac arrest in infants and children: is there a need for AEDs?

The etiology of pediatric cardiac arrest differs from cardiac arrest in adults.[61–70] Primary respiratory arrest is more common than primary cardiac arrest, and is the leading cause of cardiac arrest in children less than 5 years. The most frequent rhythm observed in patients 0–17 years old is asystole or pulseless electrical activity (PEA). Successful resuscitation rates are distressingly low (less than 10%), costs are extremely high, and permanent neurological sequelae are common.[65,67,70]

Because of the high frequency of respiratory arrest and asystole in children, the emphasis of resuscitation efforts has been on effective ventilation and oxygenation, whereas rhythm assessment and defibrillation, despite their importance, have received less emphasis. Rapid rhythm evaluation is not routinely performed in pediatric patients as[66,71] first responders evaluated rhythm in only 44% of pulseless children.[66]

We now recognize that the frequency of ventricular fibrillation may have been under-estimated during pediatric arrest. In studies of out-of-hospital pediatric arrest, ventricular fibrillation was present in 9 to 22% of those in whom an ECG was obtained.[61–66,68–70,72,73] Two out-of-hospital, population-based studies demonstrate ventricular fibrillation in 9–19% of children suffering pulseless arrest from any etiology. Mogayzel *et al.* reported ventricular fibrillation as the initial rhythm in 19% of children (5–18 years) who experienced an out-of-hospital cardiac arrest.[66] The presence of ventricular fibrillation was evenly distributed among all categories of arrest: drowning, overdose, trauma, and medical illness. Young *et al.*[70] found ventricular fibrillation in 9% of pediatric cardiac arrest victims. The disparity in frequency can probably be explained by different populations: Mogazel's study was limited to children 5–18 years; Young's study included children and infants 0–12 years as well as those diagnosed with sudden infant death syndrome (SIDS). Interestingly, 6% of the patients categorized as having SIDS had VF reported as the presenting rhythm. Two recent in-hospital studies have also documented an 11%–14% incidence of ventricular fibrillation in pediatric arrest.[72,74] Thus, ventricular fibrillation, although not common, occurs in pediatric arrest and should *not* be considered rare.

The presence of ventricular fibrillation as the initial rhythm, compared with asystole or PEA, predicts hospital discharge, improved survival, and/or neurological outcome in both in-hospital and pre-hospital situations. Long-term survival of 25%–40% has been reported in the studies cited above.[64–66,75,76]

Because of this new information, early recognition and treatment of ventricular fibrillation have been identified as one factor that could improve pediatric resuscitation rates[70,73,77] and this has also prompted the need for modification of AEDs to permit pediatric use.

Equipment design and modification for pediatric use

Potentially, adult-only AEDs could be applied to children, but there were unknown risks associated with this practice. In order to extend the new technology to children, modifications to the existing devices were necessary. The rhythm identification algorithms needed validation and a pediatric energy dose established. The rhythm identification algorithms had been validated from libraries of adult rhythms, but the rhythm algorithms from electrograms recorded from young children also needed validation. The AED energy doses were all programmed to adult energies of 150–360 J shocks and a mechanism to deliver lower energies was required. These modifications were needed without increasing the complexity of the AED operation for adult use.

Several manufacturers have tested or developed modifications of their AEDs to permit safe and effective use in children < 8 years. Adult algorithms have been validated with pediatric rhythms, or modified specifically for pediatric patients.[14,78,79] In 2001, the first pediatric pad and cable system was granted market release by the United States Food and Drug Administration and several manufacturers followed with comparable systems. Typically, the modifications utilize separate pediatric pads with an attenuator that automatically absorbs a portion of energy when the AED delivers a shock. The attenuator lowers the nominal energy delivered to the patient from 150–200 J to approximately 50 J.[80] As a result, scaled energy and current are delivered to pediatric patients. The pediatric pads are designed for use on children 0–8 years or up to 25 kg. The American Heart Association strongly recommends the use of the pediatric pads with attenuated dosing for children 1–8 years.[16,81]

Modification of energy dosing

The energy dose recommendation of 2–4 J/kg for children was derived from animal data[82,83] and one small retrospective review of in-hospital short-duration pediatric ventricular fibrillation.[84] That these doses were effective or safe in humans has not been confirmed, especially for long-duration ventricular fibrillation. Recent animal and human data indicate that 2–4 J/kg may be inadequate. Clark *et al.*[85] concluded that although biphasic waveforms were superior to monophasic waveforms in both infant and child swine models, successful biphasic defibrillation required energy doses of 3–4 J/kg. Berg *et al.* demonstrated that in 4–24 kg piglets, 2 J/kg monophasic waveforms failed to defibrillate any animal with the initial shock.[86] In a small case series from Tucson, Arizona, only 50% of children who received 2 J/kg ± 10 J were successfully defibrillated, but six had asystole and one had PEA. In the remaining 50% of children ventricular fibrillation was not terminated.

There appears to be a wide therapeutic range for energy dosing, especially with biphasic waveforms. Tang and colleagues[87] delivered 50 J to piglets weighing 3.5–25 kg. All animals were successfully defibrillated to an organized rhythm and survived for 72 hours. There were no differences in fractional area change or echocardiographic ejection fraction among the different weight groups 4 hours after the shocks. Berg *et al.* observed good survival and 24-hour neurological outcomes in 4–24 kg animals with escalating attenuated biphasic waveforms compared to monophasic doses of 2–4 J/kg.[86] Two studies of biphasic defibrillation delivered very large doses to small animals without obvious damage to the heart. Killingsworth et al. detected no abnormalities of cardiac rhythm or left ventricular function with very high-energy doses, 20–360 J delivered to animals weighing 3.8–20 kg.[88] In an animal model of *commotio cordis,* blunt trauma to the chest, small dogs received 200–360 J after ventricular fibrillation had been produced.[89] These energy doses were highly effective at terminating VF, although 17 of 26 animals died.

There are two case reports and a case series of effective pediatric defibrillation with high dosing.[90–92] Rossano *et al.* reviewed defibrillation dosing during out-of-hospital pediatric cardiac resuscitation.[92] Of 57 patients under age 18 years, the median dose for the first shock was 3.63 J/kg, range 0.67–14.29 J/kg, and 49% of patients received more than 4 J/kg as the first dose. Nineteen (33%) patients survived to hospital discharge. Energy dose did not predict survival, and some of the survivors received extremely high doses.

Is it necessary to provide attenuated energy dosing to children given the apparent wide therapeutic range?

Table 26.1. Sensitivity and specificity of AEDs for pediatric cardiac rhythms

	Philips[a]	Medtronic Physio-Control[a]	Zoll[b]
Number of patients	191	203	220
Number of rhythms	696	1561	693
Sensitivity (%)	100	99.5	99.8
Specificity VF (%)	96	99	100
Specificity VT (%)	75	70	93.9

VF Ventricular fibrillation, VT Ventricular tachycardia.
[a] Adult algorithm validated with pediatric rhythms.
[b] Algorithm developed with pediatric rhythms.

Excessive energy doses, even with biphasic waveforms, can be detrimental to myocardial tissue and may result in serious dysfunction or serologic evidence of damage.[93,94] Defibrillation with full adult dosing doubles troponin levels in small swine who receive even biphasic adult dose defibrillation compared to the animals who received the attenuated dosing. As with any other therapy, the application and energy dose should be optimized for the patient. Since pediatric pads are available and deliver an appropriate dose for children, their use should be strongly encouraged, rather than settling for adult pads that deliver larger doses than are necessary. Children deserve the same standard of care as adults receive. An adult AED should only be used if the pediatric pads are not available.[16]

Arrhythmia identification

Theoretical concerns exist concerning the capacity of AEDs to detect VF in the pediatric patient because of smaller cardiac mass in children. The American Heart Association recommends that manufacturers document the sensitivity and specificity of the algorithm for pediatric arrhythmias. Recent reports indicate high sensitivity and specificity of adult algorithms within two commercially available AEDs.[14,79] (Table 26.1) Both studies surpassed the recommendations of the AHA for specificity and sensitivity in all but one category.[95]

Analysis of the electrogram characteristics of rate, stability, and conduction as determined by one AED algorithm did demonstrate differences between shockable and non-shockable rhythms recorded from adults and children. (Fig. 26.1) Heart rate of both shockable and non-shockable rhythms and conduction scores were statistically higher in children than in adults. (Fig. 26.2) These data highlight the importance of using multiple criteria to make a shock designation in children. A third manufacturer has developed

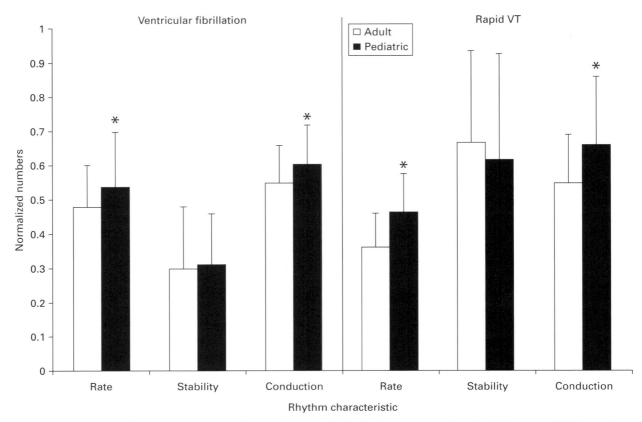

Fig. 26.1. Electrogram characteristics between pediatric and adult shockable rhythms. $P < 0.0001$. Rate is the frequency of ECG complex occurrence, stability is the morphologic stability of the ECT complexes, and conduction is a measure of rapidly conducted signals. Stability and conduction are measured from 0 to 1 and a higher number indicates less variability in the electrogram and faster conduction. The three measures are performed concurrently to make a shock decision; no one measure independently generates a shock decision. Reprinted with permission from ref. 14.

an algorithm based solely on pediatric rhythms, which is activated when the pediatric pads are attached to the device.[78] This algorithm, although not yet field-tested, also demonstrates very high sensitivity and specificity (Table 26.1).

Simplistic algorithms with only rate criteria will likely provide a lower specificity for children, potentially resulting in inappropriate shocks. It is vitally important that each manufacturer test its algorithm against a database of pediatric rhythms that includes multiple age groups, especially infants less than 1 year and rhythms with heart rates greater than 250 bpm.

Field use of AEDs in children

Field data of AED use in children has been difficult to collect, because cardiac arrest in children is an uncommon event. Thus, retrospective and postmarketing studies

become important. Using the cardiac arrest database established by the Emergency Services Learning Resource Center at the University of Iowa, we performed a retrospective study of AED use during out-of-hospital cardiac arrest in patients less than 16 years old.[76] We reviewed the years 1988–1997, when AEDs were first coming into widespread use in Iowa. Eighteen instances of AED application were reviewed. Average patient age was 12 years (range, 5–16 years). AEDs had a sensitivity of 88% and specificity of 100%. There were no instances of a shock recommendation for a non-shockable rhythm. We observed 33% survival in patients who received a shock as opposed to 11% survival with non-shockable rhythms.

More recently, the results of a postmarketing survey of the attenuated pads have established accurate rhythm detection with substantial survival. By voluntary reports of use, 27 patients with cardiac arrest (0 days to 23 years, median 2 years), were confirmed. Ventricular fibrillation was reported

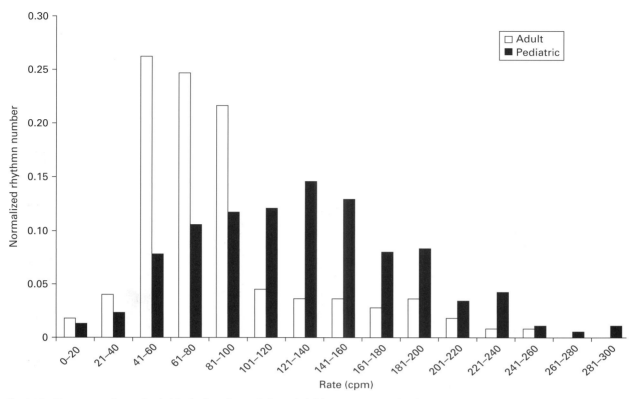

Fig. 26.2. Heart rates of non-shockable rhythms from adults and children. Data normalized to compensate for different numbers in database. Reprinted with permission from ref. 14.

in 8 cases (age range, 4.5 months to 10 years, median 3 years). Shocks were delivered to all VF patients, average shock number 1.9, range 1–4. All patients had termination of VF, were admitted to the hospital, and five survived to hospital discharge. Non-shockable rhythms were reported in 16 patients, and the AED appropriately did not advise a shock. Eleven of these patients had asystole or PEA as their initial rhythm and did not survive to hospital discharge. One report contained no additional information other than that the patient did not survive, and in two other reports, the pads were not applied to patients. More details about the youngest patient have been described in a separate report.[96]

Implications

Although children are less likely to suffer from ventricular fibrillation than are adults, it does occur in 10%–20% of pediatric cardiac arrests. The technology is now available to recognize and treat ventricular fibrillation in children as quickly as we can for adults. As this technology gains increased acceptance, resuscitation rates and outcomes for VF in children should approach those now seen in adults.

Cost-effectiveness

Introducing AEDs somewhere in the community will generate questions of cost to set up and to maintain the program. Also, questions may arise as to whether this money is wisely spent. Such questions of the relationship between the cost of a program and the effectiveness of that program, cost-effectiveness, are common in decisions in medical programs: not all decisions on AED programs are made within the framework of the medical domain. Examples are the airport act and the public building act, in which the US government enforced implementation of AEDs by law. Also, the decision of individuals acquiring an AED for their offices or home may be guided more by feelings of responsibility towards their employees or their family, without explicit or implicit cost-effectiveness considerations. After one airline showed the effectiveness of AED use on board airplanes(9), other airlines may have adopted AED programs more out of fear of litigation or consideration of marketing than consideration of cost-effectiveness.

For medical decisions regarding treatment choices, however, considerations of cost-effectiveness are more common and the principles can also be applied to AEDs in the community, especially when financial resources in a country are limited. Data are available for estimates of the costs of introduction of AEDs. These costs must be separated into the cost for the organization that purchases the AED and maintains the program, and the medical costs that will be incurred when a patient is brought to the hospital when resuscitation is successful. From the moment ambulance help is requested, the subsequent costs of emergency room care and hospital care are no longer borne by the organization that decided on the AED program. Nevertheless, these costs must be taken together for a complete analysis, because costs should be analyzed from the perspective of society.

It is difficult to attribute accurately those costs to an AED program, that are made after resuscitation and hospital admission to an AED program, even assuming the need to do so. Costs may increase: indeed, that the patient survived to admission and medical costs were incurred may be attributed to the use of the AED. Some costs may decrease: for example, earlier defibrillation may result in better neurological condition on admission and thus result in avoidance of, or a shorter stay in intensive care.[97]

The effectiveness of introducing AEDs in the community should lead to increased survival. In general, this is expressed in added quality-adjusted life–years. None of the studies that investigated the benefit of AEDs has extended the endpoint beyond discharge from the hospital, an endpoint that may not completely reflect the effect of AED use, as the cost of long-term care will not be included. When cost-effectiveness analysis is done, many components of cost or effectiveness must be derived from other studies, assumptions, or models.

When calculating effectiveness, the effect from the AED program on the survival rate observed in the specific population must be distinguished from the effect on the general population. Public Access Programs targeted to specific groups in specific places may have a significant survival benefit to that group, but may have very little effect on the survival rate for cardiac arrest in the general population. In general, PAD programs are targeted at victims in public places, where large groups are gathered and can be reached with a relatively small number of AEDs and trained rescuers: casinos, airports, public buildings, offices, sport arenas, and others. In these kinds of location, the collapse is generally witnessed, AEDs are close by and response times are short. Nonetheless, as at most 20% of victims of cardiac arrest are in these locations and 80% suffer a cardiac arrest in residential areas not suitable for PAD programs, the impact on the survival in the general population by these programs is necessarily limited. The

PAD trial included 16% of the AEDs placed in residential areas and showed no survival benefit for victims in those residential areas, although the overall survival doubled in the trial.[12] An analysis of cardiac arrests in Scotland suggested that the great majority of victims (79%) suffered their cardiac arrest in places not suitable for PAD programs.[98]

Determinants of cost-effectiveness of AED implementation

Analysis of cost-effectiveness establishes that incidence rate of cardiac arrest and response times are the main determinants of cost-effectiveness.[99] When rates are high (about > 0.5 incident per AED per year) and response times to defibrillation by rescuers with an AED are short (< 5–6 minutes), then implementing a PAD program can expected to be cost-effective.

Will AED programs designed for victims in residential areas be cost-effective? From the possible settings of AED implementation (dispatched (non-traditional) first responders, on-site responders, home use with high-risk patients and PAD), only dispatched first responders or home AEDs would potentially be suitable for victims in residential areas and therefore might be cost-effective. There are no studies published in this domain that allow a direct estimate of cost-effectiveness, but comparing key figures from the PAD trial and three controlled dispatched first responder studies may give some insight in the relative cost-effectiveness of the two strategies.

Table 26.2 compares the key resources used (number of AEDs used and number of rescuers trained) and the absolute number of victims saved (difference in survival to discharge among groups) by the institution of the AED program. Although the costs of resources may differ, the numbers suggest that dispatched first responders may be more cost-effective than PAD programs and have the added important benefit that they can reach all victims, at home and in public areas. With less than one-tenth of the rescuers required to be trained and with a few percent of the AEDs needed by dispatched first responders compared to those in the PAD study, about the same number of patients were saved by the program. Although all studies were controlled with the associated possible Hawthorne effect, they are real population-based studies, so that the comparison can be translated to routine use. Importantly, in many countries, dispatched first responders do not exist as part of EMS. In that situation, a dispatched first responder program with AED such as police, is a real addition to existing EMS and can be expected to be beneficial. When a dispatched first responder program already exists (e.g., fire fighters in the

Table 26.2. Comparison of key resources and outcome between the PAD trial and three controlled dispatched first responder studies

Study	Number of AEDs used	Number of rescuers trained	Duration of study (months)	Number of victims saved in the study period (no. experimental minus no. control)
PAD trial[12]	1650	19,376	21	15
Myerburg[8]	1900[a]	1900	20[b]	13
Capucci[50]	39	1285	22	8
Van Alem[54]	50	1650	24	11

[a] Each police officer retained his own AED, also off duty; [b] control period and experimental period not concurrent, calculated as if concurrent.

US), however, then adding another dispatched first responder may not have much added value.[100]

AEDs for home use will be purchased by individuals based on considerations other than cost-effectiveness. The effectiveness of such programs is as yet unknown and the outcome of the "HAT trial" will be the first information from a large scale study in that domain. The results are not expected before 2007. Until then, the cost-effectiveness of such a program cannot be considered.

The AED in the Guidelines 2005

In December 2005 new guidelines for cardiopulmonary resuscitation were published, with special reference to the use of the AED in several chapters.[17,101] Several changes in the guidelines are also reflected in the settings of the AED.

The defibrillation energy settings of the AED are now similar to the recommended energy settings of the manual defibrillator, both for monophasic waveform and biphasic waveform AEDs.

As one of the very important elements of the new guidelines, the significance of rapid institution of chest compressions and immediate resumption of chest compressions after a defibrillation shock, is emphasized. From experience with the AED we have learned that the modern biphasic defibrillators have a very high success rate in termination of VF, whereas immediately after the shock the probability of detecting return of perfusion is low, even when the rhythm after the shock is an organized one. As a consequence, the shock algorithm now includes only one shock, which is immediately followed by a period of chest compressions. Only after 2 minutes of uninterrupted chest compressions is the rhythm checked again, a second defibrillation shock is delivered when VF is present at that time or CPR resumed again for 2 minutes when VF is not present. There is no pulse check for lay rescuers after the shock and no lengthy assessment of signs of life. Only

when spontaneous breathing appears to be normal, are assessment of signs of life or signs of a circulation recommended, postponing chest compressions and ventilation while the signs of life or return of a pulse is confirmed.

These changes in the algorithm have profound implications for the voice prompts that guide the rescuer in the actions during the use of the AED. It is expected that these changes in the voice prompts will reduce the hands-off time as previously instructed by the voice prompts that had resulted in unnecessarily long periods without CPR.[15]

Future developments

As described in the first part of this chapter, AEDs have developed into highly sophisticated tools and can hardly be compared with the first devices of 30 years ago, which could do no more than detect and treat a shockable rhythm. It is certain, however, that developments will not stop now; some new developments are already being applied to current models.

The ability to assist the rescuer in doing Basic Life Support will become more prominent. As the importance of continued chest compressions, even when an AED is used, is now recognized, both speed of chest compressions and compression depth will be monitored by transducers and the rescuers will be aided by a metronome and voice prompts or other signals to keep the chest compressions optimal in rate and depth. As chests are not uniform in size, shape, and compliance, however, other tools to give feedback for optimal chest compressions should be developed. Potentially, feedback from blood flow resulting from chest compressions will be more informative than the mechanics of the compression. These are complex and yet unresolved biomedical problems, but the work must be done.

Finding better ways to diagnose circulatory arrest are needed. Our lay criteria of unconsciousness and absence of normal breathing are quite limited in their ability to identify a victim of circulatory arrest and tools that can identify the absence of blood flow could be very helpful, as many victims of cardiac arrest are not immediately recognized. It is possible that AEDs of the future will recognize gasping, and prompt initiation of CPR when a gasping breathing pattern is recognized.

Although AEDs are designed to shock, none is designed to pace the heart. Although asystole from prolonged VF is probably not responsive to pacing, asystole during complete heart block may well be. Also, postshock asystole may respond to pacing and it must be investigated whether this paced organized rhythm will also result in a paced perfusing rhythm, as already known and implemented in the Implantable Cardioverter Defibrillator.

There is no doubt that AEDs will be cheaper in the future. It will be important to distinguish true reduction in production costs from savings made by reducing or not including valuable features. As the volume of sales increases, larger scale production will lower these production costs. Reducing cost should then further increase their wider use. Nonetheless, as the survival rate from circulatory arrest remains low, even when AEDs are available, new developments of proven benefit should not be held back by cost considerations.

There will be many more developments not yet visible on the horizon. The hope now is that there will remain sufficient profit from AED manufacturing to provide adequate funding for the research that is needed to make the AED of the future even better than the current excellent machines.

Declared conflicts of interest

RWK is a paid advisor for and received material and financial support for research from Medtronic Emergency Response Systems and received material support from Zoll. DAC receives a grant (expenses only) from the Laerdal Foundation for his work in Cardiff. DLA received research and consultant fees from several defibrillator manufacturers to study the use of automated external defibrillators in children.

REFERENCES

1. Diack, A., Welborn, W., Rullman, R., Walter, C. & Wayne, M. An automatic cardiac resuscitator for emergency treatment of cardiac arrest. *Med. Instrum.* 1979; **13**: 78–81.

2. Jaggarao, N.S., Heber, M., Grainger, R., Vincent, R., Chamberlain, D.A. & Aronson, A.L. Use of an automated external defibrillator-pacemaker by ambulance staff. *Lancet* 1982; **2**(8289): 73–75.

3. Stults, K., Brown, D. & Kerber, R. Efficacy of an automated external defibrillator in the management of out-of-hospital cardiac arrest: validations of the diagnostic algorithm and initial experience in a rural environment. *Circulation* 1986; **73**: 701–709.

4. Weaver, W.D., Hill, D.L., Fahrenbruch, C. *et al.* Automatic external defibrillators: importance of field testing to evaluate performance. *J. Am. Coll. Cardiol.* 1987; **10**(6): 1259–1264.

5. Weaver, W.D., Hill, D., Fahrenbruch, C.E. *et al.* Use of the automatic external defibrillator in the management of out-of-hospital cardiac arrest. *N. Engl. J. Med.* 1988; **319**(11): 661–666.

6. White, R.D., Vukov, L.F. & Bugliosi, T.F. Early defibrillation by police: initial experience with measurement of critical time intervals and patient outcome. *Ann. Emerg. Med.* 1994; **23**(5): 1009–1013.

7. White, R.D., Hankins, D.G. & Atkinson, E.J. Patient outcomes following defibrillation with a low energy biphasic truncated exponential waveform in out-of-hospital cardiac arrest. *Resuscitation* 2001; **49**(1): 9–14.

8. Myerburg, R.J., Fenster, J., Velez, M. *et al.* Impact of community-wide police car deployment of automated external defibrillators on survival from out-of-hospital cardiac arrest. *Circulation* 2002; **106**(9): 1058–1064.

9. Page, R.L., Joglar, J.A., Kowal, R.C. *et al.* Use of automated external defibrillators by a U.S. airline. *N. Engl. J. Med.* 2000; **343**(17): 1210–1216.

10. Valenzuela, T.D., Roe, D.J., Nichol, G., Clark, L.L., Spaite, D.W. & Hardman, R.G. Outcomes of rapid defibrillation by security officers after cardiac arrest in casinos. *N. Engl. J. Med.* 2000; **343**(17): 1206–1209.

11. Caffrey, S.L., Willoughby, P.J., Pepe, P.E. & Becker, L.B. Public use of automated external defibrillators. *N. Engl. J. Med.* 2002; **347**(16): 1242–1247.

12. The Public Access Defibrillation Trial Investigators. Public-access defibrillation and survival after out-of-hospital cardiac arrest. *N. Engl. J. Med.* 2004; **351**: 637–646.

13. Atkins, D.L. & Jorgenson, D.B. Attenuated pediatric electrode pads for automated external defibrillator use in children. *Resuscitation* 2005; **66**(1): 31–37.

14. Cecchin, F., Jorgenson, D.B., Berul, C.I. *et al.* Is arrhythmia detection by automatic external defibrillator accurate for children? Sensitivity and specificity of an automatic external defibrillator algorithm in 696 pediatric arrhythmias. *Circulation* 2001; **103**(20): 2483–2488.

15. Van Alem, A., Sanou, B. & Koster, R. Interruption of CPR with the use of the AED in out of hospital cardiac arrest. *Med. Ann. Emerg. Med.* 2003; **42**: 449–457.

16. American Heart Association 2005 American Heart Association Guidelines for Cardiopulmonary Resuscitation and Emergency Cardiovascular Care. Part 11: Pediatric Basic Life Support. *Circulation* 2005; **112**(24 Suppl): IV-156-IV-166.

17. Handley, A.J., Koster, R., Monsieurs, K., Perkins, G.D., Davies, S. & Bossaert, L. European Resuscitation Council guidelines for resuscitation 2005. Section 2. Adult basic life support and use of automated external defibrillators. *Resuscitation* 2005; **67** Suppl 1: S7–S23.

18. Culley, L.L., Rea, T.D., Murray, J.A. *et al.* Public access defibrillation in out-of-hospital cardiac arrest: a community-based study. *Circulation* 2004; **109**(15): 1859–1863.

19. Feldman, A.M., Klein, H., Tchou, P. *et al.* Use of a wearable defibrillator in terminating tachyarrhythmias in patients at high risk for sudden death: results of the WEARIT/BIROAD. *Pacing Clin. Electrophysiol.* 2004; **27**(1): 4–9.

20. Eisenberg, M.S., Moore, J., Cummins, R.O. *et al.* Use of the automatic external defibrillator in home of survivors of out-of-hospital ventricular fibrillation. *Am. J. Cardiol.* 1989; **63**: 443–446.

21. Home Automatic External Defibrillator Trail (HAT). [cited; Available from: http://www.clinicaltrials.gov/ct/gui/show/NCT00047411]

22. O'Rourke, M.F., Donaldson, E. & Geddes, J.S. An airline cardiac arrest program. *Circulation* 1997; **96**(9): 2849–2853.

23. Goodwin, T. In-flight medical emergencies: an overview. *Br. Med. J.* 2000; **321**(7272): 1338–1341.

24. Alves, P.M., de Freitas, E.J., Mathias, H.A. *et al.* Use of automated external defibrillators in a Brazilian airline. A 1-year experience. *Arq. Bras. Cardiol.* 2001; **76**(4): 310–314.

25. Szmajer, M., Rodriguez, P., Sauval, P., Charetteur, M.P., Derossi, A. & Carli, P. Medical assistance during commercial airline flights: analysis of 11 years experience of the Paris Emergency Medical Service (SAMU) between 1989 and 1999. *Resuscitation* 2001; **50**(2): 147–151.

26. Cummins, R.O., Chapman, P.J., Chamberlain, D.A., Schubach, J.A. & Litwin, P.E. In-flight deaths during commercial air travel: how big is the problem? *J. Am. Med. Assoc.* 1988; **259**: 1983–1988.

27. FAA. 2001 [Available from: http://www.faa.govlibrary/reports/medical/fasmb/editorials_jj/assistanceact/index.cfm?print=go

28. Kaye, W., Mancini, M.E. & Richards, N. Organizing and implementing a hospital-wide first-responder automated external defibrillation program: strengthening the in-hospital chain of survival. *Resuscitation* 1995; **30**(2): 151–156.

29. Weisfeldt, M.L. & Becker, L.B. Resuscitation after cardiac arrest: a 3-phase time-sensitive model. *J. Am. Med. Assoc.* 2002; **288**(23): 3035–3038.

30. Kenward, G., Castle, N. & Hodgetts, T.J. Should ward nurses be using automatic external defibrillators as first responders to improve the outcome from cardiac arrest? A systematic review of the primary research. *Resuscitation* 2002; **52**(1): 31–37.

31. Santomauro, M., Ottaviano, L., Borrelli, A. *et al.* Role of semi-automatic defibrillators in a general hospital: "Naples Heart Project". *Resuscitation* 2004; **61**(2): 183–188.

32. Colquhoun, M. Resuscitation by primary care doctors. *Resuscitation* 2006; **70**: 229–237.

33. Fedoruk, J., Paterson, D., Hlynka, M., Fung, K., Gobet, M. & Currie, W. Rapid on-site defibrillation versus community program. *Prehosp. Disaster Med.* 2002; **17**: 102–106.

34. Whitfield, R., Colquhoun, M., Chamberlain, D., Newcombe, R., Davies, C.S. & Boyle, R. The Department of Health National Defibrillator Programme: analysis of downloads from 250 deployments of public access defibrillators. *Resuscitation* 2005; **64**(3): 269–277.

35. Jaggarao, N.S., Sless, H., Grainger, R., Vincent, R. & Chamberlain, D.A. Defibrillation at a football stadium: an experiment with Brighton and Hove Albion. *Br. Med. J. (Clin. Res. Ed.)* 1982; **284**(6327): 1451–1453.

36. Wassertheil, J., Keane, G., Fisher, N. & Leditschke, J.F. Cardiac arrest outcomes at the Melbourne Cricket Ground and shrine of remembrance using a tiered response strategy-a forerunner to public access defibrillation. *Resuscitation* 2000; **44**(2): 97–104.

37. American College of Sports Medicine and American Heart Association joint position statement: automated external defibrillators in health/fitness facilities. *Med. Sci. Sports Exerc.* 2002; **34**(3): 561–564.

38. Luiz, T., Kumpch, M., Metzger, M. & Madler, C. [Management of cardiac arrest in a German soccer stadium. Structural, process and outcome quality]. *Anaesthesist* 2005; **54**(9): 914–922.

39. Coris, E.E., Miller, E. & Sahebzamani, F. Sudden cardiac death in division I collegiate athletics: analysis of automated external defibrillator utilization in National Collegiate Athletic Association division I athletic programs. *Clin. J. Sport Med.* 2005; **15**(2): 87–91.

40. Haskell, W.L. Cardiovascular complications during exercise training of cardiac patients. *Circulation* 1978; **57**(5): 920–924.

41. Becker, L., Eisenberg, M., Fahrenbruch, C. & Cobb, L. Public locations of cardiac arrest: implications for public access defibrillation. *Circulation* 1998; **97**(21): 2106–2109.

42. De Maio, V.J., Stiell, I.G., Wells, G.A. & Spaite, D.W. Optimal defibrillation response intervals for maximum out-of-hospital cardiac arrest survival rates. *Ann. Emerg. Med.* 2003; **42**(2): 242–250.

43. de Vreede-Swagemakers, J.J., Gorgels, A.P., Dubois-Arbouw, W.I. *et al.* Out-of-hospital cardiac arrest in the 1990's: a population-based study in the Maastricht area on incidence, characteristics and survival. *J. Am. Coll. Cardiol.* 1997; **30**(6): 1500–1505.

44. Waalewijn, R.A., de Vos, R. & Koster, R.W. Out-of-hospital cardiac arrests in Amsterdam and its surrounding areas: results from the Amsterdam resuscitation study (ARREST) in 'Utstein' style. *Resuscitation* 1998; **38**(3): 157–167.

45. Norris, R.M. Circumstances of out of hospital cardiac arrest in patients with ischaemic heart disease. *Heart* 2005; **91**(12): 1537–1540.

46. Engdahl, J. Outcome after cardiac arrest outside hospital. *Br. Med. J.* 2002; **325**(7363): 503–504.

47. Herlitz, J., Andersson, E., Bang, A. *et al.* Experiences from treatment of out-of-hospital cardiac arrest during 17 years in Goteborg. *Eur. Heart J.* 2000; **21**(15): 1251–1258.

48. Kuisma, M., Repo, J. & Alaspaa, A. The incidence of out-of-hospital ventricular fibrillation in Helsinki, Finland, from 1994 to 1999. *Lancet* 2001; **358**(9280): 473–474.

49. Holmberg, M., Holmberg, S. & Herlitz, J. Effect of bystander cardiopulmonary resuscitation in out-of-hospital cardiac arrest patients in Sweden. *Resuscitation* 2000; **47**(1): 59–70.

50. Capucci, A., Aschieri, D., Piepoli, M.F., Bardy, G.H., Iconomu, E. & Arvedi, M. Tripling survival from sudden cardiac arrest via early defibrillation without traditional education in cardiopulmonary resuscitation. *Circulation* 2002; **106**(9): 1065–1070.

51. Jermyn, B.D. Response interval comparison between urban fire departments and ambulance services. *Prehosp. Emerg. Care* 1999; **3**(1): 15–18.

52. White, R.D., Asplin, B.R., Bugliosi, T.F. & Hankins, D.G. High discharge survival rate after out-of-hospital ventricular fibrillation with rapid defibrillation by police and paramedics. *Ann. Emerg. Med.* 1996; **28**(5): 480–485.

53. Ross, P., Nolan, J., Hill, E., Dawson, J., Whimster, F. & Skinner, D. The use of AEDs by police officers in the City of London. Automated external defibrillators. *Resuscitation* 2001; **50**(2): 141–146.

54. van Alem, A.P., Vrenken, R.H., de Vos, R., Tijssen, J.G. & Koster, R.W. Use of automated external defibrillator by first responders in out of hospital cardiac arrest: prospective controlled trial. *Br. Med. J.* 2003; **327**(7427): 1312.

55. Mosesso, V.N., Jr, Davis, E.A., Auble, T.E., Paris, P.M. & Yealy, D.M. Use of automated external defibrillators by police officers for treatment of out-of-hospital cardiac arrest. *Ann. Emerg. Med.* 1998; **32**(2): 200–207.

56. Groh, W.J., Lowe, M.R., Overgaard, A.D., Neal, J.M., Fishburn, W.C. & Zipes, D.P. Attitudes of law enforcement officers regarding automated external defibrillators. *Acad. Emerg. Med.* 2002; **9**(7): 751–753.

57. Cobb, L.A., Fahrenbruch, C.E., Walsh, T.R. *et al.* Influence of cardiopulmonary resuscitation prior to defibrillation in patients with out-of-hospital ventricular fibrillation. *J. Am. Med. Assoc.* 1999; **281**(13): 1182–1188.

58. Stotz, M., Albrecht, R., Zwicker, G., Drewe, J. & Ummerhofer, W. EMS defibrillation-first policy may not improve outcome in out of hospital cardiac arrest. *Resuscitation* 2003; **58**: 277–282.

59. Steen, S., Liao, Q., Pierre, L., Paskevicius, A. & Sjoberg, T. The critical importance of minimal delay between chest compressions and subsequent defibrillation: a haemodynamic explanation. *Resuscitation* 2003; **58**(3): 249–258.

60. Berg, R.A., Hilwig, R.W., Kern, K.B., Sanders, A.B., Xavier, L.C. & Ewy, G.A. Automated external defibrillation versus manual defibrillation for prolonged ventricular fibrillation: lethal delays of chest compressions before and after countershocks. *Ann. Emerg. Med.* 2003; **42**(4): 458–467.

61. Eisenberg, M., Bergner, L. & Hallstrom, A. Epidemiology of cardiac arrest and resuscitation in children. *Ann. Emerg. Med.* 1983; **12**(11): 672–674.

62. Appleton, G.O., Cummins, R.O., Larson, M.P. & Graves, J.R. CPR and the single rescuer: at what age should you "call first" rather than "call fast"? *Ann. Emerg. Med.* 1995; **25**(4): 492–494.

63. Walsh, C.K. & Krongrad, E. Terminal cardiac electrical activity in pediatric patients. *Am. J. Cardiol.* 1983; **51**(3): 557–561.

64. Safranek, D.J., Eisenberg, M.S. & Larsen, M.P. The epidemiology of cardiac arrest in young adults. *Ann. Emerg. Med.* 1992; **21**(9): 1102–1106.

65. Hickey, R.W., Cohen, D.M., Strausbaugh, S. & Dietrich, A.M. Pediatric patients requiring CPR in the prehospital setting. *Ann. Emerg. Med.* 1995; **25**(4): 495–501.

66. Mogayzel, C., Quan, L., Graves, J.R., Tiedeman, D., Fahrenbruch, C. & Herndon, P. Out-of-hospital ventricular fibrillation in children and adolescents: causes and outcomes. *Ann. Emerg. Med.* 1995; **25**(4): 484–491.

67. Ronco, R., King, W., Donley, D.K. & Tilden, S.J. Outcome and cost at a children's hospital following resuscitation for out-of-hospital cardiopulmonary arrest. *Arch. Pediatr. Adolesc. Med.* 1995; **149**(2): 210–214.

68. Sirbaugh, P.E., Pepe, P.E., Shook, J.E. *et al.* A prospective, population-based study of the demographics, epidemiology, management, and outcome of out-of-hospital pediatric cardiopulmonary arrest. *Ann. Emerg. Med.* 1999; **33**(2): 174–184.

69. Wren, C., O'Sullivan, J.J. & Wright, C. Sudden death in children and adolescents. *Heart* 2000; **83**(4): 410–413.

70. Young, K.D., Gausche-Hill, M., McClung, C.D. & Lewis, R.J. A prospective, population-based study of the epidemiology and outcome of out-of-hospital pediatric cardiopulmonary arrest. *Pediatrics* 2004; **114**(1): 157–164.

71. Gausche, M. Differences in the out-of-hospital care of children and adults: more questions than answers [editorial]. *Ann. Emerg. Med.* 1997; **29**(6): 776–779.

72. Nadkarni, V.M., Larkin, G.L., Peberdy, M.A. *et al.* First documented rhythm and clinical outcome from in-hospital cardiac arrest among children and adults. *J. Am. Med. Assoc.* 2006; **295**(1): 50–57.

73. Quan, L. Adult and pediatric resuscitation: finding common ground. *J. Am. Med. Assoc.* 2006; **295**(1): 96–98.

74. Suominen, P., Olkkola, K.T., Voipio, V., Korpela, R., Palo, R. & Rasanen, J. Utstein style reporting of in-hospital paediatric cardiopulmonary resuscitation. *Resuscitation* 2000; **45**(1): 17–25.

75. Paris, C.A., Quan, L., Fahrenbruch, C. & Copass, M.K. Predictors of survival after pediatric cardiac arrest. *Pediatrics* 1999; **45**: 63–64.

76. Atkins, D.L., Hartley, L.L. & York, D.K. Accurate recognition and effective treatment of ventricular fibrillation by automated external defibrillators in adolescents. *Pediatrics* 1998; **101**(1)(3): 393–397.

77. Quan, L. Pediatric resuscitation and emergency medical services. *Ann. Emerg. Med.* 1999; **33**(2): 214–217.

78. Atkins, D., Law, I., Scott, S. *et al.* Automated external defibrillator analysis specifically designed for pediatric patients. *JACC* 2005; **45**: 219.

79. Atkinson, E., Mikysa, B., Conway, J.A. *et al.* Specificity and sensitivity of automated external defibrillator rhythm analysis in infants and children. *Ann. Emerg. Med.* 2003; **42**(2): 185–196.

80. Jorgenson, D., Morgan, C., Snyder, D. *et al.* Energy attenuator for pediatric application of an automated external defibrillator. *Crit. Care Med.* 2002; **30**(4 Suppl.): S145–S147.

81. Samson, R.A., Berg, R.A., Bingham, R. *et al.* Use of automated external defibrillators for children: an update: an advisory statement from the pediatric advanced life support task

force, International Liaison Committee on Resuscitation. *Circulation* 2003; **107**(25): 3250–3255.

82. Babbs, C.F., Tacker, W.A., Van Vleet, J.F., Bourland, J.D. & Geddes, L.A. Therapeutic indices for transchest defibrillator shocks: effective, damaging, and lethal electrical doses. *Am. Heart J.* 1980; **99**(6): 734–738.

83. Geddes, L.A., Tacker, W.A., Rosborough, J.P., Moore, A.G. & Cabler, P.S. Electrical dose for ventricular defibrillation of large and small animals using precordial electrodes. *J. Clin. Invest.* 1974; **53**(1): 310–319.

84. Gutgesell, H.P., Tacker, W.A., Geddes, L.A., Davis, S., Lie, J.T. & McNamara, D.G. Energy dose for ventricular defibrillation of children. *Pediatrics* 1976; **58**(6): 898–901.

85. Clark, C.B., Zhang, Y., Davies, L.R., Karlsson, G. & Kerber, R.E. Pediatric transthoracic defibrillation: biphasic versus monophasic waveforms in an experimental model. *Resuscitation* 2001; **51**(2): 159–163.

86. Berg, R.A., Chapman, F.W., Berg, M.D. *et al.* Attenuated adult biphasic shocks compared with weight-based monophasic shocks in a swine model of prolonged pediatric ventricular fibrillation. *Resuscitation* 2004; **61**(2): 189–197.

87. Tang, W., Weil, M.H., Jorgenson, D. *et al.* Fixed-energy biphasic waveform defibrillation in a pediatric model of cardiac arrest and resuscitation. *Crit. Care Med.* 2002; **30**(12): 2736–2741.

88. Killingsworth, C.R., Melnick, S.B., Chapman, F.W. *et al.* Defibrillation threshold and cardiac responses using an external biphasic defibrillator with pediatric and adult adhesive patches in pediatric-sized piglets. *Resuscitation* 2002; **55**(2): 177–185.

89. Link, M.S., Maron, B.J., Stickney, R.E. *et al.* Automated external defibrillator arrhythmia detection in a model of cardiac arrest due to commotio cordis. *J. Cardiovasc. Electrophysiol.* 2003; **14**(1): 83–87.

90. Gurnett, C.A. & Atkins, D.L. Successful use of a biphasic waveform automated external defibrillator in a high-risk child. *Am. J. Cardiol.* 2000; **86**(9): 1051–1053.

91. Konig, B., Benger, J. & Goldsworthy, L. Automatic external defibrillation in a 6 year old. *Arch. Dis. Child.* 2005; **90**(3): 310–311.

92. Rossano, J.W., Quan, L., Kenney, M.A., Rea, T.D. & Atkins, D.L. Energy dosing for attempted defibrillation of out of hospital pediatric ventricular fibrillation. *Resuscitation* 2006; **70**: 80–89.

93. Berg, R.A., Chapman, F.W., Merg, M.D. *et al.* Relation between defibrillation dosage and outcome in a swine model of pediatric ventricular fibrillation. *Circulation* 2003; **108**: Suppl:IV-380.

94. Jones, J.L., Jones, R.E. & Balasky, G. Microlesion formation in myocardial cells by high-intensity electric field stimulation. *Am. J. Physiol.* 1987; **253**(2)(2): H480–H486.

95. Kerber, R.E., Becker, L.B., Bourland, J.D. *et al.* Automatic external defibrillators for public access defibrillation: recommendations for specifying and reporting arrhythmia analysis algorithm performance, incorporating new waveforms, and enhancing safety. A statement for health professionals from the American Heart Association Task Force on Automatic External Defibrillation, Subcommittee on AED Safety and Efficacy. *Circulation* 1997; **95**(6): 1677–1682.

96. Bar-Cohen, Y., Walsh, E.P., Love, B.A. & Cecchin, F. First appropriate use of automated external defibrillator in an infant. *Resuscitation* 2005; **67**(1): 135–137.

97. van Alem, A.P., Dijkgraaf, M.G., Tijssen, J.G. & Koster, R.W. Health system costs of out-of-hospital cardiac arrest in relation to time to shock. *Circulation* 2004; **110**(14): 1967–1973.

98. Pell, J.P., Sirel, J.M., Marsden, A.K., Ford, I., Walker, N.L. & Cobbe, S.M. Potential impact of public access defibrillators on survival after out of hospital cardiopulmonary arrest: retrospective cohort study. *Br. Med. J.* 2002; **325**(7363): 515.

99. Nichol, G., Valenzuela, T., Roe, D., Clark, L., Huszti, E. & Wells, G.A. Cost effectiveness of defibrillation by targeted responders in public settings. *Circulation* 2003; **108**(6): 697–703.

100. Sayre, M.R., Evans, J., White, L.J. & Brennan, T.D. Providing automated external defibrillators to urban police officers in addition to a fire department rapid defibrillation program is not effective. *Resuscitation* 2005; **66**(2): 189–196.

101. 2005 American Heart Association Guidelines for Cardiopulmonary Resuscitation and Emergency Cardiovascular Care. Part 5: Electrical Therapies: Automated External Defibrillators, Defibrillation, Cardioversion, and Pacing. *Circulation* 2005; **112**(24 Suppl): IV-35–46.

27

Public access defibrillation

Roger D. White[1], Mick Colquhoun[2], Sian Davies[3], Mary Ann Peberdy[4], and Sergio Timerman[5]

[1] College of Medicine, Mayo Clinic, Rochester, Minnesota, MN, USA
[2] Resuscitation Council, Tavistock Sq., London, UK
[3] Department of Health, London, UK
[4] Department of Medicine and Emergency Medicine, Virginia Commonwealth University, Richmond, VA, USA
[5] Resuscitation Department, Heart Institute of Sao Paolo, Brazil

Introduction

The development of automated external defibrillators (AEDs) enabled the potential life-saving benefit of rapid defibrillation to be extended into locations outside traditional boundaries. Defibrillation with these devices could now be provided by minimally medically trained persons such as firefighters and police officers. The survival benefit from AED deployment by such users led to the presumption that even more rapid defibrillation might be provided by placement of AEDs in public settings where large numbers of persons are present, and where defibrillation might be accomplished by even less-trained persons, and possibly even by persons not trained at all in AED use. And thus emerged the initiative known as public access defibrillation, or PAD. In this chapter, experience with PAD is described in several different settings, fortunately with acquisition and reporting of data to permit analysis of outcomes. Experience to date is surely encouraging, yet questions remain. Pell and colleagues have raised such questions pertaining to cost-effectiveness and have recommended expansion of first-responder defibrillation such as by police or firefighters and bystander cardiopulmonary resuscitation as more defensible options to PAD.[1-3]

In the PAD Trial reported by Peberdy in this chapter the low number of events is disheartening in light of the magnitude of the commitment in terms of numbers of persons trained and devices deployed, and the multiple locations in which AEDs were deployed. This observation may reflect yet another reality: the incidence of ventricular fibrillation (VF) as the presenting rhythm in out-of-hospital arrest settings is declining at an impressive rate, as reported now by several cardiac arrest investigators.[4-11] This reality imposes new obligations on those who advocate widespread deployment of AEDs in public settings. It will be necessary to define strategic locations where event rates are likely to confer cost-effective and life-saving benefit. The experience from the UK reported in this chapter appears to affirm that such locations can be identified.

Experience with PAD in the USA

Historical perspective

Public access defibrillation was first conceptualized by the American Heart Association's (AHA) "Future of CPR" Task Force in 1990. Although it was well recognized that the majority of cardiac arrests occur in the home, the thought of having lay persons respond with an AED to victims of cardiac arrest in public places was enticing. This model created the possibility for delivering defibrillation faster than most traditional EMS responses, and carried with it the hopes for substantial improvements in survival from out of hospital cardiac arrest. On the basis of recommendations of this task force, the AHA created an "AED Task Force" under the leadership of Dr. Myron Weisfeldt. This task force was responsible for the inclusion of the PAD concept in the 1992 AHA Guidelines on Cardiopulmonary Resuscitation and Emergency Cardiac Care. The following statement from the 1992 Guidelines provided a "large picture" view for what would be needed to begin to promote the concept of early defibrillation by non-traditional first responders.[12]

The placement of automated external defibrillators (AEDs) in the hands of large numbers of people trained in their use may be the key

Cardiac Arrest: The Science and Practice of Resuscitation Medicine. 2nd edn., ed. Norman Paradis, Henry Halperin, Karl Kern, Volker Wenzel, Douglas Chamberlain. Published by Cambridge University Press. © Cambridge University Press, 2007.

intervention to increase the survival chances of out-of-hospital cardiac arrest patients ... The widespread effectiveness and demonstrated safety of the AED have made it acceptable for nonprofessionals to effectively operate the device. Such persons must still be trained in CPR and use of defibrillators. In the near future, more creative use of AEDs by nonprofessionals may result in improved survival ... Participants in the national conference recommended that (1) AEDs be widely available for appropriately trained people, (2) all fire-fighting units that perform CPR and first aid be equipped with and trained to operate AEDs, (3) AEDs be placed in gathering places of more than 10,000 people, and (4) legislation be enacted to allow all EMS personnel to perform early defibrillation.

The first PAD conference was held in Washington, DC in 1994. Scientists, clinicians, members of the American Heart Association, representatives of the National Heart Lung and Blood Institute, and industry leadership met and collectively confirmed the need for future research and investigation in this area. Again, on the basis of the discussions during this conference, an official AHA Statement on Public Access Defibrillation was published in 1995.[13] This statement both supported the concept and began to develop a defined scope for PAD.

Early bystander cardiopulmonary resuscitation (CPR) and rapid defibrillation are the two major contributors to survival of adult victims of sudden cardiac arrest. The AHA supports efforts to provide prompt defibrillation to victims of cardiac arrest. Automatic external defibrillation is one of the most promising methods for achieving rapid defibrillation. In public access defibrillation, the technology of defibrillation and training in its use are accessible to the community. The AHA believes that this is the next step in strengthening the chain of survival. Public access defibrillation will involve considerable societal change and will succeed only through the strong efforts of the AHA and others with a commitment to improving emergency cardiac care.

Public access defibrillation will include (1) performance of defibrillation by laypersons at home and by firefighters, police, security personnel, and non-physician care providers in the community; and (2) exploration of the use of bystander-initiated automatic external defibrillation in rural communities and congested urban areas where resuscitation strategies have had little success.

The second PAD conference was held in 1997 and the recommendations published in 1998.[14] This international meeting further defined several details of implementation of the early PAD program and defined the original "four levels" of responders:

Level 1: Traditional first-responder defibrillation

This level includes defibrillation efforts by police, highway patrol personnel, and firefighter personnel. In many locations, firefighters are the first responders to cardiac emergencies, and yet they are often prohibited by regulations and state codes from providing early defibrillation.

Level 2: Non-traditional first-responder defibrillation

This level includes defibrillation efforts by lifeguards, security personnel, and airline flight attendants.

Level 3: Citizen CPR defibrillation

This level refers to citizens and laypeople that have received AED training. These individuals are interested in providing emergency cardiac care, usually in the setting of a home in which a family member who is a high-risk patient resides.

Level 4: Minimally trained witness defibrillation

This level refers to individuals who happen to witness a cardiopulmonary emergency and have an AED available (for example, through a worksite defibrillation program). In general, this level occurs most commonly in the home or at a worksite where one group of people has been trained and other groups have not. The untrained witness wants to help out and assist, but she has not yet received formal AED training. Another example of this level is possible if AEDs become accessible in the so-called "fire-extinguisher mode," in which the AED location is displayed prominently and any witness to an emergency has access to these devices. At present, both Food and Drug Administration and state regulations permit physician prescription of AEDs to individual homes. This level will become more feasible with the introduction of newer technology that provides more voice prompts to the user, automatic 911 dialing, and possibly 911 dispatcher-assisted defibrillation.

This leveling system divided potential responders into two main categories of "public safety responders" (Levels 1 and 2) and "lay citizen responders" (Levels 3 and 4). Attention was initially focused on increasing the numbers of public safety responders, since these persons may already be called upon as part of their job to respond to a potential cardiac arrest emergency. As efforts to implement widespread PAD programs at all levels continued it became clear that there were substantial regulatory barriers that negatively affected the ease and rapidity with which these programs could be developed. The Cardiac Arrest Survival Act (CASA) was passed into law in 2000. This act called for recommendations for the placement of AEDs in all Federal buildings and addressed the issue of partial immunity under the Good Samaritan Law. It also called for the publishing of training and implementation guidelines in the Federal Register, and served as the first Federal recognition of the importance of PAD. Much legal progress has been made since the passing of the CASA in the USA. Every state now has its own legislation supporting PAD, and also has specific wording in the local Good Samaritan laws for lay first responders and those acting in good faith while responding to cardiac arrest emergencies.

Other regulatory decisions have also assisted in promoting the widespread implementation of PAD throughout the USA. The Rural AED Bill was passed in 2000, which authorizes the use of up to $25 million in federal funds to help rural communities purchase AEDs and train first responders how to use them. In 2001, the Federal Aviation Administration ruled that all commercial aircraft carrying at least 30 passengers and one flight attendant are required to have an AED on board. The law also required the training of all flight attendants in how to perform CPR and use an AED. Final compliance for this ruling was in 2004. Also in 2001, the government released new guidelines for the placement of AEDs in federal facilities such as post offices, military bases, and federal parks to stress the importance of an optimal response time of less than 3 minutes.

Until recently, AEDs could only be purchased with a prescription and had to be used under the medical direction of a physician. This potential barrier for widespread placement of AEDs in public places was overcome in September, 2004 when for the first time the Food and Drug Administration granted marketing clearance for the over-the-counter sale of one manufacturer's AED designed specifically for lay users. AEDs can now be purchased and used in the USA without prescription or physician oversight.

Clinical perspective

Clinical adoption of early defibrillation with AEDs has evolved tremendously in the United States, and has demonstrated a multipronged approach to delivering defibrillation as early as possible to victims of cardiac arrest. Many EMS systems did not have first responder defibrillation capability as recently as a decade ago. One of the first mechanisms for implementation of PAD was to focus on early defibrillation by public safety personnel, such as emergency medical technicians, paramedics, and fire and police first responders, and eventually equipping nearly all ambulances throughout the country with AEDs. Fire department personnel and police are the backbone of the public safety primary response in the USA. Over 80% of police and fire agencies respond to medical emergencies and provide some level of clinical care. Adding defibrillation with AEDs theoretically should improve survival by reducing the time from collapse to first shock. White and colleagues studied the outcome of adult cardiac arrest patients in Rochester, Minnesota from 1990 through 1995.[15] The first arriving personnel delivered the shock. Of

the 84 patients in the study, 31 (37%) were initially shocked by police. Thirteen of the 31 had return of spontaneous circulation and all survived to discharge. The remaining 18 patients required ACLS and had a 27% survival to discharge. Fifty-three patients were shocked by paramedics and 14 survived without the need for ACLS. There were 9 survivors from the 38 patients who required ACLS. This study showed the effectiveness of early defibrillation with AEDs by both police and paramedics, and demonstrated that it is the rapidity with which the shock is delivered that determines the outcome, irrespective of who delivers the shock. Other results evaluating first responder defibrillation with law enforcement officials have varied, depending on factors such as the efficiency of the control systems, distance traveled to rural areas, absence of a medical response culture, unease with acting as a medical care provider, variable medical direction, and frequency of refresher training.[16,17] Most cities and larger suburban areas in the USA now use public safety personnel as first responders to deliver early defibrillation.

As the concept of PAD became more widely accepted, the effort to involve more truly "lay" first responders increased. The next level of penetration for AEDs was in equipping first responders who have a "duty to act" in public places as part of their job but not necessarily with a medical response. On-site security officials and flight attendants became the next level of personnel to be trained in the use of an AED to respond to victims of cardiac arrest. American Airlines was the first US-based airline to equip its aircraft with AEDs, train flight attendants how to use them, and publish their results. There were 36 cardiac arrests in the first 2 years of the program, with 15 in documented (13) or presumed (2) VF.[18] Forty percent (6/15) of subjects with VF survived. All 6 survivors were among the 11 VF arrests that occurred in the aircraft. One of the major dilemmas to improving survival from cardiac arrest in the air is that many cases are not acted upon quickly, because the person may be assumed to be sleeping. For further improvement of the impact of AEDs in the airline industry, AEDs began to be placed in airport terminals much in the way that fire extinguishers are distributed throughout a facility. Chicago's O'Hare and Midway airports were the first to describe their findings from placing 59 AEDs throughout their terminals spaced for a retrieval time of less than 3 minutes.[19] Although security officials were trained in how to use the AEDs, almost all of the devices were in glass-faced cabinets accessible to the public. Of the 80 million passengers that pass through these airports annually, 21 suffered a cardiac arrest (18 VF) in the first 2 years of the program. Eleven were successfully resuscitated and all but one had long-term neurologically intact survival. Half of the rescuers had no training or previous experience in the use of an AED.

Valenzuela *et al.* trained security officers in US casinos to perform CPR and use an AED.[20] They reported a survival to hospital discharge rate of 53% in the 105 patients suffering a VF arrest. Of those cases that were witnessed (86%), the mean time interval from collapse to attachment of the defibrillator was 3.5 ± 2.9 minutes, from collapse to first shock was 4.4 ± 2.9 minutes, and from collapse to arrival of EMS was 9.8 ± 4.3 minutes. This was one of the first large-scale trials of non-traditional first responders improving survival with on-site, early layperson defibrillation.

In an effort to acquire further data on more widespread use of AEDs by true laypersons in a variety of public places, the Public Access Defibrillation Trial was undertaken.[21] The PAD trial was a prospective, community-based, multi-center study that randomized public and multifamily residential locations from 24 cities throughout the United States and Canada to have lay, on-site volunteers trained in CPR alone vs. CPR plus an AED. The purpose of this trial was to determine whether or not trained laypersons without a duty to act would save more lives from out of hospital cardiac arrest by using an AED in addition to CPR compared with CPR alone. Sites qualified for participation if they had the equivalent of ≥ 250 adults over the age of 50 for 16 hours per day, or a history of one or more cardiac arrests in 2 years. Locations with on-site personnel with a duty to respond to medical emergencies, such as law enforcement officers or nurses, were excluded. Over 20 000 volunteers from 993 community units were trained to perform CPR and access EMS, with additional training in the use of the AED in the units randomized to this intervention. The AED arm received 1600 AEDs that were distributed at a density to achieve retrieval and return to the victim within 3 minutes or less. Sixteen percent of the study units were residential, and 84% were in public places and facilities. A total of 526 presumed cardiac arrests occurred during the study period, yielding 235 definite cardiac arrests after blinded review. Survival was achieved in 31 cases in the CPR + AED arm and 16 cases in the CPR only arm (RR = 2.0, CI = 1.07–3.77). Adverse events were rare and consisted mostly of device theft and varying levels of emotional distress on the part of the volunteer responder. There were no failures to shock when indicated, and no inappropriate shocks. No patient or volunteer was harmed by the use of an AED.

The PAD trial provides the first large-scale, randomized, controlled study that not only documents improved survival, but also demonstrates the safety of AEDs when used by trained lay volunteers in public locations. Evidence from the PAD trial should be generalized with caution. The sites chosen to participate had a significant percentage of people over the age of 55, who therefore were at higher risk for cardiac arrest. This, coupled with the unexpectedly low event rate, could lead to difficulties in prospectively determining the optimal public places for PAD programs. Since all volunteers were trained in both CPR and the use of an AED, when appropriate, these data should not be extrapolated to programs using untrained lay first responders. Finally, the true impact of PAD programs should be considered in relation to overall survival from cardiac arrest. Numerous studies have previously determined that approximately 80% of cardiac arrests occur in the home. PAD trial data show that only 0.6% of cardiac arrest victims in residential locations survived to hospital discharge, compared to 29.9% for those arresting in a public place. If nationwide PAD implementation occurred throughout the USA and a similar doubling of survival was seen, an add-itional 2000 to 4000 lives would be saved out of the more than 450 000 out-of-hospital cardiac arrests that occur annually.

The National Institutes of Health is currently sponsoring the Home AED Trial (HAT), scheduled to complete enrollment in late 2005 and to conclude in 2007. HAT is a randomized, controlled unblinded investigation evaluating the impact of home AED placement on survival of patients at high risk of sudden death. Eligible persons must have had a previous anterior wall myocardial infarction, no ICD placement, and have a live-in companion willing to use the AED if needed. The HAT provides first responder instruction via video, rather than traditional "hands-on" training. Information from this trial will help determine the safety and effectiveness of home AED use in high-risk patients with first responders who have not had mandatory traditional training in CPR or use of the AED.

Experience with PAD in Europe

From a technical perspective, the performance of defibrillation by minimally trained operators including laypersons became possible with the development of reliable automated external defibrillators in the late 1980s.[22,23] At that time a scheme to investigate this strategy was established in Europe by Douglas Chamberlain at Victoria Station, one of London's principal railway termini. Members of the British Transport Police working at the station were taught basic resuscitation techniques and how to use an automated defibrillator. During the first year of operation, five lives were saved by what was probably the first PAD scheme in the World.[23]

Subsequent guidance documents and position statements published by resuscitation authorities and applicable to Europe have aimed to guide the adoption of PAD 2000.[24] With the exception of England, however, progress in Europe has been limited. Several reasons have been advanced for this and are well summarized in the European Society of Cardiology – European Resuscitation Council recommendations for the use of AEDs.[25] This policy document was developed from the proceedings of an international conference on PAD held in 2002, which included resuscitation experts from most European countries. Problems with the initiation of PAD schemes and reasons for the slow initial progress in Europe identified at this conference include the following.

1. A lack of generally applicable models or defined strategies for community resuscitation schemes and their likely effectiveness.
2. Regulations in some countries that seriously limit or even forbid the use of defibrillators by lay responders. Fortunately these outdated laws are gradually being replaced by more appropriate contemporary legislation.
3. Lack of clear guidance about who should be responsible for providing equipment and for administering such programs or who should act as responders.
4. Concerns about the cost of implementing PAD schemes and a lack of evidence about cost effectiveness.
5. A lack of consensus on training requirements. Common International standards have been proposed as an ideal but have yet to be agreed or implemented.[26]
6. Uncertainty about the legal status of operators of AEDs with the possibility in some countries that a civil claim for damages might be bought against the user. These concerns have been assessed as a major problem to the implementation of PAD schemes in general and have been identified as a very important issue in Germany.[27] In contrast, a detailed analysis undertaken in England by lawyers with the help of expert medical advisors raised only minor concerns.[28,29]
7. The need for common definitions and audit standards. Although there has been little international discussion about this, the issue has been addressed in detail in England.[30,31]

Such schemes that have been reported from European centers have evolved to suit the requirements and conditions of individual countries or locations.[30–36] Other reports have investigated the feasibility and potential benefit of introducing PAD, in some cases as a prelude to their introduction.[2,8,34–40] These surveys, often based on theoretical projections based on epidemiological data, have reported variable results.

One established strategy is to place AEDs in high-risk locations where they are operated by trained lay persons who work at the site.[33,41,42] This arrangement has come to be known as "on-site" defibrillation, and dramatically successful results have been reported.[41,42]

The alternative strategy is to equip trained "first responders" who are usually despatched by ambulance control centers with AEDs.[32] This is common practice in the UK, particularly in remote rural areas of England and Wales. The responder may be a lay volunteer or a member of the police or fire service; a report from Austria has even described patrol members in alpine skiing resorts acting in this role.[43] Some workers have reported schemes that use a mixture of first responder and on-site defibrillation.[33,35] The important distinction is that "first responder" has to travel to a potential casualty; they may reach the scene more quickly than a conventional EMS response, but can only rarely match the response intervals seen with "on-site" schemes. The results have been less favorable, particularly when the response is delayed.[32,44]

Public access defibrillation in England: evolution towards a national scheme

Of importance is that there are different arrangements for the administration of health services in the individual countries that constitute the United Kingdom. The largest proportion of the population (49 million) live in England with health services administered by the Department of Health (DH) in London. In Scotland (5 million) and Wales (2.9 million) the responsibility rests with devolved national administrations. Decisions made in London for England may or may not be adopted by the other countries.

During the 1990s, PAD in the UK gradually evolved along the two major pathways described, largely through the generosity of the British Heart Foundation (BHF), a major national charity. AEDs were supplied to ambulance services for use by lay first responders, to some individual police forces, and to a few fire services. In most cases, the introduction depended on the enthusiasm of individual services, but in the fire service there was considerable opposition from one of the fire brigade trade unions that restricted deployment to a limited number of services.

At the same time AEDs were also supplied by the BHF for use in an "on-site" role. Managers of exhibition halls, concert venues, sporting stadia, shopping centers, and gymnasiums / leisure centers all installed AEDs, very often with the help of the BHF, and arranged training for their staff. This deployment was largely "reactive" and carried out according to the applications received.

During this time, the voluntary first aid societies, particularly St. John Ambulance, acquired AEDs and arranged their deployment among their trained members (usually, but not exclusively, lay first-aiders) undertaking public duties on their behalf; again the BHF provided a major source of funding. Many of these constituted an "on-site" strategy, with the operator deployed with an AED at the site of an event attended by large numbers of the general public. Many anecdotal accounts of successful resuscitation at sporting events, Remembrance Day services, and other events testified to the value of having an AED available.

Audit of these schemes was at first carried out by some individual organizations for their own purposes, and later systematic audit was established when a national scheme for the audit of all lay AED use was established by the Resuscitation Council (UK). This employs a specially designed computer database and report form described elsewhere.[31]

The English National Defibrillator Program

The major boost to PAD, and one of the principal reasons why the concept is so far advanced in the UK, came when the Government of England announced in 1999 the introduction of a scheme to place AEDs in busy public places so that some victims of sudden cardiac death could be resuscitated.[45] Funding was allocated at the outset for both the purchase of equipment and training.

The first phase of the program, which concerned the location of almost 700 AEDs, was administered by full-time staff working from central government offices in London. Considerable input to the planning, administration, and audit of the scheme came from medical advisors. The details of this scheme and its introduction have been described in detail previously.[29] Briefly, AEDs were located in busy public places identified from routine ambulance service data as sites where cardiac arrest commonly occurred. Staff who worked at these sites volunteered to be trained in basic life support and the use of an AED in classes lasting 4 hours. A standardized competency-based curriculum with adequate manikin practice is taught at each location, supplemented by the use of simulated cardiac arrest scenarios. Whereas in London, trainers from St. John Ambulance undertake the classes, at sites outside London, training is provided by the statutory ambulance services.

AEDs are located in unlocked protective cabinets at the selected locations in a density that ensures that equipment is available within notional 2 minutes' walk from any part of the premises to which the public has access.

Biphasic waveforms were used in all the defibrillators. Data about each resuscitation attempt are recorded at the location in a format compatible with the Utstein system for uniform recording of prehospital resuscitation attempts. Experience gained during this phase of auditing the program led to the design of the report form and audit methods described in detail elsewhere. The intervals between collapse and the institution of basic life support (BLS) and defibrillation are usually estimated, but are sometimes supported by data from ambulance dispatch centers or other control systems. The data on the report form is analyzed in conjunction with a download of data stored electronically in the memory chip in the AED, so that detailed analysis can be undertaken of both the electrocardiogram and the procedures undertaken during each event.

Results

The detailed audit possible with a scheme that formed a part of routine healthcare provision provided by the National Health Service has yielded valuable information.[38,39] The ambulance services consulted had indicated that the most common public places where they attended patients with cardiac arrest were transport facilities, particularly airports and mainline railway stations. Ferry terminals, underground railway stations, and bus stations were also identified. Many such sites were duly equipped with AEDs and reported every deployment of the equipment to a potential patient. In the first 250 such deployments,[41] 182 were to actual cases of cardiac arrest. The remaining 68 deployments were either as a precaution to casualties who had been taken ill for other reasons, or because initial reports had suggested the possibility of cardiac arrest. In one case, an AED was attached to a passenger who although conscious, looked very unwell. The AED subsequently documented the onset of ventricular tachycardia which degenerated into VF that responded to a single shock with the restoration of a perfusing rhythm.

As would be expected, the great majority (177/182) of arrests were witnessed. A high proportion (82%) showed VF as the first recorded rhythm; 8% showed asystole; 7% severe bradycardia; and the remainder idioventricular rhythm. The overall survival rate after defibrillation was impressive: 29% in patients presenting with VF/VT and 25% when all rhythms are considered (Table 27.1).

Of 143 cases of VF/VT where downloads were available, one or more shocks were administered (range 1–16) in 140 cases. One VF waveform was below the sensitivity of the device and equipment or operator failure occurred twice. The first shock terminated the arrhythmia at least transiently (at least 5 seconds) in 132 cases. In 74, only 1 shock was required before the patient was transferred to the

Table 27.1. Outcome of cardiac arrest by type of site and initial rhythm

| Patient group Type of site | Known VF/VT | | All rhythms |
	Proportion surviving (%)	95% confidence interval (%)	Proportion surviving (%)
Airports	21/83 (25)	17–35	22/101 (22)
Railway stations	19/50 (38)	26–52	19/58 (33)
Other	3/13 (23)	8–50	3/18 (17)
Total	43/146 (29)	23–37	44/177 (25)

Percentages are shown in parentheses, with 95% confidence intervals for survival proportions of those with known VF/VT by tape of site.

care of paramedics. None of the patients without first shock success survived to discharge. Of 44 survivors, 32 only required 1 shock on site; the remainder required 2 or more.

In most cases, the electrodes were attached to the casualties an estimated 3–5 minutes after collapse. Data obtained from ambulance services attending the sites showed average response times of 8–12 minutes. "Response time" is the interval between identification of the main complaint in the control center and the arrival of the ambulance at the scene. It does not take into account the time taken to locate a telephone and make the emergency call, interrogation by the call taker, or the time taken to reach and assess the patient after arrival (likely to be a few further minutes at a large station or airport). The use of AEDs by those working at the site is likely to have reduced the time between collapse and defibrillation considerably and is doubtless a major factor behind the excellent results achieved.

The figures presented here are the first formal evaluation of a European "on-site" PAD scheme. The results are comparable with those reported from other schemes, predominantly in the USA.[18–21] None of this evidence was published at the time that the English scheme was initiated (1999) and it represented a bold move on the part of the relevant government agencies involved.

Further evidence about the effectiveness of on-site defibrillation is available from the Resuscitation Council (UK) database.[30] This incorporates the DH data mentioned above with the results from several hundred AEDs supplied by the BHF. In 317 resuscitation attempts using AEDs placed in public places, shocks were administered in 247 (78%), ROSC occurred in 114 (36%), and 62 (20%) were discharged from hospital. Once again, the electrodes were placed on the casualty promptly, within 3–5 minutes of collapse. These figures were obtained from 138 arrests at airports, 69 at railway stations, 66 where members of the voluntary first aid societies provided an AED at a public

event, 8 at underground railway stations, 7 at other transport facilities, 11 at shopping centers, and 18 at gymnasia or other sporting facilities.

The English National Defibrillator Program (NDP): The next stages

The original proposal for the implementation of PAD on a national basis in England included the siting of a total of 3000 AEDs in the community. The second phase of the NDP began in 2004 and saw an important change of direction, with the provision of PAD becoming the responsibility of the 31 local ambulance services in the country and a core part of their NHS service provision. Funding was supplied through an award from the Big Lottery Fund (a National Lottery, some of the proceeds of which are used for community projects), and a close working relationship was established between the BHF and the DH who became partners in the administration of the next phase of the program. The funding was allocated to the procurement of the additional 2700 AEDs, to funding additional staff in ambulance services, and for administration and training.

The responsibility for implementation at a local level rests with the individual ambulance services, the additional AEDs being allocated according to a "needs assessment" undertaken by each service. Some will be used in an "on-site" role to build on the experience obtained during the first stage of the program. Others will be used by lay first responders under the control of the local ambulance service. At the time of writing, this process is at an early stage of implementation and no results are yet available. Audit is expected to be carried out as a routine in each service, however, and results should therefore be available in the future.

The partnership between the BHF and the DH also provides the opportunity to incorporate the AEDs already donated by the BHF (around 2000 by 2005) into the national strategy for PAD.

Table 27.2.

	Lay ambulance Responders	Fire service Responders	Total
Number	533	118	651
Time [a] (min)	8	12	
Shocked	186	36	222 (34%)
ROSC	68	12	80 (12%)
Discharged	21[b] (3.9%)	2 (1.7%)	23 (3.5%)

Outcome of cardiac arrests attended by first responders.

[a] Median time from receipt of call to placement of AED pads, estimated in some cases.

[b] Some arrests witnessed by a first responder dispatched to a patient judged at risk of cardiac arrest.

Percentages are shown in parentheses.

First responders in England

While there now exists a firm evidence base for the use of static AEDs installed in busy public places, the situation is less clear for their use by first responders in Europe. One prospective randomized trial in Amsterdam[32] that used police or fire personnel as first responders reported higher rates of ROSC and admission to hospital, but numbers surviving to discharge were not increased. Delays in calling for help, in handling emergency calls and in despatching were thought to have been the factors that reduced the potential effectiveness of first responders. Another study carried out in Piacenza, Italy has shown a tripling of survival (from 3.3 to 10.5%) with the introduction of 39 AEDs used by lay volunteers who achieved a reduction in response time of slightly more than 1 minute compared to that of the local EMS.[33] 12 of the AEDs were placed in lay-staffed ambulances, 15 in police cars, and 12 were installed "on-site" at high-risk locations. It is not clear how many of the arrests were actually treated by first responders and how many were treated "on-site," but the fact that 86.7% of the arrests occurred at home suggests the majority were "first responder" resuscitations.

The Resuscitation Council (UK) database contains records of arrests attended by first responders before the arrival of EMS, and a preliminary report has been presented.[44] A preliminary analysis of a more extensive series of 651 arrests attended by lay or fire service first responders dispatched by ambulance control centers, is shown in Table 27.2. In the UK, patient confidentiality issues prevent the methodical collection of hospital outcome data. Every patient in whom ROSC is achieved is followed up, but it is not always possible to establish whether or not they survived. The numbers of survivors may therefore be slightly higher than shown in the table. It is clear, however, that the results are very much poorer than those achieved by on-site responders, almost certainly related to the much longer time taken to reach the patient and attach the AED.

PAD in other locations

In 2002, Capucci and colleagues reported their first experience with deployment of AEDs in Piacenza and the surrounding region in Italy.[35] Lay responders trained in AED operation were added to those deployed by police and fire vehicles and in public assistance volunteer groups who assisted in the care and transportation of the ill. These agencies and responses were grouped collectively under the designation Piacenza Progretto Vita (PPV). During the first 22 months of this initiative, 34/143 (23%) of the patients in the PPV group were in ventricular fibrillation and 33/211 (15.6%) of those in the EMS group. Neurologically intact survival in the PPV group was 12/34 (35%) and 5/33 (15%) in the EMS group. This difference was of borderline statistical significance ($P = 0.058$), although the number of patients in each group is small.

In 2000, Wassertheil et al. published their experience with early defibrillation using a tiered response strategy in two public locations in Australia (the Melbourne Cricket Ground and the Shrine of Remembrance). Manual defibrillators were used during the first half of the study by ambulance officers and certified nurses. In all 28 arrests, VF was the presenting rhythm and 20 (71%) were discharged.[46] This study might be considered a precursor to what is now known as PAD.

Kuisma and colleagues described preliminary results in a community-based pilot study in Helsinki.[34] AEDs were placed in seven public locations where the event rate was predicted to justify inclusion in such a trial. Over the 3-year period of study there were only 7 events in the PAD locations, and only 4 of these were in VF. None were discharged from the hospital. There were 13 patients in the control group, 6 of whom were in VF on EMS arrival. Four were discharged. Obviously the numbers are very small and thus it is not possible to draw definitive conclusions. The authors pointed out an important observation: only 50% of the patients were in VF, again raising the question of cost-effectiveness in the presence of a declining incidence of VF.

In Brazil, a number of PAD initiatives are being undertaken, with legislation supporting such initiatives. At this time no patient outcome data have been reported. Varig Airlines, the Brazilian national air carrier, was one of the early commercial air carriers to equip its aircraft with AEDs. To date there is only one very preliminary reported experience with this approach, confirming the feasibility of equipping aircraft with AEDs and training flight attendants in their operation. Patient outcome data, however, are too limited to permit conclusions regarding overall cost-effective benefit.[47]

Conclusions

The results reported in this chapter provide important insights into the potential benefit of deployment of AEDs in public settings. The acquisition and reporting of accurate, credible incidence and survival data from PAD experience will provide a definitive process for assessing benefit from PAD programs in various locations. Without such data we will be left with anecdotal accounts of success, and such accounts will not in themselves be of benefit in defining the most cost-effective, durable lifesaving approaches to provision of defibrillation in various out-of-hospital cardiac arrest settings. Benefit of deployment of AEDs in home settings remains a completely unanswered question at this time. It is to be hoped that results from the Home Automated Defibrillation Trial (HAT Trial) will provide insight into this question, but that study will not be concluded until 2007.

REFERENCES

1. Pell, J.P. The debate on public place defibrillators: charged but shockingly ill informed. *Heart* 2003; **89**: 1375–1376.
2. Pell, J.P., Sirel, J.M., Marsden, A.K., Ford, I., Walker, N.L. & Cobbe, S.M. Potential impact of public access defibrillators on survival after out of hospital cardiopulmonary arrest: retrospective cohort study. *Br. Med. J.* 2002; **325**: 515.
3. Walker, A., Sirel, J.M., Marsden, A.K., Cobbe, S.M. & Pell, J.P. Cost effectiveness and cost utility model of public place

4. Cobb, L.A., Fahren bruch, C.E., Olsufka, M. & Copass, M.K. Changing incidence of out-of-hospital ventricular fibrillation, 1980–2000. *J. Am. Med. Assoc.* 2002; **288**: 3008–3013.
5. Bunch, T.J., White, R.D., Friedman, P.A., Kottke, T.E., Wu, L.A. & Packer, D.L. Trends in treated ventricular fibrillation out-of-hospital cardiac arrest: a 17-year population-based study. *Heart Rhythm.* 2004; **1**: 255–259.
6. Herlitz, J., Engdahl, J., Svensson, L., Young, M., Angquist, K.A. & Holmberg, S. Decrease in the occurrence of ventricular fibrillation as the initially observed arrhythmia after out-of-hospital cardiac arrest during 11 years in Sweden. *Resuscitation* 2004; **60**: 283–290.
7. Parish, D.C., Dinesh Chandra, K.M. & Dane, F.C. Success changes the problem: why ventricular fibrillation is declining, why pulseless electrical activity is emerging, and what to do about it. *Resuscitation* 2003; **58**: 31–35.
8. Kuisma, M. & Repo, J. The incidence of out-of-hospital ventricular fibrillation in Helsinki, Finland, from 1994 to 1999, *Lancet* 2001; **358**: 473–474.
9. Herlitz, J., Engdahl, J., Svensson, L., Young, M., Angquist, K.A. & Holmberg, S. Changes in demographic factors and mortality after out-of-hospital cardiac arrest in Sweden. *Coron. Artery Dis.* 2005; **16**: 51–57.
10. Richmond, N., Silverman, R., Kusick, M. *et al.* Survival from out-of-hospital cardiac arrest in New York city: ten years later. *Prehosp. Emerg. Care* 2005; **9**: 72.
11. Polentini, M., Pirrallo, R. & McGill, W. The changing incidence of ventricular fibrillation and cardiac arrest in Milwaukee county. *Prehosp. Emerg. Care* 2005; **9**: 103.
12. Kerber, R., Ornato, J.P., Brown, D.B. & Chandra, N.R. Emergency Cardiac Care Committee and Subcommittees, American Heart Association. Guidelines for cardiopulmonary resuscitation and emergency cardiac care, I:introduction. *J. Am. Med. Assoc.* 1992; **268**: 2172–2183.
13. Weisfeldt, M.L., Kerber, R.E., McGoldrick, R.P. *et al.* American Heart Association Report on the Public Access Defibrillation Conference December 8–10, 1994. Automatic External Defibrillation Task Force. *Circulation* 1995; **92**: 2740–2747.
14. Nichol, G., Hallstrom, A. P., Kerber, R. *et al.* American Heart Association report on the second public access defibrillation conference, April 17–19, 1997. *Circulation* 1998; **97**: 1309–1314.
15. White, R.D., Asplin, B.R., Bugliosi, T.F. & Hankins, D.G. High discharge survival rate after out-of-hospital ventricular fibrillation with rapid defibrillation by police and paramedics. *Ann. Emerg. Med.* 1996; **28**: 480–485.
16. Groh, W. J., Newman, M.M., Beal, P.E., Fineberg, N.S. & Zipes, D.P. Limited response to cardiac arrest by police equipped with automated external defibrillators: lack of survival benefit in suburban and rural Indiana – the police as responder automated defibrillation evaluation (PARADE). *Acad. Emerg. Med.* 2001; **8**: 324–330.
17. Sayre, M.R., Evans, J., White, L.J. & Brennan, T.D. Providing automated external defibrillators to urban police officers in

addition to a fire department rapid defibrillation program is not effective. *Resuscitation* 2005; **66**: 189–196.

18. Page, R.L., Joglar, J.A., Kowal, R.C. *et al.* Use of automated external defibrillators by a U.S. airline. *N. Engl. J. Med.* 2000; **343**: 1210–1216.

19. Caffrey, S.L., Willoughby, P.J., Pepe, P. E. & Becker, L.B. Public use of automated external defibrillators. *N. Engl. J. Med.* 2002; **347**: 1242–1247.

20. Valenzuela, T.D., Roe, D.J., Nichol, G., Clark, L.L., Spaite, D.W. & Hardman, R.G. *Outcomes of rapid defibrillation by security officers after cardiac arrest in casinos. N. Engl. J. Med.* 2000; **343**: 1206–1209.

21. Hallstrom, A.P., Ornato, J.P., Weisfeldt, M. *et al.* Public-access defibrillation and survival after out-of-hospital cardiac arrest. *N. Engl. J. Med.* 2004; **351**: 637–646.

22. Cummins, R.O., Eisenberg, M.S., Litwin, P.E., Graves, J.R., Hearne, T.R. & Hallstrom, A.P. Automatic external defibrillators used by emergency medical technicians. A controlled clinical trial. *J. Am. Med. Assoc.* 1987; **257**: 1605–1610.

23. Weaver, W.D., Hill, D., Fahrenbruch, C.E. *et al.* Use of the automatic external defibrillator in the management of out-of-hospital cardiac arrest. *N. Engl. J. Med.* 1988; **319**: 661–666.

24. Monsieurs, K.G., Handley, A.J. & Bossaert, L.L. European Resuscitation Council Guidelines 2000 for Automated External Defibrillation. A statement from the Basic Life Support and Automated External Defibrillation Working Group(1) and approved by the Executive Committee of the European Resuscitation Council. *Resuscitation* 2001; **48**: 207–209.

25. Priori, S.G., Bossaert, L.L., Chamberlain, D.A., *et al.* ESC-ERC recommendations for the use of automated external defibrillators (AEDs) in Europe. *Eur. Heart J.* 2004; **25**: 437–445.

26. Chamberlain, D.A. & Hazinski, M.F. Education in resuscitation. *Resuscitation* 2003; **59**: 11–43.

27. Seliger, M. & Knorr, M. Does public access to defibrillators have a chance in Germany? – On the US model, legal considerations and justification. *Gesundheitswesen*, 2000; **62**: 665–669.

28. O'Rourke, M. & Donaldson, E. Management of ventricular fibrillation in commercial airliners. *Lancet* 1995; **345**: 515–516.

29. Colquhoun, M. & Martineau, E. (2000) Resuscitation Council (UK), London.

30. Davies, C.S., Colquhoun, M., Graham, S., Evans, T. & Chamberlain, D. Defibrillators in public places: the introduction of a national scheme for public access defibrillation in England. *Resuscitation* 2002; **52**: 13–21.

31. Colquhoun, M., Davies, C.S., Harris, S., Harris, R. & Chamberlain, D. Public access defibrillation – designing a universal report form and database for a national programme. *Resuscitation* 2004; **61**: 49–54.

32. van Alem, A. P., Vrenken, R. H., de Vos, R., Tijssen, J. G. & Koster, R. W. Use of automated external defibrillator by first responders in out of hospital cardiac arrest: prospective controlled trial. *Br. Med. J.* 2003; **327**: 1312.

33. Capucci, A., Aschieri, D., Piepoli, M.F., Bardy, G.H., Iconomu, E. & Arvedi, M. Tripling survival from sudden cardiac arrest via early defibrillation without traditional education in cardiopulmonary resuscitation. *Circulation* 2002b; **106**: 1065–1070.

34. Kuisma, M., Castren, M. & Nurminen, K. Public access defibrillation in Helsinki – costs and potential benefits from a community-based pilot study. *Resuscitation* 2003; **56**: 149–152.

35. Capucci, A., Aschieri, D. & Piepoli, M.F. Out-of-hospital early defibrillation successfully challenges sudden cardiac arrest: the Piacenza Progetto Vita project. *Ital. Heart J.* 2002a; **3**: 721–725.

36. Martens, P., Calle, P. & Vanhaute, O. Theoretical calculation of maximum attainable benefit of public access defibrillation in Belgium. Belgian Cardio Pulmonary Cerebral Resuscitation Study Group. *Resuscitation* 1998; **36**: 161–163.

37. Marin-Huerta, E., Peinado, R., Asso, A. *et al.* [Sudden cardiac death out of the hospital and early defibrillation]. *Rev. Esp. Cardiol.* 2000; **53**: 851–865.

38. Katz, E., Metzger, J.T., Jaussi, A. *et al.* [What do we actually know about out-of-hospital cardiac arrest?]. *Rev. Med. Suisse* 2005; **1**: 628–630, 632–633.

39. Engdahl, J. & Herlitz, J. Localization of out-of-hospital cardiac arrest in Goteborg 1994–2002 and implications for public access defibrillation. *Resuscitation* 2005; **64**: 171–175.

40. Rortveit, S. & Meland, E. [Public access defibrillators – beneficial?]. *Tidsskr. Nor Laegeforen* 2004; **124**: 316–319.

41. Whitfield, R., Colquhoun, M., Chamberlain, D., Newcombe, R., Davies, C.S. & Boyle, R. The Department of Health National Defibrillator Programme: analysis of downloads from 250 deployments of public access defibrillators. *Resuscitation* 2005; **64**: 269–277.

42. Davies, C.S., Colquhoun, M.C., Boyle, R. & Chamberlain, D. A. A national programme for on-site defibrillation by lay people in selected high risk areas: initial results. *Heart*, 2005; **91**: 1299–1302.

43. Lienhart, H.G., Breitfeld, L. & Voelckel, W.G. [Public access defibrillation in alpine skiing areas: three case reports and a brief survey of the literature]. *Anasthesiol Intensivmed Notfallmed Schmerzther.* 2005; **40**: 150–155.

44. Colquhoun, M., Davies, C.S., Woollard, M. & Chamberlain, D. A comparison of different strategies for public access defibrillation (Abstr.) *Resuscitation* 2002; **55**: 115.

45. Department of Health The Stationery Office, London, 1999.

46. Wassertheil, J., Keane, G., Fisher, N. & Leditschke, J.F. Cardiac arrest outcomes at the Melbourne Cricket Ground and shrine of remembrance using a tiered response strategy – a forerunner to public access defibrillation. *Resuscitation* 2000; **44**: 97–104.

47. Alves, P.M., de Freitas, E.J., Mathias, H.A. *et al.* Use of automated external defibrillators in a Brazilian airline. A 1-year experience. *Arq. Bras. Cardiol.* 2001; **76**: 310–314.

28

The physiology of ventilation during cardiac arrest and other low blood flow states

Ahamed H. Idris and Andrea Gabrielli

University of Texas Southwestern Medical Center at Dallas, TX, USA
Division of Critical Care Medicine, University of Florida, Gainesville, FL, USA

Introduction

Ventilation – the movement of fresh air or other gas from the outside into the lungs and alveoli in close proximity to blood for the efficient exchange of gases – enriches blood with O_2 and rids the body of CO_2 by movement of alveolar gas out of the lungs to the outside.[1]

The importance of ventilation in resuscitation is reflected in the "ABCs" (airway, breathing, circulation), which is the recommended sequence of resuscitation practiced in a broad spectrum of illnesses including traumatic injury, unconsciousness, and respiratory and cardiac arrest. Since the modern era of cardiopulmonary resuscitation (CPR) began in the early 1960s, ventilation of the lungs of a victim of cardiac arrest has been assumed to be important for successful resuscitation.

This assumption has been questioned and the role of ventilation during resuscitation has been the subject of much research for more than a decade.[2] A number of laboratory studies of CPR have shown no clear benefit to ventilation during the early stages of cardiac arrest with ventricular fibrillation.[3–5] Furthermore, exhaled gas contains approximately 4% CO_2 and 17% O_2, thus making mouth-to-mouth ventilation the only circumstance in which a hypoxic and hypercarbic gas mixture is given as recommended therapy.[6] With the introduction of the *2000 Guidelines for Cardiopulmonary Resuscitation*, a new, evidence-based approach to the science of ventilation during CPR was introduced and continues with the publication of the 2005 edition. New evidence from laboratory and clinical science has led to less emphasis being placed on the role of ventilation following a dysrhythmic cardiac arrest (arrest primarily resulting from a cardiovascular event, such as ventricular fibrillation or asystole). Nevertheless, the classic airway patency, breathing, and circulation CPR sequence remains a fundamental factor for the immediate survival and neurological outcome of patients after asphyxial cardiac arrest (cardiac arrest primarily resulting from respiratory arrest).

This chapter reviews pulmonary anatomy and physiology, key historical studies of ventilation in respiratory and cardiac arrest, the effect of ventilation on acid–base conditions and oxygenation during low blood flow states, the effect of ventilation on resuscitation from cardiac arrest, manual, mouth-to-mouth, and newer techniques of ventilation, and current recommendations for ventilation during CPR.

History of artificial ventilation and CPR techniques

With the onset of cardiac arrest, effective spontaneous respiration quickly ceases. Attempts to provide ventilation for victims of respiratory and cardiac arrest have been described throughout history. Early descriptions are found in the Bible[7] and in anecdotal reports in the medical literature of resuscitation of victims of accidents and illness. Early examples of mouth-to-mouth ventilation are described in the resuscitation of a coal miner in 1744,[8] and in an experiment in 1796 demonstrating that expired air was safe for breathing.[9] In 1954, Elam and colleagues described artificial respiration with the exhaled gas of a rescuer using a mouth-to-mask ventilation method.[10,11]

Cardiac Arrest: The Science and Practice of Resuscitation Medicine. 2nd edn., ed. Norman Paradis, Henry Halperin, Karl Kern, Volker Wenzel, Douglas Chamberlain. Published by Cambridge University Press. © Cambridge University Press, 2007.

Descriptions of chest compression to provide circulation[12] can be found in the historical literature of more than 100 years ago. Electrical defibrillation had been applied in animal laboratory research since the early 1900s and by Kouwenhoven in 1928.[11]

The modern era of CPR began when artificial ventilation, closed-chest cardiac massage, and electrical defibrillation were combined into a set of practical techniques to initiate the reversal of death from respiratory or cardiac arrest. Resuscitation is associated with hypoperfusion and consequent ischemia. Recent studies suggest dual defects of hypoxia and hypercarbia during ischemia.[13] Thus, the primary purpose of CPR is to bring oxygenated blood to the tissues and to remove carbon dioxide from the tissues until spontaneous circulation is restored. In turn, the purpose of ventilation is to oxygenate and to remove carbon dioxide from blood. The "gold standard" of providing ventilation during CPR is direct intubation of the trachea, which not only affords a means of getting gas to the lungs, but also protects the airway from aspiration of gastric contents and prevents insufflation of the stomach. Because this technique requires skill and can be difficult during cardiac arrest, other airway adjuncts have been developed when intubation is contraindicated or impractical because of lack of user skill.

Before the arrival of an ambulance, ventilation given by bystanders must employ techniques that do not require special equipment. Manual methods of ventilation (i.e., the Sylvester method, the Shafer prone pressure method, and others) consisting of the rhythmic application and release of pressure to the chest or back and lifting of the arms had been in widespread use for 40 to 50 years prior to the rediscovery of mouth-to-mouth ventilation. These manual techniques had been taught in Red Cross classes, to lifeguards, in the military, and in the Boy Scouts as recently as the 1960s, before being replaced by mouth-to-mouth ventilation as the standard for rescue breathing. Safar and Elam first showed that obstruction of the upper airway by the tongue and soft palate occurs commonly in victims who lose consciousness or muscle tone and that ventilation with manual techniques is markedly reduced or prevented altogether by such obstruction.[14,15] Subsequently, Safar and colleagues developed techniques that prevent obstruction by extending the neck and jaw and applying this in conjunction with mouth-to-mouth ventilation.[16] Although mouth-to-mouth ventilation has been studied extensively in human respiratory arrest and has been shown to maintain acceptable oxygenation and CO_2 levels, its evaluation in laboratory models of cardiac arrest and in actual human cardiac arrest has been limited.

Pulmonary physiology during low blood flow conditions

Effects of hypoxemia and hypercarbia on pulmonary airways

During respiratory and cardiac arrest, hypoxemia and hypercarbia gradually increase over time. The concentrations of both oxygen and carbon dioxide affect ventilation and gas exchange. Hypoxemia has variable effects on airway resistance, which is the frictional resistance of the airway to gas flow and is expressed by:

$$\text{Airway resistance (cm } H_2O/l/s) = \text{pressure difference (cm } H_2O)/\text{flow rate (l/s)}$$

A number of studies in animals and humans, albeit with effective circulation, have shown that hypocapnia causes bronchoconstriction resulting in increased airway resistance, while the effect of hypercapnia on the airways is inconclusive.[17–22] In one study, when end-tidal CO_2 was increased from between 20 and 27 mmHg to between 44 and 51 mmHg, airflow resistance decreased to 29% of the initial mean.[17] Other studies have shown, however, that hypercapnia causes an increase in airflow resistance through a central nervous system effect mediated by the vagus nerve.[18–22] It appears that hypocapnia causes bronchoconstriction and increased resistance to flow through a direct local effect on airways, whereas hypercapnia causes increased airway resistance through action on the central nervous system.[18–22]

Hypoxic pulmonary vasoconstriction

Hypoxic pulmonary vasoconstriction is a physiologic mechanism that minimizes venous admixture by diverting blood from underventilated, hypoxic areas of the lung to areas that are better ventilated.[23] Pulmonary vessels perfusing underventilated alveoli are normally vasoconstricted. This effect is opposed by increases in the partial pressure of O_2. Hypoxic pulmonary vasoconstriction matches local perfusion to ventilation, increasing with low airway PO_2 and low mixed venous PO_2. The greater the hypoxia, the greater the pulmonary vasoconstriction until a point is reached where vasoconstriction becomes so intense and widespread that the response becomes pathologic and pulmonary hypertension develops.[24,25]

Hypoxic pulmonary vasoconstriction is inhibited by respiratory and metabolic alkalosis and potentiated by metabolic acidosis.[26] In addition, pulmonary vasoconstriction is more pronounced when pulmonary artery pressure is low and is attenuated by increased pulmonary vascular pressure.[26] Hence, a consequence of low inspired O_2 concentration, as occurs during mouth-to-mouth ventilation, could be decreased blood flow caused by increased pulmonary vascular resistance. Whether hypoxic pulmonary vasoconstriction occurs during cardiac arrest and CPR is unknown, and warrants evaluation because hypoxemia occurs commonly.

The ventilation/perfusion ratio ($\dot{V}/\dot{Q}$ ratio): the relationship of blood flow and ventilation during low flow conditions

During normal cardiac output, ventilation is closely matched with perfusion through a series of physiologic mechanisms exemplified by the maintenance of alveolar and arterial PCO_2 within a range close to 40 mmHg at rest. But during low blood flow states, the ventilation–perfusion relationship becomes altered.

When systemic blood flow decreases, the flow of blood through the lungs decreases as well. With less venous CO_2 delivered to the lungs, less is available for elimination via exhalation and the concentration of CO_2 in exhaled gas decreases. Because CO_2 elimination is diminished, CO_2 accumulates in venous blood and in the tissues. Mixed venous PCO_2 thus reflects primarily systemic and pulmonary perfusion and is an indicator of the tissue acid–base environment. On the other hand, during low flow conditions arterial PCO_2 and PO_2 reflect primarily the adequacy of alveolar ventilation. During low rates of blood flow, if alveolar ventilation is adequate, blood flowing through the pulmonary capillary bed is overventilated because of a large ventilation–perfusion mismatch. The relationship between alveolar ventilation and pulmonary blood flow is expressed in the ventilation–perfusion ratio equation:[27]

$$\dot{V}a/\dot{Q} = 8.63 \cdot R \cdot (CaO_2 - C\bar{v}O_2)/PaCO_2$$

where $\dot{V}a$ is alveolar ventilation; $\dot{Q}$ is the volume of blood flowing through the lungs each minute; 8.63 is a factor relating measurements made at body temperature, ambient pressure, and saturated with water vapor (BTPS) to measurements made at standard temperature, pressure, and dry (STPD); R is the respiratory exchange ratio (CO_2 minute production/O_2 consumption); CaO_2 is arterial oxygen content; $C\bar{v}O_2$ is mixed venous oxygen content and $PaCO_2$ is the partial pressure of alveolar CO_2.

This equation appears simple, but it can be solved only by numerical analysis with a computer because alveolar PO_2 is an implicit variable (i.e., alveolar PO_2 decreases when alveolar PCO_2 increases)(Fig. 28.1). The ventilation perfusion ratio equation predicts that as pulmonary blood flow

decreases (increasing $\dot{V}a/\dot{Q}$ ratio), arterial PO_2 and mixed venous PCO_2 will increase and arterial PCO_2 will decrease (Fig. 28.2). It predicts that, as pulmonary perfusion is further reduced ($\dot{V}a/\dot{Q}$ ratio approaches infinity), arterial PO_2 and PCO_2 approach the composition of inspired gas. In contrast, if blood flow is present, but alveolar ventilation is absent ($\dot{V}a/\dot{Q}$ ratio is zero), arterial PO_2 and PCO_2 approach the composition of mixed venous blood. A study of ventilation during precisely controlled low blood flow conditions found that arterial and mixed venous blood gases behaved as the equation predicts: as blood flow decreased, arterial PCO_2 decreased and PO_2 increased.[28]

Although mixed venous blood gases provide more accurate assessment of perfusion during resuscitation, it can be obtained during CPR only rarely; usually a pulmonary artery catheter is already present. Animal laboratory work seems to suggest that the intraosseous blood gas analysis can be a viable alternative to venous pH and PCO_2 measurements during cardiopulmonary resuscitation. In a swine pediatric model of hypoxic cardiac arrest, the intraosseous blood gas correlated closely to the mixed venous gas within 15 minutes of cardiopulmonary resuscitation. Beyond this time, the intraosseous blood gas reflected more local acid–base conditions or the effect of intraosseous administration of medications than mixed venous blood gas.[29]

Gas exchange and the transport of oxygen and carbon dioxide in blood

Hemoglobin is the principal protein of red blood cells and functions importantly in the transport of O_2 and in the elimination of CO_2 through the carbamate and bicarbonate pathways.[30] Although hemoglobin is usually considered solely in its role as a carrier of oxygen from the lungs to the tissues, it has an equally important role as a carrier of CO_2 from the tissues to the lungs. Deoxyhemoglobin binds about 40% more CO_2 than oxyhemoglobin and, conversely, when hemoglobin becomes oxygenated during passage through the lungs, CO_2 is actively driven off (Fig. 28.3). This mechanism is referred to as the Bohr–Haldane effect and is responsible for about 50% of the total CO_2 excreted by the lungs during each circulation cycle.[31,32] The principle mechanism of the Bohr-Haldane effect is the binding of CO_2 as carbamate compounds to the alpha-amino groups of hemoglobin.[33,34] When oxygen is released by hemoglobin in the tissues, a change takes place in the shape of the hemoglobin molecule, making binding sites available for the uptake of CO_2.[35] When hemoglobin takes up O_2 in the lungs, the change in hemoglobin conformation repels

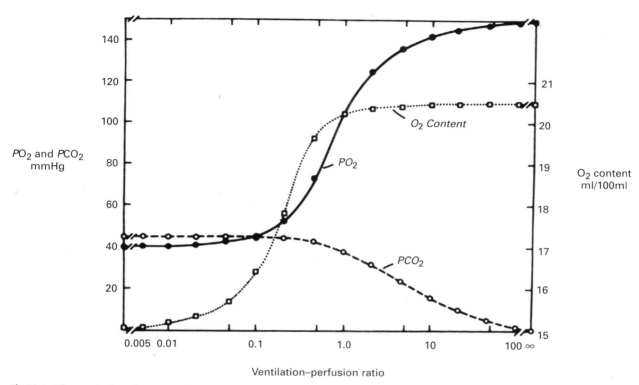

Fig.28.1. Changes in the PO_2, PCO_2, and end-capillary oxygen content in a lung unit as its ventilation-perfusion ratio is increased. The lung is assumed to be breathing air, and the PO_2, and PCO_2 of mixed venous blood are 40 and 45 mmHg, respectively. The hemoglobin concentration is 14.8 g/100 ml. (From West JB Ventilation-perfusion relationships. Am Rev Respir Dis 1977; 116: 919–943.)

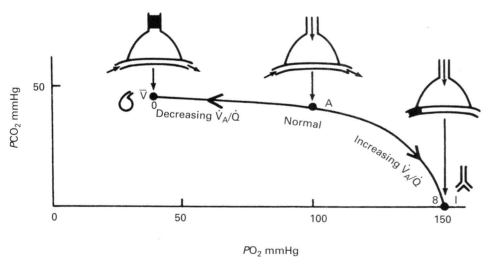

Fig.28.2. Oxygen-carbon dioxide diagram showing a ventilation-perfusion ratio $\dot{V}a/\dot{Q}$ line. The PO_2 and PCO_2 of a lung unit move along this line from the mixed venous point, $\bar{v}$, to the inspired gas point; I, as its ventilation-perfusion ratio is increased; A, alveolar gas for a lung unit with a normal ventilation-perfusion ratio. (From ref. 27.)

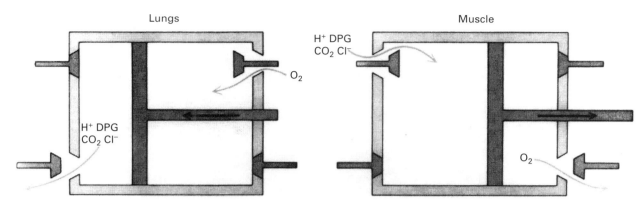

Fig.28.3 Reciprocating engine serves as a model of the cooperative effects of hemoglobin. The piston is driven to the right by the energy liberated in the reaction of hemoglobin with oxygen (O_2) and to the left by the protons (H^+) and carbon dioxide (CO_2) liberated by respiring tissues. Diphosphoglycerate (*DPG*) and chloride ions (*Cl*) are passengers riding in company with protons and carbon dioxide. (From ref. 30.)

CO_2 and promotes its excretion. Plasma proteins also function in the transport of CO_2, but have only one-eighth the buffering capacity of hemoglobin.[36]

A small amount of CO_2 dissolves in plasma (5% to 10% of total CO_2) and a much larger amount (60%) is converted to carbonic acid intracellularly in red blood cells (RBC) through catalytic hydration. Cellular membranes are extremely permeable to CO_2. As RBCs traverse the tissue capillary bed, CO_2 diffuses into them where it is converted by carbonic anhydrase to carbonic acid, which then dissociates to bicarbonate and proton. The conversion of CO_2 to bicarbonate would soon stop if protons were not buffered by hemoglobin, and bicarbonate would otherwise be trapped within the RBC because of its polarity, preventing diffusion through the RBC membrane. A membrane transport system rapidly exchanges plasma chloride for intracellular bicarbonate, however, and preserves the CO_2-carbonic acid-bicarbonate gradient.[36] Another important aspect of the interaction of proton with hemoglobin is its effect on lowering the affinity of hemoglobin for oxygen and, by the law of action and reaction, oxygenation of hemoglobin lowers its affinity for proton. When hemoglobin is exposed to higher concentrations of CO_2 from respiring tissues, the formation of protons helps to unload O_2, which becomes available to tissues. When hemoglobin is oxygenated in the pulmonary capillaries, protons are released from hemoglobin, and bicarbonate is converted back to water and CO_2, which then diffuses out of the blood into the alveoli. Thus, oxygenation of hemoglobin actively promotes excretion of CO_2 from the lungs, and CO_2 from tissues promotes the release of O_2 from hemoglobin at the tissue level.

In summary, hemoglobin is the principal protein responsible for lung-to-tissue transport of O_2 and tissue-to-lung transport of carbon dioxide. Hemoglobin transports CO_2 as

carbamino compounds and in the form of bicarbonate. These mechanisms of CO_2 exchange and O_2 transport establish that alveolar oxygenation and ventilation as well as pulmonary blood flow play crucial roles in the removal of CO_2 from the tissues. Because pH and CO_2 levels affect the affinity of hemoglobin for O_2, these factors are important during the treatment of cardiac arrest.

Ventilation during low blood flow conditions

Effect of ventilation on acid–base conditions and oxygenation

Acid–base conditions and oxygenation are important factors in resuscitation from low blood flow states such as shock[37–42] and cardiac arrest.[43–48] Hypoxemia and hypercarbic acidosis critically reduce the force of myocardial contractions,[49–53] make defibrillation difficult,[54,55] and are associated with poor outcome.[54,55] It has been observed that, during cardiac arrest, arterial blood gases do not reflect tissue conditions and that mixed venous blood has a level of CO_2 that is frequently twice the level of the arterial side.[51,52,58]

Arterial and mixed venous metabolic acidosis and mixed venous hypercarbic acidosis are associated with failure of resuscitation from cardiac arrest.[43,46,48] Studies of both human and animal cardiac arrest have shown that during CPR, the pH of blood is largely determined by the concentration of CO_2[56–71] and that arterial blood is often alkalemic whereas mixed venous blood is acidemic because of differences in CO_2 levels. A recent Norwegian study measured arterial PCO_2 and pH in patients receiving tidal volumes of 500 ml vs. 1000 ml several minutes after intubation during out-of-hospital cardiac arrest (mean time, approximately 15 minutes).[72] The study showed that mean PCO_2 was 28 and 56 mmHg with 1000 ml and 500 ml tidal volume, respectively. These results indicate that tidal volume affects arterial PCO_2 and pH significantly: larger tidal volume is associated with respiratory alkalosis and smaller tidal volume is associated with respiratory acidosis.

The arteriovenous PCO_2 gradient increases substantially during CPR and returns to near normal when spontaneous circulation is restored.[13,38,57,62,64,73–75] The CO_2 gradient likely results from reduced blood flow through the lungs, decreased pulmonary elimination of CO_2, accumulation of CO_2 on the venous side of the circulatory system, and overventilation of blood entering the arterial side (Fig. 28.4).[13,56,62,73] A recent study showed that changes in ventilation could affect excretion of CO_2 even when blood flow rate is as low as 12% of normal.[28] In addition, with decreasing blood flow, the decrease in end-tidal CO_2 parallels the decrease in arterial PCO_2. Thus, both arterial PCO_2 and end-tidal CO_2 vary directly with blood flow, while mixed venous PCO_2 varies inversely with blood flow.

Mixed venous PCO_2 and pH can be improved with proper ventilation and become worse with hypoventilation. Nevertheless, there are major interactions among the mechanics of positive pressure ventilation, intrathoracic pressure, and blood flow. Positive pressure ventilation can have such a profound effect on hemodynamics that overventilation can result in decreased blood flow and worse tissue hypoxia and hypercarbia. This issue is discussed in greater detail in the section on ventilation and hemodynamics.

Effect of ventilation on ventricular fibrillation and defibrillation

Sudden death is thought to be a primary cardiac electrical event and may not be a result of myocardial injury, although there is often underlying myocardial ischemia, which can reduce electrical stability and lead to ventricular ectopy. The event is often fatal and is probably initiated by ventricular tachycardia, or ventricular fibrillation. Investigations have shown that hypoventilation, hypoxemia, hypercarbia, and metabolic acidosis can lower the threshold for ventricular fibrillation as well as affect the tendency of the heart to develop ventricular arrhythmias. Further, arterial hypoxemia has been shown to cause arrhythmia by excitation of the autonomic nervous system and by affecting vagal tone.[76] Both hyperventilation and hypoventilation are associated with severe ventricular and supraventricular arrhythmias.[77] Hypoxemia and other factors such as hypoglycemia, hyper- and hypokalemia

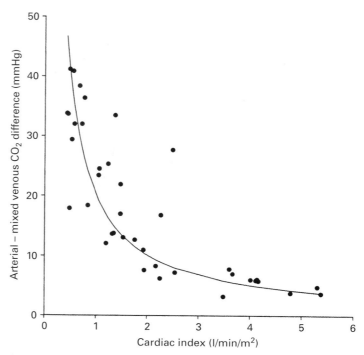

Fig.28.4. The relationship of the arteriovenous carbon dioxide gradient and cardiac index follows the form of a modified Fick equation: (mixed venous CO – arterial CO_2) $\times$ cardiac index – k, where $k < 0$. During control minute ventilation, $k = 20.2 = 2.1$ (95% confidence limits = 16.0 to 24.5), concordance n = 0.82, ($P < 0001$). (From ref. 28.)

cause ventricular fibrillation by shortening the duration of the cardiac action potential.[78] Hypercarbia without hypoxemia has been shown to lower the ventricular fibrillation threshold and respiratory alkalosis raises the ventricular fibrillation threshold and enhances spontaneous recovery from ventricular fibrillation.[79] In another study, ischemia, but not hypoxemia, lowered the ventricular fibrillation threshold.[80]

The effect of ventilation on the defibrillation threshold, which is the minimum electrical energy required for defibrillation of a fibrillating ventricle, has not been studied directly. Instead, the defibrillation threshold has been investigated under conditions of hypoxemia, and metabolic and hypercarbic acidosis, either alone or in combination.[46,48,54,81] The findings of different studies have been somewhat contradictory, but generally show that the defibrillation threshold is unaffected by acid-base conditions existing either before or during CPR. However, more recent studies using animal models of cardiac arrest suggest that hypercarbia is associated with ventricular fibrillation refractory to defibrillation.[46,52,55] Coronary perfusion pressure, duration of untreated ventricular fibrillation, and duration of CPR are critical factors known to affect success of defibrillation.[82]

A human study of factors that influenced the success of defibrillation found that arterial hypoxemia and acidemia, and delay in defibrillation attempts were associated with failure to defibrillate,[54] but it was not possible to distinguish the effect of these factors independently because they tended to occur together. A canine study, in which ischemia, ventricular hypertrophy, hypoxemia, acidosis, and alkalosis were well-controlled independent variables, did not find an adverse effect of these factors on defibrillation threshold.[81] Surprisingly, hypoxemia was found to lower the threshold for defibrillation. Another study found that metabolic acidosis, but not metabolic alkalosis or respiratory acidosis or alkalosis, lowered the threshold for ventricular fibrillation.[83] More recent laboratory CPR studies of hypercarbic acidosis found a substantial reduction in rate of resuscitation. Although the defibrillation threshold was not investigated, four of six animals ventilated with 50% CO_2 had refractory ventricular fibrillation.[46] In other studies of acid-base conditions, most animals with sufficient coronary perfusion pressure during CPR were defibrillated, but only animals without substantial hypercarbia recovered adequate cardiac output.[52,55,84–88] A recent study of human CPR also found that return of spontaneous circulation was associated with improved levels of arterial and mixed venous PO_2 and PCO_2.[44]

There are important differences in physiology during normal cardiac output and CPR that may not be widely appreciated. For example, high levels of arterial and mixed venous hypercarbia are usually tolerated by humans[89] and animals[46,90–93] when there is normal spontaneous cardiac output. Nevertheless, during cardiac arrest, hypercarbia substantially reduces success of resuscitation by adversely affecting myocardial contractility.[46,52,55,84–88] At least one laboratory study found that hypercarbia was associated with refractory ventricular fibrillation.[55] In this rat model, very high levels of inspired and thus, myocardial, PCO_2 were produced and may help explain the difference in findings of another study[81] that used more modest levels of hypercarbia and failed to find an effect on defibrillation threshold.

Among factors that can affect the likelihood of defibrillation, the duration of ventricular fibrillation is known to be of great importance.[94] In human CPR, the rate of successful defibrillation is approximately 80% or more if it is administered immediately after onset of witnessed ventricular fibrillation, but the chance of survival decreases 7 to 10% for each additional minute of ventricular fibrillation.[95,96] When

bystander CPR is provided, the decrease in survival is more gradual, about 3% to 4% per minute from collapse to defibrillation. A similar effect of duration of ventricular fibrillation is seen in laboratory CPR models[97–99] and may be explained, in part, by the gradual depletion of myocardial adenosine triphosphate, which is thought to be a marker for ischemic tissue damage and the metabolic state of the myocardium.[100] In addition, potassium uptake by myocardial cells is increased during ventricular fibrillation and is related to hydrogen ion, CO_2, and lactate production.[101] Earlier work found that the ratio of intracellular to extracellular potassium concentration affected the defibrillation threshold.[102]

In summary, hypoxemia and hypercarbia decrease the threshold for ventricular fibrillation. Hypoxemia and hypercarbia have a negligible effect on the defibrillation threshold when the duration of ventricular fibrillation is brief. Recent studies suggest that hypoxemia and hypercarbia make defibrillation more difficult when ventricular fibrillation persists for several minutes or more.

Effect of ventilation on myocardial force and rate of contraction

Studies with an isolated heart model demonstrated that hypoxia and hypercarbia caused a profound decrease in myocardial force of contraction independent of pH (Fig. 28.5).[53,103–106] In studies that examined the effect of hypercarbia on isolated spontaneously contracting myocytes, the rate and force of contraction are inhibited by modestly increased concentrations of CO_2, with pH held at 7.40 and PO_2 at 142 mmHg.[107] The model demonstrated a rapid and profound effect of CO_2 independent of pH, PO_2, vascular tone, neuroendocrine factors, or inflammatory mediators. In contrast, isolated decreased blood or perfusate pH is not associated with reduced ventricular force of contraction.[49–53] The reason for these differences in myocardial response to extracellular CO_2 and hydrogen ion is that CO_2 is a non-polar, lipid-soluble molecule that is permeable to cellular membranes and diffuses rapidly into the intracellular space. Once CO_2 enters the cell, it lowers intracellular pH by dissociating to hydrogen ion and bicarbonate. In contrast, hydrogen ion is polar, diffusing at a very slow rate through cell membranes, and this may account for its lack of effect on myocardial dynamics under most experimental conditions.[108] There is accumulating evidence that reduced intracellular pH affects calcium ion flux, exchange, and binding, and ultimately affects excitation-contraction coupling and myocardial contractility.[108]

During ventricular fibrillation, the heart continues to perform work and very likely has energy utilization

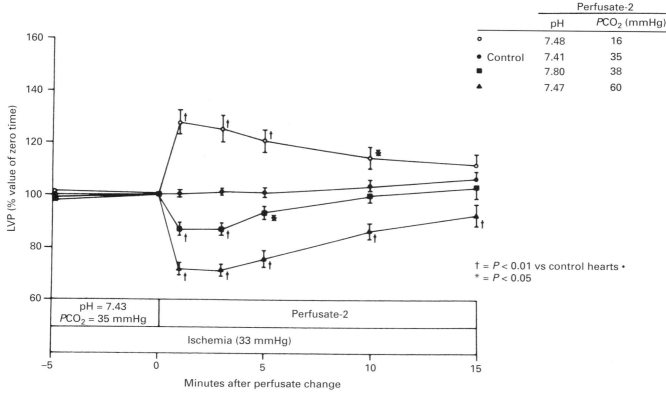

| | | Perfusate-2 | |
		pH	PCO_2 (mmHg)
○		7.48	16
●	Control	7.41	35
■		7.80	38
▲		7.47	60

† = $P < 0.01$ vs control hearts •
* = $P < 0.05$

Fig. 28.5. Peak isovolumic left ventricular pressure (*LVP*) expressed as percentage of value at zero time. Zero time is at 10 minutes of perfusion under ischemic conditions (33 mmHg) and at time of alteration of perfusate. In control hearts, perfusate was not altered (From ref. 53.)

greater than during normal contractions; metabolites in the form of hydrogen ion, lactate, and CO_2 continue to be produced. With the onset of ventricular fibrillation, myocardial CO_2 tension increases rapidly from a normal value of approximately 50 mmHg to 350 mmHg and there is a parallel increase in hydrogen ion concentration (Fig. 28.6).[74,103] As noted above, the removal of CO_2 from tissues depends upon blood flow; thus, coronary blood flow is an important co-factor influencing levels of myocardial CO_2. A coronary perfusion pressure of less than 10 mmHg was associated with myocardial CO_2 tensions >400 mmHg and failure of resuscitation, while a coronary perfusion pressure of greater than 10 mmHg was associated with myocardial CO_2 tensions <400 mmHg and successful resuscitation.[109] Decreased intracellular pH is associated with changes to the structure and function of regulatory and enzyme proteins and, if not corrected soon enough, leads to irreversible loss of cell function and cell death.[110]

In summary, both isolated hypoxemia and isolated hypercarbia have a negative inotropic effect on the heart.

Ischemia would be predicted to be a more injurious event than hypoxemia or hypercarbia alone, because ischemia causes both decreased delivery of O_2 and decreased elimination of tissue CO_2. To the extent that ventilation can affect the elimination of CO_2 and enhance tissue oxygenation, it can likely provide some benefit during cardiac arrest and CPR. There are promising therapies that perfuse the heart with oxygen-containing fluorocarbon compounds (SAPO: selective aortic arch perfusion and oxygenation) resulting in higher rates of restoration of spontaneous circulation after prolonged cardiac arrest and CPR.[111]

Interaction of hypoxemia and hypercarbia with the vasopressor effect of catecholamines

The administration of such catecholamines as epinephrine during CPR has been considered essential for successful resuscitation. Numerous studies and years of experience treating cardiac arrest have shown that adrenaline is often a pivotal factor in reversing sudden death by

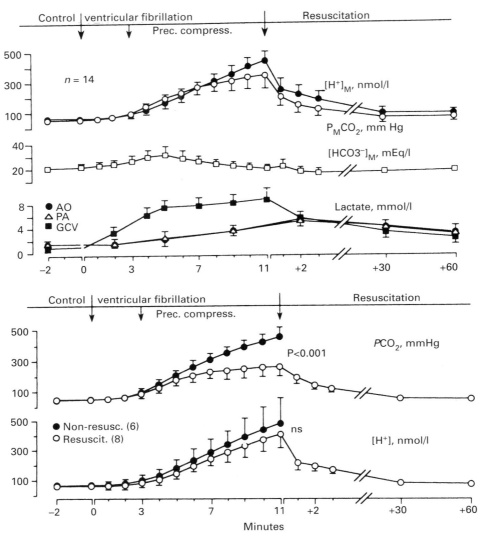

Fig.28.6. *Top:* Increases in myocardial hydrogen ion [H⁺] and myocardial PCO_2 (P_MCO_2) together with increases in lactate content in blood sampled from the great cardiac vein. More moderate increases in lactate content of systemic blood were documented. Values are mean = SD. *Bottom:* Myocardial PCO_2 and [H⁺] in resuscitated and non-resuscitated animals. *Prec. Compress,* precordial compression; [HCO_3^-], myocardial bicarbonate; *AO*, aorta; *PA*, pulmonary artery: *GCV*, great cardiac vein. (From ref. 109.)

increasing coronary perfusion pressure and the likelihood of defibrillation.[112] The efficacy of pressors on later outcome measures such as survival to discharge or neurological outcome, however, is less certain. The purpose of this section is to review and analyze the interaction of ventilation with the vasopressor activity of epinephrine and other catecholamines.

A number of studies have shown that increases in blood PCO_2 in animal models and in humans results in a

decrease in the pressor response to epinephrine and norepinephrine by more than 50%.[113–115] The mechanism for the failure of blood pressure to increase is primarily decreased peripheral vasoconstriction and vascular resistance[113–119] with a smaller contribution from a cardiac arrhythmia other than tachycardia[113–115] Metabolic acidosis (i.e., increased hydrogen ion concentration) has also been found to inhibit vasoconstriction, but to a much smaller degree than "respiratory" acidosis (i.e., increased

PCO_2).[119] With return of CO_2 to normal levels, the inhibitory effect of hypercarbia on epinephrine activity is reversed completely within 10 minutes in human volunteers with normal cardiac function.[118]

Hypoxemia also has been found to decrease the pressor response to epinephrine.[51] Hypoventilation, through simultaneous hypoxemia and retention of CO_2, causes greater peripheral vasodilation and loss of the pressor effect of epinephrine than does isolated hypercarbia or hypoxemia alone.[51] Few studies specifically examine the effect of ventilation on the pressor response to catecholamines during cardiac arrest and CPR. Successful resuscitation is associated with epinephrine-induced increases in coronary perfusion pressure, and there are data suggesting that hypoxemia and hypercarbia may modulate the increase.[120,121]

Respiratory and circulatory system interactions

Spontaneous breathing produces negative intrathoracic pressure during inspiration. Therefore, beyond respiratory functions of gas exchange, spontaneous ventilation plays an important role in maintaining cardiac output by enhancing venous return to the chest and heart.[122–124] Venous return to the heart is greatest during inspiration because negative intrathoracic pressure creates a pressure gradient between thoracic blood vessels and those outside the chest. In contrast, assisted positive pressure ventilation with mechanical ventilators and self-inflating bags produces positive intrathoracic pressure during inspiration, reducing venous return to the chest and, as a result, reducing cardiac preload and subsequent cardiac output. For a given airway pressure, pleural pressure depends on the compliance of the lung and chest wall. According to the mode of ventilation, airway pressure can be dependent on a number of variables, including inspiratory flow rate and time, tidal volume, ventilation rate, and degree of intrinsic positive end-expiratory pressure (auto-PEEP). Holding all other factors constant, the higher the ventilatory rate, the greater the proportion of time with positive intrathoracic pressure and thus the greater is the potential for hemodynamic compromise (Fig. 28.7). For example, assuming an inspiratory:expiratory ratio of 1:1, and an inspiratory time of 1 second, positive intrathoracic pressure is present 40% of the time with a ventilation rate of 12/min; 66% at 20/min; and 100% of the time with a rate of 30/min. Auto-PEEP can even occur with ventilation rates of 30 in normal lungs, or even at lower rates when the lungs are compromised from such conditions as obstructive lung disease, or other conditions with impaired expiratory flow.[125,126]

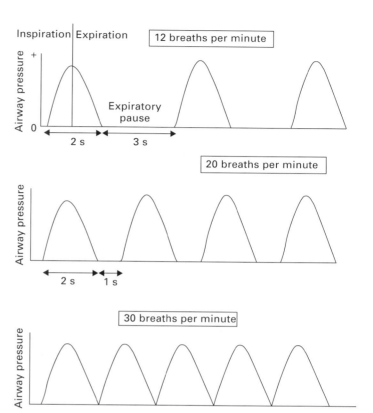

Fig. 28.7. Illustration of the effect of positive-pressure ventilation on intrathoracic pressure during ventilation rates of 12, 20, and 30 breaths per minute in a hypothetical patient with normal lungs. Positive intrathoracic pressure is present 40% of the time with a ventilation rate of 12/min, 66% of the time at a rate of 20/min, and 100% of the time at 30/min. (Original illustration by AH Idris.)

Excessive assisted ventilation can impair cardiac preload and output

The potential detrimental effects of positive pressure ventilation on hemodynamics have been well-known since the seminal description by Cournand *et al.* more than a half century ago, which demonstrated proportionate reductions in cardiac output as airway pressure increased.[127] A number of studies have shown that both intermittent PPV and positive end-expiratory pressure (PEEP) can impair cardiac output even in normally functioning hearts because of reduced venous return,[125–130] A critical factor in the development of auto-PEEP is the minute ventilation (due to excessive tidal volume, and/or increased respiratory rate) and decreased expiratory time, and it has been described as a common etiology of pulseless electrical activity during resuscitation.[125,126] Again, the major mechanism of cardiac output impairment is diminished cardiac preload, and the effects are even more pronounced in progressively hypovolemic states.[127,129,130]

Excessive assisted ventilation can lead to brain ischemia and hypoxia

In the U.S., blunt trauma accounts for approximately 80% of severe injuries, and frequently is associated with traumatic brain injury (TBI).[131] Every year, TBI results in 52 000 deaths and 90 000 people with permanent neurological disability.[132] Secondary insults such as hypoxemia and hypotension occur frequently in severe TBI, and are associated with worse outcomes. Although "therapeutic hyperventilation" has been recommended in the past to reduce intracranial pressure, it has been shown to reduce cerebral blood flow enough to cause brain tissue ischemia, especially when the patient is in shock.[133–140] Therefore, the American Association of Neurological Surgeons now recommends that hyperventilation ($PaCO_2$ < 35 mmHg) should be avoided during the first 24 hours after TBI except when signs of brain herniation are present or when specialized monitoring is available, thus excluding the prehospital setting.[141] Nevertheless, hyperventilation not only occurs very commonly in the prehospital setting, but often remains the perceived mandate for patients with TBI.[142,143] Hyperventilation during conditions of low blood flow, such as traumatic hypotension and cardiac arrest, also may further decrease blood flow to an already ischemic brain.[134,135,138,139,144–146] A number of recent studies have shown that excessive ventilation, as indicated by $ETCO_2$ levels < 30 mmHg, is associated with increased mortality rates.[147,148] Large volume crystalloid fluid resuscitation, which is used for hemorrhagic hypotension, also is associated with increased mortality in the presence of TBI.[149] Therefore, avoidance of hyperventilation may be a useful strategy to avert secondary brain injury, improve perfusion, and to decrease the volume of crystalloid necessary for resuscitation of severely injured people.

Excessive assisted ventilation during shock and cardiac arrest

Rescuers often are unable to judge appropriate timing and have a tendency to use excessive ventilation rates in stressful situations.[142,150,151] For example, although the American Heart Association had recommended about 12 breaths/minute during non-traumatic CPR, respiratory therapists have been observed to use a mean ventilation rate of 37/minute (range, 24 to 68/minute).[150] Other studies have documented ventilation rates greater than 20 breaths/minute during in-hospital CPR.[152,153] Similarly, in a recent study of cardiac arrest, the investigators observed that EMTs were using an average rate of 34 breaths/ minute despite focused training directives not to do so.[151]

Positive pressure ventilation rate during low blood flow conditions

During hemorrhagic hypotension, blood pressure is substantially affected by the rate of positive pressure ventilation. In one study, systolic blood pressure decreased significantly when ventilation rate was changed from 12 to 20 breaths/minute and decreased further with 30 breaths/ minute;[130] however, blood pressure increased when ventilation rate was decreased from 12 to 6 breaths/minute. The study emphasizes the principle that the duration of increased intrathoracic pressure is proportional to the ventilation rate when positive pressure ventilation is used. Another principle is that blood pressure is inversely proportional to ventilation rate.

A study of cardiac arrest and CPR showed that 24-hour survival was only 1 of 8 animals by using 20 breaths/ minute, and was substantially improved to 7 of 8 animals when a ventilation rate of 12 breaths/minute was used.[151] Other studies showed the best improvement in 24-hour survival from cardiac arrest occurred with ventilation rates of 4 to 6 breaths/minute and the greatest oxygen delivery to tissues occurs with a ventilation rate of 6 breaths/ minute during CPR.[154–160] A recent laboratory study of cardiac arrest compared CPR that used a compression:ventilation ratio of 15:2 with that of a ratio of 30:2. The study showed improved coronary and cerebral perfusion pressures and 24-hour survival with the 30:2 ratio without significant differences in arterial PO_2 or PCO_2.[161]

Recognition of the substantial problem of excessive ventilation rate during low blood flow conditions such as cardiac arrest, the good sense of trying to match ventilation with perfusion, and the importance of chest compressions has resulted in significant changes in guidelines for CPR. The American Heart Association Guidelines 2005 now recommend that rescuers use a compression:ventilation ratio of 30:2 during CPR when the victim does not have an advanced airway (endotracheal tube, laryngeal mask airway, Combitube, or other device) in place.[162] Once an advanced airway is placed, chest compressions should be given continuously without interruption for ventilation and no more than 8–10 ventilations/minute are now recommended.

When the victim has been resuscitated with return of a pulse, the recommended ventilation rate is 10–12 breaths/minute.

Tidal volume, pulmonary vascular resistance, and intrathoracic pressure

The effect of lung inflation on pulmonary vessels is complex. At abnormally low lung volumes, vessels are collapsed and pulmonary vascular resistance is increased.[27] When the lung is inflated, collapsed vessels open and resistance decreases. But at high inflation volumes, alveolar capillaries are compressed and resistance increases. Underventilation and ventilation perfusion mismatch at low lung volumes result in a progressive decrease in lung compliance and an increase in alveolar–arterial oxygen tension difference. Because blood flow is inversely related to pulmonary vascular resistance, if the lungs are poorly inflated during CPR, pulmonary blood flow may possibly decrease further. The alpha-adrenergic effect of adrenaline during cardiac arrest specifically depresses PaO_2 absorption and CO_2 elimination of low $\dot{V}/\dot{Q}$ lung units. Vasopressin has significantly less adverse effect on pulmonary gas exchange after CPR. It has been speculated that vasopressin could exert rehabilitation to pulmonary circulation through the agonist effect of the V2 vasopressinergic receptor,[163] but few data are available in this area.

Continuous positive airway pressure ventilation (i.e., CPAP or PEEP) given during both the compression and release phase of chest compression would be expected to interfere with venous return and to decrease blood flow just as it does during spontaneous circulation.[164] PEEP can also be the inadvertent result of excessive tidal volume, increased respiratory rate, and reduced inspiratory time (auto PEEP) and has been related to increased incidence of pulseless electrical activity during resuscitation.[125]

An impedance threshold device that causes negative intrathoracic pressure during CPR and hemorrhagic shock has been shown to increase venous return, right myocardial pre-load, blood pressure, and blood flow to the heart and brain.[165–168] It also has been shown to improve survival from cardiac arrest and hemorrhagic shock. The device is based on the physiologic principle that negative intrathoracic pressure enhances venous blood return to the chest and heart, thus making increased cardiac output possible.

Application of continuous positive airway pressure (CPAP) without active ventilation has been recently studied in CPR. In a pig model of cardiac arrest, CPAP titrated to achieve 75% of a baseline end-tidal CO_2 was compared with intermittent positive pressure ventilation.[169] A significant difference in both airway pressure and diastolic blood pressure was detected between the two techniques (27 ± 58 mmHg in CPR vs. 13 ± 11 mmHg in CPR_{CPAP}), and arterial and mixed venous pH, O_2 saturation, and CO_2 were improved in the CPR_{CPAP} animals. Cardiac output did not change significantly between the two methods. This technique has the potential advantage of simplifying CPR, decreasing pulmonary atelectasis, and improving both oxygenation and ventilation. Nevertheless, it can also have a negative effect on diastolic blood pressure and, thus, on both coronary and cerebral blood flow.

Despite the potential for decreased venous return, it is possible that very small amounts of positive airway pressure may decrease intrapulmonary shunting, pulmonary vascular collapse, and atelectasis without adverse hemodynamic effects. Indeed, recent use of a multi-slice CT scanner to allow dynamic imaging of tridimensional volume of the lung during CPR suggested that CPAP was superior to simple volume controlled ventilation or no-ventilation CPR in maintaining better lung distension and preventing atelectasis.[170]

In conclusion, movement of venous blood into the lungs takes place during the release phase of external chest compression when intrathoracic pressure is low. When the chest is compressed, intrathoracic pressure rises and blood moves out of the lungs and heart and into the systemic circulation. Negative airway pressure enhances blood flow and venous return to the chest, while continuous positive airway pressure ventilation inhibits venous return and blood flow but decreases lung atelectasis. These studies emphasize the crucial relationship between ventilation mechanics and circulation.

Effect of ventilation on outcome from resuscitation

For over 30 years, emergency ventilation has been considered an essential component of CPR. There are few studies and little direct evidence that ventilation affects outcome from cardiac arrest, although it has been assumed crucial for resuscitation. Recommendations for ventilation were based on studies performed in the 1950s and 1960s in living humans with normal cardiac output.[14–16] These studies presumed that the goal of ventilation during CPR was to achieve near "normal" tidal volumes and minute ventilation. Substantially less ventilation may be sufficient for gas exchange during CPR, however, because cardiac output and pulmonary blood flow are only 10% to 15% of normal during manual chest compression.[171] As a consequence, the amount of hemoglobin passing through the pulmonary bed is reduced and the amount of oxygen necessary to saturate hemoglobin is also reduced if there is not a large ventilation/perfusion mismatch. Because venous return and thus the quantity of CO_2 delivered to the lungs are decreased, the amount of ventilation necessary to remove CO_2 is presumably reduced as well.

The time when ventilation must be initiated during CPR and the quantity needed to achieve satisfactory results are unclear. In a canine model of cardiac arrest, arterial pH, PCO_2, and PO_2 had no significant change after 5 minutes of untreated ventricular fibrillation,[172] while arterial PO_2 decreased from 81 to 69 mmHg under similar conditions in a swine model.[173] In the canine study, there was no significant change in arterial PO_2 and PCO_2 for 30 seconds after initiation of chest compressions without ventilation. At 45 seconds, arterial PO_2 was 52 mmHg, a significant decline. Another canine study showed that chest compression alone without assisted ventilation will produce a minute ventilation of 5.2 ± 1.1 l/min and will maintain O_2 saturation $> 90\%$ for more than 4 minutes.[4] A murine study found that chest compression alone produced tidal volumes of 26% of baseline and, although arterial PCO_2 increased to 80 mmHg after 9 minutes, resuscitation rate was not impaired.[5,174] The animals were intubated in all of these studies. It is likely that ventilation induced by chest compression would be less in non-intubated models, but this would affect blood gases is unknown.

Other studies have shown that ventilation has an important role in resuscitation. An early study showed that well oxygenated dogs had better carotid artery blood flow than did asphyxiated dogs. This was attributed to loss of peripheral vascular tone.[175] Weil and colleagues showed that spontaneous gasping during cardiac arrest in a swine model favored successful resuscitation, and also showed that both the frequency and duration of gasps correlated with coronary perfusion pressure and predicted outcome.[176]

More recent studies were specifically designed to test the effect of ventilation on outcome in swine models of CPR. One study compared a group receiving mechanical ventilation during CPR with a group receiving chest compression alone and a group without chest compression or ventilation. The duration of untreated ventricular fibrillation was 30 seconds, followed by 12 minutes of CPR in the treatment groups. All animals were successfully defibrillated and entered a 2-hour intensive care period. After 24 hours, however, only two of eight animals that had no CPR survived, while all 16 animals survived in the groups receiving chest compression with and without ventilation.[3] Another study allocated 24 swine to groups with and without ventilation during 10 minutes of chest compression following 6 minutes of untreated ventricular fibrillation. Nine of 12 ventilated animals and only 1 of 12 non-ventilated animals had return of spontaneous circulation. The non-ventilated animals died with significantly

greater arterial and mixed venous hypoxemia and hypercarbia.[177] A follow-up study was done to test whether hypoxemia or hypercarbia independently affects survival from cardiac arrest. By using a swine model of isolated arterial and mixed venous hypoxemia without hypercarbia in one group, and isolated hypercarbia without hypoxemia in another group, only 1 of 10 animals had return of spontaneous circulation in each group.[121]

Other experimental work in large animals showed that survival and neurological outcome up to 48 hours were not different when ventilation was withheld during resuscitation. These initial studies, although clearly de-emphasizing the importance of ventilation during the first few minutes of CPR, were limited by the persistence of an "artificial" patent airway in the animal, which resulted from the presence of an endotracheal tube allowing exchange of ventilations from gasping and chest compressions/decompressions.[178,179]

More recent studies eliminated the possible influence of an artificial patent airway in animal models during CPR. When standard CPR was compared with compression-only CPR in a pig model in which the airway was occluded, no difference was found in 24-hour outcome.[180] Of note, a supine, unconscious dog or pig usually has a patent airway, whereas a supine, unconscious human has an obstructed airway resulting from the kinked nature of the human airway. These model differences are rarely discerned in CPR ventilation experiments, but do have fundamental clinical importance. These latest observations confirmed that ventilation for a few minutes after dysrhythmic cardiac arrest was not fundamental and suggested the need to test the no-ventilation hypothesis in humans.[181]

There are important differences among all these studies, including duration of untreated ventricular fibrillation, the use of 100% O_2 before cardiac arrest, and whether or not agonal respirations were prevented with a paralytic agent. Nonetheless, taken together, these studies provide some evidence that ventilation may possibly be withheld when chest compression is initiated promptly after cardiac arrest, but that ventilation is important for survival when chest compression is delayed.

There are even fewer human studies of the role of ventilation during cardiac arrest. Because ventilation is such a well-accepted intervention, the ethical considerations of doing a controlled study by withholding ventilation in one group have been difficult to overcome. Indirect evidence pointing to a less important role of ventilation immediately after cardiac arrest has existed since the early 1990s. For example, in Seattle, where ambulance response time is short, patients who were seen to have spontaneous agonal respiratory efforts immediately after cardiac arrest had a higher rate of successful resuscitation.[182] Another study found that hypoxemia and hypercarbia was associated with the use of the esophageal obturator airway in the field and also a lower resuscitation rate.[65] Mixed venous hemoglobin oxygen saturation is associated with prognosis for survival from cardiac arrest; mixed venous pH, PO_2, and PCO_2 measured during hemorrhagic shock and cardiac arrest were significantly better in those with return of spontaneous circulation.[44,183] In the Netherlands, clinical CPR is given in the order "CAB" (chest compression– airway–breathing) with ventilation being delayed and chest compression being initiated as soon as possible. With use of "CAB," CPR survival data from the Netherlands are comparable to those reported in the USA.[184] Human data also suggest that prompt chest compression after cardiac arrest improves brain and heart perfusion and the success of defibrillation.[185]

More human studies have become available in the last few years. In a prospective, observational study of CPR and ventilation, chest compression-only CPR, and no CPR, survival from CPR (i.e., return of spontaneous circulation) was found to be 16%, 15%, and 6%, respectively.[186] Although both forms of basic life support (BLS) were significantly better than no CPR, there were no differences between CPR with or without ventilation. Similar results were reported more recently in North America in a study of telephone dispatcher-assisted BLS–CPR in which survival of chest compression-only CPR vs. mouth-to-mouth ventilation and chest compression CPR was 14% vs. 10%, respectively, with a slight trend of survival favoring chest compression-only CPR.[187] Although this study emphasized that CPR without ventilation is better than nothing, it presents several limitations in design. Mouth-to-mouth ventilation performed by a bystander was assumed to be done and was not observed directly by the investigator at the scene; the patency of the airway was unclear in some patients, and primary respiratory arrests were excluded. In addition, if the bystander knew how to perform CPR, then the patient also was excluded from the study. Nevertheless, the study suggested a need to reconsider BLS with a goal of minimizing the time to onset of CPR in the cardiac arrest victim and maximizing the efficacy of chest compression. When the concept of this "simplified CPR" was tested in a mannequin, effective compression was achieved an average of 30 seconds earlier than with the standard technique, and the number of compressions per minute were approximately doubled.[188] Dispatcher instructions for chest compression-only CPR is quite sensible, considering the difficulty of trying to teach mouth-to-mouth ventilation in addition to chest compression over the telephone to an anxious rescuer. Also, trying to teach how to perform ventilation over the telephone takes as much as 1–2 minutes of time away from doing CPR.

Despite the overall enthusiasm for the relatively positive results of dispatcher-assisted CPR instructions without ventilation as described by the providers[186,187] it has been emphasized by independent observers that the concept of no-ventilation CPR could be a misnomer, because, provided that the airway is open, patients with ventricular fibrillation cardiac arrest often exchange a significant amount of air through gasping.[189] Therefore, the term "CPR without assisted ventilation" has been suggested. Although the North American literature seems to de-emphasize the importance of ventilation in the first few minutes after cardiac arrest, a recent Swedish report of 14 000 patients showed increased survival to 1 month for "complete CPR" (both chest compressions and ventilation) versus "incomplete CPR" (compression only) (survival, 9.7% vs. 5.1%; $P < 0.001$).[190]

In that study, ventilation, and duration of less than 2 minutes between patient collapse and the beginning of lay bystander CPR, were both powerful modifying factors on survival at 30 days, emphasizing the need for better and earlier CPR. A limitation of these out-of-hospital studies is the lack of proper neurological examination during or immediately after resuscitation. Therefore, the relative influence of ventilation on cerebral perfusion is unclear. In swine models, pupillary diameter light reaction was used and found to have a reasonable correlation with cerebral perfusion pressure. However, the animal was ventilated during resuscitation with a tidal volume of 15 ml/kg at an FiO_2 of 1.0. It is unknown whether these clinical findings could be used in a human prospective randomized study during CPR to evaluate the level of influence of ventilation on neurological outcome.[191]

It is logical that ventilation should be matched with perfusion of blood through the lungs and the systemic circulation. Thus, when blood flow is zero, ventilation is unnecessary because it would not affect tissue oxygenation and CO_2 removal. Nonetheless, with CPR techniques that improve blood flow, such as use of device adjuncts for chest compression, more ventilation may be necessary.

The duration of ventricular fibrillation before the start of chest compression is likely to be of significance regarding the need for ventilation, although the importance of ventilation in CPR has been de-emphasized in favor of the need for more effective chest compression and early defibrillation. Indeed, it is likely that time of defibrillation is an important factor in determining whether ventilation is necessary for successful resuscitation. The etiology of cardiac arrest is another very important factor related to the role of ventilation in CPR. Ventilation has primary importance when cardiac arrest occurs from asphyxia, such as in drowning, and is the most frequent cause of pediatric cardiac arrest.

In summary, recommendations for ventilation during CPR are based on numerous laboratory studies that are somewhat contradictory, computer models, and limited human studies. After evaluating the sum of available evidence, a consensus of international experts continues to recommend ventilation, although at a reduced rate and minute volume during CPR and in the postresuscitation period.[162]

Techniques of ventilation during CPR

Ventilation techniques that can be used for basic CPR by the lay public: manual, mouth-to-mouth, and mouth-to-mask ventilation

In the 1950s and early 1960s alternative methods of artificial respiration were investigated in addition to mouth-to-mouth ventilation. A number of studies showed that the application of external pressure to the chest during manual maneuvers in normal volunteers caused substantial respiratory tidal volumes that ranged from 50 to 1114 ml (Fig. 28.8).[10,14–16,192–197] The rate of manual ventilation was 10 to 12 compressions/minute and total minute ventilation (the product of tidal volume and respiratory rate per minute) provided by these techniques was 0.5 to 11.1 l/min. When these techniques were applied to patients with pre-existing pulmonary disease, tidal volumes were considerably lower (50 to 540 ml) than in healthy subjects.[197] These studies also noted that tidal volumes generated by actively expanding the chest with arm-lift or hip-lift techniques were 20 to 40% greater when compared with passive chest expansion.[195] Techniques that relied exclusively on passive chest expansion were ineffective for adequate ventilation and resulted in mean arterial oxygen saturations of 67% in normal volunteer subjects.[192] Manual techniques that included active chest expansion produced mean arterial oxygen saturations of 93% in human subjects, and thus were able to maintain acceptable gas exchange without positive pressure ventilation.[192] In contrast with the manual techniques previously mentioned, pressure applied directly over the sternum of curarized, intubated volunteers produced mean tidal volumes of only 156 ml. Furthermore, without intubation, sternal pressure produced no tidal exchange because of airway obstruction by the tongue.[15] With the head extended to prevent airway obstruction, however, five of six patients had tidal volumes greater than 340 ml and three of six had tidal volumes in excess of 500 ml.

Simultaneous with studies of manual ventilation techniques, mouth-to-mouth ventilation was also studied extensively. Several research projects were funded by the Department of the Army because of the urgency of problems of resuscitation in nerve gas poisoning. In one study, 29 volunteers were paralyzed with curare, and mouth-to-mask resuscitation was started before the onset of cyanosis.[198] The arterial oxygen saturation of the volunteers receiving artificial ventilation was never below 85% and the mean oxygen saturation was 94%. Alveolar CO_2 tensions, measured in 21 patients, were maintained at or below 50 mmHg. The mean alveolar CO_2 concentration was 5.6% before resuscitation and 3.9% during resuscitation. Expired gas resuscitation produced a fall in alveolar CO_2 concentration in all 12 patients. The authors concluded that with mild hyperventilation, the rescuer readily converted his exhaled gas to a suitable resuscitation gas. These experiments were designed to simulate a respiratory arrest and only healthy volunteers were studied. Whether exhaled gas would benefit a patient who suffers cardiac arrest was not considered and has not been investigated.

Because exhaled gas contains CO_2, it may have adverse cardiovascular effects during CPR, but few investigations have addressed this issue. A study of the effect of ventilation on resuscitation during CPR in an animal model showed that both hypoxemia and hypercarbia independently have an adverse effect on outcome from cardiac arrest. Swine were ventilated with experimental gas mixtures consisting of 85% oxygen in a control group, 95% O_2 and 5% CO_2 in a hypercarbic group, and 10% O_2 and 90% N_2 in a hypoxic group. The model succeeded in producing isolated hypoxemia without hypercarbia and isolated hypercarbia without hypoxemia. Only one of 10 (10%) animals could be resuscitated in each of the hypercarbic and hypoxic groups, while 9 of 12 (75%) animals were resuscitated in the control group.[121]

A study of the composition of gas given by mouth-to-mouth ventilation during simulated one- and two-rescuer CPR showed that the rescuers exhaled a mean concentration of CO_2 of 3.5 to 4.1% and a mean concentration of O_2 of 16.6 to 17.8%.[6] Therefore, the gas given by mouth-to-mouth ventilation has a similar concentration of CO_2 and is more hypoxic than the gas shown to be deleterious in the above-cited animal study. When compared with mouth-to-mouth ventilation, room air is a superior gas for ventilation, because it contains 21% oxygen and a negligible amount of CO_2 (0.03%).

Furthermore, when these gas concentrations were used in a swine model with 6 ml/kg ventilation, profound arterial desaturation was noted and was shortly followed by hemodynamic instability and hypotension.[199] This instability and

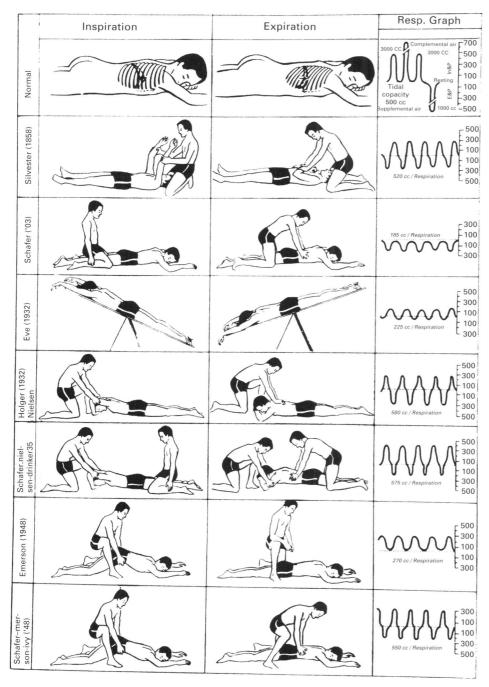

Fig. 28.8. Inspiratory and expiratory phases of normal respiration, Eve rocking method, and manual methods of artificial respiration with pneumographs produced by each. (From ref. 195.)

desaturation were not observed if the tidal volume was increased to 12 ml/kg, or if a fraction of inspired oxygen of 0.70 was used with a tidal volume of 6 ml/kg. Two main features make older human studies different from more recent animal laboratory experiences: the patients described in the original case reports were typically paralyzed, and the rescuer hyperventilated to the point of feeling dizzy, and had an arterial partial pressure of CO_2 of about 20 mmHg.[10]

These differences highlight the need for more controlled human studies before recommending withholding mouth-to-mouth ventilation during cardiac arrest.

Of note, an important factor might affect the feasibility of such studies: a widespread fear of acquiring contagious diseases from victims of cardiac arrest that has recently resulted in reluctance among the lay public, and even some health professionals, to perform mouth-to-mouth ventilation.

Infectious disease concerns published in the literature include *Helicobacter pylori, Salmonella, Herpes simplex* virus, tuberculosis, HIV, and the hepatitides.[200–203] Being repulsed by the sight of a victim in agony and the fear of doing harm may also affect the decision to provide mouth-to-mouth ventilation. Recent surveys of CPR instructors reported that all would perform mouth-to-mouth ventilation on a 4-year-old drowned child, but only 54% on a college student, 35% on a hemophiliac, 18% on a stranger in a bus in San Francisco, and 10% on a person who had overdosed on heroin.[204,205] Awareness of new infectious disease issues, if not new infectious diseases, has resulted in the current recommendation of the AHA to use barrier devices to protect the rescuer against contamination with any infective secretions.[203] Effective barriers against contamination increase efficacy and effectiveness of CPR, helping the rescuer to overcome fear of contamination and immediately to start resuscitation. The overall willingness to perform bystander CPR is disappointingly low in the United States, Europe, and Japan, however, for laypersons and healthcare providers alike. Different reasons are likely responsible for this widespread attitude. In the United States and Europe, the factor deterring performance of mouth-to-mouth ventilation by a bystander or health care provider is fear of contracting infectious diseases. This differs from the situation in Japan, where unwillingness to perform mouth-to-mouth ventilation is mostly a result of lack of confidence in a person's ability to perform CPR properly.[206] The difference may be related to the 200-fold lower incidence of HIV in Japan, as compared with the United States.[207]

Education and increased retention of proper mouth-to-mouth ventilation technique is fundamental but difficult to apply to all populations. The use of television spots as a means of teaching basic skills of CPR in at-risk populations has been explored in Brazil. Although television spots seem to increase skill retention over 1 year, mouth-to-mouth ventilation and effective external cardiac compression are recognized as skills that depend on supervised practice with mannequins. Although the study is limited, it makes sense to use an alternative methodology to promote resuscitation skills in the lay population, including the use of educational clips or scenarios in entertaining and motivating television spots.[208] Recently, a 20-minute video-based basic life support course with a new, inexpensive manikin was studied in two cities and showed skill retention rates at 2 and 6 months that were as good as those seen in students who took the standard 4-hour course.[209,210] In addition, A 5-minute course on use of an automated external defibrillator (AED), when combined with the 20-minute CPR course, showed equivalent skill retention for correct AED use 6 months after training when compared with a standard 4-hour course.[211]

While recent evidence-based literature acknowledges the importance and efficacy of CPR without ventilation, the need for assisted ventilation in cardiac arrest with asphyxia (cardiac arrest primarily resulting from respiratory arrest) or in pediatric populations (generally younger than 8 years of age) cannot be overemphasized.[212] Cardiac arrest with asphyxia was originally illustrated in the first case of external chest compressions.[213] The rationale of ventilation during CPR for cardiac arrest is based on the assumption that CPR delays brain death in no-flow situations, and that hypoxia and respiratory acidosis can aggravate the injury. A critical decrease of brain ATP of 25% below the normal level has been observed after 4 minutes in an animal model of decapitated normothermic dog.[214]

In general, arterial partial pressure of oxygen is maintained within the normal range for approximately 1 minute in a dog model of chest compressions without ventilation.[215] Furthermore, when asphyxia is the cause of cardiac arrest, oxygen consumption has reached near complete exhaustion, and CO_2 and lactate have significantly accumulated just before cardiac arrest. This is in contrast to ventricular fibrillation, in which hypoxemia and acidemia become significant only several minutes after the onset of cardiac arrest. In a model of resuscitation after asphyxia (clamping of the endotracheal tube in an anesthetized pig), the animal subjects were randomly selected to receive resuscitation with and without simulated mouth-to-mouth ventilation. Return of spontaneous circulation was noted only when ventilation was added to chest compression.[216] Successful chest compressions and mouth-to-mouth rescue breathing allowed complete neurological recovery in 90% of the animals.

The presence of a foreign body obstructing the airway is an uncommon but important cause of cardiac arrest with asphyxia, with an incidence of 0.65 to 0.9 per 100 000 cardiac arrests.[217] A recent study seems to support in part the original investigation of Ruben and MacNaughton,[218] in that abdominal thrust is not necessary in foreign body choking, and that chest compressions can achieve higher airway pressure than the Heimlich maneuver.[219] Indeed, when CPR was performed and compared with an abdominal thrust in the cadaver, median and peak airway pressure reached a value of 30 cm H_2O vs. 18 cm H_2O and 41 cm H_2O vs. 26 cm H_2O, respectively. Only in a moderately obese cadaver was the mean airway pressure produced by the Heimlich maneuver higher than that produced with chest compression. The European Resuscitation Council (ERC) also addressed acute asphyxia from airway obstruction.[220]

Despite recent knowledge that occurrence of ventricular fibrillation in children may be more frequent than was previously thought,[221] asphyxia is still the most common cause of cardiac arrest in the pediatric population. The Pediatric Resuscitation Subcommittee of the Emergency Cardiovascular Care Committee of the American Heart Association (AHA) worked with the Neonatal Resuscitation Program Steering Committee (American Academic of Pediatrics) and the Pediatric Working Group of the International Liaison Committee on Resuscitation to review recommendations on oxygenation and ventilation in neonatal resuscitation.[222] The approach to the recommendations has been the same as that described in the AHA Guidelines 2000 for adults, which uses five classes of recommendations centered on evidence-based reviews of scientific reports. Up to 10% of newborn infants require resuscitation at birth. The majority, because of meconium airway obstruction/aspiration, require immediate intervention and assisted ventilation. Because of their unique physiology, the importance of ventilation/oxygenation in newborns cannot be overemphasized. Fluid-filled lungs and intra- as well as extracardiac shunts at birth are physiologically reversed in the first few minutes of extrauterine life with either spontan-eous or assisted vigorous chest expansion. Failure to normalize this function may result in persistence of right-to-left, intra- and extracardiac shunt, pulmonary hypertension, and systemic cyanosis. Bradycardia usually follows, with severe hemodynamic instability and rapid deterioration to cardiac arrest. Although these physiologic characteristics are typical of the newborn (minutes to hours after birth), similar events can be triggered by hypoxia in neonates (first 28 days of life) and infants (up to 12 months of age). The importance of proper ventilation/ oxygenation and the small margin of safety resulting from the unique physiology and high oxygen consumption of the newborn mandate the need for immediate ventilation and the presence of skilled personnel at the bedside to perform proper basic steps of resuscitation. Clearance of meconium fluid should be immediately performed, upon birth, and providing positive pressure ventilation should be considered within 30 seconds when bradycardia or apnea is present. Tracheal intubation remains the gold standard for providing immediate ventilation/oxygenation to the newborn. European and American guidelines have essentially the same sequence of resuscitative events in neonates, recommending a chest compression–to-ventilation ratio of 3:1, with about 90 compressions and 30 breaths per minute with emphasis on quality of ventilation and compressions.[223,224]

A major change to guidelines for CPR occurred with publication of the 2005 International Consensus Conference on Cardiopulmonary Resuscitation and Emergency Cardiovascular Care Science With Treatment Recommendations.[224] It is now recommended that lay rescuers or a lone professional rescuer use a 30:2 compression:ventilation ratio for infants, children, and adults. This recommendation is intended to simplify training and reduce interruptions of chest compression, which is known to have a negative effect on outcome. When two or more professional rescuers are present, a compression:ventilation ratio of 15:2 is recommended for infants and children.[224,225] The airway patency, breathing, and circulation approach to CPR sequencing was not modified The sequence of when to call 911 (activate the EMS system) has also been modified and is now based on presumed etiology of the cardiac arrest (dysrhythmic vs. asphyxial). For *unwitnessed* or non-sudden collapse, start CPR immediately, give 5 cycles of chest compressions and ventilation, then activate EMS and get an AED. For *witnessed* sudden collapse, activate EMS/get an AED, start CPR, then attempt defibrillation.[225]

In summary, ventilation remains essential in cardiac arrest with asphyxia in both adult and pediatric patients. The need for immediate ventilation in dysrhythmic cardiac arrest is less clear, however, and has less emphasis in CPR guidelines since 2005. It is clear that future studies are needed to address the ideal compression:ventilation ratio, the ideal minute volume, and whether mouth-to-mouth ventilation during cardiac arrest is any better than chest compression without rescue breathing, and the optimal "exhaled" volume to be provided to the victim.

Positive pressure ventilation in an unprotected airway: the problem of gastric insufflation and pulmonary aspiration

Manual techniques of ventilation used for rescue breathing were in widespread use from the early 1900s to the early 1960s, when they were replaced with mouth-to-mouth ventilation. Although manual techniques were capable of providing reasonably good tidal volume and minute ventilation in patients with patent airways, a major drawback was that prevention of upper airway obstruction was not an integral part of the technique, and airway obstruction could prevent movement of air. The principal advantage of mouth-to-mouth ventilation is that providing an open airway through backward tilt of the head and lifting of the mandible is part of the technique. Also, because the provider is immediately aware of upper airway obstruction when increased resistance to

ventilation is encountered, further steps can be taken to relieve the obstruction.

Upper airway obstruction in an unconscious patient is caused by occlusion of the oropharynx by the relaxed tongue (Figs. 28.9 and 28.10). The base of the tongue is retracted against the posterior wall of the pharynx when the head is in a flexed position and occurs whether the patient is in a supine or prone position. Extension of the head can relieve obstruction in most patients and the addition of forward displacement of the mandible and/or an oropharyngeal airway opens the airway completely in 88 to 98% of subjects.[226–228] Studies of manual techniques of ventilation showed that the back-pressure-arm-lift method produced a mean tidal volume of only 126 ml when the head was allowed to remain in a natural position, but with extension of the head, tidal volume increased to 520 ml and only one of six subjects (17%) had a tidal volume that was less than dead space (Fig. 28.11).[228]

Unlike manual techniques of ventilation that produce negative intrathoracic pressure to move air into the lungs, mouth-to-mouth ventilation uses positive pressure to inflate the lungs. Because air under pressure can flow into the esophagus as well as the trachea, a frequent complication of mouth-to-mouth ventilation is gastric insufflation. Peak inflation pressure is directly related to the product of inspiratory flow rate and airways resistance. Delivering a

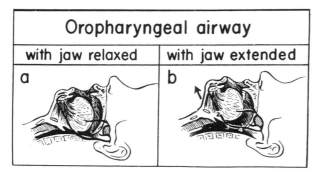

Fig. 28.9. When the mandible is extended by lifting it upward, the hyoid bone and floor of mouth are also drawn upward. This maneuver makes forward displacement of the tongue obligatory, since it is attached to the mandible, hyoid bone, and floor of mouth. (From ref. 198.)

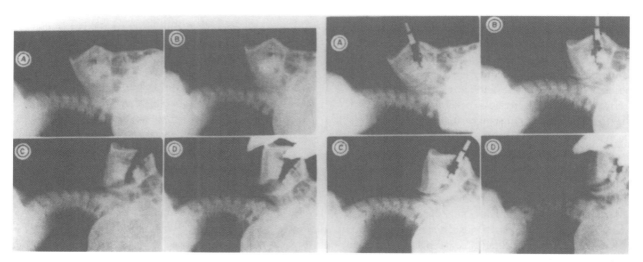

Fig. 28.10. *Left panel*. Radiographs of natural upper airway of an anesthetized spontaneously breathing adult in the supine position. *A*, neck flexed; note obstruction of oropharynx by tongue being pushed against posterior pharyngeal wall, and obstruction of nasopharynx by soft palate. *B*, head midposition; same obstruction as in *A*. *C*, neck extended; note open oropharyngeal and nasopharyngeal air spaces with tongue being lifted away from posterior pharyngeal wall. *D*, neck extended plus forward displacement of mandible; note how anteroposterior diameter of oropharynx is increased over that in *C*. *Right panel*. Radiographs of upper airway with oropharyngeal rubber airway in place. Anesthetized, spontaneously breathing adult in the supine position. *A*, neck flexed; same obstruction as without airway; *B*, head midposition; pharynx may be partially obstructed; *C*, neck extended; patent pharynx; *D*, neck extended plus forward displacement of mandible; patency further increased over that of *C*. (From ref. 14.)

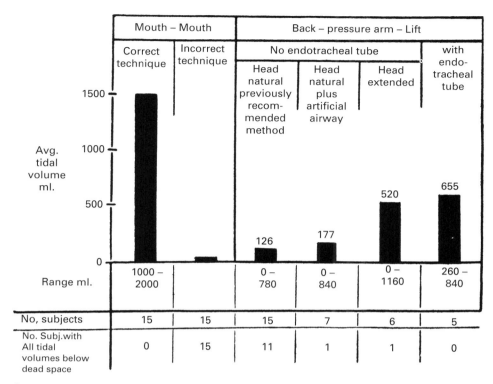

	Mouth – Mouth		Back – pressure arm – Lift			
	Correct technique	Incorrect technique	No endotracheal tube			with endo-tracheal tube
			Head natural previously recom-mended method	Head natural plus artificial airway	Head extended	
Avg. tidal volume ml.						
Range ml.	1000 – 2000		0 – 780	0 – 840	0 – 1160	260 – 840
No, subjects	15	15	15	7	6	5
No. Subj.with All tidal volumes below dead space	0	15	11	1	1	0

Fig. 28.11. Tidal volumes as influenced by upper airway obstruction. (From ref. 230.)

large tidal volume over a brief inspiratory time results in increased peak inflation pressure and leads to gastric insufflation and hypoventilation in victims with an unprotected (not intubated) airway. The volume delivered to the lungs can be increased by using a longer duration of inspiration and a lower inspiratory flow rate.[229] The pressure necessary to move gas into the lungs depends on airway resistance and total thoracic compliance, which is equal to the sum of chest and lung compliance:

$$\text{Compliance (l/cm H}_2\text{O)} = \text{change in volume (l) / change in pressure (cm H}_2\text{O)}$$

Lung compliance decreases with decreasing lung volume and the tidal volume necessary to prevent decreased compliance is approximately 7 ml/kg of body weight in patients with normal lungs. Lung compliance also is decreased by pulmonary edema and atelectasis. Chest compliance is decreased by kyphoscoliosis, scleroderma, obesity, and the supine position.

Chest compression has been shown to affect compliance during cardiac arrest and compliance decreases with each minute of chest compression.[230] Compliance becomes a crucial factor for ventilation when the upper airway is not intubated. Because the trachea, pharynx, and esophagus are all exposed to the same positive pressure during

mouth-to-mouth ventilation, or bag-mask ventilation, air could preferentially enter the stomach via the esophagus. During cardiac arrest and CPR, chest compliance decreases and thus greater pressure is needed to inflate the lungs adequately. At the same time, lower esophageal sphincter tone decreases during cardiac arrest and there is less resistance for air to enter the stomach.[231,232]

Work done in anesthetized patients found that the pressure needed to produce gastric insufflation ranged from 10 to 35 cm H_2O with a face mask technique of ventilation and the most frequent pressure needed for insufflation was 15 cm H_2O.[233] Regurgitation of gastric contents and pulmonary aspiration does not occur with chest compressions alone, but requires inflation of the stomach.[234,235] Mouth-to-mouth ventilation was shown to cause regurgitation in 48% of patients, probably because of gastric insufflation.[235] In a study of non-survivors of cardiac arrest, 46% were found to have full stomachs and at least 29% had evidence of pulmonary aspiration of gastric contents.[236] Similar complications occur with the use of a bag-mask ventilation device in patients with unprotected airways.[238] Aside from pulmonary aspiration of gastric contents, gastric insufflation, if sufficient, causes elevation and splinting of the diaphragm with consequent loss of lung volume, decreased compliance, hypoventilation, and greater risk of further gastric insufflation. Gastric insufflation can be prevented in many patients by applying pressure over the cricoid to seal off the esophagus.[237] In addition, manual techniques of ventilation would not be expected to produce gastric insufflation, because inspiratory airflow is caused by negative airway pressure and airflow during expiration is associated with very low airway pressures of approximately 0 to 1 cm H_2O.[238,239]

Effectiveness and safety of ventilation of the unprotected airway have been extensively studied in bench models. When a mechanical ventilator was used to provide tidal volumes of 500 ml and 1000 ml, respectively, in an in vitro model of an unprotected airway, significantly less stomach inflation was found when a smaller tidal volume (approximately 500 ml) was applied with a mechanical ventilator compared with a tidal volume of approximately 1000 ml.[241] For the same reason, the use of a smaller, pediatric, self-inflating bag delivering a maximal volume of 500 ml showed less gastric inflation in the same model when compared with the large adult bag.[199,241] All of these studies suggest that when the peak airway pressure exceeds lower esophageal sphincter pressure during ventilation of an unprotected airway, the stomach is likely to be inflated. As a result, a tidal volume of 6 to 7 ml/kg body weight (approximately 500 ml) and an inspiratory time of 1 second is recommended for assisted ventilation.[162,224]

The performance of the apparatus used to deliver bag-valve mask (BVM) ventilation has recently been reviewed extensively. Seven commercially available models of ventilating bags used on an advanced cardiac life support training mannequin connected to an artificial lung, in which compliance and resistance were set at normal, have been evaluated for the tidal volume achieved.[242] Interestingly, standard ventilations with one hand averaged a tidal volume between 450 to 600 ml in both genders, despite significant differences in the size of male and female hands. When the technique was modified to open palm and total squeezing of the self-inflating bag against the flexed rescuer's knee, next to the patient's head, total volume ranged from 888 to 1192 ml. This study seems to indicate that most of the commercially available ventilating bags can provide both 6 ml/kg to 12 ml/kg tidal volume, with and without available oxygen, in a reliable manner. This study was performed on a mannequin with normal compliance and resistance, however, and gastric inflation was not measured.

When ventilation is provided to a victim of cardiac arrest, proper tidal volume cannot be easily assessed. Excitement and overenthusiasm of the professional rescuer at the scene of cardiac arrest can increase the chance of gastric inflation.[243] In a recent intriguing paper from Austria, it was shown that the stomach inflation of the victim, as assessed by postresuscitation chest radiograph, was minimal and statistically lower (15%) when the lay bystander provided mouth-to-mouth ventilation versus when professional paramedics ventilated the victim with a BVM device.[244] There are many possible explanations for these results, which are partially related to the limitation of the chest radiograph as a test to assess gastric inflation and the lack of autopsy reports from the non-surviving victims. It is also possible that "extreme efficiency" of ventilation by the paramedics as compared with the bystander's mouth-to-mouth ventilation determined the difference. This finding, combined with the observation that professional rescuers tend to squeeze the bag very rapidly during the excitement of CPR (generally in < 0.5 s and with power), suggests the need for better teaching of basic manual resuscitation skills.[241]

Limiting the size of the ventilating bag to a pediatric volume could theoretically decrease the danger of delivering an exaggerated tidal volume during CPR. If oxygen is not available at the scene of an emergency, and small tidal volumes are given during BLS ventilation with a pediatric self-inflatable bag and room air (21% oxygen), insufficient oxygenation and/or inadequate ventilation may result. Recently, 80 patients were studied who were randomly allocated to receive ventilation with either an adult (maximum volume, 1500 ml) or pediatric (maximum volume, 700 ml) self-inflatable bag for 5 minutes while apneic after induction of general anesthesia and before intubation. The study used ventilation with 40% O_2 and showed no significant difference in mean arterial O_2 saturation (98% vs. 97%) or $ETCO_2$ (26 vs. 33 mmHg) with the adult or pediatric bag, respectively.[245] The investigators did a follow-up study using the same methodology, but this time they used room air instead of 40% O_2 as the ventilating gas.[246] When using an adult ($n = 20$) versus pediatric ($n = 20$) self-inflatable bag, tidal volumes and tidal volumes per kilogram (mean ± standard error) were significantly larger (719 ± 22 ml/kg vs. 455 ± 23 ml/kg and 10.5 ± 0.4 ml/kg vs. 6.2 ± 0.4 ml/kg, respectively; $P < 0.0001$). Compared with an adult self-inflatable bag, BVM ventilation with room air and use of a pediatric self-inflatable bag resulted in lower arterial PO_2 values (73 ± 4 mmHg vs. 87 ± 4 mmHg; $P < 0.01$), but comparable CO_2 elimination (40 ± 2 mmHg vs. 37 ± 1 mmHg; not significant), indicating that smaller tidal volumes of about 6 ml/kg (approximately 500 ml) given with a pediatric self-inflatable bag and room air maintain adequate CO_2 elimination, but decrease oxygenation during simulated BLS ventilation. This study confirms previous observations that if small (6 ml/kg) tidal volumes are used during BLS ventilation, supplemental oxygen is needed, and when oxygen is not available, larger tidal volumes of about 8 to 10 ml/kg should be used to maintain both sufficient oxygenation and CO_2 elimination when circulation is normal.[199]

In conclusion, proper mask ventilation is a fundamental skill of resuscitation and should receive a high priority in training of both adult and pediatric providers.[249,250] Using recommended guidelines for tidal volume and inspiratory time, pulmonary ventilation can be maximized and gastric inflation can be minimized. However, gastric inflation and pulmonary aspiration can be completely prevented only when the airway is protected with endotracheal intubation, always regarded as the "gold standard" of providing ventilation during CPR.

Ventilation caused by chest compression: standard and active chest compression–decompression

When the chest is pressed with the hands or a mechanical device, intrathoracic pressure increases above atmospheric pressure and air flows out of the lungs if the upper airway is unobstructed. Air flows back into the lungs when pressure on the chest is released and the thorax recoils passively, creating negative intrathoracic pressure. Although the tidal volume caused by chest compression usually is less than the dead space, effective gas exchange can take place under certain conditions, particularly if the frequency of compression is high enough.

Knowledge of dead space is helpful in understanding high frequency ventilation. Inhaled air passes through the conducting airways to the alveoli where gas exchange takes place. The conducting airways (the nose, mouth, pharynx, larynx, trachea, bronchi, and bronchioles) do not participate in gas exchange and have a volume, termed anatomic dead space, of about 150 to 180 ml in the adult human.[1] The total volume of alveoli not perfused with blood and thus not participating in gas exchange is called alveolar dead space. Physiologic dead space is the sum of anatomic and alveolar dead space, and is the volume of the lung that does not eliminate CO_2. Physiological dead space is a functional measurement, approximating 2.2 ml/kg of lean body weight. Physiological dead space increases during conditions of ventilation-perfusion inequality. During conventional ventilation, tidal volume must exceed physiological dead space for effective delivery of O_2 and elimination of CO_2. During high frequency ventilation, gas exchange can take place when tidal volume is less than physiologic dead space, presumably because of enhanced diffusion and mixing of gases.

Ventilation caused by chest compression is a form of high frequency ventilation, which is defined as lung ventilation at a frequency of at least four times the normal breathing frequency, usually with tidal volumes less than anatomical

dead space.[249] Gas exchange depends on several mechanisms, including bulk flow of gases, molecular diffusion, asymmetric velocity profiles where the profile is direction-dependent, cardiogenic mixing, mixing caused by turbulent airflow, and inter-regional "pendelluft" due to time-constant inequalities, which results in gas from fast-filling lung units redistributing into slow-filling units.[249,250]

High frequency ventilation has been produced by applying external pressure to the chest by means of a pressure cuff around the thorax. In a canine experiment, high frequency ventilation with use of chest compression with tidal volumes of approximately 50 ml and frequencies of 3 to 5 Hz (180 to 300 compressions per minute) produced better arterial oxygenation and elimination of CO_2 than did conventional ventilation at standard tidal volumes and rate.[251] The effectiveness of high frequency ventilation depends on where compression is applied to the body. One study found that it is more effective when applied to the abdomen.[252] High frequency ventilation was found to have equally efficient gas exchange when applied at the trachea or the chest[253] and provided enhanced ventilation in a model of airway obstruction.[254–256] Adequate gas exchange can take place with tidal volumes as low as 12% of dead space.[257]

There is a striking similarity between high frequency ventilation with chest compression and chest compression during cardiac arrest. The recommended frequency of chest compression during CPR is approximately 2 Hz (100 compressions per minute). If obstruction of the upper airway can be prevented, then tidal volume can be produced during sternal compression. In an intubated swine cardiac arrest model, a study showed that sternal compression with a mechanical device produced ventilation with a mean tidal volume of 45 ml during the first minute of resuscitation that decreased to 16 ml during the 10 minute (Fig. 28.12). Because chest compressions were given at a rate of 100 per minute, minute ventilation was 4.5 l during the first minute of resuscitation and 1.6 l during the 10 minute. When compared with conventional ventilation, however, CO_2 elimination was less with chest compression ventilation, resulting in significantly greater hypercarbic acidosis.[238]

Active compression–decompression CPR is a technique of chest compression in which force is applied to the chest during both downward compression and upward lifting decompression by means of a suction cup applied to the chest. Thus, the chest is actively re-expanded with this technique instead of passively recoiling as in conventional CPR. It has been shown that during CPR, thorax and lung compliance gradually decrease over time, thus explaining, in part, why ventilation produced by conventional chest

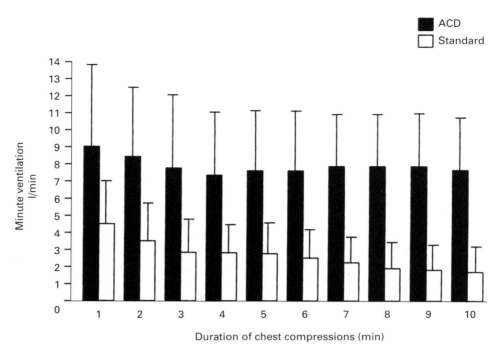

Fig. 28.12. Minute ventilation (L/min + SD) caused by external chest compression in swine without additional mechanical ventilation. Animals received either standard mechanical chest compression (*Standard*) (n = 8) or mechanical active chest compression–decompression (*ACD*) (n = 8) (Data from Idris AH. Wenzel V. Tucker KJ. Orban DJ. Chest compression ventilation: a comparison of standard CPR and active-compression/decompression CPR. Acad Emerg. Med 1994; 1: A17 refs. and 240).

compression decreases over a 10-minute period. Active compression–decompression CPR may overcome the loss of compliance because the chest is forcibly re-expanded. In another swine study of CPR, active compression–decompression chest compression was compared with conventional chest compression (Fig. 28.12).[239] The tidal volume and minute ventilation caused by active compression–decompression were twice that of standard chest compression, did not decrease during 10 minutes of CPR, and produced significantly better arterial pH, PO_2, and PCO_2.

An interesting recent application has been the use of adjunct CPAP and pressure support ventilation (CPAP-PSV) during the decompression phase. In a swine model of cardiac arrest, CPAP-PSV showed a significantly higher PaO_2 and lower A-aDO_2, maintaining moderate hypercarbia when compared with control animals. Remarkably, an unexplained increase of VO_2 was observed in all the animals with applied CPAP-PSV.[258]

Gasping ventilation

Gasping appears to be much more common than previously thought within the first few minutes of cardiac arrest.

Investigators reported the presence of gasping or agonal respiration in as many as 55% of witnessed cardiac arrest victims.[259–261] Gasping is often mistaken for normal breathing, with the unfortunate consequence that bystanders withhold CPR for up to 40% of victims with confirmed cardiac arrest. The American Heart Association Guidelines 2005 now emphasize recognition of gasping breaths and initiating CPR if the rescuer is unsure if the person is breathing normally.[162]

Current standards for ventilation during CPR and adjunct devices for ventilation

The American Heart Association has developed a set of training tools and guidelines for cardiopulmonary resuscitation and emergency cardiovascular care.[262] Control of the airway during cardiopulmonary resuscitation is divided into three general categories: basic airway management, advanced airway control, and postresuscitation airway management.

Basic management of the airway entails establishing unresponsiveness, calling for help, opening the airway with various maneuvers, maintenance of airway patency, determination of apnea, and provision of ventilation and oxygenation in conjunction with chest compression. Advanced airway control requires endotracheal intubation and use of ancillary equipment to support ventilation and oxygenation. Following successful resuscitation, the patient may remain supported by endotracheal intubation and mechanical ventilation.

Basic airway management

Basic airway management is indicated for patients who suffer respiratory and/or cardiac arrest. Primary respiratory arrest may occur during drowning, foreign body obstruction, smoke inhalation, drug overdose or anaphylactic reaction, cerebrovascular accident, thermal or electrical injury, trauma, acute myocardial infarction, epiglottitis, sepsis, and coma of whatever cause. Early initiation of rescue breathing may improve survival and prevent cardiac arrest.

The goal of basic airway management is to provide enough oxygen to the brain and heart until definitive medical treatment can restore normal heart and ventilatory activity.[262] Rescue breathing brings oxygen into the lungs while chest compression promotes oxygen transport from the lungs to vital tissues. Immediate initiation of resuscitation is necessary, because the highest rate and quality of survival are achieved when basic life support is started within 4 minutes from the time of arrest and when advanced cardiac life support is initiated within 8 minutes.[263]

Provision and maintenance of a patent upper airway

The maneuvers utilized to provide a patent upper airway in an unconscious patient are designed primarily to relieve obstruction by the tongue gravitating toward the posterior pharyngeal wall. Relaxation of the head and neck muscles supporting the mandible during loss of consciousness results in the loss of the tongue's muscular tone. When the tongue falls against the posterior pharynx, it causes obstruction of the upper airway. Airway obstruction is aggravated in a comatose patient by a semi-flexed neck, which causes narrowing of the distance from the tongue to the posterior pharynx. The epiglottis also tends to fall back onto the glottis. Furthermore, breathing against an obstructed upper airway pulls the tongue toward the airway, worsening the obstruction. The negative pressure generated in the airway during inspiration causes a ball valve type of tracheal obstruction. Even in normal, spontaneously breathing anesthetized patients, some airway obstruction occurs in 90% when the head is in neutral position and the airway is unsupported.[226]

Unless contraindicated, the victim should be properly positioned, before resuscitation is started: a firm, flat surface, with the arms alongside the body, is preferred. The patient's head should be below the level of the thorax. If the victim is prone, the patient should be moved supine as a unit to avoid twisting the head neck or back. The rescuer should kneel beside the patient's shoulder. Spontaneous breathing should be ascertained. Several maneuvers are utilized to open the airway. In Europe, it is taught that breathing should be ascertained in the position the victim is found. The victim is positioned supine if respirations cannot be assessed or if they are absent.

Head tilt/chin lift maneuver

In the absence of head and neck trauma, the head tilt/chin lift maneuver is utilized to open the airway (Fig. 28.13(a)).[264] This maneuver is also referred to as the "sniffing position" and is considered to be the most effective method of opening the airway of an unconscious victim. A roll or towel may be placed under the victim's occiput to maintain this position. The victim's mouth should be examined for dentures and debris. A piece of cloth is used to wipe out fluid or semi-liquid material. Solid materials are removed with a hooked index finger. Dentures may be left in place to maintain a normal facial shape, facilitating adequate lip seal and mouth-to-mouth breathing. But if dentures obstruct the airway, they must be removed. One hand is placed on the patient's forehead and the head is tilted backward with firm pressure. The fingers of the other hand are positioned firmly beneath the chin's bony portion, lifting it upward. This brings the chin forward and the teeth almost to occlusion, supporting the jaw and helping to tilt the head backward. Pressure on the soft tissue under the chin should be avoided because it can aggravate airway obstruction. Unless mouth-to-nose breathing is indicated, the mouth should not be completely closed. During mouth-to-nose breathing, the mouth can be closed by increasing the pressure on the hand that is already on the chin. This technique is the recommended maneuver of choice because of its simplicity, safety, effectiveness, and ease of learning. The maneuver was found to be superior in opening the airway during mouth-to-mouth resuscitation of apneic patients, achieving airway patency in 91% of cases vs. 78% with the jaw thrust and 39% with simple neck lift.[265] Greater tidal volume was also delivered during head tilt/chin lift maneuver when compared to other techniques.

In pediatric victims, airway patency is also established by maintaining the head in the sniffing position, but direct pressure on the trachea or hyperextension of the head should be avoided. The pediatric trachea is not yet fully

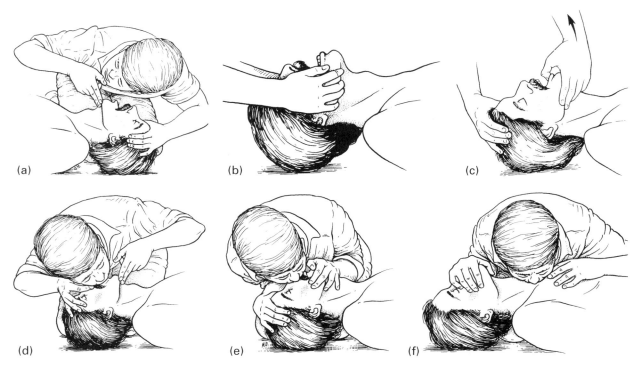

Fig. 28.13. (a) Head-tilt-chin-lift maneuver. (b) Jaw-thrust maneuver and triple airway maneuver. (c) Mandibular displacement. Arrow indicates that the mandible is pulled upward. (d) Rescue breathing. (e) Mouth-to-nose ventilation. (f) Mouth-to-stoma ventilation. (From ref. 266.)

developed and does not have a well-formed rigid cartilaginous ring. Any direct or indirect pressure on this structure causes it to collapse.

Jaw-thrust maneuver

The angles of the mandible may be displaced anteriorly by grasping the lower jaw with both hands from one side and pulling forward, and simultaneously tilting the head backwards (Fig. 28.13(b)). The elbows of the CPR provider should rest on the surface on which the patient is lying. To open the lips, the lower lip can be retracted with the thumb. Mouth-to-mouth breathing can be delivered by occluding the victim's nostrils with the rescuer's cheek pressed tightly against them. To avoid extension of the neck in patients with suspected neck injury, a modified jaw thrust maneuver is performed. Forward traction is applied on the mandible without head tilt and care must be taken to avoid moving the head from side to side. If this maneuver is unsuccessful in opening the airway, the head may be slightly tilted with care. Although jaw thrust maneuver is highly effective in providing upper airway patency, the technique may be technically problematic and the rescuer tires easily. It is considered as an ancillary method and is utilized as a secondary method by professional rescuers.

Triple airway maneuver

This is a modification of the head tilt-lift maneuver whereby the lower lip is retracted with the thumb to open the mouth after tilting the head backward and lifting the chin upward. This maneuver is usually utilized by a more experienced rescuer.

Mandibular displacement

Another method to open the upper airway is to pull the mandible forward by placing the rescuer's thumb in the patient's mouth and putting the fingers underneath the chin to pull the lower jaw upward (Fig. 28.13(c)). Although effective in opening the airway in spontaneously breathing, edentulous patients, it can cause injury to the rescuer if the patient wakes up and suddenly bites rescuer's thumb.

Determination of apnea

There are several recommended methods of determining the absence of spontaneous breathing in an unconscious patient. Spontaneous respiration may be difficult to observe unless the airway is opened. Once airway patency is established, the rescuer should place his or her ear over the victim's mouth and nose. The rise and fall of the chest should be noted. One must listen for breath sounds and feel for expired air. The absence of these signs is indicative of apnea. Frequently, gasping, gurgling, or snoring sounds or agonal respiratory efforts may be observed during cardiac arrest, especially within the first few minutes of collapse. This is not sustained, the respiratory rate is 6/minute or less, and should not be mistaken for spontaneous respiration. In some instances, the victim may show respiratory efforts but no air exchange is observed. This indicates upper airway obstruction and opening the airway facilitates resumption of air movement.

Once spontaneous respiration and pulse are established during resuscitation, the CPR provider should continue maintaining a patent airway. To reduce the likelihood of aspiration and obstruction, the patient should be rolled on his or her side. This is called the recovery position. The victim must be rolled as a unit, moving the head, shoulders and torso simultaneously without twisting. If trauma is suspected, however, the patient should not be moved unless absolutely necessary. There are several options on how the dependent arm may be placed in the recovery position: (a) it may be bent at the elbow, and alongside the victim while the other hand rests under the cheek of the victim; (b) the dependent arm may be alongside the victim; or (c) the dependent arm may be bent at the elbow with the hand under the face. The fundamental goal of the recovery position is to have the patient on his/her side so that aspiration and accidental airway obstruction is prevented.

Initiation of respiration (rescue breathing)

Delivery of an adequate tidal volume is required during rescue breathing. Usually, 500 ml to 600 ml of tidal volume is considered adequate for an adult. It is difficult for the rescuer to know exactly how much tidal volume is given during mouth-to-mouth ventilation. Therefore, it is recommended that the rescuer give just enough tidal volume with each breath to make the chest rise visibly.

The oxygen concentration of expired air is approximately 16% to 17%. With this oxygen concentration, the maximum alveolar oxygen partial pressure is about 80 mmHg, enough to meet the victim's oxygen need. It is recommended that two initial breaths should each be delivered over 1 second. Sufficient time should be allowed for exhalation between breaths. Using this inspiratory time (1 second) in conjunction with a tidal volume of about 500 ml produces a lower inspiratory flow rate, and reduces the chances of exceeding opening pressure of the esophageal sphincter, thereby decreasing the chance of gastric distention, the most common major problem associated with rescue breathing. Gastric distention elevates

the diaphragm, reduces lung volume, and promotes regurgitation and aspiration. Sellick's maneuver, the application of cricoid pressure against the cervical vertebra, helps prevent regurgitation against esophageal pressure of up to 100 cm water. This technique requires an assistant and is recommended only to be used by trained professionals. If regurgitation is observed during CPR, the victim's entire body should be turned to the side and the mouth wiped clean. The patient is then turned back to supine position and CPR is resumed. Additionally, excessive peak airway pressures may be generated during exhaled oxygenation (rescue breathing), increasing the risk of barotrauma.

Basic life support CPR can be performed either by one or two rescuers. During both one- and two-rescuer CPR, 2 breaths are given during a pause after every 30th chest compression. Exhalation occurs passively after each breath and during chest compression. Rescue breathing can be delivered through mouth-to-mouth, mouth-to-nose, mouth-to-stoma, and mouth-to-barrier devices.

After opening the airway by the head-tilt-chin lift maneuver, the rescuer can seal the nose by pinching it with the thumb and index finger of the hand on the victim's forehead (Fig. 28.13(d)). The rescuer inhales and puts his or her lips around the patient's mouth, creating an airtight seal. Two breaths are delivered at a chest compression/ventilation ratio of 30:2 with one- or two-rescuer CPR; the ratio is the same for adults, children, and infants. If two or more professional rescuers are present, the ratio is 15:2 for children and infants. Upward movement of the chest and sensing the escape of air during exhalation assure the rescuer that adequate ventilation has been delivered. *The most common cause of failure to ventilate is improper positioning of the head and chin.* If attempts to ventilate fail, the patient's head and chin should be repositioned. If after repositioning, the patient cannot be ventilated, the airway should be evaluated for the presence of foreign bodies. These maneuvers will be discussed later in this chapter. Also, it should be emphasized that pauses for ventilation pertain only to subjects with an unprotected airway (i.e., unintubated). Once the airway is intubated, chest compressions are given continuously, at a rate of 100 compressions/minute without interruption for ventilation. A ventilation rate of 8 – 10 breaths/minute should be used, which is less than was recommended prior to 2005.[162] When circulation is present with a pulse, about 10 to 12 breaths/minute should be used.[266] If an end-tidal CO_2 monitor is available, ventilation rate should be adjusted to maintain end-tidal CO_2 within a range of about 35 mmHg to 45 mmHg. In patients with obstructive pulmonary disease and increased resistance to exhalation, a lower ventilation rate should be used (e.g., 6 to 8 breaths/minute) to prevent air-trapping and to allow enough time for complete exhalation.[266] Recent studies suggest that fewer breaths/min may improve blood flow during shock or cardiac arrest and provide a better ventilation/perfusion match. This is an important area of active investigation and randomized controlled trials are currently being planned.

If it is difficult or contraindicated to deliver mouth-to-mouth breathing, mouth-to-nose breathing can be performed. It is indicated in patients with mouth trauma, trismus, or in those where a tight mouth-to-mouth seal is impossible to achieve. After the head is properly positioned and the mouth closed (as previously described), the rescuer inhales, puts his or her mouth in a tight seal around the victim's nose, and breaths out into it (Fig. 28.13(e)). The rescuer then removes his or her lips from the patient's nose and lets exhalation occur passively. The mouth may also be opened after breath delivery to allow air to escape through the mouth.

If the patient has a previous laryngectomy and has a permanent opening connecting the trachea to the front base of the neck, ventilation during CPR can be performed by delivering the breath through the stomal opening (Fig. 28.13(f)). In a similar fashion to mouth-to-mouth or mouth-to-nose breathing, the rescuer's mouth is arranged to form a tight seal around the stoma and two breaths are delivered. When the rescuer stops breathing into the stoma, air passively escapes from the opening.

The presence of vomitus and fear of infectious contamination may affect the willingness of rescuers to perform mouth-to-mouth resuscitation. Lawrence and Sivaneswaran showed that only 13% of 70 hospital staff members surveyed would use mouth-to-mouth ventilation and 59% would prefer to use mouth-to-mask ventilation.[269] Specialized masks with a one-way valve are currently utilized during CPR. The valve prevents the exhaled air from entering the rescuer's mouth. Additionally, bacterial filters are incorporated in some of the commercially available masks to prevent contamination of the rescuer. Moreover, some resuscitation masks can deliver as much as 50% oxygen.[267] Mouth-to-mask ventilation can provide adequate tidal volume at a significantly lower airway pressure when compared to mouth-to-mouth resuscitation.[9] Other barrier devices such as face shields are also available. Unlike the masks, many face shields do not have a one-way valve and air may leak around the shield. If a barrier device is used during rescue breathing, it must be placed tightly around the patient's mouth and slow, deep breaths should be delivered in a manner similar to mouth-to-mouth ventilation.

Cardiopulmonary arrest occurring in the hospital setting is often initially managed with bag-valve-mask ventilation. There are studies reporting that this device cannot deliver adequate tidal volume when only one person is doing pulmonary resuscitation.[268–271] The basic problem arises from the need to provide an adequate seal between the face and the mask while controlling the airway by head extension at the same time. Additionally, familiarity with the use of the equipment requires special training and additional manpower. It has been shown that this technique is more effective in delivering adequate ventilation when two rescuers are supporting the airway.[271,272] One rescuer effectively seals the mask to the mouth and maintains head extension while the other squeezes the bag with both hands to deliver adequate tidal volume. The central issue is that the individual providing BVM ventilation must be well-trained in the proper use of this instrument before attempting to control the airway in an arrested patient for the first time.

Oxygen supplementation can be provided during BVM ventilation, which delivers 40% to 60% O_2 without and with an oxygen reservoir, respectively.[273] Complications associated with the use of a BVM are primarily due to excessively high ventilating pressures and include pneumothorax, pneumomediastinum, pneumocephalus, and gastric rupture.[274] When oxygen is available, ventilation should be limited to approximately one-third of the total bag volume (about 600 ml in the 1.81 adult bag) and delivered (over 1 second; the recommended inspiratory time is a little faster because of the smaller tidal volume). Unless the rescuer is proficient in the use of anesthesia bags, it is preferable to use self-inflating hand-held resuscitator bags during CPR. Anesthesia bags such as the Mapleson system are not self-inflating and require a continuous oxygen source.[275] Some resuscitator bags have a pressure relief valve, a safety feature designed to limit the maximum pressure that can be delivered, thereby preventing gastric insufflation and hyperinflation of the lungs and subsequent pulmonary barotrauma. These valves may malfunction, however, and it must be emphasized that improper venting can cause inadequate ventilation. This can be recognized by the sound of air escaping through the relief valve when the bag is squeezed. Adjusting or partially occluding the valve may be life-saving.

The basic principles governing rescue breathing of pediatric patients are the same as those of adults, although the pediatric airway may be flattened by excessive extension of the cervical spine during the head tilt-chin lift maneuver. In infants and smaller children, mouth-to-nose ventilation may be necessary during CPR. Smaller breaths must be used to avoid abdominal distention, regurgitation, and pulmonary barotrauma. Ventilation in the newborn needs special consideration. Indeed, as already stated, appropriate ventilation is essential for the survival of the newborn infant.

While hypoxia before delivery can influence the time of successful resuscitation of a newborn, it is recommended that adequate ventilation should be assessed immediately and endotracheal intubations should be carried out within 30 to 60 seconds of birth.[276] This time should be reduced to <30 seconds in preterm babies, although no clear literature exists on this situation.[277] Trauma should be avoided by maintaining inflation volume at about 6 ml/kg.[278] Physiologic considerations in the newborn seem to confirm that this volume for resuscitation is probably adequate. It is known that a first breath with use of a medium tidal volume of 5 ml/kg is usually sufficient to achieve a functional residual capacity (FRC) lung volume almost immediately (reaching a total FRC volume of 28 to 30 ml/kg).[279] Furthermore, it is possible that a small tidal volume would stimulate the newborn to breathe spontaneously through a reverse Hering-Breuer reflex (called head paradoxical reflex).[280] This level of tidal volume and a real mask inflation pressure to less than 20 cm H_2O can usually limit gastric inflation.[281,282]

Adjunctive airway equipment

Airway control may be facilitated with the use of adjunctive airway devices. This equipment is generally available to the rescuing paramedics or hospital personnel. It is mandatory that people using these devices be familiar with their use and potential problems. They should be regarded as a "bridge to" rather than "alternate to" endotracheal intubation.

Oxygen source

Oxygen supplementation should be initiated as soon as possible during CPR by the trained rescuer, to avoid the adverse effects of hypoxemia. If oxygen is inadequate, all other resuscitation efforts will fail; 100% oxygen should be utilized during resuscitation. If available, pulse oximeter should be used to determine oxygen saturation.

Oxygen is generally stored either in liquid form or in cylinder reservoirs. A portable oxygen tank is color-coded green in the United States. It is provided with a regulator and flowmeter. The regulator reduces the pressure to 50 psig for delivery to the flowmeter. Most emergency medical technicians carry the smaller E cylinder. This is pressurized to 1800 to 2400 psig at 70 °F and 14.7 psig absolute pressure. The cylinder holds 659 liters of oxygen and lasts about 1 hour when the flow rate is set at 10 liters per minute. Oxygen is considered a "drug," hence its use is regulated by agencies in most states.

Face masks

A pocket facemask is the simplest adjunct beyond mouth-to-mouth resuscitation. An ideal facemask should be colorless to provide direct visualization of the mouth, lips, nose, and the presence of vomitus or secretions. It should have a soft pliable edge to create an effective seal against the face. To assure proper ventilation, an airtight seal is necessary to avoid oxygen and air escaping during supportive ventilation. The mask should provide an oxygen inlet with a standard 15 mm/22 mm coupling size. Various sizes should be available for adults and children. A reservoir bag with a one-way valve may be attached to the mask for manual ventilation of the lungs.

Placement of the face mask is best achieved when the operator is positioned at the top of the patient's head. An airtight seal can be provided by single handed or double handed technique. Single-handed technique requires that the rescuer fits the mask snugly on the victim's face, using the thumb and the index finger in a pincer grip while simultaneously displacing the mandible upward and lifting the chin with the other three fingers. The middle finger should rest on the mandible, the ring finger is positioned midway between the chin and the angle of the jaw, and the little finger is on the mandibular angle. Pressure on the soft tissue should be avoided, because it is uncomfortable and can lift the base of the tongue and cause upper airway obstruction.

Mouth-to-mask ventilation can be achieved by the rescuer sealing his/her lips around the coupling adapter of the mask. If ventilation is inadequate or if airway obstruction is unrelieved, a double-handed technique should be utilized. The fingers are placed on the same position as the single handed method but applied on both sides of the face. However, a second rescuer is necessary to deliver exhaled or manual ventilation. Care must be observed to avoid pressure damage to the eyes and soft tissues.

Manual resuscitators (bag valve devices)

Bag valve devices of various designs are available for adults and children, but a self-inflating, manually operated bag with a non-rebreathing valve is preferable because it allows ventilation even if there is no connecting oxygen supply. This device may be used in conjunction with a face mask, endotracheal tube, or other invasive airway device.

The standard parts include a delivery port with a 15 mm/22 mm adapter coupling size that can be connected to the mask or tracheal tube. It is provided with a one-way, non-jam valve that allows a minimum of 15-liter per minute oxygen flow rate for spontaneous and controlled ventilation. It should also have a system for delivering high oxygen concentration through an auxiliary oxygen inlet at the back of the bag or by an oxygen reservoir. A positive end-expiratory pressure (PEEP) valve can also be incorporated. The bag should be a self-refilling one that can be readily cleaned and sterilized. The bag usually holds a volume of up to 1600 ml. Some pediatric resuscitator bags are provided with a 25 to 30 cm H_2O pop-off valve to avoid excessive positive airway pressure. This device is expected to perform satisfactorily under all common environmental conditions and extremes of temperature.

To operate this equipment properly the operator must be positioned at the top of the victim's head. After correct head positioning as previously described, appropriate tidal volume should be delivered (6 to 7 ml/kg, sufficient to produce visible chest rise) with oxygen supplementation, if available. An oropharyngeal airway may be used to open the mouth. A single rescuer may have difficulty maintaining the head position and delivering adequate tidal volume at the same time. It is therefore recommended that two rescuers operate this device: one to hold an airtight seal over the face, the other to squeeze the bag manually. The proper use of this device requires training, practice, and familiarity with the equipment.

Oxygen-powered manually triggered devices

Oxygen-powered breathing devices have also been used by EMS personnel during CPR. These machines are expensive, and require high oxygen flow rates to overcome air leak.[267] Although they may be able to deliver adequate tidal volumes, oxygen-powered devices carry the risk of gastric distention and regurgitation. Most of these devices are time-cycled and deliver high instantaneous flow rates by a manual control button. They can be used in conjunction with a face mask, endotracheal tube, esophageal airway, or tracheostomy tube.

Parts of an oxygen-powered manually triggered device include a standard 15 mm/22 mm adapter coupling, a compact, rugged, breakable-resistant mechanical design that is easy to hold, and a trigger arranged so that both hands of the rescuer can remain on the face mask to hold it in position. It should also have the following characteristics: a constant flow rate of 100% oxygen at less than 40 liters per minute, and an inspiratory pressure relief valve that opens at approximately 60 cm H_2O and vents any remaining volume to the atmosphere or ceases gas flow. Furthermore, an alarm sound system is provided to alert the rescuer that the pressure relief valve has been activated, indicating that the patient requires high inflationary pressure and may not be receiving adequate tidal volume. It should be able to operate satisfactorily under common environmental conditions and extremes of temperature. It should be provided with a demand flow system that does not impose additional work.[217] These devices are contraindicated in children and spontaneously breathing patients. The potential for complications is high and its use requires training and familiarity.

Suction devices

A suction apparatus is essential during advanced airway support. Suction may be provided by portable battery-operated or electrically powered equipment. In the hospital, wall vacuum outlets are available for suctioning. This device should be available during resuscitation prior to airway instrumentation. Vomitus, secretions, or blood may occlude the airway and can be aspirated into the lungs, compromising the ability to adequately ventilate and oxygenate the victim. In addition to a suction apparatus, a flexible catheter or a rigid tonsillar suction tip should be attached to large bore, non-kinking suction tubing that should be 14 French or greater internal diameter. A rigid tonsillar tip can rapidly suction particulate materials or large volumes of fluid from the pharynx. Flexible catheters are available in various sizes for children and adults and are used to decompress the stomach, suction the esophagus, pharynx, and endotracheal tube.

The wall suction units should provide airflow of more than 30 l/minute at the end of the delivery tube and a vacuum of more than 300 mmHg when the tube is clamped. The suction apparatus should have an adjustable knob to control the amount of suctioning power, especially in children. It must be designed for easy cleaning and subsequent decontamination. Suctioning may damage the teeth and surrounding structures. Prolonged suctioning can cause deoxygenation. It is recommended that the procedure be limited to less than 10 seconds at a time and that the patient receive 100% O_2 in the intervals between suctioning.

Alternative methods of ventilation after successful endotracheal intubation

The relation between airway pressure, intrathoracic pressure, and circulation during CPR has been recently studied.[283] During the decompression phase of CPR, venous return is enhanced. A small inspiratory impedance valve has recently been introduced to occlude the airway selectively during the decompression phase of CPR without interfering with exhalation or active ventilation. The effect of this device on venous return, coronary perfusion pressure, and blood flow during resuscitation has been studied in animals and humans. A remarkable improvement in all of the physiologic parameters usually associated with restoration of spontaneous circulation after defibrillation was demonstrated (end-tidal CO_2, systolic blood pressure, diastolic blood pressure). Furthermore, the beneficial effect of this valve could be seen in models of both protected and unprotected ventilation.[284,285] Remarkably, when the effect of PEEP was combined with negative inspiratory pressure produced with the inspiratory threshold valve (CPAP level up to 10 cm H_2O), the increase in oxygenation was still appreciated with improved respiratory system compliance, but without the detrimental effect on hemodynamics expected with the use of CPAP.[286] Negative pressure pulmonary edema is one possible complication of that and can occur during airway obstruction or an exaggerated Mueller maneuver.[287]

Transport ventilators

Although the introduction of transport ventilators for pre-hospital and hospital care was typically aimed at providing mechanical ventilation in patients with an endotracheal tube in place, some of their features can be used to provide ventilation of the unprotected airway during and after CPR. These devices are typically compact, lightweight, time-cycled or flow-controlled, durable, pneumatically or electronically powered, easy to operate, and low maintenance. An excellent review is available in the literature.[288]

During transport of artificially ventilated patients, automatic transport ventilators (ATVs) are found to be superior at maintaining constant minute ventilation and adequate arterial blood gases when compared with BVM devices.[289] Advantages of ATVs include allowing the rescuer to do other tasks when the patient is intubated, and allowing the rescuer to use both hands to hold the mask in patients not intubated. The rescuer can also perform the Sellick maneuver with one hand while holding the mask in the other hand. ATVs can provide a specific tidal volume, respiratory rate, and minute ventilation.

It is recommended that ATVs should function as constant inspiratory flow rate generators and should have the following features: (1) a lightweight connector with a standard 15 mm/22mm adapter coupling for a mask, endotracheal tube, or other airway adjunct; (2) a lightweight (2 to 5 kg) compact, rugged design; (3) capability of operating under all common environmental conditions and extremes of temperatures; (4) a peak inspiratory pressure limiting valve set at 60 cm H_2O with an option of an 80 cm H_2O pressure that is easily accessible to the user; (5) an audible alarm that sounds when the peak inspiratory limiting pressure is generated to alert the rescuer that low compliance or high airway resistance is resulting in a diminished tidal volume delivery; (6) minimal gas consumption allowing the device to run for a minimum of 45 minutes on an E cylinder; (7) minimal gas compression volume in the breathing circuit; (8) ability to deliver 100% oxygen; (9) an inspiratory time of 1 second , and maximal inspiratory flow rates of approximately 30 l/minute in adults and 15 l/ minute in children; (10) at least two rates, 10 breaths/minute for adults and 20 breaths/minute in children. If a demand flow valve is incorporated, it should deliver a peak inspiratory flow rate on demand of at least 100 l/minute at -2 cm H_2O triggering pressure to minimize the work of breathing.[217] Additional desirable features include a pressure gauge, provision for continuous positive airway pressure, controls for rate and tidal volume, and low pressure alarms to indicate low oxygen pressure either from disconnection or depletion of the gas source. Theoretically, both time or flow cycle transport ventilators can replace BVM ventilation during CPR. One particular model, the Ohmeda HARV or pneuPAC 2-R (Ohmeda Emergency Care, Orchard Park, NY), is commercially available for either transport ventilation or assisted mask ventilation. HARV produces a rectangular flow waveform that is time-triggered, flow- or pressure-limited, and time-cycled. A single control sets one of seven rate/tidal volume combinations.[288]

Mechanically operated mask ventilation undoubtedly presents advantages during CPR, because it frees the resuscitator's hand that typically is involved in squeezing the bag. The use of a pressure-powered mechanical ventilator that operates from an external pneumatic source (wall pressured oxygen or portable oxygen tank) also has the advantages of providing constant tidal volume, flow rate, inspiratory time, and ventilation rate, once it is set. These devices may help to reduce the frequency of hyperventilation that is associated with manual bag resuscitators.

Monitoring ventilation during CPR

End-tidal carbon dioxide as a tool for monitoring the progress of CPR

A number of studies have shown that end-tidal CO_2 varies directly with cardiac output during cardiac arrest,[47,290–292] provides a useful indicator of the efficacy of resuscitation efforts, and also predicts outcome.[293–301] The presence of end-tidal CO_2 has been investigated as a guide to correct placement of endotracheal intubation.[302–305] Additionally, capnography has been used in resuscitation research as an indication of pulmonary blood flow, which serves as a proxy for the direct measurement of cardiac output.[306–309]

Aerobic and anaerobic cellular metabolism generate CO_2, which diffuses out of the cell into tissue capillaries, and is transported to the lungs, exhaled, and can be measured as end-tidal CO_2.[310,311] Under normal conditions, end-tidal CO_2 is 2 to 5 mmHg less than the $PaCO_2$. Systemic metabolism changes little during CPR, which is usually relatively brief, although ischemic hypoxia can alter the respiratory quotient.[312,314] The concentration of exhaled CO_2 changes when blood flow to the lungs changes and is an indirect indicator of cardiac output and systemic blood flow. Under conditions of constant minute ventilation, end-tidal CO_2 is linearly related to cardiac output, even during extremely low blood flow rates (Fig. 28.14).[313] The decrease in end-tidal CO_2 parallels closely the decrease in $PaCO_2$ that occurs when blood flow decreases, and is therefore useful clinically as a monitor of perfusion during shock and CPR. End-tidal CO_2 changes rapidly with changes in flow, changing one breath after a change in perfusion and almost reaching a new steady state within 30 seconds (Fig. 28.15). After administration of epinephrine, however, the prior relationships of end-tidal CO_2 may be altered because of the changes in pulmonary and peripheral vascular resistance and preferential redirection of blood flow.[302] In some instances, epinephrine may cause decreased pulmonary blood flow and end-tidal CO_2, while at the same time coronary perfusion pressure increases because of increased peripheral vascular resistance (Fig. 28.16).[314]

During the past two decades, there has been great interest in the physiology of end-tidal CO_2, especially in low blood flow states. The primary reason for this interest is the difficulty in directly measuring low rates of blood flow, particularly during human cardiac arrest. Because it is much easier to measure, end-tidal CO_2 has been used as an indicator of pulmonary blood flow, which serves as a proxy or substitute for the direct measurement of cardiac output.

In animal models of cardiac arrest and resuscitation, end-tidal CO_2 has been shown to vary directly with cardiac output.[47,290,291] Coronary artery perfusion pressure, one of the best prognostic indicators of survival in cardiac arrest,[315] correlates closely with end-tidal CO_2.[297,298] For example, end-tidal CO_2 was higher during CPR in 17 animals that survived when compared to five animals that failed resuscitation.[292] Thus, end-tidal CO_2 is correlated with blood flow and successful resuscitation from cardiac arrest.

Investigators have used end-tidal CO_2 as a substitute for the measurement of blood flow in studies of CPR techniques.[306,309] End-tidal CO_2 levels were found to increase when greater force was applied during external chest compression force in humans,[306] while changes in compression rate had little effect on end-tidal CO_2.[307] Because end-tidal CO_2 is directly related to cardiac output when minute ventilation is held constant, it is a useful tool in CPR research as a substitute for the direct measurement of cardiac output. Because lack of end tidal CO_2 may simply represent inefficient chest compression during CPR, however, new devices have been introduced to confirm endotracheal intubation in a setting of cardiac arrest. A suction bulb and a large syringe, both with standard fitting

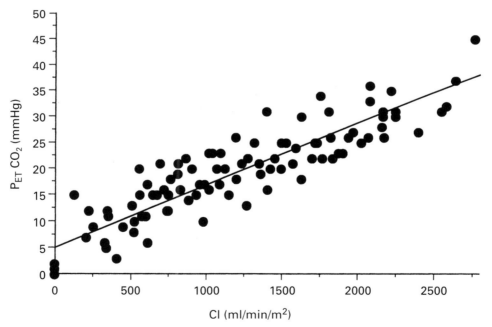

Fig. 28.14. The relationship of the partial pressure of end-tidal carbon dioxide (P_aCO_2) to cardiac index (*CI*) under conditions of constant minute ventilation (r – 0.82, *P* < 0001) in swine (n – 10) on biventricular bypass devices. (From ref.315.)

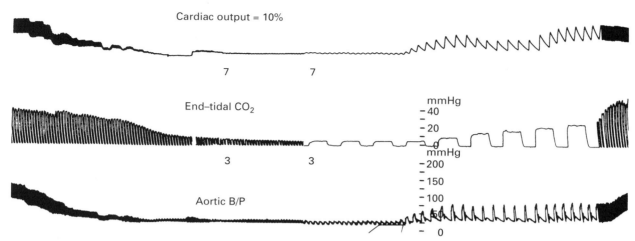

Fig. 28.15. End-tidal CO_2 (mmHg) blood flow (produced with biventricular bypass devices; cardiac output measured with a magnetic flow probe expressed as a percent of baseline; and aortic blood pressure (B/P) mmHg rate calf (125 kg). Blood flow in a rate was reduced to 10% of baseline and then back to baseline. The second half of the recording was made at a higher speed. Original data from A.H. Idris.

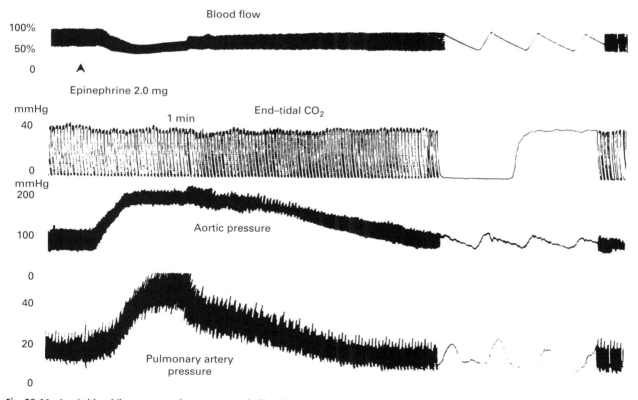

Fig. 28.16. Aortic blood flow expressed as a percent of of baseline, end-tidal CO_2 (mmHg), aortic pressure (mmHg), and pulmonary artery pressure (mmHg) in a calf (125 kg) with blood flow produced by biventricular assist devices. Epinephrine 2.0 mg was given (*arroic*) through the proximal port of the pulmonary artery catheter. Both aortic and pulmonary artery pressures increased dramatically following administration of epinephrine, probably because of increased pulmonary and peripheral vascular resistance. At the same time, aortic blood flow decreased transiently, probably because of decreased pulmonary blood flow, decreased return of blood to the left ventricular assist device, and increased peripheral vascular resistance. End-tidal CO_2 decreased approximately 5 mmHg after epinephrine. (Original data from AH Idris.)

for an endotracheal tube adaptor have been used to recognize the tracheal versus a "virtual and collapsible lumen" represented by the esophagus. At the time of this writing, the sensitivity and specificity of these devices during CPR have not been well established.[316]

Several studies of end-tidal CO_2 during low blood flow states found that levels changed significantly with changes in minute ventilation.[28,317] When minute ventilation doubled, end-tidal CO_2 decreased 50% and when minute ventilation decreased 50%, end-tidal CO_2 doubled. Thus, end-tidal CO_2 varies inversely with minute ventilation and can be used to monitor ventilation during low flow conditions. If both perfusion and ventilation are not constant, end-tidal CO_2 levels can be difficult to interpret.

The use of arterial and central venous blood gases during CPR

It has been a longstanding practice to use arterial blood pH, PO_2, PCO_2, and HCO_3 to monitor ventilation and to guide therapeutic interventions for abnormalities in acid–base conditions during CPR.[217] While $PaCO_2$ and PaO_2 are useful for monitoring pulmonary ventilation, there is mounting evidence that arterial blood may not reliably reflect tissue acid–base conditions during low blood flow states and that central venous blood more accurately reflects conditions at the tissue level.

One study showed that after 5 minutes of untreated ventricular fibrillation, arterial and mixed venous blood gases remained nearly unchanged from baseline pre-arrest values.[173] Only the PaO_2 decreased by 10 mmHg, but it was still within the normal range. This demonstrates an important relationship among blood flow, tissue perfusion, and acid–base conditions. Blood that is contained within the large arteries under no-flow conditions is static and does not reflect ongoing intracellular metabolism until some perfusion is restored so that blood at the tissue level is mobilized back into circulation. Thus, if blood flow is sufficiently low, pHa, PaO_2, and $PaCO_2$ might remain "normal" for a prolonged period of time. Moreover, if ventilation is held constant, pHa and PaO_2 will increase and $PaCO_2$ will decrease as perfusion becomes worse.[56]

A number of investigations support the view that pHa and $PaCO_2$ can be used for monitoring the effectiveness of resuscitation efforts during cardiac arrest.[28,56,318,319] Arterial PCO_2 has been shown to correlate closely with cardiac output and coronary perfusion pressure, which is known to be a good predictor of success of resuscitation. Nevertheless, changes must be interpreted differently from those in conventional practice: when perfusion improves, arterial blood becomes more acidic, $PaCO_2$ increases, and PaO_2 may decrease; when perfusion becomes worse, arterial blood becomes more alkalemic, $PaCO_2$ decreases, and PaO_2 increases.[28,66,318]

In addition, the timing of blood sampling is another variable that must be considered. If arterial blood gases are measured during CPR within 8 minutes of cardiac arrest, pH is usually normal or alkaline because significant metabolic acidosis has not yet developed and $PaCO_2$ is lower than normal. As the duration of CPR progresses, increasing blood lactate and decreasing bicarbonate concentrations ultimately cause an acidemic arterial pH.[67] Administration of sodium bicarbonate, which has been shown to cause an increased pHa and $PaCO_2$, must also be considered when interpreting blood gases.[59,68]

Another important consideration when using arterial blood gases is that $PaCO_2$ and PaO_2 values respond quickly to changes in minute ventilation. In one study, $PaCO_2$ increased by approximately 85% when minute ventilation was decreased to 25% of the previous setting; similar changes were observed with blood flow rates as low as 12% of normal.[28] Therefore, arterial blood gas analysis can be used to assess perfusion when minute ventilation is held constant, or to assess minute ventilation when perfusion is held constant. When both perfusion and minute ventilation are uncontrolled, it is difficult to interpret arterial blood gases.

Mixed venous pH, PO_2, and PCO_2 are more useful than arterial gases for assessing acid–base status and perfusion during low flow states because they more closely reflect the tissue environment.[13,46,55,56,62,64,70,320] One study of hemorrhagic shock showed that mixed venous oxygen saturation averaged 46% in survivors and only 25% in nonsurvivors;[183] others have found a similar relationship.[321,322] A study of human cardiac arrest found that mixed venous oxygen saturation was associated with prognosis for survival and mixed venous pH, PO_2, and PCO_2 measured during cardiac arrest was substantially better in those who ultimately had return of spontaneous circulation.[44] Additionally, mixed venous blood gases are more useful than arterial blood gases for assessing perfusion during CPR, because they are much less affected than arterial gases by changes in minute ventilation.[28] Because of the great difficulty in obtaining mixed venous blood samples during CPR, other venous sites may be used as a substitute. Evidence exists that central, femoral, intraosseous, and mixed venous blood gas values are very similar, even during prolonged cardiac arrest and CPR.[323–325]

In summary, $PaCO_2$, mixed venous pH and PO_2, and end-tidal CO_2 vary directly with blood flow, while mixed venous PCO_2 varies inversely with blood flow. Arterial PO_2 and pH vary directly with minute ventilation, while arterial and mixed venous PCO_2 vary inversely with minute ventilation. Both arterial and mixed venous blood gases are useful for assessing the efficacy of resuscitation efforts. Arterial PO_2 and PCO_2 are most useful for assessing the adequacy of ventilation, whereas mixed venous PO_2 and PCO_2 are most useful for assessing the adequacy of circulation. At the present time, there are no conclusive data that allow recommendations on how frequently arterial or venous gases should be monitored during resuscitation.

Conclusions

During normal cardiac activity, ventilation serves to remove CO_2 from and provide oxygen to tissues. The effect of ventilation on tissues continues even during low flow states, although its ability to provide oxygen and remove CO_2 is diminished and limited by blood flow. Ventilation during the first few minutes of dysrhythmic adult cardiac arrest has been somewhat de-emphasized in favor of more effective chest compression. Manual techniques of ventilation have a number of advantages over mouth-to-mouth ventilation, including safety from transmission of infectious diseases and a superior ventilation gas (i.e., room air). If obstruction of the airway could be prevented, manual ventilation may be a useful alternative and should be studied. In addition, chest compression alone can provide some ventilation, provided that the upper airway is unobstructed. The relationship between ventilation mechanics and circulation has been studied in cardiac arrest and hemorrhagic shock. Rescuers often inadvertently use excessively high ventilation rates. Studies have found that positive pressure ventilation may decrease blood flow by decreasing venous return to the heart. Excessive ventilation has a detrimental effect in cardiac arrest, shock, and traumatic brain injury and should be avoided. Since 2005, lower ventilation rates are now recommended.

Chest compression alone may be effective for the first few minutes of witnessed sudden cardiac arrest. This would certainly be an advantage because chest compression without ventilation could be more easily mastered by lay CPR providers and there would be less hesitation in providing bystander chest compression without mouth-to-mouth ventilation. Although the few studies of ventilation and its effect on outcome from cardiac arrest in humans are promising, they are inconclusive. The issues surrounding ventilation in resuscitation are critical and involve more than 300 000 cardiac patients per year in United States, and even more victims of severe traumatic injury. The scientific community must respond to this challenge with a targeted, multidisciplinary research effort.

REFERENCES

1. Hlastala, M.P. Ventilation. In Crystal, R.G. & West, J.B. (eds). *The Lung: Scientific Foundations*, New York: Raven Press, 1991: 1209–1214.
2. Cobb, L.A., Eliastam, M., Kerber, R.E. *et al.* Report of the American Heart Association task force on the future of cardiopulmonary resuscitation. *Circulation* 1992; **85**: 2346–2355.
3. Berg, R.A., Kern, K.B., Sanders, A.B., Otto, C.W., Hilwig, R.W. & Ewy, G.A. Bystander cardiopulmonary resuscitation: is ventilation necessary? *Circulation* 1993; **88**: 1907–1915.
4. Chandra, N.C., Gruben, K.G., Tsitlik, J.E., Guerci, A.D., Permutt, S. & Weisfeldt, M.L. Observations of ventilation during resuscitation in a canine model. *Circulation* 1994; **90**(6): 3070–3075.
5. Weil, M.H., Sun, S., Bisera, J., Tang, W. & Gazmuri, R.J. Challenge to the ABCs of cardiopulmonary resuscitation. *Chest* 1992; **102**: 127S.
6. Wenzel, V., Idris, A.H., Banner, M.J., Fuerst, R.S. & Tucker, K.J. The composition of gas given by mouth-to-mouth ventilation during CPR. *Chest* 1994; **106**(6): 1806–1810.
7. *The Bible*, II. Kings, **4**: 32–35.
8. DeBard, M.L. The history of cardiopulmonary resuscitation. *Ann. Emerg. Med.* 1980; **9**: 273–275.
9. Hermreck, A.S. The history of CPR. *Am. J. Surg.* 1988; **156**: 430–436.
10. Elam, J.O., Brown, E.S. & Elder, J.D. Jr. Artificial respiration by mouth-to-mask method: a study of the respiratory gas exchange of paralyzed patients ventilated by operator's expired air. *N. Engl. J. Med.* 1954; **250**: 749–754.
11. Safar, P. History of cardiopulmonary–cerebral resuscitation. In Kaye, W. & Bircher, N., ed. *Cardiopulmonary Resuscitation*. New York: Churchill Livingstone, 1989: 1–53.
12. Boehm, R. Ueber wiederbelebung nach vergiftungen and asphyxie. *Arch. Exp. Pathol. Pharmakol.* 1878; **8**: 68–101.
13. Johnson, B.A. & Weil, M.H. Redefining ischemia due to circulatory failure as dual defects of oxygen deficits and of carbon dioxide excesses. *Crit. Care Med.* 1991; **19**: 1432–1438.
14. Safar, P. Failure of manual respiration. *J. Appl. Physiol.* 1959; **14**: 84–88.
15. Safar, P., Brown, T.C., Holtey, W.J. & Wilder, R.J. Ventilation and circulation with closed-chest cardiac massage in man. *J. Am. Med. Assoc.* 1961; **176**: 574–576.
16. Safar, P., Escarraga, L.A. & Elam, J.O. A comparison of the mouth-to-mouth and mouth-to-airway methods of artificial respiration with the chest-pressure arm-lift methods. *N. Engl. J. Med.* 1958; **258**: 671–677.
17. Don, H.F. & Robson, J.G. The mechanics of the respiratory system during anesthesia: the effects of atropine and carbon dioxide. *Anesthesiology* 1965; **26**: 168–178.
18. Severinghaus, J.W., Swenson, E.W., Finley, T.N., Lategola, M.T. & Williams, J. Unilateral hypoventilation produced in dogs by occluding one pulmonary artery. *J. Appl. Physiol.* 1961; **16**: 53–60.

19. Nadel, J.A. & Widdicombe, J.G. Effect of changes in blood gas tensions and carotid sinus pressure on tracheal volume and total lung resistance to airflow. *J. Physiol. (Lond.)* 1962; **163**: 13–33.

20. Severinghaus, J.W. & Stupfel, M. Respiratory dead space increase following atropine in man, and atropine, vagal or ganglionic blockade and hypothermia in dogs. *J. Appl. Physiol.* 1955; **8**: 81–87.

21. Daly, M. de Burgh, Lambertsen, C.J. & Schweitzer, A. The effects upon the bronchial musculature of altering the O_2 and CO_2 tension in the blood perfusing the brain. *J. Physiol. (Lond.)* 1953; **119**: 292–314.

22. Parker, J.C., Peters, R.M. & Barnett, T.B. Carbon dioxide and the work of breathing. *J. Clin. Invest.* 1963; **42**: 1362–1372.

23. Scanlon, T.S., Benumof, J.L., Wahrenbrock, E.A. & Nelson, W.L. Hypoxic pulmonary vasoconstriction and the ratio of hypoxic lung to perfused normoxic lung. *Anesthesiology* 1978; **49**: 177–181.

24. Rodman, D.M. & Voelkel, N.F. Regulation of vascular tone. In Crystal, R.G. & West, J.B. (eds). *The Lung: Scientific Foundations*, New York: Raven Press, 1991: 1105–1119.

25. Marshall, B.E. & Marshall, C. Pulmonary hypertension. In Crystal, R.G. & West, J.B. (eds). *The Lung: Scientific Foundations*, New York: Raven Press, 1991: 1177–1187.

26. Benumof, J.L. & Wahrenbrock, E.A. Blunted hypoxic pulmonary vasoconstriction by increased lung vascular pressures. *J. Appl. Physiol.* 1975; **38**: 846–850.

27. West, J.B. *Respiratory Physiology. The Essentials*. Baltimore: Williams and Wilkins, 1974: 57–60.

28. Idris, A.H., Staples, E., O'Brian, D.J. *et al.* The effect of ventilation on acid-base balance and oxygenation in low blood-flow states. *Crit. Care Med.* 1994; **22**(11): 1827–1834.

29. Abdelmoneim, T., Kissoon, N., Johnson, L. *et al.* Acid–base status of blood from intraosseous and mixed venous sites during prolonged cardiopulmonary resuscitation and drug infusions. *Crit. Care Med.* 1999; **27**(9): 1923–1928.

30. Perutz, M.F. Hemoglobin structure and respiratory transport. *Sci. Am.* December, 1978; **239**(6): 92–125.

31. Christiansen, J., Douglas, C.G. & Haldane, J.S. The absorption of carbon dioxide by human blood. *J. Physiol.* 1914; **48**: 244–277.

32. Klocke, R.A. Mechanisms and kinetics of the Haldane effect in human erythrocytes. *J. Appl. Physiol.* 1973; **35**: 673–681.

33. Perella, M., Kilmartin, J.V., Fogg, J. & Rossi-Bernardi, L. Identification of the high and low affinity CO_2-binding sites of human hemoglobin. *Nature* 1975; **256**: 759–761.

34. Arnone, A. X-ray studies of the interaction of CO_2 with human deoxyhaemoglobin. *Nature* 1974; **247**: 143–145.

35. Kilmartin, J.V. & Rossi-Bernardi, L. Interaction of hemoglobin with hydrogen ions, carbon dioxide, and organic phosphates. *Physiol. Rev.* 1973; **53**: 836–890.

36. Klocke, R.A. Carbon dioxide, In Crystal, R.G. & West, J.B. (eds). *The Lung: Scientific Foundations*, New York: Raven Press, 1991: 1233–1239.

37. Bersin, R.M. & Arieff, A.I. Improved hemodynamic function during hypoxia with carbicarb, a new agent for the management of acidosis. *Circulation* 1988; **77**: 227–233.

38. Ducey, J.P., Lamiell, J.M. & Gueller, G.E. Arterial–venous carbon dioxide tension difference during severe hemorrhage and resuscitation. *Crit. Care Med.* 1992; **20**: 518–522.

39. Dunham, C.M., Siegal, J.H., Weireter, L. *et al.* Oxygen debt and metabolic acidemia as quantitative predictors of mortality and the severity of the ischemic insult in hemorrhagic shock. *Crit. Care Med.* 1991; **19**: 231–243.

40. Graf, H., Leach, W. & Arieff, A.I. Evidence for a detrimental effect of bicarbonate therapy in hypoxic lactic acidosis. *Science* 1984; **227**: 754–756.

41. Graf, H., Leach, W. & Arieff, A.I. Effects of dichloroacetate in the treatment of hypoxic lactic acidosis in dogs. *J. Clin. Invest.* 1985; **76**: 919–923.

42. Romeh, S.A. & Tannen, R.L. Therapeutic benefit of dichloroacetate in experimentally induced hypoxic lactic acidosis. *J. Lab. Clin. Med.* 1986; **107**: 378–383.

43. Niemann, J.T., Criley, J.M., Rosborough, J.P., Niskanen, R.A. & Alferness, C. Predictive indices of successful cardiac resuscitation after prolonged arrest and experimental cardiopulmonary resuscitation. *Ann. Emerg. Med.* 1985; **14**: 521–528.

44. Rivers, E.P., Martin, G.B., Smithline, H. *et al.* The clinical implications of continuous central venous oxygen saturation during human CPR. *Ann. Emerg. Med.* 1992; **21**: 1094–1101.

45. Steinhart, C.R., Permutt, S., Gurtner, G.H. & Traystman, R.J. B-Adrenergic activity and cardiovascular response to severe respiratory acidosis. *Am. J. Physiol.* 1983; **244**(*Heart Circ. Physiol.* 13): H46–H54.

46. von Planta, I., Weil, M.H., von Planta, M., Gazmuri, R.J. & Duggal, C. Hypercarbic acidosis reduces cardiac resuscitability. *Crit. Care Med.* 1991; **19**: 1177–1182.

47. Weil, M.H., Ruiz, C.E., Michaels, S. & Rackow, E.C. Acid–base determinants of survival after cardiopulmonary resuscitation. *Crit. Care Med.* 1985; **13**: 888–892.

48. Yakaitis, R.W., Thomas, J.D. & Mahaffey, J.E. Influence of pH and hypoxia on the success of defibrillation. *Crit. Care Med.* 1975; **3**: 139–142.

49. Cingolani, H.F., Faulkner, S.L., Mattiazzi, A.R., Bender, H.W. & Graham, T.P. Jr. Depression of human myocardial contractility with "respiratory" and "metabolic" acidosis. *Surgery* 1975; **77**: 427–432.

50. Downing, S.E., Talner, N.S. & Gardner, T.H. Cardiovascular responses to metabolic acidosis. *Am. J. Physiol.* 1965; **208**: 237–242.

51. Poole-Wilson, P.A. Is early decline of cardiac function in ischaemia due to carbon dioxide retention? *Lancet* 1975; **ii**: 1285–1287.

52. Tang, W., Weil, M.H., Gazmuri, R.J., Bisera, J. & Rackow, E.C. Reversible impairment of myocardial contractility due to hypercarbic acidosis in the isolated perfused rat heart. *Crit. Care Med.* 1991; **19**: 218–224.

53. Weisfeldt, M.L., Bishop, R.L. & Greene, H.L. Effects of pH and pCO_2 on performance of ischemic myocardium. In Roy, P.E. &

Rona, G., eds. *The Metabolism of Contraction. Recent Advances in Studies on Cardiac Structure and Metabolism.*, vol. 10. Baltimore: University Park Press, 1975: 355–364.

54. Kerber, R.E. & Sarnat, W. Factors influencing the success of ventricular defibrillation in man. *Circulation* 1979; **60**: 226–230.

55. Tang, W., Weil, M.H., Maldonado, F.A., Gazmuri, R.J. & Bisera, J. Hypercarbia decreases the effectiveness of electrical defibrillation during CPR. *Crit. Care Med.* 1992; **20** (Suppl.): S24.

56. Angelos, M.G., DeBehnke, D.J. & Leasure, J.E. Arterial pH and carbon dioxide tension as indicators of tissue perfusion during cardiac arrest in a canine model. *Crit. Care Med.* 1992; **20**: 1302–1308.

57. Benjamin, E., Paluch, T.A., Berger, S.R., Premus, G., Wu, C. & Iberti, T.J. Venous hypercarbia in canine hemorrhagic shock. *Crit. Care Med.* 1987; **15**: 516–518.

58. Beyar, R., Kishon, Y., Kimmel, E., Sideman, S. & Dinnar, U. Blood gas and acid–base balance during cardiopulmonary resuscitation by intrathoracic and abdominal pressure variations. *Basic Res. Cardiol.* 1986; **81**: 326–333.

59. Bishop, R.L. & Weisfeldt, M.L. Sodium bicarbonate administration during cardiac arrest. *J. Am. Med. Assoc.* 1976; **235**: 506–509.

60. Fillmore, S.J., Shapiro, M. & Killip, T. Serial blood gas studies during cardiopulmonary resuscitation. *Ann. Intern. Med.* 1970; **72**: 465–469.

61. Greenwood, P.V., Rossall, R.E. & Kappagoda, C.T. Acid–base changes aftercardiorespiratory arrest in the dog. *Clin. Sci.* 1980; **58**: 127–133.

62. Grundler, W., Weil, M.H. & Rackow, E.C. Arteriovenous carbon dioxide and pH gradients during cardiac arrest. *Circulation* 1986; **74**: 1071–1074.

63. Martin, G.B., Carden, D.L., Nowak, R.M. & Tomlanovich, M.C. Comparison of central venous and arterial pH and PCO_2 during open-chest CPR in the canine model. *Ann. Emerg. Med.* 1985; **14**: 529–533.

64. Nowak, R.M., Martin, G.B., Carden, D.L. & Tomlanovich, M.C. Selective venous hypercarbia during CPR. Implications regarding blood flow. *Ann. Emerg. Med.* 1987; **16**: 527–530.

65. Ornato, J.P., Gonzalez, E.R., Coyne, M.R., Beck, C.L. & Collins, C.L. Arterial pH in out-of-hospital cardiac arrest. Response time as a determinant of acidosis. *Am. J. Emerg. Med.* 1985; **3**: 498–501.

66. Ralston, S.H., Voorhees, W.D., Showen, L., Schmitz, P., Kougias, C. & Tacker, W.A. Venous and arterial blood gases during and after cardiopulmonary resuscitation in dogs. *Am. J. Emerg. Med.* 1985; **3**: 132–136.

67. Sanders, A.B., Ewy, G.A. & Taft, T.V. Resuscitation and arterial blood gas abnormalities during prolonged cardiopulmonary resuscitation. *Ann. Emerg. Med.* 1984 (part 1); **13**: 676–679.

68. Sanders, A.B., Otto, C.W., Kern, K.B., Rogers, J.N., Perrault, P. & Ewy, G.A. Acid–base balance in a canine model of cardiac arrest. *Ann. Emerg. Med.* 1988; **17**: 667–671.

69. Weil, M.H., Grundler, W., Yamaguchi, M., Michaels, S. & Rackow, E.C. Arterial blood gases fail to reflect acid–base status during cardiopulmonary resuscitation. A Preliminary report. *Crit. Care Med.* 1985; **13**: 884–885.

70. Weil, M.H., Rackow, E.C., Trevino, R., Grundler, W., Falk, J.L. & Griffel, M.I. Difference in acid–base state between venous and arterial blood during cardiopulmonary resuscitation. *N. Engl. J. Med.* 1986; **315**: 153–156.

71. Weil, M.H., von Planta, M., Gazmuri, R.J. & Rackow, E.C. Incomplete global ischemia during cardiac arrest and resuscitation. *Crit. Care Med.* 1988; **16**: 997–1001.

72. Langhelle, A., Sunde, K., Wik, L. *et al.* Arterial blood gases with 500-versus 1000-mL tidal volumes during out-of-hospital CPR. *Resus* 2000; **45**: 27–33.

73. Johnson, B.A., Maldonado, F., Weil, M.H. & Tang, W. Venoarterial carbon dioxide gradients during shock obey a modified Fick relationship. *Crit. Care Med.* 1992; **20**(Suppl.): S91.

74. von Planta, M., Weil, M.H., Gazmuri, R.J., Bisera, J. & Rackow, E.C. Myocardial acidosis associated with CO_2 production during cardiac arrest and resuscitation. *Circulation* 1989; **80**: 684–692.

75. Weil, M.H., Grundler, W., Rackow, E.C., Bisera, J., Miller, J.M. & Michaels, S. Blood gas measurements in human patients during CPR. *Chest* 1984; **86**: 282.

76. Szekeres, L. & Papp, G.Y. Effect of arterial hypoxia on the susceptibility to arrhythmia of the heart. *Acta Physiol. Academ. Scientiarum Hungaricae* 1967; **32**: 143–161.

77. Ayres, S.M. & Grace, W.J. Inappropriate ventilation and hypoxemia as causes of cardiac arrhythmias. *Am. J. Med.* 1969; **46**: 495–505.

78. Burn, J.H. & Hukovic, S. Anoxia and ventricular fibrillation; with a summary of evidence on the cause of fibrillation. *Br. J. Pharmacol.* 1960; **15**: 67–70.

79. Dong, E., Jr. Stinson, E.B. & Shumway, N.E. The ventricular fibrillation threshold in respiratory acidosis and alkalosis. *Surgery* 1967; **61**: 602–607.

80. Turnbull, A.D., MacLean, L.D., Dobell, A.R.C. & Demers, R. The influence of hyperbaric oxygen and of hypoxia on the ventricular fibrillation threshold. *J. Thorac. Cardiovasc. Surg.* 1965; **6**: 842–848.

81. Kerber, R.E., Pandian, N.G., Hoyt, R. *et al.* Effect of ischemia, hypertrophy, hypoxia, acidosis, and alkalosis on canine defibrillation. *Am. J. Physiol.* 1983; **244**(*Heart Circ. Physiol* 13): H825–H831.

82. Guerci, A.D., Chandra, N., Johnson, E. *et al.* Failure of sodium bicarbonate to improve resuscitation from ventricular fibrillation in dogs. *Circulation* 1986; **74** (Suppl IV): 75–79.

83. Gerst, P.H., Fleming, W.H. & Malm, J.R. Increased susceptibility of the heart to ventricular fibrillation during metabolic acidosis. *Circ. Res.* 1966; **19**: 63–70.

84. von Planta, M., Gudipati, C., Weil, M.H., Kraus, L.J. & Rackow, E.C. Effects of tromethamine and sodium bicarbonate buffers during cardiac resuscitation. *J. Clin. Pharmacol.* 1988; **28**: 594–599.

85. Gazmuri, R.J., von Planta, M., Weil, M.H. & Rackow, E.C. Cardiac effects of carbon dioxide-consuming and carbon

dioxide-generating buffers during cardiac resuscitation. *J. Am. Coll. Cardiol.* 1990; **15**: 482–490.

86. Kette, F., Weil, M.H., von Planta, M., Gazmuri, R.J. & Rackow, E.C. Buffer agents do not reverse intramyocardial acidosis during cardiac resuscitation. *Circulation* 1990; **81**: 1660–1666.

87. Federiuk, C.S., Sanders, A.B., Kern, K.B., Nelson, J. & Ewy, G.A. The effect of bicarbonate on resuscitation from cardiac arrest. *Ann. Emerg. Med.* 1991; **20**: 1173–1177.

88. Kette, F., Weil, M.H. & Gazmuri, R.J. Buffer solutions may compromise cardiac resuscitation by reducing coronary perfusion pressure. *J. Am. Med. Assoc.* 1991; **266**: 2121–2126.

89. Goldstein, B., Shannon, D.C. & Todres, I.D. Supercarbia in children: clinical course and outcome. *Crit. Care Med.* 1990; **18**: 166–168.

90. Holmdahl, M.H. Pulmonary uptake of oxygen, acid–base metabolism, and circulation during prolonged apnea. *Acta Chir. Scand.* 1956; **212**(Suppl): 108.

91. Graham, G.R., Hill, D.W. & Nunn, S.F. Supercarbia in the anesthetized dog. *Nature* 1959; **184**: 1071–1072.

92. Clowes, G.H.A., Hopkins, A.L. & Simeone, F.A. A comparison of the physiological effects of hypercapnia and hypoxia in the production of cardiac arrest. *Ann. Surg.* 1955; **142**: 446–460.

93. Litt, L.O., Gonzalez-Mendez, R., Severinghaus, J.W. *et al.* Cerebral intracellular changes during supercarbia: an in vivo 31P nuclear magnetic resonance study in rats. *J. Cereb. Blood Flow Metab.* 1985; **5**: 537–544.

94. Winkle, R.A., Mead, R.H., Ruder, M.A., Smith, N.A., Buch, W.S. & Gaudiani, V.A. Effect of duration of ventricular fibrillation on defibrillation efficacy in humans. *Circulation* 1990; **81**: 1477–1481.

95. Larsen, M.P., Eisenberg, M.S., Cummins, R.O. & Hallstrom, A.P. Predicting survival from out-of-hospital cardiac arrest: a graphic model. *Ann. Emerg. Med.* 1993; **22**: 1652–1658.

96. Valenzuala, T.D., Roe, D.J., Cretin, S., Spaite, D.W. & Larsen, M.P. Estimating effectiveness of cardiac arrest interventions: a logistic regression survival model. *Circulation* 1997; **96**: 3308–3313.

97. Sanders, A.B., Kern, K.B., Atlas, M., Bragg, S. & Ewy, G.A. Importance of the duration of inadequate coronary perfusion pressure on resuscitation from cardiac arrest. *J. Am. Coll. Cardiol.* 1985; **6**: 113–118.

98. Yakaitis, R.W., Ewy, G.A., Otto, C.W., Taren, D.L. & Moon, T.E. Influence of time and therapy on ventricular defibrillation in dogs. *Crit. Care Med.* 1980; **8**: 157–163.

99. Brown, C.G., Dzwonczyk, R., Werman, H.A. & Hamlin, R.L. Estimating the duration of ventricular fibrillation. *Ann. Emerg. Med.* 1989; **18**: 1181–1185.

100. Kern, K.B., Garewal, H.S., Sanders, A.B. *et al.* Depletion of myocardial adenosine triphosphate during prolonged untreated ventricular fibrillation: effect on defibrillation success. *Resus* 1990; **20**: 221–229.

101. von Planta, M., Weil, M.H., Gazmuri, R.J. & Rackow, E.C. Myocardial potassium uptake during experimental cardiopulmonary resuscitation. *Crit. Care Med.* 1989; **17**: 895–899.

102. Babbs, C.F., Whistler, S.J., Yim, G.K.W., Tacker, W.A. & Geddes, L.A. Dependence of defibrillation threshold upon extracellular/intracellular K^+ concentrations. *J. Electrocardiol.* 1980; **13**: 73–78.

103. Gremels, H. & Starling, E.H. On the influence of hydrogen ion concentration and of anoxaemia upon the heart volume. *J. Physiol. (Lond.)* 1926; **61**: 297–304.

104. Jacobus, W.E., Pores, I.H., Lucas, S.K., Weisfeldt, M.L. & Flaherty, J.T. Intracellular acidosis and contractility in the normal and ischemic heart as examined by ^{31}PNMR. *J. Mol. Cell. Cardiol.* 1982; **14**(Supp 3): 13–20.

105. Monroe, R.G., French, G. & Whittenberger, J.L. Effects of hypocapnia and hypercapnia on myocardial contractility. *Am. J. Physiol.* 1960; **199**(6): 1121–1124.

106. Tyberg, J.V., Yeatman, L.A., Parmley, W.W., Urschel, C.W. & Sonnenblick, E.H. Effects of hypoxia on mechanics of cardiac contraction. *Am. J. Physiol.* 1970; **218**(6): 1780–1788.

107. Becker, L.B., Idris, A.H., Shao, Z., Schorer, S., Art, J. & Zak, R. Inhibition of cardiomyocyte contractions by carbon dioxide. *Circulation* 1993; **88**(Suppl I): I-225.

108. Orchard, C.H. & Kentish, K.C. Effects of changes of pH on the contractile function of cardiac muscle. *Am. J. Physiol.* 1990; **258**(*Cell. Physiol.* 27); C967–C981.

109. Kette, F., Weil, M.H., Gazmuri, R.J., Bisera, J. & Rackow, E.C. Intramyocardial hypercarbic acidosis during cardiac arrest and resuscitation. *Crit. Care Med.* 1993; **21**: 901–906.

110. Grum, C.M. Tissue oxygenation in low flow states and during hypoxemia. *Crit. Care Med.* 1993; **21**(2 Suppl.): S44–S49. Review.

111. Paradis, N.A., Rose, M.I. & Gawryl, M.S. Selective aortic arch perfusion and oxygenation: an effective adjunct to external chest compression-based cardiopulmonary resuscitation. *J. Am. Coll. Cardiol.* 1994; **23**: 497–504.

112. Paradis, N., Martin, G.B., Rivers, E.P. *et al.* Coronary perfusion pressure and the return of spontaneous circulation in human cardiopulmonary resuscitation. *J. Am. Med. Assoc.* 1990; **263**: 1106–1113.

113. Weil, M.H., Houle, D.B., Brown, E.B. Jr., Campbell, G.S. & Heath, C. Influence of acidosis on the effectiveness of vasopressor agents. *Circulation* 1957; **16**: 949.

114. Houle, D.B., Weil, M.H., Brown, E.B. Jr. & Campbell, G.S. Influence of respiratory acidosis on ECG and pressor responses to epinephrine, norepinephrine and metaraminol. *Proc. Soc. Exp. Biol. Med.* 1957; **94**: 561–564.

115. Campbell, G.S., Houle, D.B., Crisp, N.W. Jr., Weil, M.H. & Brown, E.B. Jr. Depressed response to intravenous sympathicomimetic agents in human acidosis. *Dis. Chest* 1958; **33**: 18–22.

116. Köhler, E., Noack, E., Strobach, H. & Wirth, K. Effect of acidosis on heart and circulation in cats, pigs, dogs and rabbits. *Res. Exp. Med.* 1972; **158**: 308–320.

117. Bendixen, H.H., Laver, M.B. & Flacke, W.E. Influence of respiratory acidosis on circulatory effect of epinephrine in dogs. *Circ. Res.* 1963; **13**: 64–70.

118. Sechzer, P.H., Egbert, L.D., Linde, H.W., Cooper, D.Y., Dripps, R.D. & Price, H.L. Effect of CO_2 inhalation on arterial pressure,

ECG and plasma catecholamines and 17-OH corticosteroids in normal man. *J. Appl. Physiol.* 1960; **15**: 454–458.

119. Anderson, M.N. & Mouritzen, C. Effect of respiratory and metabolic acidosis on cardiac output and peripheral vascular resistance. *Ann. Surg.* 1966; **163**: 161–168.

120. Kern, K.B., Elchisak, M.A., Sanders, A.B., Badylak, S.F., Tacker, W.A. & Ewy, G.A. Plasma catecholamines and resuscitation from prolonged cardiac arrest. *Crit. Care Med.* 1989; **17**: 786–791.

121. Idris, A.H., Wenzel, V., Becker, L., Banner, M. & Orban, D. Does hypercarbia or hypoxia independently affect resuscitation from cardiac arrest? *Chest* 1995; **108**: 522–528.

122. Lenfant, C. Pulmonary circulation. In Ruch, C.R., Patton, H.D. & Scher, A.M., (eds): *Physiology and Biophysics*, edn. 20, Philadelphia: W.B. Saunders Co., 1974.

123. Nikki, P., Rasanen, J., Tahvanainen, J. & Maklainen, A. Ventilatory pattern in respiratory failure arising from acute myocardial infarction. I. Respiratory and hemodynamic effects if IMV4 vs. IPPP12 and PEEP0 vs PEEP12. *Crit. Care Med.* 1982; **10**: 75.

124. Douglas, M.E. & Downs, J.B. Cardiopulmonary effects of intermittent mandatory ventilation. *Int. Anesthesiol. Clin.* 1980; **18**: 97.

125. Woda, R.P., Dzwonczyk, R., Bernacki, B.L. *et al.* The ventilatory effects of auto-positive end-expiratory pressure development during cardiopulmonary resuscitation. *Crit. Care Med.* 1999; **27**(10): 2212–2217.

126. Pepe, P.E. & Marini, J.J. Occult positive end-expiratory pressure in mechanically ventilated patients with airflow obstruction: the auto-PEEP effect. *Am. Rev. Respir. Dis.* 1982; **126**: 166–170.

127. Cournand, A., Motley, H.L., Werko, L. & Richards, D.W. Physiological studies of the effects of intermittent positive pressure breathing on cardiac output. *Am. J. Physiol.* 1948; **152**: 162–174.

128. Sykes, M.K., Adams, A.P., Finley, W.E., McCormick, P.W. & Economides, A. The effects of variations in end expiratory inflation pressure on cardiorespiratory function in normo, hypo, and hypervolemic dogs. *Br. J. Anaesth.* 1970; **42**: 669–677.

129. Qvist, J., Pontoppidan, H., Wilson, R.S., Lowenstein, E. & Laver, M.B. Hemodynamic responses to mechanical ventilation with PEEP: The effect of hypovolemia. *Anesthesiology* 1975; **42**: 45–55.

130. Pepe, P.E., Raedler, C., Lurie, K.G. & Wigginton, J.G. Emergency ventilatory management in hemorrhagic states: elemental or detrimental? *J. Trauma* 2003; **54**(6): 1048–1055; discussion 1055–1057.

131. National Trauma Data Bank Report 2002. American College of Surgeons.

132. Management and prognosis of severe traumatic brain injury. Brain Trauma Foundation and the American Association of Neurological Surgeons. Brain Trauma Foundation, Inc. New York, 2000.

133. Coles, J.P., Minhas, P.S., Fryer, T.D. *et al.* Effect of hyperventilation on cerebral blood flow in traumatic head injury: clinical relevance and monitoring correlates. *Crit. Care Med.* 2002; **30**(9): 1950–1959.

134. Manley, G.T. Cerebral oxygenation during hemorrhagic shock: perils of hyperventilation and the therapeutic potential of hypoventilation. *J. Trauma* 2000; **48**: 1025–1033.

135. Hemphill, J.C. 3rd, Knudson, M.M., Derugin, N., Morabito, D. & Manley, G.T. Carbon dioxide reactivity and pressure autoregulation of brain tissue oxygen. *Neurosurgery* 2001; **48**(2): 377–383; discussion 383–384.

136. Imberti, R. Cerebral tissue PO_2 and $SjvO_2$ changes during moderate hyperventilation in patients with severe brain injury. *J. Neurosurg.* 2002; **96**: 97–102.

137. Robertson, C.S. Prevention of secondary ischemic insults after severe head injury. *Crit. Care Med.* 1999; **27**: 2086–2095.

138. Bullock, R. Letter to the Editor. *J. Neurosurg.* 2002; **96**: 157–158

139. Diringer, M.N. Regional cerebrovascular and metabolic effects of hyperventilation after severe traumatic brain injury. *J. Neurosurg.* 2002; **96**: 103–108.

140. Neurosurgical Forum: Letters to the Editor. *J. Neurosurg.* 2002; **96**: 155–159.

141. Gabriel, E.J., Ghajar, J., Jagoda, A., Pons, P.T., Scalea, T. & Walters, B.C. Guidelines for prehospital management of traumatic brain injury. Brain Trauma Foundation, New York, 2000.

142. Thomas, S.H., Orf, J., Wedel, S.K. & Conn, A.K. Hyperventilation in traumatic brain injury patients: inconsistency between consensus guidelines and clinical practice. *J. Trauma* 2002; **52**: 47–52.

143. Davis, D.P., Hoyt, D.B., Ochs, M. *et al.* The effect of paramedic rapid sequence intubation on outcome in patients with severe traumatic brain injury. *J. Trauma* 2003; **54**(3): 444–453.

144. Stone, H.H., MacKrell, T.N., Brandstater, B.J., Haidak, G.L. & Nemir, P. Jr. The effect of induced hemorrhagic shock on the cerebral circulation and metabolism of man. *Surg. Forum* 1955; **5**: 789–794.

145. Gotoh, F., Meyer, J.S. & Yasuyuki, T. Cerebral effects of hyperventilation in man. *Arch. Neurol.* 1965; **12**: 410–423.

146. Harper, A.M. & Glass, H.I. Effect of alterations in the arterial carbon dioxide tension on the blood flow through the cerebral cortex at normal and low arterial blood pressures. *J. Neurol. Neurosurg. Psychiatry* 1965; **28**: 449–452.

147. Davis, D.P., Dunford, J.V., Poste, J.C. *et al.* The impact of hypoxia and hyperventilation on outcome after paramedic rapid sequence intubation of severely head-injured patients. *J. Trauma* 2004; **57**(1): 1–8; discussion 8–10.

148. Shafi, S. *J. Trauma* 2004 (abstract); **57**: 448.

149. Stern, S.A., Zink, B.J., Mertz, M. *et al.* Effect of initially limited resuscitation in a combined model of fluid percussion brain injury and severe uncontrolled hemorrhagic shock. *J. Neurosurg.* 2000; **93**: 305–314.

150. Milander, M.M., Hiscok, P.S., Sanders, A.B., Kern, K.B., Berg, R.A. & Ewy, G.A. Chest compression and ventilation rates during cardiopulmonary resuscitation: the effects of audible tone guidance. *Acad. Emerg. Med.* 1995; **2**(8): 708–713.

151. Aufderheide, T.P., Sigurdsson, G., Pirrallo, R.G. *et al.* Hyperventilation-induced hypotension during cardiopulmonary resuscitation. *Circulation* 2004; **109**(16): 1960–1965.

152. Abella, B., Alvarado, J., Myklebust, H. *J. Am. Med. Assoc.* 2005; **293**(3): 363–365.

153. Losert, H., Kliegel, A., Fleischhackl, R. *et al.* Are we providing CPR according to the guidelines in in-hospital cardiac arrest? *Circulation* 2004; **110**(Suppl III): III–456.

154. Babbs, C.F. & Kern, K.B. Optimum compression to ventilation ratios in CPR under realistic, practical conditions: a physiological and mathematical analysis. *Resuscitation* 2002; **54**(2): 147–157.

155. Dorph, E., Wik, L., Stromme, T.A. *et al.* Quality of CPR with three different ventilation:compression ratios. *Resuscitation* 2003; **58**(2): 193–201.

156. Dorph, E., Wik, L., Stromme, T.L. *et al.* Oxygen delivery and return of spontaneous circulation with ventilation:compression ratio 2: 30 versus chest compressions only CPR in pigs. *Resuscitation* 2004; **60**(3): 309–318.

157. Kern, K.B., Hilwig, R.W., Berg, R.A. *et al.* Importance of continuous chest compressions during cardiopulmonary resuscitation: improved outcome during a simulated single lay-rescuer scenario. *Circulation* 2002; **105**(5): 645–649.

158. Sanders, A.B., Kern, K.B., Berg, R.A. *et al.* Survival and neurologic outcome after cardiopulmonary resuscitation with four different chest compression-ventilation ratios. *Ann. Emerg. Med.* 2002; **40**(6): 553–562.

159. Turner, I., Turner, S. & Armstrong, V. Does the compression to ventilation ratio affect the quality of CPR: a simulation study. *Resuscitation* 2002; **52**(1): 55–62.

160. Turner, I. & Turner, S. Optimum cardiopulmonary resuscitation for basic and advanced life support: a simulation study. *Resuscitation* 2004; **62**(2): 209–217.

161. Yannopoulos, D., Aufderheide, T., Gabrielli, A. *et al.* Clinical and hemodynamic comparison of 15: 2 and 30: 2 compression to ventilation ratios for cardiopulmonary resuscitation. *Crit. Care Med.* 2006, in press.

162. 2005 American Heart Association guidelines for cardiopulmonary resuscitation and emergency cardiovascular care. Part 4: Adult Basic Life Support. *Circulation* 2005; **112**: IV-18–IV-34.

163. Lockinger, A., Kleinsasser, A., Wenzeo, V. *et al.* Pulmonary gas exchange of the cardiopulmonary resuscitation with either vasopressin or epinephrine. *Crit. Care Med.* 2002; **30**: 2059–2062.

164. Hodgkin, B.C., Lambrew, C.T., Lawrence, F.H. & Angelakos, E.T. Effects of PEEP and of increased frequency of ventilation during CPR. *Crit. Care Med.* 1980; **8**: 123–126.

165. Sigurdsson, G., Yannopoulos, D., McKnite, S.H. & Lurie, K.G. Cardiorespiratory interactions and blood flow generation during cardiac arrest and other states of low blood flow. *Curr. Opin. Crit. Care* 2003; **9**(3): 183–188. Review.

166. Samniah, N., Voelckel, W.G., Zielinski, T.M. *et al.* Feasibility and effects of transcutaneous phrenic nerve stimulation combined with an inspiratory impedance threshold in a pig model of hemorrhagic shock. *Crit. Care Med.* 2003; **31**(4): 1197–1202.

167. Lurie, K.G., Zielinski, T., Voelckel, W., McKnite, S. & Plaisance, P. Augmentation of ventricular preload during treatment of cardiovascular collapse and cardiac arrest. *Crit. Care Med.* 2002; **30**(4 Suppl): S162–S165. Review.

168. Lurie, K.G., Zielinski, T., McKnite, S., Aufderheide, T. & Voelckel, W. Use of an inspiratory impedance valve improves neurologically intact survival in a porcine model of ventricular fibrillation. *Circulation* 2002; **105**(1): 124–129.

169. Hevesi, C.G., Thrush, D.N., Downs, J.B. *et al.* Cardiopulmonary resuscitation effect of CPAP on gas exchange during chest compressions. *Anesthesiology* 1999, **90**: 1078–1083.

170. Markstaller, K., Karmrodt, J., Doebrich, M. *et al.* Dynamic computed tomography: a novel technique to study lung aeration and atelectasis formation during experimental CPR. *Resuscitation* 2002; **53**: 307–313.

171. Koehler, R.C., Chandra, N., Guerci, A.D. *et al.* Augmentation of cerebral perfusion by simultaneous chest compression and lung inflation with abdominal binding after cardiac arrest in dogs. *Circulation* 1983; **67**: 266–275.

172. Meursing, B.T.J., Zimmerman, A.N.E. & van Heyst, A.N.P. Experimental evidence in favor of a reversed sequence in cardiopulmonary resuscitation. *J. Am. Coll. Cardiol.* 1983; **1**: 610 (abstr).

173. Tucker, K.J., Idris, A.H., Wenzel, V. & Orban, D.J. Changes in arterial and mixed venous blood gases during untreated ventricular fibrillation and cardiopulmonary resuscitation. *Resuscitation* 1994; **28**(2): 137–141.

174. Tang, W., Weil, M.H., Sun, S. *et al.* Myocardial function after CPR by precordial compression without mechanical ventilation. *Chest* 1991; **100**(Suppl.): 132S.

175. Pearson, J.W. & Redding, J.S. Influence of peripheral vascular tone on cardiac resuscitation. *Anesth. Analg.* 1965; **44**: 746–752.

176. Yang, L., Weil, M.H., Noc, M., Tang, W., Turner, T. & Gazmuri, R.J. Spontaneous gasping increases the ability to resuscitate during experimental cardiopulmonary resuscitation. *Crit. Care Med.* 1994; **22**: 879–883.

177. Idris, A.H., Becker, L.B., Fuerst, R.S. *et al.* The effect of ventilation on resuscitation in an animal model of cardiac arrest. *Circulation* 1994; **90**(6): 3063–3069.

178. Noc, M., Weil, M.H., Tang, W. *et al.* Mechanical ventilation may not be essential for initial cardiopulmonary resuscitation. *Chest* 1995; **108**: 821–827.

179. Berg, R.A., Kern, K.B., Hilwig, R.W. *et al.* Assisted ventilation during "bystanders" CPR in a swine acute myocardial infarction model does not improve outcome. *Circulation* 1997; **96**: 4364–4371.

180. Kern, K.B., Hilwig, R.W., Berg, R.A. *et al.* Efficacy of chest compression-only BLS CPR in the presence of an occluded airway. *Resuscitation* 1998; **39**: 179–188.

181. Kern, K.B. Cardiopulmonary resuscitation without ventilation. *Crit. Care Med.* 2000; **28**(11 Suppl.): N186–N189.

182. Clark, J.J., Larsen, M.P., Culley, L.L., Graves, J.R. & Eisenberg, M.S. Incidence of agonal respirations in sudden cardiac arrest. *Ann. Emerg. Med.* 1992; **21**: 1464–1467.

183. Kazarian, K.K. & Del Guercio, L.R.M. The use of mixed venous blood gas determinations in traumatic shock. *Ann. Emerg. Med.* 1980; **9**: 179–180.

184. Simoons, M.L., Kimman, G.P., Ivens, E.M.A., Hartman, J.A.M. & Hart, H.N. Follow up after out of hospital resuscitation. *Eur. Heart J.* 1990; **11**(Abstract Suppl.): 92.

185. Thompson, R.G., Hallstrom, A.P. & Cobb, L.A. Bystander-initiated cardiopulmonary resuscitation in the management of ventricular fibrillation. *Ann. Emerg. Med.* 1979; **9**: 737–740.

186. Van Hoeyweghen, R.J., Bossaert, L., Mullie, A. *et al.* Quality and efficiency of bystander CPR. Belgian Cerebral Resuscitation Study Group. *Resuscitation* 1993; **26**: 47–52.

187. Hallstrom, A., Cobb, L., Johnson, E. *et al.* Cardiopulmonary resuscitation by chest compression alone or with mouth-to-mouth ventilation. *N. Engl. J. Med.* 2000; **342**: 1546–1553.

188. Assar, D., Chamberlain, D., Colquhoun, M. *et al.* A rational stage of teaching basic life support. *Resuscitation* 1998; **39**: 137–143.

189. Becker, L.B., Berg, R.A., Pepe, P.E. *et al.* A reappraisal of mouth-to-mouth ventilation during bystander-initiated cardio-pulmonary resuscitation: a statement for the Healthcare Professionals from the Ventilation Working Group of Basic Life Support and Pediatric Life Support Subcommittees, American Heart Association. *Ann. Emerg. Med.* 1997; **30**: 654–666.

190. Holmberg, M., Holmberg, S. & Herlitz, J. Factors modifying the effect of bystander cardiopulmonary resuscitation on survival in out-of-hospital cardiac arrest patients in Sweden. *Eur. Heart J.* 2001; **22**: 511–519.

191. Shao, D., Weil, M.H., Tang, W. *et al.* Pupil diameter and light reaction during cardiac arrest and resuscitation. *Crit. Care Med.* 2001; **29**(4): 825–828.

192. Waters, R.M. & Bennett, J.H. Artificial respiration: comparison of manual maneuvers. *Anesth. Analg.* 1936; **15**: 151–154.

193. Gordon, A.S., Fainer, D.C. & Ivy, A.C. Artificial respiration: a new method and a comparative study of different methods in adults. *J. Am. Med. Assoc.* 1950; **144**: 1455–1464.

194. Gordon, A.S., Sadove, M.S., Raymon, F. & Ivy, A.C. Critical survey of manual artificial respiration. *J. Am. Med. Assoc.* 1951; **147**: 1444–1453.

195. Gordon, A.S., Affeldt, J.E., Sadove, M., Raymon, F., Whittenberger, J.L. & Ivy, A.C. Air-flow patterns and pulmonary ventilation during manual artificial respiration on apneic normal adults II. *J. Appl. Physiol.* 1951; **4**: 408–420.

196. Gordon, A.S., Frye, C.W., Gittelson, L., Sadove, M.S. & Beattie, E.J. Mouth-to-mouth versus manual artificial respiration for children and adults. *J. Am. Med. Assoc.* 1958; **167**: 320–328.

197. Nims, R.G., Conner, E.H., Botelho, S.Y. & Comroe, J.H. Jr. Comparison of methods for performing manual artificial respiration on apneic patients. *J. Appl. Physiol.* 1951; **4**: 486–495.

198. Elam, J.O., Greene, D.G., Brown, E.S. & Clements, J.A. Oxygen and carbon dioxide exchange and energy cost of expired air resuscitation. *J. Am. Med. Assoc.* 1958; **167**: 328–341.

199. Idris, A.H., Gabrielli, A., Caruso, L.J. *et al.* Tidal volume for bag-valve mask (BVM) ventilations: Less is more [abstract]. *Circulation* 1999; **100**(suppl): 1664.

200. Kofler, J., Sterz, F., Hofbauer, R. *et al.* Epinephrine application via an endotracheal airway and via the Combitube in esophageal position. *Crit. Care Med.* 2000; **28**: 1445–1449.

201. Saviteer, S.M., White, G.C., Cohen, M.S. *et al.* HTLV-III exposure during cardiopulmonary resuscitation. *N. Engl. J. Med.* 1985; **313**: 1606–1607.

202. Kline, S.E., Hedemark, L.L. & Davies, S.F. Outbreak of tuberculosis among regular patrons of a neighborhood bar. *N. Engl. J. Med.* 1995; **333**: 222–227.

203. Lufkin, K.C. & Ruiz, E. Mouth-to-mouth ventilation of cardiac arrested humans using a barrier mask. *Prehosp. Disaster Med.* 1993; **8**: 333–335.

204. Hew, P., Brenner, B. & Kauffman, J. Reluctance of paramedics and emergency technicians to perform mouth-to-mouth resuscitation. *J. Emerg. Med.* 1997; **15**: 279–284.

205. Ornato, J.P., Hallagan, L.F., McMahan, S.B. *et al.* Attitudes of BCLS instructors about mouth-to-mouth resuscitation during the AIDS epidemic. *Ann. Emerg. Med.* 1990; **19**: 151–156.

206. Shibata, K., Taniguchi, T., Yoshida, M. *et al.* Obstacles to bystander cardiopulmonary resuscitation in Japan. *Resuscitation* 2000; **44**: 187–193.

207. Tajima, K. & Soda, K. Epidemiology of AIDS/HIV in Japan. *J. Epidemiol.* 1996; **6**(3 Suppl): S67–S74.

208. Capone, P.L., Lane, J.C., Kerr, C.S. *et al.* Life supporting first aid (LSFA) teaching to Brazilians by television spots. *Resuscitation* 2000; **47**: 259–265.

209. Lynch, B., Einspruch, E., Nichol, G., Becker, L., Aufderheide, T. & Idris, A. Effectiveness of a 30-min CPR self-instruction program for lay responders: a controlled randomized study. *Resuscitation* 2005; **67**(1): 31–43.

210. Roppolo, L.P., Ohman, K., Pepe, P.P. & Idris, A.H. The effectiveness of a short cardiopulmonary resuscitation course for laypersons. *Circulation* 2005; **112**(Suppl II): II–325.

211. Idris, A.H., Roppolo, L.P., Kulkarni, H., Ohman, K. & Pepe, P.P. A five-minute training program for automated external defibrillator use is more effective than a 4-hour course. *Circulation* 2005, **112**(Suppl II): II–326.

212. Pepe, P.E., Gay, M., Cobb, L.A. *et al.* Action sequence for layperson cardiopulmonary resuscitation. *Ann. Emerg. Med.* 2001; **37**(4 Suppl): S17–S25.

213. Kouwenhoven, W.B., Jude, J.R. & Knickerbocker, G.G. Landmark article July 9, 1960: Closed-chest massage. *J. Am. Med. Assoc.* 1984; **251**: 3133–3136.

214. Michenfelder, J.D. & Theye, R.A. The effect of anesthesia and hypothermia on canine cerebral ATP and lactate during anoxia produced by decapitation. *Anesthesiology* 1970; **33**: 430–439.

215. Meursing, B.T.J., Zimmerman, A.N.E. & Van Huyst, A.N.P. Experimental evidence in favor of reverted sequence in cardiopulmonary resuscitations [abstract]. *J. Am. Cardiol.* 1983; **1**: 610.

216. Berg, R.A., Hilwig, R.W., Kern, K.B. *et al.* "Bystander" chest compression and assisted ventilation independently improved outcome from piglet asphyxia pulseless "cardiac arrest". *Circulation* 2000; **101**: 1743–1748.

217. Guidelines 2000 for cardiopulmonary resuscitation and emergency cardiovascular care: international consensus on science. *Circulation* 2000; **102**: I-1–I-384.

218. Ruben, H. & MacNaughton, F.I. The treatment of food choking. *Practitioner* 1978; **221**: 725–729.

219. Langhelle, A., Sunde, K., Wik, L. *et al.* Airway pressure with chest compression vs. Heimlich maneuver in recently dead adults with complete airway obstruction. *Resuscitation* 2000; **44**: 105–108.

220. Handley, A.J., Monsieurs, K.G. & Bossaert, L.L. European resuscitation council guidelines 2000 for adult basic life support. A statement from the Basic Life Support and Automated External Defibrillation Working Group (1) and approved by the Executive Committee of the European Resuscitation Council. *Resuscitation* 2001; **48**: 199–205.

221. Mogayzel, C., Quan, L., Graves, J.R. *et al.* Out-of-hospital ventricular fibrillation in children and adolescents: causes and outcomes. *Ann. Emerg. Med.* 1995; **25**: 484–491.

222. Niermeyer, S., Kattwinkel, J., Van Reempts, P. *et al.* International guidelines for neonatal resuscitations: an excerpt from the Guidelines 2000 for Cardiopulmonary Resuscitation and Emergency Cardiovascular Care: International Consensus on Science. Contributors and Reviewers for the Neonatal Resuscitation Guidelines. *Pediatrics* 2000; **106**: 1–16.

223. Biarent, D., Bingham, R., Richmond, S. *et al.* European Resuscitation Council Guidelines for Resuscitation 2005. Paediatric Life Support. *Resuscitation* 2005; **67**S1: S97–S133.

224. 2005 International Consensus Conference on Cardiopulmonary Resuscitation and Emergency Cardiovascular Care Science With Treatment Recommendations. *Circulation* 2005; **112**: III-1–III-132.

225. 2005 American Heart Association guidelines for cardiopulmonary resuscitation and emergency cardiovascular care. Part 11: Pediatric Basic Life Support. *Circulation* 2005; **112**: IV-156–IV-166.

226. Safar, P., Escarraga, L.A. & Chang, F. Upper airway obstruction in the unconscious patient. *J. Appl. Physiol.* 1959; **14**: 760–764.

227. Morikawa, S., Safar, P. & DeCarlo, J. Influence of the head-jaw position upon upper airway patency. *Anesthesiology* 1961; **22**: 265–270.

228. Safar, P. Ventilatory efficacy of mouth-to-mouth artificial respiration: airway obstruction during manual and mouth-to-mouth artificial respiration. *J. Am. Med. Assoc.* 1958; **167**: 335–341.

229. Melker, R.J. & Banner, M.J. Ventilation during CPR. Two-rescuer standards reappraised. *Ann. Emerg. Med.* 1985; **14**: 397–402.

230. Fuerst, R., Idris, A., Banner, M., Wenzel, V. & Orban, D. Changes in respiratory system compliance during cardiopulmonary

231. arrest with and without closed chest compressions. *Ann. Emerg. Med.* 1993; **22**: 931.

231. Bowman, F.P., Duckett, T., Check, B. & Menegazzi, J. Lower esophageal sphincter pressure during prolonged cardiac arrest and resuscitation. *Acad. Emerg. Med.* 1994; **1**: A18.

232. Gabrielli, A., Wenzel, V., Layon, A.J., von Goedecke, A., Verne, G.N. & Idris, A.H. Lower esophageal sphincter pressure measurement during cardiac arrest in humans: Potential implications for ventilation of the unprotected airway – a case report series. *Anesthesiology* 2005; **103**: 897–899.

233. Ruben, H., Knudsen, E.J. & Carugati, G. Gastric inflation in relation to airway pressure. *Acta Anaesth. Scand.* 1961; **5**: 107–114.

234. Ruben, A. & Ruben, H. Artificial respiration: flow of water from the lung and the stomach. *Lancet* April 14, 1962; 780–781.

235. Ruben, H. The immediate treatment of respiratory failure. *Br. J. Anaesth.* 1964; **36**: 542–549.

236. Lawes, E.G. & Baskett, P.J.F. Pulmonary aspiration during unsuccessful cardiopulmonary resuscitation. *Intens. Care Med.* 1987; **13**: 379–382.

237. Petito, S.P. & Russell, W.J. The prevention of gastric insufflation – a neglected benefit of cricoid pressure. *Anaesth. Intens. Care* 1988; **16**: 139–143.

238. Idris, A.H., Banner, M.J., Fuerst, R., Becker, L.B., Wenzel, V. & Melker, R.J. Ventilation caused by external chest compression is unable to sustain effective gas exchange during CPR: a comparison with mechanical ventilation. *Resuscitation* 1994; **28**(2): 143–150.

239. Idris, A.H., Wenzel, V., Tucker, K.J. & Orban, D.J. Chest compression ventilation: a comparison of standard CPR and active-compression/decompression CPR. *Acad. Emerg. Med.* 1994; **1**: A17.

240. Idris, A.H., Wenzel, V., Banner, M.J. *et al.* Smaller tidal volumes minimize gastric inflation during CPR with an unprotected airway [abstract]. *Circulation* 1995; **92**: 1–759.

241. Wenzel, V., Idris, A.H., Banner, M.J. *et al.* The influence of tidal volume on the distribution of gas between the lungs and stomach in the unintubated patient receiving positive pressure ventilation. *Crit. Care Med.* 1998; **26**: 364–368.

242. Wolcke, B., Schneider, T., Mauer, D. *et al.* Ventilation volumes with different self-inflating bags with reference to ERC guidelines for airway management: Comparison of two compression techniques. *Resuscitation* 2000; **47**: 175–178.

243. Wenzel, V., Dorges, V., Lindner, K.H. *et al.* Mouth-to-mouth ventilation during cardiopulmonary resuscitation: word of mouth in the street versus science. *Anesth. Analg.* 2001; **93**: 4–6.

244. Oschatz, E., Wunderbaldinger, P., Sterz, F. *et al.* Cardiopulmonary resuscitation performed by bystanders does not increase adverse effects as assessed by chest radiography. *Anesth. Analg.* 2001; **93**: 128–133.

245. Wenzel, V., Keller, C., Idris, A.H., Doerges, V., Lindner, K.H. & Brimacombe, J.R. Effects of smaller tidal volumes during basic life support ventilation in patients with respiratory

arrest: good ventilation, less risk? *Resuscitation* 1999; **43**: 25–29.

246. Dorges, V., Ocker, H., Hagelberg, S. *et al.* Smaller tidal volumes with room air are not sufficient to ensure adequate oxygenation during bag–valve–mask ventilation *Resuscitation* 2000; **44**: 37–41.

247. Cummins, R.O. & Hazinski, M.F. The most important changes in the international ECC and CPR guidelines 2000. *Resuscitation* 2000; **46**: 431–437.

248. Gausche, M., Lewis, R.J., Stratton, S.J. *et al.* Effect of out-of-hospital pediatric endotracheal intubations on survival and psychological outcome: a controlled clinical trial. *J. Am. Med. Assoc.* 2000; **283**: 783–790.

249. Froese, A.B. & Bryan, A.C. High frequency ventilation. *Am. Rev. Respir. Dis.* 1987; **135**: 1363–1374.

250. Slutsky, A.S. Nonconventional methods of ventilation. *Am. Rev. Respir. Dis.* 1988; **138**: 175–183.

251. Zidulka, A., Gross, D., Minami, H., Vartian, V. & Chang, H.K. Ventilation by high-frequency chest wall compression in dogs with normal lungs. *Am. Rev. Respir. Dis.* 1983; **127**: 709–713.

252. Fuyuki, T., Suzuki, S., Sakurai, M., Sasaki, H., Butler, J.P. & Takashima, T. Ventilatory effectiveness of high-frequency oscillation applied to the body surface. *J. Appl. Physiol.* 1987; **62**: 2410–2415.

253. Harf, A., Bertrand, C. & Chang, H.K. Ventilation by high-frequency oscillation of thorax or at trachea in rats. *J. Appl. Physiol.* 1984; **56**(1): 155–160.

254. Gross, D., Vartian, V., Minami, H., Chang, H.K. & Zidulka, A. High frequency chest wall compression and carbon dioxide elimination in obstructed dogs. *Bull. Eur. Physiopathol. Respir.* 1984; **20**: 507–511.

255. George, R.J.D., Winter, R.J.D., Flockton, S.J. & Geddes, D.M. Ventilatory saving by external chest wall compression or oral high-frequency oscillation in normal subjects and those with chronic airflow obstruction. *Clin. Sci.* 1985; **69**: 349–359.

256. Piquet, J., Isabey, D., Chang, H.K. & Harf, A. High frequency transthoracic ventilation improves gas exchange during experimental bronchoconstriction in rabbits. *Am. Rev. Respir. Dis.* 1986; **133**: 605–608.

257. Ward, H.E., Power, J.H.T. & Nicholas, T.E. High-frequency oscillations via the pleural surface: an alternative mode of ventilation? *J. Appl. Physiol.: Respirat. Environ. Exercise Physiol.* 1983; **54**: 427–433.

258. Kleinsasser, A., Lindner, K.H., Schaefer, A. *et al.* Decompression-triggered positive-pressure ventilation during cardiopulmonary resuscitation improves pulmonary gas exchange and oxygen uptake. *Circulation* 2002; **106**: 373–378.

259. Rea, T.D., Eisenberg, M.S., Culley, L.L. & Becker, L. Dispatcher-assisted Cardiopulmonary resuscitation and survival in cardiac arrest. *Circulation* 2001; **104**: 2513–2516.

260. Hauff, S.R., Rea, T.D., Culley, L.L., Kerry, F., Becker, L. & Eisenberg, M.S. Factors impeding dispatcher-assisted telephone CPR. *Ann. Emerg. Med.* 2003; **42**: 731–737.

261. Bång, A., Herlitz, J. & Martinell, S. Interaction between emergency medical dispatcher and caller in suspected out-of-hospital cardiac arrest calls with focus on agonal breathing. A review of 100 tape recordings of true cardiac arrest cases. *Resuscitation* 2003; **56**: 25–34.

262. 2005 American Heart Association guidelines for cardiopulmonary resuscitation and emergency cardiovascular care. *Circulation* 2005; **112**: IV-1–IV-205.

263. Cobb, L.A. & Hallstrom, A.P. Community based cardiopulmonary resuscitation: what have we learned? *Ann. NY Acad. Sci.* 1982; **382**: 330–342.

264. Finucane, T.B. & Santora, A.H. Basic airway management and cardiopulmonary resuscitation (CPR). In *Principles of Airway Management*. Philadelphia: FA Davis, 16: 1988.

265. Guildner, C.W. Resuscitation- opening the airway. A comparative study of techniques for opening an airway obstructed by the tongue. *JACEP* 1976; **5**(8): 588–590.

266. 2005 American Heart Association guidelines for cardiopulmonary resuscitation and emergency cardiovascular care. Part 7.**1**: Adjuncts for airway control and ventilation. *Circulation* 2005; **112**: IV-51–IV-56.

267. Lawrence, P.J. & Sivaneswaran, N. Ventilation during cardiopulmonary resuscitation: which method? *Med. J. Austr.* 1985; **143**(10): 443–446.

268. Johannigman, J.A., Branson, R.D., Davis, K. Jr. & Hurst, J.M. Techniques of emergency ventilation: a model to evaluate tidal volume, airway pressure, and gastric insufflation. *J. Trauma* 1991; **31**(1): 93–98.

269. McSwain, G.R., Garrison, W.B. & Artz, C.P. Evaluation of resuscitation from cardiopulmonary arrest by paramedics. *Ann. Emerg. Med.* 1980; **9**(7): 341–345.

270. Harrison, R.R. & Maull, K.I. Pocket mask ventilation: a superior method of acute airway management. *Ann. Emerg. Med.* 1982; **11**: 74–76.

271. Hess, D. & Baran, C. Ventilatory volumes using mouth-to-mouth, mouth-to-mask, and bag-valve-mask techniques. *Am. J. Emerg. Med.* 1985; **3**(4): 292–296.

272. Jesudian, M.C., Harrison, R.R., Keenan, R.L. & Maull, K.I. Bag-valve mask ventilation; two rescuers are better than one: preliminary report. *Crit. Care Med.* 1985; **13**(2): 122–123.

273. Hodgkin, J.E., Foster, G.L. & Nicolay, L.I. Cardiopulmonary resuscitation: development of an organized protocol. *Crit. Care Med.* 1977; **5**(2): 93–100.

274. Hirschman, A.M. & Kravath, R.E. Venting vs ventilating. A danger of manual resuscitation bags. *Chest* 1982; **82**(3): 369–370.

275. Florete, O.G. Jr. Airway devices and their application. In Kirby, R.R. & Gravenstein, N. (eds). *Clinical Anesthesia Practice*. Philadelphia: W.B. Saunders, 1994: 303.

276. Milner, A. The importance of ventilation to effective resuscitation in the term and preterm infant. *Semin. Neonatol.* 2001; **6**: 219–224.

277. Vyas, H., Field, D., Milner, A.D. & Hopkin, I.E. Determinants of the first inspiratory volume and functional residual capacity at birth. *Pediatr. Pulmonol.* 1986; **2**: 189–193.

278. Ikegami, M., Kallapur, S., Michna, J. *et al.* Lung injury and surfactant metabolism after hyperventilation of premature lambs. *Pediatr. Res.* 2000; **47**: 398–404.

279. Milner, A.D. & Saunders, R.A. Pressure and volume changes during the first breath of human neonates. *Arch. Dis. Child.* 1977; **52**: 918–924.

280. Head, H. On the regulation of respiration. *J. Physiol.* 1889; **10**: 1–70.

281. Vyas, H., Milner, A.D. & Hopkin, I.E. Efficacy of face mask resuscitation at birth. BMJ 1984; **289**: 1563–1565.

282. Vyas, H., Milner, A.D. & Hopkin, I.E. Face mask resuscitation: does it lead to gastric distension? *Arch. Dis. Child* 1983; **58**: 373–375.

283. Laurie, K., Zielinski, T., McKnit, S. *et al.* Improving the efficiency of cardiopulmonary resuscitation with an inspiratory impedance threshold valve. *Crit. Care Med.* 2000; **28**(11 Suppl.): 207–209.

284. Lurie, K.G., Mulligan, K.A., McKnite, S. *et al.* Optimizing standards of cardiopulmonary resuscitation with an inspiratory impedance threshold valve. *Chest* 1998; **113**: 1084–1090.

285. Plaisance, P., Lurie, K.G. & Payen, D. Inspiratory impedance during active compression-decompression cardiopulmonary resuscitation: a randomized evaluation in patients in cardiac arrest. *Circulation* 2000; **101**: 989–994.

286. Voelckel, W.G., Lurie, K.G., Zielinski, T. *et al.* The effect of positive end-expiratory pressure during active compression decompression cardiopulmonary resuscitation with the inspiratory threshold valve. *Anesth. Analg.* 2001; **92**: 967–974.

287. Sulek, C.A. & Kirby, R.R. The recurring problem of negative-pressure pulmonary edema. *Curr. Rev. Anesth.* 1998; **18**: 243–250.

288. Branson, R.D. Transport ventilators. In Branson, R.D., Hess, D.R. & Chatburn, R.L., eds. *Respiratory Care Equipment*, 2nd edn. Philadelphia: Lippincott Williams & Wilkins; 1999: 527–565.

289. Gervais, H.W., Eberle, B., Konietzke, D. *et al.* Comparison of blood gases of ventilated patients during transport. *Crit. Care Med.* 1987; **15**: 761.

290. Gazmuri, R.J., Weil, M.H., Bisera, J. & Rackow, E.C. End-tidal carbon dioxide tension as a monitor of native blood flow during resuscitation by extracorporeal circulation. *J. Thorac. Cardiovasc. Surg.* 1991; **101**: 984–988.

291. Gudipati, C.V., Weil, M.H., Bisera, J., Deshmukh, H.G. & Rackow, E.C. Expired carbon dioxide: a noninvasive monitor of cardiopulmonary resuscitation. *Circulation* 1988; **77**: 234–239.

292. Sanders, A.B., Atlas, M., Ewy, G.A., Kern, K.B. & Bragg, S. Expired CO_2 as an index of coronary perfusion pressure. *Am. J. Emerg. Med.* 1985; **3**: 147–149.

293. Kalenda, Z. The capnogram as a guide to the efficacy of cardiac massage. *Resuscitation* 1978; **6**: 259–263.

294. Falk, J.L., Rackow, E.C. & Weil, M.H. End-tidal carbon dioxide concentration during cardiopulmonary resuscitation. *N. Engl. J. Med.* 1988; **318**: 607–611.

295. Garnett, A.R., Ornato, J.P., Gonzalez, E.R. & Johnson, E.B. End-tidal carbon dioxide monitoring during cardiopulmonary resuscitation. *J. Am. Med. Assoc.* 1987; **257**: 512–515.

296. Grundler, W.G., Weil, M.H., Bisera, J. & Rackow, E.C. Observations on end-tidal carbon dioxide during experimental cardiopulmonary arrest. *J. Clin. Res.* 1984; **32**: 672A.

297. Sanders, A.B., Ewy, G.A., Bragg, S., Atlas, M. & Kern, K.B. Expired PCO_2 as a prognostic indicator of successful resuscitation from cardiac arrest. *Ann. Emerg. Med.* 1985; **14**: 948–952.

298. Sanders, A.B., Kern, K.B., Otto, C.W., Milander, M.M. & Ewy, G.A. End-tidal carbon dioxide monitoring during cardiopulmonary resuscitation: a prognostic indicator for survival. *J. Am. Med. Assoc.* 1989; **262**: 1347–1351.

299. Trevino, R.P., Bisera, J., Weil, M.H., Rackow, E.C. & Grundler, W.G. End-tidal CO_2 as a guide to successful cardiopulmonary resuscitation: a preliminary report. *Crit. Care Med.* 1985; **13**: 910–911.

300. Wiklund, L., Söderberg, D., Henneberg, S., Rubertsson, S., Stjernström, H. & Groth, T. Kinetics of carbon dioxide during cardiopulmonary resuscitation. *Crit. Care Med.* 1986; **14**: 1015–1022.

301. Callaham, M. & Barton, C. Prediction of outcome of cardiopulmonary resuscitation from end-tidal carbon dioxide concentration. *Crit. Care Med.* 1990; **18**: 358–362.

302. Bhende, M.S., Thompson, A.E. & Cook, D.R. Validity of a disposable end-tidal CO_2 detector in verifying endotracheal tube position in infants and children. *Ann. Emerg. Med.* 1990; **19**: 483.

303. Mickelson, K.S., Sterner, S.P. & Ruiz, E. Exhaled PCO_2 as a predictor of endotracheal tube placement. *Ann. Emerg. Med.* 1986; **15**: 657.

304. Ornato, J.P., Shipley, J.B., Racht, E.M. *et al.* Multicenter study of end-tidal carbon dioxide in the prehospital setting. *Ann. Emerg. Med.* 1992; **21**: 518–523.

305. Vukmir, R.B., Heller, M.B. & Stein, K.L. Confirmation of endotracheal tube placement: A miniaturized qualitative CO_2 detector. *Ann. Emerg. Med.* 1991; **20**: 726–729.

306. Ornato, J.P., Levine, R.L., Young, D.S., Racht, E.M., Garnett, A.R. & Gonzalez, E.R. Effect of applied chest compression on systemic arterial pressure and end-tidal carbon dioxide concentration during CPR in human beings. *Ann. Emerg. Med.* 1989; **18**: 732–737.

307. Ornato, J.P., Gonzalez, E.R., Garnett, A.R., Levine, R.L. & McClung, B.K. Effect of cardiopulmonary resuscitation compression rate on end-tidal carbon dioxide concentration and arterial pressure in man. *Crit. Care Med.* 1988; **16**: 241–245.

308. Ward, K.R., Menegazzi, J.J. & Zelenak, R.R. A comparison of mechanical CPR and manual CPR by monitoring end-tidal PCO_2 in human cardiac arrest. *Ann. Emerg. Med.* 1990; **19**: 456.

309. Ward, K.R., Sullivan, R.J., Zelenak, R.R. & Summer, W.R. A comparison of interposed abdominal compression CPR and standard CPR by monitoring end-tidal PCO_2. *Ann. Emerg. Med.* 1989; **18**: 831–837.

310. Bircher, N.G. Acidosis of cardiopulmonary resuscitation: carbon dioxide transport and anaerobiosis. *Crit. Care Med.* 1992; **20**: 1203–1205.

311. Gravenstein, J.S., Paulus, D.A. & Hayes, T.J. *Capnography in Clinical Practice.* Boston: Butterworth Publishers, 1989: 65–70.

312. Lambertsen, C.J. Transport of oxygen and carbon dioxide by the blood. In Mountcastle, V.B. (ed.). *Medical Physiology.* St. Louis, Missouri: The C.V. Mosby Co.1974: 1399–1422.

313. Idris, A., Staples, E., O'Brien, D. *et al.* End-tidal carbon dioxide during extremely low cardiac output. *Ann. Emerg. Med.* 1994; **23**: 568–572.

314. Martin, G.B., Gentile, N.T., Paradis, N.A., Moeggenberg, J., Appleton, T.J. & Nowak, R.M. Effect of epinephrine on end-tidal carbon dioxide monitoring during CPR. *Ann. Emerg. Med.* 1990; **19**: 396–398.

315. Niemann, J.T., Rosborough, J.P., Ung, S. & Criley, J.M. Coronary perfusion pressure during experimental cardiopulmonary resuscitation. *Ann. Emerg. Med.* 1982; **11**: 127–131.

316. Falk, J.L. & Sayre, M.R. Confirmation of airway placement. *Prehosp. Emerg. Care* 1999; **3**: 273–278.

317. Barton, C.W. & Callaham, M.L. Possible confounding effect of minute ventilation on ETCO$_2$ in cardiac arrest. *Ann. Emerg. Med.* 1991; **20**: 445–446.

318. Gazmuri, R.J., von Planta, M., Weil, M.H. & Rackow, E.C. Arterial PCO$_2$ as an indicator of systemic perfusion during cardiopulmonary resuscitation. *Crit. Care Med.* 1989; **17**: 237–240.

319. Angelos, M.G., DeBehnke, D.J. & Leasure, J.E. Arterial blood gases during cardiac arrest: markers of blood flow in a canine model. *Resuscitation* 1992; **23**: 101–111.

320. Tenney, S.M. A theoretical analysis of the relationship between venous blood and mean tissue oxygen pressures. *Respir. Phys.* 1974; **20**: 283–296.

321. Lee, J., Wright, F., Barber, R. *et al.* Central venous oxygen saturation in shock. *Anesth.* 1972; **36**: 472–478.

322. Kasnitz, P., Druger, G.L., Yorra, F. *et al.* Mixed venous oxygen tension and hyperlactemia. *J. Am Med. Assoc.* 1976; **236**: 570–574.

323. Emerman, C.L., Pinchak, A.C., Hagen, J.F. & Hancock, D. A comparison of venous blood gases during cardiac arrest. *Am. J. Emerg. Med.* 1988; **6**: 580–583.

324. Kissoon, N., Rosenberg, H., Gloor, J. & Vidal, R. Comparison of the acid–base status of blood obtained from intraosseous and central venous sites during steady- and low-flow states. *Crit. Care Med.* 1993; **21**: 1765–1769.

325. Kissoon, N., Idris, A., Wenzel, V., Murphey, S. & Rush, W. Intraosseous and central venous blood acid–base relationship during cardiopulmonary resuscitation. *Pediatr. Emerg. Care* 1997; **13**: 250–253.

29

Airway techniques and airway devices

Jerry P. Nolan and David A. Gabbott

Anaesthesia and Intensive Care Medicine, Royal United Hospital, Bath, UK
Department of Anaesthetics, Gloucester Royal Hospital, Gloucester, UK

". . . with a slight breath the lung will swell and the heart becomes strong . . . and as I do this and take care that the lung is inflated at intervals, the motion of the heart does not stop . . ." *Vesalius (1514–1564)*

Introduction

Maintaining a patent airway is of paramount importance if the lungs are to be inflated successfully with high inspired oxygen concentration during cardiopulmonary resuscitation (CPR) attempts. The association between delivering adequate breaths via a patent airway and maintenance of cardiac function was clearly recognized by Vesalius in the sixteenth century. Patients requiring CPR often have an obstructed airway, usually caused by loss of consciousness, but occasionally it may be the primary cause of cardiopulmonary arrest. Prompt assessment, with control of the airway and ventilation of the lungs is essential. This will help to prevent secondary hypoxic damage to the brain and other vital organs as well as maintaining cardiac function. Without adequate oxygenation it may be impossible to restore a spontaneous cardiac output from a myocardium in cardiac arrest.

An extensive review of the science behind airway management during cardiac arrest was published recently: the 2005 International Consensus on Cardiopulmonary Resuscitation and Emergency Cardiovascular Care Science with Treatment Recommendations (CoSTR).[1] The European Resuscitation Council (ERC) Basic Life Support (BLS) and Advanced Life Support (ALS) Working Parties have recently published new guidelines on management of the airway during cardiac arrest and these were based partly on the recommendations published in CoSTR.[2,3]

Airway obstruction

Causes of airway obstruction

Obstruction of the airway may be partial or complete. It may occur at any level from the nose and mouth down to the trachea (Fig. 29.1). In the unconscious patient, the commonest site of airway obstruction is at the level of the pharynx. The precise cause of airway obstruction in the unconscious state has been identified by studying patients under general anesthesia.[4–6] Until recently, this obstruction had been attributed to posterior displacement of the tongue caused by decreased muscle tone, with the tongue ultimately touching the posterior pharyngeal wall.[7,8] These studies of anesthetised patients have suggested that the site of airway obstruction is primarily at the soft palate and epiglottis and not the tongue. Obstruction may be caused also by vomit or blood, as a result of regurgitation of gastric contents or trauma, or by foreign bodies. Laryngeal obstruction may be caused by edema from burns, infection, inflammation, or anaphylaxis. Laryngeal spasm may be the result of an inappropriate response to upper airway stimulation, or caused by an inhaled foreign body. Obstruction of the airway below the larynx is less common, but it may arise from excessive bronchial secretions, mucosal edema, bronchospasm, pulmonary edema, or aspiration of gastric contents.

If airway obstruction is left unattended or allowed to progress, the consequences are progressive hypoxia, an increased work load for the patient, fatigue, hypercarbia, pulmonary edema, and ultimately complete airway obstruction leading to cardiopulmonary arrest. Furthermore, attempting to ventilate the lungs of a patient with an obstructed airway generates a cycle of gastric inflation

Cardiac Arrest: The Science and Practice of Resuscitation Medicine. 2nd edn., ed. Norman Paradis, Henry Halperin, Karl Kern, Volker Wenzel, Douglas Chamberlain. Published by Cambridge University Press. © Cambridge University Press, 2007.

and worsening respiratory system compliance as gas is forced down the esophagus and into the stomach.[9] Such an unfortunate sequence is further compounded by reduced pressure on the lower esophageal sphincter seen shortly after loss of consciousness during cardiopulmonary arrest.[10]

Assessment and recognition of airway obstruction

Airway obstruction can be subtle and is often missed by many healthcare professionals as well as by laypeople. The look, listen, and feel approach is a simple, systematic method of detecting airway obstruction:
- *look* for chest and abdominal movements
- *listen* and *feel* for airflow at the mouth and nose.

In partial airway obstruction, air entry is diminished and usually noisy. Inspiratory stridor is caused by obstruction at the laryngeal level or above. Expiratory wheeze implies obstruction of the lower airways, which tend to collapse and obstruct during expiration. Other characteristic sounds include:
- gurgling: caused by liquid or semisolid foreign material in the main airways
- snoring: arises when the pharynx is partially occluded by the soft palate or epiglottis
- crowing: is the sound of laryngeal spasm.

In a patient who is making respiratory efforts, complete airway obstruction causes paradoxical chest and abdominal movement, often described as "see–saw breathing." As the patient attempts to breathe in, the chest is drawn in and the abdomen expands, with the opposite in expiration. This is in contrast to the normal breathing pattern of synchronous movement upwards and outwards of the abdomen (pushed down by the diaphragm) with the lifting of the chest wall. During airway obstruction, other accessory muscles of respiration are used, with the neck and the shoulder muscles contracting to assist movement of the thoracic cage. Full examination of the neck, chest, and abdomen is required to differentiate the paradoxical movements that may mimic normal respiration. The examination must include listening for the absence of breath sounds in order to diagnose complete airway obstruction reliably; any noisy breathing indicates partial airway obstruction. During apnea, when spontaneous breathing movements are absent, complete airway obstruction can be recognized by failure to inflate the lungs during attempted positive pressure ventilation. Unless airway patency can be re-established to enable adequate lung ventilation within a very few minutes, neurological and other vital organ injury may occur, leading to cardiac arrest.

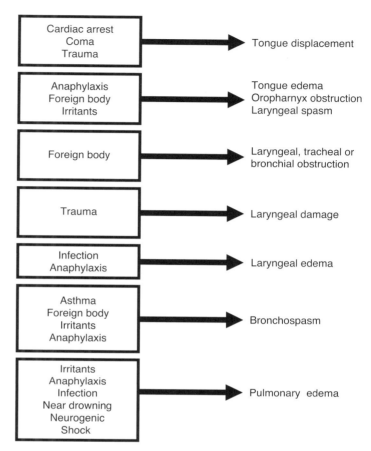

Fig. 29.1. Common causes of airway obstruction.

In patients who have complete airway obstruction, the continued uptake of oxygen from the gas remaining within the lungs can generate negative pressure within the chest cavity ("hypobaric thorax"). When airway obstruction is relieved, upper airway gases from within the mouth and pharynx may be sucked into the lungs by this negative pressure. The application of high inspired oxygen levels under these circumstances may greatly increase the pulmonary and blood oxygen levels as the airway obstruction is relieved.[11,12]

Basic airway management

Once any degree of obstruction is recognized, immediate measures must be taken to create and maintain a clear airway. There are three manoeuvres that can be used to improve an airway obstructed by the tongue or other upper airway structures: head tilt, chin lift, and jaw thrust.

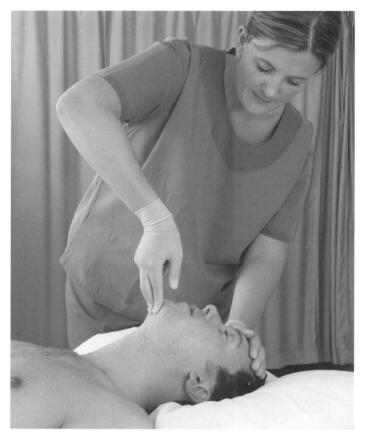

Fig. 29.2. Head tilt and chin lift. (Reproduced with permission from Dr. Mike Scott.)

Head tilt and chin lift

The rescuer's hand is placed on the patient's forehead and the head is gently tilted back; the fingertips of the other hand are placed under the point of the patient's chin, which is gently lifted to stretch the anterior neck structures (Fig. 29.2).[13–18]

Jaw thrust

Jaw thrust is an alternative maneuver for bringing the mandible forward and relieving obstruction by the soft palate and epiglottis; it was described first in 1874.[5] The rescuer's index and other fingers are placed behind the angle of the mandible, and pressure is applied upwards and forwards. Using the thumbs, the mouth is opened slightly by downward displacement of the chin (Fig. 29.3).

These simple positional methods are successful in most cases in which airway obstruction is caused by relaxation of the soft tissues. If a clear airway cannot be achieved,

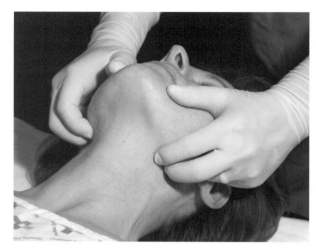

Fig. 29.3. Jaw thrust. (Reproduced with permission from Dr. Mike Scott.)

other causes of airway obstruction must be sought. A solid foreign body visible in the mouth should be removed using a finger sweep. Broken or displaced dentures should be removed, but well-fitting dentures are best left in place as they help to maintain the contours of the mouth, facilitating a good seal for ventilation.

Airway management in patients with suspected cervical spine injury

If spinal injury is suspected (e.g., if the victim has fallen, been struck on the head or neck, or has been rescued after diving into shallow water) the head, neck, chest, and lumbar region should be maintained in the neutral position during resuscitation. Excessive head tilt could aggravate the injury and damage the cervical spinal cord;[19–23] however, this complication has not been documented and the relative risk is unknown. When there is a risk of cervical spine injury, a clear upper airway should be established by using jaw thrust or chin lift in combination with manual in-line stabilization (MILS) of the head and neck by an assistant.[24,25] If life-threatening airway obstruction persists despite effective application of jaw thrust or chin lift, head tilt should be added, a little at a time, until the airway is open; establishing a patent airway takes priority over concerns about a potential cervical spine injury.

Adjuncts to basic airway techniques

Simple airway adjuncts are often helpful, and sometimes essential to maintain an open airway, particularly when resuscitation is prolonged. The position of the head and neck must be maintained to keep the airway aligned. Oropharyngeal and nasopharyngeal airways are designed to overcome backward displacement of the soft palate and tongue in an unconscious patient, but head tilt and jaw thrust may also be required.

Oropharyngeal airways

Oropharyngeal (Guedel) airways (Fig. 29.4) are available in sizes suitable for newborns to those required for large adults. An *estimate* of the size required may be obtained by selecting an airway with a length corresponding to the vertical distance between the patient's incisors and the angle of the jaw. The most common adult sizes are 2, 3, and 4.

If the glossopharyngeal and laryngeal reflexes are present, retching, vomiting, or laryngospasm may occur during insertion of an oropharyngeal airway; thus, insertion should be attempted only in comatose patients.

The procedure for insertion is as follows.

- Open the patient's mouth and insert the airway in the "upside-down" position as far as the junction between the hard and soft palate and then rotate it through 180°; it is then inserted further until it lies in the oropharynx. This rotation technique minimizes the chance of pushing the tongue backwards and downwards. A tongue depressor may also be used to facilitate insertion.
- After insertion, maintain head tilt/chin lift or jaw thrust, and check the patency of the airway.

The oropharyngeal airway can become obstructed at three possible sites:[26] part of the tongue can occlude the end of the airway, the airway can lodge in the vallecula, and it can be obstructed by the epiglottis.

Nasopharyngeal airways

In patients who are not deeply unconscious, a nasopharyngeal airway is tolerated better than an oropharyngeal airway. The nasopharyngeal airway may be life-saving in patients with clenched jaws, trismus, or maxillofacial injuries, when insertion of an oral airway is impossible. Inadvertent insertion of a nasopharyngeal airway through a fracture of the skull base and into the cranial vault is possible, but extremely rare.[27,28] In the presence of a known or suspected basal skull fracture an oral airway is preferred, but if this is not possible, and the airway is obstructed, gentle insertion of a nasopharyngeal airway may be life-saving (i.e., the benefits may far outweigh the risks).

The tubes are sized in millimeters according to their internal diameter, and the length increases with diameter.

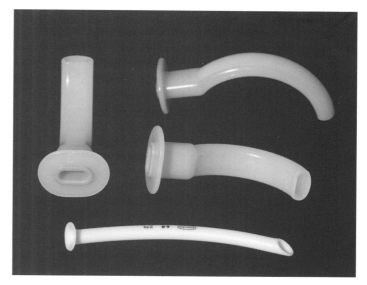

Fig. 29.4. Oropharyngeal airway. (Reproduced with permission from Dr. Mike Scott.)

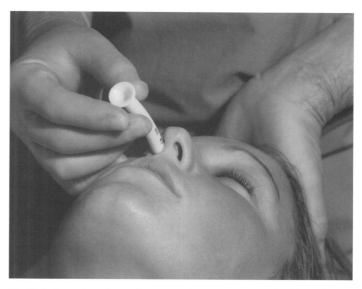

Fig. 29.5. Insertion of nasopharyngeal airway. (Reproduced with permission from Dr. Mike Scott.)

The traditional methods of sizing a nasopharyngeal airway (measurement against the patient's little finger or anterior nares) do not correlate with the airway anatomy and are unreliable.[29] Sizes 6–7 mm are suitable for adults. Insertion can damage the mucosal lining of the nasal airway, causing bleeding in up to 30% of cases.[30] If the tube is too long it may stimulate the laryngeal or glossopharyngeal reflexes to produce laryngospasm or vomiting.

The procedure for insertion is as follows (Fig. 29.5).

- Check for patency of the right nostril.
- Lubricate the airway thoroughly using water-soluble jelly
- Insert the airway bevel end first, vertically along the floor of the nose with a slight twisting action. The curve of the airway should direct it towards the patient's feet. If any obstruction is met, remove the tube and try the left nostril.
- Once in place, check the patency of the airway and adequacy of ventilation by the look, listen, and feel technique. Chin lift or jaw thrust may still be required to maintain airway patency. When there is suspicion of an injury to the cervical spine, maintain correct alignment of the head and neck.

Supraglottic airway devices

The tracheal tube has generally been considered as the optimal method of managing the airway during cardiac arrest. But there is evidence that, without adequate training and experience, the incidence of complications, such as unrecognized esophageal intubation (6%–14% in some studies)[31–34] and dislodgement, is unacceptably high.[35] Prolonged attempts at tracheal intubation are harmful: the cessation of chest compressions during this time will compromise coronary and cerebral perfusion. Several alternative airway devices have been considered for airway management during CPR.[36] Many of these devices are designed to enable ventilation through apertures situated above the laryngeal inlet. Some have perilaryngeal cuffs and some have pharyngeal cuffs. Many also have

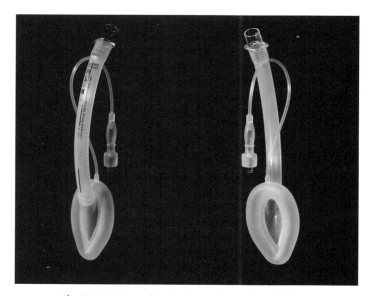

Fig. 29.6. Laryngeal mask airway. (Reproduced with permission from Dr. Mike Scott.)

esophageal drain tubes, whereas others are simply placed as esophageal obturators.

The Combitube, the classic laryngeal mask airway (cLMA), and the laryngeal tube (LT) are the only alternative devices that have been studied during CPR, but none of these studies has been powered adequately to enable survival to be studied as a primary endpoint; instead, most researchers have studied insertion and ventilation success rates. There are no data supporting the routine use of any specific approach to airway management during cardiac arrest. The best technique depends on the precise circumstances of the cardiac arrest and the competence of the rescuer.

Laryngeal mask airway and variants

Classic LMA

The cLMA was introduced in 1988 and comprises a wide bore tube with an elliptical inflated cuff designed to seal around the laryngeal opening (Fig. 29.6). When positioned correctly, the cLMA tip lies within the top of the esophagus. Experience with its use is extensive, with 2500 publications and an estimated 200 million insertions worldwide.[36] The cLMA is easier to insert than a tracheal tube.[37–43]

On the basis of data from anesthetic practice, the cLMA establishes an airway in more than 99% of cases; when attempted bag-mask ventilation fails, the cLMA will resolve airway obstruction in more than 95% of cases.[44]

The LMA has been studied during CPR but none of these studies has compared it directly with the tracheal tube. During CPR, successful ventilation was achieved with the LMA in 72%–98% of cases (Table 29.1).[45–51]

Ventilation with the LMA is more efficient and easier than with a bag-mask.[52] When an LMA can be inserted without delay it is preferable to avoid bag-mask ventilation altogether. When used for intermittent positive pressure ventilation, provided that high inflation pressures (>20 cm H_2O) are avoided, gastric inflation can be minimized. In comparison with bag-mask ventilation, use of a self-inflating bag and LMA during cardiac arrest reduces the incidence of regurgitation from 12% to 3%.[53] In cases of suspected neck injury, the cLMA can be inserted easily with the head and neck maintained in a neutral position.[54,55]

In comparison with tracheal intubation, the perceived disadvantages of the LMA are the increased risk of aspiration and inability to provide adequate ventilation in patients with low lung and/or chest wall compliance. There are remarkably few cases of pulmonary aspiration reported in the studies of the LMA during CPR. Rumball and MacDonald reported 1 aspiration out of 15 cases that were autopsied,[45] Tanigawa and Shigematsu reported six

Table 29.1. The success rates for insertion and/or ventilation with the LMA during CPR

Study	In-/out-of-hospital	n	Insertion (%)	Ventilation (%)
Baskett, 1994[48]	In	164	100	86
Kokkinis, 1994[50]	In	50	N/A	98
Leach et al., 1993[51]	In	40	N/A	95
Verghese et al., 1994[46]	In	64	100	N/A
Grantham et al., 1994[49]	Out	156	N/A	90
Rumball & MacDonald, 1997[45]	Out	108	N/A	73
Tanigawa & Shigematsu, 1998[47]	Out	2701	89.5	71.5

cases of aspiration (almost certainly under-reported), [47] and Baskett reported just one case and this patient survived to discharge.[48] There are no data demonstrating whether or not it is possible to provide adequate ventilation via an LMA without interruption of chest compressions. The ability to ventilate the lungs adequately while continuing to compress the chest may be one of the main benefits of a tracheal tube. There has been one case report describing gastric rupture associated with use of the LMA during CPR;[56] however, this complication is more likely to have been caused during the period of layperson CPR before arrival healthcare professionals.[57]

Although often taught as a method for helping to protect the airway from esophageal and gastric sources of aspiration, cricoid pressure is problematic when used with the LMA. Evidence clearly suggests that application of cricoid pressure impairs the correct positioning and function of the LMA.[58–60] The tip of the LMA normally sits within the upper esophageal sphincter where studies on cadavers have shown that acts as an "obturator" preventing, to a certain degree, overspill of esophageal contents into the larynx. This position is important when the LMA is used as a ventilation device. The application of cricoid pressure prevents the LMA from adopting its correct location in relation to the larynx, and the aperture of the LMA is pushed out towards the base of the tongue.

Technique for insertion of a laryngeal mask airway
- Select an LMA of appropriate size for the patient and deflate the cuff fully. A size 5 will be correct for most men and a size 4 for most women. Lubricate the outer face of the cuff area (the part that will not be in contact with the larynx) with water-soluble gel.

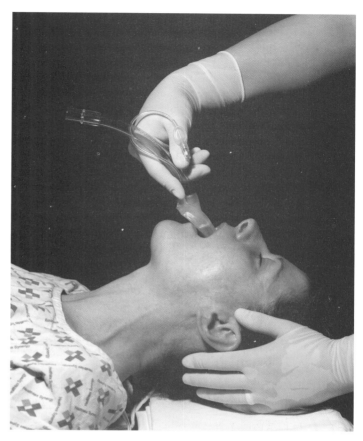

Fig. 29.7. Technique for insertion of laryngeal mask airway. (Reproduced with permission from Dr. Mike Scott.)

- Flex the patient's neck slightly and extend the head (try to maintain neutral alignment of the head neck if there is suspicion of cervical spine injury).
- Holding the LMA like a pen, insert it into the mouth (Fig. 29.7). Advance the tip behind the upper incisors with the upper surface applied to the palate until it reaches the posterior pharyngeal wall. Press the mask backwards and downwards around the corner of the pharynx until resistance is felt as it locates in the back of the pharynx. If possible, get an assistant to apply a jaw thrust after the LMA has been inserted into the mouth – this increases the space in the posterior pharynx and makes successful placement easier.
- Connect the inflating syringe and inflate the cuff with air (40 ml for a size 5 LMA and 30 ml for a size 4 LMA); alternatively, inflate the cuff to a pressure of 60 cm H_2O. If insertion is satisfactory, the tube will lift 1–2 cm out of the mouth as the cuff finds its correct position and the larynx is pushed forward.

- If the LMA has not been inserted successfully after 30 seconds, oxygenate the patient by using a pocket mask or bag-mask before reattempting LMA insertion.
- Confirm a clear airway by listening over the chest during inflation and observing bilateral chest movement. A large, audible leak suggests malposition of the LMA, but a small leak is acceptable provided that chest rise is adequate.
- Insert a bite block alongside the tube if available and secure the LMA with a bandage or tape.

Single-use LMA

The cLMA can be reused up to 40 times after sterilization. After the patent for the basic design of the cLMA expired in 2003, several companies have manufactured single-use versions, many of which are currently available. All differ slightly from the cLMA. Several reports indicate slightly increased difficulty with insertion of the single-use variants,[61–63] although seal pressure may be slightly higher in some models.[62–64] There are no studies of single-use laryngeal masks during resuscitation either in or out of hospital and their routine use during CPR cannot necessarily be extrapolated from the data acquired when using the cLMA. Single-use airway devices may have advantages when they are likely to be used infrequently and where there are problems accessing sterilizing services, e.g., out-of-hospital.

ProSeal LMA

The ProSeal LMA (PLMA) is a modified version of the original LMA. It has an additional posterior cuff and a gastric

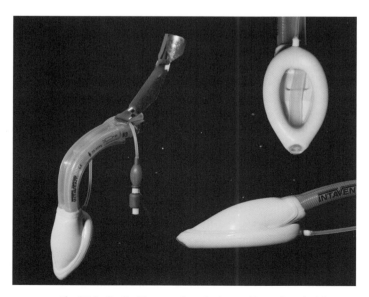

Fig. 29.8. ProSeal laryngeal mask airway. (Reproduced with permission from Dr. Mike Scott.)

drain tube (Fig. 29.8). The device has been studied extensively in anesthetized patients,[65] but there are no studies of its function and performance during CPR. It has several attributes that, in theory, make it more suitable than the original LMA for use during CPR. Nine comparative studies of 1470 patients indicate that the airway seal pressure is approximately 50% higher with the PLMA than the cLMA (PLMA 27–31 cm H_2O vs. cLMA 16–22 cm H_2O).[65] The inclusion of a gastric drain tube enables venting of liquid gastric contents regurgitated from the upper esophagus and passage of a gastric tube to drain liquid gastric contents. The in-built bite block prevents occlusion of the airway tube. The higher seal pressures achieved with the ProSeal may enable ventilation volume to be maintained during uninterrupted chest compressions. At pressures above 30 cm H_2O, leak-free ventilation should be achievable in 48% of patients with the PLMA, but in only 4% with the cLMA.[66] Potential weaknesses of the ProSeal LMA as an airway device for CPR are that it is slightly more difficult to insert than is the original LMA, it is not available in disposable form at present (although expected to be available in 2007), it is relatively expensive, and that solid regurgitated gastric contents could block the gastric drainage tube. There are no data on its performance during CPR in humans, but the cLMA, PLMA, intubating LMA (ILMA), LMA Unique (single-use), facemask and tracheal tube have been evaluated in a manikin with chest compressions given by a mechanical chest thumper.[67] Ventilation was measured both during interrupted and uninterrupted chest compressions. When chest compressions were paused for ventilation, all airway devices performed adequately. When chest compressions were uninterrupted, only the PLMA, ILMA, and tracheal tube (TT) enabled effective ventilation of the manikin; excessive gastric inflation occurred with the other airway devices. The Proseal LMA is also inserted easily with the head and neck maintained in a neutral position, making it useful in suspected cases of cervical spine injury.[68]

Intubating LMA

The intubating LMA (ILMA) is valuable for managing the difficult airway during anesthesia, but it has not been studied during CPR. Although it is relatively easy to insert the ILMA,[69,70] reliable, blind insertion of a tracheal tube requires considerable training[71] and, for this reason, it is not an ideal technique for the inexperienced provider. The ILMA provides a slightly higher airway seal pressure than the cLMA (ILMA 34 cm H_2O vs. cLMA 27 cm H_2O) enabling leak-free ventilation in a higher proportion of patients.[70] Further improvements in the seal pressure are possible by pushing the ILMA onto the laryngeal inlet after first optimizing its position. The device can also be inserted successfully with the head and neck maintained in a neutral position in suspected cases of cervical spine injury.[72] Concerns surrounding the pressure applied to the cervical spine by the rigid metal tube of the ILMA have not been substantiated and there are no case reports of neurological deterioration after ILMA insertion in patients with known cervical spine injury.[73,74] Like the cLMA, cricoid pressure significantly impairs the ability to place the ILMA correctly.[75] A single-use version of the ILMA is now available, which may make it a useful option for managing the airway during CPR.

Combitube

The Combitube is a double-lumen airway available in two sizes (37F SA and 41F).[76] It is passed blindly into the mouth, over the tongue and into the pharynx. It enables ventilation of the patient's lungs whether the tube enters the esophagus or trachea. The tracheal channel has an open distal end. The esophageal tube has no terminal opening, but has several small side-holes located between two cuffs. A large volume pharyngeal cuff (85–100 ml) and a small volume distal cuff (12–15 ml) are used to create seals so that the device may function correctly. Each cuff has an independent pilot balloon. The Combitube is positioned by opening the mouth and manually lifting the jaw. Prior bending of the device into a "hockey stick" configuration aids placement. A laryngoscope is not necessary and, if the Combitube is inserted correctly, no fixation is required. When introduced blindly, the tube usually enters the esophagus (in 95% of cases), and the patient's lungs are ventilated through the esophageal channel via the side holes located at, or above, the larynx (Fig. 29.9(a)). Gas cannot pass down the esophagus because of the blind end of the esophageal channel, and the distal cuff, which is positioned just proximal to the blind end. If the tube enters the trachea, ventilation is achieved via the tracheal port through its open distal end (Fig. 29.9(b)).

The Combitube may have some distinct advantages over other available airway adjuncts. It occludes the esophagus with a distal cuff and allows "venting" of esophageal and gastric contents via one of the two lumens. This may also protect against gastric rupture. Ventilation with high airway pressures is possible, furthermore, the Combitube functions well with the neck maintained in a neutral position making it potentially useful in victims of trauma.[77]

Early published data with use of the device showed an improvement in arterial oxygenation when compared with ventilation via a tracheal tube at equivalent oxygen concentrations.[78] This is probably a consequence of positive end expiratory pressure in the trachea generated via increased

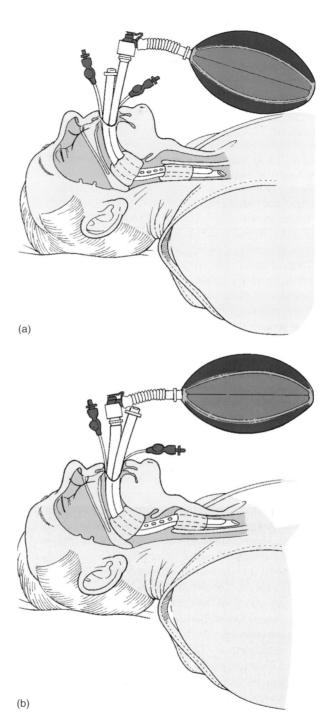

(a)

(b)

Fig. 29.9. Combitube in (a) esophageal and, (b) tracheal positions.

resistance to expiration through the small supraglottic apertures. There may also be some degree of glottic closure.

There are many studies of the Combitube in CPR and successful ventilation was achieved in 79%–98% of patients

Table 29.2. The success rates for insertion and/or ventilation with the Combitube during CPR. All except that of Staudinger *et al.** are out-of-hospital studies

Study	*n*	Insertion (%)	Ventilation (%)
Lefrancois & Dufour, 2002[80]	831	95.4	91.4
Ochs *et al.*, 2000[81]	195	N/A	79
Rabitsch *et al.*, 2003[85]	89	98	98
Rumball & McDonald, 1997[45]	77	N/A	86
Rumball *et al.*, 2004[84]	95	N/A	65.2
Tanigawa & Shigematsu, 1998[47]	1594	93.1	78.9
*Staudinger *et al.*, 1993[79]	20	94	94

(Table 29.2).[47,79–85] All except one[79] of these studies involved out-of-hospital cardiac arrest, which reflects the infrequency with which the Combitube is used in hospitals. The Combitube has been compared directly with the tracheal tube during CPR in four controlled studies (Table 29.3). On the basis of these studies, the Combitube appears as safe and effective as tracheal intubation for airway management during cardiac arrest; however, there are inadequate survival data to permit us to comment with certainty on the impact on outcome. The relatively poor success rates in both studies by Rumball and colleagues' probably reflects the relatively short period of manikin-only training;[45,84] however, the physicians in the Rabitsch study received just 2 hours of manikin training with the Combitube (they were already skilled in tracheal intubation).[85] It is possible to attempt to ventilate the lungs through the wrong port of the Combitube (2.2% in one study):[80] this is equivalent to unrecognized esophageal intubation with a standard tracheal tube.

Recent work has suggested that higher airway pressures (up to 30 cm H_2O) can be generated with the Combitube than with the cLMA.[87] Furthermore, drug access to the trachea via the Combitube has been demonstrated successfully with both lidocaine and adrenaline.[88] One other major advantage of the Combitube is the ability to deflate the pharyngeal balloon while keeping the esophageal balloon inflated. The trachea can thus be safely intubated and protected from esophageal contents when the device needs to be exchanged for a tracheal tube. Finally, it appears that the Combitube protects the larynx well from soiling above the larynx. A study of methylene blue instilled above the inflated pharyngeal balloon has demonstrated little staining of the trachea.[89]

Limitations of the Combitube

Much of the recent work has also highlighted problems with the Combitube. The device may be difficult to insert without correct training. Since it is not in daily use for non-emergencies, teaching is limited to manikins. It also causes a degree of pharyngeal or laryngeal trauma during insertion. In two studies, the incidence of blood staining the Combitube after removal was 24% and 45%.[89,90] Some trauma may be related to overdistension of the pharyngeal balloon and consequent stretching of the pharyngeal mucosa. It would seem prudent therefore to recommend that the proximal cuff is inflated sufficiently only to create the best pharyngeal seal possible. More recently this suggestion has been supported with pharyngeal cuff volumes for the Combitube correlating well with patient height when titrated to leak pressure.[87,91] Furthermore, esophageal rupture,[82,92] mucosal tears and hematomas[91] have been reported after Combitube insertion. Studies in cadavers have demonstrated significant distortion to the esophagus by the Combitube, thought to be due to pressure exerted by its tip which is angulated anteriorly.[93] This may, in part, explain some of the reported cases of esophageal perforation.

There are also reports of a complete inability to ventilate the lungs by using the Combitube. This is usually caused by the device being inserted too far, with the pharyngeal cuff sitting directly over the laryngeal inlet. Withdrawing the tube a small distance easily overcomes the problem. Finally, while it has been shown that ventilation in the presence of a cervical collar is adequate, insertion of the Combitube with the patient wearing a cervical collar is very difficult. One study demonstrated a complete inability to insert the device in 10/15 patients when a rigid cervical collar was in place.[77] This was probably caused by poor mouth opening and the size of the device. In half of these failures insertion was possible with the aid of a laryngoscope. Other studies have demonstrated that, in comparison with several other supraglottic airway devices, the Combitube potentially causes the most cervical spine movement.[23]

Laryngeal tube

The laryngeal tube (LT) is a relatively new airway device (Fig. 29.10); its function in anesthetized patients has been reported in several studies.[94,95] The performance of the LT is favorable in comparison with the classic LMA and ProSeal LMA[96–99] and successful insertion rates have been reported even in studies of paramedics and emergency medical technicians.[100,101] There are sporadic case reports relating to use of the LT during CPR.[102,103] In a recent study, the LT was placed in 30 patients in cardiac arrest out-of-hospital by minimally trained nurses.[104] Insertion of the laryngeal tube was successful within two attempts in 90% of patients, and ventilation was adequate in 80% of cases. No regurgitation occurred in any patient.

Table 29.3. Controlled studies comparing the Combitube with the tracheal tube during CPR

Study	n	Ventilation success Combitube	Ventilation success Tracheal tube	Comments
Staudinger *et al.*, 1993[79]	37	16/17 (94%)	19/20 (95%)	In-hospital, better PaO_2 with Combitube
Staudinger *et al.*, 1994[86]	86	N/A	N/A	Inadequate data in German abstract
Rabitsch *et al.*, 2003[85]	172	87/89 (98%)	78/83 (94%)	5 intubation fails had Combitube OK 2, Combitube fails were intubated Insertion time shorter with Combitube (12 s vs. 18 s) – Physicians
Rumball *et al.*, 2004[84]	357	62//95 (65%)	175/250 (70%)	Minimal training

There are three other modified versions of the LT: the single-use LT, the LT-Suction II, and the single-use LT-Suction II.[95] The LT-Suction II has a suction tube located behind the airway tube. Two studies of the first version of this device in anesthetized patients indicate that its performance is similar to the ProSeal LMA[105,106], but one study concluded that the quality of the airway achieved with the LT-Suction was inferior to that achieved with the ProSeal LMA.[107] The LT-Suction II has yet to be studied during CPR.

Other new supraglottic airway devices

There are now a large variety of commercially available new airway devices. All are designed in some way to be placed above the larynx and allow a blind insertion technique. Current manufacturing legislation allows such devices to be sold for clinical use without any properly conducted human trial data as to their efficacy. Many of the new devices are marketed for use during cardiopulmonary resuscitation, but until reliable data are available, they should be used with caution. Recent work and subsequent correspondence concerning where some of these new devices are positioned within the pharynx has highlighted some of the issues.[108,109]

Tracheal intubation

There is insufficient evidence to support or refute the use of any specific technique to maintain an airway and provide ventilation in adults with cardiopulmonary arrest. Despite this, tracheal intubation is perceived as the optimal method of providing and maintaining a clear and secure airway. It should be used only when highly skilled, confident personnel are available to carry out the procedure. The only

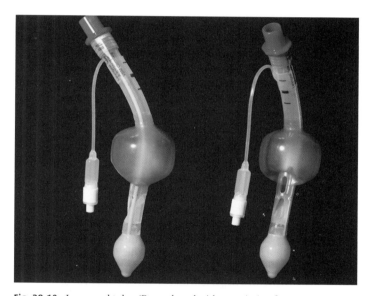

Fig. 29.10. Laryngeal tube. (Reproduced with permission from Dr. Mike Scott.)

randomized controlled trial comparing tracheal intubation with bag-mask ventilation (BMV) was undertaken in children requiring airway management out-of-hospital.[110] There was no difference in survival to discharge: 123/404 (30%) in the bag-mask group vs. 110/416 (26%) in the intubation group (OR 0.82 (95% CI 0.61–1.11)). In the children with a diagnosis of cardiopulmonary arrest ($n = 591$) the survival to hospital discharge was 24/290 (8%) in the bag-mask group vs. 24/301 (8%) in the tracheal intubation group. Of the 420 children in the intubation group, paramedics attempted intubation in 305 (73%) and, of these, 174 (57%) were intubated successfully. There were three

(2%) unrecognized esophageal intubations and 12 (6%) unrecognized tube dislodgements. The incidence of vomiting (14%) and aspiration (14%–15%) was no different between the groups, but gastric distention was more common in the bag-mask group (31% vs. 7%). It is very difficult to extrapolate these data to adult cardiac arrest: children are more difficult to intubate and tube dislodgement is probably more likely, paramedic training was suboptimal (6 h of classroom training in pediatric airway management; they were already trained in and practiced adult tracheal intubation), and the etiology of cardiac arrest in children is different from that in adults. Two studies compared outcomes from out-of-hospital cardiac arrest in adults when treated by either emergency medical technicians or paramedics.[111,112] The skills provided by the paramedics, including intubation and intravenous cannulation[111,112] and drug administration,[112] made no difference to survival to hospital discharge.

The perceived advantages of tracheal intubation over bag-mask include: maintenance of a patent airway, which is protected from aspiration of gastric contents or blood from the oropharynx; ability to provide an adequate tidal volume reliably, even when chest compressions are uninterrupted; the ability to generate high airway pressures where significant resistance is encountered, e.g., asthma; the potential to free the rescuers' hands for other tasks; the ability to suction airway secretions; and the provision of a route for giving drugs. Use of the bag-mask is more likely to cause gastric distention, which, theoretically, is more likely to cause regurgitation with risk of aspiration; however, the higher incidence of regurgitation occurred in a study of the laryngeal mask airway vs. bag-mask.[53] Nonetheless, there are no reliable data to indicate that the incidence of aspiration is any lower in cardiac arrest Patients ventilated with bag-mask versus those who are ventilated via tracheal tube.

The perceived disadvantages of tracheal intubation over the bag-mask include: the risk of an unrecognized misplaced tracheal tube, which in patients with out-of-hospital cardiac arrest is as high as 6%[31–33] to 14% (Table 29.4);[34] a prolonged time without chest compressions while intubation is attempted; and a comparatively high failure rate. Intubation success rates correlate with the intubation experience attained by individual paramedics.[113] Rates for failure to intubate are as high as 50% in prehospital systems with a low patient volume and providers who do not perform intubation frequently.[33] The cost of training prehospital staff to undertake intubation should also be considered. Healthcare personnel who undertake prehospital intubation should do so only within a structured, monitored program, which should include comprehensive com-

Table 29.4. Reported rates of unrecognized esophageal intubation after out-of-hospital cardiac arrest

Study	Number (%)
Sayre, M.R., 1998[33]	3/103 (2.9)
Rumball, C., 2004[84]	7/208 (3.0)
Pelucio, M., 1997[32]	10/168 (6.0)
Jones, J.H., 2004[31]	10/160 (6.3)
Katz, S.H., 2001[34]	18/108 (16.7)

petency-based training and regular opportunities to refresh skills.

In some cases, laryngoscopy and attempted intubation may prove impossible or cause life-threatening deterioration in the patient's condition. Such circumstances include acute epiglottitis, pharyngeal pathology, head injury (where straining may occur, further raising intracranial pressure), or in patients with cervical spine injury. In these circumstances, specialist skills such as the use of anesthetic drugs or fiberoptic laryngoscopy may be required. These techniques require a high level of skill and training.

Rescuers must weigh the risks and benefits of intubation against the need to provide effective chest compressions. The intubation attempt will require interruption of chest compressions, but once an advanced airway is in place, ventilation will not require interruption of chest compressions. Personnel skilled in advanced airway management should be able to perform laryngoscopy without stopping chest compressions – a brief pause in chest compressions will be required as the tube is passed through the vocal cords. Alternatively, to avoid any interruptions in chest compressions, the intubation attempt may be deferred until return of spontaneous circulation. No intubation attempt should take longer than 30 seconds: if intubation has not been achieved after this time, bag-mask ventilation should be restarted.[3] After intubation, tube placement must be confirmed and the tube secured adequately.

Aids to intubation

Alternative laryngoscope blades
The Macintosh blade is a good general-purpose blade and size 3 is suitable for most adults. Occasionally a longer (size 4) blade is better for very large, long-necked patients. The McCoy levering laryngoscope has a hinged tip, and will often improve the view at laryngoscopy.[114] Use of the straight blade is occasionally necessary and often preferred by some, particularly in the United States.[115,116]

Introducers

If visualization is difficult, a gum elastic bougie may be helpful to guide the tracheal tube into the larynx.[117–120] It is best inserted into the larynx separately – the tube is then passed over it into the trachea. When correctly placed, a bougie will demonstrate "hold up" within the bronchial tree.[121] A bougie placed accidentally in the esophagus will pass without obvious resistance.

Newer single-use bougies are now widely available. They do not possess the same memory, i.e., retain the shape into which they are preformed before insertion into the trachea, and their performance is inferior to the reusable device.[122,123]

Confirmation of correct placement of the tracheal tube

Unrecognized esophageal intubation is the most serious complication of attempted tracheal intubation – routine use of primary and secondary techniques to confirm correct placement of the tracheal tube should reduce this risk. Primary assessment includes observation of chest expansion bilaterally, auscultation over the lung fields bilaterally in the axillae (breath sounds should be equal and adequate) and over the epigastrium (breath sounds should not be heard). Clinical signs of correct tube placement (condensation in the tube, chest rise, breath sounds on auscultation of lungs, and inability to hear gas entering the stomach) are not completely reliable. Secondary confirmation of tracheal tube placement by an exhaled CO_2 or esophageal detection device should reduce the risk of unrecognized esophageal intubation. If there is doubt about correct tube placement, the laryngoscope should be used to see if the tube passes through the vocal cords.

None of the secondary confirmation techniques will differentiate a tube placed in a main bronchus from one placed correctly in the trachea. Data are currently inadequate to identify the optimal method of confirming tube placement during cardiac arrest and all devices should be considered as adjuncts to other confirmatory techniques.[1,124]

Esophageal detector device

The esophageal detector device creates a suction force at the tracheal end of the tracheal tube, either from pulling back the plunger on a large syringe or releasing a compressed flexible bulb. Air is aspirated easily from the lower airways through a tracheal tube placed in the cartilage-supported rigid trachea. When the tube is in the esophagus, air cannot be aspirated because the esophagus collapses when aspiration is attempted. The esophageal detector device is generally reliable in patients with both a perfusing and a non-perfusing rhythm, but it may be misleading in patients with morbid obesity, late pregnancy, or severe asthma, or when there are copious tracheal secretions; in these conditions the trachea may collapse when aspiration is attempted.[33,125–129]

The esophageal detector device is highly sensitive for detecting misplaced tracheal tubes in the esophagus.[129–133] But in two studies of patients in cardiac arrest, the esophageal detector device had poor sensitivity for confirming tracheal placement of a tracheal tube:[125,126] up to 30% of correctly placed tubes may have been removed because the esophageal detector device suggested esophageal placement of a tube.[134]

Carbon dioxide detector devices

Carbon dioxide detector devices (waveform, colorimetry, or digital) measure the concentration of CO_2 exhaled from the lungs and may be useful as adjuncts to confirm tracheal tube placement during cardiac arrest.[124,126,134–144] The persistence of exhaled CO_2 after six ventilations indicates placement of the tracheal tube in the trachea or a main bronchus.[135] Confirmation of correct placement above the carina will require auscultation of the chest bilaterally in the mid-axillary lines. In patients with a spontaneous circulation, a lack of exhaled CO_2 indicates that the tube is in the esophagus. During cardiac arrest, pulmonary blood flow may be so low that there is insufficient exhaled CO_2, so the detector does not identify a correctly placed tracheal tube. When exhaled CO_2 is detected in cardiac arrest, it indicates reliably that the tube is in the trachea or main bronchus, but when it is absent, placement of the tracheal tube is best confirmed with an esophageal detector device. A variety of electronic as well as simple, inexpensive, colorimetric CO_2 detectors are available for both in-hospital and out-of-hospital use. Again data from cardiac arrests are insufficient to enable any firm recommendations for any particular one of these techniques.

If there is a perfusing rhythm, detection of exhaled CO_2 can be used to monitor tracheal tube position during transport.[145]

Cricoid pressure

During bag-mask ventilation and attempted intubation, cricoid pressure applied by a trained assistant should prevent passive regurgitation of gastric contents and the consequent risk of pulmonary aspiration.[146–150]

The cricoid cartilage is identified immediately below the thyroid cartilage where it forms a complete ring at the upper end of the trachea. A pressure of 30 newtons (3 kg) is

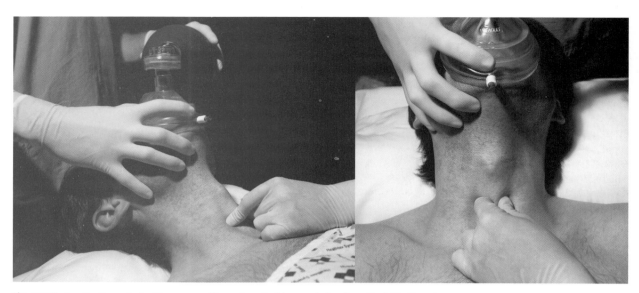

Fig. 29.11. Application of cricoid pressure. (Reproduced with permission from Dr. Mike Scott.)

applied anteroposteriorly, forcing the cricoid ring backwards to press the esophagus against the vertebral column (Fig. 29.11).[151,152] Pressure should be maintained continuously until a tracheal tube is inserted through the vocal cords and the cuff has been inflated. Although effective at preventing passive regurgitation, cricoid pressure should not be used in cases of active vomiting or retching, as it could result in damage/rupture to the esophagus, particularly in the presence of esophageal pathology.[153] In patients with suspected cervical spine injury, counter-pressure may be applied to the back of the neck to reduce movement of the cervical spine.[154] If the technique is applied imprecisely or with excessive force, ventilation with a bag–valve–mask and tracheal intubation can be made significantly more difficult. Application of cricoid pressure at 30 N causes airway obstruction in 3% of patients compared with 35% when 40 N are applied.[155] If ventilation of the patient's lungs is not possible, reduce the pressure applied to the cricoid cartilage or remove it completely.

It is also important to apply the cricoid pressure in the correct direction. If the true perpendicular anterior–posterior position is not used, significant problems may occur. Pushing the larynx in an upward direction (a technique often used to improve the view at laryngoscopy) will cause closure of the vocal cords and worsen any attempts at ventilation.[152] If the patient's head and neck are not aligned correctly, e.g., during lateral tilting of the pregnant patient, the view at laryngoscopy may be made worse if the cricoid is displaced to the left.

Securing the tracheal tube

Accidental dislodgement of a tracheal tube can occur at any time, but may be more likely during resuscitation and during transport. There are no studies comparing different strategies for securing the tracheal tube during CPR. Two studies undertaken in intensive care units,[156,157] comparing commercial devices with traditional taping for securing tracheal tubes, reported no difference in rates of accidental tube displacement. Thus, either conventional tapes or ties, or purpose-made tracheal tube holders can be used to secure the tracheal tube during CPR.

Cricothyroidotomy

Occasionally it will be impossible to ventilate an apnoeic patient with a bag-mask, or to pass a tracheal tube or alternative airway device. This may occur in patients with extensive facial trauma or laryngeal obstruction caused by edema or foreign material. In these circumstances, delivery of oxygen through a needle or surgical cricothyroidotomy may be life-saving.[158–160] A tracheostomy is contraindicated in an emergency as it is time-consuming, hazardous, and requires considerable surgical skill and equipment.

Surgical cricothyroidotomy provides a definitive airway that can be used to ventilate the patient's lungs until semielective intubation or tracheostomy is performed. Needle cricothyroidotomy is a much more temporary procedure providing only short term oxygenation.[161] It requires a wide-bore non-kinking cannula, a high pressure oxygen source, runs the risk of barotrauma, and can be particularly ineffective in patients with chest trauma. It is also prone to failure because of kinking of the cannula, and is unsuitable for patient transfer. A recent cadaver study indicated that a Seldinger technique cricothyroidotomy was quicker to achieve than a standard surgical technique;[162] however, an animal study indicated that a cannula-over-needle technique (Quicktrach) was better than a wire-guided technique (Mini-trach).[163]

Several new purpose-built cricothyroidotomy devices are now available, e.g., PCT (Portex), Quicktrach II (VBM), cuffed Melker (Cook). These are manufactured to enable quick and easy insertion, they have a short wide-bore tube permitting ventilation with a self-inflating bag, and they have cuffs to enable both high airway pressure ventilation and airway protection.

Summary

Airway obstruction is common during cardiopulmonary arrest; establishing and maintaining a patent airway is a fundamental component of cardiopulmonary resuscitation. Basic airway maneuvers with or without the use of simple adjuncts will often enable airway patency to be established. In the hands of highly skilled personnel, tracheal intubation should provide the most reliable protection of the airway and route for ventilation of the lungs during cardiac arrest. The time taken to insert the tracheal tube and the risk of unrecognized esophageal intubation, however, are significant disadvantages. Supraglottic airway devices, such as the LMA and Combitube, are easier to insert than a tracheal tube and may be a better option for personnel who are not skilled in tracheal intubation. Several other supraglottic devices are available, but there are insufficient data to recommend their use during CPR.

REFERENCES

1. International Liaison Committee on Resuscitation. Part 4. Advanced Life Support. 2005 International Consensus on Cardiopulmonary Resuscitation and Emergency Cardiovascular Care Science with Treatment Recommendations. *Resuscitation* 2005; **67**: 213–247.

2. Handley, A.J., Koster, R.W., Monsieurs, K., Perkins, G.D., Davies, S. & Bossaert, L. European Resuscitation Council Guidelines for Resuscitation 2005. Section 2: Adult basic life support and use of automated external defibrillators. *Resuscitation* 2005; **67** Suppl. 1: S7–S24.

3. Nolan, J.P., Deakin, C.D., Soar, J., Bottiger, B.W. & Smith, G. European Resuscitation Council Guidelines for Resuscitation 2005. Section 4: Adult advanced life support. *Resuscitation* 2005; **67** Suppl. 1: S39–S86.

4. Hillman, D.R., Platt, P.R. & Eastwood, P.R. The upper airway during anaesthesia. *Br. J. Anaesth.* 2003; **91**: 31–39.

5. Boidin, M.P. Airway patency in the unconscious patient. *Br. J. Anaesth.* 1985; **57**: 306–310.

6. Nandi, P.R., Charlesworth, C.H., Taylor, S.J., Nunn, J.F. & Dore, C.J. Effect of general anaesthesia on the pharynx. *Br. J. Anaesth.* 1991; **66**: 157–162.

7. Safar, P., Escarraga, L.A. & Chang, F. Upper airway obstruction in the unconscious patient. *J. Appl. Physiol.* 1959; **14**: 760–764.

8. Safar, P. Ventilatory efficacy of mouth-to-mouth artificial respiration; airway obstruction during manual and mouth-to-mouth artificial respiration. *J. Am. Med. Assoc.* 1958; **167**: 335–341.

9. Wenzel, V., Idris, A.H., Banner, M.J. *et al.* Respiratory system compliance decreases after cardiopulmonary resuscitation and stomach inflation: impact of large and small tidal volumes on calculated peak airway pressure. *Resuscitation* 1998; **38**: 113–118.

10. Wenzel, V., Idris, A.H., Dorges, V. *et al.* The respiratory system during resuscitation: a review of the history, risk of infection during assisted ventilation, respiratory mechanics, and ventilation strategies for patients with an unprotected airway. *Resuscitation* 2001; **49**: 123–134.

11. Hardman, J.G., Wills, J.S. & Aitkenhead, A.R. Factors determining the onset and course of hypoxemia during apnea: an investigation using physiological modelling. *Anesth. Analg.* 2000; **90**: 619–624.

12. Hardman, J.G., Wills, J.S. & Aitkenhead, A.R. Investigating hypoxemia during apnea: validation of a set of physiological models. *Anesth. Analg.* 2000; **90**: 614–618.

13. Guildner, C.W. Resuscitation: opening the airway. A comparative study of techniques for opening an airway obstructed by the tongue. *J. Am. Coll. Emerg. Phys.* 1976; **5**: 588–590.

14. Safar, P. & Aguto-Escarraga, L. Compliance in apneic anesthetized adults. *Anesthesiology* 1959; **20**: 283–289.

15. Greene, D.G., Elam, J.O., Dobkin, A.B. & Studley, C.L. Cinefluorographic study of hyperextension of the neck and upper airway patency. *J. Am. Med. Assoc.* 1961; **176**: 570–573.

16. Morikawa, S., Safar, P. & Decarlo, J. Influence of the headjaw position upon upper airway patency. *Anesthesiology* 1961; **22**: 265–270.

17. Ruben, H.M., Elam, J.O., Ruben, A.M. & Greene, D.G. Investigation of upper airway problems in resuscitation, 1: studies of pharyngeal X-rays and performance by laymen. *Anesthesiology* 1961; **22**: 271–279.

18. Elam, J.O., Greene, D.G., Schneider, M.A. *et al.* Head-tilt method of oral resuscitation. *J. Am. Med. Assoc.* 1960; **172**: 812–815.

19. Aprahamian, C., Thompson, B.M., Finger, W.A. & Darin, J.C. Experimental cervical spine injury model: evaluation of

airway management and splinting techniques. *Ann. Emerg. Med.* 1984; **13**: 584–587.

20. Donaldson, W.F., 3rd, Heil, B.V., Donaldson, V.P. & Silvaggio, V.J. The effect of airway maneuvers on the unstable C1–C2 segment. A cadaver study. *Spine* 1997; **22**: 1215–1218.

21. Donaldson, W.F., 3rd, Towers, J.D., Doctor, A., Brand, A. & Donaldson, V.P. A methodology to evaluate motion of the unstable spine during intubation techniques. *Spine* 1993; **18**: 2020–2023.

22. Hauswald, M., Sklar, D.P., Tandberg, D. & Garcia, J.F. Cervical spine movement during airway management: cinefluoroscopic appraisal in human cadavers. *Am. J. Emerg. Med.* 1991; **9**: 535–538.

23. Brimacombe, J., Keller, C., Kunzel, K.H., Gaber, O., Boehler, M. & Puhringer, F. Cervical spine motion during airway management: a cinefluoroscopic study of the posteriorly destabilized third cervical vertebrae in human cadavers. *Anesth. Analg.* 2000; **91**: 1274–1278.

24. Majernick, T.G., Bieniek, R., Houston, J.B. & Hughes, H.G. Cervical spine movement during orotracheal intubation. *Ann. Emerg. Med.* 1986; **15**: 417–420.

25. Lennarson, P.J., Smith, D.W., Sawin, P.D., Todd, M.M., Sato, Y. & Traynelis, V.C. Cervical spinal motion during intubation: efficacy of stabilization maneuvers in the setting of complete segmental instability. *J. Neurosurg. Spine* 2001; **94**: 265–270.

26. Marsh, A.M., Nunn, J.F., Taylor, S.J. & Charlesworth, C.H. Airway obstruction associated with the use of the Guedel airway. *Br. J. Anaesth.* 1991; **67**: 517–523.

27. Schade, K., Borzotta, A. & Michaels, A. Intracranial malposition of nasopharyngeal airway. *J. Trauma* 2000; **49**: 967–968.

28. Muzzi, D.A., Losasso, T.J. & Cucchiara, R.F. Complication from a nasopharyngeal airway in a patient with a basilar skull fracture. *Anesthesiology* 1991; **74**: 366–368.

29. Roberts, K. & Porter, K. How do you size a nasopharyngeal airway? *Resuscitation* 2003; **56**: 9–23.

30. Stoneham, M.D. The nasopharyngeal airway. Assessment of position by fibreoptic laryngoscopy. *Anaesthesia* 1993; **48**: 575–580.

31. Jones, J.H., Murphy, M.P., Dickson, R.L., Somerville, G.G. & Brizendine, E.J. Emergency physician-verified out-of-hospital intubation: miss rates by paramedics. *Acad. Emerg. Med.* 2004; **11**: 707–709.

32. Pelucio, M., Halligan, L. & Dhindsa, H. Out-of-hospital experience with the syringe esophageal detector device. *Acad. Emerg. Med.* 1997; **4**: 563–568.

33. Sayre, M.R., Sakles, J.C., Mistler, A.F., Evans, J.L., Kramer, A.T. & Pancioli, A.M. Field trial of endotracheal intubation by basic EMTs. *Ann. Emerg. Med.* 1998; **31**: 228–233.

34. Katz, S.H. & Falk, J.L. Misplaced endotracheal tubes by paramedics in an urban emergency medical services system. *Ann. Emerg. Med.* 2001; **37**: 32–37.

35. Nolan, J.P. Prehospital and resuscitative airway care: should the gold standard be reassessed? *Curr. Opin. Crit. Care* 2001; **7**: 413–421.

36. Cook, T.M. & Hommers, C. New airways for resuscitation? *Resuscitation* 2006; In press.

37. Davies, P.R., Tighe, S.Q., Greenslade, G.L. & Evans, G.H. Laryngeal mask airway and tracheal tube insertion by unskilled personnel. *Lancet* 1990; **336**: 977–979.

38. Flaishon, R., Sotman, A., Ben-Abraham, R., Rudick, V., Varssano, D. & Weinbroum, A.A. Antichemical protective gear prolongs time to successful airway management: a randomized, crossover study in humans. *Anesthesiology* 2004; **100**: 260–266.

39. Ho, B.Y., Skinner, H.J. & Mahajan, R.P. Gastro-oesophageal reflux during day case gynaecological laparoscopy under positive pressure ventilation: laryngeal mask vs. tracheal intubation. *Anaesthesia* 1998; **53**: 921–924.

40. Reinhart, D.J. & Simmons, G. Comparison of placement of the laryngeal mask airway with endotracheal tube by paramedics and respiratory therapists. *Ann. Emerg. Med.* 1994; **24**: 260–263.

41. Rewari, W. & Kaul, H.L. Regurgitation and aspiration during gynaecological laparoscopy: Comparison between laryngeal mask airway and tracheal intubation. *J. Anaesth. Clin. Pharmacol.* 1999; **15**(1): 67–70.

42. Pennant, J.H. & Walker, M.B. Comparison of the endotracheal tube and laryngeal mask in airway management by paramedical personnel. *Anesth. Analg.* 1992; **74**: 531–534.

43. Maltby, J.R., Beriault, M.T., Watson, N.C., Liepert, D.J. & Fick, G.H. LMA-Classic and LMA-ProSeal are effective alternatives to endotracheal intubation for gynecologic laparoscopy. *Can. J. Anaesth.* 2003; **50**: 71–77.

44. Parmet, J.L., Colonna-Romano, P., Horrow, J.C., Miller, F., Gonzales, J. & Rosenberg, H. The laryngeal mask airway reliably provides rescue ventilation in cases of unanticipated difficult tracheal intubation along with difficult mask ventilation. *Anesth. Analg.* 1998; **87**: 661–665.

45. Rumball, C.J. & MacDonald, D. The PTL, Combitube, laryngeal mask, and oral airway: a randomized prehospital comparative study of ventilatory device effectiveness and cost-effectiveness in 470 cases of cardiorespiratory arrest. *Prehosp. Emerg. Care* 1997; **1**: 1–10.

46. Verghese, C., Prior-Willeard, P.F. & Baskett, P.J. Immediate management of the airway during cardiopulmonary resuscitation in a hospital without a resident anaesthesiologist. *Eur. J. Emerg. Med.* 1994; **1**: 123–125.

47. Tanigawa, K. & Shigematsu, A. Choice of airway devices for 12,020 cases of nontraumatic cardiac arrest in Japan. *Prehosp. Emerg. Care* 1998; **2**: 96–100.

48. Baskett, P.J. The laryngeal mask in resuscitation. *Resuscitation* 1994; **28**: 93–95.

49. Grantham, H., Phillips, G. & Gilligan, J.E. The laryngeal mask in prehospital emergency care. *Emerg. Med.* 1994; **6**: 193–197.

50. Kokkinis, K. The use of the laryngeal mask airway in CPR. *Resuscitation* 1994; **27**: 9–12.

51. Leach, A., Alexander, C.A. & Stone, B. The laryngeal mask in cardiopulmonary resuscitation in a district general hospital: a preliminary communication. *Resuscitation* 1993; **25**: 245–248.

52. Alexander, R., Hodgson, P., Lomax, D. & Bullen, C. A comparison of the laryngeal mask airway and Guedel airway, bag and face mask for manual ventilation following formal training. *Anaesthesia* 1993; **48**: 231–234.

53. Stone, B.J., Chantler, P.J. & Baskett, P.J. The incidence of regurgitation during cardiopulmonary resuscitation: a comparison between the bag valve mask and laryngeal mask airway. *Resuscitation* 1998; **38**: 3–6.

54. Pennant, J.H., Pace, N.A. & Gajraj, N.M. Role of the laryngeal mask airway in the immobile cervical spine. *J. Clin. Anesth.* 1993; **5**: 226–230.

55. Brimacombe, J. & Berry, A. Laryngeal mask airway insertion. A comparison of the standard versus neutral position in normal patients with a view to its use in cervical spine instability. *Anaesthesia* 1993; **48**: 670–671.

56. Haslam, N., Campbell, G.C. & Duggan, J.E. Gastric rupture associated with use of the laryngeal mask airway during cardiopulmonary resuscitation. *Br. Med. J.* 2004; **329**: 1225–1226.

57. Nolan, J.P., Colquhoun, M. & Deakin, C.D. Gastric rupture and laryngeal mask airway: laryngeal mask airway was not likely cause of gastric rupture. *Br. Med. J.* 2005; **330**: 538; author reply.

58. Asai, T., Barclay, K., Power, I. & Vaughan, R.S. Cricoid pressure impedes placement of the laryngeal mask airway. *Br. J. Anaesth.* 1995; **74**: 521–525.

59. Asai, T., Barclay, K., McBeth, C. & Vaughan, R.S. Cricoid pressure applied after placement of the laryngeal mask prevents gastric insufflation but inhibits ventilation. *Br. J. Anaesth.* 1996; **76**: 772–776.

60. Ansermino, J.M., & Blogg, C.E. Cricoid pressure may prevent insertion of the laryngeal mask airway. *Br. J. Anaesth.* 1992; **69**: 465–467.

61. Brimacombe, J., von Goedecke, A., Keller, C., Brimacombe, L. & Brimacombe, M. The laryngeal mask airway Unique versus the Soft Seal laryngeal mask: a randomized, crossover study in paralyzed, anesthetized patients. *Anesth. Analg.* 2004; **99**: 1560–1563.

62. Paech, M.J., Lain, J., Garrett, W.R., Gillespie, G., Stannard, K.J. & Doherty, D.A. Randomized evaluation of the single-use SoftSeal and the re-useable LMA Classic laryngeal mask. *Anaesth. Intens. Care* 2004; **32**: 66–72.

63. Cook, T.M., Trumpelmann, P., Beringer, R. & Stedeford, J.A randomised comparison of the Portex Softseal laryngeal mask airway with the LMA-Unique during anaesthesia. *Anaesthesia* 2005; **60**: 1218–1225.

64. Van Zundert, A.A., Fonck, K., Al-Shaikh, B. & Mortier, E. Comparison of the LMA-classic with the new disposable soft seal laryngeal mask in spontaneously breathing adult patients. *Anesthesiology* 2003; **99**: 1066–1071.

65. Cook, T.M., Lee, G. & Nolan, J.P. The ProSealTM laryngeal mask airway: a review of the literature: [Le masque larynge ProSealTM : un examen des publications]. *Can. J. Anaesth.* 2005; **52**: 739–760.

66. Cook, T.M., Nolan, J.P., Verghese, C. *et al.* Randomized crossover comparison of the proseal with the classic laryngeal mask airway in unparalysed anaesthetized patients. *Br. J. Anaesth.* 2002; **88**: 527–533.

67. Genzwurker, H., Hundt, A., Finteis, T. & Ellinger, K. Comparison of different laryngeal mask airways in a resuscitation model. *Anasth. Intens. Notfallmedi. Schmerzther.* 2003; **38**: 94–101.

68. Asai, T., Murao, K. & Shingu, K. Efficacy of the ProSeal laryngeal mask airway during manual in-line stabilisation of the neck. *Anaesthesia* 2002; **57**: 918–920.

69. Burgoyne, L. & Cyna, A. Laryngeal mask vs intubating laryngeal mask: insertion and ventilation by inexperienced resuscitators. *Anaesth Intens. Care* 2001; **29**: 604–608.

70. Choyce, A., Avidan, M.S., Shariff, A., Del Aguila, M., Radcliffe, J.J. & Chan, T. A comparison of the intubating and standard laryngeal mask airways for airway management by inexperienced personnel. *Anaesthesia* 2001; **56**: 357–360.

71. Baskett, P.J., Parr, M.J. & Nolan, J.P. The intubating laryngeal mask. Results of a multicentre trial with experience of 500 cases. *Anaesthesia* 1998; **53**: 1174–1179.

72. Asai, T., Wagle, A.U. & Stacey, M. Placement of the intubating laryngeal mask is easier than the laryngeal mask during manual in-line neck stabilization. *Br. J. Anaesth.* 1999; **82**: 712–714.

73. Keller, C., Brimacombe, J. & Keller, K. Pressures exerted against the cervical vertebrae by the standard and intubating laryngeal mask airways: a randomized, controlled, cross-over study in fresh cadavers. *Anesth. Analg.* 1999; **89**: 1296–1300.

74. Ferson, D.Z., Rosenblatt, W.H., Johansen, M.J., Osborn, I. & Ovassapian, A. Use of the intubating lma-fastrach in 254 patients with difficult-to-manage airways. *Anesthesiology* 2001; **95**: 1175–1181.

75. Harry, R.M. & Nolan, J.P. The use of cricoid pressure with the intubating laryngeal mask. *Anaesthesia* 1999; **54**: 656–659.

76. Frass, M., Frenzer, R., Mayer, G., Popovic, R. & Leithner, C. Mechanical ventilation with the esophageal tracheal combitube (ETC) in the intensive care unit. *Arch. Emerg. Med.* 1987; **4**: 219–225.

77. Mercer, M.H. & Gabbott, D.A. Insertion of the Combitube airway with the cervical spine immobilised in a rigid cervical collar. *Anaesthesia* 1998; **53**: 971–974.

78. Frass, M., Frenzer, R., Rauscha, F., Schuster, E. & Glogar, D. Ventilation with the esophageal tracheal combitube in cardiopulmonary resuscitation: promptness and effectiveness. *Chest* 1988; **93**: 781–784.

79. Staudinger, T., Brugger, S., Watschinger, B. *et al.* Emergency intubation with the Combitube: comparison with the endotracheal airway. *Ann. Emerg. Med.* 1993; **22**: 1573–1575.

80. Lefrancois, D.P. & Dufour, D.G. Use of the esophageal tracheal combitube by basic emergency medical technicians. *Resuscitation* 2002; **52**: 77–83.

81. Ochs, M., Vilke, G.M., Chan, T.C., Moats, T. & Buchanan, J. Successful prehospital airway management by EMT-Ds using the combitube. *Prehosp. Emerg. Care* 2000; **4**: 333–337.

82. Vezina, D., Lessard, M.R., Bussieres, J., Topping, C. & Trepanier, C.A. Complications associated with the use of the

esophageal–tracheal Combitube. *Can. J. Anaesth.* 1998; **45**: 76–80.

83. Richards, C.F. Piriform sinus perforation during esophageal-tracheal Combitube placement. *J. Emerg. Med.* 1998; **16**: 37–39.

84. Rumball, C., Macdonald, D., Barber, P., Wong, H. & Smecher, C. Endotracheal intubation and esophageal tracheal Combitube insertion by regular ambulance attendants: a comparative trial. *Prehosp. Emerg. Care* 2004; **8**: 15–22.

85. Rabitsch, W., Schellongowski, P., Staudinger, T. *et al.* Comparison of a conventional tracheal airway with the Combitube in an urban emergency medical services system run by physicians. *Resuscitation* 2003; **57**: 27–32.

86. Staudinger, T., Brugger, S., Roggla, M. *et al.* [Comparison of the Combitube with the endotracheal tube in cardiopulmonary resuscitation in the prehospital phase]. *Wien Klin. Wochenschr.* 1994; **106**: 412–415.

87. Hartmann, T., Krenn, C.G., Zoeggeler, A., Hoerauf, K., Benumof, J.L. & Krafft, P. The oesophageal-tracheal Combitube Small Adult. *Anaesthesia* 2000; **55**: 670–675.

88. Kofler, J., Sterz, F., Hofbauer, R. *et al.* Epinephrine application via an endotracheal airway and via the Combitube in esophageal position. *Crit. Care Med.* 2000; **28**: 1445–1449.

89. Mercer, M. The role of the Combitube in airway management. *Anaesthesia* 2000; **55**: 394–395.

90. Mercer, M.H. & Gabbott, D.A. The influence of neck position on ventilation using the Combitube airway. *Anaesthesia* 1998; **53**: 146–150.

91. Oczenski, W., Krenn, H., Dahaba, A.A. *et al.* Complications following the use of the Combitube, tracheal tube and laryngeal mask airway. *Anaesthesia* 1999; **54**(12): 1161–1165.

92. Klein, H., Williamson, M., Sue-Ling, H.M., Vucevic, M. & Quinn, A.C. Esophageal rupture associated with the use of the Combitube. *Anesth. Analg.* 1997; **85**: 937–939.

93. Vezina, D., Trepanier, C.A., Lessard, M.R. & Bussieres, J. Esophageal and tracheal distortion by the esophageal–tracheal Combitube: a cadaver study. *Can. J. Anaesth.* 1999; **46**: 393–397.

94. Dorges, V., Ocker, H., Wenzel, V. & Schmucker, P. The laryngeal tube: a new simple airway device. *Anesth. Analg.* 2000; **90**: 1220–1222.

95. Asai, T. & Shingu, K. The laryngeal tube. *Br. J. Anaesth.* 2005; **95**: 729–736.

96. Asai, T., Kawashima, A., Hidaka, I. & Kawachi, S. The laryngeal tube compared with the laryngeal mask: Insertion, gas leak pressure and gastric insufflation. *Br. J. Anaesth.* 2002; **89**(5): 729–732.

97. Ocker, H., Wenzel, V., Schmucker, P., Steinfath, M. & Dorges, V. A comparison of the laryngeal tube with the laryngeal mask airway during routine surgical procedures. *Anesth. Analg.* 2002; **95**(4): 1094–1097.

98. Cook, T.M., McCormick, B. & Asai, T. Randomized comparison of laryngeal tube with classic laryngeal mask airway for anaesthesia with controlled ventilation. *Br. J. Anaesth.* 2003; **91**(3): 373–378.

99. Cook, T.M., McKinstry, C., Hardy, R. & Twigg, S. Randomized crossover comparison of the ProSeal laryngeal mask airway with the laryngeal tube during anaesthesia with controlled ventilation. *Br. J. Anaesth.* 2003; **91**: 678–683.

100. Asai, T. & Kawachi, S. Use of the laryngeal tube by paramedic staff. *Anaesthesia* 2004; **59**: 408–409.

101. Kurola, J.O., Turunen, M.J., Laakso, J.P., Gorski, J.T., Paakkonen, H.J. & Silfvast, T.O. A comparison of the laryngeal tube and bag-valve mask ventilation by emergency medical technicians: a feasibility study in anesthetized patients. *Anesth. Analg.* 2005; **101**: 1477–1481.

102. Asai, T., Moriyama, S., Nishita, Y. & Kawachi, S. Use of the laryngeal tube during cardiopulmonary resuscitation by paramedical staff. *Anaesthesia* 2003; **58**: 393–394.

103. Genzwuerker, H.V., Dhonau, S. & Ellinger, K. Use of the laryngeal tube for out-of-hospital resuscitation: *Resuscitation* 2002; **52**: 221–224.

104. Kette, F., Reffo, I., Giordani, G. *et al.* The use of laryngeal tube by nurses in out-of-hospital emergencies: preliminary experience. *Resuscitation* 2005; **66**: 21–25.

105. Gaitini, L.A., Vaida, S.J., Somri, M., Yanovski, B., Ben-David, B. & Hagberg, C.A. A randomized controlled trial comparing the ProSeal laryngeal mask airway with the laryngeal tube suction in mechanically ventilated patients. *Anesthesiology* 2004; **101**: 316–320.

106. Roth, H., Genzwuerker, H.V., Rothhaas, A., Finteis, T. & Schmeck, J. The ProSeal laryngeal mask airway and the laryngeal tube suction for ventilation in gynaecological patients undergoing laparoscopic surgery. *Eur. J. Anaesthesiol.* 2005; **22**: 117–122.

107. Cook, T.M. & Cranshaw, J. Randomized crossover comparison of ProSeal laryngeal mask airway with laryngeal tube Sonda during anaesthesia with controlled ventilation. *Br. J. Anaesth.* 2005; **95**: 261–266.

108. Cook, T.M. & Lowe, J.M. An evaluation of the Cobra perilaryngeal airway: study halted after two cases of pulmonary aspiration. *Anaesthesia* 2005; **60**: 791–796.

109. Cook, T.M. & Lowe, J. More on the CobraPLA. *Anaesthesia* 2005; **60**: 1144–1145; author reply 5–7.

110. Gausche, M., Lewis, R.J., Stratton, S.J. *et al.* Effect of out-of-hospital pediatric endotracheal intubation on survival and neurological outcome: a controlled clinical trial. *J. Am. Med. Assoc.* 2000; **283**: 783–790.

111. Guly, U.M., Mitchell, R.G., Cook, R., Steedman, D.J. & Robertson, C.E. Paramedics and technicians are equally successful at managing cardiac arrest outside hospital. *Br. Med. J.* 1995; **310**: 1091–1094.

112. Stiell, I.G., Wells, G.A., Field, B. *et al.* Advanced cardiac life support in out-of-hospital cardiac arrest. *N. Engl. J. Med.* 2004; **351**: 647–656.

113. Garza, A.G., Gratton, M.C., Coontz, D., Noble, E. & Ma, O.J. Effect of paramedic experience on orotracheal intubation success rates. *J. Emerg. Med.* 2003; **25**: 251–256.

114. McCoy, E.P. & Mirakhur, R.K. The levering laryngoscope. *Anaesthesia* 1993; **48**: 516–519.

115. Arino, J.J., Velasco, J.M., Gasco, C. & Lopez-Timoneda, F. Straight blades improve visualization of the larynx while

curved blades increase ease of intubation: a comparison of the Macintosh, Miller, McCoy, Belscope and Lee-Fiberview blades. *Can. J. Anaesth.* 2003; **50**: 501–506.

116. Henderson, J.J. The use of paraglossal straight blade laryngoscopy in difficult tracheal intubation. *Anaesthesia* 1997; **52**: 552–560.

117. Dogra, S., Falconer, R. & Latto, I.P. Successful difficult intubation: tracheal tube placement over a gum-elastic bougie. *Anaesthesia* 1990; **45**: 774–776.

118. Latto, I.P., Stacey, M., Mecklenburgh, J. & Vaughan, R.S. Survey of the use of the gum elastic bougie in clinical practice. *Anaesthesia* 2002; **57**: 379–384.

119. Nolan, J.P. & Wilson, M.E. Orotracheal intubation in patients with potential cervical spine injuries. An indication for the gum elastic bougie. *Anaesthesia* 1993; **48**: 630–633.

120. Nolan, J.P. & Wilson, M.E. An evaluation of the gum elastic bougie. Intubation times and incidence of sore throat. *Anaesthesia* 1992; **47**: 878–881.

121. Kidd, J.F., Dyson, A. & Latto, I.P. Successful difficult intubation. Use of the gum elastic bougie. *Anaesthesia* 1988; **43**: 437–438.

122. Hames, K.C., Pandit, J.J., Marfin, A.G., Popat, M.T. & Yentis, S.M. Use of the bougie in simulated difficult intubation. 1. Comparison of the single-use bougie with the fibrescope. *Anaesthesia* 2003; **58**: 846–851.

123. Marfin, A.G., Pandit, J.J., Hames, K.C., Popat, M.T. & Yentis, S.M. Use of the bougie in simulated difficult intubation. 2. Comparison of single-use bougie with multiple-use bougie. *Anaesthesia* 2003; **58**: 852–855.

124. Li, J. Capnography alone is imperfect for endotracheal tube placement confirmation during emergency intubation. *J. Emerg. Med.* 2001; **20**: 223–229.

125. Tanigawa, K., Takeda, T., Goto, E. & Tanaka, K. Accuracy and reliability of the self-inflating bulb to verify tracheal intubation in out-of-hospital cardiac arrest patients. *Anesthesiology* 2000; **93**: 1432–1436.

126. Takeda, T., Tanigawa, K., Tanaka, H., Hayashi, Y., Goto, E. & Tanaka, K. The assessment of three methods to verify tracheal tube placement in the emergency setting. *Resuscitation* 2003; **56**: 153–157.

127. Baraka, A., Khoury, P.J., Siddik, S.S., Salem, M.R. & Joseph, N.J. Efficacy of the self-inflating bulb in differentiating esophageal from tracheal intubation in the parturient undergoing cesarean section. *Anesth. Analg.* 1997; **84**: 533–537.

128. Davis, D.P., Stephen, K.A. & Vilke, G.M. Inaccuracy in endotracheal tube verification using a Toomey syringe. *J. Emerg. Med.* 1999; **17**: 35–38.

129. Bozeman, W.P., Hexter, D., Liang, H.K. & Kelen, G.D. Esophageal detector device versus detection of end-tidal carbon dioxide level in emergency intubation. *Ann. Emerg. Med.* 1996; **27**: 595–599.

130. Sharieff, G.Q., Rodarte, A., Wilton, N. & Bleyle, D. The self-inflating bulb as an airway adjunct: is it reliable in children weighing less than 20 kilograms? *Acad. Emerg. Med.* 2003; **10**: 303–308.

131. Wee, M.Y. & Walker, A.K. The oesophageal detector device: an assessment with uncuffed tubes in children. *Anaesthesia* 1991; **46**: 869–871.

132. Williams, K.N. & Nunn, J.F. The oesophageal detector device: a prospective trial on 100 patients. *Anaesthesia* 1989; **44**: 412–424.

133. Zaleski, L., Abello, D. & Gold, M.I. The esophageal detector device. Does it work? *Anesthesiology* 1993; **79**: 244–247.

134. Tanigawa, K., Takeda, T., Goto, E. & Tanaka, K. The efficacy of esophageal detector devices in verifying tracheal tube placement: a randomized cross-over study of out-of-hospital cardiac arrest patients. *Anesth. Analg.* 2001; **92**: 375–378.

135. Grmec, S. Comparison of three different methods to confirm tracheal tube placement in emergency intubation. *Intens. Care Med.* 2002; **28**: 701–704.

136. Anton, W.R., Gordon, R.W., Jordan, T.M., Posner, K.L. & Cheney, F.W. A disposable end-tidal CO_2 detector to verify endotracheal intubation. *Ann. Emerg. Med.* 1991; **20**: 271–275.

137. Bhende, M.S., Thompson, A.E., Cook, D.R. & Saville, A.L. Validity of a disposable end-tidal CO_2 detector in verifying endotracheal tube placement in infants and children. *Ann. Emerg. Med.* 1992; **21**: 142–145.

138. Bhende, M.S. & Thompson, A.E. Evaluation of an end-tidal CO_2 detector during pediatric cardiopulmonary resuscitation. *Pediatrics* 1995; **95**: 395–399.

139. Hayden, S.R., Sciammarella, J., Viccellio, P., Thode, H. & Delagi, R. Colorimetric end-tidal CO_2 detector for verification of endotracheal tube placement in out-of-hospital cardiac arrest. *Acad. Emerg. Med.* 1995; **2**: 499–502.

140. MacLeod, B.A., Heller, M.B., Gerard, J., Yealy, D.M. & Menegazzi, J.J. Verification of endotracheal tube placement with colorimetric end-tidal CO_2 detection. *Ann. Emerg. Med.* 1991; **20**: 267–270.

141. Ornato, J.P., Shipley, J.B., Racht, E.M. *et al.* Multicenter study of a portable, hand-size, colorimetric end-tidal carbon dioxide detection device. *Ann. Emerg. Med.* 1992; **21**: 518–523.

142. Varon, A.J., Morrina, J. & Civetta, J.M. Clinical utility of a colorimetric end-tidal CO_2 detector in cardiopulmonary resuscitation and emergency intubation. *J. Clin. Monit.* 1991; **7**: 289–293.

143. Sayah, A.J., Peacock, W.F. & Overton, D.T. End-tidal CO_2 measurement in the detection of esophageal intubation during cardiac arrest. *Ann. Emerg. Med.* 1990; **19**: 857–860.

144. Sum Ping, S.T., Mehta, M.P. & Symreng, T. Accuracy of the FEF CO_2 detector in the assessment of endotracheal tube placement. *Anesth. Analg.* 1992; **74**: 415–419.

145. Campbell, R.C., Boyd, C.R., Shields, R.O., Odom, J.W. & Corse, K.M. Evaluation of an end-tidal carbon dioxide detector in the aeromedical setting. *J. Air Med. Transp.* 1990; **9**: 13–15.

146. Sellick, B.A. Cricoid pressure to control regurgitation of stomach contents during induction of anaesthesia. *Lancet* 1961; **2**: 404–406.

147. Salem, M.R., Wong, A.Y., Mani, M. & Sellick, B.A. Efficacy of cricoid pressure in preventing gastric inflation during

bagmask ventilation in pediatric patients. *Anesthesiology* 1974; **40**: 96–98.

148. Moynihan, R.J., Brock-Utne, J.G., Archer, J.H., Feld, L.H. & Kreitzman, T.R. The effect of cricoid pressure on preventing gastric insufflation in infants and children. *Anesthesiology* 1993; **78**: 652–656.

149. Petito, S.P. & Russell, W.J. The prevention of gastric inflation – a neglected benefit of cricoid pressure. *Anaesth. Intens. Care* 1988; **16**: 139–143.

150. Wenzel, V., Lindner, K.H. & Prengel, A.W. Ventilation during cardiopulmonary resuscitation: a review of the literature and an analysis of ventilation strategies. [German]. *Anaesthesist* 1997; **46**: 133–141.

151. Vanner, R.G. Mechanisms of regurgitation and its prevention with cricoid pressure. *Int. J. Obstet. Anesth.* 1993; **2**: 207–215.

152. Vanner, R.G. & Asai, T. Safe use of cricoid pressure. *Anaesthesia* 1999; **54**: 1–3.

153. Vanner, R.G. & Pryle, B.J. Regurgitation and oesophageal rupture with cricoid pressure: a cadaver study. *Anaesthesia* 1992; **47**: 732–735.

154. Gabbott, D.A. The effect of single-handed cricoid pressure on neck movement after applying manual in-line stabilisation. *Anaesthesia* 1997; **52**: 586–588.

155. Hartsilver, E.L. & Vanner, R.G. Airway obstruction with cricoid pressure. *Anaesthesia* 2000; **55**: 208–211.

156. Levy, H. & Griego, L. A comparative study of oral endotracheal tube securing methods. *Chest* 1993; **104**: 1537–1540.

157. Tasota, F.J., Hoffman, L.A., Zullo, T.G. & Jamison, G. Evaluation of two methods used to stabilize oral endotracheal tubes. *Heart Lung* 1987; **16**: 140–146.

158. Jacobson, L.E., Gomez, G.A., Sobieray, R.J., Rodman, G.H., Solotkin, K.C. & Misinski, M.E. Surgical cricothyroidotomy in trauma patients: analysis of its use by paramedics in the field. *J. Trauma* 1996; **41**: 15–20.

159. Bair, A.E., Panacek, E.A., Wisner, D.H., Bales, R. & Sakles, J.C. Cricothyrotomy: a 5-year experience at one institution. *J. Emerg. Med.* 2003; **24**: 151–156.

160. Fortune, J.B., Judkins, D.G., Scanzaroli, D., McLeod, K.B. & Johnson, S.B. Efficacy of prehospital surgical cricothyrotomy in trauma patients. *J. Trauma* 1997; **42**: 832–836; discussion 7–8.

161. Peak, D.A. & Roy, S. Needle cricothyroidotomy revisited. *Pediatr. Emerg. Care* 1999; **15**: 224–226.

162. Schaumann, N., Lorenz, V., Schellongowski, P. *et al.* Evaluation of Seldinger technique emergency cricothyroidotomy versus standard surgical cricothyroidotomy in 200 cadavers. *Anesthesiology* 2005; **102**: 7–11.

163. Fikkers, B.G., van Vugt, S., van der Hoeven, J.G., van den Hoogen, F.J. & Marres, H.A. Emergency cricothyrotomy: a randomised crossover trial comparing the wire-guided and catheter-over-needle techniques. *Anaesthesia* 2004; **59**: 1008–1011.

External chest compression: standard and alternative techniques

30

Manual cardiopulmonary resuscitation techniques

Henry R. Halperin and Barry K. Rayburn

Johns Hopkins University School of Medicine, Baltimore, MD, USA
University of Alabama School of Medicine, Birmingham, AL, USA

The standard technique of external chest compression in cardiopulmonary resuscitation (CPR) has changed little since the landmark paper of Kouwenhoven et al. in 1960 (Fig. 30.1).[1] This is despite the fact that a variety of alternate techniques have been proposed as providing an advantage over the standard method. The rhythmic application of force to the body of the patient is fundamental to the process of generating blood flow in CPR, but there is little agreement as to the optimal technique for applying that force. There is a great need for improved external chest compression techniques since only an average of 15% of patients treated with standard CPR survive cardiac arrest,[2,3] and it is widely agreed that increasing the blood flow generated by chest compression will improve survival.

This chapter will review the standard external chest compression technique as it is currently taught, including its origins and its rather scant scientific basis. It will also explore in detail the origins, physiology, and applicability of some alternate manual techniques that have been proposed.

Standard external chest compression

According to the most recently published guidelines of the Emergency Cardiac Care Committee of the American Heart Association,[4] external chest compressions are applied by the rescuer who places the heel of one hand over the victim's sternum. The second hand is placed on top of the first in such a way that the fingers do not touch the chest. The fingers may be interlocked if desired. Force is applied straight down with the elbows locked and the shoulders in line with the hands. The goal is to displace the sternum

1 1/2 to 2 inches for an average sized adult victim. The compressions are repeated at a rate of 100 times/minute regardless of whether there are one or two rescuers. Compression is maintained for 50% of each cycle to maximize arterial pressures, but is released completely between cycles without removing the hands from the chest. The Emergency Cardiac Care Committee guidelines provide specific recommendations for the integration of compressions with artificial respiration. Without endotracheal intubation, it is recommended that there be cycles of 30 compressions followed by two ventilations. With endotracheal intubation, it is recommended that compressions not be interrupted for ventilation. Additional guidelines specify the optimal method for two rescuers to switch roles during a resuscitation and also for the introduction of a second rescuer to ongoing one-rescuer CPR. Readers are referred to the latest published manuals on basic and advanced life support for full details and the most up-to-date recommendations regarding the performance of CPR. Although training programs in CPR are widespread, little is known about how often chest compressions are performed correctly in actual resuscitations or how this affects survival.

Origin

In the article by Kouwenhoven et al.,[1] two earlier investigators were cited who described external chest compression in a limited fashion. Boehm in 1878 described a study in which he applied pressure to the thorax of cats by wrapping his hands around the chest (analogous to the current recommendations for infant external chest compression).[5] In 1934, Tournade et al. described the hemodynamic

Cardiac Arrest: The Science and Practice of Resuscitation Medicine. 2nd edn., ed. Norman Paradis, Henry Halperin, Karl Kern, Volker Wenzel, Douglas Chamberlain. Published by Cambridge University Press. © Cambridge University Press, 2007.

Fig. 30.1. (**a**) Illustration from the original article by
Kouwenhoven *et al.* describing the technique of external chest
compression. (**b**) Illustration from the latest published guidelines
for the performance of chest compressions. Note the similarity
between the illustrations even though they were published over
30 years apart. (**a**) From ref. 1 (**b**) From ref. 4.

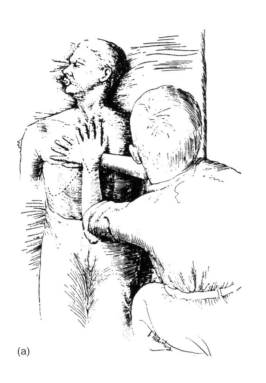

(a)

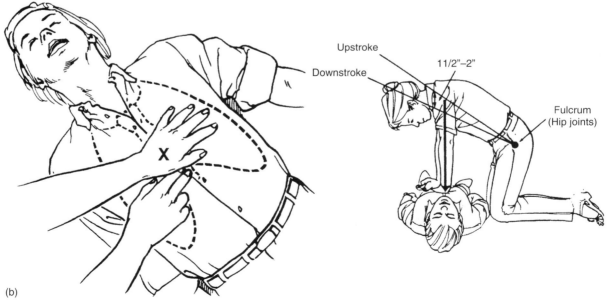

(b)

results of a sudden compression of the chest in a dog.[6] The
extent to which Kouwenhoven was influenced by these
studies is unclear. In a review of the history of cardiopulmonary resuscitation research, Criley *et al.* described
Kouwenhoven's discovery of closed-chest massage as "the
serendipitous by-product of defibrillation studies in
animals."[7] Regardless of these earlier studies, 1960 was the
dawn of modern CPR and specifically of the standard technique of external chest compression as it is currently used.

In the many years since the article by Kouwenhoven and
colleagues, the details of how external chest compressions
are integrated into the technique we know as CPR have
changed somewhat in response both to anecdotal observations and to sound research in the field. In general,
changes have become accepted into standard practice by
their adoption by an organization, and incorporated into
that organization's teaching standards for CPR.

The first widely disseminated guidelines for the performance of CPR, including external chest compression, were
published in 1966,[8] a mere 6 years after the original
description of CPR in the literature. These guidelines were
written by an ad hoc committee of the National Academy
of Sciences – National Research Council. Widespread interest in CPR prompted rapid, national attention. The salient
points for chest compression in these first guidelines were
(*a*) compression to a depth of 1 1/2 to 2 inches over the
lower half of the sternum; (*b*) avoidance of compression
over the xiphoid process; (*c*) a firm support behind the
patient; and finally (*d*) equal duration of compression and
relaxation phases. Although these guidelines were not
specifically referenced, many stem from the original article

of Kouwenhoven et al. and seem to be based mostly on empiric observations.[1]

The guidelines that were published in 1974 introduced the American Heart Association (AHA) as a cosponsor,[9] by which time the AHA and the American Red Cross had already become leaders in education in the technique of CPR. The guidelines for external chest compression changed only minimally in this publication, with new emphasis placed on moving the victim to a horizontal position before initiating compressions and a more refined technique for identifying the correct position of the hands while avoiding compression of the xiphoid. These guidelines were the first to instruct the rescuer not to remove his hands from the chest wall during relaxation, a variance from the original technique introduced by Kouwenhoven et al. Once again, this suggestion was not specifically referenced and its origin is uncertain. In 1979 a conference to update these guidelines was convened, and the results were published in 1980;[10] external chest compression was codified into 11 steps, but few changes were added to the existing recommendations. These guidelines were the first to mention the importance of keeping the fingers off the chest while performing compressions but again do not cite a reference for this recommendation. All of the published guidelines up to this point had maintained a recommended compression rate of 60 per minute for two-person CPR and 80 per minute for one-person CPR (the latter yielding 60 actual compressions because of the mandatory pause for ventilation). In 1986, the guidelines were again revised, but the only change made was an increase in the recommended rate of compressions to 80 to 100 per minute for both one- and two-rescuer CPR.[11] This change was made based on the basis of strong recommendations from several researchers in the field. Despite a disagreement on the exact mechanism of blood flow during CPR (Chapter 17), most researchers agreed that a faster compression rate would improve blood flow. Those who favored direct cardiac compression as the dominant mechanism of blood flow believed that more compressions per minute would yield more blood flow. Likewise, those who favored changes in intrathoracic pressure as the dominant mechanism sought to assure that compression and relaxation were equal in duration. This was much more easily accomplished by rescuers at a rate of 80 to 100 per minute than at 60 per minute. The most recent guidelines for the performance of CPR, joint publication by the American Heart Association and the International Liaison Committee on Resuscitation (ILCOR), were published in 2005.[4] Those latter guidelines had a number of changes: (1) The rate of compressions should be 100/min, (2) During the decompression phase of the chest compression cycle, there should be complete recoil of the chest with no residual force being applied by the rescuer, (3) There should be as few interruptions as possible, and (4) The hands should be placed over the mid sternum, rather than trying to measure the placement with respect to the xiphoid.[4]

Physiology

Developments in the field of closed-chest defibrillation served as a driving force in the rapid acceptance of external chest compression as a beneficial technique. Kouwenhoven and others recognized that closed-chest defibrillation provided an opportunity to reverse a process that was previously irreversible. Further, it was recognized in early studies of defibrillation that it was only successful if applied during the first few minutes after the onset of ventricular fibrillation, which was assumed to be due to the effects of lack of blood flow to the heart itself during fibrillation. Thus, the primary physiologic goal of external chest compression was to maintain the heart in a state where external defibrillation would be effective for as long as possible.

In their original paper, Kouwenhoven et al. stated that chest compression "compresses the heart between [the sternum] and the spine, forcing out blood."[1] From the data presented in that paper, it is clear that this statement was fundamentally an assumption on the part of the investigators, based on the anatomical relationships of the heart and bony thoracic structures. Despite this lack of rigorous scientific data, and a certain amount of skepticism, the concept of direct cardiac compression as the sole explanation for the movement of blood during standard external chest compression was widely taught for nearly two-and-a-half decades. In the last 20 years, this assumption has come under rigorous investigation. It is now apparent that the exact mechanism by which blood moves in response to externally applied force is complicated, and probably involves a combination of mechanisms. A detailed discussion of the controversies surrounding the mechanisms of blood flow in CPR is presented in Chapter 17.

Discussions of the efficacy of various techniques of CPR usually focus on either hemodynamic considerations (blood flow, perfusion pressures, and others), on initial survival (also known as return of spontaneous circulation), or on long-term survival (survival to hospital discharge and beyond). In order to provide a basis of comparison for alternative techniques of external chest compression, we will briefly review the results of the standard technique in these terms. Much of the available data regarding the hemodynamics and outcome of standard CPR come from the control groups of studies of various alternate techniques, raising concern that some bias against the standard

Table 30.1. Hemodynamic results of standard external chest compression in dogs

Author	Number of dogs studied	Peak or systolic aortic pressure (mm Hg)	Myocardial perfusion pressure (mm Hg)	Myocardial blood flow (% control)	Cerebral blood flow (% control)	Sternal force (N)
Chandra *et al.*	6	22 ± 3	5[a]	NA[b]	4	NA
Voorhees *et al.*	9	65	19[a]	15	12	NA
Walker *et al.*	8	NA	NA	NA	11	NA
Michael *et al.*	6	NA	14 ± 6	9	44	667 N
Halperin *et al.*	7	45 ± 8	5 ± 2	4[a]	31[a]	300 N
Kern *et al.*	10	66 ± 6	22 ± 3	NA	NA	NA
Halperin *et al.*	8	95 ± 6	26 ± 4	30	59	400 N
Cohen *et al.*	8	44 ± 11	8 ± 6	NA	NA	NA

[a] Information derived from data in publication.

[b] NA, not available.

technique may be present. Some investigators have attempted to minimize bias by measuring and controlling the amount of compression force or displacement.

Although small amounts of data are available for a wide variety of species, the dog model of cardiac arrest is most widely used in CPR research. Table 30.1 lists the results obtained by several investigators during standard external chest compression in dogs. The wide variation in the data highlights the difficulty in comparing CPR studies; "conventional" or "standard" external chest compression is described in a similar fashion in all the publications. It has been shown that critical determinants of blood flow during chest compression include the sternal compression force (or depth of compression; Chapter 17)[12,13], the duration of compression (percent of the compression cycle during which compression occurs),[12] and the use of vasopressors.[14] Not all authors, however, control for or even measure these variables. In addition, even the methods used for determining perfusion pressures and flows differ greatly. While such ambiguities make direct comparisons difficult, some general conclusions can be drawn from the data. The very highest coronary perfusion pressure in these studies resulted in only 30% of control myocardial blood flow. Most of the results were, or would be expected to be, considerably worse than this (based on lower perfusion pressures). Cerebral blood flow is likewise poor, attaining less than 60% of control level in all dog studies of standard external chest compression reviewed. The wide variation among peak or systolic aortic pressures in these studies likely reflects variations in the force applied during compression as well as the effects of using epinephrine. This suggests that an improvement in perfusion pressures and flow could be attained by applying higher force in standard external chest compression. In both animals and man,

trauma becomes the limiting factor in applying excessive force to the sternum. Fig. 30.2 shows several pressure tracings of standard external chest compression in dogs. The differences in these tracings further illustrate the difficulty in comparing studies and the need for rigorous standardization of external chest compression in laboratory models of CPR.

Survival studies in animal models of CPR have been performed, but are of somewhat limited utility. True long-term survival is not an available endpoint in an instrumented animal model. At best, 24-hour survival has been measured with an attempt to look at some type of neurologic outcome. Available 24-hour survival studies with standard external chest compression demonstrate that between 14 and 50% of animals survive.[15–18] Again, differences in the experimental protocols as well as subtle differences in the application of "standard" CPR likely account for this variability. In any case, 24-hour survival in animal models of cardiac arrest receiving standard external chest compression is probably better than can be expected in large populations of human cardiac arrest patients, simply because of the inherent absence of underlying pathology in the study animals, and less time between the onset of arrest and the start of CPR. Animal survival data are perhaps most useful in estimating the best possible human outcome from a CPR technique. These studies are done by highly motivated and trained investigators in well-equipped laboratories, and it is unlikely that most human resuscitation efforts will have such advantages.

All of the difficulties that exist in comparing one animal study to another are magnified in studies of human CPR. When considering hemodynamic outcomes and survival data, it is critical to take into account that the exact method of applied force is only one of many variables that may

Table 30.2. Hemodynamic results of standard external chest compression in humans

Author	Number studied	Peak or systolic arterial pressure (mm Hg)	Myocardial perfusion pressure (mm Hg)	Cerebral perfusion pressure (mm Hg)	Sternal force (N)
MacKenzie *et al.*	3	120[a]	31[a]	NA[b]	NA
Martin *et al.*	20	74 ± 20	8 ± 9	NA	NA
Swenson *et al.*	9	61 ± 29	9 ± 11	NA	NA
Paradis *et al.*	22	48 ± 16	7 ± 9	9 ± 10	NA
Chandra *et al.*	8	60 ± 4	11 ± 2	NA	NA
Paradis *et al.*	100	NA	12[a]	NA	NA
Cohen *et al.*	10	53 ± 14	NA	NA	NA
Halperin *et al.*	15	78 ± 26	15 ± 8	NA	400

[a] Information derived from data in publication.

[b] NA, not available.

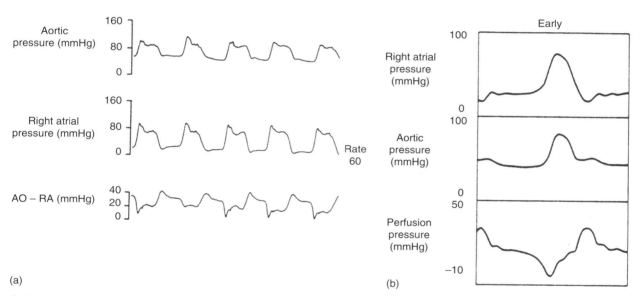

(a)

(b)

Fig. 30.2. Two examples of pressures recorded during manual external chest compressions in dogs, using standard CPR. Both illustrations also show the myocardial perfusion pressure determined by subtracting the right atrial pressure from the aortic pressure. (**a**) Reproduced with permission from ref. 15. Copyright 1986 American Heart Association. (**b**) Reproduced with permission from ref. 18. (Copyright 1988 American Heart Association.)

influence the results. The population studied, other components of the resuscitation protocol, the time between arrest and intervention, and a host of other factors influence the final outcome.

Unlike comparable animal studies, direct measurements of myocardial and cerebral blood flow are not available in human CPR. Surrogate measures of efficacy include peak compression-phase (systolic) pressure, myocardial and cerebral perfusion pressures, and direct and indirect measures of cardiac output (Table 30.2; Fig. 30.3). Several animal studies have shown that the myocardial perfusion pressure (typically defined as the difference between aortic

release phase (diastolic) pressure and right atrial pressure) is a predictor of return of spontaneous circulation.[19–22] Paradis *et al.* were also able to demonstrate this in humans undergoing CPR.[23] In their study of 100 patients, only patients who could achieve a maximum myocardial perfusion pressure of greater than or equal to 15 mm Hg had return of spontaneous circulation. This finding is consistent with the results from animal studies and serves as a useful benchmark for assessing alternative external compression techniques.

The clinically important results from human CPR studies are long-term survival and neurologic function.

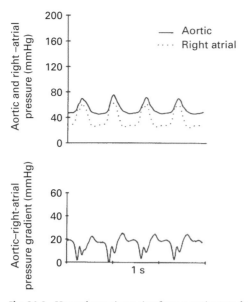

Fig. 30.3. Hemodynamic tracing from a patient undergoing standard external chest compressions. Note the relatively low coronary perfusion pressure despite similar compression phase pressures when compared with Fig. 30.2 in a dog model. (From Halperin, H.R., Tsitlik, .J.E., Gelfand, M., *et al.* A preliminary study of cardiopulmonary resuscitation by circumferential compression of the chest with the use of a pneumatic vest. *N Engl J Med* 1993; **329**: 762–768. Reprinted by permission of *The New England Journal of Medicine.* Copyright 1993 *Massachusetts Medical Society.* All rights reserved.)

Notably, despite the large number of variables that play a role in the outcome of CPR, several studies have achieved similar results. Schneider *et al.* have provided one of the most comprehensive reviews on survival following in-hospital standard CPR (including standard external chest compression).[2] Their review of 98 reports of clinical outcomes in CPR includes nearly 20 000 patients. A meta-analysis of these reports showed that overall survival-to-hospital discharge in this group of patients was 15%. An additional 3765 patients reported from a British registry had a survival-to-hospital discharge of approximately 20% with a 1-year survival of 15%.[3] Among the noteworthy findings of the analysis by Schneider et al. was the absence of any significant trend in survival-to-hospital discharge across the years from 1960 to 1990. This disputes individual, smaller reports that concluded that there was a generalized decrease in success rates of resuscitation over time,[24–27] possibly attributable to a change in the composition of in-hospital populations over time. Several reports, including the metaanalysis conducted by Schneider *et al.*, have concluded that the success rate of in-hospital resuscitation declines in an elderly population.[25,26,28] Data for out-of-hospital cardiac arrests suggest that, for large, unselected populations, the overall survival-to-hospital discharge is lower than for in-hospital arrests. Several large studies report survival-to-hospital discharge rates of 8 to 10% of all patients receiving CPR in the pre-hospital setting.[29–36] In a study performed in King County, Washington, 2043 patients cared for by paramedics in the prehospital setting were found to have a survival-to-discharge rate of 18%.[35]

Complications

Trauma is the major complication from manual CPR. The reported incidence of trauma, as the result of manual CPR, ranges from 21% to more than 65%.[37–45] The most frequent thoracic injuries, occurring more than 20% of the time, include chest abrasions or contusions, defibrillator burns, sternal and rib fractures, gastric dilation, and pulmonary edema. Even properly executed manual CPR can lead to injury. A comprehensive list of the types of trauma associated with standard CPR is presented in Table 30.3.

Applicability

The single most striking feature of standard external chest compression is its inherent ability to be applied in cardiac arrest. Thousands of people are saved each year by standard CPR, but this represents only a small fraction of the patients who suffer a cardiac arrest. Manual CPR has the disadvantage that its effectiveness can be compromised by misapplication of the technique resulting from such factors as operator fatigue and operator error. Standard CPR can be difficult to apply correctly, since in most instances a gauge is not available to assure that the operator applies the recommended 1 1/2 to 2 inches of sternal displacement. In addition, there are a significant number of manual CPR-related injuries. Despite these limitations, however, any CPR is probably better than no CPR.[30,34,35] The detrimental effects of trauma are unclear, since most research on the incidence of CPR-related trauma has focused on non-survivors of CPR, who might have died even if no trauma had occurred. Improvements in outcome may be achieved by external CPR techniques that improve blood flow; these external techniques could be available to larger numbers of rescuers than are those requiring invasive measures. Some alternative manual techniques have been studied, and are discussed below. Alternative techniques that use mechanical devices are discussed in Chapter 31.

Table 30.3. Complications reported for standard cardiopulmonary resuscitation

Thorax (42%)
  Rib fracture (31–52%)
  Sternal fracture (21–22%)
  Anterior mediastinal hemorrhage (18%)
  Pneumothorax (3%)
  Hemothorax (1%)
  Flail chest (0.5%)
  C-spine fracture (0.1%)[a]
  Lacerations of the diaphragm
Abdomen (31%)
  Gastric dilation (29%)
  Liver rupture (2%)
  Other liver injury (1%)
  Spleen rupture (0.3%)
  Gastric rupture (0.1%)
  Omentum hemorrhage (0.1%)
  Abdominal distension
  Ischemic bowel
Lung (13%)
  Pulmonary edema (44–46%)
  Aspiration (11%)
  Interstitial emphysema (1%)
  Contusion/puncture (1%)
  Infiltrates (0.6%)
  Atelectasis (0.6%)
  Pulmonary embolus
  Pulmonary hemorrhage

Heart and great vessels (11%)
  Pericardial sac blood (8%)
  Epicardial hematoma (3%)
  Myocardial contusion (1%)
  Vena cava injury (1%)
  Myocardial laceration (0.1%)
Upper airway (20%)
  Oropharynx vomitus (10%)
  Tracheal vomitus (9%)
  Endotracheal tube misplacement (4%)
  Tongue laceration
Oropharynx injury (2%)
  Larynx injury (2%)
  Dental injury (1%)
  Tracheal injury (1%)
  Hemorrhage of vocal cords (0.5%)
  Misplaced nasogastric tube (0.5%)
  Fractured thyroid cartilage (0.1%)
  Contusion – epiglottis/esophagus (0.1%)
  Hypopharyngeal hematoma (0.1%)
  Hemorrhage of cricoid (0.1%)
  Lip injury (8%)
  Dislocated mandible
  Dislocated C-spine/neck strain
  Esophageal rupture

Skin (66%)
  Chest abrasion/contusion (59%)
  Defibrillator burns (31%)
Miscellaneous
  Air embolus to coronary (1%)
  Air – other locations (1%)
  Retroperitoneal hemorrhage (0.1%)
  Bladder wall hemorrhage (0.1%)
  Bone marrow embolus
  Vertebral fractures
  Ruptured tympanic membrane

[a] C-spine, cervical spine.

Interposed abdominal compression

Interposed abdominal compression (IAC)-CPR (or abdominal counterpulsation CPR) includes an additional rescuer (for a total of two or three) positioned alongside or opposite the rescuer applying chest compressions. This additional rescuer places his or her hands on the abdomen, usually near the umbilicus, and compresses the abdomen during the relaxation-phase of chest compression (Fig. 30.4). The ratio of abdominal to chest compressions is one to one, so the rate of abdominal compressions is also 100/min. Some authors place a blood pressure cuff or another measuring device between the hands and the abdominal wall in order to measure the amount of force applied to the abdomen. Exact guidelines as to how much to compress the abdomen, or how much force to apply if measured, have not been proposed. In studies of this technique, the forces measured from air-filled measuring devices have ranged from 20 to 150 mm Hg. Most authors describe abdominal compression as lasting through the entire release phase of chest compression, resulting in a 50% compression duration for each.

Ohomoto *et al.* first published a description of interposed abdominal compression using a mechanical device with two pistons (one for the chest, one for the abdomen) in 1976[46]. Since that time, there has been ongoing and extensive research into this method[47–74].

Physiology

IAC-CPR may improve blood flow in CPR by a number of mechanisms. First and foremost, IAC-CPR may act in a fashion analogous with intraaortic balloon pumping, where abdominal and aortic compressions would result in greater retrograde aortic flow into the chest and greater aortic pressure between chest compressions, with greater coronary flow and survival. Second, abdominal pressure by itself increases intrathoracic pressure, even without chest compression. Interposed abdominal compression could therefore either (a) optimize the duration of the rise in intrathoracic pressure since durations of compression longer than those usually present during manual CPR are known to improve flow, or (b) increase the rise of

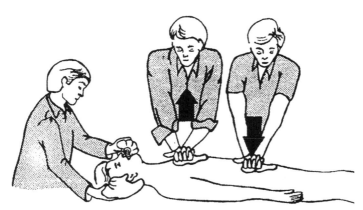

Fig. 30.4. IAC-CPR with three rescuers. This technique could also be performed by two rescuers with one rescuer performing both chest compressions and artificial ventilation. The arrows depict how one rescuer pushes while the other relaxes and vice versa. (From ref. 65. Copyright 1992, American Medical Association.)

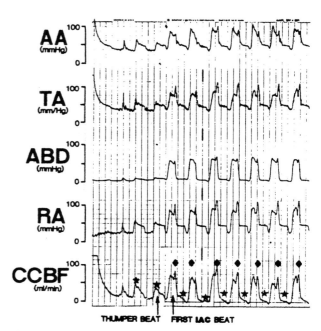

Fig. 30.5. Hemodynamic tracings in a dog undergoing CPR. Beginning about halfway across the recording, mechanical CPR was augmented with IAC-CPR. Abdominal aorta (*AA*), thoracic aorta (*TA*), intra-abdominal (*ABD*) and right atrial (*RA*) pressures, and common carotid blood flow (*CCBF*) are shown. Note that the majority of intravascular pressure as well as carotid flow seems to occur coincident with abdominal compression rather than with thoracic compression in this model. (From ref. 70.)

intrathoracic pressure as a result of moving the diaphragm and abdominal contents upward. In addition, during the diastolic phase (i.e., relaxation of chest compression), compression of the abdomen "charges" the intrathoracic compliance in preparation for the next chest-compression cycle. This coincides with work in our laboratory that shows, in a model of the canine circulation, that an intrathoracic pump would be optimized by minimizing the compliance of the vessels inside the thorax and maximizing the compliance of vessels in the abdomen during compression. During the relaxation phase, this extrathoracic compliance would then discharge into the intrathoracic vessels, thus maintaining myocardial blood flow during diastole. Of potential concern is that compression of the abdomen during the relaxation phase of chest compression can raise the pressure inside the thorax, since the abdominal and thoracic compartments are contiguous. This rise in intrathoracic pressure could raise right atrial and aortic pressures to an equal extent, which could actually decrease coronary perfusion pressure[14]. A pressure waveform during IAC-CPR is shown in Fig. 30.5.

Ralston *et al.* compared standard CPR with mechanical (Piston) external chest compression, with and without the addition of IAC.[75] They showed that with no other changes in the technique, the addition of IAC increased cardiac output, and systolic and diastolic arterial pressures in 10 dogs. Eight of 10 dogs had an increase in the arteriovenous difference (myocardial perfusion pressure). Walker *et al.*,[76] Voorhees *et al.*,[77] and Einagle *et al.*[70] all demonstrated an increase in either brain or carotid blood flow with IAC-CPR. Despite the similarity of conclusions among these studies, however, these data are somewhat difficult to interpret.

Studies by Walker and Voorhees and colleagues do show a statistically significant increase in brain blood flow versus standard CPR, but in the study by Voorhees *et al.* this difference is physiologically trivial (0.03 ml/min/g). Alternatively, the study by Walker *et al.* showed a substantial increase in brain blood flow (0.21 ml/min/g), but had extremely low brain blood flow in the standard CPR group, raising concern about the quality of the standard CPR. Of note, no study looking at myocardial blood flow showed a statistically significant difference between standard CPR and IAC-CPR. Kern *et al.* studied 24-hour survival in a dog model of cardiac arrest comparing standard external chest compression, IAC-CPR, and high-impulse CPR and found no difference among the groups.

Several trials have looked at human hemodynamics or survival with IAC-CPR. Studies by Berryman and Phillips[69] and Howard *et al.*[78] at the end of conventional resuscitation showed an increase in mean arterial pressure with the addition of IAC-CPR. Despite these increases, Howard *et al.* did not find a significant difference in the myocardial perfusion pressure. Berryman and Phillips reported this information in only a single patient in whom it was increased.

McDonald[79] reported on six patients, also late in resuscitation, in whom there was no difference in any measured variable with the addition of IAC. Mateer et al.[68] described a large field trial of IAC-CPR conducted by paramedics in Milwaukee: no difference in initial resuscitation was found after randomizing medical arrest patients to either standard external chest compression or IAC-CPR after intubation. In an in-hospital trial of IAC-CPR, Sack et al.[65] reported the results of 135 resuscitation attempts in 103 patients who had been randomized on admission to the hospital to receive either IAC-CPR or standard CPR should they arrest. In this study, they reported an increase in initial resuscitation (51% vs. 27%), discharge from the hospital (25% vs. 7%), and discharge neurologically intact (17% vs. 6%) with IAC-CPR. Conducting this type of randomized trial in a hospital setting is in itself a considerable accomplishment. Obviously a CPR trial cannot be a blind study, and this is one of the self-criticisms mentioned by the investigators. In addition, no attempt was made to control for the force of sternal compression used in either group, which may account in part for the rather marked difference seen in this study. Of greater concern is the relatively low survival rate of the standard CPR group. Only 7% of these patients survived to hospital discharge, which is roughly half the survival-to-discharge rate typically reported by large studies of CPR in hospitalized patients. Again, this may reflect a subtle difference in the standard CPR technique utilized during the study, or may reflect some bias in the group of patients included in the study. In a follow-up study of 143 hospitalized patients with either pulseless electrical activity or asystole, the same group demonstrated improved initial resuscitation and 24-hour survival with IAC-CPR compared with standard CPR.[64] Survival-to-hospital discharge was not an endpoint in this study, although the investigators noted that no patients survived to discharge neurologically intact. These results from a technique that is easy to apply should encourage ongoing investigation.

Although the incidence of abdominal trauma could be increased with IAC-CPR, specific data are limited. Kern et al. in one trial compared three methods of manually applied CPR, including IAC-CPR, and noted no difference in the incidence of trauma with the addition of abdominal counterpulsations.[63] In their most recent study, Sack et al. noted no clinically obvious difference in abdominal trauma between the groups, and none of the five IAC-CPR patients who underwent autopsy had any abdominal trauma.[64]

Applicability

IAC-CPR requires at least two rescuers. Beyond this requirement, it is a manually applied technique that requires no specialized equipment. The ability of rescuers in general to perform the technique correctly has not been determined. Hemodynamic data in humans are less convincing than those in animals, although this may reflect a limited ability to look at brain blood flow in humans. If IAC-CPR does improve brain perfusion as suggested by animal models, then it may well have clinical utility. Provided that it does not adversely affect the myocardial perfusion and therefore the chances of establishing return of spontaneous circulation, additional brain blood flow may improve the neurologic outcome of those patients who do survive resuscitation. The study reported by Sack et al., despite its limitations, may address these facts.[65] They showed a survival-to-hospital discharge of 25%, which is higher than historical controls, suggesting a benefit over standard CPR. Larger trials of IAC-CPR will be needed, however, before its true clinical utility can be determined.

High-impulse external chest compression

High-impulse external chest compression is performed by placing the hands in a position identical with that of standard external chest compression. The compression itself, however, is done at a higher rate (typically 120 to 150/minute) and with a very quick, jabbing onset and offset. Ventilation is provided as with standard CPR, at a rate of 12/minute.

Investigators at Duke University first proposed high-impulse chest compression as a replacement for standard external chest compressions in 1984.[80] Despite one reference cited for rapid compressions from the 1890s, these authors were clearly the major force that brought this technique into the modern era of CPR research. High-impulse CPR became one of the focal points of the debate between the two schools of thought (direct cardiac compression vs. intrathoracic pressure fluctuations) on the mechanism of blood flow in CPR.[12,18,80–87] Those investigations led to a significantly improved understanding of the physiology of blood movement during chest compression.

Physiology

In studies of the physiology of blood flow during external chest compression in dogs, Maier et al. noted that increasing the rate of compressions resulted in increased cardiac output and increased coronary flow compared with slower rates.[80] They showed that stroke volume stayed constant, while cardiac output rose. Coronary blood flow tended to be higher, although not significantly, at a compression rate of 150/minute vs. 60/minute.[80] These data were

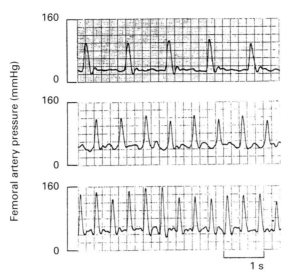

Fig. 30.6. Hemodynamic tracings from a patient undergoing CPR. The top tracing shows CPR at a rate of 60/min, the middle at 100/min, and the bottom at 150/min or high-impulse CPR. Note on each tracing the amount of time spent during the compression and relaxation phases. Only the third tracing appears consistent with the recommended 50% compression duration. (Reproduced with permission from ref. 80. Copyright 1984 American Heart Association.)

interpreted as showing that direct cardiac compression was the predominant mechanism of blood flow since stroke volume was constant for each compression, and cardiac output rose at higher rates as more stroke volumes were delivered per unit time. The investigators attempted to control compression force by measuring intrapleural pressure with micromanometers in the intrapleural space. This was one of the two major criticisms of the work since measurements of intrapleural pressure are difficult and often inaccurate. Nevertheless, they did achieve the same reading in a given animal for each compression rate.

The second major criticism is illustrated in Fig. 30.6: a variable not controlled by the investigators in these initial studies was the compression duration, or the percent of the compression–decompression cycle during which compression occurs. At low compression rates, the duration of compression appeared to be approximately 20% of the cycle; at high rates, it was much closer to 50%, the currently recommended standard. This provided a potential mechanism for the increase in cardiac output, even if an intrathoracic pump mechanism was operative since compression duration does affect blood flow in the intrathoracic pump model. Subsequent animal studies examined survival differences between high-impulse external chest compression and standard CPR. Kern *et al.* found no dif-

ference in 24-hour survival between a group receiving standard external chest compression and a group receiving high-impulse CPR.[63] A later study by Feneley *et al.* did show improved survival in a group of animals receiving high-impulse CPR compared with standard manual CPR.[18] In this latter study, the authors attempted to control for duty cycle between the two groups. Compression force was not quantitatively reported, however, and pressures generated in the control group were substantially lower than in other studies of standard external compression done by the same research group.[80]

A number of case-report type studies of high-impulse CPR have been published.[80,88] Minimal quantitative analysis of these data are available, however, and no controlled trials of standard vs. high-impulse CPR in humans have been reported.

Applicability

High-impulse CPR requires little more than an alteration in training from that in standard external chest compression. None of the data reported for high-impulse CPR, however, provide convincing evidence that this technique would provide substantial benefit over standard CPR in the general population. There may be subsets of patients in whom the jabbing chest compressions of high-impulse CPR are beneficial. These chest compressions may alter airway mechanics in these patients to produce higher intrathoracic pressure, or alternatively, may enhance cardiac compression. If these groups can be identified, it is conceivable that high-impulse CPR could provide a hemodynamic benefit over standard external chest compression.

Future directions

Research aimed at improving survival from cardiac arrest both in- and out-of-hospital continues. The first 30 years of external chest compression have been marked by enthusiasm, disappointment, innovation, and speculation, but to date no technique has convincingly positioned itself to replace standard CPR as we now know it. Research has contributed a great deal to the science of CPR and set the stage for real advancement in the resuscitation of cardiac arrest victims. The critical importance of early defibrillation is now clearly recognized. Likewise, the criteria used to judge a new CPR method have been defined. These measures – coronary perfusion pressure (important in predicting return of spontaneous circulation), systolic arterial pressure (predictive of cerebral blood flow and likely of neurologic recovery), and ultimately survival-to-hospital discharge – will drive the search for the best method or methods of applying force to the human body over the next several years. The future may lie not so much in a replacement of current CPR as in evolution to differing types of CPR under different circumstances. Resuscitation initiated by lay persons will by necessity remain a manual technique, but some other form of CPR may be used once qualified rescuers are on the scene. The use of gauges to assure that manual CPR is performed correctly, and a reduction in interruptions in chest compression, may improve the efficacy of manual CPR dramatically. Currently the distinction between basic and advanced life support involves the availability of drugs, mechanical airways, and defibrillation. It is very possible that the form of CPR utilized may also become part of this distinction.

Finally, with several of the techniques discussed in this chapter providing some promise for improved survival from cardiac arrest, we are entering an era where small trials will be unlikely to add significantly to our knowledge. For a new technique of external chest compression to be widely accepted, it will need to be tested in a sufficiently large population to produce statistically significant as well as clinically significant data, much as thrombolytic therapy and angiotensin-converting enzyme inhibitors have been tested in mega-trials. These trials, both in-hospital and in the field, should provide the information needed for a technique to be judged for its long-term benefits. Smaller trials can be useful, as still other alternate techniques are developed. In small human survival trials, it is critical for authors to know and report the baseline survival data from their institution by using standard CPR in a nearly identical population *before* the onset of the study. Control groups are always subject to bias in studies that are not performed blind. Knowing the existing survival data from standard CPR at the same institution before the study begins will allow the investigators to judge whether a bias was introduced into their control group during the study.

REFERENCES

1. Kouwenhoven, W.B., Jude, J.R. & Knickerbocker, G.G. Closed chest cardiac massage. *J. Am. Med. Assoc.* 1960; **173**: 1064–1067.

2. Schneider, A.P., 2nd, Nelson, D.J. & Brown, D.D. In-hospital cardiopulmonary resuscitation: a 30-year review. *J. Am. Board. Fam. Pract.* 1993; **6**: 91–101.

3. Tunstall-Pedoe, H., Bailey, L., Chamberlain, D.A., Marsden, A.K., Ward, M.E. & Zideman, D.A. Survey of 3765 cardiopulmonary resuscitations in British hospitals (the BRESUS Study): methods and overall results. *Br. Med. J.* 1992; **304**: 1347–1351.

4. 2005 American Heart Association Guidelines for Cardiopulmonary Resuscitation and Emergency Cardiovascular Care. *Circulation* 2005; **112**: IV1–IV203.

5. Boehm, R.V. Arbeiten aus dem pharmakologischen Institute der Universitat Dorpat: 13. Ueber weiderbelebung nach vergiftungen und asphyxie. *Arch. Exp. Path. Pharmakol.* 1878; **8**: 68–101.

6. Tournade, A., Rocchisani, L. & Mely, G. Etude experimentale des effets circulatoires qu'entrainent la respiration artificielle et la compression asccadee du thorax chez le chien. *Comput. Rend. Soc. Biol.* 1934; **117**: 1123–1126.

7. Criley, J.M., Niemann, J.T. & Rosborough, J.P. Cardiopulmonary resuscitation research 1960–1984: discoveries and advances. *Ann. Emerg. Med.* 1984; **13**: 756–758.

8. Cardiopulmonary resuscitation: statement by the *ad hoc* committee on cardiopulmonary resuscitation of the division of medical sciences, National Academy of Sciences–National Research Council. *J. Am. Med. Assoc.* 1966; **198**: 372–379.

9. Standards for cardiopulmonary resuscitation (CPR) and emergency cardiac care (ECC). I. Introduction. *J. Am. Med. Assoc.* 1974; **227**:Suppl: 837–840.

10. Standards and guidelines for cardiopulmonary resuscitation (CPR) and emergency cardiac care (ECC). *J. Am. Med. Assoc.* 1980; **244**: 453–509.

11. Standards and guidelines for Cardiopulmonary Resuscitation (CPR) and Emergency Cardiac Care (ECC). National Academy of Sciences – National Research Council. *J. Am. Med. Assoc.* 1986; **255**: 2905–2989.

12. Halperin, H.R., Tsitlik, J.E., Guerci, A.D. *et al.* Determinants of blood flow to vital organs during cardiopulmonary resuscitation in dogs. *Circulation* 1986; **73**: 539–550.

13. Babbs, C.F., Voorhees, W.D., Fitzgerald, K.R., Holmes, H.R. & Geddes, L.A. Relationship of blood pressure and flow during CPR to chest compression amplitude: evidence for an effective compression threshold. *Ann. Emerg. Med.* 1983; **12**: 527–532.

14. Michael, J.R., Guerci, A.D., Koehler, R.C. *et al.* Mechanisms by which epinephrine augments cerebral and myocardial perfusion during cardiopulmonary resuscitation in dogs. *Circulation* 1984; **69**: 822–835.

15. Halperin, H.R., Guerci, A.D., Chandra, N. *et al.* Vest inflation without simultaneous ventilation during cardiac arrest in dogs: improved survival from prolonged cardiopulmonary resuscitation. *Circulation* 1986; **74**: 1407–1415.

16. Kern, K.B., Carter, A.B., Showen, R.L. *et al.* Comparison of mechanical techniques of cardiopulmonary resuscitation: survival and neurologic outcome in dogs. *Am. J. Emerg. Med.* 1987; **5**: 190–195.

17. Kern, K.B., Carter, A.B., Showen, R.L. *et al.* Twenty-four hour survival in a canine model of cardiac arrest comparing three methods of manual cardiopulmonary resuscitation. *J. Am. Coll. Cardiol.* 1986; **7**: 859–867.

18. Feneley, M.P., Maier, G.W., Kern, K.B. *et al.* Influence of compression rate on initial success of resuscitation and 24 hour survival after prolonged manual cardiopulmonary resuscitation in dogs. *Circulation* 1988; **77**: 240–250.

19. Kern, K.B., Ewy, G.A., Voorhees, W.D., Babbs, C.F. & Tacker, W.A. Myocardial perfusion pressure: a predictor of 24-hour survival during prolonged cardiac arrest in dogs. *Resuscitation* 1988; **16**: 241–250.

20. Niemann, J.T., Criley, J.M., Rosborough, J.P., Niskanen, R.A. & Alferness, C. Predictive indices of successful cardiac resuscitation after prolonged arrest and experimental cardiopulmonary resuscitation. *Ann. Emerg. Med.* 1985; **14**: 521–528.

21. Niemann, J.T. Differences in cerebral and myocardial perfusion during closed-chest resuscitation. *Ann. Emerg. Med.* 1984; **13**: 849–853.

22. Sanders, A.B., Ewy, G.A. & Taft, T.V. Prognostic and therapeutic importance of the aortic diastolic pressure in resuscitation from cardiac arrest. *Crit. Care Med.* 1984; **12**: 871–873.

23. Paradis, N.A., Martin, G.B., Rivers, E.P. *et al.* Coronary perfusion pressure and the return of spontaneous circulation in human cardiopulmonary resuscitation. *J. Am. Med. Assoc.* 1990; **263**: 1106–1113.

24. McGrath, R.B. In-house cardiopulmonary resuscitation – after a quarter of a century. *Ann. Emerg. Med.* 1987; **16**: 1365–1368.

25. Taffet, G.E., Teasdale, T.A. & Luchi, R.J. In-hospital cardiopulmonary resuscitation. *J. Am. Med. Assoc.* 1988; **260**: 2069–2072.

26. Murphy, D.J., Murray, A.M., Robinson, B.E. & Campion, E.W. Outcomes of cardiopulmonary resuscitation in the elderly. *Ann. Intern. Med.* 1989; **111**: 199–205.

27. Dans, P.E., Nevin, K.L., Seidman, C.E., McArthur, J.C. & Kariya, S.T. Inhospital CPR 25 years later: why has survival decreased? *South Med. J.* 1985; **78**: 1174–1178.

28. Van Hoeyweghen, R.J., Bossaert, L.L., Mullie, A. *et al.* Survival after out-of-hospital cardiac arrest in elderly patients. Belgian Cerebral Resuscitation Study Group. *Ann. Emerg. Med.* 1992; **21**: 1179–1184.

29. Myerburg, R.J., Kessler, K.M., Estes, D. *et al.* Long-term survival after prehospital cardiac arrest: analysis of outcome during an 8 year study. *Circulation* 1984; **70**: 538–546.

30. Roth, R., Stewart, R.D., Rogers, K. & Cannon, G.M. Out-of-hospital cardiac arrest: factors associated with survival. *Ann. Emerg. Med.* 1984; **13**: 237–243.

31. Earnest, M.P., Yarnell, P.R., Merrill, S.L. & Knapp, G.L. Long-term survival and neurologic status after resuscitation from out-of-hospital cardiac arrest. *Neurology* 1980; **30**: 1298–1302.

32. Bachman, J.W., McDonald, G.S. & O'Brien, P.C. A study of out-of-hospital cardiac arrests in northeastern Minnesota. *J. Am. Med. Assoc.* 1986; **256**: 477–483.

33. Weaver, W.D., Cobb, L.A., Hallstrom, A.P., Fahrenbruch, C., Copass, M.K. & Ray, R. Factors influencing survival after out-of-hospital cardiac arrest. *J. Am. Coll. Cardiol.* 1986; **7**: 752–757.

34. Ritter, G., Wolfe, R.A., Goldstein, S. *et al.* The effect of bystander CPR on survival of out-of-hospital cardiac arrest victims. *Am. Heart J.* 1985; **110**: 932–937.

35. Cummins, R.O., Eisenberg, M.S., Hallstrom, A.P. & Litwin, P.E. Survival of out-of-hospital cardiac arrest with early initiation of cardiopulmonary resuscitation. *Am. J. Emerg. Med.* 1985; **3**: 114–119.

36. Eisenberg, M.S., Bergner, L. & Hallstrom, A. Survivors of out-of-hospital cardiac arrest: morbidity and long-term survival. *Am. J. Emerg. Med.* 1984; **2**: 189–192.

37. Himmelhoch, S.R., Dekker, A., Gazzaniga, A.B. & Like, A.A. Closed-chest cardiac resuscitation. A prospective clinical and pathological study. *N. Engl. J. Med.* 1964; **270**: 118–122.

38. Gallagher, J.T., Holmes, W. & Cunningham, J.D. Tympanic injury and cardiopulmonary resuscitation. *Trans. Pa. Acad. Ophthalmol. Otolaryngol.* 1986; **38**: 464–467.

39. Silberberg, B. & Rachmaninoff, N. Complications following external cardiac massage. *Surg. Gynecol. Obstet.* 1964; **111**: 6–10.

40. Wolfe, W.G., Dudley, A.W. & Wallace, A.G. A pathologic study of unsuccessful cardiac resuscitation. *Arch. Surg.* 1968; **96**: 123–126.

41. Nadel, E.L., Fine, E.G., Krischer, J.P. & Davis, J.H. Complications of CPR. *Crit. Care.* 1981; **9**: 424.

42. Bedell, S.E. & Fulton, E.J. Unexpected findings and complications at autopsy after cardiopulmonary resuscitation (CPR). *Arch. Intern. Med.* 1986; **146**: 1725–1728.

43. Powner, D.J., Holcombe, P.A. & Mello, L.A. Cardiopulmonary resuscitation-related injuries. *Crit. Care Med.* 1984; **12**: 54–55.

44. Krischer, J.P., Fine, E.G., Davis, J.H. & Nagel, E.L. Complications of cardiac resuscitation. *Chest* 1987; **92**: 287–291.

45. Sommers, M.S. The shattering consequences of C.P.R. *Nursing* 1992; **22**: 34–41.

46. Ohomoto, T., Miura, I. & Konno, S. A new method of external cardiac massage to improve diastolic augmentation and prolong survival time. *Ann. Thorac. Surg.* 1976; **21**: 284–290.

47. Badylak, S.F., Kern, K.B., Tacker, W.A., Ewy, G.A., Janas, W. & Carter, A. The comparative pathology of open chest vs. mechanical closed chest cardiopulmonary resuscitation in dogs. *Resuscitation* 1986; **13**: 249–264.

48. Babbs, C.F., Ralston, S.H. & Geddes, L.A. Theoretical advantages of abdominal counterpulsation in CPR as demonstrated in a simple electrical model of the circulation. *Ann. Emerg. Med.* 1984; **13**: 660–671.

49. Babbs, C.F., Weaver, J.C., Ralston, S.H. & Geddes, L.A. Cardiac, thoracic, and abdominal pump mechanisms in cardiopulmonary resuscitation: studies in an electrical model of the circulation. *Am. J. Emerg. Med.* 1984; **2**: 299–308.

50. Babbs, C.F. Abdominal counterpulsation in cardiopulmonary resuscitation: animal models and theoretical considerations. *Am. J. Emerg. Med.* 1985; **3**: 165–170.

51. Babbs, C.F. Preclinical studies of abdominal counterpulsation in CPR. *Ann. Emerg. Med.* 1984; **13**: 761–763.

52. Babbs, C.F. & Tacker, W.A. Jr. Cardiopulmonary resuscitation with interposed abdominal compression. *Circulation* 1986; **74**: IV37–IV41.

53. Babbs, C.F. & Blevins, W.E. Abdominal binding and counter-pulsation in cardiopulmonary resuscitation. *Crit. Care Clin.* 1986; **2**: 319–332.

54. Babbs, C.F. Hemodynamic mechanisms in CPR: a theoretical rationale for resuscitative thoracotomy in non-traumatic cardiac arrest. *Resuscitation* 1987; **15**: 37–50.

55. Babbs, C.F. Interposed abdominal compression – CPR. Low technology for the clinical armamentarium. *Circulation* 1992; **86**: 2011–2012.

56. Babbs, C.F. Interposed abdominal compression – cardiopulmonary resuscitation: are we missing the mark in clinical trials? *Am. Heart J.* 1993; **126**: 1035–1041.

57. Babbs, C.F. Interposed abdominal compression–CPR: a case study in cardiac arrest research. *Ann. Emerg. Med.* 1993; **22**: 24–32.

58. Babbs, C.F. The evolution of abdominal compression in cardiopulmonary resuscitation. *Acad. Emerg. Med.* 1994; **1**: 469–477.

59. Babbs, C.F., Sack, J.B. & Kern, K.B. Interposed abdominal compression as an adjunct to cardiopulmonary resuscitation. *Am. Heart J.* 1994; **127**: 412–421.

60. Babbs, C.F. CPR techniques that combine chest and abdominal compression and decompression: hemodynamic insights from a spreadsheet model. *Circulation* 1999; **100**: 2146–2152.

61. Babbs, C.F. & Thelander, K. Theoretically optimal duty cycles for chest and abdominal compression during external cardiopulmonary resuscitation. *Acad. Emerg. Med.* 1995; **2**: 698–707.

62. Babbs, C.F. Efficacy of interposed abdominal compression – cardiopulmonary resuscitation (CPR), active compression and decompression – CPR and Lifestick CPR: basic physiology in a spreadsheet model. *Crit. Care Med.* 2000; **28**: N199–N202.

63. Kern, K.B., Carter, A.B., Showen, R.L. *et al.* CPR-induced trauma: comparison of three manual methods in an experimental model. *Ann. Emerg. Med.* 1986; **15**: 674–679.

64. Sack, J.B., Kesselbrenner, M.B. & Jarrad, A. Interposed abdominal compression-cardiopulmonary resuscitation and resuscitation outcome during asystole and electromechanical dissociation. *Circulation* 1992; **86**: 1692–1700.

65. Sack, J.B., Kesselbrenner, M.B. & Bregman, D. Survival from in-hospital cardiac arrest with interposed abdominal counterpulsation during cardiopulmonary resuscitation. *J. Am. Med. Assoc.* 1992; **267**: 379–385.

66. Sack, J.B. & Kesselbrenner, M.B. Hemodynamics, survival benefits, and complications of interposed abdominal compression during cardiopulmonary resuscitation. *Acad. Emerg. Med.* 1994; **1**: 490–497.

67. Mateer, J.R., Stueven, H.A., Thompson, B.M., Aprahamian, C. & Darin, J.C. Interposed abdominal compression CPR versus standard CPR in prehospital cardiopulmonary arrest: preliminary results. *Ann. Emerg. Med.* 1984; **13**: 764–766.

68. Mateer, J.R., Stueven, H.A., Thompson, B.M., Aprahamian, C. & Darin, J.C. Pre-hospital IAC-CPR versus standard CPR: paramedic resuscitation of cardiac arrests. *Am. J. Emerg. Med.* 1985; **3**: 143–146.

69. Berryman, C.R. & Phillips, G.M. Interposed abdominal compression-CPR in human subjects. *Ann. Emerg. Med.* 1984; **13**: 226–229.

70. Einagle, V., Bertrand, F., Wise, R.A., Roussos, C. & Magder, S. Interposed abdominal compressions and carotid blood flow during cardiopulmonary resuscitation. Support for a thoracoabdominal unit. *Chest* 1988; **93**: 1206–1212.

71. Voorhees, W.D., 3rd, Ralston, S.H. & Babbs, C.F. Regional blood flow during cardiopulmonary resuscitation with abdominal counterpulsation in dogs. *Am. J. Emerg. Med.* 1984; **2**: 123–128.

72. Babbs, C.F. Design of near-optimal waveforms for chest and abdominal compression and decompression in CPR using computer-simulated evolution. *Resuscitation* 2006; **68**: 277–293.

73. Babbs, C.F. Relative effectiveness of interposed abdominal compression CPR: sensitivity analysis and recommended compression rates. *Resuscitation* 2005; **66**: 347–355.

74. Babbs, C.F. Interposed abdominal compression CPR: a comprehensive evidence based review. *Resuscitation* 2003; **59**: 71–82.

75. Ralston, S.H., Babbs, C.F. & Niebauer, M.J. Cardiopulmonary resuscitation with interposed abdominal compression in dogs. *Anesth. Analg.* 1982; **61**: 645–651.

76. Walker, J.W., Bruestle, J.C., White, B.C., Evans, A.T., Indreri, R. & Bialek, H. Perfusion of the cerebral cortex by use of abdominal counterpulsation during cardiopulmonary resuscitation. *Am. J. Emerg. Med.* 1984; **2**: 391–393.

77. Voorhees, W.D., Niebauer, M.J. & Babbs, C.F. Improved oxygen delivery during cardiopulmonary resuscitation with interposed abdominal compressions. *Ann. Emerg. Med.* 1983; **12**: 128–135.

78. Howard, M., Carrubba, C., Foss, F., Janiak, B., Hogan, B. & Guinness, M. Interposed abdominal compression-CPR: its effects on parameters of coronary perfusion in human subjects. *Ann. Emerg. Med.* 1987; **16**: 253–259.

79. McDonald, J.L. Effect of interposed abdominal compression during CPR on central arterial and venous pressures. *Am. J. Emerg. Med.* 1985; **3**: 156–159.

80. Maier, G.W., Tyson, G.S., Jr., Olsen, C.O. *et al.* The physiology of external cardiac massage: high-impulse cardiopulmonary resuscitation. *Circulation* 1984; **70**: 86–101.

81. Halperin, H.R., Tsitlik, J.E., Beyar, R., Chandra, N. & Guerci, A.D. Intrathoracic pressure fluctuations move blood during CPR: comparison of hemodynamic data with predictions from a mathematical model. *Ann. Biomed. Eng.* 1987; **15**: 385–403.

82. Halperin, H.R., Weiss, J.L., Guerci, A.D. *et al.* Cyclic elevation of intrathoracic pressure can close the mitral valve during cardiac arrest in dogs. *Circulation* 1988; **78**: 754–760.

83. Halperin, H.R., Brower, R., Weisfeldt, M.L. *et al.* Air trapping in the lungs during cardiopulmonary resuscitation in dogs. A mechanism for generating changes in intrathoracic pressure. *Circ. Res.* 1989; **65**: 946–954.

84. Maier, G.W., Newton, J.R., Jr., Wolfe, J.A. *et al.* The influence of manual chest compression rate on hemodynamic support

during cardiac arrest: high-impulse cardiopulmonary resuscitation. *Circulation* 1986; **74**: IV51–IV59.

85. Feneley, M.P., Maier, G.W., Gaynor, J.W. *et al.* Sequence of mitral valve motion and transmitral blood flow during manual cardiopulmonary resuscitation in dogs. *Circulation* 1987; **76**: 363–375.

86. Newton, J.R., Jr., Glower, D.D., Wolfe, J.A. *et al.* A physiologic comparison of external cardiac massage techniques. *J. Thorac. Cardiovasc. Surg.* 1988; **95**: 892–901.

87. Wolfe, J.A., Maier, G.W., Newton, J.R., Jr. *et al.* Physiologic determinants of coronary blood flow during external cardiac massage. *J. Thorac. Cardiovasc. Surg.* 1988; **95**: 523–532.

88. Swenson, R.D., Weaver, W.D., Niskanen, R.A., Martin, J. & Dahlberg, S. Hemodynamics in humans during conventional and experimental methods of cardiopulmonary resuscitation. *Circulation* 1988; **78**: 630–639.

31

Mechanical devices for cardiopulmonary resuscitation

Henry R. Halperin

Johns Hopkins University School of Medicine, Baltimore, MD, USA

The rhythmic application of force to the body of the patient is fundamental to the process of generating blood flow in CPR, but there is little agreement as to the optimal technique for applying that force. There is a great need for improved external chest compression techniques since only an average of 5%–15% of patients treated with standard CPR survive cardiac arrest,[1,2] and it is widely agreed that increasing the blood flow generated by chest compression will improve survival. Given the potential importance of newer devices and techniques that may augment blood flow, this chapter will explore several alternate devices and techniques that have been studied.

Piston chest compression

According to the most recently published guidelines of the Emergency Cardiac Care Committee of the American Heart Association,[3] external chest compressions are applied by the rescuer who places the hands over the victim's sternum. Force is applied straight down with the rescuer's elbows locked and the shoulders in line with the hands. The goal is to displace the sternum 1 1/2 to 2 inches for an average-sized adult victim, 100 times per minute, with compression maintained for 50% of each cycle. Unfortunately, compressions are often done incorrectly,[4,5] and incorrect chest compression can compromise survival.[6,7] One way of improving the quality of chest compression is with automatic mechanical devices, which can potentially apply compression more consistently than by manual compression. Another way of potentially improving the quality of chest compression is to use gauges that provide feedback to the rescuer on the depth and rate of compressions, allowing the

rescuer to adjust the application of force to produce compressions that have the correct depth and rate.

One type of automatic mechanical device uses a pneumatic piston (Fig. 31.1) to administer external chest compressions at a specified rate, compression depth, and duty cycle (percent of time compression is held during each cycle). The piston is located at the end of an arm that extends over the patient's chest, and is based on a board which provides a firm surface under the patient's back. In addition, a ventilation circuit is integrated into the device, which allows for continuous CPR with minimal operator input once the device is set up. Although there are some differences between mechanical and manual external chest compression in the time course of application of force, which may affect hemodynamics,[8,9] one small study showed no difference in survival with use of the two techniques.[9] Two additional small studies suggested a slight hemodynamic benefit to CPR performed by the pneumatic piston, one using end-tidal CO_2 as a surrogate measure for cardiac output,[10] and the other showing a slight improvement in mean arterial pressure (25 versus 31 mm Hg), although no statistical analysis was provided.[9] An updated version of the piston compression device moves the piston with higher velocity, and in an animal model produces increased vascular pressures compared to the earlier version.[11] Despite these slight differences in hemodynamics, chest compression performed by a pneumatic device probably has the same physiology as manual chest compression and is generally considered an extension of the standard technique.

Trauma is the major complication from piston CPR. The reported incidence of trauma, as the result of piston CPR, can be as high as 65%.[12,13] The most frequent thoracic

Cardiac Arrest: The Science and Practice of Resuscitation Medicine. 2nd edn., ed. Norman Paradis, Henry Halperin, Karl Kern, Volker Wenzel, Douglas Chamberlain. Published by Cambridge University Press. © Cambridge University Press, 2007.

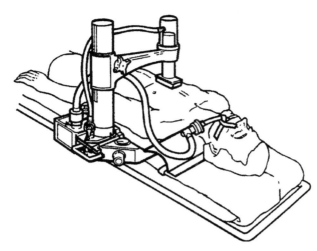

Fig. 31.1. Piston device used for performing mechanical external chest compressions. (Thumper, Courtesy of Michigan Instruments, Grand Rapids, MI.)

injuries, occurring more than 20% of the time, include chest abrasions or contusions, defibrillator burns, sternal and rib fractures, gastric dilation, and pulmonary edema. Even properly executed CPR can lead to injury.

Despite the substantial amount of trauma, however, the detrimental effects of trauma are unclear, because most research on the incidence of CPR-related trauma has focused on non-survivors of CPR, who might have died even if no trauma had occurred. Improvements in outcome may be achieved by external CPR techniques that enhance blood flow; but such improvement has not been convincingly demonstrated for piston-type devices. These devices do, however, allow CPR to be performed in situations where standard manual CPR would be difficult, such as in moving ambulances, and where personnel are limited.

Simultaneous compression and ventilation

Simultaneous compression and ventilation (SCV), as originally described, requires the subject to be endotracheally intubated or to have a tracheostomy.[14–16] Compressions are administered as with standard external chest compression, but at a slower rate (typically 40 compressions/minute). Instead of interposed ventilation between appropriate compressions, ventilation to a high airway pressure (typically 60 to 100 mm Hg) is performed synchronously with each compression. Some authors have modified this technique slightly, compressing at faster rates or adding an abdominal binder.[14,16,17] Most studies of this technique in both animal models and humans were performed using a mechanical compression device with an integrated system to deliver ventilation to the endotracheal tube.

In 1967 Wilder *et al.* reported an increase in blood flow in dogs by using simultaneous ventilation and external chest compression at low airway pressures.[18] This phenomenon was left unexplained and largely unexplored, however, until the late 1970s when it was studied by a group of investigators at Johns Hopkins,[14,15] and subsequently by other groups.[17,19–21]

Physiology

Simultaneous compression–ventilation CPR (SCV-CPR) was a direct by-product of the theory that intrathoracic pressure fluctuations are responsible for blood movement during CPR. The assumption was that if blood flow is due to fluctuations in intrathoracic pressure, then anything that makes those fluctuations larger should increase blood flow. Many authors went a step beyond this and added abdominal binding to the technique, assuming that binding the abdomen would restrict the motion of the diaphragm, and thus result in higher intrathoracic pressure for a given applied force.[14,16,22,23]

Animal studies of the hemodynamics of SCV-CPR resulted in a number of observations that were unanticipated by the investigators, but ultimately led to an increased understanding of the determinants of blood flow during chest compression. For example, when electromagnetic flow probes around the carotid artery were used as an estimate of cerebral blood flow in animals,[16] administration of epinephrine resulted in a paradoxical decrease in carotid flow, despite an increase in cerebral perfusion pressure. This observation led investigators to seek alternative techniques for measuring cerebral blood flow and resulted in the routine use of radioactive microspheres during animal studies of CPR. Such studies showed that carotid flow measurements in dogs estimate blood flow to the facial muscles and tongue, and not to the brain.[14] Brain flow was actually augmented by epinephrine, as was myocardial blood flow.[24] Another observation that resulted from animal studies of SCV-CPR was that excessively high airway pressures (100 mm Hg) could cause carotid collapse, which can reduce blood flow,[24] and that negative airway pressure in-between compressions can augment blood flow.[16] Although not recognized at the time, this latter mechanism may be operative in other forms of CPR that induce negative intrathoracic pressure in-between compressions.

Another somewhat surprising observation was that abdominal binding can actually reduce coronary perfusion pressure.[23,25] The mechanism of this phenomenon remains incompletely understood, but it is probably the result of an alteration of the distribution of vascular compliance (see Chapter 17). During the compression phase of CPR, blood moves out of the thorax into a relatively compliant set of vessels, mostly in the abdomen. This blood is then readily available for redistribution to the thoracic vasculature to provide for coronary blood flow during the release phase. Abdominal binding seems to reduce this extrathoracic arterial compliance, thus reducing the amount of blood available for coronary perfusion.

In human studies of SCV-CPR, Chandra et al. reported an increase in radial artery pressure and carotid flow velocity in a hemodynamic study of 11 patients at the end of failed conventional resuscitation.[15] Martin *et al.* examined hemodynamics in five patients and found a decrease in coronary perfusion pressure with SCV-CPR.[21] These patients were very late in resuscitation, which may have adversely affected the outcome. A major clinical trial of SCV-CPR was reported by Krischer et al., where 994 patients with out-of-hospital cardiac arrest were treated with either SCV-CPR or standard CPR.[26] The ambulance crews, rather than the patients, were randomized, so that the crews knew which form of CPR was going to be administered prior to arrival at the scene of the arrest. This block randomization method was criticized for its potential for adding bias. The survival (to hospital admission) was greater with standard CPR than with SCV-CPR (26% vs. 19%). This study did utilize abdominal binding with the SCV-CPR, which as noted could have had a deleterious effect on coronary perfusion. Because of the lack of significant resuscitation survival benefit in any study, there is little active research on this technique.

Active compression–decompression (ACD) CPR

In this technique, CPR is applied by using a compression device (either manual or mechanical) with an integral suction cup (Fig. 31.2). The suction cup allows for active decompression of the chest in-between compressions. Investigators studying this technique have used standard guidelines for the rate and duration of compressions. The decompression phase actively returns the chest wall to its expanded position without breaking contact. In human studies, ventilation has been performed according to the usual guidelines, but some animal studies have omitted ventilation except that caused by the compression–decompression itself.

ACD-CPR research began with a report of an elderly man resuscitated by his uninitiated son with a bath-

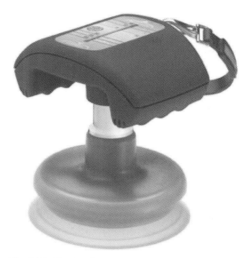

Fig. 31.2. Device for performing active compression–decompression CPR. The upper part is a handle, while the lower part is a suction cup. (Courtesy AMBU Corporation).

room plunger.[27] Lurie *et al.* at the University of California at San Francisco then began active research into the technique in both humans and an animal model. A device to perform ACD-CPR was developed by Ambu International (Copenhagen, Denmark), and numerous investigations have been performed with this technique.[28–48]

Physiology

ACD-CPR likely works in a fashion not dissimilar to interposed abdominal CPR where the active decompressions serve to prime the intrathoracic pump mechanism.[49–52] The active decompressions could result in greater chest expansion and filling with air between compressions, so that the next compression results in a greater rise in intrathoracic pressure and greater flow. A greater rise in intrathoracic pressure could be mediated through increased trapping of air in the lungs,[53] or simply increased application of force. Of note, chest compression force has not been measured in control groups undergoing standard manual CPR. Even if the peak compression forces used during active-decompression CPR and standard CPR were comparable, it would still not be known whether the reported benefit for active-decompression CPR results from the active decompressions, or from the increased force change (peak compression-to-peak decompression force) applied. For example, if 400 N compression force and 100 N decompression force were applied to the chest, is it equivalent simply to applying 500 N of compression force, or does the decompression force have unique physiologic effects that improve blood flow?

The active decompressions could produce negative intrathoracic pressure between compressions and greater venous return, even without increasing the right atrial pressure relative to aortic pressure, which would impede coronary flow. Alternatively, there may be better right heart flow into the pulmonary bed between compressions. Additionally, the design of the device used for ACD-CPR results in the potential for a mechanism in the application of compression force that is slightly different from that in conventional CPR. In standard external chest compression, the hands never lose contact with the thorax, and therefore the onset of application of force is gradual. The ACD-CPR device provides an air space of a few inches between the location of the hands and the chest wall. This allows some acceleration to take place before the force of compression actually reaches the chest, resulting in a slight impact on the chest wall. The significance of this with regard to the physiology of ACD-CPR is unknown. Studies reported to date have not resolved these issues. One study in pigs showed, in the absence of vasoconstrictors, increased coronary blood flow for active-decompression CPR for a standardized amount of chest compression from a mechanical chest compressor.[54] Nevertheless, that same study showed no difference in coronary flow when vasoconstrictors were used.

A number of clinical trials have been reported with ACD-CPR. In the first clinical study, it was reported that 18 of 29 (62%) patients treated with active-decompression CPR had return of spontaneous circulation, compared with 10 of 33 (30%) patients treated with standard CPR. A number of larger clinical trials have been reported since that time. Most of the trials have shown no difference in survival for patients treated with standard CPR or ACD-CPR.[38,55-58]

In one trial of 512 patients in Paris, France,[43] there was an improvement in survival (ACD vs. standard CPR) at 1 hour (36.6% vs. 24.8%, $P = 0.003$), 24 hours (26% vs. 13.6%, $P = 0.002$), and at hospital discharge (5.5% vs. 1.9%, $P = 0.03$). Mean time from collapse to basic cardiac life support CPR was 9 minutes and from collapse to ACLS CPR was 21 minutes. A more recent report of 750 patients from that latter group showed that survival was also improved at 1 year (5% vs. 2%, $P=0.03$).[45] All patients who survived to 1 year had cardiac arrests that were witnessed.

It is unclear why most trials showed no benefit for ACD-CPR over standard CPR, and that there was a statistically significant, albeit small, benefit in the Paris study. It has been speculated that ACD-CPR may be of more benefit if administered relatively late in the course of cardiac arrest, as was done in Paris, and that the level of training and retraining is important.

There is a possibility that the high velocity of impact of the device at the start of chest compression could cause additional trauma as compared to conventional chest compressions.[59,60] In addition, the increased chest excursions produced by the active decompressions could cause increased flexing of the ribs, and increased trauma.

Applicability

ACD-CPR shares the advantages of all manual techniques in that it is readily applied in a wide variety of circumstances. The device required to perform this technique could be made widely available should it prove significantly beneficial. The technique itself is not appreciably more difficult than standard external chest compression, although it may prove substantially more tiring, given that the rescuer is required to be active during both phases (compression and decompression) of each cycle.[61] The disadvantages of manual devices, however, are that an operator can perform the compressions incorrectly and chest compression must be interrupted for defibrillation. Finally, the combination of the Impedance Threshold Device (see below) with the Active Compression Decompression Device seems to improve its hemodynamics and efficacy substantially.

Impedance threshold device

The impedance threshold device (valve), is placed in the airway circuit to impede the flow of air into the chest during chest decompression (Fig. 31.3). Its goal is to increase the level of negative intrathoracic pressure generated during chest decompression, and thereby augment the beneficial effects of that negative intrathoracic pressure.

The impedance threshold device (ITD) has been studied with standard CPR in a porcine model of cardiac arrest. In one study, coronary perfusion pressure (CPP) (diastolic aortic minus right atrial pressure) was the primary endpoint. After 2 minutes of CPR, mean +/− SEM CPP was 14 +/− 2 mm Hg with a sham valve versus 20 +/− 2 mm Hg in the ITD group ($P < 0.006$).[62] Significantly higher CPPs were maintained throughout the study when the ITD was used. In another study, microsphere-measured myocardial blood flow was higher with the use of the impedance threshold valve (0.32 +/− 0.04 vs. 0.23 +/− 0.03 ml/min per g, $P<0.05$), as was cerebral blood flow (0.23 +/− 0.02 vs. 0.19 +/− 0.02; $P<0.05$).[63] In a third study, the use of the ITD was evaluated to determine the potential to improve 24-hour survival and neurological function in a pig model of cardiac arrest. That study used a randomized, prospective, and blinded design, where the effect of a sham versus

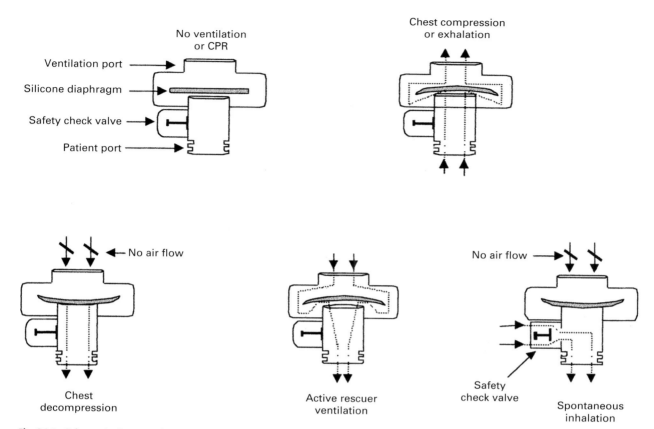

Fig. 31.3. Schematic diagram of impedance threshold device. The components of the device are shown on the upper left panel. During chest compression or exhalation(upper right panel) air moves freely through the valve. During chest decompression (lower left panel) airflow is impeded by the device to increase the level of negative intrathoracic pressure generated. During rescuer ventilation or spontaneous inhalation (lower middle and right panels) air also moves freely through the valve. (From ref. 63.)

active ITD was evaluated on 24-hour survival and neurological function. After 6 minutes of ventricular fibrillation, followed by 6 minutes of standard CPR with either a sham or an active valve, advanced life support was performed. A total of 11 of 20 pigs (55%) in the sham vs. 17 of 20 (85%) in the active valve group survived for 24 hours ($P<0.05$). Neurological scores were significantly higher with the active valve; the cerebral performance score (1 = normal, 5 = brain death) was $2.2+/-0.2$ with the sham ITD versus $1.4+/-0.2$ with the active valve ($P<0.05$).[64] Thus, with standard CPR in animal models, the ITD improved coronary perfusion pressure, microsphere-determined myocardial and cerebral blood flows, and 24-hour survival and neurologic function.

Similar to the animal studies, clinical studies during manual cardiopulmonary resuscitation have shown a hemodynamic benefit for the impedance threshold device,[65] as well as improved short-term survival for patients with pulseless electrical activity with use of the ITD.[66]

The impedance threshold device has also been studied in conjunction with active compression–decompression cardiopulmonary resuscitation.[64,67,68] In a prospective, randomized, blinded trial performed in Paris, France, patients in non-traumatic cardiac arrest received ACD-CPR plus the valve or ACD-CPR alone for 30 minutes during advanced cardiac life support.[67] With the use of the impedance threshold device (Fig. 31.4) there were increases in end tidal carbon dioxide pressure ($19.1+/-1.0$ vs. $13.1+/-0.9$ mm Hg, $P<0.001$), diastolic blood pressure ($56.4+/-1.7$ vs. $36.5+/-1.5$ mmHg, $P<0.001$), and coronary perfusion pressure ($43.3+/-1.6$ vs. $25.0+/-1.4$ mmHg, $P<0.001$). In addition, return of spontaneous circulation was observed in 2 of 10 patients with ACD-CPR alone after $26.5+/-0.7$ minutes versus 4 of 11 patients with ACD-CPR plus the impedance threshold device after $19.8+/-2.8$ minutes ($P<0.05$).

A prospective trial of ACD-CPR with the ITD vs. standard CPR was performed in Mainz, Germany. Patients with

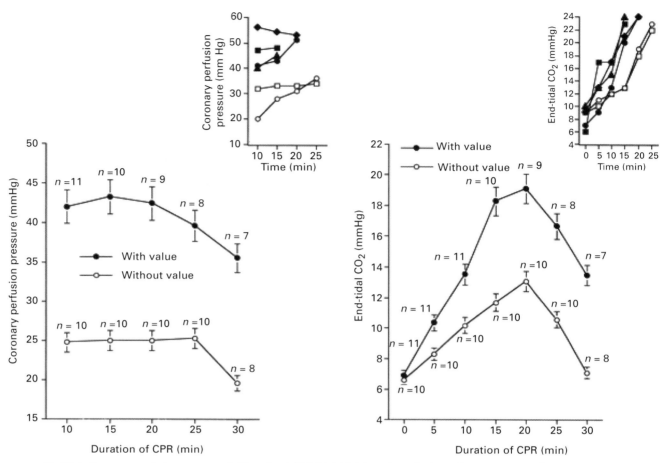

Fig. 31.4. Coronary perfusion pressures (left), and end tidal CO_2(right) in patients during active compression–decompression CPR without (lower tracing) and with (upper tracing) the use of the impedance threshold device. (From ref. 67.)

out-of-hospital arrest of presumed cardiac pathogenesis were randomized to ACD+ITD CPR or standard-CPR. The randomization was by rescuer crews, not individual patients. With ACD+ITD CPR (n=103), return of spontaneous circulation and 1- and 24-hour survival rates were 55%, 51%, and 37% vs. 37%, 32%, and 22% with standard-CPR (n=107) (P=0.016, 0.006, and 0.033, respectively). One- and 24-hour survival rates in witnessed arrests were 55% and 41% with ACD+ITD CPR vs. 33% and 23% in control subjects (P=0.011 and 0.019), respectively. One- and 24-hour survival rates in patients with a witnessed arrest in ventricular fibrillation were 68% and 58% after ACD+ITD CPR vs. 27% and 23% after standard-CPR (P=0.002 and P=0.009), respectively. Hospital discharge rates were 18% after ACD+ITD CPR versus 13% in control subjects (P=0.41). In witnessed arrests, overall neurological function trended higher with ACD+ITD CPR vs. control subjects (P=0.07).[69]

A subsequent, blinded, multicenter study was done to determine whether an inspiratory impedance threshold device, when used in combination with active compression–decompression cardiopulmonary resuscitation, would improve survival rates in patients with out-of-hospital cardiac arrest. Patients were randomized to receive either a sham (n=200) or an active impedance threshold device (n=200) during advanced cardiac life support performed with active compression–decompression cardiopulmonary resuscitation. The primary endpoint of this study was 24-hour survival. The 24-hour survival rates were 44/200 (22%) with the sham valve and 64/200 (32%) with the active valve (P=0.02). The number of patients who had return of spontaneous circulation (ROSC), intensive care unit (ICU) admission, and hospital discharge rates was 77 (39%), 57 (29%), and 8 (4%) in the sham valve group vs. 96 (48%) (P=0.05), 79 (40%) (P=0.02), and 10 (5%) (P=0.6) in the active valve group.[70] Thus, whether the control group was standard CPR or ACD-CPR, the use of the ITD improved short-term survival.

Thus, the results with the impedance threshold device are very promising, particularly since the device can be used with standard CPR as well as more advanced forms of CPR. There appears to be a clear hemodynamic benefit and short-term survival benefit with use of the device. Further studies are needed to determine if the valve can be used successfully in larger studies of cardiac arrest, and whether the improved hemodynamics and short term survival will translate into improved long-term survival.

Phased chest and abdominal compression

A mechanical device is being developed that allows for active compression and decompression of the chest as well as for active compression and decompression of the abdomen. The device consists of two adhesive pads that are connected to a mechanical linkage. The pads are attached to the chest and abdomen, respectively. The linkage has two handles that are held by the rescuer. The rescuer pushes or pulls on the chest handle to compress or decompress the chest, and alternately pushes or pulls on the abdominal handle to compress or decompress the abdomen.

Laboratory studies of phased chest and abdominal compression has shown an increase in coronary perfusion pressure, as well as an increase in the number of animals resuscitated over that with standard cardiopulmonary resuscitation.[71] Kern *et al.* studied different types of ventilation, and showed that the type of ventilation could have a serious impact on the hemodynamics produced by this type of resuscitation.[72]

In a clinical study of phased chest and abdominal compression CPR, 54 patients were studied.[73] More patients treated with standard CPR survived to hospital discharge (7 vs. 0), but fewer patients treated with phased chest and abdominal compression had significant trauma at autopsy.

Since there are only small studies of phased chest and abdominal compression, further studies are needed to determine if this device will be useful in the treatment of cardiac arrest victims.

Vest cardiopulmonary resuscitation

With vest CPR, a bladder-containing vest (analogous to a large blood pressure cuff) is placed circumferentially around the patient's chest (Fig. 31.5) and cyclically inflated and deflated by an automated pneumatic system. In this manner, the chest is compressed cyclically. The device permits control of rate, compression duration, and inflation pressure. The vest also maintains a small amount of positive pressure on the chest between compressions to keep the vest snugly against the chest, except during the built-in pause for ventilation, at which time the vest completely deflates. The vest is generally inflated to a pressure of approximately 250 mm Hg, 60 times/ minute, with 40% to 50% of each cycle in compression. Adherent defibrillation pads are placed on the chest before applying the vest to allow for defibrillation without having to remove the vest or interrupt CPR.

As with SCV-CPR, vest CPR was developed as a means for augmenting intrathoracic pressure over that which could be produced by standard CPR. Vest CPR was largely developed by a group of investigators at Johns Hopkins University,[53,74–84] although other groups also made contributions.[23,85–93]

Physiology

Vest CPR is designed to maximize the intrathoracic pressure rises generated for a given force applied to the chest. By encircling the chest (Fig. 31.5), force can be applied evenly, thus resulting in a large decrement in the volume of the chest with minimal displacement of an individual point on the chest wall. This circumferential compression allows for large increases in intrathoracic pressure without the trauma inherent in applying force to a single point, as with standard chest compression.

Many generations of vest CPR systems have been developed and tested. Studies with an early vest device reported by Luce *et al.* in 1983 and 1984 showed that hemodynamics in a dog model of CPR were only minimally if at all improved with vest CPR compared with mechanically performed standard external chest compression.[92,93] Niemann *et al.*[91] and Halperin *et al.*[74] used an improved system and showed augmentation of perfusion pressures and blood flows with vest CPR either with or without simultaneous ventilation. In the study by Halperin's group, survival was also better in the group of dogs receiving vest CPR. At high vest pressures, they produced myocardial and brain blood flows equivalent to that in control animals, although they noted some trauma. At somewhat lower vest pressures, myocardial blood flow was 40% of prearrest flow, and cerebral blood flow was essentially equal to prearrest flow, with no trauma. These latter flows were greater than had been reported previously with standard external chest compression by any author.

Swenson et al. reported a study of vest CPR in 10 patients late in cardiac arrest[85]; they found no improvement in

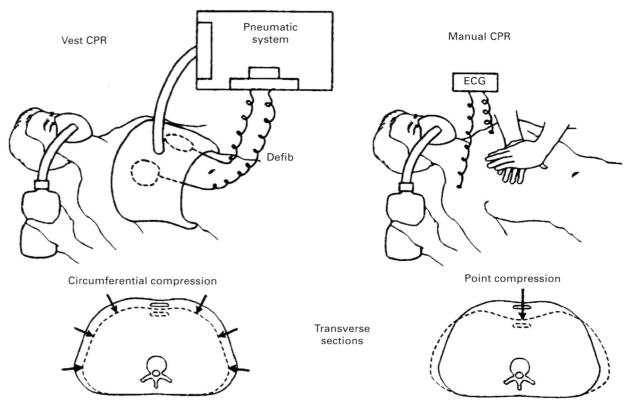

Fig. 31.5. Comparison of vest CPR and manual CPR. The vest is like a large blood pressure cuff that encircles the chest. A pneumatic system inflates and deflates the vest to compress and release the chest. Flat defibrillator (defib) pads can be placed beneath the vest so that defibrillation can be performed during compressions. The vest compresses most of the circumference of the chest (lower panels), compared with a point compression of standard CPR. (From ref. 78.) Copyright 1993, *N. Engl. J. Med.*

coronary perfusion pressure produced with that vest CPR system. Halperin et al. subsequently reported a two-phase study of vest CPR using an improved vest CPR system, which incorporated a vest that covered more of the chest than did previous systems.[78] This system also included a small positive pressure on the chest in-between compressions to keep the vest tight against the chest. With the improved vest CPR system, hemodynamics in humans were significantly improved over those of standard external chest compression. Peak aortic pressure was nearly doubled (up to an average of 138 mm Hg), and coronary perfusion pressure increased by 50%. A hemodynamic tracing during manual and vest CPR in a patient is shown in Fig. 31.6. In addition, 4 of the 29 patients had return of spontaneous circulation during vest CPR despite being treated late (50 ± 22 min) in resuscitation. The second phase of the study randomized patients to either vest CPR or standard external chest compression after initial (11 ± 4 min) advanced cardiac life support failed to resuscitate the patients. There was a trend toward improved initial resus-

citation in the vest CPR group, but the trial was too small to show a statistically significant benefit.

If the vest is applied below the desired thoracic region, increased abdominal trauma could be expected. The vest does not, however, appear to increase the incidence of trauma over that of manual CPR,[78] although only limited data are available.

Applicability

Vest CPR requires a sophisticated device for its administration, which limits its use to locations where the device would be readily available. Application of the vest itself is not difficult and can be performed successfully by nurses, given only a few minutes instruction in its use. It is likely that, if vest CPR proves successful in improving survival from cardiac arrest, it will remain predominantly in the hands of health care professionals. It will serve as a supplement, therefore, to the best form of standard CPR available for out-of-hospital arrests. Both animal and

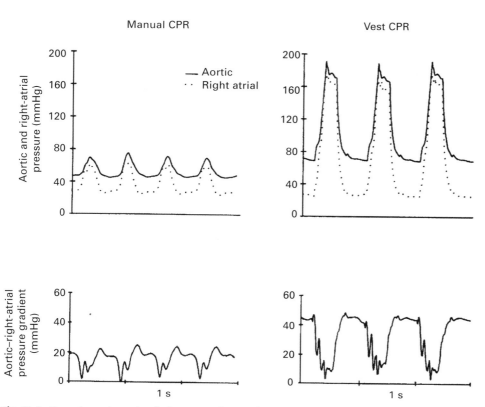

Fig. 31.6. Hemodynamic tracing during vest and manual CPR. Aortic, right atrial, and aortic minus right atrial pressures are shown. (From ref. 78.) Copyright 1993, *N. Engl. J. Med.*

human data show rather dramatic improvements in hemodynamics with vest CPR. If vest CPR can routinely raise the coronary perfusion gradient above the threshold required for late defibrillation to be successful, then it could make a measurable impact on the ability to achieve return of spontaneous circulation. Until sufficient human studies are done, however, we will not know whether or not this will result in improved long-term survival and neurologic recovery.

Load distributing band (LDB) cardiopulmonary resuscitation

It had previously been shown that the circumferential vest device, analogous to a large blood pressure cuff that was inflated and deflated, could generate pressures during CPR that were substantially improved over those generated by standard CPR.[74,78] That vest device, however, was too large, and consumed too much power to be easily portable, and it has not been tested in large clinical trials. An improved device, based on a band that distributed the compression load over the entire anterior chest (load distributing band, LDB) was subsequently developed.

Physiology

The LDB device probably has similar physiology to the vest CPR device, given that the compressive load is distributed over a large portion of the chest with both devices. An initial animal trial showed that the LDB device generated peak aortic and coronary perfusion pressures that were improved over those generated with standard CPR.[94] An improved device was subsequently developed and was named the AutoPulse™ (Fig. 31.7). In a study with an improved LDB device, 30 pigs (16 ± 4 kg) were investigated, comparing LDB-CPR to conventional CPR with the piston device (C-CPR). LDB-CPR improved coronary perfusion pressure without epinephrine (LDB-CPR 21 ± 8 vs. C-CPR 14 ± 6 mmHg, mean ± SD, $P<0.0001$) and with epinephrine (LDB-CPR 45 ± 11 vs. C-CPR 17 ± 6 mmHg, $P<0.0001$). LDB-CPR improved myocardial flow without epinephrine, and cerebral and myocardial flow with epinephrine ($P<0.05$). LDB-CPR also produced greater myocardial flow at every coronary perfusion pressure ($P<0.01$). One of the mechanisms for the improved hemodynamics with LDB-CPR appears to be airway collapse (Fig. 31.8) that occurs with LDB-CPR, trapping air in the lungs resulting in higher and more sustained intrathoracic pressure generation, and not present with C-CPR.[95]

In a preliminary trial in terminally ill patients, after a minimum of 10 minutes of failed advanced life support, subjects received alternating periods of manual and LDB chest compressions for 90 seconds each. Peak aortic pressures were higher with LDB CPR when compared with manual CPR (150 ± 8 vs. 122 ± 11 mm Hg, $P<0.05$, mean $\pm$ SEM), as was coronary perfusion pressure (20 ± 3 vs. 15 ± 3 mm Hg, $P<0.02$), even though the manual chest compressions were of consistently high quality (51 ± 20 kg) and in all cases met or exceeded American Heart Association guidelines for depth of compression.[96] In that latter study, coronary perfusion pressure was raised above the level generally associated with improved survival.[97]

In a case control study of LDB-CPR, a retrospective chart review was undertaken where a manual CPR comparison group was case-matched for age, gender, initial presenting ECG rhythm, and the number of doses of ACLS medications as a proxy for treatment time. Matching was performed by an investigator blinded to outcome and treatment group. Sixty-nine LDB-CPR cases were matched to 93 manual CPR only cases. LDB-CPR showed improvement in the primary outcome of survival to arrival at the emergency department, when compared to manual CPR with any presenting rhythm (LDB-CPR 39%, manual 29%, $P=0.003$). When patients were classified by first presenting rhythm, shockable rhythms showed no difference in outcome (LDB-CPR 44%, manual 50%, $P=0.340$). Outcome was improved with LDB-CPR in initial presenting asystole and approached significance with pulseless electrical activity (asystole: A-CPR 37%, manual 22%, $P=0.008$; PEA: A-CPR 38%, manual 23%, $P=0.079$).[98]

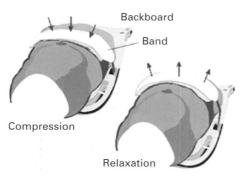

Fig. 31.7. Operation of the load distributing band device. During compression (left) the band is tightened by a motor, and compression force is directed inward. During relaxation (right), the band is released, and the chest expands.

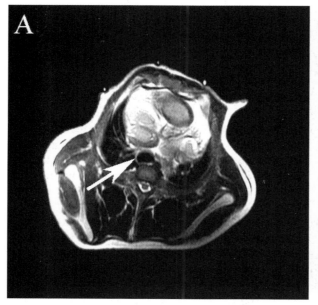
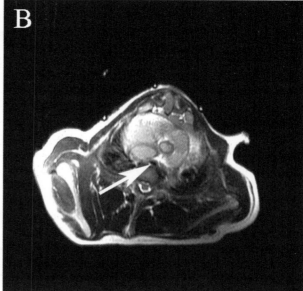

Fig. 31.8. Magnetic resonance imaging of the thorax during Load Distributing Band cardiopulmonary resuscitation in a pig. The trachea is widely patent in the uncompressed state (A, arrow) but is nearly fully collapsed during peak compression (B, arrow). (From ref. 95.)

A prospective trial (ASPIRE trial) compared resuscitation outcomes following out-of-hospital cardiac arrest when an automated LDB-CPR device was added to standard emergency medical services (EMS) care with manual CPR. The trial included 5 centers and enrolled 1071 patients. Block randomization was done, in which a specific EMS crew would perform either LDB-CPR or manual CPR on a specific number of patients (block size), then perform the other type on a subsequent block of patients. In addition, the crews had the discretion of whether or not to enroll specific patients. The primary end point was survival to 4 hours after the 911 call. Following the first planned interim monitoring conducted by an independent data and safety monitoring board, study enrollment was terminated. No difference existed in the primary end point of survival to 4 hours between the manual CPR group and the LDB-CPR group overall ($N = 1071$; 30% vs. 29%; $P = 0.74$). However, among the patients who were felt to have primary cardiac arrests, survival to hospital discharge was 9.9% in the manual CPR group and 5.8% in the LDB-CPR group ($P = 0.06$, adjusted for covariates and clustering). A cerebral performance category of 1 or 2 at hospital discharge was recorded in 7.5% of patients in the manual CPR group and in 3.1% of the LDB-CPR group ($P = 0.006$).[99]

There are a number of issues that make interpretation of the results of the ASPIRE trial problematic. Statistical analysis showed that the study sites were not statistically homogeneous, in that one site was statistically different from the other four sites. The statistically different site had much higher survival rates for both manual CPR and LDB-CPR than the other four sites, prior to a protocol change that occurred in the middle of the trial. The survival with LDB-CPR and manual CPR were similar before the protocol change, but the survival with LDB-CPR decreased dramatically after the protocol change. The one statistically different site was responsible for the overall decrease in survival noted in the study. In addition to the change in protocol, other factors that could explain the decreased survival with LDB-CPR in the ASPIRE include: (1) bias that could be introduced by the block randomization and crew enrollment discretion, (2) delays in performing defibrillation, and (3) inadequate training.

A prospective and retrospective trial (Richmond trial) was conducted in Richmond, Virginia, comparing LDB-CPR with manual CPR after the emergency medical services system there switched from manual cardiopulmonary resuscitation (CPR) to load-distributing band (LDB) CPR. A total of 499 patients were included in the manual CPR phase (January 1, 2001, to March 31, 2003) and 284 patients in the LDB-CPR phase (December 20, 2003, to March 31, 2005); of these patients, the LDB device was applied in 210 patients. Patients in the manual CPR and LDB-CPR phases were comparable except for a faster response time interval (mean difference, 26 seconds) and more EMS-witnessed arrests (18.7% vs. 12.6%) with LDB. Rates for ROSC and survival were increased with LDB-CPR compared with manual CPR (for ROSC, 34.5% vs. 20.2%; and for survival to hospital discharge, 9.7%; 95% CI, 6.7%–13.8% vs. 2.9%; 95% CI, 1.7%–4.8%; adjusted OR, 2.27; 95% CI, 1.11–4.77). In a secondary analysis of the 210 patients in whom the LDB device was applied, 38 patients (18.1%) survived to hospital admission (95% CI, 13.4%–23.9%) and 12 patients (5.7%) survived to hospital discharge (95% CI, 3.0%–9.3%).[100] A weakness of the Richmond trial is that there is a historical control group. A major strength is that all patients treated for cardiac arrest were included.

Applicability

Like vest CPR, LDB-CPR requires a sophisticated device for its administration, which limits its use to locations where the device would be readily available. The LDB device is, however, readily portable and can be applied in as little as 30 seconds. The LDB device will likely serve as a supplement, therefore, to the best form of standard CPR available for out-of-hospital arrests. Both animal and human data show rather dramatic improvements in hemodynamics with LDB-CPR, and there are mechanistic explanations for those improvements. If LDB-CPR can routinely raise the coronary perfusion pressure above the threshold required for resuscitation, then it could make a measurable impact on the ability to achieve return of spontaneous circulation. LDB-CPR significantly improved survival in the Richmond trial, but not in the ASPIRE trial. The reasons that these two trials showed such differences in survival are unclear. There are likely to be implementation and training issues that have to be addressed. In addition, one site was responsible for the overall decrease in survival noted for the ASPIRE trial, which was probably due to that site's change in protocol midway through the trial. Another trial is commencing that will address the issues noted in the previous trials and should be large enough to determine the true clinical utility of LDB-CPR.

The future

Research aimed at improving survival from cardiac arrest both in- and out-of-hospital continues. The first 45 years of external chest compression have been marked by enthusiasm, disappointment, innovation, and speculation, but to date no technique has convincingly positioned itself to replace standard CPR as we now know it. Research has contributed a great deal to the science of CPR and set the stage for real advancement in the resuscitation of cardiac arrest victims. The critical importance of early defibrillation is now clearly recognized, as is the importance of improved blood flow. Likewise, the criteria used to judge a new CPR method have been defined. These measures – coronary perfusion pressure (important in predicting return of spontaneous circulation), systolic arterial pressure (predictive of cerebral blood flow and likely of neurologic recovery), and ultimately survival-to-hospital discharge – will drive the search for the best method or methods of applying force to the human body over the next several years. The future may lie not so much in a replacement of current CPR as in evolution to differing types of CPR under different circumstances, as well as improving the quality of standard CPR. Small hand-held devices are already under development that measure chest compression depth and compression rate to provide even lay rescuers with feedback to help them perform chest compressions at the specified 1.5–2 in of displacement and 100 compressions/ minute. Resuscitation initiated by lay persons will by necessity remain a manual technique, but some other form of CPR may be used once qualified rescuers are on the scene. Currently the distinction between basic and advanced life support involves the availability of drugs, mechanical airways, and defibrillation. It is very possible that the form of CPR utilized may also become part of this distinction, as well as the concomitant use of more advance strategies such as hypothermia.

REFERENCES

1. Schneider, A.P., 2nd, Nelson, D.J. & Brown, D.D. In-hospital cardiopulmonary resuscitation: a 30-year review. *J. Am. Board Fam. Pract.* 1993; **6**: 91–101.

2. Tunstall-Pedoe, H., Bailey, L., Chamberlain, D.A., Marsden, A.K., Ward, M.E. & Zideman, D.A. Survey of 3765 cardiopulmonary resuscitations in British hospitals (the BRESUS Study): methods and overall results. *Br. Med. J.* 1992; **304**: 1347–1351.

3. Guidelines 2000 for Cardiopulmonary Resuscitation and Emergency Cardiovascular Care. Part 3: Adult basic life support. The American Heart Association in collaboration with the International Liaison Committee on Resuscitation. *Circulation* 2000; **102**: I22–I59.

4. Ochoa, F.J., Ramalle-Gomara, E., Lisa, V. & Saralegui, I. The effect of rescuer fatigue on the quality of chest compressions. *Resuscitation* 1998; **37**: 149–152.

5. Hightower, D., Thomas, S.H., Stone, C.K., Dunn, K. & March, J.A. Decay in quality of closed-chest compressions over time. *Ann. Emerg. Med.* 1995; **26**: 300–303.

6. Gallagher, E.J., Lombardi, G. & Gennis, P. Effectiveness of bystander cardiopulmonary resuscitation and survival following out-of-hospital cardiac arrest. *J. Am. Med. Assoc.* 1995; **274**: 1922–1925.

7. Van Hoeyweghen, R.J., Bossaert, L.L., Mullie, A. *et al.* Quality and efficiency of bystander CPR. Belgian Cerebral Resuscitation Study Group. *Resuscitation* 1993; **26**: 47–52.

8. Newton, J.R., Jr., Glower, D.D., Wolfe, J.A. *et al.* A physiologic comparison of external cardiac massage techniques. *J. Thorac. Cardiovasc. Surg.* 1988; **95**: 892–901.

9. McDonald, J.L. Systolic and mean arterial pressures during manual and mechanical CPR in humans. *Ann. Emerg. Med.* 1982; **11**: 292–295.

10. Ward, K.R., Menegazzi, J.J., Zelenak, R.R., Sullivan, R.J. & McSwain, N.E., Jr. A comparison of chest compressions between mechanical and manual CPR by monitoring end-tidal PCO_2 during human cardiac arrest. *Ann. Emerg. Med.* 1993; **22**: 669–674.

11. Betz, A.E., Menegazzi, J.J., Logue, E.S., Callaway, C.W. & Wang, H.E. A randomized comparison of manual, mechanical and high-impulse chest compression in a porcine model of prolonged ventricular fibrillation. *Resuscitation* 2006.

12. Nagel, E.L., Fine, E.G., Krischer, J.P. & Davis, J.H. Complications of CPR. *Crit. Care Med.* 1981; **9**: 424.

13. Krischer, J.P., Fine, E.G., Davis, J.H. & Nagel, E.L. Complications of cardiac resuscitation. *Chest* 1987; **92**: 287–291.

14. Koehler, R.C., Chandra, N., Guerci, A.D. *et al.* Augmentation of cerebral perfusion by simultaneous chest compression and lung inflation with abdominal binding after cardiac arrest in dogs. *Circulation* 1983; **67**: 266–275.

15. Chandra, N., Rudikoff, M. & Weisfeldt, M.L. Simultaneous chest compression and ventilation at high airway pressure during cardiopulmonary resuscitation. *Lancet* 1980; **1**: 175–178.

16. Chandra, N., Weisfeldt, M.L., Tsitlik, J. *et al.* Augmentation of carotid flow during cardiopulmonary resuscitation by ventilation at high airway pressure simultaneous with chest compression. *Am. J. Cardiol.* 1981; **48**: 1053–1063.

17. Sanders, A.B., Ewy, G.A., Alferness, C.A., Taft, T. & Zimmerman, M. Failure of one method of simultaneous chest compression, ventilation, and abdominal binding during CPR. *Crit. Care Med.* 1982; **10**: 509–513.

18. Wilder, R., Weir, D., Rush, B.F. & Ravitch, M.M. Method of coordinating ventilation and closed chest massage in the dog. *Surgery* 1963; **53**: 186–194.

19. Kern, K.B., Carter, A.B., Showen, R.L. *et al.* Comparison of mechanical techniques of cardiopulmonary resuscitation: survival and neurologic outcome in dogs. *Am. J. Emerg. Med.* 1987; **5**: 190–195.

20. Ralston, S.H., Babbs, C.F. & Niebauer, M.J. Cardiopulmonary resuscitation with interposed abdominal compression in dogs. *Anesth. Analg.* 1982; **61**: 645–651.

21. Martin, G.B., Carden, D.L., Nowak, R.M., Lewinter, J.R., Johnston, W. & Tomlanovich, M.C. Aortic and right atrial pressures during standard and simultaneous compression and ventilation CPR in human beings. *Ann. Emerg. Med.* 1986; **15**: 125–130.

22. Chandra, N., Snyder, L.D. & Weisfeldt, M.L. Abdominal binding during cardiopulmonary resuscitation in man. *J. Am. Med. Assoc.* 1981; **246**: 351–353.

23. Niemann, J.T., Rosborough, J.P., Ung, S. & Criley, J.M. Coronary perfusion pressure during experimental cardiopulmonary resuscitation. *Ann. Emerg. Med.* 1982; **11**: 127–131.

24. Michael, J.R., Guerci, A.D., Koehler, R.C. *et al.* Mechanisms by which epinephrine augments cerebral and myocardial perfusion during cardiopulmonary resuscitation in dogs. *Circulation* 1984; **69**: 822–835.

25. Niemann, J.T., Rosborough, J.P., Ung, S. & Criley, J.M. Hemodynamic effects of continuous abdominal binding during cardiac arrest and resuscitation. *Am. J. Cardiol.* 1984; **53**: 269–274.

26. Krischer, J.P., Fine, E.G., Weisfeldt, M.L., Guerci, A.D., Nagel, E. & Chandra, N. Comparison of prehospital conventional and simultaneous compression–ventilation cardiopulmonary resuscitation. *Crit. Care Med.* 1989; **17**: 1263–1269.

27. Lurie, K.G., Lindo, C. & Chin, J. CPR: the P stands for plumber's helper. *J. Am. Med. Assoc.* 1990; **264**: 1661.

28. Sack, J.B., Gerber, R.S. & Kesselbrenner, M.B. Active compression–decompression cardiopulmonary resuscitation. *J. Am. Med. Assoc.* 1992; **268**: 3200–3201.

29. Cohen, T.J., Goldner, B.G., Maccaro, P.C. *et al.* A comparison of active compression–decompression cardiopulmonary resuscitation with standard cardiopulmonary resuscitation for cardiac arrests occurring in the hospital. *N. Engl. J. Med.* 1993; **329**: 1918–1921.

30. Tucker, K.J., Khan, J.H. & Savitt, M.A. Active compression–decompression resuscitation: effects on pulmonary ventilation. *Resuscitation* 1993; **26**: 125–131.

31. Carli, P.A., De La Coussaye, J.E., Riou, B., Sassine, A. & Eledjam, J.J. Ventilatory effects of active compression–decompression in dogs. *Ann. Emerg. Med.* 1994; **24**: 890–894.

32. Chang, M.W., Coffeen, P., Lurie, K.G., Shultz, J., Bache, R.J. & White, C.W. Active compression–decompression CPR improves vital organ perfusion in a dog model of ventricular fibrillation. *Chest* 1994; **106**: 1250–1259.

33. Sachs, F.L. Active compression–decompression cardiopulmonary resuscitation. *N. Engl. J. Med.* 1994; **330**: 1391.

34. Wik, L., Naess, P.A., Ilebekk, A. & Steen, P.A. Simultaneous active compression–decompression and abdominal binding increase carotid blood flow additively during cardiopulmonary resuscitation (CPR) in pigs. *Resuscitation* 1994; **28**: 55–64.

35. Schwab, T.M., Callaham, M.L., Madsen, C.D. & Utecht, T.A. A randomized clinical trial of active compression–decompression CPR vs standard CPR in out-of-hospital cardiac arrest in two cities. *J. Am. Med. Assoc.* 1995; **273**: 1261–1268.

36. Wenzel, V., Fuerst, R.S., Idris, A.H., Banner, M.J., Rush, W.J. & Orban, D.J. Automatic mechanical device to standardize active compression–decompression CPR. *Ann. Emerg. Med.* 1995; **25**: 386–389.

37. Weston, C.F. Cardiopulmonary resuscitation with active compression–decompression. *Br. Heart J.* 1995; **74**: 212–214.

38. Wik, L., Mauer, D. & Robertson, C. The first European pre-hospital active compression–decompression (ACD) cardiopulmonary resuscitation workshop: a report and a review of ACD-CPR. *Resuscitation* 1995; **30**: 191–202.

39. Kern, K.B., Figge, G., Hilwig, R.W. *et al.* Active compression–decompression versus standard cardiopulmonary resuscitation in a porcine model: no improvement in outcome. *Am. Heart J.* 1996; **132**: 1156–1162.

40. Malzer, R., Zeiner, A., Binder, M. *et al.* Hemodynamic effects of active compression–decompression after prolonged CPR. *Resuscitation* 1996; **31**: 243–253.

41. Schneider, T., Wik, L., Baubin, M. *et al.* Active compression–decompression cardiopulmonary resuscitation – instructor and student manual for teaching and training. Part I: The workshop. *Resuscitation* 1996; **32**: 203–206.

42. Baubin, M., Schirmer, M., Nogler, M. *et al.* Active compression–decompression cardiopulmonary resuscitation in standing position over the patient: pros and cons of a new method. *Resuscitation* 1997; **34**: 7–10.

43. Plaisance, P., Adnet, F., Vicaut, E. *et al.* Benefit of active compression–decompression cardiopulmonary resuscitation as a prehospital advanced cardiac life support. A randomized multicenter study. *Circulation* 1997; **95**: 955–961.

44. Mauer, D.K., Nolan, J., Plaisance, P. *et al.* Effect of active compression–decompression resuscitation (ACD-CPR) on survival: a combined analysis using individual patient data. *Resuscitation* 1999; **41**: 249–256.

45. Plaisance, P., Lurie, K.G., Vicaut, E. *et al.* A comparison of standard cardiopulmonary resuscitation and active compression–decompression resuscitation for out-of-hospital cardiac arrest. French Active Compression–Decompression Cardiopulmonary Resuscitation Study Group. *N. Engl. J. Med.* 1999; **341**: 569–575.

46. Steen, S., Liao, Q., Pierre, L., Paskevicius, A. & Sjoberg, T. Evaluation of LUCAS, a new device for automatic mechanical compression and active decompression resuscitation. *Resuscitation* 2002; **55**: 285–299.

47. Rubertsson, S. & Karlsten, R. Increased cortical cerebral blood flow with LUCAS; a new device for mechanical chest compressions compared to standard external compressions during experimental cardiopulmonary resuscitation. *Resuscitation* 2005; **65**: 357–363.

48. Babbs, C.F. Design of near-optimal waveforms for chest and abdominal compression and decompression in CPR using computer-simulated evolution. *Resuscitation* 2006; **68**: 277–293.

49. Lurie, K.G., Shultz, J.J., Callaham, M.L. *et al.* Evaluation of active compression–decompression CPR in victims of out-of-hospital cardiac arrest. *J. Am. Med. Assoc.* 1994; **271**: 1405–1411.

50. Babbs, C.F. Circulatory adjuncts. Newer methods of cardiopulmonary resuscitation. *Cardiol. Clin.* 2002; **20**: 37–59.

51. Babbs, C.F. CPR techniques that combine chest and abdominal compression and decompression: hemodynamic insights from a spreadsheet model. *Circulation* 1999; **100**: 2146–2152.

52. Babbs, C.F. & Thelander, K. Theoretically optimal duty cycles for chest and abdominal compression during external cardiopulmonary resuscitation. *Acad. Emerg. Med.* 1995; **2**: 698–707.

53. Halperin, H.R., Brower, R., Weisfeldt, M.L. *et al.* Air trapping in the lungs during cardiopulmonary resuscitation in dogs. A mechanism for generating changes in intrathoracic pressure. *Circ. Res.* 1989; **65**: 946–954.

54. Lindner, K.H., Pfenninger, E.G., Lurie, K.G., Schurmann, W., Lindner, I.M. & Ahnefeld, F.W. Effects of active compression–decompression resuscitation on myocardial and cerebral blood flow in pigs. *Circulation* 1993; **88**: 1254–1263.

55. Nolan, J., Smith, G., Evans, R. *et al.* The United Kingdom prehospital study of active compression–decompression resuscitation. *Resuscitation* 1998; **37**: 119–125.

56. Panzer, W., Bretthauer, M., Klingler, H., Bahr, J., Rathgeber, J. & Kettler, D. ACD versus standard CPR in a prehospital setting. *Resuscitation* 1996; **33**: 117–124.

57. Stiell, I.G., Hebert, P.C., Wells, G.A. *et al.* The Ontario trial of active compression–decompression cardiopulmonary resuscitation for in-hospital and prehospital cardiac arrest. *J. Am. Med. Assoc.* 1996; **275**: 1417–1423.

58. Luiz, T., Ellinger, K. & Denz, C. Active compression–decompression cardiopulmonary resuscitation does not improve survival in patients with prehospital cardiac arrest in a physician-manned emergency medical system. *J. Cardiothorac. Vasc. Anesth.* 1996; **10**: 178–186.

59. Rabl, W., Baubin, M., Broinger, G. & Scheithauer, R. Serious complications from active compression–decompression cardiopulmonary resuscitation. *Int. J. Legal Med.* 1996; **109**: 84–89.

60. Baubin, M., Rabl, W., Pfeiffer, K.P., Benzer, A. & Gilly, H. Chest injuries after active compression–decompression cardiopulmonary resuscitation (ACD-CPR) in cadavers. *Resuscitation* 1999; **43**: 9–15.

61. Shultz, J.J., Mianulli, M.J., Gisch, T.M., Coffeen, P.R., Haidet, G.C. & Lurie, K.G. Comparison of exertion required to perform standard and active compression–decompression cardiopulmonary resuscitation. *Resuscitation* 1995; **29**: 23–31.

62. Lurie, K.G., Voelckel, W.G., Zielinski, T. *et al.* Improving standard cardiopulmonary resuscitation with an inspiratory impedance threshold valve in a porcine model of cardiac arrest. *Anesth. Analg.* 2001; **93**: 649–655.

63. Lurie, K.G., Mulligan, K.A., McKnite, S., Detloff, B., Lindstrom, P., & Lindner, K.H. Optimizing standard cardiopulmonary resuscitation with an inspiratory impedance threshold valve. *Chest* 1998; **113**: 1084–1090.

64. Lurie, K.G., Zielinski, T., McKnite, S., Aufderheide, T., & Voelckel, W. Use of an inspiratory impedance valve improves neurologically intact survival in a porcine model of ventricular fibrillation. *Circulation* 2002; **105**: 124–129.

65. Pirrallo, R.G., Aufderheide, T.P., Provo, T.A., & Lurie, K.G. Effect of an inspiratory impedance threshold device on hemodynamics during conventional manual cardiopulmonary resuscitation. *Resuscitation* 2005; **66**: 13–20.

66. Aufderheide, T.P., Pirrallo, R.G., Provo, T.A., & Lurie, K.G. Clinical evaluation of an inspiratory impedance threshold device during standard cardiopulmonary resuscitation in patients with out-of-hospital cardiac arrest. *Crit. Care Med.* 2005; **33**: 734–740.

67. Plaisance, P., Lurie, K.G. & Payen, D. Inspiratory impedance during active compression–decompression cardiopulmonary resuscitation: a randomized evaluation in patients in cardiac arrest. *Circulation* 2000; **101**: 989–994.

68. Lurie, K., Voelckel, W., Plaisance, P. *et al.* Use of an inspiratory impedance threshold valve during cardiopulmonary resuscitation: a progress report. *Resuscitation* 2000; **44**: 219–230.

69. Wolcke, B.B., Mauer, D.K., Schoefmann, M.F. *et al.* Comparison of standard cardiopulmonary resuscitation versus the combination of active compression–decompression cardiopulmonary resuscitation and an inspiratory impedance threshold device for out-of-hospital cardiac arrest. *Circulation* 2003; **108**: 2201–2205.

70. Plaisance, P., Lurie, K.G., Vicaut, E. *et al.* Evaluation of an impedance threshold device in patients receiving active compression–decompression cardiopulmonary resuscitation for out-of-hospital cardiac arrest. *Resuscitation* 2004; **61**: 265–271.

71. Tang, W., Weil, M.H., Schock, R.B. *et al.* Phased chest and abdominal compression–decompression. A new option for cardiopulmonary resuscitation. *Circulation* 1997; **95**: 1335–1340.

72. Kern, K.B., Hilwig, R.W., Berg, R.A., Schock, R.B. & Ewy, G.A. Optimizing ventilation in conjunction with phased chest and abdominal compression–decompression (Lifestick) resuscitation. *Resuscitation* 2002; **52**: 91–100.

73. Arntz, H.R., Agrawal, R., Richter, H. *et al.* Phased chest and abdominal compression–decompression versus conventional cardiopulmonary resuscitation in out-of-hospital cardiac arrest. *Circulation* 2001; **104**: 768–772.

74. Halperin, H.R., Guerci, A.D., Chandra, N. *et al.* Vest inflation without simultaneous ventilation during cardiac arrest in dogs: improved survival from prolonged cardiopulmonary resuscitation. *Circulation* 1986; **74**: 1407–1415.

75. Halperin, H.R., Tsitlik, J.E., Guerci, A.D. *et al.* Determinants of blood flow to vital organs during cardiopulmonary resuscitation in dogs. *Circulation* 1986; **73**: 539–550.

76. Beattie, C., Guerci, A.D., Hall, T. *et al.* Mechanisms of blood flow during pneumatic vest cardiopulmonary resuscitation. *J. Appl. Physiol.* 1991; **70**: 454–465.

77. Eleff, S.M., Schleien, C.L., Koehler, R.C. *et al.* Brain bioenergetics during cardiopulmonary resuscitation in dogs. *Anesthesiology* 1992; **76**: 77–84.

78. Halperin, H.R., Tsitlik, J.E., Gelfand, M. *et al.* A preliminary study of cardiopulmonary resuscitation by circumferential

compression of the chest with use of a pneumatic vest. *N. Engl. J. Med.* 1993; **329**: 762–768.

79. Rudikoff, M.T., Maughan, W.L., Effron, M., Freund, P. & Weisfeldt, M.L. Mechanisms of blood flow during cardiopulmonary resuscitation. *Circulation* 1980; **61**: 345–352.

80. Weisfeldt, M.L. & Chandra, N. Physiology of cardiopulmonary resuscitation. *Annu. Rev. Med.* 1981; **32**: 435–442.

81. Weisfeldt, M.L. Recent advances in cardiopulmonary resuscitation. *Jpn. Circ. J.* 1985; **49**: 13–24.

82. Weisfeldt, M.L. & Halperin, H.R. Cardiopulmonary resuscitation: beyond cardiac massage. *Circulation* 1986; **74**: 443–448.

83. Halperin, H.R. & Weisfeldt, M.L. New approaches to CPR. Four hands, a plunger, or a vest. *J. Am. Med. Assoc.* 1992; **267**: 2940–2941.

84. Weisfeldt, M.L. Challenges in cardiac arrest research. *Ann. Emerg. Med.* 1993; **22**: 4–5.

85. Swenson, R.D., Weaver, W.D., Niskanen, R.A., Martin, J. & Dahlberg, S. Hemodynamics in humans during conventional and experimental methods of cardiopulmonary resuscitation. *Circulation* 1988; **78**: 630–639.

86. Ben-Haim, S.A., Anuchnik, C.L. & Dinnar, U. A computer controller for vest cardiopulmonary resuscitation (CPR). *IEEE Trans. Biomed. Eng.* 1988; **35**: 413–416.

87. Ben-Haim, S.A., Shofti, R., Ostrow, B. & Dinnar, U. Effect of vest cardiopulmonary resuscitation rate on cardiac output and coronary blood flow. *Crit. Care Med.* 1989; **17**: 768–771.

88. Raessler, K.L., Kern, K.B., Sanders, A.B., Tacker, W.A., Jr. & Ewy, G.A. Aortic and right atrial systolic pressures during cardiopulmonary resuscitation: a potential indicator of the mechanism of blood flow. *Am. Heart J.* 1988; **115**: 1021–1029.

89. Criley, J.M., Niemann, J.T., Rosborough, J.P. & Hausknecht, M. Modifications of cardiopulmonary resuscitation based on the cough. *Circulation* 1986; **74**: IV42–IV50.

90. Criley, J.M. The thoracic pump provides a mechanism for coronary perfusion. *Arch. Intern. Med.* 1995; **155**: 1236.

91. Niemann, J.T., Rosborough, J.P., Niskanen, R.A. & Criley, J.M. Circulatory support during cardiac arrest using a pneumatic vest and abdominal binder with simultaneous high-pressure airway inflation. *Ann. Emerg. Med.* 1984; **13**: 767–770.

92. Luce, J.M., Ross, B.K., O'Quin, R.J. *et al.* Regional blood flow during cardiopulmonary resuscitation in dogs using simultaneous and nonsimultaneous compression and ventilation. *Circulation* 1983; **67**: 258–265.

93. Luce, J.M., Rizk, N.A. & Niskanen, R.A. Regional blood flow during cardiopulmonary resuscitation in dogs. *Crit. Care Med.* 1984; **12**: 874–878.

94. Halperin, H., Berger, R., Chandra, N. *et al.* Cardiopulmonary resuscitation with a hydraulic–pneumatic band. *Crit. Care Med.* 2000; **28**: N203–N206.

95. Halperin, H.R., Paradis, N., Ornato, J.P. *et al.* Cardiopulmonary resuscitation with a novel chest compression device in a porcine model of cardiac arrest: improved hemodynamics and mechanisms. *J. Am. Coll. Cardiol.* 2004; **44**: 2214–2220.

96. Timerman, S., Cardoso, L.F., Ramires, J.A. & Halperin, H. Improved hemodynamic performance with a novel chest compression device during treatment of in-hospital cardiac arrest. *Resuscitation* 2004; **61**: 273–280.

97. Paradis, N.A., Martin, G.B., Rivers, E.P. *et al.* Coronary perfusion pressure and the return of spontaneous circulation in human cardiopulmonary resuscitation. *J. Am. Med. Assoc.* 1990; **263**: 1106–1113.

98. Casner, M., Andersen, D. & Isaacs, S.M. The impact of a new CPR assist device on rate of return of spontaneous circulation in out-of-hospital cardiac arrest. *Prehosp. Emerg. Care* 2005; **9**: 61–67.

99. Hallstrom, A., Rea, T.D., Sayre, M.R. *et al.* Manual chest compression vs use of an automated chest compression device during resuscitation following out-of-hospital cardiac arrest: a randomized trial. *J. Am. Med. Assoc.* 2006; **295**: 2620–2628.

100. Ong, M.E., Ornato, J.P., Edwards, D.P. *et al.* Use of an automated, load-distributing band chest compression device for out-of-hospital cardiac arrest resuscitation. *J. Am. Med. Assoc.* 2006; **295**: 2629–2637.

32

Invasive reperfusion techniques

Mark G. Angelos

Department of Emergency Medicine, The Ohio State University, OH, USA

Standard external cardiopulmonary resuscitation (CPR) generates at best, 20% to 25% of normal cardiac output and is frequently inadequate to restore initial cardiac activity. Furthermore, this limited blood flow during CPR decreases as either the time of arrest is prolonged[1] or the time of CPR is increased.[2] When sudden death is the result of ventricular fibrillation, immediate countershock is very effective not only in defibrillating the heart but also in restoring effective myocardial contractions.[3] As the time in which the heart fibrillates in a non-perfused state increases, however, the likelihood of successful defibrillation with restoration of adequate contractile function diminishes.[4] At some point, the heart reaches an irreversible resuscitation state. It is this limited reperfusion capability of standard CPR techniques that continues to drive the search for newer reperfusion techniques following cardiac arrest.

Cardiopulmonary bypass in animal models

Cardiopulmonary bypass has been investigated as a means to reperfuse the non-working heart in cardiac arrest. Cardiopulmonary bypass can generate much higher flows than traditional external chest compression, allowing for resuscitation after prolonged cardiac arrest. Even with the capability of restoring full flow, there are still limits to myocardial resuscitability after long periods of cardiac arrest. In the canine model, normal levels of reperfusion flow generated by cardiopulmonary bypass after 15 and 20 minutes of untreated ventricular fibrillation resulted in successful resuscitation in all animals.[5] After 30 minutes of non-perfused ventricular fibrillation, however, full flow cardiopulmonary bypass was successful in restoring ROSC

in only 50% of animals.[5] During cardiac arrest, coronary perfusion pressure has been noted to correlate with myocardial blood flow.[6,7] The minimum coronary perfusion pressures necessary for ROSC have been estimated at greater than 18 mm Hg in canine models,[8] and greater than 15 mm Hg in humans.[9] With cardiopulmonary bypass, much higher coronary perfusion pressures can be achieved. In a ventricular fibrillation model, coronary perfusion pressure was noted to improve from 18 ± 8 mmHg during standard external CPR, to 27 ± 10 mmHg after adrenaline administration, to 58 ± 6 mmHg after institution of cardiopulmonary bypass (Fig. 32.1).[10]

Although high flows can be achieved, perfusion pressures while subjects are on cardiopulmonary bypass generally do not return to baseline levels unless an adrenergic agent is used, particularly after prolonged ischemia. The previously reported correlation between coronary perfusion pressure and myocardial blood flow seems to be lost with cardiopulmonary bypass reperfusion following cardiac arrest. Despite normal flows, coronary perfusion pressure may be subnormal. This is similar to the intraoperative experience of central cardiopulmonary bypass, where the mean arterial pressure is noted to fall after the patient is placed on cardiopulmonary bypass. Perfusion pressures of 40 to 60 mm Hg are tolerated without adverse consequences.[11] The significance of subnormal coronary perfusion pressures in the face of normal or supranormal organ blood flow during acute resuscitation is unclear. When epinephrine, either as a bolus or continuous infusion, is given in conjunction with cardiopulmonary bypass, normal or even supranormal coronary perfusion pressures can be generated while the heart is fibrillating.[12,13] In "high flow" reperfusion states after prolonged

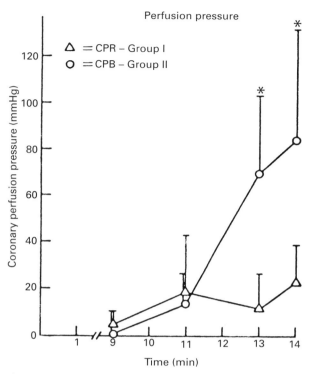

Fig. 32.1. Coronary perfusion pressure with standard external CPR (*Group I*) and cardiopulmonary bypass (*Group II*). All animals received adrenaline 0.05 mg/kg at 10 minutes. (From Angelos, M.G., Gaddis, M., Gaddis, S., Leasure, J.E. Improved survival and reduced myocardial necrosis with cardiopulmonary bypass reperfusion in a canine model of coronary occlusion and cardiac arrest. *Ann. Emerg. Med.* 1990;**19**:1126.)

cardiac arrest, the β-adrenergic effects of adrenaline may be more important in reversing postresuscitation myocardial dysfunction than α-adrenergic effects in raising coronary perfusion pressure.[13, 14]

The main benefit of cardiopulmonary bypass in cardiac arrest seems to be its ability to restore flow. Cardiopulmonary bypass can provide flows that approximate baseline cardiac output. During reperfusion of ventricular fibrillation, flows of 80 to 100 ml/kg per min have been reported in canine cardiac arrest models[15] and flows above 200 ml/kg per min have been reported in swine cardiac arrest models.[12,16] These flows far exceed those generated by standard CPR and its variations. With the use of peripheral cardiopulmonary bypass during ventricular fibrillation, there is retrograde perfusion of the aorta from the femoral arteries and antegrade perfusion of the coronary and cerebral arteries.[17,18] Organ blood flow patterns seem to be altered when cardiopulmonary bypass is instituted after the global ischemia of cardiac arrest. An early hyperemia is seen in some organs, particularly the brain and the heart, and is probably secondary to ischemic vasodilation with loss of vascular autoregulation.[19]

In canine cardiac arrest models, cardiopulmonary bypass has shown improved ROSC rates when compared to standard CPR with advanced life support after non-perfused ventricular fibrillation of 10 minutes,[20] 12 minutes,[21] 12.5 minutes,[22] and 4 minutes of ventricular fibrillation plus 30 minutes of CPR.[23] Cardiopulmonary bypass survivors in these studies showed improved neurologic outcome at 72 hours, when compared to survivors of CPR and advanced life support. Similar results have been reported in the swine model. Cardiopulmonary bypass was successful in achieving ROSC in 8/8 swine after 10 minutes of ventricular fibrillation and 5 minutes of failed conventional CPR therapy.[12] The utilization of an adrenaline infusion (3 μg/kg per min) during cardiopulmonary bypass resulted in normalization of coronary perfusion pressure and re-establishment of spontaneous circulation after an average of 23 minutes compared to 152 minutes without adrenaline.[12]

In a comparison of cardiopulmonary bypass with open-chest CPR and closed-chest CPR (in a canine ventricular fibrillation model), improved rates of ROSC were obtained with cardiopulmonary bypass.[24] Furthermore, cardiopulmonary bypass showed improved ROSC rates when compared with standard and high-dose adrenaline in a canine postcountershock model of pulseless electrical activity.[25] In both of these studies, however, there was no statistical improvement in 2-hour survival. Safar *et al.* reviewed their work with cardiopulmonary bypass in cardiac arrest animal models at the University of Pittsburgh Resuscitation Center from 1982 to 1988. Of 221 dogs from six cardiac arrest studies, 179 received cardiopulmonary bypass during ventricular fibrillation. All animals receiving cardiopulmonary bypass achieved ROSC after ventricular fibrillation times ranging from 10 to 30 minutes prior to the onset of cardiopulmonary bypass.[15]

Human resuscitation applications of percutaneous cardiopulmonary bypass

Currently, there is growing experience with the use of cardiopulmonary bypass for the acute resuscitation of cardiac arrest patients. This has been facilitated by the availability of smaller, more portable centrifugal pumps and the utilization of percutaneous cardiopulmonary bypass performed by cannulation of the femoral vessels. Reference to the most recent American Society for Artificial Internal Organs Registry indicates a trend toward centrifugal pumps even for the more standard indication of postcardiotomy cardiogenic shock cases, with about 70% of cases treated with centrifugal pumps.[26] To date, no controlled studies have examined the use of cardiopulmonary bypass in cardiac arrest, but there are a growing number of case series.[27–34]

The first successful complete bypass of the heart and lungs in a human was reported by Gibbon in 1954.[35] For acute resuscitation, the use of cardiopulmonary bypass was first reported in 1961 for successful pulmonary thrombolectomy.[36] In 1967, two cases of hypothermia treated with cardiopulmonary bypass were reported.[37,38] In 1976, Mattox and Beal reported a series of 39 moribund patients resuscitated with portable cardiopulmonary bypass by using femoral artery and vein access.[27] Etiologies of shock or arrest state included massive pulmonary embolus, trauma, drug overdose, myocardial infarction, and cardiac arrest of unclear origin. Of the 39 patients, 15 were long-term survivors, 13 of whom were patients with pulmonary embolus.

Utilizing femorofemoral bypass, Phillips et al. reported on five patients with cardiac arrest who, after failing conventional therapy, achieved ROSC with cardiopulmonary bypass.[28] Three patients survived. The investigators reported flows on bypass of 2.0 to 2.5 l/min. Interestingly, they reported that the procedure took less than 5 minutes in all patients. The ease and speed of cannulation for femorofemoral bypass seems to be quite variable, with other groups reporting much longer cannulation and set-up times. In a later report, Phillips et al. reported on 22 additional patients, of whom 15 were in cardiac arrest at the time of femorofemoral cardiopulmonary bypass. All cardiac arrest patients except the four trauma patients were initially resuscitated and six were long-term survivors.[29] Again they noted application times of less than 5 minutes.

Attempts have been made to use cardiopulmonary bypass in out-of-hospital cardiac arrest patients once they arrive in the emergency department.[30] Key elements in successful resuscitation with cardiopulmonary bypass are the ischemia time prior to institution of cardiopulmonary bypass, time and success of cannulae placement, and availability of an on-call bypass team within the hospital.

The most extensive experience with the use of cardiopulmonary bypass in cardiac arrest has been with in-hospital cardiac arrests. Reported outcomes have been variable. In a series of 11 patients in cardiac arrest who received percutaneous cardiopulmonary bypass, 2 patients were long-term survivors. The two survivors were significantly younger and without atherosclerotic heart disease when compared with the non-survivors.[31] In another series of 32 patients receiving cardiopulmonary bypass, the overall survival rate was 12.5%, and only 1 (3.4%) of the 29 patients presenting in cardiac arrest left the hospital.[32] In this series, cardiopulmonary bypass was instituted within 15 minutes of cardiac arrest in 10/29 patients, within 15 to 30 minutes in 9 patients, and in more than 30 minutes in 10 patients. The time to place patients on bypass after the request was received ranged from 5 to 35 minutes.

In another series of patients from Sharp Memorial Hospital in San Diego, California, the experience of 38 hospitalized patients receiving emergent cardiopulmonary bypass was reported. Patients had cardiac arrest and failure of standard CPR prior to the onset of portable cardiopulmonary bypass. Thirty-six of 38 patients were successfully resuscitated to a stable heart rhythm. Two patients could not be cannulated. Bypass support allowed eight diagnostic angiographic procedures to be performed. Twenty-four of the 36 patients underwent operative procedures and 18 of the 36 patients were successfully weaned from bypass. Six (17%) of 36 were long-term survivors.[33]

In the largest series to date, the National Cardiopulmonary Support Registry for Emergency Applications in 1992 reported a total of 187 patients from 17 institutions who were treated with emergent portable cardiopulmonary bypass.[34] Of the 187 patients, 116 patients had witnessed cardiac arrest and 14 had unwitnessed cardiac arrest. In the witnessed cardiac arrests, the time in arrest before bypass ranged from 5 to 272 minutes, with a mean time of 45 ± 43 minutes. Other emergent indications for bypass were cardiogenic shock, profound hypothermia, and pulmonary insufficiency. The registry defined successful bypass as a mean arterial pressure of >60 mm Hg together with flows >2.0 l/m². One of the key advantages to the use of bypass in these patients appeared to be the capability of supporting the patient so that various diagnostic and therapeutic procedures could be performed. This occurred in 74.9% of the total patients. Bypass times ranged from 5 to 4,500 minutes, with 36 patients having bypass times of more than 8 hours. In patients suffering cardiac arrest, 30-day survival was 15.5%, with overall survival in all patients of 21.4%. The authors concluded that patients with unwitnessed cardiac arrest and patients with refractory cardiac arrest who have received more than 30 minutes of CPR are poor candidates for emergent cardiopulmonary bypass. Good candidates for emergent cardiopulmonary bypass are patients with anatomically correctable problems and patients for whom therapeutic procedures such as angioplasty can be performed. The other small but important group that should benefit from emergency cardiopulmonary bypass are patients with hypothermic cardiac arrest.

Both femorofemoral bypass[39] and central cardiopulmonary bypass with median sternotomy have been used[40] in the successful treatment of hypothermic cardiac arrest patients. A number of case studies and reports in the literature describe successful outcome with bypass-assisted perfusion and rewarming.[41,42] Such cases include the resuscitation of a child submersed for 66 minutes in cold water, with subsequent normal neurologic outcome.[43] A case series from Finland of 23 patients with hypothermia-generated cardiac arrest (mean temperature, 24.4 °C) were placed on cardiopulmonary bypass after a mean of 106 min of CPR. Fourteen of the 23 patients (61%) were resuscitated and discharged from the hospital.[44] A recent follow-up report on 15 young, severely hypothermic patients (core temperature 17.1 °C–25 °C) in cardiac arrest who were resuscitated using cardiopulmonary bypass found minimal or no cerebral impairment, despite the long cardiac arrest times.[45] There is general consensus that severe hypothermia with refractory cardiac arrest is an indication for emergent cardiopulmonary bypass. Nevertheless, no controlled studies have been performed, nor are they likely to be done, given the small number of available cases at single institutions.

Percutaneous cardiopulmonary bypass has also been used in elective high-risk coronary intervention, including valvuloplasty, coronary arthrectomy, or coronary angioplasty.[46] Patients are instrumented for bypass before the procedure. If cardiovascular collapse or cardiac arrest should occur during the procedure, bypass can be initiated immediately. There are reports of successful implementation of cardiopulmonary bypass in cardiac arrest patients who fail to respond to advanced cardiac life support allowing transfer to the operating room for coronary artery bypass graft surgery or emergent coronary angioplasty.[47] Shawl et al. reported that 4 of 7 patients had good long-term survival.[47] The location of the cardiac arrest has been noted to be a significant factor, with the best survival rates in patients suffering cardiac arrest near the cardiac catheterization laboratory.[48] Presumably, the coronary anatomy of these patients was rapidly defined and could be followed by a therapeutic procedure if a reversible lesion were present. In the National Cardiopulmonary Support Registry report of 187 patients (125 patients in cardiac arrest), bypass was initiated in the cardiac catheterization laboratory in 33% of the total patients. Another 28% of these patients had bypass started in the operating room, 26% in the intensive care unit, 5% in the emergency department, and 5% on the hospital floor.[34]

In pediatric patients, veno-arterial extracorporeal membrane oxygenation (ECMO) has been used successfully for resuscitation from shock and cardiac arrest. Although analogous to cardiopulmonary bypass, generally lower flows are used to assist the intact but dysfunctional circulatory system. In a report of more than 600 children receiving ECMO, specific indications for instituting ECMO included cardiopulmonary arrest unresponsive to standard therapy, inability to wean from cardiopulmonary bypass following surgery, and refractory hypotension with blood pressure <50 mm Hg.[49] The University of Michigan reported their experience with either veno-venal bypass or veno-arterial bypass in severe pediatric respiratory failure in which 15/25 patients were long-term survivors.[50] Veno-venous bypass was used for respiratory failure without concomitant cardiac failure. This has little, if any, application during cardiac arrest. Flow rates were titrated to maintain arterial oxyhemoglobin saturation around 90%. Required flows were generally similar to full cardiopulmonary bypass flows, ranging from 100 to 150 ml/kg per min for veno-arterial bypass and 80 to 100 ml/kg per min for veno-venal bypass. The hematocrit was maintained at 45% and continuous heparinization was used to maintain anticoagulation. The Children's Hospital of Pittsburgh reported their experience with ECMO in 33 children between 1981 to 1991. Eleven of these patients suffered sudden cardiac arrest after open-heart surgery and were placed on ECMO after unsuccessful CPR; there were 7/11 early survivors, 6 (55%) of whom were long-term neurologically intact. Overall long-term survival in all patients receiving ECMO was 14/33 (42%). The duration of CPR prior to institution of ECMO ranged from 20 to 110 minutes, with an average time of 65 ± 9 minutes.[51] The application of ECMO to cardiac arrest patients is limited by the time needed to institute therapy. The authors report the time required to set up and prime an ECMO circuit is 20 to 30 minutes with a separate perfusion team on call at all times for ECMO.

Recently a combination of therapies has shown a surprisingly high resuscitation rate with good neurologic outcome. Two recent series from Japan in out-of-hospital cardiac arrest patients combined the use of cardiopulmonary bypass for resuscitation with emergent percutaneous coronary intervention (PCI) in suspected acute coronary syndrome (ACS) and then mild induced hypothermia to 34 °C.[52,53] Both noted higher resuscitation rates in patients found to have coronary lesions amenable to PCI than cardiac arrest of undetermined cardiac etiology. The survival rate was 40% with 25% having good neurologic outcome in one study[53] and 30% survival with 24% good neurologic outcome in the other study.[52]

In summary, percutaneous cardiopulmonary bypass for resuscitation from cardiac arrest can provide near normal flow even after prolonged cardiac arrest periods, with improved outcome compared with standard CPR and ALS.

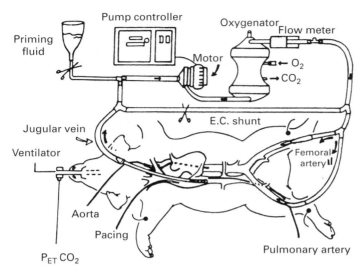

Fig. 32.2. Cardiopulmonary bypass system for use in humans. (From Ott RA, Gutfinger DE, Gazzaniga AB, eds. Cardiac surgery: state of arts review. Philadelphia: Hanley & Belfus, 1993.)

Nonetheless, based on work to date, this methodology is likely to be successful only under specific cardiac arrest situations, namely profound hypothermia or cardiac arrest due to ACS responsive to PCI, or another surgical emergency such as valvular dysfunction. Non-discriminate use of percutaneous cardiopulmonary bypass is unlikely to improve outcome and becomes cost- and labor-prohibitive.

Implementation of emergent cardiopulmonary bypass

Much of what we know about the technical considerations of providing emergent cardiopulmonary extracorporeal support to cardiac arrest patients comes from cardiopulmonary bypass-supported angioplasty.[54–59] Although it might be possible to use the equipment and techniques found in the open-heart surgical arena for elective high-risk angioplasty procedures, emergency support requires alterations in traditional techniques. For example, the preparation time required to set up equipment and devices associated with conventional bypass surgery would prohibit success in emergency procedures. Cannulation techniques resulting in a large diameter, unrestricted venous outflow into hard-shell or collapsible reservoirs make the use of gravity venous drainage possible in the operating room, but impractical to use in emergency situations. Bulky equipment and devices also make adaptability and portability to sites outside the operating room difficult.

Many of the limitations of conventional bypass techniques have been resolved with the use of preassembled

membrane oxygenator circuits, percutaneous cannulation, and centrifugal pumps (see schematic Fig. 32.2). Preassembled circuits, with only the devices and connections required to perform emergency bypass support, have allowed preparation time to be shortened to as little as 5 minutes.[28,60,61] Centrifugal pumps not only move the blood forward through the membrane oxygenator and into the patient, but also serve to aspirate the venous blood from the patient. This allows venous cannulation to be performed with smaller diameter cannulae, which would be unsuitable for gravity venous drainage. As a result, both arterial and venous cannulae can be inserted percutaneously in a time frame suitable for emergency situations.

Circuits used for emergency support, therefore, are typically simple, closed non-compliant systems, but with this lack of complexity comes an element of risk if they are operated by personnel who are unaware of the inherent dangers (e.g., massive air embolism, hemolysis, thrombotic incident, or disseminated intravascular coagulopathy). It is essential that the team assembled to provide emergency support include perfusionists who have experience with operating the pump and oxygenator and monitoring the hemodynamic, oxygenation, and anticoagulation status of patients undergoing extracorporeal circulation.[55,61–63] Careful attention must be given to the development of protocols for each application of these devices and for each potential complication. These techniques can only be successful if all team members have a clear understanding of their role and responsibility in the initiation and maintenance of emergent cardiopulmonary bypass.

Equipment and circuit

The hardware and circuits needed for successful emergency support can be either designed and constructed by the institution or commercially purchased. A centrifugal pump is required both to aspirate venous blood from the patient and to drive the blood through the oxygenator to the patient. Currently, centrifugal pumps are found in a constrained vortex or impeller design. Both can provide full bypass flow as long as the cannulae selected are appropriate for the size of the patient and oxygen delivery requirement. A calibrated flow meter, either electromagnetic or ultrasonic, must be included in the line distal to the pump to allow blood flow to be monitored and adjusted. The pump console (Fig. 32.3) consists of a magnetic coupling drive motor and measures both flow and revolutions per minute (rpm) of the pump head. Each of the pump designs has safety features that are helpful in emergency support applications. They appear to be less traumatic to blood over extended support periods and air locks will form if they are deprimed with large quantities of air. They are also considered to be afterload- and preload-dependent pumps. As an afterload-dependent pump, if the resistance to outflow is increased by any means (e.g., a change in patient vascular resistance), the flow will decrease. This adds an important safety element. If the bypass line returning blood to the patient should kink or inadvertently be clamped, the line will not be disrupted. As a preload-dependent pump, the volume must be continuously provided in an unrestricted way to the pump head in order for outflow to occur. The perfusionist must continuously monitor the rpm of the pump and patient flow in order to adjust for probable changes in pump afterloading (change in arterial vascular resistance) or preloading (change in venous volume).

A second hardware item required is a water bath system designed to deliver thermoregulated water to the heat exchanger of the circuit. This is necessary in order to maintain or adjust the patient's blood temperature. This system may be either a simple water bath that heats to a narrow normothermic temperature range with no potential for adjustment, or a more complicated heating/cooling system with an adjustable water temperature ranging from normothermia to deep hypothermia. For many emergency procedures, maintaining normal body temperature will be all that is required. For emergency support procedures involving rewarming the core of hypothermic patients, some option in the adjustment of water temperature for heat exchange will be desired. In these situations, careful regulation of the temperature gradient between the water and inlet blood temperature will allow for controlled rewarming.[43,64]

A gas supply is also required for emergency support systems. Although some adaptation of wall gas supply is desired, portability of the equipment necessitates that E or D cylinders be available. Oxygen can be used alone as a gas source, but mixing of oxygen and compressed air allows adjustment of the fractional inspiratory oxygen (FIO_2) of the gas source to the membrane oxygenator. A flowmeter and gas blender must be used to adjust and monitor both total gas flow and FIO_2.

Additional equipment includes arterial and venous temperature probes that are inserted into thermowells in the circuit for temperature monitoring. External battery systems must be integral to all of the equipment to make portability to other areas of the hospital possible (e.g., intensive care unit, catheterization laboratory, or operating room). All of this equipment should be housed in a cart that allows portability and provides storage space for disposable supplies for circuit construction and replacement.

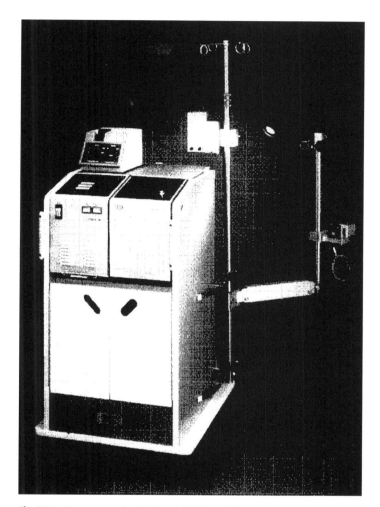

Fig. 32.3. Pump console. *Medtronic* PBS portable bypass system (Courtesy of Medtronic Inc., Anaheim, CA.)

The disposable circuit is made up of a membrane oxygenator and centrifugal pump head (Fig. 32.4) connected with appropriate lengths of polyvinyl chloride tubing. This tubing also makes up an arteriovenous loop, which connects to the vascular cannulae. The membrane lung is often a polypropylene or polyethylene hollow fiber design that directs blood flow around the outside of a fiber bundle and gas flow to the inside of each fiber. This outside fiber blood flow design provides excellent gas exchange and minimizes resistance to blood flow from the centrifugal pump. The membrane oxygenator may have a heat exchanger, proximal to or integral with the fiber bundle, to maintain or adjust the patient's blood temperature. If not part of the oxygenator, the heat exchanger must be added as a separate device in the circuit. In some cases, a membrane oxygenator is chosen

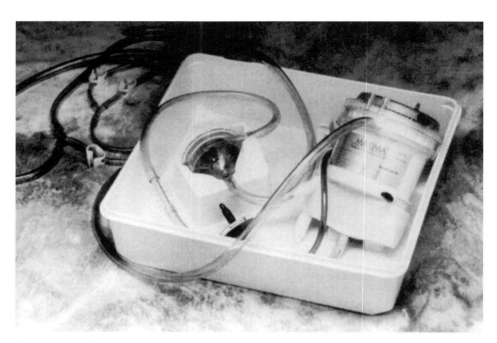

Fig. 32.4. Centrifugal pump. Need updated photo of Medtronic Biopump Plus Centrifugal Blood Pump. (Courtesy of Medtronic Inc., Anaheim, CA.)

with design features that allow it to act as a safety device in case of accidental introduction of air. It is possible that air, inadvertently introduced into the venous side of a membrane oxygenator, can be trapped in the device and perhaps be eliminated by diffusing to the gas path. This eliminates the need for air-trapping devices placed distal to the oxygenator, which would add complexity to the circuit design and priming procedures.

A fluid administration line is located proximal to the centrifugal pump head. This is used to prime the circuit prior to bypass and may be opened during the procedure for rapidly administering replacement volume to the patient. Approximately 350 ml of fluid are required to prime most systems. Sampling sites should be provided for access to arterial and venous blood. Often a tubing bridge, located close to the patient, connects the arterial and venous lines. This bridge is helpful in the priming procedure, for oxygenator change-out procedures, to eliminate air that may enter the circuit after bypass has begun, and often is used to circulate the circuit volume to minimize stasis at times when bypass is discontinued. Lastly, a line pressure monitoring device may be incorporated in the circuit at the oxygenator or at some point in the arterial line. This is usually a small piece of tubing connecting the circuit to an aneroid pressure gauge.

Concerns about the use of anticoagulants in these patients has led to attempts to provide support with circuits that have been precoated with heparin.[65,66] This likely reduces the risk of heparin-induced hemorrhage and the complications associated with heparin reversal requiring protamine.

Patient preparation and management with cardiopulmonary bypass

Rapid cannulation and initiation of cardiopulmonary bypass is key to the success of extracorporeal emergency support. Thin-walled polyurethane cannulae are available that can be inserted percutaneously into the femoral artery and vein by the Seldinger technique or directly inserted by a modified Seldinger technique or complete cutdown.[28,57] The more direct approach, with some level of cutdown, may be required in patients with complete circulatory collapse.[67] Other cannulation sites (e.g., the internal jugular vein) may be used if needed. The venous cannula is available in 17 to 30 F sizes and is long enough (50 to 60 cm) to advance the tip to the venocaval-atrial junction. The end of the cannula is multiholed to minimize tissue obstruction to venous flow. The arterial cannula is available in 12 to 21 F (15 to 30 cm) sizes and is advanced to the common iliac artery (Fig. 32.5) Both cannulae must be sized to the patient in order to ensure minimal obstruction to preloading and afterloading of the centrifugal pump. Iliofemoral angiography is helpful in elective cases (e.g., angioplasty)

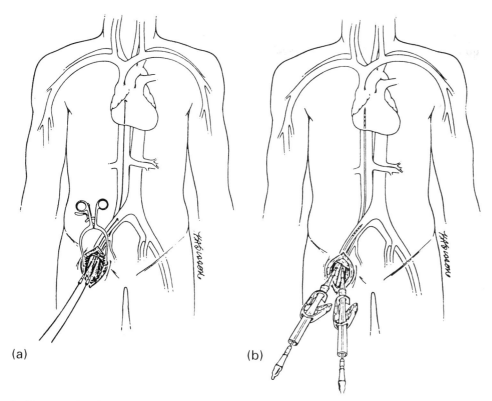

(a)   (b)

Fig. 32.5. Peripheral cannulation of femoral vessels for CPB. A. A right groin cutdown is followed by systemic heparinization. 18-gauge femoral venipuncture and arterial puncture are performed with insertion of guidewires. B. A 20F, thin-walled cannula is placed with end holes in the right atrium and a short 20F cannula is placed into the common iliac artery. (Reprinted with permission from the Society of Thoracic Surgeons from Hartz R, LoCicero J, Sanders JH, Frederiksen JW, Joob AW, Michaelis LL. Clinical experience with portable cardiopulmonary bypass in cardiac arrest patients. Ann Thorac Surg 1990;50:438.)

to ensure an unobstructed course for arterial cannula advancement and blood flow, but is not practical for emergent procedures. Heparin is administered (300 U/kg) to the patient after guidewire placement but before vessel dilatation and cannula insertion.[28,61,68,69]

Since the venous volume is aspirated from the patient with the centrifugal pump, it is essential that all central and peripheral venous infusion and monitoring lines be checked for proper functioning prior to initiation of bypass.[67] Central monitoring catheters must be closed systems and peripheral administration lines must be closed or placed on occlusive infusion pumps. It is possible that an open peripheral line used for drug delivery could be rapidly emptied of its volume because of the aspiration that will occur in the venous vascular system. Venipuncture during the bypass procedure could result in a massive venous air embolism. All venous cannulae must be properly secured in the patient to avoid movement of

the cannula and exposure of the end holes to air, which would lead to depriming of the circuit.

Initiation of bypass is performed slowly, especially in patients who are conscious. This minimizes sudden shifts in temperature or the consequences of hemodilution.[62] The circuit bypass is clamped and the venous and arterial cannulae are unclamped (in that order) with the centrifugal pump operating at low rpm to ensure displacement of the prime volume to the patient. If the centrifugal pump is not on, or is set at an rpm value too low to overcome the afterload of the patient and circuit, retrograde flow will occur from arterial to venous cannula. Flow should be increased to the predetermined target over several minutes. As the speed of the pump increases, flow will also increase until there is insufficient preload of the centrifugal pump head with volume. At this point, further increases in rpm will not produce increases in flow and the perfusionist will note decreased flow if the rpm is further adjusted upward. A vibration in the venous line and low or negative central venous pressures are additional signs that the pump head is not adequately preloaded. If additional flow is required, volume may be administered to determine if the problem is inadequate preload or obstruction of the venous cannula.[55,61] Fluid additions through the administration line proximal to the pump must be monitored carefully since fluid will be aspirated into the circuit at a rapid rate. When fluid bags are being changed, all air must be evacuated from the bag and administration line before they are opened to the patient. Only collapsible fluid containers are acceptable for use.

Full flow may not be required if the patient is able to provide some cardiac output and does not show symptoms of hypoxia or hypotension. If this is the case, some pulsatility in the arterial pressure waveform will be noted and some ventilation of the patient's lungs must be maintained in order to ensure that the blood that is ejected to the proximal aorta is arterial. The ventilation of the membrane lung can be adjusted downward to avoid hypocarbia. If, however, bypass is supporting the entire cardiac output, no pulsatility will be noted in the arterial waveform. It is likely that the pulmonary artery and capillary wedge pressures will also be low under these circumstances. Flow rates achieving full support should be possible as long as the cannulae are properly sized to the patient and aspiration of the venous volume is unobstructed.

Typical measures that are monitored to assess bypass flow include arterial and central venous pressures, systemic vascular resistance, venous oxygen saturation, and rpm. As patients regain consciousness, systemic vascular resistance may increase. High rpm values with low flow may suggest a high systemic vascular resistance.[70] Blood gases, activated clotting time, hematocrit, electrolytes, and urinary output are also monitored. Changing the flow rate and FIo_2 on the gas source to the membrane oxygenator will affect arterial Pco_2 and Po_2, respectively. Arterial Pco_2 is inversely related to gas flow rate. As the gas flow rate is increased, more carbon dioxide is removed from the gas path of the membrane oxygenator, thus increasing the gradient for carbon dioxide transfer and lowering arterial Pco_2. Gas flow should be initiated at a rate equal to blood flow (a 1:1 ratio) with subsequent adjustments made based on blood gas analysis. Arterial Po_2 is directly related to ventilating gas Fio_2. Precise control of arterial blood gases, acid–base balance, electrolyte levels, and volume is possible with extracorporeal support. This precision is a distinct advantage over other techniques used to resuscitate the arrest patient or rewarm the hypothermic patient.[71,72] The activated clotting time should be maintained at levels in excess of 400 seconds,[56,58,61,68,69] which can be accomplished with inter-mittent administration of heparin. Since most emergency support procedures are performed at normothermia, heparin metabolism will likely be more rapid than is found in conventional open-heart bypass. Frequent measurements of activated clotting time are required by the perfusionist to avoid a thrombotic incident.

As flow is reduced, more volume will enter the right side of the heart with eventual ejection from the left side. Arterial waveform pulsatility will reappear. Volume can be added to the patient by aspirating through the administration line until the central venous or pulmonary capillary wedge pressures are increased to predetermined targets. As the flow is decreased below 0.5 l/min, the arterial line will require clamping to avoid retrograde flow through the arterial line from the patient. Once the patient is off bypass and the line leading to the centrifugal pump is clamped, additional volume can be administered from the administration line into the venous cannula. When the arterial and venous cannulae are both clamped, the bypass bridge can be opened to recirculate the blood slowly through the circuit to avoid stasis while the patient's hemodynamic stability is assessed. Residual volume in the bypass circuit can be drained into blood transfusion bags or centrifuged to recover the cells for later infusion to the patient.

Open chest cardiac massage

Despite improved hemodynamics during cardiac arrest with open chest cardiac massage in animal models, at present open chest cardiac massage is mainly of historical interest. The current indications for opening the chest during cardiac arrest in order to perform direct cardiac massage are limited to very specific traumatic arrests. Current recommendations advocate emergency thoracotomy only for trauma patients with recent loss of vital signs (cardiac arrest within approximately 5 minutes) and penetrating chest injury. While thoracotomy and open chest cardiac massage have been done after longer cardiac arrests and following blunt trauma, no survival benefit has been noted. Earlier reported series of cardiac arrest patients who received open chest cardiac massage involved primarily intraoperative patients who arrested[73] many predating the seminal work of Kouwenhoven et al.[74] describing closed chest CPR. More recently a few small series have been described in which open chest cardiac massage was performed on out-of-hospital cardiac arrests. In a study from Brussels in which a physician-staffed mobile intensive care unit was dispatched to the scene of the cardiac arrest victim, over a 12-year period (1984–1996) open chest CPR was instituted at the scene in 33 of 2212 patients who received out-of-hospital closed chest CPR.[75] In these 33 patients ROSC was obtained in 13 (39%) and survival to hospital discharge in 2 patients. At present, efforts to improve CPR outcome continue to be directed away from open chest cardiac massage except in very specific and infrequent situations.

Ventricular assist devices

A number of left, right, and biventricular assist devices have been used for support in profound heart failure after various cardiac surgical procedures, and cardiogenic shock following acute myocardial infarction.[76–78] These devices have demonstrated the ability to sustain circulation even during ventricular fibrillation. Because of the technical difficulty in applying these devices, however, such devices are not currently viewed as a therapeutic option for cardiac arrest patients, unless some degree of circulatory support is already present. The time constraints of global ischemia induced by cardiac arrest do not allow for application of these devices in a reasonable time period.

Ventricular assist devices that have been utilized in cardiac arrest are known as direct mechanical ventricular assistance (DMVA) devices. DMVA was first described in 1966[79] and consists of a heart assist cup and a pneumatic driving system. The heart assist cup is constructed of a rigid translucent shell containing an inner elastic diaphragm which is placed around the ventricles after a thoracotomy has been performed. The outer portion of the cup communicates with the pneumatic drive system through two ports. A sustained negative pressure exerted from the driving system holds the cup securely in place on the ventricles. Through the second port, alternating positive and negative pressures are pulsed to actuate the myocardium in systole and diastole. DMVA has shown increased perfusion pressures and cardiac output in canine cardiac arrest models when compared with both closed- and open-chest CPR.[80,81] Myocardial blood flow was measured in a swine model of 10-minute ventricular fibrillation arrest and reperfusion with 3 minutes of external CPR, followed by DMVA. Myocardial blood flow was significantly elevated above CPR levels and probably approached baseline levels, although the study did not report baseline levels or controls.[82] Four of the seven animals were successfully defibrillated.

Potential advantages of DMVA when compared to cardiopulmonary bypass include no interface of blood with a foreign surface, which precludes the need for anticoagulation, and perfusion with pulsatile flow, which may be more beneficial than non-pulsatile cardiopulmonary bypass flow. Moreover, since the DMVA device is placed directly over the ventricles after a thoracotomy is performed, the technique does not rely on obtaining vascular access.

Comparisons between DMVA and cardiopulmonary bypass in the canine model have not shown one technique to be clearly superior over the other. In a comparison of 20 dogs with 10 in each group, 4 hours of DMVA was compared to 4 hours of cardiopulmonary bypass while the heart remained in ventricular fibrillation. Time-to-peak contracture at the end of the 4-hour perfusion period was longer in the DMVA group. High-energy phosphate depletion was assessed through myocardial biopsies. A significant delay in depletion of left ventricular subendocardial adenosine phosphate (ATP) was noted in the DMVA animals. There were no significant changes in ATP between groups in left ventricular epicardial, right ventricular, or septal regions of the heart.[83] Although both groups received 4 hours of augmented perfusion, there were differences in perfusion between groups. Mean arterial pressure during perfusion was significantly higher in the DMVA group than in the cardiopulmonary bypass group.[83] Central venous pressures were higher in the DMVA group, however, so that the arteriovenous pressure difference was similar in the two groups. In assessing organ blood flow during the 4-hour perfusion period, organ flows with cardiopulmonary bypass were increased significantly over DMVA (cardiopulmonary bypass 110% of normal versus DMVA 75% of control), while at the same time the DMVA group had a mean arterial pressure significantly higher than did the cardiopulmonary bypass group.[84]

Clinical experience with use of DMVA is very limited. A single trial with DMVA in human cardiac arrests has been reported.[85] Twenty-two patients had institution of DMVA after failure of conventional cardiac arrest therapy. Twenty of the 22 patients presented to the emergency department in cardiac arrest. The average time in cardiac arrest until application of DMVA was 81 ± 9 minutes. Four of the 22 patients were initially defibrillated; however, two died within the first hour. The other two died in hospital before discharge. The authors noted that DMVA could be applied within 2 to 3 minutes, including thoracotomy time. Because the time of cardiac arrest before application of DMVA is not known, it is difficult to determine whether the device conferred any clinical benefit.

The future

The greatest laboratory and clinical experience to date with perfusion-augmenting devices and therapy has been with cardiopulmonary bypass. Both laboratory and clinical studies have demonstrated the ability to restore normal levels of circulation after prolonged periods of cardiac arrest. What has become clear, however, is that successful restoration of perfusion is not always sufficient to restart the heart or ensure good neurologic outcome. There are time limits to global ischemia beyond which normal or even greater than normal reperfusion and circulatory support are insufficient to reverse ischemic damage. When therapy is started late, the efficiency of treatment in reversing the arrest state to a good long-term outcome cannot be evaluated accurately. Late therapy, no matter how good, is never effective once the ischemic capability of the heart and brain is exceeded. Nevertheless, the window for recovery may be lengthened by circulatory support, thereby allowing the administration of reperfusion agents that may be important in ameliorating ischemic and reperfusion injury. Cardiopulmonary bypass and other circulation assist therapies may facilitate delivery of such agents and compensate for any hypotensive effects or reduced perfusion that these agents might cause.

The future use of cardiopulmonary bypass in the setting of cardiac arrest depends on being able to institute cardiopulmonary bypass quickly after the onset of cardiac arrest refractory to initial treatment. The best outcomes in cardiac arrest with this therapy seem to be in patients with cardiac arrest due to profound hypothermia or secondary to acute coronary syndrome with coronary lesions amenable to PCI or surgical repair. Given that specific subpopulations of cardiac arrest patients may be more likely to respond to this therapy and it is not feasible to institute such therapy in every cardiac arrest patient, strict criteria for patient selection are needed. Criteria for starting and stopping these therapies after both successful and unsuccessful ROSC must also be developed.

Future use of cardiopulmonary bypass early in cardiac arrest may be effective with only partial reperfusion support, rather than requiring flows equivalent to normal cardiac output. Early partial circulatory assistance may permit the attainment of ROSC with continued partial assistance after circulation has returned. Partial circulatory support would allow the use of much smaller cannulae, which would greatly facilitate placement. Lower flow requirements would permit further modification and presumably miniaturization of current pumping systems. In order to utilize this technology effectively, future cardiopulmonary bypass systems must be smaller, more mobile and allow for easy set-up and rapid insertion of percutaneous cannulas. Eventually this technology must be capable of transport to the patient's side in the field prior to arrival to the hospital, to maximize outcome success. Currently the time to implement cardiopulmonary bypass and the resources required constitute the foremost obstacles hindering the utilization of this methodology in cardiac arrest.

Summary

Generally global ischemia of >10 minutes is thought to be universally fatal. Earlier large animal cardiac arrest studies, however, have shown good neurologic and cardiac recovery after cardiac arrests of 12–30 minutes duration prior to any resuscitative attempts. The key determinant of successful reperfusion in these prolonged cardiac arrest situations is controlled reperfusion with use of cardiopulmonary bypass. Cardiopulmonary bypass allows for much higher reperfusion flows, reperfusion pressures, and oxygen delivery than any available CPR methods. Although this level of reperfusion clearly seems to be superior to the much lower reperfusion provided by CPR techniques, there are very significant limitations of the technique, which continue to preclude its widespread use. The primary limitations of cardiopulmonary bypass with cardiac arrest consist of: (a) the duration of time necessary to bring a portable device to the patient's side; (b) time and difficulty to cannulate the patient's large vessels under arrest conditions; (c) time to prime the circuit; (d) large expenditure of resources for this equipment; (e) the availability of adequately trained personnel to monitor and run the equipment; and (f) determining the subpopulation of cardiac arrest victims that might benefit from this intervention. At present, we are not able to overcome these limitations on a widespread scale, although it is likely these obstacles can be overcome in the future. The promise of this therapy is the capability of providing controlled, near normal circulation despite the absence of functional cardiac pumping.

REFERENCES

1. Lee, S.K., Vaagenes, P., Safar, P., Stezoski, S.W. & Scanlon, M. Effect of cardiac arrest time on cortical cerebral blood flow during subsequent standard external cardiopulmonary resuscitation in rabbits. *Resuscitation* 1989; **17**: 105–117.

2. Scharff, J.A., Pantley, G. & Noel, E. Effect of time on regional organ perfusion during two methods of cardiopulmonary resuscitation. *Ann. Emerg. Med.* 1984; **13**: 649–656.

3. Weaver, W.D., Cobb, L.A., Hallstrom, A.P., Fahrenbruch, C., Copass, M.K. & Ray, R. Factors influencing survival after out-of-hospital cardiac arrest. *J. Am. Coll. Cardiol.* 1986; **7**: 752–757.

4. Yakaitis, R.W., Ewy, G.A., Otto, C.W., Taren, D.L. & Moon, T.E. Influence of time and therapy on ventricular defibrillation in dogs. *Crit. Care Med.* 1980; **8**: 157–163.

5. Reich, H., Angelos, M., Safar, P., Sterz, F. & Leonov, Y. Cardiac resuscitability with cardiopulmonary bypass after increasing ventricular fibrillation times in dogs. *Ann. Emerg. Med.* 1990; **19**: 887–890.

6. Michael, J.R., Guerci, A.D., Koehler, R.C. *et al.* Mechanisms by which epinephrine augments cerebral and myocardial perfusion during cardiopulmonary resuscitation in dogs. *Circulation* 1984; **69**: 822–835.

7. Halperin, H.R., Tsitlik, J.E., Guerci, A.D. *et al.* Determinants of blood flow to vital organs during cardiopulmonary resuscitation in dogs. *Circulation* 1986; **73**: 539–550.

8. Niemann, J.T., Criley, J.M., Rosborough, J.P., Niskanen, R.A. & Alferness, C. Predictive indices of successful cardiac resuscitation after prolonged arrest and experimental cardiopulmonary resuscitation. *Ann. Emerg. Med.* 1985; **14**: 521–528.

9. Paradis, N.A., Martin, G.B., Rivers, E.P. *et al.* Coronary perfusion pressure and the return of spontaneous circulation in human cardiopulmonary resuscitation. *J. Am. Med. Assoc.* 1990; **263**: 1106–1113.

10. Angelos, M., Safar, P. & Reich, H. A comparison of cardiopulmonary resuscitation with cardiopulmonary bypass after prolonged cardiac arrest in dogs. Reperfusion pressures and neurologic recovery. *Resuscitation* 1991; **21**: 121–135.

11. Taylor, K.M., ed. *Cardiopulmonary Bypass Principles and Management.* Baltimore: Williams & Wilkins, 1986.

12. Gazmuri, R.J., Weil, M.H., von Planta, M., Gazmuri, R.R., Shah, D.M. & Rackow, E.C. Cardiac resuscitation by extracorporeal circulation after failure of conventional CPR. *J. Lab. Clin. Med.* 1991; **118**: 65–73.

13. Angelos, M.G. & DeBehnke, D.J. Epinephrine and high flow reperfusion after cardiac arrest in a canine model. *Ann. Emerg. Med.* 1995; **26**: 208–215.

14. Wanchun, T., Weil, M.H., Sun, S., Gazmuri, R.J. & Bisera, J. Progressive myocardial dysfunction after cardiac resuscitation. *Crit. Care Med.* 1993; **21**: 1046–1050.

15. Safar, P., Abramson, N.S., Angelos, M.G. *et al.* Emergency cardiopulmonary bypass for resuscitation from prolonged cardiac arrest. *Am. J. Emerg. Med.* 1990; **8**: 55–67.

16. Gazmuri, R.J., Weil, M.H., Terwilliger, K., Shah, D.M., Duggal, C. & Tang, W. Extracorporeal circulation as an alternative to open-chest cardiac compression for cardiac resuscitation. *Chest* 1992; **102**: 1846–1852.

17. Angelos, M.G., Gaddis, M., Gaddis, G. & Leasure, J.E. Cardiopulmonary bypass in a model of acute myocardial infarction and cardiac arrest. *Ann. Emerg. Med.* 1990; **19**: 874–880.

18. Angelos, M.G., Gaddis, M., Gaddis, G. & Leasure, J.E. Improved survival and reduced myocardial necrosis with cardiopulmonary bypass reperfusion in a canine model of coronary occlusion and cardiac arrest. *Ann. Emerg. Med.* 1990; **19**: 1122–1128.

19. Angelos, M.G., Ward, K.R., Hobson, J. & Beckley, P.D. Organ blood flow following cardiac arrest in a swine low flow cardiopulmonary bypass model. *Resuscitation* 1994; **27**: 245–254.

20. Martin, G.B., Nowak, R.M., Carden, D.L., Eisiminger, R.A. & Tomlanovich, M.C. Cardiopulmonary bypass vs CPR as treatment for prolonged canine cardiopulmonary arrest. *Ann. Emerg. Med.* 1987; **16**: 628–636.

21. Carden, D.L., Martin, G.B., Nowak, R.M., Foreback, C.C. & Tomlanovich, M.C. The effect of cardiopulmonary bypass resuscitation on cardiac arrest induced lactic acidosis in dogs. *Resuscitation* 1989; **17**: 153–161.

22. Pretto, E., Safar, P., Saito, R., Stezoski, W. & Kelsey, S. Cardiopulmonary bypass after prolonged cardiac arrest in dogs. *Ann. Emerg. Med.* 1987; **16**: 611–619.

23. Levine, R., Gorayeb, M., Safar, P., Abramson, N., Stezoski, W. & Kelsey, S. Cardiopulmonary bypass after cardiac arrest and prolonged closed-chest CPR in dogs. *Ann. Emerg. Med.* 1987; **16**: 620–627.

24. DeBehnke, D.J., Angelos, M.G. & Leasure, J.E. Comparison of standard external CPR, open-chest CPR, and cardiopulmonary by pass in a canine myocardial infarct model. *Ann. Emerg. Med.* 1991; **20**: 754–760.

25. DeBehnke, D.J., Angelos, M.G. & Leasure, J.E. Use of cardiopulmonary bypass, high-dose epinephrine, and standard-dose epinephrine in resuscitation from post-counter-shock electromechanical dissociation. *Ann. Emerg. Med.* 1992; **21**: 1051–1057.

26. Takatani, S. Guest editorial: second-generation cardiopulmonary bypass pump and beyond: dedication to Dr. Michael, E. Debakey. *Artif. Organs* 1993; **17**: 585–586.

27. Mattox, K.L. & Beall, A.C. Resuscitation of the moribund patient using portable cardiopulmonary bypass. *Ann. Thorac. Surg.* 1976; **22**: 436–442.

28. Phillips, S.J., Ballentine, B., Slonine, D. *et al.* Percutaneous initiation of cardiopulmonary bypass. *Ann. Thorac. Surg.* 1983; **36**: 223–225.

29. Phillips, S.J., Zeff, R.H., Kontahworn, C. *et al.* Percutaneous cardiopulmonary bypass: application and indication for use. *Ann. Thorac. Surg.* 1989; **47**: 121–123.

30. Martin, G.B., Paradis, N.A., Rivers, E.P. *et al.* Femoro-femoral cardiopulmonary bypass in the treatment of cardiac arrest in human beings. *Chest* 1998; **113**: 743–751.

31. Sugimoto, J.T., Baird, E. & Bruner, C. Percutaneous cardiopulmonary support in cardiac arrest. *ASAIO Trans.* 1991; **37**: M282–M283.

32. Hartz, R., LoCicero, J., Sanders, J.H., Frederiksen, J.W., Joob, A.W. & Michaelis, L.L. Clinical experience with portable cardiopulmonary bypass in cardiac arrest patients. *Ann. Thorac. Surg.* 1990; **50**: 437–441.

33. Reichman, R.T., Joyo, C.I., Dembitsky, W.P. *et al.* Improved patient survival after cardiac arrest using a cardiopulmonary support system. *Ann. Thorac. Surg.* 1990; **49**: 101–105.

34. Hill, J.G., Bruhn, P.S., Cohen, S.E. *et al.* Emergent applications of cardiopulmonary support: a multiinstitutional experience. *Ann. Thorac. Surg.* 1992; **54**: 699–704.

35. Gibbon, J.H. Application of a mechanical heart and lung apparatus to cardiac surgery. *Minn. Med.* 1954; **37**: 171–185.

36. Cooley, D.A., Beall, A.C. & Alexander, J.K. Acute massive pulmonary embolism: successful surgical treatment using temporary cardiopulmonary bypass. *J. Am. Med. Assoc.* 1961; **177**: 283–286.

37. Kugelberg, J., Schuller, H., Berg, B. *et al.* Treatment of accidental hypothermia. *Scand. J. Thorac. Cardiovasc. Surg.* 1967; **1**: 142–146.

38. Davies, D.M., Millar, E.J. & Miller, I.A. Accidental hypothermia treated by extracorporeal blood-warming. *Lancet* 1967; **1**: 1036–1037.

39. Baumgartner, F.J., Janusz, M.T., Jamieson, W.R.E., Winkler, T., Burr, L.H. & Vestrup, J.A. Cardiopulmonary bypass for resuscitation of patients with accidental hypothermia and cardiac arrest. *Can. J. Surg.* 1992; **35**: 184–187.

40. Letsou, G.V., Kopf, G.S., Elefteriades, J.A., Carter, J.E., Baldwin, J.C. & Hammond, G.L. Is cardiopulmonary bypass effective for treatment of hypothermic arrest due to drowning or exposure? *Arch. Surg.* 1992; **127**: 525–528.

41. Maresca, L. & Vasko, J.S. Treatment of hypothermia by extracorporeal circulation and internal rewarming. *J. Trauma* 1987; **27**: 89–90.

42. Hauty, M.G., Esrig, B.C., Hill, J.G. & Long, W.B. Prognostic factors in severe accidental hypothermia: experience from the Mt. Hood tragedy. *J. Trauma* 1987; **27**: 1107–1112.

43. Bolte, R.G., Black, P.G., Bowere, R.S., Thorne, J.K. & Corneli, H.M. The use of extracorporeal rewarming in a child submerged for 66 minutes. *J. Am. Med. Assoc.* 1988; **260**: 377–379.

44. Silfvast, T. & Pettila, V. Outcome from severe accidental hypothermia in Southern Finland-a 10 year review. *Resuscitation* 2003; **59**: 285–290.

45. Walpoth, B.H., Walpoth-Aslan, B.N., Mattle, H.P. *et al.* Outcome of survivors of accidental deep hypothermia and circulatory arrest treated with extracorporeal blood warming. *N. Engl. J. Med.* 1997; **337**: 1500–1505.

46. Vogel, R.A. The Maryland experience: angioplasty and valvuloplasty using percutaneous cardiopulmonary support: *Am. J. Cardiol.* 1988; **62**: 11K–14K.

47. Shawl, F.A., Domanski, M.J., Wish, M.H., Davis, M., Sudhakar, P. & Hernandez, T.J. Emergency cardiopulmonary bypass support in patients with cardiac arrest in the catheterization laboratory. *Cathet. Cardiovasc. Diagn.* 1990; **19**: 8–12.

48. Mooney, M.R., Arom, K.V., Joyce, L.D. *et al.* Emergency cardiopulmonary bypass support in patients with cardiac arrest. *J. Thorac. Cardiovasc. Surg.* 1991; **101**: 450–454.

49. Butt, W. & Beca, J. Extracorporeal circulatory support in children in intensive care. *Crit. Care Med.* 1993; **21**(Suppl): S381–S382.

50. Molar, F.W., Custer, J.R., Bartlett, R.H. *et al.* Extracorporeal life support for pediatric respiratory failure. *Crit. Care Med.* 1992; **20**: 1112–1118.

51. del Nido, P.J., Dalton, H.J., Thompson, A.E. & Siewers, R.D. Extracorporeal membrane oxygenator rescue in children during cardiac arrest after cardiac surgery. *Circulation* 1992; **86**: (Suppl 2): II-300–II-304.

52. Nagao, K., Hayashi, N., Kanmatsuse, K. *et al.* Cardiopulmonary cerebral resuscitation using emergency cardiopulmonary bypass, coronary reperfusion therapy and mild hypothermia in patients with cardiac arrest outside of hospital. *JACC* 2000; **36**: 776–783.

53. Hase, M., Tsuchihashi, K., Fujii, N. *et al.* Early defibrillation and circulatory support can provide better long-term outcomes through favorable neurological recovery in patients with out-of-hospital cardiac arrest of cardiac origin. *Circ J.* 2005; **69**: 1302–1307.

54. Riley, J.B. & Litzie, A.K. Supported angioplasty: a new contribution for extra-corporeal circulation technology. *J. Extracorporeal. Technol.* 1988; **20**: 134–137.

55. Gundry, S.R., Brinkley, J., Wolk, M. *et al.* Percutaneous cardiopulmonary bypass to support angioplasty and valvuloplasty. Technical considerations. *ASAIO Trans.* 1989; **35**: 725–727.

56. Hedlund, K.D., Sanford, D.M. & Dattilo, R. Percutaneous cardiopulmonary support during high risk coronary angioplasty: a case report. *Proc. Am. Acad. Cardiovasc. Perf.* 1989; **10**: 100–103.

57. Shawl, F.A. Percutaneous cardiopulmonary support in high risk angioplasty. *Cardiol. Clin.* 1989; **7**: 865–875.

58. Harloff, M. Supportive angioplasty utilizing the Bard cardiopulmonary support device. *Perfusion* 1990; **5**: 53–56.

59. Shawl, F.A., Domanski, M.J., Wish, M.H. & Davis, M. Percutaneous cardiopulmonary bypass support in the catheterization laboratory: technique and complications. *Am. Heart J.* 1990; **120**: 195–203.

60. Litzie, K. & Roberts, C.P. Emergency femorofemoral cardiopulmonary bypass. *Proc. Am. Acad. Cardiovasc. Perf.* 1987; **8**: 60–65.

61. Vogel, R.A. Supported angioplasty. In Topol, E.J., ed. *Textbook of Interventional Cardiology.* Philadelphia: WB Saunders, 1990; 467–476.

62. Achorn, N.L. Cardiopulmonary support techniques and dilemmas. *Proc. Am. Soc. Extracorporeal Technol.* 1990.

63. Mooney, M.R., Arom, K.V., Joyce, L.D. *et al.* Emergency cardiopulmonary bypass support in patients with cardiac arrest. *J. Thorac. Cardiovasc. Surg.* 1991; **101**: 450–454.

64. Bolgiano, E., Sykes, L., Barish, R.A., Zickler, R. & Eastridge, B. Accidental hypothermia with cardiac arrest: recovery following rewarming by cardiopulmonary bypass. *J. Emerg. Med.* 1992; **10**: 427–433.

65. von Segesser, L.K., Garcia, E. & Turina, M. Perfusion without systemic heparinization for rewarming in accidental hypothermia. *Ann. Thorac. Surg.* 1991; **52**: 560–561.

66. DelRossi, A.J., Cernaianu, A.C., Vertrees, R.A. *et al.* Heparinless extracorporeal bypass for treatment of hypothermia. *J. Trauma* 1990; **30**: 79–82.

67. Aufiero, T.X. & Pae, W.E. Extracorporeal cardiopulmonary support for resuscitation and invasive cardiology outside the operating suite. In Gravlee, G.P., Davis, R.F. & Utley, J.R., eds. *Cardiopulmonary Bypass: Principles and Practice.* Baltimore: Williams & Wilkins, 1993; 682–692.

68. Lowinger, T., Shawl, F., Diffee, G. & Richmond, J. Percutaneous cardiopulmonary (by pass) support in the cardiac catheterization laboratory: a new application of perfusion. *Proc. Am. Soc. Extracorporeal Technol.* 1989; 9–10.

69. Whittaker, S., Rees, M.R., Hick, D.G. *et al.* Percutaneous cardiopulmonary bypass. *Proc. Am. Soc. Extracorporeal Technol.* 1992; 134–139.

70. Justison, G.A. & Pelley, W. Hemodynamic management during closed circuit percutaneous cardiopulmonary bypass. *Proc. Am. Soc. Extracorporeal. Technol.* 1989; 88–95.

71. Cohen, D.J., Cline, J.R., Lepinski, S.M., Bowman, H.M. & Ireland, K. Resuscitation of the hypothermic patient. *Am. J. Emerg. Med.* 1988; **6**: 475–478.

72. Baumgartner, F.J., Junusz, M.T., Jamieson, W.R.E., Winkler, T., Burr, L.H. & Vestrup, J.A. Cardiopulmonary bypass for resuscitation of patients with accidental hypothermia and cardiac arrest. *Can. J. Surg.* 1992; **35**: 184–187.

73. Stephenson, H.E. Jr., Reid, L.C. & Hinton, J.W. Some common denominators in 1200 case of cardiac arrest. *Ann. Surg.* 1953; **137**: 731–744.

74. Kouwenhoven, W.B., Jude, J.R. & Knickerbocker, G.G. Closed-chest cardiac massage. *J. Am. Med. Assoc.* 1960; **173**: 1064–1067.

75. Hachimi-Idrissi, S., Leeman, J., Hubloue, Y., Huyghens, L. & Corne, L. Open chest cardiopulmonary resuscitation in out-of-hospital cardiac arrest. *Resuscitation* 1997; **35**: 151–156.

76. Rose, D.M., Connolly, M., Cunningham, J.N. Jr. & Spencer, F.C. Technique and results with a roller pump left and right heart assist device. *Ann. Thorac. Surg.* 1989; **47**: 124–129.

77. Farrar, D.J., Hill, J.D., Gray, L.A. Jr., Galbraith, I.A., Chow, E. & Hershon, J.J. Successful biventricular circulatory support as a bridge to cardiac transplantation during prolonged ventricular fibrillation and asystole. *Circulation* 1989; **80**: III 147–151.

78. Shahian, D.M., St. Ledger, S., Kimmel, W., Bogosian, M., Abraham, W. & Johnson, M.E. Successful recovery of postischemic stunned myocardium using centrifugal left ventricular assist. *J. Cardiothorac. Anesth.* 1990; **4**: 84–88.

79. Anstadt, G.L., Schiff, P. & Baue, A.E. Prolonged circulatory support by direct mechanical ventricular assistance. *Trans. Am. Soc. Artif. Intern. Organs.* 1966; **12**: 72–79.

80. McCabe, J.B., Ventriglia, W.J., Anstadt, G.L. & Nolan, D.J. Direct mechanical ventricular assistance during ventricular fibrillation. *Ann. Emerg. Med.* 1983; **12**: 739–744.

81. Bartlett, R.L., Stewart, N.J., Raymond, J., Anstadt, G.L. & Martin, S.D. Comparative study of three methods of resuscitation: closed-chest, open-chest manual, and direct mechanical ventricular assistance. *Ann. Emerg. Med.* 1984; **13**: 773–777.

82. Brown, C.G., Schlaifer, J., Jenkins, J. *et al.* Effect of direct mechanical ventricular assistance on myocardial hemodynamics during ventricular fibrillation. *Crit. Care Med.* 1989; **17**: 1175–1180.

83. Anstadt, M.P., Hendry, P.J., Plunkett, M.D., Menius, J.A., Pacifico, A.D. & Lowe, J.E. Mechanical myocardial actuation during ventricular fibrillation improves tolerance to ischemia compared with cardiopulmonary bypass. *Circulation* 1990; **82**:(Suppl. 4):IV-284–IV-290.

84. Anstadt, M.P., Hendry, P.J., Plunkett, M.D., Menius, J.A., Pacifico, A.D. & Lowe, J.E. Mechanical cardiac actuation achieves hemodynamics similar to cardiopulmonary by pass. *Surgery* 1990; **108**: 442–451.

85. Anstadt, M.P., Bartlett, R.L., Malone, J.P. *et al.* Direct mechanical ventricular actuation for cardiac arrest in humans: a clinical feasibility trial. *Chest* 1991; **100**: 86–92.

33

Routes of drug administration

Thomas Kerz[1], Gideon Paret[2], and Holger Herff[3]

[1] Department of Neurosurgery, Intensive Care Unit, Johannes Gutenberg-Universität Klinikum, Mainz, Germany
[2] Department of Pediatic Critical Care, Chaim Sheba Medical Center Safra Children's Hospital, Israel
[3] Department of Anesthesiology and Critical Care Medicine, Innsbruck Medical University, Austria

Historical review of routes of drug administration

Baggellardus, a contemporary of Columbus, observed Indians applying fumigation to the mouth or anus of apparently dead persons and brought the technique to Europe.[1] In the aftermath, during the seventeenth and eighteenth century, scientific societies all over Europe recommended warmth, artificial respiration, rectal fumigation with tobacco smoke, friction, and bleeding for resuscitation purposes.[2,3] Insufflation of air, tobacco smoke, or vaporized aromatic plants either by mouth, the nostrils, or the rectum was common,[4] stimulants were administered by nasogastric or rectal tubes, and topical application with "spirits of wine, hartshorn, or, which is perhaps the most powerful, the spirits of sal ammoniac" were used .[5] Eventually, tobacco insufflation was abandoned when Brodie in 1811 published his observations that even a dog was easily killed by injection of smoke into the rectum.[2]

History of intravenous techniques

Bronze syringes had been known since antiquity,[6] when Heron of Alexandria had recommended his pus extractor for injection of fluids.[7] Blood circulation was discovered in 1616 by William Harvey,[8] and in 1656 the British astronomer Sir Percival Christopher Wren (1632 to 1723) first demonstrated intravenous therapy by injecting wine and beer into a dog.[9] He noted that "the opium. . . did within a short time stupefy, though not kill the dog." Three other physicians, acting independently of Wren, described intravenous (iv) therapy: Johann Sigismund Elsholtz (1623 to 1688), who infused water into the brachial artery of a drowned woman in 1661, the surgeon Carlo Fracassati (ar. 1630 to 1672), and lastly Johann David Major (1634 to 1693), a medical doctor. Intravenous drug injection was supposedly first attempted in man in the failed execution of a servant of the French envoy to London in 1657.[10] A silver syringe and cannula were first described by Elsholtz in 1667.[11] In the years following, Richard Lower (1631 to 1691) performed the first transfusion from animal to animal in 1666, while Jean-Baptiste Denis (ar. 1615 to 1704) attempted animal to human transfusion. As Denis' patient died one night after the transfusion, the court of Paris interdicted all transfusions in 1670. Because of the observed complications (thrombosis, hemolysis, embolism), intravenous techniques played only a marginal role until the nineteenth century. Intra-arterial injections for the purpose of resuscitation were then performed by Moritz Schiff.[12] In 1891, Arnaud injected blood directly into the coronary arteries and showed that defibrinated and oxygenated blood could revive an arrested heart.[13]

In 1929, Forssmann started percutaneous techniques when he catheterized his own right ventricle.[14] Intravenous catheters were tested by Cournand and Ranges[15] and Meyers.[16] Duffy described the use of the external jugular vein in 1949,[17] Aubaniac[18] reported cannulation of the subclavian vein in 1952, and in 1953 Seldinger described his technique for catheterization.[19] Despite all these advances, Kouwenhoven, Jude, and Knickerbocker[20,21] in the 1960s still recommended a venous cut-down for drug therapy after emergency treatment with intracardiac injections. Swan *et al.*[22] reported on the use of pulmonary artery catheters in 1970, when Jernigan et al. also published their experiences with the internal jugular vein approach.[23]

History of intracardiac injection

The anatomical features of intracardiac injections were described by Steiner[24] in 1871. Intracardiac injection of epinephrine probably was first done by Latzko[12] in 1904 and Crile and Dolley[25] in 1906. In 1919, von den Velden[26] reported on 45 cases of intracardiac injections that he had performed since 1906. Intracardiac (or intraarterial) injections were used mainly for blood transfusion, however, until 1921 when several authors reported the successful use of intracardiac epinephrine.[27–29] In their important papers, Kouwenhoven et al.[21,21] recommended intracardiac vasopressor injections "since the drug should be injected into the blood stream for immediate effect."[20] The common perception was that peripheral iv injections had no effect in the low flow state of CPR, although sparse data supported this view:[12] "Many physicians are under the impression that intracardiac injections should be more effective than intravenous. . . they are reluctant to use them intravenously even with an intravenous route immediately available."[30] In addition to the pharmacologic effect, insertion of the needle itself was deemed to affect the heart.[24,26,31] Fontana[32] in 1775 had provoked a heart beat simply by inserting a needle, and in 1829 Krimer[33] combined the technique with electricity to resuscitate drowned patients, thereby introducing some sort of intracardiac pacemaker for the first time. In 1871, Steiner[24] published extensive historical, anatomical, and physiologic studies recommending "electropuncture" of the heart for cardiac arrest during chloroform anesthesia. By the end of the nineteenth century, however, electrical therapy of cardiac arrest was no longer practiced.

History of endotracheal administration

Endotracheal (ET) intubation was first performed by the Belgian anatomist Andreas Vesalius[34] in 1543. The absorption capacity of the lungs was demonstrated by the french physiologist Claude Bernard[35] in 1857 with the administration of curare to dogs by way of tracheostomy. Several years later, resorption of many more drugs administered by the ET-route was reported[36,37] Kline and Winternitz in 1915 were the first to recommend the ET route for administering medication.[38] In 1935, Graeser and Rowe[39] recommended inhalation of epinephrine for treatment of bronchial asthma, and direct aerosolized drug delivery was broadly used for antibiotic therapy of lung infections.[40–45] From the 1940s until the 1970s, numerous reports established that substantial uptake of local anesthetics occurs during topical anesthesia of the larynx and trachea, as even occasional deaths were reported.[46–52]

History of intraosseous routes

The intraosseous route was introduced after the description of the circulation within mammalian bone by Drinker et al.[53] and Doan in 1922.[54] The first site chosen was the sternum, but this was quickly abandoned in preference for the tibia or femur. In 1940, Tocantins showed that substances injected into the bone marrow appeared almost immediately in the circulation.[55] The intraosseous technique fell from favor, however, with the introduction and improvement of intravascular catheters that allowed for more permanent peripheral intravenous access but was reinstated in 1983 after a letter to the editor about intraosseous infusion by Turkel,[56] which was followed by a plethora of clinical and experimental reports.

Peripheral venous routes

Basic physiology

In animal studies with indocyanine green dye, the time from dye injection to appearance at the aortic root was 94 seconds.[57] Peak dye concentration following peripheral injection was lower than that following central injection and time-to-peak concentration was delayed. In another study, lidocaine time-to-peak following peripheral injection was 42 seconds, with therapeutic lidocaine levels persisting for 9.6 minutes.[58] Peak lidocaine levels averaged 22 μg/ml following peripheral injection compared to 34.5 μg/ml when given by central venous injection. Open-chest massage reduced circulation time compared to closed-chest compression.[57] For example, while circulation time after peripheral injection during closed-chest CPR averaged 94 seconds, it was only 31 seconds with open-chest massage. Dye concentration curves obtained during open-chest CPR have a sharp peak with rapid decay, comparable to those observed during spontaneous circulation and in contrast to those obtained during closed-chest CPR (Fig. 33.1). The route of administration is probably less critical during open-chest CPR as there are only small differences in circulation times between sites. For example, there is an average difference of only 10 seconds in circulation time between central and femoral injection during open-chest CPR in dogs. It is unlikely that there are clinically significant differences in man. Although peripheral injection somehow delays the drug effect, one clinical study suggests that this does not alter clinical outcome.[59] Gueugniaud et al. reviewed 233 patients given either peripheral epinephrine (175 patients) or central injection of

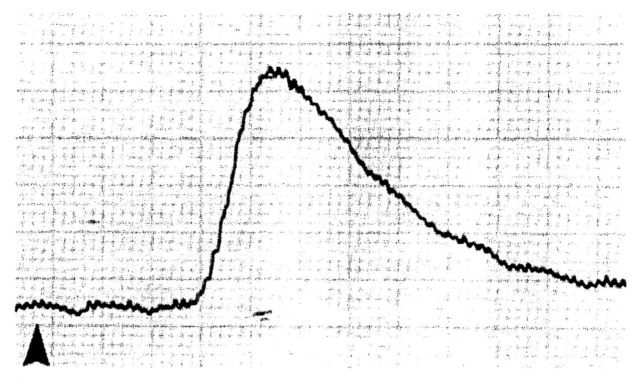

Fig. 33.1. Dye dilution curve after central venous injection during open chest CPR (paper speed 1 mm/s). *Arrow* indicates dye injection.

epinephrine (58 patients). Of these patients, 51% receiving peripheral injection had temporary return of spontaneous circulation (ROSC) compared to 38% of patients receiving central injection; 13 patients were alive after 21 days, including 12 who received peripheral injection and 1 who received central injection. With this sample size, this study would have a power of 36% to detect a difference in survival.

Drug delivery after peripheral injection is enhanced by following the injection with a saline flush.[60] After a 20-ml flush, circulation times are 40% shorter than those without a saline flush (Fig. 33.2),[61] and correspond to those seen after central injection.[62,63] Yet peak dye concentrations show no differences.[60] Varying the bolus size from 10 to 30 ml also was without significant effect on either circulation time or peak dye concentration. Virtually all of the studies have been performed in animal models and there are no data providing a reliable basis for clinical use. Nevertheless, since preliminary results in dogs have indicated that 10- to 30-ml boluses result in similar circulation times, it seems reasonable to assume that, for clinical use, a bolus of about 20 ml is appropriate. Peripheral

venous access is the least invasive and safest means of administering medication during cardiac arrest and does not interfere with CPR.

Drugs

Injection of epinephrine into the antecubital vein has been demonstrated to lead to a marked rise in epinephrine levels within 2 minutes after injection.[64] Quinton *et al.* randomized 12 patients to receive intravenous epinephrine administered either in an antecubital vein or via an endotracheal tube. The injection of 1 mg of epinephrine IV increased serum epinephrine levels up to three times the level before administration. By comparison, the maximal increase in levels after ET administration was less than half the minimal increase in epinephrine levels after iv administration. In dogs, an increase in coronary perfusion pressure occurs within 1 minute after injection and reaches a peak around 3 minutes, after which the coronary perfusion pressure begins to return to baseline.[65] iv Injection of 0.015 mg/ kg of epinephrine was found to increase coronary perfusion pressure from 16.9 mmHg to a peak of 22.5 mmHg.

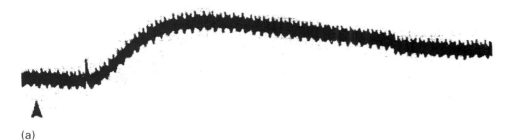

(a)

Fig 33.2 (a). Dye dilution curve after central venous injection during closed chest CPR (paper speed 0.25 mm/s). *Arrow* indicates dye injection.

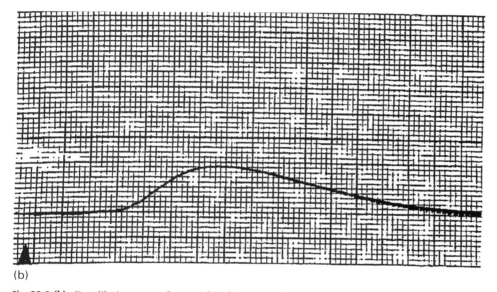

(b)

Fig. 33.2 (b). Dye dilution curve after peripheral injection of indocyanine green dye, followed by injection of a 20 ml saline bolus (paper speed 0.25 mm/s).

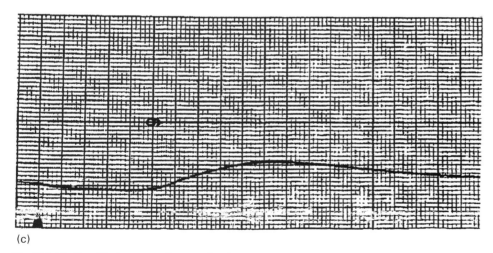

(c)

Fig. 33.2 (c). Dye dilution curve after peripheral injection of indocyanine green dye with no saline bolus injection (paper speed 0.25 mm/s).

For further data, comparing peripheral vs. central venous, endotracheal or intraosseous routes the reader is referred to the relevant chapters.

Femoral injection

There is broad, especially military, experience in using the femoral vein for resuscitation. These lines can provide a route for fluid administration, although the incidence of complications increases the longer the line is in place. Experience during the Vietnam war showed that the femoral vein could be catheterized successfully 95% of the time even in patients without palpable pulses.[66] The technique was associated with arterial puncture in approximately 6% of patients, hematoma formation in 1%, and wound infection in 1%. No instances of retroperitoneal hematoma formation in this large series were observed. At least one civilian study has demonstrated that 89% of attempts at femoral vein catheterization in patients either in cardiac arrest or requiring fluid perfusion for shock were successful.[67] Femoral venous access was particularly useful for rapid fluid infusion, although this is not a consideration, and indeed may be deleterious, in cardiac resuscitation.

There has been some concern that drugs administered near the femoral route may not circulate to the central compartment during CPR.[68] A canine CPR model did not demonstrate a pressure gradient between the inferior vena cava and right atrium, and cineangiographic studies revealed significant reflux into the inferior vena cava during compression. In another canine arrest model, measurements with radioisotopes established that the time-to-reach half-peak count over both the right and left ventricles was markedly delayed for injection into the inferior vena cava compared to superior vena cava injection. When corrected for cardiac output during CPR, the times to right and -left ventricle peaks and half-peaks were all significantly delayed after inferior vena cava injection.[69]

In two studies of femoral vein catheterization during human cardiac arrest, the success rate for correct placement was low. Jastremski et al. found that physicians of various backgrounds correctly placed catheters in the femoral vein in only 31% of cases.[70] In a larger study with injection of radiopaque dye to verify catheter placement, femoral vein catheters were placed correctly 77% of the time as compared to 94% of subclavian vein catheters.[71] The femoral route has never been compared to other routes during CPR in humans. An older study compared dogs given epinephrine by a variety of routes: ROSC-time was 127 seconds for the femoral route, compared to 139 seconds for the intracardiac route, and 116 seconds for endotracheal administration.[30] Recently, Chiang and Baskin reported that in 121 critically ill infants, children, or young adults, placement of femoral central venous catheters was successful in 83% of all cases. Twenty of their patients were in cardiac/respiratory arrest.[72] In summary, femoral venous injection during cardiac arrest is limited by a low chance of successful cannulation as well as prolonged circulation times. Its use should be limited to situations in which other routes of administration are unavailable.

Central venous injection

Peak dye concentrations after central injection in animal studies were 40%[57] or 270%[73] greater than those seen after peripheral injection. Circulation times after central venous injection are 30%–50% shorter compared to peripheral injection. In human studies, peak lidocaine levels were four times greater after central injection than after peripheral injection.[74] Lidocaine levels reached a peak 30 seconds after central injection, whereas lidocaine was not detected until 90 seconds after peripheral injection and did not reach a peak during the 5-minute study period after peripheral injection. In a review of 554 catheterizations, including shock patients, the overall complication rate was 13.7%.[75] Normally, the complication rate of placing subclavian catheters can be as low as 1%,[76] and differences may be related to the higher accuracy of prospective studies, urgency of the situation, and level of physician training.[75] Most of these studies have been performed when circulation was spontaneous and the results may not be directly applicable to the difficult situation of central vein catheterization during ongoing CPR.

Few studies have examined central venous catheterization during human CPR. Dronen et al. compared the superior and inferior approaches to the subclavian vein in 76 patients undergoing CPR, and found no difference in the overall success rate, although malpositioning was more frequent with the inferior approach.[77] Moreover, the inferior approach led to more frequent interruptions in chest compression. Emerman et al. found that 94% of attempts at infraclavicular approaches to the subclavian vein were successful in human CPR.[71] In that study, 11% of catheters were malpositioned in the venous system, and 6% of the catheters were inadvertently placed into the arterial system. Our personal experience is that the supraclavicular approach to the subclavian vein provides less interference with ongoing CPR with a high rate of success. Nevertheless, the approach chosen should be related to the individual operator's personal experience and expertise. There is little evidence to suggest that any one approach is mandated during CPR.

An alternative approach to the central circulation is cannulation of the external jugular vein, which is generally engorged during CPR and is easily cannulated. If desired, a wire can be passed through the catheter allowing subsequent placement of a longer catheter into the superior vena cava, although venous valves occasionally limit the success of this maneuver.

Intraosseous injection

Rationale

Successful resuscitation has been shown to depend on the time to achieve intravascular access, but this is a major problem, especially in pediatric CPR. Rossetti and coworkers[78] reported that placement of an intravenous catheter required at least 10 minutes in 24% of the children in cardiac arrest. Lillis and Jaffe[79] found that more than half of the children younger than 6 years who required intravascular access did not receive an IV line in the prehospital setting, and that only 4% of children under 6 years with absent vital signs had successful placement of an IV line. Unlike iv access, studies of intraosseous infusions have shown overall success rates of 76%, and 85% of infusions were achieved in less than 1 minute.[80] Therefore, it is recommended that in children under 3 years old, attempts at peripheral access not be sustained beyond 90 seconds before an alternative route for drug administration is sought.[81] Although intraosseous infusion is generally considered a technique for pediatric resuscitation, it can also be used in adults. Valdes reported no complications in 15 adults, none of whom were in cardiac arrest, who received 2–42 liters via the intraosseous route over a period of 3.5–30 days.[82] Iserson used the intraosseous route successfully in 22 adults who were in cardiac arrest.[83] Temporally related pharmacologic effects were observed after administration of sodium bicarbonate, lidocaine, atropine, and vasopressors. Based on experience on adult cadavers, Clem and Tierney recommended using the calcaneus as the preferred site for intraosseous infusion in adults.[84]

Flow rates of 10 ml/min with gravity and 41 ml/min with 300 mmHg pressure have been demonstrated with a 13-gauge needle in the medial malleolus of calves.[85] In vivo flow rates depend on the flow through the bone marrow, e.g., the characteristics of the medullary space, rather than on the size of the needle.[86] Similar flow rates were also attained in humans.[87] Laspada and coworkers used a piglet model to compare the extravasation rates and insertion complications under gravity and 300 mmHg pressure infusion of threaded and nonthreaded needles and found no significant differences.[88]

Physiology

A rich network of medullary sinusoids in the long bones is drained by numerous venous channels that empty into a solitary longitudinal central venous sinus. From there, the blood enters the central venous circulation.[89] The marrow cavity functions as a rigid vein and does not collapse during hypovolemia or circulatory shock.[90] After intraosseous injection, the distribution of drugs and fluids appears to be very similar to that after iv injection.

Technique

The proximal tibia is the optimal site for the insertion of the intraosseous needle in children. This site is approximately 1 cm below the tibial tuberosity and medially on the tibial plateau, and it permits concomitant ventilation or chest compression during placement.

Other sites for intraosseous infusions include the sternum, humerus, clavicle, distal tibia, iliac crests, and femur. Drug absorption and fluid infusion are equally effective from either site.[91] If the distal tibia is used, the optimal location is in the medial surface of the tibia proximal to the medial malleolus.[89] The distal femur site is just about 1 cm above the patella and in the midline. The sternum, humerus, and clavicle cannot be used during CPR.

A number of commercially available bone marrow needles exist for intraosseous access and infusion.[92,93]. In the absence of a bone marrow needle, a strong, large bore needle with a stylet, such as a lumbar puncture needle, should be used[94] and inserted perpendicular to the bone, with the bevel pointing away from the joint space. Entry into the marrow space is confirmed by noting a lack of resistance after passing through the cortex.[95] Aspiration of blood marrow with a syringe confirms the correct position. After conventional vascular access is established, the intraosseous infusion should be discontinued.

Complications

The complication rate for this technique is low. Difficulty or inability to enter the marrow cavity is the most common problem, whereby, the needle is accidentally forced through the opposite site of the bone. Extravasation of fluid around the puncture site is a minor but frequently reported problem and can occur at any site where there has been a break in the cortex, e.g., around the puncture site, or from holes from unsuccessful attempts or fractures in the cortex.[89]

Potential hazards include fat embolization, cellulitis, abscess, subperiosteal infiltration or hematoma, and subcutaneous infiltration. Risk of osteomyelitis is low: of 4270 cases reported between 1942–1977, only 27 cases of infections were reported.[89] Bowley *et al.* reported an iatrogenic fracture of the proximal tibia caused by the use of a bone injection gun device, and suggested performing follow-up radiographs for all children in whom intraosseous insertion had been attempted.[96] Damage to the epiphyseal plate is at least of theoretical concern, although it has never been reported and may be avoided by placing the needle several centimeters away, and pointed away from the joint space.[89] Follow-up studies after intraosseous infusion have shown only short-term periostitis and no long-term sequelae. One study reported 72 patients followed-up with radiographs and showed no adverse effects 1–2 years after intraosseous infusions.[97] Fatalities attributed to intraosseous infusions were all related to sternal puncture with associated mediastinitis or injury to the heart or great vessels.[98] Therefore, the sternal site should be avoided altogether. Multiple insertion attempts can significantly decrease vascular drug levels, presumably due to extravasation.

Clinical applications

Only a few human studies are available, most of which compared intraosseous, intravenous, and endotracheal drug administration.

Orlowski *et al.* studied the pharmacokinetics of epinephrine hydrochloride, sodium bicarbonate, calcium chloride, hydroxyethyl starch, 50% dextrose in water, and lidocaine hydrochloride in normotensive anesthetized dogs.[99] Each animal was treated with all three routes of administration (central iv, peripheral iv, and intraosseous) in a randomized sequence. Effects of adrenaline were also assessed in a shock model. The IO route was comparable with the central and peripheral iv routes for all drugs, with equivalent magnitudes of peak effect or drug level and equal or longer durations of action.

Time-to-peak plasma concentration of atropine in anesthetized monkeys was shortest with iv administration and longest with endotracheal administration, with intraosseous administration in-between.[100] The mean concentration of atropine in plasma was significantly higher in the iv group than in the endotracheal group at 0.75 and 2 minutes, and the concentration was sig-

nificantly higher only at 0.75 minute compared to intraosseous administration. Its mean plasma concentration was, however, significantly higher than that of endotracheal administration at 5 minutes and it was greater than that of iv and endotracheal administrations for the samples collected over 5–30 minutes.

In another study, Orlowski *et al.* compared central iv, peripheral iv, intraosseous, and intratracheal administration of epinephrine in both normotensive and hemorrhagic shock dogs.[101] Epinephrine was equally effective by the intraosseous, central iv, and peripheral iv routes in terms of time-to-onset of action, time-to-peak effect, and magnitude of effect on systolic, diastolic, and mean arterial pressures in both the shock and non-shock animals. The duration of effect was significantly longer for the intraosseous route of administration.

Several studies used radioactive isotopes to compare peripheral and central delivery times by iv and intraosseous infusion. Cameron et al. injected a radionuclide tracer and showed that intraosseous infusion achieved peripheral and central circulation transit times comparable to those achieved by the iv route during both normovolemic and hypovolemic states.[102] Warren and coworkers studied the pharmacokinetics from multiple intraosseous sites, including tibial, medial malleolar, distal femoral, and humeral, as well as from peripheral iv site injections in normovolemic and hypovolemic pigs. They demonstrated similarly rapid transit times and proportions of bicarbonate and radioactive tracers from all sites.[103]

In summary, the above-cited studies demonstrate that intraosseous drug delivery is comparable to both the peripheral and central venous routes, with equivalent magnitudes of peak drug effect and levels, and equal or longer durations of action. Most of these studies, however, were performed when circulation was spontaneous and therefore the results may not be directly applicable to a cardiac arrest setting.

Cardiac arrest

There are only isolated case reports describing successful resuscitation after intraosseous infusion of epinephrine, albumin, and bicarbonate in humans.[104–106] Ryder *et al.* reported on an 11-week-old infant who suffered cardiac arrest secondary to gastrointestinal hemorrhage and was successfully treated by intraosseous infusion and discharged with no apparent neurological deficit.[105]

McNamara *et al.* reported on a 3-month-old in asystole who achieved a stable rhythm and blood pressure before iv access had been obtained following after administration of epinephrine and atropine via the endotracheal route and sodium bicarbonate through intraosseous infusion.[106]

In a porcine resuscitation model, Spivey compared intraosseous and central and peripheral iv bicarbonate injection after CPR. The peak increase in pH after intraosseous administration was greater than that after peripheral iv injection, although both were somewhat lower than that after central iv injection.[107] In another swine CPR study, intraosseous injection of 0.01 mg/kg of epinephrine increased plasma epinephrine levels without effects on diastolic or mean blood pressure. Injection of a 10-fold dose led to an increase in blood pressure, suggesting that intraosseous administration requires larger than currently recommended doses to produce a significant change in blood pressure.[108] Similarly, injection of epinephrine via both the intraosseous and central venous route in a lamb CPR model led to significant increases in plasma epinephrine levels. Peak concentrations were similar for both routes, although the peak for the intraosseous route was delayed by 15 seconds compared with that following central venous injection.[109]

Recommendations and summary

Intraosseous drug administration offers an alternative means of administering drugs, and is now standard emergency care. The technique is simple, rapid and rarely associated with major complications. Considering the difficulty in securing vascular access during low-flow states, current recommendations of the European Resuscitation Council consider intraosseous administration the method of choice of emergency drugs and fluids when iv access cannot be achieved.[110]

Endotracheal administration

Advantages

Endobronchial drug administration is a simple and rapid alternative during CPR when intubation is performed before intravenous cannulation,[111] when the time interval to intravenous access is prolonged, or when attempts to establish intravenous access are unsuccessful.[112]

Basic physiology

The lung with its capillary surface of about $70 \, m^2$ plays a major role in drug uptake.[113] Absorption of water occurs at all levels of the upper airway and lungs, but drug absorp-

tion[114] depends on particle size, thickness of absorption membrane, area of membrane surface, drug conversion or degradation by lung tissue, the ventilation/perfusion ratio, drug dilution with saline or water, volume of dilution carrier, and depth of drug administration into the bronchial tree.[115–120] Small particles, up to a diameter of 6 μm or a molecular weight of 75 000,[121] are absorbed similarly to gas molecules by a simple diffusion process, and drugs have to be aerosolized to particles of 1 to 10 μm in diameter to reach the presumed site of absorption.[122] Larger molecules (more than 6 μm) are absorbed via the bronchial mucosa (Fig. 33.3). A small amount of drug may be resorbed by the lymphatic system.[123]

Method of application

It would be expected that deep endobronchial injection close to the alveoli would result in a more rapid absorption than shallow injection. Unfortunately, study data are contradictory, and several studies suggest varying tracheal or bronchial uptake of non-aerosolized drugs; e.g., after injection of 4 ml of dye in 12 cadavers via a specially designed catheter, followed by three-to-five manual hyperinflations, (Fig. 33.4) all right main bronchi and 90% of the left main bronchi are stained by the dye within 24 hours.[124]

Likewise, shallow injection results in drug delivery only to the main bronchi, even when followed by manual hyperinflation.[117,125] Even when the saline solution was administered into the proximal aperture of the tube, the results were similar to those seen with injection under bronchoscopic control into the trachea, right main bronchus, or the right lower lobe bronchus.[117] Arterial lidocaine or epinephrine levels tended to be higher after shallow administration.[119,126]

Therefore, adequate drug dilution may be more important than the method of application. Dilution of lidocaine with normal saline to a total volume of 6 ml is more effective than any other application method.[127,128] Lidocaine levels in anesthetized adults are higher with 10 ml of fluid than with 3 or 5 ml.[115] More recent studies recommend dilution of epinephrine in at least 5 ml of saline.[129]

Results in patients with low pulmonary blood flow may be different. In the study by Ralston et al. on dogs in ventricular fibrillation (VF), 0.2 mg/kg of epinephrine diluted in 10 ml of saline produced no change in blood pressure after shallow injection.[130] Conversely, a lower dose of 0.1 mg/kg of epinephrine in 10 ml of saline, injected via a catheter wedged deep into the bronchial tree and followed by three hyperinflations, elevated both systolic and diastolic blood pressure. Therefore, the guidelines in 2000

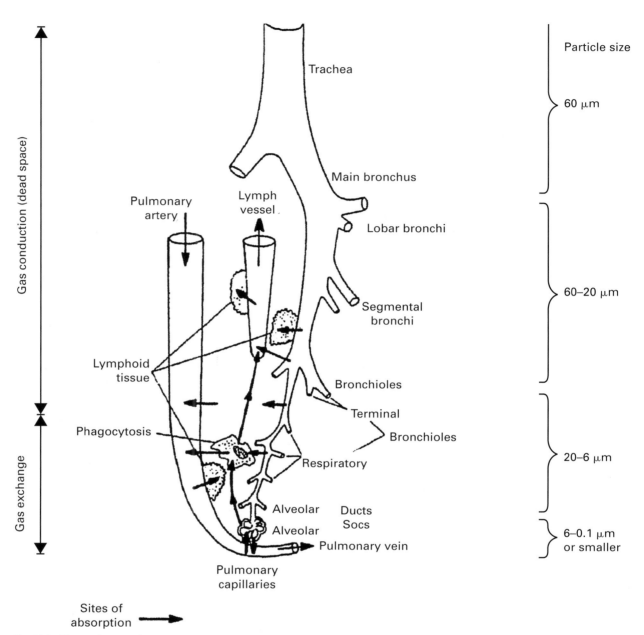

Fig. 33.3. Upper airway and respiratory units. Absorption rate of particles depends on their nature and size, as well as on ventilation and conditions of the respiratory tract. (from ref. 23.)

recommend passing a catheter beyond the tip of the tube and hyperventilating the patient after administration via the catheter, although this is estimated to interrupt oxygen supply and chest compressions significantly longer.[131] To avoid this, in neonatal cardiac arrest, direct drug application into the tube is recommended by some authors.[132]

Diluent

For choosing the ideal type and amount of diluent for ET therapy, the effects on blood gases, pulmonary surfactant, and rapidity of absorption, as well as possible short- and long-term sequelae should be considered. Some investigators have advocated the use of normal saline.[133] In one study in dogs, arterial PCO_2 increased and PO_2 was depressed after water was used, whereas no significant change was observed after ET instillation of normal saline.[134] Yet, as 2 ml/kg of endotracheal fluid were used which correspond to 140 ml in humans, the results might not be transferable to humans. No adverse effects of up to 25 ml of normal saline on blood gases were reported.[135] Gas exchange is not impaired during CPR in dogs when 10 ml of saline are instilled endobronchially.[130]

In contrast, Redding *et al.* in 1967 found that dilution of 1 mg of epinephrine in 10 ml of water achieved ROSC faster than in 10 ml of normal saline, which was similar to iv or intracardiac injection.[136] Naganobu *et al.* reported that in dogs, 20 µg/kg of epinephrine given endobronchially in 2 ml of distilled water increased both levels of epinephrine in plasma and blood pressure significantly better than did 2 ml of normal saline as diluent, indicating that distilled water provided a "solvent drag" for endobronchial epinephrine.[137] Although distilled water administered into the endobronchial tree may decrease partial pressure oxygen significantly more than normal does saline, these changes could be judged to be acceptable.[138] As a compromise, Orlowski *et al.* suggested one-fourth or one-half normal saline. In their study, intrapulmonary shunt increased to almost 50% with the use of water and to a lesser extent with normal saline, whereas use of 0.225% NaCl solution was least injurious and approximated the control with no fluid in the trachea.[133]

There are no data analyzing the adequate volume of diluent for pediatric patients, and only case reports exist for this group of patients.[111,139] It is possible that the volume administered to children should be correlated to alveolar surface size, but this requires further investigation.

Drugs

Epinephrine

As early as 1967, Redding and colleagues reported on the endotracheal route for systemic administration of epinephrine during resuscitation.[30] The onset of action for ET therapy starts after seconds and lasts for 18 to 20 minutes, whereas onset of IV therapy starts after seconds and lasts for 2 to 3 minutes.[140] When blood levels from the femoral artery are compared, maximal epinephrine concentrations are achieved 15 seconds after either iv or ET administration. Schuettler *et al.* observed maximal heart rate 0.5 minute after IV and 1 to 2 minutes after ET administration.[141]

In a study by Crespo[142] standard dosing of epinephrine through the endotracheal tube (0.01 mg/kg) produced only a small rise of epinephrine blood levels. When common iv-doses are used endotracheally, the beta-receptor effect is unopposed by alpha-adrenergic vasoconstriction which

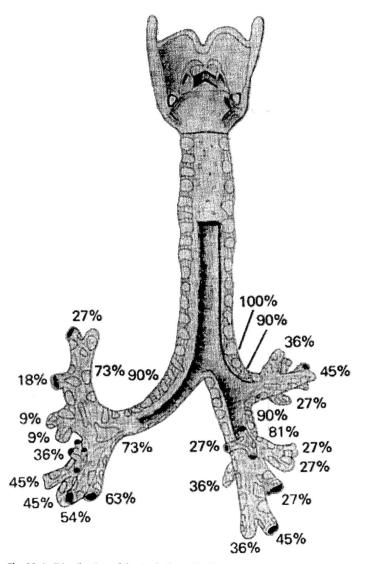

Fig. 33.4. Distribution of dye in the bronchial tree.

can result in decreases in blood pressure[143,144] In models with spontaneous circulation, a ten-fold higher dose usually is necessary to produce effects similar to iv therapy.[141] During CPR, the "equipotent epinephrine dose" administered endobronchially is approximately 3 to 10 times higher than the intravenous dose.[145,146]

Schuettler *et al.* prospectively compared peripheral venous plasma epinephrine levels after intravenous or deep endobronchial drug therapy in patients with out-of-hospital ventricular fibrillation, (Fig. 33.5). Intravenous epinephrine resulted in mean plasma levels 70% higher than endobronchial therapy, was more rapidly detected, and fell more rapidly below therapeutic levels than did epinephrine

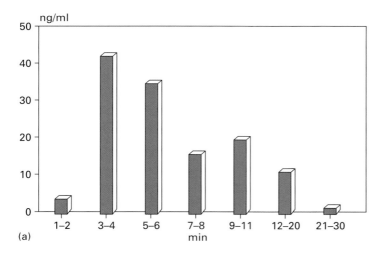

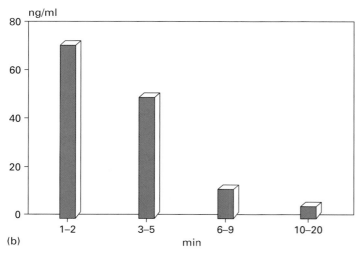

Fig. 33.5 (a) Mean plasma concentration in 28 out-of-hospital patients in VF after endobronchial administration of 2.5 mg epinephrine in 5–10 ml of normal saline. (b) Mean plasma concentration in 8 out-of-hospital patients in VF after intravenous administration of 1 mg epinephrine (From ref. 147)

20% of the initial maximal concentration was detected 5 minutes after iv injection.[151] This may provide evidence of poor initial absorption as lung perfusion is only approximately 10%–30% of normal during CPR. With restoration of spontaneous circulation, perfusion improves and a washout effect occurs, resulting in arterial hypertension, malignant arrhythmias, and recurrence of ventricular fibrillation. Therefore, some investigators advise against repeated administration of ET epinephrine.[112]

Accordingly, intravenous drug administration remains the first-line strategy during CPR. Administration of drugs via an endotracheal tube during CPR is only a second-line approach.

Vasopressin

When endobronchial vasopressin is diluted with normal saline,[152] identical dosages of vasopressin result in comparable blood pressure responses, irrespective of endobronchial, intraosseous,[153] or intravenous administration.[154] Coronary perfusion pressure increased 2 to 3 minutes later after endobronchial than after intravenous vasopressin.[154] In animal studies, vasopressin accomplished its effect on diastolic blood pressure more rapidly, vigorously, and protractedly compared to epinephrine.[155] To avoid bradycardia after cardiopulmonary resuscitation, some authors propose to use vasopressin with atropine.[156] The ILCOR guidelines 2000[150] called for vasopressin as an alternative to epinephrine in shock-refractory ventricular fibrillation, and the 2005 guidelines concluded that there is insufficient evidence to support or refute the use of vasopressin as an alternative to adrenaline.[157]

Lidocaine

Use of lidocaine during CPR is debatable, yet many studies have documented its rapid uptake from the respiratory tract.[147] In animal studies, bioavailability of ET lidocaine is 90%. In patients undergoing elective surgery, lidocaine levels reached therapeutic plasma levels comparable to iv administration, albeit more slowly, but within minutes.[158] Endotracheal administration of 2 mg/kg of lidocaine, diluted with normal saline to a total volume of 10 ml, resulted in therapeutic action after 30 seconds.[159] One of the few studies undertaken under CPR conditions was Elam's bradycardia/ventricular standstill model in which ET lidocaine suppressed premature ventricular contractions (PVCs) after 11 seconds, while the same dose of IV lidocaine took 43 seconds.[140] The duration of action was 43 versus 17 minutes, respectively. Therapeutic levels were not achieved in plasma in all animals treated with ET lidocaine.[160] In a human study of 17 patients with ET therapy, 14 were found to have insufficient plasma levels of lidocaine (below

given endobronchially.[147] The investigators considered endobronchial administration a reliable alternative to iv injection. Earlier, Schuettler *et al.* had reported successful resuscitation of 7 of 19 out-of-hospital cardiac arrest victims who received only ET epinephrine.[146] Several case reports document the feasibility of ET therapy in children as well as in adults, recommending an ET dose of 0.1 mg/kg of epinephrine.[148–150]

A side effect of endotracheal epinephrine therapy is the "depot-like" effect.[146] Five minutes after ET administration, blood concentrations were 80% of the initial value, and this high level persisted for 30 minutes, whereas only

1.5 mg/ml), whereas 1 patient had more than the therapeutic value of 5 mg/ml.[161]

In summary, clinically significant lidocaine levels can be achieved by ET therapy when a large bolus is administered, but plasma lidocaine levels are not exactly predictable. The ILCOR Guidelines 2000 recommended a 2 to 2.5 times larger bolus endotracheally than intravenously (2–3.2 mg/kg).[150] Endotracheal application of other antiarrythmics, e.g., amiodarone, is not feasible.

Atropine

Elam found that ET administration of 2 mg of atropine in 10 ml of water produced an ECG-response after 16 seconds, compared to 54 seconds for IV delivery. This effect lasted for 10 vs. 6 minutes.[140] Nevertheless, ET atropine doses were up to 0.8 mg higher than those given iv. Fifteen minutes after endobronchial application, atropine levels were almost four times higher than after IV application. As a clinical response can be found even with low plasma atropine levels, the clinical significance of measuring atropine levels is not clear.

Bray et al.[162] administered 0.6 mg of atropine to anesthetized patients either iv or ET (1 ml of solution deep endobronchially followed by five manual hyperinflations). The maximal increase in heart rate was similar in ET- or iv-treated patients. The effect of endobronchial atropine persisted for only 4 minutes in contrast to 9 minutes after IV application.

A few case reports are available on the ET use of atropine in human CPR,[163] but prospective studies did not demonstrate any efficacy of atropine.[164] In one study with 170 patients in asystole, 43 patients received atropine. Six (14%) were resuscitated, compared with none of 37 patients in the control group.[165]

Even though atropine is recommended early in the treatment of cardiac arrest, it is usually not given until 2 to 3 minutes into resuscitation.[150] Consequently, in most cases an iv line will be established when administration of atropine is considered, and this route should be used. Alternatively, 2 to 3 mg can be given ET, but few data support this method of application. Use of atropine for treatment of bradycardia or heart block, however, is strongly recommended.[150]

Sodium bicarbonate

In one study by Bauer in an animal model, as reported by Elam, inactivation of surfactant by alkalinization rendered the lung atelectatic. High levels of positive end-expiratory pressure resulted in circulatory deterioration, and the endotracheal application of sodium bicarbonate was discouraged.[140]

Summary

Whenever possible, iv or io application is favored because there is no evidence of benefit by endotracheal drug administration.[166,167] In congruence with ILCOR and ERC guidelines, we recommend this method of drug administration during CPR whenever an iv line is not in place before the arrest and the establishment of other routes is delayed.[110,150,157]

Intracardiac administration

Advantages

Promoters of this technique have stressed the ease of injection[168] and the low risk.[169,170] There are no clinical outcome data, however, that have demonstrated an advantage for the IC route over intravascular or ET routes[30,171] in spite of the extensive use of IC routes for CPR over many years. Administration of drugs to the left ventricle should reduce the time-to-peak interval to a minimum, but autopsy studies in 18 cadavers after CPR with 46 intracardiac (IC) injections (5 subxiphoid punctures) revealed left ventricular puncture in only 5 (11%) cases. All other injections ended either in the right ventricule in (28%), the pulmonary trunk, the ascending aorta, the lung, or were untraceable.[172] Thus, in most instances the effect at best will be similar to central venous administration. In the few cases of successful left ventricular injection, this means of drug administration might be superior to administration to the right side of the heart.[173]

Techniques

Either the subxiphoid or the left sternal approach are commonly recommended for intracardiac injections.

Subxiphoid

The subxiphoid injection is considered safer than a transthoracic injection. A long needle is inserted from 1 cm left of the xiphoid process at a 20°- to 30°-angle in both the sagittal and vertical plane, with continuous withdrawal of the plunger on needle insertion. If no blood appears as the needle is fully inserted, the needle is withdrawn under suction and redirected in another angle. No injections should be performed without prior aspiration of blood, as it is essential to inject into the ventricular lumen.

Left sternal

In the left sternal approach, the needle is inserted from the fourth or fifth left intercostal space, immediately left of the sternum. It should be directed toward the vertebral column of the patient. Laceration of the left anterior descending artery or the internal mammary artery is a special hazard of this approach.[174,175]

Complications

Intramyocardial injections of epinephrine or sodium bicarbonate inevitably lead to extensive myocardial necrosis. Interestingly, Forssman's development of right ventricle catheterization in 1929 was originally stimulated by the need to replace IC injections because of the high rates of laceration of the coronary artery and subsequent hemopericardium associated with the method.[14] Because of difficulties in placing the needle in a ventricular cavity, there is a possibility for delay.[30] In one study, all patients developed serosanguineous pericardial fluid after ic injections, whereas patients without this route of drug delivery exhibited almost no pericardial fluid after CPR.[176] In that study, cardiac puncture was documented in only 3 of 65 cases at autopsy. With right ventricular puncture, there is no self-sealing as occurs with left ventricular puncture.[177] Even when only a small amount of fluid is present in the cardiac sac, hemopericardium can further compromise the already reduced cardiac output.[170] Other complications include pneumothorax,[178] pneumopericardium, cardiac tamponade[179] and successive death,[180] laceration of the myocardium, coronary artery, and internal mammary artery, intramyocardial injection with ventricular arrhythmia,[181] intractable ventricular fibrillation,[182] persisting total arteriovenous block after injection into the interventricular septum,[183] and bacterial endocarditis.

Animal studies

Three well-performed studies have been published claiming the superiority of left ventricular injection of epinephrine. Showen _et al._ demonstrated a faster onset of action for the left vs. the right ventricular route for dogs with pulseless electrical activity.[184] Left ventricular but not aortic injection of epinephrine in dogs was superior with respect to time to reach a 20% increase in heart rate and a 10% increase in mean arterial pressure, but not in peak mean artery pressure itself when compared to right ventricular injection.[185] In mongrel dogs, injection of 1 mg of epinephrine into the descending aortic arch during CPR resulted in a doubling of coronary perfusion pressure within 10 seconds, whereas administration to the superior vena cava was not followed by a detectable change.[173] Nevertheless, this approach is highly impracticable in the CPR setting as most ic injections result in right ventricular drug delivery,[172] whereas left ventricular catheterization would result

in an unacceptable delay compared to ET or IV routes. In addition, in another study on dogs, time-to-therapeutic level in the aorta during CPR was about 30 seconds after both right and left ventricular injection.[58]

Human studies

Several older studies in patients with out-of-hospital CPR have claimed that IC injections can be done with an acceptable rate of (noted) side effects, but none has prospectively demonstrated the superiority of this method over another.[169,170,186,187] In one study, as many as 24% of patients with intracardiac medication developed pneumothoraces, compared to only 3% in the group with iv therapy.[186] Davison _et al._[170] reported that 31% of patients developed hemopericardium after ic injection.

Comparisons with intravenous/endotracheal access

In dogs, the time from intracardiac administration of 1 mg of epinephrine to ROSC was marginally slower than with peripheral intravenous injection (139 ± 34 vs. 127 ± 76 seconds).[30] ET access resulted in a mean time to ROSC of 132 ± 44 seconds when 1 mg of epinephrine was diluted with water and 217 ± 142 seconds when it was diluted with saline. The investigators' conclusion was that "intratracheal (diluted), intravenous, and intracardiac routes are equally effective." When central venous administration of lidocaine in dogs with open-chest CPR was compared to left ventricular and peripheral venous administration, there were no differences in the appearance of significant amounts at the level of the coronary artery ostia.[58,106]

Recommendations/summary

AHA guidelines indicate that the intracardiac route should be used during open chest massage or when other routes are unavailable.[188] In our opinion, IV, ET, and intraosseous routes with well-documented effectiveness have fewer side effects, and IC injections during CPR should be avoided.

Other routes of drug administration

Oral transmucosal drug absorption (sublingual and buccal)

Systemic effects are known to occur quickly following sublingual drug administration. Captopril, beta agonists, and benzodiazepines have all been shown to enter the central circulation rapidly when placed in liquid form under the tongue.[189] Several transmucosally administered cardiovascular drugs have been studied extensively, e.g., nitroglycerin.[190] Research on captopril, verapamil, nifedipine, propafenone, and others has proven promising.[191–193] Arnold *et al.* used intraglossal atropine in a large series of children undergoing strabismus surgery, and have shown better effects through this route than through the intravenous route.[194]

Epinephrine

Limited data are available on intralingual administration of epinephrine. Ordog and coworkers[195] used a goat model to simulate the effect of sublingual injections on pediatric patients. Sublingual injection of Cardio-Green in kid goats undergoing internal cardiac massage is associated with a tenfold lower central blood level compared to that after peripheral injection, and the authors recommended obtaining a central line. Rothrock *et al.* reported on a 7-month-old successfully resuscitated with intralingual epinephrine and atropine injected into the midline of the sublingual tissues.[196] Redding and coworkers reported that the injection of 1 mg/1ml of epinephrine into the tongues of dogs undergoing CPR resulted in ROSC in only 2 of 10 animals, whereas injection into the thigh muscles saved 4 of 10 dogs. The mean time from injection to ROSC was 292 (intralingual) versus 50 (intramuscular) seconds.[30]

Given the ease of administration of epinephrine via the endotracheal and intraosseous routes, the potential necrosis of sublingual tissues, and the limited experience with intralingual epinephrine, this route cannot be recommended as an alternative for drug administration.

Vasopressin

A synthetic form of vasopressin, desmopressin, has been used to treat diabetes insipidus. The sublingual route of administration has been suggested as an alternative to the usual one via intranasal administration.[197] In a study comparing pharmacokinetics and biological effects of vasopressin in eight healthy volunteers who were administered desmopressin by several routes, including sublingual, bioavailability was found to be 3.4% after intranasal administration and 0.1% after oral administration.[198]

De Groot and coworkers assessed the bioavailability and pharmacokinetics of oxytocin in six male subjects after sublingual dose of 400 IU (684 μg) and after an intravenous dose of 1 IU (1.71 μg).[199]After sublingual administration, poor bioavailability with 10-fold variation between 0.007%–0.07% was observed. The authors suggested that the sublingual route of administration with its "long" lag time and "long" absorption half-life does not seem to provide reliable, accurate high dosing for immediate prevention of postpartum hemorrhage.

Naloxone

A rapid effect of intralingual naloxone was demonstrated in dogs by Maio *et al.*[200] Ventilation increased well above baseline and control levels at 1 minute after administration. In a human study, Maio *et al.* reported a reversal of narcotic-induced respiratory depression in a 25-year-old man following the administration of intralingual naloxone.[201] Wasserberger *et al.* recommended intralingual naloxone injections only when patients are in shock, have a systolic blood pressure <80 mmHg, and there is no iv line or endotracheal tube in place.[202]

Midazolam

Buccal administration of midazolam has been shown to be very effective when compared with nasal and rectal formulations. High bioavailability and reliable plasma concentrations after buccal administration of midazolam have been reported in healthy volunteers by Schwagmeier *et al.*[203] Scott *et al.* aimed to determine whether there are differences in efficacy and adverse events between buccal administration of liquid midazolam and rectal administration of liquid diazepam in the acute treatment of seizures.[204] They found the buccal cavity easy to reach safely, and suggest that the buccal administration of midazolam seems to have some distinct advantages over rectal administration of diazepam. Geldner and coworkers[205] found plasma concentrations of midazolam were significantly higher following sublingual administration compared with nasal administration with better acceptance by patients.

Intranasal drug delivery

The nasal mucosal surface provides a suitable route for many drugs with molecular weights <1000.[206] Drugs sprayed into the nasal mucosa are rapidly absorbed by three routes: the olfactory neurons, the supporting cells and the surrounding capillary bed, and by the transneuronal route through the cerebrospinal fluid. Transneuronal absorption is generally slow, whereas absorption by the supporting cells and the capillary bed is rapid.[207]

For some drugs, administration by nasal spray results in a greater CSF-to-plasma concentration than does iv administration, providing evidence for diffusion of these compounds through the perineural space around the olfactory nerves, a compartment known to be continuous with the subarachnoid space.[208,209] In one study, drops were found to cover the wall of the nasal cavity more effectively than nasal sprays, independent of the volume administered, while another study reported that both forms were equally effective.[210] Absorption rates are also influenced by the site of deposition and by concomitant pathologic conditions, such as rhinitis.[211]

Vasopressin and corticosteroids were among the first drugs to be administered by this route.[212,213] Sedatives,[214–216] potent narcotics, and a variety of drugs that are used in emergency medicine such as ketamine,[217] sufentanil, verapamil, metoclopramide,[218] nitroglycerin, salbutamol,[219] digoxin,[220] atropine,[221] and anticonvulsants[222] have been employed.

Drug administration

Epinephrine

Early animal studies found that sympathomimetics, such as adrenaline and ephedrine, did not penetrate the nasal mucosa of the frontal sinuses of cats and dogs.[223] Similarly, Myers and Iazzetta found no significant changes in heart rate and blood pressure in humans after intranasal administration of phenylephrine.[224] Shapiro and Grenvik, however, described a patient with C1 tetraplegia who responded to nasal phenylephrine,[225] and differing results from several other animal studies have also been published. Yamada demonstrated that epinephrine plasma concentrations increased substantially following administration of epinephrine in the nasal septal mucosa:[226] the mean peak value of the plasma epinephrine (20.1 ± 12.4 ng/ml) was obtained after 15 seconds, and the peak systolic pressure was 200% of the control value after 60 seconds.

In a dog model of closed chest CPR, intranasal delivery of epinephrine (28 mg) produced the same increase in aortic systolic and aortic diastolic perfusion pressures as did 0.015 mg/kg of iv epinephrine.[65] Further studies by the same group suggested that the optimal combinations of nasally administered epinephrine and phentolamine to improve coronary perfusion pressure in a canine model were 0.25 and 7.5 mg/kg/nostril, respectively.[227] In addition, continuous nasal absorption of epinephrine maintained pressures over a prolonged period of time.

Naloxone

Loimer *et al.* compared intranasal naloxone to other routes (intravenous/intramuscular) in 17 opiate-dependent patients and found the nasal route to be as effective as the iv route.[228] In the study by Barton *et al.*, a total of 30 patients received intranasal naloxone by paramedics in the field: 11 responded to either intranasal or iv naloxone. Ten of these 11 (91%) patients responded to intranasal naloxone alone, with an average response time of 3.4 minutes and seven (7/11, 64%) did not require an iv line.[229]

When intranasal was compared to intramuscular naloxone for treatment of respiratory depression due to suspected opiate overdose in the prehospital setting, intranasal delivery was less effective as than intramuscular treatment.[230]

Further research and recommendations

The sublingual/intralingual and the intranasal routes offer a variety of opportunities for drug delivery, including bypassing the gastrointestinal tract and first-pass metabolism in the liver. There are, however, no validated studies addressing the pharmacokinetic and pharmacodynamic issues, such as optimal injection site, circulation times, time-to-peak effect, duration of action, and ROSC. Optimal volume and concentration levels need to be determined. The nasal route could be important for drugs that are used in crisis treatments, such as for pain, and for centrally acting drugs where the putative pathway from the nose to the brain might provide a more rapid and more specific effect. Explorations for novel nasal and transmucosal drug delivery systems, drug carriers and their exploitation for their administration of drugs are being actively pursued.[231] The products developed will first comprise products for crisis management, such as sleep induction, acute pain, nausea, and heart attacks.[232] Until appropriate studies have been completed, however, it is advisable not to administer resuscitation drugs through this route.

Experimental techniques

Several additional routes that are not currently in clinical use are available for drug administration during CPR. In animal studies, selective perfusion of the aortic arch has been shown to improve aortic pressures and carotid artery flow.[233] By occluding the distal aorta with a balloon catheter and infusing normal saline, the aortic arch to right atrial pressure gradient increased from 2 mmHg before infusion to 9 mmHg after 60 seconds. The investigators concluded that solutions that could improve cardiac and cerebral function can be delivered by this method. In another study, aortic arch instillation of epinephrine led to greater improvement in coronary perfusion pressures than did administration by superior vena cava.[173] The time to achieve a postarrest systolic blood pressure of 60 mmHg was shortest for the animals given aortic epinephrine, and the aortic arch pressure consistently rose within 10 seconds to a plateau after 40 to 60 seconds. ROSC was seen in all eight animals given epinephrine via the aortic arch, and time-to-ROSC was short-

Table 33.1. Cardiopulmonary drugs: routes of administration and recommended dosages

	Intravenous/Intraosseous	Endobronchial	Sub-/intralingual	Intranasal
Epinephrine	1 mg	2–3 mg	1 mg[a]	Not recommended
Lidocaine	1.5 mg/kg	400–500 mg[a]	Not recommended	Not recommended
Atropine	1 mg	2.5 mg[a]	Not recommended	Not recommended
Naloxone	0.4–0.8 mg	1.2–2.4 mg[a]	0.4 mg[a]	Not recommended

[a] Insufficient data, not routinely recommended.

est with epinephrine given via the aortic arch rather than via the superior vena cava. In contrast, Rubertsson *et al.* found no difference in coronary perfusion pressures or survival in dogs when 100 μg/kg of intra-aortic or central venous epinephrine was given combined with aortic occlusion during experimental CPR.[234] When central venous and left atrial infusion of norepinephrine were compared in a canine model of cardiopulmonary bypass,[235] there was no difference in hemodynamic efficacy over a wide range of three doses in a model with normal lungs. In one study by Fullerton's *et al.*, on aorto-coronary bypass patients, left atrial administration of epinephrine produced a 35% greater cardiac output, 25% lower pulmonary artery pressure, and 32% lower pulmonary vascular resistance than did central venous administration.[236] Cardiopulmonary bypass has been utilized in canine resuscitation models,[237] which provides another mechanism to administer medication to the central circulation. Notably, these techniques, while interesting, remain experimental and have not been proven outside of the laboratory at this time.

Summary (Table 33.1)

The choice of route for drug administration during CPR must be made on an individual basis and requires consideration of the speed with which access can be obtained, the technical difficulties with performing the procedure, associated risk of complications, delays in drug delivery to the central circulation, duration of effective drug levels following their injection, and magnitude of peak drug levels. The peripheral venous route is the safest method and drug delivery can be enhanced by saline bolus after medication injection. Central venous cannulation provides more direct access to the central circulation, although with some risk of complications. Circulation time is shortest and drug concentrations are highest when this route is used. The femoral route is associated with delays in drug delivery and a higher incidence of unsuccessful catheterization. Its use should be reserved for instances when other routes of drug

administration are not available. The endotracheal tube is a route for administration of most drugs, but peak concentrations are lower than those obtained by other routes. The intraosseous route should be utilized in resuscitation of children when iv access cannot be obtained promptly. Intraosseous injection can also be an option in adults.

The ultimate goal of vascular access during CPR should be to contribute to oxygen delivery to the cardiac and cerebral circulation at a sufficiently high pressure to ensure perfusion. Although almost all administration routes can deliver drugs to the central circulation, there are only limited human data comparing the effectiveness of one route over another and at establishing ROSC. The few available studies either had limited numbers of subjects or had not controlled for confounding variables. Even adequate animal models comparing resuscitation rates among different routes of venous access are lacking. The information given above can provide some guidelines to aid in the choice of routes for administration. The goal of future studies should be to determine which routes of administration provide the best opportunity for ROSC. New techniques such as aortic arch perfusion, combined with the development of resuscitation fluids and medications that can establish critical coronary and cerebral perfusion, offer other promising areas for research.

Recommendations

We prefer to initiate drug therapy with the first available route. In adults this generally means administering endotracheal drugs while peripheral access is attempted. Endotracheal administration is accompanied by a 10-ml flush with either saline or water and followed by forceful hyperinflations. Peripheral catheterization is attempted during or immediately after intubation. Administration by this route is followed by a 20-ml saline bolus. If peripheral access is not rapidly accomplished after intubation, an attempt is made to cannulate the external jugular vein. Central venous cannulation is almost always unwarranted in the acute setting. Very exceptionally, a venous cutdown will be needed. Percutaneous cannulation of the femoral vein has a low success rate but may also be used if no other route is available. Finally, in the patient with no other access, medications may be administered by intraosseous injection.

In children, drug therapy is initiated through the endotracheal tube, while attempts are made to obtain peripheral placement. If peripheral access is not obtained within a few minutes, an intraosseous line is placed. Central venous and external jugular lines or venous cutdown are used rarely in children and only when the peripheral and intraosseous routes cannot be used.

The above constitutes our personal preferences. The more invasive procedures carry risks that some practitioners would not consider justifiable. Given the lack of evidence to establish the importance of utilizing a particular protocol for venous access, it is difficult to argue against another, less invasive approach. Finally, even more aggressive approaches exist, such as the use of intraaortic injection, along with balloon counterpulsation or cardiopulmonary bypass, but these approaches currently remain within the investigator's domain.

REFERENCES

1. Schechter, D.C. Role of humane societies in the history of resuscitation. *Surg. Gynecol. Obstet.* 1969; **129**: 811–815.
2. Keith, A. Three hunterian lectures on the various mechanisms underlying the various methods of artificial respiration. *Lancet* 1909; **1**: 748.
3. Luckhardt, A.B. Instruction on the manner in which one can be of help in saving the life of the drowned. Published at the command of the high-magistrates in the year 1779, 1938.
4. Cary, R.I. A brief history of the methods of resuscitation of the apparently drowned. *Johns Hopkins Hosp. Bull* 1913; **24**: 243–251.
5. Hosack, D. An enquiry into the causes of suspended animation from drowning with the means of restoring life. New York, 1792.
6. Sudhoff, K. Eine Bronzespritze aus dem Altertum. *Arch. Ges. Med.* 1908; **1**: 75–78.
7. Alexandria, Ho. Opera quae supersunt omnia. Leipzig: Schmidt W, 1899.
8. Harvey, W. Exercitatio anatomica de motu cordis et sanguinis in animalibus. 1628.
9. Wren, C. An account of the rise and attempts of a way to conveigh liquors immediately into the mass of blood. *Phil. Trans.* 1665; **1**: 128–130.
10. Clarck, T. A letter, written to the publisher by the learned and experienced Dr. TC, concerning some anatomical inventions and observations, particularly the origin of the injections into veins, the transfusion of blood, and the parts of generation. *Phil. Trans. R. Soc. Lond. [Biol.]* 1668; **35**: 672–682.
11. Elsholtz, JS. Clysmatica nova; 1667.
12. Morris, N. The history of cardiac resuscitation, vol. 15. St. Louis: CV Mosby; 1958.
13. Arnaud, H. Experiences pour décider si le coeur et le centre respiratoire, ayant cessé d'agir, sont irrevocablement morts. *Arch. Physiol. Norm. Path.* 1891; **3**: 396–400.
14. Forssmann, W. Die Sondierung des rechten Herzens. *Klin. Wschr.* 1929; **8**: 2085–2086.
15. Cournand, A.F. & Ranges, H.S. Catheterization of the right auricle in man. *Proc. Soc. Exp. Biol. Med.* 1941; **46**: 462–466.
16. Meyers, L. Intravenous catheterization. *Am. J. Nurs.* 1945; **45**: 930.
17. Duffy, B.J., Jr. The clinical use of polyethylene tubing for intravenous therapy; a report on 72 cases. *Ann. Surg.* 1949; **130**(5): 929–936.
18. Aubaniac, R. Une nouvelle voie d'injection ou de poncture veineuse: la voie claviculare. *Sem. Hop. Paris.* 1952; **28**: 3445.
19. Seldinger, S.I. Catheter replacement of the needle in percutaneous arteriography: a new technique. *Acta Radiol.* 1953; **39**(5): 368–376.
20. Jude, J.R., Kouwenhoven, W.B., & Knickerbocker, G.G. External cardiac resuscitation. *Monogr. Surg. Sci.* 1964; **1**: 59–117.
21. Kouwenhoven, W.B., Jude, J.R. & Knickerbocker, G.G. Closed chest cardiac massage. *J. Am. Med. Assoc.* 1960; **173**: 1064–1067.
22. Swan, H.J., Ganz, W., Forrester, J., Marcus, H., Diamond, G. & Chonette, D. Catheterization of the heart in man with the use of a flow-guided balloon-tipped catheter. *N. Engl. J. Med.* 1970; **283**(9): 447–451.
23. Jernigan, W.R., Gardner, W.C., Mahr, M.M. & Milburn, J.L. Use of the internal jugular vein for placement of central venous catheter. *Surg. Gynecol. Obstet.* 1970; **130**(3): 520–524.
24. Steiner, F. Ueber die Electropunctur des Herzens als Wiederbelebungsmittel in der Chloroformsyncope, zugleich eine Studie ueber Stichwunden des Herzens. *Arch. Klin. Chir.* 1871; **12**: 741–790.
25. Crile, G.W. & Dolley, D.H. An experimental research into the resuscitation of dogs killed by anesthetics and asphyxia. *J. Exp. Med.* 1906: 713–715.
26. von den Velden, R. Die intrakardiale Injektion. *Muenchner Med. Wochenschr.* 1919; **66**: 274–275.
27. Vogt, E. Anatomische und technische Fragen zur intrakardialen Injektion. *Deutsche Med. Wochenschr.* 1921; **47**: 1491–1492.
28. Greuel, W. Zur intrakardialen Injektion. *Berl. Klin. Wchnschr.* 1921; **58**: 1381–1384.
29. Kneier, G. Ueber initiale Adrenalininjektion bei akuter Herzlaehmung. *Deutsche Med. Wochenschr.* 1921; **47**: 1490–1491.
30. Redding, J.S., Asuncion, J.W. & Pearson J.W. Effective routes of drug administration during cardiac arrest. *Anesth. Analg.* 1967; **46**: 253–258.
31. Holzmann, M. Der kardiale Zusammenbruch, vol. 20: Hippokrates, 1961.

32. Rothschuh, K.E. Geschichte der Physiologie. Berlin, Göttingen, Heidelberg: Springer, 1953.

33. Krimer, W. Die Acupunctur als Belebungsmittel bei Ersaeuften und durch Steinkohlendampf Erstickten. *J. Chir. Augenheilk.* 1829; **13**: 520–523.

34. Vesalius, A. De humanis corporis fabricia. Basel; 1543.

35. Bernard, C. Lecons sur les effets des substances toxiques et medicamenteuses. Paris: Baillière, 1857.

36. Mutch, N. Inhalation of chemotherapeutic substances. *Lancet* 1944; **2**: 775–780.

37. Meltzer, S.J. & Auer, J. Eine Vergleichung der "Volhardschen Methode der kuenstlichen Atmung" mit der von Meltzer und Auer in der kontinuierlichen Respiration ohne respiratorische Bewegung verwendeten Methode. *Zentralbl. Physiol.* 1909; **23**: 210–213.

38. Kline, B.S. & Winternitz, M.C. Studies upon experimental pneumonia in rabbits. VIII. Intra vitam staining in experimental pneumonia, and the circulation in the pneumonic lung. *J. Exp. Med.* 1915; **21**: 311–319.

39. Graeser, J.B. & Rowe, A.H. Inhalation of epinephrine for the relief of asthmatic symptoms. *J. Allergy Clin. Immunol.* 1935; **6**: 415–420.

40. Barach, A.L., Molomut, N. & Soroka, M. Inhalation of nebulized promin in experimental tuberculosis. *Am. Rev. Tuberculosis* 1942; **46**: 268–276.

41. Bryson, V., Sansome, E. & Laskin, S. Aerosolisation of penicillin solutions. *Science* 1944; **100**: 33–35.

42. May, H.B. & Floyer, M.A. Infected bronchiectasis treated with intratracheal penicillin. *Br. Med. J.* 1945; **1**: 907–908.

43. Norris, C.M. Sulfonamides in bronchial secretion. *J. Am. Med. Assoc.* 1943; **123**: 667–670.

44. Segal, M.S., Levinson, L. & Miller, D. Penicillin inhalation therapy in respiratory infections. *J. Am. Med. Assoc.* 1947; **143**: 762–770.

45. Stacey, J.W. The inhalation of nebulized solutions of sulfonamides in the treatment of bronchiectasis. *Dis. Chest* 1943; **9**: 302–306.

46. Adilani, F.H. & Campbell, O. Fatalities following topical applications of local anesthetics to mucous membranes. *J. Am. Med. Assoc.* 1956; **162**: 1527–1530.

47. Campbell, D. & Adriani, J. Absorption of local anesthetics. *J. Am. Med. Assoc.* 1958; **168**: 873–877.

48. Chin, S.S., Rah, K.H., Brannan, M.D. & Cohen, J.L. Plasma concentrations of lidocaine after endotracheal spray. *Anesth. Analg.* 1974; **54**: 438–441.

49. Curran, J., Hamilton, C. & Taylor, T. Topical analgesia before tracheal intubation. *Anaesthesia* 1975; **30**(6): 765–768.

50. Derbes, V.J. & Engelhardt, H.T. Deaths following the use of local anesthetics in transcricoid therapy: a critical review. *J. Lab. Clin. Med.* 1944; **29**: 478–482.

51. Rubin, H.J. & Kully, B.M. Speed of administration as related to the toxicity of certain topical anesthetics. *Ann. Otol. Rhinol. Laryngol.* 1951; **69**: 627–630.

52. Steinhaus, J.E. A comparative study of the experimental toxicity of local anesthetic agents. *Anesthesiology* 1952; **13**: 577–586.

53. Drinker, C.K., Drinker, K.R. & Lund, C.C. The circulation in the mammalian bone marrow. *Am. J. Physiol.* 1922; **62**: 1–92.

54. Doan, C. The circulation of bone marrow. *Contrib. Embryol.* 1922; **14**: 27.

55. Tocantins, L.M. Rapid absorption of substances injected into the bone marrow. *Proc. Soc. Exp. Biol. Med.* 1940; **45**: 292–296.

56. Turkel, H. Intraosseous infusion. *Am. J. Dis. Child.* 1983; **137**(7): 706.

57. Emerman, C.L., Pinchak, A.C., Hancock, D. & Hagen, J.F. Effect of injection site on circulation times during cardiac arrest. *Crit. Care Med.* 1988; **16**: 1138–1141.

58. Barsan, W.G., Levy, R.C. & Weir, H. Lidocaine levels during CPR: differences after peripheral venous, central venous, and intracardiac injections. *Ann. Emerg. Med.* 1981; **10**: 73–78.

59. Gueugniaud, P.Y., Theurey, O., Vaudelin, T., Rochette, M. & Petit, P. Peripheral versus central intravenous lines in emergency cardiac care. *Lancet* 1987; **2**(8558): 573.

60. Emerman, C.L., Pinchak, A.C., Hancock, D. & Hagen, J.F. The effect of bolus injection on circulation times during cardiac arrest. *Am. J. Emerg. Med.* 1990; **8**(3): 190–193.

61. Fontanarosa, P.B. Superbolusing: an intravenous technique in advanced cardiac life support. New Orleans, 1982.

62. Dolister, M., Gaddis, G.M. & Gaddis, M.L. A comparison of effects of central versus peripheral drug administration plus different sized postinfusion flushes on drug delivery to the aortic root in a canine cardiac arrest model. *Ann. Emerg. Med.* 1993; **22**: 930.

63. Gaddis, G.M., Dolister, M. & Gaddis, M.L. Mock drug delivery to the proximal aorta during cardiopulmonary resuscitation: central vs peripheral intravenous infusion with varying flush volumes. *Acad. Emerg. Med.* 1995; **2**(12): 1027–1033.

64. Quinton, D.N., O'Byrne, G. & Aitkenhead, A.R. Comparison of endotracheal and peripheral intravenous adrenaline in cardiac arrest. *Lancet* 1987: 828–829.

65. Bleske, B.E., Warren, E.W., Rice, T.L., Shea, M.J., Amidon, G. & Knight, P. Comparison of intravenous and intranasal administration of epinephrine during CPR in a canine model. *Ann. Emerg. Med.* 1992; **21**(9): 1125–1130.

66. Getzen, L.C. & Pollak, E.W. Short-term femoral vein catheterization. A safe alternative venous access? *Am. J. Surg.* 1979; **138**(6): 875–878.

67. Swanson, R.S., Uhlig, P.N., Gross, P.L. & McCabe, C.J. Emergency intravenous access through the femoral vein. *Ann. Emerg. Med.* 1984; **13**(4): 244–247.

68. Niemann, J.T., Rosborough, J.P., Hausknecht, M., Garner, D. & Criley, J.M. Pressure-synchronized cineangiography during experimental cardiopulmonary resuscitation. *Circulation* 1981; **64**(5): 985–991.

69. Dalsey, W.C., Barsan, W.G., Joyce, S.M., Hedges, J.R., Lukes, S.J. & Doan, L.A. Comparison of superior vena caval and inferior vena caval access using a radioisotope technique during normal perfusion and cardiopulmonary resuscitation. *Ann. Emerg. Med.* 1984; **13**(10): 881–884.

70. Jastremski, M.S., Matthias, H.D. & Randell, P.A. Femoral venous catheterization during cardiopulmonary resusci-

tation: a critical appraisal. *J. Emerg. Med.* 1984; **1**(5): 387–391.

71. Emerman, C.L., Bellon, E.M., Lukens, T.W., May, T.E. & Effron, D. A prospective study of femoral versus subclavian vein catheterization during cardiac arrest. *Ann. Emerg. Med.* 1990; **19**(1): 26–30.

72. Chiang, V.W. & Baskin, M.N. Uses and complications of central venous catheters inserted in a pediatric emergency department. *Pediatr. Emerg. Care* 2000; **16**(4): 230–232.

73. Talit, U., Braun, S., Halkin, H., Shargorodsky, B. & Laniado, S: Pharmacokinetic differences between peripheral and central drug administration during cardiopulmonary resuscitation. *J. Am. Coll. Cardiol.* 1985; **6**(5): 1073–1077.

74. Kuhn, G.J., White, B.C., Swetnam, R.E., *et al.* Peripheral vs central circulation times during CPR: a pilot study. *Ann. Emerg. Med.* 1981; **10**(8): 417–419.

75. Eisenhauer, E.D., Derveloy, R.J. & Hastings, P.R. Prospective evaluation of central venous pressure (CVP) catheters in a large city-county hospital. *Ann. Surg.* 1982; **196**(5): 560–564.

76. Rubio, P.A. & Farrell, E.M. Percutaneous infraclavicular subclavian catheterization. *Am. Surg.* 1982; **48**(5): 230–231.

77. Dronen, S., Thompson, B., Nowak, R. & Tomlanovich, M. Subclavian vein catheterization during cardiopulmonary resuscitation. A prospective comparison of the supraclavicular and infraclavicular percutaneous approaches. *J. Am. Med. Assoc.* 1982; **247**(23): 3227–3230.

78. Rossetti, V., Thompson, B. & Aprahamian, C. Difficulty and delay in intravascular access in pediatric patients. *Ann. Emerg. Med.* 1984; **13**: 406.

79. Lillis, K.A. & Jaffe, D.M. Prehospital intravenous access in children. *Ann. Emerg. Med.* 1992; **21**(12): 1430–1434.

80. Fuchs, S., LaCovey, D. & Paris, P. A prehospital model of intraosseous infusion. *Ann. Emerg. Med.* 1991; **20**(4): 371–374.

81. Zaritsky, A. Drug therapy of cardiopulmonary resuscitation in children. *Drugs* 1989; **37**(3): 356–374.

82. Valdes, M.M. Intraosseous fluid administration in emergencies. *Lancet* 1977; **1**(8024): 1235–1236.

83. Iserson, K.V. Intraosseous infusions in adults. *J. Emerg. Med.* 1989; **7**(6): 587–591.

84. Clem, M. & Tierney, P. Intraosseous infusions via the calcaneus. *Resuscitation* 2004; **62**(1): 107–112.

85. Shoor, P.M., Berryhill, R.E. & Benumof, J.L. Intraosseous infusion: pressure-flow relationship and pharmacokinetics. *J. Trauma* 1979; **19**(10): 772–774.

86. Hodge, D., 3rd, Delgado-Paredes, C. & Fleisher, G. Intraosseous infusion flow rates in hypovolemic "pediatric" dogs. *Ann. Emerg. Med.* 1987; **16**(3): 305–307.

87. Iserson, K.V. & Criss, E. Intraosseous infusions: a usable technique. *Am. J. Emerg. Med.* 1986; **4**(6): 540–542.

88. LaSpada, J., Kissoon, N., Melker, R., Murphy, S., Miller, G. & Peterson, R. Extravasation rates and complications of intraosseous needles during gravity and pressure infusion. *Crit. Care Med.* 1995; **23**(12): 2023–2028.

89. Spivey, W.H. Intraosseous infusions. *J. Pediatr.* 1987; **111**(5): 639–643.

90. Rosetti, V.A., Thompson, B.M., Miller, J., Mateer, J.R. & Aprahamian, C. Intraosseous infusion: an alternative route of pediatric intravascular access. *Ann. Emerg. Med.* 1985; **14**(9): 885–888.

91. Fiser, D.H. Intraosseous infusion. *N. Engl. J. Med.* 1990; **322**(22): 1579–1581.

92. Calkins, M.D., Fitzgerald, G., Bentley, T.B. & Burris, D. Intraosseous infusion devices: a comparison for potential use in special operations. *J. Trauma* 2000; **48**(6): 1068–1074.

93. Curran, A. & Sen, A. Best evidence topic report. Bone injection gun placement of intraosseous needles. *Emerg. Med. J* 2005; **22**(5): 366.

94. Orlowski, J.P. Emergency alternatives to intravenous access. Intraosseous, intratracheal, sublingual, and other-site drug administration. *Pediatr. Clin. North Am.* 1994; **41**(6): 1183–1199.

95. Arbeiter, H. & Greengrad, J. Tibial bone marrow infusions in infancy. *J. Pediatr* 1944; **25**: 1–12.

96. Bowley, D.M., Loveland, J. & Pitcher, G.J. Tibial fracture as a complication of intraosseous infusion during pediatric resuscitation. *J. Trauma* 2003; **55**(4): 786–787.

97. Heinild, S., Sondergaard, T. & Tudvad, F. Bone marrow infusion in childhood: experiences from a thousand infusions. *J. Pediatr.* 1947; **30**: 400–412.

98. Fortner, J.G. & Moss, E.S. Death following sternal puncture: report of two cases. *Ann. Intern. Med.* 1951; **34**(3): 809–815.

99. Orlowski, J.P., Porembka, D.T., Gallagher, J.M., Lockrem, J.D. & VanLente, F. Comparison study of intraosseous, central intravenous, and peripheral intravenous infusions of emergency drugs. *Am. J. Dis. Child.* 1990; **144**(1): 112–117.

100. Prete, M.R., Hannan, C.J., Jr. & Burkle, F.M., Jr. Plasma atropine concentrations via intravenous, endotracheal, and intraosseous administration. *Am. J. Emerg. Med.* 1987; **5**(2): 101–104.

101. Orlowski, J.P., Gallagher, J.M. & Porembka, D.T. Endotracheal epinephrine is unreliable. *Resuscitation* 1990; **19**(2): 103–113.

102. Cameron, J.L., Fontanarosa, P.B. & Passalaqua, A.M. A comparative study of peripheral to central circulation delivery times between intraosseous and intravenous injection using a radionuclide technique in normovolemic and hypovolemic canines. *J. Emerg. Med.* 1989; **7**(2): 123–127.

103. Warren, D.W., Kissoon, N., Mattar, A., Morrissey, G., Gravelle, D., & Rieder, M.J. Pharmacokinetics from multiple intraosseous and peripheral intravenous site injections in normovolemic and hypovolemic pigs. *Crit. Care Med.* 1994; **22**(5): 838–843.

104. Glaser, P. & Losek, J. Emergency intraosseous infusions in children. *Am. J. Emerg. Med.* 1986; **4**(1): 34–36.

105. Ryder, I.G., Munro, H.M. & Doull, I.J. Intraosseous infusion for resuscitation. *Arch. Dis. Child* 1991; **66**(12): 1442–1443.

106. McNamara, R.M., Spivey, W.H. & Sussman, C. Pediatric resuscitation without an intravenous line. *Am. J. Emerg. Med.* 1986; **4**: 31–33.

107. Spivey, W.H., Lathers, C.M., Malone, D.R. *et al.* Comparison of intraosseous, central, and peripheral routes of sodium bicar-

bonate administration during CPR in pigs. *Ann. Emerg. Med.* 1985; **14**(12): 1135–1140.

108. Spivey, W.H., Crespo, S.G., Fuhs, L.R. & Schoffstall, J.M. Plasma catecholamine levels after intraosseous epinephrine administration in a cardiac arrest model. *Ann. Emerg. Med.* 1992; **21**(2): 127–131.

109. Andropoulos, D.B., Soifer, S.J. & Schreiber, M.D. Plasma epinephrine concentrations after intraosseous and central venous injection during cardiopulmonary resuscitation in the lamb. *J. Pediatr.* 1990; **116**(2): 312–315.

110. Nolan, J., Deakin, C., Soar, J., Böttiger, B. & Smith, G. European Resuscitation Council Guidelines for Resuscitation 2005. Section 4. Adult advanced life support. *Resuscitation* 2005; **67**S1: S39–S86.

111. Lindemann, R. Endotracheal administration of epinephrine during cardiopulmonary resuscitation. *Am. J. Dis. Child.* 1982; **136**(8): 753–754.

112. Hahnel, J., Lindner, K.H. & Ahnefeld, F.W. Endobronchial administration of emergency drugs. *Resuscitation* 1989; **17**(3): 261–272.

113. Fishman, A. & Pietra, G. Handling of bioactive material by the lung. *N. Engl. J. Med.* 1974; **291**(17): 884–889; 953–959.

114. Rebuck, A.S. & Braude, A.C. Assessment of drug disposition in the lung. *Drugs* 1984; **28**(6): 544–553.

115. Hahnel, J.H., Lindner, K.H., Schurmann, C., Prengel, A. & Ahnefeld, F.W. Plasma lidocaine levels and PaO_2 with endobronchial administration: dilution with normal saline or distilled water? *Ann. Emerg. Med.* 1990; **19**(11): 1314–1317.

116. Prengel, A.W., Lindner, K.H., Hahnel, J.H. & Georgieff, M. Pharmacokinetics and technique of endotracheal and deep endobronchial lidocaine administration. *Anesth. Analg.* 1993; **77**(5): 985–989.

117. Prengel, A.W., Lindner, K.H., Hahnel, J. & Ahnefeld, F.W. Endotracheal and endobronchial lidocaine administration: effects on plasma lidocaine concentration and blood gases. *Crit. Care Med.* 1991; **19**(7): 911–915.

118. Ralston, S.H., Tacker, W.A., Showen, L., Carter, A. & Babbs, C.F. Endotracheal versus intravenous epinephrine during electromechanical dissociation with CPR in dogs. *Ann. Emerg. Med.* 1985; **14**(11): 1044–1048.

119. Hahnel, J.H., Lindner, K.H., Schurmann, C., Prengel, A. & Ahnefeld, F.W. Endobronchial drug administration: does deep endobronchial delivery have advantages in comparison with simple injection through the endotracheal tube? *Resuscitation* 1990; **20**(3): 193–202.

120. Hahnel, J.H., Lindner, K.H., Schurmann, C., Prengel, A. & Ahnefeld, F.W. What is the optimal volume of administration for endobronchial drugs? *Am. J. Emerg. Med.* 1990; **8**(6): 504–508.

121. Schanker, L.S. Drug absorption from the lung. *Biochem. Pharmacol.* 1978; **27**(4): 381–385.

122. Bates, D.V., Fish, B.R., Hatch, T.F., Mercer, T.T. & Morrow, P.E. Deposition and retention models for internal dosimetry of the human respiratory tract. Task group on lung dynamics. *Health Phys.* 1966; **12**(2): 173–207.

123. dal Santo, G. Absorption capacity of the airway and lungs. *Int. Anesthesiol. Clin.* 1977; **15**(4): 61–90.

124. Sefrin, P. & Finkenzeller, A. [Endobronchial drug administration in resuscitation]. *Med. Klin. (Munich)* 1991; **86**(1): 20–23.

125. Hanley, M., Rudd, T. & Butler, J. What happens to ontratracheal saline instillations? *Am. Rev. Resp. Dis.* 1978; **117**: 124.

126. Jasani, M.S., Nadkarni, V.M., Finkelstein, M.S., Mandell, G.A., Salzman, S.K. & Norman, M.E. Effects of different techniques of endotracheal epinephrine administration in pediatric porcine hypoxic-hypercarbic cardiopulmonary arrest. *Crit. Care Med.* 1994; **22**(7): 1174–1180.

127. Mace, S.E. Effect of technique of administration on plasma lidocaine levels. *Ann. Emerg. Med.* 1986; **15**(5): 552–556.

128. Mace, S.E. Differences in plasma lidocaine levels with endotracheal drug therapy secondary to total volume of diluent administered. *Resuscitation* 1990; **20**(3): 185–191.

129. Paret, G., Vaknin, Z., Ezra, D. *et al.* Epinephrine pharmacokinetics and pharmacodynamics following endotracheal administration in dogs: the role of volume of diluent. *Resuscitation* 1997; **35**(1): 77–82.

130. Ralston, S.H., Voorhees, W.D. & Babbs, C.F. Intrapulmonary epinephrine during prolonged cardiopulmonary resuscitation: improved regional blood flow and resuscitation in dogs. *Ann. Emerg. Med.* 1984; **13**(2): 79–86.

131. Mielke, L.L., Lanzinger, M.J., Entholzner, E.K., Hargasser, S.R. & Hipp, R.F. The time required to perform different methods for endotracheal drug administration during CPR. *Resuscitation* 1999; **40**(3): 165–169.

132. Rehan, V.K., Garcia, M., Kao, J., Tucker, C.M. & Patel, S.M. Epinephrine delivery during neonatal resuscitation: comparison of direct endotracheal tube vs catheter inserted into endotracheal tube administration. *J. Perinatol.* 2004; **24**(11): 686–690.

133. Orlowski, J.P., Abulleil, M.M. & Phillips, J.M. Effects of tonicities of saline solutions on pulmonary injury in drowning. *Crit. Care Med.* 1987; **15**(2): 126–130.

134. Greenberg, M.I., Baskin, S.I., Kaplan, A.M. & Urrichio, F.J. Effects of endotracheally administered distilled water and normal saline on the arterial blood gases of dogs. *Ann. Emerg. Med.* 1982; **11**(11): 600–604.

135. Mace, S.E. The effect of dilution on plasma lidocaine levels with endotracheal administration. *Ann. Emerg. Med.* 1987; **16**(5): 522–526.

136. Redding, J.S., Asuncion, J.S. & Pearson, J.W. Effective routes of drug administration during cardiac arrest. *Anesth. Analg.* 1967; **46**(2): 253–258.

137. Naganobu, K., Hasebe, Y., Uchiyama, Y., Hagio, M. & Ogawa, H. A comparison of distilled water and normal saline as diluents for endobronchial administration of epinephrine in the dog. *Anesth. Analg.* 2000; **91**(2): 317–321.

138. Yang, L.Y., He, C.Q. & Zhang, Z.G. Endotracheal administration of epinephrine during cardiopulmonary resuscitation. *Chin. Med. J. (Engl.)* 1991; **104**(12): 986–991.

139. Greenberg, M.I., Roberts, J.R. & Baskin, S.I. Use of endotracheally administered epinephrine in a pediatric patient. *Am. J. Dis. Child.* 1981; **135**(8): 767–768.

140. Elam, J. The Intrapulmonary Route for CPR Drugs. New York: Springer, 1977.

141. Schuttler, J., Hornchen, U., Stoeckel, H. & Hahn, N. [Endobronchial administration of adrenaline in cardiopulmonary resuscitation: pharmacokinetic and dynamic studies in the dog]. *Langenbecks Arch. Chir.* 1987; **370**(2): 119–127.

142. Crespo, S.G., Schoffstall, J.M., Fuhs, L.R. & Spivey, W.H. Comparison of two doses of endotracheal epinephrine in a cardiac arrest model. *Ann. Emerg. Med.* 1991; **20**(3): 230–234.

143. Manisterski, Y., Vaknin, Z., Ben-Abraham, R. *et al.* Endotracheal epinephrine: a call for larger doses. *Anesth. Analg.* 2002; **95**(4): 1037–1041, table of contents.

144. Vaknin, Z., Manisterski, Y., Ben-Abraham, R. *et al.* Is endotracheal adrenaline deleterious because of the beta adrenergic effect? *Anesth. Analg.* 2001; **92**(6): 1408–1412.

145. Hornchen, U., Schuttler, J., Stoeckel, H., Eichelkraut, W. & Hahn, N. Endobronchial instillation of epinephrine during cardiopulmonary resuscitation. *Crit. Care Med.* 1987; **15**(11): 1037–1039.

146. Schuttler, J., Bartsch, A., Ebeling, B.J. *et al.* [Endobronchial administration of adrenaline in preclinical cardiopulmonary resuscitation]. *Anasth. Intensivther. Notfallmed.* 1987; **22**(2): 63–68.

147. Schuttler, J., Bremer, F., & Hornchen, U. [Pharmacotherapy of ventricular fibrillation. A prospective study in an emergency medical service]. *Anaesthesist* 1991; **40**(3): 172–179.

148. Ornato, J.P. Use of adrenergic agonists during CPR in adults. *Ann. Emerg. Med.* 1993; **22**(2 Pt 2): 411–416.

149. Polin, K., Brown, D.H. & Leikin, J.B. Endotracheal administration of epinephrine and atropine. *Pediatr. Emerg. Care.* 1986; **2**(3): 168–169.

150. Babbs, C.F., Berg, R.A., Kette, F. *et al.* Use of pressors in the treatment of cardiac arrest. *Ann Emerg. Med.* 2001; **37**(4 Suppl.): S152–S162.

151. Roberts, J.R., Greenberg, M.I., Knaub, M.A., Kendrick, Z.V. & Baskin, S.I. Blood levels following intravenous and endotracheal epinephrine administration. *JACEP* 1979; **8**(2): 53–56.

152. Wenzel, V., Lindner, K.H., Prengel, A.W., Lurie, K.G. & Strohmenger, H.U. Endobronchial vasopressin improves survival during cardiopulmonary resuscitation in pigs. *Anesthesiology* 1997; **86**(6): 1375–1381.

153. Wenzel, V., Lindner, K.H., Augenstein, S. *et al.* Intraosseous vasopressin improves coronary perfusion pressure rapidly during cardiopulmonary resuscitation in pigs. *Crit. Care Med.* 1999; **27**(8): 1565–1569.

154. Wenzel, V., Lindner, K.H., Prengel, A.W. *et al.* Vasopressin improves vital organ blood flow after prolonged cardiac arrest with postcountershock pulseless electrical activity in pigs. *Crit. Care Med.* 1999; **27**(3): 486–492.

155. Efrati, O., Barak, A., Ben-Abraham, R. *et al.* Should vasopressin replace adrenaline for endotracheal drug administration? *Crit. Care Med.* 2003; **31**(2): 572–576.

156. Efrati, O., Modan-Moses, D., Ben-Abraham, R., Bibi, H. & Paret, G. Atropine aborts bradycardic effect of endotracheally administered vasopressin. *Med. Sci. Monit.* 2005; **11**(9): CR410–CR414.

157. Part 4: Advanced life support. *Resuscitation* 2005; **67**: 213–247.

158. Benowitz, N.L. & Meister, W. Clinical pharmacokinetics of lignocaine. *Clin. Pharmacokinet.* 1978; **3**(3): 177–201.

159. McBurney, A., Jones, D.A., Stanley, P.J. & Ward, J.W. Absorption of lignocaine and bupivacaine from the respiratory tract during fibreoptic bronchoscopy. *Br. J. Clin. Pharmacol.* 1984; **17**(1): 61–66.

160. Yealy, D., Manegaxzi, J., Klain, M., Molner, R., James, W. & Stezoski, W. Endobronchial drug absorption during CPR in a canine model. *Ann. Emerg. Med.* 1991; **20**(9): 949.

161. McDonald, J.L. Serum lidocaine levels during cardiopulmonary resuscitation after intravenous and endotracheal administration. *Crit. Care Med.* 1985; **13**(11): 914–915.

162. Bray, B.M., Jones, H.M. & Grundy, E.M. Tracheal versus intravenous atropine. A comparison of the effects on heart rate. *Anaesthesia* 1987; **42**(11): 1188–1190.

163. Greenberg, M.I., Mayeda, D.V., Chrzanowski, R., Brumwell, D., Baskin, S.I. & Roberts, J.R. Endotracheal administration of atropine sulfate. *Ann. Emerg. Med.* 1982; **11**(10): 546–548.

164. Coon, G.A., Clinton, J.E. & Ruiz, E. Use of atropine for brady-asystolic prehospital cardiac arrest. *Ann. Emerg. Med.* 1981; **10**(9): 462–467.

165. Stueven, H.A., Tonsfeldt, D.J., Thompson, B.M., Whitcomb, J., Kastenson, E. & Aprahamian, C. Atropine in asystole: human studies. *Ann. Emerg. Med.* 1984; **13**(9 Pt 2): 815–817.

166. Niemann, J.T., & Stratton, S.J. Endotracheal versus intravenous epinephrine and atropine in out-of-hospital "primary" and postcountershock asystole. *Crit. Care Med.* 2000; **28**(6): 1815–1819.

167. Niemann, J.T., Stratton, S.J., Cruz, B. & Lewis, R.J. Endotracheal drug administration during out-of-hospital resuscitation: where are the survivors? *Resuscitation* 2002; **53**(2): 153–157.

168. Barsan, W.G., Hedges, J.R., Nishiyama, H. & Lukes, S.T. Differences in drug delivery with peripheral and central venous injections: normal perfusion. *Am. J. Emerg. Med.* 1986; **4**(1): 1–3.

169. Jespersen, H.F., Granborg, J., Hansen, U., Torp-Pedersen, C. & Pedersen, A. Feasibility of intracardiac injection of drugs during cardiac arrest. *Eur. Heart. J.* 1990; **11**(3): 269–274.

170. Davison, R., Barresi, V., Parker, M., Meyers, S.N. & Talano, J.V. Intracardiac injections during cardiopulmonary resuscitation. A low-risk procedure. *J. Am. Med. Assoc.* 1980; **244**(10): 1110–1111.

171. Pentel, P. & Benowitz, N. Pharmacokinetic and pharmacodynamic considerations in drug therapy of cardiac emergencies. *Clin. Pharmacokinet.* 1984; **9**(4): 273–308.

172. Sabin, H.I., Coghill, S.B., Khunti, K. & McNeill, G.O. Accuracy of intracardiac injections determined by a post-mortem study. *Lancet* 1983; **2**(8358): 1054–1055.

173. Manning, J.E., Murphy, C.A., Jr., Batson, D.N., Perretta, S.G., Mueller, R.A. & Norfleet, E.A. Aortic arch versus central

venous epinephrine during CPR. *Ann. Emerg. Med.* 1993; **22**(4): 703–708.

174. Hao-Hui, C. Closed-chest intracardiac injection. *Resuscitation* 1981; **9**(1): 103–106.

175. Hao-Hui, C. On the intracardiac use of combined adrenaline, isoprenaline and noradrenaline in the resuscitation of the heart beat: a review of resuscitation, Part II. *Resuscitation* 1981; **9**(1): 53–59.

176. Steinberg, J.J. Intracardiac injection of inotropic agents. *Lancet* 1984; **1**(8370): 218.

177. Schechter, D. Transthoracic epinephrine injection in heart resuscitation is dangerous. *J. Am. Med. Assoc.* 1975; **234**: 1184.

178. Harrison, E. Intracardiac injections. *J. Am. Med. Assoc.* 1981; **245**(13): 1315.

179. Martens, P. Intracardiac injection. *Resuscitation* 1994; **27**: 177.

180. Pun, K.K. Cardiac tamponade after intracardiac injection. *Anaesth. Intens. Care* 1984; **12**(1): 66–67.

181. Vijay, N.K. & Schoonmaker, F.W. Cardiopulmonary arrest and resuscitation. *Am. Fam. Phys.* 1975; **12**(2): 85–90.

182. Hasegawa, E. The endotracheal administration of drugs. *Heart Lung* 1986; **15**: 60–63.

183. Lehman, J.S., Lykens, H.D. & Musser, B.G. Cardiac ventriculography; direct transthoracic needle puncture opacification of the left (or right) ventricle. *Am. J. Roentgenol. Radium Ther. Nucl. Med.* 1957; **77**(2): 207–234.

184. Showen, R.L., Tacker, W.A. & Ralston, S.H. Treatment of electromechanical dissociation with intracardiac epinephrine. *Ann. Emerg. Med.* 1986; **4**: 422.

185. Varat, M.A., Jetty, P., Michelson, E.A. & Schneider, S.M. Effects of alternate routes of epinephrine delivery in experimental bradycardia-hypotension. *Resuscitation* 1991; **21**(2–3): 239–246.

186. Amey, B.D., Harrison, E.E., Straub, E.J. & McLeod, M. Paramedic use of intracardiac medications in prehospital sudden cardiac death. *JACEP* 1978; **7**(4): 130–134.

187. Glasser, S.P., Harrison, E.E., Amey, B.D. & Straub, E.J. Echocardiographic incidence of pericardial effusion in patients resuscitated by emergency medical technicians. *JACEP* 1979; **8**(1): 6–8.

188. Part 6: Advanced Cardiovascular Life Support: Section 6: Pharmacology II: Agents to Optimize Cardiac Output and Blood Pressure. *Circulation* 2000; **102**, Suppl. I(8): I-129-I-135.

189. Motawani, J.G. & Lipworth, B.J. Clinical pharmacokinetics of drugs administered bucally and sublingually. *Clin. Pharmacokinet.* 1991; **21**: 83–94.

190. Armstrong, P.W., Armstrong, J.A. & Marks, G.S. Blood levels after sublingual nitroglycerin. *Circulation* 1979; **59**(3): 585–588.

191. Hamilton, R.J., Carter, W.A. & Gallagher, E.J. Rapid improvement of acute pulmonary edema with sublingual captopril. *Acad. Emerg. Med.* 1996; **3**(3): 205–212.

192. Fort, S., Lewis, M.J., Luscombe, D.K. & John, D.N. Preliminary investigation of the efficacy of sublingual verapamil in the

management of acute atrial fibrillation and flutter. *Br. J. Clin. Pharmacol.* 1994; **37**(5): 460–463.

193. Sasaki, S., Koumi, S., Sato, R. *et al.* Kinetics of buccal absorption of propafenone single oral loading dose in healthy humans. *Gen. Pharmacol.* 1998; **31**(4): 589–591.

194. Arnold, R.W., Farah, R.F. & Monroe, G. The attenuating effect of intraglossal atropine on the oculocardiac reflex. *Binocul. Vis. Strabismus Q.* 2002; **17**(4): 313–318.

195. Ordog, G.J., Wasserberger, J., Jones, J., Rouzier, R., Elstin, D. & Balasubramaniam, S. Efficacy of absorption of sublingual and intravenous Cardio-Green. *Ann. Emerg. Med.* 1984; **13**(6): 426–428.

196. Rothrock, S.G., Green, S.M., Schafermeyer, R.W., & Colucciello, S.A. Successful resuscitation from cardiac arrest using sublingual injection for medication delivery. *Ann. Emerg. Med.* 1993; **22**(4): 751–753.

197. Laczi, F., Mezei, G., Julesz, J. & Lazlo, F.A. Effects of vasopressin analogues (DDAVP, DVDAVP) in the form of sublingual tablets in central diabetes insipidus. *Int. J. Clin. Pharmacol. Ther. Toxicol.* 1981; **19**(2): 63–68.

198. Fjellestad-Paulsen, A., Hoglund, P., Lundin, S. & Paulsen, O. Pharmacokinetics of 1-deamino-8-D-arginine vasopressin after various routes of administration in healthy volunteers. *Clin. Endocrinol. (Oxf.)* 1993; **38**(2): 177–182.

199. De Groot, A.N., Vree, T.B., Hekster, Y.A. *et al.* Bioavailability and pharmacokinetics of sublingual oxytocin in male volunteers. *J. Pharm. Pharmacol.* 1995; **47**(7): 571–575.

200. Maio, R.F., Griener, J.C., Clark, M.R., Gifford, G. & Wiegenstein, J.G. Intralingual naloxone reversal of morphine-induced respiratory depression in dogs. *Ann. Emerg. Med.* 1984; **13**(12): 1087–1091.

201. Maio, R.F., Gaukel, B. & Freeman, B. Intralingual naloxone injection for narcotic-induced respiratory depression. *Ann. Emerg. Med.* 1987; **16**(5): 572–573.

202. Wasserberger, J., Ordog, G.J. & Kolodny, M. Intralingual naloxone injections. *Ann. Emerg. Med.* 1988; **17**(8): 874–875.

203. Schwagmeier, R., Alincic, S. & Striebel, H.W. Midazolam pharmacokinetics following intravenous and buccal administration. *Br. J. Clin. Pharmacol.* 1998; **46**(3): 203–206.

204. Scott, R.C., Besag, F.M. & Neville, B.G. Buccal midazolam and rectal diazepam for treatment of prolonged seizures in childhood and adolescence: a randomised trial. *Lancet* 1999; **353**(9153): 623–626.

205. Geldner, G., Hubmann, M., Knoll, R. & Jacobi, K. Comparison between three transmucosal routes of administration of midazolam in children. *Paediatr. Anaesth.* 1997; **7**(2): 103–109.

206. McMartin, C., Hutchinson, L.E., Hyde, R. & Peters, G.E. Analysis of structural requirements for the absorption of drugs and macromolecules from the nasal cavity. *J. Pharm. Sci.* 1987; **76**(7): 535–540.

207. Gopinath, P., Gopinath, G. & Kumar, T. Target size of intranasally sprayed substances and their transport across the nasal mucosa: a new insight into the intranasal route of drug delivery. *Curr. Ther. Res.* 1978; **23**: 596–607.

208. Alternative routes of drug administration – advantages and disadvantages (subject review). American Academy of Pediatrics. Committee on Drugs. *Pediatrics* 1997; **100**(1): 143–152.

209. Sakane, T., Akizuki, M. Yoshida, M. *et al.* Transport of cephalexin to the cerebrospinal fluid directly from the nasal cavity. *J. Pharm. Pharmacol.* 1991; **43**(6): 449–451.

210. Hardy, J.G., Lee, S.W. & Wilson, C.G. Intranasal drug delivery by spray and drops. *J. Pharm. Pharmacol.* 1985; **37**(5): 294–297.

211. Olanoff, L.S., Titus, C.R., Shea, M.S., Gibson, R.E. & Brooks, C.D. Effect of intranasal histamine on nasal mucosal blood flow and the antidiuretic activity of desmopressin. *J. Clin. Invest.* 1987; **80**(3): 890–895.

212. Harris, A.S., Hedner, P. & Vilhardt, H. Nasal administration of desmopressin by spray and drops. *J. Pharm. Pharmacol.* 1987; **39**(11): 932–934.

213. Mabry, R.L. Corticosteroids in the management of upper respiratory allergy: the emerging role of steroid nasal sprays. *Otolaryngol. Head Neck Surg.* 1992; **107**(6 Pt 2): 855–859; discussion 859–860.

214. Walbergh, E.J., Wills, R.J. & Eckhert, J. Plasma concentrations of midazolam in children following intranasal administration. *Anesthesiology* 1991; **74**(2): 233–235.

215. Wilton, N.C., Leigh, J., Rosen, D.R. & Pandit, U.A. Preanesthetic sedation of preschool children using intranasal midazolam. *Anesthesiology* 1988; **69**(6): 972–975.

216. Theroux, M.C., West, D.W., Corddry, D.H., *et al.* Efficacy of intranasal midazolam in facilitating suturing of lacerations in preschool children in the emergency department. *Pediatrics* 1993; **91**(3): 624–627.

217. Aldrete, J.A., Russell, L.J. & Davis, F.A. Intranasal administration of ketamine: possible applications. *Acta Anaesthesiol. Belg.* 1988; **39**(3 Suppl. 2): 95–96.

218. Citron, M.L., Reynolds, J.R., Kalra, J. *et al.* Pharmacokinetic comparison of intranasal, oral, and intramuscular metoclopramide in healthy volunteers. *Cancer Treat. Rep.* 1987; **71**(3): 317–319.

219. Weksler, N., Brill, S., Tarnapolski, A. & Gurman, G.M. Intranasal salbutamol instillation in asthma attack. *Am. J. Emerg. Med.* 1999; **17**(7): 686–688.

220. Kato, Y., Yagi, N., Yamada, S., Sato, M. & Kimura, R. Nasal absorption of digoxin in rats. *J. Pharmacobiodyn.* 1992; **15**(1): 1–6.

221. Wood, C.C., Fireman, P., Grossman, J., Wecker, M. & MacGregor, T. Product characteristics and pharmacokinetics of intranasal ipratropium bromide. *J. Allergy Clin. Immunol.* 1995; **95**(5 Pt 2): 1111–1116.

222. Li, L., Gorukanti, S., Choi, Y.M. & Kim, K.H. Rapid-onset intranasal delivery of anticonvulsants: pharmacokinetic and pharmacodynamic evaluation in rabbits. *Int. J. Pharm.* 2000; **199**(1): 65–76.

223. Childrey, J. & Essex, H. Absorption from the mucosa of the frontal sinus. *Arch. Otolaryngol. Head Neck Surg.* 1931; **14**: 564.

224. Myers, M.G. & Iazzetta, J.J. Intranasally administered phenylephrine and blood pressure. *Can. Med. Assoc. J.* 1982; **127**(5): 365–368.

225. Shapiro, M.J. & Grenvik, A. Enteral and intranasal treatment for vasopressor-dependent hypotension in C1 tetraplegia. *Neurosurgery* 1988; **22**(1 Pt 1): 147–148.

226. Yamada, T. The potential of the nasal mucosa route for emergency drug administration via a high-pressure needleless injection system. *Anesth. Prog.* 2004; **51**(2): 56–61.

227. Bleske, B.E., Rice, T.L., Warren, E.W. *et al.* Effect of dose on the nasal absorption of epinephrine during cardiopulmonary resuscitation. *Am. J. Emerg Med.* 1996; **14**(2): 133–138.

228. Loimer, N., Hofmann, P. & Chaudhry, H.R. Nasal administration of naloxone is as effective as the intravenous route in opiate addicts. *Int. J. Addict.* 1994; **29**(6): 819–827.

229. Barton, E.D., Ramos, J., Colwell, C., Benson, J. & Baily, J., Dunn, W. Intranasal administration of naloxone by paramedics. *Prehosp Emerg. Care* 2002; **6**(1): 54–58.

230. Kelly, A.M., Kerr, D., Dietze, P., Patrick, I., Walker, T. & Koutsogiannis, Z. Randomised trial of intranasal versus intramuscular naloxone in prehospital treatment for suspected opioid overdose. *Med. J. Aust.* 2005; **182**(1): 24–27.

231. Sarkar, M.A. Drug metabolism in the nasal mucosa. *Pharm. Res.* 1992; **9**(1): 1–9.

232. Illum, L. Nasal drug delivery: new developments and strategies. *Drug Discov. Today* 2002; **7**(23): 1184–1189.

233. Manning, J., Murphy, C. & Hertz, C. Selective aortic arch perfusion: description of a technique with potential benefit in cardiopulmonary and cerebral resuscitation. *Ann. Emerg. Med.* 1990; **19**: 1226.

234. Rubertsson, S., Bircher, N.G., Smarik, S.D., Young, M.C., Alexander, H. & Grenvik, A. Intra-aortic administration of epinephrine above aortic occlusion does not alter outcome of experimental cardiopulmonary resuscitation. *Resuscitation* 1999; **42**(1): 57–63.

235. Lee, R., Neya, K., Svizzero, T.A., Koski, G., Mitchell, J.D. & Vlahakes, G.J. Norepinephrine infusion following cardiopulmonary bypass: effect of infusion site. *J. Surg. Res.* 1995; **58**(2): 143–148.

236. Fullerton, D.A., St Cyr, J.A., Albert, J.D. & Grover, F.L. Hemodynamic advantage of left atrial epinephrine administration after cardiac operations. *Ann. Thorac. Surg.* 1993; **56**(6): 1263–1266.

237. Safar, P., Abramson, N.S., Angelos, M. *et al.* Emergency cardiopulmonary bypass for resuscitation from prolonged cardiac arrest. *Am. J. Emerg. Med.* 1990; **8**(1): 55–67.

Vasopressor therapy during cardiac arrest

34

Adrenergic agonists

Max Harry Weil, Shijie Sun, and Wanchun Tang

Weil Institute of Critical Care Medicine, Rancho Mirage, CA and
Keck School of Medicine of the University of Southern California, Los Angeles, CA, USA

Introduction

Although there is persuasive evidence that the administration of adrenaline during CPR favors the success of electrical defibrillation as well as the return of pulsatile rhythm, its more ultimate benefit on survival is unproven. To the contrary, the more recent discovery of reversible myocardial dysfunction after successful resuscitation from cardiac arrest initially in experimental models[1] and subsequently in human patients[2] led to a re-examination of its role. Although there is only indirect evidence that impaired myocardial function accounts for early death, the high correlation between the severity of myocardial impairment and decreased survival supports this assumption. Accordingly, postresuscitation myocardial dysfunction may therefore explain, at least in part, the high fatality rate within the initial 72 hours after successful resuscitation from cardiac arrest such that fewer than 5% of victims recover to be discharged from the hospital without major impairment.[3]

The immediate effort during CPR is to restore blood flows to sustain the functions of vital organs, and most especially, to the heart and the brain prior to successful restoration of spontaneous circulation. Blood flow to the vital organs during CPR is contingent primarily on the cardiac output generated by precordial or direct cardiac compression and by the resistance in the systemic arterial bed. Yet the cardiac output that is generated by precordial compression represents only approximately 25% to 30% of normal values.[4] Vasopressor drugs increase arterial and arteriolar vasoconstriction, and thereby produce increases in aortic diastolic pressure. The increases in aortic diastolic pressure in turn produce increases in coronary and cerebral perfusion pressures, in part "borrowing" from blood flow to viscera and muscle.[5] Restoration of threshold levels of coronary perfusion pressure with corresponding augmentation of myocardial blood flow has been a consistent predictor of successful restoration of spontaneous circulation during CPR.[1,6] Electrical defibrillation is itself facilitated after coronary perfusion pressures are increased above such thresholds, especially after prolonged, untreated cardiac arrest.[7] Cerebral "survival" in relation to vasopressor therapy during CPR has been less intensely studied, but it is also an ultimate criterion of outcome following cardiac arrest. Although the focus of this chapter is on the role of adrenergic vasopressor agents for resuscitation of the heart, including effects on postresuscitation myocardial function and survival, we recognize that long term survival is appropriately defined in terms of *both* cardiac and cerebral survival.

Epinephrine

Pharmacological actions of epinephrine are mediated by adrenergic receptors. Ahlquist first demonstrated in 1948 that epinephrine, and endogenous catecholamines more generally, act through alpha- and beta-adrenergic receptors.[8] In the years that followed, alpha$_1$ and alpha$_2$ subtype receptors and beta$_1$, beta$_2$, and beta$_3$ subtype receptors were identified.[9] Currently available adrenergic vasopressor agonists are summarized in Table 34.1 in relation to their receptor function.[10]

Epinephrine has both alpha- and beta-adrenergic actions, and has been the preferred adrenergic agent for the management of cardiac arrest for almost 40 years.[11,12] The pressor effects of epinephrine follow alpha-adrenergic

Cardiac Arrest: The Science and Practice of Resuscitation Medicine. 2nd edn., ed. Norman Paradis, Henry Halperin, Karl Kern, Volker Wenzel, Douglas Chamberlain. Published by Cambridge University Press. © Cambridge University Press, 2007.

Table 34.1. Adrenergic vasopressor agents in relation to their receptor function

Agent	Receptors
Epinephrine	Alpha, beta
Methoxamine	Alpha$_1$
Phenylephrine	
Clonidine (crosses blood–brain barrier, vasodilator)	Alpha$_2$
Alpha-methylnorepinephrine (selective peripheral vasoconstrictor)	

receptor activation.[13–17] Beta-adrenergic effects, which are inotropic and chronotropic, have unfavorable actions in that they produce substantial increases in myocardial oxygen consumption. Epinephrine therefore increases the severity of ischemic injury of the myocardium during resuscitation. If the patient is subsequently resuscitated, it increases the severity of postresuscitation myocardial dysfunction.[18,19] The chronotropic effects of epinephrine are equally striking. They account for both increases in heart rate and ectopic ventricular arrhythmias leading to recurrent ventricular tachycardia and ventricular fibrillation.[19,20] Quite apart from its cardiac action, epinephrine also reduces arterial oxygen saturation and therefore oxygen delivery. This phenomenon has been studied by our group, which identified ventilation-perfusion mismatch as accounting for pulmonary arteriovenous shunting.[18]

The issue is especially important because during the chaotic and disorganized contraction of the heart during VF, there are dramatic increases in the myocardial demands for oxygen. Human data reported in a paper by Holmberg *et al.*[21] were based on 14 065 patients during cardiac arrest. Among 10 966 resuscitated patients, epinephrine had been administered to 4566 or 42.4% of cases, but only 156 (3.4%) patients survived for 1 month. This contrasted with 6207 patients who received no epinephrine of whom 388 (6.3%) were survivors. Treatment with epinephrine was an independent predictor of lower likelihood of survival ($P < 0.0001$), independently of gender, incidence of arrhythmias, witnessed or unwitnessed arrest, and bystander CPR. These data are supported by those of Laurent *et al.*,[22] who reported that administration of epinephrine was associated with a lower postresuscitation cardiac output in survivors of out-of-hospital cardiac arrest. Gonzales *et al.*[23] confirmed decreases in end-tidal carbon dioxide with increased doses of epinephrine, a finding explained by both pulmonary arteriovenous shunting produced by epinephrine and decreases in pulmonary blood flow also observed by our group.[18]

Objective evidence of the failure of epinephrine to improve the balance between myocardial oxygen supply and demand during closed-chest cardiopulmonary resuscitation in dogs was reported in 1988 by Ditchey and Lindenfeld.[17] The late Dr. Joseph S. Redding in collaboration with Pearson in 1963 had already identified potential benefits of more selective alpha-adrenergic agonists including phenylephrine and methoxamine when compared to epinephrine.[5] In 1990, Roberts *et al.*[24] further demonstrated that methoxamine, a selective alpha$_1$-agonist, produced significantly greater myocardial and cerebral blood flows during CPR in dogs than did epinephrine, with more optimal postresuscitation cardiac output and greater survival.

Beta-adrenergic blocking agents

Studies by Ditchey *et al.*[19] demonstrated improved resuscitability and better postresuscitation myocardial function in dogs after pretreatment with a non-specific β-adrenergic blocking agent, namely, propranolol.[25] Propranolol has also been shown by Maroko *et al.*[26,27] to decrease electrocardiographic evidence of ischemic myocardial cell damage in both experimental and clinical settings. Ischemic cells had less mitochondrial swelling in propranolol-pretreated animals. Obeid *et al.*[28] reported that propranolol preserved ATP stores in ischemic myocardium. In brief, we can now conclude that beta-adrenergic stimulation is adverse to the globally ischemic heart and this concept applies to the global ischemic injury during cardiac arrest and resuscitation.

In subsequent animal studies, a short acting beta$_1$-selective adrenergic blocking agent, esmolol, was administered during cardiopulmonary resuscitation. Esmolol significantly improved initial cardiac resuscitation, minimized postresuscitation myocardial dysfunction, and increased the duration of postresuscitation survival.[29] Current evidence suggests that there is likely to be an important role for beta-adrenergic blockade during CPR as it is now used for routine management of acute coronary syndromes and acute myocardial infarction.

With special focus on postresuscitation myocardial dysfunction, major decreases in myocardial contractile function followed successful restoration of spontaneous circulation. When the effects of epinephrine were compared with a more selective alpha-adrenergic agonist, phenylephrine, outcomes of cardiac resuscitation were improved with phenylephrine.[20] In experiments on a rat model of cardiac arrest and CPR, epinephrine was combined with the beta$_1$-adrenergic blocking agent, esmolol. Restoration of spontaneous circulation, postresuscitation myocardial function, and survival were each improved,[20] and these benefits were subsequently confirmed in a cardiac arrest-CPR model in pigs.[30]

It is now apparent that beta-adrenergic effects of adrenergic agonists administered during CPR are detrimental. Although this is now established in both experimental and clinical settings of coronary artery disease with regional myocardial ischemia, there was relatively slow acceptance of the practice. While epinephrine improves the success of initial resuscitation attempts, the evidence that it is adverse to ultimate survival is persuasive to us and that this dichotomy is best explained by its detrimental effects on postresuscitation myocardial function cited above. It is these adverse pharmacological actions of epinephrine that have increasingly called into question the highly traditional and widely accepted use of epinephrine as the preferred adrenergic vasopressor agent for management of advanced cardiac life support. The current American Heart Association Guidelines specifically point to the unproven value of epinephrine.[31]

Both experimental studies and a small series of clinical reports first published in the mid-1980s held that as much as 10-fold higher doses of epinephrine yielded greater coronary perfusion pressure, myocardial and cerebral blood flows, and the success rates of initial resuscitation. Nevertheless, no improvement in long-term survival was confirmed.[32–34] Three large, randomized clinical studies were subsequently reported in which the effects of high-dose epinephrine were compared with standard-dose epinephrine on outcomes of CPR.[35–37] In one study, either 1- or 7-mg bolus doses of epinephrine were administered during both in-hospital and out-of-hospital settings of cardiac resuscitation. There were no significant differences in initial return of spontaneous circulation, neurological outcomes, and hospital survivals. In two additional studies in which standard and high doses of epinephrine were compared during out-of-hospital CPR, again there were no statistically significant differences in the return of spontaneous circulation and no difference in in-hospital survival. On the basis of these reports, the recommended dose of epinephrine has been maintained as 1.0 mg administered intravenously (or by intraosseous route) every 3 to 5 minutes during resuscitation. High-dose epinephrine (0.1 mg/kg) in adults would best be reserved for treatment of overdose of beta-adrenergic blocking agents or calcium channel blockers.[11]

Alpha₁-adrenergic agonists

After the adverse effects of beta-adrenergic agonists on cardiopulmonary resuscitation were exposed, the more selective role of alpha-adrenergic receptors with respect to CPR were explored. The extent to which peripheral vascular resistance, and therefore myocardial and cerebral perfusion pressure and blood flows, could be increased by alpha-adrenergic agonists during resuscitation was investigated. The favorable effects of non-specific alpha-agonists were confirmed in part.[19,20,24] Observations on the relatively selective alpha₁-adrenergic agonists methoxamine and phenylephrine had earlier indicated diminished effectiveness in comparison with epinephrine in settings of prolonged cardiac arrest.[38] These observations pointed to selectively lesser effects, especially on alpha₁-adrenergic receptor responses, in settings of myocardial ischemia.[39,40] This loss of effectiveness was subsequently traced to desensitization of the alpha₁-receptor after prolongation of cardiac arrest.[41] It was also recognized that alpha₁-adrenergic receptors reside in the myocardium and, like beta-receptors, account for inotropic effects.[42] Alpha₁-agonists therefore also increased myocardial oxygen requirements at the very time that supply was reduced and consequently that they increased the severity of global ischemic injury during cardiac arrest. When alpha₁-adrenergic receptors were blocked by either a selective or non-selective alpha-adrenergic blocking agent when cardiac arrest was induced following experimental coronary occlusion, myocardial function was significantly improved.[43] Alpha₁-adrenergic agonists have also been shown to constrict coronary arteries such that additional reductions in myocardial perfusion may be superimposed on already reduced coronary blood flows.[43]

Alpha₂-adrenergic agonists

After the limitations of epinephrine for management of cardiac resuscitation were recognized, and specifically the adverse effects of beta- and to a lesser extent alpha₁-receptor agonists, the role of selective alpha₂-adrenoceptor agonists was investigated by our group. Three subtypes of alpha₂-receptors are now identified, namely alpha₂A, alpha₂B, and alpha₂C as shown in Table 34.2.[45] Alpha₂A-agonists act centrally on the medulla and mediate a tonic sympatho-inhibitory effect. These central effects account for reductions in arterial blood pressure, myocardial contractility, and heart rate. This contrasts with alpha₂B actions which are primarily arterial and arteriolar vasoconstrictor. Alpha₂B subtype receptors are also present but are less abundant in brain tissue and do not appear to diminish a predominant peripheral vasoconstrictor response.[46,47] Alpha₂C is a third subclass which, like alpha₂A, has a predominant central nervous system effect, including a so-called stress response, but as yet it has no defined cardiovascular actions.[48] As of the

Table 34.2. Subgroup classification of alpha-adrenergic receptors

	Site	Action	Additional effects
Alpha $_1$	Arterial Myocardial Coronary	Vasoconstriction Inotropic Vasoconstriction	Early desensitization
Alpha$_{2A}$	CNS (medulla) (Crosses blood-brain barrier)	Vasodilatation	Reduced heart rate and arterial pressure, reduced myocardial contractility
Alpha$_{2B}$	Arterial, arteriolar (Does not cross into CNS)	Vasoconstriction	
Alpha$_{2C}$	CNS	Stress response	No overt cardiovascular effects

present writing, we identify only alpha$_2$ receptors as a group pertinent to the management of CPR. The potential roles of individual alpha$_2$ subtypes have not yet been addressed in these settings.

When alpha$_2$-receptor agonists act centrally and produce vasodilator effects, they may override peripherally acting vasoconstrictor effects. Accordingly, only the peripheral actions are regarded as beneficial for the initial management of cardiac arrest. This prompted a search for a selective alpha$_2$-adrenergic agonist that had peripheral vasoconstrictor actions and led our group to identify alpha-methylnorepinephrine (alpha-MNE). Alpha-MNE does not cross the blood-brain barrier.[49] The vasoconstrictor effects of alpha-MNE were associated with significant improvement in the likelihood of initial resuscitation, better postresuscitation myocardial function, and increased postresuscitation survival when tested in a rat model of cardiac arrest and resuscitation (Fig. 34.1). Alpha$_2$-MNE produced neither transient hypoxemia nor did it increase the incidence of postresuscitation ventricular arrhythmias in comparison with epinephrine. Accordingly, a selective alpha$_2$-agonist proved to be as effective as epinephrine for initial cardiac resuscitation and there was evidence that this occurred without disproportionate increases in myocardial oxygen consumption, without compromise of postresuscitation myocardial function, or of survival. More recent evidence that alpha$_2$-adrenergic agonists increase endothelial nitric oxide production is also of interest since such activity would mitigate any alpha$_2$-adrenergic vasoconstrictor effects on coronary arteries.[44] At the time of this writing, alpha-MNE is not commercially available nor is it an approved drug in the United States.

The effects of epinephrine on microvascular cerebral blood flow were more recently reported from studies in anesthetized pigs. When epinephrine was administered during CPR, there was a striking decrease in capillary blood flow but not in the carotid artery flow. Decreases in capillary flow were documented in both sublingual sites[50] and at the surface of the frontoparietal cortex.[51] The preliminary experimental observations indicate surprising dissociation between large vessel and microcirculatory flow. For the present, we cannot assume that large vessel and, specifically, arterial blood flow is itself predictive of flow to sustain microvascular blood flow and delivery of substrates to the capillary exchange beds.

Adrenergic vasopressors compared to vasopressin

The relationships between equipressor doses of epinephrine, vasopressin, and epinephrine after alpha$_1$- and beta-adrenergic blockade have also been examined. Each was comparably effective for restoring spontaneous circulation in a pig model of cardiac arrest.[51] Combined alpha$_1$- and beta-adrenergic blockade, however, which represented the equivalent of administering selective alpha$_2$ vasopressor agonists, resulted in better postresuscitation cardiac and neurological recovery. In these experiments, we identified an adverse effect in the postresuscitation period, by which vasopressin produced more myocardial dysfunction. This may be explained by its prolonged action, in which increases in afterload impose more prolonged increases in workloads on the stunned heart and after postresuscitation contractile function has already been impaired.

Discussion

A large number of pharmaceuticals were initially recommended for routine use during CPR. Except for selective management of hypocalcemia, hyperkalemia, heart block, or other unique mechanisms of cardiac arrest, only agents that increase peripheral vasoconstriction are of proven

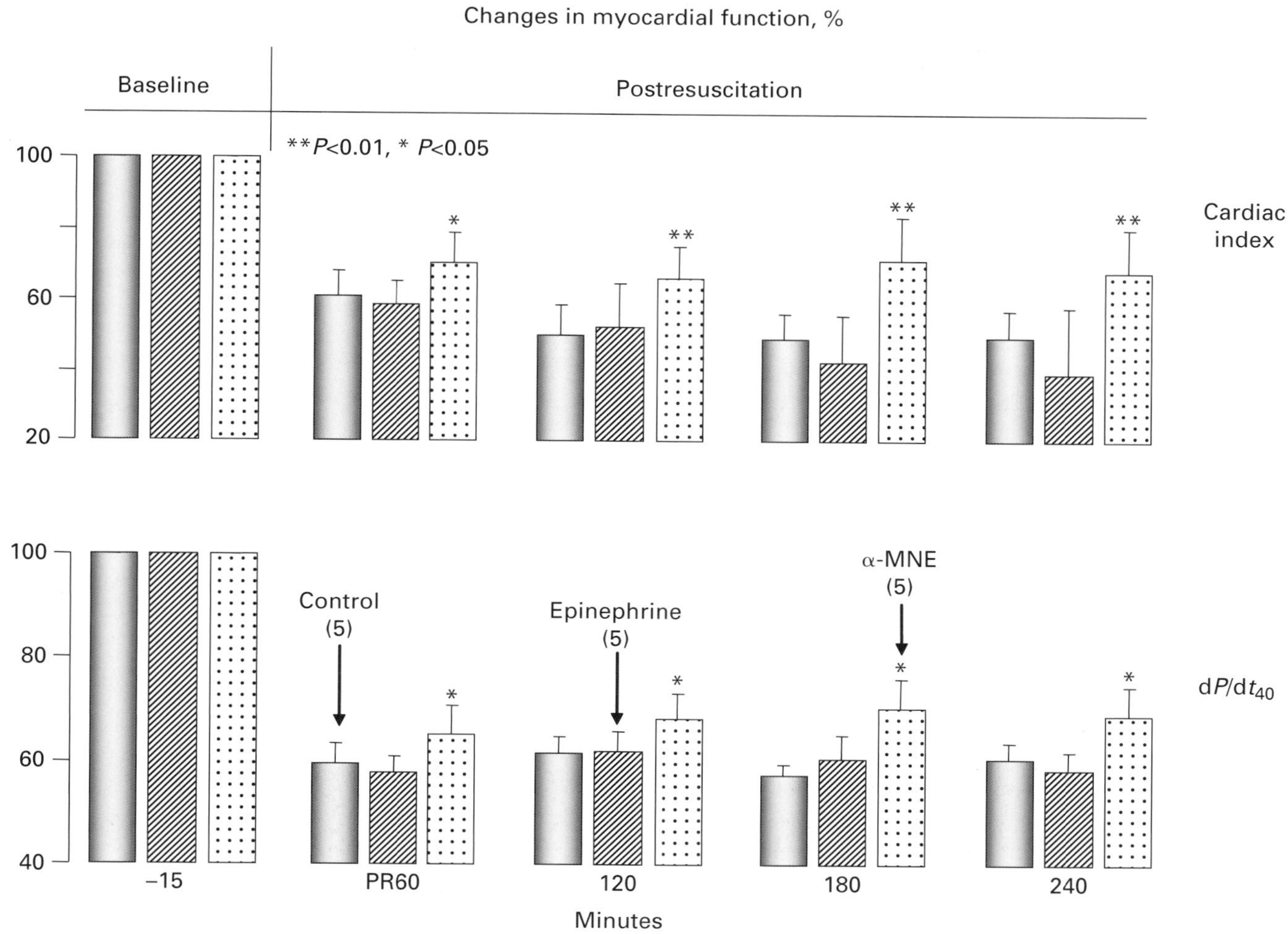

Changes in myocardial function, %

Fig. 34.1. A comparison of changes in cardiac index and dP/dt_{40} compared to precardiac arrest (baseline) values when measured at the indicated intervals postresuscitation with re-establishment of spontaneous circulation, i.e., PR. Ventricular fibrillation was untreated for 8 minutes. (From ref. 48.)

benefit and in most instances only for initial resuscitation. Adrenergic vasopressors, which increase myocardial oxygen consumption by their beta and alpha$_1$ actions, increase ectopic ventricular arrhythmias, and transient hypoxemia. Although epinephrine may improve initial resuscitation and return of spontaneous circulation, there is no secure evidence of improved postresuscitation outcomes in terms of survival, as cited above. The major adverse effects are admittedly the inotropic and chronotropic beta-adrenergic actions of epinephrine. Although alpha$_1$ and alpha$_2$-adrenergic agonists increase peripheral vascular resistance and therefore favor myocardial coronary and cerebral perfusion, the inotropic and chronotropic actions of alpha$_1$-adrenergic agonists also increase myocardial oxygen consumption. To that extent,

they act much like beta-adrenergic agonists, whereby postresuscitation myocardial dysfunction is increased. Alpha$_2$-adrenoceptor agonists that do not cross the blood brain–barrier are promising. These agonists acting peripherally have improved outcomes of CPR, based entirely on experimental studies, however. In comparison, vasopressin is also effective for initial resuscitation, but its prolonged vasopressor action after successful restoration of spontaneous circulation has potential adverse effects when it imposes increased workloads on the heart at a time when work capability is already impaired.

The primary goal of chest compression or open chest cardiac message is to re-establish the flow of blood to vital organs until spontaneous circulation is restored to these organs. Blood flow to the heart itself, and specifically the restoration of blood flow to the coronary arteries to sustain myocardial blood flow, is of predominant import for successful restoration of spontaneous circulation. When adrenergic vasopressor agents produce systemic vasoconstriction they are intended to increase aortic diastolic pressure and consequently coronary and cerebral perfusion pressures. We have described in detail the pharmacological actions of adrenergic agents and how they are mediated by receptors and specifically alpha, including alpha$_1$ and alpha$_2$, and beta, including beta$_1$, beta$_2$, and beta$_3$. Epinephrine has each of these adrenergic actions, and was the predominant adrenergic drug used during CPR for more than a century. Its primary effect is alpha-adrenergic vasoconstriction. This contrasts with its beta-adrenergic actions, which are mildly vasodilatory and more strikingly inotropic and chronotropic. Beta-adrenergic actions result in increases in myocardial oxygen demands and consumption, and increases in heart rate and ventricular premature beats. The beta-adrenergic effects of epinephrine also account for transient hypoxemia caused by pulmonary arteriovenous shunting. There is no evidence that epinephrine improves ultimate survival in human victims of cardiac arrest.

More selective alpha-adrenergic agonists have been investigated to minimize these adverse beta-adrenergic effects. Both alpha$_1$- and alpha$_2$-agonists have peripheral vasopressor actions. Nevertheless, desensitization of alpha$_1$-adrenergic receptors during CPR may account for lesser vasopressor potency. In addition, alpha$_1$-adrenergic receptors in the myocardium, like beta-adrenergic agonists, increase myocardial oxygen demands. Alpha$_2$-adrenoceptor agonists act in the central nervous system where they produce vasodilatory effects, but only if they cross the blood–brain barrier. If an alpha$_2$-agonist does not have central nervous system access, it produces selective peripheral vasoconstrictive effects. Experimentally, during CPR, selective alpha$_2$-agonists that do not gain entrance into the brain therefore may produce more optimal systemic vasoconstriction. Selective alpha$_2$-agonists have as a major advantage that they do not increase myocardial oxygen consumption and thereby increase ischemic injury during the reduced low flow state of cardiac resuscitation. Myocardial ischemic injury during CPR is therefore minimized and myocardial function after successful restoration of spontaneous circulation is better preserved with improved survival in animals. The issues are of substantial clinical importance, for clinical studies have as yet failed to confirm neither an optimal drug nor an optimal dose of either adrenergic vasopressor amines or vasopressin of proven benefit for increased survival in settings of cardiac resuscitation.

These observations prompt re-examination of adrenergic agents for routine management of cardiac resuscitation and invite clinical studies on the patented benefits of selective alpha$_2$-agonists.

REFERENCES

1. Niemann, J.T., Rosborough, J.P. & Ung, S. Coronary perfusion pressure during experimental cardiopulmonary resuscitation. *Ann. Emerg. Med.* 1982; **11**: 127–131.
2. Deantonio, H.J., Kaul, S. & Lerman, B.B. Reversible myocardial depression in survivors of cardiac arrest. *Pacing Clin. Electrophysiol.* 1990; **13**: 982–985.
3. Weil, M.H. & Tang, W. Cardiopulmonary resuscitation: a promise that is as yet largely unfulfilled. *Dis. Mon.* 1997; **43**: 431–501.
4. Sun, S.J., Weil, M.H., Tang, W., Povoas, H.P. & Mason, E. Combined effects of buffer and adrenergic agents on postresuscitation myocardial function. *J. Pharm. Exp. Ther.* 1999; **291**: 773–777.
5. Redding, J.S. & Pearson, J.W. Evaluation of drugs for cardiac resuscitation. *Anesthesiology* 1963; **24**: 203–207.
6. Paradis, N.A., Martin, G.B. & Rivers, E.P. Coronary perfusion pressure and the return of spontaneous circulation in human cardiopulmonary resuscitation. *J. Am. Med. Assoc.* 1990; **263**: 1106–1113.
7. Tang, W., Weil, M.H., Sun, S.J. *et al.* The effects of biphasic and conventional monophasic defibrillation on postresuscitation myocardial function. *J. Am. Coll. Cardiol.* 1999; **4**: 815–822.
8. Ahlquist, R.P. A study of the adrenotropic receptors. *Am. J. Physiol.* 1948; **153**: 586.
9. Bylund, D.B. Subtypes of α_2-adrenoceptors: pharmacological and molecular biological evidence converge. *Trends Pharmacol. Sci.* 1988; **9**: 356–361.
10. Standards and guidelines for cardiopulmonary resuscitation (CPR) and emergency care (ECC). *J. Am. Med. Assoc.* 1947; **227** Suppl: 833–886.
11. AHA Guidelines 2000 for Cardiopulmonary Resuscitation and Emergency Cardiovascular Care. *Circulation* 2000; **8**(Suppl): I-129–135.
12. Pearson, J.W. & Redding, J.S. Peripheral vascular tone in cardiac resuscitation. *Anesth. Analg.* 1965; **44**: 746–752.
13. Otto, C.W., Yakaitis, R.W. & Blitt, C.D. Mechanism of action of epinephrine resuscitation from asphyxial arrest. *Crit. Care Med.* 1981; **9**: 321–324.
14. Otto, C.W., Yakaitis, R.W. The role of epinephrine in CPR: a reappraisal. Part 2. *Ann. Emerg. Med.* 1984; **13**: 840–843.
15. Paradis, N.A. & Koscove, E.M. Epinephrine in cardiac arrest: a critical review. *Ann. Emerg. Med.* 1990; **19**: 1288–1301.
16. Emergency Cardiac Care Committee and Subcommittees, American Heart Association. Guidelines for cardiopulmonary resuscitation and emergency cardiac care. *J. Am. Med. Assoc.* 1992; **268**: 2172–2241.

17. Ditchey, R.V. & Lindenfeld, J. Failure of epinephrine to improve the balance between myocardial oxygen supply and demand during closed-chest resuscitation in dogs. *Circulation* 1988; **78**: 382–389.

18. Tang, W., Weil, M.H., Gazmuri, R.J., Sun, S.J., Duggal, C. & Bisera, J. Pulmonary ventilation/perfusion defects induced by epinephrine during cardiopulmonary resuscitation. *Circulation* 1991; **84**: 2101–2107.

19. Ditchey, R.V., Rubio-Perez, A. & Slinker, B.K. Beta-adrenergic blockade reduces myocardial injury during experimental cardiopulmonary resuscitation. *J. Am. Coll. Cardiol.* 1994; **24**: 804–812.

20. Tang, W., Weil, M.H., Sun, S.J., Noc, M., Yang, L. & Gazmuri, R.J. Epinephrine increase the severity of postresuscitation myocardial dysfunction. *Circulation* 1995; **92**: 3089–3093.

21. Holmberg, M., Holmberg, S. & Herlitz, J. Low chance of survival among patients requiring adrenaline (epinephrine) or intubation after out-of-hospital cardiac arrest in Sweden. *Resuscitation* 2002; **54**: 37–45.

22. Laurent, I., Monchi, M., Chiche, J. *et al.* Reversible myocardial dysfunction in survivors of out-of-hospital cardiac arrest. *Am. J. Coll. Cardiol.* 2002; **40**: 2110–2116.

23. Gonzalez, E.R., Ornato, J.P. & Garnet, A.R. Dos-dependent vasopressor response to phenylephrine during CPR in human beings. *Ann. Emerg. Med.* 1989; **18**: 920–926.

24. Roberts, D., Landolfo, K., Dobson, K. & Light, B.R. The effects of methoxamine and epinephrine on survival and regional distribution of cardiac output in dogs with prolonged ventricular fibrillation. *Chest* 1990; **98**: 999–2205.

25. Huang, L., Weil, M.H., Cammarata, G., Sun, S. & Tang, W. Nonselective β-blocking agent improves the outcome of cardiopulmonary resuscitation in a rat model. *Crit. Care Med.* 2004; **32**: S378–S380.

26. Gold, H.K., Leinbach, R.C. & Maroko, P.R. Propranolol-induced reduction of signs of ischemic injury during acute myocardial infarction. 1972; **38**: 689–695.

27. Maroko, P.R., Libby, P., Covell, J.W. *et al.* Precordial S-T elevation mapping: an atraumatic method for assessing alteration in the extent of myocardial ischemic injury *Am. J. Cardiol.* 1972; **29**: 223–230.

28. Obeid, A., Spear, R., Mookherjee, S. *et al.* The effect of propranolol on myocardial energy stores during myocardial ischemia in dogs. *Circulation* 1976; **54**(Suppl II): II-159.

29. Cammarata, G., Weil, M.H., Sun, S., Tang, W., Wang, J. & Huang, L. β$_1$-blockade during cardiopulmonary resuscitation improves survival. *Crit. Care Med.* 2004; **32**: S440–S443.

30. Gazmuri, R.J., Weil, M.H., Bisera, J., Tang, W., Fukui, M. & McKee, D. Myocardial dysfunction after successful resuscitation from cardiac arrest. *Crit. Care Med.* 1996; **24**: 992–1000.

31. Lindner, K., Ahnefeld, F. & Bowdler, I. Comparison of different doses of epinephrine on myocardial perfusion and resuscitation in a pig model. *Am. J. Emerg. Med.* 1991; **9**: 27–31.

32. Gonzalez, E.R. & Ornato, J.P. The dose of epinephrine during cardiopulmonary resuscitation in humans: what should it be? *DICP Ann. Pharmacol.* 1991; **25**: 773–777.

33. Stiell, I.G., Hebert, P.C., Weitzman, B.N. *et al.* High-dose epinephrine in adult cardiac arrest. *N. Engl. J. Med.* 1992; **327**: 1045–1050.

34. Lindner, K.H., Ahnefeld, F.W. & Prengel, A.W. Comparison of standard and high-dose adrenaline in the resuscitation of asystole and electromechanical dissociation. *Acta. Anaesthesiol. Scand.* 1991; **35**: 253–256.

35. Brown, C.G., Martin, D.R., Pepe, P.E. *et al.* The Multicenter High-Dose Epinephrine Study Group. A comparison of standard-dose and high-dose epinephrine in cardiac arrest outside the hospital. *N. Engl. J. Med.* 1992; **327**: 1051–1055.

36. Callaham, M., Madsen, C.D., Barton, C.W., Saunders, C.E. & Pointer, J. A randomized clinical trial of high-dose epinephrine and norepinephrine vs. standard-dose epinephrine in prehospital cardiac arrest. *J. Am. Med. Assoc.* 1992; **268**: 2667–2772.

37. Brown, C.G., Birinyi, F., Werman, H.A., Davis, E.A. & Hamlin, R.L. The comparative effects of epinephrine versus phenylephrine on regional cerebral blood flow during cardiopulmonary resuscitation. *Resuscitation* 1986; **14**: 171–183.

38. Schnabel, P., Nohr, T., Nickenig, G., Paul, M. & Bohm, M. Alpha-adrenergic signal transduction in renin transgenic rats. *Hypertension* 1997; **30**(6): 1356–1361.

39. Hashimi, M.W., Thornton, J.D., Downey, J.M. & Cohen, M.V. Loss of myocardial protection from ischemic preconditioning following chronic exposure to R(-)-N$_6$-(2-phenylisopropyl) adenosine is related to defect at the adenosine A$_1$ receptor. *Mol. Cell. Biochem.* 1998; **186**(1–2): 19–25.

40. Sun, S., Tang, W., Fang, X., Huang, L. & Weil, M.H. Decreased sensitivity of 1-adrenergic receptors after prolonged cardiac arrest. *Crit. Care Med.* 2004; **32**(Suppl. 12): A8.

41. Grupp, I.L., Lorenz, J.N., Walsh, R.A., Boivin, G.P. & Rindt, H. Overexpression of alpha 1B-adrenergic receptor induces left ventricular dysfunction in the absence of hypertrophy. *Am. J. Physiol.* 1998; **275**: H1338–H1350.

42. Gregorini, L., Marco, J., Kozakova, M. *et al.* Alpha-adrenergic blockade improves recovery of myocardial perfusion and function after coronary stenting in patients with acute myocardial infarction. *Circulation* 1999; **99**: 482–490.

43. Ishibashi, Y., Duncker, D.J. & Bache, R.J. Endogenous nitric oxide masks alpha$_2$-adrenergic coronary vasoconstriction during exercise in the ischemic heart. *Circ. Res.* 1997; **80**: 196–207.

44. Lomasney, J.W., Cotecchia, S., Lefkowitz, R.J. & Caron, M.G. Molecular biology of alpha-adrenergic receptors: implications for receptor classification and for structure-function relationships. *Biochim. Biophys. Acta.* 1991; **1095**: 127–139.

45. Link, R.E., Desai, K., Hein, L. *et al.* Cardiovascular regulation in mice lacking α$_2$-adrenergic receptor subtypes b and c. *Science* (Wash. DC) 1996; **273**: 803–805.

46. Kable, J.W., Murrin, L.C. & Bylund, D.B. In vivo gene modification elucidates subtype-specific function of α$_2$-adrenergic receptors. *J. Pharmacol. Exp. Ther.* 2000; **293**(1): 1–7.

47. Gavras, I. & Gavras, H. Role of alpha$_2$-adrenergic receptors in hypertension. 1: *Am. J. Hypertens* 2001; **14**(6 Pt 2): 171S–177S.

48. Sun, S.J., Weil, M.H., Tang, W., Kamohara, T. & Klouche, K. Alpha-methylnorepinephrine, a selective alpha$_2$-adrenergic agonist for cardiac resuscitation. *J. Am. Coll. Cardiol.* 2001; **37**(3): 951–956.

49. Fries, M., Tang, W., Chang, Y.T., Castillo, C. & Weil, M.H. Detrimental effects of epinephrine on microcirculatory blood flow in a porcine model of cardiac arrest. *Crit. Care Med.* 2004; **32**(Suppl. 12): A56.

50. Ristagno, G., Sun, S.J., Chang, Y.T. *et al.* Epinephrine reduces cerebral microcirculatory blood flow during CPR. *Crit. Care Med.* 2005; **33**(Suppl. 12): A24.

51. Pellis, T., Weil, M.H., Tang, W., Sun, S.J., Xie, J. & Song, L. Comparison of vasopressin, epinephrine, and epinephrine after combined alpha$_1$ and beta adrenergic blockade for CPR. *Circulation* 2002; **106**(19): II496.

35

Vasopressin and other non-adrenergic vasopressors

Anette C. Krismer, Martin Dunser, Karl H. Stadlbauer, Karl H. Lindner and Volker Wenzel

Department of Anesthesiology and Critical Care Medicine, Innsbruck Medical University, Austria

Basic science

The importance of arterial vascular tone in resuscitation from cardiac arrest has been described in detail in the previous chapters of this book.

Efficacy of non-adrenergic pressors

There is a longstanding concern that administration of adrenaline during resuscitation may result in detrimental effects during the postresuscitation period. For example, laboratory studies with adrenaline during cardiopulmonary resuscitation (CPR) showed increased myocardial oxygen consumption,[1] ventricular arrhythmias,[2] ventilation–perfusion defects,[3] and postresuscitation myocardial dysfunction.[4] Therefore, non-adrenergic vasoactive peptides such as vasopressin hold considerable promise, since they may raise perfusion pressure without the β-receptor-mediated side effects of adrenergic vasopressors. Another intriguing possibility is that they may act synergistically when administered together with catecholamines, and that concomitant use of adrenergic drugs and nonadrenergic vasoactive peptides may allow lowering of the dose of each agent.

Vasopressin, an endogenous stress hormone

A number of fundamental endocrine responses of the human body to cardiac arrest and CPR have been investigated in past years,[5–8] and are summarized in another chapter of this book. Circulating endogenous vasopressin concentrations were high in patients undergoing CPR, and levels in successfully resuscitated patients have been shown to be significantly higher than those in patients who died.[5] This may indicate that the human body discharges vasopressin as an adjunct endogenous vasopressor to epinephrine in life-threatening situations such as cardiac arrest in order to preserve homeostasis. In a clinical study of 60 out-of-hospital cardiac arrest patients, parallel increases in plasma vasopressin and endothelin during CPR were found only in surviving patients.[6] Thus, plasma concentrations of vasopressin may have a more important effect on CPR outcome than was previously thought. These observations prompted several investigations to assess the role of arginine vasopressin in the management of CPR in order to improve patient outcome.

Arginine vasopressin physiology

Arginine vasopressin is an endogenous hormone with osmoregulatory, vasopressor, hemostatic, endocrinologic, thermoregulatory, and central nervous effects (Fig. 35.1). The hormone is produced in the magnocellular nuclei of the hypothalamus, and stored in neurosecretory vesicles of the neurohypophysis. It is secreted upon osmotic, hemodynamic, and endocrinologic stimuli. Although only 10%–20% of the total hormonal pool of arginine vasopressin in the neurohypophysis can be readily released, the time from synthesis to secretion into the circulation is ~1.5 hours.[9] Once released, the plasma half-life of arginine vasopressin is 5–15 minutes. Dose-dependent clearance occurs through vasopressinases in the liver and the kidneys.[10]

The most important hemodynamic signals for secretion are reduced atrial filling and lower arterial blood pressure.

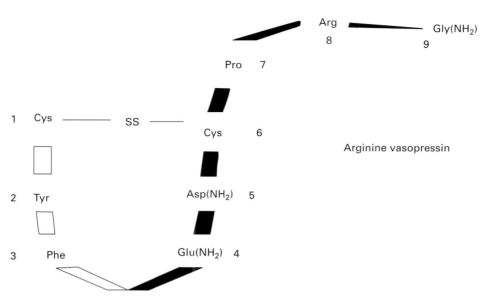

Fig. 35.1. Amino acid sequence of arginine-vasopressin. (From ref. 107.)

Any reduction in blood volume or venous return stimulates secretion of arginine vasopressin *via* activation of stretch receptors located in the left atrium and pulmonary arteries (Gauer–Henry reflex). Activation of baroreceptors in the aortic arch and carotid sinus further augments secretion of arginine vasopressin *via* the glossopharyngeus and vagal nerves. Baroreceptor stimulation is the primary and most important mechanism for release of this hormone in hypotensive states and cardiac arrest.[11] In acute hypotension, there is an exponential relationship between levels of arginine vasopressin in plasma and the decrease in arterial blood pressure. Whereas small reductions in blood pressure (~5–10% from baseline) usually have only minor or no effect on arginine vasopressin levels in plasma, a 20%–30% decline in arterial pressure results in arginine vasopressin concentrations that are severalfold higher.[12] Similarly, volume depletion produces little elevation in plasma levels of this hormone unless blood volume decreases by more than 10% and results in diminished arterial blood pressure.[11,13] Nevertheless, secretion of argin-ine vasopressin can also be directly stimulated by hypoxia, endotoxin, low concentrations of norepinephrine and angiotensin, or hypoglycemia.[14]

Pharmacological effects of arginine vasopressin

Peripheral effects of arginine vasopressin are mediated by different vasopressin receptors: namely V_{1a}, V_{1b}, and V_2 arginine vasopressin receptors. V_{1a} receptors are located on smooth muscle cells in arterial blood vessels, and induce vasoconstriction by an increase in cytoplasmic ionized calcium *via* the phosphatidyl-inositol-bisphosphonate cascade.[15] On a molar basis, arginine vasopressin was shown to be a severalfold more potent vasoconstrictor than were norepinephrine and angiotensin II.[16] In contrast to catecholamine-mediated vasoconstriction, effects of arginine vasopressin are preserved during hypoxia and severe acidosis.[17]

Vascular effects mediated by vasopressin differ substantially within particular vascular beds, however. Physiologically, most arterial beds exhibit vasoconstriction in response to vasopressin.[18,19] Vasopressor effects are strongest in the muscular, adipose, cutaneous, and probably also the splanchnic vasculature. In a porcine CPR model, Voelckel *et al.*[20] found a significantly lower blood flow in the superior mesenteric artery in pigs resuscitated with arginine vasopressin when compared to epinephrine; there were no differences in hepatic or renal blood flow. Similar to oxytocin-mediated paradoxical vasodilatation of vascular smooth muscle, vasodilatation after arginine vasopressin has not only been described in the pulmonary, coronary, and vertebrobasilar circulation, but interestingly also in the mesenteric vascular bed, suggesting a dose-dependent response.[21–24] The underlying mechanisms for such an arginine vasopressin-mediated vasodilatation seem to be nitric oxide dependent.[22] Russ and Walker reported that stimulation of V_1-receptors can release nitric oxide, presumably from the endothelium of some vascular regions.[25] There is increasing evidence of hemodynamically relevant V_1-receptors on cardiomyocytes. In vitro and animal experi-ments have demonstrated an increase of intracellular calcium concentration and inotropy after stimulation of myocardial V_1-receptors.[26,27]

In the kidney, V_2-receptors are located on distal tubules and collecting ducts. Upon stimulation, they facilitate integration of aquaporines into the luminal cell membrane of the collecting ducts, leading to increased resorption of free water *via* an adenylate cyclase-dependent mechanism.[28] Despite its antidiuretic effect, a paradoxical increase of urine output has been reported during continuous infusion of arginine vasopressin in patients with advanced vasodilatory shock.[29–31] It is hypothesized that together with increased renal perfusion pressure, arginine vasopressin selectively constricts efferent glomerular arterioles, whereas it dilates afferent vessels, thus increasing effective filtration pressure in the glomerulus.[29]

V_{1b} receptors are located on the anterior hypophysis; stimulation induces liberation of ACTH and prolactin.[32] Accordingly, Kornberger *et al.*[33] reported significantly higher ACTH and cortisol concentrations in serum from animals resuscitated from cardiac arrest with arginine vasopressin when compared to epinephrine. In patients with advanced vasodilatory shock, however, a continuous infusion of arginine vasopressin at dosages of 4 IU/h affected neither serum ACTH nor cortisol concentrations.[34] A complex dysfunction of the hypophyseal–adrenal axis in critical illness may explain the lack of effects of the potent stimulator arginine vasopressin on ACTH-producing cells. Nonetheless, arginine vasopressin seems to be able to promote prolactin excretion by V_{1b} receptor stimulation. Additional V_{1b} receptors are expressed on pancreatic islet cells where they enhance insulin secretion in the presence of high glycemic levels.[35]

Arginine vasopressin during CPR in laboratory models

In a porcine model simulating ventricular fibrillation, a dose–response investigation of three arginine vasopressin dosages (0.2; 0.4; 0.8 U/kg) compared with the maximum effective dose of 200 µg/kg epinephrine showed that 0.8 U/kg of arginine vasopressin was the most effective drug for increasing blood flow to vital organs and coronary perfusion pressure (Figs. 35.2 and 35.3).[36] Correspondingly, arginine vasopressin significantly improved cerebral oxygen delivery, and mean frequency of ventricular fibrillation during CPR when compared with a maximum dose of epinephrine[37] (Fig. 35.4). Furthermore,

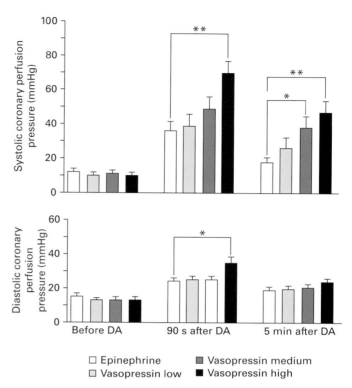

Fig. 35.2. Effects of different doses of vasopressin vs. high dose epinephrine on systolic and diastolic blood pressure. (From ref. 36.)

the effects on vital organ blood flow lasted longer after administration of arginine vasopressin than after treatment with epinephrine (~4 vs. ~1.5 min); significantly more arginine vasopressin animals could be resuscitated.[38] The same dose of intravenous and endobronchial arginine vasopressin resulted in similar coronary perfusion pressures 4 minutes after drug administration.[39,40] Intraosseous vs. intravenous arginine vasopressin lead to comparable levels of arginine vasopressin in plasma, hemodynamic variables, coronary perfusion pressure, and rates of return of spontaneous circulation (Fig. 35.5).[41] Therefore, the intraosseous route might be a valuable alternative for administration of arginine vasopressin during CPR, when intravenous access is delayed, or not available.

After repeated dosages of arginine vasopressin vs. epinephrine were administered in a porcine model, coronary perfusion pressure increased only after the first of three epinephrine injections, but increased after each of three arginine vasopressin injections; accordingly, all arginine vasopressin-treated animals survived, whereas all pigs resuscitated with epinephrine died (Fig. 35.6).[42] In the early postresuscitation phase of the same model, arginine

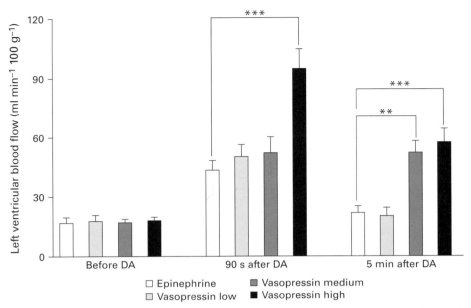

Fig. 35.3. Effects of different doses of vasopressin vs. high dose epinephrine on left ventricular blood flow. (From ref. 36.)

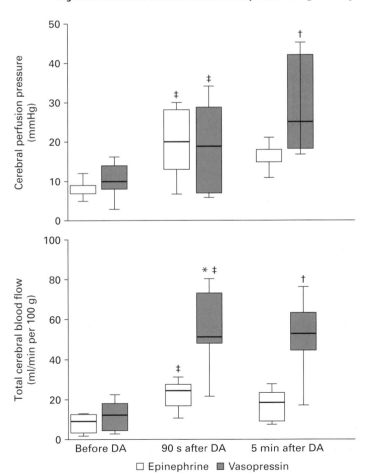

Fig. 35.4. Effects of different doses of vasopressin vs. high dose epinephrine on total cerebral blood flow and cerebral perfusion pressure. (From ref. 37.)

vasopressin administration resulted in higher arterial blood pressure, but a lower cardiac index; a reversible depressant but not critical effect on myocardial function by arginine vasopressin was observed when compared with epinephrine.[43] Renal and splanchnic perfusion may be impaired during[44] and after[45] successful resuscitation from cardiac arrest. Arginine vasopressin impaired mesenteric blood flow during CPR and in the early postresuscitation phase.[20] Neither renal blood flow, nor renal function, however, was influenced by arginine vasopressin or epinephrine in this investigation.[20]

In a model of prolonged advanced cardiac life support (22 minutes), all arginine vasopressin animals had return of spontaneous circulation, whereas all pigs in the epinephrine and saline placebo group died. Twenty-four hours after return of spontaneous circulation, the only neurological deficit of pigs resuscitated with arginine vasopressin was an unsteady gait, which disappeared within another 3 days. Subsequently performed magnetic resonance imaging revealed no cerebral cortical or subcortical edema, intraparenchymal hemorrhage, ischemic brain lesions, or cerebral infarction, indicating that arginine vasopressin- but not epinephrine-treated pigs recovered fully from cardiac arrest in both anatomical and physiological terms even after prolonged CPR.[46]

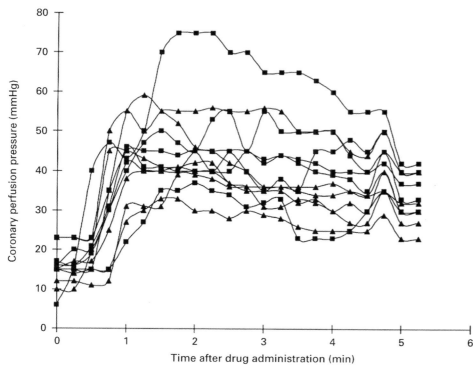

Fig. 35.5. Intravenous vs. intraosseous vasopressin during CPR. Individual coronary perfusion pressure tracings after intravenous (■) and intraosseous (▲) vasopressin administration during CPR. No statistical analysis was performed for this figure. Some tracings may be superimposed on each other; defibrillation was performed approximately at 5 min and 15 s after drug administration. (From ref. 41.)

Clinical studies with arginine vasopressin during cardiac arrest

In patients with refractory cardiac arrest, arginine vasopressin induced an increase in arterial blood pressure, and in some cases, return of spontaneous circulation, where standard therapy with chest compressions, ventilation, defibrillation, and epinephrine had failed.[47] In a small ($n = 40$) prospective, randomized investigation of patients with shock-refractory out-of-hospital ventricular fibrillation, a significantly larger proportion of patients treated with arginine vasopressin were successfully resuscitated and survived for 24 hours compared with patients treated with epinephrine.[48] In 1999, a Chinese study group reported a prospective, randomized trial comparing two different dosages of arginine vasopressin and two different dosages of epinephrine in 83 patients with in-hospital cardiac arrest. Their findings indicated that high-dose arginine vasopressin (1 IU/kg) significantly increased the rate of return of spontaneous circulation, and improved the survival rate compared with standard (1 mg) and high dosages

(5 mg) of epinephrine.[49] In a large ($n = 200$) in-hospital CPR trial from Ottawa, Canada, comparable short-term survival was found in both groups treated with either arginine vasopressin or epinephrine, indicating that these drugs may be equipotent when response times of rescuers are short.[50] In another clinical evaluation in Detroit, Michigan, 4 of 10 patients responded to arginine vasopressin administration after ~45 minutes of unsuccessful advanced cardiac life support, and had a mean increase in coronary perfusion pressure of 28 mmHg.[51] This is surprising, because an increase in arterial blood pressure with any drug after such a long period of ineffective CPR management is expected to be minimal.

From June 1999 to March 2002, we conducted a large multicenter trial in Austria, Germany, and Switzerland, and randomized 1219 out-of-hospital cardiac arrest patients to be treated with epinephrine or arginine vasopressin[52] (Fig. 35.7). Hospital admission and discharge rates were comparable between treatment arms for patients with ventricular fibrillation and for pulseless electrical activity, but patients with asystole were more likely

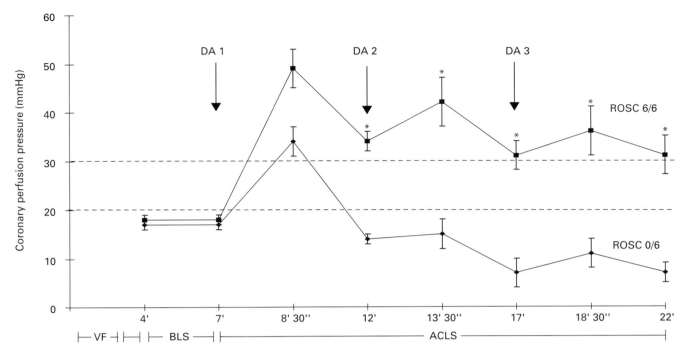

Fig. 35.6. Vasopressin vs. epinephrine during prolonged CPR. Administration of repeated doses of vasopressin (■), but not epinephrine (◆) given early during basic life support CPR maintained mean ± SEM CPP above the threshold of ∼ 20 to 30 mmHg (dashed lines) that is needed for successful defibrillation with return of spontaneous circulation. DA 1 indicates drug administration of 0.4 U/kg of vasopressin vs. 45 μg/kg of epinephrine; DA 2, 0.4 U/kg of vasopressin vs. 45 μg/kg of epinephrine; DA 3, 0.8 U/kg of vasopressin vs. 200 μg/kg of epinephrine; *$P < 0.05$ vs. epinephrine; ROSC, return of spontaneous circulation; VF, ventricular fibrillation; and ACLS, advanced cardiac life support. Time is given in minutes (') and seconds ("). (From ref. 53.)

to survive when primarily treated with arginine vasopressin (Table 35.1, Fig. 35.8). If patients could not be successfully resuscitated with two injections of arginine vasopressin, however, additional epinephrine significantly improved hospital admission ($p = 0.002$) and discharge rates ($p = 0.002$) when compared to epinephrine-treated patients (Table 35.2, Fig. 35.9). There was no difference in cerebral performance between groups for the entire trial.

These results did not confirm earlier data suggesting that arginine vasopressin was more effective than epinephrine as a first-line vasopressor drug in the treatment of ventricular fibrillation, pulseless electrical activity, or asystole.[36–38,46,48,53] Criticism has been raised that arginine vasopressin may improve coronary and cerebral perfusion pressures during CPR with refractory ventricular fibrillation and pulseless electrical activity, but not outcome. Unfortunately, we are unable to state whether this phenomenon may be similar to the observations described with high-dose epinephrine during CPR, when increasing epinephrine dosages were effective in the laboratory,[54] but not in clinical practice.[55] It is clearly a virtually impossible

problem to extrapolate laboratory CPR to the clinical setting since species differences, comparing diseased patients with healthy laboratory animals, or differences in out-of-hospital CPR compared to laboratory conditions cannot be controlled adequately.

In contrast to ventricular fibrillation and pulseless electrical activity, in the multicenter study, arginine vasopressin improved the likelihood of asystolic patients reaching the hospital alive by about 40% over epinephrine. A possible explanation may be profound ischemia which is frequently present in asystolic patients. This is in accordance with a study *in vitro*, where it was demonstrated that arginine vasopressin has vasoconstricting efficacy even in severe acidosis, when catecholamines are less potent.[17] Thus, arginine vasopressin seems to be more effective than epinephrine in asystolic patients, thereby resulting in better coronary perfusion pressure during cardiac resuscitation. Since improved coronary perfusion pressure during CPR improves survival,[56] arginine vasopressin may be a better option than epinephrine for asystolic patients, who normally have the worst chance of survival. Also, improvement

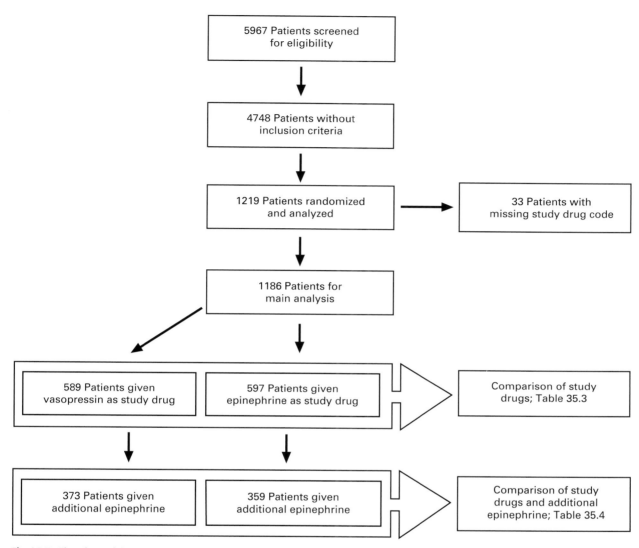

Fig. 35.7. Flowchart of the European multicenter study and analysis. (From ref. 52.)

in hospital discharge after treatment with epinephrine following arginine vasopressin may indicate that interactions among arginine vasopressin, epinephrine, and the underlying degree of ischemia during CPR may be more complex than was previously thought. When prolonged asphyxia had depleted endogenous epinephrine levels and caused profound ischemia in pigs, arginine vasopressin combined with epinephrine tripled coronary perfusion pressure over either epinephrine or arginine vasopressin alone (Fig. 35.10).[57] This suggests that the presence of arginine vasopressin may enhance the effects of epinephrine or *vice versa*, especially during prolonged ischemia.[57,58]

In an in-hospital CPR study reporting comparable effects of arginine vasopressin and epinephrine, 87%

of arginine vasopressin patients received additional epinephrine.[50] The concept of deliberate administration of arginine vasopressin combined with epinephrine during CPR is also supported by clinical observations that epinephrine followed by arginine vasopressin significantly improved coronary perfusion pressure,[51] return of spontaneous circulation,[47,58] and 24-hour survival rates.[59] This was also confirmed by a retrospective review that compared arginine vasopressin after epinephrine *vs.* epinephrine only, in a subset of patients with out-of-hospital cardiac arrest who did not respond to immediate therapy with epinephrine (Fig. 35.11).[58]

Although half of the survivors in the multicenter study with good neurological outcome received the combi-

Table 35.1. Outcome data of all patients (*N* = 1186), and cerebral performance category of all patients at hospital discharge (*N* = 115)[52]

	Vasopressin 589 of 1186 (49.7%)	Epinephrine 597 of 1186 (50.3%)	*P*	OR	CI
All cardiac rhythms					
ROSC after study drugs	145 of 589 (24.6%)	167 of 597 (28.0%)	0.19	1.2	0.9–1.5
Hospital admission	214 of 589 (36.3%)	186 of 597 (31.2%)	0.06	0.8	0.6–1.0
Hospital discharge [a]	57 of 578 (9.9%)	58 of 588 (9.9%)	0.99	1.0	0.7–1.5
Ventricular fibrillation					
ROSC after study drugs	82 of 223 (36.8%)	106 of 249 (42.6%)	0.20	1.3	0.9–1.8
Hospital admission	103 of 223 (46.2%)	107 of 249 (43.0%)	0.48	0.9	0.6–1.3
Hospital discharge	39 of 219 (17.8%)	47 of 245 (19.2%)	0.70	1.1	0.7–1.8
Pulseless electrical activity					
ROSC after study drugs	21 of 104 (20.2%)	17 of 82 (20.7%)	0.93	1.0	0.5–2.1
Hospital admission	35 of 104 (33.7%)	25 of 82 (30.5%)	0.65	0.8	0.5–1.6
Hospital discharge	6 of 102 (5.9%)	7 of 81 (8.6%)	0.47	1.4	0.5–4.7
Asystole					
ROSC after study drugs	42 of 262 (16.0%)	44 of 266 (16.5%)	0.87	1.0	0.7–1.6
Hospital admission	76 of 262 (29.0%)	54 of 266 (20.3%)	0.02	0.6	0.4–0.9
Hospital discharge	12 of 257 (4.7%)	4 of 262 (1.5%)	0.04	0.3	0.1–1.0
All cardiac rhythms – cerebral performance [b]					
Good cerebral performance	15 of 46 (32.6%)	16 of 46 (34.8%)	0.99	. . .	. . .
Moderate cerebral disability	7 of 46 (15.2%)	12 of 46 (26.1%)	0.30	. . .	. . .
Severe cerebral disability	9 of 46 (19.6%)	7 of 46 (15.2%)	0.78	. . .	. . .
Coma	15 of 46 (32.6%)	11 of 46 (23.9%)	0.49	. . .	. . .

European multicenter study.

OR denotes odds ratio; CI, 95% confidence interval; ROSC, return of spontaneous circulation; [a] lost to follow-up, 11 (1.9%) vasopressin vs. 9 (1.5%) epinephrine patients; [b] lost to follow-up, 11 (9.6%) vasopressin vs. 12 (10.4%) epinephrine patients; . . ., not calculated; *P* values are not adjusted for multiple comparisons.

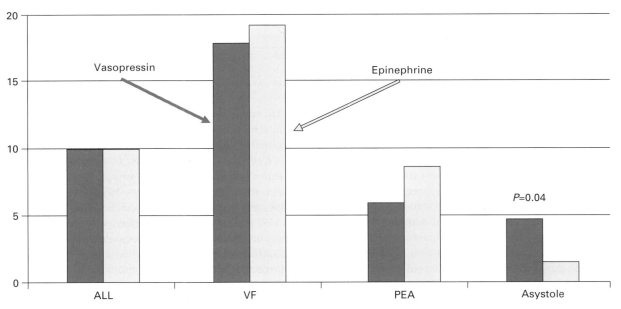

Fig. 35.8. Hospital-discharge of all patients (*n* = 1186) of the European multicenter study. (From ref. 52.)

Table 35.2. Outcome data of patients who received vasopressin or epinephrine initially, and subsequently additional epinephrine ($N = 732$); and cerebral performance category at hospital discharge ($N = 29$)

	Vasopressin 373 of 732 (51.0%)	Epinephrine 359 of 732 (49.0%)	P	OR	CI
All cardiac rhythms					
ROSC	137 of 373 (36.7%)	93 of 359 (25.9%)	0.002	0.6	0.4–0.8
Hospital admission	96 of 373 (25.7%)	59 of 359 (16.4%)	0.002	0.6	0.4–0.8
Hospital discharge [a]	23 of 369 (6.2%)	6 of 355 (1.7%)	0.002	0.3	0.1–0.6
Ventricular fibrillation					
ROSC	58 of 122 (47.5%)	40 of 122 (32.8%)	0.02	0.5	0.3–0.9
Hospital admission	37 of 122 (30.3%)	25 of 122 (20.5%)	0.08	0.6	0.3–1.1
Hospital discharge	13 of 121 (10.7%)	6 of 121 (5.0%)	0.09	0.4	0.2–1.2
Pulseless electrical activity					
ROSC	18 of 64 (28.1%)	14 of 56 (25.0%)	0.70	0.8	0.4–1.8
Hospital admission	17 of 64 (26.6%)	10 of 56 (17.9%)	0.25	0.6	0.2–1.4
Hospital discharge	3 of 64 (4.7%)	0 of 55 (0.0%)	0.10	. . .	. . .
Asystole					
ROSC	61 of 187 (32.6%)	39 of 181 (21.5%)	0.02	0.6	0.4–0.9
Hospital admission	42 of 187 (22.5%)	24 of 181 (13.3%)	0.02	0.5	0.3–0.9
Hospital discharge	7 of 184 (3.8%)	0 of 179 (0.0%)	0.008	. . .	. . .
All cardiac rhythms – cerebral performance [b]					
Good cerebral performance	8 of 20 (40.0%)	2 of 5 (40.0%)	1.00	. . .	. . .
Moderate cerebral disability	2 of 20 (10%)	2 of 5 (40.0%)	0.17	. . .	. . .
Severe cerebral disability	2 of 20 (10%)	1 of 5 (20.0%)	0.50	. . .	. . .
Coma	8 of 20 (40%)	0 of 5 (0.0%)	0.14	. . .	. . .

OR denotes odds ratio; CI, 95% confidence interval; ROSC, return of spontaneous circulation; [a] patients lost to follow-up, 4 (1.1%) vasopressin vs. 4 (1.1%) epinephrine patients; [b] patients lost to follow-up, 3 (10.3%) vasopressin vs. 1 (3.4%) epinephrine patients; . . . , not calculated; P values are not adjusted for multiple comparisons.
European multicenter study.

nation of arginine vasopressin and epinephrine, this strategy also resulted in more, albeit not statistically significant, patients in coma than after epinephrine alone. This indicates that the combination of arginine vasopressin and epinephrine effectively resuscitated the heart, but was too late to resuscitate the brain in some patients. When starting CPR, it is difficult to predict postresuscitation brain function.[60] Although our hospital discharge rate (9.7%) compares favorably with that in other reports, 2.2% of our patients had severe neurological impairment. Thus, combining arginine vasopressin and epinephrine improved survival rates, but resulted in unfavorable neurological outcome in some patients. In patients treated with arginine vasopressin, unfavorable neurological outcome was observed in 5 of 10 patients who were first found to be in asystole or pulseless electrical activity; in contrast, no asystole or pulseless electrical activity patient receiving ≥ 3 mg epinephrine had unfavorable neurological outcome since all died before being discharged.

While an unfavorable ECG diagnosis upon starting CPR, such as asystole, may be one important surrogate for unfavorable neurological outcome, we should not forget that duration of ischemia reflects vital organ injury, and the required vasopressor dosage reflects the organism's ability to respond to CPR efforts. For example, both witnessed cardiac arrest and basic life support within 10 min was highly significant ($p < 0.001$) in predicting hospital admission in the European multicenter study. Patients who needed only one or two injections of the study drugs had a hospital discharge rate of 19.5%, whereas patients requiring two injections of either one of the study drugs and additional epinephrine had a hospital discharge rate of only 4%. A final judgment whether combining arginine vasopressin and epinephrine is beneficial, especially when administered earlier, as in our investigation, requires confirmation in a prospective study, which is currently under way in France. More than 1500 patients have already been randomized (PY Gueugniaud, personal communication, 2005).

Table 35.3. Meta-analysis comparing vasopressin vs. epinephrine. Death before hospital admission[61]

Study	Vasopressin (*n*/*N*)	Epinephrine (*n*/*N*)	RR (random) (95% Cl)	Weight (%)	RR (random) (95% Cl)
Lindner 1997	6/20	13/20		35.45	0.46 [0.22, 0.97]
Wenzel 2004	375/589	411/597		64.55	0.92 [0.85, 1.00]
Total (95% Cl)	609	617		100.00	0.72 [0.38, 1.39]

Total events: 381 (vasopressin), 424 (epinephrine)
Test for heterogeneity: Chi^2 = 3.36, df = 1 (*P* = 0.07), I^2 = 70.2%
Test for overall effect Z = 0.97 (*P* = 0.33)

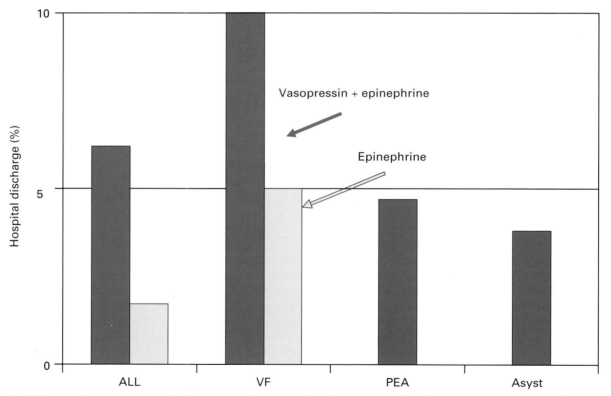

Fig. 35.9. In a subgroup analysis of the European multicenter study, patients treated with arginine-vasopressin after epinephrine (*n* = 732) had a better long-term outcome compared to patients treated with epinephrine only. Asyst, asystole. (From ref. 52.)

Limitations of arginine vasopressin during CPR

The promising news about vasopressin CPR studies cannot disguise the fact that many issues have not been addressed as of today. For example, there is still lack of large clinical studies. This may be the reason why a recently conducted meta-analysis[61] did not show statistically significant differences between arginine vasopressin and epinephrine in return of spontaneous circulation, hospital admission, and discharge rates (Tables 35.3–35.5). It is to be hoped that the ongoing French vasopressin study will answer these questions decisively.

Further, extrapolating experience with arginine vasopressin from the adult to the pediatric setting is difficult, and needs to be investigated.[62] Preliminary laboratory

Table 35.4. Meta-analysis comparing vasopressin vs. epinephrine. Death within 24 hours[61]

Study	Vasopressin (n/N)	Epinephrine (n/N)	RR (random) (95% CI)	Weight (%)	RR (random) (95% CI)
Lindner 1997	8/20	16/20		41.40	0.50 [0.28, 0.89]
Stiell 2001	77/104	73/96		58.60	0.97 [0.83, 1.14]
Total (95% CI)	124	116		100.00	0.74 [0.38, 1.43]

Total events: 85 (vasopressin), 424 (epinephrine)
Test for heterogeneity: Chi^2 = 4.99, df = 1 (P = 0.03), I^2 = 80.0%
Test for overall effect Z = 0.90 (P = 0.37)

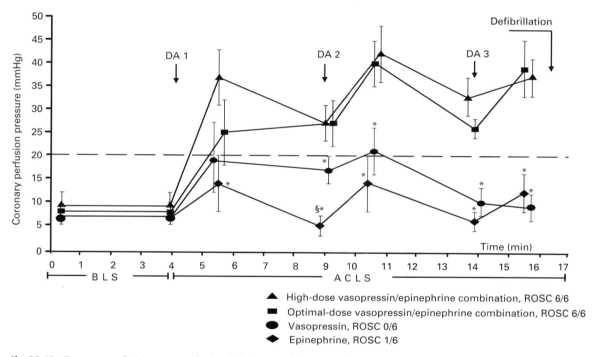

Fig. 35.10. Coronary perfusion pressure during CPR. Repeated doses of high-dose (▲) and optimal-dose (■) vasopressin/epinephrine combinations, but not vasopressin alone (●) or epinephrine alone (◆), maintained mean ± SEM coronary perfusion pressure at a level of 35 to 45 mmHg, which makes successful defibrillation more likely. *P < 0.05 vs. vasopressin alone and epinephrine alone; §P < 0.05 vs. epinephrine alone. BLS indicates basic life support; ACLS, advanced cardiac life support; DA 1, administration of 0.4 U/kg of vasopressin/45 µg/kg of epinephrine combinations vs. 0.4 U/kg of vasopressin alone vs. 45 µg/kg of epinephrine alone; DA 2, administration of 0.8 U/kg of vasopressin/200 µg/kg of epinephrine combination vs. 0.8 U/kg of vasopressin/45 µg/kg of epinephrine combination vs. 0.8 U/kg of vasopressin alone vs. 200 µg/kg of epinephrine alone; and DA 3, administration of 0.8 U/kg of vasopressin/200 µg/kg of epinephrine combination vs. 0.8 U/kg of vasopressin/45 µg/kg of epinephrine combination vs. 0.8 U/kg of vasopressin alone vs. 200 µg/kg of epinephrine alone. Area below the dashed line indicates coronary perfusion pressure that usually does not correlate with return of spontaneous circulation. (From ref. 57.)

evidence suggests beneficial effects of a combination of arginine vasopressin with epinephrine in asphyxic cardiac arrest; however, this observation is inconsistent with reports in a postcountershock, pulseless electrical activity preparation. Although preliminary experimental data suggest coronary vasodilatation after arginine vasopressin, this model may not reflect diffuse coronary artery disease of humans with possibly different physiology of the

Table 35.5. Meta-analysis comparing vasopressin *vs.* epinephrine. Death before hospital discharge[61]

Study	Vasopressin (n/N)	Epinephrine (n/N)	RR (random) (95% Cl)	Weight (%)	RR (random) (95% Cl)
Lindner 1997	12/20	17/20		5.25	0.71 [0.47, 1.06]
Li 1999	30/40	39/43		15.79	0.83 [0.68, 1.01]
Lee 2000	2/5	4/5		0.70	0.50 [0.16, 1.59]
Stiell 2001	92/104	83/96		31.64	1.02 [0.92, 1.14]
Wenzel 2004	521/578	530/588		46.62	1.00 [0.96, 1.04]
Total (95% Cl)	747	752		100.00	0.96 [0.87, 1.05]

Total events: 657 (vasopressin), 673 (epinephrine)
Test for heterogeneity: Chi^2 = 8.05, df = 4 (P = 0.09), I^2 = 50.3%
Test for overall effect Z = 0.92 (P = 0.36)

0.1 0.2 0.5 1 2 5 10
Favors vasopressin   Favors epinephrine

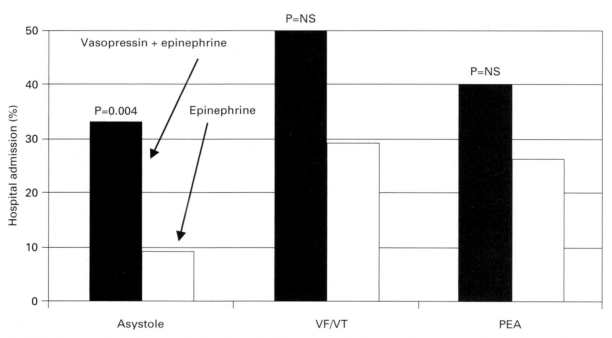

Fig. 35.11. Retrospective study comparing the effects of arginine vasopressin after epinephrine vs. epinephrine only. Asystolic patients treated with arginine-vasopressin after epinephrine had a better short-term survival compared to patients treated with epinephrine only. (From ref. 58.)

coronary arteries.[63,64] Currently, we do not know whether arginine vasopressin acts simply as a back-up for the vasopressor epinephrine during life-threatening shock states, whether arginine vasopressin or epinephrine alone is better in certain situations, or whether these two hormones have unique adjunct features that we are only beginning to understand. Better knowledge of these underlying mechanisms would most likely save many

patients, who at this point in time have relatively little chance of survival.[65]

Arginine vasopressin in hemorrhagic shock

In 1990, about 5 million people died worldwide as a result of injury, and it seems likely that the global epidemic of deadly trauma is only beginning. By 2020, deaths from injury are expected to increase to 8 million worldwide,[66] and 30% of these fatalities will be attributable to uncontrolled hemorrhagic shock.[67] Resuscitation of patients in uncontrolled hemorrhagic shock remains one of the most challenging aspects of emergency care, and trauma patients with complete cardiovascular collapse have an extremely poor chance of survival. For example, in a 1993 study of 138 trauma patients requiring cardiopulmonary resuscitation at the accident scene or during transport, none of the initially successfully resuscitated patients survived to hospital discharge.[68] Accordingly, prevention of cardiac arrest has been considered to be the primary goal of trauma care.[69] Unfortunately, trauma-related cardiac arrest is only the tip of the iceberg. Because hemorrhage-induced hypotension in trauma patients is predictive of frequent mortality and morbidity, managing prolonged hypotension aggressively may be equally important.

For hemodynamic stabilization of critically injured patients with uncontrolled hemorrhagic shock, current trauma guidelines recommend infusion of crystalloid or colloid solutions in addition to catecholamine vasopressors. In a large clinical study of penetrating torso trauma, patients receiving delayed fluid resuscitation had better survival rates than did those receiving immediate fluid resuscitation.[70] Roberts *et al.*[71] further found no scientific evidence for the effectiveness of immediate fluid resuscitation in uncontrolled hemorrhagic shock. Also, a Cochrane review of randomized controlled trials found no evidence either for or against early or large volume IV fluid administration in uncontrolled hemorrhage.[72] At present, therefore, we have no clearly proven fluid resuscitation strategy for uncontrolled hemorrhagic shock, and it seems expedient to consider alternative strategies to prevent immediate or delayed cardiac arrest in these patients. Moreover, during the late phase of hemorrhagic shock when cardiac arrest may occur at any time, replacement of fluids and blood may become ineffective even when supported by conventional vasopressors such as norepinephrine.[73] In an experimental shock model in dogs, arginine vasopressin has been shown effectively to restore circulation in the late phase of hemorrhagic shock that was unresponsive to blood replacement and catecholamines.[73] Furthermore, arginine vasopressin enabled short- and long-term survival in a porcine model of uncontrolled hemorrhagic shock after penetrating liver trauma (Fig. 35.12)[74–77] and after traumatic brain injury.[78] Arginine vasopressin has also been used in a small number of non-trauma patients with upper gastrointestinal bleeding and subsequent shock that was unresponsive to volume replacement.[79] In the clinical setting, positive effects of arginine vasopressin were observed in some patients with life-threatening hemorrhagic shock with collapsing arterial blood pressure, who did not continue to respond to adrenergic catecholamines and fluid resuscitation (Fig. 35.13).[80–83] Interestingly, all patients in these case reports received a combination of vasopressin and catecholamines during the late phase of uncontrolled hemorrhagic shock, which may be more effective than either drug alone. This enhancing effect of a combination of vasopressin and catecholamines is in accord with our evidence in settings of severe shock such as cardiac arrest and septic shock.[52,57,80,82,84] Furthermore, these case reports demonstrate that prolonged hemorrhagic shock with severe hypotension managed with vasopressin can result in fully conscious patients with intact cardiocirculatory function and full neurological recovery. This is in agreement with a case report[80] of a patient with multiple fractures of the pelvis, spine, and legs, as well as a severe head trauma after a fall from a roof (fourth floor), resulting in uncontrolled hemorrhagic shock and severe hypotension that was refractory to massive infusion of fluids, blood products and norepinephrine. Subsequent infusion of vasopressin prevented cardiocirculatory collapse, resulted in a stable hemodynamic function, and enabled emergency surgery. This patient made a full neurological recovery (Fig. 35.13).[80]

The case reports also provide valuable information, because the successful treatment of uncontrolled hemorrhagic shock with vasopressin was reproducible and reported by different observers. We believe that in patients with uncontrolled hemorrhagic shock, infusing vasopressin may be an option for stabilizing cardiocirculatory function and prevent cardiac arrest. In the absence of randomized controlled trials investigating the role of vasopressin in uncontrolled hemorrhagic shock today, even the currently limited clinical data available may support treatment decisions in selected patients who would otherwise die rapidly. In the future, we need to assess whether the existing laboratory[74–78] and limited clinical data[80–83] on treating uncontrolled hemorrhagic shock successfully with vasopressin can be confirmed in a randomized controlled clinical trial. In addition, the best timing of application and optimal dose of this form of therapy need to be addressed.

Angiotensin II

Angiotensin II is a potent vasoconstricting octapeptide. As an intermediary in the renin-angiotensin-aldosterone system, angiotensin II has received much attention as a mediator of hypertension and congestive heart failure.

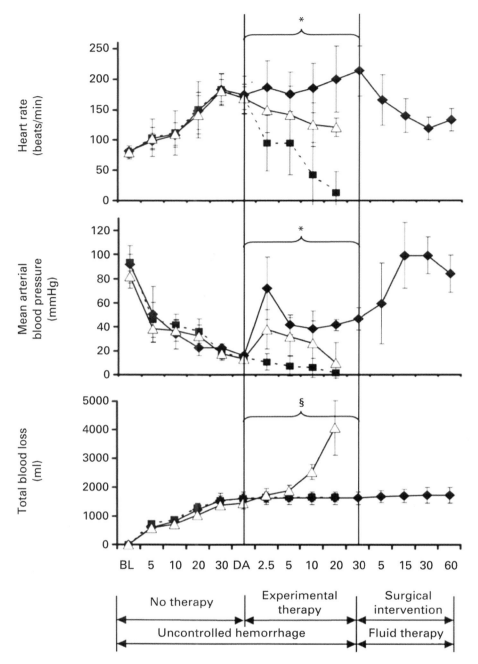

Fig. 35.12. Mean ± SD heart rate, mean arterial blood pressure, and total blood loss before, during, and after administration of a 0.4 U/kg bolus dose, and 0.08 U/kg/min continuous infusion of vasopressin (closed diamond, continuous line) vs. fluid resuscitation (closed triangle, continuous line) with 25 ml/kg lactated Ringer's solution and 25 ml/kg 3% gelatin solution vs. saline placebo (closed square, dotted line). Uncontrolled hemorrhage = the non-intervention interval after liver injury; experimental therapy = vasopressin or fluid resuscitation or saline placebo administration without bleeding control; surgical intervention = surgical management of the liver lobe to control bleeding; fluid therapy = infusion of lactated Ringer's solution, 3% gelatin solution, and transfusion of blood; BL = baseline; DA = drug administration; *$P < 0.05$ between groups for differences between all groups during the experimental protocol; §$P < 0.05$ for differences between the fluid resuscitation, and vasopressin and saline placebo group during the experimental protocol. No statistical comparison was performed after 20 min of experimental therapy because of death of all fluid resuscitation and saline placebo pigs, respectively. (From ref. 74.)

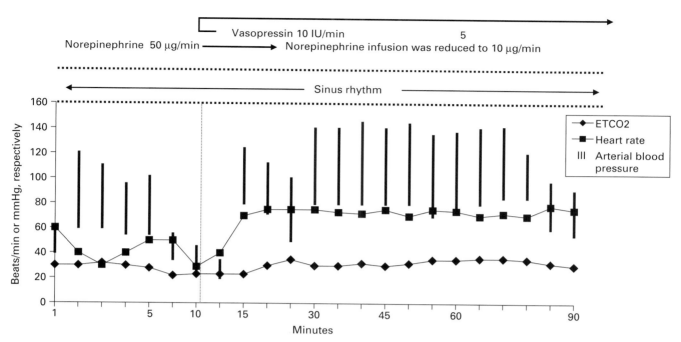

Fig. 35.13. A 41-year-old woman fell off a roof (height ~15 m), and was transported to the next county hospital. Because of an unstable pelvic fracture, the patient became hemodynamically unstable; therefore, an arterial cannula, and a large-bore central venous catheter were placed, and four units of packed red cells and coagulation factors were administered, and the patient was airlifted to a university hospital. After arrival in the emergency room of the level one trauma center, hemodynamic stability could not be maintained despite massive infusion of fluids and norepinephrine (50 μg/min). The patient had a TRISS score-predicted death rate of 84.9%. An infusion of vasopressin was then started (10 IU/min), and blood pressure was stabilized, thus allowing emergent angiography and application of a pelvic clamp. Angiography revealed a ruptured left internal iliac, and left pudendal artery; both blood vessels were successfully coiled and the patient was stabilized. Subsequent CT scanning revealed an injury pattern consisting of complex facial injuries, subdural hematoma, diffuse edema of the brain, spine and rib fractures, hemothorax and hemomediastinum, rupture of the right bronchus, central hematoma of the liver, massive retroperitoneal hematoma, pelvic fractures, open fracture of the left femur, open fractures of both tibias, and fractures of both ankles, and the right upper arm. The patient underwent several surgical procedures to repair fractures, developed a systemic inflammatory response and a multiple organ dysfunction syndrome, but was discharged from the critical care unit to the ward without neurological damage 39 days after the accident. (From ref. 80.)

Renin, on secretion by the renal juxtaglomerular cells, catalyzes the cleavage of angiotensinogen to angiotensin I, which is only a weak vasopressor.[85] Angiotensin II is formed by cleavage of angiotensin I by angiotensin-converting enzyme. Angiotensin II is then converted to angiotensin III, which stimulates aldosterone release by the adrenal cortex. Angiotensin II has a very short serum half-life as it is quickly converted to angiotensin III and broken down by serum and tissue peptidases.[85]

Angiotensin II has unique receptors, designated AT_1 and AT_2, of which AT_1-receptors mediate the vasopressor and chronotropic effects of angiotensin II.[86,87] The second-messenger system of the AT_1-receptor appears to involve activation of phospholipases C and D leading to increased inositol phosphates.[85,87,88] This increase in inositol phosphates increases intracellular calcium and leads to smooth muscle contraction. The second-messenger system is distinct from that of the adrenergic system, which utilizes cyclic adenosine monophosphate (cAMP).

The vascular response to angiotensin II infusion is generalized vasoconstriction. On a molar basis, angiotensin II is approximately 30 times more potent than norepinephrine.[85] It produces a dose-dependent increase in blood pressure in humans and animals.[88–90] It acts in conjunction with the adrenergic system and vasopressin to maintain mean arterial pressure during a variety of physiologic insults, including hemorrhage, sepsis, adrenal insufficiency, and other hypotensive states.[91–95]

Angiotensin II has been used experimentally as a vasopressor since the 1950s. The effect of pharmacologic doses of angiotensin II in the setting of hypotension and shock, however, has not been well studied. There are case reports of use of angiotensin II in individual patients, but no comprehensive physiologic assessment. Much of the use of angiotensin II occurred before invasive hemodynamic monitoring became routine. The relative contribution of direct vasoconstriction by angiotensin II compared to its effects on adrenal catecholamine release was not examined. The effects of angiotensin II on myocardial blood flow have been tested in a swine model of cardiac arrest with open-chest cardiac compressions. After administration of angiotensin II, myocardial blood flow was 118 ml/min per 100 g, which is near normal, compared to 56 ml/min per 100 g for the placebo group. Myocardial oxygen delivery and oxygen-extraction ratio were improved in the angiotensin II group.[96] Cerebral oxygen delivery and extraction ratios were also improved by angiotensin II in a porcine cardiac arrest model.[97] A porcine study described the effects of angiotensin II (50 μg/kg) compared to epinephrine (20 μg/kg), and a group receiving the two agents in combination.[98] All groups had a significant increase in myocardial blood flow during CPR following drug administration, but there was a trend toward higher flows in the epinephrine-treated animals. Furthermore, both groups that received epinephrine had significantly higher myocardial blood flow after return of spontaneous circulation when compared with those treated with angiotensin II.[98] Further studies will be needed to determine whether angiotensin II may have a role as a vasopressor in the therapy of cardiac arrest. At this time, clinical evidence is not sufficient to support use of angiotensin II during CPR.

Endothelin

Endothelin has been identified as a powerful vasoconstricting hormone secreted by endothelial cells.[99–101] DeBehnke *et al.*[102] reported that compared with endothelin or epinephrine, the combination of endothelin-1 plus epinephrine improved coronary perfusion pressure in a canine model of CPR. It was further shown that endothelin may significantly improve cerebral perfusion.[103,104] Another porcine model studied the effects of a combination of epinephrine and endothelin.[105] Although more animals that received the combination of endothelin-1 plus epinephrine had return of spontaneous circulation, fewer animals survived to 1 or 24 hours.[105] This was the result of a marked vasoconstricting effect of the combination of epinephrine and endothelin-1 in the doses used. There was a marked increase in the coronary perfusion pressure, but a dramatic narrowing of the pulse pressure, and a marked drop in the end-tidal carbon dioxide level, indicating a marked

decrease in forward blood flow. Results from a canine study suggested that endothelin-1 may contribute to the failure of cerebral circulation after cardiac arrest.[106]

In summary, it had been axiomatic that increased vasoconstriction during CPR improves coronary perfusion pressure, and thereby immediate resuscitation success; however, data indicate that vasoconstriction can be excessive. Postresuscitation left ventricular dysfunction is well documented, and is difficult to manage in the intensive care unit. Accordingly, the stunned left ventricle may be unable to tolerate the increased systemic vascular resistance immediately after resuscitation and, therefore, heart failure and malignant ventricular arrhythmias may occur. Accordingly, use of endothelin during CPR is not beneficial.

Practice points

CPR

Both angiotensin II and endothelin should not be administered during CPR. According to the new data from the European arginine vasopressin study,[52] we recommend administering first, 1 mg of epinephrine followed alternately by 40 IU of vasopressin and 1 mg of epinephrine

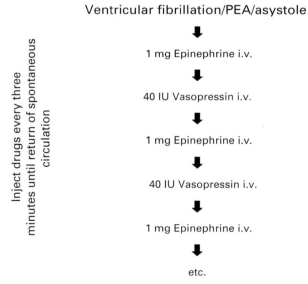

Fig. 35.14. Algorithm according to the new data from the European arginine vasopressin study.[52] We recommend administering 1 mg of epinephrine first, followed alternately by 40 IU vasopressin and 1 mg epinephrine every 3 minutes in adult cardiac arrest victims, regardless of the initial ECG rhythm. (From ref. 52.)

every 3 minutes in adult cardiac arrest victims, regardless of the initial ECG rhythm (Fig. 35.14).

Hemorrhagic shock

Although promising at present observations made with arginine vasopressin in hemorrhagic shock and collapsing blood pressure in the laboratory and in individual patients, need to be confirmed in future prospective, randomized clinical trials. In selected patients with massive bleeding and intractable hemorrhagic shock resulting in collapsing blood pressure despite advanced trauma life support, 5–10 IU vasopressin may be injected; the cumulative dose should be titrated according to arterial blood pressure.

REFERENCES

1. Ditchey, R.V. & Lindenfeld, J. Failure of epinephrine to improve the balance between myocardial oxygen supply and demand during closed-chest resuscitation in dogs. *Circulation* 1988; **78**: 382–389.

2. Niemann, J.T., Haynes, K.S., Garner, D. *et al.* Postcountershock pulseless rhythms: response to CPR, artificial cardiac pacing, and adrenergic agonists. *Ann. Emerg. Med.* 1986; **15**: 112–20.

3. Tang, W., Weil, M.H., Gazmuri, R.J. *et al.* Pulmonary ventilation/perfusion defects induced by epinephrine during cardiopulmonary resuscitation. *Circulation* 1991; **84**: 2101–2107.

4. Tang, W.C., Weil, M.H., Sun, S.J. *et al.* Epinephrine increases the severity of postresuscitation myocardial dysfunction. *Circulation* 1995; **92**: 3089–3093.

5. Lindner, K.H., Strohmenger, H.U., Ensinger, H. *et al.* Stress hormone response during and after cardiopulmonary resuscitation. *Anesthesiology* 1992; **77**: 662–668.

6. Lindner, K.H., Haak, T., Keller, A., Bothner, U. & Lurie, K.G. Release of endogenous vasopressors during and after cardiopulmonary resuscitation. *Br. Heart J.* 1996; **75**: 145–150.

7. Strohmenger, H.U., Lindner, K.H., Keller, A. *et al.* Concentrations of prolactin and prostaglandins during and after cardiopulmonary resuscitation. *Crit. Care Med.* 1995; **23**: 1347–1355.

8. Schultz, C.H., Rivers, E.P., Feldkamp, C.S. *et al.* A characterization of hypothalamic–pituitary–adrenal axis function during and after human cardiac arrest. *Crit. Care Med.* 1993; **21**: 1339–1347.

9. Sklar, A.H. & Schrier, R.W. Central nervous system mediators of vasopressin release. *Physiol. Rev.* 1983; **63**: 1243–1280.

10. Mutlu, G.M. & Factor, P. Role of vasopressin in the management of septic shock. *Intens. Care Med.* 2004; **30**: 1276–1291.

11. Thrasher, T.N. & Keil, L.C. Systolic pressure predicts plasma vasopressin responses to hemorrhage and vena caval constriction in dogs. *Am. J. Physiol. Regul. Integr. Comp. Physiol.* 2000; **279**: R1035–R1042.

12. Berl, T. & Robertson, G.L. Pathophysiology of water metabolism. In Brenner, B.M., ed. Brenner & Rector's *The Kidney* Philadelphia: Saunders, 2000: 866–924.

13. Callahan, M.F., Ludwig, M., Tsai, K.P., Sim, L.J. & Morris, M. Baroreceptor input regulates osmotic control of central vasopressin secretion. *Neuroendocrinology* 1997; **65**: 238–245.

14. Kasting, N.W., Mazurek, M.F. & Martin, J.B. Endotoxin increases vasopressin release independently of known physiological stimuli. *Am. J. Physiol.* 1985; **248**: E420–E424.

15. Birnbaumer, M. Vasopressin receptors. *Trends Endocrinol. Metab.* 2000; **11**: 406–410.

16. Reid, I.A. & Schwartz, J. Role of vasopressin in the control of blood pressure. In Martini, L. & Ganong, W.F., eds. *Frontiers in Neuroendocrinology.* New York: Raven Press, 1976: 177–197.

17. Fox, A.W., May, R.E. & Mitch, W.E. Comparison of peptide and nonpeptide receptor-mediated responses in rat tail artery. *J. Cardiovasc. Pharmacol.* 1992; **20**: 282–289.

18. Garcia-Villalon, A.L., Garcia, J.L., Fernandez, N. *et al.* Regional differences in the arterial response to vasopressin: role of endothelial nitric oxide. *Br. J. Pharmacol.* 1996; **118**: 1848–1854.

19. Moursi, M.M., van Wylen, D.G. & D'Alecy, L.G. Regional blood flow changes in response to mildly pressor doses of triglycyl desamino lysine and arginine vasopressin in the conscious dog. *J. Pharmacol. Exp. Ther.* 1985; **232**: 360–368.

20. Voelckel, W.G., Lindner, K.H., Wenzel, V. *et al.* Effects of vasopressin and epinephrine on splanchnic blood flow and renal function during and after cardiopulmonary resuscitation in pigs. *Crit. Care Med.* 2000; **28**: 1083–1088.

21. Martinez, M.C., Vila, J.M., Aldasoro, M. *et al.* Relaxation of human isolated mesenteric arteries by vasopressin and desmopressin. *Br. J. Pharmacol.* 1994; **113**: 419–424.

22. Wallace, A.W., Tunin, C.M. & Shoukas, A.A. Effects of vasopressin on pulmonary and systemic vascular mechanics. *Am. J. Physiol.* 1989; **257**: H1228–H1234.

23. Okamura, T., Ayajiki, K., Fujioka, H. & Toda, N. Mechanisms underlying arginine vasopressin-induced relaxation in monkey isolated coronary arteries. *J. Hypertens.* 1999; **17**: 673–678.

24. Suzuki, Y., Satoh, S., Oyama, H. *et al.* Vasopressin mediated vasodilation of cerebral arteries. *J. Auton. Nerv. Syst.* 1994; **49** Suppl: S129–S132.

25. Russ, R.D. & Walker, B.R. Role of nitric oxide in vasopressinergic pulmonary vasodilatation. *Am. J. Physiol.* 1992; **262**: H743–H74.

26. Xu, Y.J. & Gopalakrishnan, V. Vasopressin increases cytosolic free [Ca^{2+}] in the neonatal rat cardiomyocyte. Evidence for V1 subtype receptors. *Circ. Res.* 1991; **69**: 239–45.

27. Fujisawa, S. & Iijima, T. On the inotropic actions of arginine vasopressin in ventricular muscle of the guinea pig heart. *Jpn. J. Pharmacol.* 1999; **81**: 309–12.

28. Wuttke, T. Endocrinology. In Schmidt, R.F. & Thews, G., eds. *Human Physiology.* Berlin Heidelberg, New York: Springer, 1993: 390–420.

29. Landry, D.W., Levin, H.R., Gallant, E.M. *et al.* Vasopressin pressor hypersensitivity in vasodilatory septic shock. *Crit. Care Med.* 1997; **25**: 1279–1282.

30. Tsuneyoshi, I., Yamada, H., Kakihana, Y. *et al.* Hemodynamic and metabolic effects of low-dose vasopressin infusions in vasodilatory septic shock. *Crit. Care Med.* 2001; **29**: 487–493.

31. Holmes, C.L., Walley, K.R., Chittock, D.R., Lehman, T. & Russell, J.A. The effects of vasopressin on hemodynamics and renal function in severe septic shock: a case series. *Intens. Care Med.* 2001; **27**: 1416–1421.

32. Bilezikjian, L.M. & Vale, W.W. Regulation of ACTH secretion from corticotrophs: the interaction of vasopressin and CRF. *Ann. N Y Acad. Sci.* 1987; **512**: 85–96.

33. Kornberger, E., Prengel, A.W., Krismer, A. *et al.* Vasopressin-mediated adrenocorticotropin release increases plasma cortisol concentrations during cardiopulmonary resuscitation. *Crit. Care Med.* 2000; **28**: 3517–3521.

34. Dunser, M.W., Hasibeder, W.R., Wenzel, V. *et al.* Endocrinologic response to vasopressin infusion in advanced vasodilatory shock. *Crit. Care Med.* 2004; **32**: 1266–1271.

35. Lee, B., Yang, C., Chen, T.H., al-Azawi, N. & Hsu, W.H. Effect of AVP and oxytocin on insulin release: involvement of V1b receptors. *Am. J. Physiol.* 1995; **269**: E1095–E1100.

36. Lindner, K.H., Prengel, A.W., Pfenninger, E.G. *et al.* Vasopressin improves vital organ blood flow during closed-chest cardiopulmonary resuscitation in pigs. *Circulation* 1995; **91**: 215–221.

37. Prengel, A.W., Lindner, K.H. & Keller, A. Cerebral oxygenation during cardiopulmonary resuscitation with epinephrine and vasopressin in pigs. *Stroke* 1996; **27**: 1241–1248.

38. Wenzel, V., Lindner, K.H., Prengel, A.W. *et al.* Vasopressin improves vital organ blood flow after prolonged cardiac arrest with postcountershock pulseless electrical activity in pigs. *Crit. Care Med.* 1999; **27**: 486–492.

39. Wenzel, V., Lindner, K.H., Prengel, A.W., Lurie, K.G. & Strohmenger, H.U. Endobronchial vasopressin improves survival during cardiopulmonary resuscitation in pigs. *Anesthesiology* 1997; **86**: 1375–1381.

40. Wenzel, V., Prengel, A.W. & Lindner, K.H. A strategy to improve endobronchial drug administration. *Anesth. Analg.* 2000; **91**: 255–256.

41. Wenzel, V., Lindner, K.H., Augenstein, S. *et al.* Intraosseous vasopressin improves coronary perfusion pressure rapidly during cardiopulmonary resuscitation in pigs. *Crit. Care Med.* 1999; **27**: 1565–1569.

42. Wenzel, V., Lindner, K.H., Krismer, A.C. *et al.* Repeated administration of vasopressin but not epinephrine maintains coronary perfusion pressure after early and late administration during prolonged cardiopulmonary resuscitation in pigs. *Circulation* 1999; **99**: 1379–1384.

43. Prengel, A.W., Lindner, K.H., Keller, A. & Lurie, K.G. Cardiovascular function during the postresuscitation phase after cardiac arrest in pigs: a comparison of epinephrine versus vasopressin. *Crit. Care Med.* 1996; **24**: 2014–2019.

44. Lindner, K.H., Brinkmann, A., Pfenninger, E.G. *et al.* Effect of vasopressin on hemodynamic variables, organ blood flow, and acid–base status in a pig model of cardiopulmonary resuscitation. *Anesth. Analg.* 1993; **77**: 427–435.

45. Prengel, A.W., Lindner, K.H., Wenzel, V., Tugtekin, I. & Anhaupl, T. Splanchnic and renal blood flow after cardiopulmonary resuscitation with epinephrine and vasopressin in pigs. *Resuscitation* 1998; **38**: 19–24.

46. Wenzel, V., Lindner, K.H., Krismer, A.C. *et al.* Survival with full neurologic recovery and no cerebral pathology after prolonged cardiopulmonary resuscitation with vasopressin in pigs. *J. Am. Coll. Cardiol.* 2000; **35**: 527–533.

47. Lindner, K.H., Prengel, A.W., Brinkmann, A. *et al.* Vasopressin administration in refractory cardiac arrest. *Ann. Intern. Med.* 1996; **124**: 1061–1064.

48. Lindner, K.H., Dirks, B., Strohmenger, H.U. *et al.* A Randomised comparison of epinephrine and vasopressin in patients with out-of-hospital ventricular fibrillation. *Lancet* 1997; **349**: 535–537.

49. Li, P.F., Chen, T.T. & Zhang, J.M. Clinical study on administration of vasopressin during closed-chest cardiopulmonary resuscitation. *Chin. Crit. Care Med.* 1999; **11**: 28–31.

50. Stiell, I.G., Hebert, P.C., Wells, G.A. *et al.* Vasopressin versus epinephrine for inhospital cardiac arrest: a randomised controlled trial. *Lancet* 2001; **358**: 105–109.

51. Morris, D.C., Dereczyk, B.E., Grzybowski, M. *et al.* Vasopressin can increase coronary perfusion pressure during human cardiopulmonary resuscitation. *Acad. Emerg. Med.* 1997; **4**: 878–883.

52. Wenzel, V., Krismer, A.C., Arntz, H.R. *et al.* A comparison of vasopressin and epinephrine for out-of-hospital cardiopulmonary resuscitation. *N. Engl. J. Med.* 2004; **350**: 105–113.

53. Wenzel, V., Lindner, K.H., Krismer, A.C. *et al.* Repeated administration of vasopressin but not epinephrine maintains coronary perfusion pressure after early and late administration during prolonged cardiopulmonary resuscitation in pigs. *Circulation* 1999; **99**: 1379–1384.

54. Callaham, M. High dose epinephrine in cardiac arrest. *West. J. Med.* 1991; **155**: 289–290.

55. Paradis, N.A., Wenzel, V. & Southall, J. Pressor drugs in the treatment of cardiac arrest. *Cardiol. Clin.* 2002; **20**: 61–78.

56. Paradis, N.A., Martin, G.B., Rivers, E.P. *et al.* Coronary perfusion pressure and the return of spontaneous circulation in human cardiopulmonary resuscitation. *J. Am. Med. Assoc.* 1990; **263**: 1106–1113.

57. Mayr, V.D., Wenzel, V., Voelckel, W.G. *et al.* Developing a vasopressor combination in a pig model of adult asphyxial cardiac arrest. *Circulation* 2001; **104**: 1651–1656.

58. Guyette, F.X., Guimond, G.E., Hostler, D. & Callaway, C.W. Vasopressin administered with epinephrine is associated with a return of a pulse in out-of-hospital cardiac arrest. *Resuscitation* 2004; **63**: 277–282.

59. Grmec, S., Kamenik, B. & Mally, S. Vasopressin in refractory out-of-hospital ventricular fibrillation: preliminary results. *Crit. Care Med.* 2002; **6**: P162 (Abstract).

60. Anonymous. Mild therapeutic hypothermia to improve the neurologic outcome after cardiac arrest. *N. Engl. J. Med.* 2002; **346**: 549–556.

61. Aung, K. & Htay, T. Vasopressin for cardiac arrest: a systematic review and meta-analysis. *Arch. Intern. Med.* 2005; **165**: 17–24.

62. Lienhart, H.G., John, W. & Wenzel, V. Cardiopulmonary resuscitation of a near-drowned child with a combination of epinephrine and vasopressin. *Pediatr. Crit. Care Med.* 2005; **6**: 486–488.

63. Mayr, V.D., Wenzel, V., Muller, T. *et al.* Effects of vasopressin on left anterior descending coronary artery blood flow during extremely low cardiac output. *Resuscitation* 2004; **62**: 229–235.

64. Wenzel, V., Kern, K.B., Hilwig, R.W. *et al.* Effects of intravenous arginine vasopressin on epicardial coronary artery cross sectional area in a swine resuscitation model. *Resuscitation* 2005; **64**: 219–226.

65. Wenzel, V. & Lindner, K.H. Employing vasopressin during cardiopulmonary resuscitation and vasodilatory shock as a life-saving vasopressor. *Cardiovasc. Res.* 2001; **51**: 529–541.

66. Murray, C.J. & Lopez, A.D. Alternative projections of mortality and disability by cause 1990–2020: Global Burden of Disease Study. *Lancet* 1997; **349**: 1498–1504.

67. Deakin, C.D. & Hicks, I.R. AB or ABC: pre-hospital fluid management in major trauma. *J. Accid. Emerg. Med.* 1994; **11**: 154–157.

68. Rosemurgy, A.S., Norris, P.A., Olson, S.M., Hurst, J.M. & Albrink, M.H. Prehospital traumatic cardiac arrest: the cost of futility. *J. Trauma* 1993; **35**: 468–473; discussion 73–74.

69. Shoemaker, W.C., Peitzman, A.B., Bellamy, R. *et al.* Resuscitation from severe hemorrhage. *Crit. Care Med.* 1996; **24** Suppl.: S12–S23.

70. Bickell, W.H., Wall, M.J., Jr., Pepe, P.E. *et al.* Immediate versus delayed fluid resuscitation for hypotensive patients with penetrating torso injuries. *N. Engl. J. Med.* 1994; **331**: 1105–1109.

71. Roberts, I., Evans, P., Bunn, F., Kwan, I. & Crowhurst, E. Is the normalisation of blood pressure in bleeding trauma patients harmful? *Lancet* 2001; **357**: 385–387.

72. Kwan, I., Bunn, F. & Roberts, I. Timing and volume of fluid administration for patients with bleeding. *Cochrane Database Syst. Rev.* 2003: CD002245.

73. Morales, D., Madigan, J., Cullinane, S. *et al.* Reversal by vasopressin of intractable hypotension in the late phase of hemorrhagic shock. *Circulation* 1999; **100**: 226–229.

74. Stadlbauer, K.H., Wagner-Berger, H.G., Raedler, C. *et al.* Vasopressin, but not fluid resuscitation, enhances survival in a liver trauma model with uncontrolled and otherwise lethal hemorrhagic shock in pigs. *Anesthesiology* 2003; **98**: 699–704.

75. Voelckel, W.G., Raedler, C., Wenzel, V. *et al.* Arginine vasopressin, but not epinephrine, improves survival in uncontrolled hemorrhagic shock after liver trauma in pigs. *Crit. Care Med.* 2003; **31**: 1160–1165.

76. Voelckel, W.G., von Goedecke, A., Fries, D. *et al.* Treatment of hemorrhagic shock. New therapy options. *Anaesthesist* 2004; **53**: 1151–1167.

77. Raedler, C., Voelckel, W.G., Wenzel, V. *et al.* Treatment of uncontrolled hemorrhagic shock after liver trauma: fatal effects of fluid resuscitation versus improved outcome after vasopressin. *Anesth. Analg.* 2004; **98**: 1759–1766, table of contents.

78. Feinstein, A.J., Patel, M.B., Sanui, M. *et al.* Resuscitation with pressors after traumatic brain injury. *J. Am. Coll. Surg.* 2005; **201**: 536–545.

79. Shelly, M.P., Greatorex, R., Calne, R.Y. & Park, G.R. The physiological effects of vasopressin when used to control intra-abdominal bleeding. *Intens. Care Med.* 1988; **14**: 526–531.

80. Krismer, A.C., Wenzel, V., Voelckel, W.G. *et al.* Employing vasopressin as an adjunct vasopressor in uncontrolled traumatic hemorrhagic shock. Three cases and a brief analysis of the literature. *Anaesthesist* 2005; **54**: 220–224.

81. Sharma, R.M. & Setlur, R. Vasopressin in hemorrhagic shock. *Anesth. Analg.* 2005; **101**: 833–834.

82. Haas, T., Voelckel, W.G., Wiedermann, F., Wenzel, V. & Lindner, K.H. Successful resuscitation of a traumatic cardiac arrest victim in hemorrhagic shock with vasopressin: a case report and brief review of the literature. *J. Trauma* 2004; **57**: 177–179.

83. Yeh, C.C., Wu, C.T., Lu, C.H., Yang, C.P. & Wong, C.S. Early use of small-dose vasopressin for unstable hemodynamics in an acute brain injury patient refractory to catecholamine treatment: a case report. *Anesth. Analg.* 2003; **97**: 577–579.

84. Dunser, M.W., Mayr, A.J., Ulmer, H. *et al.* The effects of vasopressin on systemic hemodynamics in catecholamine-resistant septic and postcardiotomy shock: a retrospective analysis. *Anesth. Analg.* 2001; **93**: 7–13.

85. Garrison, J.C. & Peach, M.J. Renin and angiotensin. In Gilman, A.G., ed. *The Pharmacological Basis of Therapeutics.* Pergamon Press, 1990: 749–763.

86. Griendling, K.K., Murphy, T.J. & Alexander, R.W. Molecular biology of the renin-angiotensin system. *Circulation* 1993; **87**: 1816–1828.

87. Vallotton, M.B., Capponi, A.M., Johnson, E.I. & Lang, U. Mode of action of angiotensin II and vasopressin on their target cells. *Horm. Res.* 1990; **34**: 105–110.

88. Doursout, M.F., Chelly, J.E., Hartley, C.J. *et al.* Regional blood flows and cardiac function changes induced by angiotensin II in conscious dogs. *J. Pharmacol. Exp. Ther.* 1988; **246**: 591–596.

89. Scroop, G.C., Walsh, J.A. & Whelan, R.F. A comparison of the effects of intra-arterial and intravenous infusions of angiotensin and noradrenaline on the circulation in man. *Clin. Sci* 1965; **29**: 315–326.

90. Heyndrickx, G.R., Boettcher, D.H. & Vatner, S.F. Effects of angiotensin, vasopressin, and methoxamine on cardiac function and blood flow distribution in conscious dogs. *Am. J. Physiol.* 1976; **231**: 1579–1587.

91. Brooks, V.L. Vasopressin and ANG II in the control of ACTH secretion and arterial and atrial pressures. *Am. J. Physiol.* 1989; **256**: R339–R347.

92. Downing, S.W., Edmunds, L.H., Jr. Release of vasoactive substances during cardiopulmonary bypass. *Ann. Thorac. Surg.* 1992; **54**: 1236–1243.

93. Ishikawa, S., Okada, K. & Saito, T. Increases in cellular sodium concentration by arginine vasopressin and endothelin in cultured rat glomerular mesangial cells. *Endocrinology* 1992; **131**: 1429–1435.

94. Paller, M.S. & Linas, S.L. Role of angiotensin II, alpha-adrenergic system, and arginine vasopressin on arterial pressure in rat. *Am. J. Physiol.* 1984; **246**: H25–H30.

95. Schaller, M.D., Waeber, B., Nussberger, J. & Brunner, H.R. Angiotensin II, vasopressin, and sympathetic activity in conscious rats with endotoxemia. *Am. J. Physiol.* 1985; **249**: H1086–H1092.

96. Lindner, K.H., Prengel, A.W., Pfenninger, E.G. & Lindner, I.M. Effect of angiotensin II on myocardial blood flow and acid–base status in a pig model of cardiopulmonary resuscitation. *Anesth. Analg.* 1993; **76**: 485–492.

97. Little, C.M. & Brown, C.G. Angiotensin II administration improves cerebral blood flow in cardiopulmonary arrest in swine. *Stroke* 1994; **25**: 183–186.

98. Little, C.M., Angelos, M.G. & Paradis, N.A. Compared to angiotensin II, epinephrine is associated with high myocardial blood flow following return of spontaneous circulation after cardiac arrest. *Resuscitation* 2003; **59**: 353–359.

99. Luscher, T.F. Endothelin: systemic arterial and pulmonary effects of a new peptide with potent biologic properties. *Am. Rev. Respir. Dis.* 1992; **146**: S56–S60.

100. Luscher, T.F., Boulanger, C.M., Dohi, Y. & Yang, Z.H. Endothelium-derived contracting factors. *Hypertension* 1992; **19**: 117–130.

101. Marsden, P.A. & Brenner, B.M. Nitric oxide and endothelins: novel autocrine/paracrine regulators of the circulation. *Semin. Nephrol.* 1991; **11**: 169–185.

102. DeBehnke, D.J., Spreng, D., Wickman, L.L. & Crowe, D.T. The effects of endothelin-1 on coronary perfusion pressure during cardiopulmonary resuscitation in a canine model. *Acad. Emerg. Med.* 1996; **3**: 137–141.

103. DeBehnke, D. The effects of graded doses of endothelin-1 on coronary perfusion pressure and vital organ blood flow during cardiac arrest. *Acad. Emerg. Med.* 2000; **7**: 211–221.

104. Holzer, M., Sterz, F., Behringer, W. *et al.* Endothelin-1 elevates regional cerebral perfusion during prolonged ventricular fibrillation cardiac arrest in pigs. *Resuscitation* 2002; **55**: 317–327.

105. Hilwig, R.W., Berg, R.A., Kern, K.B. & Ewy, G.A. Endothelin-1 vasoconstriction during swine cardiopulmonary resuscitation improves coronary perfusion pressures but worsens postresuscitation outcome. *Circulation* 2000; **101**: 2097–2102.

106. Takasu, A., Yagi, K. & Okada, Y. Role of endothelin-1 in the failure of cerebral circulation after complete global cerebral ischemia. *Resuscitation* 1995; **30**: 69–73.

107. Schmittinger, C.A., Wenzel, V., Herff, H. *et al.* Drug therapy during CPR. *Anasthesiol. Intensivmed. Notfallmed. Schmerzther.* 2003; **38**: 651–672.

36

Antiarrhythmic therapy during cardiac arrest and resuscitation

Markus Zabel[1], Douglas Chamberlain[2], Paul Dorian[3], Peter Kudenchuk[4], Edward Platia[5], and Hans-Richard Arutz[6]

[1] Division of Cardiology, University of Göttingen, Germany
[2] Prehospital Research Unit, School of Medicine, Cardiff University, UK
[3] Division of Cardiology, St Michael's Hospital, Toronto, Canada
[4,5] University of Washington Medical Center, Seattle, WA, USA
[6] Division of Cardiology, Charité Campus Benjamin Franklin, Berlin, Germany

Most cases of sudden cardiac death (SCD) are due to malignant ventricular tachyarrhythmias, such as ventricular tachycardia (VT) and ventricular fibrillation (VF)(see Fig. 36.1).[1,2] Both VF and pulseless VT require defibrillation as definitive therapy. If these or other arrhythmias persist despite basic life support and defibrillation, the current international advanced cardiac life support guidelines (ILCOR 2005)[3] recommend administration of pharmacologic agents to help stabilize rhythm and restore cardiac output.

The pathophysiologic substrate of cardiac arrest: therapeutic implications

The pathophysiology of sudden cardiac death is relevant to both acute and long-term management. In most instances, the underlying cardiac pathology is ischemia and coronary artery disease. For instance, Liberthson and coworkers[4] reported that 81% of a series of SCD victims had significant coronary artery disease. In another series, up to 50% of the victims of out-of-hospital cardiac arrest had suffered a recent acute myocardial infarction.[5] Although the majority have a coronary disease etiology, numerous other pathologies can be involved in the genesis of sudden cardiac death, such as ventricular hypertrophy, cardiomyopathies, congenital disorders of ion channels ("channelopathies"), but also massive pulmonary embolism, as well as coronary dissection, and coronary inflammation or embolism to the coronary arteries. From a clinical perspective, it is appropriate to assume that the cause of sudden death is coronary artery disease unless circumstances suggest otherwise.

Although the creatine kinase (CK) and its MB fraction may not be diagnostic of acute myocardial ischemia, cardiac troponins can identify myocardial ischemic damage and thus prompt invasive coronary studies, which may make long-term antiarrhythmic treatment irrelevant. A study by Spaulding et al.[6] demonstrated that even without positive cardiac markers, significant coronary disease and coronary occlusions are frequently found in patients with cardiac arrest. These authors reported that 60 of 84 (71%) patients they investigated after out-of-hospital cardiac arrest had significant coronary artery disease and that 40 patients (47%) had coronary occlusions – supporting a more general application of coronary angiography in this situation. In addition to acute myocardial ischemia due to coronary artery disease, hypertrophic or dilated cardiomyopathy are relatively frequent causes of unexpected malignant arrhythmias.

All antiarrhythmics have the potential to increase the risk of cardiac arrest; those that affect repolarization are particularly important in this regard, especially if the substrate for which they are used also involves ion channels. This has been shown for the Class I sodium channel blocking agents encainide and flecainide in the CAST study,[7] which found a significant excess mortality in patients with chronic coronary artery disease, mostly due to ventricular fibrillation. Moreover, Class III drugs that prolong the action potential – such as sotalol, dofetilide, or ibutilide – can directly cause torsades de pointes that may then degenerate into ventricular fibrillation.[8–13] Whether or not patients have received antiarrhythmics, channelopathies have to be considered if no coronary or myocardial abnormality can be identified. They comprise the congenital long QT syndrome,[14] the Brugada syndrome,[15] and other less well recognized

Cardiac Arrest: The Science and Practice of Resuscitation Medicine. 2nd edn., ed. Norman Paradis, Henry Halperin, Karl Kern, Volker Wenzel, Douglas Chamberlain. Published by Cambridge University Press. © Cambridge University Press, 2007.

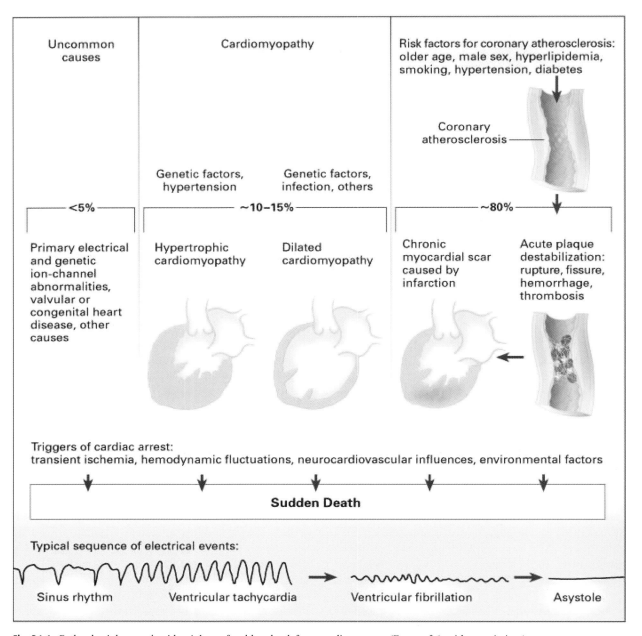

Fig. 36.1. Pathophysiology and epidemiology of sudden death from cardiac causes. (From ref. 1, with permission.)

disorders.[16] Not only patients, but also their siblings, should be investigated if a channelopathy is likely, so that their genotype and phenotype can be characterized. Other specific causes for VT/VF and consecutive cardiac arrest are severe electrolyte abnormalities that are of particular risk in individuals who are vulnerable for other reasons.

Non-cardiac causes that lead to cardiac arrest are usually associated with electromechanical dissociation, which is the most profound form of pulseless electrical activity, rather than to ventricular fibrillation or fast and degenerating ventricular tachycardia.

Irrespective of the pathophysiology, the patient's long-term risk of malignant ventricular arrhythmias needs to be assessed after hemodynamic stabilization and successful management of the acute hospital phase. Treatment with an automatic implantable cardioverter-defibrillator

(ICD) should generally be considered to be mandatory following a clinical event such as resuscitation from cardiac arrest. An exception is the acute phase of myocardial infarction. If VT/VF occurs within the first 48 hours of a transmural acute myocardial infarction, then the long-term risk of sudden cardiac death for a given patient is not increased compared with that in other similar patients.[17-19]

Other rhythms during cardiac arrest and resuscitation

Pulseless electrical activity (PEA) is defined as cardiac electrical activity in the absence of any palpable pulses. It occurs not only in cases without a primary cardiac cause, but also in patients with very severe underlying myocardial disease. If PEA or asystole is seen, or even if bradycardic rhythms are present, antiarrhythmic agents should be avoided because of their side effects including negative inotropic effects and further exacerbation of bradycardia and asystole. Intravenous administration of atropine (3 mg) is recommended,[3] because its strong vagal blocking effect offers a clear benefit in bradycardia, and an occasional apparent beneficial effect in an asystolic patient. Human studies have failed, however, to demonstrate a systematic advantage in cardiac arrest with PEA or asystole.[20,21] Similarly, the phosphodiesterase inhibitor aminophylline has shown some positive clinical effects in asystole, but cannot be generally recommended on the basis of the available clinical evidence.[22-24]

Amiodarone treatment during cardiac arrest and resuscitation

Amiodarone is an antiarrhythmic drug with multiple complex actions that may potentiate each other. It is one of the most powerful antiarrhythmic drugs both at atrial and ventricular levels. It is highly lipophilic and has a very long half-life. It prolongs the cardiac action potential and the QT interval on the surface ECG (Class III in the Vaughan-Williams classification), and in addition exerts conduction-prolonging effects (Class I), non-competitive beta-blocking activity (Class II), and calcium antagonism (Class IV). A central line should be available for intravenous use, because the solvent (polysorbate 80) is an irritant as well as having some antiarrhythmic and negative inotropic activity of its own.

The amiodarone in resuscitation of refractory sustained ventricular tachyarrhythmias (ARREST) study,[25] was the first to investigate an antiarrhythmic drug in a double-blind placebo-controlled trial in the setting of cardiac arrest. In this study, patients with shock-refractory ventricular fibrillation were given amiodarone or matching placebo during continued CPR efforts. Three shocks were delivered before randomization. Survival to discharge was similar in both groups (13.4% vs. 13.2%, P=NS, see Fig. 36.2), but there was a highly significant advantage in survival to hospital admission (44% vs. 34%, P= 0.03).

A second important randomized study, the amiodarone vs. lidocaine in prehospital ventricular fibrillation evaluation trial (ALIVE)[26] randomized 347 patients with cardiac arrest and ventricular fibrillation to lidocaine or amio-

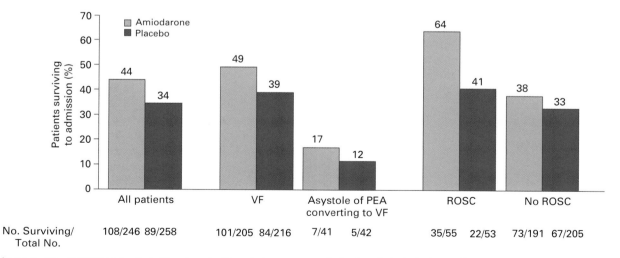

Fig. 36.2. The ARREST trial: effect of treatment with amiodarone on survival to hospital admission in all patients and subgroups of patients. VF = ventricular fibrillation, PEA = pulseless electrical activity, ROSC = return of spontaneous circulation before the study. (From ref. 25, with permission.)

darone given intravenously. With a primary endpoint of survival to hospital admission, a clear advantage for amiodarone was found for the main study population but also within many subgroups. For example, patients with asystole recorded as the initial rhythm and ventricular fibrillation later showed a benefit similar to patients with ventricular fibrillation as the initial rhythm on the scene. Survival to admission in the amiodarone-treated patients was 23% compared with 12% in patients treated with lidocaine (P = 0.009)(see Fig. 36.3). Survival to discharge, however, was only 5% and 3%, respectively, in the two groups (P=NS). The results of this study significantly changed the practice of using lidocaine as the primary antiarrhythmic agent in patients with cardiac arrest and ventricular fibrillation.

Thus, conclusion from the ARREST and ALIVE trials is that for refractory ventricular fibrillation the administration of intravenous lidocaine may be an alternative only if amiodarone is not available at the resuscitation scene. Importantly, however, the data do not show a survival benefit for amiodarone beyond hospital discharge. Consequently, administration of amiodarone during resuscitation is considered useful but not mandatory, and the decision is at the discretion of the emergency physician. Since data were accumulated in patients with VF refractory to three shocks, they may not apply to VF resistant to a single shock. The 2005 ILCOR consensus[3] recommends amiodarone as a possible and useful antiarrhythmic agent in shock-refractory VF. Lidocaine, however, is not recommended in the consensus document.

The administration of amiodarone or other antiarrhythmic agents should not interfere with other CPR efforts. In addition to the advantages shown in the randomized studies, amiodarone may have theoretical advantages in cardiac arrest patients. First, it has no negative inotropic action in contrast to Class I antiarrhythmic agents (although its solvent does); and secondly it is not a vasodilator, unlike procainamide, for example.

Treatment with other antiarrhythmic agents

Lidocaine

Lidocaine is an antiarrhythmic agent with Class Ib action that prolongs conduction and has a membrane-stabilizing effect without a major influence on the cardiac action potential. Because of its ease of administration, its rapid onset and short action, and a good side effect profile, it was previously considered the antiarrhythmic agent of first choice in patients undergoing resuscitation from cardiac arrest due to ventricular fibrillation. This widely

accepted practice was first questioned by a meta-analysis of a number of previous studies of lidocaine in this setting.[27] In a subsequent study by Weaver *et al.*[28] 199 patients with prehospital cardiac arrest due to ventricular fibrillation were randomized to lidocaine 100 mg vs. adrenaline (epinephrine). Initial resuscitation and discharge alive from the hospital were not significantly different in this study. Interestingly, the number of patients discharged from the hospital alive was higher if *no* pharmacologic therapy was administered between repetitive defibrillation shocks in these patients.

Procainamide and bretylium

Because procainamide is an antiarrhythmic agent that prolongs action-potential activity (class III of the Vaughan Williams classification), it should not be given in addition to amiodarone. Another disadvantage is that it can only be infused slowly at a rate of 30 mg/min. Although procainamide has major antiarrhythmic activity, clinical evidence is at best anecdotal and not nearly as strong as that for amiodarone. Previously the guidelines recommended procainamide as an alternative agent if amiodarone is unavailable, but the new ILCOR consensus[3] no longer includes it. Similarly, bretylium (also with class III antiarrhythmic action), which had been widely used in the United States for the treatment of ventricular fibrillation is no longer recommended for lack of favorable evidence.

Intravenous administration of magnesium

Magnesium plays a role in many enzyme systems, for neurochemical transmission, and for myocardial contraction. The acute administration of intravenous magnesium may therefore exert a number of beneficial effects in the patient with VT/VF. There is a direct beneficial effect on afterdepolarizations associated with QT prolongation that can precipitate torsades de pointes type of arrhythmias, and in arrhythmias caused by digitalis toxicity. There may also be stabilizing effects in arrhythmias due to hypokalemia and hypomagnesemia, both of which occur quite frequently in resuscitated patients. The only transient side effect may be hypotension. In several controlled and randomized trials in the cardiac arrest setting, magnesium has failed, however, to demonstrate a clear-cut clinical advantage except for one study in shock-refractory VF[29–32]. Therefore, the new ILCOR consensus[3] recommends intravenous magnesium only for torsades de pointes arrhythmias, in arrhythmias due to digitalis toxicity, and in VT/VF that is shock-refractory or due to possible hypomagnesemia.

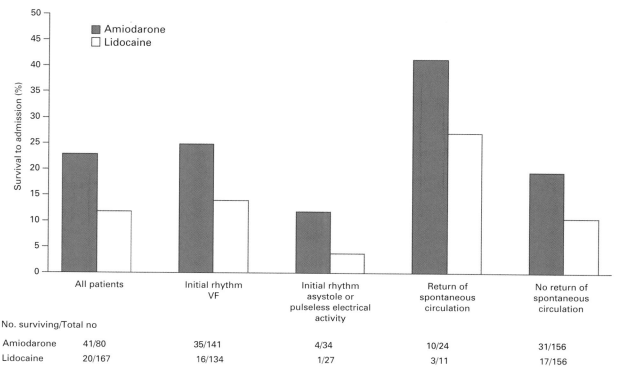

Fig. 36.3. The ALIVE study: effect of treatment with amiodarone or lidocaine on survival to hospital admission in all patients and in selected subgroups. VF = ventricular fibrillation. (From ref. 26, with permission.)

Effects of concomitant adrenaline and vasopressin treatment

Vasopressor agents such as adrenaline or vasopressin, which may be used concomitantly with antiarrhythmics, may influence their efficacy or have proarrhythmic effects. Notably, high dose adrenaline does not compare favorably with conventional doses when given for cardiac arrest outside the hospital.[33] These data should be considered together with the study by Weaver et al.[28] that showed no benefit from adrenaline or lidocaine treatment during cardiac arrest. Since patients receiving no drugs showed improved survival, it was concluded that the delay in resuscitation efforts caused by drug preparation and drug administration was detrimental.

A recent randomized study by Wenzel et al.[34] compared the effect of intravenous vasopressin and intravenous adrenaline in 1219 patients with prehospital cardiac arrest. Overall, there was a similar survival in the two groups; but in a post-hoc subgroup analysis of those with asystole, survival to admission (29% vs. 20%) as well as survival to discharge (4.7% vs. 1.5%) was significantly improved by vasopressin compared with adrenaline. Furthermore, if patients were treated with additional non-randomized adrenaline after

the trial vasopressin, there was also a survival benefit both to admission (26% vs. 16%, $P=0.002$) and survival to discharge (4.7% vs. 1.5%, $P=0.002$) suggesting that the combination of the two drugs is potentially useful.

Vasopressin is a non-adrenergic vasopeptide with significant vasoconstricting activity that might be responsible for a lower incidence of arrhythmias during resuscitation efforts.

Cardiac arrest and resuscitation in ICD patients

Although the ICD was designed specifically to detect and to provide immediate treatment for malignant ventricular arrhythmias, these devices cannot prevent their occurrence.[35] Even when they are in place, repetitive arrhythmias may be associated with a high mortality,[36] and therefore immediate antiarrhythmic treatment and admission to an intensive care monitoring unit is justified before cardiac arrest and the need for resuscitation is reached. The term "electrical storm" or "arrhythmic storm" has been defined as a series of two or more shocks for different arrhythmic episodes within any 24 hours. The situation is similar to shock-refractory cardiac arrest discussed above. Generally, intravenous amiodarone is recommended,[37–39] while class I antiarrhythmics may be detrimental. The administration of beta-blockers has also proved to be useful if the hemodynamic state permits their use.[38]

Acute treatment of supraventricular arrhythmias

On rare occasions, supraventricular arrhythmias may play an important role in cardiac arrest. For this reason, the 2000 guidelines called for cardioversion of patients with narrow complex supraventricular tachycardia at a rate of more than 250 bpm. Such underlying rhythms may be explained by atrial flutter with 1:1 conduction to the ventricles, by fast AV reciprocating tachycardias in patients with accessory pathways, and by fast AV nodal reentry tachycardias. In the absence of a bypass tract, atrial fibrillation is unable to generate such rapid ventricular rates. No definite rate, however, is set as a marker in the European Resuscitation 2005 guidelines:[40] the markers of instability relate to consciousness levels, hypotension, failure, or cardiac pain. Supraventricular arrhythmia may also present as broad complex tachycardia as a result of aberrant conduction or pre-existing bundle branch block, and constitute an important differential diagnosis to ventricular tachycardia. If a broad complex tachycardia is seen in an emergency setting with acute hemodynamic compromise, however, time should not be wasted in attempting to differentiate between SVT and VT: instead, ventricular tachycardia should be assumed and the appropriate algorithm should be followed. If, however, the rate is less than 250 bpm in suspected SVT and hemodynamic collapse has not yet occurred, vagal maneuvers such as the Valsalva maneuver or carotid massage may be attempted. Such treatment may terminate the arrhythmia directly or slow the rate and thereby unmask the underlying rhythm. If unsuccessful, intravenous adenosine in increasing doses is the agent of choice and is recommended in the 2005 consensus document.[3] The administration of adenosine will result in the prompt termination of the SVT (AVNRT, AVRT) at no major risk because of the short half-life of the agent, or at least provide a clue to the diagnosis. As an alternative to intravenous adenosine, the consensus document also mentions verapamil or diltiazem if adenosine is not successful, and cardioversion if the patient is unstable. Where the rates of SVT are sufficiently slow to permit hemodynamic stability, the use of i.v. beta blockers, digoxin, or amiodarone may also be appropriate.

Summary

Amiodarone has several advantages as an antiarrhythmic agent for use during cardiac arrest. Importantly, it improves survival to hospital admission, although it has not been shown to have a survival advantage to discharge. Other antiarrhythmic drugs may also be used empirically on an individual basis. Lidocaine has the advantages of ease of use and wide availability. Magnesium has beneficial actions without doing harm and can be useful in some situations. Procainamide and bretylium have little scientific support and should no longer be used. The administration of antiarrhythmics should never be allowed to hinder other resuscitation efforts. As a vasopressor agent, vasopressin has the advantage of lack of proarrhythmic activity, but its role has not yet been well defined.

REFERENCES

1. Huikuri, H.V., Castellanos, A. & Myerburg, R.J. Sudden death due to cardiac arrhythmias. *N. Engl. J. Med.* 2001; **345**(20): 1473–1482.

2. Zipes, D.P. & Wellens, H.J. Sudden cardiac death. *Circulation* 1998; **98**(21): 2334–2351.

3. International Liaison Committee on Resuscitation. Nolan, J. & Hazinski, M.J. eds. 2005 International consensus on cardiopulmonary resuscitation and emergency cardiovascular care science with treatment recommendations. *Resuscitation* 2005; **67**: 157–341.

4. Liberthson, R.R., Nagel, E.L., Hirschman, J.C., Nussenfeld, S.R., Blackbourne, B.D. & Davis, J.H. Pathophysiologic observations in prehospital ventricular fibrillation and sudden cardiac death. *Circulation* 1974; **49**(5): 790–798.

5. Cobbe, S.M., Redmond, M.J., Watson, J.M., Hollingworth, J. & Carrington, D.J. "Heartstart Scotland"– initial experience of a national scheme for out-of-hospital defibrillation. *Br. Med. J.* 1991; **302**(6791): 1517–1520.

6. Spaulding, C.M., Joly, L.M., Rosenberg, A. *et al.* Immediate coronary angiography in survivors of out-of-hospital cardiac arrest. *N. Engl. J. Med.* 1997; **336**(23): 1629–1633.

7. Preliminary report: effect of encainide and flecainide on mortality in a randomized trial of arrhythmia suppression after myocardial infarction. The Cardiac Arrhythmia Suppression Trial (CAST) Investigators. *N. Engl. J. Med.* 1989; **321**(6): 406–412.

8. Habbab, M.A. & el-Sherif, N. Drug-induced torsades de pointes: role of early afterdepolarizations and dispersion of repolarization. *Am. J. Med.* 1990; **89**(2): 241–246.

9. Roden, D.M. Early afterdepolarizations and torsade de pointes: implications for the control of cardiac arrhythmias by prolonging repolarization. *Eur. Heart J.* 1993; **14**(Suppl. H): 56–61.

10. Buchanan, L.V., Kabell, G., Brunden, M.N. & Gibson, J.K. Comparative assessment of ibutilide, D-sotalol, clofilium, E-4031, and UK-68, 798 in a rabbit model of proarrhythmia. *J. Cardiovasc. Pharmacol.* 1993; **22**(4): 540–549.

11. Chen, Y.J., Hsieh, M.H., Chiou, C.W. & Chen, S.A. Electropharmacologic characteristics of ventricular proarrhythmia induced by ibutilide. *J. Cardiovasc. Pharmacol.* 1999; **34**(2): 237–247.

12. Hohnloser, S.H. Proarrhythmia with class III antiarrhythmic drugs: types, risks, and management. *Am. J. Cardiol.* 1997; **80**(8A): 82G–89G.

13. Waldo, A.L., Camm, A.J., deRuyter, H. *et al.* Effect of d-sotalol on mortality in patients with left ventricular dysfunction after recent and remote myocardial infarction. The SWORD Investigators. Survival With Oral d-Sotalol. *Lancet* 1996; **348**(9019): 7–12.

14. Towbin, J.A. New revelations about the long-QT syndrome. *N. Engl. J. Med.* 1995; **333**(6): 384–385.

15. Brugada, P., Brugada, J. & Brugada, R. The Brugada syndrome. *Cardiovasc. Drugs Ther.* 2001; **15**(1): 15–17.

16. Veldkamp, M.W., Viswanathan, P.C., Bezzina, C., Baartscheer, A., Wilde, A.A. & Balser, J.R. Two distinct congenital arrhythmias evoked by a multidysfunctional Na(+) channel. *Circ. Res.* 2000; **86**(9): E91–E97.

17. Volpi, A., Cavalli, A., Santoro, L. & Negri, E. Incidence and prognosis of early primary ventricular fibrillation in acute myocardial infarction–results of the Gruppo Italiano per lo Studio della Sopravvivenza nell'Infarto Miocardico (GISSI-2) database. *Am. J. Cardiol.* 1998; **82**(3): 265–271.

18. Behar, S., Goldbourt, U., Reicher-Reiss, H. & Kaplinsky, E. Prognosis of acute myocardial infarction complicated by primary ventricular fibrillation. Principal Investigators of the SPRINT Study. *Am. J. Cardiol.* 1990; **66**(17): 1208–1211.

19. Tofler, G.H., Stone, P.H., Muller, J.E. *et al.* Prognosis after cardiac arrest due to ventricular tachycardia or ventricular fibrillation associated with acute myocardial infarction (the MILIS Study). Multicenter Investigation of the Limitation of Infarct Size. *Am. J. Cardiol.* 1987; **60**(10): 755–761.

20. Stiell, I.G., Wells, G.A., Hebert, P.C., Laupacis, A. & Weitzman, B.N. Association of drug therapy with survival in cardiac arrest: limited role of advanced cardiac life support drugs. *Acad. Emerg. Med.* 1995; **2**(4): 264–273.

21. Engdahl, J., Bang, A., Lindqvist, J. & Herlitz, J. Factors affecting short- and long-term prognosis among 1069 patients with out-of-hospital cardiac arrest and pulseless electrical activity. *Resuscitation* 2001; **51**(1): 17–25.

22. Viskin, S., Belhassen, B., Roth, A. *et al.* Aminophylline for bradyasystolic cardiac arrest refractory to atropine and epinephrine. *Ann. Intern. Med.* 1993; **118**(4): 279–281.

23. Mader, T.J., Smithline, H.A., Durkin, L. & Scriver, G. A randomized controlled trial of intravenous aminophylline for atropine-resistant out-of-hospital asystolic cardiac arrest. *Acad. Emerg. Med.* 2003; **10**(3): 192–197.

24. Abu-Laban, R.B., McIntyre, C.M., Christenson, J.M. *et al.* Aminophylline in bradysystolic cardiac arrest: a randomised placebo-controlled trial. *Lancet* 2006; **367** (9522): 1577–1584.

25. Kudenchuk, P.J., Cobb, L.A., Copass, M.K. *et al.* Amiodarone for resuscitation after out-of-hospital cardiac arrest due to ventricular fibrillation. *N. Engl. J. Med.* 1999; **341**(12): 871–878.

26. Dorian, P., Cass, D., Schwartz, B., Cooper, R., Gelaznikas, R. & Barr, A. Amiodarone as compared with lidocaine for shock-resistant ventricular fibrillation. *N. Engl. J. Med.* 2002; **346**(12): 884–890.

27. Hine, L.K., Laird, N., Hewitt, P. & Chalmers, T.C. Meta-analytic evidence against prophylactic use of lidocaine in acute myocardial infarction. *Arch. Intern. Med.* 1989; **149**(12): 2694–2698.

28. Weaver, W.D., Fahrenbruch, C.E., Johnson, D.D., Hallstrom, A.P., Cobb, L.A. & Copass, M.K. Effect of epinephrine and lidocaine therapy on outcome after cardiac arrest due to ventricular fibrillation. *Circulation* 1990; **82**(6): 2027–2034.

29. Thel, M.C., Armstrong, A.L., McNulty, S.E., Califf, R.M. & O'Connor, C.M. Randomised trial of magnesium in in-hospital cardiac arrest. Duke Internal Medicine Housestaff. *Lancet* 1997; **350**(9087): 1272–1276.

30. Fatovich, D.M., Prentice, D.A. & Dobb, G.J. Magnesium in cardiac arrest (the magic trial). *Resuscitation* 1997; **35**(3): 237–241.

31. Allegra, J., Lavery, R., Cody, R. *et al.* Magnesium sulfate in the treatment of refractory ventricular fibrillation in the prehospital setting. *Resuscitation* 2001; **49**(3): 245–249.

32. Hassan, T.B., Jagger, C. & Barnett, D.B. A randomised trial to investigate the efficacy of magnesium sulfate for refractory ventricular fibrillation. *Emerg. Med. J.* 2002; **19**(1): 57–62.

33. Gueugniaud, P.Y., Mols, P., Goldstein, P. *et al.* A comparison of repeated high doses and repeated standard doses of epinephrine for cardiac arrest outside the hospital. European Epinephrine Study Group. *N. Engl. J. Med.* 1998; **339**(22): 1595–1601.

34. Wenzel, V., Krismer, A.C., Arntz, H.R., Sitter, H., Stadlbauer, K.H. & Lindner, K.H. A comparison of vasopressin and epinephrine for out-of-hospital cardiopulmonary resuscitation. *N. Engl. J. Med.* 2004; **350**(2): 105–113.

35. Pinter, A. & Dorian, P. Approach to antiarrhythmic therapy in patients with ICDs and frequent activations. *Curr. Cardiol. Rep.* 2005; **7**(5): 376–381.

36. Exner, D.V., Pinski, S.L., Wyse, D.G. *et al.* Electrical storm presages nonsudden death: the antiarrhythmics versus implantable defibrillators (AVID) trial. *Circulation* 2001; **103**(16): 2066–2071.

37. Kowey, P.R., Levine, J.H., Herre, J.M. *et al.* Randomized, double-blind comparison of intravenous amiodarone and bretylium in the treatment of patients with recurrent, hemodynamically destabilizing ventricular tachycardia or fibrillation. The Intravenous Amiodarone Multicenter Investigators Group. *Circulation* 1995; **92**(11): 3255–3263.

38. Credner, S.C., Klingenheben, T., Mauss, O., Sticherling, C. & Hohnloser, S.H. Electrical storm in patients with transvenous implantable cardioverter- defibrillators: incidence, management and prognostic implications. *J. Am. Coll. Cardiol.* 1998; **32**(7): 1909–1915.

39. Nademanee, K., Taylor, R., Bailey, W.E., Rieders, D.E. & Kosar, E.M. Treating electrical storm: sympathetic blockade versus advanced cardiac life support-guided therapy. *Circulation* 2000; **102**(7): 742–747.

40. Nolan, J.P. & Baskett, P., eds. European Resuscitation Council Guidelines for Resuscitation 2005. *Resuscitation* 2005; **67** (Suppl. 1): S1–S186.

37

Acid–base considerations and buffer therapy

Gad Bar-Joseph[1], Fulvio Kette[2], Martin von Planta[3], Lars Wiklund[4]

[1] Pediatric Intensive Care, Meyer Children's Hospital, Rambam Medical Center, The Ruth and Bruce Rappaport Faculty of Medicine, Technion Israel Institute of Technology, Haifa, Israel
[2] Emergency Department and Intensive Care Unit, S. Vito al Tagliamento Hospital, Italy
[3] Internal Medicine, University of Basel, Switzerland
[4] Department of Surgical Sciences/Anesthesiology and Intensive Care Medicine, Uppsala University Hospital, Sweden

Introduction

Both respiratory (hypercarbic) and metabolic acidosis are important components of cardiac arrest pathophysiology, and resuscitation measures aim to ameliorate or to counteract their potentially harmful effects. The acid–base derangements of cardiac arrest and CPR are exceptionally complicated because of the distinctive kinetics of carbon dioxide during the low-flow state of CPR. On the basis of this physiology, far-reaching hypotheses regarding buffer therapy in general and bicarbonate in particular have been considered and have profoundly affected clinical practice for the past two decades. These hypotheses, however, have not been substantiated by firm published data, resulting in rather ambiguous official recommendations and an atmosphere of uncertainty in the field.

The main objectives of this chapter are to discuss the complicated acid–base derangements of cardiac arrest and CPR and their effects on critical body systems, and to clarify ambiguities regarding buffer therapy.

The discussion in this chapter is limited to acid–base considerations in the context of cardiac arrest and CPR, and not in other contexts of metabolic acidosis, such as hypoxia with adequate tissue perfusion, shock, or ketoacidosis. Despite some similarities, the pathophysiology of these conditions differs markedly from that of cardiac arrest and direct extrapolation might lead to erroneous conclusions.

Historical perspectives

In their original 1961 "Report of Application of External Cardiac Massage in 118 Patients"[1] Jude, Kouwenhoven and Knickerbocker wrote: "Continued cardiac arrest, even though the circulation is artificially maintained, will result in metabolic acidosis. Sodium bicarbonate is beneficial in maintaining blood pH close to the normal value . . ." Since the accompanying metabolic acidosis was believed to be detrimental to outcome, sodium bicarbonate (SB) – the prime representative of buffer therapy – has become part of the basic therapeutic armamentarium of modern CPR. Subsequently, SB was introduced in 1974 as a first line drug in the first Standards for Cardiopulmonary Resuscitation and Emergency Cardiac Care of the American Heart Association.[2]

Reservations about the necessity, efficacy, and side effects of SB and a newly drafted hypothesis on the kinetics of carbon dioxide in very low-flow states resulted in a rather drastic change towards the use of SB in the 1986 update of the Standards and Guidelines for CPR and ACLS.[3] The "low-flow state" hypothesis postulated that the very limited tissue perfusion generated by external cardiac massage is insufficient to transport all of the CO_2 produced from the tissues to the lungs. Hence, CO_2 remains "trapped" at the tissue level, and tissue perfusion – rather than alveolar ventilation – limits its elimination. It was further hypothesized that the administration of "CO_2 producing" buffers, such as SB, will further increase tissue CO_2 concentrations, and CO_2 molecules will rapidly diffuse into the cells, cause "paradoxical" intracellular acidosis and thus might worsen CPR outcome.[3–7] This attractive, although (at best) only partially substantiated hypothesis, prompted the 1986 Guidelines no longer to recommend the use of SB, but rather left its use to "the discretion of the team leader".[3]

This approach was only slightly modified in the 1992 version of the AHA ACLS Guidelines[8] and by the 1998

European Resuscitation Council Guidelines.[9] The 2000 International ACLS Guidelines did not offer any new discussion of buffer therapy and this section was basically copied from the 1992 version.[10]

Thus, the 2000 Guidelines regarding buffer therapy state: "In certain circumstances, such as patients with pre-existing metabolic acidosis, hyperkalemia, or tricyclic or phenobarbitone overdose, bicarbonate can be beneficial. After protracted arrest or long resuscitative efforts, bicarbonate possibly benefits the patient. However, bicarbonate therapy should be considered only after confirmed interventions, such as defibrillation, cardiac compression, intubation, ventilation and vasopressor therapy, have been ineffective".[10]

Acid–base changes during cardiac arrest and CPR

Definitions of acid–base changes

Acidity of the blood (and of other body fluids) is customarily expressed as pH, which represents the negative logarithm of the measured hydrogen ion, or proton, concentration $[H^+]$. $[H^+]$ can also be conveniently expressed in nanomoles (10^{-9} mol) per liter. Normal values of arterial pH and of $[H^+]$ are 7.42 ± 0.04 and 40 ± 4 nmol/l, respectively. Any increase in measured blood $[H^+]$ (i.e., a decrease in blood pH value) is termed acidemia, and any decrease in blood $[H^+]$ (i.e., an increase in its pH) is termed alkalemia. Acidosis and alkalosis are the processes that change hydrogen ion concentrations: acidosis will increase, whereas alkalosis will decrease $[H^+]$.

Respiratory processes change $[H^+]$ through changes in carbon dioxide concentrations (conveniently expressed as PCO_2). Thus, any increase in PCO_2 (normal arterial values are 40 ± 4 torr) will be interpreted as respiratory acidosis, and any decrease in PCO_2 as respiratory alkalosis.

Metabolic changes in $[H^+]$ are mediated through changes in fixed (non-volatile) acids or bases. Conventionally, metabolic processes are assessed by the readily calculated value of bicarbonate ion concentration $[HCO_3^-]$. Such a straightforward assessment is inaccurate, however, since $[HCO_3^-]$ is also directly influenced by changes in PCO_2. According to the formula

$$CO_2 + H_2O \leftrightarrow H_2CO_3 \leftrightarrow H^+ + HCO_3^-$$

every molecule of CO_2 that reacts with H_2O will produce one ion of HCO_3^- (and one H^+). This represents a respiratory, rather than a metabolic, change in HCO_3^-. Several methods were devised to dissociate the respiratory effects from the "true" metabolic effects on HCO_3^-, one of which is the calculation of base excess (BE).[11,12] Although BE has been recently criticized,[13,14] it can be conveniently used in the cardiac arrest/CPR scenario as it is automatically calculated with every blood gas analysis. "Normal" BE is 0 ± 2 mmol/L: a positive BE denotes metabolic alkalosis and a negative BE ("base deficit") denotes metabolic acidosis.

Nature of acidosis of cardiac arrest and CPR and its rate of development

CO_2 and lactic acid are the predominant determinants of extra- and intracellular pH during CPR. Extracellular HCO_3^- (such as $NaHCO_3$ intravenously) increases intracellular pH only after some delay because of its slow distribution by low blood flow and the transfer time from the blood into the intracellular space.

Metabolic (lactic) acidosis in the cardiac arrest setting

At what rate does significant metabolic (lactic) acidosis develop during arrest and CPR? This question is not academic as it has a direct impact on the issue of buffer therapy and its timing.

The development rate of lactic acidosis depends on both severity and duration of tissue hypoxia. During circulatory arrest, acids remain confined to the tissues, and will not be detected in peripheral blood.[15–18] Only after the establishment of at least some tissue perfusion by CPR or after return of spontaneous circulation (ROSC), will acidemia be detected in peripheral blood.[15–18] The magnitude of the detected acidemia depends on the degree of tissue acidosis, the rate of acid washout, and the timing of blood sampling. These complicated dynamics partly explain the marked variability in the reported data about both severity of metabolic acidosis and the effectiveness of buffer therapy in treating it.[15]

Retrospective clinical studies reporting acid–base data are difficult to interpret as major variables, such as "downtimes," location of arrest, duration and quality of CPR, buffers administration, and timing of blood sampling, were not controlled. During in-hospital resuscitations with relatively short response times, rapid increases in serum lactate[19] and in the metabolic component of acidosis[20] were observed. Serum $[HCO_3^-]$ of 14–15 mmol/l and $[H^+]$ of 68–85 nmol/l were found in patients undergoing CPR in the emergency department, even though most patients received large bicarbonate doses within 10 minutes of CPR.[21] Children presenting to the emergency department in respiratory or cardiac arrest had initial mean arterial pH values of 7.05 and base deficits of −15 mmol/l in survivors, and 6.94 and −18 mmol/l, respectively, in non-survivors.[22]

More rigorous data were provided by controlled laboratory experiments. pH values <7.10 and base deficits of −17 mmol/l were demonstrated after 10 minutes of ventricular fibrillation (VF) and 5 minutes of CPR.[17] Serum base deficits increased by 1.1 to 1.5 mmol/l for every minute of circulatory arrest.[17,18,23,24] Arterial lactate increased by 0.3 mmol/l for every minute of cardiac arrest and CPR when epinephrine was used,[17,24] and by almost 0.6 mmol/l when epinephrine was not used.[23] In the fibrillating heart, myocardial lactate concentrations, as reflected in great cardiac vein blood, increased approximately three times faster than systemic lactate concentrations.[16,23,25] Myocardial lactate increased about tenfold in 10 minutes of untreated VF.[26]

Carbon dioxide and acid–base physiology during the low-flow state of ACLS

In 1976, Bishop and Weisfeldt[27] showed in a canine model that arterial pH could be maintained at approximately normal levels during the initial 13 minutes of cardiac arrest and CPR with hyperventilation to a $PaCO_2$ of around 15 torr. Similarly, Sanders *et al.*[28] documented almost normal arterial pH during the initial 18 minutes of ventricular fibrillation (VF) and CPR by hyperventilating dogs to $PaCO_2$ values of 10 to 18 torr.

Subsequently, Weil and his group highlighted the exceptional acid–base and carbon dioxide dynamics during the very-low-flow state of CPR. In a porcine model, Grundler *et al.*[5] demonstrated that arterial pH remained alkalemic during 11 minutes of cardiac arrest and CPR by maintaining $PaCO_2$ of 20–23 torr. Nevertheless, mixed venous blood disclosed pH values lower by 0.27–0.3 units compared to prearrest and to the concurrent arterial values. These differences were mainly due to increases in venous PCO_2, resulting in widening of the veno-arterial PCO_2 differences to 34.2–39.4 torr.[5]

The same investigators supported these experimental findings with clinical observations in a group of 16 patients during CPR.[29] Over a median interval of 23 minutes from onset of cardiac arrest and blood sampling, the patients received on average 130 meq of SB. At the time of sampling, arterial pH and PCO_2 averaged 7.41 and 32 torr, respectively, while mixed venous pH and PCO_2 averaged 7.15 and 74 torr, respectively. Calculated bicarbonate concentrations were equal in arterial and venous samples. Thus, arterial blood tended towards alkalemia and venous blood showed acidemia.

These findings were explained by the unique physiology of the "very low flow state":[6,10,29] with normal or moderately reduced tissue perfusion, CO_2 elimination depends only on alveolar ventilation; whereas under conditions of very low flow, tissue perfusion becomes the rate-limiting step of CO_2 elimination. External chest compressions generate at best only 25%–30% of normal cardiac output,[30,31] insufficient to carry all of the produced CO_2 to the pulmonary circulation. CO_2 remains partly "trapped" at the tissue level, and the increased tissue PCO_2 is reflected as increased venous PCO_2 ($Pvco_2$). Pulmonary blood flow and CO_2 transport to the lungs are very low, as detected by decreased end-tidal CO_2.[32–34] The high ventilation:perfusion ratio leads to arterial hypocarbia and to elevated arterial pH,[29,35–38] which further widens the veno-arterial differences. This phenomenon of hypercarbic venous acidemia coincident with normo- to hypocarbic arterial alkalemia was termed the "arterio-venous paradox."[5,29]

This phenomenon was subsequently demonstrated in other clinical studies[39] and in various models of cardiac arrest and CPR[18,23,37,38,40] (Fig. 37.1), and was investigated thoroughly by Adrogue *et al.*[35,36] The phenomenon was also observed, but to a somewhat lesser degree, in dogs during hemorrhagic shock.[41,42] In an experimental model of progressive pericardial tamponade, arterial-venous pH and PCO_2 gradients increased proportionally with the reduction in cardiac output.[43] Venous hypercarbia developed

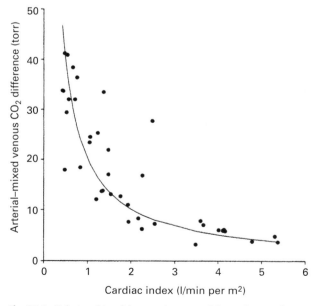

Fig. 37.1. Relationship of the arteriovenous CO_2 gradient and cardiac index follows the form of a modified Fick equation. (From ref. 38. Copyright Williams & Wilkins.)

during septic shock with systemic hypoperfusion.[44–46] By using tissue electrodes, tissue hypercarbia was demonstrated during shock in the kidney,[46,47] liver, and brain.[46] In the myocardial circulation, cardiac venous PCO_2 and the cardiac venous to arterial PCO_2 differences were greater than were the concurrent systemic differences.[16,23,25,48]

Of note, however, there is nothing really "paradoxical" about this phenomenon, and it can be accurately predicted by the Fick principle.[15,40] Tissue and venous hypercarbia are common pathophysiological phenomena, and basically characterize any global or regional ischemia.[38,40,49] The magnitudes of the veno-arterial pH and PCO_2 gradients are inversely related to the cardiac output[18,38–40] (Fig. 37.1) and they may actually provide an index of the severity of the perfusion defect.[35,36,38,39,49]

Of note, in CPR animal models, markedly increased $Pvco_2$ and veno-arterial PCO_2 gradients were observed mainly when no epinephrine was used and tissue perfusion pressures were extremely low.[5,50–53] When epinephrine or other measures were used to produce higher perfusion pressures, P_vco_2 increased only moderately.[17,54–56]

Hypothesis regarding bicarbonate and other alkalinizing agents in the low flow state

On the basis of these observations, Weil's group postulated a far-reaching, encompassing hypothesis regarding buffer therapy during CPR.[4,5,16,29,57] The hypothesis consisted basically of four consecutive elements: (1) During the very low flow state of CPR, CO_2 elimination is determined mainly by tissue perfusion rather than by alveolar ventilation. (2) SB administration will result in excessive carbon dioxide production, which cannot be eliminated effectively and will accumulate in the tissues. (3) As CO_2 penetrates cellular membranes more rapidly than bicarbonate ions, it will accumulate intracellularly and will paradoxically aggravate intracellular acidosis by enhancing its hypercarbic ("respiratory") component. (4) Intracellular (myocardial) hypercarbic acidosis is detrimental and therefore SB administration might worsen CPR outcome.[3–10,16,29,57,58]

In the mid-1980s this hypothesis triggered the controversy around the use of SB and had a profound clinical impact, causing a sharp decline in the utilization SB in both out- and in-hospital resuscitations. In the early 1980s, SB was the most frequently used medication during CPR – administered to 84.7% of patients undergoing in-hospital CPR.[59] Aufderheide et al. found a 79.9% bicarbonate usage rate among resuscitated patients in a single emergency medical service during 1982–1984.[60] In a large, multicenter clinical trial performed between 1989 and 1992, Bar-Joseph et al. reported that SB was administered in only 54.5% of the

resuscitations,[61] and its usage rate by the various study sites ranged between 3.9% and 98.3% of CPR attempts.[62] Levy et al. audited SB usage for CPR in a single district hospital in England, and found that it decreased progressively from 1986 to no usage at all by 1991.[63]

Nevertheless, as will be described later (Buffer Therapy in CPR), steps 2, 3, and 4 of this far-reaching hypothesis were not really supported by the available evidence, which points out that SB either increases or does not decrease intracellular pH and that it does not worsen CPR outcome.

Role of (arterial) blood gas monitoring during CPR

Historically, arterial blood gas (ABG) determination during CPR was recommended, as it may provide information on the adequacy of ventilation and oxygenation, the magnitude of metabolic acidosis, and an indirect estimate of tissue perfusion. Our current understanding of the pathophysiology of the low-flow-state, however, has greatly modified the practical value of ABG determination.

The high pO_2 measured in ABGs in patients ventilated with supplemental oxygen does not reflect tissue hypoxia and the very low venous pO_2.[21,23,29,35]

Although ABGs accurately reflect "adequacy" of ventilation in arterial blood,[64] they do not reflect conditions at the tissue level, as evidenced by the large differences between arterial and venous values of PCO_2 and pH because of the low tissue perfusion and the high ventilation:perfusion ratios characterizing CPR.[5,16,21,23,25,29,39]

Arterial PCO_2 was shown to correlate well with end-tidal CO_2 ($EtCO_2$) which in turn correlates with coronary perfusion pressure – the major determinant of tissue (myocardial) perfusion.[65,66] It was therefore thought that $PaCO_2$ could provide an indirect estimate of the perfusion generated during CPR. Although $PaCO_2$ correlated well with $EtCO_2$ during CPR in animals,[65] it did not correlate well in humans.[67] Furthermore, while in some animal studies $PaCO_2$ correlated to a certain degree with coronary perfusion pressure,[65,68,69] Barton et al.[70] failed to demonstrate such a positive correlation in humans undergoing CPR, and $PaCO_2$ could not differentiate between resuscitated and non-resuscitated patients. Thus, ABGs apparently do not provide a useful estimate of tissue perfusion.

What about metabolic acidosis? We are used to thinking of serum bicarbonate $[HCO_3^-]$ as the marker of metabolic acidosis. $[HCO_3^-]$ changes by 1 to 2 meq/l for every 10 torr change in PCO_2. The markedly elevated venous PCO_2, "elevates" the calculated venous $[HCO_3^-]$ and the arteriovenous $[HCO_3^-]$ differences are numerically less prominent than the PCO_2 differences.[16,21,23,25,35,40,71,72] This "respiratory" contribution may be misleading if we regard $[HCO_3^-]$ as the only marker of metabolic acidosis. This phenomenon was even more prominent in the coronary venous blood, where despite extreme combined acidosis (pH 6.62 and 6.75, lactate 7.6 and 8.2 mmol/l) and extreme hypercarbia (PCO_2 177 and 150 torr), the $[HCO_3^-]$ values were 18 and 20 meq/l.[25]

Base excess (or deficit), on the other hand, provides a straightforward estimate of the metabolic component of the acid–base imbalance and it does not vary markedly between arterial and venous blood.[54,73,74] Base excess was shown to be an excellent predictor of resuscitability in dogs undergoing CPR.[17]

Lactate concentrations are equal in arterial and in mixed venous blood.[16,23,25,52,75] Many modern blood gas analyzers measure lactate concentration. Nevertheless, changes in blood lactate are also flow-dependent and do not necessarily reflect concurrent tissue concentrations. It should be kept in mind that the physiologic effects of (metabolic) acidosis are determined by H^+ ion concentrations and the lactate anion has no significant physiologic effect. H^+ ion concentration is obviously affected by other factors, such as ventilation, natural buffer systems, and buffer therapy. Therefore, the clinical applicability of "lactate concentration" during CPR is rather limited (Fig. 37.2).

Thus, the use of ABGs to monitor or guide therapy during CPR is of very limited, if any, clinical value, as they do not reflect tissue hypoxia, pH, or PCO_2. The question of whether the measurement of ABGs has any effect on the clinical management of CPR or on CPR outcome, however, was never subjected to a proper clinical trial.

Effects of acidosis on critical organs – is the acidosis of cardiac arrest detrimental?

This is a highly controversial question. On the one hand, intuitively and "teleologically," the answer should be "yes": if our organism functions optimally at an extracellular $[H^+]$ of 40 nmol/l, and exquisite mechanisms are utilized to maintain it within a very narrow range, why should it be expected to function even better (i.e., resume sinus rhythm and effective spontaneous circulation) under the extremely unfavorable conditions of both tissue hypoxia and much higher acidity? As mentioned, this was the basic approach during the first 25 years of modern CPR.

On the other hand, researchers have claimed that acidosis is not detrimental,[76] and may even be protective.[7,57,77]

This ambiguity is seemingly reflected in the text of the 2000 Guidelines,[8,10] which state that "laboratory and clinical data fail to conclusively show that low blood pH adversely affects ability to defibrillate, ability to restore spontaneous circulation, or short-term survival. Adrenergic responsiveness also appears to be unaffected by tissue acidosis."[10] The same Guidelines, however,

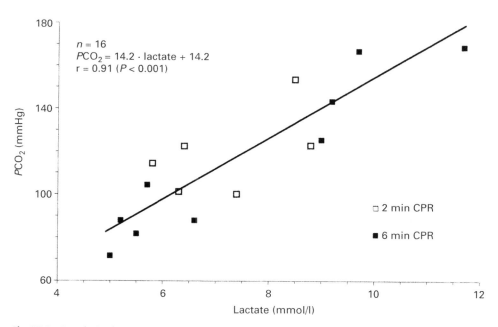

Fig. 37.2. Correlation between great cardiac vein PCO_2 and lactate. (Adapted from ref. 48. Copyright American Physiological Society).

recommend bicarbonate (Class IIa recommendation) for pre-existing metabolic acidosis and upon return of spontaneous circulation[78] – apparently because metabolic acidosis is considered harmful. Furthermore, the postulation that bicarbonate paradoxically worsens intracellular acidosis (and therefore outcome) is obviously based on the premise that acidosis is harmful and will impede resuscitation.

The ambiguity surrounding the potential detrimental effects of acidosis in CPR has several sources. One is the inability to differentiate precisely the detrimental effects of hypoxia from those of acidosis. Second, attempts to resolve the issue in experimental studies by comparing the effects of buffers to those of placebo yielded equivocal results, as they depend largely on the model and study design (see below, under "Buffer therapy in CPR").

The following discussion of the effects of acidosis in cardiac arrest and CPR will concentrate mainly on the two major "target organs" – the heart and the brain.

Cardiac acid–base changes

Myocardial acidosis

During CPR, anaerobic myocardial metabolism generates hydrogen ions, CO_2, and lactate. Myocardial CO_2 accumulation stems from local CO_2 production, dissociation of endogenous myocardial bicarbonate when buffering anaerobically generated hydrogen ions, and from reduced clearance of CO_2 due to low blood flow. Therefore, intramyocardial CO_2 ($PmCO_2$) increases when coronary blood flow (CBF) is impaired and is negatively correlated to the coronary perfusion pressure (CPP) during CPR (Fig. 37.3).

Capparelli et al.[23] and Gudipati et al.[48] demonstrated that changes in the cardiac venous pH and PCO_2 are much more prominent than the concurrent changes in mixed venous blood. After 5 minutes of VF and 7 minutes of CPR, great cardiac vein pH declined from 7.3 to 6.7 and PCO_2 increased from 50 to 140 mmHg with marked increases in the arterial-coronary vein pH and PCO_2 gradients.[48] After ROSC, cardiac venous pH and PCO_2 returned to near normal levels within minutes. It was hypothesized that such high CO_2 levels may reflect an even more profound acidosis within myocardial tissue.[16]

This was indeed confirmed by von Planta et al.[16] who used a miniature electrode to measure intramyocardial tissue pH. Following 3 minutes of untreated VF and 8 minutes of CPR, intramyocardial pH declined from 7.27 to 6.88, and returned to pre-arrest levels 60 minutes after ROSC.

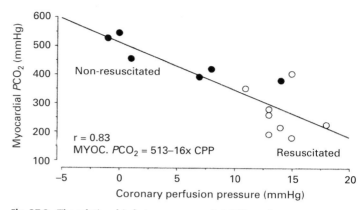

Fig. 37.3. The relationship between myocardial PCO_2 and coronary perfusion pressure (CPP) documented a critical threshold for myocardial PCO_2 of approximately 400 torr and for CPP of approximately 10 mmHg which predicted failure of successful resuscitation. (From ref. 25. Copyright Williams & Wilkins).

Subsequently, Kette et al.[25] measured both myocardial pH and $PmCO_2$ in the same model. Myocardial pH decreased to 7.05 and $PmCO_2$ increased to 97 torr following 3 minutes of untreated VF. Eight minutes after initiation of CPR, myocardial pH declined further to 6.38 and $PmCO_2$ increased to 346 torr. $PmCO_2$ returned to normal levels 30 minutes after ROSC (Fig. 37.4).

Lactate production is the second cause of myocardial acidosis. In the same VF models, great cardiac vein lactate increased approximately three times faster than systemic lactate.[16,23,25,48] Myocardial content of lactate increased about tenfold by 10 minutes of untreated VF.[26]

With initiation of chest compressions, a sharp increase in lactate concentration is observed, reflecting myocardial washout of lactate. Subsequently, cardiac venous lactate concentrations, as well as PCO_2, increase slowly and tend to reach a plateau.[16,25,48,50] Possibly the minimal perfusion and oxygenation generated by CPR result in partial aerobic metabolism, mitigating further lactate production. That CO_2 and H^+ continue to accumulate in the myocardium[25] supports this possibility of incomplete myocardial ischemia.

Coronary perfusion pressure, myocardial acidosis and resuscitability

Myocardial blood flow correlates closely with CPP which is considered the most important determinant of cardiac resuscitability.[79] CPP levels above 20 mmHg in dogs,[80] 20 mmHg in rats,[81] 10 mmHg in minipigs,[51,52] and 15 mmHg in human patients[82] predicted outcome. Kette et al. showed an inverse correlation between CPP and $PmCO_2$, and

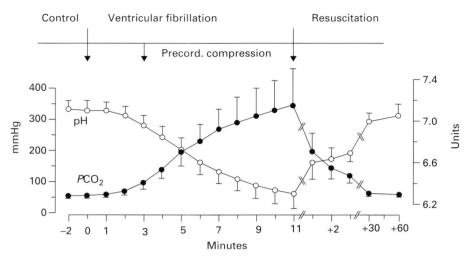

Fig. 37.4. Marked hypercarbia is associated with low pH levels within the myocardium. Restoration of spontaneous circulation is followed by prompt return of pH and PCO_2 to normal levels. (Adapted from ref. 25. Copyright Williams & Wilkins).

demonstrated a threshold level of CPP and $PmCO_2$ for ROSC in pigs[25] (Fig. 37.3): resuscitated animals had CPP >10 mmHg and $PmCO_2$ <400 torr, while non-resuscitated animals had CPP <10 mmHg and $PmCO_2$ >400 torr.

Likewise, MacGregor *et al.*[83] demonstrated in a canine anoxic arrest model, a critical $PmCO_2$ threshold of 416 torr as predicting failure of cardiac resuscitation.

Effects of acidosis on the heart

Multiple adverse effects of severe acidosis – either hypercarbic ("respiratory") or metabolic – on cardiac function, resuscitability, and viability were reported and reviewed,[84–88] many of them relevant to the cardiac arrest/CPR scenario. It has been known for well over 100 years that acidosis decreases cardiac contractility.[89] Extensive review pointed out that acidosis interferes with almost every step in the excitation–contraction coupling, and that H^+ metabolism is intimately linked to the cellular handling of Na^+ and Ca^{2+}.[84] Acidosis can lead to arrhythmias, mainly to slow heart rates, by interfering with both pacemaker activity and the conduction system.[88,90] Recently, a direct correlation between low pH and induction of apoptosis in cardiac samples from human patients and porcine subjects was reported.[91]

Assessing the effects of acidosis on CPR outcome in uncontrolled, retrospective clinical studies is basically impossible, as the intensity of metabolic acidosis correlates directly with the duration and magnitude of tissue hypoxia, which determines CPR outcome. For this reason, the presence of acidosis or the need for buffer therapy was repeatedly found to be associated with worse CPR outcome.[92–96] In a prospective clinical trial, Tribonate® failed to improve

survival.[97] In a recent post-hoc analysis of the BRCT III trial data, SB use in association with epinephrine resulted in better resuscitability and long-term outcomes.[62]

In the laboratory, the effects of acidosis on hemodynamics, response to epinephrine, and resuscitability depend largely on the model.[98] The effects of metabolic and respiratory acidosis are not necessarily identical. Metabolic acidosis arising from cellular hypoxia during cardiac arrest differs substantially from acidosis induced by external administration of acids[98,99] or from hypoxic lactic acidosis with normal circulation.[100]

Gerst *et al.* showed that metabolic acidosis lowered the cardiac fibrillation threshold, whereas respiratory acidosis had no effect.[101] Defibrillation threshold was not affected by mild (pH < 7.25)[102] or moderate (pH = 7.12)[103] respiratory or metabolic acidosis induced by external administration of acid, although in the latter study fewer animals with metabolic acidosis resumed spontaneous circulation.[103] In isolated, perfused rat hearts, Morimoto *et al.*[104] found that extramyocardial metabolic acidosis (pH < 7.1) decreased resuscitability and cardiac performance after VF. No hearts recovered after perfusion below pH 6.5. Mandolano *et al.* found that hypercarbic acidosis, induced during reperfusion in a ventricular fibrillation model, reduced early resuscitability.[105] Administration of buffer during CPR improved resuscitability[17,54,55,106] and postresuscitation myocardial dysfunction.[107]

Response to catecholamines

Several reports have shown that, in states of acidosis, the ability of catecholamines to attenuate or reverse the contractile impairment induced by acidosis is substantially reduced.[108–111]

In the cardiac arrest setting, the reports are equivocal: whereas one study[54] found higher systemic and coronary perfusion pressures in dogs treated with SB during CPR, others did not show an enhanced vasopressor effect of epinephrine following administration of buffers.[17,52,112]

These discrepancies may be explained by the model (spontaneously beating hearts vs. hearts in VF)[98], by the epinephrine dosage, or by the combination of hypoxia and acidosis. Preziosi et al.[113] found that induced metabolic acidemia had no effect on the hemodynamic response to epinephrine, but when animals were made hypoxic, acidemia attenuated the vasopressor response to epinephrine, which was restored only after correction of hypoxia.

Acid–base changes and the brain

Since the introduction of modern CPR in the 1960s, survival with good neurological activity of patients not responding to early defibrillation remains a most yearned for, but still unaccomplished goal.

Cerebral tissue pH and bicarbonate, as well as cerebrospinal fluid pH, decrease sharply after cessation of blood flow to the brain.[114,115] This occurs parallel to decreases in cerebral tissue pO_2, cerebral oxygen metabolic rate, and cellular adenylate charge (i.e., decrease in ATP and increase in AMP), and to increases in cerebral tissue lactate and Pco_2.[114–116] These processes depend mainly on the duration of the hypoxic-ischemic event and on its intensity (i.e., complete cessation of blood flow vs. variable degrees of low blood flow, such as those generated during CPR).[114,116]

An intriguing aspect of the acid–base status of the brain is concerned with the different permeability characteristics of carbon dioxide and bicarbonate ions through the blood–brain barrier.[117] This relates to the discussion of acid–base and buffer therapy in CPR, as cerebrospinal fluid (CSF) acid–base status is thought to represent intracellular acid–base status. This basic premise, however, may be wrong.[118,119]

An excellent review of pH-associated brain injury in cerebral ischemia and circulatory arrest was published by Hurn and Traystman.[120] Energy depletion is the most critically damaging event in brain ischemia/hypoxia. Protons (H^+) are generated in large amounts through hydrolysis of ATP, unbalanced by the normal uptake of H^+ during formation of new ATP in the creatine kinase reaction, and through (anaerobic) lactate production.

Intracellular brain pH (pHi) decreases to approximately 6.2 within 6 minutes[115,121] and to 6.0 by 10–12 minutes[122] of complete ischemia (circulatory arrest), and extracellular pH (pHe) decreases generally in parallel to pHi.[123]

Severe cerebral acidosis enhances ischemic brain damage,[124,125] and these effects are intensified by the "glucose paradox of cerebral ischemia":[126] as brain metabolism depends largely on glucose oxidation, increased tissue glucose content or continued glucose delivery to hypoxic, energy-depleted brain tissue exacerbates lactic acidosis. Originally, Siesjo's group[127,128] showed that a high blood glucose during hypoxia simultaneously decreased cerebral tissue pH and the cellular content of ATP, and Myers and Yamaguchi[129] showed that administration of glucose just before arrest markedly augments the severity of brain injury and alters its distribution.

It is now well established that hyperglycemia or increased tissue glycogen stores or the administration of glucose-containing solutions before, during, or after the ischemic insult (in both cardiac arrest and stroke models) result in significantly elevated cerebral lactate and lower tissue pH. This profound brain acidosis causes reduction of ATP synthesis and impaired energy metabolism,[130,131] endothelial and glial swelling,[132] and enhanced brain edema[132–134] which hampers postischemic perfusion and recovery of regional blood flow,[132,135,136] and worsens histopathologic damage[133,137] and neurological outcome.[134,138,139] In patients, a strong association exists between hyperglycemia and poor neurologic outcome following cardiac arrest[140,141] and stroke.[142,143]

The next question is whether buffer therapy can enhance recovery of brain acidosis and improve cellular function and neurological outcome. Restoration of circulation sets the stage for recovery of pHi and pHe by removing accumulated CO_2 and lactate and by providing oxygen to promote oxidative phosphorylation and ATP production.[144] ATP reactivates energy-dependent transmembrane ion exchange mechanisms, particularly H^+ extrusion by Na^+/H^+ exchange.[145] This high capacity antiporter system is operating below its maximal capacity when pHe is very low, as H^+ competes with Na^+ at the external side of the exchanger. Thus, measures that reduce pHe are expected to facilitate normalization of pHi.[145,146]

Buffers were shown to correct cerebral acidosis in various CPR models.[68,146–148] Using a pH/PCO_2 electrode, Liu et al.[148] confirmed that the profound acidosis developing during circulatory arrest was associated with a rapid increase of cerebral tissue PCO_2. Buffer (SB or Tribonate®) administration during CPR increased cerebral cortical blood flow during the initial reperfusion phase after ROSC, and prevented the development of secondary cerebral tissue acidosis during the subsequent period of low systemic perfusion pressure.

Hyperventilation to counteract metabolic acidosis

ACLS Guidelines[3,8,10] stressed the importance of "adequate alveolar ventilation," which, together with restoration of tissue perfusion "are the mainstays of control of acid–base balance during cardiac arrest." Guidelines also state that hyperventilation corrects respiratory acidosis by removing carbon dioxide, which is freely diffusible across cellular and organ membranes.[3,8,10] These statements imply that acidosis of cardiac arrest is mainly respiratory and not metabolic, and that hyperventilation can correct the entire acid–base derangements,[6,27,28,76,149] despite the official recommendation to ventilate at 12–15 times per minute.

Clearly, "adequate" ventilation can effectively eliminate CO_2 from the diminished blood flow reaching the pulmonary circulation. To correct arterial academia temporarily, Bishop and Weisfeldt, in their often-quoted study,[27] hyperventilated dogs to $PaCO_2$ below 20 torr. Sanders *et al.* "adequately" ventilated dogs to $PaCO_2$ of 10 torr[28] and Capparelli *et al.* to 16.6 torr.[23] Still, concomitant mixed venous pH and PCO_2 were 7.09 and 72 torr and cardiac venous pH and PCO_2 were 6.76 and 128 torr, respectively.[23] Thus, hyperventilation cannot correct whole body acidosis when tissue perfusion becomes the limiting step in CO_2 elimination.[15,68,69]

Moreover, hyperventilation may be deleterious during CPR: Aufderheide *et al.* observed that professional rescuers ventilated patients excessively during out-of-hospital CPR.[150] Subsequent animal studies demonstrated that similar excessive ventilation rates resulted in significantly increased positive intrathoracic pressures and markedly decreased coronary perfusion pressures and survival rates.[150] Aside from potential detrimental mechanical effects,[151] hyperventilation causes cerebral vasoconstriction and can reduce cerebral perfusion, which may be particularly deleterious in low flow states. This was demonstrated in traumatic brain injury,[152] and may also be applicable to the cardiac arrest victim. A human study suggested that cerebrovascular reactivity to changes in $PaCO_2$ is preserved in comatose adults following CPR.[153]

Buffer therapy during cardiopulmonary resuscitation

The discussion of buffer therapy during CPR should address several issues: first, is the metabolic acidosis detrimental? This issue was discussed above. Second, does buffer therapy improve CPR outcome? Third, is buffer therapy safe, especially with SB, as so many concerns about putative deleterious effects have been raised. And finally, how do various buffer agents compare in the context of CPR outcome?

Does buffer therapy improve CPR outcome?

An attempt to answer this question is severely hampered by the paucity of adequate clinical studies. Therefore, most of the evidence available is based on animal experiments, which varied markedly in their design. To appraise correctly their results careful attention should be paid to details such as arrest time, timing and dosage of buffer administration, the use of epinephrine, and other measures affecting tissue perfusion and outcome endpoints.

Clinical studies

No large, prospective randomized clinical trial (RCT) on buffers during CPR has ever been conducted.

Several retrospective studies attempted to analyze the outcome effects of buffers (mainly SB), administered in an uncontrolled fashion.[60,94–96,154,155] These studies were all inconclusive because of an inherent bias: patients who had longer resuscitation attempts and had worse outcome also received buffers more frequently. Thus, buffer administration was an epiphenomenon of prolonged arrest and CPR.

The only prospective RCT was published by Dybvik *et al.*[97] 502 patients received either Tribonat® (a mixture of SB, tromethanol, phosphate, and acetate, used frequently in Scandinavia) or normal saline during out-of-hospital CPR. Buffer therapy did not improve immediate resuscitability or long-term outcome. However, the response time in this study was short, only moderate acidosis was detected in both treatment arms on hospital admission, the number of patients was relatively small, and the odds ratio was very wide.[156]

Bar-Joseph *et al.* recently reported a post hoc analysis of bicarbonate usage among 16 emergency medical services (EMS) systems that participated in the BRCT III trial – a clinical trial that compared primarily standard-dose and high-dose epinephrine.[62] SB usage was optional and its usage rates and timing of administration varied widely among the EMS systems. A total of 2122 patients undergoing out-of-hospital CPR were analyzed. SB usage rates correlated inversely with the sites' timing of bicarbonate administration (Fig. 37.5). Study sites were divided according to their SB usage profile: "high SB user" sites administered SB in over 50% of CPRs and within 10 minutes of the first epinephrine dose, while "low SB user" sites administered SB in < 50% of CPRs and beyond 10 minutes of the first epinephrine. "High SB user" sites had significantly higher ROSC and hospital discharge rates and better long-term neurological outcome.

This study, however, was not a randomized controlled trial of buffer use, and it suffered from some expected limitations of a post-hoc analysis.[157] The information it provides can, and should, be used to set up a proper prospective clinical trial.[62,157]

Laboratory studies

At least eight animal studies demonstrated a clear beneficial effect of SB or other buffers on ROSC, post-resuscitation myocardial function, or neurological outcome,[17,54,55,106,107,158–160] while a significant number of other studies were "neutral," i.e., not showing such beneficial effects.[37,50–52,56,73,161–165] Study design plays a major role. The more "mechanism"-oriented studies utilized models with relatively brief untreated arrest times, administered unrealistically large buffer doses, and did not use vasopressors. The "outcome"-oriented studies utilized experimental protocols better resembling realistic cardiac arrest and CPR conditions. Some of the studies included only 5 animals in each group, a number too small to permit conclusions to be drawn.

In their "classical" studies on resuscitation drugs, Redding and Pearson[106] found that the combination of SB and epinephrine yielded significantly better short- and long-term outcome than no drugs or either drug alone. Interestingly, they administered large sodium SB doses (approximately 1.5 to 3 meq/kg) and their animals had rather extreme arterial alkalemia.

Vukmir et al.[54] demonstrated higher survival rates and reduced neurological deficit with the combination of SB and epinephrine in dogs resuscitated after 5 and 15 minutes of VF.

Bar-Joseph et al.[17] found that SB, and to a somewhat lesser degree Carbicarb (a mixture of sodium carbonate and sodium bicarbonate), increased resuscitability rate and shortened the time to ROSC in dogs subjected to 10 minutes of VF. Arterial pH and base deficit were the best predictors of ROSC. In a similar model, Leong et al.[55] found that administration of epinephrine and SB before defibrillation attempts was associated with increased ROSC rates compared to administration of epinephrine and saline. ROSC was achieved with fewer shocks and in a shorter time. Coronary perfusion pressures were significantly higher in SB-treated animals than in controls.

Katz et al.[160] compared the effects of "low dose" Carbicarb, "high-dose" Carbicarb, and saline on neurological outcome in a rat asphyxial arrest model. Importantly, the buffer dose administered as a bolus in the "low" and "high dose" Carbicarb groups was equivalent to approximately 1.3 and 2.6 meq/kg of SB, respectively. "Low dose" Carbicarb attenuated acidosis,

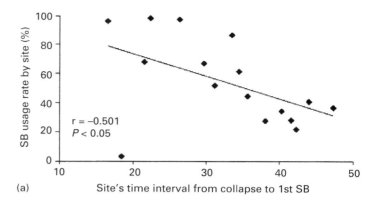

(a)

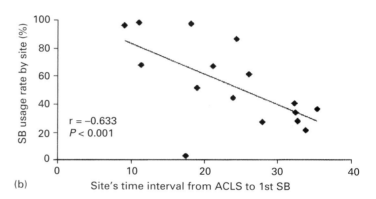

(b)

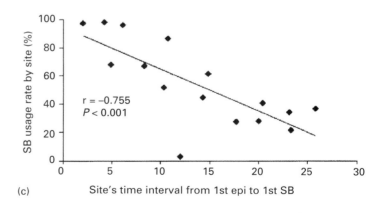

(c)

Fig. 37.5. Sodium bicarbonate (SB) usage rates for each of the 16 Brain Resuscitation Clinical Trial III (BRCT III) study sites vs. time intervals to sodium bicarbonate (SB) administration: (a) from collapse, (b) from initiation of advanced cardiac life support (ACLS), and (c) from administration of the first epinephrine (Epi) dose. Significant inverse correlations were found between SB usage rates and the timing of its administration: Study sites with higher SB usage rates administered it significantly earlier. (From ref. 62. Copyright Blackwell Publishing).

improved resuscitation, reduced neurologic deficits, and reduced the number of dead hippocampal neurons. Neutralization of cerebral acidosis with "high-dose" Carbicarb increased the number of dead hippocampal neurons and neurologic deficits.

In a rat VF model, Sun *et al.*[107] found that buffers administered during CPR reduced coronary perfusion pressure due to their hypertonicity and did not affect immediate resuscitability ($n = 5$ in each group). Nevertheless, buffers ameliorated postresuscitation myocardial dysfunction and increased postresuscitation survival. "CO_2 consuming" buffers (Tromethamine and Carbicarb) were more effective than SB. Of note: no vasopressors were used and animals received a buffer dose of 2.5 meq/kg.

Kette *et al.*[51] studied the effects of SB, Carbicarb, and hypertonic saline on myocardial acid–base status. Defibrillation attempts were successful in each animal, but spontaneous circulation was reestablished in a smaller number of animals treated with SB compared to those treated with Carbicarb or saline. This was a typical "mechanism"-oriented study: buffer doses were very large, no vasopressors were used, and the coronary perfusion pressures (CPP) during CPR were very low.

Liu *et al.*[148] explored the effects of SB, Tribonat®, and hypertonic saline on cerebral perfusion and cerebral acidosis during CPR. ROSC was achieved in a significantly smaller proportion of piglets treated with SB. During CPR and following ROSC, buffer-treated animals had significantly higher arterial, mixed venous, internal jugular, and cerebral tissue pH values compared to saline. Cerebral cortical blood flow following ROSC was higher and of longer duration in the buffer-treated animals (Fig. 37.6).

Other laboratory studies found neither beneficial nor detrimental effects of buffer therapy on CPR outcome.[37,50,52,56,73,161–165] In most of these studies, cardiac arrest with no CPR was rather brief[37,50,52,73,161,162] and buffers were administered very early in the course of CPR.[50,52,73] Such experimental protocols deviate markedly from actual timeline of the common clinical scenario[61] and have a rather unsound physiologic logic: i.e., with no significant metabolic acidosis, buffer therapy is not indicated and cannot be expected to prove beneficial. In most of these studies a very large dose of buffer (2.5–3 meq/kg) was administered[50,52,73,162,163] and in some[50,52,163] epinephrine was not used, resulting in extremely low perfusion pressures. The combination of large doses (2.5 meq/kg) of hypertonic buffers or NaCl with no epinephrine was shown to decrease CPP,[163] which has been repeatedly shown to be an important determinant of ROSC.[163]

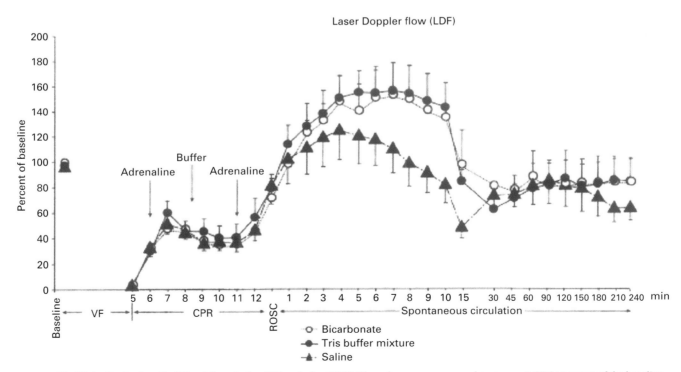

Fig. 37.6. Cerebral cortical blood flow during CPR and after ROSC. The values were expressed as means ± SD in percent of the baseline values. O Bicarbonate group; • Tribonat® Group: ▲ Saline group. (From ref. 148. Copyright Elsevier).

Is SB therapy during CPR detrimental?

Since 1986,[3] a rather long list of presumptive detrimental effects of buffer therapy in general and SB in particular has been repeatedly cited,[3,6–10,58,99,166,167] and consequently it has been "insinuated" that SB therapy worsens CPR outcome. The 2000 Guidelines assert that bicarbonate "can compromise coronary perfusion pressure; may cause adverse effects due to extracellular alkalosis, including shifting the oxyhemoglobin saturation curve or inhibiting the release of oxygen; may induce hyperosmolarity and hypernatremia; produces carbon dioxide, which is freely diffusible into myocardial and cerebral cells and may paradoxically contribute to intracellular acidosis; exacerbates central venous acidosis; and may inactivate simultaneously administered catecholamines."[10] The following section analyzes the evidence underlying these assertions.

"SB can compromise coronary perfusion pressure"

This variably seen effect is apparently "model-dependent:" CPP decreased only when no vasopressor preceded buffer and when the buffer dose was very large (2.5–3 meq/kg)[51,52,107,163,168] but not when either a vasopressor preceded SB or when clinically "reasonable" SB doses (i.e. 1–1.5 meq/kg) were administered.[17,54,73,159,161,162,165,168] Sun et al. showed that both SB and tromethamine decreased CPP when given before vasopressor, but not when vasopressor preceded the buffers.[168] The hypotensive effect of the large SB doses is secondary to the high sodium load rather than to the alkalinizing effect, as equivalent loads of hypertonic saline resulted in the same effect.[163]

"Bicarbonate may induce alkalosis which may shift oxyhemoglobin saturation curve to the left or inhibit oxygen release"

This repeatedly mentioned claim[3,7,8,10,76,169] was postulated based on the physiologic leftward shift of the oxyhemoglobin saturation curve with alkalemia. A single reference[170] is mentioned (in ref. 8) as presumably supporting this hypothesis. In this study, investigators used a "near drowning" (not CPR) hypoxemia model, where swine received massive SB loading (8 meq/kg over 1 minute). Arterial pH increased to 7.75, arterial saturation increased from 38.2% to 65.3% and venous saturation decreased from 34.3% to 28.4%. Thus, the calculated oxygen extraction increased almost tenfold, from 3.9% before to 36.9% after SB. Using an indirect, convoluted reasoning, however, the authors concluded that "these findings suggest that bicarbonate caused a distinct leftward shift . . . which could impair tissue oxygenation."[170]

In cardiac arrest/CPR models, increased oxygen release and oxygen uptake at the tissue level were observed following administration of SB or other buffers.[17,171] Other data on oxygen extraction, mixed venous PO_2, or saturation did not support the notion that buffer therapy impairs tissue oxygenation.[54,68,112] Moreover, buffer therapy, and specifically SB, did not increase arterial or coronary sinus lactate in CPR models.[17,50–52] Cerebral oxygen extraction did not change after SB, but tended to decrease after Tribonate®.[148]

"SB may induce hyperosmolarity and hypernatremia"

This can certainly happen – depending on the amount of SB given. In the often-quoted paper by Mattar et al.[172] patients became severely alkalemic, hypernatremic, and hyperosmotic following massive doses of SB during prolonged CPR (mean of 338 meq SB per patient). Bishop and Weisfeldt[27] found transient increases in serum osmolarity (from 308–309 to 343–349 mOsm/kg) 2 minutes after the administration of 0.7–1 meq/kg of SB. Serum osmolarity declined rapidly within the next 3 minutes. Other clinical[60,173] and experimental[165] studies showed no significant increases in serum sodium if recommended doses (ca. 1 meq/kg) of SB were used.

"SB may inactivate simultaneously administered adrenaline"

This was never shown to be true: mixing epinephrine with SB (or Tris buffer) in the same syringe caused a slight decrease in its biological activity.[174] After administering a very high SB dose (3 meq/kg) and making the animals extremely alkalotic (pH 7.7), the response to epinephrine did not differ from that of the control group.[175]

"SB produces carbon dioxide, which is freely diffusible into myocardial and cerebral cells and may paradoxically contribute to intracellular acidosis; exacerbates central venous acidosis"

Based on the findings of increased central venous PCO_2 ($PvCO_2$) in the "low flow state", this postulation has stirred up the "SB controversy" during CPR.[3,4,6,8,16,58]

No RCT reported values of $PvCO_2$ following SB administration. In the original reports by Weil et al.[29] and Nowak et al.[39] $PvCO_2$ values were elevated, but most of the patients received SB during CPR and no comparison with patients not receiving SB was reported. In previously ventilated patients undergoing CPR, Adrogue' et al. actually found lower $PvCO_2$ in those who received SB than in those who did not.[36] In previously unventilated patients, both $PaCO_2$ and $PvCO_2$ were higher in those who received SB during CPR. The authors concluded that hypoventilation on top of severe circulatory failure is required for CO_2

accumulation.[36] Barton and Callaham[70] found similar arterial PCO_2 values in patients who received SB during CPR and in those who did not.

In animal studies, $PvCO_2$ transiently increased when SB doses ≥2 meq/kg were administered[51,52,55,107,162,163,54] but not when doses < 2 meq/kg were used.[17,54,73,176] These increased $PvCO_2$ values were observed only within 3 minutes of SB administration.[17,50–52,54,161–163,148,176,177] CO_2 elimination during CPR follows a bi-exponential function, with an initial fast phase representing elimination from the lung's FRC and a slow phase, with a half-time of 108 seconds, representing elimination from the pulmonary capillary blood and from peripheral tissues.[177] Therefore, a single, early sampling will fail to depict the transitory nature of the rise in $PvCO_2$. Increases in $PvCO_2$ were more pronounced when no epinephrine was used,[26,50–52,54,162] but not when epinephrine was used to improve tissue perfusion pressures.[17,54,73,148]

Most important, in none of these studies did pH values decrease after SB administration. Even when $PvCO_2$ transiently increased – arterial,[17,27,51–53,56,107,148,159,162–164,176] central venous,[17,25,51–54,56,73,107,161,162,164] cardiac venous,[50–52] or cerebral venous[26,148] pH significantly increased following SB administration. Thus, SB was never shown to exacerbate venous acidemia.

The notion that SB "paradoxically contribute to intracellular acidosis" is consistently traced back to the study by Berenyi *et al.*[178] After 4 minutes of VF, still with no metabolic acidosis, dogs received during 20 minutes of CPR approximately 10 meq/kg of SB (!). Epinephrine was not used and ventilation was unchanged. At 20 minutes, arterial PCO_2 was 64 torr, pH 7.81, and $[HCO_3^-]$ 120 meq/l! Cerebrospinal fluid, supposedly reflecting intracellular acid–base status, had a PCO_2 of 81 torr and a pH of 7.24, which was not significantly different from that of the control group. This "SB loading" model – with no relevance to clinical buffer therapy during CPR – is repeatedly cited as the evidence for "worsening of intracellular acidosis."

No other study that used a cardiac arrest/CPR model supported this hypothesis: intracellular pH either increased[68,146–148] (Fig. 37.7) or did not change,[48,89,91,96] following SB administration.

In a hypoxic lactic acidosis model, Sessler *et al.* showed that a very large SB dose did not produce paradoxical intracellular acidosis in the brain.[179] Multiple other *in vivo* "non-CPR" and *in vitro* models investigated this issue, with models of hypercarbic acidosis, cell suspensions, isolated heart preparations, and more.[180–186] Results are equivocal and depend on experimental design, model, initial intracellular pH, amount and mode of SB administration, and timing of intracellular pH measurements.[185,187]

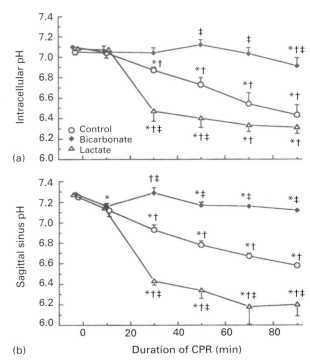

Fig. 37.7. Cerebral intracellular pH and sagittal sinus blood pH during prolonged cardiopulmonary resuscitation. Dogs were placed in a control group or received sodium bicarbonate or lactate at 14 minutes of CPR. *P <0.05 vs. prearrest P<0.05 vs. values at 10 minutes of CPR; ‡ p<0.05 vs. control group at the same time point. (From ref. 146. Copyright American Heart Association).

Timing of buffer administration

ALS Guidelines repeatedly stated that "after protracted arrest or long resuscitative efforts, SB possibly benefits the patient. However, SB therapy should be considered only after the confirmed interventions, such as defibrillation, cardiac compression, intubation, ventilation, and vasopressor therapy, have been ineffective."[3,8–10] It was estimated that these interventions are accomplished within the first 10 minutes of CPR.[3]

What is the actual timing of buffer administration in CPR? In a systematic analysis of SB usage in a large clinical trial, Bar-Joseph *et al.*[61] found that in the out-of-hospital setting, the time from collapse to ACLS was 11.4 minutes and to the first epinephrine 20.4 minutes. SB was administered 11.4 minutes after the first epinephrine, i.e., over 31 minutes after the patients' collapse.[61,62] A similar timeline for the first epinephrine dose was found in other large clinical trials.[188,189]

The long time intervals to administration of buffers should be related to the development rate of metabolic acidosis, as discussed above. If buffers are thought to be effective in promoting return of spontaneous circulation, there is no "physiologic" sense in delaying their administration by 11 minutes beyond the first epinephrine.[62]

Comparison of different buffers during CPR

The controversy surrounding the use of the "CO_2-producing" SB, has led to the development and testing of other "CO_2-consuming" buffers. As of today, three buffers were considered as alternatives to SB during CPR: Tromethamine (THAM), Carbicarb®, and Tribonate®.

Tromethamine (THAM, Tris buffer)

Tromethamine is an organic H^+ ion acceptor, which crosses cell membranes and acts both as an extracellular and intracellular buffer.[190,191] With a pK = 7.84 it is a stronger buffer compared to SB (pK = 6.10), binding H^+ ions according to the formula

$$(CH_2OH)_3 C - NH_2 + HA \leftrightarrow (CH_2OH)_3 C - NH_3^+ + A^-$$

which leads to a right shift of the reaction

$$CO_2 + H_2O \leftrightarrow H_2CO_3 \leftrightarrow HCO_3^- + H^+$$

and thereby decreases CO_2 and increases HCO_3^- concentrations.[192,193] THAM markedly reduced CO_2 in arterial, mixed venous, and great cardiac vein blood.[17,50] Interestingly, THAM was previously thought to bind CO_2 directly,[194] but this was disputed later.[193] In animal experiments, THAM was less effective than SB in promoting ROSC.[17,50] This may be related to its vasodilating effect, resulting in lower CPPs.[17,50] Therefore, THAM cannot be recommended for routine use as a buffer during CPR.

Carbicarb

Carbicarb® is an equimolar mixture of sodium carbonate (Na_2CO_3) and sodium SB ($NaHCO_3$), devised to capitalize on the "CO_2-consuming" effects of sodium carbonate without the hazards of its very alkaline pH of 11.[195] Carbicarb® was originally reported as capable of buffering H^+ ions with no net production of CO_2.[195,196] In the setting of hypoxic lactic acidosis, Carbicarb® provided greater hemodynamic stability compared to normal saline or SB, increased arterial pH without increasing $PaCO_2$, increased tissue oxygen utilization, and prevented further increases of lactate.[196,197] In cardiac arrest/CPR models, results depend on experimental details: Carbicarb® decreased while SB increased both $PaCO_2$ and $PvCO_2$ 2 minutes after the administration of large doses (2–2.5 meq/kg) of buffer.[51,52] When clinically rel-

evant doses (1 meq/kg) were given, Carbicarb® administration resulted in slightly (though not significantly) higher $PvCO_2$ compared to SB administration.[17] Blecic *et al.*[56] found no difference between Carbicarb® and SB (1 meq/kg) in either $PaCO_2$ or $PvCO_2$ at 5 minutes post ROSC. In all of the studies, both buffers corrected blood pH effectively. In fact, arterial pH values of 7.90 and 8.21 were measured after the administration of the large Carbicarb® doses.[51,52] Intramyocardial pH did not increase and was not different 2 minutes after either Carbicarb® or SB administration.[51] No significant differences in resuscitability, or arterial or coronary perfusion pressures were found between these buffers during CPR.[17,51,52,163] Carbicarb® and SB were equally effective in ameliorating postresuscitation myocardial dysfunction following prolonged VF.[107]

Overall, despite a theoretical advantage, Carbicarb® was not shown to be superior to SB during CPR in any of the clinically relevant parameters.

Tribonat®

This is a mixture of SB, THAM, phosphate, and acetate, that was introduced in 1985 by Wiklund *et al.*[166,198,199] and is used clinically mainly in Scandinavia. Tribonat® was designed to overcome previously reported disadvantages of both sodium SB and THAM: compared to SB it has a lower sodium content, a significant intracellular buffering capacity, and it was hypothesized that it causes less metabolic alkalosis.[166,198,199]

In two cardiac arrest models, Tribonat® resulted in better ROSC rates than did SB.[73,148]

In a cardiac arrest model, neither arterial nor CSF pH and PCO_2 differed between Tribonat®- and SB-treated piglets.[68] A recent, large and well-designed animal study compared Tribonat®, SB, and saline in piglets undergoing CPR.[148] No differences were found between Tribonat® and SB effects on arterial, mixed venous, and internal jugular pH and PCO_2 – although both buffers improved these variables compared to saline. No differences were found between the effects of these buffers on cerebral cortical blood flow, cerebral oxygen extraction ratio, and cerebral tissue pH both during CPR and following ROSC.

The hemodynamic responses to epinephrine during CPR were compared:[112] while SB-treated animals had higher systemic blood pressures before epinephrine administration, Tribonat® (as well as THAM and saline) resulted in larger systemic pressure increases following epinephrine, so that there were no differences between the groups at this point. No differences were found between the effects of Tribonat® and SB on myocardial energy metabolism during CPR.[26,73]

Thus, in cardiac arrest models, Tribonat® was more effective than SB in restoring early resuscitability, but despite theoretical expectations, no other differences between the two buffers were found. Tribonat® seems to be an acceptable alternative to SB.

Buffer therapy postresuscitation

Guidelines[8,10] recommended the use of sodium SB after ROSC, especially following prolonged CPR. Lacking any specific published evidence, however, this may be supported only by rational conjunctures or common practices.

Sun *et al.* reached contradictory conclusions regarding the effects of buffers on postresuscitation myocardial dysfunction in two studies using the same rat CPR model.[107,168] The first study[107] concluded that buffers administered during CPR may ameliorate postresuscitation myocardial dysfunction and thereby improve postresuscitation survival. Their later study,[168] which added epinephrine and esmolol (to block the beta1 effect of epinephrine) to buffers, concluded that buffers caused greater impairment of postresuscitation myocardial function and decreased postresuscitation survival. Unfortunately, the authors provided no hypothesis to explain these differences. Both of these studies compared multiple small ($n = 5$ each) groups, limiting their statistical power.

Buffer therapy for cardiac arrest and CPR under special circumstances

Cardiac arrest associated with pre-existing metabolic acidosis

ACLS Guidelines[2,3,8,10] recommended SB for patients with "preexisting metabolic acidosis" (Level IIa recommendation). Neither the Guidelines nor the background text[169] specify to which type of "preexisting metabolic acidosis" it relates, and at what degree of acidosis is buffer indicated. Obviously, the basic presumption of this downright indication is that metabolic acidosis is detrimental, yet the same Guidelines are very reserved regarding buffer therapy for metabolic acidosis developing during arrest and CPR. Are these lactic acidoses really different?

There is practically no literature to support this longstanding recommendation, which may be supported by inference from other situations and rational conjecture. Since buffer therapy – including SB – is not detrimental, however, there seems to be no clinical logic in changing this recommendation.

This indication for buffer treatment may be especially important in pediatric advanced life support (PALS), as pediatric cardiac arrest is usually secondary to on-going respiratory or circulatory failure resulting from wholebody hypoxia and lactate production.[22] In adults, pulseless electrical activity is also secondary to deteriorating primary conditions with metabolic (lactic) acidosis developing before the final cardiac arrest.[92,214]

Cardiac arrest associated with hyperkalemia

The use of SB for "cardiac arrest associated with hyperkalemia" is another longstanding, seemingly undisputed recommendation (Level I or Level IIa)[2,3,8–10] The origins of this recommendation date back to a 1959 paper by Bellet[200] and to a dramatic case report by Stewart *et al.*[201] Nevertheless, literature search for hyperkalemia, CPR and SB found only nine case reports, which do not allow drawing any unequivocal conclusions, as patients were treated with various means, including SB, to reduce serum potassium levels.[202–210] No animal studies on hyperkalemia in cardiac arrest models were reported. Evidence suggests that SB is not very effective in the initial management of hyperkalemia in patients who are stable, not acidotic and not in cardiac arrest.[211,212] One small case series[213] reported on a significant reduction of elevated serum potassium (associated with ECG changes) following SB therapy in four profoundly acidotic patients. Since the potassium-lowering effect of sodium SB is not large and not immediate, it cannot be relied upon as a sole therapy to treat hyperkalemia during CPR. SB should be combined with other measures such as calcium, insulin/glucose, or hemodialysis.[211,212]

Cardiac arrest associated with tricyclic antidepressant toxicity

SB has been indicated as a Class IIa recommendation in cardiac arrest associated with tricyclic antidepressant toxicity.[8–10,214] Surprisingly, only a single case report involving the use of SB in the treatment of cardiac arrest following tricyclic antidepressant intoxication was published.[215] Nevertheless, vast literature exists on the efficacy of SB in treating the cardiovascular toxicity of tricyclics and other sodium channel blockers such as type 1a antiarrhythmics and cocaine. No randomized clinical trials are available, but observational studies,[216] case reports,[217–219] and animal studies[220–228] demonstrated rapid improvement in hypotension and cardiac arrhythmias following SB administration. It remains controversial whether it is the alkalinization or the administration of extra sodium that causes these beneficial effects.[225,227–232] As SB is readily available, however, its toxicity is low and its benefit is high, it can be safely recommended for tricyclic antidepressant toxicity. No clear-cut recommendations concerning dosing and the duration of therapy can be provided from the published literature.[233]

Conclusions

1. Both CO_2 accumulation and lactate production contribute to the rapidly developing acidosis during cardiac arrest and CPR.

2. As a result of the low tissue perfusion generated by external cardiac massage, CO_2 and H^+ accumulate at the tissue level. This phenomenon is responsible for the large veno-arterial differences in PCO_2 and pH consistently found during CPR.

3. The hypothesis derived from this finding, suggesting that SB – a typical "CO_2-producing" buffer – paradoxically aggravates intracellular acidosis was not substantiated.

4. Acidosis, especially when coupled with hypoxia, decreases cardiac contractility and reduces the chances for successful defibrillation. Profound cerebral acidosis develops within minutes of cardiac arrest, further impairing brain energy metabolism, enhancing brain edema, and worsening histopathologic and neurological damage.

5. Hyperventilation cannot effectively compensate for metabolic acidosis, and, at least theoretically, may have detrimental effects.

6. No large, prospective RCT of buffer therapy in CPR was performed. One relatively small prospective RCT found no outcome benefit of buffer therapy. A recent retrospective analysis found that EMS systems with frequent and earlier use of SB had better CPR outcome than did EMS systems with infrequent and late use of SB.

7. At least eight animal studies found a beneficial outcome effect of buffers (mainly SB), whereas 10 other studies did not find such an effect.

8. Careful review of the literature does not confirm any of the claims previously raised against SB when it is used in a clinically appropriate manner during CPR:
   - When used in combination with vasopressors and in clinically relevant dosages, SB does not compromise coronary perfusion pressure.
   - Buffer therapy does not worsen, but rather improves tissue oxygenation.
   - SB only rarely increases serum Na^+ and osmolarity during CPR and the clinical importance of these changes is rather minimal in light of the extremely grave prognosis of prolonged CPR.
   - SB does not exacerbate central venous acidosis. Early after administration of large SB doses, $PvCO_2$ may transiently increase, but arterial, central venous, and cardiac venous pH always increase significantly.
   - No "paradoxical intracellular acidosis" was proven in cardiac arrest/CPR models, even when very large SB doses were used. Most data suggest that intracellular pH increases following SB administration.
   - SB does not inactivate simultaneously administered epinephrine.

9. Clinical data show that SB administration is often delayed and administered at a stage when little or no benefit can be expected.

10. Although logical, there is no evidence for a beneficial effect of SB for "pre-existing metabolic acidosis." Similarly, there is very little, rather contradictory evidence, on the effects of buffers "upon return of spontaneous circulation."

11. None of the other buffers tested as an alternative to SB have proven to be superior or to have less clinically important side effects.

12. There is only weak evidence for a beneficial effect of SB in cardiac arrest associated with hyperkalemia. SB cannot be relied upon as a sole therapy to treat hyperkalemia and should be combined with other measures such as calcium, insulin/glucose, or hemodialysis.

13. SB can be safely recommended for cardiovascular emergencies associated with tricyclic antidepressant toxicity.

14. What are our current knowledge gaps?
    - There is an urgent need for a proper prospective randomized clinical trial of SB in ACLS. Until this is accomplished, it seems unjustified to discard a potentially useful, and rather harmless, drug from use in a clinical emergency that has an extremely unfavorable outcome and no other viable alternatives are available.
    - There are no published clinical data on pediatric use of buffers.
    - Recommendations for dosage and timing of repeated buffer doses are not supported by sufficient factual data.
    - There is a need to clarify the cause–effect relationship between correction of acidosis and CPR outcome.

Addendum

The new Guidelines for Cardiopulmonary and Cerebral Resuscitation (CPR) 2005[236] were published after completion of this chapter. The paragraph relating to Buffers is very succinct, and is copied here in its entirety (reference numbers relate to this text):

Consensus on science

There were no published LOE 1, 2, or 3 studies on the use of sodium bicarbonate during CPR. One LOE 2 study[97] showed no advantage of Tribonate over placebo (neutral), and 5 retrospective analyses of uncontrolled clinical use of sodium bicarbonate were inconclusive (LOE 4).[4,60,94,96,154] One LOE 4 study[62] suggested that emergency medical services (EMS) systems using sodium bicarbonate earlier and more frequently had significantly higher rates of ROSC and hospital discharge and better long-term neurologic outcome.

Results of animal studies are conflicting and inconclusive. Sodium bicarbonate was effective for treating the cardiovascular toxicity (hypotension, cardiac arrhythmias) caused by tricyclic antidepressants and other fast sodium channel blockers (see "Drug overdose and poisoning," below). Only 1 LOE 5 publication[215] reported the successful treatment of VF cardiac arrest caused by tricyclic poisoning using sodium bicarbonate.

Treatment recommendation

Giving sodium bicarbonate routinely during cardiac arrest and CPR (especially in out-of-hospital cardiac arrest) or after ROSC is not recommended. Sodium bicarbonate may be considered for life-threatening hyperkalemia or cardiac arrest associated with hyperkalemia, pre-existing metabolic acidosis, or tricyclic antidepressant overdose.

REFERENCES

1. Jude, J.R., Kouwenhoven, W.B. & Knickerbocker, G.G. Cardiac arrest. Report of application of external cardiac massage on 118 patients. *J. Am. Med. Assoc.* 1961; **178**: 1063–1070.
2. Standards for cardiopulmonary resuscitation (CPR) and emergency cardiac care (ECC). *J. Am. Med. Assoc.* 1974; **227**: 833–868.
3. Standards and guidelines for cardiopulmonary resuscitation and emergency cardiac care. *J. Am. Med. Assoc.* 1986; **255**: 2843–2989.
4. Weil, M.H., Trevino, R.P. & Rackow, E.C. Sodium bicarbonate during CPR – does it help or hinder? *Chest* 1985; **88**: 487.
5. Grundler, W., Weil, M.H. & Rackow, E.C. Arteriovenous carbon dioxide and pH gradients during cardiac arrest. *Circulation* 1986; **74**: 1071–1074.
6. Jaffe, A.S. New and old paradoxes: Acidosis and cardiopulmonary resuscitation. *Circulation* 1989; **80**: 1079–1083.
7. Arieff, A.I. Efficacy of buffers in the management of cardiac arrest. *Crit. Care Med.* 1998; **26**: 1311–1313.
8. Adult Advanced Cardiac Life Support, in Guidelines for Cardiopulmonary Resuscitation and Emergency Cardiac Care. *J. Am. Med. Assoc.* 1992; **268**: 2199–2241.
9. Working Group on Advanced Life Support of the European Resuscitation Council: The 1998 European Resuscitation Council Guidelines for Adult Advanced Life Support. *Resuscitation* 1998; **37**: 81–90.
10. Agents to optimize cardiac output and blood pressure. In Guidelines for Cardiopulmonary Resuscitation and Emergency Cardiac Care. *Circulation* 2000; **102/8** (suppl I): 129–135.
11. Astrup, P., Jorgensen, K., Siggaard-Andersen, O. & Engel, K. The acid–base metabolism. A new approach. *Lancet* 1960; **1**: 1035–1039.
12. Schwartz, W.B. & Relman, A.S. A critique of the parameters used in evaluation of acid–base disorders. *N. Eng. J. Med.* 1963; **268**: 1382–1388.
13. Sirker, A.A., Rhodes, A., Grounds, R.M. & Bennett, E.D. Acid base physiology: the 'traditional' and the 'modern' approaches. *Anaesthesia* 2002; **57**: 348–356.
14. Balasubramanyan, N., Havens, P.L. & Hoffman, G.M. Unmeasured anions identified by the Fencl–Stewart method predict mortality better than base excess, anion gap, and lactate in patients in the pediatric intensive care unit. *Crit. Care. Med.* 1999; **27**: 1577–1581.
15. Bircher, N.G. Acidosis of cardiopulmonary resuscitation: carbon dioxide transport and anaerobiosis. *Crit. Care. Med.* 1992; **20**: 1203–1205.
16. von Planta, M., Weil, M.H., Gazmuri, R.J., Bisera, J. & Rackow, E.C. Myocardial acidosis associated with CO_2 production during cardiac arrest and resuscitation. *Circulation* 1989; **80**: 684–692.
17. Bar-Joseph, G., Weinberger, T., Castel, T. *et al.* Comparison of sodium bicarbonate, Carbicarb and THAM during cardiopulmonary resuscitation in dogs. *Crit. Care. Med.* 1998; **26**: 1397–1408.
18. Angelos, M.G. & DeBehnke, D.J. Epinephrine-mediated changes in carbon dioxide tension during eperfusion of ventricular fibrillation in a canine model. *Crit. Care. Med.* 1995; **23**: 925–930.
19. Fillmore, S.J., Shapiro, M. & Killip, T. serial blood gas studies during cardiopulmonary resuscitation. *Ann. Int. Med.* 1970; **72**: 465–469.

20. Chazan, J.A., Stenson, R. & Kurland, G.S. The acidosis of cardiac arrest. *N. Engl. J. Med.* 1968; **278**: 360–364.

21. Steedman, D.J. & Robertson, C.E. Acid base changes in arterial and central venous blood during cardiopulmonary resuscitation. *Arch. Emerg. Med.* 1992; **9**: 169–176.

22. Schindler, M.B., Bohn, D., Cox, P.N. *et al.* Outcome of out-of-hospital cardiac or respiratory arrest in children. *N. Engl. J. Med.* 1996; **335**: 1473–1479.

23. Capparelli, E.V., Chow, M.S.S., Kluger, J. & Fieldman, A. Differences in systemic and myocardial acid–base status during cardiopulmonary resuscitation. *Crit. Care Med.* 1989; **17**: 442–446.

24. Carden, D.L., Martin, G.B., Nowak, R.M., Foreback, C.C. & Tomlanovich, M.C. Lactic acidosis during closed-chest CPR in dogs. *Ann. Emerg. Med.* 1987; **16**: 1317–1320.

25. Kette, F., Weil, M.H., Gazmuri, R.J., Bisera, J. & Rackow, E.C. Intramyocardial hypercarbic acidosis during cardiac arrest and resuscitation. *Crit. Care. Med.* 1993; **21**: 901–906.

26. Wiklund, L., Ronquist, G. Roomans, G.M., Rubertsson, S. & Waldenstrom, A. Response of myocardial cellular energy metabolism to variation of buffer composition during open-chest experimental cardiopulmonary resuscitation in the pig. *Eur. J. Clin Invest.* 1997; **27**: 417–426.

27. Bishop, R.L. & Weisfeldt, M.L. Sodium bicarbonate administration during cardiac arrest: Effect on arterial pH, pCO_2 and osmolarity. *J. Am. Med. Assoc.*1976; **235**: 506–509.

28. Sanders, A.B., Ewy, G.A. & Taft, T.V. Resuscitation and arterial gas abnormalities during prolonged cardiopulmonary resuscitation. *Ann. Emerg. Med.* 1984; **13**: 676–679.

29. Weil, M.H., Rackow, E.C., Trevino, R., Grundler, W., Falk, J.L. & Griffel, M.I. Differences in acid–base state between venous and arterial blood during cardiopulmonary cardiopulmonary resuscitation. *N. Engl. J. Med.* 1986; **315**: 153–156.

30. Bellamy, R.F., DeGuzman, L.R. & Pedersen, D.C. Coronary blood flow during cardiopulmonary resuscitation in swine. *Circulation* 1984; **69**: 174–180.

31. Fitzgerald, K.R., Babbs, C.F., Frissora, H.A., Davis, R.W. & Silver D.I. Cardiac output during cardiopulmonary resuscitation at various compression rates and durations. *Am. J. Physiol.* 1981; **241**: H442–H448.

32. Weil, M.H., Bisera, J., Trevino, R.P. & Rackow, E.C. Cardiac output and end-tidal carbon dioxide. *Crit. Care Med.* 1985; **13**: 907–909.

33. Falk, J.L., Rackow, E.C. & Weil, M.H. End-tidal carbon dioxide concentration during cardiopulmonary resuscitation. *N. Engl. J. Med.* 1988; **318**: 607–611.

34. Idris, A.H., Staples, E.D., O'Brien, D.J. *et al.* End-tidal carbon dioxide during extremely low cardiac output. *Ann. Emerg. Med.* 1994; **23**: 568–572.

35. Adrogue, H.J., Rashad, M.N., Gorin, A.B., Yacoub, J. & Madias N.E. Assessing acid–base status in circulatory failure. Differences between arterial and central venous blood. *N. Engl. J. Med.* 1989; **320**: 1312–1316.

36. Adrogue, H.J., Rashad, M.N., Gorin, A.B., Yacoub, J. & Madias, N.E. Arteriovenous acid–base disparity in circulatory failure:

studies on mechanism. *Am. J. Physiol.* 1989; **257**: F1087–F1093.

37. Wiklund, L., Jorfeldt, L., Stjernstrom, H. & Rubertsson, S. Gas exchange as monitored in mixed venous and arterial blood during experimental cardiopulmonary resuscitation. *Acta Anaesthesiol. Scand.* 1992; **36**: 427–435.

38. Idris, A.H., Staples, E.D., O'Brian, D.J. *et al.* Effect of ventilation on acid–base balance and oxygenation in low blood-flow states. *Crit. Care Med.* 1994; **22**: 1827–1834.

39. Nowak, R.M., Martin, G.B., Carden, D.L. & Tomlanovich, M.C. Selective venous hypercarbia during human CPR: Implications regarding blood flow. *Ann. Emerg. Med.* 1987; **16**: 527–530.

40. Johnson, B.A. & Weil, M.H. Redefining ischemia due to circulatory failure as dual effects of oxygen deficits and of carbon dioxide excesses. *Crit. Care Med.* 1991; **19**: 1432–1438.

41. Halmagyi, D.F.J., Kennedy, M. & Varga, D. Hidden hypercapnia in hemorrhagic hypotension. *Anesthesiology* 1970; **33**: 594–601.

42. Benjamin, E., Paluch, T.A., Berger, S.R., Premus, G., Wu, C. & Iberti, T.J. Venous hypercarbia in canine hemorrhagic shock. *Crit. Care. Med.* 1987; **15**: 516–518.

43. Mathias, D.W., Clifford, P.S. & Klopfenstein, H.S. Mixed venous blood gases are superior to arterial blood gases in assessing acid–base status and oxygenation during acute cardiac tamponade in dogs. *J. Clin. Invest.* 1988; **82**: 833–838.

44. Mecher, C.E., Rackow, E.C., Astiz, M.E. & Weil, M.H. Venous hypercarbia associated with severe sepsis and systemic hypoperfusion. *Crit. Care. Med.* 1990; **18**: 585–589.

45. Rackow, E.C., Astiz, M.E., Mecher, C.E. & Weil, M.H. Increased venous-arterial carbon dioxide tension difference during severe sepsis in rats. *Crit. Care Med.* 1994; **22**: 121–125.

46. Desai, V.S., Weil, M.H., Tang, W., Gazmuri, R. & Bisera, J. Hepatic, renal, and cerebral tissue hypercarbia during sepsis and shock in rats. *J. Lab. Clin. Med.* 1995; **125**: 456–461.

47. Nelimarkka, O. & Niinikoski, J. Oxygen and carbon dioxide tensions in the canine kidney during arterial occlusion and hemorrhagic hypotension. *Surg. Gynecol. Obstet.* 1984; **158**: 27–32.

48. Gudipati, C.V., Weil, M.H., Gazmuri, R.J., Deshmukh, H.G., Bisera, J. & Rackow, E.C. Increases in coronary vein CO_2 during cardiac resuscitation. *J. Appl. Physiol.* 1990; **68**: 1405–1408.

49. Bergman, K.S. & Harris, B.H. Arteriovenous pH difference – a new index of perfusion. *J. Pediatr. Surg.* 1988; **23**: 1190–1192.

50. Von Planta, M., Gudipati, C., Weil, M.H., Kraus, L.J. & Rackow, E.C. Effects of tromethamine and sodium bicarbonate buffers during cardiac resuscitaion. *J. Clin. Pharmacol.* 1988; **28**: 594–599.

51. Kette, F., Weil, M.H., von Planta, M., Gazmuri, R.J. & Rackow, E.C. Buffer agents do not reserve intramyocardial acidosis during cardiac resuscitation. *Circulation* 1990; **81**: 1660–1666.

52. Gazmuri, R.J., von Planta, M., Weil, M.H. & Rackow, E.C. Cardiac effects of carbon dioxide-consuming and carbon

dioxide-generating buffers during cardiopulmonary resuscitation. *J. Am. Coll. Cardiol.* 1990; **15**: 482–490.

53. Sanders, A.B., Otto, C.W., Kern, K.B., Rogers, J.N., Perrault, P. & Ewy, G.A. Acid–base balance in a canine model of cardiac arrest. *Ann. Emerg. Med.* 1988; **17**: 667–671.

54. Vukmir, R.B., Bircher, N.G., Radovsky, A. & Safar, P. Sodium bicarbonate may improve outcome in dogs with brief or prolonged cardiac arrest. *Crit. Care Med.* 1995; **23**: 515–522.

55. Leong, E.C.M., Bendall, J.C., Boyd, A.C. & Einstein, R. Sodium bicarbonate improves the chance of resuscitation after 10 minutes of cardiac arrest in dogs. *Resuscitation* 2001; **51**: 309–315.

56. Blecic, S., De Backer, D., Deleuze, M., Vachiery, J.L. & Vincent, J.L. Correction of metabolic acidosis in experimental CPR: a comparative study of sodium bicarbonate, carbicarb, and dextrose. *Ann. Emerg. Med.* 1991; **20**: 235–238.

57. Weil, M.H. Is there a role for buffer administration during CPR? Cardiopulmonary and *Crit. Care Letter*, 1999 (Spring) 7–12.

58. Koster, R. & Carli, P. Acid–base management, a statement for the Advanced Life Support Working Party of the European Resuscitation Council. *Resuscitation* 1992; **24**: 143–146.

59. Batenhorst, R.L., Clifton, G.D., Booth, D.C., Hendrickson, N.M. & Ryberg, M.L. Evaluation of 516 cardiopulmonary resuscitation attempts. *Am. J. Hosp. Pharm.* 1985; **42**: 2478–2483.

60. Aufderheide, T.P., Martin, D.R., Olson, D.W. Prehospital bicarbonate use in cardiac arrest: a 3-year experience. *Am. J. Emerg. Med.* 1992; **10**: 4–7.

61. Bar-Joseph, G., Abramson, N.S., Jansen-McWilliams, L. *et al.* for the Brain Resuscitation Clinical Trial III Study Group: Clinical use of sodium bicarbonate during cardiopulmonary resuscitation – is it used sensibly? *Resuscitation* 2002; **54**: 47–55.

62. Bar-Joseph, G., Abramson, N.S., Kelsey, S.F., Mashiach, T., Craig, M.T. & Safar, P. for the Brain Resuscitation Clinical Trial III Study Group: Improved resuscitation outcome in emergency medical systems with increased usage of sodium bicarbonate during cardiopulmonary resuscitation. *Acta Anaesthesiol. Scand.* 2005; **49**(1): 6–15.

63. Hevy, R.D., Rhoden, W.E., Shearer, K., Varley, E. & Brooks, N.H. An audit of drug usage for in-hospital cardiopulmonary resuscitation. *Eur. Heart J.* 1992; **13**: 1665–1668.

64. Langhelle, A., Sunde, K., Wik, L. & Steen, P.A. Arterial blood-gases with 500- versus 1000-ml tidal volumes during out-of-hospital CPR. *Resuscitation* 2000; **45**: 27–33.

65. Gazmuri, R.J., von Planta, M., Weil, M.H. & Rackow, E.C. Arterial PCO_2 as an indicator of systemic perfusion during cardiopulmonary resuscitation. *Crit. Care Med.* 1989; **17**: 237–240.

66. Blumenthal, S.R. & Voorhees, W.D. The relationship of carbon dioxide excretion during cardiopulmonary resuscitation to regional blood flow and survival. *Resuscitation.* 1997; **35**: 135–143.

67. Prause, G., Hetz, H., Lauda, P., Pojer, H., Smolle-Juettner, F. & Smolle, J. A comparison of the end-tidal-CO_2 documented by capnometry and the arterial PCO_2 in emergency patients. *Resuscitation* 1997; **35**: 145–148.

68. Wiklund, L., Soderberg, D., Henneberg, S., Rubertsson, S., Stjernstrom, H. & Groth, T. Kinetics of carbon dioxide during cardiopulmonary resuscitation. *Crit. Care Med.* 1986; **14**: 1015–1022.

69. Angelos, M.G. & DeBehnke, D.J. Arterial pH and carbon dioxide as indicators of tissue perfusion during cardiac arrest in a canine model. *Crit. Care Med.* 1992; **20**: 1302–1308.

70. Barton, C. & Callaham, M. Lack of correlation between end-tidal carbon dioxide concentrations and $PaCO_2$ in cardiac arrest. *Crit. Care Med.* 1991; **19**: 108–110.

71. Idris, A.H., Becker, L.B., Fuerst, R.S. *et al.* Effect of ventilation on resuscitation in an animal model of cardiac arrest. *Circulation* 1994; **90**: 3063–3069.

72. Engoren, M., Severyn, F., Fenn-Bruderer, N. & DeFrank, M. Cardiac output, coronary blood flow, and blood gases during open-chest standard and compression-active-decompression cardiopulmonary resuscitation. *Resuscitation* 2002; **55**: 309–316.

73. Wiklund, L., Ronquist, G., Stjernstrom, H. & Waldenstrom, A. Effects of alkaline buffer administration on survival and myocardial energy metabolism in pigs subjected to ventricular fibrillation and closed chest CPR. *Acta Anesthesiol. Scand.* 1990; **34**: 430–439.

74. McGill, J.W. & Ruiz, E. Central venous pH as a predictor of arterial pH in prolonged cardiac arrest. *Ann. Emerg. Med.* 1984; **13**: 684–687.

75. Carden, D.L., Martin, G.B., Nowak, R.M., Foreback, C.C. & Tomlanovich, M.C. Lactic acidosis as a predictor of downtime during cardiopulmonary arrest in dogs. *Am. J. Emerg. Med.* 1985; **3**: 120–124.

76. Young, G.P. Reservations and recommendations regarding sodium bicarbonate administration in cardiac arrest. *J. Emerg. Med.* 1988; **6**: 321–323.

77. Kitakaze, M., Weisfeldt, M.L. & Marban, E. Acidosis during early reperfusion prevents myocardial stunning in perfused ferret hearts. *J. Clin. Invest.* 1988; **82**: 920–927.

78. A guide to the International ACLS algorithms. In Guidelines for Cardiopulmonary Resuscitation and Emergency Cardiac Care. *Circulation* 2000; **102/8** (Suppl I): 142–157.

79. Ralston, S.H., Voorhees, W.D. & Babbs, C.F. Intrapulmonary epinephrine during prolonged cardiopulmonary resuscitation: Improved regional blood flow and resuscitation in dogs. *Ann. Emerg. Med.* 1984; **13**: 79–86.

80. Sanders, A.B., Ewy, G.A. & Taft, T.V. Prognostic and therapeutic importance of the aortic diastolic pressure in resuscitation from cardiac arrest. *Crit. Care Med.* 1984; **12**: 871–873.

81. von Planta, I., Weil, M.H., von Planta, M. *et al.* Cardiopulmonary resuscitation in the rat. *J. Appl. Physiol.* 1988; **65**: 2641–2647.

82. Paradis, N.A., Martin, G.B., Rivers, E.P. *et al.* Coronary perfusion pressure and the return of spontaneous circulation in human cardiopulmonary resuscitation. *J. Am. Med. Assoc.* 1990; **263**: 1106–1113.

83. MacGregor, D.C., Wilson, G.J., Holness, D.E. *et al.* Intramyocardial carbon dioxide tension. A guide to the safe period of anoxic arrest of the heart. *J. Thor. Cardiovasc. Surg.* 1974; **68**: 101–107.

84. Orchard, C.H. & Kentish, J.C. Effects of changes of pH on the contractile function of cardiac muscle. *Am. J. Physiol.* 1990; **258**: C967–C981.

85. Vukmir, R.B., Bircher, N. & Safar, P. Sodium bicarbonate in cardiac arrest: a reappraisal. *Am. J. Emerg. Med.* 1996; **14**: 192–206.

86. Adrogue, H.J. & Madias, N.E. Management of life-threatening acid–base disorders. *N. Engl. J. Med.* 1998; **338**: 26–34.

87. Alberts, B., Bray, D., Lewis, J. *et al.* Membrane transport of small molecules and the ionic basis of membrane excitability. In *The Molecular Biology of the Cell*, 3rd edn. New York, Garland Publishing, 1994: 518–519.

88. Orchard, C.H. & Cingolani, H.E. Acidosis and arrhythmias in cardiac muscle. *Cardiovasc. Res.* 1994; **28**: 1312–1319.

89. Gaskel, W.H. On the tonicity of the heart and blood vessels. *J. Physiol, Lond.* 1880; **3**: 48–75.

90. McElroy, W.T., Gedes, A.J. & Brown, F.B. Effects of CO_2, bicarbonate and pH on the performance of isolated perfused guinea pig hearts. *Am. J. Physiol.* 1958; **195**: 412–416.

91. Thatte, H.S., Rhee, J.H., Zagarins, S.E. *et al.* Acidosis-induced apoptosis in human and porcine heart. *Ann. Thorac. Surg.* 2004; **77**: 1376–1383.

92. Camarata, S.J., Weil, M.H., Hanashiro, P.K. & Shubin, H. Cardiac arrest in the critically ill. I. A study of predisposing causes in 132 patients. *Circulation* 1971; **44**: 688–695.

93. Kerber, R.E. & Sarnat, W. Factors influencing the success of ventricular defibrillation in man. *Circulation* 1979; **60**: 226–230.

94. Suljaga-Pechtel, K., Goldberg, E., Strickon, P., Berger, M. & Skovron, M.L. Cardiopulmonary resuscitation in a hospitalized population: prospective study of factors associated with outcome. *Resuscitation* 1984; **12**: 77–95.

95. Weil, M.H., Ruiz, C.E., Sybil, M. & Rackow, E.C. Acid–base determinants of survival after cardiopulmonary resuscitation. *Crit. Care Med.* 1985; **13**: 888–892.

96. Roberts, D., Landolfo, K., Light, R.B. & Dobson, K. Early predictors of mortality for hospitalized patients suffering cardiopulmonary arrest. *Chest* 1990; **97**: 413–419.

97. Dybvik, T., Strand, T. & Steen, P.A. Buffer therapy during out-of-hospital cardiopulmonary resuscitation. *Resuscitation* 1995; **29**: 89–95.

98. Zaritski, A.L. & Gomez, R. Acidosis, epinephrine, and the model. *Crit. Care Med.* 1993; **21**: 1821–1823.

99. Levi, M.M. An evidence-based evaluation of the use of sodium bicarbonate during cardiopulmonary resuscitation. *Crit. Care Clin.* 1998; **14**: 457–483.

100. Graf, H., Leach, W. & Arieff, A.I. Evidence for a detrimental effect of bicarbonate therapy in hypoxic lactic acidosis. *Science* 1985; **227**: 754–756.

101. Gerst, P.H., Fleming, W.H. & Malm, J.R. A quantitative evaluation of the effects of acidosis and alkalosis upon the ventricular fibrillation threshold. *Surgery* 1966; **59**: 1050–1060.

102. Kerber, R.E., Pandian, N.G., Hoyt, R. *et al.* Effect of ischemia, hypertrophy, hypoxia, acidosis, and alkalosis on canine defibrillation. *Am. J. Physiol.* 1983; **244**: H825–H831.

103. Yakaitis, R.W., Thomas, J.D. & Mahaffey, J.E. Influence of pH and hypoxia on the success of defibrillation. *Crit. Care. Med.* 1975; **3**: 139–142.

104. Morimoto, Y., Kemmotsu, O. & Morimoto, Y. Extramyocardial acidosis impairs cardiac resuscitability in isolated, perfused, rat hearts. *Crit. Care Med.* 1996; **24**: 1719–1723.

105. Maldonado, F.A., Weil, M.H., Tang, W. *et al.* Myocardial hypercarbic acidosis reduces cardiac resuscitability. *Anesthesiology* 1993, **78**: 343–352.

106. Redding, J.S. & Pearson, J.W. Resuscitation from ventricular fibrillation. Drug therapy. *J. Am. Med. Assoc.* 1968; **203**: 255–260.

107. Sun, S., Weil, M.H., Tang, W. & Fukui, M. Effects of buffer agents on postresuscitation myocardial dysfunction. *Crit. Care Med.* 1996; **24**: 2035–2041.

108. Wildenthal, K., Mierzwiak, D.S., Myers, R.W. & Mitchell, J.H. Effects of acute lactic acidosis on ventricular performance. *Am. J. Physiol.* 1968; **214**: 1352–1359.

109. Cingolani, H.E., Maas, A.J., Zimmerman, A.N. & Meijler, F.L. Hydrogen ion changes and contractile behavior in the perfused rat heart. *Eur. J. Cardiol.* 1975; **3**: 329–336.

110. Huang, Y.G., Wong, K.C., Yip, W.H., McJames, S.W. & Pace, N.L. Cardiovascular responses to graded doses of three catecholamines during lactic and hydrochloric acidosis in dogs. *Br. J. Anaesth.* 1995; **74**: 583–590.

111. Toller, W., Wolkart, G., Stranz, C., Metzler, H. & Brunner, F. Contractile action of levosimendan and epinephrine during acidosis. *Eur. J. Pharm.* 2005; **507**: 199–209

112. Rubertsson, S. & Wiklund, L. Hemodynamic effects of epinephrine in combination with different alkaline buffers during experimental, open-chest, cardiopulmonary resuscitation. *Crit. Care Med.* 1993; **21**: 1051–1057.

113. Preziosi, M.P., Roig, J.C., Hargrove, N. & Burchfield, D.J. Metabolic acidemia with hypoxia attenuates the hemodynamic responses to epinephrine during resuscitation in lambs. *Crit. Care Med.* 1993; **21**: 1901–1907.

114. Eleff, S.M., Schleien, C.L., Koehler, R.C. *et al.* Brain bioenergetics during cardiopulmonary resuscitation in dogs. *Anesthesiology* 1992; **76**: 77–84.

115. Eleff, S.M., Kim, H., Shaffner, D.H., Traystman, R.J. & Koehler, R.C. Effect of cerebral blood flow generated during cardiopulmonary resuscitation in dogs on maintenance versus recovery of ATP and pH. *Stroke* 1993; **24**: 2066–2073.

116. Posner, J.B. & Plum, F. Spinal fluid pH and neurologic symptoms in systemic acidosis. *N. Engl. J. Med.* 1967; **277**: 605–613.

117. Javaheri, S., Weyne, J. & Demeester, G. Changes in the brain surface pH and cisternal cerebrospinal fluid acid–base variables in respiratory arrest. *Respir. Physiol.* 1983; **51**: 31–43.

118. Javaheri, S., Clendening, A., Papadakis, N. & Brody, J.S. PH changes on the surface of brain and in cisternal fluid in dogs in cardiac arrest. *Stroke* 1984; **15**: 553–557.

119. Hurn, P.D., Koehler, R.C., Norris, S.E., Schwentker, A.E. & Traystman. R.J. Bicarbonate conservation during incomplete cerebral ischemia with superimposed hypercapnia. *Am. J. Physiol.* 1991; **261**: H853–H859.

120. Hurn, P.D. & Traytsman, R.J. pH associated brain injury in cerebral ischemia and circulatory arrest. *J. Intens. Care Med.* 1996; **11**: 205–218.

121. Eleff, S.M., Maruki, Y., Monsein, L.H., Traystman, R.J., Bryan, R.N. & Koehler, R.C. Sodium, ATP, and intracellular pH transients during reversible complete ischemia of dog cerebrum. *Stroke* 1991; **22**: 233–241.

122. Maruki, Y., Koehler, R.C., Eleff, S.M. & Traystman, R.J. Intracellular pH during reperfusion influences evoked potential recovery after complete cerebral ischemia. *Stroke* 1993; **24**: 697–703.

123. Kraig, R.P. & Chesler, M. Astrocytic acidosis in hyperglycemic and complete ischemia. *J. Cereb. Blood Flow Metab.* 1990; **10**: 104–114.

124. Kraig, R.P., Petito, C.K., Plum, F. & Pulsinelli, W.A. Hydrogen ions kill brain at concentrations reached in ischemia. *J. Cereb. Blood Flow Metab.* 1987; **7**: 379–386.

125. Goldman, S.A., Pulsinelli, W.A., Clarke, W.Y., Kraig, R.P. & Plum, F. The effects of extracellular acidosis on neurons and glia in vitro. *J. Cereb Blood Flow Metab.* 1989; **9**: 471–477.

126. Payne, R.S., Tseng, M.T. & Schurr, A. The glucose paradox of cerebral ischemia: evidence for corticosterone involvement. *Brain Res.* 2003; **971**: 9–17.

127. Ljunggren, B., Norberg, K. & Siesjo, B.K. Influence of tissue acidosis upon restitution of brain energy metabolism following total ischemia. *Brain Res.* 1974; **77**: 173–186.

128. Gardiner, M., Smith, M.L., Kagstrom, E., Shohami, E. & Siesjo, B.K. Influence of blood glucose concentration on brain lactate accumulation during severe hypoxia and subsequent recovery of brain energy metabolism. *J. Cereb. Blood Flow Metab.* 1982; **2**: 429–438.

129. Myers, R.E. & Yamaguchi, S. Nervous system effects of cardiac arrest in monkeys. Preservation of vision. *Arch. Neurol.* 1977; **34**: 65–74.

130. Welsh, F.A., Ginsberg, M.D., Rieder, W. & Budd, W.W. Deleterious effect of glucose pretreatment on recovery from diffuse cerebral ischemia in the cat. II. Regional metabolite levels. *Stroke* 1980; **11**: 355–363.

131. Wagner, K.R., Kleinholz, M. & Myers, R.E. Delayed onset of neurologic deterioration following anoxia/ischemia coincides with appearance of impaired brain mitochondrial respiration and decreased cytochrome oxidase activity. *J. Cereb. Blood Flow Metab.* 1990; **10**: 417–423.

132. Paljarvi, L., Rehncrona, S., Soderfeldt, B., Olsson, Y. & Kalimo, H. Brain lactic acidosis and ischemic cell damage: quantitative ultrastructural changes in capillaries of rat cerebral cortex. *Acta Neuropathol.* (Berl.) 1983; **60**: 232–240.

133. Pulsinelli, W.A., Waldman, S., Rawlinson, D. & Plum, F. Moderate hyperglycemia augments ischemic brain damage: a neuropathologic study in the rat. *Neurology* 1982; **32**: 1239–1246.

134. Warner, D.S., Smith, M.L. & Siesjo, B. Ischemia in normo- and hyperglycemic rats: effects on brain water and electrolytes. *Stroke* 1987; **18**: 464–471.

135. Ginsberg, M.D., Welsh, F.A. & Budd, W.W. Deleterious effect of glucose pretreatment on recovery from diffuse cerebral ischemia in the cat. I. Local cerebral blood flow and glucose utilization. *Stroke* 1980; **11**: 347–354.

136. Paljarvi, L. Brain lactic acidosis and ischemic cell damage: a topographic study with high-resolution light microscopy of early recovery in a rat model of severe incomplete ischemia. *Acta Neuropathol.* (Berl.) 1984; **64**: 89–98.

137. Lanier, W.L., Stangland, K.J., Scheithauer, B.W., Milde, J.H. & Michenfelder, J.D. The effects of dextrose infusion and head position on neurologic outcome after complete cerebral ischemia in primates: examination of a model. *Anesthesiology* 1987; **66**: 39–48.

138. D'Alecy, L.G., Lundy, E.F., Barton, K.J. & Zelenock, G.B. Dextrose containing intravenous fluid impairs outcome and increases death after eight minutes of cardiac arrest and resuscitation in dogs. *Surgery* 1986; **100**: 505–511.

139. Nakakimura, K., Fleischer, J.E., Drummond, J.C. *et al.* Glucose administration before cardiac arrest worsens neurologic outcome in cats. *Anesthesiology* 1990; **72**: 1005–1011.

140. Longstreth, W.T. Jr., & Inui, T.S. High blood glucose level on hospital admission and poor neurological recovery after cardiac arrest. *Ann. Neurol.* 1984; **15**: 59–63.

141. Longstreth, W.T. Jr., Diehr, P., Cobb, L.A., Hanson, R.W. & Blair, A.D. Neurologic outcome and blood glucose levels during out-of-hospital cardiopulmonary resuscitation. *Neurology* 1986; **36**: 1186–1191.

142. Pulsinelli, W.A., Levy, D.E., Sigsbee, B., Scherer, P. & Plum, F. Increased damage after ischemic stroke in patients with hyperglycemia with or without established diabetes mellitus. *Am. J. Med.* 1983; **74**: 540–544.

143. Berger, L. & Hakim, A.M. The association of hyperglycemia with cerebral edema in stroke. *Stroke* 1986; **17**: 865–871.

144. Martin, G.B., Nowak, R.M., Paradis, N. *et al.* Characterization of cerebral energetics and brain pH by 31P spectroscopy after graded canine cardiac arrest and bypass reperfusion. *J. Cereb. Blood Flow Metab.* 1990; **10**: 221–226.

145. Siesjo, B.K. Mechanisms of ischemic brain damage. *Crit. Care Med.* 1988; **16**: 954–963.

146. Ellef, S.M., Sugimoto, H., Shaffner, D.H., Traytsman, R.J. & Koehler, R.C. Acidemia and brain pH during prolonged cardiopulmonary resuscitation in dogs. *Stroke* 1995; **26**: 1028–1034.

147. Rosenberg, J.M., Martin, G.B., Paradis, N.A. *et al.* The effects of CO_2 and non-CO_2 – generating buffers on cerebral acidosis after cardiac arrest: a 31P NMR study. *Ann. Emerg. Med.* 1989; **18**: 341–347.

148. Liu, X., Nozari, A. Rubertsson, S. & Wiklund, L. Buffer administration during CPR promotes cerebral reperfusion after return of spontaneous circulation and mitigates post-resuscitation cerebral acidosis. *Resuscitation* 2002; **55**: 45–55.

149. Weisfeldt, M.L. & Guerci, A.D. Sodium bicarbonate in CPR (Editorial). *J. Am. Med. Assoc.* 1991; **266**: 2129–2130.

150. Aufderheide, T.P., Sigurdsson, G., Pirrallo, R.G. *et al.* Hyperventilation-induced hypotension during cardiopulmonary resuscitation. *Circulation* 2004; **109**: 1960–1965.

151. Pitts, S. & Kellermann, A.L. Hyperventilation during cardiac arrest. *Lancet* 2004; **364**: 313–315.

152. Skippen, P., Seear, M., Poskitt, K. *et al.* Effect of hyperventilation on regional cerebral blood flow in head-injured children. *Crit. Care Med.* 1997; **25**: 1402–1402.

153. Buunk, G., van der Hoeven, J.G. & Meinders, A.E. Cerebrovascular reactivity in comatose patients resuscitated from a cardiac arrest. *Stroke* 1997; **28**: 1569–1573.

154. Delooz, H.H. & Lewi, P.J. Are inter-center differences in EMS-management and sodium bicarbonate administration important for the outcome of CPR? The Cerebral Resuscitation Study Group. *Resuscitation* 1989; **17** Suppl: S161–S172.

155. van Walraven, C., Stiell, I.G., Wells, G.A., Herbert, P.C., Vandemheen, K. for the OTAC Study Group: Do advanced cardiac life support drugs increase resuscitation rates from in-hospital cardiac arrests? *Ann. Emerg. Med.* 1998; **32**: 544–553.

156. Koster, R.W. Correction of acidosis during cardio-pulmonary resuscitation. *Resuscitation* 1995; **29**: 87–88.

157. Steen, P.A. Post-hoc analysis of sodium bicarbonate use in EMS systems? A caveat in resuscitation research. *Acta Anaesthesiol. Scand.* 2005; **49**: 1–3.

158. Kirimli, B., Harris, L.C. & Safar, P. Evaluation of sodium bicabonate and epinephrine in cardiopulmonary resuscitation. *Anesth. Analg.* 1969; **48**: 649–658.

159. Sanders, A.B., Kern, K.B., Fonken, S., Otto, C.W. & Ewy, G.A. The role of bicarbonate and fluid loading in improving resuscitation from prolonged cardiac arrest with rapid manual chest compression CPR. *Ann. Emerg. Med.* 1990; **19**: 1–7.

160. Katz, L.M., Wang, Y., Rockoff, S. & Bouldin, T.W. Low-dose Carbicarb improves cerebral outcome after asphyxial cardiac arrest in rats. *Ann. Emerg. Med.* 2002; **39**: 359–365.

161. Guerci, A.D., Chandra, N., Johnson, E. *et al.* Failure of sodium bicarbonate to improve resuscitation from ventricular fibrillation in dogs. *Circulation* 1986; **74**(Suppl IV): 75–79.

162. Federiuk, C.S., Sanders, A.B., Kern, K.B., Neslon, J. & Ewy, G.A. The effects of bicarbonate on resuscitation from cardiac arrest. *Ann. Emerg. Med.* 1991; **20**: 1173–1177.

163. Kette, F., Weil, M.H. & Gazmuri, R.J. Buffer solutions may compromise cardiac resuscitaion by reducing coronary perfusion pressure. *J. Am. Med. Assoc.* 1991; **266**: 2121–2126.

164. Bleske, B.E., Rice, T.L., Warren, E.W., De La Alas, V.R., Tait, A.R. & Knight, P.R. The effect of sodium bicarbonate administration on the vasopressor effect of high-dose epinephrine during cardiopulmonary resuscitation in swine. *Am. J. Emerg. Med.* 1993; **11**: 439–443.

165. Neumar, R.W., Bircher, N.G. Sim, K.M. *et al.* Epinephrine and sodium bicarbonate during CPR following asphyxial cardiac arrest in rats. *Resuscitation* 1995; **29**: 249–263.

166. Bjerneroth, G. Tribonat – a comprehensive summary of its properties. *Crit. Care Med.* 1999; **27**: 1009–1013.

167. Gazmuri, R.J. Buffer treatment for cardiac resuscitation: putting the cart before the horse? *Crit. Care Med.* 1999; **27**: 875–876.

168. Sun, S., Weil, M.H., Tang, W., Povoas, H.P. & Mason, E. Combined effects of buffer and adrenergic agents on postresuscitation myocardial function. *J. Pharmacol. Exp. Ther.* 1999; **291**: 773–777.

169. Von Planta, M., Bar-Joseph, G., Wiklund, L., Bircher, N.G. Falk, J.L. & Abramson, N.S. Pathophysiologic and therapeutic implications of acid–base changes during CPR. *Ann. Emerg. Med.* 1993; **22** (2): 404–410.

170. Douglas, M.E., Downs, J.B., Mantini, E.L. & Ruiz, B.C. Alteration of oxygen tension and oxyhemoglobin saturation, a hazard of sodium bicarbonate administration. *Arch. Surg.* 1979; **114**: 326–329.

171. Rubertsson, S., Karlsson, T. & Wiklund, L. Systemic oxygen uptake during experimental closed-chest cardiopulmonary resuscitation using air or pure oxygen ventilation. *Acta Anaesthesiol. Scand.* 1998; **42**: 32–38.

172. Mattar, J.A., Weil, M.H., Shubin, H. & Stein, L. Cardiac arrest in the critically ill. II. Hyperosmolal states following cardiac arrest. *Am. J. Med.* 1974; **56**: 162–168.

173. White, B.C. & Tintinalli, J.E. Effects of sodium bicarbonate administration during cardiopulmonary resuscitation. *JACEP* 1977; **6**: 187–190.

174. Gedeborg, R. & Wiklund, L. The biological activity of adrenaline after injection through an intravenous cannula containing alkaline buffer. *Resuscitation* 1989; **18**: 49–58.

175. Bleske, B.E., Warren, E.W., Rice, T.L., Gilligan, L.J. & Tait, A.R. Effect of high-dose sodium bicarbonate on the vasopressor effects of epinephrine during cardiopulmonary resuscitation. *Pharmacotherapy* 1995; **15**: 660–664.

176. Bleske, B.E., Chow, M.S.S., Zhao, H., Kluger, J. & Fieldman, A. Effects of different dosages and modes of sodium bicarbonate administration during cardiopulmonary resuscitation. *Am. J. Emerg. Med.* 1992; **10**: 525–532.

177. Dohi, S., Takeshima, R. & Matsumiya, N. Carbon dioxide elimination during circulatory arrest. *Crit. Care Med.* 1987; **15**: 944–946.

178. Berenyi, K.J., Wolk, M. & Killip, T. Cerebrospinal fluid acidosis complicating therapy of experimental cardiopulmonary arrest. *Circulation* 1975; **52**: 319–324.

179. Sessler, D., Mills, P., Gregory, G., Litt, L. & James, T. Effects of bicarbonate on arterial and brain intracellular pH in neonatal rabbits recovering from hypoxic lactic acidosis. *J. Pediatr.* 1987; **111**(6 Pt 1): 817–823.

180. Ritter, J.M., Doktor, H.S. & Bejamin, N. Paradoxical effect of bicarbonate on cytoplasmic pH. *Lancet* 1990; **335**: 1243–1246.

181. Li, Y.C., Wiklund, L., Tarkkila, P. & Bjerneroth, G. Influence of alkaline buffers on cytoplasmic pH in myocardial cells exposed to metabolic acidosis. *Resuscitation* 1996; **32**: 33–44.

182. Bjerneroth, G., Sammeli, O., Li, Y.C. & Wiklund, L. Effects of alkaline buffers on cytoplasmic pH in lymphocytes. *Crit. Care Med.* 1994; **22**: 1550–1556.

183. Sonett, J., Pagani, F.D., Baker, L.S. *et al.* Correction of intramyocardial hypercarbic acidosis with sodium bicarbonate. *Circ. Shock* 1994; **42**: 163–173.

184. Rao, R.S., Graver, M.L., Urivetsky, M. & Scharf, S.M. Mechanisms of myocardial depression after bolus injection of sodium bicarbonate. *J. Crit. Care* 1994; **9**: 255–261.

185. Goldsmith, D.J., Forni, L.G. & Hilton, P.J. Bicarbonate therapy and intracellular acidosis. *Clin. Sci.* 1997; **93**: 593–598.

186. Levraut, J., Giunti, C., Ciebiera, J.P., de Sousa, G., Ramhani, R., Payan, P. & Grimaud, D. Initial effect of sodium bicarbonate on intracellular pH depends on the extracellular nonbicarbonate buffering capacity. *Crit. Care Med.* 2001; **29**: 1033–1039.

187. Cuhaci, B., Lee, J. & Ahmed, A. Sodium bicarbonate and intracellular acidosis: myth or reality? *Crit. Care Med.* 2001; **29**: 1088–1090.

188. Brown, C.G., Martin, D.R., Pepe, P.E. *et al.* A comparison of standard-dose and high-dose epinephrine in cardiac arrest outside the hospital. *N. Engl. J. Med.* 1992; **327**: 1051–1055.

189. Gueugniaud, P.Y., Mols, P., Goldstein, P. *et al.* A comparison of repeated high doses and repeated standard doses of epinephrine for cardiac arrest outside the hospital. *N. Engl. J. Med.* 1998; **339**: 1595–1561.

190. Rothe, K.F. & Diedler, J. Comparison of intra- and extracellular buffering of clinically used buffer substances: Tris and bicarbonate. *Acta Anaesth. Scand.* 1982; **26**: 194–198.

191. Nahas, G.G., Sutin, K.M., Fermon, C. *et al.* Guidelines for the treatment of acidaemia with THAM. *Drugs* 1998; **55**: 191–224.

192. Bleich, H.L. & Schwartz, W.B. Tris buffer (THAM). An appraisal of its physiologic effects and clinical usefulness. *N. Engl. J. Med.* 1966; **274**: 782–787.

193. Brown, E.S., Greene, D.G., Elam, J.O., Evers, J.L., Bunnell, I.L. & Lowe, H.J. Effects of 2-amino 2-hydroxymethyl-1,3-propanediol on CO_2 elimination and production in normal man. *Ann. NY Acad. Sci.* 1961; **92**: 508–519.

194. Minuck, M. & Sharma, G.P. Comparison of THAM and sodium bicarbonate in resuscitation of the heart after ventricular fibrillation in dogs. *Anesth. Analg.* 1977; **56**: 38–45.

195. Filley, G.F. & Kindig, N.B. Carbicarb. An alkalinizing ion-generating agent of possible clinical usefulness. *Trans. Am. Clin. Climat. Assoc.* 1984; **96**: 141–153.

196. Bersin, R.M. & Arieff, A.I. Improved hemodynamic function during hypoxia with Carbicarb, a new agent for the management of acidosis. *Circulation* 1988; **77**: 227–233.

197. Rhee, K.H., Toro, L.O., McDonald, G.G., Nunnally, R.L. & Levin, D.L. Carbicarb, sodium bicbonate and sodium chloride in hypoxic lactic acidosis. *Chest* 1993; **104**: 913–918.

198. Wiklund, L., Oequist, L., Skoog, G. *et al.* Clinical buffering of metabolic acidosis: Problems and a solution. *Resuscitation* 1985; **12**: 279–293.

199. Bjerneroth, G. Alkaline buffers for correction of metabolic acidosis during cardiopulmonary resuscitation with focus on Tribonat® – a review. *Recuscitation* 1998; **37**: 161–171.

200. Bellet, S. The cardiotoxic effects of hyperpotassemia and its treatment. *Postgrad. Med.* 1959; **25**: 602–609.

201. Stewart, J.S.S., Stewart, W.K. & Gillies, H.G. Cardiac arrest and acidosis. *Lancet* 1962; **2**: 964–967.

202. Roth, F. & Saidi, M. Dangerous increase in serum potassium following succinylcholine administration. *Anaesthesist* 1971; **20**: 35–38.

203. Hoy, R.H. Accidental systemic exposure to sodium hypochlorite (Chlorox) during hemodialysis. *Am. J. Hosp. Pharm.* 1981; **38**: 1512–1514.

204. Zobel, G., Haim, M., Ritschl, E. & Muller, W. Continuous arteriovenous hemofiltration as emergency procedure in severe hyperkalemia. *Child Nephrol. Urol.* 1988; **9**: 236–238.

205. Werba, A. & Spiss, C.K. Atrial arrest and intraventricular conduction disorders due to accidental hyperkalemia during kidney transplantation. *Anaesthesist* 1989; **38**: 375–378.

206. Lin, J.L., Lim, P.S., Leu, M.L. & Huang, C.C. Outcomes of severe hyperkalemia in cardiopulmonary resuscitation with concomitant hemodialysis. *Intens. Care Med.* 1994; **20**: 287–290.

207. Griner, R.L. 2nd & Tobin, J.R. Probable succinylcholine-induced hyperkalemia in a trauma victim after recent benign anesthetics with succinylcholine. *CRNA.* 1994; **5**: 151–155.

208. Voelckel, W. & Kroesen, G. Unexpected return of cardiac action after termination of cardiopulmonary resuscitation. *Resuscitation* 1996; **32**: 27–29.

209. Wu, C.C., Tseng, C.S., Shen, T.H., Yang, T.C., Chi, K.P. & Ho, W.M. Succinylcholine-induced cardiac arrest in unsuspected becker muscular dystrophy – a case report. *Acta Anaesthesiol. Sin.* 1998; **36**: 165–168.

210. Kao, K.C., Huang, C.C., Tsai, Y.H., Lin, M.C. & Tsao, T.C.I. Hyperkalemic cardiac arrest successfully reversed by hemodialysis during cardiopulmonary resuscitation: case report. *Changgeng Yi Xue Za Zhi* 2000; **23**: 555–559.

211. Greenberg, A. Hyperkalemia: treatment options. *Semin. Nephrol.* 1998; **18**: 46–57.

212. Gennari, F.J. Disorders of potassium homeostasis. Hypokalemia and hyperkalemia. *Crit. Care Clin.* 2002; **18**: 273–288, vi.

213. Schwarz, K.C. & Cohen, B.D. Severe acidosis and hyperpotassemia treated with sodium bicarbonate infusion. *Circulation* 1959; **19**: 215–220.

214. A Guide to the International ACLS algorithms. In Guidelines for Cardiopulmonary Resuscitation and Emergency Cardiac Care. *Circulation* 2000; **102/8** (suppl I): 151–152.

215. Sandeman, D. J., Alahakoon, T.I. & Bentley, S.C. Tricyclic poisoning – successful management of ventricular fibrillation following massive overdose of imipramine. *Anaesth. Intens. Care* 1997; **25**: 542–545.

216. Brown, T.C. Sodium bicarbonate treatment for tricyclic antidepressant arrhythmias in children. *Med. J. Aust.* 1976; **2**: 380–382.

217. Molloy, D.W., Penner, S.B., Rabson, J. & Hall, K.H. Use of sodium bicarbonate to treat tricyclic antidepressant-induced arrhythmias in a patient with alkalosis. *Can. Med. Assoc. J.* 1984; **130**: 1457–1459.

218. Hodes, D. Sodium bicarbonate and hyperventilation in treating an infant with severe overdose of tricyclic antidepressant. *Br. Med. J. (Clin. Res. Ed.)* 1984; **288**: 1800–1801.

219. Graudins, A., Vossler, C. & Wang, R. Fluoxetine-induced cardiotoxicity with response to bicarbonate therapy. *Am. J. Emerg. Med.* 1997; **15**: 501–503.

220. Brown, T.C. Tricyclic antidepressant overdosage: experimental studies on the management of circulatory complications. *Clin. Toxicol.* 1976; **9**: 255–272.

221. Pentel, P. & Benowitz, N. Efficacy and mechanism of action of sodium bicarbonate in the treatment of desipramine toxicity in rats. *J. Pharmacol. Exp. Ther.* 1984; **230**: 12–19.

222. Hedges, J.R., Baker, P.B., Tasset, J.J., Otten, E.J., Dalsey, W.C. & Syverud, S.A. Bicarbonate therapy for the cardiovascular toxicity of amitriptyline in an animal model. *J. Emerg. Med.* 1985; **3**: 253–260.

223. Levitt, M.A., Sullivan, J.B. Jr., Owens, S.M., Burnham, L. & Finley, P.R. Amitriptyline plasma protein binding: effect of plasma pH and relevance to clinical overdose. *Am. J. Emerg. Med.* 1986; **4**: 121–125.

224. Sasyniuk, B.I., Jhamandas, V. & Valois, M. Experimental amitriptyline intoxication: treatment of cardiac toxicity with sodium bicarbonate. *Ann. Emerg. Med.* 1986; **15**: 1052–1059.

225. Bou-Abboud, E. & Nattel, S. Relative role of alkalosis and sodium ions in reversal of class I antiarrhythmic drug-induced sodium channel blockade by sodium bicarbonate. *Circulation* 1996; **94**: 1954–1961.

226. Knudsen, K. & Abrahamsson, J. Epinephrine and sodium bicarbonate independently and additively increase survival in experimental amitriptyline poisoning. *Crit. Care Med.* 1997; **25**: 669–674.

227. McCabe, J.L., Cobaugh, D.J., Menegazzi, J.J. & Fata, J. Experimental tricyclic antidepressant toxicity: a randomized, controlled comparison of hypertonic saline solution, sodium bicarbonate, and hyperventilation. *Ann. Emerg. Med.* 1998; **32**(1): 329–333.

228. Liebelt, E.L. Targeted management strategies for cardiovascular toxicity from tricyclic antidepressant overdose: the pivotal role for alkalinization and sodium loading. *Pediatr. Emerg. Care* 1998; **14**: 293–298.

229. Mackway-Jones, K. Towards evidence based emergency medicine: best BETs from the Manchester Royal Infirmary. Alkalinisation in the management of tricyclic antidepressant overdose. *J. Accid. Emerg. Med.* 1999; **16**: 139–140.

230. Kerr, G.W., McGuffie, A.C. & Wilkes, G.J. Tricyclic antidepressant overdose: a review. *Emerg. Med. J.* 2001; **18**: 236–241.

231. Blackman, K., Brown, S.G. & Wilkes, G.J. Plasma alkalinization for tricyclic antidepressant toxicity: a systematic review. *Emerg. Med. (Fremantle)* 2001; **13**: 204–210.

232. Vrijlandt, P.J., Bosch, T.M., Zijlstra, J.G., Tulleken, J.E., Ligtenberg, J.J. & van der Werf, T.S. Sodium bicarbonate infusion for intoxication with tricyclic antidepressives: recommended inspite of lack of scientific evidence. *Ned. Tijdschr. Geneeskd.* 2001; **145**: 1686–1689.

233. Seger, D.L., Hantsch, C., Zavaral, T. & Wrenn, K. Variability of recommendations for serum alkalinization in tricyclic antidepressant overdose: a survey of U.S. Poison Center medical directors. *J. Toxicol. Clin. Toxicol.* 2003; **41**: 331–338.

234. Holger, J.S., Harris, C.R. & Engebretsen, K.M. Physostigmine, sodium bicarbonate, or hypertonic saline to treat diphenhydramine toxicity. *Vet. Hum. Toxicol.* 2002; **44**: 1–4.

235. Glauser, J. Tricyclic antidepressant poisoning. *Cleve. Clin. J. Med.* 2000; **67**: 704–706, 709–713, 717–719.

236. International Liaison Committee On Resuscitation (ILCOR): Part 4: Advanced life support. *Resuscitation* 2005; **67**: 213–247.

38

Cardiac arrest resuscitation monitoring

Kevin R. Ward and Joseph Bisera

Department of Emergency Medicine, Virginia Commonwealth University and Virginia Commonwealth University Reanimation Engineering Shock Center
The Weil Institute of Critical Care Medicine, Rancho Mirage, California

Introduction

Shock is a complex entity traditionally defined as a state in which the oxygen utilization or consumption needs of tissues are not matched by sufficient delivery of oxygen. This mismatch commonly results from states of altered tissue perfusion. From this perspective, cardiopulmonary arrest represents the most extreme of shock states.

Figure 38.1 represents the basic relationship between oxygen consumption (VO_2) and oxygen delivery (DO_2) that is pertinent to individual organs as well as to the whole body.[1–3] VO_2 can remain constant over a wide range of DO_2, because most tissue beds are capable of efficiently increasing the extraction of oxygen. This will be reflected by decreasing venous oxygen saturation from each organ. When DO_2 reaches a critical threshold, however, tissue extraction of oxygen cannot be further increased to meet tissue demands. At this point VO_2 becomes directly dependent on DO_2 (DO_2crit) and cells begin to convert to anaerobic metabolism, as manifested by increases in certain metabolic products such as lactate, NADH, and reduced cytochrome oxidase. The point of DO_2crit is the point of dysoxia or ischemia at which tissue DO_2 cannot meet tissue oxygen demand.[2] Oxygen debt can be defined as the amount of cumulative difference of VO_2 between baseline and that spent below DO_2crit. As discussed later, the level of accumulated oxygen debt in shock states is critically linked with survival.[4,5]

Several unique physiologic aspects and principles of cardiac arrest and CPR exist that limit the usefulness of many monitoring modalities, some of which will be more useful in the postresuscitation period.[6] These include the following.

1. Cardiac arrest produces a global state of ischemia wherein all organ systems, especially those most metabolically active (heart and brain), experience severe ischemia within minutes. DO_2crit is immediately surpassed. As opposed to other shock states, such as those produced by hemorrhage or sepsis, there is no compensatory state prior to sudden death cardiac arrest. Thus every minute of cardiac arrest results in a greater temporal based oxygen debt than other etiologies of shock. This state of profound whole body ischemia is further complicated because the brain and heart, which are usually globally spared from dysoxia until the late stages of other forms of shock, reach dysoxia almost immediately (within minutes) in cardiac arrest. Additionally, depending on the cause of the arrest, individual organ regions may have undergone significant ischemia (such as occurs in acute myocardial infarction) before arrest, or globally (such as occurs in asphyxial arrest) and thus accumulated a significant degree of regional or whole body oxygen debt before the actual arrest.

2. Traditional CPR is incapable of restoring DO_2 to a point of VO_2 independence. This is especially true of the brain, in which high-energy phosphate depletion occurs within minutes and cannot be restored with CPR. Only ROSC or alternative methods of CPR such as open chest cardiac massage or cardiopulmonary bypass can produce this.

3. Optimal outcomes from cardiac arrest are, for the most part, directly linked to pre-arrest events and the duration of arrest. Thus the goal of CPR is to achieve hemodynamic changes capable of producing ROSC within seconds to minutes, as opposed to the minutes to hours

Cardiac Arrest: The Science and Practice of Resuscitation Medicine. 2nd edn., ed. Norman Paradis, Henry Halperin, Karl Kern, Volker Wenzel, Douglas Chamberlain. Published by Cambridge University Press. © Cambridge University Press, 2007.

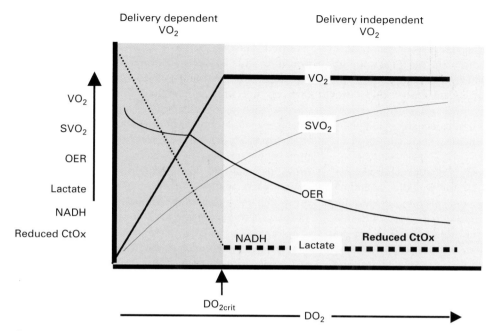

Fig. 38.1. Biphasic relationship between oxygen delivery (DO_2) and oxygen consumption (VO_2). Oxygen extraction ratio (OER) increases and mixed venous oxygen saturation (SvO_2) decreases in response to decreased DO_2. Below a critical DO_2 (DO_2crit), VO_2 becomes delivery-dependent. DO_2 below DO_2crit results in the beginning of anaerobic metabolism as noted by an increase in a variety of cellular products including lactate, NADH, and reduced cytochrome oxidase (CtOx). The DO_2crit of various organ systems can occur at points either above or below whole body DO_2crit, depending on the metabolic and blood flow regulatory characteristics of the organ system and the rapidity of the reductions in DO_2. $DO_2 = CO \times CaO_2$ (normal range: 460-650 ml/min/m²); $VO_2 = CO \times (CaO_2 - CvO_2)$ (normal range: 96-170 ml/min/m²); CaO_2 (arterial oxygen content) $= (Hb \times 1.39 \times SaO_2) + (0.003 \times PaO_2)$; $CvO_2 = (Hb \times 1.39 \times SvO_2) + (0.0003 \times PvO_2)$. CO, Cardiac output; PaO_2, arterial oxygen tension; Hb, hemoglobin; SvO_2 normal range 70%–80%.

time frame that can be used to effect favorable hemodynamic changes during the postresuscitation period. To date, the major hemodynamic factor determining the ability to produce ROSC is coronary perfusion pressure (CPP).

Therefore, it is apparent that the most immediate goal of CPR is to restart the heart as soon as possible so as to limit the total time of ischemia especially to the brain, and the heart itself. Because of this compressed time frame, selected monitoring end-points must have the ability to detect targeted processes or parameters that are linked with ROSC and are capable of changing within seconds of interventions (i.e., coronary perfusion pressure). Consequently, monitors must have corresponding response times and be capable of being applied to the patient and reporting data within seconds.

Monitoring during CPR

Traditional monitoring

Monitoring during CPR has traditionally consisted of carotid or femoral pulse palpation along with ECG evaluation in one or more leads. Although the lack of a palpable pulse during CPR may indicate inadequate forward flow, quantification of forward flow cannot be estimated in the presence of a palpable CPR-generated pulse since pressures generated by chest compressions may be transmitted equally to both the major arterial and venous vessels.[7] In addition, inability to palpate a pulse has not been demonstrated conclusively to rule out spontaneous forward flow in certain rhythms such as pulseless electrical activity.[8] Myocardial blood flow is not dependent on palpated arterial systolic pressure, but depends instead on CPP, which is defined as the difference between aortic diastolic and coronary sinus (or right atrial) diastolic pressure.[9] ECG monitoring during CPR will indicate the electrical status of the heart, but not mechanical activity. Although perhaps the best attainable in certain circumstances, these two monitoring modalities do not provide reliable information about the effectiveness of CPR (both mechanical and pharmacologic interventions) or prognosis given current treatment recommendations.

In the absence of immediate defibrillation it is now clear that the essential menu of CPR interventions, including chest compression, management of the airway, and breathing for the victim take priority. In the out-of-hospital setting, only a small minority of witnessed cardiac arrests receive successful defibrillation with an AED within 3 minutes after collapse. Thus, in the lay setting, monitoring challenges exist that may affect outcome.

The first challenge encountered by the bystander/lay rescuer is the limited capability to *detect* cardiac arrest promptly. The detection, and indeed, the definition of cardiac arrest that then prompts CPR is now based solely on the observer's capability to observe or sense breathing and/or detect a pulse in an unresponsive individual. Yet, the very specificity of the pulse check, including the carotid pulse, by lay persons under stress, even after completion of the Basic Life Support Course (BLS), is no better than random. Since 1968 the pulse check has been the "gold standard" for determining whether the heart is beating. Evidence indicated that the pulse check by lay rescuers failed to identify a pulse as present or absent 50% of the time and it was therefore random.[10,11] Since 1992, however, the validity of the pulse check has been called into question and in the American Heart Association Guidelines the pulse check was deleted as a basis for establishing that the victim has cardiac arrest triggering CPR, including immediate defibrillation.[12,13]

Prompt distinction between the presence of heartbeat and the absence of breathing would allow the A, B, C, and D (airway, breathing, chest compression, and defibrillation) to be optimally prioritized, and even quality-controlled, contingent on real-time measurements.[14–17] Failure to restore breathing and circulation with chest compression compromises survival in some patients.

In a recent study, CPR before delivery of the initial shock increased survival (to hospital discharge) from 24% to 30%.[18] Significantly better outcomes followed chest compression when it preceded electrical defibrillation, although delaying defibrillation can compromise successful defibrillation.[18–20] Under experimental conditions, successful resuscitation by defibrillation is reduced to 40% if the delay is 15 seconds and < 5% if defibrillation is delayed by as much as 20 seconds.[21]

Current versions of AEDs, which analyze rhythm, do provide the intelligence and prompting for electrical defibrillation during ventricular fibrillation. As yet, however, they do not provide real-time measurements of the mechanical heartbeat, breathing, blood circulation, or the intelligence for optimizing and sequencing of CPR in real-time, especially for the nonprofessional and occasional professional rescuer. These new insights add incentive to providing real-time diagnosis during cardiac arrest for optimal guidance for sequencing of the essential airway, breathing, and chest compression intervention as well as electrical defibrillation.

An example of how this might be done is with the use of simple transthoracic impedance. Measurement of transthoracic impedance has evolved over more than a century with impedance plethysmography described as early as 1897 for physiological measurements.[22] Circulation and respiration were both quantified by impedance measurements.[23–26] Impedance monitoring as a clinical application for management of the critically ill and injured for estimating cardiac output followed the demonstration of Kubicek that changes in transthoracic impedance were indicative of changes in intrathoracic blood volume.[27] More recently, these techniques have been incorporated into commercial devices for estimation of stroke volumes and therefore cardiac output in the critically ill and injured.[28] The applicability of impedance methods during CPR has been shown to be a useful alternative for detection of breathing, or heart beat, or both.[29] The same electrodes that sense the electrocardiogram for diagnosis of the ECG rhythm and for delivery of a defibrillating shock were employed for the impedance measurements. Indeed, the impressive correlation between the arterial pulse pressure and impedance (Fig. 38.2) indicates that the impedance signal serves as a surrogate not only for "pulse check" but also to quantify arterial pressure produced by cardiac injection. Concurrent measurement of ECG and impedance would enable prompt detection and interpretation of cardiac or respiratory arrest, and therefore, guide more appropriate priority interventions for either (1) artificial breathing or (2) chest compressions, or both, preceded or followed by automated defibrillation.

Central hemodynamic or global monitoring

Coronary perfusion pressure

Laboratory data have clearly demonstrated the relationship between CPP and myocardial blood during CPR and the need to reach a certain threshold of CPP in order to

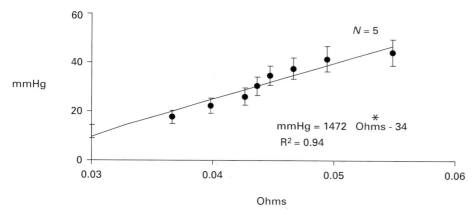

Fig. 38.2. The relationship between pulse pressure and thoracic impedance demonstrates the potential for AEDs to detect spontaneous circulation and thus provide first responders better direction in the initial care of the collapsed victim. (From ref. 29.).

achieve ROSC.[9,30,31] Clinical studies have confirmed the link between CPP and ROSC and have established that using current resuscitative treatment modalities as recommended by the American Heart Association, a minimum CPP of 15 mmHg is necessary to achieve ROSC if initial defibrillation attempts fail.[32,33] This is necessary, although not always sufficient, to achieve ROSC, and factors such as significant coronary artery lesions, downtime, and others have shown that despite reaching a CPP of 15 mmHg, ROSC is not possible. For example, not only are myocardial oxygen requirements of ventricular fibrillation higher than for example the asystolic heart, fibrillation has been demonstrated to cause mechanical compression of subendocardial vessels.[34,35] Higher opening pressures and flow may be required to achieve ROSC in these circumstances.[36,37] In addition, vasopressors such as epinephrine have been shown in some instances to increase further the imbalance between myocardial oxygen demand and delivery despite increasing myocardial blood flow.[30]

Clinical studies have demonstrated that CPP can be positive or negative during CPR and are indistinguishable by palpation of a pulse alone (Fig. 38.3).[38] Although monitoring of CPP is the most directly reliable indicator of adequacy of chest compression and pharmacological interventions, its major drawbacks are that it requires time and resources (both equipment and human), because access to both the arterial and central venous vasculature is needed to determine arterial diastolic and central venous diastolic pressure. In addition, pressure transduction supplies and equipment are necessary to verify pressure tracings and calculate CPP since most pressure monitors, while capable of reporting systolic and diastolic arterial pressure, report central venous pressure as a mean value.

Animal data indicate that the ability to achieve a diastolic arterial pressure of at least 40 mmHg is predictive of ROSC and is likely to be related to achieving a threshold CPP; however, clinical CPP data to substantiate this are lacking and critical CPPs can be achieved in humans without a diastolic arterial blood pressure of 40 mmHg.[39] Furthermore, it may be impossible to achieve a diastolic arterial pressure of 40 mmHg in some individuals by traditional closed chest compressions.

Measurement of CPP in the manner described above is possible in the hospital, especially in intensive care units where patients may already be instrumented. Unfortunately, this important variable is often ignored. Measurement is also possible in most emergency departments with proper staffing and preparation, and should be utilized, especially in circumstances in which central vascular access is obtained for drug administration. Nonetheless, it does not appear that simply monitoring diastolic CVP alone can predict CPP. In reality, since it is becoming increasingly popular to carry out cardiac arrest resuscitations in their entirety in the prehospital setting, it is unlikely that real-time direct CPP monitoring will ever become standard in emergency departments or other settings. Its application in the prehospital setting is simply not feasible from a technical and time standpoint.

Arterial blood pressure monitoring

Use of the oscillometer or other non-invasive blood pressure monitoring techniques are unreliable in their ability to measure true arterial blood pressure during CPR. These

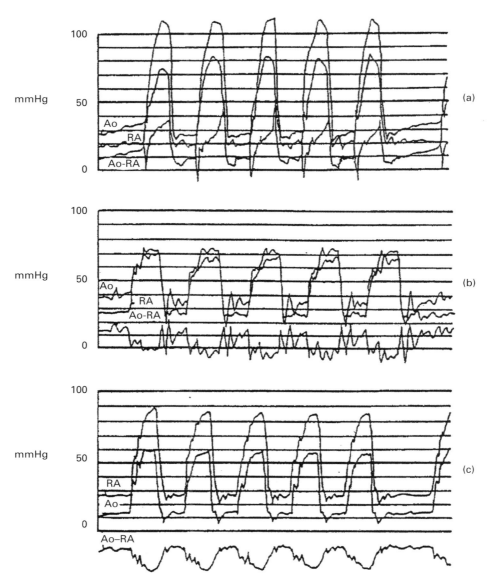

Fig. 38.3. Aortic (Ao), right atrial (RA), and coronary perfusion (Ao-RA) pressure tracings during human CPR. (a) Positive coronary perfusion pressure (CPP) generated during both compression and relaxation phases of chest compressions. (b) Positive CPP generated only during relaxation phase of chest compressions. (c) Negative CPP throughout compression cycle. The degree of CPP cannot be predicted by palpation of CPR-produced peripheral pulses. (From ref. 38.).

methods require detection of pulsations in the cuff or other detector transmitted by the artery. Although these techniques provide acceptable levels of variance from intra-arterial measures in stable patients, levels of variance are greatly increased in states of critical illness. Motion produced during CPR as well as the low pressure produced will require sensitivity not required of standard applications of the technology.[40] If knowledge of systolic pressure is desired, use of a manually inflated pressure cuff along with a Doppler device is recommended, with the caveat that diastolic pressure cannot be determined in this manner. It must be emphasized, however, that achieving a target systolic pressure alone during CPR has never been associated with ROSC; thus, use of non-invasive blood pressure monitoring will be of little value during CPR. Because of the physiology of cardiac arrest and

CPR-induced perfusion pressures, significant changes in systolic blood pressure may occur without favorable changes in CPP. Direct arterial blood pressure monitoring will be useful in distinguishing true electromechanical dissociation (EMD) from pseudo-EMD in which patient body habitus or significantly low pulse pressure prevents detection of pulsatile flow by pulse detection or end-tidal CO_2 monitoring (discussed later).[8]

During the postresuscitation phase, invasive arterial blood pressure monitoring is recommended because of the noted unreliability of non-invasive measures during labile states.[40] Since to stay in the autoregulatory range of the brain and to maintain coronary perfusion pressure a minimal perfusion pressure of 70 mmHg is recommended, invasive arterial pressure will be helpful in ensuring this. Invasive monitoring will also make acquisition of arterial blood gases easier.

Laboratory testing

Intermittent venous and arterial blood sampling for gas or chemistry analysis is of limited utility during CPR and basically has no application in the out-of-hospital setting. Use of whole blood gas and electrolyte measurements (now available at many institutions and in point of care testing kits) can provide both hemoglobin and potassium levels within minutes. These may be helpful in excluding hyperkalemia and severe anemia as a cause of arrest or of inhibiting attempts at resuscitation. Co-oximetry measurement of hemoglobin for evidence of carbon monoxide poisoning would be helpful in certain circumstances. Severely elevated carboxyhemoglobin levels are likely to preclude successful resuscitation by standard resuscitation techniques since a state of functional anemia will exist in combination with the poor perfusion produced by CPR, thus further reducing DO_2.

Typical blood gas findings during CPR include severe venous respiratory acidosis and arterial respiratory alkalosis, which reflect the large dead space created in the lungs by cardiac arrest and the poor forward blood flow produced by chest compressions as compared to the normal circulation (Fig. 38.4).[41–44] SaO_2 is usually 99% with PO_2 levels well above 100 mmHg.

Lactate monitoring during CPR itself has been examined as a means to determine the duration of cardiac arrest, the so-called "down time" and to titrate therapy.[45–47] Normal lactate levels (in the absence of liver failure) are less than 2–3 mmol/L. Lactic acidosis existing during CPR and the initial postresuscitation period is due to inadequate DO_2 (Type A lactic acidosis). However, single measurements have limited value. Changes in lactate will not occur rapidly enough during CPR to allow changes in therapy.

Indeed, it can be argued that better CPR may result in increasing lactate levels because of washout phenomena (removal of lactate sequestered in tissue beds into the central circulation) and/or because of enhanced delivery of substrate to cells that are still below the point of DO_2crit, thus resulting in additional lactate production. Moreover, lactate levels at the beginning of CPR may differ among individuals, depending on the etiology of arrest. For example, an asthmatic who experienced significant hypoxemia before arrest will have higher levels of lactate and a higher oxygen debt than will the victim of sudden death. Lactate levels during CPR have not been demonstrated in humans to correlate with neurologic outcome.[48]

The major utility of lactate monitoring is in the postresuscitation setting as a useful endpoint to guide hemodynamic management. Lactate levels are universally elevated immediately after ROSC; therefore, use of lactate as a postresuscitation endpoint to assess adequacy of DO_2 will require serial measurements. It is thus not the absolute level of lactate that is prognostic in shock, but the ability to halt dysoxic lactate production and clear it.[49–52] Lactate clearance of at least 5%–10% an hour should be a goal. Rising lactate levels or the inability to clear lactate indicates continuing accumulation of oxygen debt and thus DO_2 levels below DO_2crit or significant regional dysoxia.[3,50] Therapies aimed at increasing DO_2 or reducing VO_2 should be instituted.

It is not uncommon to observe elevated or rising lactate levels in the postresuscitation period despite normal or elevated systemic blood pressures. This should be interpreted as an indication of severe microcirculatory shunting, which may be secondary to excessive circulating levels of catecholamines or other vasoactive mediators.[53] In this setting, the presence of elevated lactate levels concomitant with elevated central or mixed venous hemoglobin oxygen saturation again indicates severe microcirculatory injury and portends a poor outcome.[53,54] Non-intuitive therapies such as vasodilator therapy may be required to reverse this state.

Although lactic acid and base deficit are highly correlated, hyperlactemia (levels 2–5 mmol/L) may be observed in the latter phases of postresuscitation care in the absence of metabolic acidosis as a consequence of processes that increase the glycolytic flux of glucose to lactate, such as catecholamine administration.[55] Nevertheless, clinicians should aggressively rule out occult hypoperfusion as a cause of elevated lactate levels.

Postresuscitation laboratory testing of other markers or compounds as indicators of myocardial function, neuronal injury, immune and inflammatory function, and others will inevitably be developed as our ability to treat cardiac arrest and the postresuscitation syndrome

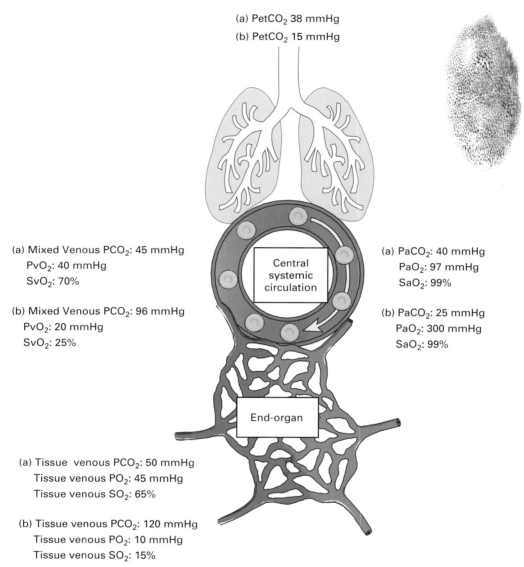

(a) PetCO$_2$ 38 mmHg
(b) PetCO$_2$ 15 mmHg

(a) Mixed Venous PCO$_2$: 45 mmHg
   PvO$_2$: 40 mmHg
   SvO$_2$: 70%

(b) Mixed Venous PCO$_2$: 96 mmHg
   PvO$_2$: 20 mmHg
   SvO$_2$: 25%

Central systemic circulation

(a) PaCO$_2$: 40 mmHg
   PaO$_2$: 97 mmHg
   SaO$_2$: 99%

(b) PaCO$_2$: 25 mmHg
   PaO$_2$: 300 mmHg
   SaO$_2$: 99%

End-organ

(a) Tissue venous PCO$_2$: 50 mmHg
   Tissue venous PO$_2$: 45 mmHg
   Tissue venous SO$_2$: 65%

(b) Tissue venous PCO$_2$: 120 mmHg
   Tissue venous PO$_2$: 10 mmHg
   Tissue venous SO$_2$: 15%

Fig. 38.4. Representative blood and tissue gas levels of the normal circulation (a) and during cardiac arrest and CPR (b). Mixed venous values represent aggregate values from all organ systems. Thus tissue venous values are not necessarily identical to mixed venous values but can be higher or lower depending on the individual organ system's level of metabolic activity. The majority of blood volume at the level of the tissue is contained in the venous compartment. Because of the tremendous reductions in blood flow produced by CPR, a deadspace in the lungs is created thus producing gaps between mixed venous PCO$_2$, PetCO$_2$, and PaCO$_2$. The severe reductions in DO$_2$ to each organ system result in very high oxygen extraction at the level of the tissue, which produces very low tissue venous PO$_2$ and thus SO$_2$ levels. The very high venous PCO$_2$ levels are due to decreased removal of both aerobically and anaerobically produced CO$_2$ (see Fig. 38.5).

evolves. Much of this will be as a result of advances in our understanding of the molecular basis and complex interplay between systems in the pathology and treatment of the disease. It is possible to envision performing bedside genomic and proteomic profiling in the postresuscitation period to obtain better understanding of prognosis or to develop individual pharmacogenomic approaches to therapy for the patient.

Pulse oximetry

The technique of pulse oximetry utilizes two wavelengths of light (red and infrared) to determine the percentages of oxy- and deoxyhemoglobin. This is determined by isolating the small increase in blood volume occurring at the site of measurements in response to systole and comparing it to background absorption, which includes blood, bone, skin, and other tissue components. The technique thus requires pulsatile flow. There has been confusion with respect to the role of pulse oximetry during CPR. Because of the physiology of CPR, which produces low systemic blood flow and significant increases in physiologic deadspace, along with ventilation that uses high flow oxygen, arterial blood gases reveal hemoglobin oxygen saturations of 99%, as PaO_2 levels are uniformly above 100 mmHg.[41,56] Thus, in the absence of significant anemia, obtaining maximum arterial oxygen content during CPR is rarely a problem. For monitoring the effectiveness of chest compressions, use of SpO_2 to observe the produced plethysmograph is unreliable because of various factors, including presence of nail polish, temperature-induced vasoconstriction of digits, shunting due to reductions in CPR blood flow, and others. In addition, studies have demonstrated that very low pulsatile blood flow is capable of producing a plethysmograph.[57,58] Various manufacturers have developed very bright light-emitting diodes and sensitive detectors that can pick up very weak signals. They have even developed sensitive motion artifact rejection software. Most manufacturers "auto scale" the detected plethysmograph for the user so that information on signal intensity is not available. Thus, the ability to detect a peripheral SpO_2-produced plethysmograph is not indicative of adequate CPR.

The characteristics of the plethysmograph determined by pulse oximetry have not been examined for its ability to correlate with central hemodynamics produced by closed chest compressions and pharmacologic interventions, although it may warrant study. It is likely, however, that interpatient variations produced by arterial vascular disease and other factors will preclude its use as a sensitive guide to resuscitation.

End-tidal CO_2 monitoring

Capnometry is the measurement of the concentration of CO_2 in the airway during inspiration and expiration. Capnography refers to the graphic display of this measurement over time. Measurement of CO_2 concentrations at the very end of expiration is termed end-tidal CO_2 ($PetCO_2$). CO_2 in respiratory gases can be measured by several methods, with infrared spectroscopy being the most common. $PetCO_2$ can also be measured qualitatively and semiquantitatively by using pH-sensitive filter papers containing metacresol purple, which changes color in response to varying concentrations of CO_2 owing to the formation of hydrogen ions.[59,60]

Beginning with the work of Kalenda and Smallhout, the value of $PetCO_2$ monitoring for resuscitation of victims of cardiac arrest has been demonstrated repeatedly.[61] The value of $PetCO_2$ monitoring lies in its ability to reflect closely alveolar CO_2. Alveolar CO_2 is determined by the combination of CO_2 production (VCO_2), pulmonary capillary blood flow (i.e., cardiac output), and alveolar ventilation. As such, alveolar CO_2 and $PetCO_2$ are linearly related to VCO_2. VCO_2 depends on two different factors: pulmonary excretion and metabolic production of CO_2. In low flow states with steady-state ventilation, VCO_2 declines secondary to decreased delivery of CO_2 to the lungs and to ventilation/perfusion mismatches in the lung resulting in an enormous increase in deadspace (up to 0.7 in the setting of CPR).[62] This results in a widening of the arterial PCO_2 to $PetCO_2$ gradient and is further reflected by mixed venous hypercarbia. Although difficult to measure, VCO_2 also declines secondary to reductions in actual CO_2 production from decreases in DO_2.[42,63,64] Although sometimes described as logarithmic, VCO_2 and thus $PetCO_2$ basically have almost the same biphasic relationship with DO_2 as does VO_2 (Fig. 38.5). Thus, DO_2crit determined by following changes in VCO_2 and $PetCO_2$ does not significantly differ from determinations using changes in VO_2 or lactate production.[63,65] Concomitant with reductions in DO_2 will be increases in tissue CO_2, as decreases in blood flow will reduce the amount of aerobically produced CO_2 removed from tissue, creating a tissue respiratory acidosis.[66–68] Additional tissue CO_2 will be produced after DO_2crit is reached, as metabolic acids such as lactic acid are buffered by tissue bicarbonate, although tissue CO_2 production as a whole will be decreased in accordance with decreases in VO_2.[69]

VCO_2 and thus $PetCO_2$ are linearly related to DO_2 during metabolic states dependent on oxygen supply. Since during CPR, oxygen content does not change significantly, then the major component of DO_2 tracked by VCO_2 or $PetCO_2$ is cardiac output. This is advantageous during CPR since, as discussed earlier, CPR is a state where VO_2 is directly dependent upon DO_2.

Again, in order for this to be valid, both alveolar ventilation (minute ventilation) and VCO_2 must be assumed to be relatively constant. If this is assumed, changes in $PetCO_2$ will reflect changes in pulmonary capillary blood flow or cardiac output. Of note, in this setting, although $PetCO_2$ correlates with cardiac output, it does not correlate with actual $PaCO_2$ during CPR in humans,

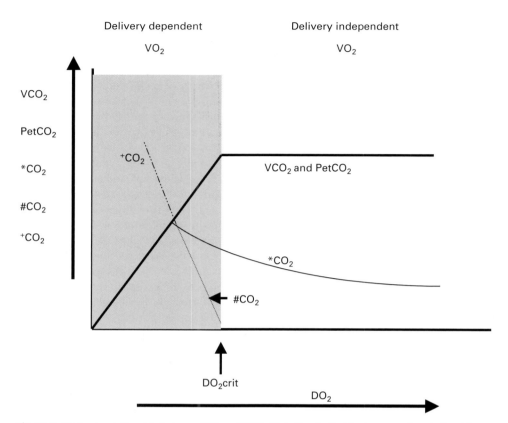

Fig. 38.5. Biphasic relationship between DO_2 and VCO_2. Note the similarities between the relationships as compared to Fig. 38.1. When minute ventilation is held constant, DO_2crit can be determined by reductions in VCO_2 and thus $PetCO_2$. This corresponds to the point of delivery-dependent VO_2. $*CO_2$ represents CO_2 that accumulates as a result of decreased removal of aerobically produced CO_2 secondary to decreases in flow (respiratory acidosis). $\#CO_2$ represents additional tissue CO_2 production and accumulation due to buffering of metabolic acids produced by anaerobic metabolism after DO_2crit is reached, and would correspond to the production of lactate at the point of DO_2crit (see Fig. 38.1). $+CO_2$ represents the combination of aerobically and an aerobically derived CO_2. Overall VCO_2 is decreased due to declines in VO_2. Quantities of CO_2 as depicted on the Y axis are not drawn to scale, but instead are depicted to demonstrate their temporal relationship to each other in reference to changes in DO_2.

because of the large increase in pulmonary deadspace produced.

Although VCO_2 production during CPR is difficult to measure, there are not likely to be wide swings. In addition, the extremely high concentrations of CO_2 in the mixed venous blood pool (> 60 mmHg) and large pulmonary deadspace ensure that small changes in VCO_2 do not cause appreciable changes in $PetCO_2$.[42] Only ROSC or improved artificial circulation (e.g., with open chest massage) will result in a dramatic and sustained increase in $PetCO_2$. Minute ventilation should be held relatively constant if $PetCO_2$ is to be used as an indicator of cardiac output.

Both animal and human data have demonstrated that $PetCO_2$ correlates with CPP and cerebral perfusion pressure (CePP) during CPR.[70–72] The correlation between $PetCO_2$, CPP, and CePP is due to its relationship with cardiac output in the low-flow setting of CPR. This can be predicted on the basis of the known relationship between mean arterial pressure and cardiac output when peripheral vascular resistance (PVR) is constant. Thus when PVR is not significantly changing, increases in cardiac output will result in increases in organ blood flow; the increased cardiac output will result in an increase in $PetCO_2$ if minute ventilation and VCO_2 are held constant.

These correlations between $PetCO_2$, CPP, CePP, and cardiac output may be uncoupled by epinephrine and other vasopressors administered during CPR. Animal and human studies have shown that $PetCO_2$ decreases when large doses of epinephrine are used during cardiac arrest, despite significant increases in CPP and myocardial and cerebral blood flow.[31,73] Initially thought to be due to increases in shunt fraction, it has been found that this effect is due to actual decreases in CPR-produced cardiac output as a result of increases in afterload.[31] Thus, although cardiac output is decreased, DO_2 to the myocardium and cerebrum are increased because of the redistribution of blood volume, much of which lies in the aorta. Although consistently shown in animals, the effect of epinephrine administration during CPR on reducing $PetCO_2$ in humans has been variable.[74,75] When decreases in $PetCO_2$ occur after epinephrine administration, they correlate with the timing of increases in central arterial levels of epinephrine and the concomitant vasopressor effect. The duration of these changes, if they occur clinically, has not been well quantified. Interestingly, such changes in $PetCO_2$ may be potentially useful for timing subsequent epinephrine or other vasopressor dosing or in understanding if CPR is producing enough forward flow to distribute intravenously administered vasopressors to the systemic circulation.

Because sodium bicarbonate contains and produces CO_2, its bolus administration during CPR will cause a variable but significant transient rise in $PetCO_2$. The timing of this increase is within 1 minute of administration, and it usually lasts for <2 minutes depending on whether minute ventilation changes.[76]

End-tidal CO_2 can be used as a feedback to optimize chest compressions during CPR. Monitoring $PetCO_2$ during cardiac arrest may detect unrecognized fatigue in the CPR provider.[61,77] Since an effective threshold for chest compressions has been demonstrated, $PetCO_2$ may be of value in detecting compression thresholds, with either manual or mechanical chest compressions.[78,79] Changes in pulse pressure as detected by palpation of CPR-produced peripheral pulses do not necessarily correlate with flow.[7] $PetCO_2$ on the other hand provides evidence of improvements or deterioration in real-time forward flow, given that the possible effects of bicarbonate and vasopressor agents on $PetCO_2$ are recognized. One effective strategy might be to perform CPR at a rate and compression depth to produce maximum $PetCO_2$ values. Chest compressions need not be halted during CPR to palpate pulses if $PetCO_2$ monitoring is performed.

In cases of mechanical causes of PEA, $PetCO_2$ monitoring should be valuable in indicating the immediate success of such therapeutic maneuvers as needle decompression of tension pneumothorax, pericardiocentesis for relief of cardiac tamponade, or fluid resuscitation for hypovolemia. $PetCO_2$ monitoring might also be (deemed to be) helpful in determining which patients with PEA have true electromechanical dissociation versus those with significant cardiac contractions, but in whom a pulse cannot be palpated due to obesity, vasoconstriction, or hypothermia. Paradis *et al.* found that a significant number of patients with PEA had arterial pulse pressures when monitored invasively, with several patients having systolic blood pressures of 90 mmHg.[8] $PetCO_2$ monitoring would have demonstrated values significantly greater than 0 mmHg in these patients when no chest compressions were performed.

Several investigators have reported $PetCO_2$ values during CPR that may offer prognostic information concerning chances of obtaining ROSC. These include averaging $PetCO_2$ values over 20 minutes of resuscitation, taking initial and maximal $PetCO_2$ values, measuring $PetCO_2$ changes after epinephrine administration, and measuring $PetCO_2$ values during resuscitation of various presenting rhythms such as asystole or PEA.[80–85] Levine and colleagues have demonstrated that a $PetCO_2$ value of <10 mmHg after 20 minutes of resuscitation in out-of-hospital cardiac arrest with PEA has a 100% predictive value of no ROSC.[84] Similar results have been observed in other out-of-hospital studies, as well as in the in-hospital setting.[74,75,81,82] Others have demonstrated that an initial $PetCO_2$ value of <15 mmHg has a 91% predictive value for no ROSC. The use of high-dose epinephrine (>10 mg) changes, but does not eliminate, the ability of $PetCO_2$ to predict ROSC. Two studies have demonstrated that reductions in $PetCO_2$ after epinephrine administration result in positive predictive values for ROSC ranging from 29% to 53% and negative predictive value ranging from 92% to 100%.[74,75] Nonetheless, it should be remembered that epinephrine doses of ≥ 1 mg may decrease or have no effect on $PetCO_2$.[75]

Although no formal guidelines or recommendations have been made by any organization concerning the use of $PetCO_2$ to guide CPR efforts, the following is suggested. For $PetCO_2 < 10$ mmHg, the clinician should modify the ongoing resuscitation. Standard CPR should be enhanced (e.g., by increased rate or depth of compression). If, despite optimal performance of CPR, $PetCO_2$ values remain <10 mmHg and the clinical scenario warrants aggressive intervention, the clinician should consider an alternative method of CPR, such as open chest cardiac massage. If, despite optimal resuscitative efforts, the $PetCO_2$ cannot be raised to ≥ 10 mmHg and the patient's dysrhythmia is not amenable to electrical therapy, ceasing resuscitation efforts in a normothermic arrest patient should be considered.[76]

Because values are low during CPR and mixed venous PCO_2 is so high, ROSC should be immediately detected by significant increases in $PetCO_2$. Indeed, $PetCO_2$ values have been shown to be the first changes noted after ROSC.[76,86,87] Upon ROSC, there is a rapid rise in $PetCO_2$ that will generally overshoot values of 40 mmHg. This overshoot stems from the large tissue and venous respiratory acidosis that has existed since the onset of arrest. Elevated $PetCO_2$ may persist for some time as CO_2 is washed out of various tissue beds. $PetCO_2$ monitoring can be helpful at this time in adjusting minute ventilation as a guide to bringing $PaCO_2$ back to baseline, because ROSC will reduce deadspace back to levels where $PetCO_2$ can be used to estimate $PaCO_2$. This will assist in using ventilation to control systemic pH. Similarly, $PetCO_2$ monitoring can help detect deterioration in perfusion after resuscitation. Sudden reductions in $PetCO_2$ after ROSC when no changes in ventilation have been made can be interpreted as significant deterioration in cardiac output, consistent with returning to a state below DO_2crit.[63,65] In these instances, re-arrest is likely to be imminent if no action is taken.

In summary, $PetCO_2$ monitoring is an ideal tool for use during CPR and in the postresuscitation period because of its linear relationship with cardiac output in low flow states and the relationship between cardiac output and critical perfusion pressures such as CPP and CePP. Its link with these central hemodynamic events during CPR allows real-time changes to be detected within seconds of interventions, given current cardiac arrest treatment protocols. For diagnostic and treatment decisions, $PetCO_2$ monitoring during CPR should be carried out with devices that use infrared technology, so that quantitative values can be obtained and the capnogram can be inspected. Figure 38.6 provides several examples of $PetCO_2$ monitoring during cardiac arrest by use of time-compressed capnography.

Cardiac output and oxygen consumption monitoring

There are now numerous invasive and non-invasive means to monitor cardiac output, ranging from traditional thermodilution methods with the pulmonary artery catheter to less invasive methods that utilize impedance (impedance cardiography), esophageal Doppler technology, rebreathing of CO_2 (CO_2 Fick method), and others.[88–91] Although the use of non-invasive methods to measure cardiac output during CPR is tempting, the efficacy of such an approach is questionable, especially in light of the proven utility of $PetCO_2$ monitoring described above. If the goal of CPR is to produce the highest cardiac output and CPP to achieve ROSC in the shortest period of time, it would be difficult to justify actual cardiac output monitoring during CPR. Furthermore, given the low cardiac outputs and motion that CPR produces, it is doubtful that any cardiac output readings obtained with these techniques would have the required accuracy and precision to be useful.

Cardiac output monitoring may be more useful in the postresuscitation setting as a means to recognize cardiac dysfunction and to optimize global DO_2. Use of cardiac output as an end-point *per se* is ill-advised since significant end-organ hypoperfusion can exist despite normal and even supernormal cardiac output.[92–98] Instead, cardiac output monitoring may be more appropriately used as a guide to volume resuscitation in determining optimal preload (volume challenges provided until no further increase in cardiac output is obtained). In addition, its use in conjunction with markers of end-organ perfusion (discussed below) may assist in identifying the points in which pharmacologic therapy to increase cardiac output have been maximized and, in turn, the need to institute additional circulatory adjuncts such as intra-aortic balloon pumping. The method of cardiac output monitoring used is less important than how and when it is used.

Measurement of VO_2 in states of critical illness is very underutilized. Although its use during CPR will be uninformative since a state of severe DO_2-dependent VO_2 is present, its use during the postresuscitation phase of care has shown promise in predicting survival. There are two major methods of measuring VO_2: 1; the use of the indirect or reverse Fick method which requires insertion of a pulmonary artery catheter for determination of cardiac output and the arterial to mixed venous difference in oxygen content; and 2, the use of indirect calorimetry. The latter is believed to be more accurate, because it eliminates the potential for mathematical coupling of VO_2 with cardiac output that is thought to occur.[1] In addition, it takes into account actual oxygen utilization of the lung itself, which can be substantial in some situations.[99]

Rivers *et al.* have reported the use of VO_2 monitoring after cardiac arrest and found that failure to achieve of VO_2 greater than 90 ml/min per m^2 within the first 6 hours of arrest was associated with 100% mortality at 24 hours after ROSC.[53] There appear to be two reasons for this. First there is as expected a component of cardiogenic shock in which DO_2 is impaired in relation to the amount of cardiac output. Importantly but under-recognized, however, is that the oxygen extraction ratio in these individuals is lower than expected and is accompanied by venous hyperoxia.[53,54] This indicates the likely presence of an impairment in microcirculatory DO_2 because of microcirculatory occlusion or shunting, which contributes to the accumulation of a fatal level of oxygen debt.

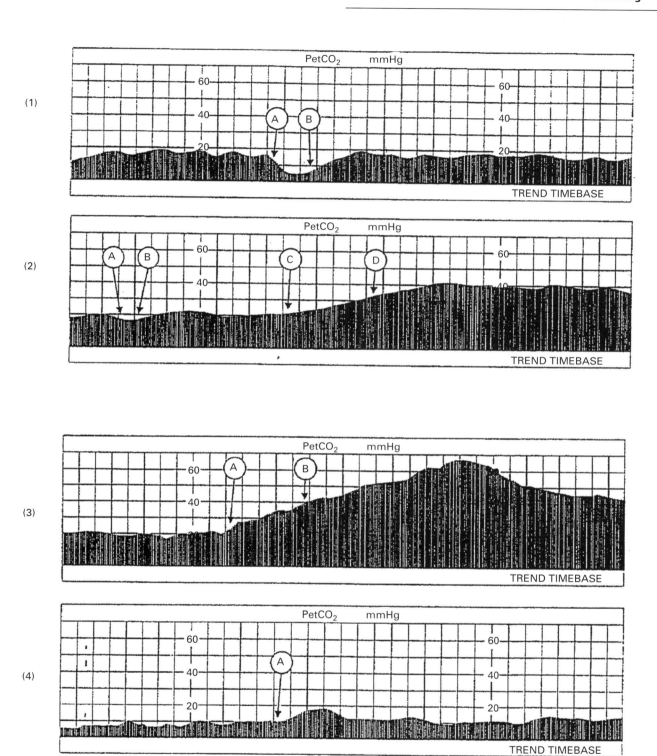

Fig. 38.6. Capnogram tracings of PetCO$_2$ during cardiac arrest and CPR. (1) Effect of rescuer fatigue is demonstrated at point A. Point B demonstrates the effect of changing to a new chest compression provider. (2) Patient with pseudo-EMD. At point A the patient is pulsless but has persistent PetCO$_2$ value of 20 mmHg without chest compressions; at point B, chest compression is restarted; at point C, a dopamine infusion is begun; and at point D, chest compressions are stopped and a pulse is palpated. (3) Sudden rise in PetCO$_2$ (A) heralds ROSC and pulses are palpated at point B. (4) Point A shows a transient rise in PetCO$_2$ just after an intravenous bolus of sodium bicarbonate.[60,76]

A very valuable surrogate of VO_2 monitoring is mixed venous (SvO_2) or central venous ($ScvO_2$) hemoglobin oxygen saturation monitoring. The use of mixed venous hemoglobin oxygen saturation (SvO_2) has long been advocated as a means to detect tissue hypoxia in the critically ill or injured patient since it is a reflection of oxygen extraction which, in turn, reflects the adequacy of DO_2.[93] Normal values average 75%. SvO_2 reflects the aggregate balance between tissue oxygen delivery and consumption or the extraction ratio of all tissues, and thus reflects global DO_2 (Fig. 39.1). It is not difficult to understand the potential value of such a measure as an early warning system in identifying reductions in DO_2 before DO_2crit, as well as the need for increasing DO_2 even after a state of VO_2-independent DO_2 is reached. Nevertheless, placement of a pulmonary artery catheter is difficult in the immediate postresuscitation period (and may not be needed) and impossible during CPR. Although not truly mixed, a suitable surrogate of SvO_2 may be $ScvO_2$ monitoring.[100–103] $ScvO_2$ has been advocated for use during CPR.[100] Similar to tissue CO_2 measurements, $ScvO_2$ values will be significantly below baseline, demonstrating maximum oxygen extraction. Rivers and colleagues have found that similar to CPP thresholds, there appears to be a $ScvO_2$ threshold below which patients undergoing CPR cannot be resuscitated. In their studies, no patient with an $ScvO_2$ of less than 30% could be resuscitated. All but one patient who achieved ROSC obtained an $ScvO_2$ during CPR of at least 40%. These findings should reflect the adequacy of DO_2 from a cardiac output produced during CPR. Unfortunately, the study by Rivers did not report simultaneous PetCO_2 levels and thus it is unclear if $ScvO_2$ monitoring would have any significant advantage over PetCO_2 monitoring during cardiac arrest that would justify its use.

Similar, however, to some of the tissue-specific methods of monitoring discussed below, the real value of $ScvO_2$ or SvO_2 monitoring will likely be in the postresuscitation setting as a means to exclude occult tissue hypoxia and to determine the adequacy of DO_2. Of special note is the ability of the technique to detect venous hyperoxia as a manifestation of severe microcirculatory injury, especially after high dose vasopressor use.[53] In this setting, $ScvO_2$ levels are noted to be significantly elevated in the presence of elevated lactate levels, indicating that significant shunting is likely.[53,104] In this setting, the body is not consuming oxygen (again likely to be due to problems with microcirculatory DO_2) and measures that increase microcirculatory DO_2 must be considered quickly before fatal levels of oxygen debt are reached. Such measures might include intra-aortic balloon pumping, use of vasodilators, or use of extracorpreal circulation techniques. Although studies examining the use of both SvO_2 and tissue-specific indicators of oxygenation, for example, gastric tonometry in other shock states such as trauma and sepsis (discussed below), have demonstrated the superiority of tissue-specific measures over SvO_2, these studies have not applied the techniques very early. It is therefore unclear whether there would be cases in the immediate post-arrest period where $ScvO_2$ would be normal, but tissue-specific measures would be abnormal. The transition from perfusion-limited shock states (hemorrhage, cardiogenic) to those associated with significant inflammation (sepsis) make the interpretation of SvO_2, $ScvO_2$, and tissue-specific measures such as gastric tonometry more difficult.[92,93,105] Recent evidence suggests, however, that early use of $ScvO_2$ will be able to identify significant tissue hypoxia (much of it occult) and will be useful as an end-point to guide treatment, in addition to identifying states of venous hyperoxia after cardiac arrest.[53,103,106] The technique has the added advantage of allowing the user to monitor central venous pressure and thus assist in optimizing preload.

Ultrasound

Rapid access and use of ultrasound in the emergent setting is becoming more common, given advances in the quality and portability of devices. In the setting of cardiac arrest, ultrasound can rapidly assist the clinician in distinguishing between true electromechanical dissociation (EMD) and pseudo-EMD during treatment of PEA. It will also assist the clinician in diagnosing other causes of PEA or arrest, such as pericardial tamponade (in addition to guiding pericardiocentesis), and in diagnosing exsanguinating intra-abdominal or intrathoracic hemorrhage. Special ultrasound variations such as transesophageal echocardiography, which provide higher resolution visualization of the heart and mediastinal structures, may be useful in identifying other causes of cardiac arrest, such as pulmonary embolism or aortic dissection and in detecting severe valvular abnormalities.[107] Lastly, the use of ultrasound for echocardiography in the postresuscitation period could be extremely helpful in judging the degree of post-arrest myocardial dysfunction and in making decisions on how to assist the failing heart. Ultrasound may also assist in vascular cannulation of central vessels, when "blind" cannulation by use of anatomical landmarks, is unsuccessful.[108,109] The major limitations to the use of ultrasound in the settings above are the experience and skills of the operator. Making the diagnosis of pericardial tamponade or intraabdominal hemorrhage will require less skill than determining the degree of myocardial dysfunction in the postresuscitation setting.

Tissue-specific monitoring

Figures 38.1 and 38.5 demonstrate that the biphasic relationship between VO_2 and VCO_2 with DO_2 exists not only for the whole body, but also for individual organ systems, which may have DO_2 crit values that differ from whole body DO_2crit. Studies have demonstrated, for example in hemorrhagic shock, that the DO_2 crit of the splanchnic bed occurs at a higher global DO_2 than the DO_2crit of the whole body.[69,110,111] As noted earlier, however, cardiac arrest immediately results in a state of profound delivery-dependent VO_2, so that all organ systems are immediately past their DO_2crit values. Therefore, each would show evidence of profound tissue hypoxia and flow stagnation as represented by very low venous hemoglobin oxygen saturations and elevated venous or tissue CO_2 levels. The advantage of monitoring one tissue over another in this setting is difficult to defend. Nevertheless, tissue-specific monitoring in the postresuscitation setting may make sense based on the characteristics of the tissue and the goals to be achieved.

Tissue CO_2 monitoring

Several options that are available to monitor tissue CO_2 have been studied in various shock states. These include transcutaneous CO_2 ($PtcCO_2$) skin monitoring, interstitial fiberoptic PCO_2, gastric mucosal CO_2 via gastric tonometry ($PgCO_2$), and most recently sublingual tonometry ($PslCO_2$).[93,112-120] $PtcCO_2$, $PgCO_2$, and $PslCO_2$ are non-invasive, whereas interstitial PCO_2 monitoring requires insertion of a probe into tissue parenchyma. Details of how CO_2 is actually measured by these techniques have been well described.[93] All of these methods are based on the diffusion of CO_2 from tissue: each will reflect the balance among supply of CO_2 to the tissue, CO_2 production by the tissue, and CO_2 removal of the tissue. This balance does not mean all tissue compartments contribute equally. Values are a composite of vascular and interstitial levels in the immediate environment of the sensor. Since the majority of blood volume in tissues is venous (approximately 70%), the tissue CO_2 concentrations will mainly reflect venous PCO_2 concentrations.[121,122] The ability of these measures, however, to reflect the balance between DO_2 and VO_2 or to reflect perfusion pressures or other real-time hemodynamic changes during CPR has not been studied. The highest CO_2 concentrations that can be reached in each tissue after cardiac arrest in humans are not known, but in animal models, some tissue beds reach levels well over 100 mmHg.[123] The majority of CO_2 accumulation in each tissue will be secondary to the inability to remove CO_2 that was being produced aerobically prior to ischemia. As mentioned previously, additional CO_2 will be produced in response to

metabolic acids (mainly lactate) produced after the onset of ischemia by the cells as they are buffered by endogenous bicarbonate stores. Interpretation of real-time changes in tissue PCO_2 in response to interventions will be challenging compared to use in other shock settings in which there is significantly more flow and more time for trending. If improvements in forward flow are not accompanied by an increase in minute ventilation, arterial PCO_2 will be increased; thus, more CO_2 will be delivered to the tissue.[44] Use of vasopressors to improve CPP and CePP will most likely result in decreases in peripheral tissue flow, thus potentially further reducing removal of CO_2 during CPR. It is doubtful that tracking tissue CO_2 changes will be meaningful during the short duration of cardiac arrest, especially given the redistribution of blood flow that occurs during CPR and in response to vasopressor administration. Response times are unlikely to be rapid enough to guide the resuscitation effort. Although this seems counterintuitive on the basis of the previous discussion of $PetCO_2$ monitoring, it must be remembered that $PetCO_2$ reflects CO_2 at the end of its journey from the tissue beds. Its rapid breath-by-breath analysis makes its response time to interventions difficult to improve upon. The only thing that can be said with certainty is that, upon ROSC, tissue PCO_2 should decline rapidly as CO_2 is removed from previously stagnant tissue beds and aerobic metabolism is reestablished.

The real value of tissue CO_2 monitoring will be in the postresuscitation phase of care, where it can assist in assuring resolution of end-organ perfusion abnormalities. $PgCO_2$ and perhaps $PslCO_2$ may be particularly helpful. It is known that the splanchnic bed is particularly sensitive to reductions in systemic blood flow, in part because the responsiveness of its vasculature to the myriad of vasoactive mediators associated with shock.[124,125] Of special concern in the victim of cardiac arrest are the mediators angiotensin II, vasopressin, endothelin, and epinephrine. Endogenous levels of these agents are significantly elevated during shock and will be even higher in the postresuscitation phase, if vasopressin and epinephrine are administered during the arrest to achieve ROSC or in the postresuscitation period to maintain blood pressure.[126,127] These and other vasopressor agents provided for blood pressure support in shock states have been shown to contribute to ischemia in intestinal mucosa.[124,128] This, in turn, has been hypothesized to lead to a breach of the intestinal mucosal barrier, allowing bacteria and other toxic mediators into the systemic circulation, which leads to sepsis and multisystem organ failure.[129-133] This paradigm, which is generally accepted in other shock states, has not been well studied in the setting of cardiac arrest.[125] The postresuscitation experience of patients who received vasopressin during CPR has not been well described and no clinical studies regardless of vasopressin use have been reported that have examined the incidence of splanchnic hypoperfusion or ischemia as determined by $PgCO_2$ monitoring. Nonetheless, the need for vasopressor support in the postresuscitation phase is high and will be complicated by significant cardiogenic shock. Monitoring of splanchnic blood flow by either $PgCO_2$ or $PslCO_2$ as performed in other shock states makes sense, especially in the very early stages of postresuscitation care since, as with other shock states, there is clear evidence that occult splanchnic ischemia can exist in the presence of normal systemic variables, such as blood pressure, heart rate, cardiac output, and mixed venous hemoglobin oxygen saturation.[92,134,135]

$PgCO_2$ monitoring has been used successfully to guide resuscitation of trauma patients and those with septic and cardiogenic shock.[95,115,136] This technique essentially monitors intraluminal CO_2 that has diffused into the stomach from the stomach mucosa. A modified nasogastric tube containing a CO_2-permeable balloon is placed in the stomach. Air is intermittently circulated through the balloon. CO_2 diffuses from the mucosa into the balloon where it is circulated proximally and measured via an infrared detector in the same manner as $PetCO_2$. This CO_2 value has been used previously to estimate the intramucosal pH (pHi) by substituting it for arterial CO_2 in the Henderson-Hasselbalch equation. Use of this formula assumes that arterial HCO_3^- and mucosal HCO_3^- are equivalent. pHi values of less than 7.32 are considered abnormal. The technique also assumes constant minute ventilation. A more robust use of the technology involves $PgCO_2 - PaCO_2$ or $PgCO_2 - PetCO_2$ gap to detect abnormalities in perfusion since this does not require the previous assumptions regarding HCO_3^- and, in addition, does not require strict maintenance of normocapnia, because since hypo- or hyperventilation, although affecting $PgCO_2$, will not affect the gap. Given that the arterial to alveolar PCO_2 gap is approximately 4 mmHg, it is thought that a $PgCO_2 - PaCO_2$ or $PgCO_2 - PetCO_2$ gap of 11–14 mmHg is abnormal and reflects perfusion abnormalities.[116] Although the response time of current $PgCO_2$ methodologies will not permit their use during CPR, they should prove to be quite valuable during the postresuscitation period. As with other shock states, normalization of the $PgCO_2 - PaCO_2$ or $PgCO_2 - PetCO_2$ gap will help ensure that occult tissue hypoxia is not present, thus helping to avoid further accumulation of oxygen debt and its associated complications.

$PslCO_2$ monitoring as a substitute for $PgCO_2$ monitoring to detect shock and guide its treatment is a recent development. Several studies appear to support the premise that the sublingual surface of the tongue may be as sensitive to disturbances in perfusion as the rest of the GI tract, perhaps because it shares the same embryonic origin as the rest of the gut.[66,67,117,137–140] This technique uses fiberoptic determination of CO_2 within a disposable cover (similar to an oral electronic thermometer) which allows diffusion of CO_2 from the sublingual surface into the space between the cover and sensor. The advantage of this technique is that the response time is faster since the sensor is more or less in direct contact with the tissue surface as opposed to $PgCO_2$ balloon, which is in the middle of a large lumen (the stomach). The disadvantage is that it is currently still difficult to perform continuous monitoring. As with $PgCO_2$, or any other tissue CO_2 monitoring technique, the gap of the measure with either $PaCO_2$ or $PetCO_2$ should be utilized in order to avoid misinterpretation of $PslCO_2$ in the setting of hyper- or hypocarbia. Definitive values of this gap or of absolute $PslCO_2$ levels have not been determined, but it is likely that they will not differ from those of the $PgCO_2 - PaCO_2$ or $PgCO_2 - PetCO_2$ gap. Although use of the $PslCO_2 - PetCO_2$ gap may have potential value in monitoring during actual CPR, it is not likely that it will have an advantage over simple $PetCO_2$ monitoring. As suggested above, it is plausible that the use of vasopressors would actually increase $PslCO_2$, despite increasing CPP above a critical threshold for ROSC.

Similarly, $PtcCO_2$ monitoring of the skin and/or interstitial tissue PCO_2 monitoring of tissues such as skeletal muscle may be useful in assuring resolution of end-organ tissue perfusion abnormalities in the postresuscitation setting. Both should be used similarly to that described for $PgCO_2$ and $PslCO_2$. Continued elevations of CO_2 as measured by these methods in the presence of normocapnia have been associated with increased mortality.[112,119,120,141,142] Of note, the technology used to measure interstitial PCO_2 is the same as that used in the development of continuous arterial blood gas monitoring and is thus also capable of simultaneous measurement of PO_2 and pH. The disadvantage of the technique is that it is slightly invasive, and can only sense the environment several micrometers from the sensor. It also requires a considerable calibration time (about 30 minutes).

Tissue oxygen monitoring

Similar to tissue CO_2 monitoring, several options exist for monitoring tissue oxygenation, which provides information on the balance between DO_2 and VO_2 of the tissue. These include transcutaneous PO_2 ($PtcO_2$) monitoring from the skin, interstitial PO_2 monitoring from tissue parenchyma, and tissue hemoglobin oxygen saturation (StO_2) by using near infrared absorption spectroscopy (NIRS). The general principles making tissue oxygenation monitoring potentially helpful are the same as those discussed above for tissue PCO_2.

Of special interest is the use of StO_2 monitoring by NIRS. Visible light (450–700 nm) penetrates tissue for only short distances, because it is usually strongly attenuated by various tissue components that absorb and scatter at these wavelengths. In the NIR spectrum (700–1100 nm), however, photons are capable of deeper penetration (several centimeters or more) even through bone. It is also within this spectral region that oxygen-dependent electronic transitions of the metalloproteins hemoglobin and cytochrome oxidase (the terminal electron acceptor in the mitochondrial electron transport chain) absorb light. These chromophores absorb NIR radiation differentially based on their concentration and interaction with oxygen. These changes in absorption can be measured by using NIRS technology. The Beer–Lambert law provides the physical and mathematical basis for NIRS, although it is modified to account for the inhomogeneous media that the NIR light traverses. The depth of penetration and volume of tissue being interrogated by NIRS depends on the distance between optodes. The technique of NIRS differs from that of pulse oximetry, because pulse oximetry targets only the arterial component of blood flow.

The basis for using NIRS to monitor the state of tissue oxygenation is similar to that of tissue PCO_2 monitoring in that it relies on the compartmentalization of blood volume, which in most systems is believed to be proportioned among the arteriolar, capillary, and venular compartments in a ratio of 10:20:70, respectively.[121,122] Thus, the values obtained by NIRS closely parallel those of venous hemoglobin leaving the tissue. This essentially allows it to be used in the same manner as SvO_2 and $ScvO_2$, except that instead of representing an aggregate reflection of the balance between DO_2 and VO_2 for the entire body, it reflects the balance in an individual organ (skeletal muscle, brain, and others). In addition to being non-invasive, the use of StO_2 monitoring may prove more sensitive than $ScvO_2$ or SvO_2 if the organ being interrogated is sensitive to changes in DO_2. Figure 38.7 depicts the use of NIRS for monitoring StO_2 of a skeletal muscle bed.

The vast majority of NIRS technology has been used to monitor the oxygenation status of the brain in neonates and in adults undergoing operative procedures that may affect the brain, such as carotid endarterectomy or cardiopulmonary bypass.[143] It is also being aggressively studied in the setting of trauma by using skeletal muscle or GI tract as the end-organ of interest.[144–148] Normal NIRS-derived StO_2 values for brain and skeletal muscle range from 60% to 80%. Use of NIRS during both cardiac arrest and in the postresuscitation phase has only been reported

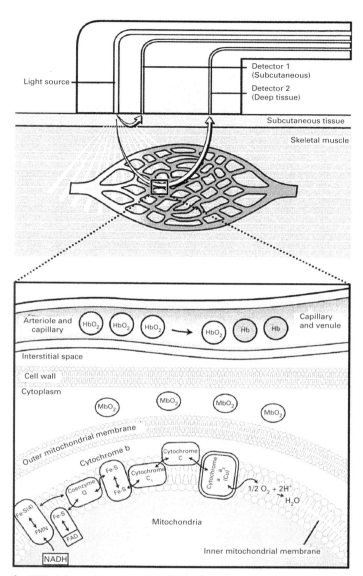

Fig. 38.7. Schematic representing NIRS in the reflectance mode overlying skin and skeletal muscle. NIRS is capable of providing information about the balance between oxygen delivery and consumption of an organ(s) by assessing the state of hemoglobin oxygen saturation in the microvasculature, as well as intracellular oxygen utilization via the redox state of cytochrome oxidase. The value and measure of StO_2 lies in the distribution of blood in the organ of interest with approximately 70% of blood volume being in the venous compartment under normal conditions. When NIRS is used to assess skeletal muscle perfusion, the contribution of myoglobin must be taken into account. Note that the technology diagrammed here might allow differentiation of the NIRS radiation returning from the subcutaneous tissue versus deeper underlying tissues such as skeletal muscle. Light follows an elliptical pathway, thus spacing of detectors at various distances from the light source assist in determining the origin of the returning signal.[148]

for the brain,[149–152] where special bilateral probes are placed on the forehead. This is necessary because it reduces the amount of skeletal muscle that the NIR light must traverse. The NIRS spectra between hemoglobin and myoglobin cannot be distinguished from each other. This is important since myoglobin and hemoglobin are present in almost equal proportions in skeletal muscle, with the p50 for myoglobin being only 5 mmHg.[153,154] There is some evidence that, when used as an indicator of skeletal muscle oxygenation, the NIRS signal is derived mainly from myoglobin and not from hemoglobin within the tissue.[155] This would limit its use during CPR and potentially the postresuscitation period, if skeletal muscle were chosen as the end-organ to guide resuscitation efforts. On the basis of these issues, when used for brain oxygenation monitoring, the NIRS signal is reported to derive from the frontal lobes. The bilateral probes were developed to allow comparison between the cerebral circulations of both hemispheres during surgical procedures in which the circulation to one hemisphere may be compromised. As expected, in many instances, StO_2 values are so low they cannot be registered. There is some evidence, however, that during CPR, higher cerebral StO_2 values are associated with ROSC.[149] This is not surprising given the redistribution of blood flow during cardiac arrest and the relationship between myocardial and cerebral blood flow with CPR-produced cardiac output described earlier. Similar to $PetCO_2$ monitoring, StO_2 values should immediately increase upon ROSC. Additional studies will be needed to include a larger number of patients to determine whether, as with $PetCO_2$ monitoring, there is a threshold cerebral StO_2 value below which victims cannot achieve ROSC. Unfortunately, no studies to date have measured cerebral StO_2 values concomitantly with $PetCO_2$ monitoring to assess whether StO_2 values are simply a reflection of cardiac output and therefore CPP and CePP, similar to $PetCO_2$. If this is the case, it may be hard to justify StO_2 monitoring during CPR over the technology of $PetCO_2$ monitoring, which can also provide information about proper airway management and sudden hemodynamic collapse after ROSC.

It is tempting to suggest the use of cerebral StO_2 monitoring in the postresuscitation phase to guide therapy. Whereas it may be a valid assumption that the circulation to the frontal lobes during cardiac arrest is indicative of blood flow to the rest of the brain (since the cerebral circulation is maximally dilated), use of cerebral StO_2 monitoring during the postresuscitation phase may be more complicated. It is well known that the brain undergoes a complicated pattern of heterogeneous blood flow and oxygen extraction in the postresuscitation period along with the potential for decreased global cerebral DO_2.[156–160] Although there is

potential for use of cerebral oximetry in this setting, it gave mixed results.[149,152] When compared to jugular venous bulb oximetry (a measure of global cerebral oxygen utilization), NIR cerebral oximetry values are higher, indicating that they may not reflect global cerebral blood flow and oxygenation, especially given that the majority of blood flow heterogeneity and damage will occur in the regions of the hippocampus and basal ganglia, which are supplied by circulation different from that of the frontal lobes. Because of blood flow heterogeneity and differences in regional cerebral metabolic activity, it may be difficult to conclude that changes in cerebral StO_2 values are secondary to changes in blood flow vs. extraction due to increased metabolism. Infarction of a region of brain tissue being interrogated may result in increases in StO_2.[150] It is unclear how the use of therapeutic hypothermia will affect the potential for NIRS use in the brain in the postresuscitation period.

As mentioned earlier, NIR StO_2 monitoring of skeletal muscle as an end-organ during CPR or in the postresuscitation period will require further study. Use of NIR StO_2 monitoring of the GI tract is still in the experimental stages of development.

Although the potential exists to use NIRS to determine the redox status of the cytochrome oxidase (the terminal electron acceptor in the mitochondrial transport chain) and thus the point of DO_2crit for the organ being monitored, this has proven to be extraordinarily challenging, in part because the reduced form of cytochrome oxidase does not have an absorption spectrum, and because the amount of cytochrome oxidase is so much smaller compared to hemoglobin. Thus, in order to use NIRS to monitor the redox state of the mitochondria, monitoring must take place before changes in the redox state. This obviously limits its value for monitoring during cardiac arrest or postresuscitation.

Direct visualization of the microcirculation

The ability to visualize microcirculatory blood flow directly and non-invasively has recently been introduced to clinical practice through the technique of orthogonal polarization spectral imaging (OPSI).[161] Linearly polarized light is used to illuminate the tissue. Because of the wavelength used, the light is reflected by the background, and is absorbed by hemoglobin.[161–164] Optical filtration allows elimination of the light reflected at the surface of the tissue to produce high-contrast-reflected light images of the microcirculation. Red cells appear dark (due to absorption of light by hemoglobin), but vessels are not visible unless they contain red cells. The technique works best on mucosal surfaces. With experience, semiquantitative information on microcirculatory hemodynamics is possible by assessing the density of functional (perfused) vessels within the field of view, as well as the flow of red cells. Unfortunately, automated software is not yet available for real-time quantitative analysis. OPSI of the sublingual area has been used in the evaluation of the microcirculation in patients with sepsis, cardiogenic shock, and during transfusions.[164–166] The technique establishes that the sublingual mucosal surface is very sensitive to changes in blood flow and that these changes reflect what may be occurring at a more global level. Manipulation of hemodynamic variables has been shown to improve microcirculatory flow. These have included both transfusion and vasodilation, indicating that rapid feedback can be obtained at a local tissue level in response to acute interventions.[167,168]

Its study and use in cardiac arrest is only beginning. Whether or not it will have clinical utility during arrest and CPR is unclear. Nevertheless, similar to its use in sepsis and cardiogenic shock, it may have a significant role as a monitoring endpoint in the postresuscitation care of the patient. This may be particularly helpful in understanding and optimizing the effects of postresuscitation hypothermia. Figure 38.8 demonstrates the sublingual circulation of a pig in ventricular fibrillation and during CPR.

Ventricular waveform analysis

It has long been held that ventricular fibrillation (VF) represented a simple chaotic dysrhythmia with little structure. It had been observed that the initial VF rhythm appeared "coarse" and later became "fine" in appearance as the arrest continued and that coarse VF seemed to be more amenable to treatment than fine VF. Often defibrillation of fine VF resulted in postcountershock asystole or PEA, which was difficult to resuscitate. Several studies seem to clearly indicate that deterioration of the VF waveform occurs in response to depletion of intramyocardial high energy phosphates, which may make it more prone to injury from the countershock itself. Indeed, several studies have demonstrated that treatment of VF with chest compressions and epinephrine before countershock appears to increase the chances of successful defibrillation into a perfusing rhythm.[18,19,169,170] Before the last decade, little had been done to objectively analyze the rhythm for patterns, which could predict response to treatment.

Currently endorsed guidelines for applying a defibrillation shock, namely those proposed by the American Heart Association and European Resuscitation Council, propose a three-shock sequence at the earliest practical moment when there is no detectable sign of consciousness after

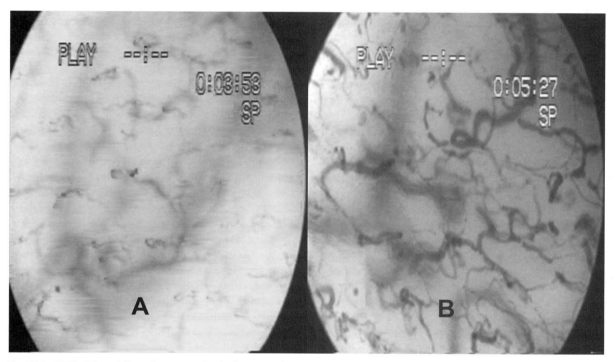

Fig. 38.8. OPSI of the sublingual mucosa of a pig during cardiac arrest (A) and during CPR (B). An increase in functional capillary density can be seen as produced by CPR. The vessel population in the field of view represents a combination of arterioles, capillaries, and venules.

management of airway and breathing. Thus the very nature of these guidelines promotes delivery of defibrillation countershock without consideration of its potential harm. Such a defibrillation procedure may ultimately result in excessive application of electrical energy with low likelihood of successful ROSC and increase in myocardial injury.[14,16,17,171,172]

Optimally, only a single electric shock should be effective. Implementing this approach would require methods by which the success of defibrillation may be predicted before delivery of the shock. This would allow delivery of the least total energy at the earliest time with high probability of success.

Electrocardiographic rhythm analysis for estimating success of defibrillation has been under investigation for several decades as a method to minimize the risk of defibrillation injury and as a potential method to prioritize interventions for early terminations of VF. The rationale for the analysis of the VF waveform is that if VF is likely to be terminated by defibrillation shock; it would be of benefit to shock immediately. In contrast, an indicator of poor success of defibrillation would guide rescue intervention toward alternate therapies, such as precordial compression, that may improve resuscitation outcomes.

Studies linking properties of VF to defibrillation success were demonstrated by Weaver as early as 1985.[173] Weaver's study found an inversely proportional relationship between the duration of VF and the amplitude and further correlation of the survival rates of victims of cardiac arrest to the amplitude. Weaver's study also pointed out potential pitfalls in associating VF properties to defibrillation success. For example, electrode size, location, and chest dimension may affect the signal amplitude, which will adversely affect the amplitude as a reliable, single parameter measure.

Other investigators adopted alternative approaches characterizing VF frequency properties, which alleviated many of the problems associated with reliance on amplitude alone.[174–179] These "frequency domain" approaches share a common background in decomposing the electrocardiogram into a spectrum by orthogonal transformation, such as Fourier or Wavelet. Still other investigators implemented methods that deviated from quantification by transform or pure amplitude. Menegazzi and Callaway recently developed a fractal technique of "scaling exponents" to predict defibrillation success. A VF signal is analyzed for its relatedness to minute changes in VF. The more random and unrelated an incoming VF signal is in relation to its present position in "time," the higher the score will be and less likely the success of defibrillation.[180,181] This is consistent with anecdotal observations that coarse VF, a more easily convertible rhythm, is somewhat less random and more predictable than is fine VF.

Eftestol demonstrated a method of incorporating multivariate information to a *single variable* ((P_{ROSC} (v)), the probability of successful defibrillation).[176,182] This method selects a combination of features such as centroid frequency, peak power frequency, spectral flatness and energy that would produce the highest prediction of sensitivity and specificity. The usefulness of P_{ROSC} may be improved by adding new features to existing sets and searching for the combination that provides the best predictable performance.

Similarly, amplitude spectrum area (AMSA) combines amplitude and frequency in the frequency domain according to the following equation:

$$AMSA = \sum AiFi$$

Ai is defined as the magnitude of the complex Fourier coefficient of the transformed VF waveform. Fi is defined as the frequency of the complex Fourier coefficient.[177, 178]

In a retrospective study by Eftestol, positive changes in P_{ROSC} were observed in patients who were successfully defibrillated to ROSC while there were no increases in P_{ROSC} in patients who were defibrillated but were not resuscitated.[183] AMSA derived by Marn-Pernat on experimental animals without interrupting precordial compression was confirmed by Povoas, who utilized real-time monitoring with sensitivity and specificity of 0.90.[177,178] During CPR, a progressive increase in the AMSA was observed and correlated well with coronary perfusion pressure (Fig. 38.9).[178]

Both P_{ROSC} and AMSA therefore support the notion that VF waveform analyses and especially the trend of sequential values can identify thresholds for predicting the success of electrical defibrillation. These indicators can also serve as quality control for cardiopulmonary resuscitation during uninterrupted chest compression, with the anticipation of achieving more successful defibrillation. These objective measurements integrated in existing AEDs would then eliminate the current empiricism of delivering repetitive electrical shocks that cause myocardial injury. If the likelihood of successful defibrillation is remote, the rescuer can be guided accordingly and especially emphasize the importance of precordial compression to improve myocardial blood flow and myocardial oxygen delivery before the next attempt at defibrillation.

The attractiveness of using spectral analysis of the VF waveform is its apparent direct link to myocardial blood flow (demonstrated in animal models).[184] This will be particularly important in humans where significant coronary artery occlusions may exist that impede myocardial blood flow, despite what appears to be good CPR-produced cardiac output and CPP based on PetCO$_2$ analysis.

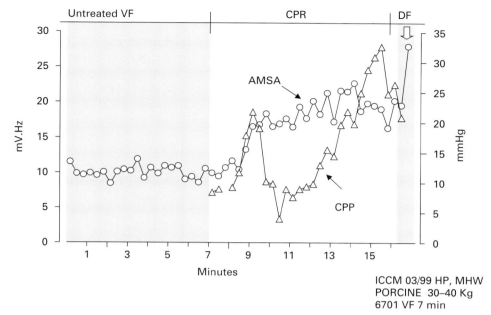

Fig. 38.9. The amplitude spectrum area (AMSA) depicted during cardiac arrest and CPR is shown to correlate well with coronary perfusion pressure (CPP) without interrupting CPR. The AMSA predicted successful ROSC with a sensitivity and specificity of 0.9.[177]

Use of VF analysis tools is limited to VF and will thus not be helpful in gauging the response of asystole, PEA, or pulseless ventricular tachycardia to treatment, nor will it predict outcome. An important aspect of VF waveform analysis technology that requires study is its performance in settings where VF is not the initial rhythm encountered, or in which patients have repetitive episodes of VF with intervening rhythms, including ROSC followed by refibrillation. Despite this, incorporation of this type of technology in defibrillators including AEDs holds great potential to improve outcomes from VF. Although the data are compelling, this technology awaits a definitive prospective trial. The major impediment to use of such technology will be the mammoth re-education of health care providers who have been taught for decades to defibrillate first and then provide adjunctive treatments.

Postresuscitation monitoring

Resuscitation of the cardiac arrest victim does not end with ROSC. The immediate post-ROSC period represents a complex shock state with components of both traditional cardiogenic shock from ischemia, and microvascular shunting due to vasopressor use and occurrence of microthrombi. It is during this time that rapid institution of both global and tissue-specific goal-directed measures

of oxygen transport should take place to optimize the potential for both satisfactory cardiovascular and neurologic outcomes. The reader is again referred to Figs. 38.1, 38.4, and 38.5. The time of ROSC does not ensure that a state of VO_2-independent DO_2 exists. Thus, the clinician must institute such monitoring techniques that can assist in assuring that both overt and occult tissue hypoxia is being resolved. The importance of this cannot be overemphasized. Both animal and clinical studies have demonstrated the effect of cumulative oxygen debt on mortality or in developing significant morbidity including multisystem organ failure. Studies in critically ill surgery patients demonstrate little or no mortality when oxygen debt is less than $4100\,ml/m^2$. Mortality increases to 50% and 95% when cumulative oxygen debt is $4900\,ml/m^2$ and $5800\,ml/m^2$, respectively.[4,5] In contrast, for a 70-kg individual with a baseline VO_2 of $120\,ml/min/m^2$, a 30-minute cardiac arrest would create an oxygen debt of only $3600\,ml/m^2$. Rivers has shown that significant additional oxygen debt that cannot be quantified by blood pressure and other conventional means can accumulate after ROSC.[53,54] It is thus apparent that significant ongoing accumulation of oxygen debt is possible during the postresuscitation period. Deferring aggressive postresuscitation care until, for example, the patient is moved from the emergency department into the intensive care unit is ill-conceived and could allow patients to develop cumu-

Table 38.1. Monitoring goals during CPR and postresuscitation

Monitoring end points during CPR	
CPP:	≥ 15 mmHg
PetCO$_2$	> 10 mmHg (prior to vasopressor administration)
ScvO$_2$	$> 40\%$
Postresuscitation monitoring goals	
Global end points	
Mean arterial pressure	70–90 mmHg
CVP/PCWP	10–15/15–18 mmHg (or pressure which results in no further improvement in CO$_2$)
Hemoglobin	≥ 10 g/dL
Lactate	< 2.0 mM
SaO$_2$	94–99%
ScvO$_2$/SvO$_2$	70–80%
VO$_2$	> 90 mL/min per m^2
Tissue-specific end points	
pHi	> 7.32
PgCO$_2$–PaCO$_2$ gap	< 15 mmHg
PgCO$_2$ – PetCO$_2$ gap	<15 mmHg
PslCO$_2$–PaCO$_2$ gap	<15 mmHg
PslCO$_2$–PetCO$_2$ gap	<15 mmHg
StO$_2$	$> 65\%$ (skeletal muscle, brain, or GI tract)

lative oxygen debts, which are not consistent with prolonged survival.

Although there are many end-points to choose from, those that can be instituted rapidly within the first minutes of ROSC are preferred, and may be able to guide the clinical team as to whether additional monitoring and therapy are warranted. Our preference is to use a combination of global and tissue-specific techniques in a goal-directed fashion. The techniques and principles discussed are applicable to all forms of initial resuscitation including trauma. Table 38.1 lists those end-points that should be considered during CPR to gauge the effectiveness of the resuscitation, as well as end-points that might be considered to optimize the postresuscitation effort. Although many may consider these experimental, they are far more objective and sensitive than the use of traditional heart rate and blood pressure monitoring. The effect of therapeutic hypothermia on these variables has not been well studied. Reduced global oxygen demand should be one favorable aspect, thus making it potentially easier to reach a state of VO$_2$-independent DO$_2$, especially in the face of reduced myocardial function.

Acknowledgments

Supported in part by the US Office of Naval Research (Grants N00014-02-10344, N00014-02-1-0642, and N00014-03-1-0253) and in part by Grants from the US Army Medical Research and Material Command (Grants: USAMRMC W81K00-04-0998 and DAMD17-03-1-0172).

REFERENCES

1. Chittock, D.R., Ronco, J. & Russel, J. Monitoring of oxygen transport and oxygen consumption. In Tobin, M.J. ed. *Principles and Practice of Intensive Care Monitoring*. New York: McGraw-Hill, 1998: 317–343.

2. Schumacker, P.T. & Cain, S.M. The concept of a critical oxygen delivery. *Intens. Care Med.* 1987; **13**(4): 223–229.

3. Vincent, J.L. Lactate and biochemical indexes of oxygenation. In Tobin, M.J., ed. *Principles and Practice of Intensive Care Monitoring*. New York: McGraw-Hill, 1998: 369–376.

4. Shoemaker, W.C., Appel, P.L. & Kram, H.B. Tissue oxygen debt as a determinant of lethal and nonlethal postoperative organ failure. *Crit. Care Med.* 1988; **16**(11): 1117–1120.

5. Shoemaker, W.C., Appel, P.L. & Kram, H.B. Role of oxygen debt in the development of organ failure sepsis, and death in high-risk surgical patients. *Chest* 1992; **102**(1): 208–215.

6. Ward, K.R., Barbee, R.W. & Ivatury, R.R. Monitoring techniques during resuscitation. In Ornato, J.P. & Peberdy, M.A., eds. *Cardiopulmonary Resuscitation*. Totowa: Humana Press, 2005: 475–502.

7. McDonald, J.L. Systolic and mean arterial pressures during manual and mechanical CPR in humans. *Ann. Emerg. Med.* 1982; **11**(6): 292–295.

8. Paradis, N.A., Martin, G.B., Goetting, M.G., Rivers, E.P., Feingold, M. & Nowak, R.M. Aortic pressure during human cardiac arrest. Identification of pseudo-electromechanical dissociation. *Chest* 1992; **101**(1): 123–128.

9. Kern, K.B. & Niemann, J.T. Coronary perfusion pressure during cardiopulmonary resuscitation. In Paradis, N.A., Halperin, H. & Nowak, R.M., eds. *Cardiac Arrest: The Science and Practice of Resuscitation Medicine*. Baltimore: Williams and Wilkins, 1996: 270–284.

10. Mather, C. & O'Kelly, S. The palpation of pulses. *Anaesthesia* 1996; **51**(2): 189–191.

11. Bahr, J., Klingler, H., Panzer, W., Rode, H. & Kettler, D. Skills of lay people in checking the carotid pulse. *Resuscitation* 1997; **35**(1): 23–26.

12. AHA guidelines 2000 for cardiopulmonary resuscitation and emergency cardiovascular care. *Circulation* 2000; **108**(8): I-1–I-384.

13. Cummins, R.O. & Hazinski, M.F. Cardiopulmonary resuscitation techniques and instruction: when does evidence justify revision? *Ann. Emerg. Med.* 1999; **34**(6): 780–784.

14. Tang, W., Weil, M.H., Sun, S. *et al.* The effects of biphasic and conventional monophasic defibrillation on postresuscitation myocardial function. *J. Am. Coll. Cardiol.* 1999; **34**(3): 815–822.

15. Weil, M.H., Tang, W. & Bisera, J. Cardiopulmonary resuscitation: one size does not fit all. *Circulation* 2003; **107**(6): 794.

16. Xie, J., Weil, M.H., Sun, S. *et al.* High-energy defibrillation increases the severity of postresuscitation myocardial dysfunction. *Circulation* 1997; **96**(2): 683–688.

17. Yamaguchi, H., Weil, M., Tang, W., Kamohara, T., Jin, X. & Bisera, J. Myocardial dysfunction after electrical defibrillation. *Resuscitation* 2002; **54**(3): 289–296.

18. Wik, L., Hansen, T.B., Fylling, F. *et al.* Delaying defibrillation to give basic cardiopulmonary resuscitation to patients with out-of-hospital ventricular fibrillation: a randomized trial. *J. Am. Med. Assoc.* 2003; **289**(11): 1389–1395.

19. Cobb, L.A., Fahrenbruch, C.E., Walsh, T.R. *et al.* Influence of cardiopulmonary resuscitation prior to defibrillation in patients with out-of-hospital ventricular fibrillation. *J. Am. Med. Assoc.* 1999; **281**(13): 1182–1188.

20. Kern, K.B., Hilwig, R.W., Berg, R.A., Sanders, A.B. & Ewy, G.A. Importance of continuous chest compressions during cardiopulmonary resuscitation: improved outcome during a simulated single lay-rescuer scenario. *Circulation* 2002; **105**(5): 645–649.

21. Yu, T., Weil, M.H., Tang, W. *et al.* Adverse outcomes of interrupted precordial compression during automated defibrillation. *Circulation* 2002; **106**(3): 368–372.

22. Powers, S.R., Jr., Schaffer, C., Boba, A. & Nakamura, Y. Physical and biologic factors in impedance plethysmography. *Surgery* 1958; **44**(1): 53–62.

23. Geddes, L.A., Hoff, H.E., Mello, A. & Palmer, C. Continuous measurement of ventricular stroke volume by electrical impedance. *Cardiovasc. Res. Cent. Bull.* 1966; **4**(4): 118–131.

24. Baker, L.E., Hill, D.W. & Pate, T.D. Comparison of several pulse-pressure techniques for monitoring stroke volume. *Med. Biol. Eng.* 1974; **12**(1): 81–89.

25. Allison, R.D., Holmes, E.L. & Nyboer, J. Volumetric dynamics of respiration as measured by electrical impedance plethysmography. *J. Appl. Physiol.* 1964; **19**: 166–173.

26. Hamilton, L.H., Beard, J.D. & Kory, R.C. Impedance measurement of tidal volume and ventilation. *J. Appl. Physiol.* 1965; **20**(3): 565–568.

27. Kubicek, W.G., Karnegis, J.N., Patterson, R.P., Witsoe, D.A. & Mattson, R.H. Development and evaluation of an impedance cardiac output system. *Aerosp. Med.* 1966; **37**(12): 1208–1212.

28. Shoemaker, W.C., Wo, C.C., Chan, L. *et al.* Outcome prediction of emergency patients by noninvasive hemodynamic monitoring. *Chest.* 2001; **120**(2): 528–537.

29. Pellis, T., Bisera, J., Tang, W. & Weil, M.H. Expanding automatic external defibrillators to include automated detection of cardiac, respiratory, and cardiorespiratory arrest. *Crit. Care Med.* 2002; **30**(4 Suppl): S176–S178.

30. Ditchey, R.V. & Lindenfeld, J. Failure of epinephrine to improve the balance between myocardial oxygen supply and demand during closed-chest resuscitation in dogs. *Circulation* 1988; **78**(2): 382–389.

31. Chase, P.B., Kern, K.B., Sanders, A.B., Otto, C.W. & Ewy, G.A. Effects of graded doses of epinephrine on both noninvasive and invasive measures of myocardial perfusion and blood flow during cardiopulmonary resuscitation. *Crit. Care Med.* 1993; **21**(3): 413–419.

32. Paradis, N.A., Martin, G.B., Rivers, E.P. *et al.* Coronary perfusion pressure and the return of spontaneous circulation in human cardiopulmonary resuscitation. *J. Am. Med. Assoc.* 1990; **263**(8): 1106–1113.

33. Paradis, N.A., Martin, G.B., Rosenberg, J. *et al.* The effect of standard- and high-dose epinephrine on coronary perfusion pressure during prolonged cardiopulmonary resuscitation. *J. Am. Med. Assoc.* 1991; **265**(9): 1139–1144.

34. Downey, J. Compression of the coronary arteries by the fibrillating canine heart. *Circ. Res.* 1976; **39**(1): 53–57.

35. Downey, J.M., Chagrasulis, R.W. & Hemphill, V. Quantitative study of intramyocardial compression in the fibrillating heart. *Am. J. Physiol.* 1979; **237**(2): H191–H196.

36. Kern, K.B., Lancaster, L., Goldman, S. & Ewy, G.A. The effect of coronary artery lesions on the relationship between coronary perfusion pressure and myocardial blood flow during cardiopulmonary resuscitation in pigs. *Am. Heart J.* 1990; **120**(2): 324–333.

37. Kern, K.B., de la Guardia, B. & Ewy, G.A. Myocardial perfusion during cardiopulmonary resuscitation (CPR): effects of 10, 25 and 50% coronary stenoses. *Resuscitation* 1998; **38**(2): 107–111.

38. Martin, G.B., Carden, D.L., Nowak, R.M., Lewinter, J.R., Johnston, W. & Tomlanovich, M.C. Aortic and right atrial pressures during standard and simultaneous compression and ventilation CPR in human beings. *Ann. Emerg. Med.* 1986; **15**(2): 125–130.

39. Niemann, J.T., Criley, J.M., Rosborough, J.P., Niskanen, R.A. & Alferness, C. Predictive indices of successful cardiac resuscitation after prolonged arrest and experimental cardiopulmonary resuscitation. *Ann. Emerg. Med.* 1985; **14**(6): 521–528.

40. Lodato, R.F. Arterial pressure monitoring. In Tobin, M.J., ed. *Principles and Practice of Intensive Care Monitoring*. New York: McGraw-Hill, 1998: 733–749.

41. Angelos, M.G., DeBehnke, D.J. & Leasure, J.E. Arterial blood gases during cardiac arrest: markers of blood flow in a canine model. *Resuscitation* 1992; **23**(2): 101–111.

42. Weil, M.H., Rackow, E.C., Trevino, R., Grundler, W., Falk, J.L. & Griffel, M.I. Difference in acid–base state between venous and arterial blood during cardiopulmonary resuscitation. *N. Engl. J. Med.* 1986; **315**(3): 153–156.

43. von Planta, M. Acid–base and electrolyte management. In Weil, M.H. & Tang, W., eds. *CPR: Resuscitation of the Arrested Heart*. Philadelphia: W.B. Saunders, 1999: 37–52.

44. Gazmuri, R.J., von Planta, M., Weil, M.H. & Rackow, E.C. Arterial PCO_2 as an indicator of systemic perfusion during cardiopulmonary resuscitation. *Crit. Care Med.* 1989; **17**(3): 237–240.

45. Carden, D.L., Martin, G.B., Nowak, R.M., Foreback, C.C. & Tomlanovich, M.C. Lactic acidosis as a predictor of downtime during cardiopulmonary arrest in dogs. *Am. J. Emerg. Med.* 1985; **3**(2): 120–124.

46. Carden, D.L., Martin, G.B., Nowak, R.M., Foreback, C.C. & Tomlanovich, M.C. Lactic acidosis during closed-chest CPR in dogs. *Ann. Emerg. Med.* 1987; **16**(12): 1317–1320.

47. Prause, G., Ratzenhofer-Comenda, B., Smolle-Juttner, F. *et al.* Comparison of lactate or BE during out-of-hospital cardiac arrest to determine metabolic acidosis. *Resuscitation* 2001; **51**(3): 297–300.

48. Mullner, M., Sterz, F., Domanovits, H., Behringer, W., Binder, M. & Laggner, A.N. The association between blood lactate concentration on admission, duration of cardiac arrest, and functional neurological recovery in patients resuscitated from ventricular fibrillation. *Intens. Care Med.* 1997; **23**(11): 1138–1143.

49. Tuchschmidt, J.A. & Mecher, C.E. Predictors of outcome from critical illness. Shock and cardiopulmonary resuscitation. *Crit. Care Clin.* 1994; **10**(1): 179–195.

50. Vincent, J.L., Dufaye, P., Berre, J., Leeman, M., Degaute, J.P. & Kahn, R.J. Serial lactate determinations during circulatory shock. *Crit. Care Med.* 1983; **11**(6): 449–451.

51. Bakker, J., Coffernils, M., Leon, M., Gris, P. & Vincent, J.L. Blood lactate levels are superior to oxygen-derived variables in predicting outcome in human septic shock. *Chest* 1991; **99**(4): 956–962.

52. Bakker, J., Gris, P., Coffernils, M., Kahn, R.J. & Vincent, J.L. Serial blood lactate levels can predict the development of multiple organ failure following septic shock. *Am. J. Surg.* 1996; **171**(2): 221–226.

53. Rivers, E.P., Rady, M.Y., Martin, G.B. *et al.* Venous hyperoxia after cardiac arrest. Characterization of a defect in systemic oxygen utilization. *Chest* 1992; **102**(6): 1787–1793.

54. Rivers, E.P., Wortsman, J., Rady, M.Y., Blake, H.C., McGeorge, F.T. & Buderer, N.M. The effect of the total cumulative epinephrine dose administered during human CPR on hemodynamic, oxygen transport, and utilization variables in the postresuscitation period. *Chest* 1994; **106**(5): 1499–1507.

55. Luchette, F.A., Robinson, B.R., Friend, L.A., McCarter, F., Frame, S.B. & James, J.H. Adrenergic antagonists reduce lactic acidosis in response to hemorrhagic shock. *J. Trauma* 1999; **46**(5): 873–880.

56. Tucker, K.J., Idris, A.H., Wenzel, V. & Orban, D.J. Changes in arterial and mixed venous blood gases during untreated ventricular fibrillation and cardiopulmonary resuscitation. *Resuscitation* 1994; **28**(2): 137–141.

57. Jay, G.D., Hughes, L. & Renzi, F.P. Pulse oximetry is accurate in acute anemia from hemorrhage. *Ann. Emerg. Med.* 1994; **24**(1): 32–35.

58. Severinghaus, J.W. & Spellman, M.J., Jr. Pulse oximeter failure thresholds in hypotension and vasoconstriction. *Anesthesiology* 1990; **73**(3): 532–537.

59. Hess, D.R. Capnometry. In Tobin, M.J., ed. *Principles and Practice of Intensive Care Monitoring.* New York: McGraw-Hill, 1998: 377–400.

60. Ward, K.R. & Yealy, D.M. End-tidal carbon dioxide monitoring in emergency medicine, Part 1: Basic principles. *Acad. Emerg. Med.* 1998; **5**(6): 628–636.

61. Kalenda, Z. The capnogram as a guide to the efficacy of cardiac massage. *Resuscitation* 1978; **6**(4): 259–263.

62. Hindman, B.J. Sodium bicarbonate in the treatment of sub-types of acute lactic acidosis: physiologic considerations. *Anesthesiology* 1990; **72**(6): 1064–1076.

63. Dubin, A., Murias, G., Estenssoro, E. *et al.* End-tidal CO_2 pressure determinants during hemorrhagic shock. *Intens. Care Med.* 2000; **26**(11): 1619–1623.

64. Relman, A.S. Letter. *N. Engl. J. Med.* 1986; **315**: 1618.

65. Guzman, J.A., Lacoma, F.J., Najar, A. & Kruse, J.A. End-tidal partial pressure of carbon dioxide as a noninvasive indicator of systemic oxygen supply dependency during hemorrhagic shock and resuscitation. *Shock* 1997; **8**(6): 427–431.

66. Sato, Y., Weil, M.H. & Tang, W. Tissue hypercarbic acidosis as a marker of acute circulatory failure (shock). *Chest* 1998; **114**(1): 263–274.

67. Jin, X., Weil, M.H., Sun, S., Tang, W., Bisera, J. & Mason, E.J. Decreases in organ blood flows associated with increases in sublingual PCO_2 during hemorrhagic shock. *J. Appl. Physiol.* 1998; **85**(6): 2360–2364.

68. Schlichtig, R., Mehta, N. & Gayowski, T.J. Tissue-arterial PCO_2 difference is a better marker of ischemia than intramural pH (pHi) or arterial pH-pHi difference. *J. Crit. Care* 1996; **11**(2): 51–56.

69. Schlichtig, R. & Bowles, S.A. Distinguishing between aerobic and anaerobic appearance of dissolved CO_2 in intestine during low flow. *J. Appl. Physiol.* 1994; **76**(6): 2443–2451.

70. Sanders, A.B., Atlas, M., Ewy, G.A., Kern, K.B. & Bragg, S. Expired PCO_2 as an index of coronary perfusion pressure. *Am. J. Emerg. Med.* 1985; **3**(2): 147–149.

71. Kern, K.B., Sanders, A.B., Voorhees, W.D., Babbs, C.F., Tacker, W.A. & Ewy, G.A. Changes in expired end-tidal carbon dioxide during cardiopulmonary resuscitation in dogs: a prognostic guide for resuscitation efforts. *J. Am. Coll. Cardiol.* 1989; **13**(5): 1184–1189.

72. Lewis, L.M., Stothert, J., Standeven, J., Chandel, B., Kurtz, M. & Fortney, J. Correlation of end-tidal CO_2 to cerebral perfusion during CPR. *Ann. Emerg. Med.* 1992; **21**(9): 1131–1134.

73. Martin, G.B., Gentile, N.T., Paradis, N.A., Moeggenberg, J., Appleton, T.J. & Nowak, R.M. Effect of epinephrine on end-tidal carbon dioxide monitoring during CPR. *Ann. Emerg. Med.* 1990; **19**(4): 396–398.

74. Cantineau, J.P., Merckx, P., Lambert, Y., Sorkine, M., Bertrand, C. & Duvaldestin, P. Effect of epinephrine on end-tidal carbon dioxide pressure during prehospital cardiopulmonary resuscitation. *Am. J. Emerg. Med.* 1994; **12**(3): 267–270.

75. Callaham, M., Barton, C. & Matthay, M. Effect of epinephrine on the ability of end-tidal carbon dioxide readings to predict initial resuscitation from cardiac arrest. *Crit. Care Med.* 1992; **20**(3): 337–343.

76. Ward, K.R. & Yealy, D.M. End-tidal carbon dioxide monitoring in emergency medicine, Part 2: Clinical applications. *Acad. Emerg. Med.* 1998; **5**(6): 637–646.

77. Ward, K.R., Menegazzi, J.J., Zelenak, R.R., Sullivan, R.J. & McSwain, N.E., Jr. A comparison of chest compressions between mechanical and manual CPR by monitoring end-tidal PCO_2 during human cardiac arrest. *Ann. Emerg. Med.* 1993; **22**(4): 669–674.

78. Babbs, C.F., Voorhees, W.D., Fitzgerald, K.R., Holmes, H.R. & Geddes, L.A. Relationship of blood pressure and flow during CPR to chest compression amplitude: evidence for an effective compression threshold. *Ann. Emerg. Med.* 1983; **12**(9): 527–532.

79. Ornato, J.P., Gonzalez, E.R., Garnett, A.R., Levine, R.L. & McClung, B.K. Effect of cardiopulmonary resuscitation compression rate on end-tidal carbon dioxide concentration and arterial pressure in man. *Crit. Care Med.* 1988; **16**(3): 241–245.

80. Callaham, M. & Barton, C. Prediction of outcome of cardiopulmonary resuscitation from end-tidal carbon dioxide concentration. *Crit. Care Med.* 1990; **18**(4): 358–362.

81. Sanders, A.B., Kern, K.B., Otto, C.W., Milander, M.M. & Ewy, G.A. End-tidal carbon dioxide monitoring during cardiopulmonary resuscitation. A prognostic indicator for survival. *J. Am. Med. Assoc.* 1989; **262**(10): 1347–1351.

82. Cantineau, J.P., Lambert, Y., Merckx, P. *et al.* End-tidal carbon dioxide during cardiopulmonary resuscitation in humans presenting mostly with asystole: a predictor of outcome. *Crit. Care Med.* 1996; **24**(5): 791–796.

83. Asplin, B.R. & White, R.D. Prognostic value of end-tidal carbon dioxide pressures during out-of-hospital cardiac arrest. *Ann. Emerg. Med.* 1995; **25**(6): 756–761.

84. Levine, R.L., Wayne, M.A. & Miller, C.C. End-tidal carbon dioxide and outcome of out-of-hospital cardiac arrest. *N. Engl. J. Med.* 1997; **337**(5): 301–306.

85. Wayne, M.A., Levine, R.L. & Miller, C.C. Use of end-tidal carbon dioxide to predict outcome in prehospital cardiac arrest. *Ann. Emerg. Med.* 1995; **25**(6): 762–767.

86. Sanders, A.B., Ewy, G.A., Bragg, S., Atlas, M. & Kern, K.B. Expired PCO_2 as a prognostic indicator of successful resuscitation from cardiac arrest. *Ann. Emerg. Med.* 1985; **14**(10): 948–952.

87. Garnett, A.R., Ornato, J.P., Gonzalez, E.R. & Johnson, E.B. End-tidal carbon dioxide monitoring during cardiopulmonary resuscitation. *J. Am. Med. Assoc.* 1987; **257**(4): 512–515.

88. De Maria, A.N. & Raisinghani, A. Comparative overview of cardiac output measurement methods: Has impedance cardiography come of age? *Congest. Heart Fail.* 2000; **6**(2): 60–73.

89. Valtier, B., Cholley, B.P., Belot, J.P., de la Coussaye, J.E., Mateo, J. & Payen, D.M. Noninvasive monitoring of cardiac output in critically ill patients using transesophageal Doppler. *Am. J. Respir. Crit. Care Med.* 1998; **158**(1): 77–83.

90. Botero, M. & Lobato, E.B. Advances in noninvasive cardiac output monitoring: an update. *J. Cardiothorac. Vasc. Anesth.* 2001; **15**(5): 631–640.

91. Murias, G.E., Villagra, A., Vatua, S. *et al.* Evaluation of a noninvasive method for cardiac output measurement in critical care patients. *Intens. Care Med.* 2002; **28**(10): 1470–1474.

92. Ivatury, R.R., Simon, R.J., Havriliak, D., Garcia, C., Greenbarg, J. & Stahl, W.M. Gastric mucosal pH and oxygen delivery and oxygen consumption indices in the assessment of adequacy of resuscitation after trauma: a prospective, randomized study. *J. Trauma* 1995; **39**(1): 128–134; discussion 134–126.

93. Ward, K.R., Ivatury, R.R. & Barbee, R.W. Endpoints of resuscitation for the victim of trauma. *J. Intens. Care Med.* 2001; **16**: 55–75.

94. Porter, J.M. & Ivatury, R.R. In search of the optimal end points of resuscitation in trauma patients: a review. *J. Trauma* 1998; **44**(5): 908–914.

95. Maynard, N., Bihari, D., Beale, R. *et al.* Assessment of splanchnic oxygenation by gastric tonometry in patients with acute circulatory failure. *J. Am. Med. Assoc.* 1993; **270**(10): 1203–1210.

96. Gutierrez, G., Bismar, H., Dantzker, D.R. & Silva, N. Comparison of gastric intramucosal pH with measures of oxygen transport and consumption in critically ill patients. *Crit. Care Med.* 1992; **20**(4): 451–457.

97. Gutierrez, G., Palizas, F., Doglio, G. *et al.* Gastric intramucosal pH as a therapeutic index of tissue oxygenation in critically ill patients. *Lancet* 1992; **339**(8787): 195–199.

98. Marik, P.E. Gastric intramucosal pH. A better predictor of multiorgan dysfunction syndrome and death than oxygen-derived variables in patients with sepsis. *Chest* 1993; **104**(1): 225–229.

99. Light, R.B. Intrapulmonary oxygen consumption in experimental pneumococcal pneumonia. *J. Appl. Physiol.* 1988; **64**(6): 2490–2495.

100. Rivers, E.P., Martin, G.B., Smithline, H. *et al.* The clinical implications of continuous central venous oxygen saturation during human CPR. *Ann. Emerg. Med.* 1992; **21**(9): 1094–1101.

101. Rady, M.Y., Rivers, E.P., Martin, G.B., Smithline, H., Appelton, T. & Nowak, R.M. Continuous central venous oximetry and shock index in the emergency department: use in the evaluation of clinical shock. *Am. J. Emerg. Med.* 1992; **10**(6): 538–541.

102. Scalea, T.M., Hartnett, R.W., Duncan, A.O. *et al.* Central venous oxygen saturation: a useful clinical tool in trauma patients. *J. Trauma* 1990; **30**(12): 1539–1543.

103. Ander, D.S., Jaggi, M., Rivers, E. *et al.* Undetected cardiogenic shock in patients with congestive heart failure presenting to the emergency department. *Am. J. Cardiol.* 1998; **82**(7): 888–891.

104. Nguyen, B., Rivers, E. & Muzzin, A. Central venous oxygen saturation/lactic acid index as an earlier indicator of survival of patients in shock (abstract). *Acad. Emerg. Med.* 2000; **7**: 586–587.

105. Gomersall, C.D., Joynt, G.M., Freebairn, R.C., Hung, V., Buckley, T.A. & Oh, T.E. Resuscitation of critically ill patients based on the results of gastric tonometry: a prospective, randomized, controlled trial. *Crit. Care Med.* 2000; **28**(3): 607–614.

106. Rivers, E., Nguyen, B., Havstad, S. *et al.* Early goal-directed therapy in the treatment of severe sepsis and septic shock. *N. Engl. J. Med.* 2001; **345**(19): 1368–1377.

107. Ma, M.H., Huang, G.T., Wang, S.M. *et al.* Aortic valve disruption and regurgitation complicating CPR detected by trans-

esophageal echocardiography. *Am. J. Emerg. Med.* 1994; **12**(5): 601–602.

108. Hilty, W.M., Hudson, P.A., Levitt, M.A. & Hall, J.B. Real-time ultrasound-guided femoral vein catheterization during cardiopulmonary resuscitation. *Ann. Emerg. Med.* 1997; **29**(3): 331–336; discussion 337.

109. Hrics, P., Wilber, S., Blanda, M.P. & Gallo, U. Ultrasound-assisted internal jugular vein catheterization in the ED. *Am. J. Emerg. Med.* 1998; **16**(4): 401–403.

110. Schlichtig, R., Kramer, D.J. & Pinsky, M.R. Flow redistribution during progressive hemorrhage is a determinant of critical O_2 delivery. *J. Appl. Physiol.* 1991; **70**(1): 169–178.

111. Bowles, S.A., Schlichtig, R., Kramer, D.J. & Klions, H.A. Arteriovenous pH and partial pressure of carbon dioxide detect critical oxygen delivery during progressive hemorrhage in dogs. *J. Crit. Care* 1992; **7**: 95–105.

112. Tremper, K.K., Mentelos, R.A. & Shoemaker, W.C. Effect of hypercarbia and shock on transcutaneous carbon dioxide at different electrode temperatures. *Crit. Care Med.* 1980; **8**(11): 608–612.

113. Tremper, K.K., Shoemaker, W.C., Shippy, C.R. & Nolan, L.S. Transcutaneous PCO_2 monitoring on adult patients in the ICU and the operating room. *Crit. Care Med.* 1981; **9**(10): 752–755.

114. Shoemaker, W.C., Thangathurai, D., Wo, C.C. *et al.* Intraoperative evaluation of tissue perfusion in high-risk patients by invasive and noninvasive hemodynamic monitoring. *Crit. Care Med.* 1999; **27**(10): 2147–2152.

115. Ivatury, R.R., Simon, R.J., Islam, S., Fueg, A., Rohman, M. & Stahl, W.M. A prospective randomized study of end points of resuscitation after major trauma: global oxygen transport indices versus organ-specific gastric mucosal pH. *J. Am. Coll. Surg.* 1996; **183**(2): 145–154.

116. Hurley, R., Chapman, M.V. & Mythen, M.G. Current status of gastrointestinal tonometry. *Curr. Opin. Crit. Care.* 2000; 6.

117. Weil, M.H., Nakagawa, Y., Tang, W. *et al.* Sublingual capnometry: a new noninvasive measurement for diagnosis and quantitation of severity of circulatory shock. *Crit. Care Med.* 1999; **27**(7): 1225–1229.

118. Nakagawa, Y., Weil, M.H., Tang, W. *et al.* Sublingual capnometry for diagnosis and quantitation of circulatory shock. *Am. J. Respir. Crit. Care Med.* 1998; **157**(6 Pt 1): 1838–1843.

119. McKinley, B.A., Parmley, C.L. & Butler, B.D. Skeletal muscle PO_2, PCO_2, and pH in hemorrhage, shock, and resuscitation in dogs. *J. Trauma* 1998; **44**(1): 119–127.

120. McKinley, B.A., Ware, D.N., Marvin, R.G. & Moore, F.A. Skeletal muscle pH, $P(CO_2)$, and $P(O_2)$ during resuscitation of severe hemorrhagic shock. *J. Trauma* 1998; **45**(3): 633–636.

121. Guyton, A.C. The systemic circulation. In Guyton, A.C., ed. *Textbood of Medical Physiology.* 6th edn. Philadelphia: W.B. Saunders, 1981: 219.

122. Shepherd, J.T. Circulation to skeletal muscle. In Shepherd, J.T., Abboud, F.M. & Geiger, S.R., eds. *Handbook of Physiology.* Vol 3. Bethesda, MD: American Physiology Society, 1983: 319–370.

123. von Planta, M., Weil, M.H., Gazmuri, R.J., Bisera, J. & Rackow, E.C. Myocardial acidosis associated with CO_2 production during cardiac arrest and resuscitation. *Circulation* 1989; **80**(3): 684–692.0

124. Reilly, P.M. & Bulkley, G.B. Vasoactive mediators and splanchnic perfusion. *Crit. Care Med.* 1993; **21**(2 Suppl): S55–S68.

125. Ward, K.R. Visceral organ ischemia and reperfusion in cardiac arrest. In Paradis, N.A., Halperin, H. & Nowak, R.M., eds. *Cardiac Arrest: The Science and Practice of Resuscitation Medicine.* Baltimore: Williams and Wilkins, 1996: 160–184.

126. Morris, D.C., Dereczyk, B.E., Grzybowski, M. *et al.* Vasopressin can increase coronary perfusion pressure during human cardiopulmonary resuscitation. *Acad. Emerg. Med.* 1997; **4**(9): 878–883.

127. Wortsman, J., Paradis, N.A., Martin, G.B. *et al.* Functional responses to extremely high plasma epinephrine concentrations in cardiac arrest. *Crit. Care Med.* 1993; **21**(5): 692–697.

128. Toung, T., Reilly, P.M., Fuh, K.C., Ferris, R. & Bulkley, G.B. Mesenteric vasoconstriction in response to hemorrhagic shock. *Shock* 2000; **13**(4): 267–273.

129. Abello, P.A., Buchman, T.G. & Bulkley, G.B. Shock and multiple organ failure. *Adv. Exp. Med. Biol.* 1994; **366**: 253–268.

130. Baron, P., Traber, L.D., Traber, D.L. *et al.* Gut failure and translocation following burn and sepsis. *J. Surg Res.* 1994; **57**(1): 197–204.

131. Deitch, E.A., Bridges, W., Berg, R., Specian, R.D. & Granger, D.N. Hemorrhagic shock-induced bacterial translocation: the role of neutrophils and hydroxyl radicals. *J. Trauma* 1990; **30**(8): 942–951; discussion 951–942.

132. Deitch, E.A. The role of intestinal barrier failure and bacterial translocation in the development of systemic infection and multiple organ failure. *Arch. Surg.* 1990; **125**(3): 403–404.

133. Deitch, E.A. Multiple organ failure. Pathophysiology and potential future therapy. *Ann. Surg.* 1992; **216**(2): 117–134.

134. Guzman, J.A. & Kruse, J.A. Splanchnic hemodynamics and gut mucosal-arterial PCO(2) gradient during systemic hypocapnia. *J. Appl. Physiol.* 1999; **87**(3): 1102–1106.

135. Guzman, J.A., Lacoma, F.J. & Kruse, J.A. Relationship between systemic oxygen supply dependency and gastric intramucosal PCO_2 during progressive hemorrhage. *J. Trauma* 1998; **44**(4): 696–700.

136. Janssens, U., Graf, J., Koch, K.C., vom Dahl, J. & Hanrath, P. Gastric tonometry in patients with cardiogenic shock and intra-aortic balloon counterpulsation. *Crit. Care Med.* 2000; **28**(10): 3449–3455.

137. Sato, Y., Weil, M.H., Tang, W. *et al.* Esophageal PCO_2 as a monitor of perfusion failure during hemorrhagic shock. *J. Appl. Physiol.* 1997; **82**(2): 558–562.

138. Povoas, H.P., Weil, M.H., Tang, W., Moran, B., Kamohara, T. & Bisera, J. Comparisons between sublingual and gastric tonometry during hemorrhagic shock. *Chest* 2000; **118**(4): 1127–1132.

139. Povoas, H.P., Weil, M.H., Tang, W., Sun, S., Kamohara, T. & Bisera, J. Decreases in mesenteric blood flow associated with increases in sublingual PCO_2 during hemorrhagic shock. *Shock* 2001; **15**(5): 398–402.

140. Marik, P.E. Sublingual capnography: a clinical validation study. *Chest* 2001; **120**(3): 923–927.

141. Tatevossian, R.G., Wo, C.C., Velmahos, G.C., Demetriades, D. & Shoemaker, W.C. Transcutaneous oxygen and CO_2 as early warning of tissue hypoxia and hemodynamic shock in critically ill emergency patients. *Crit. Care Med.* 2000; **28**(7): 2248–2253.

142. McKinley, B.A. & Butler, B.D. Comparison of skeletal muscle PO_2, PCO_2, and pH with gastric tonometric $P(CO_2)$ and pH in hemorrhagic shock. *Crit. Care Med.* 1999; **27**(9): 1869–1877.

143. Owen-Reece, H., Smith, M., Elwell, C.E. & Goldstone, J.C. Near infrared spectroscopy. *Br. J. Anaesth.* 1999; **82**(3): 418–426.

144. Cairns, C.B., Moore, F.A., Haenel, J.B. *et al.* Evidence for early supply independent mitochondrial dysfunction in patients developing multiple organ failure after trauma. *J. Trauma* 1997; **42**(3): 532–536.

145. McKinley, B.A., Marvin, R.G., Cocanour, C.S. & Moore, F.A. Tissue hemoglobin O2 saturation during resuscitation of traumatic shock monitored using near infrared spectrometry. *J. Trauma* 2000; **48**(4): 637–642.

146. Crookes, B.A., Cohn, S.M., Bloch, S. *et al.* Can near-infrared spectroscopy identify the severity of shock in trauma patients? *J. Trauma* 2005; **58**(4): 806–813; discussion 813–806.

147. Cohn, S.M., Crookes, B.A. & Proctor, K.G. Near-infrared spectroscopy in resuscitation. *J. Trauma* 2003; **54**(5 Suppl): S199–S202.

148. Ward, K.R., Ivatury, R.R., Barbee, R.W. *et al.* Near infrared spectroscopy for evaluation of the trauma patient: A technology review. *Resuscitation* 2005, **68**(1): 27–44.

149. Mullner, M., Sterz, F., Binder, M., Hirschl, M.M., Janata, K. & Laggner, A.N. Near infrared spectroscopy during and after cardiac arrest – preliminary results. *Clin. Intens. Care* 1995; **6**(3): 107–111.

150. Nemoto, E.M., Yonas, H. & Kassam, A. Clinical experience with cerebral oximetry in stroke and cardiac arrest. *Crit. Care Med.* 2000; **28**(4): 1052–1054.

151. Newman, D.H., Callaway, C.W., Greenwald, I.B. & Freed, J. Cerebral oximetry in out-of-hospital cardiac arrest: standard CPR rarely provides detectable hemoglobin-oxygen saturation to the frontal cortex. *Resuscitation* 2004; **63**(2): 189–194.

152. Buunk, G., van der Hoeven, J.G. & Meinders, A.E. A comparison of near-infrared spectroscopy and jugular bulb oximetry in comatose patients resuscitated from a cardiac arrest. *Anaesthesia* 1998; **53**(1): 13–19.

153. Moller, P. & Sylven, C. Myoglobin in human skeletal muscle. *Scand. J. Clin. Lab. Invest.* 1981; **41**(5): 479–482.

154. Nemeth, P.M. & Lowry, O.H. Myoglobin levels in individual human skeletal muscle fibers of different types. *J. Histochem. Cytochem.* 1984; **32**(11): 1211–1216.

155. Tran, T.K., Sailasuta, N., Kreutzer, U. *et al.* Comparative analysis of NMR and NIRS measurements of intracellular PO_2 in human skeletal muscle. *Am. J. Physiol.* 1999; **276**(6 Pt 2): R1682–1690.

156. Sterz, F., Leonov, Y., Safar, P. *et al.* Multifocal cerebral blood flow by Xe-CT and global cerebral metabolism after prolonged cardiac arrest in dogs. Reperfusion with open-chest CPR or cardiopulmonary bypass. *Resuscitation* 1992; **24**(1): 27–47.

157. Wolfson, S.K., Jr., Safar, P., Reich, H. *et al.* Dynamic heterogeneity of cerebral hypoperfusion after prolonged cardiac arrest in dogs measured by the stable xenon/CT technique: a preliminary study. *Resuscitation* 1992; **23**(1): 1–20.

158. Leonov, Y., Sterz, F., Safar, P., Johnson, D.W., Tisherman, S.A. & Oku, K. Hypertension with hemodilution prevents multifocal cerebral hypoperfusion after cardiac arrest in dogs. *Stroke* 1992; **23**(1): 45–53.

159. Oku, K., Kuboyama, K., Safar, P. *et al.* Cerebral and systemic arteriovenous oxygen monitoring after cardiac arrest. Inadequate cerebral oxygen delivery. *Resuscitation* 1994; **27**(2): 141–152.

160. Mullner, M., Sterz, F., Domanovits, H., Zeiner, A. & Laggner, A.N. Systemic and cerebral oxygen extraction after human cardiac arrest. *Eur. J. Emerg. Med.* 1996; **3**(1): 19–24.

161. Groner, W., Winkelman, J.W., Harris, A.G. *et al.* Orthogonal polarization spectral imaging: a new method for study of the microcirculation. *Nat. Med.* 1999; **5**(10): 1209–1212.

162. De Backer, D. OPS techniques. *Minerva Anestesiol.* 2003; **69**(5): 388–391.

163. De Backer, D., Creteur, J., Dubois, M.J., Sakr, Y. & Vincent, J.L. Microvascular alterations in patients with acute severe heart failure and cardiogenic shock. *Am. Heart J.* 2004; **147**(1): 91–99.

164. De Backer, D., Creteur, J., Preiser, J.C., Dubois, M.J. & Vincent, J.L. Microvascular blood flow is altered in patients with sepsis. *Am. J. Respir. Crit. Care Med.* 2002; **166**(1): 98–104.

165. Harris, A.G., Sinitsina, I. & Messmer, K. Validation of OPS imaging for microvascular measurements during isovolumic hemodilution and low hematocrits. *Am. J. Physiol. Heart Circ. Physiol.* 2002; **282**(4): H1502–H1509.

166. Sakr, Y., Dubois, M.J., De Backer, D., Creteur, J. & Vincent, J.L. Persistent microcirculatory alterations are associated with organ failure and death in patients with septic shock. *Crit. Care Med.* 2004; **32**(9): 1825–1831.

167. Spronk, P.E., Ince, C., Gardien, M.J., Mathura, K.R., Oudemans-van Straaten, H.M. & Zandstra, D.F. Nitroglycerin in septic shock after intravascular volume resuscitation. *Lancet* 2002; **360**(9343): 1395–1396.

168. Genzel-Boroviczeny, O., Christ, F. & Glas, V. Blood transfusion increases functional capillary density in the skin of anemic preterm infants. *Pediatr. Res.* 2004; **56**(5): 751–755.

169. Niemann, J.T., Cruz, B., Garner, D. & Lewis, R.J. Immediate countershock versus cardiopulmonary resuscitation before countershock in a 5-minute swine model of ventricular fibrillation arrest. *Ann. Emerg. Med.* 2000; **36**(6): 543–546.

170. Niemann, J.T., Cairns, C.B., Sharma, J. & Lewis, R.J. Treatment of prolonged ventricular fibrillation. Immediate countershock versus high-dose epinephrine and CPR preceding countershock. *Circulation* 1992; **85**(1): 281–287.

171. DiCola, V.C., Freedman, G.S., Downing, S.E. & Zaret, B.L. Myocsrdial uptake of technetium-99m stannous pyrophos-

phate following direct current transthoracic countershock. *Circulation* 1976; **54**(6): 980–986.

172. Osswald, S., Trouton, T.G., O'Nunain, S.S., Holden, H.B., Ruskin, J.N. & Garan, H. Relation between shock-related myocardial injury and defibrillation efficacy of monophasic and biphasic shocks in a canine model. *Circulation* 1994; **90**(5): 2501–2509.

173. Weaver, W.D., Cobb, L.A., Dennis, D., Ray, R., Hallstrom, A.P. & Copass, M.K. Amplitude of ventricular fibrillation waveform and outcome after cardiac arrest. *Ann. Intern. Med.* 1985; **102**(1): 53–55.

174. Brown, C.G. & Dzwonczyk, R. Signal analysis of the human electrocardiogram during ventricular fibrillation: frequency and amplitude parameters as predictors of successful countershock. *Ann. Emerg. Med.* 1996; **27**(2): 184–188.

175. Noc, M., Weil, M.H., Tang, W., Sun, S., Pernat, A. & Bisera, J. Electrocardiographic prediction of the success of cardiac resuscitation. *Crit. Care Med.* 1999; **27**(4): 708–714.

176. Eftestol, T., Sunde, K. & Steen, P.A. Effects of interrupting precordial compressions on the calculated probability of defibrillation success during out-of-hospital cardiac arrest. *Circulation* 2002; **105**(19): 2270–2273.

177. Marn-Pernat, A., Weil, M.H., Tang, W., Pernat, A. & Bisera, J. Optimizing timing of ventricular defibrillation. *Crit. Care Med.* 2001; **29**(12): 2360–2365.

178. Povoas, H.P., Weil, M.H., Tang, W., Bisera, J., Klouche, K. & Barbatsis, A. Predicting the success of defibrillation by electrocardiographic analysis. *Resuscitation* 2002; **53**(1): 77–82.

179. Reed, M.J., Clegg, G.R. & Robertson, C.E. Analysing the ventricular fibrillation waveform. *Resuscitation* 2003; **57**(1): 11–20.

180. Menegazzi, J.J., Callaway, C.W., Sherman, L.D. *et al.* Ventricular fibrillation scaling exponent can guide timing of defibrillation and other therapies. *Circulation* 2004; **109**(7): 926–931.

181. Callaway, C.W., Sherman, L.D., Mosesso, V.N., Jr., Dietrich, T.J., Holt, E. & Clarkson, M.C. Scaling exponent predicts defibrillation success for out-of-hospital ventricular fibrillation cardiac arrest. *Circulation* 2001; **103**(12): 1656–1661.

182. Eftestol, T., Sunde, K., Ole Aase, S., Husoy, J.H. & Steen, P.A. Predicting outcome of defibrillation by spectral characterization and nonparametric classification of ventricular fibrillation in patients with out-of-hospital cardiac arrest. *Circulation* 2000; **102**(13): 1523–1529.

183. Eftestol, T., Sunde, K., Aase, S.O., Husoy, J.H. & Steen, P.A. "Probability of successful defibrillation" as a monitor during CPR in out-of-hospital cardiac arrested patients. *Resuscitation* 2001; **48**(3): 245–254.

184. Brown, C.G., Griffith, R.F., Van Ligten, P. *et al.* Median frequency – a new parameter for predicting defibrillation success rate. *Ann. Emerg. Med.* 1991; **20**(7): 787–789.

39

Special considerations in the therapy of non-fibrillatory cardiac arrest

Tom P. Aufderheide, Todd M. Larabee, Norman A. Paradis

Medical College of Wisconsin Milwaukee, WI, USA and
University of Colorado Health Science Center, Denver, CO, USA

Non-fibrillatory cardiac arrest is a term used to encompass the defined cardiac arrest rhythms, pulseless electrical activity (PEA) and asystole, arrest rhythms that are distinct from ventricular fibrillation or pulseless ventricular tachycardia. Until recently, the term electromechanical dissociation (EMD) was used in place of PEA. EMD was defined as the presence of electrical complexes without accompanying mechanical contractions of the heart. Several studies have demonstrated that often during EMD arrest there actually is mechanical cardiac activity associated with the electrical complexes seen on a cardiac monitor.[1,2] PEA, defined as organized electrical activity with the absence of clinically detectable pulses, is thus a physiologically more appropriate terminology. Patients in asystole, by definition, have no discernible ventricular activity by electrocardiography or ultrasonography, and no associated perfusion. This chapter will focus on the diagnosis and treatment of PEA subsets.

The incidence of PEA during cardiac arrest appears to be changing. Prior to 1990, PEA was reported to be the initial presenting rhythm in approximately 20% of hospitalized patients who are monitored at the onset of cardiac arrest and 16.5% of patients who present to a prehospital system in cardiac arrest.[3,4] Several recent studies have reported the incidence of PEA to be 35%–40% of all in-hospital resuscitation events.[5–7] Data from the Ontario province advanced life support (OPALS) study found over a 4-year study period an increasing PEA incidence of 19.9% to 24.5%, with a coexisting shortened EMS system response time.[8] The OPALS group further demonstrated a 50.1% incidence of PEA arrests in the subgroup of patients that arrested after the arrival of EMS.[9] A Swedish longitudinal study demonstrated that the incidence of PEA increased from 6 to 26% over a 17-year study period (1980–1996) with an associated shorter EMS response time and an increased rate of bystander cardiopulmonary resuscitation.[10] Approximately 20% of PEA patients are successfully resuscitated, and 2–4.4% are discharged from the hospital alive.[11,12]

The reasons for the changes in incidence of PEA are unclear, but may be related to our improved diagnostic capabilities for detecting coronary artery disease.[13] Ventricular fibrillation (VF) is the most common presenting rhythm in patients with sudden cardiac death due to CAD. As our abilities to detect previously undiagnosed CAD improve, the incidence of sudden death related to this disease decreases. One theory, then, is that the decline in the rate of VF may be leading to a relative increase in the incidence of alternative cardiac arrest rhythms such as PEA.

Patients in PEA present with a spectrum of perfusion states that range from hypotension to complete absence of perfusion.[1] Approximately 80% of patients have visible echocardiographic myocardial wall motion correlated with electrocardiographic (ECG) complexes.[2] Between 40 and 50% of patients may have demonstrable aortic pressure if invasive central monitoring is accomplished.[1]

Pseudo- and true pulseless electrical activity

One of the most significant advances in understanding the spectrum of perfusion states in PEA is the recognition of pseudo- and true PEA.[1] Pseudo-PEA patients tend to be younger, have a shorter time from onset of cardiac arrest, and a higher frequency of witnessed arrests.[1,11] Patients

Cardiac Arrest: The Science and Practice of Resuscitation Medicine. 2nd edn., ed. Norman Paradis, Henry Halperin, Karl Kern, Volker Wenzel, Douglas Chamberlain. Published by Cambridge University Press. © Cambridge University Press, 2007.

in pseudo-PEA receiving cardiopulmonary resuscitation also have a higher measured coronary perfusion-pressure when compared with patients in true PEA.[1] This information supports the contention that patients in pseudo-PEA have a less deranged pathophysiologic state and may be more amenable to resuscitation. Patients with pseudo-PEA are more likely to have a return of spontaneous circulation with standard doses of epinephrine than are patients in true PEA.[4] In one study, 14 (77%) of 18 patients with pseudo-PEA who received high-dose epinephrine had return of spontaneous circulation.[1]

For these reasons, rapid differentiation of pseudo- and true PEA may assist the clinician in the choice, duration, and intensity of therapeutic intervention, possibly improving patient outcome. Consideration of electrocardiographic characteristics may assist differentiation. PEA patients who are resuscitated successfully have average QRS widths less than or equal to 0.09 +/- 0.04 second and frequently have normal initial Q-R deflection (Fig. 39.1, Tables 39.1–39.3 from past chapter).[1,11] Furthermore, no patient in pseudo-PEA had a QRS interval or initial deflection in the QRS of greater than 0.2 second.[1] Despite the strong correlation between normal duration of the QRS and pseudo-PEA, there is significant overlap.[1] Immediate emergency department echocardiography, placing a Doppler probe over the femoral artery, or rapid placement of a peripheral arterial line or central monitoring arterial catheter, can differentiate true from pseudo-PEA.

Causes of pulseless electrical activity

PEA frequently results from a primary condition that profoundly decreases preload or afterload, or causes severe inflow or outflow obstruction. The primary disorder results in hypoxia, acidosis, and increased vagal tone, which, if not rapidly reversed, affect the strength of myocardial contraction, resulting in PEA. The most common cause of PEA is severe respiratory insufficiency or respiratory arrest, reported in as many as 53% of PEA cases.[4] Mechanical causes of PEA are so classified because their etiology is related to anatomical structure and their resolution requires mechanical intervention. Tension pneumothorax causes a reduction in venous return to the heart and may be resolved with needle or tube thoracostomy. Cardiac tamponade may critically reduce left ventricular filling and may resolve with pericardiocentesis. Auto-positive end-expiratory pressure (PEEP) results in increased alveolar pressure and air trapping in ventilated patients with bronchospastic pulmonary disease. Under these circumstances, decreasing inspiratory volumes and respiratory rates decreases excessively high intrathoracic pressure (which impedes venous blood return to the heart) and may circumvent cardiovascular collapse.

Hypovolemia is the primary cause of PEA in 4%–5% of patients.[4] Massive pulmonary embolism is responsible in 1%–5%.[4,14] Numerous causes of direct myocardial dysfunction result in PEA. Acute myocardial ischemia can cause ventricular "stunning," or acute myocardial infarction may result in a critical loss of myocardial contraction. This has

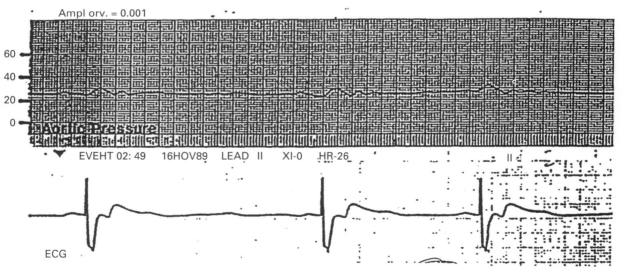

Fig. 39.1. Simultaneous aortic arch pressure (expressed in millimeters of mercury) and lead II ECG from patient in pseudo-PEA. Total QRS duration of 0.12 msec or less and especially a normal duration of initial QR deflection are more frequently seen in patients with pseudo-PEA. (From ref. 1.)

Table 39.1. Unsuccessful vs. successful resuscitations

Group [a]	Rate	Presence of P waves (%)	QT interval (s)	QRS interval (s)
Group I (n = 405)	55 ± 27 }[b]	21.0 }[b]	0.56 ± 0.2 }[b]	0.12 ± 0.06 }[b]
Group II initial (n = 98)	75 ± 45 {	42.9 {	0.46 ± 0.21 {	0.09 ± 0.04 {
Group II final (n = 98)	114 ± 36 }[b]	60.0 }[c]	0.40 ± 0.11 }[c]	0.09 ± 0.03

[a] Group I, unsuccessful resuscitations; group II, successful resuscitations.
[b] $P \leq 0.01$.
[c] $P \leq 0.04$.

Table 39.2. Duration of ECG components in patients with true PEA and pseudo-PEA[a]

	True PEA	Pseudo-PEA	P
QR	0.19 ± 0.13 (0.04–0.56)	0.07 ± 0.05 (0.02–0.20)	0.0004
RS	0.12 ± 0.08 (0.05–0.24)	0.09 ± 0.05 (0.04–0.24)	0.5
QRS	0.24 ± 0.12 (0.11–0.56)	0.12 ± 0.06 (0.04–0.26)	0.006

[a] Values are durations expressed in seconds, with range in parentheses.

Table 39.3. Characteristics of patients with true PEA and pseudo-PEA

Characteristic	True PEA	Pseudo-PEA	P
Age (yr)	71 ± 15	65 ± 15	0.7
Total arrest time (min)	25 ± 11	21 ± 13	0.44
Witnessed arrests	22/55	26/39	0.01
PO_2 (mm Hg)	237 ± 168	310 ± 134	0.03
PCO_2 (mm Hg)	34 ± 23	24 ± 16	0.04
pH	7.23 ± 0.25	7.23 ± 0.25	0.7
Coronary perfusion pressure (mm Hg)	9.9 ± 11.5	19.2 ± 9.5	<0.0001

been variably reported in 13% to 60% of non-fibrillatory arrest patients.[4,15,16] Decreased left ventricular contraction from severe congestive heart failure may produce hypotension, causing decreased coronary perfusion that further impairs myocardial function, resulting in greater hypotension and onset of PEA. Ingestion of drugs such as tricyclic antidepressants, β-blockers, calcium channel blockers, and digitalis, all of which have direct cardiotoxic effects, may result in PEA. Hyperkalemia reduces cardiac conduction and decreases inotropic activity of the heart. Hypothermia has similar effects.

Postdefibrillation pulseless electrical activity and asystole

Patients who experience immediate PEA after counter-shock from ventricular fibrillation were thought to have a better prognosis than patients in whom defibrillation fails to produce any organized rhythm.[17] The development of postdefibrillation PEA was thought to represent a transient recovery rhythm that in many cases improved spontaneously, leading to the appearance of pulses, supraventricular activity, stabilization of hemodynamic status, and possible long-term survival.[17] More recent data, however, suggest that the outcome of these patients is actually worse than in those found in primary PEA or asystole. In a 5-year retrospective study, Niemann et al. compared the outcome of a group of patients found in VF and defibrillated into PEA

or asystole to a group of patients found in PEA or asystole prior to EMS interventions.[18] Return of spontaneous circulation and survival to hospital admission was more likely in those found in primary PEA and asystole. Survival to hospital discharge was not significantly different between the groups.

Initial diagnostic maneuvers

Rapid identification of PEA subsets and reversible causes of non-fibrillatory cardiac arrest

A rapid search for reversible causes of PEA should be undertaken while resuscitative efforts are being initiated. Potentially reversible causes include: severe respiratory insufficiency, tension pneumothorax, cardiac tamponade, auto-PEEP, hypovolemia, pulmonary embolus, acute myocardial infarction, congestive heart failure, drug ingestions such as tricyclic antidepressants, β-blockers, calcium channel blockers, and digitalis, hyperkalemia, and hypothermia.

Hints to the etiology of the arrest may be obtained through the history and physical examination, and should be acted upon aggressively in order to restore coronary perfusion pressure and spontaneous circulation.

Clinical approach

History

Prehospital providers, the patient's family, medical records if immediately available, and the patient's family physician are all potential sources of information for the emergency physician caring for a patient with PEA. An estimate of time from onset of cardiac arrest and whether it was witnessed or unwitnessed may assist clinical decision-making. Witnesses or family may be able to relate the patient's symptoms before onset of arrest, such as an extended period of shortness of breath that would indicate a pulmonary cause or chest pain that would indicate a cardiac cause.

The patient's past medical history may be helpful in uncovering a possible cause for PEA. A prior history of coronary artery disease may indicate myocardial ischemia or possible myocardial infarction. Renal dialysis patients are at risk to develop severe hyperkalemia. Patients who have undergone prolonged immobilization, such as those placed in casts following an orthopedic procedure, are at risk for developing pulmonary embolus. Patients with a prior history of peptic ulcer disease or esophageal varices may have depletion of intravascular volume secondary to gastrointestinal bleeding. A history of chronic obstructive pulmonary disease (COPD) or smoking may lead the clinician to consider tension pneumothorax. A prior history of psychiatric illness or depression may lead to the consideration of a drug overdose. Documentation of severe peripheral arterial vascular disease may indicate the possibility of a false-positive diagnosis of PEA. Current medications, including tricyclic antidepressants, β-blockers, calcium channel blockers, and digitalis, should be determined and assessed for potential cardiac toxicity.

Physical examination

Airway, breathing, and circulation (ABC) should be assessed or reassessed immediately on the patient's arrival to the Emergency Department. The airway should be evalu-ated for obstruction, equal and bilateral breath sounds, and the presence of a midline trachea. The airway should be secured or prior endotracheal placement confirmed by auscultation and capnography. Initially, the patient should be ventilated with 100% oxygen to restore maximal systemic oxygenation, although excessive ventilation (resulting in increased intrathoracic pressure and impeding venous blood return to the heart) should be strictly avoided. The possibility of auto-PEEP PEA should be considered in patients with COPD or bronchospastic pulmonary disease, and the frequency and duration of ventilation further decreased accordingly.

Bilateral femoral and carotid pulses should be rapidly and carefully assessed, with and without CPR, particularly if the patient has no clinically detectable pulse. Femoral or carotid pulses should be present with adequate CPR. Immediate use of Doppler ultrasound, while briefly interrupting CPR, may reveal blood flow that was not detected by simple arterial palpation. Rapid placement of a peripheral arterial line may also be helpful. Auscultation for heart tones may also assist the clinician in determining the presence of underlying myocardial contractility.

If the patient continues in PEA, the American Heart Association advanced cardiac life support (ACLS) protocol for PEA should be initiated or continued (Fig. 39.2). While resuscitative efforts progress, further physical examination should be undertaken to identify causes that may be reversible. Evidence of deep venous thrombosis in the lower extremities may indicate a pulmonary embolus, whereas evidence of an arteriovenous fistula may indicate a renal dialysis patient who is at risk for hyperkalemia. A rectal examination should be performed, a nasogastric tube placed, and a gastric aspirate acquired to uncover signs of gastrointestinal bleeding. A core temperature should also be obtained, if appropriate, before discontinuing resuscitation efforts.

Ancillary evaluation

Ancillary data should be gathered in an expeditious and directed fashion. As soon as the patient is placed on a cardiac monitor, a rhythm strip or 12-lead electrocardiogram should be acquired to determine Q-R and QRS duration. A Q-R or QRS duration of less than or equal to 0.2 second is highly correlated with pseudo-PEA.[1] If not already accomplished, Doppler ultrasound should be performed in all patients with PEA to detect blood flow not revealed by arterial palpation. Immediate emergency department echocardiography, where available, may greatly assist in identifying the PEA subtype. Normal echocardiographic wall motion indicates PEA possibly due to a readily reversible cause, such as hypovolemia or tension pneumothorax. Wall motion that is present but decreased may indicate pseudo-PEA, whereas absent wall motion represents true PEA. Immediate echocardiography also may identify acute cardiac tamponade, pulmonary embolus, ruptured intraventricular septum or ventricle, or pericardial effusion and tamponade. Rapid placement of central arterial monitoring catheters may also help to identify subsets of PEA patients, differentiating pseudo- and true PEA. Chest radiography is useful for diagnosis of pneumothorax, congestive heart failure, or, in the presence of an enlarged cardiac silhouette, possible cardiac tamponade.

Specific therapies for reversible etiologies

Figures 39.2 and 39.3 summarize the therapeutic interventions in PEA.

As previously stated, an aggressive initial evaluation should be undertaken in a patient who presents with PEA arrest to discern any immediately reversible etiologies for the arrest. This section will focus on the therapeutic interventions for these reversible causes.

Hypovolemia

Hypovolemia is the primary cause of PEA in 4 to 5% of patients.[4] Reports of bloody stools, fevers or possible sepsis, or signs of recent trauma can all direct the provider to consider hypovolemia as a potential cause of the PEA arrest. Physical examination may show guaiac-positive stools in support of the history. Aggressive intravenous fluid resuscitation is warranted in all patients presenting with PEA arrest to ensure adequate preload.

Hypoxia

There are many etiologies for hypoxemic states, all of which can result in PEA cardiac arrest. Obvious causes such as asphyxiation and strangulation will be apparent by history and physical examination. Patients with a history of COPD or asthma are at risk for hypoxemia and hypercarbia as well as associated complications, such as tension pneumothorax. Severe hypoxemia may also be related to infection or to coagulation disorders resulting in pulmonary embolism. Information obtained from available history and medical records may help discern the underlying etiology for hypoxemic states. Physical examination should focus on symmetry of breath sounds and adventitious sounds, as well as jugular venous pulsations and distention. Skin crepitus may be helpful in diagnosing pneumothorax. Chest radiography is useful early during resuscitation for cases of tension pneumothorax that are not clinically apparent or other pulmonary causes. Pulse oximetry is rarely useful because of low or absent peripheral perfusion and arterial vasoconstriction. Depending on the primary cause, patient management in all hypoxemic situations should be directed at securing a permanent airway through endotracheal intubation and appropriate ventilatory management. For example, patients with COPD may have a high degree of auto-PEEP due to increased air trapping that results in elevated intrathoracic pressures, decreased venous blood return to the heart, and decreased forward blood flow.[19,20] Management of ventilation for any patient with PEA should focus on maximizing coronary perfusion pressure (forward blood flow) during CPR. Following establishment of an advanced airway, ventilation rates should not exceed 8–10 breaths per minute and each breath should be limited to 1 second. Even lower ventilation rates for patients with auto-PEEP may be required to achieve adequately reduced intrathoracic pressure at the necessary expense of permissive hypercapnia.

Cardiac tamponade

Cardiac tamponade is an uncommon etiology in the presentation of non-fibrillatory arrest. A patient with a history of cancer, recent cardiothoracic surgery, renal failure and dialysis, coagulopathy, platelet disorder, or chest trauma may suggest this diagnosis. Physical findings such as distended neck veins, muffled heart tones, and pulsus paradoxus are helpful if they can be reliably determined, but are difficult to establish during the initial phases of resuscitation and may be absent. Cardiac tamponade is best diagnosed with early bedside ultrasonography on patient arrival in the emergency department.[21,22] Electrical alternans may be apparent on the electrocardiogram in cases of pseudo-PEA owing to the "swinging of the heart while beating," usually associated with effusions of 300–600 ml.[23,24] Specific therapy for cardiac tamponade includes fluid administration, pericardiocentesis, thoracostomy, and, if required, resuscitative thoracotomy.

Volume expansion with crystalloid infusion may be used as a temporizing maneuver while the clinician is preparing for pericardiocentesis or thoracotomy. Gascho *et al.* studied the effects of volume expansion and vasodilation in a canine non-arrest model of acute pericardial tamponade.[25] They found that volume expansion alone, and in conjunction with vasodilation with nitroprusside, improved tissue blood flow. Vasodilation should not be used during cardiac arrest secondary to pericardial tamponade; drainage of the tamponade is the therapy of choice. The subxiphoid technique is best used for pericardiocentesis since it avoids injury to the coronary arteries. The subxiphoid region should be quickly prepared with a povidine-iodine solution and a 16- to 18-gauge catheter over needle introduced between the xiphoid process and the left subcostal angle at a 30 to 45 degree angle to the skin. The tip of the needle should be directed at the inferior tip of the left scapula. This procedure may be difficult and dangerous while CPR is in progress and the clinician should discontinue CPR for 30 seconds while attempts at drainage are made. If unsuccessful, CPR should resume for several minutes and another attempt at drainage should be made. When fluid is aspirated, the catheter is advanced into the pericardial space and the needle

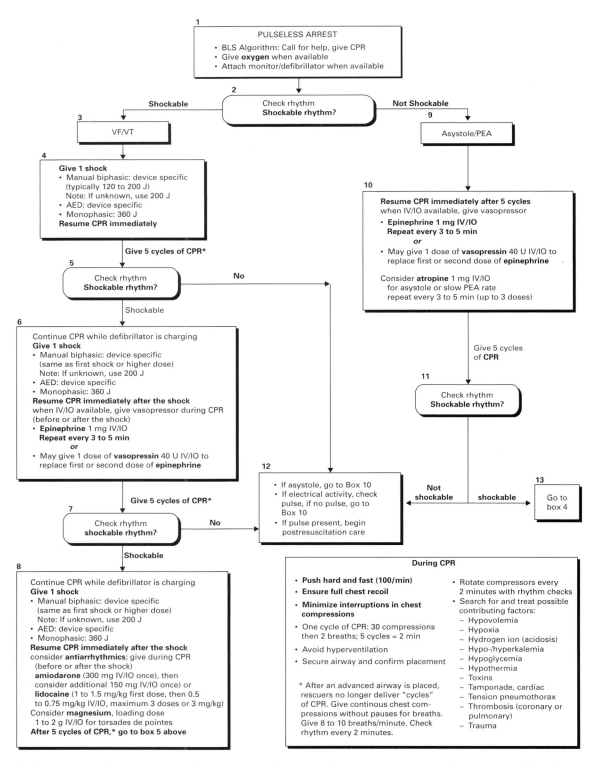

Fig. 39.2. American Heart Association Algorithm for Pulseless Arrest. (From the American Heart Association Guidelines for Cardiopulmonary Resuscitation and Emergency Cardiovascular Care Pt 7.2: Management of Cardiac Arrest. *Circulation* 2005; **112** (Suppl I): IV-59.

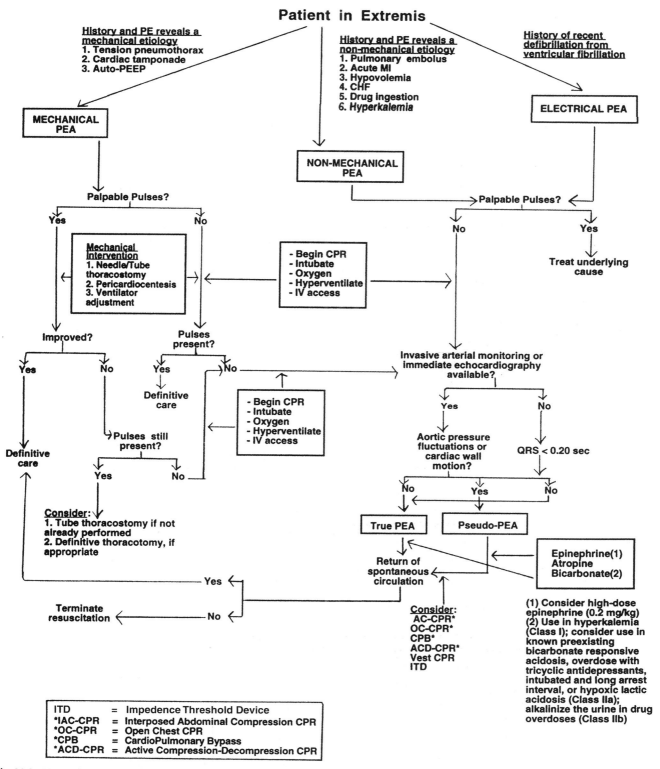

Fig. 39.3. PEA patient management algorithm. *PE*, physical examination; *MI*, myocardial infarction; *CHF*, congestive heart failure; *IV*, intravenous.

removed. A three-way stopcock should be attached to permit repeated aspirations if necessary.[26]

If this technique is unsuccessful and cardiac tamponade is still highly suspected, a resuscitative thoracotomy can be performed. The benefit of this approach is unclear because there have been no outcome studies of thoracotomy in non-traumatic PEA cardiac arrest. The clinician must weigh the benefits of direct pericardial drainage and open cardiac massage with the possible long-term morbidity from instituting this invasive technique in the presence of prolonged, low flow cardiac arrest. Conversely, thoracotomy may be both diagnostic and therapeutic in PEA arrest: the clinician can directly observe the myocardium for signs of mechanical activity (allowing differentiation of pseudo- and true PEA) and, with internal massage, amplify the ineffectual contractions in pseudo-PEA.

When performing thoracotomy, a left anterolateral incision over the fourth interspace provides the best access to the heart. Once the chest is entered, the pericardium should be inspected for evidence of pericardial tamponade. If tamponade is present, the pericardium should be opened via an incision anterior and parallel to the phrenic nerve.[27] Once the pericardial fluid is drained, and if return of spontaneous circulation occurs, the thoracotomy must be closed in the operating room.

Tension pneumothorax

Pirolo *et al.* reviewed the autopsy files of 50 patients who had died after documented episodes of PEA and found a 4% (2 of 50) incidence of pneumothorax.[3] This condition is suggested by unilateral decreased breath sounds after endotracheal intubation, jugular venous distention, devi-ation of the trachea away from the side of pneumothorax, and hyperresonance to percussion over the affected hemithorax. The clinician should first determine appropriate placement of the endotracheal tube by auscultating the epigastrium to rule out esophageal intubation. Bilateral breath sounds should also be assessed, and, if unilaterally reduced, the endotracheal tube should be withdrawn slightly to rule out endobronchial intubation. Proper placement of the endotracheal tube can also be confirmed by end-tidal CO_2 capnography. Since the esophagus can have low levels of CO_2 present, the end-tidal CO_2 should be monitored over several breaths. Continued presence of CO_2 confirms proper endotracheal tube placement.[28] If decreased breath sounds persist after these maneuvers, needle thoracostomy should be performed, followed by tube thoracostomy. Needle thoracostomy may be performed with a large catheter over needle system (14 to 18 gauge). The system should be attached to a syringe and the insertion site

quickly prepared with povidine-iodine (1 to 2 seconds). The needle should be introduced in the second intercostal interspace in the midclavicular line. Once the pleural space is entered, the catheter should be advanced over the needle and air aspirated through the syringe. A three-way stopcock should be attached to the catheter to permit repeated aspirations as necessary.[29] Once time permits (usually after return of spontaneous circulation), tube thoracostomy should be performed. If the clinician still suspects pneumothorax following unsuccessful needle thoracostomy, however, definitive tube thoracostomy should be performed immediately. Of note, needle thoracostomy should only be performed when pneumothorax is suspected by history or physical examination. The cavalier performance of bilateral needle thoracostomy in all patients in PEA is not warranted and may increase postresuscitation morbidity.

Hypothermia

There are numerous documented cases of accidental hypothermia and prolonged cardiac arrest that have been successfully resuscitated after instituting re-warming protocols. The lowest recorded temperature in a patient who suffered from accidental hypothermia with successful resuscitation is 13.7 °C (56.7 °F) in an adult[30] and 14.4 °C (57.9 °F) in a child.[31] It may be difficult to determine by history and physical if the initial event leading to cardiac arrest was due to hypothermia or to another etiology with resulting hypothermia. History and physical should be undertaken to determine primary from secondary accidental hypothermia. Cold-reading thermometers are needed to record core body temperatures accurately in this population. The characteristic Osborn waves on the electrocardiogram in patients with a cardiac rhythm appears as a deflection at the J-point in the direction of the QRS complex.

Passive rewarming techniques (warm packs, warming blankets) are not indicated in hypothermic patients in cardiac arrest. Treatment of severely hypothermic patients (core temperature <30 °C (86 °F)) in arrest should be directed at active core rewarming techniques, including warm humidified air via endotracheal tube, warm peritoneal lavage, warm intravenous fluids, and extracorporeal cardiopulmonary bypass. Forced air rewarming techniques have been described[32,33] as well as intrathoracic lavage.[34] Walpoth *et al.* examined the long-term outcomes of 32 patients who underwent extracorporeal cardiopulmonary bypass for severe accidental hypothermia.[35] Of the 15 long-term survivors, no adverse neurologic sequelae were documented, and the group had an average time from discovery to extracorporeal warming of 141 + /− 50 minutes. Owing to the need for prolonged periods of CPR in these patients, a mechanical compression device is advocated to ensure consistent delivery of compressions.[36] Resuscitation efforts may be withheld for patients with associated lethal body injuries, those found with an ice mask, and those who are so frozen as to hinder chest compressions.[37] Rewarming efforts in the remainder of the population should continue until body temperature approaches normal and there is no response to ACLS protocols. In patients who are refractory to rewarming, efforts should also be discontinued.

Pulmonary embolism

Pulmonary embolism is a less common cause of cardiac arrest. The overall incidence of disease is debatable, but estimates of 1%–5% are reported in the literature.[2,104,123] For those patients who present primarily as PEA arrest, however, the incidence may be >50%.[37,38] Sudden cardiac arrest in a young, otherwise healthy patient should raise suspicion for this cause. History should probe for causes of hypercoagulability including use of oral contraceptives, prolonged immobility, recent orthopedic surgeries, and cancer, among others. Physical examination should focus on pulmonary auscultation and examination of the lower extremities for signs of deep venous thrombosis, such as unilateral edema or palpable posterior cords. These physical findings, however, are unreliable and may be absent. For those patients with a presenting rhythm, the 12-lead electrocardiogram may show evidence of right ventricular strain or right atrial enlargement (P-pulmonale in lead II). The classically described S1, Q3, T3 pattern is related to the axis shift associated with right ventricular strain, but is present in less than 5% of patients with pulmonary embolus. Tachycardia and non-specific ST-T changes are the most common presenting finding on the electrocardiogram, but 25% of patients will have no change in their EKG from baseline.[39] Bedside echocardiography may show evidence of a dilated right ventricle, indicating elevated pulmonary arterial pressures. In patients without evidence of an alternative diagnosis following history, physical examination, ECG and chest radiography, and in those for whom the clinician has a high suspicion for embolism without contraindications, thrombolytic therapy should be initiated empirically. It should be started as soon as possible while high quality CPR continues. CPR should continue for a time sufficient for the thrombolytic therapy to dislodge the clot (at least 45 minutes to 1 hour).

Hyperkalemia

Hyperkalemia as the etiology of non-fibrillatory arrest should be suspected in patients with renal dysfunction. Any patient with a history of end stage renal disease or dialysis who presents in arrest should be immediately treated for presumed hyperkalemia. Other etiologies for hyperkalemia include excessive use of salt substitute, rhabdomyolysis, tumor lysis syndrome, adrenal insufficiency, and multiple recent transfusions. Hyperkalemia is also extensively described associated with the use of succinylcholine and related rhabdomyolysis.[40,41] In patients with a presenting cardiac rhythm, the electrocardiogram is the most useful diagnostic tool. The earliest electrocardiographic sign of hyperkalemia is tall symmetric T waves in the anterior leads.[42] There is a progression of further EKG changes that correlate poorly with serum potassium levels.[43] These include prolongation of the PR interval or QRS interval, P-wave flattening with eventual disappearance, a sinusoidal wave pattern, and eventually ventricular fibrillation. Since hyperkalemic patients die as a resut of an arrhythmia, immediate cardiac membrane stabilization should be undertaken by intravenous administration of calcium chloride (8–16 mg/kg) (unless a contraindication exists such as coexisting use of digoxin). This should be followed by intravenous sodium bicarbonate (1 mEq/kg bolus), often with repeated doses until electrocardiographic changes are evident. This should then be followed by 10 units of regular intravenous insulin and one ampule of intravenous D50. Onset of therapeutic action of insulin is about 30 minutes. Emergency dialysis should be considered once the patient has been resuscitated.

Metabolic acidosis

Severe metabolic acidosis exerts a negative inotropic effect on the heart. In particular, severe acidosis can impair cardiac contractility, increase pulmonary vascular resistance, sensitize the myocardium to arrhythmia, and lower the threshold for ventricular fibrillation. These changes in myocardial function occur in conjunction with an associated hyperkalemia that can accompany severe acidosis because of action of the potassium-hydrogen ion exchange pump at the cellular level. The causes of metabolic acidosis are categorized into non-anion gap and high-anion gap. Acute severe metabolic acidosis leading to cardiac dysfunction and arrest is more commonly due to the high-anion gap etiology, including diabetic ketoacidosis, uremia, lactic acidosis, and multiple toxic ingestions including salicylates, methanol, paraldehyde, and isopropranol. Multiple medications have been associated with the development of a severe metabolic acidosis, including metformin, colchicine, arginine, and herbicides.[44–47] Starvation and physical restraint have also been documented as etiologies of severe metabolic acidosis and arrest.[48,49] Attempting to determine whether metabolic acidosis is the etiology of cardiac arrest can be difficult, as prolonged arrest can lead to a lactic acidosis. Laboratory evaluation should include a basic chemistry panel, a serum lactate level, and an arterial blood gas. Treatment should be directed at the underlying etiology of the acidosis. Bicarbonate therapy for acidosis is controversial because of acid-base shifts in the cerebral spinal fluid, but is generally recommended for a serum pH less than 6.9 and should be considered if the serum pH is less than 7.1.

Myocardial infarction/ischemia

Although the largest contributing disease among all causes of sudden cardiac death, the incidence of myocardial infarction as a primary cause of non-fibrillatory arrest appears lower, with reported ranges from 13% to 60% of all causes.[4,15,16] The diagnosis should be considered in all patients with a past medical history of coronary artery disease or those who have the known risk factors for the disease. A history from EMS workers, family, or other witnesses of patient symptoms preceding arrest is also helpful. An early 12-lead electrocardiogram should be obtained in all patients with a presenting cardiac rhythm, as acute ischemic changes may be evident and will direct further therapy. If the diagnosis of acute myocardial infarction is made, therapy must be directed at thrombus disruption or removal. Depending upon the institution, the patient can be transported to the cardiac catheterization laboratory for emergent intervention while resuscitative efforts are continued, or thrombolytic therapy can be initiated in the emergency department. The use of thrombolytic therapy during resuscitation from cardiac arrest remains controversial. An initial study of thrombolytics in patients presenting with cardiac arrest showed significantly increased rates of return of spontaneous circulation and ICU admission,[50] while a second study in patients with PEA cardiac arrest demonstrated no benefit,[51] but was possibly confounded by patient selection criteria and timing of thrombolytic therapy during the study.[52,53] The use of thrombolytics for patients with non-fibrillatory cardiac arrest, in whom resuscitative efforts are initially unsuccessful, is an appropriate area for ongoing research.[54]

Non-specific therapy for non-fibrillatory cardiac arrest

In many cases of non-fibrillatory cardiac arrest, the clinical presentation does not clearly indicate any immediately reversible etiology. Although the overall goal during a resuscitation is to treat any reversible etiology, non-specific pharmacologic therapies should be initiated quickly in an effort to improve coronary perfusion pressure, cardiac output, and perfusion of other vital organs. This section will address the role of various pharmacologic agents in accomplishing this task.

Adrenergic agents

Adrenergic agents have long been known to improve resuscitation because of their vasoactive properties, specifically α-adrenergic stimulation. The specific physiologic response to adrenergic stimulation is improved coronary perfusion pressure (coronary diastolic arteriovenous perfusion gradient). Increased coronary perfusion pressure has been shown experimentally and clinically to predict return of spontaneous circulation.[55,56] Adrenaline has been the adrenergic agent of choice in cardiac arrest, but appropriate dosing has been questioned. Higher doses of epinephrine have been shown to improve regional myocardial blood flow, coronary perfusion pressure, and defibrillation rates in animal models of ventricular fibrillation arrest,[57–60] but clinical studies have not confirmed this benefit.

Some studies have been undertaken which address the use on high-dose epinephrine in non-fibrillatory cardiac arrest. As previously noted, a subgroup of patients present in pseudo-PEA cardiac arrest, with aortic pressure fluctuations detectable by aortic catheter. This subgroup of patients possibly would benefit from high-dose epinephrine. Paradis *et al.* studied the administration of standard or high-dose epinephrine to patients with pseudo- and true PEA and found the best response to resuscitative efforts (e.g., return of spontaneous circulation) in patients with pseudo-PEA who received high-dose epinephrine (14 of 18 [78%]). Nevertheless, no patient in this study survived to hospital discharge.[1] Lindner *et al.* performed a clinical study comparing high-dose epinephrine (5 mg) to standard dose epinephrine (1 mg) in PEA and asystolic cardiac arrest.[61] Return of spontaneous circulation was achieved in 56% (5 of 9) patients with high-dose epinephrine and 7% (1 of 14) standard dose epinephrine patients ($P<0.05$). Hospital discharge rates were 22% (2 of 9) in the high-dose epinephrine group and 7% (1 of 14) in the standard dose epinephrine group. This difference in hospital discharge rates was not statistically significant.[61] In a multicenter study of high-dose epinephrine (0.2 mg/kg) in prehospital cardiac arrest, Brown *et al.* found that patients presenting with PEA had higher rates of return of spontaneous circulation compared to patients receiving standard dose epinephrine (0.02 mg/kg) (47% versus 33%, respectively; $P<0.05$).[62] The hospital discharge rates and neurologic outcomes for this subgroup of patients were not reported.[62] In another multicenter study of high-dose epinephrine, Stiell *et al.* found no difference in resuscitation and discharge rates in patients receiving high-dose epinephrine (7 mg) or standard dose epinephrine (1 mg).[63] Since this study included in-hospital cardiac arrests, the results are difficult to compare with those in other studies. Furthermore, prehospital arrest patients did not receive epinephrine in the prehospital setting; instead, they received their epinephrine after hospital arrival, approximately 21 minutes after arrest.

Adverse effects associated with use of adrenaline, including increased myocardial oxygen consumption and ventricular dysrryhthmia, have been a stimulus to find the best vasoactive agent for use during cardiac arrest. Various adrenergic agents have been compared, with equivocal results.[57,60,64–68] Most previous work with adrenergic agent dose response and comparisons of various adrenergic agents has been performed in ventricular fibrillation models of cardiac arrest,[57,60,64–67] whereas the dose and type of adrenergic agents used in PEA cardiac arrest have not been extensively studied. Ralston *et al.* studied a postcountershock model of PEA and found the median effective dose (ED 50) of epinephrine to be 14 μg/kg intravenously and 130 μg/kg endotracheally.[69] Lindner and Ahnefeld compared epinephrine and norepinephrine (45 mg/kg) in an asphyxiation PEA model and found a resuscitation rate of 100% with both drugs.[70] Epinephrine resulted in resuscitation earlier than did norepinephrine, but no hemodynamic differences were noted between the drugs. DeBehnke *et al.* compared standard dose epinephrine (0.02 mg/kg) and high-dose epinephrine (0.2 mg/kg) in a postcountershock model of PEA and found no difference in return of spontaneous circulation rates between groups; however, coronary perfusion pressure was higher in the high-dose epinephrine group.[71]

Methoxamine is a pure α-adrenergic agonist and therefore lacks β-adrenergic activity, which may be detrimental during cardiac resuscitation.[72] In an asphyxial model of PEA, Redding *et al.* found a 100% resuscitation rate with use of methoxamine (20 mg).[73] In a clinical study of PEA arrest, methoxamine (10 mg) and epinephrine (1 mg) were compared in 80 cases of prehospital and in-hospital PEA arrest. A resuscitation rate of 55% (22 of 40) was found in each group, with only one patient who received epinephrine being discharged from the hospital.[74] Notably, the dose of methoxamine in this clinical study (10 mg or approximately 0.14 mg/kg in a 70-kg patient) was substantially lower than the dose used in the animal experiment (20 mg or approximately 1 mg/kg in a 20-kg dog). Patrick *et al.* performed a clinical study with higher doses of methoxamine.[75] Sixty-eight PEA patients received 20 mg of methoxamine followed by 40 mg 4 minutes later and were compared to 77 patients who received 2 mg of epinephrine followed by 2 mg every 4 minutes during resuscitation. They found no differences in return of spontaneous circulation, survival to hospital discharge, or neurologic status of those patients discharged between the two groups. Similarly, Olson *et al.* performed a prospective, randomized, double-blind out-of-hospital clinical trial administering equipressor doses of epinephrine (0.5 mg) and methoxamine (5 mg) to 102 patients in ventricular fibrillation refractory to initial defibrillations. The rates of return of spontaneous circulation and admission to the emergency department with a pulse did not differ between the two groups. There was an insignificant trend toward improved survival to hospital discharge in the epinephrine group (19.6% vs. 7.8%, $P = 0.07$).[76]

Phenylephrine, another pure α-adrenergic agonist, has been investigated for use in cardiac arrest. When 1 mg of epinephrine was compared to 10 mg of phenylephrine in 13-kg dogs, there were no differences in hemodynamics, resuscitation rates, and neurologic deficit scores.[77] There also was no difference in resuscitation on 24-hour survival between epinephrine and phenylephrine in a canine ventricular fibrillation cardiac arrest model.[78] Brown *et al.* compared 0.2 mg/kg epinephrine, with 0.1 mg/kg and 1 mg/kg phenylephrine in a swine ventricular fibrillation model and found improved defibrillation rates, myocardial blood flow, and oxygen extraction ratios in animals receiving epinephrine.[60] In a similar study, some of these investigators showed that 10 mg/kg of phenylephrine was no different from 0.2 mg/kg of epinephrine in improving regional cerebral blood flow in a swine model.[64] One clinical study of out-of-hospital cardiac arrest compared 1 mg of phenylephrine to 0.5 mg of epinephrine and found no difference in the return of spontaneous circulation rates.[67] In total, these studies investigated the use of phenylephrine in cardiac arrest and found equivocal results.

β_1-Stimulation with agents such as isoproterenol produce improved chronotropy. β-Stimulation also causes vasodilation, however, which will decrease cerebral and myocardial blood flow. Until further research on the use of β-agonists in PEA arrest is performed, this potentially detrimental physiologic effect precludes its use for this condition.[79]

The literature on the use of adrenergic agents in non-fibrillatory arrest is mixed. Problems with previous experimental models include the diversity of models chosen (postcountershock versus asphyxial), variability of adrenergic doses used, and lack of a neurologic outcome model. From the available data, it is reasonable to recommend standard dose epinephrine (1 mg) as an initial dose in non-fibrillatory arrest. In a patient with pseudo-PEA, either documented through invasive monitoring or suspected by ECG analysis or echocardiography, a trial of high-dose epinephrine appears reasonable. Further studies evaluating long-term survival and neurologic recovery in pseudo-PEA arrest are required before a stronger recommendation for high-dose epinephrine can be made.

Vasopressin

Vasopressin is a peptide hormone naturally produced in the pituitary gland whose main physiologic function is related to free water balance (antidiuretic hormone) with actions at the level of the kidney. At concentrations above normal physiologic levels, it has been found to have direct effects at the level of the arterioles as a potent vasoconstrictor. In this regard, some authors have advocated its use during resuscitation in conjunction with, or in place of, epinephrine.[80–85] Several studies have been undertaken to address these issues. Wenzel, *et al.*[68] in a randomized comparison of vasopressin and epinephrine for out-of-hospital cardiac resuscitation, analyzed 1186 patients, of whom 589 received vasopressin and 597 received epinephrine. They found no significant differences between the groups related to return of spontaneous circulation, hospital admission, or hospital discharge. The authors performed a subset analysis of 104 PEA patients in the vasopressin group as compared to 82 patients in the epinephrine group. Again, no significant differences were found in the rates of return of spontaneous circulation, hospital admission, or hospital discharge between the groups. In a meta-analysis of 1519 cardiac arrest patients from five randomized controlled trials comparing vasopressin and epinephrine, Aung and Htay[86] found no significant differences between the vasopressin and epinephrine groups related to return of spontaneous circulation, death before hospital admission, death within 24 hours, death before hospital discharge, or combination of number of deaths and neurologically impaired survivors. In the PEA subset analysis (145 patients in the vasopressin group and 133 patients in the epinephrine group), no significant difference was found between groups with respect to the rate of death before hospital discharge.

Although the data are limited, there appears to be no specific beneficial effect of vasopressin on outcomes of patients in PEA arrest as compared to those treated with epinephrine. No studies have been implemented to examine this drug's effect on outcomes from patients found in PEA cardiac arrest, nor have studies examined the effect of vasopressin on the outcomes of patients who have pseudo-PEA.

Atropine

Atropine has been recommended in cases of bradycardic PEA owing to its cardioacceleratory properties. The effects of atropine in PEA have been less than convincing. Redding *et al.* studied atropine (0.5 mg), comparing it to methoxamine (20 mg) and calcium chloride (5 ml of a 10% solution), and found that methoxamine significantly improved resuscitation compared to atropine and calcium chloride.[73] Atropine was found to be no different from calcium chloride in this model of PEA arrest.[73] The only clinical study of atropine in PEA compared 2 mg of atropine with placebo in patients with slow, pulseless idioventricular rhythms and found no difference in resuscitation rates.[87] Currently, ACLS guidelines recommend a total atropine dose of 0.04 mg/kg as a vagolytic dose in bradycardic PEA (<60 beats/ minute) and asystole.[88] This dose of atropine is based on several studies of patients undergoing spinal anesthesia or healthy volunteers.[89,90] None of the patients in these studies were in cardiac arrest or a low cardiac output state. DeBehnke has questioned the dose of atropine in PEA arrest.[91] He studied the effects of surgical vagolysis in asphyxial PEA arrest and found improved return of spontaneous circulation rates in animals that received vagotomy. This study supports the contention that vagolysis is important in resuscitation from PEA arrest. In a second animal study, Debehnke *et al.* compared standard and high dose atropine in a canine model of PEA arrest.[92] No differences in resuscitation rates were observed between the groups, and the rates tended to decrease in the higher dose groups. Currently, administration of 0.04 mg/kg of atropine in bradycardic PEA and asystolic arrest is recommended.

Sodium bicarbonate

Past data indicated that bicarbonate administration in cardiac arrest was detrimental because of paradoxical cerebrospinal fluid acidosis, inability to reverse myocardial acidosis, and potential decreases in coronary perfusion pressure.[93–95] Further study of this issue remained controversial, as some experimental and clinical studies of the use of bicarbonate in cardiac arrest had not shown any benefit,[96] and other investigators demonstrated benefit during cardiac arrest.[97–99] Most recent data support the use of sodium bicarbonate or a buffering solution during cardiac arrest.[100–103] No study has specifically addressed the issue of bicarbonate use in non-fibrillatory cardiac arrest. Vanags *et al.* retrospectively studied various interventions in out-of-hospital PEA cardiac arrest and found that administration of bicarbonate was as effective as epinephrine and atropine in generating pulses.[104] Since this study was retrospective, only a temporal relationship to drug administration could be observed. Patients whose last drug administered was bicarbonate had similar return of spontaneous circulation and save rates compared to those whose last drug administered was epinephrine or atropine. A prospective randomized clinical trial of bicarbonate use in cardiac arrest and in non-fibrillatory arrest is necessary to determine definitively the optimal role for bicarbonate during cardiac arrest. The use of bicarbonate has been shown to be beneficial in patients with shock secondary to tricyclic antidepressant, aspirin, and phenobarbital overdose and in cases of hyperkalemia.[105–107] Hence, bicarbonate therapy might also be useful in cases of PEA arrest secondary to these causes.[105–107] In these situ-ations, the initial dose of bicarbonate should be 1 mEq/kg intravenously, followed by 0.5 mEq/kg 10 minutes later. If arterial blood gas values are available, the bicarbonate dosing should be titrated based on the calculated base deficit.[107]

Other agents

Calcium

Older ACLS guidelines have included calcium in the PEA resuscitation protocol.[108] This was based on the hypothesis that calcium ions would enhance myocardial contraction and aid in resuscitation. In the early 1980s, the effectiveness of calcium use during cardiac arrest was questioned. Animal and clinical studies demonstrate that calcium does not improve resuscitation in PEA arrest.[109–112] There may be a subgroup of patients in PEA, however, who would benefit from calcium administration. Stueven et al. retrospectively divided PEA patients by QRS morphology and found that patients with wide QRS complexes (<0.12 second) or peaked T waves and ST-segment elevation were more easily resuscitated when calcium was administered (8 of 39 vs. 1 of 31; $P<0.028$).[112]

When hyperkalemia, hypocalcemia (such as seen following massive blood transfusion), or calcium-channel blocker overdose is the cause of PEA cardiac arrest, calcium administration may be life-saving. A 10% solution of calcium chloride provides 27.3 mg of elemental calcium/ml. The recommended dose of calcium chloride is 2 to 4 mg of elemental calcium/kg, which equals approximately 10 ml of the calcium chloride solution. A 10% solution of calcium gluconate provides 18 mg of elemental calcium/ml, so that 10 to 15 ml of the solution will be needed to provide 2 to 4 mg of elemental calcium/kg. These doses can be repeated every 10 minutes as needed.[107]

Glucagon

Glucagon has been shown to have chronotropic and inotropic properties because of its non-adrenergically mediated stimulation of myocardial adenyl cyclase.[113,119] Niemann et al. studied the effects of 1 mg of glucagon on resuscitation from postdefibrillation PEA and found a significant improvement in return of spontaneous circulation rates in animals receiving glucagon.[115] No clinical study of glucagon use in PEA arrest has been performed, and its use cannot be recommended. Glucagon has been shown to be beneficial in cases of β-blocker overdose, however, and should be considered in cases of PEA arrest secondary to overdose with these agents.[106] The dose is 3 to 10 mg intravenously and an infusion of 2 to 5 mg/hour after return of spontaneous circulation is achieved.[106]

Naloxone

There is speculation that naloxone may increase arterial pressure in various shock states. Rothstein et al. administered naloxone (5 mg/kg) after postcountershock PEA and showed return of spontaneous circulation in 100% of animals (4 of 4).[116] There has been no clinical study of naloxone use in PEA arrest. Nevertheless, naloxone should be used in dosages of 2 to 10 mg intravenously in patients with narcotic-induced PEA arrest.[106] A case report documents the use of naloxone in asystolic out-of-hospital arrest due to opioid ingestion with return of spontaneous circulation.[117]

Aminophylline

Aminophylline is a competitive antagonist of adenosine and has been used to treat conduction disturbances and bradycardia in stable patients.[118–120] Viskin et al. administered 250 mg of aminophylline in patients with bradyasystolic arrest refractory to atropine and epinephrine and achieved return of spontaneous circulation in 73% (11 of 15) of patients, but only one patient was discharged from the hospital alive.[121] A recent review of 16 previous articles describing the use of aminophylline in PEA and asystole suggests that the drug may be useful in some cases of non-fibrillatory arrest refractory to epinephrine and atropine.[122] Mader et al. have reported the most recent article related to the use of aminophylline in non-fibrillatory arrest.[123] In a randomized controlled trial of aminophylline vs. placebo as an adjunct to atropine-resistant prehospital asystolic cardiac arrest, they reported a trend towards improvement in ROSC and reversal of asystole in the aminophylline group. Fewer patients in the aminophylline group survived to hospital admission, and none were alive at 24 hours. The benefits for use of this drug during non-fibrillatory cardiac arrest require further investigation.

Improved hemodynamics during CPR in non-fibrillatory cardiac arrest

One of the most promising interventions in patients with PEA and asystole is improved hemodynamics during CPR. There is an inversely proportional relationship between mean intrathoracic pressure, coronary perfusion pressure, and survival from cardiac arrest.[124,126] Increased ventilation rates and increased ventilation duration impede venous blood return to the heart, decreasing forward blood flow to the heart and brain during CPR.[124–127] Conversely, generation of negative intrathoracic pressure on the upstroke of CPR augments venous blood return to the heart, significantly improving hemodynamics and outcome.[128–130] This hemodynamic principle of intrathoracic pressure is a fundamental physiologic concept applying to states of profound shock[124,126–128,131–136] and defines cardiopulmonary interactions during CPR.

The impedance threshold device (ITD)

The impedance threshold device (ITD) is a CPR hemodynamic adjunct based on the principle of intrathoracic pressure changes.[128] Placed on any airway (facemask, ET tube, combitube, LMA, and others), it impedes entry of air into the lungs during the upstroke of CPR without impeding normal positive pressure ventilations. This creates relatively negative intrathoracic pressure on the upstroke of CPR, thereby augmenting venous blood return to the heart and increasing hemodynamics during CPR.[128] Aufderheide *et al.* performed a prospective, double-blind trial in adult patients with cardiac arrest randomized to receive standard CPR with a sham ITD or standard CPR with a functional ITD.[129] In a substudy of 20 patients, systolic blood pressure was recorded at the scene of cardiac arrest by using invasive femoral arterial monitoring.[131] The hemodynamic substudy demonstrated an average systolic blood pressure of about 85 mmHg during CPR with the active device and a systolic blood pressure of about 40 mmHg during CPR with the sham device, thus more than doubling the hemodynamics and effectiveness of CPR.[131] In this initial feasibility study of only 230 patients, proximal outcome in all patients was insignificantly improved. Nevertheless, nearly half the patients had PEA as an initial cardiac arrest rhythm or had PEA at some time

during cardiac arrest. In these patients, return of spontaneous circulation, ICU admission, and 24-hour survival was significantly increased compared to control.[129] Reviewing invasive hemodynamic monitoring demonstrated that 68% of episodes of PEA were pseudo-PEA with an average invasive systolic blood pressure of 28.6 ± 11.6 mmHg.[175] These data indicate that the majority of patients with PEA have some myocardial contraction and that improved hemodynamics during CPR is an effective intervention for patients with PEA.

Use of the ITD during CPR in patients with out-of-hospital cardiac arrest in Staffordshire, England demonstrates similar benefits for patients with asystole.[130] Thayne *et al.* implemented ITD use in the Staffordshire Ambulance System comparing survival (defined in this study as admitted to the emergency department with a sustained pulse) with historical controls. Survival in all patients receiving an ITD (61/181 [34%]) improved by 50% compared to historical controls (180/808 [22%]) ($P<0.01$). Survival in patients presenting with asystole tripled in the group receiving an ITD (26/76 [34%]) compared with controls (39/351 [11%]) ($P=0.001$). In this study, presumed improvement in CPR hemodynamics resulted in markedly improved short-term survival for all patients, especially patients with asystole.[130]

There have been no interventions studied (pharmacological or mechanical) in non-fibrillatory cardiac arrest that hold as much promise for improved outcome as augmenting hemodynamics during CPR. As a result, early administration of basic life support with the impedance threshold device is strongly recommended by the National American Heart Association (IIa Recommendation). Other methods for improving hemodynamics during CPR exist, but have not demonstrated significant benefit in prospective, randomized clinical trials or are limited by the technical logistics of their application.

Interposed abdominal compression cardiopulmonary resuscitation (IAC-CPR)

IAC-CPR has been shown to improve coronary perfusion pressures and blood flow compared to standard CPR.[137–141] Two clinical studies from 1992 showed improved return of spontaneous circulation and long-term survival rates when IAC-CPR is used during in-hospital PEA arrest.[141,143] Conversely, a prospective, randomized trial of standard CPR versus IAC-CPR in the out-of-hospital setting failed to demonstrate improved cardiac resuscitation rates.[144] Given the mixed results from multiple trials, a meta-analysis of all IAC-CPR animal, preclinical and clinical trials advocates for early implementation of this technique during resuscitative efforts.[145]

Active compression–decompression cardiopulmonary resuscitation (ACD-CPR)

The ResQPUMP®, a device designed to apply active compression–decompression CPR, was developed after an ordinary bathroom plunger was applied to the chest of a patient during cardiopulmonary arrest. With active decompression as well as compression, spontaneous circulation was restored and the patient was discharged from the hospital neurologically intact.[144] Studies in both a dog model of ventricular fibrillation and in a small number of humans in cardiopulmonary arrest, active compression–decompression (ACD)-CPR resuscitation with a hand-held suction device improved cardiopulmonary circulation in comparison to standard CPR.[147,148] Lindner et al. found that ACD-CPR significantly increased myocardial and cerebral blood flow during cardiac arrest in a swine model in the absence of vasopressor therapy as compared with standard CPR.[149] The largest human study to date was reported by Plaisance et al. in 1999.[126] They found that both the rate of hospital discharge without neurologic impairment and the 1-year survival rate were significantly higher among patients who received active compression–decompression CPR as compared to patients who received standard CPR. The majority of these patients presented in asystole.

Pneumatic vest CPR and other mechanical adjuncts

Pneumatic vest CPR is based on the thoracic pump theory: increases in intrathoracic pressure produce forward blood flow during cardiac arrest and higher vascular pressures can be achieved with circumferential compression of the thorax compared with manual CPR. Halperin et al. demonstrated significantly improved myocardial and cerebral blood flow with vest CPR compared with manual CPR in a ventricular fibrillation dog model.[150] This study also demonstrated improved survival after ventricular fibrillation cardiac arrest in animals receiving vest CPR compared with those receiving manual CPR.[150] In a preliminary study in humans, Halperin and colleagues have also demonstrated increased aortic pressure and coronary perfusion pressure with vest CPR compared with standard CPR and an insignificant trend toward a greater likelihood of return of spontaneous circulation.[151]

A retrospective review comparing prehospital adult cardiac arrest patients assigned to receive either manual CPR or CPR using an Autopulse device (Revivant Corporation) was undertaken by Casner et al. with the primary endpoint of arrival to the ED with measurable spontaneous pulses.[152] This study demonstrated a significant difference in the primary outcome with use of the Autopulse device. When subgroup analysis was undertaken to compare the outcomes for the different presenting rhythms, only those patients with an initial arrest rhythm of asystole were found to benefit from the use of the Autopulse device. In those whose initial arrest rhythm was PEA, the difference approached, but did not achieve, significance. A larger, prospective randomized multicenter clinical trial (the ASPIRE Trial) found no significant difference in outcome with the device compared to standard CPR. Further studies are required to characterize the benefits of this approach.

LUCAS is a new device for mechanical compression and decompression of the chest during CPR.[153–155] Hemodynamic studies in a porcine model of ventricular fibrillation demonstrate significantly higher cardiac output, carotid artery blood flow, end-tidal CO_2, and coronary perfusion pressure compared with standard CPR.[153] Ongoing clinical trials will characterize the benefits of this new hemodynamic adjunct.

Open chest CPR

Improved blood flow has been reported when open-chest cardiac massage is used for resuscitation from cardiac arrest.[156] Before recommending open-chest CPR for resuscitation in PEA arrest, definitive prospective, randomized clinical trials should be performed that establish safety and efficacy of this technique.

Cardiopulmonary bypass

Cardiopulmonary bypass is an excellent reperfusion technique that has been shown to improve resuscitation rates in ventricular fibrillation cardiac arrest.[157–162] Only one study has investigated the use of cardiopulmonary bypass in PEA arrest (postdefibrillation animal model) and found improved return of spontaneous circulation rates when cardiopulmonary bypass was compared to standard CPR with standard dose epinephrine and high-dose epinephrine.[71] DeBehnke investigated the use of cardiopulmonary bypass after increasing intervals of prolonged asphyxial PEA arrest and found cardiopulmonary bypass significantly increased 1-hour survival when applied early (<15 minutes after PEA arrest).[163] The largest human study in out-of-hospital cardiac arrest patients was published by Nagao et al. in 2000.[164] The majority of these 36 patients presented with ventricular fibrillation due to acute coronary syndrome, with no data available regarding the PEA subset. Of the 23 survivors to hospital discharge, only 12 patients had good cerebral performance scores, and 10 patients were reported with significant neurological deficits. Interpretation of the study results is challenged by uncontrolled use of post-resuscitation hypothermia. Thus, cardiopulmonary bypass appears to be a reperfusion technique in its infancy. Appropriate application to patients who suffer out-of-hospital cardiac arrest, and in particular, to those found in PEA or pseudo-PEA remains to be defined.

Aortic balloon counterpulsation

Aortic balloon counterpulsation during CPR may enhance coronary perfusion pressure and coronary and cerebral blood flow. Inflation of an intraaortic balloon (IAB) during CPR may raise aortic diastolic blood pressure (AODP), increasing coronary perfusion pressure. In an early animal study comparing the use of IAB vs. epinephrine-only during VF arrest, 10 of 10 animals were resuscitated in the IAB groups, while 1 of 5 was resuscitated in the epinephrine-only group.[165] Although other animal studies have shown benefits with IAB use,[166,167] no human clinical trials have been performed. A case report of 2 patients who suffered cardiac arrest while being maintained on an intraaortic balloon pump (IABP) documents augmented coronary perfusion pressure measurements with the IAB use during CPR.[168]

Transvenous and transthoracic cardiac pacing

In the middle 1980s, transcutaneous and transvenous cardiac pacing were studied as an adjunctive therapy for patients during non-fibrillatory cardiac arrest unresponsive to pharmacologic interventions. Although found to be somewhat successful in patients with symptomatic bradycardia not in arrest, no survival benefit was demonstrated in patients with PEA or asystolic cardiac arrest unless the technique was used early in resuscitative treatment.[169–174] Current ACLS guidelines continue to allow consideration of cardiac pacing early during resuscitative efforts from non-fibrillatory arrest.

Postresuscitation issues

Following return of spontaneous circulation in non-fibrillatory cardiac arrest, attention should be directed at continued treatment of the underlying etiology of arrest, and assurance of adequate tissue perfusion and oxygenation. Excessive ventilation rates, prolonged duration of ventilation, and high tidal volumes should be avoided. The resulting increase in intrathoracic pressure will impede venous blood return to the heart and compromise hemo-

dynamics. Despite normalization of blood pressure, central venous pressure, and heart rate postresuscitation, some patients may have continued myocardial dysfunction and poor tissue oxygenation or perfusion. Central venous oximetry, lactate levels, and calculation of the shock index (heart rate/systolic arterial pressure) can be utilized to assess the adequacy of tissue oxygenation and cardiac dysfunction.[175] If the underlying etiology was mechanical, therapy should be specifically directed at that cause. Patients with pneumothorax relieved by needle thoracostomy should have tube thoracostomy performed for definitive treatment. Patients with pericardial tamponade should have definitive drainage of their tamponade or closure of the emergency thoracotomy if performed. All patients should have adequate oxygenation and tissue perfusion assured, with use of volume expansion and pressor therapy as needed. Right heart catheterization, central venous oximetry, and lactate levels should guide therapy in these cases. In patients whose PEA arrest was caused by pump failure secondary to acute myocardial infarction, emergent cardiac catheterization with angioplasty has been shown to improve patient outcomes. These patients may develop profound myocardial dysfunction and require circulatory assist with balloon counterpulsation. In situations where cardiac catheterization or angioplasty is not available, thrombolytic therapy should be administered if the CPR time was less than 10 minutes and no other contraindications exist.[176] The acid–base status should be optimized through increased alveolar ventilation for primary respiratory acidosis and judicious bicarbonate use for metabolic acidosis. Electrolyte abnormalities should be identified and corrected during this postresuscitation period.

Future of directions in the therapy of non-fibrillatory arrest

Patients with pseudo-PEA and reversible causes of PEA should be rapidly identified, as they are most likely to benefit from aggressive therapeutic intervention. Q-R and QRS duration along with immediate use of Doppler ultrasound applied in all PEA patients hold the potential for quick and non-invasive identification of the pseudo-PEA subgroup. Spreng *et al.* described an audible esophageal Doppler probe that non-invasively detects pseudo-PEA.[177] The availability of emergency echocardiography may rapidly and accurately distinguish pseudo-PEA from true PEA. Enhancing hemodynamics by delivering high quality CPR (e.g., compression rate of 100 compressions/minute, depth of 1½ to 2 inches per compression, minimal interruption of chest compressions, allowing the chest to completely recoil after each compression, avoiding excessive ventilation rates) and use of the impedance threshold device (ITD) (IIa Recommendation by the American Heart Association) remains one of the most promising interventions for this patient population. The use of thrombolytic therapy in cardiac arrest and PEA remains controversial.[50,51–53] The identification of PEA patient subgroups by non-invasive and immediately available methods, combined with delivering significantly improved hemodynamics during CPR, may substantially improve patient outcomes.

REFERENCES

1. Paradis, N.A., Martin, G.B., Goetting, M.G., Rivers, E.P., Feingold, M. & Nowak, R.M. Aortic pressure during human cardiac arrest: identification of pseudo-electromechanical dissociation. *Chest* 1992; **101**: 123–128.

2. Bocka, J.J., Overton, D.T. & Hauser, A. Electromechanical dissociation in human beings: an echocardiographic evaluation. *Ann. Emerg. Med.* 1988; **17**: 450–452.

3. Pirolo, J.S., Hutchins, G.M. & Moore, G.W. Electromechanical dissociation: pathologic explanations in 50 patients. *Hum. Pathol.* 1985; **16**: 485–487.

4. Stueven, H.A., Aufderheide, T.P., Waite, E.M. & Mateer, J.R. Electromechanical dissociation: six years prehospital experience. *Resuscitation* 1989; **17**: 173–182.

5. Parish, D.C., Dane, F.C., Montgomery, M., Wynn, L.J., Durham, M.D. & Brown, T.D. Resuscitation in the Hospital: relationship of year and rhythm to outcome. *Resuscitation* 2000; **47**: 219–229.

6. Cooper, S. & Cade, J. Predicting survival, in-hospital cardiac arrests: resus survival variables and training effectiveness. *Resuscitation* 1997; **35**: 17–22.

7. VanWalraven, C., Forster, A.J. & Steill, I.G. Derivation of a clinical decision rule for the discontinuation of in-hospital cardiac arrest resuscitations. *Arch. Int. Med.* 1999; **159**: 129–134.

8. Stiell, I.G., Wells, G.A., Field, B.J. *et al.* Improved out-of-hospital cardiac arrest survival through the inexpensive optimization of an existing defibrillation program. *J. Am. Med. Assoc.* 1999; **281**: 1175–1181.

9. DeMaio, V.J., Steill, I.G., Wells, G.A. & Spaite, D.W. Cardiac arrest witnessed by emergency medical services personnel: descriptive epidemiology, prodromal symptoms, and predictors of survival. *Ann. Emerg. Med.* 2000; **35**: 138–146.

10. Herlitz, J., Andersson, E., Bang, A. *et al.* Experiences from treatment of out-of-hospital cardiac arrest during 17 years in Goteborg. *Eur. Heart J.* 2000; **21**: 1251–1258.

11. Aufderheide, T.P., Thakur, R.K., Stueven, H.A. *et al.* Electrocardiographic characteristics in PEA. *Resuscitation* 1989; **17**: 183–193.

12. Herlitz, J., Estrom, L., Wennerblom, B. *et al.* Survival among patients with out-of-hospital cardiac arrest found in electromechanical dissociation. *Resuscitation* 1995; **29**: 97–106.

13. Parish, D.C., Dinesh Chandra, K.M. & Dane, F.C. Success changes the problem: Why ventricular fibrillation is declining, why pulseless electrical activity is emerging, and what to do about it. *Resuscitation* 2003; **58**: 31–35.

14. Kurkiciyan, L., Meron, G., Sterz, F. *et al.* Pulmonary Embolism as a cause of cardiac arrest: presentation and outcome. *Arch. Intern. Med.* 2000; **160**: 1529–1535.

15. Fozzard, H.A. Electromechanical dissociation and its possible role in sudden cardiac death. *J. Am. Coll. Cardiol.* 1985; **5**: 31B–34B.

16. Engdahl, J., Bang, A., Lidqvist, J. & Herlitz, J. Factors affecting short-and long-term prognosis among 1069 patients with out-of-hospital cardiac arrest and pulseless electrical activity. *Resuscitation* 2001; **51**: 17–25.

17. Hoffman, J.R. & Stevenson, L.W. Postdefibrillation idioventricular rhythm – a salvageable condition. *West. J. Med.* 1987; **146**: 188–191.

18. Niemann, J.T., Stratton, S.J., Cruz, B. & Lewis, R.J. Outcome of out-of-hospital asystole and pulseless electrical activity versus primary asystole and pulseless electrical activity. *Crit. Care Med.* 2001; **29**: 2366–2370.

19. Rogers, P.L., Schlichtig, R., Miro, A. & Pinsky, M. Auto-PEEP during CPR: an "Occult" cause of electromechanical dissociation? *Chest* 1991; **99**: 492–493.

20. Wiener, C. Ventilatory management of respiratory failure in asthma. *J. Am. Med. Assoc.* 1993; **269**: 2128–2131.

21. Spodick, D.H. Acute cardiac tamponade. *N. Engl. J. Med.* 2003; **349**: 684–690.

22. Berger, B.C. Pericardiocentesis using echocardiography. *Cardiovasc Clin.* 1985; **15**: 269.

23. Spodick, D.H. Electrical alternans of the heart: its relation to the kinetics and physiology of the heart during cardiac tamponade. *Am. J. Cardiol.* 1962; **10**: 155–165.

24. D'Cruz, I., Rehman, A.U. & Hancock, H.I. Quantitative echocardiographic assessment in pericardial disease. *Echocardiography* 1997; **14**: 207–214.

25. Gascho, J.A., Martins, J.B., Marcus, M.L. & Kerber, R.E. Effects of volume expansion and vasodilators in acute pericardial tamponade. *Am. J. Physiol.* 1981; **240**: H49–H53.

26. Harper, R.J. & Callaham, M.L. Pericardiocentesis. In Roberts, J.R. & Hedges, J.R., eds. *Clinical Procedures in Emergency Medicine.* Philadelphia: W.B. Saunders, 1998: 231–253.

27. Bartlett, R.L. Resuscitative thoracotomy. In Roberts, J.R. & Hedges, J.R., eds. *Clinical Procedures in Emergency Medicine.* Philadelphia: W.B. Saunders, 1998: 264–280.

28. Sanders, A.B. Capnometry in emergency medicine. *Ann. Emerg. Med.* 1989; **18**: 1287–1290.

29. Ross, D.S. Thoracentesis. In Roberts, J.R. & Hedges, J.R., eds. *Clinical Procedures in Emergency Medicine.* Philadelphia: W.B. Saunders, 1991: 116–117.

30. Gilbert, P., Busund, R., Skagseth, A., Nilsen, P.A. & Solbo, J.P. Resuscitation from accidental hypothermia of 13.7 degrees C with circulatory arrest. *Lancet* 2000; **355**: 375–376.

31. Lloyd, E.L. Accidental hypothermia. *Resuscitation* 1996; **32**: 111–124.

32. Kornberger, E., Schwarz, B., Lindner, K.H. & Mair, P. Forced air surface rewarming in patients with severe accidental hypothermia. *Resuscitation* 1999; **41**: 105–111.

33. Koller, R., Schnider, T.W. & Neidhart, P. Deep accidental hypothermia and cardiac arrest-rewarming with forced air. *Acta Anaesthesiol. Scand.* 1997; **41**: 1359–1364.

34. Plaiser, B.R. Thoraciclavage in accidental hypothermia with cardiac arrest-report of a case and review of the literature. *Resuscitation* 2005; **66**: 99–104.

35. Walpoth, B.H., Walpoth-Aslan, B.N., Mattle, H.P. *et al.* Outcomes of survivors of accidental deep hypothermia and circulatory arrest treated with extracorporeal blood warming. *N. Engl. J. Med.* 1997; **337**: 1500–1505.

36. Wik, L. & Kiil, S. Use of an automatic mechanical chest compression device (LUCAS) as a bridge to establishing cardiopulmonary bypass for a patient with hypothermic cardiac arrest. *Resuscitation* 2005; **66**: 391–394.

37. Courtney, D.M. & Kline, J.A. Prospective use of a clinical decision rule to identify pulmonary embolism as likely cause of outpatient cardiac arrest. *Resuscitation* 2005; **65**: 57–64.

38. Kurkciyan, I., Meron, G., Sterz, F. *et al.* Pulmonary embolism as a cause of cardiac arrest: presentation and outcome. *Arch. Int. Med.* 2000; **160**: 1529–1535.

39. Bell, W.R., Simon, T.L. & DeMets, D.L. The clinical features of submassive and massive pulmonary embolism. *Am. J. Med.* 1977; **62**: 355.

40. Huggins, R.M., Kennedy, W.K., Melroy, M.J., Tollerton, D.G. Cardiac arrest from succinylcholine-induced hyperkalemia. *Am. J. Health Syst. Pharm.* 2003; **119**: 740–748.

41. Gronert, G.A. Cardiac arrest after succinylcholine: mortality greater with rhabdomyolysis than receptor upregulation. *Anesthesiology* 2001; **94**: 523–529.

42. Wagner, G.S. Miscellaneous conditions – electrolyte abnormalities In *Marriott's Practical Electrocardiography* 9th edn, Williams and Wilkins, 1994:182–183.

43. Surawicz, B. Relationship between electrocardiogram and electrolytes. *Am. Heart J.* 1967; **73**: 814–834.

44. von Mach, M.A., Sauer, O. & Sacha Weilemann, L. Experiences of a poison center with metformin-associated lactic acidosis. *Exp. Clin. Endocrinol. Diabetes* 2004; **112**: 187–190.

45. Miller, M.A., Hung, Y.M., Haller, C., Galbo, M. & Levsky, M.E. Colchicine-related death presenting as an unknown case of multiple organ failure. *J. Emerg. Med.* 2005; **28**: 445–448.

46. Gerard, J.M. & Luisiri, A. A fatal overdose of arginine hydrochloride. *J. Toxicol. Clin. Toxicol.* 1997; **35**: 621–625.

47. Legras, A., Skrobala, D., Furet, Y. *et al.* Herbicide: fatal ammonium thiocyanate and animotriazole poisoning. *J. Toxicol. Clin. Toxicol.* 1996; **34**: 441–446.

48. Toth, H.L., Greenbaum, L.A. Severe acidosis caused by starvation and stress. *Am. J. Kid. Dis.* 2003; **42**: E16.

49. Hick, J.L., Smith, S.W. & Lynch, M.T. Metabolic acidosis in restraint-associated cardiac arrest: a case series. *Acad. Emerg. Med.* 1999; **6**: 239–243.

50. Bottinger, B.W., Bode, C., Kern, S. *et al.* Efficacy and safety of thrombolytic therapy after initially unsuccessful cardiopulmonary resuscitation: a prospective clinical trial. *Lancet* 2001; **357**: 1583–1585.

51. Abu-Ladan, R.B., Christenson, J.M., Innes, G.O. *et al.* Tissue plasminogen activator in cardiac arrest with pulseless electrical activity. *N. Engl. J. Med.* 2002; **346**: 1522–1528.

52. Paradis, N.A., Knaut, A. & Halperin, H. Tissue plasminogen activator in cardiac arrest with pulseless electrical activity (correspondence). *N. Engl. J. Med.* 2002; **347**: 1281–1282.

53. Bottinger, B.W., Padosch, S.A. & Wenzel, V. Tissue plasminogen activator in cardiac arrest with pulseless electrical activity (correspondence). *N. Engl. J. Med.* 2002; **347**: 1281–1282.

54. Spohr, F., Arntz, H.R., Bluhmki, E. *et al.* International multi-center trial protocol to assess the efficacy and safety of tenecteplase during cardiopulmonary resuscitation in patients with out-of-hospital cardiac arrest: the Thrombolysis in Cardiac Arrest (TROICA) Study. *Eur. J. Clin. Invest.* 2005; **35**: 315–323.

55. Paradis, N.A., Martin, G.B., Rivers, E.P. *et al.* Coronary perfusion pressure and the return of spontaneous circulation in human cardiopulmonary resuscitation. *J. Am. Med. Assoc.* 1990; **263**: 1106–1113.

56. Sanders, A.B., Ogle, M. & Ewy, G.A. Coronary perfusion pressure during cardiopulmonary resuscitation. *Am. J. Emerg. Med.* 1985; **3**: 11–14.

57. Brown, C.G., Katz, S.E., Werman, H.A., Luu, T., Davis, E.A. & Hamlin, R.L. The effect of epinephrine versus methoxamine on regional myocardial blood flow and defibrillation rates following a prolonged cardiorespiratory arrest in a swine model. *Am. J. Emerg. Med.* 1987; **5**: 362–369.

58. Brown, C.G., Werman, H.A., Davis, E.A., Hobson, J. & Hamlin, R.L. The effects of graded doses of epinephrine on regional myocardial blood flow during cardiopulmonary resuscitation in swine. *Circulation* 1987; **75**: 491–497.

59. Lindner, K.H., Strohmenger, H., Prengel, A.W., Ensinger, H., Goertz, A. & Weichel, T. Hemodynamic and metabolic effects of epinephrine during cardiopulmonary resuscitation in a pig model. *Crit. Care Med.* 1992; **20**: 1020–1026.

60. Brown, C.G., Taylor, R.B., Werman, H.A., Luu, T., Ashton, J. & Hamlin, R.L. Myocardial oxygen delivery/consumption during cardiopulmonary resuscitation: a comparison of epinephrine and phenylephrine. *Ann. Emerg. Med.* 1988; **17**: 302–308.

61. Lindner, K.H., Ahnefeld, F.W. & Prengel, A.W. Comparison of standard and high-dose adrenaline in the resuscitation of asystole and electromechanical dissociation. *Acta Anaesthesiol. Scand.* 1991; **35**: 253–256.

62. Brown, C.G., Martin, D.R., Pepe, P.E. *et al.* A comparison of standard-dose and high-dose epinephrine in cardiac arrest outside the hospital. *N. Engl. J. Med.* 1992; **327**: 1051–1055.

63. Stiell, I.G., Hebert, P.C., Weitzman, B.N. *et al.* High-dose epinephrine in adult cardiac arrest. *N. Engl. J. Med.* 1992; **327**: 1045–1050.

64. Brown, C.G., Werman, H.A., Davis, E.A., Katz, S. & Hamlin, R.L. The effect of high-dose phenylephrine versus epineph-

rine on regional cerebral blood flow during CPR. *Ann. Emerg. Med.* 1987; **16**: 743–748.

65. Brown, C.G., Davis, E.A., Werman, H.A. & Hamlin, R.L. Methoxamine versus epinephrine on regional cerebral blood flow during cardiopulmonary resuscitation. *Crit. Care Med.* 1987; **15**: 682–686.

66. Robinson, L.A., Brown, C.G., Jenkins, J. *et al.* The effect of norepinephrine versus epinephrine on myocardial hemodynamics during CPR. *Ann. Emerg. Med.* 1989; **18**: 336–340.

67. Silfvast, T., Saarnivaara, L., Kinneunen, A. *et al.* Comparison of adrenaline and phenylephrine in out-of-hospital cardiopulmonary resuscitation: a double-blind study. *Acta Anaesthesiol. Scand.* 1985; **29**: 610–613.

68. Wenzel, V., Krismer, A.C., Arntz, H.R. *et al.* A comparison of vasopressin and epinephrine for out-of-hospital cardiopulmonary resuscitation, *N. Engl. J. Med.* 2004; **350**: 105–113.

69. Ralston, S.H., Tacker, W.A., Showen, L., Carter, A. & Babbs, C.F. Endotracheal versus intravenous epinephrine during electromechanical dissociation with CPR in dogs. *Ann. Emerg. Med.* 1985; **14**: 1044–1048.

70. Lindner, K.H. & Ahnefeld, F.W. Comparison of epinephrine and norepinephrine in the treatment of asphyxial or fibrillatory cardiac arrest in a porcine model. *Crit. Care Med.* 1989; **17**: 437–441.

71. DeBehnke, D.J., Angelos, M.G. & Leasure, J.E. Use of cardiopulmonary bypass, high-dose epinephrine, and standard-dose epinephrine in resuscitation from post-counter-shock electromechanical dissociation. *Ann. Emerg. Med.* 1992; **21**: 1051–1057.

72. Brown, C.G. & Werman, H.A. Adrenergic agonists during cardiopulmonary resuscitation. *Resuscitation* 1990; **19**: 1–16.

73. Redding, J.S., Haynes, R.R. & Thomas, J.D. Drug therapy in resuscitation from electromechanical dissociation. *Crit. Care Med.* 1983; **11**: 681–684.

74. Turner, L.M., Parsons, M., Luetkemeyer, R.C., Ruthman, J.C., Anderson, R.J. & Aldag, J.C. A comparison of epinephrine and methoxamine for resuscitation from electromechanical dissociation in human beings. *Ann. Emerg. Med.* 1988; **17**: 443–449.

75. Patrick, W.D., Freeman, J., McEwen, T. *et al.* A randomized, double-blind comparison of methoxamine and epinephrine in human cardiopulmonary arrest. *Am. J. Respir. Crit. Care Med.* 1995; **152**: 519–523.

76. Olson, D.W., Thakur, R.K., Stueven, H.A. *et al.* Randomized study of epinephrine versus methoxamine in prehospital ventricular fibrillation. *Ann. Emerg. Med.* 1989; **18**(11): 1258–1259.

77. Brillman, J., Sanders, A., Otto, C., Fahmy, H., Bragg, S. & Ewy, G. Comparison of epinephrine and phenylephrine for resuscitation and neurologic outcome of cardiac arrest in dogs. *Ann. Emerg. Med.* 1987; **16**: 11–17.

78. Redding, J.S. & Pearson, J.W. Resuscitation from ventricular fibrillation. *J. Am. Med. Assoc.* 1968; **203**: 93–98.

79. Evans, T.R. & Mogensen, L. Pharmacological treatment of asystole and electromechanical dissociation. *Resuscitation* 1991; **22**: 167–172.

80. Lindner, K.H., Prengel, A.W., Pfenninger, E.G. *et al.* Vasopressin improves vital organ blood flow during closed-chest cardiopulmonary resuscitation in pigs. *Circulation* 1995; **91**: 215–221.

81. Prengel, A.W., Lindner, K.H. & Keller, A. Cerebral oxygenation during cardiopulmonary resuscitation with epinephrine and vasopressin in pigs. *Stroke* 1996; **27**: 1241–1248.

82. Wenzel, V., Lindner, K.H., Prengel, A.W. *et al.* Vasopressin improves vital organ blood flow after prolonged cardiac arrest with postcountershock pulseless activity in pigs. *Crit. Care Med.* 1999; **27**: 486–492.

83. Wenzel, V., Lindner, K.H., Krismer, A.C. *et al.* Repeated administration of vasopressin but not epinephrine maintains coronary perfusion pressure after early and late administration during cardiopulmonary resuscitation in pigs. *Circulation* 1999; **99**: 1379–1384.

84. Wenzel, V., Lindner, K.H., Krismer, A.C. *et al.* Survival with full neurologic recovery and no cerebral pathology after prolonged cardiopulmonary resuscitation and vasopressin in pigs. *J. Am. Cardiol.* 2000; **35**: 527–533.

85. Wenzel, V., Dirks, B., Strohmenger, H.U., Prengel, A.W., Lindner, I.M. & Lurie, K.G. Randomized comparison of epinephrine and vasopressin in patients with out-of-hospital ventricular fibrillation. *Lancet* 1997; **349**: 535–537.

86. Aung, K. & Htay, T. Vasopressin for cardiac arrest: a systematic review and meta-analysis. *Arch. Int. Med.* 2005; **165**: 17–24.

87. Coon, G.A., Clinton, J.E. & Ruiz, E. Use of atropine for bradyasystolic prehospital cardiac arrest. *Ann. Emerg. Med.* 1981; **10**: 462–467.

88. American Heart Association Guidelines for Cardiopulmonary Resuscitation and Emergency Cardiovascular Care: Management of Cardiac Arrest Pt 7.2. *Circulation* 2005; 112 (Suppl 1): IV-58–66.

89. O'Rourke, G.W. & Greene, N.M. Autonomic blockade and the resting heart rate in man. *Am. Heart J.* 1970; **80**: 469–474.

90. Chamberlain, D.A., Turner, P. & Sneddon, J.M. Effects of atropine on heart rate in healthy man. *Lancet* 1967; **2**: 12–15.

91. DeBehnke, D.J. The effects of vagal tone on resuscitation from experimental electromechanical dissociation. *Ann. Emerg. Med.* 1993; **22**: 1789–1794.

92. Debehnke, D.J., Swart, G.L., Spreng, D. & Aufderheide, T.P. Standard and higher doses of atropine in a canine model of pulseless electrical activity. *Acad. Emerg. Med.* 1995; **2**: 1034–1041.

93. Berenyi, K.J., Wolk, M. & Killip, T. Cerebrospinal fluid acidosis complicating therapy of experimental cardiopulmonary arrest. *Circulation* 1975; **52**: 319–324.

94. Kette, F., Weil, M.H., von Planta, M., Gazmuri, R.J. & Rackow, E.C. Buffer agents do not reverse intramyocardial acidosis during cardiac resuscitation. *Circulation* 1990; **81**: 1660–1666.

95. Kette, F., Weil, M.H. & Gazmuri, R.J. Buffer solutions may compromise cardiac resuscitation by reducing coronary perfusion pressure. *J. Am. Med. Assoc.* 1991; **266**: 2121–2126.

96. Federiuk, C.S., Sanders, A.B., Kern, K.B., Nelson, J. & Ewy, G.A. The effect of bicarbonate on resuscitation from cardiac arrest. *Ann. Emerg. Med.* 1991; **20**: 1173–1177.

97. Aufderheide, T.P., Martin, D.R., Olson, D.W. *et al.* Prehospital bicarbonate use in cardiac arrest: a 3-year experience. *Am. J. Emerg. Med.* 1992; **10**: 1–4.

98. Vukmir, R.B., Bircher, N.G., Radovsky, A. & Safar, P. Sodium bicarbonate improves hemodynamics and perfusion in canine cardiac arrest. *Crit. Care Med.* 1993; **21**: S272.

99. Bircher, N., Vukmir, R. & Safar, P. Increasing arrest interval increases and sodium bicarbonate decreases post-resuscitation nor-epinephrine requirements [Abstract]. *Crit. Care Med.* 1994; **22**: A131.

100. Bar-Joseph, G., Weinberger, T., Castel, T. *et al.* Comparison of sodium bicarbonate, Carbicarb, and THAM during cardiopulmonary resuscitation in dogs. *Crit. Care Med.* 1998; **26**: 1397–1408.

101. Leong, E.C., Bendall, J.C., Boyd, A.C. & Einstein, R. Sodium bicarbonate improves the chance of resuscitation after 10 minutes of cardiac arrest in dogs. *Resuscitation* 2001; **51**: 309–315.

102. Liu, X., Nozari, A., Rubertsson, S. & Wiklund, L. Buffer administration during CPR promotes cerebral perfusion after return of spontaneous circulation and mitigates post-resuscitation cerebral acidosis. *Resuscitation* 2002; **55**: 45–55.

103. Bar-Joseph, G., Abramson, N.S., Kelsey, S.F. *et al.* Improved resuscitation outcome in emergency medical systems with increased usage of sodium bicarbonate during cardiopulmonary resuscitation. *Acta Anaesthiol. Scand.* 2005; **49**: 6–15.

104. Vanags, B., Thakur, R.K., Stueven, H.A., Aufderheide, T. & Tresch, D.D. Interventions in the therapy of electromechanical dissociation. *Resuscitation* 1989; **17**: 163–171.

105. Callaham, M. Cyclic antidepressant overdose. In Rosen, P. & Barkin, R.M., eds. *Emergency Medicine: Concepts and Clinical Practice.* St. Louis: Mosby-Year Book, 1992: 2566–2567.

106. Eilers, M.A. & Garrison, T.E. General management principles. In Rosen, P. & Barkin, R.M., eds. *Emergency Medicine: Concepts and Clinical Practice.* St. Louis: Mosby-Year Book, 1992: 2497.

107. Janson, C.L. & Marx, J.A. Fluid and electrolyte balance. In Rosen, P. & Barkin, R.M., eds. *Emergency Medicine: Concepts and Clinical Practice.* St. Louis: Mosby-Year Book, 1992: 2146.

108. American Heart Association. Standards for cardiopulmonary resuscitation and emergency cardiac care. *J. Am. Med. Assoc.* 1974; **227**: 833–868.

109. Stueven, H., Thompson, B., Aprahamian, C. *et al.* Use of calcium chloride in prehospital cardiac arrest. *Ann. Emerg. Med.* 1983; **12**: 136–139.

110. Blecic, S., De Backer, D., Huynh, C.H. *et al* Calcium chloride in experimental electromechanical dissociation: a placebo-controlled trial in dogs. *Crit. Care Med.* 1987; **15**: 324–327.

111. Harrison, E.E. & Amey, B.D. Use of calcium in electromechanical dissociation. *Ann. Emerg. Med.* 1984; **13**: 844–845.

112. Stueven, H.A., Thompson, B., Aprahamian, C., Tonsfeldt, D. & Kastenson, E.H. The effectiveness of calcium chloride in refractory electromechanical dissociation. *Ann. Emerg. Med.* 1985; **14**: 626–629.

113. Parmley, W.W. & Sonnenblick, E.H. Glucagon: a new agent in cardiac therapy. *Am. J. Cardiol.* 1971; **27**: 298–303.

114. Jones, R.J. & Phillips, J.H. Glucagon: present status in cardiovascular disease. *Clin. Pharmacol. Ther.* 1971; **12**: 427–444.

115. Niemann, J.T., Haynes, K.S., Garner, D., Jagels, G. & Rennie, C.J. Postcountershock pulseless rhythms: hemodynamic effects of glucagon in a canine model. *Crit. Care Med.* 1987; **15**: 554–558.

116. Rothstein, R.J., Niemann, J.T., Rennie, C.J. & Suddath, W.O. Use of naloxone during cardiac arrest and CPR: potential adjunct for postcountershock electrical-mechanical dissociation. *Ann. Emerg. Med.* 1985; **14**: 198–203.

117. Marsden, A.K. & Mora, F.M. Case report-the successful use of naloxone in an asystolic pre-hospital arrest. *Resuscitation* 1996; **32**: 109–110.

118. Belardinelli, L., Fenton, R.A., West, A., Linden, J., Althaus, J.S. & Berne, R.M. Extracellular action of adenosine and the antagonism by aminophylline on the atrioventricular conduction of isolated perfused guinea pig and rat hearts. *Circ. Res.* 1982; **51**: 569–579.

119. Wesley, R.C., Lerman, B.B., DiMarco, J.P., Berne, R.M. & Belardinelli, L. Mechanism of atropine-resistant atrioventricular block during inferior myocardial infarction: possible role of adenosine. *J. Am. Coll. Cardiol.* 1986; **8**: 1232–1234.

120. Strasberg, B., Bassevich, R., Mager, A., Kusniec, J., Sagie, A. & Sclarovsky, S. Effects of aminophylline on atrioventricular conduction in patients with late atrioventricular block during inferior wall acute myocardial infarction. *Am. J. Cardiol.* 1991; **67**: 527–528.

121. Viskin, S., Belhassen, B., Roth, A. *et al.* Aminophylline for bradyasystolic cardiac arrest refractory to atropine and epinephrine. *Ann. Intern. Med.* 1993; **118**: 279–281.

122. Marder, T.J., Bertolet, B., Ornato, J. & Gutterman, J.M. Aminophylline in the treatment of atropine-resistant bradyasystole. *Resuscitation* 2000; **47**: 105–112.

123. Mader, T.J., Smithline, H.A., Durkin, L. & Scriver, G. A randomized controlled trial of intravenous aminophylline for atropine-resistant out-of-hospital asystolic cardiac arrest. *Acad. Emerg. Med.* 2003; **10**: 192–197.

124. Aufderheide, T.P., Sigurdsson, G., Pirrallo, R.P. *et al.* Hyperventilation-induced hypotension during cardiopulmonary resuscitation. *Circulation* 2004; **109**: 1960–1965.

125. Aufderheide, T.P. & Lurie, K.G. Death by hyperventilation: a common and life-threatening problem during CPR. *Crit. Care. Med.* 2004; **32**(9)[Suppl]: S345–S351.

126. Plaisance, P., Lurie, K.G., Vicaut, E. *et al.* A comparison of standard cardiopulmonary resuscitation and active compression-decompression resuscitation for out-of-hospital cardiac arrest. *N. Engl. J. Med.* 1999; **341**: 569–575.

127. Yannopoulos, D., Tang, W., Ruossos, C. *et al.* Reducing ventilation frequency during cardiopulmonary resuscitation in a porcine model of cardiac arrest. *Resp. Care* 2005; **50**(5): 628–635.

128. Lurie, K.G., Zielinski, T., McKnite, S. *et al.* Use of an inspiratory impedance valve improves neurologically intact survival in a porcine model of ventricular fibrillation. *Circulation* 2002; **105**: 124–129.

129. Aufderheide, T.P., Pirrallo, R.G., Provo, T.A. & Lurie, K.G. Clinical evaluation of an inspiratory impedance threshold device during standard cardiopulmonary resuscitation in patients with out-of-hospital cardiac arrest. *Crit. Care Med.* 2005; **33**: 734–740.

130. Thayne, R.C., Thomas, D.C., Neville, J.D. & Van Dellen, A. Use of an impedance threshold device improves short-term outcomes following out-of-hospital cardiac arrest. *Resuscitation* 2005; **67**(1): 103–108.

131. Pirrallo, R.G., Aufderheide, T.P., Provo, T.A. & Lurie, K.G. Effect of an inspiratory impedance threshold device on hemodynamics during conventional manual cardiopulmonary resuscitation. *Resuscitation* 2005; **66**(1): 13–20.

132. Pepe, P.E., Lurie, K.G., Wigginton, J.G. *et al.* Detrimental hemodynamic effects of assisted ventilation in hemorrhagic states. *Crit. Care Med.* 2004; **32**(Suppl.): S414–S420.

133. Marino, B.S., Yannopoulos, D., Sigurdsson, G. *et al.* Spontaneous breathing through an inspiratory impedance threshold device augments cardiac index and stroke volume index in a pediatric porcine model of hemorrhagic hypovolemia. *Crit. Care Med.* 2004; **32**(Suppl): S398–S405.

134. Lurie, K.G., Zielinski, T., McKnite, S. *et al.* Treatment of hypotension in pigs with an inspiratory impedance threshold device: a feasibility study. *Crit. Care Med.* 2004; **32**(7): 1555–1562.

135. Pepe, P.E., Roppolo, L.P. & Fowler, R.L. The detrimental effects of ventilation during low-blood-flow states. *Curr. Opin. Crit. Care.* 2005; **11**: 212–218.

136. Lurie, K.G., Mulligan, K.A., McKnite, S. *et al.* Optimizing standard cardiopulmonary resuscitation with an impedance threshold valve. *Chest* 1998; **113**: 1048–1090.

137. Lindner, K.H., Ahnefeld, F.W. & Bowdler, I.M. Cardiopulmonary resuscitation with interposed abdominal compression after asphyxial or fibrillatory cardiac arrest in pigs. *Anesthesiology* 1990; **72**: 675–681.

138. Ralston, S.H., Babbs, C.F. & Niebauer, M.J. Cardiopulmonary resuscitation with interposed abdominal compression in dogs. *Anesth. Analg.* 1982; **61**: 645–651.

139. Voorhees, W.D., Niebauer, M.J. & Babbs, C.F. Improved oxygen delivery during cardiopulmonary resuscitation with interposed abdominal compressions. *Ann. Emerg. Med.* 1983; **12**: 128–135.

140. Einagle, V., Bertrand, F., Wise, R.A., Roussos, C. & Magder, S. Interposed abdominal compressions and carotid blood flow during cardiopulmonary resuscitation: support for a thoracoabdominal unit. *Chest* 1988; **93**: 1206–1212.

141. Walker, J.W., Bruestle, J.C., White, B.C., Evans, A.T., Indreri, R. & Bialek, H. Perfusion of the cerebral cortex by use of abdominal counterpulsation during cardiopulmonary resuscitation. *Am. J. Emerg. Med.* 1984; **2**: 391–393.

142. Sack, J.B., Kesselbrenner, M.B. & Bregman, D. Survival from in-hospital cardiac arrest with interposed abdominal counterpulsation during cardiopulmonary resuscitation. *J. Am. Med. Assoc.* 1992; **267**: 379–385.

143. Sack, J.B., Kesselbrenner, M.B. & Jarrad, A. Interposed abdominal compression—cardiopulmonary resuscitation and resuscitation outcome during asystole and electromechanical dissociation. *Circulation* 1992; **86**: 1692–1700.

144. Mateer, J.R., Stueven, H.A., Thompson, B.M., Aprahamian, C. & Darin, J.C. Pre-hospital IAC-CPR versus standard CPR: paramedic resuscitation of cardiac arrest. *Am. J. Emerg. Med.* 1985; **3**(2): 143–146.

145. Babbs, C.F. Interposed abdominal compression CPR: a comprehensive evidence based review. *Resuscitation* 2003; **59**: 71–82.

146. Lurie, K.G., Lindo, C. & Chin, J. CPR: the P stands for plumber's helper (Letter). *J. Am. Med. Assoc.* 1990; **264**: 1661.

147. Cohen, T.J., Tucker, K.J., Lurie, K.G. *et al.* Active compression-decompression: a new method of cardiopulmonary resuscitation. *J. Am. Med. Assoc.* 1992; **267**: 2916–2923.

148. Cohen, T.J., Tucker, K.J., Redberg, R.F. *et al.* Active compression-decompression resuscitation: a novel method of cardiopulmonary resuscitation. *Am. Heart J.* 1992; **124**: 1145–1150.

149. Lindner, K.H., Pfenninger, E.G., Lurie, K.G., Schürmann, W., Lindner, I.M. & Ahnefeld, F.W. Effects of active compression-decompression resuscitation on myocardial and cerebral blood flow in pigs. *Circulation* 1993; **88**: 1254–1263.

150. Halperin, H.R., Guerci, A.D., Chandra, N. *et al.* Vest inflation without simultaneous ventilation during cardiac arrest in dogs: improved survival from prolonged cardiopulmonary resuscitation. *Circulation* 1986; **74**(6): 1407–1415.

151. Halperin, H.R., Tsitlik, J.E., Gelfand, M. *et al.* A preliminary study of cardiopulmonary resuscitation by circumferential compression of the chest with use of a pneumatic vest. *N. Engl. J. Med.* 1993; **329**: 762–768.

152. Casner, M., Andersen, D. & Isaacs, S.M. The impact of a new CPR assist device on the rate of return of spontaneous circulation in out-of-hospital cardiac arrest, *Prehosp. Emerg. Care.* 2005; **9**: 61–67.

153. Steen, S., Liao, Q., Paskevicius, A. & Sjoberg, T. Evaluation of LUCAS, a new device for automatic mechanical compression and active decompression resuscitation. *Resuscitation* 2002; **55**(3): 285–299.

154. Rubertsson, S. & Karlsten, R. Increased cortical cerebral blood flow with LUCAS: a new device for mechanical chest compressions compared to standard external compressions during experimental cardiopulmonary resuscitation. *Resuscitation* 2005; **65**(3): 357–363.

155. Vatsgar, T.T., Ingebrigtsen, O., Fjose, L.O., Wikstrom, B., Nilsen, J.E. & Wik, L. Cardiac arrest and resuscitation with an automatic mechanical chest compression device (LUCAS) due to anaphylaxis of a woman receiving caesarean section because of pre-eclampsia. *Resuscitation* 2006; **68**(1): 155–159.

156. del Guercio, L., Feins, N.R., Cohn, J.D., Coomaraswamy, R.P., Wollman, S.B. & State, D. Comparison of blood flow during external and internal cardiac massage in man. *Cardiovasc. Surg.* 1964; (**Suppl** I): I171–I180.

157. Pretto, E., Safar, P., Saito, R., Stezoski, W. & Kelsey, S. Cardiopulmonary bypass after prolonged cardiac arrest in dogs. *Ann. Emerg. Med.* 1987; **16**: 611–619.

158. Martin, G.B., Nowak, R.M., Garden, D.L., Eisiminger, R.A. & Tomlanovich, M.C. Cardiopulmonary bypass vs. CPR as treatment for prolonged canine cardiopulmonary arrest. *Ann. Emerg. Med.* 1987; **16**: 628–636.

159. Levine, R., Gorayeb, M., Safar, P., Abramson, N., Stezoski, W. & Kelsey, S. Cardiopulmonary bypass after cardiac arrest and prolonged closed-chest CPR in dogs. *Ann. Emerg. Med.* 1987; **16**: 620–627.

160. DeBehnke, D.J., Angelos, M.G. & Leasure, J.E. Comparison of standard external CPR, open-chest CPR, and cardiopulmonary bypass in a canine myocardial infarct model. *Ann. Emerg. Med.* 1991; **20**: 754–760.

161. Tisherman, S.A., Grenvik, A. & Safar, P. Cardiopulmonary-cerebral resuscitation: advanced and prolonged life support with emergency cardiopulmonary bypass. *Acta Anaesthesiol. Scand.* 1990; **94**: 63–72.

162. Angelos, M., Safar, P. & Reich, H. A comparison of cardiopulmonary resuscitation with cardiopulmonary bypass after prolonged cardiac arrest in dogs. Reperfusion pressures and neurologic recovery. *Resuscitation* 1991; **21**: 121–135.

163. DeBehnke, D.J. Resuscitation time limits in experimental pulseless electrical activity cardiac arrest using cardiopulmonary bypass. *Resuscitation* 1994; **27**: 221–229.

164. Nagao, K., Hayashi, N., Kanmatsuse, K. *et al.* Cardiopulmonary cerebral resuscitation using emergency cardiopulmonary bypass, coronary reperfusion therapy and mild hypothermia inpatients with cardiac arrest outside the hospital. *J. Am. Coll. Cardiol.* 2000; **36**: 776–783.

165. Tang, W., Weil, M.H., Noc, M., Sun, S., Gazmuri, R.J. & Bisera, J. Augmented efficacy of external CPR by intermittent occlusion of ascending aorta. *Circulation* 1993; **88**: 1916–1921.

166. Paradis, N.A., Rose, M.I. & Gawryl, M.S. Selective aortic perfusion and oxygenation: an effective adjunct to external chest compression-based cardiopulmonary resuscitation. *J. Am. Coll. Cardiol.* 1994; **23**: 497–504.

167. Spence, P.A., Lust, R.M., Chitwood, W.R. *et al.* Transfemoral balloon aortic occlusion during open cardiopulmonary resuscitation improves myocardial and cerebral blood flow. *J. Surg. Res.* 1990; **49**: 217–221.

168. Deakin, C.D. & Barron, D.J. Haemodynamic effects of descending aortic occlusion during cardiopulmonary resuscitation. *Resuscitation* 1996; **33**: 49–52.

169. Clinton, J.E., Zoll, P.M., Zoll, R. & Ruiz, E. Emergency noninvasive external cardiac pacing. *J. Emerg. Med.* 1985; **2**: 155–162.

170. Hedges, J.R., Syverud, S.A., Dalsey, W.C., Ferro, S., Easter, R. & Shultz, B. Prehospital trial of emergency transcutaneous cardiac pacing. *Circulation* 1987; **76**: 1337–1343.

171. Olson, C.M., Jastremski, M.S., Smith, R.W. *et al.* External cardiac pacing for out-of-hospital bradyasystolic arrest. *Am. J. Emerg. Med.* 1985; **3**: 129–131.

172. White, J.M., Nowak, R.M., Martin, G.B. *et al.* Immediate emergency department external cardiac pacing for prehospital bradyasystolic arrest. *Ann. Emerg. Med.* 1985; **14**: 298–301.

173. Syverud, S.A., Dalsey, W.C. & Hedges, J.R. Transcutaneous and transvenous cardiac pacing for bradyasystolic cardiac arrest. *Ann. Emerg. Med.* 1986; **15**: 121–124.

174. Cummins, R.O., Graves, J.R., Larsen, M.P. *et al.* Out-of-hospital transcutaneous pacing by emergency medical technicians in patients with asystolic cardiac arrest. *N. Engl. J. Med.* 1993; **328**: 1377–1382.

175. Rady, M.Y., Rivers, E.P., Martin, G.B., Smithline, H., Appleton, T. & Nowak, R.M. Continuous central venous oximetry and shock index in the emergency department: use in the evaluation of clinical shock. *Am. J. Emerg. Med.* 1992; **10**: 538–541.

176. Tenaglia, A.N., Califf, R.M., Candela, R.J. *et al.* Thrombolytic therapy in patients requiring cardiopulmonary resuscitation. *Am. J. Cardiol.* 1991; **68**: 1015–1019.

177. Spreng, D., DeBehnke, D.J., Crowe, D. & Swart, G. Evaluation of an esophageal Doppler probe for the identification of experimental pseudo-electromechanical dissociation: a preliminary study. *Resuscitation* 1995; **29**: 153–156.

40

Cardiocerebral resuscitation: a new approach to out-of-hospital cardiac arrest

Gordon A. Ewy and Michael J. Kellum

University of the Arizona Sarver Heart Center, University of Arizona College of Medicine, Tucson, AZ, USA
Emergency Department, Mercy Walworth Medical Center, Lake Geneva, WI, USA

Introduction

Prehospital treatment of cardiac arrest became practical in 1960 when the technique of closed chest cardiac massage was demonstrated effectively to prolong the time for successful defibrillation following cessation of circulation due to cardiac arrest.[1] Closed chest massage was merged with externally applied defibrillation and mouth-to-mouth ventilation to form what is today known as cardiopulmonary resuscitation or CPR.[2–5] By 1966 standardized training and performance criteria had been developed and published.[5] A few years later the American Heart Association (AHA) adopted CPR and spearheaded the campaign to disseminate it to both professionals and the public. The AHA periodically reviews the science, practice and implementation of CPR and publishes updated "guidelines."[6–10]

As an organizational model, CPR can be considered an outstanding public health achievement; but its success in this realm is marred by its failure as a treatment modality for patients who sustain an out-of-hospital cardiac arrest (OOH-CA). When the currently recommended guideline-driven CPR is used to treat patients with an OOH-CA, survival rates have been and continue to be dismal. These poor and unchanged survival rates, in spite of periodic updates, may in part be explained because CPR was conceived as and is currently promulgated as an appropriate intervention for what turns out to be two pathophysiologically entirely different disorders: respiratory arrest and cardiac arrest.

A new approach to the resuscitation of individuals with out-of-hospital cardiac arrest due to ventricular fibrillation or pulseless ventricular tachycardia was developed by the University of Arizona Sarver Heart Center CPR Research Group in Tucson, Arizona.[11–13] Many of the changes were based on animal experimentation. This new approach, now called Cardiocerebral Resuscitation (CCR), was implemented in Tucson in late 2003 and a modified version was instituted in 2004 in Rock and Walworth Counties of Wisconsin.[14] At the time of its implementation, it was a dramatic departure from the existing technique of cardiopulmonary resuscitation (CPR) endorsed by the American Heart Association and the international community in "Guidelines 2000."[10]

Data from the Emergency Medical Services (EMS) quality control observational study in Rock and Walworth counties of Wisconsin showed that this new approach is clinically sound, for when the principles of Cardiocerebral Resuscitation were utilized in the prehospital care of adults with a witnessed arrest and an initially shockable rhythm, a 300% improvement in survival was observed.[14]

The purpose of this chapter is to describe cardiocerebral resuscitation (CCR) and its implementation, to review its scientific rationale and to promote its acceptance by emergency care providers worldwide.

Survival

The definition of "survival" is relevant for both statistical and clinical reasons. Both the return of spontaneous circulation and being alive at hospital admission were initially used as "survival" endpoints. But because many such "survivors" ultimately died before being discharged from the hospital, a more clinically relevant definition of "survival" has been introduced: neurologically intact survival at hospital discharge.[15,16]

Cardiac Arrest: The Science and Practice of Resuscitation Medicine. 2nd edn., ed. Norman Paradis, Henry Halperin, Karl Kern, Volker Wenzel, Douglas Chamberlain. Published by Cambridge University Press. © Cambridge University Press, 2007.

Comparisons of survival rates are often difficult to interpret because of differences in the definition of survival and the inclusion/exclusion criteria that exist in any given report. But when survival rates for OOH-CA are examined, it is clear that they are very low and, with few exceptions, that they have remained stagnant over the last few decades.[17,18] Overall survival rates from non-traumatic OOH-CA in Tucson, Arizona have been unchanged at about 6% over the past decade.[19] Overall survival in larger cities such as Chicago, Los Angeles, and New York is closer to 1%.[17] Most survivors are found in the subset of patients with a witnessed arrest and an initially shockable rhythm. In this group, survival in Tucson, Arizona has been 10 ± 2% for the past decade,[19] while survival in Los Angeles in 2002 was 6%,[17] and in Rock and Walworth counties in Wisconsin during 2000–2003 it was 20%.[14]

Three phases of ventricular fibrillation

The three-phase time-sensitive model of cardiac arrest due to ventricular fibrillation, articulated by Weisfeldt and Becker, is helpful in understanding some of the problems with CPR that are overcome with cardiocerebral resuscitation.[20]

The first or electrical phase lasts for about 4 or 5 minutes from the onset of collapse. During this period the most important intervention is prompt defibrillation. Although the heart is fibrillating, the myocardium has not yet used up its energy stores nor has it undergone serious cellular damage and is therefore not only responsive to the defibrillation shock but, if defibrillated, is also able to generate a perfusing rhythm. This is why automated external defibrillators (AEDs) have been utilized so successfully in a wide variety of settings, including airplanes, airports, casinos, and in the community where prompt defibrillation could be accomplished.[21–24]

The second or circulatory phase lasts for a variable period of time, but probably from minute 4 or 5 to minute 10 after the onset of a VF arrest. Within this time, the lack of myocardial perfusion during active myocyte contractions results in waning cardiac energy stores and the accumulation of toxic metabolites. Immediate defibrillation is inappropriate in this phase because the dysfunctional ventricles seldom generate a perfusing rhythm. The shock usually results in ventricular asystole or pulseless electrical activity (PEA). Therefore, the most crucial intervention during this phase is to restore myocardial blood flow by the generation of adequate coronary perfusion pressure with chest compressions prior to defibrillation. Although not proven, myocardial perfusion is assumed to help replenish energy stores and to remove toxic metabolites to the point that the heart can respond adequately to the defibrillation shock. These changes are assumed to occur as chest compressions during the circulatory phase have been shown to increase the amplitude of the electrocardiographically recorded fibrillation wave forms and improve the chances of successful defibrillation with a perfusing rhythm.[25–27] It is very probable that restoring perfusion to the brain during this time period is also of critical importance for neurologically intact survival.

The third or "metabolic" phase follows the "circulatory" phase. Defibrillation first during this phase is almost universally unsuccessful and survival rates for individuals first treated at this stage are uniformly very poor. In theory, both the provision of adequate cerebral and coronary perfusion, as well as adequate oxygenation and ventilation would be a necessary prerequisite to survival. Multiple interacting detrimental factors are operant during this phase. Innovative therapies are needed. As noted above, an appreciation of these three phases helps put into context some of the recent findings in resuscitation research.

Cardiocerebral resuscitation

Cardiocerebral resuscitation, as its name implies, was developed to improve neurologically normal survival of patients with cardiac arrest by advocating continuous cerebral and cardiac perfusion by early and near continuous chest compressions.[12,13] Its recommendations for defibrillation are also guided by the three-phase time-dependent model of ventricular fibrillation.[20] Its primary focus is amelioration of the global effects of the lack of perfusion that follow the cessation of effective cardiac activity. It is this lack of perfusion that initiates, perpetuates, and intensifies the pathophysiological derangements that thwart the effectiveness of interventions such as defibrillation and ultimately leads to disability or death. The perfusion pressures generated by chest compressions are typically quite marginal relative to those developed by the beating heart; any interruption of chest compressions has a marked effect on perfusion and therefore the chance of neurologically intact survival. The performance of near continuous appropriately delivered chest compressions is therefore a fundamental tenet of cardiocerebral resuscitation (CCR).

The emphasis on limiting interruptions of chest compressions is based on the findings that the major determinant of neurologically normal survival from prolonged cardiac arrest is not the blood gas composition, the acid–base balance, or the frequency or strength of defibrillation shocks, but rather the cardiac and cerebral perfusion pressures generated during chest compressions.[13,33–37] Adequate perfusion must be generated relatively early in the arrest, because delays in its establishment results in few, if any, favorable outcomes.[38]

Chest compressions generate perfusion; and when they are stopped, blood flow is immediately curtailed. This in itself is detrimental; but equally important is that such interruptions also transiently diminish the effectiveness of subsequent chest compressions. It takes several compressions to regenerate the perfusion pressures that existed before the interruption.[39] This effect is magnified by repeated interruptions for activities such as rescue breathing or assisted ventilations. But it is also relevant to interruptions for any reason, including those for pulse checks, rhythm analysis, stacked shocks, intubation, patient reassessment, intravenous line placements, and pacing without perfusion. This is a major reason why cardiocerebral resuscitation advocates near continuous uninterrupted chest compressions and recommends that they only be interrupted for rhythm analysis and defibrillation.

It should be emphasized once more that cardiocerebral resuscitation was not developed for use in patients whose arrest is non-cardiac in origin (even though many of its principles might well be applicable in the management of patients with respiratory arrest as well).

Cardiocerebral resuscitation summary

Cardiocerebral resuscitation is recommended for adults with witnessed unexpected collapse without normal breathing – a condition that is almost always due to cardiac and not respiratory arrest or for patients with witnessed collapse and a ventricular arrhythmia that might respond to defibrillation or cardioversion.

There are three components of cardiocerebral resuscitation or CCR. The first is directed toward the public to emphasize the importance of activating the EMS system (calling 911 in the United States), chest-compression-only bystander CPR, and using an AED early in witnessed arrest if a unit is readily available. Notably, the major difference between CCR and CPR for this component is that CCR discourages rescue breathing. This lay component has been called "Be a Lifesaver" in Tucson and "Call and Pump" in Rock and Walworth counties of Wisconsin.[12–14] The most appropriate name is probably, "Be a lifesaver – call and pump." The second component of cardiocerebral resuscitation consists of new recommendations for EMS systems and personnel (Fig. 40.1.).[12–14] This component will be discussed in detail in the following sections. The third

component of cardiocerebral resuscitation is similar to the second, but is for in-hospital personnel and encourages the use of mild hypothermia and other therapies that improve survival in comatose patients following a cardiac arrest.[28–32]

Cardiocerebral resuscitation guidelines

Laypersons are taught to "Be a lifesaver – call and pump." They are to call 911 as soon as possible and then begin continuous chest compressions (CCC) – that is pump on the chest. Rescue breathing is not recommended. The technique of CCC is ideally taught with emphasis on a metronome-guided rate of 100 per minute. Additionally, full chest recoil after each compression is specifically emphasized. Dispatchers answering 911 calls give CCC-only instructions to callers and it is recommended that they also provide metronome guidance.

Law officers and other EMS rescuers who are equipped with AEDs are to defibrillate immediately *only* if they personally witness the collapse or if good continuous-chest compressions are being provided by a bystander. Otherwise, they are to perform CCC for 2 minutes (200 compressions so they do not have to be concerned about the time) before defibrillation. To assure prompt defibrillation after the chest compressions, if only one rescuer is on scene, AED pads are attached before continuous chest compressions are initiated. If two rescuers are available, one initiates chest compressions while the other attaches the defibrillator pads. If a shockable rhythm is present, a single shock is delivered, by using maximum joules and biphasic waveforms if possible, and chest compressions are immediately resumed for another 200 compressions. Therefore, most of the voice instructions on the AEDs available at the time of this writing are to be ignored. During training, emphasis is placed on minimizing the hands-off period between cessation of CCC and delivery of the shock and between the shock and resumption of CCC. Pulse checks are not to be done following the shock, but rather are performed after the 200 postshock chest compressions during the rhythm analysis period. Establishment of intravenous access is encouraged as soon as possible, but again without interruption of CCC.

Initial airway management consists of insertion of an oropharyngeal airway and provision of high flow oxygen by non-rebreather mask. Rescue breaths and assisted ventilations (positive pressure ventilations that increase intrathoracic pressure and decrease venous return to the heart) are not encouraged until either the return of spontaneous circulation or until after three cycles of "200 CCC/rhythm analysis/± shock" are completed.

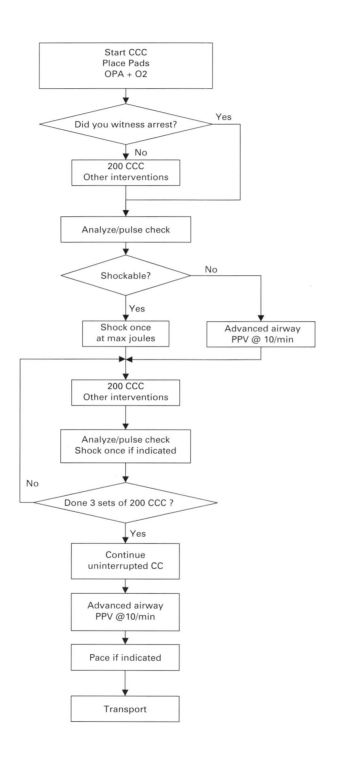

(1) If single rescuer - place pads **before** beginning CCC

Interrupt chest compressions **only** for
(1) Switching pumpers
(2) Analysis/shock

Pulse check procedure
(1) Do near end of 200 CCC
(2) Find carotid pulse during CC
(3) Check pulse during analysis

Priority for "other interventions"
(1) CCC
(2) Metronome @100/min for CC
(3) Switch pumper every minute
(4) OPA + oxygen
(5) Start IV or IO
(6) IV Epi (repeat every 3 minutes)
(7) IV Vasopressin (one dose)
(8) Glucagon (one dose of 2–4 mg)
(9) Atropine (brady PEA, asystole)
(10) Amiodarone 300 mg bolus (if recurrent or refractory Vfib)
(11) Advanced airway(combitube or Endotracheal tube)
(12) Airway valve (ResQ Pod)
(13) Ventilate at 10–12/minute (one every 5–6 seconds)

Positive pressure ventilations
Do **during** CCC
Deliver each breath in 1 second

Code monitor responsibilities
(1) Metronome must be used
(2) CC done properly: full recoil after compression
(3) Switch CC person every minute
(4) Ensure uninterrupted CC
(5) Interventions done as prioritized above
(6) Notify dispatch at moment
   (a) shock given first
   (b) ROSC
(6) Amiodarone used if recurrent or persistent Vfib
(7) Assisted ventilation rate is10–12/minute
(8) Pulse checks done properly
(9) Note changes in spontaneous respirations
(10) Note change(s) associated with ROSC
(11) ResQ Pod is removed if pulse returns or CPR is discontinued

Fig. 40.1. Adult cardiac arrest.

If the first analysis after 200 CCC reveals a non-shockable rhythm, chest compressions are resumed and ventilation and advanced airway interventions are initiated with emphasis upon minimal, if any, interruptions of CCC. Hyperventilation is to be avoided. Individual ventilations are to be performed at a rate of no more than 10 per minute. Each breath is to be delivered over a 2-second interval.

Of note, recommendations for ventilation after prolonged periods of chest-compression-only are not well established and are the subject of ongoing investigations.

This protocol is only applicable to individuals with a presumed cardiac arrest, i.e., an adult with unexpected sudden collapse without normal breathing.

Defibrillation

Immediate defibrillation is the treatment of choice during the first or "electrical" phase of a VF arrest; that is during the first 4 minutes or so. Unfortunately, rescuers equipped with defibrillators seldom arrive during this phase. As mentioned above, immediate defibrillation during the "circulatory" phase is counterproductive, producing either asystole or PEA. Two human studies and animal studies have demonstrated that this detrimental effect of defibrillation can be avoided if the heart is perfused before delivering the shock.[25–27] During this phase, adequate coronary perfusion is a prerequisite to successful defibrillation and currently this can only be achieved by chest compressions.

Therefore, CCR advocates 2 minutes of CCC prior to defibrillation in all cases except those where the AED-equipped rescuer actually witnesses the collapse. This recommendation simplifies the EMS decision-making process for a rescuer. It was developed for two reasons. First, it is very often difficult to ascertain an accurate down-time in real-life circumstances and thereafter to calculate the minute interval. Second, the studies cited above did not demonstrate a detrimental effect of performing compressions (actually CPR) during the first or electrical phase of VF arrest.[26,27]

Single shocks

Stacked shocks and their associated preshock analysis and postshock pulse check activities interrupt chest compressions for significant periods of time. Stacked shocks are therefore not advocated in CCR. Instead, single shocks

immediately followed by resumption of chest compression without a pulse check are recommended. In a recent study from Seattle, a median interruption of 29 seconds was observed when stacked shocks were utilized.[40] This interruption of perfusion to the heart and brain is significant, because studies have shown that interruptions as brief as 10–15 seconds significantly reduce the efficacy of a shock and increase the incidence of postresuscitation myocardial dysfunction.[41,42] In man, the group in Seattle found that rhythm reanalysis and subsequent shocks generated a pulse in only 1 of 50 individuals studied. This meager benefit came at a cost of no perfusion for median periods of 45 and 55 seconds, respectively, for 2nd and 3rd shocks.[40] These authors concluded, "Because the activities of rhythm reanalyzes, stacked shock, and initial postshock pulse checks had low yield with regard to the balance between achieving or detecting a pulse and initiating CPR, one consideration would be to eliminate these activities from the resuscitation algorithm."[40] It is reasonable to conclude, especially with the increasing percentage of defibrillators having biphasic design, that the cardiocerebral resuscitation approach of delivering single instead of stacked shocks is credible.[12,13]

Postshock activities

A pulse is rarely present immediately after a shock that is delivered during the circulatory phase of VF arrest. A recent study reported that a pulse was detected during the initial postshock interval in only 2.5% of cardiac arrest victims.[40] Pulse checks immediately after a shock are therefore not advocated. They seldom provide useful information and they routinely interrupt chest compressions. Instead, CCR recommends that pulse checks be performed during the rhythm analysis period, when cessation of compression is mandatory. The pulse site is ascertained during the last few seconds of the 200 compression cycle.

The Sarver Heart Center CPR Research Group of the University of Arizona noted in their experimental laboratory that following prolonged VF arrest, that is, in the circulatory phase of VF arrest, the shock almost always defibrillated the subject into a non-perfusing rhythm. Because researchers had immediate access to the hemodynamics of the instrumented swine, they would immediately restart chest compressions to restore coronary perfusion pressures. With this approach, pulseless electrical activity was likely to revert to a perfusing rhythm.[12,13] This is why a second set of 200 chest compressions is recommended immediately after the defibrillator shock.

Chest compression technique

Cardiocerebral Resuscitation recommends a chest compression rate of 100 per minute, the upper rate of that currently recommended by Guidelines for CPR.[9] Metronome guidance is advocated, because in the out-of-hospital setting chest compression rates are very commonly above 120 per minute and not infrequently approach 150 per minute (Kellum *et al.* personal communication). The impact of rapid rates on perfusion has not been well studied in man. In experimental animals, compression rates of 120 were found to be more effective than chest compression rates of 60 per minute.[43] These findings were instrumental in the AHA Guidelines change from compression rates of 60 per minute to 80 to 100 compressions a minute in 1992.[9] Compression rates of 150 in experimental studies are associated with diminished cardiac output.[44]

Recently, the importance of full chest recoil during the release phase of each compression has been highlighted.[45] Incomplete chest recoil compromises perfusion, because it interferes with the generation of a negative pressure in the chest cavity and therefore is associated with decreased venous blood returning to the heart. As a consequence, cardiac output is reduced. These authors noted incomplete chest recoil to occur in 46% of simulated resuscitations performed by paramedics. In a companion study, they found significant decreases in both coronary perfusion pressure and cerebral blood flow when incomplete chest recoil occurred.[45] Accordingly, lifting the hands from the chest after each chest compression is essential to assure complete chest recoil.

Furthermore, when incomplete chest recoil was combined with excessive ventilations, perfusion was severely compromised.[45] Excessive ventilation rates (see below) are extremely common features reported by both in-hospital staff and out-of-hospital paramedics.

Airway ventilations

The three recommendations that CCR makes concerning airway management and ventilations in OOH-CA are summarized as follows. (1) Bystander and first responder CPR is simplified to continuous-chest compression-only CPR. (2) Initial EMS airway management is limited to assuring an open airway and administration of high flow supplemental oxygen. (3) Advanced airway management and assisted ventilations should be initiated only when appropriate and performed in a manner that minimizes their negative impact on perfusion pressures.

Although each of these three recommendations represents a deviation from the CPR guidelines 2000, and each is counterintuitive to the "ABCs" that have been taught for decades, the reasoning for each is presented below. Cardiocerebral Resuscitation does not advocate the elimination of ventilations; instead, it emphasizes the beneficial effects of negative intrathoracic pressure, e.g., normal breathing, chest recoil, gasping or agonal breathing, and deemphasizes the use of positive intrathoracic pressure ventilation from "rescue breathing," bag-mouth ventilation, and endotracheal intubation with positive pressure ventilation.[46]

Bystander "CPR"

Bystander and most first EMS responder should provide continuous-chest-compression only, without rescue breathing. At the onset of primary ventricular fibrillation, the pulmonary veins, left side of the heart, and entire arterial system are filled with oxygenated blood. Hence, the traditional CPR-recommended initial step of positive pressure "rescue" breathing with oxygen-poor exhaled breaths never seemed reasonable. What is critical is that the existing oxygenated blood be delivered to the tissues. Because of this logic, years ago, the Dutch recommended replacing the ABCs of CPR with CBA.[47]

It is well documented that bystander CPR saves lives when coupled with advanced cardiac life support.[48–51] A significant problem contributing to the less than optimal survival rates in OOH-CA, however, is the failure of citizens to initiate bystander CPR, predominantly because they do not want to do mouth-to-mouth rescue breathing on a stranger.[52–56] In some cultures the reluctance is even greater.[57] In Japan, only 2% of students and 3% of nurses said they were willing to perform mouth-to-mouth rescue breathing on a stranger.[57] Other reasons include fear of harming the victim or the complicated psychomotor skills necessary. The requirement for "rescue breathing" is a major problem. The AHA "Guidelines 2000" state that, "If a person is unwilling or unable to perform mouth-to-mouth ventilation for an adult victim, chest-compression-only CPR should be provided rather than no attempt at CPR being made."[58] Nonetheless, in our areas, before the institution of cardiocerebral resuscitation, this approach was seldom if ever mentioned or taught.

But the major reason for recommending continuous-chest-compression CPR for single bystander is that rescue breathing, when performed the way it has been taught for the past few decades, e.g., two breaths before each 15 chest compressions, is actually harmful.[59] Each recommended breath is taught to be delivered over at least 2 seconds. This recommendation assumes a short time to deliver the two recommended breaths before each 15 chest compressions. But, by the time the would-be rescuer stops chest compressions, lifts the victim's chin, pinches their nose, takes a deep breath, makes a seal with their mouth over the victim's mouth, blows, watches the chest rise and fall, repeats this sequence a second time, and then finds the location to reposition their hands and resume chest compressions, the recommended "two quick breaths" interrupts chest compression an average of 16 seconds.[60] By using a simulated single rescuer protocol, continuous-chest-compression BLS was compared with "standard" BLS in the experimental laboratory where the two breaths were given over 16 seconds before each of the15 compressions.[59] In this study, Kern and associates found that the survival rate was 13%.[59] The survival rate of 13% was of intense interest, for in Tucson, Arizona the average survival of individuals with OOH-CA due to ventricular fibrillation over the past decade was similar.[19]

Abella and associates reported that in-hospital suboptimal compression rates correlated with poor return of spontaneous circulation and thus initial survival.[61] Initial survival rates were significantly higher for patients receiving more than 87 compressions per minute than were those receiving fewer than 72 compressions per minute.[61] Obviously, if every set of 15 compressions is interrupted for 14 to 16 seconds to deliver the recommended two ventilations, the individual will not receive enough chest compressions to survive.

Unfortunately, any changes in the guidelines that alter the 2:15 rescue breathing to chest compression ratio might improve survival, but only in those who receive prompt bystander-initiated resuscitation. "Further, any change in the ratio will not change the reluctance of bystanders to perform bystander-initiated CPR."[62] One can only conclude that the recommendation of chest-compression-only CPR for bystanders of cardiac arrest as recommended by cardiocerebral resuscitation is logical.

What is the role of gasping or agonal respirations?

Another observation is that, if a subject collapses with ventricular fibrillation, gasping lasts for a variable period of time. Gasping is both fortunate and unfortunate. It is fortunate because, when chest compressions are promptly initiated, the subject is likely to continue to gasp and provide self-ventilation. Indeed, Kouwenhoven, Jude, and Knickerbocker in one of their early programs indicated that ventilation was not necessary during chest compression because the subject gasped.[1] (Demonstration of the

technique of CPR for New York Society of Anesthesiologist 1960s. Copy of demonstration provided on CD by J.R. Jude). Nevertheless, gasping may be unfortunate, as most lay individuals interpret this as an indication that the individual is still breathing, and do not initiate bystander CPR or activate the EMS as soon as they should. Education will be essential to improving prompt initiation of bystander chest compressions in patients with cardiac arrest.

Ventilations by emergency medical systems personnel can be deadly!

The two major problems with assisted ventilations by the Emergency Medical Services are the deleterious effects of early intubation and hyperventilation.

As noted above, any interruption of chest compressions during the circulatory phase of VF arrest markedly decreases the chances of survival. In addition to the excessive delays caused by AEDs, when the delay time for the average intubation is added, the victim has little chance of survival. Even in children, where respiratory arrest is more common, it has been shown that the use of bag-mask ventilation is better than intubation.[63]

As also noted above, however, all positive pressure ventilations increase intrathoracic pressures and thereby reduce venous return. In the setting of cardiac arrest, this can result in a significant reduction of cardiac output that, in turn, compromises both cardiac and cerebral perfusion.[64] This is more than a theoretical issue; studies in trained and retrained paramedics showed that once assisted ventilations are initiated, they are almost always performed at rates that severely compromise perfusion. Indeed, a recent publication by Aufderheide and Lurie entitled "Death by hyperventilation" highlighted this real problem.[65] In-hospital as well as field observations documented that these personnel delivered an average of 37 breaths per minute rather than the 12–15 minutes recommended by the guidelines.[66]

Even when one is on the scene, it is difficult to get the excited individual to "slow down" when it comes to delivering ventilations. Cardiocerebral resuscitation protocols minimize the chances for excessive ventilations. Cardiocerebral resuscitation advocates placement of an oropharyngeal device and oxygenation by non-rebreather mask in the initial phases of treatment and deliberately delay positive pressure ventilations in patients with an initially shockable rhythm. Assisted ventilations are not started until ROSC or three series of 200 chest compressions and shock (if necessary) are completed.[14] While the first person with a duty to respond applies the defibrillator pads and begins chest compressions, the second emergency-trained and equipped EMS person places an oropharyngeal airway and a non-rebreather mask with high flow oxygen.

The optimal type of ventilation by EMS personnel for patients who have only had bystander-chest-compressions prior to their arrival is unknown, and is the subject of intense investigation.

Conclusions

This chapter describes cardiocerebral resuscitation, a new approach to out-of-hospital witnessed arrest due to ventricular fibrillation or pulseless ventricular tachycardia in adults. We reviewed the studies that led the University of Arizona Sarver Heart Center CPR Research Group and the Tucson Fire Department and the EMS systems of Rock and Walworth counties in Wisconsin to advocate and to help institute this new methodology for witnessed unexpected sudden cardiac arrest in adults. It is dramatically different from Guidelines 2000 and is significantly different from Guidelines 2005. Compared to historical controls, where Guidelines 2000 CPR was used, cardiocerebral resuscitation resulted in significant improvement in neurologically normal survival in patients with out-of-hospital cardiac arrest and shockable arrhythmias.[14] In patients with witnessed cardiac arrest and a shockable rhythm on arrival of EMS system, survival was increased 300%.[14] Although these findings were in an observational study, they were so dramatic and in accordance with our animal research studies that we recommend this approach for all out-of-hospital cardiac arrests with a shockable rhythm until a different protocol is proven to be better.

Note added in proof

Since this chapter was initially submitted, preliminary data on the effect of initiating Cardiocerebral Resuscitation in a large metropolitan area has become available. Survival of adults with cardiac arrest was compared for 6 months before and after training of medics in two EMS agencies to perform Cardiocerebral Resuscitation. The primary endpoint was survival of patients with VF to hospital discharge. Survival to hospital discharge was 3.5% (3/85) prior to initiation of Cardiocerebral Resuscitation and 21% (21 of 97) after (<0.001).[67]

Acknowledgments

We wish to acknowledge the invaluable editorial and research assistance of Dr. Ronald Hilwig. We also gratefully acknowledge the past and continuing research of our colleagues in the University of Arizona Sarver Heart Center CCR Research Group. The men and women of the EMS systems in Tucson and Rock and Walworth counties of Wisconsin are also gratefully acknowledged.

REFERENCES

1. Kouwenhoven, W.B., Jude, J. & Knickerbocker, G.G. Closed-chest cardiac massage. *J. Am. Med. Assoc.* 1960; **173**: 1064–1067.
2. Zoll, P.M., Linethal, A.J. & Gibson, W. Termination of ventricular fibrillation in man by externally applied electric counter-shock. *N. Engl. J. Med.* 1956; **254**: 727–732.
3. Lown, B., Amarasingham, R. & Neuman, J. New method for terminating cardiac arrhythmias; use of synchronized capacitor discharge. *J. Am. Med. Assoc.* 1962; **182**: 548–555.
4. Safar, P. Ventilatory efficacy of mouth-to-mouth artificial respiration. *J. Am. Med. Assoc.* 1958(May): 335–341.
5. Statement by the Ad Hoc Committee on Cardiopulmonary Resuscitation of the Division of Medical Sciences NAoS-NRC. *J. Am. Med. Assoc.* 1966; **198**: 138–145.
6. AHA. Standards for cardiopulmonary resuscitation (CPR) and emergency cardiac care (ECC). II: Basic life support. *J. Am. Med. Assoc.* 1974; **227**(Suppl 7): 833–868.
7. AHA. Standards and guidelines for cardiopulmonary resuscitation (CPR) and emergency cardiac care (ECC). *J. Am. Med. Assoc.* 1980; **244**(5): 453–509.
8. AHA. Standards and guidelines for cardiopulmonary resuscitation (CPR) and emergency cardiac care (ECC). *J. Am. Med. Assoc.* 1986; **255**(21): 2905–2989.
9. AHA. Guidelines for cardiopulmonary resuscitation and emergency cardiac care. Emergency Cardiac Care Committee and Subcommittees, American Heart Association. Part, I. Introduction. *J. Am. Med. Assoc.* 1992; **268**: 2171–2241.
10. AHA. American Heart Association in collaboration with International Liaison Committee on Resuscitation. Guidelines 2000 for Cardiopulmonary Resuscitation and Emergency Cardiovascular Care: International Consensus on Science, Part **6**: Advanced Cardiovascular Life Support. *Circulation* 2000; **102**(Suppl. I (8)): I-1–I-403.
11. Ewy, G. A new approach for out-of-hospital CPR: a bold step forward. *Resuscitation* 2003; **58**(3): 271–272.
12. Kern, K.B., Valenzuela, T., Clark, L.L. *et al.* An alternative approach to advancing resuscitation science. *Resuscitation.* 2005; **64**: 261–268.
13. Ewy, G. Cardiocerebral resuscitation: The new cardiopulmonary resuscitation. *Circulation* 2005; **111**(16): 2134–2142.
14. Kellum, M.J., Kennedy, K.W. & Ewy, GA. Cardiocerebral resuscitation improves survival of patients with out-of-hospital cardiac arrest. *Am. J. Med.* 2006; **119**: 335–340.
15. Jacobs, I., Nadkarni, V., Bahr, J. *et al.* International Liaison Committee on Resuscitation. Cardiac arrest and cardiopulmonary resuscitation outcome reports: update and simplification of the Utstein templates for resuscitation registries. A

statement for healthcare professionals from a task force of the international liaison committee on resuscitation (American Heart Association, European Resuscitation Council, Australian Resuscitation Council, New Zealand Resuscitation Council, Heart and Stroke Foundation of Canada, InterAmerican Heart Foundation, Resuscitation Council of Southern Africa). *Resuscitation* 2004; **63**(3): 233–249.

16. Safar, P. Prevention and therapy of postresuscitation neurologic dysfunction and injury. In Cardiac Arrest: The Science and Practice of Resuscitation Medicine. Baltimore: Williams & Wilkins, 1966.

17. Eckstein, M., Stratton, S.J. & Chan, L.S. Cardiac arrest resuscitation evaluation in Los Angeles: CARE-LA. *Ann. Emerg. Med.* 2005; **45**: 504–509.

18. Valenzuela, T.D., Roe, D.J., Cretin, S., Spaite, D.W. & Larsen, M.P. Estimating effectiveness of cardiac arrest interventions: a logistic regression survival model. *Circulation* 1997; **96**(10): 3308–3313.

19. Valenzuela, T.D., Kern, K.B., Clark, L.L. *et al.* Interruptions of chest compressions during emergency medical systems resuscitations. *Circulation.* 2005; **112**: 1259–1265.

20. Weisfeldt, M.L. & Becker, L. Resuscitation after cardiac arrest: a 3-phase time-sensitive model. *J. Am. Med. Assoc.* 2002; **288**(23): 3035–3038.

21. Page, R.L., Joglar, J.A., Kowal, R.C. *et al.* Use of automated external defibrillators by a U.S. airline. *N. Engl. J. Med.* 2000; **343**(17): 1210–1216.

22. Caffrey, S.L., Willoughby, P.J., Pepe, P.E. & Becker, L.B. Public use of automated external defibrillators. *N. Engl. J. Med.* 2002; **347**(16): 1242–1247.

23. Valenzuela, T.D., Roe, D.J., Nichol, G., Clark, L.L., Spaite, D.W. & Hardman, R.G. Outcomes of rapid defibrillation by security officers after cardiac arrest in casinos. *N. Engl. J. Med.* 2000; **343**(17): 1206–1209.

24. O'Rourke, M.F., Donaldson, E. & Geddes, J.S. An airline cardiac arrest program (see comments) *Circulation* 1997; **96**(9): 2849–2853.

25. Berg, R.A., Hilwig, R.W., Kern, K.B. & Ewy, G.A. Precountershock cardiopulmonary resuscitation improves ventricular fibrillation median frequency and myocardial readiness for successful defibrillation from prolonged ventricular fibrillation: a randomized controlled swine study. *Ann. Emerg. Med.* 2002; **40**: 563–570.

26. Cobb, L.A., Fahrenbruch, C.E., Walsh, T.R., Compass, M.K. & Olsufka, M. Influence of cardiopulmonary resuscitation prior to defibrillation in patients wtih out-of-hospital ventricular fibrillation. *J. Am. Med. Assoc.* 1999; **281**: 1182–1188.

27. Wik, L., Hansen, T.B., Fylling, F. *et al.* Delaying defibrillation to give basic cardiopulmonary resuscitation to patients with out-of-hospital ventricular fibrillation: a randomized trial. *J. Am. Med. Assoc.* 2003; **289**(11): 1389–1395.

28. Bernard, S., Gray, T.W., Buist, M.D. *et al.* Treatment of comatose survivors of out-of-hospital cardiac arrest with induced hypothermia. *N. Engl. J. Med.* 2002; **346**(8): 557–563.

29. Holzer, M. for The hypothermia after cardiac arrest study group. Mild therapeutic hypothermia to improve the neurologic outcome after cardiac arrest. *N. Engl. J. Med.* 2002; **346**(8): 549–556.

30. Holzer, M., Bernard, S., Hachimi-Idrissi, S., Roine, R.O., Sterz, F. & Mullner, M. on behalf of the Collaborative Group on Induced Hypothermia for Neuroprotection After Cardiac Arrest Hypothermia for neuroprotection after cardiac arrest: systematic review and individual patient data meta-analysis. *Crit. Care. Med.* 2005; **33**(2): 414–418.

31. Bernard, S., Buist, M., Monteiro, O. & Smith, K. Induced hypothermia using large volume, ice-cold intravenous fluid in comatose survivors of out-of-hospital cardiac arrest: a preliminary report. *Resuscitation* 2003; **56**: 9–13.

32. Holzer, M., Bernard, S., Hachimi-Idrissi, S., Roine, R.O., Sterz, F. & Mullner, M. Hypothermia for neuroprotection after cardiac arrest: systematic review and individual patient data meta-analysis. *Crit. Care Med.* 2005; **33**(2): 414–418.

33. Sanders, A.B., Ewy, G.A. & Taft, T.V. Prognostic and therapeutic importance of the aortic diastolic pressure in resuscitation from cardiac arrest. *Crit. Care Med.* 1984; **12**: 871–873.

34. Paradis, N.A., Martin, G.B., Rivers, E.P. *et al.* Coronary perfusion pressure and the return of spontaneous circulation in human cardiopulmonary resuscitation. *J. Am. Med. Assoc.* 1990; **263**: 1106–1113.

35. Kern, K.B., Ewy, G.A., Voorhees, W.D., Babbs, C.F. & Tacker, W.A. Myocardial perfusion pressure; a predictor of 24-hour survival during prolonged cardiac arrest in dogs. *Resuscitation* 1988; **16**: 241–250.

36. Sanders, A.B., Kern, K.B., Atlas, M., Bragg, S. & Ewy, G.A. Importance of the duration of inadequate coronary perfusion pressure on resuscitation from cardiac arrest. *J. Am. Coll. Cardiol.* 1985; **6**: 113–118.

37. Sanders, A.B., Olge, M. & Ewy, G.A. Coronary perfusion pressure during cardiopulmonary resuscitation. *Am. J. Emerg. Med.* 1985; **3**: 11–14.

38. Sanders, A.B., Kern, K.B., Bragg, S. & Ewy, G.A. Neurological benefits from the use of early cardiopulmonary resuscitation. *Ann. Emerg. Med.* 1987; **16**: 142–146.

39. Berg, R.A., Sanders, A.B., Kern, K.B. *et al.* Adverse hemodynamic effects of interrupting chest compressions for rescue breathing during cardiopulmonary resuscitation for ventricular fibrillation cardiac arrest. *Circulation* 2001; **104**(20): 2465–2470.

40. Rea, T.D., Sachita, S., Kudenchuck, P.J., Copass, M.K. & Cobb, L.A. Automated external defibrillators: to what extend does the algorithm delay CPR? *Ann. Emerg. Med.* 2005; **46**(2): 132–141.

41. Yu, T., Weil, M.H., Tang, W. *et al.* Adverse outcomes of interrupted precordial compression during automated defibrillation. *Circulation.* 2002; **106**(3): 368–372.

42. Yamaguchi, H., Weil, M.H., Tang, W., Kamohara, T., Jin, X. & Bisera, J. Myocardial dysfunction after electrical defibrillation. *Resuscitation* 2002; **54**(3): 289.

43. Feneley, M.P., Maier, G.W., Kern, K.B. *et al.* Influence of compression rate on initial success of resuscitation and 24 hour

survival after prolonged manual cardiopulmonary resuscitation in dogs. *Circulation.* 1988; **77**(1): 240–250.

44. Fitzgerald, K.R., Babbs, C.F., Frissora, H.A., Davis, R.W. & Silver, D.I. Cardiac output during cardiopulmonary resuscitation at various compression rates and durations. *Am. J. Physiol.* 1981; **241**(3): H442–H448.

45. Aufderheide, T.P., Pirrallo, R.G., Yannopoulos, D. *et al.* Incomplete chest wall decompression: a clinical evaluation of CPR performance by EMS personnel and assessment of alternative manual chest compression-decompression techniques. *Resuscitation* 2005; **64**: 353–362.

46. Becker, L.B., Berg, R.A., Pepe, P.E. *et al.* A reappraisal of mouth-to-mouth ventilation during bystander-initiated cardiopulmonary resuscitation. A statement for healthcare professionals from the Ventilation Working Group of the Basic Life Support and Pediatric Life Support Subcommittees, American Heart Association. *Circulation* 1997; **96**(6): 2102–2112.

47. Meursing, B.T.J., Wulterkens, D.W. & van Kesteren, R.G. The ABC of resuscitation and the Dutch (re)treat. *Resuscitation* 2005; **64**: 279–286.

48. Herlitz, J.E.I., Wennerblom, B., Axelsson, A., Bang, A. & Holmberg, S. Effects of bystander initiated cardiopulmonary resuscitation on ventricular fibrillation and survival after witnessed cardiac arrest outside hospital. *Br. Heart J.* 1994; **72**: 408–412.

49. Stiell, I.G., Wells, G.A., Field, B. *et al.* for the Ontario Prehospital Advanced Life Support Study Group. Advanced cardiac life support in out-of-hospital cardiac arrest *N. Engl. J. Med.* 2004; **351**: 647–656.

50. Eisenberg, M.S., Bergner, L. & Hallstrom, A. Cardiac resuscitation in the community: Importance of rapid provision and implication of program planning. *J. Am. Med. Assoc.* 1979; **241**: 1905–1907.

51. Cummins, R.O., Ornato, J.P., Thies, W.H. & Pepe, P.E. Improving survival from sudden cardiac arrest: The "chain of survival" concept. A statement for health professionals from the Advanced Cardiac Life Support Subcommittee and Emergency Cardiac Care Committee, American Heart Association. *Circulation* 1991; **83**: 1832–1847.

52. Locke, C.J., Berg, R.A., Sanders, A.B. *et al.* Bystander cardiopulmonary resuscitation. Concerns about mouth-to-mouth contact. *Arch. Intern. Med.* 1995; **155**(9): 938–904.

53. Ornado, J.P., Hallagan, L.F., McMahan, S.B., Peeples, E.H. & Rostafinski, A.G. Attitudes of BCLS instructors about mouth-to-mouth resuscitation during the AIDS epidemic. *Ann. Emerg. Med.* 1990; **19**: 151–156.

54. Brenner, B.E. & Kaufmann, J. Reluctance of internist and medical nurses to perform mouth-to-mouth resuscitation. *Arch. Intern. Med.* 1993; **153**: 1763–1769.

55. Brenner, B.E., Stark, B. & Kauffman, J. The reluctance of house staff to perform mouth-to-mouth resuscitation in the inpatient setting: what are the considerations? *Resuscitation* 1994; **28**: 185–193.

56. Brenner, B.E., Kaufmann, J. & Sachter, J.J. Comparison of the reluctance of house staff of metropolitan and suburban hospitals to perform mouth-to-mouth resuscitation. *Resuscitation* 1996; **32**: 5–12.

57. Shibata, K., Taniguchi, T., Yoshida, M. & Yamamoto, K. Obstacles to bystander cardiopulmonary resuscitation in Japan. *Resuscitation* 2000; **44**: 187–193.

58. AHA. American Heart Association, in collaboration with the International Liaison Committee on Resuscitation. Guidelines for cardiopulmonary resuscitation and emergency cardiac care: international consensus on science. *Circulation* 2000; **102**(Suppl. I): I-1–I-403.

59. Kern, K.B., Hilwig, R.W., Berg, R.A., Berg, M.D., Sanders, A.B. & Ewy, G.A. Importance of continuous chest compressions during cardiopulmonary resuscitation: improved outcome during a simulated single lay-rescuer scenario. *Circulation* 2002; **105**(5): 645–649.

60. Assar, D., Chamberlain, D., Colquhoun, M. *et al.* Randomized controlled trials of staged teaching for basic life support: 1. skill acquisition at bronze stage. *Resuscitation* 2000; **45**: 7–15.

61. Abella, B.S., Sandbo, N., Vassilatos, P. *et al.* Chest compression rates during cardiopulmonary resuscitation are suboptimal. A prospective study during in-hospital cardiac arrest. *Circulation* 2005; **111**: 428–434.

62. Sanders, A.B. & Ewy, G.A. Cardiopulmonary resuscitation in the real world: When will the guidelines get the message? *J. Am. Med. Assoc.* 2005; **293**: 363–365.

63. Gausche, M., Lewis, R.J., Strattton, S.J. *et al.* Effect of out-of-hospital pediatric endotracheal intubation on survival and neurological outcome: a controlled clinical trial. *J. Am. Med. Assoc.* 2000; **283**: 783–790.

64. Aufderheide, T.P., Sigurdsson, G., Pirrallo, R.G. *et al.* Hyperventilation-induced hypotension during cardiopulmonary resuscitation. *Circulation* 2004; **109**: 1960–1965.

65. Aufderheide, T.P. & Lurie, K. Death by hyperventilation: a common and life-threatening problem during cardiopulmonary resuscitation. *Crit. Care Med.* 2004; 2004(32 (Suppl):) S345–S351.

66. Milander, M.M., Hiscok, P.S., Sanders, A.B., Kern, K.B., Berg, R.A. & Ewy, G.A. Chest compression and ventilation rates during cardiopulmonary resuscitation: the effects of audible tone guidance. *Acad. Emergency Medicine.* 1995; **2**(8): 708–713.

67. Bobrow, B., Clark, L. Sanders, A.B., Kern, K.B., Berg, R.A., & Ewy, G.A. Cardiocerebal resuscitation (CCR), improves survival from out-of-hospital cardiac arrest. Abstract submitted to Society of American Emergency Medicine 2007.

41

Thrombolysis during resuscitation from cardiac arrest

Fabian Spöhr and Bernd W. Böttiger

Department of Anaesthesiology, University of Heidelberg, Heidelberg, Germany

Cardiac arrest has been associated with a very poor prognosis. It has been estimated that 15%–37% of patients suffering in-hospital cardiac arrest, and only 5%–14% of patients suffering out-of-hospital cardiac arrest are expected to be discharged from hospital.[1–3] Unfortunately, the prognosis of these patients has hardly changed during the last 20 years,[4] which may be explained in part by the lack of specific therapeutic strategies for cardiac arrest. Several promising drug therapies have failed to improve long-term survival.[5,6] For example, administration of amiodarone in patients with shock-refractory ventricular fibrillation has been demonstrated to increase the number of patients admitted to hospital,[7] but no drug therapy has shown a positive impact on long-term survival.

Coronary artery disease resulting in acute myocardial infarction (MI) or ischemia-related arrhythmia and massive pulmonary embolism (PE) are the causes of sudden cardiac arrest in more than 70% of patients.[8–10] Systemic thrombolysis is an established and effective therapy for acute MI or PE occurring with hemodynamic instability.[11] The fear of causing life-threatening bleeding complications, however, has been a major drawback for using thrombolytic drugs during CPR. Consequently, thrombolytic agents have historically been withheld in the setting of cardiac arrest. According to the international guidelines for the therapy of acute MI, prolonged or traumatic CPR has been regarded as a relative contraindication for thrombolytic treatment.[12,13] In the recent international guidelines for cardiopulmonary resuscitation, however, CPR is no longer a general contraindication to thrombolysis.[14,15] A high incidence of fatal bleeding complications, however, may outweigh the potential therapeutic benefit of thrombolysis during CPR.

In the first part of this chapter, we will outline the pathophysiological background for the use of thrombolytic drugs during CPR. In the second part, data from clinical studies will be presented and discussed. In the third part, safety concerns will be highlighted.

Pathophysiological considerations and mechanisms of action

Thrombolytic therapy initiated during resuscitation after acute MI or massive PE aims to treat the cause of cardiac arrest while the patient is still being stabilized. Direct thrombolysis at the site of coronary or pulmonary occlusion may resolve the underlying cause of cardiac arrest in a majority of patients and may increase the chance for restoration of spontaneous circulation (ROSC) and the maintenance of spontaneous circulation substantially.[16] This is the most intuitive mechanism of thrombolytic agents administered during cardiopulmonary resuscitation (CPR). All thrombolytic agents, except for streptokinase which is rarely used nowadays, directly activate plasmin by stimulating the conversion of plasminogen to plasmin. Plasmin has proteolytic activity on prothrombin and thrombin, thereby resolving the vascular obstruction (Fig. 41.1).

In addition, thrombolytic drugs may have an important effect on the microcirculation, especially cerebral reperfusion, after ROSC. Microcirculatory reperfusion disorders are known to be one of the major reasons for cerebral dysfunction after cardiac arrest.[17–19] It has been demonstrated that 30 minutes after cardiac arrest lasting 15 minutes, 30% of the cerebral microcirculation was not adequate.[18]

Cardiac Arrest: The Science and Practice of Resuscitation Medicine. 2nd edn., ed. Norman Paradis, Henry Halperin, Karl Kern, Volker Wenzel, Douglas Chamberlain. Published by Cambridge University Press. © Cambridge University Press, 2007.

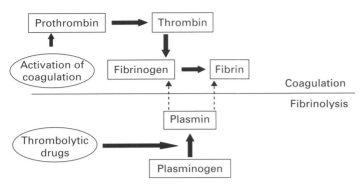

Fig. 41.1. Simplified diagram demonstrating the action of thrombolytic drugs. Thrombolytic drugs activate the enzymatic conversion of plasminogen to plasmin. Plasmin has a proteolytic activity on fibrinogen and fibrin which are the final substances resulting from the activation of coagulation.

Although the pathophysiology of cerebral reperfusion disorders is not completely understood, increased blood viscosity, endothelial cell swelling, leukocyte–endothelial interactions, and capillary fibrin deposition caused by activation of coagulation, may play an important role for the impaired cerebral reperfusion, also referred to as "no-reflow" phenomenon, after cardiac arrest.[20,21] The degree of the "no-reflow" phenomenon probably translates into neurological outcome after cerebral reperfusion. After cardiac arrest, a marked imbalance between activation of coagulation and fibrinolysis has been demonstrated. In out-of-hospital cardiac arrest, blood coagulation was significantly activated in all patients and was demonstrated until 8 to 48 hours after ROSC. In contrast, in most patients, the plasma levels of d-dimer, an indicator of endogenous fibrinolytic activity, were not increased during CPR.[22] These data suggested that in patients after cardiac arrest, a marked activation of blood coagulation was not counterbalanced by an appropriate activation of endogenous fibrinolysis. An impairment of fibrinolysis during and after CPR caused by massive generation of fibrin in patients who suffered out-of-hospital cardiac arrest was reported in another study.[23] Activation of coagulation during reperfusion after cardiac arrest may be caused by hypoxia, stasis of the blood, endothelial cell damage, and high levels of catecholamines in the blood.[16] In addition, significant activation of thrombocytes was reported during and after CPR in humans.[24,25] Therefore, thrombolytic treatment during CPR aims at adjusting the balance of coagulation and fibrinolysis in order to reduce microcirculatory reperfusion deficits after the arrest.

In an early observation, Crowell *et al.* found beneficial dose-dependent effects on survival and neurological outcome when heparin or streptokinase were administered *before* cardiac arrest in dogs.[26] Consistently, a combination of heparin, dextran, and hypertensive perfusion 12 minutes *after* cardiac arrest, resulted in an improved neurological outcome in dogs.[27] Whereas activation of coagulation may be prevented by heparin, an intravascular deposition of fibrin is not likely to be resolved by heparin alone. Thrombolytic treatment started *during* CPR and continued for 5 hours improved the recovery of cerebral perfusion and neurological performance in dogs compared to untreated controls.[28] The effect of thrombolytic therapy administered during CPR on cerebral "no-reflow" was investigated by fluorescent microscopy in cats.[20] In that trial, animals that received a bolus of alteplase and heparin after 15 minutes of cardiac arrest showed a significant reduction in the cerebral "no-reflow" in the entire forebrain compared to animals that had received no thrombolytic treatment. These experimental data suggested that the poor prognosis of patients suffering cardiac arrest after fulminant PE or acute MI is caused by pathophysiological changes that are not influenced by conventional resuscitation efforts. Thrombolytic treatment may have two beneficial effects in these patients: while the direct actions of thrombolytics are aimed at treating the cause of cardiac arrest, the effect of thrombolytics on microcirculatory reperfusion after cardiac arrest may contribute to a good neurological performance of patients even after prolonged resuscitation.[16]

Clinical studies

The first report on thrombolysis during CPR in a patient with fulminant PE was published more than 30 years ago.[29] In the years following, many other case reports have been published, most of them demonstrating an exceptionally high rate of ROSC after unsuccessful conventional treatment and a high rate of neurologically intact survivors even after prolonged CPR.[30] The promising results of case reports and case studies have led to a number of clinical studies in the in-hospital and out-of-hospital setting.

In-hospital studies

Several small in-hospital studies on thrombolytic therapy during CPR have been performed (Table 41.1). In an early study, 20 cardiac arrest patients with fulminant PE diagnosed by pulmonary angiography received streptokinase via the pulmonary artery catheter. ROSC was achieved in 11 patients (55%).[31] In a retrospective analysis,[32] seven of nine patients with acute angiographically proven PE showed hemodynamic stabilization after administration of a

Table 41.1. Thrombolysis during CPR. In-hospital studies

Reference	Study type	Number of patients	Underlying disease	Thrombolytic agent	CPR-related bleeding	Number of survivors
31	prospective	20	PE	SK	–	11
32	retrospective	9	PE	SK / UK / rt-PA	pectoral / sternal hemorrhage, liver laceration	5
34	prospective	28	AMI	SK / rt-PA	pericardial / sternal hemorrhage (4)	3
49	retrospective	6	AMI	SK / UK / rt-PA	–	3
33	retrospective	21	PE	rt-PA	2 liver ruptures, mediastinal bleeding	2
35	prospective	30	n.r.	TNK	–	2
36	randomized, placebo-controlled	19	n.r.	TNK	–	1
Total		133			9 (6.7%)	27 (20.3)

AMI = myocardial infarction, CPR = cardiopulmonary resuscitation, n.r. = not reported, PE = pulmonary embolism, rt-PA = recombinant tissue plasminogen activator (alteplase), SK = streptokinase, TNK = tenecteplase, UK = urokinase.

thrombolytic drug during CPR (streptokinase, urokinase, or alteplase), and five patients survived. Some of these patients received CPR for up to 90 minutes to achieve ROSC. Another retrospective study found ROSC to be achieved significantly more frequently in 21 patients presenting with cardiac arrest after massive PE who were treated with a bolus dose of recombinant tissue plasminogen activator (alteplase) during CPR compared to a control group of 21 patients receiving standard treatment. Survival rates, however, were not significantly different in the two groups.[33] In patients suffering cardiac arrest after acute MI, Gramann and colleagues prospectively treated 28 patients with thrombolytics during CPR after conventional resuscitation had been unsuccessful. Nine patients were stabilized initially (32%), but only three patients (11%) survived.[34] In a prospective observational study,[35] 30 patients with out-of-hospital (83%) and in-hospital (17%) cardiac arrest of unknown origin received in-hospital treatment with tenecteplase after failure of conventional resuscitation efforts. ROSC was achieved in 30% of these patients, 17% were admitted to, and 7% were discharged from hospital. A recent prospective, double-blind, placebo-controlled pilot study[36] randomized 35 patients who were transferred to hospital after out-of-hospital cardiac arrest to either treatment with tenecteplase or standard treatment. Patients treated with tenecteplase achieved ROSC more frequently compared to standard treatment, but there was no difference in survival at hospital discharge. Unfortunately,

that study was not powered to show a significant difference in long-term outcome between the standard and thrombolytic treatment. In summary, clinical studies on thrombolysis during CPR have shown a significantly improved rate of ROSC compared to standard treatment in patients with cardiac arrest after massive PE or acute MI. In addition, most survivors who recovered were neurologically intact after CPR even after prolonged resuscitation (> 90 minutes). The recent guidelines on CPR recommend considering thrombolytic therapy in patients with proven or suspected PE and performing CPR up to 60–90 minutes when thrombolytic agents have been given.[14,15] More studies, however, are necessary to determine if an improved short-term survival can translate into an improved long-term survival in these patients.

Out-of-hospital studies

As already stated, out-of-hospital cardiac arrest is known to be associated with an extremely poor prognosis, and only 5%–14% of patients suffering out-of-hospital cardiac arrest are expected to be discharged from hospital.[1–3] Four studies on out-of-hospital thrombolysis have been performed (Table 41.2). An inclusion criterion in all studies was a suspected cardiac cause of cardiac arrest, i.e., acute MI or massive PE, which account for more than 70% of causes for sudden cardiac arrest.[8–10] In 34 out-of-hospital cardiac arrest patients refractory to conventional advanced cardiac

Table 41.2. Thrombolysis during CPR. Out-of-hospital studies

Reference	Study type	Number of patients	Thrombolytic agent	CPR-related bleeding	Number of survivors
Klefisch 1995[37]	prospective	34	SK	hemothorax	5
Böttiger 2001[38]	prospective, controlled	40	rt-PA	–	6
Lederer 2001[39]	retrospective, controlled	108	rt-PA	2 pericardial tamponades, 1 hemothorax	27
Abu-Laban 2002[40]	prospective, randomized, controlled	117	rt-PA	1 pulmonary hemorrhage, 1 major hemorrhage (not clearly specified)	1
Total		299		6 (2.0%)	39 (13.0%)

CPR = cardiopulmonary resuscitation, rt-PA = recombinant tissue plasminogen activator (alteplase), SK = streptokinase.

life support, "rescue" thrombolytic treatment was administered.[37] Five patients survived longer than 3 weeks, and three of them were neurologically intact. In the first controlled prospective study on thrombolysis in out-of-hospital cardiac arrest,[38] 40 patients received thrombolytic treatment (alteplase) and heparin during CPR after resuscitation had been unsuccessful for more than 15 minutes. Compared to conventionally treated patients, significantly more patients were hemodynamically stabilized in the thrombolysis group (ROSC, 68% vs. 44%), and admitted to an intensive care unit (58% vs. 30%); 15% of the patients treated with alteplase were discharged from the hospital alive, whereas only 8% of patients from the control group were discharged. These results were confirmed by a retrospective chart review[39] comparing 108 patients who received alteplase during CPR with 216 control patients. ROSC was achieved significantly more frequently after thrombolytic treatment (70.4% vs. 51.0%). Survival after 24 hours (48.1% vs. 32.9%) and survival to discharge (25.0% vs. 15.3%) were significantly improved in the thrombolysis group. In contrast to these studies, the first randomized, double-blind, placebo-controlled trial in patients presenting with pulseless electrical activity of the heart did not show improved survival of patients who were treated with alteplase during CPR.[40] The results of that trial have been difficult to interpret, however, since a population with an extremely poor prognosis (no survivor among 116 patients in the control group) was studied. Therefore, the study was not powered to show any difference in a group of patients with such a poor prognosis.[41] In summary, early thrombolytic therapy may improve the outcome of patients suffering out-of-hospital cardiac arrest of cardiac origin, but more data from a large multicentre trial, which is currently under way in Europe (see below), are required. The success of any measure in these patients appears to depend on the initial EKG rhythm; in patients presenting with asystole or pulseless electrical activity, only studies with an extraordinary high number of patients can be powered to show a possible difference.

Safety of thrombolysis during CPR

The major safety concern associated with the use of thrombolytics is the risk of severe intracranial or systemic hemorrhagic complications. It is well known that thrombolysis is associated with the risk of bleeding. The risk for major bleeding, defined as bleeding that required transfusion or was life-threatening within the first 35 days after thrombolysis for treatment of acute myocardial infarction, is estimated to be about 1.1%, compared to 0.4% in the control group, as shown in a large meta-analysis.[42] The incidence of intracranial bleeding after thrombolysis for acute myocardial infarction is estimated to be 0.8% compared to 0.1% in the control group without thrombolysis.[42] In patients receiving thrombolysis for massive PE, the incidence of episodes of intracranial bleeding, one-third of which are fatal, has been reported to be up to 1.9%.[43] In summary, the risk for severe bleeding in patients with acute MI or PE who received thrombolytics is thought to range between 1.9% and 3.0% as compared to 0.5% in patients not receiving thrombolytics.[44] In addition, conventional resuscitation efforts are frequently associated with relevant bleeding complications,[45] among which hemorrhages of the heart and the great vessels, the lung, and abdominal bleeding are most common.[46,47] An overall incidence for hemorrhagic complications in patients after CPR of more than 15% has been suggested by autopsy studies.[44]

Although the incidence of severe CPR-related bleeding complications associated with thrombolysis after CPR is similar to the incidence of severe hemorrhage reported in the large studies on thrombolysis for acute myocardial infarction or PE,[44,48] the risk of severe bleeding caused by thrombolysis *during* CPR may be higher. As shown in Table 41.1, the incidence of CPR-related bleeding complications reported by several in-hospital studies on thrombolysis *during* CPR appears to be about 6.7%. Although these hemorrhages were severe, all of them were treated successfully by blood transfusion or urgent surgical intervention.

Out-of-hospital thrombolytic treatment during CPR may be expected to be associated with a significantly higher incidence of bleeding, as history-taking and physical examination of the patient are often limited. The overall incidence of severe bleeding complications related to CPR reported in out-of-hospital studies on thrombolysis during CPR, however, was 2.0% (Table 41.2) and therefore, similar to the overall incidence of bleeding following thrombolytic therapy without CPR. In the retrospective study by Lederer *et al.*,[39] autopsy was performed in a subgroup of non-surviving patients which revealed 6 severe bleeding incidents in 45 patients who had received thrombolytic treatment, 3 of them directly related to CPR. Interestingly, 7 cases of severe bleeding were identified in the corresponding control group of 46 patients. Therefore, thrombolytic treatment did not appear to have influenced the incidence of severe hemorrhagic events. Consequently, the recent CPR guidelines do not regard ongoing CPR as a contraindication to thrombolytic therapy.[14,15] In summary, recent data do not suggest that thrombolysis during out-of-hospital resuscitation is associated with a critically increased bleeding risk. Nevertheless, more data are necessary to assess the exact risk and the benefit/risk ratio of thrombolysis during CPR.

Outlook

A large randomized, double-blind, placebo-controlled multicenter trial on thrombolysis during CPR after out-of-hospital cardiac arrest has been recently performed in Europe. The Thrombolysis in Cardiac Arrest (TROICA) trial was designed to enroll more than 1000 patients in 10 European countries who suffer witnessed cardiac arrest of presumed cardiac origin. The primary endpoint was survival at 24 hours and 30 days; additional endpoints include neurological performance of surviving patients and the incidence of bleeding complications. The study showed an increase in survival at the primary endpoints by addition of tenecteplase to standard therapy. Interestingly, thermolytic therapy also did not increase symptomatic intracranial hemorrhage and major bleeding rates. A detailed presentation of these results that were presented at the World Congress of Cardiology 2006 is expected for 2007.

Conclusions

The poor prognosis of patients suffering cardiac arrest has not changed. No drug therapy has been found to improve the long-term survival of patients undergoing CPR. Thrombolytic therapy administered during CPR has been shown not only to eliminate the coronary thrombosis or pulmonary vascular obstruction, but also to improve microcirculatory reperfusion after ROSC. Clinical studies on thrombolytic treatment of patients suffering cardiac arrest of presumed cardiac origin have shown improved short-term outcome and a trend towards improved long-term outcome. The risk of causing critical bleeding complications does not appear to outweigh the potential benefit in patients with suspected massive PE. In addition, thrombolytic therapy may also be considered in patients with acute MI in whom conventional CPR has been unsuccessful. A large, randomized, placebo-controlled study which has recently been performed in Europe is expected to yield more detailed evidence for or against a generalized use of thrombolytic drugs in patients suffering cardiac arrest of presumed cardiac origin.

REFERENCES

1. Bedell, S.E., Delbanco, T.L., Cook, E.F. *et al.* Survival after cardiopulmonary resuscitation in the hospital. *N. Engl. J. Med.* 1983; **309**: 569–576.
2. Böttiger, B.W., Grabner, C., Bauer, H. *et al.* Long term outcome after out-of-hospital cardiac arrest with physician staffed emergency medical services: the Utstein style applied to a midsized urban/suburban area. *Heart* 1999; **82**: 674–679.
3. Newman, D.H., Greenwald, I. & Callaway, C.W. Cardiac arrest and the role of thrombolytic agents. *Ann. Emerg. Med.* 2000; **35**: 472–480.
4. Herlitz, J., Bang, A., Gunnarsson, J. *et al.* Factors associated with survival to hospital discharge among patients hospitalised alive after out of hospital cardiac arrest: change in outcome over 20 years in the community of Goteborg, Sweden. *Heart* 2003; **89**: 25–30.

5. Brain Resuscitation Clinical Trial I Study Group. Randomized clinical study of thiopental loading in comatose survivors of cardiac arrest. *N. Engl. J. Med.* 1986; **314**: 397–403.

6. Brain Resuscitation Clinical Trial II Study Group. A randomized clinical study of a calcium-entry blocker (lidoflazine) in the treatment of comatose survivors of cardiac arrest. Brain Resuscitation Clinical Trial II Study Group. *N. Engl. J. Med.* 1991; **324**: 1225–1231.

7. Kudenchuk, P.J., Cobb, L.A., Copass, M.K. *et al.* Amiodarone for resuscitation after out-of-hospital cardiac arrest due to ventricular fibrillation. *N. Engl. J. Med.* 1999; **341**: 871–878.

8. Silfvast, T. Cause of death in unsuccessful prehospital resuscitation. *J. Intern. Med.* 1991; **229**: 331–335.

9. Spaulding, C.M., Joly, L.M., Rosenberg, A. *et al.* Immediate coronary angiography in survivors of out-of-hospital cardiac arrest. *N. Engl. J. Med.* 1997; **336**: 1629–1633.

10. Zipes, D.P. & Wellens, H.J. Sudden cardiac death. *Circulation* 1998; **98**: 2334–2351.

11. Arcasoy, S.M. & Kreit, J.W. Thrombolytic therapy of pulmonary embolism: a comprehensive review of current evidence. *Chest* 1999; **115**: 1695–1707.

12. Antman, E.M., Anbe, D.T., Armstrong, P.W. *et al.* ACC/AHA guidelines for the management of patients with ST-elevation myocardial infarction – executive summary: a report of the American College of Cardiology/American Heart Association Task Force on Practice Guidelines (Writing Committee to Revise the 1999 Guidelines for the Management of Patients With Acute Myocardial Infarction). *Circulation* 2004; **110**: 588–636.

13. Van de Werf, F., Ardissino, D., Betriu, A. *et al.* Management of acute myocardial infarction in patients presenting with ST-segment elevation. The Task Force on the Management of Acute Myocardial Infarction of the European Society of Cardiology. *Eur. Heart. J.* 2003; **24**: 28–66.

14. American Heart Association 2005 guidelines for cardiopulmonary resuscitation. Part 4: Advanced Life Support. *Circulation* 2005; **112**: III-25–III-54.

15. Nolan, J.P., Deakin, C.D., Soar, J. *et al.* European Resuscitation Council Guidelines for Resuscitation 2005 Section 4. Adult advanced life support. *Resuscitation* 2005; **67** Suppl 1: S39–S86.

16. Böttiger, B.W. & Martin, E. Thrombolytic therapy during cardiopulmonary resuscitation and the role of coagulation activation after cardiac arrest. *Curr. Opin. Crit. Care* 2001; **7**: 176–183.

17. Fischer, E.G., Ames, A. & Lorenzo, A.V. Cerebral blood flow immediately following brief circulatory stasis. *Stroke* 1979; **10**: 423–427.

18. Fischer, M. & Hossmann, K. No reflow after cardiac arrest. *Intens. Care Med.* 1995; **21**: 132–141.

19. Hossmann, K.A. Ischemia-mediated neuronal injury. *Resuscitation* 1993; **26**: 225–235.

20. Fischer, M., Böttiger, B.W., Popov-Cenic, S. *et al.* Thrombolysis using plasminogen activator and heparin reduces cerebral no-reflow after resuscitation from cardiac arrest: an experimental study in the cat. *Intens. Care Med.* 1996; **22**: 1214–1223.

21. Böttiger, B. Thrombolysis during cardiopulmonary resuscitation. *Fibrinolysis* 1997; **11**: 93–100.

22. Böttiger, B.W., Motsch, J., Böhrer, H. *et al.* Activation of blood coagulation after cardiac arrest is not balanced adequately by activation of endogenous fibrinolysis. *Circulation* 1995; **92**: 2572–2578.

23. Gando, S., Kameue, T., Nanzaki, S. *et al.* Massive fibrin formation with consecutive impairment of fibrinolysis in patients with out-of-hospital cardiac arrest. *Thromb. Haemost.* 1997; **77**: 278–282.

24. Böttiger, B.W., Böhrer, H., Böker, T. *et al.* Platelet Factor 4 release in aptients undergoing cardiopulmonary resuscitation: can reperfusion be impaired by platelet aggregation? *Acta Anaesthesiol. Scand.* 1996; **40**: 631–635.

25. Gando, S., Kameue, T., Nanzaki, S. *et al.* Platelet activation with massive formation of thromboxane A2 during and after cardiopulmonary resuscitation. *Intens. Care Med.* 1997; **23**: 71–76.

26. Crowell, J., Sharpe, G., Lambright, R. *et al.* The mechanism of death after resuscitation following acute circulatory failure. *Surgery* 1955; **38**: 696–702.

27. Safar, P., Stezoski, W. & Nemoto, E.M. Amelioration of brain damage after 12 minutes' cardiac arrest in dogs. *Arch. Neurol.* 1976; **33**: 91–95.

28. Lin, S.R., O'Connor, M.J., Fischer, H.W. *et al.* The effect of combined dextran and streptokinase on cerebral function and blood flow after cardiac arrest: and experimental study on the dog. *Invest. Radiol.* 1978; **13**: 490–498.

29. Renkes-Hegendörfer, U. & Herrmann, K. Successful treatment of a case of fulminant massive pulmonary embolism with streptokinase. *Anaesthesist* 1974; **23**: 500–501.

30. Padosch, S.A., Motsch, J. & Böttiger, B.W. Thrombolysis during cardiopulmonary resuscitation. *Anaesthesist* 2002; **51**: 516–532.

31. Köhle, W., Pindur, G., Stauch, M. *et al.* Hochdosierte Streptokinasetherapie bei fulminanter Lungenarterienembolie. *Anaesthesist* 1984; **33**: 469.

32. Scholz, K.H., Hilmer, T., Schuster, S. *et al.* Thrombolysis in resuscitated patients with pulmonary embolism. *Dtsch Med Wochenschr* 1990; **115**: 930–935.

33. Kürkciyan, I., Meron, G., Sterz, F, et al. Pulmonary embolism as a cause of cardiac arrest: presentation and outcome. *Arch. Intern. Med.* 2000; **160**: 1529–1535.

34. Gramann, J., Lange-Braun, P., Bodemann, T. *et al.* Der Einsatz von Thrombolytika in der Reanimation als Ultima ratio zur Überwindung des Herztodes. *Intens. Notfallbehandl.* 1991; **16**: 134–137.

35. Kleiner, D.M., Ferguson, K.L., King, K. *et al.* Empiric tenecteplase use in cardiac arrest refractory to standard advanced cardiac life support interventions. *Circulation* 2003; **108**: 318–319.

36. Fatovich, D.M., Dobb, G.J. & Clugston, R.A. A pilot randomised trial of thrombolysis in cardiac arrest (The TICA trial). *Resuscitation* 2004; **61**: 309–313.

37. Klefisch, F., Gareis, R., Störk, T. *et al.* Präklinische ultima-ratio Thrombolyse bei therapierefraktärer kardiopulmonaler Reanimation. *Intensivmedizin* 1995; **32**: 155–162.

38. Böttiger, B.W., Bode, C., Kern, S. *et al.* Efficacy and safety of thrombolytic therapy after initially unsuccessful cardiopulmonary resuscitation: a prospective clinical trial. *Lancet* 2001; **357**: 1583–1585.

39. Lederer, W., Lichtenberger, C., Pechlaner, C. *et al.* Recombinant tissue plasminogen activator during cardiopulmonary resuscitation in 108 patients with out-of-hospital cardiac arrest. *Resuscitation* 2001; **50**: 71–76.

40. Abu-Laban, R.B., Christenson, J.M., Innes, G.D. *et al.* Tissue plasminogen activator in cardiac arrest with pulseless electrical activity. *N. Engl. J. Med.* 2002; **346**: 1522–1528.

41. Böttiger, B.W., Padosch, S.A., Wenzel, V. *et al.* Tissue plasminogen activator in cardiac arrest with pulseless electrical activity. *N. Engl. J. Med.* 2002; **17**: 1281–1282.

42. Indications for fibrinolytic therapy in suspected acute myocardial infarction: collaborative overview of early mortality and major morbidity results from all randomised trials of more than 1000 patients. Fibrinolytic Therapy Trialists' (FTT) Collaborative Group. *Lancet* 1994; **343**: 311–322.

43. Kanter, D.S., Mikkola, K.M., Patel, S.R. *et al.* Thrombolytic therapy for pulmonary embolism. Frequency of intracranial hemorrhage and associated risk factors. *Chest* 1997; **111**: 1241–1245.

44. Spöhr, F. & Böttiger, B.W. Safety of thrombolysis during cardiopulmonary resuscitation. *Drug Saf.* 2003; **26**: 367–379.

45. Krischer, J.P., Fine, E.G., Davis, J.H. *et al.* Complications of cardiac resuscitation. *Chest* 1987; **92**: 287–291.

46. Bedell, S.E. & Fulton, E.J. Unexpected findings and complications at autopsy after cardiopulmonary resuscitation (CPR). *Arch. Intern. Med.* 1986; **146**: 1725–1728.

47. Nagel, E.L., Fine, E.G., Krischer, J.P. *et al.* Complications of CPR. *Crit. Care Med.* 1981; **9**: 424.

48. Kürkciyan, I., Meron, G., Sterz, F. *et al.* Major bleeding complications after cardiopulmonary resuscitation: impact of thrombolytic treatment. *J. Intern. Med.* 2003; **253**: 128–135.

49. Scholz, K.H., Tebbe, U., Herrmann, C. *et al.* Frequency of complications of cardiopulmonary resuscitation after thrombolysis during acute myocardial infarction. *Am. J. Cardiol.* 1992; **69**: 724–728.

42

Percutaneous coronary intervention (PCI) after successful reestablishment of spontaneous circulation and during cardiopulmonary resuscitation

Marko Noc[1], Bjørn Bendz[2] and Karl B. Kern[3]

[1] University Medical Center, Ljubljana, Slovenia
[2] Rikshospitalet University Hospital, Oslo, Norway
[3] University of Arizona Sarver Heart Center, Tucson, Arizona, USA

Introduction

Coronary artery disease represents the most important cause of out-of-hospital cardiac arrest. Immediate coronary angiography in patients after reestablishment of spontaneous circulation demonstrated angiographic evidence of coronary artery disease in 80% of patients, with the majority (90%) having significant obstructive stenoses of one or more coronary arteries.[1] Experimental animal models have shown that coronary obstructions have a profound effect on the utility of cardiopulmonary resuscitation to perfuse the myocardium during cardiac arrest.[2] We found that coronary diameter stenoses as little as 33% decreased distal perfusion by more than half (see Chapter 18 for more details).[2] Postmortem examinations of sudden cardiac death victims indicate that unstable plaque with associated coronary thrombosis may be documented in more than 80% of the cases.[3] Accordingly, acute coronary thrombotic events leading to critical narrowing or complete coronary obstruction and possibly distal microembolization may be a main trigger of sudden arrhythmic cardiac arrest.

Current strategy for management of acute coronary syndromes

Acute coronary syndrome (ACS), based on 12-lead electrocardiogram, is traditionally divided into evolving ST segment elevation acute myocardial infarction (STEMI) and unstable angina/non-ST elevation myocardial infarction (UA/NSTEMI) (Fig. 42.1). More than 90% of the patients with STEMI have a complete thrombotic occlusion of the epicardial part of one of the coronary arteries without adequate collateral flow to the distal part of the affected artery. The mechanisms of coronary obstruction in patients with UA/NSTEMI are more heterogeneous. Pre-existing chronic coronary narrowing, plaque inflammation, thrombosis and spasm, alone or in combination, lead to critical stenosis rather than complete occlusion of the culprit artery.

Immediate, complete, and sustained recanalization of the culprit coronary artery, preferably by primary percutaneous coronary intervention (PCI), is crucial for survival of patients with evolving STEMI. This is also true for a small subgroup of patients presenting with an isolated posterior wall acute myocardial infarction. In these patients the ECG often shows both ST depression and a tall R wave in the second and third (V2–V3) precordial leads in this subgroup.

Patients with UA/NSTEMI, on the other hand, undergo early risk stratification and those with high risk features (positive troponin, ST depression, recurrent ischemia/heart failure/malignant arrhythmia despite adequate medical therapy) qualify for an early invasive approach including coronary angiography and revascularization within 24 to 48 hours after admission.[4]

Immediate coronary angiography and PCI after resuscitated cardiac arrest

Since acute coronary syndrome is the underlying event in the majority of the patients with sudden arrhythmic

Cardiac Arrest: The Science and Practice of Resuscitation Medicine. 2nd edn., ed. Norman Paradis, Henry Halperin, Karl Kern, Volker Wenzel, Douglas Chamberlain. Published by Cambridge University Press. © Cambridge University Press, 2007.

cardiac arrest, immediate coronary angiography, followed by PCI, after reestablishment of spontaneous circulation is ideally suited to define and treat the culprit coronary event. By adequate percutaneous treatment of the coronary culprit, greater electrical stability and myocardial salvage leading to reduction in recurrent arrhythmias, hemodynamic stabilization and reduction in infarct size may be expected. The American College of Cardiology and American Heart Association in their guidelines for Coronary Angiography[5] suggest that adult patients successfully resuscitated from sudden cardiac arrest are at high risk for recurrence and should undergo coronary angiography to identify coronary artery disease for potential revascularization therapy (Class I recommendation). Although they recognize that immediate coronary angiography in survivors of out-of-hospital cardiac arrest can reveal acute coronary occlusion in nearly 50% of patients, and that successful emergency PCI of an acute occlusion is an independent predictor of survival,[1] no specific recommendation concerning timing of such angiography is provided. The most common approach has been to perform coronary angiography on cardiac arrest survivors before implantation of an ICD before hospital discharge. If the patient is deemed not a candidate for the ICD (usually secondary to central nervous system injury), coronary angiography is likewise not usually performed. An AHA statement from 1997 further addresses this issue.[6]

An alternative approach is to submit all resuscitated victims of cardiac arrest to coronary angiography upon presentation at the hospital. Most will not have regained consciousness by that time, making assessment of their long-term neurological prognosis uncertain. Some European centers have championed this approach,[1] but at the present time the data supporting such treatment are limited.[7,8] There are no current recommendations from either American Heart Association/American College of Cardiology[7,9] or the European Society of Cardiology[4] with respect to such an immediate invasive approach. Accordingly, immediate coronary angiography and PCI for all resuscitated cardiac arrest victims is routinely performed in only a few PCI centers. It is becoming more common to perform early postresuscitation angiography and PCI in patients showing evidence of a STEMI (showing persistent ST elevation after resuscitation). In contrast, for patients with UA/NSTEMI, coronary angiography and percutaneous or surgical revascularization is usually delayed for several days until more accurate information regarding their neurological outcome can be obtained.[10] It is, important to notice, however, that acute chest pain and ST-segment elevation may be less predictive for acute coronary occlusion after resuscitated cardiac arrest. Even

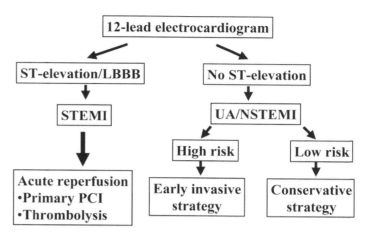

Fig. 42.1. Classification of acute coronary syndrome and principles of treatment based on 12-lead electrocardiogram. STEMI = ST-segment elevation acute myocardial infarction; LBBB = new left bundle branch block; UA = unstable angina pectoris; NSTEMI-acute myocardial infarction without ST-segment elevation; PCI = percutaneous coronary intervention.

though the positive predictive value for coronary occlusion in the presence of both signs is 87%, the negative predictive value is only 61%.[1] The absence of localizing electrocardiogram changes may indicate that the occlusion may be old and is not necessarily causally related to the fatal arrhythmia. Moreover, interpretation of the 12-lead electrocardiogram is further complicated because transient broad QRS complexes often appear immediately after reestablishment of spontaneous circulation and may resolve spontaneously by the time the next 12-lead electrocardiogram is obtained. Several 12-lead electrocardiograms are warranted after resuscitation to ensure that such transient changes are not mistaken for a STEMI.

An immediate invasive approach with coronary angiography and PCI would make sense if improvements not only in survival but also in survival with acceptable neurological outcome (Cerebral Performance Scale 1 and 2) could be expected. Except for patients with short intervals of cardiac arrest who have already regained consciousness on reaching the emergency department (Figs. 42.2 and 42.3), neurological outcome is impossible to predict accurately in unconscious patients at the time when decision for immediate coronary angiography and PCI has to be made. Since patients with unwitnessed cardiac arrest, no basic life support, long delay between call and arrival of the ambulance, and non-shockable rhythms on first electrocardiogram are unlikely to regain consciousness despite initially successful cardiac resuscitation,[11] they generally have not been treated with an immediate invasive

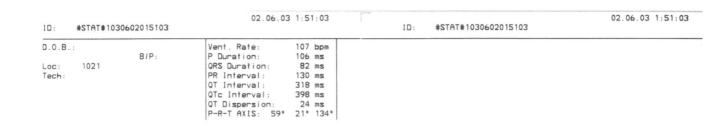

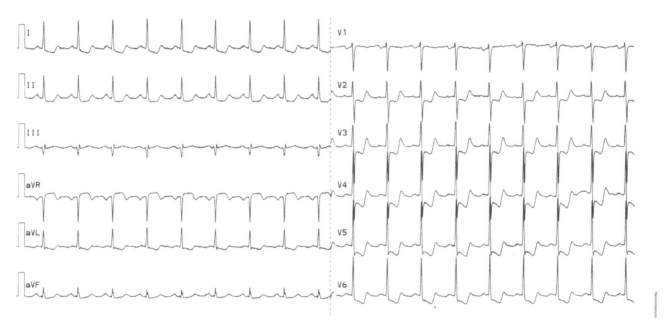

Fig. 42.2. Electrocardiogram of 41-year-old patient who had emergency personnel-witnessed ventricular fibrillation and regained consciousness after short period of chest compression and successful defibrillation on the field.

approach. The decision for such an approach is therefore largely made on an individual basis and may vary significantly according to interventional and acute cardiac care hospital facilities and practice.

Primary PCI in STEMI after resuscitated cardiac arrest

During primary percutaneous coronary intervention, the thrombotic occlusion in the infarct-related artery is first-passed by a guidewire introduced via the guiding catheter (Figs. 42.4 and 42.5). A PCI balloon is then advanced over the wire and filled with the contrast medium under high pressure to compress and fragment the thrombus and restore coronary patency and flow. Alternatively, a dedicated suction device can be used to aspirate the

thrombotic burden. In a great majority of the current patients (≥80%), a coronary stent is deployed to secure a good and stable angiographic result with epicardial patency and normal epicardial coronary blood flow in excess of 90%.

Even though primary PCI is considered both a better and safer reperfusion strategy than thrombolysis in evolving STEMI,[12] data on the use of such mechanical reperfusion in the subgroup of patients with resuscitated cardiac arrest are very limited. Kahn and coworkers were the first to report 11 selected patients with out-of-hospital ventricular fibrillation and STEMI after reestablishment of spontaneous circulation.[7] Four of their patients had regained consciousness before arrival in the emergency department. The infarct-related arteries were the left anterior descending artery (LAD) in 9 patients and the right coronary artery (RCA) in 2 patients. PCI was successful in 7 out of

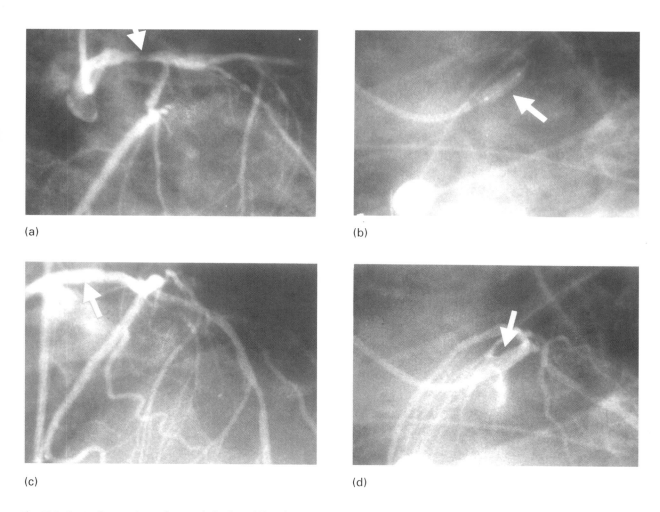

(a)

(b)

(c)

(d)

Fig. 42.3. Immediate angiography revealed subtotal "hazy" stenosis of the midshaft of the left main coronary artery (a). Direct stenting with a drug-eluting stent was successfully performed under hemodynamic support of intraaortic balloon counterpulsation (b). Finally angiography revealed widely patent left main coronary artery in both angiographic views (c) and (d).

11 patients; 6 patients survived to hospital discharge. Complete neurological recovery was documented in 4 patients and mild disability in 2 patients.

Recently, Bendz and coworkers reported long-term survival in 40 STEMI patients with less than 10 minutes of untreated ventricular fibrillation before reestablishment of spontaneous circulation in the field.[8] A great majority of the patients (90%) were unconscious at the time of coronary angiography. The infarct-related arteries were LAD in 50%, left circumflex (LCX) in 5%, RCA in 30% and an unprotected left main coronary artery (LMCA) in 15%. Contemporary techniques of primary PCI, including coronary stenting and glycoprotein IIb/IIIa inhibitor, resulted in much better angiographic results than were reported by Kahn and coworkers.[7] Optimal angiographic results in the culprit artery were obtained in 95% of the patients. In-hospital and 2-year mortality of this very high risk STEMI subgroup of patients was only 28%. Accordingly, with contemporary technology, primary PCI is both feasible and highly successful in selected STEMI patients after resuscitation from cardiac arrest.

The recent advances in preserving central nervous system function after resuscitation by using mild therapeutic hypothermia in comatose survivors of cardiac arrest[13,14] makes an interesting theoretical basis for more aggressive use of primary PCI in resuscitated victims of cardiac arrest with persistent ST elevation. Thus, a combination of primary PCI preceded or followed by induction of hypothermia (32° to 34° Celsius) may be an important future approach. At the moment, however, there are no specific data in the literature showing improved outcome with this combined approach.

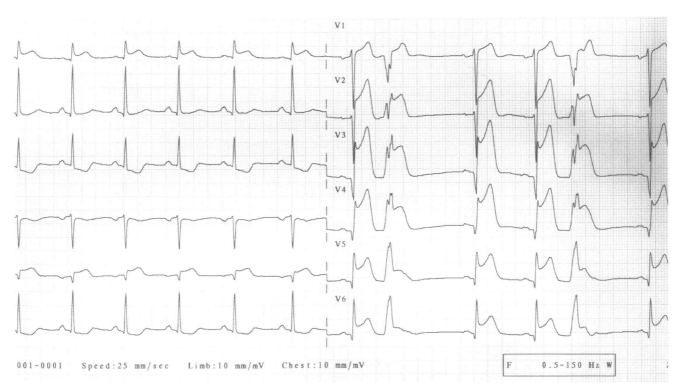

Fig. 42.4. 12-lead electrocardiogram of 56-year-old still unconscious patient after resuscitated out-of-hospital ventricular fibrillation on arrival to emergency department. ST-segment elevation in precordial leads together with multiple ventricular ectopic beats is seen.

PCI during cardiopulmonary resuscitation

Cardiac arrest can occur during coronary angiography or PCI or both procedures. This complication, although rare, must be dealt with expeditiously if the patient is to be resuscitated and survive long-term with intact neurological function. An important part of therapy is to deal with the underlying cause of cardiac arrest during angiography or PCI.[15]

In the majority of the cases, interventions such as cardioversion/defibrillation, intravenous pacing, pharmacological agents such as epinephrine and amiodarone, as well as mechanical support by intraaortic balloon counterpulsation at least temporarily restore spontaneous circulation, which allows a lifesaving PCI attempt. If these stabilizing measures fail, PCI may be attempted *during* ongoing cardiopulmonary resuscitation (CPR). Such a combined PCI/CPR procedure requires not only extraordinary skills, but close cooperation and coordination between the interventional cardiologist and the CPR team. Intermittent pauses in chest compressions during different phases of PCI (placement of guiding catheter, passage of a guidewire, balloon inflation, stent deployment) may be required, but the more chest compressions and hence circulatory support to the central nervous system, the less likely will irreversible neurological damage result. Continuous monitoring of aortic pressure is very valuable for assessing the adequacy of chest compression because it provides an invasive and fair estimate of coronary perfusion. If at all possible an aortic diastolic pressure of at least 25–30 mmHg should be maintained during CPR.[16] If an intraaortic balloon counterpulsation is in place, continuous balloon inflation during chest compression may further increase vital perfusion pressures by centralizing the flow generated by chest compression to the heart and head.[17] Fast and successful PCI of the culprit lesion may, in addition to the previously described measures, result in reestablishment of spontaneous circulation.

A review of Anglo-Saxon literature revealed reports of 11 patients who underwent a combined PCI/CPR procedure either in the setting of ongoing acute coronary syndrome or due to complications during elective coronary angiography or PCI.[18–22] In 10 patients, the culprit event was a severe stenosis or occlusion of unprotected LMCA. One patient presented with ongoing STEMI due to ostial occlusion of LAD. Since an ostial spasm with complete occlusion

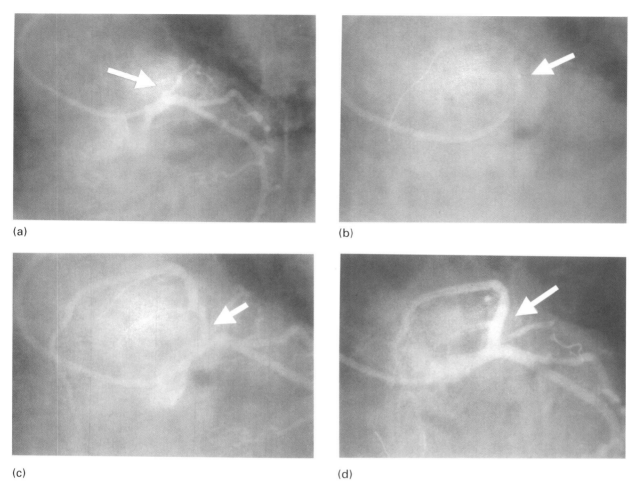

(a)

(b)

(c)

(d)

Fig. 42.5. Immediate coronary angiography revealed complete thrombotic occlusion of left anterior descending artery (a). Guidewire was easily advanced across the occlusion. The PCI balloon was positioned at the site of thrombus and filled by contrast medium under thigh pressure (b). Following balloon deflation, antegrade flow was re-established (c). Because of dissection and residual thrombosis at the culprit lesion, a bare metal stent was successfully implanted with optimal angiographic result (d). The patient was then transferred to the intensive care unit for temporary mechanical ventilation and hemodynamic support, regained consciousness 3 days later, and was discharged in normal neurological condition.

of LCX occurred during the LAD stenting, this patient may be regarded as having the equivalent of an unprotected LMCA occlusion as well. Accordingly, there was an extremely large amount of ischemic myocardium in each of these 11 patients who developed cardiac arrest on the angiography table. PCI with balloon predilatation or direct stenting during interruptions of chest compression was successful in every patient, and 9 out of 11 patients survived at least to hospital discharge.

It is, however, very important to emphasize that only successful cases are likely to be reported in the medical literature and actual survival of such patients is probably much worse. Nevertheless, these case reports underscore

the notion that combined PCI/CPR intervention should be attempted, because the patient may survive long term with complete neurological recovery if the catastrophic coronary problem can be resolved quickly and adequate cerebral perfusion is maintained during PCI.

But what if cardiac arrest preceded the patient's entry into the cardiac catheterization suite? What if ongoing resuscitation efforts have been underway without success for a while? Is PCI possible and efficacious in such dire circumstances? This is perhaps the most difficult situation since long-term central nervous system outcomes depend on both the quality of resuscitation effort and its duration. Each individual case must be carefully and quickly evaluated before preceding with an attempt at PCI.

Observations of the coronary anatomy at the onset of cardiac arrest may also explain, at least in part, why even timely CPR may not be effective in a considerable number of patients in the field. A major coronary event such as severe stenosis or occlusion of an unprotected LMCA, unless resolving spontaneously, most likely precludes adequate myocardial perfusion during CPR and hence failure to reestablish spontaneous circulation. In such patients, use of thrombolytics *during* CPR for refractory cardiac arrest may be a preferred approach. Thrombolytics given during CPR in an attempt to use chemical reperfusion means and reestablish spontaneous circulation in the field, may at least theoretically represent the only option of achieving reperfusion of such a culprit sentinel artery[23–25] before the coronary anatomy can be defined and PCI performed.

Summary

Percutaneous coronary intervention after successful resuscitation is becoming more common, particularly for those cardiac arrest victims manifesting evidence of a STEMI post resuscitation. The greatest challenge is determining the most appropriate candidates, because the majority of such patients are comatose and their long-term neurological function is not easily determined before the time such intervention is contemplated and performed. Percutaneous coronary intervention can be attempted during resuscitation, but great care in needed to ensure that adequate chest compressions are performed throughout the effort to avoid damage to the central nervous system even if the myocardium is reperfused.

REFERENCES

1. Spaulding, C.M., Joly, L.-M., Rosenberg, A. *et al.* Immediate coronary angiography in survivors of out-of hospital cardiac arrest. *N. Engl. J. Med.* 1997; **336**: 1629–1633.
2. Kern, K.B., Lancaster, L., Goldman, S. & Ewy, G.A. The effect of coronary artery lesions on the relationship between coronary perfusion pressure and myocardial flow during cardiopulmonary resuscitation in pigs. *Am. Heart J.* 1990; **120**: 324–333.
3. Davies, M.J. Anatomic features in victims of sudden coronary death: coronary artery pathology. *Circulation* 1992; **85**: (Suppl I): I-19–I-24.
4. Silber, S., Albertsson, P., Aviles, F.F. *et al.* Task Force for Percutaneous Coronary Interventions of the European Society of Cardiology. *Eur. Heart J.* 2005; **26**: 804–847.
5. Scanlon, P.J., Faxon, D.P., Audet, A.M. *et al.* ACC/AHA guidelines for coronary angiography: executive summary and recommendations: a report of the American College of Cardiology/American Heart Association Task Force on Practice Guidelines (Committee on Coronary Angiography). *Circulation* 1999; **99**: 2345–2357.
6. Survivors of out-of-hospital cardiac arrest with apparently normal heart: need for definition and standardized clinical evaluation. Consensus Statement of the Joint Steering Committees of the Unexplained Cardiac Arrest Registry of Europe and of the Idiopathic Ventricular Fibrillation Registry of the United States. *Circulation* 1997; **95**: 265–272.
7. Kahn, J.K., Glazier, S., Swar, R., Savas, V. & O'Neill, W.W. Primary coronary angioplasty for acute myocardial infarction complicated by out-of-hospital cardiac arrest. *Am. J. Cardiol.* 1995; **75**: 1069–1070.
8. Bendz, B., Eritsland, J., Nakstad, A.R. *et al.* Long term prognosis after out-of-hospital cardiac arrest and primary percutaneous coronary intervention. *Resuscitation* 2004; **63**: 49–53.
9. Smith, S.C. Jr, Feldman, T.E., Hirshfeld, J.W. Jr *et al.* ACC/AHA/SCAI 2005 guideline update for percutaneous coronary intervention: a report of the American College of Cardiology/American Heart Association Task Force on Practice Guidelines (ACC/AHA/SCAI Writing Committee to Update the 2001 Guidelines for Percutaneous Coronary Intervention). American Heart Association Web Site. Available at: http://www.americanheart.org/
10. Borger van der Burg, A.E., Bax, J.J., Boersma, E. *et al.* Impact of percutaneous coronary intervention or coronary artery bypass grafting on outcome after nonfatal cardiac arrest outside hospital. *Am. J. Cardiol.* 2003; **91**: 785–789.
11. Herlitz, J., Engdahl, Svensson, L., Young, M., Angquist, K.-A. & Holmberg, S. Can we define patients with no chance of survival after out-of-hospital cardiac arrest? *Heart* 2004; **90**: 114–118.
12. Keeley, E.C., Boura, J.A. & Grins, C.L. Primary angioplasty versus intravenous thrombolytics therapy for acute myocardial infarction: a quantitative review of 23 randomized trials. *Lancet* 2003; **361**: 13–20.
13. The Hypothermia After Cardiac Arrest (HACA) study group. Mild therapeutic hypothermia to improve the neurological outcome after cardiac arrest. *N. Engl. J. Med.* 2002; **346**: 549–556.
14. Bernard, S.A., Gray, T.W., Buist, M.D. *et al.* Treatment of comatose survivors of out-of-hospital cardiac arrest with induced hypothermia. *N. Engl. J. Med.* 2002; **346**: 557–563.
15. Kern, K.B. & Thai, H.M. Cardiac Arrest and Resuscitation During Percutaneous Coronary Interventions. In Butman, S.M., ed. *Complications of Percutaneous Coronary Interventions*, New York: Springer, 2005:141–151.
16. Paradis, N.A., Martin, G.B., Rivers, E.P. *et al.* Coronary perfusion pressure and return of spontaneous circulation in human cardiopulmonary resuscitation. *J. Am. Med. Assoc.* 1990; **263**: 1106–1113.

17. Tang, W., Weil, M.H., Noc, M., Sun, S., Gazmuri, R.J. & Bisera, J. Augumented efficacy of external CPR by intermittent occlusion of the ascending aorta. *Circulation* 1993; **88**: 1916–1921.

18. Ramondo, A., Favero, L. & Chioin, R. Emergency stenting of the unprotected left main coronary artery. *Ital. Heart J.* 2002; **3**: 72–74.

19. Sanz, A.J., Hernandez, F. & Tascon, J.C. Thrombotic occlusion of the left main coronary artery during coronary angiography. *J. Invas. Cardiol.* 2002; **14**: 426–429.

20. Phillipe, F., Bouabdallah, K., Dibie, A. & Laborde, F. Left main artery dissection during 4 French coronary angiography in elderly patient with severe aortic stenosis: "speedy recovery" using emergency primary stenting. *J. Interv. Cardiol.* 2002; **15**: 219–221.

21. Azman, K.J., Gorjup, V. & Noc, M. Rescue percutaneous coronary intervention during cardiopulmonary resuscitation. *Resuscitation* 2004; **61**: 231–236.

22. Teirstein, P.S. A chicken in every pot and a drug eluting stent in every lesion. *Circulation* 2004; **109**: 1906–1910.

23. Bottiger, B.W., Bode, C., Kern, S. *et al.* Efficacy and safety of thrombolytic therapy after initially successful cardiopulmonary resuscitation: a prospective clinical trial. *Lancet* 2001; **357**: 1583–1585.

24. Kern, K.B. Thrombolytic therapy during cardiopulmonary resuscitation. *Lancet* 2001; **357**: 1549.

25. Lederer, W., Lichtenberger, C., Pechlaner, C., Kroesen, G. & Baubin, M. Recombinant tissue plasminogen activator during cardiopulmonary resuscitation in 108 patients with out-of-hospital cardiac arrest. *Resuscitation* 2001; **50**: 71–76.

43

Emergency medical services systems and out-of-hospital cardiac arrest

Matthias Fischer[1], Thomas Krafft[2], Luis García-Castrillo Riesgo[3], Freddy Lippert[4], Jerry Overton[5] and Iain Robertson-Steel[6]

[1] Department of Anaesthesiology and Intensive Care Medicine, Klinik am Eichert, Göppingen, Germany
[2] Ludwig-Maximilians-Universität München, Germany
[3] Universidad de Cantabria, Hospital Universitario Marqués de Valdecilla, Santander, Spain
[4] Copenhagen Hospital Corporation, Copenhagen University Hospital, Denmark
[5] Richmond Ambulance Authority, Richmond, Virginia, USA
[6] West Midlands Ambulance Service NHS Trust, Dudley, W. Midlands, UK

Introduction

Emergency Medical Services (EMS) constitute a unique component of health care in the prehospital setting. Prehospital EMS systems are commonly understood as the resources used for planning and providing medical care for patients who experience an unpredicted need for emergency or urgent medical care outside a hospital. The EMS system's primary role is to provide care for patients whose lives are at immediate or imminent risk. In the beginning of organized prehospital care, most emergencies were of traumatic origin but in the last decades this has changed to include medical problems. In 2002 at the conference of the European Resuscitation Council in Florence the *First Hour Quintet* (FHQ) was defined, a set of five major medical problems of prehospital care on which EMS can have a significant impact on the outcome; these are:

- out-of-hospital cardiac arrest (OHCA)
- severe respiratory difficulties
- severe trauma
- chest pain, including acute coronary syndrome
- stroke.

Together these conditions are among the four leading causes of death in the European Union (EU). Cardiovascular problems, cancer, external causes, and respiratory diseases represent the top four leading causes of death and morbidity: 80% of all deaths are attributable to these common causes. Cardiovascular disease (CVD) is the number one cause of death in all EU countries, resulting in 4 million deaths per

year in Europe or 1.5 million in the EU, respectively. CVD also accounts for the largest amount of years of life lost by early death in Europe and in the European Union, contributing significantly to the escalating costs of health care. Coronary Heart Disease (CHD) is the most important cause of death in the adult population, comprising 55% of all CVD deaths. Acute coronary syndromes (ACS) include acute myocardial infarction (AMI), unstable angina, and sudden cardiac death. This diagnostic group represents the most severe forms of CHD. With this group, rapid access to the health system and prompt definitive care are vital. Mortality from ACS is extremely common outside the hospital, with 52% of deaths occurring before the patient reaches the hospital (World Health Organization (2004): The World Health Report 2004. Changing History. Geneva). Out-of-hospital cardiac arrest with prehospital cardiopulmonary resuscitation is the most time-critical emergency. Chance of survival from this event decreases every minute by 5%–10% that passes without treatment.[1-3] The design of EMS systems significantly influences survival rates.[4,5] On the basis of data from different EMS systems across the world, the annual incidence of resuscitation for out-of-hospital cardiopulmonary arrest of cardiac aetiology is 5–119 per 100 000 population[5-7] with an average incidence of 38 CPR attempts per 100 000 per year.[7]

In cases of OHCA therefore, EMS systems are the only organised providers bringing professional care to patients. Success of resuscitation measures is closely linked to minimizing the time without treatment and delivering definitive care as fast as possible. To reach these targets, each

Cardiac Arrest: The Science and Practice of Resuscitation Medicine. 2nd edn., ed. Norman Paradis, Henry Halperin, Karl Kern, Volker Wenzel, Douglas Chamberlain. Published by Cambridge University Press. © Cambridge University Press, 2007.

Chain of survival

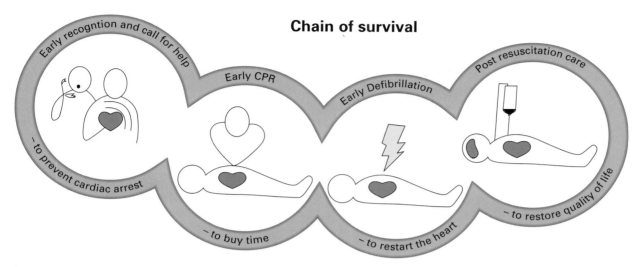

Fig. 43.1. ERC chain of survival.

link of the Chain of Survival (Fig. 43.1) must be analyzed and optimized by the provider of EMS. This includes early recognition of the emergency and activation of the EMS, early CPR, early defibrillation, and early advanced life support.

First link: Early recognition and call for help

Early recognition and call for help is the first link in the chain of survival. This step is a complex task for EMS and dispatch providers, however, because it encompasses multiple requirements.[8,9]

1. Recognition of sudden cardiac arrest by lay persons, which will be improved by training programs[10–12]
2. Call for help, knowledge of the "common" emergency number, comprehensive transfer of essential information to the dispatch center
3. Early receipt of the call in the dispatch center
4. Ability to differentiate calls into categories, including immediately life-threatening, urgent, and non-life-threatening (prioritization)[13–17]
5. Recognition of sudden cardiac arrest as an emergency of highest priority (criteria-based dispatch)[8,18,19]
6. Localization of emergency (calling line identity)
7. Localization of nearest ambulance and dispatching the appropriate response (Global Positioning System (GPS), computer-aided dispatch of Emergency Life Support (ELS), Basic Life Support (BLS), Advanced Life Support Units (ALS))[20]
8. Telephone-guided CPR[8,21–25]
9. Fastest possible drive to the place of emergency (GPS-guided)[26]

EMS providers are involved in all of these requirements. For example, to improve the ability of lay persons to recognize sudden cardiac arrest, public training programs have to be organized. These programs should start at primary school, but they must be continued during secondary school, high school, and university, and other job training.[12,27–31] Lay rescuers should be taught how to call for help, as well as basic life support skills and the use of automated external defibrillators (AED).[32,33] By using geographic information systems (GIS) it is possible to identify clusters of OHCAs in which the patients did not receive bystander CPR and where direct educational programs should be started.[34]

The provision of organized prioritization and dispatching systems is the crucial first step in the delivery of any emergency medical support, especially in sudden cardiac arrest.[9,35] Dispatch procedures have an important gatekeeper role in sorting, streaming, and directing resources. While dispatch centers may take a wide range of calls, it is vitally important that they are able to differentiate calls into categories, including *Immediately Life-Threatening*: like sudden cardiac arrest, or *Urgent* and *Non-Life-Threatening*. They must have the alternative to respond immediately to emergencies of CPR with ALS-units and to pass non-urgent minor illness calls to alternative resources, such as General Practice or ELS/BLS units.[14] This allows them to avoid down-grading the responsiveness of the resource-limited system. The best strategy for prioritization of the calls is still under discussion. A distinction is drawn between computer-aided criteria-based dispatch.[36–40] and having highly qualified personnel at the dispatch centers, like physicians in France[41,42] or paramedics and highly trained dispatchers in other parts of Europe.[43–47] Independent of the employed personnel at the dispatch centers, it is commonly accepted that improvement of dispatch techniques needs a supervisory quality assurance program.[35,48–51]

After identification of OHCA, dispatch personnel must localize the place of emergency and send out the nearest ambulance unit. These tasks will be supported best by computer-aided dispatch, including caller line identification and GPS.[26,52,53]

Second link: Early CPR, to buy time

After ischemia, the recovery of the brain is related to the duration of no-flow. In the clinical situation it is widely accepted that after more than 5 minutes of ischemia, full recovery of brain function is almost impossible. Experimental studies, however, clearly demonstrated that after 11 minutes[54] or even 60 minutes[55,56] of cerebral ischemia under normothermic conditions, neurological recovery to nearly normal function is possible. These studies, therefore, emphasize the hypothesis that there is still a chance for survival after sudden cardiac arrest beyond the 5-minute limit. But with increasing time of no-flow, the chance of survival after OHCA dramatically decreases:[57–59] this is a clear request for optimized EMS design. Many clinical studies consistently show that the early initiation of BLS measures – cardiac massage and ventilation – will improve neurological recovery and increase survival rates two- or threefold.[2,60–62]

To buy time, basic life support should be started when the first contact to EMS is made. Telephone-guided CPR[8,63–65] organized by the dispatch center therefore should be considered, because early bystander CPR can double or triple survival from OHCA.[2,60,61] The new guidelines of CPR recommend – especially for telephone-guided CPR – that laypeople should be encouraged to perform compression-only CPR if they are unable or unwilling to provide rescue breaths, although combined chest compression and ventilation is the better method of CPR.[33,65] To minimize duration of layperson CPR, the ambulance units bringing professional help to the OHCA victim should arrive in the shortest time. This could be attained by training the EMS drivers[66,67] and the implementation of GPS and GIS assisted dispatch.[26]

The providers of EMS therefore are challenged to reduce the time interval without professional treatment to a minimum.[68,69] However, this medical need is limited by financial resources and legal requirements. The response time interval, which is one of the main determinants of EMS costs, is often defined by law, but the definition across

Europe differs widely. The European Emergency Data Project (EED).[9] (www.eed-project.de) defined the response time interval uniformly as time interval from receiving the call at the dispatch center to arrival of the ambulance on scene. For comparing and benchmarking EMS systems a uniform format must be used. The response time interval should be expressed as a percentage of highest priority calls that were reached within 8 minutes. By using this format the ability of the EMS system to meet the widely accepted 8-minute response-time standard will be measured. The data must be provided as percentiles. Average response times are not only misleading, they are also clinically inappropriate. The EED-group found the response time to be a valuable indicator of EMS system performance across Europe. In 2004, 22 out of 31 UK Ambulance trusts reached the nation-wide key target defined by getting a first EMS response in 75% of category A calls within 8 minutes (http://ratings 2004.health carecommission. org. uk/). In some European and US high performance EMS systems, up to 85%–90% of all highest priority calls were read within 8 minutes (www.eed-project.de).

To reduce the time interval of no-flow and to optimize the response time interval, EMS providers should review and implement the following measures.

1. Training of laypersons in BLS skills beginning in primary schools[27,28,30,70–72]
2. Telephone-guided CPR[8,21–25]
3. First responder unit organized by professional care providers (fire fighters, police, patient transport ambulance)[69,73–79]
4. First responder units initialized by volunteer aid organizations[73,80]
5. Strategy of the nearest ambulance unit[81]
6. Computer-aided dispatch, caller line identification, GPS localization and guidance of ambulance units[18,26,52,82]
7. Ambulance base paging[83,84]
8. Improved deployment of ambulances by using Geographic Information Systems and the Global Positioning System[85,86]
9. Predictive analysis for localization of highest priority calls

Third link: early defibrillation, to restart the heart

Public access defibrillation, first responder units with AEDs

Early defibrillation is a key link in the Chain of Survival. In ventricular fibrillation after cardiac arrest it is a class 1 recommendation of the 2005 guidelines of CPR,[87,88] because it has been shown that early defibrillation improved outcome from VF/VT cardiac arrest.[73,89–92] EMS providers therefore are responsible for implementing early defibrillation programs. They have to equip BLS- as well as ALS-units with manual or automated defibrillators; they have to consider public access defibrillation[93–95] or first responder AED programs. The latter could be organized with the fire department, police, transporting ambulances, or volunteers. Depending on local or national standards or within the regulations by law EMS providers are responsible for the medical education of first responder units, their connection to the professional EMS, and debriefing and quality improvement programs. Medical direction of the EMS systems, therefore, should be an integrated part of quality assurance.[96] The logistic problem that occurs if first responders did not arrive before the professional EMS-teams at the scene must be overcome by intelligent deployment of all resources including BLS-, ALS- and first responder units. Geographic Information Systems and the Global Positioning System are modern tools for solving these multivariate problems of deployment.[34,85] Mobile EMS-units, on the other hand, should be controlled by a computer-based dispatch technology, including calling line identity, GPS-aided automatic vehicle location, digital mapping, predictive analysis, real-time system status management, and digital data transmission.

In introducing public access defibrillation programs to their communities,[95] EMS providers should manage the whole process, including positioning of PADs, training of anticipated lay rescuers, linking PAD initiative to the professional EMS, and programs of continuous audit. PAD programs will increase survival from OHCA most effectively if defibrillators are located where witnessed cardiac arrest occurs most frequently, but because 80% of OHCA occur in private or residential settings, PAD programs have only limited impact on survival rates. Currently, no studies have documented effectiveness of home AED deployment. Therefore some studies conclude that it might be better to establish an increased number of mobile first responder units than to start a PAD program.[97,98]

Fourth link: advanced life support and postresuscitation care to restore quality of life

Immediately after arrival at the scene, professional EMS teams will adopt and continue BLS-skills from lay- or volunteer-rescuers and continue cardiopulmonary resuscitation by starting ALS measures. Basic life support – compression and ventilation with a ratio of 30:2 – is the fundamental measure for successful CPR, because nutritive blood flow to the heart and brain depends crucially on effective heart massage.[33] The most effective performance of compression and ventilation, however, is only achieved with periodic drill and training, which cannot be expected from lay rescuers. Professional rescuers therefore take over BLS skill immediately, and reduce hand-off time to a minimum during CPR. EMS providers have to decide whether to implement mechanical devices to increase myocardial blood flow during CPR such as "active compression–decompression CPR" in combination with "impedance threshold device" (ACD+ITD),[99] load-distributing band CPR (AutoPulse™[100,101] or mechanical piston device/Lund University Cardiac Arrest System (LUCAS[102]).[88,103]

The new guidelines for adult advanced cardiac life support were published in 2005 in the journals Circulation and Resuscitation.[88,103] These guidelines were developed by clinical experts around the world who followed precisely defined procedures for searching and evaluating medical evidence. The recommendations were grouped as follows: (1) causes and prevention, (2) airway and ventilation, (3) drugs and fluids given during cardiac arrest, (4) techniques and devices to monitor and assist the circulation, (5) periarrest arrhythmias, (6) cardiac arrest in special circumstances, (7) postresuscitation care, and (8) prognostication.

The advanced life support skills discussed and recommended in previous chapters are listed as follows.

1. Defibrillation
2. Endotracheal intubation and confirmation of tube placement
3. Monitoring of CPR efficiency by end-tidal CO_2
4. Intravenous access and alternatives (intraosseous route, via tracheal tube)
5. Application of drugs (adrenaline, vasopressin, amiodarone, atropine, thrombolytics and others see below)
6. Electrical stimulation of the heart (pacemaker)
7. Treatment of periarrest arrhythmias (vagal maneuvers, magnesium, ß-blockers, diltiazem, amiodarone, propafenone, digoxin, clonidine, sotalol, isoproterenol, atropine, dopamine, adrenaline, ventricular pacing, electrical therapy, defibrillation)
8. Search for and treat possible contributing factors
   - Hypovolemia → adequate volume replacement
   - Hypoxia → reoxygenation, tracheal intubation
   - Hydrogen ion → buffers (acidosis)
   - Hypokalemia → potassium
   - Hyperkalemia → Ca and buffers, glucose, and insulin

- Hypoglycemia → glucose
- Hypothermia → appropriate rewarming
- Toxins → specific antidotes
- Tamponade, cardiac → drainage of pericardium
- Tension pneumothorax → thoracic drainage
- Thrombosis (coronary or pulmonary) → thrombolytics (after 12-lead ECG)
- Trauma → diagnosis, sedation, analgesia, intubation, infusion therapy (colloids, crystalloids), immobilization, transportation – advanced trauma life support (ATLS)

9. Induction of therapeutic hypothermia after ROSC in comatose patients
10. Cardiac arrest in special circumstances (hypothermia, drowning, electrocution, pregnancy, asthma)
11. Documentation of findings, diagnosis and CPR measures according to the "Utstein Style"

All these recommended ALS skills must be performed during resuscitation from out-of-hospital cardiac arrest under enormous pressure of time. To increase and optimize survival after OHCA, EMS providers and their BLS/ALS teams should follow the recently published CPR guidelines in detail. From the medical point of view, it cannot be accepted to withhold from a patient BLS, defibrillation, or ALS measures if sudden cardiac arrest occurred outside the hospital. Best results can only be achieved if the chain of survival is implemented in all links. Because CPR is a complex and demanding medical treatment, which requires detailed knowledge about the pathophysiology and pharmacology of sudden cardiac arrest and the underlying diseases, it is common sense that CPR has to be performed by the best trained ALS-teams. In hospitals around the world Medical Emergency Teams and Cardiac Arrest Teams have been established or are under consideration in order to avoid or to treat cardiac arrest. These teams consist of physicians and nurses with critical care training. In many European countries, this concept was rolled out years ago to the pre-clinical situation and the emergency physician on scene is an integrated participant in those high quality EMS systems. Therefore, many European citizens today expect to have a specialized emergency physician performing the whole ALS-treatments outside the hospitals (www.eed-project.de)[37,43,104–109] Recently published clinical studies comparing and benchmarking resuscitation success after OHCA clearly established that survival rates of greater than 7 patients discharged alive per 100 000 inhabitants annually were found only in EMS-systems with emergency physicians operating in the field.[7,43] It was demonstrated that compared to a paramedic EMS system, the preclinical treatment by an emergency physician increased vital scores and the probability of survival after CPR.[43]

Conclusions

EMS system design has to address these medical needs and the public expectation on the provision of best medical response to life-threatening emergencies. Each component of the EMS process depicted in the "EMS Patient Journey Template" (Fig. 43.2) developed by the European Emergency Data Project has to be carefully designed according to its crucial role within the chain of survival described above.[9,110] The advances in communication and information technologies (including GPS and GIS) have opened up new opportunities to minimize call to scene time systematically, while simultaneously maximizing the effective use of the available resources, both clinical and fiscal. Nonetheless, there is an urgent need to harmonize and standardize the emergency dispatch process. Utstein-like standards of reporting the EMS dispatch process and guidelines for rapid assessments and decision-making in the dispatch center could lead the way for further improvements.

Throughout the world, it would be reasonable to suggest that all citizens should have access to organized EMS with basic life support (BLS) provided to their community as a minimum standard. BLS, as defined by the European Resuscitation Council in 2005, is the ability to deliver cardiopulmonary resuscitation (CPR) and to provide a defibrillator to treat ventricular fibrillation in cardiac emergencies. BLS needs to be supported by the knowledge and the ability of first responders to carry out Emergency Life Support (ELS) on the citizens of the community to bridge the time gap until a BLS provider arrives on scene. The ideal standard for any EMS system is to aim towards the capability of providing early advanced life support (ALS) and advanced trauma life support. The first hour Quintet conditions – as defined by the European Resuscitation Council – require early delivery of full ALS skills.

Acknowledgments

Steering Committee of the European Emergency Data Project – EMS Data-based Health Surveillance

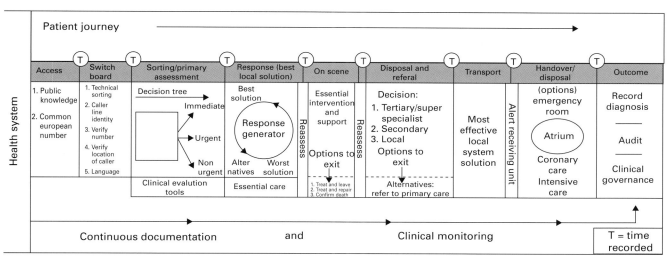

Fig.43.2 "Patient journey"

System. Grant Agreement No. SPC.2002299 under the European Community Health Monitoring Programme 1997–2002.

REFERENCES

1. Karch, S.B., Graff, J., Young, S. & Ho, C.H. Response times and outcomes for cardiac arrests in Las Vegas casinos. *Am. J. Emerg. Med.* 1998; **16**(3): 249–253.

2. Valenzuela, T.D., Roe, D.J., Cretin, S., Spaite, D.W. & Larsen, M.P. Estimating effectiveness of cardiac arrest interventions: a logistic regression survival model. *Circulation* 1997; **96**(10): 3308–3313.

3. Waalewijn, R.A., de Vos, R., Tijssen, J.G. & Koster, R.W. Survival models for out-of-hospital cardiopulmonary resuscitation from the perspectives of the bystander, the first responder, and the paramedic. *Resuscitation* 2001; **51**(2): 113–122.

4. Eisenberg, M.S., Horwood, B.T., Cummins, R.O., Reynolds-Haertle, R. & Hearne, T.R. Cardiac arrest and resuscitation: a tale of 29 cities. *Ann. Emerg. Med.* 1990; **19**(2): 179–186.

5. Herlitz, J., Bahr, J., Fischer, M., Kuisma, M., Lexow, K. & Thorgeirsson, G. Resuscitation in Europe: a tale of five European regions. *Resuscitation* 1999; **41**(2): 121–131.

6. Fischer, M., Fischer, N.J. & Schüttler, J. One-year survival after out-of-hospital cardiac arrest in Bonn city: outcome report according to the "Utstein style". *Resuscitation* 1997; **33**(3): 233–243.

7. Atwood, C., Eisenberg, M.S., Herlitz, J. & Rea, T.D. Incidence of EMS-treated out-of-hospital cardiac arrest in Europe. *Resuscitation* 2005; **67**(1): 75–80.

8. Kuisma, M., Boyd, J., Vayrynen, T., Repo, J., Nousila-Wiik, M. & Holmstrom, P. Emergency call processing and survival from out-of-hospital ventricular fibrillation. *Resuscitation* 2005; **67**(1): 89–93.

9. Krafft, T., Castrillo-Riesego, L.G., Edwards, S. *et al.* European Emergency Data Project (EED Project), EMS data-based Health Surveillance System. *Eur. J. Public Health* 2003, **13**(3 Suppl): 85–90.

10. Fong, Y.T., Anantharaman, V., Lim, S.H., Leong, K.F. & Pokkan, G. Mass cardiopulmonary resuscitation 99 – survey results of a multi-organisational effort in public education in cardiopulmonary resuscitation. *Resuscitation* 2001; **49**(2): 201–205.

11. Rasmus, A. & Czekajlo, M.S. A national survey of the Polish population's cardiopulmonary resuscitation knowledge. *Eur. J. Emerg. Med.* 2000; **7**(1): 39–43.

12. Gagliardi, M., Neighbors, M., Spears, C., Byrd, S. & Snarr, J. Emergencies in the school setting: are public school teachers adequately trained to respond? *Prehospital Disaster Med.* 1994; **9**(4): 222–225.

13. Cady, G. 200 city survey. JEMS 2001 annual report on EMS operational & clinical trends in large, urban areas. *J. Emerg. Med. Serv.* 2002; **27**(2): 46–65, 68–70.

14. Schmidt, T., Neely, K.W., Adams, A.L. *et al.* Is it possible to safely triage callers to EMS dispatch centers to alternative resources? *Prehosp. Emerg. Care* 2003; **7**(3): 368–374.

15. Neely, K.W., Eldurkar, J.A. & Drake, M.E. Do emergency medical services dispatch nature and severity codes agree with paramedic field findings? *Acad. Emerg. Med.* 2000; **7**(2): 174–180.

16. Neely, K.W., Eldurkar, J. & Drake, M.E. Can current EMS dispatch protocols identify layperson-reported sentinel conditions? *Prehosp. Emerg. Care* 2000; **4**(3): 238–244.

17. Neely, K.W., Norton, R.L. & Schmidt, T.A. The strength of specific EMS dispatcher questions for identifying patients with important clinical field findings. *Prehosp. Emerg. Care* 2000; **4**(4): 322–326.

18. Curka, P.A., Pepe, P.E., Ginger, V.F., Sherrard, R.C., Ivy, M.V. & Zachariah, B.S. Emergency medical services priority dispatch. *Ann. Emerg. Med.* 1993; **22**(11): 1688–1695.

19. Heward, A., Damiani, M. & Hartley-Sharpe, C. Does the use of the Advanced Medical Priority Dispatch System affect cardiac arrest detection? *Emerg. Med. J.* 2004; **21**(1): 115–118.

20. Campbell, J.P., Gridley, T.S. & Muelleman, R.L. Measuring response intervals in a system with a 911 primary and an emergency medical services secondary public safety answering point. *Ann. Emerg. Med.* 1997; **29**(4): 492–496.

21. Dorph, E., Wik, L. & Steen, P.A. Dispatcher-assisted cardiopulmonary resuscitation. An evaluation of efficacy amongst elderly. *Resuscitation* 2003; **56**(3): 265–273.

22. Bang, A., Ortgren, P.O., Herlitz, J. & Wahrborg, P. Dispatcher-assisted telephone CPR: a qualitative study exploring how dispatchers perceive their experiences. *Resuscitation* 2002; **53**(2): 135–151.

23. Rea, T.D., Eisenberg, M.S., Culley, L.L. & Becker, L. Dispatcher-assisted cardiopulmonary resuscitation and survival in cardiac arrest. *Circulation* 2001; **104**(21): 2513–2516.

24. Hallstrom, A.P. Dispatcher-assisted "phone" cardiopulmonary resuscitation by chest compression alone or with mouth-to-mouth ventilation. *Crit. Care Med.* 2000; **28**(11 Suppl): N190–N192.

25. Culley, L.L., Clark, J.J., Eisenberg, M.S. & Larsen, M.P. Dispatcher-assisted telephone CPR: common delays and time standards for delivery. *Ann. Emerg. Med.* 1991; **20**(4): 362–366.

26. Ota, F.S., Muramatsu, R.S., Yoshida, B.H. & Yamamoto, L.G. GPS computer navigators to shorten EMS response and transport times. *Am. J. Emerg. Med.* 2001; **19**(3): 204–205.

27. Eisenburger, P. & Safar, P. Life supporting first aid training of the public: review and recommendations. *Resuscitation* 1999; **41**(1): 3–18.

28. Lewis, R.M., Fulstow, R. & Smith, G.B. The teaching of cardiopulmonary resuscitation in schools in Hampshire. *Resuscitation* 1997; **35**(1): 27–31.

29. Starc, B. & Pecan, M. Training of medical students in resuscitation at the University of Ljubljana. *Resuscitation* 1996; **32**(1): 19–22.

30. Lafferty, C., Larsen, P.D. & Galletly, D. Resuscitation teaching in New Zealand schools. *N Z Med. J.* 2003; **116**(1181): U582.

31. Altintas, K.H., Aslan, D., Yildiz, A.N. *et al.* The evaluation of first aid and basic life support training for the first year university students. *Tohoku J. Exp. Med.* 2005; **205**(2): 157–169.

32. Nolan, J.P., Handley, A., Soar, J., Biarent, D. & Richmond, S. European Resuscitation Council Guidelines for Resuscitation 2005 Section 9. Principles of training in resuscitation. *Resuscitation* 2005, **67** Suppl 1: S181–S189.

33. Handley, A.J., Koster, R., Monsieurs, K., Perkins, G.D., Davies, S. & Bossaert, L. European Resuscitation Council Guidelines for Resuscitation 2005 Section 2. Adult basic life support and use of automated external defibrillators. *Resuscitation* 2005; **67** (Suppl 1): S7–S23.

34. Lerner, E.B., Fairbanks, R.J. & Shah, M.N. Identification of out-of-hospital cardiac arrest clusters using a geographic information system. *Acad. Emerg. Med.* 2005; **12**(1): 81–84.

35. Rossi, R. The role of the dispatch centre in preclinical emergency medicine. *Eur. J. Emerg. Med.* 1994; **1**(1): 27–30.

36. Shah, M.N., Bishop, P., Lerner, E.B., Fairbanks, R.J. & Davis, E.A. Validation of using EMS dispatch codes to identify low-acuity patients. *Prehosp. Emerg. Care* 2005; **9**(1): 24–31.

37. Langhelle, A., Lossius, H.M., Silfvast, T. *et al.* International EMS Systems: the Nordic countries. *Resuscitation* 2004; **61**(1): 9–21.

38. Thakore, S., McGugan, E.A. & Morrison, W. Emergency ambulance dispatch: is there a case for triage? *J. Roy. Soc. Med.* 2002; **95**(3): 126–129.

39. Wilson, S., Cooke, M., Morrell, R., Bridge, P. & Allan, T. A systematic review of the evidence supporting the use of priority dispatch of emergency ambulances. *Prehosp. Emerg. Care* 2002; **6**(1): 42–49.

40. Bailey, E.D., O'Connor, R.E. & Ross, R.W. The use of emergency medical dispatch protocols to reduce the number of inappropriate scene responses made by advanced life support personnel. *Prehosp. Emerg. Care* 2000; **4**(2): 186–189.

41. Nemitz, B. Advantages and limitations of medical dispatching: the French view. *Eur. J. Emerg. Med.* 1995; **2**(3): 153–159.

42. Renier, W. & Seys, B. Emergency medical dispatching by general practitioners in Brussels. *Eur. J. Emerg. Med.* 1995; **2**(3): 160–171.

43. Fischer, M., Krep, H., Wierich, D. *et al.* [Comparison of the emergency medical services systems of Birmingham and Bonn: process efficacy and cost effectiveness]. *Anasthesiol Intensivmed Notfallmed Schmerzther* 2003; **38**(10): 630–642.

44. Handschu, R., Poppe, R., Rauss, J., Neundorfer, B. & Erbguth, F. Emergency calls in acute stroke. *Stroke* 2003; **34**(4): 1005–1009.

45. Moecke, H. Emergency medicine in Germany. *Ann. Emerg. Med.* 1998; **31**(1): 111–115.

46. Gijsenbergh, F., Nieuwenhof, A. & Machiels, K. Improving the first link in the chain of survival: the Antwerp experience. *Eur. J. Emerg. Med.* 2003; **10**(3): 189–194.

47. Calle, P.A., Lagaert, L., Vanhaute, O. & Buylaert, W.A. Do victims of an out-of-hospital cardiac arrest benefit from a training program for emergency medical dispatchers? *Resuscitation* 1997; **35**(3): 213–218.

48. Garza, A.G., Gratton, M.C., Chen, J.J. & Carlson, B. The accuracy of predicting cardiac arrest by emergency medical services dispatchers: the calling party effect. *Acad. Emerg. Med.* 2003; **10**(9): 955–960.

49. Sobo, E.J., Andriese, S., Stroup, C., Morgan, D. & Kurtin, P. Developing indicators for emergency medical services (EMS) system evaluation and quality improvement: a statewide demonstration and planning project. *Jt Comm. J. Qual. Improv.* 2001; **27**(3): 138–154.

50. Clawson, J.J., Cady, G.A., Martin, R.L. & Sinclair, R. Effect of a comprehensive quality management process on compliance

with protocol in an emergency medical dispatch center. *Ann. Emerg. Med.* 1998; **32**(5): 578–584.

51. National Heart Attack Alert Program Coordinating Committee Access to Care Subcommittee: Emergency medical dispatching: rapid identification and treatment of acute myocardial infarction. *Am. J. Emerg. Med.* 1995; **13**(1): 67–73.

52. Yang, X. & Clarke, A.M. A computer/GPS guidance system for emergency rescue vehicle location. *Biomed. Instrum. Technol.* 1995; **29**(1): 34–38.

53. Ott, W.E. Electronic and data management issues: global positioning system and EMS. *Jems* 2003; **28**(8): 94–97.

54. Safar, P., Xiao, F., Radovsky, A. *et al.* Improved cerebral resuscitation from cardiac arrest in dogs with mild hypothermia plus blood flow promotion. *Stroke* 1996; **27**(1): 105–113.

55. Hossmann, K.A. & Zimmermann, V. Resuscitation of the monkey brain after 1 h complete ischemia, I: physiological and morphological observations. *Brain Res.* 1974; **81**(1): 59–74.

56. Hossmann, K.A., Schmidt-Kastner, R. & Grosse Ophoff, B. Recovery of integrative central nervous function after one hour global cerebro-circulatory arrest in normothermic cat. *J. Neurol. Sci.* 1987; **77**(2–3): 305–320.

57. Fischer, M. & Hossmann, K.A. No-reflow after cardiac arrest. *Intens. Care Med.* 1995; **21**(2): 132–141.

58. Safar, P., Behringer, W., Böttiger, B.W. & Sterz, F. Cerebral resuscitation potentials for cardiac arrest. *Crit. Care Med.* 2002; **30**(4 Suppl): S140–S144.

59. De Maio, V.J., Stiell, I.G., Wells, G.A. & Spaite, D.W. Optimal defibrillation response intervals for maximum out-of-hospital cardiac arrest survival rates. *Ann. Emerg. Med.* 2003; **42**(2): 242–250.

60. Holmberg, M., Holmberg, S., Herlitz, J. & Gardelov, B. Survival after cardiac arrest outside hospital in Sweden. Swedish Cardiac Arrest Registry. *Resuscitation* 1998; **36**(1): 29–36.

61. Holmberg, M., Holmberg, S. & Herlitz, J. Effect of bystander cardiopulmonary resuscitation in out-of-hospital cardiac arrest patients in sweden. *Resuscitation* 2000; **47**(1): 59–70.

62. Herlitz, J., Bang, A., Gunnarsson, J. *et al.* Factors associated with survival to hospital discharge among patients hospitalised alive after out of hospital cardiac arrest: change in outcome over 20 years in the community of Goteborg, Sweden. *Heart* 2003; **89**(1): 25–30.

63. Kern, K.B. Cardiopulmonary resuscitation without ventilation. *Crit. Care Med.* 2000; **28**(suppl)(11): N186–N189.

64. Bang, A., Herlitz, J. & Holmberg, S. Possibilities of implementing dispatcher-assisted cardiopulmonary resuscitation in the community: an evaluation of 99 consecutive out-of-hospital cardiac arrests. *Resuscitation* 2000; **44**(1): 19–26.

65. Roppolo, L.P., Pepe, P.E., Cimon, N. *et al.* Modified cardiopulmonary resuscitation (CPR) instruction protocols for emergency medical dispatchers: rationale and recommendations. *Resuscitation* 2005; **65**(2): 203–210.

66. Levick, N.R. & Swanson, J. An optimal solution for enhancing ambulance safety: implementing a driver performance feed-

back and monitoring device in ground emergency medical service vehicles. *Annu. Proc. Assoc. Adv. Automot. Med.* 2005; **49**: 35–50.

67. Elling, R. Dispelling myths on ambulance accidents. *Jems* 1989; **14**(7): 60–64.

68. Blackwell, T.H. & Kaufman, J.S. Response time effectiveness: comparison of response time and survival in an urban emergency medical services system. *Acad. Emerg. Med.* 2002; **9**(4): 288–295.

69. Stiell, I.G., Wells, G.A., DeMaio, V.J. *et al.* Modifiable factors associated with improved cardiac arrest survival in a multicenter basic life support/defibrillation system: OPALS Study Phase I results. Ontario Prehospital Advanced Life Support. *Ann. Emerg. Med.* 1999; **33**(1): 44–50.

70. Uray, T., Lunzer, A., Ochsenhofer, A. *et al.* Feasibility of life-supporting first-aid (LSFA) training as a mandatory subject in primary schools. *Resuscitation* 2003; **59**(2): 211–220.

71. Rosafio, T., Cichella, C., Vetrugno, L., Ballone, E., Orlandi, P. & Scesi, M. Chain of survival: differences in early access and early CPR between policemen and high-school students. *Resuscitation* 2001; **49**(1): 25–31.

72. Gasco, C., Avellanal, M. & Sanchez, M. Cardiopulmonary resuscitation training for students of odontology: skills acquisition after two periods of learning. *Resuscitation* 2000; **45**(3): 189–194.

73. Capucci, A., Aschieri, D., Piepoli, M.F., Bardy, G.H., Iconomu, E. & Arvedi, M. Tripling survival from sudden cardiac arrest via early defibrillation without traditional education in cardiopulmonary resuscitation. *Circulation* 2002; **106**(9): 1065–1070.

74. Myerburg, R.J., Fenster, J., Velez, M. *et al.* Impact of community-wide police car deployment of automated external defibrillators on survival from out-of-hospital cardiac arrest. *Circulation* 2002; **106**(9): 1058–1064.

75. Ross, P., Nolan, J., Hill, E., Dawson, J., Whimster, F. & Skinner, D. The use of AEDs by police officers in the City of London. Automated external defibrillators. *Resuscitation* 2001; **50**(2): 141–146.

76. Groh, W.J., Newman, M.M., Beal, P.E., Fineberg, N.S. & Zipes, D.P. Limited response to cardiac arrest by police equipped with automated external defibrillators: lack of survival benefit in suburban and rural Indiana – the police as responder automated defibrillation evaluation (PARADE). *Acad. Emerg. Med.* 2001; **8**(4): 324–330.

77. Davis, E.A., McCrory, J. & Mosesso, V.N., Jr. Institution of a police automated external defibrillation program: concepts and practice. *Prehosp. Emerg. Care* 1999; **3**(1): 60–65.

78. Davis, E.A. & Mosesso, V.N., Jr. Performance of police first responders in utilizing automated external defibrillation on victims of sudden cardiac arrest. *Prehosp. Emerg. Care* 1998; **2**(2): 101–107.

79. Kellermann, A.L., Hackman, B.B., Somes, G., Kreth, T.K., Nail, L. & Dobyns, P. Impact of first-responder defibrillation in an urban emergency medical services system. *J. Am. Med. Assoc.* 1993; **270**(14): 1708–1713.

80. Jermyn, B.D. Cost-effectiveness analysis of a rural/urban first-responder defibrillation program. *Prehosp. Emerg. Care* 2000; **4**(1): 43–47.

81. Peters, J. & Hall, G.B. Assessment of ambulance response performance using a geographic information system. *Soc. Sci. Med.* 1999; **49**(11): 1551–1566.

82. Pons, P.T. Advances in pre-hospital care: the technology of emergency medical services. *Med. Instrum.* 1988; **22**(3): 143–145.

83. Stiell, I.G., Wells, G.A., Field, B.J. *et al.* Improved out-of-hospital cardiac arrest survival through the inexpensive optimization of an existing defibrillation program: OPALS study phase II. Ontario Prehospital Advanced Life Support. *J. Am. Med. Assoc.* 1999; **281**(13): 1175–1181.

84. Jermyn, B.D. Reduction of the call-response interval with ambulance base paging. *Prehosp. Emerg. Care* 2000; **4**(4): 318–321.

85. Peleg, K. & Pliskin, J.S. A geographic information system simulation model of EMS: reducing ambulance response time. *Am. J. Emerg. Med.* 2004; **22**(3): 164–170.

86. Stout, J., Pepe, P.E. & Mosesso, V.N.J. All-advanced life support vs tiered-response ambulance systems. *Prehosp. Emerg. Care* 2000; **4**(1): 1–6.

87. Deakin, C.D. & Nolan, J.P. European Resuscitation Council Guidelines for Resuscitation 2005 Section 3. Electrical therapies. automated external defibrillators, defibrillation, cardioversion and pacing. *Resuscitation* 2005; **67** (Suppl 1): S25–S37.

88. 2005 American Heart Association Guidelines for Cardiopulmonary Resuscitation and Emergency Cardiovascular Care. *Circulation* 2005; **112**(24 Suppl): IV1–203.

89. Cappato, R., Curnis, A., Marzollo, P. *et al.* Prospective assessment of integrating the existing emergency medical system with automated external defibrillators fully operated by volunteers and laypersons for out-of-hospital cardiac arrest: the Brescia Early Defibrillation Study (BEDS). *Eur. Heart J.* 2005.

90. Choi, S. Does early defibrillation improve long-term survival and quality of life after cardiac arrest? *Can. Med. Assoc. J.* 2003; **169**: N586–N587.

91. Gottschalk, A., Burmeister, M.A., Freitag, M., Cavus, E. & Standl, T. Influence of early defibrillation on the survival rate and quality of life after CPR in prehospital emergency medical service in a German metropolitan area. *Resuscitation* 2002; **53**(1): 15–20.

92. Koster, R.W. Automatic external defibrillator: key link in the chain of survival. *J. Cardiovasc. Electrophysiol.* 2002; **13**(1 Suppl): S92–S95.

93. Clare, C. Do public access defibrillation (PAD) programmes lead to an increase of patients surviving to discharge from hospital following out of hospital cardiac arrest? – a literature review. *Int. J. Nurs. Stud.* 2006.

94. Hallstrom, A.P., Ornato, J.P., Weisfeldt, M. *et al.* Public-access defibrillation and survival after out-of-hospital cardiac arrest. *N. Engl. J. Med.* 2004; **351**(7): 637–646.

95. Richardson, L.D., Gunnels, M.D., Groh, W.J. *et al.* Implementation of community-based public access defibrillation in the PAD trial. *Acad. Emerg. Med.* 2005; **12**(8): 688–697.

96. Stone, R.M., Seaman, K.G. & Bissell, R.A. A statewide study of EMS oversight: medical director characteristics and involvement compared with national guidelines. *Prehosp. Emerg. Care* 2000; **4**(4): 345–351.

97. Pell, J.P., Sirel, J.M., Marsden, A.K., Ford, I., Walker, N.L. & Cobbe, S.M. Potential impact of public access defibrillators on survival after out of hospital cardiopulmonary arrest: retrospective cohort study. *Br. Med. J.* 2002; **325**(7363): 515.

98. Walker, A., Sirel, J.M., Marsden, A.K., Cobbe, S.M. & Pell, J.P. Cost effectiveness and cost utility model of public place defibrillators in improving survival after prehospital cardiopulmonary arrest. *Br. Med. J.* 2003; **327**(7427): 1316.

99. Wolcke, B.B., Mauer, D.K. & Schoefmann, M.F. Comparison of standard cardiopulmonary resuscitation versus the combination of active compression-decompression cardiopulmonary resuscitation and an inspiratory impedance threshold device for out-of-hospital cardiac arrest. *Circulation* 2003; **108**(18): 2201–2205.

100. Timerman, S., Cardoso, L.F., Ramires, J.A. & Halperin, H. Improved hemodynamic performance with a novel chest compression device during treatment of in-hospital cardiac arrest. *Resuscitation* 2004; **61**(3): 273–280.

101. Halperin, H.R., Paradis, N., Ornato, J.P. *et al.* Cardiopulmonary resuscitation with a novel chest compression device in a porcine model of cardiac arrest: improved hemodynamics and mechanisms. *J. Am. Coll. Cardiol.* 2004; **44**(11): 2214–2220.

102. Steen, S., Liao, Q., Pierre, L., Paskevicius, A. & Sjoberg, T. Evaluation of LUCAS, a new device for automatic mechanical compression and active decompression resuscitation. *Resuscitation* 2002; **55**(3): 285–299.

103. Nolan, J.P., Deakin, C.D., Soar, J., Böttiger, B.W. & Smith, G. European Resuscitation Council Guidelines for Resuscitation 2005 Section 4. Adult advanced life support. *Resuscitation* 2005; **67** (Suppl 1): S39–S86.

104. Ringburg, A.N., Frissen, I.N., Spanjersberg, W.R., Jel, G., Frankema, S.P. & Schipper, I.B. Physician-staffed HEMS dispatch in the Netherlands: Adequate deployment or minimal utilization? *Air. Med. J.* 2005; **24**(6): 248–251.

105. BEPS Collaborative Group. Prehospital thrombolysis in acute myocardial infarction: the Belgian eminase prehospital study (BEPS). *Eur. Heart J.* 1991; **12**(9): 965–967.

106. Thierbach, A., Piepho, T., Wolcke, B., Kuster, S. & Dick, W. [Prehospital emergency airway management procedures. Success rates and complications]. *Anaesthesist* 2004; **53**(6): 543–550.

107. Naess, A.C. & Steen, P.A. Long term survival and costs per life year gained after out-of-hospital cardiac arrest. *Resuscitation* 2004; **60**(1): 57–64.

108. Adnet, F. & Lapostolle, F. International EMS systems: France. *Resuscitation* 2004; **63**(1): 7–9.

109. Platz, E., Bey, T. & Walter, F.G, International report: current state and development of health insurance and emergency medicine in Germany. The influence of health insurance laws on the practice of emergency medicine in a European country. *J. Emerg. Med.* 2003; **25**(2): 203–210.

110. Krafft, T., Garcia-Castrillo Riesgo, L., Fischer, M., Lippert, F., Overton, J. & Robertson-Steel, I. Health Monitoring and Benchmarking of European EMS Systems: Components, Indicators and Recommendations. Project Report of the European Emergency Data Project – EMS Data-based Health Surveillance System. Grant Agreement No. SPC.2002299. Bonn/München; 2005

44

In-hospital resuscitation

Mary Ann Peberdy[1], Johan Herlitz[2] and Michelle Cretikos[3]

[1] Department of Medicine and Emergency Medicine, Virginia Commonwealth University Health System, Richmond, Virginia, USA
[2] Division of Cardiology, Sahlgrenska University Hospital, Goteborg, Sweden
[3] Simpson Centre for Health Services Research, University of New South Wales, Sydney, Australia

Introduction

In-hospital resuscitation practices have changed very little despite significant advances in resuscitation science. Unlike pre-hospital providers, hospital personnel have been slow to focus on resuscitation practices and even slower to adopt evolving science and technology to improve outcomes. Consequently, there has been no improvement in survival over time for hospitalized patients suffering a cardiorespiratory arrest, where overall survival remains approximately 18%.[1]

Hospitalized patients have different comorbidities from persons who arrest outside of the hospital. In a large series of cardiorespiratory arrests occurring in hospitalized patients in the United States, many arrest patients had electrocardiographic or oximetry monitoring, an invasive airway, or were receiving an intravenous vasoactive drug prior to their arrest, suggesting that this population has varying degrees of underlying instability.[1] Nevertheless, to stop here and suggest that survival will always be poor because the patients are "sick" and cannot be expected to do well leads to a self-fulfilling prophecy. Although the hospitalized patient population may inherently be more acutely ill, the hospital also has potential resources that far outweigh those in the pre-hospital setting.

Different strategies may be necessary to improve survival in the hospital environment. One of the most significant changes that must occur is within the hospital culture. Attention needs to be focused on the science of resuscitation, and on the process of care delivery. The importance of administrative and organizational support is paramount to achieving success. Traditionally, hospitals focus only on the arrest event itself when planning their resuscitation practices. Little attention is given to prevention or the specific care the patient receives after return of spontaneous circulation (ROSC).

There is an emerging concept of a "bow-tie" strategy to encompass the entire spectrum of hospital-based resuscitation practices (Fig. 44.1). In this schematic, the arrest event represents only a small part of the time and resources that a hospital needs to commit to the resuscitation program. It illustrates that there is a substantial period of time prior to the majority of arrests when easily identifiable physiological triggers can be identified and intervention implemented to decrease the likelihood of cardiorespiratory arrest. This shifts the hospital response from a "reactive" one that merely responds to patients once they have had an arrest, to a "pro-active" one where prevention of the arrest is the primary goal. There is no better way to improve survival from cardiorespiratory arrest than to prevent it from occurring in the first place. For those patients who do suffer an arrest, the schematic also demonstrates that the resuscitation process does not end with ROSC, but suggests that targeted care of the recently resuscitated patient is needed.

The purpose of this chapter is to present a comprehensive strategy, beginning with early intervention and prevention, and ending with targeted postresuscitation therapies.

Prearrest rapid response systems

In-hospital cardiac arrests,[2-7] intensive care unit (ICU) admissions,[8-10] and unexpected deaths[11] are often preceded by warning signs for clinically significant periods of time prior to the event. Evidence of deterioration is

Cardiac Arrest: The Science and Practice of Resuscitation Medicine. 2nd edn., ed. Norman Paradis, Henry Halperin, Karl Kern, Volker Wenzel, Douglas Chamberlain. Published by Cambridge University Press. © Cambridge University Press, 2007.

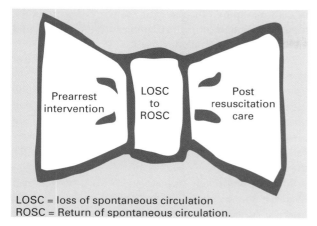

LOSC = loss of spontaneous circulation
ROSC = Return of spontaneous circulation.

Fig. 44.1. "Bow-tie concept".

typically present for up to 6–8 hours, but in some studies up to 72 hours prior to the event. Nearly 80% of patients suffering an in-hospital cardiac arrest have a heart rate, respiratory rate, or oxygen saturation out of the normal range within the 8 hours prior to the event. This suggests that many of these events are predictable and therefore potentially preventable.

A better understanding of the organizational factors that provide the conditions in which adverse events occur is required. The identification of both active errors (errors of omission and commission) and latent errors caused by inadequate systems has led to an appreciation that serious events are commonly preceded by multiple failures within the hospital system.[12–17] Examples of such failures include evidence that the majority of potentially avoidable arrests or unplanned ICU admissions had a delay in diagnosis or errors in diagnosis, and most patients had inadequate treatment prior to their event.[13] There is evidence that junior physicians are insufficiently trained or experienced to respond appropriately to patients with critical illness, but are commonly the only doctors who review patients with potentially preventable arrests in the hours prior to their event. Some cardiac arrests classified as potentially preventable occur in patients nursed in an area inappropriate for their primary illness, even though it is known that mortality is higher where patients are admitted to an inappropriate level of care for their illness.[13] Once a cardiac arrest has occurred, most patients will still die despite the intensive level of care and resources provided after the event, with approximately 18% surviving to discharge. Compare this to a 60% survival in non-arrest patients admitted urgently to the ICU from the floor. Outcomes are clearly better when the arrest is prevented and aggressive care occurs early.

These findings have directed attention towards prevention of these serious events by using a systems approach. Critical care medicine has been using systems to improve patient care for decades, with trauma systems now well developed in most health services, and the chain of survival for out-of-hospital cardiac arrests providing a system-type response similar to those now advocated for in-hospital critical events.

The most effective approach to identifying and responding to in-hospital clinical deterioration is the Medical Emergency Team (MET).[18–20] This is a team-based system response to patients identified as being at risk of clinical deterioration. The MET system is designed to recognize and respond rapidly and appropriately to any patient within the hospital displaying signs of instability. The MET system comprises the Medical Emergency Team itself, ongoing education and awareness campaigns, and monitoring and feedback processes.[21,22] The ICU or Emergency Department of the hospital generally provide the Medical Emergency Team members. The team is composed of at least two people, a physician and a nurse with advanced diagnosis and resuscitation skills. The team may be called by any member of the clinical staff to any of the units in the hospital to obtain immediate assistance in caring for an unstable patient. The team is available at all times, and is activated by calling an emergency number. The response is immediate. The team will attend a call with equipment required for advanced resuscitation, including drugs, fluids, intravenous access, intubation and ventilation equipment, and a cardiac monitor and defibrillator. The aim is to be able to evaluate and treat the patient immediately, with the goal of preventing cardiac or respiratory arrest or transfer to the ICU.

The MET calling criteria are specified clearly and based on abnormal clinical observations in addition to a subjective "seriously worried" criterion. These criteria are used as a screening tool, to help clinical staff recognize and respond to patients at risk of acute decompensation. "Calling criteria" posters are typically displayed throughout the hospital, and all members of staff are educated on the specific calling criteria used in their hospital.

The functions of the team include diagnosis, critical intervention, and resuscitation, as well as decision making. Decisions include not only the treatment decisions, but also decisions about the need for transfer to a higher level of care or even another institution, notification and consultation with the responsible consultant and team, and institution of "do not attempt resuscitation" (DNAR) orders where appropriate. Although the MET is capable of a range of responses, it is often required to perform only relatively simple interventions, such as the administration of oxygen and nasopharyngeal suctioning, obtaining IV access and administering fluids or basic medications.[22,23] The MET also provides support to clinical staff on the wards, and may also provide training on the appropriate management of patients at risk for clinical deterioration.

The MET system has been associated with many beneficial outcomes. These include a 17%–65% reduction in the rates of cardiac arrest in three single-center "before and after" studies, although one other smaller before-and-after study did not show any effect.[2,24–26] The MERIT trial is the only randomized controlled clinical trial evaluating the effects of MET vs. no-MET within the same hospital.[27] This was a neutral trial; however, the event rate was underpowered to detect a difference between the two groups. The MET has also been associated with reductions in unplanned ICU admissions, reductions in morbidity and mortality postsurgery, reductions in length of ICU admissions and reductions in length of stay, as well as reductions in total in-hospital mortality.[23–25,28] In addition, the MET may facilitate increased rates of appropriate DNAR documentation, as well as an improvement in the process and planning of critical care admissions.[22]

The effectiveness of the MET not only depends on the activities of the team, but on the cohesive activities of the entire system. The MET system includes initial and ongoing education of physician and nursing staff to raise awareness, and improve identification, of patients at risk and to increase appreciation of the urgency of response required for such patients. This process includes regular MET education sessions on the ward, department meetings and active support of the system by both administration and clinicians, calling card ID badges, posters of the calling criteria, an overhead address system or paging system for calling the MET, formal MET reviews, and other informal feedback processes. Hospitals that have implemented the MET usually require a dedicated coordinator to ensure these activities are organized and occurring continuously. This coordinator may also be responsible for the MET databases, the incorporation of the MET outcomes into the quality system as outcome indicators, and to provide feedback to all involved in a MET response.

The implementation of the MET requires attention to cultural and structural factors within the hospital that may prevent the system from being used effectively. These may include concerns about the resources required to run the system and about loss of control over patient care, and fears of retribution for bypassing the hierarchy or crossing the boundaries of the hospital organization in calling the MET, as well as fear of negative comments from the MET members when a call is attended. Implementation should take account of the time needed for the necessary change

in culture required for the MET system to become fully functional, and the ongoing training and support required for the system's optimal function.

The success of the MET system also depends on the frequent and complete documentation of clinical observations and vital signs in all patients admitted to the hospital. Clearly, if the observations are not measured, the MET will not be called even though the signs of deterioration are present. Many studies have provided evidence that observations are often missing or incomplete, in particular for the respiratory rate.[5,22]

When appropriately implemented, MET systems can decrease the incidence of in-hospital cardiac arrests, improve survival from arrests, and lower the number of urgent transfers to the ICU. The development of a MET system has been identified as a patient safety issue in the United States by both the Joint Commission for the Accreditation of Hospitals and the Institute for Healthcare Improvement, and is endorsed by organizations such as the American Heart Association and the Society of Critical Care Medicine.

Cardiac arrest event

Process issues: administrative structure

Despite the most meticulous attention to patient safety and attempts to prevent catastrophic events in hospitals, cardiorespiratory arrests will occur. Most hospitals have a committee or some sort of oversight mechanism responsible for governing resuscitation practices. With rapidly accruing new science, new defibrillator technology, and devices for improving hemodynamics during CPR, hospitals are now faced with potentially needing more frequent equipment updates. Because most resuscitation programs have no independent budget, many resuscitation committees are finding it increasingly more difficult to maintain the quality of their programs. Political and financial support is often quite variable. Committees must have the authority to act on their findings and recommendations. Resuscitation committees are often caught between having all of the responsibility and none of the authority to do what is best for patient care. This culture of "delegation to the powerless" must change for hospitals to be able to adopt evolving technologies more readily.

The members of the resuscitation committee can vary widely among hospitals. It is important to have representation from groups that are related to the local resuscitation practices. With the advent of the MET system, hospitals will need to decide if the MET committee will be part of the overall resuscitation committee or will be politically and financially separate. Committees will also need to expand their focus to assure optimal postresuscitation management.

Organized response to cardiac arrest

First responder

The most critical period of a cardiac arrest is the first few minutes after collapse, regardless of whether the arrest occurs inside or outside of the hospital. Therefore, improvement in very early treatment (mostly prior to admission of the rescue team) has the potential to have the most marked influence on the chance of survival after in-hospital cardiac arrest. Thus, the single most important issue is to secure optimal preparedness for a cardiac arrest, regardless of place within the hospital. This preparedness involves all health care providers within the hospital and includes various aspects of training (see below).

The consequences of increased preparedness for a cardiac arrest within the hospital has recently been highlighted. Thus, it has been shown that a program including widespread education of use of defibrillators with AED-function all over the hospital was associated with an improved survival to discharge after in-hospital cardiac arrest.[29] Furthermore, in agreement with findings in out-of-hospital cardiac arrest,[30] it has been suggested that among patients found in ventricular fibrillation, those who were defibrillated within 3 minutes after collapse have a very high survival (maybe as high as 70%), regardless of where the arrest took place.[31] Thus, the goal for every hospital should be to defibrillate all patients who suffer from ventricular fibrillation within 3 minutes after collapse. This goal can only be achieved by having defibrillators on each ward that are easy to handle and therefore can be used by a large proportion of health care providers.

Technical personnel training includes education and skills development in the recognition of a cardiac arrest, chest compression and ventilation, the use of simple devices such as mouth to mask ventilation and the use of suction devices, how to call for the rescue team, the use of medication and intubation, and the use of automated external defibrillators as well as manual defibrillators.

The appointment of a resuscitation training officer has enhanced the survival rate after in-hospital cardiac arrest.[32] This indicates that organized training of the hospital staff in CPR might improve survival after in-hospital cardiac arrest. In the UK, all public hospitals are obliged to have an appointed Resuscitation Training Officer supervising and organizing CPR-related activities.

In 2003, 60% of hospitals in Sweden had a service assigned to CPR education and other CPR-related activities; the corresponding figure for Finland was 75%.[33] Data from Finland indicate that nurses seem to receive more training than physicians.[33] In the United States, physician training in CPR is not mandatory. Some hospitals in the UK documented an increase in the survival rate of patients resuscitated from VF/VT that was linked to improvements in resuscitation training.

Because rapid defibrillation is of major importance, it would be helpful to have defibrillation performed by first responders.[34,35] With appropriate training, nurses can use an automated external defibrillator (AED) appropriately and can retain the actual skill. Nurses trained in basic life support can often use AED in a simulated cardiac arrest situation, even without prior training.[36] Nonetheless, when not under supervision, they are often reluctant to use the AED and fail to deliver defibrillation prior to arrival of more advanced care providers.[37] There are no specific recommendations for either manual or automated defibrillation in the hospital. What is important is that the shock gets delivered by the fastest mechanism in a given environment.

Skills retention

Skills retention has been shown to be limited.[38] Thus, repetition courses are required. The optimal interval between courses are not known, but an interval of 1 year has been considered to be appropriate. Nonetheless, with respect to defibrillation, skill retention has been reported to be good.[39]

Rescue team

There is no clear definition of how a rescue team should deal with in-hospital cardiac arrest. The three major aspects are quantity (number of persons), quality (competence), and proximity (how soon the rescue team will appear on scene). Local factors will influence the structure of the rescue team. In large university hospitals outside the United States, for example, it is common to have a rescue team consisting of multiple senior physicians. An anesthesiologist, a cardiologist, and an internist may all respond to resuscitation calls. In large training hospitals in the United States it is more common to have the resuscitation care delivered by junior physicians in training. In small hospitals there may be no resuscitation teams. In these instances, there is often an anesthesiologist who, in collaboration with the ward or emergency physician, performs resuscitation.[33] In many hospitals one rescue team may cover the whole hospital, whereas in other hospitals multiple teams may exist. Whereas there is no one correct way to structure the emergency response to in-hospital cardiac arrest, the program must assure that enough trained and experienced people respond in a timely fashion.

Before the arrival of the advanced rescue team, there must be an organized response on the ward where the event occurs. Policies and procedures should be in place to ensure a rapid local response with quality CPR and early defibrillation prior to arrival of the team.

Despite the presence of a dedicated team working under appropriate protocols, the cardiac arrest response is often chaotic, loud, and inefficient. While most hospitals focus on assuring adequate technical skills of the responders, there is typically little focus on non-technical issues such as communication and overall team performance. Crisis Resource Management (CRM) training is used in other medical settings, such as trauma team response and subspecialty practices, particularly anesthesia.[40–42] CRM focuses on improving interpersonal skills and team building to make medical responses more efficient. Instead of a disorganized response with all team members trying to do the same thing, there is a clear team leader who directs all clinical activities. Every responder has a specific job to perform, knows what that job is, uses checklists to assure accuracy, repeats and confirms all activities with the team leader, and effectively communicates with other team members. Focus on non-technical training of resuscitation teams may be an important way to improve patient care and decrease medical errors.

Ethical issues and outcomes reporting

Multiple comorbidities are linked with poor survival, including cancer,[43] septicemia,[44,45] renal failure,[46,47] and neurological disease.[48,49] The question of whether old age alone predicts mortality is not clear, with some studies supporting this assumption[50,51] and others not doing so.[52,53] Several prediction models for poor survival exist; however, using them on an individual patient to make decisions on withholding care is not widely practiced, since it is difficult to predict individual outcome from aggregate data.

Prearrest DNAR practices differ widely among hospitals. Aggressive resuscitation efforts indicate that CPR is initiated on a high proportion of patients suffering from cardiac arrest. When this occurs, the risk of starting CPR on a patient with a very low chance of survival is higher. A non-aggressive approach assigns DNAR status to more patients and indicates that CPR is started on a relatively low proportion of patients suffering from cardiac arrest, resulting in a greater chance of survival when resuscitation attempts are made. Percent survival of patients suffering from in-hospital cardiac arrest will depend on whether an aggressive or non-aggressive approach is used, and can influence reported quality improvement data as well as research outcomes.

Science

The American Heart Association's National Registry of Cardiopulmonary Resuscitation (NRCPR) is an international quality improvement database of over 75 000 in-hospital cardiac arrests.[1] Persons who experienced an arrest in the NRCPR dataset are typically male (57%) in their mid to late 60s. Over one-third of arrest events occur on medical-cardiac services. Several pre-existing conditions are associated with cardiac arrest. Myocardial infarction, congestive heart failure, respiratory insufficiency, diabetes mellitus, and infection are the most prominent comorbidities. Cardiac arrhythmia, acute respiratory insufficiency, and hypotension are the most common precipitating factors. Nearly half of all arrests occur in the ICU. Only 25% of in-hospital arrest victims had ventricular fibrillation (VF) as the initial pulseless rhythm, despite 86% of patients being either monitored or witnessed at the time of the arrest. This suggests that a delay in rhythm recognition alone may not completely explain the infrequent presence of VF. Forty-four percent of all patients had ROSC, while only 17% survived to hospital discharge. Survival was higher with VF as the presenting rhythm (34%) compared to asystole (10%) and pulseless electrical activity (PEA) (10%). Use of the term "overall survival" to describe outcome may be misleading. The 34% survival rate from VF that occurs in only 25% of arrests is diluted by the 10% survival rate for asystole and PEA that occurs in 66% of arrests. Future descriptions of cardiac arrest outcomes should be based on the initial arrest rhythms, not overall survival from all rhythms combined. Of those patients who died prior to discharge, 63% were made DNAR after ROSC. The average length of stay after an arrest is nearly 2 weeks for survivors and less than 2 days for those who die in the hospital, suggesting that care is being withdrawn very early after an event. Of those who survived to discharge, 86% of patients with a cerebral performance category (CPC) scale of 1 on admission had a CPC scale of 1 at the time of discharge, suggesting that survivors have relatively well-preserved neurological function.

Correct performance of chest compressions and ventilations is associated with a significant survival benefit in both animal and human studies. Abella and colleagues performed quantitative recordings of actual CPR during in-hospital cardiac arrest and found that the quality of CPR was deficient, according to guideline recommendations.[54] Chest compression rates and depth were lower than recommended, ventilation was significantly faster than recommended, and there were prolonged periods of no chest compression activity at all, resulting in long "no-flow" states. Experience from a single hospital in Sweden indicates that when CPR is started within 1 minute after collapse there is a marked improvement in survival compared to later initiation of CPR.[55] These findings suggest the need for rescuer feedback and more intensive monitoring of the quality of CPR during in-hospital resuscitation.

Postresuscitation care

All patients surviving a cardiac arrest ultimately receive the rest of their care in the hospital. It is the final common denominator for patients who arrest both in and outside the hospital setting. Care delivered and decisions made after ROSC will have a significant impact on outcome. In an era in which scientific, clinical, and regulatory communities demand improved long-term outcomes before recommending and adopting changes in practice, optimization and standardization of postresuscitation care is necessary to ensure that survival is more likely to reflect the intervention being studied rather than the quality and type of care delivered after ROSC. The science defining optimal postresuscitation care is in its infancy, yet is growing rapidly. Therapies such as therapeutic hypothermia and tight blood glucose control have been identified as providing benefit. The challenge faced by hospitals to implement new diagnostic and therapeutic initiatives in these patients is multifaceted. Hospitals must have a person who is responsible for the identification of new science and who is empowered to implement clinical change. Disseminating new scientific information to the end-user at individual hospitals is a formidable task, only to be surpassed by changing behavior. A survey performed in the United States by Abella *et al.* documented that nearly 90% of physician responders had never induced hypothermia in a comatose cardiac arrest survivor 18 months after the publication of two large randomized controlled clinical trials documenting benefit.[56] Literature documenting that change in practice does not parallel change in knowledge is abundant. It is often not until algorithms, standardized protocols, and flow-sheets are developed to help physicians and nurses operationalize the science that extensive changes in behavior occur. This is especially true of low volume clinical occurrences such as survival from cardiac arrest, and where care is often performed by clinicians unfamiliar with evolving postresuscitation science. In many teaching hospitals, cardiac arrest events and postresuscitation therapies are often delivered primarily by physicians at various levels of training, without direct or immediate supervision by a senior physician. Hospitals must begin to move away from delegating the decisions to junior inexperienced doctors in training.

Therapeutic hypothermia

The 2005 International Consensus on Cardiopulmonary Resuscitation and Emergency Cardiovascular Care Science states that "Unconscious adult patients with spontaneous circulation after out-of-hospital cardiac arrest should be cooled to 32 °C–34°C for 12–24 hours when the initial rhythm was VF. Cooling to 32 °C–34 °C for 12–24 hours may be considered for unconscious adult patients with spontaneous circulation after out-of-hospital cardiac arrest from any other rhythm or cardiac arrest in the hospital. The supporting science for therapeutic hypothermia in these populations is discussed in detail elsewhere in this book. This section focuses on issues pertinent to program development and implementation.

A systematic, comprehensive approach to the delivery of therapeutic hypothermia to comatose survivors of cardiac arrest must be implemented to assure optimal support, development, and utilization. It is imperative to gather individual "thought leaders" in resuscitation and have representation from physicians, nurses, administrators, and whatever ancillary services will be needed to provide the therapy. Decisions must be made regarding which units in the hospital will provide the hypothermia. Optimally, all units receiving post-non-traumatic arrest patients should be capable of delivering hypothermia. Decisions to centralize the location of these patients within an intensive care area, however, may decrease the resources needed to initiate and maintain the program. Resuscitation committees need to be armed with as much information as possible to educate those less familiar with evolving postresuscitation practices. Once a hospital-wide decision has been made to provide therapeutic hypothermia, appropriate policies and procedures require development. Inclusion and exclusion criteria can be somewhat subjective and decisions need to be made as to whether or not the therapy will be provided to in-hospital patients as well as those that arrest out of the hospital. Because hypothermia is a relatively new therapy, hospitals are required to develop their own criteria for its implementation and monitoring; however, decisions can be assisted by criteria used in the randomized clinical trials of hypothermia in comatose survivors of cardiac arrest.

Two types of educational programs are helpful before program implementation. Widespread education of all clinical providers is crucial to more rapid acceptance and application of the process. All physician and nursing staff, including doctors in training or house officers who may be caring for or covering these patients while in the ICU, must be educated. More detailed education on the physiological effects and potential complications of therapeutic hypothermia, as well as instruction on how to deliver the therapy is required for the specific groups of nurses and physicians primarily responsible for care delivery. An understanding of the physiology, and knowing how to expect a typical patient to behave, is helpful in alleviating the stress and uncertainty of providing a new therapy.

There are several mechanisms by which therapeutic hypothermia can be delivered. Cooling can be done externally or internally. Readily available ice packs, iced saline and gastric lavage, and conventional cooling blankets found in most hospitals can be used. Specific equipment is also available for temperature regulation that uses both endovascular and external methods. There is no current recommendation of one type of delivery mechanism over another. Hospitals should consider personnel requirements, ease and accuracy of induction, maintenance and reversal, and patient accessibility when deciding the technique by which hypothermia will be provided.

As with all new therapies, there is much to be learned about the optimal approach to providing care and minimizing complications. There are many specific clinical details that remain suboptimally understood in patients treated with therapeutic hypothermia. This should not deter a hospital from implementing a therapy shown to be of benefit, but should encourage meticulous observation and evaluation of these patients to assure that new clinical information is identified and shared.

Much practical information has been gathered since the implementation of this therapy. Program coordinators need to consider several details in order to develop a successful program. Attempting to reach the target temperature within the shortest amount of time possible is a common goal. Decrease in temperature may be slowed by the presence of overhead lights shining down on the patient, heated air in the ventilator, an elevated ambient room temperature, and by several pieces of electronic equipment in the room each giving off heat. Temperature should be monitored frequently and overshoot of the target temperature should be avoided, since temperatures less than 30°C may cause complications. Local protocols should be developed with specific sets of routine laboratory tests to evaluate for possible complications, such as renal insufficiency, infection, coagulopathy, or pancreatitis. Neurological examination should be documented before the initiation of hypothermia. Modified Rankin and CPC data are needed to document the patient's baseline. The Glasgow Coma Scale and brainstem reflexes should be documented before, during, and after therapy.

Many patients treated with hypothermia are therapeutically paralyzed to decrease shivering and may remain paralyzed throughout the duration of the hypothermia. It is impossible to detect focal or generalized seizure activity in these patients since they cannot move. Since seizure activity is common in postarrest patients who have suffered a global ischemic insult, there is an increasing concern that seizures may be undetected until paralytic agents are discontinued. This has prompted some centers to perform routine electroencephalographic monitoring during the hypothermia or only to use paralytic agents until the target temperature is reached.

Metabolic management

Tight control of blood glucose with insulin lowers hospital mortality in critically ill adults. Although this has not been studied specifically in the cardiac arrest population, there is a strong association between postarrest hyperglycemia and poor neurological outcome. The optimal blood glucose level in these patients has not been determined, but frequent monitoring of glucose, treatment with insulin, and avoidance of hypoglycemia should be part of a comprehensive postresuscitation protocol.

Postresuscitation decision making

The decision to stop resuscitation efforts or to withdraw care after ROSC from cardiac arrest is one that is often made very early after the event and is commonly based more on emotion than on physiology. Data from the NRCPR show that 63% of patients who initially survive an in-hospital cardiac arrest are declared DNAR.[1] With an average hospital length of stay for those who die of 2 days, this documents that the decision to withdraw care is frequently being made very early. Good clinical indicators exist for predicting poor outcome in patients who remain in persistent coma after arrest. They include a lack of papillary reflex at day 3, extensor posturing or worse at day 3, absence of certain-wave in cortical evoked response within 72 hours to 1 week, and the occurrence of status myoclonic seizures (not to be confused with simple myoclonus). The neurological literature supports waiting for a 3-day period to be able more accurately predict neurological outcome on postarrest patients who are not treated with therapeutic hypothermia. Making decisions to withdraw or not provide care prior to this time may be premature. The optimal timeframe for decision making on DNAR status in patients treated with hypothermia is unknown. It remains unclear how quickly the brain is expected to gain near maximal benefit from the hypothermia, and when is it reasonable to assume that no significant improvement will occur. Although no recommendations are available based on data, it may be reasonable to wait an additional few days beyond the 3-day recommendation when evaluating neurological status in comatose patients treated with mild hypothermia.

The aggressiveness with which an individual hospital withdraws care and withholds future resuscitation attempts has significant bearing on individual and aggregate survival data and can have a tremendous impact on clinical trial data, where survival to discharge after cardiac arrest is an end point.

Summary

The hospital provides a unique setting for pre-, intra-, and postresuscitation care. The burden of prevention and optimal postresuscitation management, in addition to acute resuscitation, poses unique opportunities not recognized in the past. With a focus on patient safety and implementation of medical emergency teams/rapid response systems, prevention of cardiopulmonary arrest and improved outcomes is a reality. For patients who ultimately suffer an arrest, opportunities for improved care delivery come from crisis management training, skilled responders, and optimal performance of both CPR and advanced care delivery. The sequence of events that begins with the ischemic insult from the arrest and the global reperfusion that accompanies return of circulation create a cascade of metabolic activity that can be treated with such therapies as therapeutic mild hypothermia. Hospitals must develop programs that focus specifically on postresuscitation care, and more effort is needed to remain abreast of this rapidly evolving area, so that new advances can be rapidly incorporated into clinical practice. The in-hospital chain of survival needs to be expanded by an additional two links from both a systems and clinical perspective. The first link begins with rapid response systems that prevent clinical deterioration in a significant number of patients, followed by the traditional links of early access in summoning the appropriate clinical team and equipment, early and good quality CPR, early defibrillation by whatever mechanism gets the shock delivered as quickly as possible within individual hospital settings, early advanced life support delivered in a consistent manner by healthcare providers experienced in resuscitation practices, and ending with the final link of optimal postresuscitation care. The clasp that holds this enhanced in-hospital chain of survival together is a comprehensive quality review program that includes mechanisms for the rapid adoption of new science as well as appropriate process and outcomes review. Perhaps this broader focus will be the key to improving survival for in-hospital cardiac arrest.

REFERENCES

1. Peberdy, M.A., Kaye, W., Ornato, J.P. *et al.* Cardiopulmonary resuscitation of adults in the hospital: a report of 14720 cardiac arrests from the National Registry of Cardiopulmonary Resuscitation. *Resuscitation* 2003; **58**(3): 297–308.

2. Buist, M.D., Moore, G.E., Bernard, S.A., Waxman, B.P., Anderson, J.N., & Nguyen, T.V. Effects of a medical emergency team on reduction of incidence of and mortality from unexpected cardiac arrests in hospital: preliminary study. *Br. Med. J.* 2002; **324**(7334): 387–90.

3. Fieselmann, J.F., Hendryx, M.S., Helms, C.M. & Wakefield, D.S. Respiratory rate predicts cardiopulmonary arrest for internal medicine inpatients. *J. Gen. Intern. Med.* 1993; **8**(7): 354–360.

4. Franklin, C. & Mathew, J. Developing strategies to prevent inhospital cardiac arrest: analyzing responses of physicians and nurses in the hours before the event. *Crit. Care Med.* 1994; **22**(2): 244–247.

5. Hodgetts, T.J., Kenward, G., Vlachonikolis, I.G., Payne, S. & Castle, N. The identification of risk factors for cardiac arrest and formulation of activation criteria to alert a medical emergency team. *Resuscitation* 2002; **54**(2): 125–131.

6. Schein, R.M., Hazday, N., Pena, M., Ruben, B.H. & Sprung, C.L. Clinical antecedents to in-hospital cardiopulmonary arrest. *Chest* 1990; **98**(6): 1388–1392.

7. Smith, A.F. & Wood, J. Can some in-hospital cardio-respiratory arrests be prevented? A prospective survey. *Resuscitation* 1998; **37**(3): 133–137.

8. Garrard, C. & Young, D. Suboptimal care of patients before admission to intensive care is caused by a failure to appreciate or apply the ABCs of life support. *Br. Med. J.* 1998; **316**(7148): 1841–1842.

9. Goldhill, D.R., White, S.A. & Sumner, A. Physiological values and procedures in the 24 h before ICU admission from the ward. *Anaesthesia* 1999; **54**(6): 529–534.

10. McQuillan, P., Pilkington, S., Allan, A. *et al.* Confidential inquiry into quality of care before admission to intensive care. *Br. Med. J.* 1998; **316**(7148): 1853–1858.

11. Hillman, K.M., Bristow, P.J., Chey, T. *et al.* Antecedents to hospital deaths. *Intern. Med. J.* 2001; **31**(6): 343–348.

12. Chassin, M.R. & Galvin, R.W. The urgent need to improve health care quality. Institute of Medicine National Roundtable on Health Care Quality. *J. Am. Med. Assoc.* 1998; **280**(11): 1000–1005.

13. Hodgetts, T., Kenward, G., Vlackonikolis, I. *et al.* Incidence, location and reasons for avoidable in-hospital cardiac arrest in a district general hospital. *Resuscitation* 2002; **54**(2): 115.

14. Koeck, C. Time for organisational development in healthcare organisations. Improving quality for patients means changing the organisation. *Br. Med. J.* 1998; **317**(7168): 1267–1268.

15. Leape, L.L. Error in medicine. *J. Am. Med. Assoc.* 1994; **272**(23): 1851–1857.

16. McNeil, B.J. Shattuck Lecture – hidden barriers to improvement in the quality of care. *N. Engl. J. Med.* 2001; **345**(22): 1612–1620.

17. Vincent, C., Neale, G. & Woloshynowych, M. Adverse events in British hospitals: preliminary retrospective record review. *Br. Med. J.* 2001; **322**(7285): 517–519.

18. Cretikos, M. & Hillman, K. The medical emergency team: does it really make a difference? *Intern. Med. J.* 2003; **33**(11): 511–514.

19. Daly, F.F., Sidney, K.L. & Fatovich, D.M. The Medical Emergency Team (MET): a model for the district general hospital. *Aust. N Z J. Med.* 1998; **28**(6): 795–798.

20. Lee, A., Bishop, G., Hillman, K.M. & Daffurn, K. The Medical Emergency Team. *Anaesth. Intens. Care* 1995; **23**(2): 183–186.

21. Hillman, K., Parr, M., Flabouris, A., Bishop, G. & Stewart, A. Redefining in-hospital resuscitation: the concept of the medical emergency team. *Resuscitation* 2001; **48**(2): 105–110.

22. Parr, M.J., Hadfield, J.H., Flabouris, A., Bishop, G. & Hillman, K. The Medical Emergency Team: 12 month analysis of reasons for activation, immediate outcome and not-for-resuscitation orders. *Resuscitation* 2001; **50**(1): 39–44.

23. Bellomo, R., Goldsmith, D., Uchino, S. *et al.* Prospective controlled trial of effect of medical emergency team on postoperative morbidity and mortality rates. *Crit. Care Med.* 2004; **32**(4): 916–921.

24. Bellomo, R., Goldsmith, D., Uchino, S. *et al.* A prospective before-and-after trial of a medical emergency team. *Med. J. Aust.* 2003; **179**(6): 283–287.

25. Bristow, P.J., Hillman, K.M., Chey, T. *et al.* Rates of in-hospital arrests, deaths and intensive care admissions: the effect of a medical emergency team. *Med. J. Aust.* 2000; **173**(5): 236–240.

26. DeVita, M.A., Braithwaite, R.S., Mahidhara, R., Stuart, S., Foraida, M. & Simmons, R.L. Use of medical emergency team responses to reduce hospital cardiopulmonary arrests. *Qual. Saf. Health Care* 2004; **13**(4): 251–254.

27. Hillman, K., Chen, J., Cretikos, M. *et al.* Introduction of the medical emergency team (MET) system: a cluster-randomised controlled trial. *Lancet* 2005; **365**(9477): 2091–2097.

28. Salamonson, Y., Kariyawasam, A., van Heere, B. & O'Connor, C. The evolutionary process of Medical Emergency Team (MET) implementation: reduction in unanticipated ICU transfers. *Resuscitation* 2001; **49**(2): 135–141.

29. Zafari, A.M., Zarter, S.K., Heggen, V. *et al.* A program encouraging early defibrillation resulsts in improved in-hospital resuscitation efficacy. *J. Am. Coll. Cardiol.* 2004; **44**(4): 846–852.

30. Valenzuela, T.D., Roe, D.J., Nichol, G., Clark, L.L., Spaite, D.W. & Hardman, R.G. Outcomes of rapid defibrillation by security officers after cardiac arrest in casinos. *N. Engl. J. Med.* 2000; **343**(17): 1206–1209.

31. Herlitz, J., Aune, S., Bång, A. *et al.* Very high survival among patients defibrillated at an early stage after in-hospital ventricular fibrillation on wards with and without monitoring facilities. *Resuscitation* 2005; **66**: 159–166.

32. McGowan, J., Graham, C.A. & Gordon, M.W. Appointment of a Resuscitation Training Officer is associated with improved survival from in-hospital ventricular fibrillation/ventricular tachycardia cardiac arrest. *Resuscitation* 1999; **41**(2): 169–173.

33. Skrifvars, M.B., Rosenberg, P.H., Finne, P. *et al.* Evaluation of the in-hospital Utstein template in cardiopulmonary resuscitation in secondary hospitals. *Resuscitation* 2003; **56**(3): 275–282.

34. Cummins, R.O., Sanders, A., Mancini, E. & Hazinski, M.F. In-hospital resuscitation: executive summary. *Ann. Emerg. Med.* 1997; **29**(5): 647–649.

35. Parr, M. In-hospital resuscitation: review and revise. *Resuscitation* 2001; **50**(1): 13–14.

36. Domanovits, H., Meron, G., Sterz, F. *et al.* Successful automatic external defibrillator operation by people trained only in basic life support in a simulated cardiac arrest situation. *Resuscitation* 1998; **39**(1–2): 47–50.

37. Coady, E.M. A strategy for nurse defibrillation in general wards. *Resuscitation* 1999; **42**(3): 183–186.

38. Chamberlain, D., Smith, A., Wollard, M. *et al.* Trials of teaching methods in basic life support (3): Comparison of simulated CPR performance after first training and at 6 months, with a note on the value of re-training. *Resuscitation* 2002; **53**: 179–187.

39. Warwick, J.P., Mackie, K. & Spencer, I. Towards early defibrillation – a nurse training programme in the use of automated external defibrillators. *Resuscitation* 1995; **30**: 231–235.

40. Blum, R.H., Raemer, D.B., Carroll, J.S., Sunder, N., Felstein, D.M. & Cooper, J.B. Crisis resource management training for an anaesthesia faculty: a new approach to continuing education. *Med. Educ.* 2004; **38**(1): 45–55.

41. Flanagan, B., Nestel, D. & Joseph, M. Making patient safety the focus: crisis resource management in the undergraduate curriculum. *Med. Educ.* 2004; **38**(1): 56–66.

42. Rall, M. & Dieckmann, P. Safety culture and crisis resource management in airway management: general principles to enhance patient safety in critical airway situations. *Best Pract. Res. Clin. Anaesthesiol.* 2005; **19**(4): 539–557.

43. Taffet, G.E., Teasdale, T.A. & Luchi, R.J. In-hospital cardiopulmonary resuscitation. *J. Am. Med. Assoc.* 1988; **260**(14): 2069–2072.

44. Ballew, K.A., Philbrick, J.T., Caven, D.E. & Schorling, J.B. Predictors of survival following in-hospital cardiopulmonary resuscitation. A moving target. *Arch. Intern. Med.* 1994; **154**(21): 2426–2432.

45. Schultz, S.C., Cullinane, D.C., Pasquale, M.D., Magnant, C. & Evans, S.R. Predicting in-hospital mortality during cardiopulmonary resuscitation. *Resuscitation* 1996; **33**(1): 13–17.

46. de Vos, R., Koster, R.W., de Haan, R.J., Oosting, H., van der Wouw, P.A. & Lampe-Schoenmaeckers, A.J. In-hospital cardiopulmonary resuscitation: prearrest morbidity and outcome. *Arch. Intern. Med.* 1999; **159**(8): 845–850.

47. George, A.L., Jr., Folk, B.P., 3rd, Crecelius, P.L. & Campbell, W.B. Pre-arrest morbidity and other correlates of survival after in-hospital cardiopulmonary arrest. *Am. J. Med.* 1989; **87**(1): 28–34.

48. Bedell, S.E., Delbanco, T.L., Cook, E.F. & Epstein, F.H. Survival after cardiopulmonary resuscitation in the hospital. *N. Engl. J. Med.* 1983; **309**(10): 569–576.

49. O'Keeffe, S. & Ebell, M.H. Prediction of failure to survive following in-hospital cardiopulmonary resuscitation: comparison of two predictive instruments. *Resuscitation* 1994; **28**(1): 21–25.

50. de Vos, R., Koster, R.W. & de Haan, R.J. Impact of survival probability, life expectancy, quality of life and patient preferences on do-not-attempt-resuscitation orders in a hospital. Resuscitation Committee. *Resuscitation* 1998; **39**(1–2): 15–21.

51. Weerasinghe, D.P., MacIntyre, C.R. & Rubin, G.L. The epidemiology of cardiac arrests in a Sydney hospital. *Resuscitation* 2002; **53**(1): 53–62.

52. Berger, R. & Kelley, M. Survival after in-hospital cardiopulmonary arrest of noncritically ill patients. A prospective study. *Chest* 1994; **106**(3): 872–879.

53. Ravakhah, K., Khalafi, K., Bathory, T. & Wang, H.C. Advanced cardiac life support events in a community hospital and their outcome: evaluation of actual arrests. *Resuscitation* 1998; **36**(2): 95–99.

54. Abella, B.S., Alvarado, J.P., Myklebust, H. *et al.* Quality of cardiopulmonary resuscitation during in-hospital cardiac arrest. *J. Am. Med. Assoc.* 2005; **293**(3): 305–310.

55. Herlitz, J., Bang, A., Alsen, B. & Aune, S. Characteristics and outcome among patients suffering from in hospital cardiac arrest in relation to the interval between collapse and start of CPR. *Resuscitation* 2002; **53**(1): 21–27.

56. Abella, B.S., Rhee, J.W., Huang, K.N., Vanden Hoek, T.L. & Becker, L.B. Induced hypothermia is underused after resuscitation from cardiac arrest: a current practice survey. *Resuscitation* 2005; **64**(2): 181–186.

45

Complications of CPR

Michael Baubin[1], Walter Rabl[2] and Robert Sebastian Hoke[3]

[1] Department of Anesthesiology and Critical Care, Innsbruck Medical University, Austria
[2] Institute of Legal Medicine, Innsbruck Medical University, Austria
[3] Department of Cardiology–Angiology, University of Leipzig, Germany

Introduction

Cardiopulmonary resuscitation is an invasive medical treatment. Its measures can cause more or less severe complications, which often remain unrevealed unless autopsy is performed.

Performing sufficient chest compressions needs regular thumps with force up to 392 N (40 kp). The human thorax, the ribs, and especially the sternum are not built for such force and will frequently suffer iatrogenic injuries. If the patient's biological age is unknown, the occurrence of some of these injuries cannot be avoided. In the last decades, a number of chest compression devices have been developed to increase cardiac output and to replace the rescuer's hands and his/her manpower. Although some of these devices are already commercially available, there is a general lack of information on their adverse effects in comparison to manual chest compression.

Defibrillation constitutes one of the most invasive resuscitative measures. Complications of defibrillation may affect the patient, the rescuers, and the immediate environment. Although systematic investigations have rarely been conducted, the available evidence will be discussed in the corresponding paragraph.

Time is critical in CPR, and medical personnel as well as lay rescuers generally work under emotional pressure. Moreover, CPR is frequently performed under challenging conditions, such as at night, in uncomfortable weather conditions, environmental dangers, inadequate manpower, noise, in a confined space, and other adverse circumstances, which in particular, are found in the prehospital setting. Therefore, it is understandable that, for example, endotracheal intubation has to be performed under conditions that are considerably worse than in the OR and therefore cause harm more frequently. Meticulous autopsy can find macro- and micro-lesions caused by intubation maneuvers.

This chapter will provide detailed information on typical complications of chest compression (including use of new CPR devices), defibrillation, and airway management.

Complications of chest compressions

Chest compression is a blunt thoracic trauma with defined localization and force. It is reasonable to assume that these complications can be reduced by proper hand position and technique. The following complications are described in the literature, but are too numerous to all be discussed in this chapter: rib and sternal fractures, fractures of clavicles, scapulae, and vertebral column, flail chest, skin trauma, subcutaneous emphysema, pulmonary edema, pulmonary hematoma, pneumothorax, hemothorax, embolization, lung laceration, pneumomediastinum, mediastinitis, cardiac contusion/rupture, pericarditis, liver laceration, and bowel injury.

Precordial thump

A solitary precordial thump is sometimes used in the pulseless victim.[1] The potential to convert the patient from ventricular tachycardia to fibrillation, however, has led most authorities to consider one immediate precordial thump manoever after a monitored cardiac arrest if an electrical defibrillator is not immediately available.

Cardiac Arrest: The Science and Practice of Resuscitation Medicine. 2nd edn., ed. Norman Paradis, Henry Halperin, Karl Kern, Volker Wenzel, Douglas Chamberlain. Published by Cambridge University Press. © Cambridge University Press, 2007.

Transient complete atrioventricular block,[2] pleomorphic ventricular tachycardia,[3] induction of re-entrant ventricular tachycardia after supraventricular tachycardia,[4] and a faster ventricular tachycardia rate[5] are conditions that have been described during the treatment of ventricular tachycardia with a chest thump. Thus, monitoring the patient during the chest thump maneuver is recommended.

Manual chest compression

Skeletal injuries

The incidence reported for rib fractures after conventional closed-chest compression in the treatment of cardiac arrest ranges from 13% to 97%; the incidence of sternal fractures ranges from 1% to 43%.[6] In a retrospective review of forensic records of 499 deaths (343 males, 156 females) in patients who had received CPR before death, rib fractures were described in 29% and sternal fractures in 14%.[7] The best method to detect fractures of the thorax is by autopsy that prospectively reveals such fractures. However, only five studies are available that have employed this method.[8–12] These studies report rib fractures in 32% to 60% and sternal fractures in 19% to 43%.

For the very rare situation of CPR with the patient in the prone position, e.g., in the operating room for a vertebral operation, no complications or injuries are described in the literature.[13]

Other complications

Chest wall bruising is among the most common adverse effects of CPR – it is reported for up to 59% of all resuscitated patients.[10] Pulmonary fat emboli can be detected in almost all cardiopulmonary resuscitated patients when special attempts are made to detect this complication.[14,15] Bone marrow emboli are found in 11% to 27%.[8,16–20] The clinical relevance of these findings is undetermined.

Critical internal organ damage can also result from chest compressions. Table 45.1 provides an overview of all those soft-tissue injuries that may worsen outcome and that, according to research, have an apparent incidence of at least 1%. Further, tracheal, esophageal, gastric, renal, and diaphragmatic ruptures, and various internal hemorrhages have been described in case reports.

Chest compressions with chest compression devices

All chest compression assist devices, reported in the literature, have only been studied in adults; moreover, the complication rates have not been studied in a standardized manner. Sternal and/or rib fractures are sometimes reported or excluded by external examination of the

Table 45.1. Incidence of internal organ damage seen after CPR.

Complication	Incidence reported	References
Left ventricular hemorrhage	0 to 8%	11, 16, 17
Pneumothorax	1 to 3.0%	9, 15, 45
Hemothorax	1 to 9%	15, 16, 45
Hepatic laceration/rupture	1 to 4.3%	9, 10, 15
Hemopericarditis	1 to 8%	7, 9, 15, 17, 18
Aortic laceration	0.5 to 1.6%	15, 46
Splenic laceration/rupture	0.3 to 2.6%	9, 15, 16, 28

Modified from ref. 6.

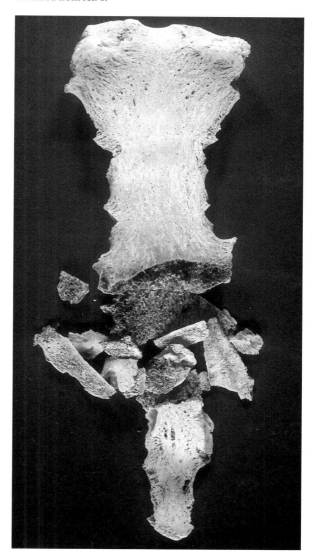

Fig. 45.1. Sternal fragments after ACD-CPR preceded by standard CPR.

thorax, by X-ray, rarely by autopsy, very rarely by special autopsy focusing on skeletal injuries, and never by computed tomography or magnetic resonance imaging.

Active compression–decompression (ACD) CPR

Only one randomized ACD-CPR trial included assessment of skeletal injuries in fatal cases by thorough autopsy.[9] This trial was halted by the local ethics committee because of an unexpectedly high rate of rib and sternal fractures (13/15, 87%, and 14/15, 93%). Earlier studies had suggested that ACD-CPR is associated with rib fractures in 4% to 87% and sternal fractures in 0% to 93%.[21–25]

Another study that specifically addressed skeletal injuries after ACD-CPR alone, as well as after standard CPR followed by ACD-CPR revealed rib fractures in 11/16 and 14/15 patients, respectively, and sternal fractures in 11/16 and 9/15 patients, respectively.[26] This study included cases in which multiple rib and comminuted sternal fractures (Fig. 45.1) were associated with aortic laceration or atrial or ventricular rupture. The authors concluded that sternal fractures with its saw-like fragments might pose a particular threat to intrathoracic organs. The same authors investigated biomechanical aspects of ACD-CPR complications.[27] The shape of the patient's chest seems to have a considerable influence on the way in which forces are transmitted to the thorax.

Accordingly, to date, the frequency of skeletal chest injuries after ACD-CPR cannot be specified with certainty. A Cochrane review from 2002[28] and a combined analysis[29] from eight trials stated that ACD-CPR is as safe as standard CPR.

LUCAS-CPR

LUCAS, Lund University Cardiopulmonary Assist System, is a device for standardized, gas-driven automatic chest compression and decompression up to the physiological level.[30] The first report on 100 consecutive cases of out-of-hospital cardiac arrest treated with LUCAS failed to assess the occurrence of traumatic sequelae.[31]

AutoPulse

Revivant AutoPulse is an automatic, battery-driven, circumferential chest compression device. A study of AutoPulse application in 31 in-hospital cardiac arrests did not disclose adverse effects associated with this device.[32] In an autopsy report of three patients who had been treated with Revivant AutoPulse, the following complications were reported: unusual cutaneous abrasions in all three cases, bilateral confluent paravertebral hemorrhages of the midthoracic spine in one patient with preceding manual CPR, abrasions on one breast in a female patient, non-

displaced bilateral parasternal rib fractures, and upper arm contusions.[33] According to the authors of this study, all of these findings appear to be associated with the CPR device.

Minimal invasive direct cardiac massage (mid-cm)

Only one study exists where the minimal invasive direct cardiac massage device[34] was used in humans;[35] in one out of 25 patients a heart rupture was caused by the device.

Open-chest CPR

Open-chest CPR is a heroic procedure that may improve vital organ perfusion and the outcome of selected patients. Because it is invasive, open-chest CPR places both the patient and the clinician at a significantly greater risk than does external chest compression.

Injury to the chest wall is inevitable during performance of this procedure, and should not be considered a complication. Lacerations of the intercostal or internal mammary arteries are avoidable and, as such, are complications. Hemodynamic control of an injured intercostal artery can be obtained by placing a suture through the next intercostal space lateral to the incision and looping it around the artery and rib. Gaining control of a torn internal mammary artery is often difficult and requires at least initial placement of a hemostat.

Because entry into the chest must be made expeditiously under emergency conditions, pulmonary lacerations are common. Care must be taken not to enter the chest with the knife, but to use scissors that are placed superficially to a protecting finger.

Fracture of the ribs is an avoidable but common complication of open-chest CPR. In cases of non-traumatic cardiac arrest, the operator needs an opening large enough to permit cross-clamping of the aorta and to provide cardiac compression. In older patients, fractures may occur despite minimal opening of the rib space. Care must be taken by the operator not to lacerate the hand or wrist on a jagged bone fragment.[36]

Except in patients who have penetrating trauma to the chest, it is not necessary to incise the pericardium. Some authorities believe that more effective compressions of the myocardium can be performed with an intact pericardium, and the myocardium is protected. Properly performed internal cardiac massage has a pattern of injury similar to that in external cardiac compression.

Blind attempts to place an aortic cross-clamp may result in injury to the mediastinum. It is not necessary to include the whole aorta within the clamp to occlude flow to distal structures significantly. If the aortic cross-clamp is placed too tightly, aortic injury may occur. If the clamp is left in place for too long, abdominal or retroperitoneal structures may be injured. During spontaneous circulation, cross-clamps should not be left in place for more than 20 minutes in normothermic patients. It is not known whether this also applies to patients in cardiac arrest. The state of emergency of this procedure does not allow adequate time to disinfect the skin before the incision is made. Despite this, the incidence of infection among survivors is low.[36]

Once the chest has been opened, there is significant risk of exposure to aerosolized blood. This occurs more frequently when there is a pulmonary laceration. All personnel should use universal precautions.

Methodology of detecting skeletal injuries

As discussed by Hoke *et al.*, most of the studies reporting on skeletal injuries after CPR cannot be compared to one another,[6] because of essential differences in inclusion and exclusion criteria, protocols, methods of data collection and presentation. Further, evaluation of clinical records, clinical examination, and chest radiographs must be considered inadequate for assessing the incidence of chest fractures. Plain chest radiographs have frequently been used to assess thoracic fractures, especially in studies of active compression–decompression CPR.[23,24,37] Nevertheless, the sensitivity of plain chest radiographs is poor. In a prospective study comparing postmortem findings of X-ray and forensic results in 19 patients after attempted cardiopulmonary resuscitation, no correlation was found between the X-ray and the autopsy findings and it was shown that postmortem autopsy is more accurate in detecting rib and sternum fractures as compared to X-ray.[38] It is possible that computed tomography or magnetic resonance imaging can play a future role in unravelling skeletal injuries and could replace autopsy in this regard.

Differences in gender, age, and location

In a forensic autopsy records report of 499 records of patients who had received CPR before death, rib fractures were found in 29% and sternal fracture in 14%.[7] More females than males sustained rib fractures (37% vs. 26%; $P < 0.05$). There was no significant gender difference for sternal fractures. In addition, the incidence of rib fractures increased with age ($P < 0.001$). While the positive correlation between age and rib fracture incidence is in accordance with another large autopsy study,[9] the latter found no difference in relation to gender.

A study on 27 human corpses showed a significant correlation between sternal fractures and gender ($P=0.008$) and between rib fractures and age ($P=0.008$) after ACD-CPR was performed on the corpses for 60 seconds.[39] Female corpses were found to have a higher risk for sternal fractures, whereas corpses of older patients had a higher risk for rib fractures. Maximal compression force (measured by a built-in force transducer in the ACD device) was another factor associated with a higher risk for rib and sternal fractures ($P= 0.48$). In 20 of the 27 corpses either the sternum fractured or the ribs fractured parasternally or medioclavicularly. Sternum fractures do not seem to protect against rib fractures and vice versa. The sternum fragments tilted inwards at the time of the fracture, and only moved inwards thereafter.

Chest injuries in children

According to the literature available, rib fractures occurred in 0% to 2.1% of all children in whom CPR was attempted.[40–44] In contrast, sternal fractures have never been reported. All in all, 770 pediatric CPR cases were included in the five aforementioned studies, only three of which exhibited skeletal injuries attributable to CPR. In addition, a few case reports have been published. In a retrospective review of autopsy records for deceased children under 12 years of age who had been given CPR without historical or physical evidence of preceding trauma, 211 children (mean age 19.0 months) met the inclusion criteria.[42] The mean duration of CPR was 45 minutes. Fifteen children (7%) showed at least one injury as a result of CPR, including retroperitoneal hemorrhage ($n=2$), pneumothorax ($n=1$), pulmonary hemorrhage ($n=1$), epicardial hematoma ($n=1$), and gastric perforation ($n=1$). Only one patient was noted to have rib fractures.

Thus, although significant iatrogenic injuries are rare in children who receive CPR, recognizing the possibility of a complication may be critical in the management of children who survive cardiac arrest. Regardless of resuscitation history, physical abuse should be considered whenever traumatic injuries are encountered.

Conclusions

In conclusion, organ injuries after CPR maneuvres must be seen as serious complications. Rib fractures are common adverse effects especially in elderly patients. Sternal fractures are more dangerous than rib fractures as these may cause direct organ injuries in the thorax; sternal fractures may occur more frequently in females. Correct CPR technique is likely to reduce the risk of skeletal injuries.

New CPR methods with CPR assist devices should be evaluated for their pressure pattern and compared with standard manual chest compressions in regard to skeletal and organ injuries. Chest X-ray is inadequate as a method for investigating the incidence of rib or sternal fractures. Only autopsy with detailed focus on CPR-related injuries provides adequate evidence.

Complications of external defibrillation

Electric defibrillation and cardioversion are irreplaceable as first-line interventions to terminate ventricular fibrillation (VF) and hemodynamically unstable ventricular tachycardias. They are vigorous procedures, however. Currents up to 70 amperes at voltages above 1000 volts are applied to the chest, depending on energy selected, waveform technology, and transthoracic impedance. Such electric shocks would, under different circumstances, be considered a high-tension electrical accident. There are dangers for the person being defibrillated as well as for the person carrying out the procedure and in the immediate environment. The main issues, including burns, skeletal muscle damage, myocardial injury, pacemakers and implantable cardioverter-defibrillators, and hazards for responders are discussed in the following paragraphs.

Complications for the patient

Burns

Skin burns at the site of electrode attachment to the chest are frequent adverse effects of defibrillation and probably the best recognized among health care professionals. Their severity ranges from transient faint erythema to deep serious lesions. Affections of the skin are typically more intense at the edge of the electrode mark, referred to as the "perimeter effect" (Fig. 45.2). It is not established whether manual paddles and self-adhesive pads differ with respect to skin burns. It is known, however, that commercially available self-adhesive pads vary significantly both in their own intrinsic impedance and thermal affection of the skin.[47] In cardioversion sequences, higher cumulative shock energies cause more damage.[48] Evidence suggests that prophylactic use of topical 5 % ibuprofen, but not 0.1% betamethasone, cream reduces pain and inflammation after external cardioversion.[49]

Superficial burns are most probably due to thermal effects at the electrode-skin interface, although electroporation of dermal cells with subsequent local inflammatory reaction may contribute. Basically, heating of the skin results from conversion of electrical to thermal energy. The

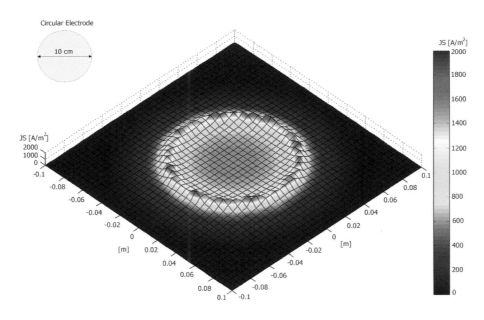

Fig. 45.2. Current density distribution under a defibrillation electrode modeled by a finite-element method. This so-called perimeter effect accounts for greater skin affection at the edges of electrodes. (Courtesy of Vessela Krasteva, Sofia, Bulgaria.).

energy converted to heat is linearly related to the resistance of the electrode-skin interface, which comprises the electrode surface, the conduction gel, and the skin itself. Three factors contribute to this resistance and hence influence heating of the skin: electrode contact, paddle force, and hairiness.

The importance of complete paddle contact to the chest is emphasized by both international resuscitation guidelines and defibrillator manufacturers. Indeed, when using hand-held paddles operators should ensure that the paddles are in full contact with the skin. Use of a sufficient amount of an approved conductive gel or paste and gel-pads, respectively, is obligatory. Ultrasound gel or other clinical lubricants are inappropriate, as their conductivity is usually too low. During attachment of self-adhesive pads it must be ensured that no air bubbles are trapped underneath the electrode pads. Such disposable pads must be checked further for their expiration date and for leaks in the hermetic packaging.

Paddle force is another important determinant of resistance of the paddle-skin interface. In adults, increasing paddle force decreases transthoracic impedance (TTI) exponentially. This is largely due to a decrease of the resistance at the paddle-skin interface.[50] Although difficult to control for the operator, an optimal paddle force of 78 N (8 kg) has been suggested for adult patients on the basis of a clinical study.[51]

A hairy chest is another important source of high resistance at the electrode-skin interface. Transthoracic impedance (TTI) is significantly higher in hirsute subjects compared to non-hirsute subjects, both with manual defibrillation paddles and self-adhesive electrode pads.[52,53] This most probably reflects a higher resistance between the electrodes and the skin. In one study, shaving of hirsute patients resulted in a remarkable mean TTI decrease of 35%.[52] Interestingly, even shaving of non-hirsute skin is associated with a significant TTI reduction as well.[53] If the reason was creation of numerous tiny epidermal lesions functioning as low-impedance pathways, these lesions would pose a particular risk for further injury to the skin, because low-impedance pathways are transited by high currents. Therefore, it has been proposed that – if circumstances permit – it may be better to clip hair close to the chest with scissors.

In summary, skin burns are frequent and seem to be unavoidable after multiple defibrillations. The major determinant of heat production is high resistance at the electrode–skin interface. Following common rules for defibrillation as well as manufacturer advice will help to minimize local resistance. No direct evidence exists, however, that these measures actually reduce the extent or intensity of defibrillatory skin burns. Postprocedural anti-inflammatory and analgesic treatment may be necessary.

Skeletal muscle damage

Substantial pectoral muscle necrosis as a result of multiple defibrillations has been demonstrated pathologically.[54,55] Also, elevated serum levels of creatine kinase (CK) are common findings after CPR both in patients with and without electrocardiographic evidence of myocardial infarction. This could reflect skeletal or cardiac cell damage, or both. Although after CPR, cardiac-specific enzymes often increase as well, upper-normal CK levels are seen with and without concurrent elevations of myocardial cell markers, thus indicating skeletal muscle damage. Whereas about 90% of cardiac arrest survivors exhibit serum CK levels > 80 U/l, serum CK-MB concentrations > 10 U/l have been reported in 78%, and elevations of troponin T above 0.1 μg/l in 90%.[56,57] Concerns about myocardial injury secondary to defibrillations are discussed later in this chapter.

Three possible causes may account for muscle damage demonstrated: (1) mechanical injury as the result of chest compressions; (2) electroporation or thermal injury caused by defibrillation; and (3) ischemia and accompanying metabolic consequences arising from circulatory arrest. Indeed, increases in serum CK levels correlate positively with both cumulative defibrillation energy administered and the duration of chest compressions during the course of CPR.[56–58] The independent contribution of these interdependent factors to CK release, however, is unknown. Several studies investigated whether electric shocks alone are capable of producing a significant CK release. In summary, total creatine kinase levels above the upper normal limit are seen after approximately 50% of elective direct current transthoracic cardioversions of arrhythmia, whereas troponin levels are largely unaffected. Further, similar to the effect of CPR, the maximum CK rise correlates with the cumulated energy dose administered during therapeutic cardioversion.

In conclusion, evidence of damage to skeletal muscles is common after CPR. Multiple electric countershocks are likely to play a major causative role for this finding and chest compressions may contribute. Patients undergoing prolonged or recurrent resuscitation attempts, including repeated defibrillations, may even be at risk for complications of rhabdomyolysis.

Myocardial injury

Defibrillation and cardioversion are achieved by means of a current flow through the myocardium, which alters the transmembrane potential. Concerns have been expressed that this life-saving current may at the same time cause an electric injury to the heart. Damage to myocardial cells has been assessed by microscopic and macroscopic examination, and determination of serum levels of myocardial enzymes.

Early histologic studies demonstrated that repetitive defibrillation with high energy doses can cause myocardial damage. In a dog model of VF, defibrillated with a damped sine waveform, an energy dose of 30 J/kg (which corresponded to a peak current of 5.8 A/kg) caused pathologically detectable damage in 50% of cases.[59] Also in a dog model of VF, conduction abnormalities were induced by voltage gradients greater than 64 V/cm for monophasic and 71 V/cm for biphasic shocks ($P<0.005$).[60] In contrast, the intracardiac voltage gradients produced by common commercial monophasic and biphasic defibrillators are substantially lower; in a recent study they did not exceed 33 V/cm, even with 360 J shock energy at very low impedances of 35 ± 3 Ω.[61] Likewise, the peak current delivered by common defibrillators is substantially lower than current levels previously described as being harmful.[62] These findings are in accordance with earlier reports that had established that the ratio of the voltage/current necessary to cause myocardial damage or dysfunction to the voltage/current that defibrillates the heart (referred to as the safety factor) is about 4 to 10 for monophasic and even greater for biphasic waveforms.[59,60,63]

Another approach for studying myocardial damage is determination of serum levels of cardiac troponins I (cTnI) or T (cTnT). Their release into the bloodstream is specific for cardiac cell death and, since 2000, constitutes the biochemical basis for the diagnosis of myocardial infarction. In approximately 90% of all out-of-hospital cardiac arrest (OOHCA) survivors, cTnT will be elevated.[56] This may reflect: (1) implication of a causal myocardial infarction (MI); (2) ischemic damage due to lack of perfusion during cardiac arrest; (3) mechanical injury of the heart as a result of chest compressions; and (4) electrical injury caused by defibrillation attempts. When measured after elective cardioversion for atrial fibrillation, cTnT levels are not or only minimally elevated above the detection threshold of 0.01 µg/l, indicating no or only minimal myocardial injury.[64] In cardiac arrests, however, the interrelations are far more complex. While it has been established that cTnT is elevated in 80% to 85% of all survivors of OOHCA without evidence of acute MI, the extent to which hypoxia, chest compression, and defibrillation contribute to troponin release from cardiac cells is largely unknown.

Another approach to estimating the impact of defibrillation on myocardial integrity is the study of postshock functional parameters, such as arterial pressure, indices of systolic and diastolic function, or electrocardiographic indices of ischemia. When delivered during sinus rhythm or after short periods of VF in animal models, transthoracic shocks cause only modest and transient myocardial dysfunction and normal function is usually restored within seconds or a few minutes. Experimental data suggest, however, that ischemic hearts, as in cardiac arrests, are more susceptible to detrimental effects of defibrillatory countershocks. In animal models of resuscitation after 7 min of untreated pediatric VF, certain defibrillation protocols resulted in systolic dysfunction that lasted longer than 4 hours and a reduced 24-hour survival with good neurologic outcome.[65,66] In contrast, another animal study of prolonged pediatric VF did not find impaired postresuscitation cardiac function or reduced survival with different defibrillation schemes.[67] In a rat model that simulated cumulative shock energy by delivering one defibrillation with excess energy, a strict relationship between shock energy and both cardio-circulatory impairment and survival time was demonstrated.[68]

In summary, excessive defibrillation energies can cause structural damage to and functional impairment of the heart. In adult resuscitation, however, clinically relevant defibrillation energies are unlikely to result in myocardial injury in addition to that caused by the underlying condition. In infants, transthoracic defibrillation may precipitate cardiac dysfunction under specific circumstances, the extent and impact of which has yet to be demonstrated. With respect to adverse effects, biphasic defibrillation waveforms seem to be safer compared to monophasic impulses.

Pacemakers (PM) and implantable cardioverter-defibrillators (ICD)

Nowadays, an increasing number of patients at high-risk for cardiac arrest are implanted with an ICD or a pacemaker. The safety concerns with regard to these devices are twofold. First, myocardial damage may occur at the site of endocardial insertion of the PM/ICD lead. Second, externally applied electric countershocks may interfere with such a device.

Two mechanisms have been suggested that may result in tissue modifications at the electrode-endocardium interface.[69] First, ICD and PM leads are excellent conductors. Consequently, a considerable proportion of the transthoracic current may travel along the lead producing a detrimentally high current density when entering the heart at the electrode-endocardium interface. Second, a process called capacitive coupling may occur, i.e., the transthoracic current induces an additional current in the intrathoracic lead capable of causing micro-cauterizations to the heart.

Even with the defibrillation paddles attached as far as possible from the pectoral implantation pocket, transient loss of PM capture, sensing failure, and lead dislocation can occur. Postcardioversion ventricular stimulation thresholds in patients with a unipolar PM implanted have been demonstrated to be more than six times the baseline value – associated with a transient loss of capture in 50% of patients.[69] In this study, duration of capture failure ranged from 5 s to 30 minutes (mean approx. 1.5 min). Therefore, immediate external pacing should be attempted in all those PM carriers who exhibit asystole after defibrillation or show electrocardiographic evidence of an exit block of the internal PM.

Finally, the possibility of electromagnetic interference of defibrillation with implanted devices is generally acknowledged. The spectrum of interference ranges from reprogramming and malfunction to total breakdown of the device. After every resuscitation, a functional check of PMs and ICDs by a specialist is mandatory. During and after resuscitation, alterations in the mode of functioning of the PM and the ICD should be considered in interpretation of ECG readings. Furthermore, paddles or pads, for external defibrillation must not be placed on the skin directly over the device. Concrete recommendations for the distance between the hard lump beneath the skin (where the device can be expected) and the external electrodes differ considerably, ranging between > 1 inch (> 2.5 cm) and 6 inches (15 cm).

Hazards for responders

Current advanced life support courses attach great importance to a safe defibrillation procedure.[70] In spite of very few critical incidents reported, the possibility of harm to any of the rescuers involved is evidently taken very seriously. The following paragraph discusses the evidence regarding electric shock to the rescuer and the danger of fire as well as explosions in conjunction with transdermal medication patches.

Electric shock to the rescuer

Considering that a defibrillator discharge delivers several thousand volts to the patient it is not surprising that there are concerns that deleterious electrical injuries may be inflicted on responding medical personnel who are in close contact with the patient or adjacent material while defibrillation is carried out. In fact, numerous minor incidents are documented in the literature. These incidents can be divided in two groups: (1) intentional shocks to subjects without therapeutic indication, thus based on carelessness, ignorance, or intention to harm; and (2) accidental

shocks as complications of regular medical or maintenance procedures.

Intentional shocks

Reports on intentional shocks in the medical literature include suicide attempts, confusion with training devices, a few cases of people who had "fooled around", and finally, one case of a child who played with a defibrillator. One report included a 23-year-old man who self-administered a 200-J defibrillation to his chest.[71] The first postshock ECG recorded showed polymorphic ventricular tachycardia which, after defibrillation, degenerated to VF. The patient eventually died. Two other incidents comprised deliberate transthoracic defibrillator discharges, neither of which resulted in arrhythmia or in long-term disability.[71]

As described, a full-capacity transthoracic discharge may prove fatal. It has long been known that electric shocks applied for cardioversion of tachyarrhythmias can result in VF. A vulnerable phase exists within the cardiac cycle, during which VF can be induced by external electric stimuli. Occasionally, appropriately R-wave-triggered cardioversion shocks also cause VF. Morbid circumstances, such as a structural heart disease, drug abuse, and ischemia, facilitate degeneration of arrhythmias into VF.

Defibrillatory countershocks applied to the head have also been reported. They cause tonic-clonic seizures, altered vigilance, amnesia, confusion, dissociative symptoms, changes in affect, paresthesias, local burns, and pain. This is in accordance with observations made after electroconvulsive therapy (ECT), a therapeutic option in severe psychiatric disorders that deliberately exposes the patient's head to electric shocks. But ECT impulses and defibrillation can only be compared in a limited manner, because of substantial differences in electrical shock parameters. Nevertheless, in the three cases of "cranial defibrillation" cited above, no long-term complications have been noted apart from memory loss for the event itself. Restriction of accessibility of defibrillators for suicidal patients, persons who behave irrationally, and, obviously, children is indicated.

Accidental shocks

Accidental electric shocks to medical personnel may occur during standard procedures, such as resuscitation attempts or device maintenance. They are either due to neglect of safety precautions by the operator or failure of or damage to the defibrillator. Gibbs *et al.* reported 8 incidents observed in King County, WA, USA, between 1979 and 1988 along with 13 incidents that were reported to the Food and Drug Administration in the USA within a 45-month period between 1984 and 1987.[72] Of these 21 episodes, 3 were caused by equipment failure while 17 were caused by improper handling and neglected safety precautions, respectively; the reason for the remaining episode could not be determined. Based on the records of the Emergency Medical Services in King County, where paramedics had treated more than 3000 cardiac arrest patients at that time, the authors estimated the incidence of electrical shocks to ambulance personnel at approximately 1 injury per 1700 shocks. In most cases, the physical consequences of such accidental shocks are minor. Short-term discomfort and local tingling have been described. More serious sequelae included burns and one case of hospital admission for frequent premature ventricular contractions. To the best of our knowledge, there are no case reports of death or long-term impairment in personnel after suffering an electric shock during defibrillation or cardioversion of a patient. Likewise, we are not aware that such an accidental shock to bystanders has ever resulted in a critical medical condition or even cardiac arrest. It is a popular but erroneous belief that a current always travels the path of least resistance. Unless there is arcing of electricity from the electrodes, the majority of the total current produced by the defibrillator will travel through the chest. The current to which a bystander may be exposed can only be a fraction of the total current, being indirectly proportional to the resistance of the bodies, the bystander's shoes, the floor and the bed. It has yet to be investigated whether such shunt currents are at all capable of reaching the fibrillation threshold and thus inducing VF. The safety precautions advocated by the medical authorities and manufacturers to prevent electrical accidents include standard device maintenance procedures, avoidance of excessive amounts of conduction gel during resuscitation (and preferential use of gel pads), giving announcements aloud, checking that everybody stands clear before defibrillator discharge, and ensuring that manual paddles are placed only on either the patient's chest or in the defibrillator pockets. Although the actual risk of being harmed by shunt currents during defibrillation is very low it seems reasonable to follow these rules.

Danger of fire

Defibrillation may set the patient, rescuers, the bed, and medical equipment on fire. Severe burns, considerable material damage, and the exigency of ward evacuation have been described repeatedly. Such fires are no mysteries of resuscitation; circumstances that may culminate in this hazardous complication are well known and precautions for its prevention are available. Three prerequisites must be fulfilled to ignite a fire by defibrillation: (1) an oxygen-enriched atmosphere must exist in the vicinity of the defibrillator electrodes; (2) an electric spark is needed

for ignition; and (3) an agent that is combustible must be present. If any of these three "ingredients" is absent, a fire is very unlikely.

1. An oxygen-enriched atmosphere (OEA) appears to be the basis for ignition. Ventilation bags with an oxygen-flow of $\geq 10\,l/min$ put next to the patient's head increase the oxygen concentration of the ambient air at several points around the head and chest of the patient.[73] The same finding applies to mechanical ventilator tubes when they are disconnected from the tracheal tube, left close to the patient, and continue to deliver oxygen. Also, oxygen masks left on the patient's face during defibrillation are sufficient to establish an OEA – probably by leakage of oxygen under the edges of the mask.[74] Evidence suggests that keeping the ventilation devices 1 m off the patient's head is safe. Clearly, a mechanical ventilator that is left connected to a tracheal tube poses no threat. It is a matter of controversy, however, whether a manual ventilation bag that remains connected to a tracheal airway with oxygen leaking from the overflow valve is safe or not. Since increased ambient oxygen concentrations have been demonstrated in a corresponding manikin model, it appears prudent to consider this condition as dangerous as well.[75] The highest oxygen concentration on the body surface is usually measured in the axilla. Indeed, oxygen, being slightly denser than room air, may accumulate in swales and cavities as, for instance, those provided by crumpled sheets or clothing.

2. An electric arc or spark is essential to set combustible material on fire by defibrillation. Sparks are more likely if resistance of the electrode–skin junction is high. This condition occurs when electrode paddles or pads are not in proper contact with the chest across their entire surface, when inadequate conductive gel is used, or when adhesive electrode pads are dried out. Case reports have also suggested that too much gel (smeared across the chest) and ECG electrodes next to the defibrillator electrodes may have contributed to fire incidents in the past.

3. Oxygen itself is not flammable. To feed a fire it needs an agent that is combustible. Some agents present during resuscitation are particularly prone to be ignited by a spark in an oxygen-enriched atmosphere. These include fine body hair, surface nap fibres found on most fabrics, dust, and others. Once one of these easily flammable materials has been ignited, other adjacent matter may catch fire. Often, the flame flashes instantaneously over the surface of the bed or patient in a phenomenon referred to as "surface-fibre flame propagation."[76] Spreading of the fire front towards the oxygen source is common, and damage of devices such as the mechanical ventilator have been described.

Table 45.2. Safeguards to minimize the risk of fire during defibrillation

1. *Prevention of an oxygen-enriched atmosphere*

   Always connect an airway adjunct to oxygen supplies properly.

   Before defibrillation, leave a mechanical ventilator tube properly connected to the tracheal airway, but remove manual ventilation bags and oxygen masks as far away from the patient as practical (at least 1 m).

   During resuscitation never leave an open oxygen source next to the patient.

2. *Prevention of sparks*

   Avoid electrode placement over an irregular chest surface. If contact gaps, e.g., caused by depressed intercostal spaces, are inevitable, consider anterior-posterior electrode position.

   Do not place paddles or pads over or close to ECG wires or ECG electrodes.

   Shave or, if time permits, clip excessive chest hair under the area of electrode contact.

   (a) Use of manual paddles:

      Use an appropriate amount of conductive gel. Make sure the gel is approved for defibrillation. Consider gel-pads as a substitute for jelly.

      Apply firm and even paddle force according to the guidelines. Make sure the whole paddle surface is in contact with the skin.

   (b) Use of self-adhesive pads:

      Check date of expiration and integrity of the pad packaging before application.

      When attaching the pads to the chest wall, make sure that they are not folded, air bubbles are not trapped underneath, and adherence to the skin is complete.

      Remember to change dried-out pads during long-term or repetitive resuscitation according to manufacturer's advice.

3. *Removal of flammable material*

   If feasible, move gowns, patient's clothing, bedding, drapes, curtains, etc. from the resuscitation area.

In conclusion, fires ignited by defibrillation are not rare, but adherence to a few simple rules can prevent this potentially devastating complication (Table 45.2).

Danger of explosions

In the past, attempted defibrillation through nitroglycerin (glyceryl trinitrate) patches has occasionally resulted in "explosions" including arcing, a loud noise, and smoke. This was first interpreted as an actual explosion of the pharmacologic agent. In contrast, further investigations concluded that this phenomenon only occurred in medication patches containing metal foil or mesh, and that it appeared to be due to a voltage breakdown resulting from the high resistance of such patches.[77–79] This voltage-breakdown follows the same principles as were discussed above in conjunction with burns and may be accompanied by an arc between the defibrillator electrode and the metal foil in the patch. As a consequence, perforation of the patch is common. Modern transdermal medication patches no longer contain a metal foil. Nonetheless, as such patches may increase the resistance at the electrode–skin interface, with the subsequent risk of sparks, burns, and dissipation of defibrillation energy as discussed above, it is reasonable to advise defibrillating personnel not to place defibrillator paddles or pads over any kind of medication patches. Patches should be removed.

Conclusions

Most patients who undergo multiple defibrillation attempts will develop at least first-degree burns at the site of electrode attachment. Higher cumulative energy will cause more severe burns. Repetitive countershocks may be accompanied by a considerable degree of skeletal muscle decomposition, including the risk of rhabdomyolysis. At least in adults, clinically relevant postresuscitative impairment of myocardial function so far has not conclusively been shown to be attributable to defibrillation. In pacemaker or ICD carriers, medical personnel must be aware that defibrillation can result in temporary or permanent malfunction or breakdown of the device. Minor electric shocks may be inflicted to rescue personnel during defibrillation of a patient. No case of long-term impairment or lethal outcome of such accidental shocks has been reported in the medical literature, however. In contrast, non-therapeutic full capacity transthoracic shocks can be fatal. Defibrillation can ignite a fire at the bedside if an oxygen-enriched atmosphere is present; preventive measures are available. Safety precautions for defibrillation are discussed above.

Complications of artificial respiration

Universal complications of artificial respiration

Injuries associated with reclination of the cervical spine
To keep the airway patent and protected is one of the first steps in resuscitation of collapsed patients.

The patency of the airway can be maintained by chin lift (performed with one hand at the side of the patient) and jaw thrust (Esmarch maneuver performed with both hands above the patient) and additional head tilt, with or without the assistance of airway device, for example, oropharyngeal or nasopharyngeal airway devices.

Airway management can be particularly complex when there are facial bone fractures, head injuries, and cervical spine instability.[80]

Whereas results of some authors indicate that the chin lift technique provides the most consistently adequate airway,[81,82] other authors stated that the jaw thrust maneuver is more effective in improving airway patency and ventilation, especially in children.[83]

During head tilt and the assistance for intubation, the patient's neck is put in an extreme reclination and maximal straightening, which leads to a high tension load on the cervical column. Typical complications are intimal lesions in the vessels[84] and retropharyngeal hemorrhage.

When the maneuvres are conducted with high force and velocity, the risk is high for injury to the cervical spine itself. Elderly people have a higher risk for such osseous lesions, because of degenerative and osteoporotic alterations. Spinal cord injury and dislocation of the cervical spine may occur, especially in patients with preexisting trauma.

Pneumoperitoneum
Mechanical ventilation and cardiopulmonary resuscitation can be specific causes of non-surgical pneumoperitoneum. Pneumothorax has also been associated with pneumoperitoneum. A direct passage through pleural and diaphragmatic defects and a passage via the mediastinum along perivascular connective tissue or major diaphragmatic portals to the retroperitoneum and finally to the peritoneum are considered as mechanisms. The management of pneumoperitoneum of suspected thoracic etiology can be conservative when there are no peritoneal signs or a suspicious ruptured viscus.[85]

Regurgitation and aspiration
The risk of gastric regurgitation and subsequent pulmonary aspiration is a recognized complication of cardiac arrest – a risk, that may be further increased by the resuscitative procedure itself. A study comparing bag valve mask (BVM) and laryngeal mask airway (LMA) confirmed that when an LMA is used as a first line airway device, regurgitation is relatively uncommon.[86]

Despite orotracheal intubation, aspiration around the tracheal tube may be a complication provoked by frequent swallowing movements.[87]

Artificial respiration without devices: gastric distension and rupture

Air insufflation in the stomach is a frequent complication of mouth-to-mouth ventilation promoted in the case of airway obstruction. The gastric distension interferes with ventilation by elevating the diaphragm, resulting in a decreased lung volume. Constant cricoid pressure – the Sellick maneuver – during artificial breathing could prevent gastric distension in these instances and should be recommended.[88] Rupture of the stomach is a rare complication of cardiopulmonary resuscitation. An incidence of 0.1% has been reported in the literature.[69] Between 1970 and 2000 the number of cases referred in the literature did not exceed 30.[90]

The majority of reported cases have been associated with difficulty in airway management or esophageal intubation (Fig. 45.3).[91]

In an experimental study design, the mean rupture pressure of the human stomach was $73 +/- 13$ mmHg $(9.7 +/- 1.7$ kPa$)$ and the mean rupture volume was $2670 +/- 410$ ml. A viscoelastic model can be used for representing the relations between pressure and volume as well as pressure and time. The site of main ruptures coincides with mesenteric insertion at the lesser gastric curvature. The effusion of gastric contents into the lesser omentum and the mediastinum may be responsible for an occasional lack of abdominal symptoms.[92]

Artificial respiration with devices

Tracheal intubation
Securing the airway with an endotracheal tube is the gold standard, but excellent success in emergency airway management depends on initial training, retraining, and actual frequency of a given procedure in routine.[93]

Intubation may result in further injury of oral and/or cervical soft tissue by mechanical damage during the manipulations, especially in a sequence of multiple attempts.[94]

Undesirable incidents or complications are seen in about 20% of prehospital emergency airway management procedures. The most common complications (n=201) are: more than one attempt of intubation (14.4%), vomiting and/or aspiration (6.8%), esophageal intubation (3.2%), and mucosal injuries (1.7%).[95]

Multiple endotracheal intubation attempts are associated with significant complications, offer limited advantage over bag valve mask, and may possibly affect outcome. Indications for field intubations may require review, especially in rural pediatric trauma. In the field, more attempts of intubation were necessary compared to planned intubation in operation rooms. Airway complications and multiple intubations were associated with transport delay, lower GCS, longer hospital stay, and lower discharge GCS, but were independent of injury severity score, sex, age, and survival.[96]

In elective intubation, the teeth most likely to be injured are the upper incisors. In most cases dental injury is not associated with a pre-event prediction of difficult intubation.[97] Compared to metal laryngoscopes plastic blades do not fracture any dental model materials; therefore, plastic laryngoscope blades are less likely to cause dental fracture compared with metal blades.[98]

Chewing on an endotracheal tube may be another cause of tooth damage.[99] Such factors must be taken into account in cases of claiming iatrogenic damage.

Tapia's syndrome (paralysis of the hypoglossal and recurrent laryngeal nerves) is due to extracranial involvement of the hypoglossal nerve and the recurrent laryngeal branch of the vagal nerve and may be a complication of intubation.[100] Use of more than one tube, a narrow laryngeal space, and accidental flexion of the neck contribute to a bilateral recurrent paralysis of the laryngeal nerve.[101]

Although tracheal rupture is a rare complication of endotracheal intubation,[102] if it does occur, the mortality is 75%[103]. Tracheal rupture leads to pneumothorax and emphysema of subcutaneous tissue and infections. Lesions from intubation are always located in the membraneous part and follow the longitudinal axis of the trachea.[104] Even the hypopharyngeal tissue can be perforated during intubation.[105]

Esophageal intubation

Cardiac arrest during emergency tracheal intubation is a relatively common problem. Airway-related complications play a prominent role in these cases. Out of 3035 critically ill patients suffering from cardiopulmonary, traumatic, septic, metabolic, or neurological-based deterioration and requiring emergency airway management, 60 suffered from cardiac arrest. Esophageal intubation was a frequent complication ($n = 38$; 63%), often leading to hypoxemia (97%) and regurgitation (67%). Immediate access to advanced airway devices and endotracheal tube-verifying

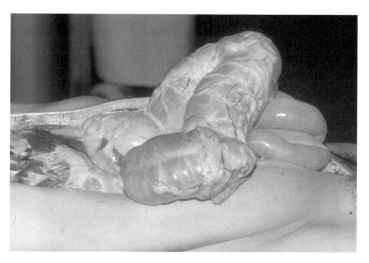

Fig. 45.3. Intestinal insufflation after esophageal intubation.

devices appears to have a significant impact on the incidence of hypoxemia-driven cardiac arrest.[106]

Nasotracheal and nasopharyngeal airway

Complications such as hemorrhage occur more frequently with the nasotracheal than with the orotracheal route.[107] On the other hand, the orotracheal intubation route was significantly associated with a higher frequency of aspiration compared with nasotracheal intubation in children. These results suggest that the nasotracheal intubation route is recommended as the first choice for reducing this potential clinical complication.[87]

Blind nasopharyngeal airway insertion may result in lethal iatrogenic injury when used in a head-injured patient. Even an intracranial insertion of a nasopharyngeal airway during resuscitation after trauma has been reported. Oropharyngeal airways may be used to assist with ventilation.[108]

In patients with lesions of the cervical spine, direct laryngoscopy for endotracheal intubation entails the risk of injuring the spinal cord. In an attempt to avoid this complication, flexible fiberoptic nasal intubation can be used.[109]

Alternative airway devices

Alternative airway devices have been developed, especially for emergency care systems when the use of endotracheal intubation by prehospital care personnel is restricted by policy or statute, or as a second line airway device. These alternative airway devices include Laryngeal Mask Airway (LMA), the Esophageal Obturator Airway (EOA) and Esophageal Gastric Tube Airway (EGTA), the

Pharyngeotracheal Lumen Airway (PTL), and the Esophageal-Tracheal Combitube (ETC). The EGTA adds a Levine tube to the EOA to relieve gastric pressure.

Ventilation and oxygenation can, in some circumstances, be achieved equally well with the EOA/EGTA device or with endotracheal intubation. Alternative airway devices can be inadequate and the complication rate is relatively high. The PTL and the ETC seem to provide adequate ventilation and oxygenation with few complications.[110]

Laboratory and clinical evidence supports the important role of alternative airway devices to mask ventilation and endotracheal intubation in the chain of survival. In particular, the laryngeal mask airway (LMA) and ETC proved to be effective alternatives in providing oxygenation and ventilation to the patient in cardiac arrest.[111]

In a comparative study of patients in cardiopulmonary arrest with ventricular fibrillation, endotracheal tube airway and EGTA were compared. Complication rates and success of intubation were similar in the two groups, although only training time was longer for endotracheal intubation.[112]

The esophageal–tracheal Combitube (ETC) is a ventilatory device consisting of a twin lumen tube with proximal and distal inflatable cuffs. The major benefit of the Combitube is that its design and function allow for ventilation through non-laryngoscope-assisted insertion into either the trachea or esophagus.[113]

Although visualized endotracheal intubation remains the preferred method of airway control, the ETC may be an effective prehospital airway device as both a backup to the endotracheal tube and a primary airway. Although the ETC does not require visualization with a laryngoscope, comprehensive training and continuing education are key factors in maintaining skill retention.[114]

Complications of ETC include subcutaneous emphysema, pneumomediastinum, and pneumoperitoneum. In a cadaver study, a protrusion of the anterior wall of the esophagus and distension resulting from inflation of the distal cuff was found, which could lead to esophageal injuries.[115,116]

In another study[118], the serious or potentially lethal complication rate was 3.3 times more common with the use of the EOA/EGTA than with the tracheal tube.

In a direct comparison of LMA, ETC, and the tracheal tube, the use of the tracheal tube by medical students was difficult and the skills acquired deteriorated significantly over time. The LMA, the LT and the ETC seemed to have an advantage over the tracheal tube insofar as the techniques were more easily learned and the skills better retained. For the LMA and the ETC, the authors recommended that

these alternative devices be included in the medical school curriculum for airway management.[118]

Insufflation of the stomach with air can be a complication of face mask ventilation in the case of airway obstruction. Although the laryngeal mask airway (LMA) has proven of value in airway resuscitation, it has two major failings: a relatively low seal pressure, and lack of access to the alimentary tract. These problems led to the development of the LMA-ProSeal, which permits ventilation with higher airway pressures.[119] The placement of the ProSeal laryngeal mask airway is said to be significantly easier than for the laryngeal mask airway.[120]

Cricothyrotomy and tracheotomy

Percutaneous transtracheal ventilation has proven useful in emergency airway management. Its speed and ease of performance are offset by the need for specialized equipment to accomplish it.[121] There is a tendency toward carbon dioxide retention and poor alveolar washout. The most common complication is subcutaneous emphysema caused by incorrect placement of the catheter.[122]

Infections are a rare complication of percutaneous transtracheal ventilation. In a reported case, the contamination of the deep neck spaces facilitated by pressure dissection of the fascial planes led to cervical osteomyelitis.[123]

Tracheotomy and coniotomy are procedures that cause frequent early and later complications; therefore, there must be a rigorous indication that they are necessary. If emergency airway access is needed and translaryngeal intubation is not possible, a cricothyroidotomy should be considered.[124] Careful management and expert nursing support can prevent many later complications.

"Minimally invasive" cricothyroidotomy devices are now available for the professional health care provider who is not proficient or comfortable with performing an emergency surgical tracheotomy or cricothyroidotomy.[111]

The main indication for cricothyroidotomy is the inability to establish an airway by intubation, usually in a situation of possible neck injury or severe facial trauma. The use of emergency cricothyroidotomy is supported in situations in which intubation is not successful or thought not to be safe. Tracheostomy subsequent to emergency cricothyroidotomy does not necessarily reduce airway-related morbidity in these patients.[125]

Conclusions

Ventilation with the objective of oxygenating the blood is a decisive step in resuscitation. For this purpose the airway must be kept patent and protected. First, the indication for artificial airway management must be examined carefully. Depending on preexisting conditions like head and cervical spine injuries, airway management can be particularly complex.

Any action taken – even mouth-to-mouth resuscitation – is subject to more or fewer complications, some of them life-threatening. The rescuer should be aware of these hazards and minimize their frequency by continuing education and comprehensive training. Concomitantly, refraining from indicated airway management and artificial ventilation leads to a lethal outcome in every patient.

New advanced airway devices can be helpful and are increasingly included in the medical staff training for airway management. Professional skills have to be achieved and sustained: practice makes perfect.

REFERENCES

1. 2005 International Consensus on Cardiopulmonary Resuscitation and Emergency Core Science with Treatment Recommendations. *Resuscitation* 2000; **67**: 203–204.

2. Katz, A., Henkin, J. & Ovsyshcher, I.A. Transient complete atrioventricular block induced by a chest thump in a patient with ventricular tachycardia. *Int. J. Cardiol.* 1989; **23**: 395–396.

3. Sclarovsky, S., Kracoff, O., Arditi, A. & *et al.* Ventricular tachycardia "pleomorphism" induced by chest thump. *Chest* 1982; **81**: 97–99.

4. Cotoi, S. Precordial thump and termination of cardiac re-entrant tachyarrythmias. *Am. Heart J.* 1981; **101**: 675–677.

5. Penneington, J.E., Taylor, J. & Lown, B. Chest thump for reverting ventricular tachycardia. *N. Engl. J. Med.* 1970; **26**: 1192–1195.

6. Hoke, R.S. & Chamberlain, D. Skeletal chest injuries secondary to cardiopulmonary resuscitation. *Resuscitation* 2004; **63**: 327–338.

7. Black, C.J., Busuttil, A. & Robertson, C. Chest wall injuries following cardiopulmonary resuscitation. *Resuscitation* 2004; **63**: 339–343.

8. Himmelhoch, S.R., Dekker, A., Gazzaniga, A.B. & Like, A.A. Closed-chest cardiac resuscitation. A prospective clinical and pathological study. *N. Engl. J. Med.* 1964; **270**: 118–122.

9. Baubin, M., Sumann, G., Rabl, W., Eibl, G., Wenzel, V. & Mair, P. Increased frequency of thorax injuries with ACD-CPR. *Resuscitation* 1999; **41**: 33–38.

10. Krischer, J.P., Fine, E.G., Davis, J.H. & Nagel, E.L. Complications of cardiac resuscitation. *Chest* 1987; **92**: 287–291.

11. Saternus, K.S. Direkte und indirekte Traumatisierung bei der Reanimation. *Z. Rechtsmed* 1981; **86**: 161–174.

12. Kloss, T., Puschel, K., Wischhusen, F., Welk, I., Roewer, N. & Jungck, E. Reanimationsverletzungen. *Anaesth. Intensivther. Notfallmed.* 1983; **18**: 199–203.

13. Brown, J., Rogers, J. & Soar, J. Cardiac arrest during surgery and ventilation in the prone position: a case report and a systematic review. *Resuscitation* 2001; **50**: 233–238.

14. Jackson, C.T. & Greendyke, R.M. Pulmonary and cerebral fat embolism after closed-chest cardiac massage. *Surg. Gynec. Obstet.* 1965; **120**: 25–27.

15. Yarnoff, M. Incidence of bone marrow embolism due to closed-chest cardiac massage. *N. Engl. J. Med.* 1963; **269**: 837.

16. Patterson, R.H., Burns, W.A. & Jannotta, F.S. Complications of external cardiac resuscitation: a retrospective review and survey of the literature. *Med. Ann. Distr. Columb.* 1974; **43**: 389–393.

17. Bynum, W.R., Connell, R.M. & Hawk, W.A. Causes of death after external cardiac massage: analysis of observations on fifty consecutive autopsies. *Cleve. Clin. Q.* 1963; **30**: 147–151.

18. Baringer, J.R., Salzman, E.W., Jones, W.A. & Friedlich, A.L. External cardiac massage. *N. Engl. J. Med.* 1961; **265**: 62–65.

19. Powner, D.J., Holcombe, P.A. & Mello, L.A. Cardiopulmonary resuscitation-related injuries. *Crit. Care Med.* 1984; **12**: 54–55.

20. Winkel, E.C. & Brown, W.G. Bone marrow embolism following closed chest cardiac message. *J. Am. Med. Assoc.* 1961; **178**: 329–331.

21. Lurie, K.G., Shultz, J.J., Callaham, M.L. *et al.* Evaluation of active compression–decompression CPR in victims of out-of-hospital cardiac arrest. *J. Am. Med. Assoc.* 1994; **271**: 1405–1411.

22. Mauer, D., Schneider, T., Dick, W., Withelm, A., Elich, D. & Mauer, M. Active compression-decompression resuscitation: a prospective, randomized study in a two-tiered EMS system with physicians in the field. *Resuscitation* 1996; **33**: 125–134.

23. Cohen, T.J., Goldner, B.G., Maccaro, B.C., *et al.* A comparison of active compression–decompression cardiopulmonary resuscitation with standard cardiopulmonary resuscitation for cardiac arrests occurring in the hospital. *N. Engl. J. Med.* 1993; **329**: 1918–1921.

24. Plaisance, P., Adnet, F., Vicaut, E. *et al.* Benefit of active compression–decompression cardiopulmonary resuscitation as a prehospital advanced cardiac life support. A randomized multicenter study. *Circulation* 1997; **95**: 955–961.

25. Luiz, T., Ellinger, K. & Denz, C. Active compression–decompression cardiopulmonary resuscitation does not improve survival in patients with prehospital cardiac arrest in a physician-manned emergency medical system. *J. Cardiothorac. Vasc. Anesth.* 1996; **10**: 178–186.

26. Rabl, W., Baubin, M., Broinger, G. & Scheithauer, R. Serious complications from active compression–decompression cardiopulmonary resuscitation. *Int. J. Legal Med.* 1996; **109**: 84–89.

27. Rabl, W., Baubin, M., Haid, C., Pfeiffer, K.P. & Scheithauer, R. Review of active compression–decompression cardiopulmonary resuscitation (ACD-CPR). Analysis of iatrogenic complications and their biomechanical explanation. *Forens. Sci. Int.* 1997; **89**: 175–183.

28. Lafuente-Lafuente, C. & Melero-Bascones, M. Active chest compression–decompression for cardiopulmonary resuscitation. *Cochrane Database Syst. Rev.* 2002;(3):CD002751.

29. Mauer, D.K., Nolan, J., Plaisance, P *et al.* Effect of active compression–decompression resuscitation (ACD-CPR) on survival: a combined analysis using individual patient data. *Resuscitation* 1999; **41**: 249–256.

30. Steen, S., Liao, Q., Pierre, L., Paskevicius, A. & Sjöberg, T. Evaluation of LUCAS, a new device for automatic mechanical compression and active decompression resuscitation. *Resuscitation* 2002; **55**: 285–299.

31. Steen, S., Sjöberg, T., Olsson, P. & Young, M. Treatment of out-of-hospital cardiac arrest with LUCAS, a new device for automatic mechanical compression and active decompression resuscitation. *Resuscitation* 67; **2005**: 25–30.

32. Timerman, S., Luis Francisco Cardoso, L.F., Ramires, J.A. & Halperin, H. Improved hemodynamic performance with a novel chest compression device during treatment of in-hospital cardiac arrest. *Resuscitation* 2004; **61**: 273–280.

33. Hart, A.P., Azar, V.J., Hart, K.R. & Stephens, B.G. Autopsy artifact created by the Revivant AutoPulse resuscitation device. *J. Forens. Sci.* 2005; **50**: 1–5.

34. Buckman, R.F. Jr., Badellino, M.M., Eynon, C.A. *et al.* Open-chest cardiac massage without major thoracotomy: metabolic indicators of coronary and cerebral perfusion. *Resuscitation* 1997; **34**: 247–253.

35. Rozenberg, A., Incagnoli, P., Delpech, P. *et al.* Prehospital use of minimally invasive direct cardiac massage (MID-CM): a pilot study. *Resuscitation* 2001; **50**: 257–262.

36. Moore, E.E., Mattox Kl & Feliciano, D.V. Trauma. 2nd edn. New York: McGraw-Hill, 1991: 181–193.

37. Schwab, T.M., Callaham, M.L., Madsen, C.D. & Utecht, T.A. A randomized clinical trial of active compression–decompression CPR vs standard CPR in out-of-hospital cardiac arrest in two cities. *J. Am. Med. Assoc.* 1995; **273**: 1261–1268.

38. Lederer, W., Mair, D., Rabl, W. & Baubin, M. Frequency of rib and sternum fractures associated with out-of-hospital cardiopulmonary resuscitation is underestimated by conventional chest X-ray. *Resuscitation* 2004; **60**: 157–162.

39. Baubin, M., Rabl, W., Pfeiffer, K.P., Benzer, A. & Gilly, H. Chest injuries after active compression–decompression cardiopulmonary resuscitation in cadavers. *Resuscitation* 1999; **43**: 9–15.

40. Spevak, M.R. Cardiopulmonary resuscitation and rib fractures in infants. A post-mortem radiologic-pathologic study. *J. Am. Med. Assoc.* 1994; **272**: 617–618.

41. Feldman, K.W. & Brewer, D.K. Child abuse, cardiopulmonary resuscitation, and rib fractures. *Pediatrics* 1984; **73**: 339–342.

42. Bush, C.M., Jones, J.S., Cohle, S.D. & Johnson, H. Pediatric injuries from cardiopulmonary resuscitation. *Ann. Emerg. Med.* 1996; **28**: 40–44.

43. Price, E.A., Rush, L.R., Perper, J.A. & Bell, M.D. Cardiopulmonary resuscitation-related injuries and homicidal blunt abdominal trauma in children. *Am. J. Forens. Med. Pathol.* 2000; **21**: 307–310.

44. Betz, P. & Liebhardt, E. Rib fractures in children – resuscitation or child abuse? *Int. J. Leg. Med.* 1994; **106**: 215–218.

45. Paaske, F., Hart Hansen, J.P., Koudahl, G. & Olsen, J. Complications of closed-chest cardiac massage in a forensic autopsy material. *Dan. Med. Bull.* 1968; **15**: 225–230.

46. Bjork, R.J., Snyder, B.D., Campion, B.C. & Loewenson, R.B. Medical complications of cardiopulmonary arrest. *Arch. Intern. Med.* 1982; **142**: 500–503.

47. Meyer, P.F., Gadsby, P.D., Van Sickle, D., Schoenlein, W.E., Foster, K.S. & Graber, G.P. Impedance-gradient electrode reduces skin irritation induced by transthoracic defibrillation. *Med. Biol. Eng. Comput.* 2005; **43**: 225–229.

48. Pagan-Carlo, L.A., Stone, M.S. & Kerber, R.E. Nature and determinants of skin "burns" after transthoracic cardioversion. Am. J. Cardiol. 1997 **79**: 689–691.

49. Ambler, J.J., Zideman, D.A. & Deakin, C.D. The effect of topical non-steroidal anti-inflammatory cream on the incidence and severity of cutaneous burns following external DC cardioversion. *Resuscitation* 2005; **65**: 173–178.

50. Deakin, C.D., Sado, D.M., Petley, G.W. & Clewlow, F. Differential contribution of skin impedance and thoracic volume to transthoracic impedance during external defibrillation. *Resuscitation* 2004; **60**: 171–174.

51. Deakin, C.D., Sado, D.M., Petley, G.W. & Clewlow, F. Determining the optimal paddle force for external defibrillation. Am. J. Cardiol. 2002 **90**: 812–813.

52. Bissing, J.W. & Kerber, R.E. Effect of shaving the chest of hirsute subjects on transthoracic impedance to self-adhesive defibrillation electrode pads. Am. J. Cardiol. 2000 **86**: 587–589.

53. Sado, D.M., Deakin, C.D., Petley, G.W. & Clewlow, F. Comparison of the effects of removal of chest hair with not doing so before external defibrillation on transthoracic impedance. Am. J. Cardiol. 2004 **93**: 98–100.

54. Corbitt. J.D. Jr., Sybers, J. & Levin, J.M. Muscle changes of the anterior chest wall secondary to electrical countershock. *Am. J. Clin. Pathol.* 1969; **51**: 107–112.

55. Vogel, U., Wanner, T. & Bultmann, B. Extensive pectoral muscle necrosis afterdefibrillation: nonthermal skeletal muscle damage caused by electroporation. *Intensive Care Med.* 1998; **24**: 743–745.

56. Grubb, N.R., Fox, K.A. & Cawood, P. Resuscitation from out-of-hospital cardiac arrest: implications for cardiac enzyme estimation. *Resuscitation* 1996; **33**: 35–41.

57. Mullner, M., Sterz, F., Binder, M. *et al.* Creatine kinase and creatine kinase-MB release after nontraumatic cardiac arrest. Am. J. Cardiol. 1996 **77**: 581–585.

58. Mattana, J. & Singhal, P.C. Determinants of elevated creatine kinase activity and creatine kinase MB-fraction following cardiopulmonary resuscitation. *Chest* 1992; **101**: 1386–1392.

59. Babbs, C.F., Tacker, W.A., VanVleet, J.F., Bourland, J.D. & Geddes, L.A. Therapeutic indices for transchest defibrillator shocks: effective, damaging, and lethal electrical doses. *Am. Heart J.* 1980; **99**: 734–738.

60. Yabe, S., Smith, W.M., Daubert, J.P., Wolf, P.D., Rollins, D.L. & Ideker, R.E. Conduction disturbances caused by high current density electric fields. *Circ. Res.* 1990; **66**: 1190–1203.

61. Niemann, J.T., Walker, R.G. & Rosborough, J.P. Intracardiac

voltage gradients during transthoracic defibrillation: implications for postshock myocardial injury. *Acad. Emerg. Med.* 2005; **12**: 99–105.

62. Walker, R.G., Melnick, S.B., Chapman, F.W., Walcott, G.P., Schmitt, P.W. & Ideker, R.E. Comparison of six clinically used external defibrillators in swine. *Resuscitation* 2003; **57**: 73–83.

63. Jones, J.L., Lepeschkin, E., Jones, R.E. & Rush, S. Response of cultured myocardial cells to countershock-type electric field stimulation. *Am. J. Physiol.* 1978; **235**: H214–H222.

64. Morrow, D.A. & Antman, E.M. Cardiac marker elevation after cardioversion: sorting out chicken and egg. *Eur. Heart J.* 2000; **21**: 171–173.

65. Berg, R.A., Chapman, F.W., Berg, M.D., *et al.* Attenuated adult biphasic shocks compared with weight-based monophasic shocks in a swine model of prolonged pediatric ventricular fibrillation. *Resuscitation* 2004; **61**: 189–197.

66. Berg, R.A., Samson, R.A., Berg, M.D. *et al.* Better outcome after pediatric defibrillation dosage than adult dosage in a swine model of pediatric ventricular fibrillation. *J. Am. Coll. Cardiol.* 2005 **45**: 786–789.

67. Niemann, J.T., Burian, D., Garner, D. & Lewis, R.J. Monophasic versus biphasic transthoracic countershock after prolonged ventricular fibrillation in a swine model. *J. Am. Coll. Cardiol.* 2000; **36**: 932–938.

68. Xie, J., Weil, M.H., Sun, S. *et al.* High-energy defibrillation increases the severity of postresuscitation myocardial dysfunction. *Circulation* 1997; **96**: 683–688.

69. Altamura, G., Bianconi, L., Lo Bianco, F. *et al.* Transthoracic DC shock may represent a serious hazard in pacemaker dependent patients. *Pacing Clin. Electrophysiol.* 1995; **18**: 194–198.

70. Bullock, I. & Colquhoun, M. *Advanced Life Support Instructor Manual.* Resuscitation Council UK, London, 2001.

71. Montauk, L. Lethal defibrillator mishap. *Ann. Emerg. Med.* 1997; **29**: 825.

72. Gibbs, W., Eisenberg, M. & Damon, S.K. Dangers of defibrillation: injuries to emergency personnel during patient resuscitation. *Am. J. Emerg. Med.* 1990; **8**: 101–104.

73. Robertshaw, H. & McAnulty, G. Ambient oxygen concentrations during simulated cardiopulmonary resuscitation. *Anaesthesia* 1998; **53**: 634–637.

74. Miller, P.H. Potential fire hazard in defibrillation. *J. Am. Med. Assoc.* 1972; **221**: 192.

75. Cantello, E., Davy, T.E. & Koenig, K.L. The question of removing a ventilation bag before defibrillation. *J. Accid. Emerg. Med.* 1998; **15**:286.

76. Bruley, M. & Lavanchy, C. Oxygen-enriched fires during surgery of the head and neck. In Stoltzfus, J., Benz, F. & Stradling, J. (eds.) *Flammability and Sensitivity of Materials in Oxygen-Enriched Atmospheres.* Vol. 4. ASTM STP 1040. Philadelphia, PA: American Society for Testing and Materials, 1989: 392–405.

77. Babka, J.C. Does nitroglycerin explode? N. Engl. J. Med. 1983; **309**: 379.

78. Kuhnen, R., Nitsch, J. & Luderitz, B. Explosion von Nitropflastern bei Defibrillation. *Deutsche Medizinische Wochenschrift* 1985; **110**: 37.

79. Liddle, R. & Richmond, W. Investigation into voltage breakdown in glyceryl trinitrate patches. *Resuscitation* 1998; **37**: 145–148.

80. Lim, B.L. Airway management – when and how? *Singapore Med. J.* 2001; Suppl. **1**: 43–45.

81. Guildner, C.W. Resuscitation – opening the airway. A comparative study of techniques for opening an airway obstructed by the tongue. *JACEP* 1976; **5**: 588–590.

82. Roth, B., Magnusson, J., Johansson, I., Holmberg, S. & Westrin, P. Jaw lift – a simple and effective method to open the airway in children. *Resuscitation* 1998; **39**: 171–174.

83. Bruppacher, H., Reber, A., Keller, J.P., Geiduschek, J., Erb, T.O. & Frei, F.J. The effects of common airway maneuvers on airway pressure and flow in children undergoing adenoidectomies. *Anesth. Analg.* 2003; **97**: 29–34.

84. Saternus, K.S. & Fuchs, V. Verletzungen der A. carotis communis durch Reanimationsmaflnahmen. *Z. Rechtsmed.* 1982; **88**: 305–311.

85. Mularski, R.A., Sippel, J.M. & Osborne, M.L. Pneumoperitoneum: a review of nonsurgical causes. *Crit. Care Med.* 2000; **28**: 2638–2644.

86. Stone, B.J., Chantler, P.J. & Baskett, P.J. The incidence of regurgitation during cardiopulmonary resuscitation: a comparison between the bag valve mask and laryngeal mask airway. *Resuscitation* 1998; **38**: 3–6.

87. Amantea, S.L., Piva, J.P., Sanches, P.R. & Palombini, B.C. Oropharyngeal aspiration in pediatric patients with endotracheal intubation. *Pediatr. Crit. Care Med.* 2004; **5**: 152–156.

88. Ghirga, G., Ghirga, P., Palazzi, C., Pipere, M. & Colaiacomo, M. Bag-mask ventilation as a temporizing measure in acute infectious upper-airway obstruction: does it really work? *Pediatr. Emerg. Care* 2001; **17**: 444–446.

89. Reiger, J., Eritscher, C., Laubreiter, K., Trattnig, J., Sterz, F., Grimm, G. Gastric rupture – an uncommon complication after successful cardiopulmonary resuscitation: report of two cases. *Resuscitation* 1997; **35**: 175–178.

90. Piardi, T., D'Adda, F., Palmieri, F., Vettoretto, N., Lanzi, S. & Pouche, A. Shock and dyspnea after cardiopulmonary resuscitation: a case of iatrogenic gastric rupture. *Chir. Ital.* 2000; **52**: 593–596.

91. Offerman, S.R., Holmes, J.F. & Wisner, D.H. Gastric rupture and massive pneumoperitoneum after bystander cardiopulmonary resuscitation. *J. Emerg. Med.* 2001; **21**: 137–139.

92. Rabl, W., Ennemoser, O., Tributsch, W. & Ambach, E. Iatrogenic ruptures of the stomach after balloon tamponade. Two case reports: viscoelastic model. *Am. J. Forens. Med. Pathol.* 1995; **16**: 135–139.

93. Von Goedecke, A., Keller, C., Voelckel, W.G., *et al.* Mask ventilatation as an exit strategy of endotracheal intubation. *Anaethesist* 2005; in press.

94. Darok, M. Injuries resulting from resuscitation procedures. In Tsokos, M. (Ed.) *Forensic Pathology Reviews.* Vol 1. Humana Press Inc.; Totowa,NJ Chapter 13: 293–303.

95. Thierbach, A., Piepho, T., Wolcke, B., Küster, S. & Dick, W. Präklinische Sicherung der Atemwege. Erfolgsraten und Komplikationen. *Anaesthesist* 2004; **53**: 543–550.

96. Ehrlich, P.F., Seidman, P.S., Atallah, O., Haque, A. & Helmkamp, J. Endotracheal intubations in rural pediatric trauma patients. *J. Pediatr. Surg.* 2004; **39**: 1376–1380.

97. Givol, N., Gershtansky, Y., Halamish-Shani, T., Taicher, S., Perel, A. & Segal, E. Perianesthetic dental injuries: analysis of incident reports. *J. Clin. Anesth.* 2004; **16**: 173–176.

98. Itoman, E.M., Kajioka, E.H. & Yamamoto, L.G. Dental fracture risk of metal vs plastic laryngoscope blades in dental models. *Am. J. Emerg. Med.* 2005; **23**: 186–189.

99. Quinn, J.B., Schultheis, L.W. & Schumacher, G.E. A tooth broken after laryngoscopy: unlikely to be caused by the force applied by the anesthesiologist. *Anesth. Analg.* 2005; **100**: 594–596.

100. Cinar, S.O., Seven, H., Cinar, U. & Turgut, S. Isolated bilateral paralysis of the hypoglossal and recurrent laryngeal nerves (Bilateral Tapia's syndrome) after transoral intubation for general anesthesia. *Acta Anaesthesiol. Scand.* 2005; **49**: 98–99.

101. Hattori, S., Ohata, H. & Dohi, S. [Bilateral recurrent laryngeal nerve paralysis in a child following a neurosurgical operation] [Article in Japanese]. *Masui.* 2005; **54**: 683–686.

102. Schonfelder, K., Thieme, V. & Olthoff, D. Iatrogenic injuries of the trachea. *Anaesthesiol. Reanim.* 2004; **29**: 8–11.

103. Doherty, K.M., Tabaee, A., Castillo, M. & Cherukupally, S.R. Neonatal tracheal rupture complicating endotracheal intubation: a case report and indications for conservative management. *Int. J. Pediatr. Otorhinolaryngol.* 2005; **69**: 111–116.

104. Kaloud, H., Smolle-Juettner, F.M., Prause, G. & List, W.F. Iatrogenic ruptures of the tracheobronchial tree. *Chest* 997; **112**: 774–778.

105. Koscielny, S. & Gottschall, R. Perforation of the hypopharynx as a rare life-threatening complication of endotracheal intubation. *Anaesthesist* 2005 in press.

106. Mort, T.C. The incidence and risk factors for cardiac arrest during emergency tracheal intubation: a justification for incorporating the ASA Guidelines in the remote location. *J. Clin. Anesth.* 2004; **16**: 508–516.

107. Piepho, T., Thierbach, A. & Werner, C. Nasotracheal intubation: look before you leap. *Br. J. Anaesth.* 2005; **94**: 859–860.

108. Martin, J.E., Mehta, R., Aarabi, B., Ecklund, J.E., Martin, A.H. & Ling, G.S. Intracranial insertion of a nasopharyngeal airway in a patient with craniofacial trauma. *Mil. Med.* 2004; **169**: 496–497.

109. Fuchs, G., Schwarz, G., Baumgartner, A., Kaltenbock, F., Voit-Augustin, H. & Planinz, W. Fiberoptic intubation in 327 neurosurgical patients with lesions of the cervical spine. *J. Neurosurg. Anesthesiol.* 1999; **11**: 11–16.

110. Pepe, P.E., Zachariah, B.S. & Chandra, N.C. Invasive airway techniques in resuscitation. *Ann. Emerg. Med.* 1993; **22**: 393–403.

111. Gabrielli, A., Layon, A.J., Wenzel, V., Dorges, V. & Idris, A.H. Alternative ventilation strategies in cardiopulmonary resuscitation. *Curr. Opin. Crit. Care* 2002; **8**: 199–211.

112. Shea, S.R., MacDonald, J.R. & Gruzinski, G. Prehospital endotracheal tube airway or esophageal gastric tube airway: a critical comparison. *Ann. Emerg. Med.* 1985; **14**: 102–112.

113. Stoppacher, R., Teggatz, J.R. & Jentzen, J.M. Esophageal and pharyngeal injuries associated with the use of the esophageal-tracheal Combitube. *J. Forens. Sci.* 2004; **49**: 586–591.

114. Atherton, G.L. & Johnson, J.C. Ability of paramedics to use the Combitube in prehospital cardiac arrest. *Ann. Emerg. Med.* 1993; **22**: 1263–1268.

115. Vezina, D., Lessard, M.R., Bussieres, J., Topping, C. & Trepanier, C.A. Complications associated with the use of the esophageal–tracheal combitube. *Can. J. Anaesth.* 1998; **45**: 76–80.

116. Vezina, D., Trepanier, C.A., Lessard, M.R. & Bussieres, J. Esophageal and tracheal distortion by the esophageal–tracheal combitube: a cadaver study. *Can. J. Anaesth.* 1999; **46**: 393–397.

117. Hankins, D.G., Carruthers, N., Frascone, R.J., Long, L.A. & Campion, B.C. Complication rates for the esophageal obturator airway and endotracheal tube in the prehospital setting. *Prehosp. Disaster Med.* 1993; **8**: 117–121.

118. Tiah, L., Wong, E., Chen, M.F. & Sadarangani, S.P. Should there be a change in the teaching of airway management in the medical school curriculum? *Resuscitation* 2005; **64**: 87–91.

119. Rosenblatt, W.H. The use of the LMA-ProSeal in airway resuscitation. *Anesth. Analg.* 2003; **97**: 1773–1775.

120. Asai, T., Murao, K. & Shingu, K. Efficacy of the ProSeal laryngeal mask airway during manual in-line stabilisation of the neck. *Anaesthesia* 2002; **57**: 918–920.

121. Jorden, R.C. Percutaneous transtracheal ventilation. *Emerg. Med. Clin. North Am.* 1988; **6**: 745–752.

122. Dunlap, L.B. & Oregon, E. A modified, simple device for the emergency administration of percutaneous transtracheal ventilation. *JACEP* 1978; **7**: 42–46.

123. Newlands, S.D. & Makielski, K.H. Cervical osteomyelitis after percutaneous transtracheal ventilation and tracheotomy. *Head Neck* 1996; **18**: 295–8.

124. Heffner, J.E. The technique of tracheotomy and cricothyroidotomy. When to operate and how to manage complications. *J. Crit. Illn.* 1995; **10**: 561–568.

125. DeLaurier, G.A., Hawkins, M.L., Treat, R.C. & Mansberger, A.R. Jr. Acute airway management. Role of cricothyroidotomy. *Am. Surg.* 1990; **56**: 12–15.

46

Bringing it all together: state-of-the-art therapy for cardiac arrest

Max Harry Weil and Wanchun Tang

Weil Institute of Critical Care Medicine, Rancho Mirage, CA, USA

Introduction

The history of CPR is in part documented in the Old Testament,[1] but the science of CPR is but a half century old and is still emerging from its infancy.[2] Accordingly, it is not unexpected and certainly not shameful that as the science of resuscitation goes forward, we must sometimes retreat as often as we advance. Yet, that is indeed progress and inevitably the path that is characteristic of meaningful achievements in science and medicine.

Airway techniques and devices

One size does not fit all[3]

The vast majority of sudden deaths in children and, indeed, in victims under the age of 40 years are attributable to failure of ventilation. Accordingly, either mechanical obstruction by foreign body, laryngospasm, or laryngeal edema, or bronchoconstriction, constrains air exchange. Neuromuscular or skeletal injury, including intrathoracic crises such as pneumothorax, may account for death, though typically *not* sudden death. It is in these settings that the priority is establishment and maintenance of a patent airway and external ventilation. Since a majority of the foreign bodies that are swallowed by children and adults lodge in the posterior pharynx, the rescuer is the person best prepared to remove these promptly. Hence, the traditional (A) of the ABC survives, especially for children and young adults and in settings of witnessed cardiac arrest when respiratory distress with paradoxical chest and abdominal movements and especially stridor precedes loss of consciousness.

There has been an appropriate re-examination of the role of routine endotracheal intubation during CPR, whether in the field or in the hospital. For practical purposes, endotracheal intubation interrupts chest compression. The predominance of evidence now favors clearance of the airway, but coincident with starting chest compression. Even among professional rescuers, there is an unduly high incidence of initially failed intubation and potentially fatal esophageal intubation. There is trauma to the airway with bleeding after emergency intubations out-of-hospital in as many as 30% of attempted intubations. Routine endotracheal intubation during CPR is therefore now disadvised. The alternative is that of a more reliable and less traumatic method of airway control, namely the use of a laryngeal mask airway (LMA). The LMA may be inserted rapidly and securely by a minimally trained professional rescuer with initial benefits comparable to those of endotracheal tubes.[4]

Drug administration

The routine of establishing a route by which resuscitative drugs may be delivered into the central circulation was prompted, in part, by the priority and essentially universal use of epinephrine, atropine, sodium bicarbonate, calcium gluconate or chloride, and lidocaine beginning in the 1960s. Intracardiac injection lost favor because it had questionable effectiveness and a risk of serious injury. Endotracheal administration survived as an alternative. Yet none of these drugs nor any routine pharmaceutical intervention can now be regarded as of proven benefit, even treatment with epinephrine. This is more directly

Cardiac Arrest: The Science and Practice of Resuscitation Medicine. 2nd edn., ed. Norman Paradis, Henry Halperin, Karl Kern, Volker Wenzel, Douglas Chamberlain. Published by Cambridge University Press. © Cambridge University Press, 2007.

addressed below. Accordingly, the assumption that there is a high priority for establishment of a route for drug administration routinely *during* CPR is now not sustained. Nevertheless, there are major exceptions. Intravenous access is required for volume repletion after volume depletion and especially exsanguinations, for administration of specific antidotes to drug intoxication, and for emergency management of major electrolyte or endocrine abnormalities, especially hyperkalemia.

Ready access to the central circulation may be gained through the internal jugular or subclavian veins. Although the supraclavicular approach to the jugular or the subclavian vein has been utilized during CPR, this is inevitably a challenging procedure during chest compression. Femoral vein cannulation may be accomplished without interruption of CPR, but the site is less predictable. Evidence favoring endobronchial administration of drugs is quite controversial. As stated above, the evidence favoring its use is not persuasive. Absorption is erratic and drugs accumulate such that effects are of unpredictable onset and duration. This route would best be viewed as a last resort in instances in which venous access for specific indications becomes a priority.

A new development has been intraosseous access to the central circulation. Employed initially with high success, in children, the technique has been expanded for use in adults. Commercial kits are now available. Ease of insertion by trained operators, usually into the tibia, and confirmation of appropriate placement provides a highly effective option for reliable and minimally invasive access to the central circulation.[5]

Ventilation

Methods by which pulmonary gas exchange is restored by artificial ventilation represent the very foundation of resuscitation medicine. Yet objective evidence of its lifesaving value during routine CPR after sudden death has greatly diminished. Most important, delays in instituting or maintaining chest compression for external ventilation have been shown to have adverse effects on outcomes. There is persuasive physiological rationale and experimental confirmation that in settings of cardiac arrest due to sudden death and therefore in the absence of asphyxia, chest compressions without ventilation do not compromise outcomes. To the contrary, positive pressure breathing, whether by mouth-to-mouth, mouth-to-nose, valved bag and mask, or mechanical ventilators increases intrathoracic pressure and thereby impedes cardiac filling

in close relationship to the tidal volumes and the rates at which breaths are delivered. Accordingly, the greater the tidal volumes and the higher the frequency, the less is the cardiac output generated by chest compression. Hyperventilation resulting in extremes of hypocapnia also may compromise the success of resuscitation.[6] There is some optimism that these adversities may be mitigated by use of the impedance threshold valve. Greatly reduced pulmonary blood flow requires greatly reduced minute volumes for adequate alveolar ventilation. Hence, as little as 300 mL of tidal volume may be adequate for the average adult patient when cardiac output is likely to be less than 20% of normal during CPR. Whether hyperventilation-induced hypocapnia and specifically the marked reduction in arterial PCO_2 is itself detrimental has not as yet been secured.

The demotion of ventilations as a priority intervention, however, does not apply to asphyxial cardiac arrest due to drowning or airway obstruction or to pediatric and neonatal resuscitation. Whereas there is no secure proof that increasing the inspired oxygen concentrations delivered into or near the airway improves outcomes, there is sufficient rationale and no adverse effects have been identified.

Public access defibrillation

The enthusiasm for early use of automated external defibrillators (AEDs) was understandably ignited by remarkably successful experiences in Rochester, Minnesota, especially by police first responders; in the Las Vegas casinos; in the Chicago airports, in part by untrained rescuers; and by Basic Life Support/AED trained cabin attendants in flight.[7] The ultimate life-saving benefits have been less impressive, however, for at least three reasons. First, there is persuasive evidence of benefit in public settings, but the preponderance of cardiac arrests occur in the home. Second, there is a remarkable decrease in the incidence of sudden death presenting as ventricular fibrillation (VF) both in- and out-of-hospital. The overall incidence has decreased below 50%. Third, it is now apparent that the non-professional rescuer's initial resuscitation effort may have been distracted by prioritizing defibrillation therefore engendering delays in initiating and maintaining uninterrupted chest compression.

Accordingly, chest compression has once again become the primary and initial intervention for both lay and professional rescuers during out-of-hospital CPR, except perhaps for witnessed sudden death during the initial 3 to 5 minutes and asphyxial cardiac arrest.

Sequencing CPR

There is much merit in the proposal by Weisfeldt and Becker[8] to identify three time-sensitive phases of resuscitation after cardiac arrest. Nonetheless, these apply primarily to sudden death of cardiac cause, in contrast to either cardiac arrest in settings of asphyxia or exsanguination. The first is the electrical phase which the authors estimate to be 4 minutes. It is the phase during which electrical conversion takes precedence. The second phase extends from 4 to 10 minutes and this is the time window for restoring blood flow that currently is performed almost entirely with precordial compression or, in uncommon instances of chest surgery or trauma to the thorax, open chest direct cardiac compression. The third and final phase is the metabolic phase in which there is myocardial (and cerebral) ischemic injury with progression to cell death. The heart itself loses compliance and there is evidence of progression to a stone heart. As highlighted by Cobb,[9] chest compression with effort to restore circulation promptly continues to take the lead as the *initial* intervention in all instances of sudden death, except for opening of the airway and restoring breathing in settings of asphyxial cardiac arrest, in addition to precordial compression.

Prevention

Sudden cardiac death is epidemic, and the predominant cause of cardiac arrest in industrialized nations is cardiovascular disease, specifically atherosclerosis. A remarkable 70% of all deaths in the United States are now attributed to coronary or cerebral vascular diseases which terminate in myocardial infarction or stroke.

Prevention of sudden death therefore appropriately focuses on prevention of identifiable risk factors. Though family history may in part account for as many as 50% of fatal atherosclerotic vascular events, evidence favors lifestyle interventions and, when that alone is of limited effectiveness, appropriate pharmacological interventions.

It is likely that understanding of a "metabolic syndrome"[10] has been both a conceptual and a pragmatic advance. The hallmarks include a combination of abdominal obesity, hypertension, hypertriglyceridemia, fasting hyperglycemia, and a disproportionately higher LDL cholesterol and a lower HDL cholesterol. Lifestyle interventions include diet, exercise, and cessation of smoking. Pharmacological interventions include control of hypertension, hyperglycemia, and hyperlipidemia and, in some instances, the administration of antiplatelet agents.

Relatively rare causes of sudden death, especially in children and younger adults, are genetic causes of heart disease. These are now better identified by genotyping[11] and include hypertrophic (subaortic, septal) cardiomyopathies, long QT syndromes, Brugada syndrome, so-called catecholaminogenic polymorphic ventricular tachycardia and arrhythmogenic right ventricular dysplasia. Syncope is an important warning sign.

Perhaps the largest cause of cardiac death is that of end-stage heart failure when ejection fractions decline to less than 30%. Both survivors of cardiac arrest and individuals who are identifiably at high risk of sudden death are candidates for internally implanted defibrillators and this has proven to be a major advance for prolonging survival in such patients.

Vasopressor agents and sodium bicarbonate

Perhaps no two subjects bearing on CPR have been debated more vigorously and, from our vantage point, with greater emotional fervor than the use of vasopressor agents and sodium bicarbonate. Epinephrine has been the singularly most prominent resuscitative drug for more than a century and for good reason. It improves the success of initial resuscitation with the likelihood of restoring spontaneous circulation. In experimental animals, it has been shown to increase survival, but there is no secure evidence of survival benefit in human patients. Unfortunately, the same applies to vasopressins. Theoretically, vasopressin has advantages over epinephrine in that it may diminish the severity of postresuscitation myocardial dysfunction, especially in patients with ischemic heart disease, in whom beta adrenergic blockade has reduced the risk of fatal ischemic episodes. There is experimental evidence of protection by the administration of a beta adrenergic blocking agent during CPR. Hence, there has been interest in alternative non-adrenergic vasoconstrictor drugs, including angiotensin II, endothelin for which no secure data of benefit exist, and arginine vasopressin. At the time of this writing, vasopressin has advantages over epinephrine, but there is no secure proof that any vasopressor drug improves long-term outcomes.

With respect to bicarbonate or other buffer agents, there is no persuasive evidence of improved outcomes but instead the potential of serious adverse effects.

Drug management of arrhythmias

Two dicta emerge. The first is that the routine administration of any antiarrhythmic drug during CPR has not been proven to increase long-term survival. The second is that almost all antiarrhythmic drugs are also proarrhythmic. Of all agents currently available, amiodarone remains the best option for drug management of recurrent ventricular tachycardia and ventricular fibrillation other than those due to electrolyte abnormalities. Admittedly, no survival benefit beyond hospital discharge has been demonstrated. There is now no secure evidence favoring the administration of lidocaine, bretylium, and procainamide. Administration of atropine, though still widely practiced for management of bradyarrhythmias or agonal rhythms, also has no proven survival benefit. Accordingly, present data prompt us to conclude that antiarrhythmic agents, like other routine pharmacological interventions, have so far failed to improve outcomes of sudden death. Moreover, these drugs unfortunately have the potential for serious adverse effects.

Postresuscitation care

Hypothermia was widely used in conjunction with cardiac surgery in the 1950s and later in conjunction with cardiopulmonary bypass. The recent demonstration that modest hypothermia in the range of 32°C to 35°C produces impressive improvement in neurological outcomes has prompted widespread enthusiasm for its routine use. The rationale for its use, and especially the pioneering of the late Peter Safar, have established both the rationale and benefits of its routine use. As yet, however, there is need for agreement on preferred methods of cooling, methods of monitoring core temperature, and the rationale for and interpreting measurements such as blood gases during hypothermia. Prevention of adverse effects of hypothermia, including thrombocytopenia and platelet dysfunction, which compromises blood clotting, is being actively explored.

Complications include cold diuresis, hypernatremia with hyperosmolal states, probable pancreatic dysfunction with increases in serum amylase and hyperglycemia, and decreased insulin effectiveness. The risks of infection, especially pneumonia and wound infections, are increased. Better understanding of these complications is sought as a basis for patient selection. The technique is promising and important. The goal is to mitigate the devastation that follows irreversible ischemic injury to the brain and major neurological deficits after successful initial resuscitation.

Monitoring and measurements

It is clear that the detection of cardiac arrest cannot be achieved reliably by palpation of the carotid or femoral pulses, especially by non-professional providers. Accordingly, the pulse check is appropriately deleted from the armamentariam of the BLS provider. Even for the professional provider, it is unlikely that palpation is reliable, especially during uninterrupted chest compression. Most important, however, is the consensus that chest compression should not be delayed for a pulse check. The possibility that the presence or absence of the heart beat may be detected by measurements of transthoracic impedance is attractive.

The most consistent guide for predicting the likelihood of defibrillation and restoration of spontaneous circulation is the coronary perfusion pressure (CPP). Except for patients who are invasively monitored in the hospital prior to cardiac arrest in the operating suite, cardiac catheterization laboratory, or intensive care unit, this is not applicable in other settings and especially out-of-hospital. End-tidal PCO_2 (EtPCO$_2$), however, is an excellent surrogate of both coronary perfusion pressure and cardiac output generated by chest compression.[12] EtPCO$_2$ is also useful for guiding effective chest compression and for the decision to discontinue CPR. Chest compression should consistently increase and maintain EtPCO$_2$ at levels exceeding 15 mm Hg. Although there are only observational clinical data to secure the proposed rule that CPR efforts may be abandoned absent EtPCO$_2$ values exceeding 10 mm Hg for more than 10 minutes in normothermic patients, this deserves consideration.

Pulse oximetry fails during cardiac arrest when peripheral blood flow is critically reduced or ceases. Measurements of cardiac output and oxygen consumption during CPR are both impractical and of no proven value. Blood gases, oximetry, serum electrolytes, and arterial blood lactate are potentially useful measurements including detection of carbon monoxide intoxication, life-threatening hypoglycemia, some drug intoxications, and electrolyte abnormalities. Sublingual tissue CO_2 is also of unproven value for guiding cardiac resuscitation. Nevertheless, each of these measurements is of substantial value primarily for postresuscitation management rather than during CPR.

There are important advances in the search for a predictor to guide the timing and predict the success of a defibrillating shock.[12] These include electrocardiographic measurements based on voltage (amplitude), frequency, and an algorithm that represents a combination of amplitude and frequency (AMSA).

Thrombolysis

The therapeutic value of anticoagulants and thrombolysis in settings of acute myocardial ischemia and following pulmonary embolization is undisputed. There is also evidence of impaired microvascular blood flow with stasis during and following resuscitation from cardiac arrest. The potential value of anticoagulants and of thrombolytic agents that have proteolytic activity acting on prothrombin and thrombin in settings of CPR have been based on experimental data, but as yet have gained no clear clinical support. Observational studies project a five-fold greater likelihood of bleeding including intracranial hemorrhage. The incidence of serious bleeding is only 3%, however, which is best viewed in relation to the current national estimate of greater than 95% overall mortality after out-of-hospital cardiac arrest. Though the rationale for anticoagulants and thrombolysis is conceptually attractive, clinical data are insufficient to support its use as adjunctive therapy during CPR at this time.

In-hospital resuscitation

The overall survival is largely contingent on co-morbidities. Better outcomes are likely if preventive measures are instituted by which the incidence of cardiac arrest is reduced. Proactive Medical Emergency Teams (METs) have been organized to identify patients at risk, arrange prompt transfer of such patients to more intensive observation and management in monitored beds, or transfer into intensive care units. The success of the MET, the organized early response team, which typically includes a Critical Care or Emergency Medicine specialist and a Critical Care/Emergency Medicine RN specialist, is likely to be contingent on the local hospital setting. There is lesser need in teaching hospitals and greater benefit in non-teaching hospitals in the absence of in-house physicians. Hospitalists increasingly provide in-house services, including MET equivalents. The effectiveness of a MET is also contingent on the geographic location of patients and availability of monitored beds. Finally, much is determined by the culture of the institution and the extent to which physicians and other health providers share responsibility without undue fear of intrusion or perceived liabilities.

A special issue relates to the perceived obsolescence of manual defibrillators that do not deliver biphasic waveform, lower energy shocks, and escalating energies up to 360 joules. The likelihood that such compromise outcomes is now of lesser concern, however. The new and now more appropriate routine is delivery of only one shock with brief interruption of chest compressions. A single shock will therefore be at the lowest power setting, typically 200 joules.

Complications

As yet unsettled are the possible benefits and the adverse effects of the "precordial thump" delivered after witnessed cardiac arrest. There is persuasive evidence that a mechanically induced chest wall impact so timed that it immediately precedes the peak of the T wave may induce ectopic ventricular arrhythmias including ventricular fibrillation, so-called COMMOTIO CORDIS. Defibrillation produces skin burns, the so-called perimeter effect.[13]

Electrical shocks produce increases in both total creatine phosphokinase (CPK) principally from striated muscle and in the cardiac CPK-MB fraction together with Troponin T of myocardial source. If the rescuer is shocked, it is an unpleasant experience but quite remarkably, there has never been documentation of serious injury.

In a majority of victims, manual precordial compression fractures ribs. This applies also to mechanical chest compression, including the LUCAS® and the Autopulse®, together with a minority incidence of sternal fractures.

In contrast to primary cardiac causes of cardiac arrest in older adults, the predominant causes of cardiac arrest in pediatric patients are not cardiac. They are associated with asphyxia and especially foreign body aspiration and drowning or traumatic blood loss with exsanguination. More recent experimental studies nevertheless provide persuasive evidence that opening the airway and starting ventilation do not alone result in optimal outcomes. After onset of cardiac arrest, conventional precordial compression would best be part of initial management.

Ventricular fibrillation occurs in fewer than 10% of pediatric patients. If VF evolves during resuscitation from pulseless rhythms or asystole, the likelihood of a favorable outcome is diminished. The empirical decision to "dose" the energy delivered at 2 joules/kg proves 90% effective. Newer versions of AEDs that deliver biphasic waveform shocks provide pediatric cables and electrodes that attenuate the delivered shock to between 50 and 80 joules, an appropriate dose for children.

The routine of airway intubation for pediatric patients with cardiac arrest in out-of-hospital settings has been largely abandoned because of the dual detriments of delayed ventilation and precordial compression and the high incidence of both airway trauma and esophageal intubation.

As in adults, substantially lower tidal volumes are now delivered to avoid hyperventilation. Also as in adults, there is currently no proof that routine administration of drugs is of proven value. Calcium gluconate or chloride is administered on specific indication, including calcium channel blockade overdose, hyperkalemia, and hypocalcemia.

Sodium bicarbonate is administered for management of hyperkalemia and tricyclic antidepressant overdose.

Vascular access is now most predictably obtained by the intraosseous route. Neurological recovery is compromised by fever. We anticipated major benefits of hypothermia, but for pediatric patients additional objective clinical confirmation is awaited.

In pediatric patients who sustain cardiac arrest after cardiac surgery, early implementation of extracorporeal oxygenation (ECMO) has survival value.

Concluding comments

Though a preponderance of controlled clinical studies have failed to establish survival benefits, especially for drugs, the absence of proven benefit is not to be interpreted that there is no potential for benefits. There are extraordinary ethical and legal limitations that typically impose serious restraints on the enrollment of patients during cardiac arrest, and equally formidable challenges in the implementation of such human experiments. Accordingly, we must not despair of what may appear to be a see-saw of progress, but maintain appreciation and optimism for the progress that is being achieved.

REFERENCES

1. II Kings, Chapter 4, verses 34-35, *Bible, King James Version.*
2. Weil, M.H. & Tang, W. Cardiopulmonary resuscitation: A promise as yet largely unfulfilled. *Disease-a-Month* 1997; **43**(7): 429–504.
3. Weil, M.H., Tang, W. & Bisera, J. Cardiopulmonary resuscitation. One size does not fit all. *Circulation* 2003; **107**: 794 (Editorial).
4. Nolan, J.P. & Gabbott, D.A. Airway techniques and airway devices, Chapter 29, this volume.
5. Kerz, T., Paret, G. & Herff, H. Routes of drug administration, Chapter 33, this volume.
6. Idris, A.H. & Gabrielli, A. The physiology of ventilation during cardiac arrest and other low blood flow states, Chapter 28, this volume.
7. White, R.D., Colqhoun, M., Davies, S., Peberdy, M.A. & Timerman, S. Public access defibrillation, Chapter 27, this volume.
8. Weisfeldt, M.L. & Becker, L.B. Resuscitation after cardiac arrest. A 3-phase time-sensitive model. *J. Am. Med. Assoc.* 2002; **288**: 3035–3038.
9. Cobb, L.A. Sequence of therapies during resuscitation: defibrillation vs compressions, Chapter 24, this volume.
10. Kohli, P. & Greenland, P. Role of the metabolic syndrome in risk assessment for coronary heart disease. *J. Am. Med. Assoc.* 2006; **295**: 819–821.
11. Campbell, C., Gluckman, T., Henrikson, C., Ashen, D. & Blumenthal, R. Prevention of sudden cardiac death, Chapter 23, this volume.
12. Ward, K.R. & Bisera, J. Cardiac arrest resuscitation monitoring, Chapter 38, this volume.
13. Baubin, M., Rabl, W. & Hoke, R. Complications of CPR, Chapter 45, this volume.

Part V

Postresuscitation disease and its care

47

Postresuscitation syndrome

Erga L. Cerchiari

Department of Anaesthesia and Critical Care,
Ospedale Maggiore, and Area of Anaesthesia and Critical Care,
Surgical Department, Provincial Health Care Structure, Bologna, Italy

The postresuscitation syndrome (PRS) has been defined as a condition of an organism resuscitated following prolonged cardiac arrest, caused by a combination of whole body ischemia and reperfusion, and characterized by multiple organ dysfunction, including neurologic impairment.[1]

Background

Following resuscitation from cardiac arrest, patients either recover consciousness or remain unconscious, depending on the duration of cardiac arrest and the effectiveness of any CPR, but also on prearrest conditions such as age and comorbidities.[2]

Shortening no-flow times by timely interventions that can maintain some perfusion and promote the restoration of spontaneous circulation (e.g., bystander CPR, early defibrillation, and other means) improves the possibility of a successful outcome with the patient recovering consciousness.[3]

The wider availability of resuscitation techniques to reverse clinical death, however, has led to increasingly frequent observations of a pathological condition occurring in patients who remain unconscious, involving multiple organ injury or failure following reperfusion after prolonged cardiac arrest.

The concept of postresuscitation disease as a unique and new nosological entity was introduced by Negovsky in 1972;[4,5] the most interesting aspect of this innovative concept was the recognition that the etiology depended on a combination of severe circulatory hypoxia with the unintended sequelae of measures used for resuscitation.

On the basis of the wide variety of ischemic/hypoxic mechanisms that can trigger its development, the disease was redefined by Safar as a syndrome in which pathogenetic processes triggered by cardiac arrest were exacerbated by reperfusion, causing damage to the brain and other organs, the complex interactions of which combine to determine overall outcome (see early experimental findings summary).[6,7]

The evidence of features common to the postresuscitation syndrome and multiple organ dysfunction syndrome led to the hypothesis that a systemic inflammatory response of the entire organism was triggered by ischemia and reperfusion, adding to the damage directly induced by ischemia during cardiac arrest.[8]

Two landmark studies, showing that mild therapeutic hypothermia started after reperfusion can improve recovery after cardiac arrest, confirm that outcome is determined not only by events occurring during arrest and CPR but also by pathogenetic processes continuing after reperfusion.[9,10]

Recent reports confirm the occurrence of a "sepsis-like syndrome" after resuscitation from cardiac arrest,[11,12] although the mechanistic relationship to the direct damage induced by ischemia during cardiac arrest has yet to be clarified.

Early Experimental Findings

Negovsky[4,5] and his group of Russian investigators pioneered the concept of postresuscitation disease as a unique nosological entity, caused by the combination of severe hypoxia and resuscitation, on the basis of hundreds of experimental observations that fall into three groups:

1. Phasic Pattern of Postresuscitation Recovery

Independent of the type of insult, alterations in cerebral and extracerebral organs occur starting with reperfusion and developing over time.

From insult to 6 to 9 hours postinsult: rapid changes in cerebral and systemic hemodynamics, metabolism, and rheology (clotting disturbances, increased viscosity), increase levels of biologically active substances and prostaglandin derivatives; alterations of the immune system (increased bactericidal activity, depressed reticuloendothelial system, and hyperreactivity of B- and T-lymphocytes), and toxic factors in the blood (peptide fraction 800 to 2000 Daltons and endotoxin secondary to gram-negative bacteremia).

From 10 to 24 hours postinsult: normalization of cardiovascular variables and progression of metabolic derangements ensue. During this time, 50% of deaths occur as a result of recurrent cardiac arrest.

From 1 to 3 days postinsult: stable cardiovascular variables and improvement in cerebral function associated with increased intestinal permeability leading to bacteremia.

The stabilization phase (more than 3 days postinsult): characterized by the prevalence of localized or generalized infection that represents the major cause of delayed deaths. The degree of cerebral and extracerebral organ derangements is reported to be more severe and prolonged the longer the duration of the hypoxic–ischemic insult.

2. Interactions between Cerebral and Extracerebral Postischemic Damage on Outcome

The severity of systemic and hemodynamic derangements after 20 minutes of isolated brain ischemia is comparable to that recorded after only 12–15 minutes of total circulatory arrest with ventricular fibrillation, suggesting that cerebral postischemic damage plays a role in development of extracerebral dysfunction, probably by inducing changes in neurohumoral regulation.

Cerebral function recovers better after bloodless global brain ischemia than after the same duration of circulatory arrest from ventricular fibrillation, leading to the conclusion that extracerebral factors account for about half of the pathological findings in the brain induced by cardiac arrest.

3. Benefical Effect of Trials with Detoxification Techniques

A series of trials aimed at removing toxins and normalizing homeostasis by various detoxification techniques showed that all the techniques can improve neurological recovery and survival compared with concurrent controls; cross-circulation was the most effective, in which circulation in the body of the resuscitated dog was maintained for 30 minutes post-ROSC by the heart of a healthy donor dog, aided by an extracorporeal circulation system.

Safar and his group in Pittsburgh, in parallel with – but subsequent to – the Russian experimental work, confirmed that extracerebral organ dysfunction may hamper cerebral recovery following resuscitation from cardiac arrest, based on the observations that (a) cerebral function after isolated global brain ischemia recovers better than after comparable durations of total body ischemia[13,14] and (b) the use of cardiopulmonary bypass for resuscitation and for short-term postresuscitation assistance improves myocardial performance after weaning, and significantly increases neurological outcome and survival.[15] Extracerebral organ dysfunction following resuscitation from cardiac arrest of increasing durations was studied in animal experimental models:[1,6,7,14–19]

- cardiac output and arterial oxygen transport, after a transient increase, showed a prolonged and profound decrease associated with increased peripheral resistance; this starts sooner and is more severe and prolonged after longer durations of VF, resolving by 12 to 24 hours postresuscitation
- pulmonary gas exchange, with assisted ventilation for 6 to 24 hours postresuscitation, is well maintained even after extubation (normoxia, normocarbia, and rapid pH normalization)
- coagulation disturbances with hypocoagulability start during resuscitation, with prolonged clotting times and decreased platelets and fibrinogen, and normalize at 24 hours after resuscitation; elevated fibrin-degradation products and decreased platelet counts were observed to 72 hours postresuscitation.

- erythrocyte count decreases significantly
- renal function (blood urea nitrogen, serum creatinine, osmolarity, sodium, potassium, and calcium) remain normal after a transient reduction in urine output with positive fluid balance, normalizing at 3 to 6 hours
- hepatic function is altered transiently; plasma ammonia and branched chain and aromatic amino acids increase, with higher levels in the animals with poor outcome, suggesting an alteration of liver-detoxifying function
- bacteremia is a constant feature after cardiac arrest, with transient leukocytosis but without hyperthermia (90% were constituents of the intestinal flora, suggesting postischemic bacterial translocation).

In summary, following resuscitation from cardiac arrest, multiorgan dysfunction occurs, but the abnormalities have different time patterns (Fig. 47.1).

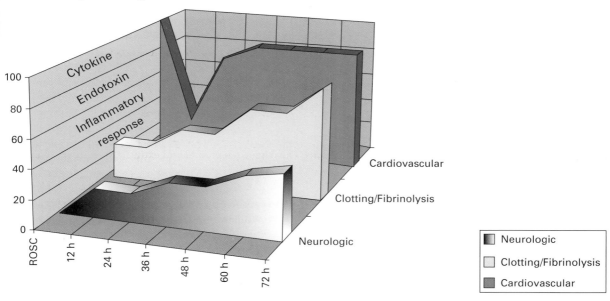

Fig. 47.1. Time pattern of organ dysfunction after resuscitation from cardiac arrest from the early experimental work.[1,4–7]

Incidence and prevalence

The incidence of out-of-hospital cardiac arrest is estimated to be 49.5–66 per 100 000 cases per year:[2] in these, return of spontaneous circulation can be achieved in 17% to 33%, depending on the efficiency of the emergency response system.[20]

The incidence of in-hospital cardiac arrest has been estimated as 1.4/100 admissions/year:[21] in these cases, restoration of spontaneous circulation occurs in 40%–44%.[22]

Of the patients resuscitated from cardiac arrest, a small proportion (variable as a function of timeliness and effectiveness of response) achieve early recovery, with restoration of spontaneous respiration and consciousness. Identification and treatment of the cause of arrest is the main or only therapeutic challenge for this group of subjects.

But most survivors of cardiac arrest (80%) are comatose postresuscitation, and are admitted to the ICU where they represent the population of patients with postresuscita-

tion syndrome (PRS), amounting to about 15%–20% of all cardiac arrest victims (Fig. 47.2).

Among the PRS patients, mortality has been reported to be very high, reaching 80% by 6 months postresuscitation:[23–25] approximately one-third of the deaths are due to cardiac causes (early deaths usually < 24 hours), one-third to malfunction of extracerebral organs, and one-third to neurologic causes (late deaths).

The prevalence of the postresuscitation syndrome can only be inferred, because of the bias of data resulting from decisions to limit treatment, including instructions for "do not attempt resuscitation," in cases of recurrent cardiac arrest.[22–26]

Etiology

Following resuscitation from cardiac arrest of less than 5 minutes, recovery is rapid and complete. After prolonged arrest, ROSC is impossible or only transient.

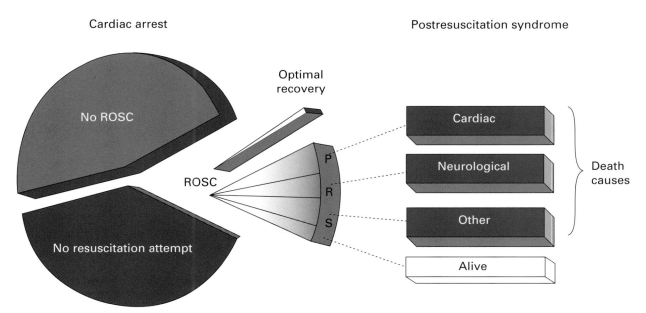

Fig. 47.2. Estimated fate for cardiac arrest patients.

Therefore, the postresuscitation syndrome only develops following resuscitation given during an intermediate duration of ischemia (the limits of which are affected by prearrest conditions) and depending on the circumstances of resuscitation, leading to the "*reperfusion paradox.*"

The insult induced by cardiac arrest and CPR is multifaceted, encompassing several contributing factors occurring during cardiac arrest, during CPR, and following restoration of spontaneous circulation:[1,6,7]

- *ischemia – anoxia* occurring during the cardiac arrest with no-flow
- *hypoperfusion – hypoxia* during the low-flow of external cardiac compressions (inducing at best a cardiac output of 25% baseline)
- *reperfusion*, which, although potentially permitting survival, adds to the ischemic-hypoxic–hypoperfusion insult, inducing a variety of mechanisms that continue to evolve subsequently, including reperfusion failure and injury, altered coagulation, and activation of a systemic inflammatory response.

Pathogenesis

Two major pathways have been identified
1. a direct insult to the brain, which is particularly sensitive to ischemia; and to the heart, which may suffer postresuscitation myocardial stunning leading in turn

to a secondary insult from postreperfusion impairment of cardiac output and hypoperfusion.
2. postreperfusion activation of the systemic inflammatory response syndrome, with hypoperfusion and/or altered perfusion as one pathological mechanism;[12] in this pathway, the PRS shares many features with severe sepsis, including elevation of plasma cytokines with dysregulated cytokine production, endothelial injury, complement activation, coagulation and fibrinolysis abnormalities, endotoxemia, disturbed modulation of the immune response, and adrenal dysfunction.

Organ function postresuscitation

The postresuscitation syndrome occurs in patients resuscitated after cardiac arrest of more than 5 minutes' duration and is characterized by different components: neurologic functional impairment, cardiovascular functional impairment – both well characterized – and the extracerebral extracardiac functional impairment comprising a complex picture of determinants and interactions.

The three major components variously contribute to the complex clinical picture of the patient resuscitated from cardiac arrest and admitted to ICU. Rapidly occurring early post-resuscitation changes create an acute phase of instability during which specific and aggressive treatments may favorably affect outcome. After the first

24 hours the clinical picture stabilizes and treatment becomes less specific, and is not different from that of a comatose ICU patient.

For purposes of clarity, the three components are described separately, with analysis of the relative contribution of the two pathogenetic pathways, functional derangement interactions, and contributions to outcome and specific early treatments.

Neurologic function postresuscitation

The best defined component of the postresuscitation syndrome is neurologic functional impairment.

With the increased application of resuscitation interventions, postcardiac arrest unconsciousness has become the third most common cause of coma. Almost 80% of patients who initially survive cardiac arrest remain comatose for variable lengths of time, approximately 40% enter a persistent vegetative state, while 10% to 30% of survivors achieve a meaningful recovery.[27]

Cardiac arrest causes a global ischemic insult to the brain. The extent of cerebral damage is a function of the duration of interrrupted blood flow. Accordingly, minimizing both the arrest (no-flow) time and the cardiopulmonary resuscitation (low-flow) time, is critical.

Even in selected patients with a witnessed cardiac arrest after ventricular fibrillation and an estimated arrest to ALS intervention interval no longer than 15 minutes, mortality at 6 months was 55% and of the survivors, 61% had an unfavorable neurological outcome.[9] With reperfusion, extracerebral factors may hamper neurological recovery, requiring interventions aimed at mitigating secondary postischemic anoxic encephalopathy.[7]

Pathophysiology

The mechanisms of cerebral damage following ischemia and reperfusion have been studied in detail (for detailed reviews see refs. 7,27).

Changes induced by ischemia set the stage for reoxygenation-induced, free radical-triggered injury cascades, exacerbated by reduced cardiac output and local circulatory impairment that starts during cardiac arrest with altered blood–brain barrier permeability and systemic changes such as activation of complement, coagulation, platelet aggregation, and adhesion of white blood cells.[28]

The pattern of prolonged global and multifocal cerebral hypoperfusion is associated with variations of regional cerebral blood flow both in the cortex and in the basal ganglia[29] with regional anoxic cerebral anaerobic metabolism.

Posthypoxic encephalopathy has been shown to be associated with a marked decrease of cerebral metabolic activity and of glucose uptake, even 24 hours after resuscitation.[30]

A significant activation of inflammatory mediators (Interleukin 8, soluble elastin, and polymorphonuclear elastase) immediately postinsult and lasting about 12 hours has recently been reported following both cardiac arrest and isolated brain trauma, suggesting an inflammatory response as a common pathogenetic pathway activated by cerebral damage.[31]

Clinical features and prognostic evaluation

A variety of methods have been proposed to monitor the evolution of the depth of coma and its prognosis, including neurological examination, electrophysiologic techniques, and biochemical tests.

A recent meta-analysis, including nearly 2000 patients, assessed the reliability of neurological examination, including Glasgow Coma Scale (GCS) and brainstem reflexes, reviewed at different time intervals after resuscitation; it concluded that patients who lack pupillary and corneal reflexes at 24 hours and have no motor response to pain at 72 hours have an extremely small chance of meaningful recovery.

The most reliable signs of prognosis occur at 24 hours after cardiac arrest: earlier assessment should not be based on clinical evidence alone.[32]

A systematic review of 18 studies analyzed the predictive ability of somatosensory evoked potentials (SSEP) acquired early after the onset of coma (1–3 days) in 1136 adult patients with hypoxic-ischemic encephalopathy: the results showed that patients with absent cortical SSEP responses have a less than 1% chance of regaining consciousness.[33]

A recent study tested the value of serial measurement of serum neuron-specific enolase (NSE) at admission and daily postinsult, in combination with GCS and SSEP measurements, to predict neurological prognosis in unconscious patients admitted to the ICU after resuscitation from cardiac arrest. High serum NSE levels at 24 and 48 hours after resuscitation predict a poor neurological outcome. Addition of NSE to GCS and SSEP increases predictability.[34]

By 48–72 hours postresuscitation, predictability of unfavorable long-term neurologic outcome may guide decisions to curtail treatment, because only patients with lighter levels of coma or who have regained consciousness by this time have any realistic prospect of long-term survival.[32]

Treatment

Research into cardiopulmonary cerebral resuscitation has attempted to mitigate the postischemic–anoxic encephalopathy but, until recently, experimental results had never been replicated in patients.[7]

Mild therapeutic hypothermia induced following reperfusion in patients who have been successfully resuscitated from ventricular fibrillation cardiac arrest is the only postresuscitation intervention that has proved effective in increasing the rate of favorable neurologic outcome in two different randomized studies conducted in Europe and Australia[9,10] and in reducing mortality in one of them.[9] Clinical and experimental results show a multifactorial neuroprotective effect of hypothermia during and after ischemic situations by influencing several damaging pathways.[27]

Thrombolytics, administered during arrest or early after reperfusion, have been shown in animal experiments to improve the microcirculation in the brain and may, by this mechanism, contribute to the favorable neurological outcome of patients as described in many case reports and small case series with predominantly positive results.[35] The first properly designed, large, randomized, double-blind multicenter study of thrombolytics was stopped before completion of recruitment because the data safety monitoring board judged it unlikely that, in the population in study, tenecteplase would demonstrate superiority over placebo. These results, presented at a 2006 conference, should be considered preliminary until a detailed analysis is performed and published.[36]

Cardiovascular function postresuscitation

Following successful resuscitation from prolonged cardiac arrest, a typical component of the postresuscitation syndrome is prolonged myocardial contractile failure, associated with life-threatening ventricular arrhythmias and hemodynamic instability.[37,38]

Cardiac complications are stated to occur in 50% of resuscitated patients, ranging from transient – but sometimes severe – impairment of myocardial function (occurring early and normalizing several days later) to permanent malfunction and fatal rearrest. The severe impairment of myocardial function in the early hours following resuscitation accounts for 25% to 45% of early postresuscitation deaths.[23–25]

The global nature of ischemic myocardial dysfunction[38] and also its occurrence following resuscitation from respiratory arrest[39] or electroconvulsive treatment[40] strongly support its role during cardiac arrest and cardiopulmonary resuscitation as the primary etiological determinant, as opposed to the role of the primary cause of arrest which is cardiac in 55%–65% of cases.[41]

The severity and duration of postresuscitation myocardial impairment is a function of both duration of cardiac arrest and subsequent resuscitation efforts,[16–42] with a contribution from adrenaline (epinephrine) used during CPR,[43,44] and the energy and waveform required for defibrillation.[45,46] In humans, the dose of adrenaline used during CPR has been reported to be the only variable independently associated with postresuscitation myocardial dysfunction.[44]

Pathophysiology

The mechanisms responsible for myocardial stunning after global myocardial ischemia remain unclear, but several hypothesis have been proposed. Among these are the postreperfusion long-lasting depletion of the total adenine nucleotide pool, the generation of oxygen-derived free radicals, calcium overload, and uncoupling of excitation-contraction due to sarcoplasmic reticulum dysfunction.[37,38]

Recently, a correlation has been established between levels of proinflammatory cytokines, synthesized and released in response to the stress of global ischemia, and the depression of myocardial function in the early postresuscitation period.[47]

Clinical features

In animal studies, postresuscitation myocardial dysfunction is characterized by increased filling pressures, impaired contractile function, decreased cardiac index, decrease in both systolic and diastolic right ventricular function,[16,38] starting at 2–6 hours and returning to normal at 24 hours postresuscitation.

These findings were confirmed initially by anedoctal observations of prolonged reversible myocardial dysfunction in human cardiac arrest survivors[50,51] and, later, were better defined in systematic studies in patients.[44,52]

The global nature of postresuscitation dysfunction has been demonstrated with echocardiography and ventriculography, which show a decrease in ejection fraction and in fractional shortening.

Myocardial dysfunction in patients may improve at 24–48 hours postresuscitation with return to normal values; persistently low cardiac index at 24 hours postresuscitation is associated with early death by multiple organ failure.[44] In the same study, despite the significant improvement of cardiac index at 24 hours, persisting vasodilatation was described, delaying the discontinuation of vasoactive drugs.

In parallel with the failure of the heart to sustain normal circulation, a condition of altered peripheral oxygen utilization has been described.[44] These two mechanisms together account for the persistent anaerobic metabolism characteristic of the early postresuscitation phase.

Relationship to neurological recovery and outcome

The cardiovascular impairment in the early postresuscitation hours has been reported to correlate with impaired cerebral recovery from the ischemic insult of cardiac arrest.[16]

Indirect evidence of the role of impaired perfusion on cerebral recovery comes from the beneficial effect of cardiopulmonary bypass in augmenting flow after cardiac arrest.[15]

In cardiac arrest survivors, good functional neurological recovery has been independently and positively associated with arterial blood pressure during the first 2 hours postresuscitation, whereas hypotensive episodes correlate with poor cerebral outcome.[52] The latter finding could be explained by the loss or impairment of cerebral autoregulation in comatose patients resuscitated from cardiac arrest, causing a reduction in cerebral blood flow if blood pressure is low.[54,55]

The finding of a correlation between low cardiac index and neurologic outcome, however, has not been confirmed in a recent study in humans.[44]

Treatment

Successful treatment of myocardial dysfunction could reduce or prevent the cardiac causes of death that are the major determinants of early postresuscitation deaths.

Treatment with dobutamine has proved effective in supporting output and pressure during the postresuscitation phase prior to return to baseline function.[56] A dobutamine dose of 5 mcg/kg min has been shown to be better than a dose of 2 or 7.5 mcg/kg min, and better than placebo or aortic counterpulsation in sustaining cardiovascular performance for 6 hours postresuscitation.[56–58]

The similarities in cardiovascular status between septic and postresuscitation patients have suggested that in addition to the inotropic support with dobutamine the 'early goal-directed therapy' that has proved effective in severe sepsis should be included[59] – namely normalization of intravascular volume, of blood pressure by vasoactive drugs, and of oxygen transport by red cell transfusion during the first 6 hours postresuscitation.[11,12] Data on its effectiveness in cardiac arrest patients are not yet available.

Extracerebral extracardiac function postresuscitation

The extracerebral extracardiac function derangements, accounting for one-third of deaths,[23–25] represent the less specific component of the postresuscitation syndrome.[11,12]

In patients surviving the early postresuscitation phase, cardiovascular function improves, neurologic function may show gradual improvement or remain severely compromised, but conditions facilitating the development of sepsis are created, leading ultimately to multiorgan dysfunction.

Systemic findings and pathogenesis

The direct effect of cardiac arrest, besides its role in neuronal injury and myocardial dysfunction, is also involved in the genesis of coagulation disturbances,[60] endothelial injury,[60,61] and in triggering the cascades of inflammatory responses.[7,63]

A variety of changes and findings, which still need to be clearly classified and systematized, have been described following resuscitation from cardiac arrest:
- a considerable increase in various acute phase response proteins[64]
- a sharp rise in plasma cytokines and soluble receptors within the blood compartment as early as 3 hours postarrest[31,46,65–69]
- endothelial injury and release of intracellular adhesion molecules
- marked activation of complement, polymorphonuclear (PMN) leukocytes, and an increased PMN-endothelial interaction[61–64]
- marked activation of blood coagulation and fibrinolysis[60]
- leukocyte dysregulation[11,12]
- evidence of the presence of endotoxin in plasma

The complex interaction of endothelial injury, inflammatory and procoagulant host responses, intravascular fibrin formation, and microvascular thrombosis contribute to reperfusion defects,[7,60,64] which augment systemic hypoperfusion induced by cardiovascular dysfunction to trigger a secondary insult of persisting anerobic metabolism.

The altered systemic oxygen utilization, together with circulating endotoxin and immune hyporeactivity, may facilitate development of infection.[11,12]

Extracerebral and extracardiac organs, however, can tolerate periods of ischemia much longer than those generally occurring in cardiac arrest and resuscitation: thus, the impairment of function in these organs appears to be the combined result of the mechanisms triggered by ischemia but compounded by reperfusion.

Derangements of organ function

Clotting and fibrinolytic function
Starting during cardiopulmonary resuscitation, marked activation of coagulation has been demonstrated, without adequate concomitant activation of endogenous fibrinolysis,[60,70] suggesting that intravascular fibrin formation and microvascular thrombosis after cardiac arrest may contribute to organ dysfunction, including neurological impairment. With restoration of spontaneous circulation and reperfusion, coagulation activity (thrombin-antithrombin complex) increases, anticoagulation (antithrombin, protein C, and protein S) decreases, and

fibrinolysis (plasmin–antiplasmin complex) is activated or in some cases inhibited (increased plasminogen activator inhibitor-1 with a peak on day 1). These abnormalities are more severe in patients dying within 2 days and most severe in patients dying from early refractory shock. Protein C and S levels are low compared with those in healthy volunteers and discriminated OHCA survivors from non-survivors.[66]

Marked activation of complement, polymorphonuclear leukocytes, and an increased PMN-endothelieal interaction have been clearly demonstrated during cardiopulmonary resuscitation and early reperfusion after cardiac arrest in humans.[62]

Adrenal function

Serum cortisol levels have been reported consistently to be high in all patients resuscitated from cardiac arrest for up to 36 hours postresuscitation,[74–76] with lower levels in non-survivors,[74] particularly in those who died of early refractory shock.[76]

Relative adrenal insufficiency as assessed by corticotropin tests was observed in 42% of patients but showed no association with arrest duration variables or with outcome.[76]

Renal function

Renal dysfunction,[77] was recently confirmed in patients presenting with hemodynamic instability and was characterized by significant increases in plasma creatinine and by a decrease in the International Normalized Ratio.[44]

Intestinal function

Following cardiac arrest and reperfusion, severe intestinal ischemia occurs, showing a pattern of metabolic extracellular changes similar to those recorded in the brain.[78] It is associated with early intestinal dysfunction and/or endoscopic lesions identified in 60% of patients.[79]

A role for ischemia-reperfusion-mediated increase in intestinal permeability has been proposed as predisposing the patient to the sepsis syndrome.

Endotoxin and infection

The finding of plasma endotoxin detected in 46% of patients 1–2 days after resuscitation (although with no relation to outcome), and of endotoxin-dependent hyporeactivity of patients' leukocytes, with high levels of circulating cytokines and dysregulated production of plasma cytokines, delineates an immunological pattern similar to the profile characterizing patients with sepsis. Half of endotoxin-positive patients have been found to develop secondarily acquired bacterial infection 3–4 days postresuscitation (mostly pulmonary, occasionally bacteremia).[11,12]

The finding of bacteremia, generally associated with pathogens of intestinal origin, occurring in 39% of patients within the first 24 hours of admission postresuscitation associated with increased mortality,[80] was not confirmed in a subsequent study in which bacteremia was encountered only sporadically.[12]

The incidence of pneumonia in patients admitted to the ICU following cardiac arrest has been reported to vary from 24% to 45% of patients.[9,81]

In a systematic study,[82] newly acquired infection developed in 46% of patients resuscitated from cardiac arrest and admitted to the ICU, the most common being pneumonia (65% of infections). Compared with cardiac arrest survivors without infection, patients with infection had longer mechanical ventilation and ICU length of stay, but mortality was similar.

A possible role for procalcitonin has been proposed for the early identification of post-resuscitation patients with an acute phase response and bacterial complications: it was the only marker higher in patients with ventilator-acquired pneumonia.[83]

Hyperthermia not associated with positive blood cultures has been reported frequently during the first 24 hours following CPR, suggesting that mechanisms other than infection may contribute to the development of fever in cardiac arrest survivors.[82,84]

Correlation with outcome

The peak level and the time of occurrence of many of the above-mentioned mediators of the inflammatory response have been reported to correlate with outcome (differently defined as: early death, early death from cardiac causes, death at 1 month, and others) in different case series from single centers and without precise standardization of resuscitation procedures and postresuscitation treatments.[61–72]

The data now available suggest the opportunity for a reassessment and systematic analysis of the interactions involving various cascades and of their role in determining outcome in a well-designed multicenter study adopting a standardized treatment and evaluation protocol.

The better characterization of PRS in its early phase is confirmed by the high predictive value of cerebral impairment, the severity of which can be quantified, allowing a reliable prognostication of outcome.[47,52]

In the later phase of PRS, when secondary multiple organ derangement syndrome (MODS) becomes apparent, the existing limitations of prognostic evaluation based on severity scoring systems[85] inherent to MODS are further complicated by the persisting postischemic impairment of cerebral function.

Treatment

Similar to the treatment of patients with impaired cardiovascular function, in PRS patients showing extracerebral and extracadiac impairment, the standard treatment encompasses mild hypothermia induced after reperfusion from cardiac arrest to improve neurological outcome[9,10] and dobutamine to sustain transient myocardial dysfunction.[56–58] Mild hypothermia has been hypothesized to interfere with the inflammatory cascades of cardiac arrest in its effect on survival.

One interesting trial studied the effect of isovolumic high-volume hemofiltration (HF) (200 ml/kg/h over 8 hours) with and without hypothermia, in an attempt to remove circulating molecules believed to be responsible for ischemia-reperfusion injury.[86] Compared with controls, the high-volume hemofiltration with and without hypothermia decreased the relative risk of death from intractable shock and improved survival. Nonetheless, definite conclusions must await larger randomized clinical trials testing the combination of HF with hypothermia in a larger cohort of cardiac arrest survivors.

The relevance of the quality of in-hospital treatment and its impact on overall outcome after resuscitation from cardiac arrest has been confirmed in two studies showing that factors associated with better outcome encompassed: the condition of patients prearrest (age under median 71 years old and better overall performance category prearrest); prehospital care (shorter time from emergency call to CPR initiation and no use of adrenaline); and in-hospital care (no seizure activity, temperature under 37.8 °C (median), S-glucose under 10.6 mmol/l 24 hours after admission (median), and BE over >3.5 mmol/l 12 hours (median) after admission).[87,88]

Summary

Widespread implementation of adequate system responses and application of resuscitation techniques to reverse clinical death increase both the rate of optimal recovery and, by raising the number of patients with restored spontaneous circulation, the occurrence of PRS.

Reduction of the duration of ischemia is the most obvious intervention to prevent development of PRS; nevertheless, strengthening the "chain of survival," may also restore spontaneous circulation in patients who otherwise would not have been revived and are at high risk for the development of this complex condition.

During the first 24 hours postresuscitation, the PRS is well characterized and requires aggressive treatment, aimed at reducing the progression of cerebral injury and the effects of the secondary insult determined by impaired cardiovascular performance. Besides standard intensive care support of impaired function, the gold standard includes mild hypothermia maintained for at least 12 hours and optimization of perfusion and oxygen delivery.

After the first 24 hours postresuscitation, the clinical picture is not different from that of a comatose intensive care patient. The role of the quality of treatment administered in this phase has been shown and includes brain-oriented care (prevention of hyperthermia and seizures, optimization of perfusion, glucose and metabolic control), and standard intensive care oriented to prevention of infection and support of impaired organ function.

It is of paramount importance to optimize postresuscitation treatment in the first 2–3 days after the arrest, until reliable prognostic instruments permit the prediction of an unfavorable neurologic outcome, in order to exclude self-fulfilling prophecies and provide sound information to families, but also to plan the continuation of appropriate treatment strategies.

Promising prognostic markers of the acute phase response and treatment strategies, aimed at improving disturbances in microcirculation and reducing the impact of the specific inflammatory response, deserve further evaluation in systematic, well-controlled studies.

REFERENCES

1. Safar, P. Effects of the postresuscitation syndrome on cerebral recovery from cardiac arrest. *Crit. Care Med.* 1985; **13**: 932–935.
2. Pell, J.P., Sirel, J.M., Marsden, A.K., Ford, I., Walker, N.L. & Cobbe, S.M. Presentation, management, and outcome of out of hospital cardiopulmonary arrest: comparison by underlying aetiology. *Heart* 2003; **89**: 839–42.
3. Cummins, R.O., Ornato, J.P., Thies, W.H. & Pepe, P.E. Improving survival from sudden cardiac arrest: the 'chain of survival' concept: a statement for health professionals from the Advanced Cardiac Life Support Subcommittee and the Emergency Cardiac Care Committee. American Heart Association. *Circulation* 1991; **83**: 1832–1847.
4. Negovsky, V.A. The second step in resuscitation: the treatment of the post-resuscitation disease. *Resuscitation* 1972; **1**: 1–7.
5. Negovsky, V.A., Gurvitch, A.M. & Zolo-tokrylina, E.S. *Postresuscitation Disease*. Amsterdam: Elsevier, 1983.
6. Safar, P. Resuscitation from clinical death. *Crit. Care Med.* 1988; **16**: 923–941.

7. Safar, P., Behringer, W., Böttiger, B.W. *et al*. Cerebral resuscitation potentials for cardiac arrest. *Crit. Care Med.* 2002, **30**(Suppl): 140–144.

8. Cerchiari, E.L. & Ferrante, M. Postresuscitation syndrome. In Paradis, N.A., Halperin, H.R. & Novak, R.M. *Cardiac Arrest. The Science and Practice of Resuscitation Medicine*. Baltimore: Williams and Wilkins, 1996; 837–949.

9. The Hypothermia After Cardiac Arrest study group: Mild therapeutic hypothermia to improve the neurologic outcome after cardiac arrest. *N. Engl. J. Med.* 2002, **346**: 549–556.

10. Bernard, S.A., Gray, T.W., Buist, M.D. *et al*. Treatment of comatose survivors of out-of-hospital cardiac arrest with induced hypothermia. *N. Engl. J. Med.* 2002, **346**: 557–563.

11. Adrie, C., Adib-Conquy, M., Laurent, I. *et al*. Successful cardiopulmonary resuscitation after cardiac arrest as a "sepsis-like" syndrome. *Circulation* 2002; **106**: 562–568.

12. Adrie, C., Laurent, I., Monchi, M. *et al*. Postresuscitation disease after cardiac arrest: a sepsis-like syndrome? *Curr. Opin. Crit. Care* 2004; **10**: 208–212.

13. Pulsinelli, W.A., Brierley, J.B. & Plum, F. Temporal profile of neuronal damage in a model of transient forebrain ischemia. *Ann. Neurol.* 1982; **11**: 491–498.

14. Vaagenes, P., Cantadore, R., Safar, P. *et al*. Amelioration of brain damage by lidoflazine after prolonged ventricular fibrillation cardiac arrest in dogs. *Crit. Care Med.* 1984; **12**: 846–855.

15. Safar, P., Abramson, N.S., Angelos, M. *et al*. Emergency cardiopulmonary bypass for resuscitation from prolonged cardiac arrest. *Am. J. Emerg. Med.* 1990; **8**: 55–67.

16. Cerchiari, E.L., Safar, P., Klein, E., Cantadore, R. & Pinsky, M. Cardiovascular function and neurologic outcome after cardiac arrest in dogs: the cardiovascular post-resuscitation syndrome. *Resuscitation* 1993; **25**: 9–33.

17. Cerchiari, E.L., Safar, P., Klein, E. & Diven, W. Visceral post-resuscitation syndrome and neurologic outcome. *Resuscitation* 1993; **25**: 119–136.

18. Hossmann, K.A. & Hossmann, V. Coagulopathy following experimental cerebral ischemia. *Stroke* 1977; **8**: 249–253.

19. Sterz, F., Safar, P., Diven, W., Leonov, Y., Radovsky, A. & Oku, K. Detoxification with hemabsorption after cardiac arrest does not improve neurologic recovery. *Resuscitation* 1993; **25**: 137–160.

20. Rea, T.D., Eisenberg, M.S., Sinibaldi, G. & White, R.D. Incidence of EMS-treated out-of-hospital cardiac arrest in the United States. *Resuscitation* 2004; **63**: 17–24.

21. Parish, D.C., Dane, F.C., Montgomery, M. *et al*. Resuscitation in the hospital: differential relationships between age and survival across rhythms. *Crit. Care Med.* 1999; **27**: 2137–2141.

22. Peberdy, M.A., Kaye, W., Ornato, J.P. *et al*. Cardiopulmonary resuscitation of adults in the hospital: a report of 14,720 cardiac arrests from the National Registry of Cardiopulmonary Resuscitation. *Resuscitation* 2003; **58**: 297–308.

23. Brain Resuscitation Clinical Trial I Study Group. Randomized clinical study of thiopental loading in comatose survivors of cardiac arrest. *N. Engl. J. Med.* 1986; **314**: 397–403.

24. Brain Resuscitation Clinical Trial 2 Study Group. A randomized clinical study of calcium-entry blocker in the treatment of comatose survivors of cardiac arrest. *N. Engl. J. Med.* 1991; **324**: 1125–1131.

25. Becker, L.B., Ostrander, M.P., Barrett, J. *et al*. Outcome of cardiopulmonary resuscitation in a large metropolitan area: where are the survivors? *Ann. Emerg. Med.* 1991; **20**: 355–361.

26. Niemann, J.T. & Stratton, S.J. The Utstein template and the effect of in-hospital decisions: the impact of do-not-attempt resuscitation status on survival to discharge statistics. *Resuscitation* 2001; **51**: 233–237.

27. Madl, C. Holzer, M. Brain function after resuscitation from cardiac arrest *Curr. Opin. Crit. Care* 2004; **10**: 213–217.

28. Bottiger, B.W., Motsch, J., Bohrer, H. *et al*. Activation of blood coagulation following cardiac arrest is not balanced adequately by activation of endogenous fibrinolysis. *Circulation* 1995; **92**: 2572–2578.

29. Krep, H., Bottiger, B.W., Bock, C. *et al*. Time course of circulatory and metabolic recovery of cat brain after cardiac arrest assessed by perfusion- and diffusion weighted imaging and MR-spectroscopy. *Resuscitation* 2003; **58**: 337–348.

30. Schaafsma, A., de Jong, B.M., Bams, J.L. *et al*. Cerebral perfusion and metabolism in resuscitated patients with severe posthypoxic encephalopathy. *J. Neurol. Sci.* 2003; **210**: 23–30.

31. Mussack, T. & Peter Biberthaler, P.A., Cornelia Gippner-Steppert, C. *et al*. Early cellular brain damage and systemic inflammatory response after cardiopulmonary resuscitation or isolated severe head trauma: a comparative pilot study on common pathomechanisms. *Resuscitation* 2001; **49**: 193–199.

32. Booth, C.M., Boone, R.H., Tomlinson, G. & Detsky, A.S. Is this patient dead, vegetative, or severely neurologically impaired? Assessing outcome for comatose survivors of cardiac arrest. *J. Am. Med. Assoc.* 2004; **291**: 870–879.

33. Robinson, L.R., Micklesen, P.J., Tirschwell, D.L. *et al*. Predictive value of somatosensory evoked potentials for awakening from coma. *Crit. Care Med.* 2003; **31**: 960–967.

34. Meynaar, I.A., Oudemans-van Straaten, H.W., Wetering, J. *et al*. Serum neuron-specific enolase predicts outcome in postanoxic coma: a prospective cohort study. *Intens. Care Med.* 2003; **29**: 189–195.

35. Böttiger, B.W., Bode, C., Kern, S. *et al*. Efficacy and safety of thrombolytic therapy after initially unsuccessful cardiopulmonary resuscitation: a prospective clinical trial. *Lancet* 2001; **357**: 1583–1585.

36. Spohr, H.R., Bluhmki, E. *et al*. International multicentre trail protocol to assess the efficacy and safety of tneecteplase during cardiopulmonay resiscitation in patients with out-of-hospital cardiac arrest: the Thrombolysis in Cardiac Arrest (TROICA) Study. *Eur. J. Clin. Invest.* 2005; **35**: 315–323.

37. Elmenyar, A.A. Postresuscitation myocardial stunning and its outcome. *Crit. Pathways Cardiol.* 2004; **3**: 209–215.

38. Kern, K.B. Postresuscitation myocardial dysfunction. *Cardiol. Clin.* 2002; **20**: 89–101.

39. Bashir, R., Padder, F.A. & Khan, F.A. Myocardial stunning following respiratory arrest. *Chest.* 1995; **108**: 1459–1460.

40. Wei, X. Myocardial stunning electroconvulsive therapy. *Ann. Intern. Med* 1995; **117**: 914–915.

41. Engdahl, J., Holmberg, M., Karlson, B.W., Luepker, R. & Herlitz, J. The epidemiology of out-of-hospital 'sudden' cardiac arrest. *Resuscitation* 2002; **52**(3): 235–245.

42. Kern, K.B., Hilwig, R.W., Rhee, K.H. & Berg, R.A. Myocardial dysfunction after resuscitation from cardiac arrest: an example of global myocardial stunning. *J. Am. Coll. Cardiol.* 1996; **28**: 232–240.

43. Tang, W., Weil, M.H., Sun, S. *et al.* Epinephrine increases the severity of postresuscitation myocardial dysfunction. *Circulation* 1995; **92**: 3089–3093.

44. Laurent *et al.* Myocardial dysfunction after cardiac arrest. *J. Am. Coll. Cardiol.* 2000; **40**(12): 2110–2116.

45. Xie, J., Weil, M.H., Sun, S.J. *et al.* High-energy defibrillation increases the severity of postresuscitation myocardial dysfunction. *Circulation* 1997; **96**: 683–688.

46. Tang, W., Weil, M.H., Sun, S. *et al.* The effects of biphasic waveform design on post-resuscitation myocardial function. *J. Am. Coll. Cardiol.* 2004; **43**: 1228–1235.

47. Jennings, R.B., Murry, C.E. & Steenbergen, C. Jr. Development of cell injury in sustained acute ischemia. *Circulation* 1990; **82**(Suppl 3): 2–12.

48. Bolli, R. & Marban, E. Molecular and cellular mechanisms of myocardial stunning. *Physiol. Rev.* 1999; **79**: 609–634.

49. Niemann, J.T., Garner, D. & Lewis, R.J. Tumor necrosis factor is associated with early postresuscitation myocardial dysfunction. *Crit. Care Med.* 2004; **32**: 1753–1758.

50. De Antonio, A.J., Kaul, S. & Lerman, B.B. Reversible myocardial depression in survivors of cardiac arrest. *PACE* 1990; **13**: 982–986.

51. Rivers, E.P., Rady, M.Y., Martin, G.B., Smithline, H.A., Alexander, M.E. & Nowak, R.M. Venous hyperoxia after cardiac arrest: characterization of a defect in systemic oxygen utilization. *Chest* 1992; **102**: 1787–1793.

52. Mullner, M., Domanovits, H., Sterz, F. *et al.* Measurement of myocardial contractility following successful resuscitation: quantitated left ventricular systolic function utilising non-invasive wall stress analysis. *Resuscitation* 1998; **39**: 51–59.

53. Mullner, M., Sterz, F., Binder, M. *et al.* Arterial blood pressure after human cardiac arrest and neurological recovery. *Stroke* 1996; **27**: 59–62.

54. Nishizawa, H. & Kudoh, I. Cerebral autoregulation is impaired in patients resuscitated after cardiac arrest. *Acta Anaesthesiol. Scand.* 1996; **40**: 1149–1153.

55. Sundgreen, C., Larsen, F.S., Herzog, T.M., Knudsen, G.M., Boesgaard, S. & Aldershvile, J. Autoregulation of cerebral blood flow in patients resuscitated from cardiac arrest. *Stroke* 2001; **32**: 128–132.

56. Tennyson, H., Kern, K.B., Hilwig, R.W., Berg, R.A. & Ewy, G.A. Treatment of post resuscitation myocardial dysfunction: aortic counterpulsation versus dobutamine. *Resuscitation* 2002; **54**: 69–75.

57. Vasquez, A., Kern, K.B., Hilwig, R.W., Heidenreich, J., Berg, R.A. & Ewy, G.A. Optimal dosing of dobutamine for treating post-resuscitation left ventricular dysfunction. *Resuscitation* 2004; **61**: 199–207.

58. Meyer, R.J., Kern, K.B., Berg, R.A., Hilwig, R.W. & Ewy, G.A. Postresuscitation right ventricular dysfunction: delineation and treatment with dobutamine. *Resuscitation* 2002; **55**: 187–191.

59. Rivers, E., Nguyen, B., Havstad, S. *et al.* Early goal-directed therapy in the treatment of severe sepsis and septic shock. *N. Engl. J. Med.* 2001; **345**: 1368–1377.

60. Böttiger, B.W., Motsch, J., Böhrer, H. *et al.* Activation of blood coagulation after cardiac arrest is not balanced adequately by activation of endogenous fibrinolysis *Circulation* 1995; **92**: 2572–2578.

61. Gando, S., Nanzaki, S., Morimoto, Y. *et al.* Out-of-hospital cardiac arrest increases soluble vascular endothelial adhesion molecules and neutrophil elastase associated with endothelial injury. *Intens. Care Med.* 2000; **26**: 38–44.

62. Böttiger, B.W., Motsch, J., Braun, V. *et al.* Marked activation of complement and leukocytes and an increase in the concentrations of soluble endothelial adhesion molecules during cardiopulmonary resuscitation and early reperfusion after cardiac arrest in humans. *Crit. Care Med.* 2002; **30**: 2473–2480.

63. Geppert, A., Zorn, G., Karth, G.D. *et al.* Soluble selectins and the systemic inflammatory response syndrome after successful cardiopulmonary resuscitation. *Crit. Care Med.* 2000; **28**: 2360–2365.

64. Geppert, A., Zorn, G., Delle-Karth, G. *et al.* Plasma concentrations of von Willebrand factor and intracellular adhesion molecule-1 for prediction of outcome after successful cardiopulmonary resuscitation. *Crit. Care Med.* 2003; **31**: 805–811.

65. Oppert, M., Gleiter, C.H., Müller, C. *et al.* Kinetics and characteristics of an acute phase response following cardiac arrest. *Intens. Care Med.* 1999; **25**: 1386–1394.

66. Adrie, C., Monchi, M., Laurent, I. *et al.* Coagulopathy after successful cardiopulmonary resuscitation following cardiac arrest – implication of the protein C anticoagulant pathway. *J. Am. Coll. Cardiol.* 2005; **46**: 21–28.

67. Gando, S., Nanzaki, S., Morimoto, Y., Kobayashi, S. & Kemmotsu, O. Tissue factor and tissue factor pathway inhibitor levels during and after cardiopulmonary resuscitation. *Thromb. Res.* 1999; **96**: 107–113.

68. Kempski, O. & Behmanesh, S. Endothelial cell swelling and brain perfusion. *J. Trauma.* 1997; **42**: S38–S40.

69. Ito, T., Saitoh, D., Fukuzuka, K. *et al.* Significance of elevated serum interleukin-8 in patients resuscitated after cardiopulmonary arrest. *Resuscitation* 2001; **51**: 47–53.

70. Shyu, K., Chang, H., Likn, C. *et al.* Concentrations of serum interleukin-8 after successful cardiopulmonary resuscitation in patients with cardiopulmonary arrest. *Am. Heart. J.* 1997; **134**: 551–556.

71. Gando, S., Nanzaki, S., Morimoto, Y. *et al.* Alterations of soluble L- and P-selectins during cardiac arrest and CPR. *Intens. Care Med.* 1999; **25**: 588–593.

72. Fries, M., Kunz, D., Gressner, A.M. *et al.* Procalcitonin serum levels after out-of-hospital cardiac arrest. *Resuscitation* 2003; **59**: 105–109.

73. Gando, S., Kameue, T., Nanzaki, S. *et al.* Massive fibrin formation with consecutive impairment of fibrinolysis in patients with out-of-hospital cardiac arrest. *Thromb. Haemost.* 1997; **77**: 278–282.

74. Schultz, C.H., Rivers, E.P., Feldkamp, C.S. *et al.* A characterization of hypothalamic-pituitaryadrenal axis function during and after human cardiac arrest. *Crit. Care Med.* 1993; **21**: 1339–1347.

75. Ito, T., Saitoh, D., Takasu, A. *et al.* Serum cortisol as a predictive marker of the outcome in patients resuscitated after cardiopulmonary arrest arrest *Resuscitation* 2004; **62**: 55–60.

76. Hékimian, G., Baugnon, T., Thuong, M. *et al.* Cortisol levels and adrenal reserve after successful cardiac arrest resuscitation. *SHOCK*, 2004; **22** (2): 116–119.

77. Mattana, J. & Singhal, P.C. Prevalence and determinants of acute renal failure following cardiopulmonary resuscitation. *Arch. Intern. Med.* 1993; **153**: 235–239.

78. Korth, U., Krieter, H., Denz, C. *et al.* Intestinal ischaemia during cardiac arrest and resuscitation: comparative analysis of extracellular metabolites by microdialysis, *Resuscitation* 2003; **58**: 209–217.

79. L'Her, E., Cassaz, C., Le Gal, G. *et al.* Gut dysfunction and endoscopic lesions after out-of-hospital cardiac arrest *Resuscitation* 2005; **66**: 331–334.

80. Gaussorgues, P., Gueugniaud, P.Y., Vedrinne, J.M. *et al.* Bacteraemia following cardiac arrest and cardiopulmonary resuscitation. *Intens. Care Med.* 1998; **14**: 575–577.

81. Rello, J., Valles, J., Jubert, P. *et al.* Lower respiratory tract infections following cardiac arrest and cardiopulmonary resuscitation. *Clin. Infect. Dis.* 1995; **21**: 310–314.

82. Gajic, O., Emir Festic, E. & Afessa, B. Infectious complications in survivors of cardiac arrest admitted to the medical intensive care unit, *Resuscitation* 2004; **60**: 65–69.

83. Oppert, M., Albrecht Reinicke, A., Christian Muller, C. *et al.* Elevations in procalcitonin but not C-reactive protein are associated with pneumonia after cardiopulmonary resuscitation *Resuscitation* 2002; **53**: 167–170.

84. Takino, M. & Okada, Y. Hyperthermia following cardiopulmonary resuscitation. *Intens. Care Med.* 1991; **17**: 419–420.

85. Bone, R.C., Balk, R.A., Cerra, F.B. *et al.* (The ACCP/SCCM Consensus Conference Committee). Definitions for sepsis and organ failure and guidelines for the use of innovative therapies in sepsis. *Chest* 1992; **101**: 1644–1655.

86. Laurent, I., Adrie, C., Vinsonneau, C. *et al.* High-volume hemofiltration to improve prognosis after cardiac arrest – a randomised study *J. Am. Coll. Cardiol.* 2005; **46**: 432–437.

87. Langhelle, A., Tyvold, S.S., Lexow, K. *et al.* In-hospital factors associated with improved outcome after out-of-hospital cardiac arrest. A comparison between four regions in Norway. *Resuscitation* 2003; **56**: 247–263.

88. Skrifvars, M.B., Rosenberg, P.H., Finne, P. *et al.* Evaluation of the in-hospital Utstein template in cardiopulmonary resuscitation in secondary hospitals *Resuscitation* 2003; **56**: 275–282.

48

Prevention and therapy of postresuscitation myocardial dysfunction

Raúl J. Gazmuri[1], Max Harry Weil[2], Karl B. Kern[3], Wanchun Tang[4],
Iyad M. Ayoub[5], Julieta Kolarova[6], Jeejabai Radhakrishnan[7]

[1] North Chicago VA Medical Center, IL, USA, [2] Rancho Springs, CA, [3] Tucson, AZ, [4] Palm Springs, CA, [5] North Chicago, IL, [6] North Chicago, IL, [7] North Chicago, IL

Introduction

It is estimated that between 400 000 and 460 000 individuals suffer an episode of sudden cardiac arrest every year in the United States.[1] Yet, the percentage of individuals who are successfully resuscitated and leave the hospital alive with intact neurological function averages less than 10% nationwide.[2-4] Efforts to restore life successfully are formidably challenging. They require not only that cardiac activity be initially restored but that injury to vital organs be prevented or minimized. A closer examination of resuscitation statistics reveals that efficient Emergency Medical Services systems are able to re-establish cardiac activity in 30% to 40% of sudden cardiac arrest victims at the scene.[5-7] Yet, close to 40% die before admission to a hospital presumably from recurrent cardiac arrest or complications during transport.[8] Of those admitted to the hospital nearly 60% succumb before discharge, such that only one in four initially resuscitated victims leaves the hospital alive.

Although the causes of postresuscitation deaths have not been systematically investigated, the available information suggests that postresuscitation myocardial dysfunction, hypoxic brain damage, systemic inflammatory responses, intercurrent illnesses, or a combination thereof are the main culprits.[8-10] The core pathogenic process driving such poor outcome is the intense ischemia of variable duration that organs suffer after cessation of blood flow and the subsequent reperfusion injury that accompanies the resuscitation effort. In addition, the precipitating event of cardiac arrest may also play a role in the post-resuscitation phase.

This chapter focuses on the effects of cardiac arrest and resuscitation on the myocardium, mindful that many other organs are concomitantly affected by similar mechanisms of cell injury. The chapter is organized to describe: (1) the functional myocardial abnormalities that occur during and after resuscitation from cardiac arrest; (2) the underlying cellular mechanisms of such injury; (3) factors that may contribute to myocardial injury; (4) therapies that have been shown in the laboratory to prevent or ameliorate myocardial injury; and (5) the management of postresuscitation myocardial dysfunction. As the chapter develops the reader will learn that postresuscitation myocardial dysfunction is largely a reversible phenomenon such that support of the failing heart during the critical postresuscitation interval is fully justified.

Functional myocardial manifestations

The working heart is a highly metabolically active organ that consumes close to 10% of the total body oxygen consumption and extracts nearly 70% of the oxygen supplied by the coronary circuit. Nevertheless, it has minimal capability for extracting additional oxygen such that increased metabolic demands are met through coronary vasodilation with augmentation of blood flow and oxygen delivery.[11,12] Consequently, a severe energy imbalance develops immediately after cardiac arrest supervenes and coronary blood flow ceases. The severity of the energy deficit is contingent on the metabolic requirements and is particularly high in the setting of ventricular fibrillation (VF) when the oxygen requirements are comparable to or exceed that of the normally beating heart.[13,14] A lesser energy deficit is anticipated when cardiac arrest occurs in a quiescent or minimally active heart (i.e., asystole or pulseless electrical activity as a result of asphyxia or exsanguination).[15] Because most experimental studies have examined the myocardial manifestations of cardiac arrest and resuscitation in animal models of VF, caution should be exercised when extrapolating these findings to cardiac arrest settings precipitated by mechanisms other than VF.

With cessation of coronary blood flow and oxygen availability, the mitochondrial capability for regenerating ATP through oxidative phosphorylation stops, prompting anaerobic regeneration of limited amounts of ATP at the substrate level from breakdown of creatine phosphate and oxidation of pyruvate to lactate.[16–18] Hence, there is rapid depletion of creatine phosphate, marked elevation in lactate, and a relatively slow depletion of ATP.[17] In one recent study in a rat model of VF, 10 minutes of untreated VF were accompanied by decreases in myocardial creatine phosphate and ATP to levels 7% and 19% of baseline, respectively, whereas the lactate content increased by more than 50-fold.[19] Coincident with the energy deficit, accumulation of CO_2 and H^+ account for profound myocardial acidosis.[18,20]

When conventional closed-chest resuscitation is used, the coronary blood flow generated rarely exceeds 20% of the normal flow,[21] thus failing to reverse myocardial ischemia. In addition, reperfusion of ischemic myocardium activates multiple pathogenic mechanisms, leading to what is known as reperfusion injury. Accordingly, resuscitation typically proceeds during and in spite of severe myocardial ischemia and in the midst of reperfusion injury compounded by specific interventions, such as electrical shocks and adrenergic vasopressor agents, that can also contribute to myocardial injury. As a result, various functional myocardial abnormalities develop that may themselves compromise resuscitability and survival. These myocardial abnormalities represent a continuum along the injury process that can be grouped into those that manifest during the resuscitation effort and those that manifest after the return of spontaneous circulation. The former include ischemic contracture and increased resistance to electrical defibrillation; the latter include reperfusion arrhythmias and myocardial dysfunction.

Ischemic contracture

Ischemic contracture refers to progressive left ventricular wall thickening with parallel reductions in cavity size consequent to myocardial ischemia. Ischemic contracture was first reported in the early 1970s during open heart surgery when operations were conducted under normothermic conditions and in the fibrillating heart to render a bloodless surgical field.[22,23] The onset of ischemic contracture in this setting was associated with reductions in myocardial ATP levels to < 10% of normal.[24] An extreme manifestation of ischemic contracture is the so-called "stony heart" and typically heralds irreversible ischemic injury.

More recent studies in animal models of VF and closed chest resuscitation have demonstrated a phenomenon akin to ischemic contracture, but of earlier onset and associated with less ATP depletion.[25,26] This form of ischemic contracture is likely to represent a manifestation of reperfusion injury[27] such that withholding chest compression (and hence coronary blood flow) markedly delays the onset of contracture.[28,29] The resulting left ventricular thickening with reductions in cavity size compromises ventricular preload and the amount of blood that can be ejected by chest compression.[14,27,30] Thus, ischemic contracture may partly explain the characteristic time-dependent reductions in the hemodynamic efficacy of chest compression.[31] Moreover, recent studies in a porcine model of VF demonstrate that the severity of ischemic contracture is proportional to the preceding interval of untreated VF.[26] In humans, ischemic contracture has been described as myocardial "firmness" during open-chest resuscitation after failure of closed-chest attempts and found also to compromise resuscitability.[32] Studies in the research laboratory have shown that ischemic contracture can be attenuated by pharmacologic interventions targeting reperfusion injury, resulting in hemodynamically more stable closed-chest resuscitation.[27,33] The possibility that ischemic contracture might increase coronary vascular resistance by extrinsic compression of the coronary circuit[14,34] has not been substantiated.[33,35]

Resistance to defibrillation

Electrical shocks delivered immediately after onset of VF are consistently effective in re-establishing cardiac activity. Even short delays (i.e., up to 3 minutes) may not be substantially detrimental and result in more than 50% likelihood of successful resuscitation.[36] Longer intervals of untreated VF – as usually occurs in out-of-hospital settings – predict decreased effectiveness of defibrillation attempts, however, in which electrical shocks may fail to reverse VF or may precipitate asystole or pulseless electrical activity.[37] Under these conditions, additional resuscitation interventions are required to restore myocardial conditions favorable for successful defibrillation. New approaches are being developed to optimize the effectiveness of electrical defibrillation by identifying the proper timing for shock delivery and by using safer and more effective defibrillation waveforms.[38,39]

Reperfusion arrhythmias

Electrical instability manifested by premature ventricular complexes and episodes of ventricular tachycardia and VF commonly occurs during the early minutes after return of cardiac activity. Episodes of VF have been reported to occur in up to 79% of patients, with the number of episodes inversely correlated with ultimate survival.[40] The mechanism responsible for postresuscitation arrhythmias is complex and probably involves prominent cytosolic Ca^{2+} overload with afterdepolarizations triggering ventricular ectopic activity.[41] In addition, there are repolarization abnormalities that include shortening of the action potential (AP) duration, decreased AP amplitude, and development of AP duration alternans creating conditions for re-entry.[42] Experimentally, these repolarization abnormalities are short-lived (5 to 10 minutes) and coincide with the interval of increased propensity for ventricular arrhythmias and recurrent VF.[27] They are in part related to opening of sarcolemmal K^{+}_{ATP} channels;[43] however, recent evidence suggests that activation of the sarcolemmal Na^{+}-H^{+} exchanger isoform-1 (NHE-1) may also play a role.[44]

Postresuscitation myocardial dysfunction

Variable degrees of left ventricular systolic and diastolic dysfunction develop after resuscitation from cardiac arrest, despite full restoration of coronary blood flow. Left ventricular dysfunction is largely reversible, conforming to the definition of myocardial stunning.[45–48]

Systolic dysfunction has been documented by using load-independent indices of contractility, which demonstrates decreases in the slope of the end-systolic pressure-volume relationship (elastance) and increases in the volume intercept at a left ventricular pressure of 100 mm Hg (V_{100}).[46] Impaired contractility leads to reductions in indices of global ventricular performance, such as cardiac index, ejection fraction, and left ventricular stroke work,[8,47,49] and renders the heart susceptible to afterload increases during the postresuscitation phase. In a pig model of VF and closed chest resuscitation, the administration of vasopressin during cardiac resuscitation was associated with decreased left ventricular performance, with reversal by administration of a specific antagonist of the V_1 receptor.[50]

Diastolic dysfunction is characterized by left ventricular wall thickening with reductions in end-diastolic volume and impaired relaxation,[27] and appears to be maximal immediately after restoration of spontaneous circulation. The magnitude of diastolic dysfunction correlates closely with the magnitude of ischemic contracture,[51] suggesting a common pathogenic thread with diastolic dysfunction being a manifestation of resolving ischemic contracture. From a functional perspective, diastolic dysfunction may limit the compensatory ventricular dilatation required to overcome decreased contractility according to the Frank-Starling mechanism.

Postresuscitation myocardial dysfunction was first documented in humans by Deantonio and colleagues.[45] They reported on three female patients who were successfully resuscitated following transthoracic defibrillation after approximately 3, 10, and 30 minutes of cardiac arrest and who developed prominent left ventricular dilatation with reduction in fractional shortening within 3 days postresuscitation. None of these patients had coronary artery disease and ventricular function normalized within 2 weeks. Likewise, Ruiz-Bailen and coworkers reported severe postresuscitation myocardial dysfunction with reductions in left ventricular ejection fraction to 0.42 in 29 patients within the initial 24 hours postresuscitation.[52] In a subset of 20 patients who had left ventricular dysfunction, the ejection fraction decreased to 0.28 ($P < 0.05$). Patients who died had a significantly lower ejection fraction. Patients who survived gradually normalized their ejection fraction within an interval of approximately 4 weeks postresuscitation (Fig. 48.1).

Laurent and colleagues stratified 165 patients successfully resuscitated from out-of-hospital cardiac arrest based on whether hemodynamic instability was present within the initial 72 hours postresuscitation.[8] Hemodynamic instability was defined as hypotension requiring vasoactive drugs after fluid resuscitation. It occurred in 55% of the patients and was associated with longer resuscitation times, greater number of electrical shocks, larger amounts of adrenaline, and worse left ventricular function (Table 48.1). The incidence and severity of coronary artery disease was comparable between groups; however, a trend was noted towards a higher incidence of recent coronary occlusion in patients with hemodynamic instability. Myocardial dysfunction was initially accompanied by a low cardiac index (2.05 l/min per m²) with elevated systemic vascular resistance (2908 dynes s/cm⁵ per m²). However, a hyperdynamic state developed during the ensuing 72 hours, characterized by increased cardiac index, decreased systemic vascular resistance, and the need for large amounts of fluids to maintain adequate filling pressures (Fig. 48.2).

The late hyperdynamic state reported by Laurent and coworkers is consistent with the development of a systemic inflammatory response akin to that observed during sepsis but precipitated by cardiac arrest and resuscitation.[53–55] Adrie and colleagues measured circulating cytokines in 61 victims of out-of-hospital cardiac arrest who were successfully resuscitated.[55] Measurements obtained at approximately 3 hours

Table 48.1. Factors associated with postresuscitation hemodynamic instability

	Hemodynamic stability ($n = 75$)	Hemodynamic instability ($n = 73$)	P
Resuscitation data			
Collapse to ROSC, min	15 (7–30)	25 (14–28)	< 0.01
Countershocks, *n*	2 (1–3)	3 (1–6)	< 0.01
Total epinephrine, mg	2 (0–10)	10 (3–15)	< 0.01
Angiography/ventriculography data			
Heart rate, beats/min	85 (48–118)	105 (75–143)	< 0.05
LVEF	0.43 (0.35–0.50)	0.32 (0.25–0.40)	< 0.01
LVEDP, mmHg	12 (5–25)	19 (10–32)	< 0.01
Recent coronary occlusion, %	37	51	0.06

ROSC = Return of spontaneous circulation; LVEF = Left ventricular ejection fraction; LVEDP = Left ventricular end diastolic pressure. Median (interquartile range). (Adapted from ref. 8.)

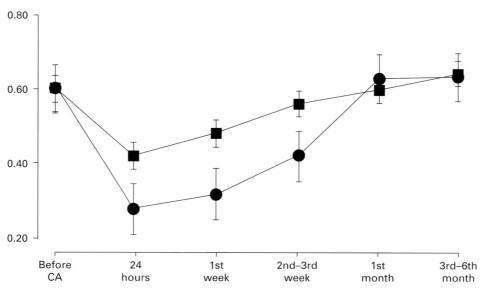

Fig. 48.1. Serial measurements of left ventricular ejection fraction by echocardiography in 29 patients successfully resuscitated from cardiac arrest (CA) without known cardiovascular disease – except for hypertension – and who survived a minimum of 72 hours. Patients had a median age of 65 years and 41% were females. Prearrest echocardiograms were available in 16 patients demonstrating a mean left ventricular ejection fraction of 0.60. Squares represent the entire cohort of 29 patients; circles represent a subset of 20 patients who had myocardial dysfunction. (Adapted from ref. 52.)

postresuscitation demonstrated prominent increases in plasma levels of tumor necrosis factor (TNF)-α, interleukin (IL)-6, IL-8, IL-10, soluble TNF receptor type II (sTNFII), IL-1 receptor antagonist (IL-1ra), and regulated on activation, normal T-cell expressed and secreted (RANTES). In a subset of 35 patients, increased endotoxin levels were detected in 46% within the initial 48 hours postresuscitation.

Underlying cell mechanisms: role of mitochondria

The underlying mechanism of cell injury is complex and probably time-sensitive. There are processes that develop shortly after onset ischemia and during reperfusion that lead to abnormalities in energy metabolism, acid base status, and intracellular ion homeostasis. Other processes develop at a slower pace and encompass signaling mechanisms, leading to sustained disruption of energy production and contractile function with activation of apoptotic pathways. Discussion on the various cell mechanisms responsible for cell injury is beyond the scope of this chapter. Nonetheless, pertinent to our discussion is the growing evidence placing the mitochondria at the center of myocardial preservation, reperfusion injury, and postischemic dysfunction. Better understanding of mitochondrial injury may also serve to identify novel therapeutic strategies.[56–66]

Energy production

The mitochondria are organelles present in all eukaryotic cells that play an essential role in aerobic metabolism and generation of ATP. Mitochondria have an inner membrane that is highly impermeable and folds inwardly into the mitochondrial matrix, forming multiple cristae where proteins responsible for oxidative phosphorylation reside. The outer mitochondrial membrane is more porous and surrounds the inner mitochondrial membrane. Generation of energy in the form of ATP results from oxidation of NADH in the electron transport chain. This chain is composed of protein complexes assembled along the inner mitochondrial membrane where electrons are transferred down their redox potential while H^+ are pumped into the intermembrane space. The accumulation of H^+ establishes an electromotive force, which is used by F_oF_1 ATP synthase to form ATP from ADP and inorganic phosphate. ATP is then exported into the cytosol in exchange for ADP by the adenine nucleotide translocase (Fig. 48.3).

Disruption of the inner membrane permeability leads to reduction of the H^+ gradient, compromising the electromotive force required for ATP synthesis. Factors that may contribute to such injury during ischemia and reperfusion include mitochondrial Ca^{2+} overload and generation of reactive oxygen species (ROS) explaining decreased mitochondrial capability for regeneration of ATP.

Apoptotic signaling

In addition to the key role on energy production, mitochondria can also signal cell death by activation of the intrinsic apoptotic pathway through release of cytochrome *c*. Cytochrome *c* is a 14-kDa hemoprotein normally present in the intermembrane mitochondrial space that plays a key role by transferring electrons from complex III to complex IV (Fig. 48.3). Cytochrome *c* can be released to the cytosol, prompting the formation of an oligomeric complex with dATP and the apoptotic protease activating factor-1 (Apaf-1).[57] This complex recruits procaspase-9, forming the so-called apop-

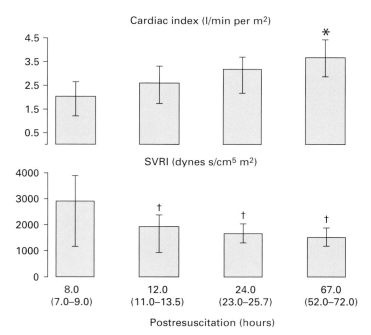

Fig. 48.2. Serial measurements of cardiac index and systemic vascular resistance index (SVRI) in a subset of 73 patients who had hemodynamic instability after resuscitation from out-of-hospital cardiac arrest. A cumulative amount of 8,000 ml was required to maintain a pulmonary artery occlusive pressure > 12 mmHg. The mortality was 19 %. Median (interquartile range) *$P < 0.05$; † $P < 0.001$. (Adapted from ref. 8.)

tosome. In the apoptosome, procaspase-9 is activated and then released as caspase-9, which in turn, activates the executioner caspases 3, 6, and 7.[67,68] Active executioner caspases cleave several cytoplasmic proteins, including α-spectrin and actin, and nuclear proteins including poly (ADP-ribose) polymerase (PARP), lamin A, and the inhibitor of caspase-activated DNase (ICAD). Cleavage of ICAD leads to activation of caspase activated DNase (CAD), which in turn cleaves chromatin into 180 to 200 bp fragments. Other substrates activated during apoptosis include components of DNA repair machinery and a number of protein kinases,[67] ultimately culminating in cell death.

Various mechanisms have been proposed to explain cytochrome *c* release. One mechanism involves opening of a high-conductance mega channel formed by apposition of transmembrane proteins from the inner and the outer mitochondrial membrane known as the mitochondrial permeability transition pore (MPTP).[59] Opening of the pore allows molecules up to 1.5 kDa to enter the mitochondrial matrix along with water and solutes, leading to mitochondrial swelling with stretching and disruption of the outer mitochondrial membrane, ultimately causing

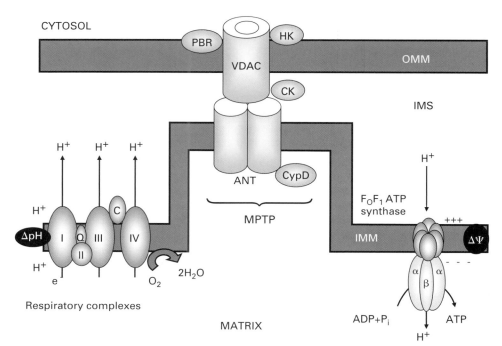

Fig. 48.3. Scheme depicting the structural organization of the electron transport chain, the mitochondrial permeability transition pore (MPTP), and the F_oF_1 ATP synthase in relation to the inner and outer mitochondrial membranes. PBR = peripheral benzodiazepine receptor; VDAC = voltage dependent anion channel; HK = hexokinase; CK = creatine kinase; ANT = adenine nucleotide translocase; CypD = cyclophilin-D; I, II, III, and IV = respiratory complexes; Q = coenzyme Q; C = cytochrome *c*; OMM = outer mitochondrial membrane; IMS = intermembrane space; IMM = inner mitochondrial membrane; ΔpH = pH gradient; $\Psi\Delta$ = mitochondrial membrane potential. (Adapted from Gross A *et al. Genes Dev* 1999;13:1899 and Kim JS *et al. Biochem Biophys Res Commun* 2003;304:463.)

release of cytochrome *c*.[59] Pathophysiological conditions responsible for opening of the MPTP include Ca^{2+} overload, production of reactive oxygen species (ROS), depletion of ATP and ADP, increases in inorganic phosphate, and acidosis.[59] Cytochrome *c* can also be released without MPTP opening through formation of pores in the outer mitochondrial membrane. This is best explained by permeabilization of the outer membrane by pro-apoptotic proteins such as Bcl-2–associated X protein (Bax), Bcl-2 homologous antagonist killer (Bak), or truncated BH3 interacting domain death agonist (Bid).[69] Anti-apoptotic proteins such as Bcl-2, Bcl-x, and Bcl-w, however, may play important roles by counterbalancing the aforementioned pro-apoptotic effects.[70]

Mitochondrial Ca^{2+}

Mitochondrial Ca^{2+} overload plays a critical role during ischemia and reperfusion. Ca^{2+} normally enters the mitochondria through a Ca^{2+} uniporter and leaves through a

Na^+-Ca^{2+} exchanger located in the inner mitochondrial membrane. This transport mechanism enables changes in cytosolic Ca^{2+} to be relayed to the mitochondrial matrix and thus regulate the activity of various enzymes of the tricarboxylic acid cycle. Increases in cytosolic Ca^{2+} during ischemia prompt mitochondrial Ca^{2+} increases leading to production of reactive oxygen species (ROS). ROS cause peroxidation of cardiolipin, which is the principal lipid constituent of the inner mitochondrial membrane and to which a fraction of cytochrome *c* is bound. Peroxidation decreases the binding affinity of cardiolipin for cytochrome *c*,[71] facilitating its release out of the mitochondria. Modest increases in extramitochondrial Ca^{2+} (i.e., 2 μM) cause cytochrome *c* release without MPTP opening. At higher Ca^{2+} levels (i.e., 20 μM), ROS and Ca^{2+} acting together prompt MPTP opening, presumably through oxidative injury of the adenine nucleotide translocase. Both mechanisms of cytochrome *c* release can be prevented by blocking the mitochondrial Ca^{2+} uniporter with ruthenium red.[72]

Link to myocardial dysfunction

Mounting evidence suggests that acute modifications of regulatory proteins of the contractile apparatus occur through cleavage of specific components[73,74] following intracellular Ca^{2+} increase and activation of proteases such as calpain-1 and caspase-3.[75–78] Communal and colleagues reported that activated caspase-3 cleaves α-actin and α-actinin but not myosin heavy chain, myosin light chain 1/2, and tropomyosin.[77] Incubation of recombinant troponin (Tn) complex with caspase-3 selectively cleaved cardiac TnT, resulting in 25-kDa fragments. Functionally, activated caspase-3 decreases maximal Ca^{2+}-activated force and myofibrillar ATPase activity, suggesting that activation of apoptotic pathways may lead to contractile dysfunction. Radhakrishnan and coworkers recently demonstrated activation of caspase-3 in left ventricular homogenates of rat hearts harvested at 4 hours postresuscitation coincident with left ventricular dysfunction.[79] In models of VF and coronary occlusion, Ca^{2+} overload was associated with decreases in the Ca^{2+}-force relationship presumably following modifications in the interaction between proteins of the troponin complex.[80,81] Zaugg and coworkers specifically demonstrated, in a model of prolonged untreated VF, prominent cytosolic Ca^{2+} increases leading to reduced Ca^{2+} sensitivity of troponin, TnC and impaired contractility.[82] Similarly, Barta and coworkers demonstrated cleavage of TnI and TnT following activation of calpain-1.[78] In addition, these proteases have also been shown to cleave structural proteins such as titin, α-actinin, α-fodrin, and desmin.[83–85]

Various novel pharmacological interventions that have been investigated in the setting of cardiac arrest (and are discussed below) seem to protect the myocardium by limiting mitochondrial Ca^{2+} overload. Postresuscitation myocardial dysfunction, as pointed out earlier, is largely a reversible phenomenon. It is less clear, however, whether dysfunction and cell death represent part of a continuum manifesting varying degrees of severity. Much work remains before we can fully elucidate the process of ischemic injury and postischemic dysfunction. Meanwhile, understanding the mechanisms that affect mitochondrial function and its signaling of apoptosis may provide an opportunity for developing new resuscitation therapies.

Factors contributing to myocardial injury

Factors that contribute to myocardial injury during cardiac resuscitation include the duration of cardiac arrest, the delivery of electrical shocks, and the use of adrenergic vasopressor agents. Efforts to shorten the duration of the cardiac arrest by prompt recognition and rapid intervention are thus important to minimize injury. Likewise, delivery of quality cardiopulmonary resuscitation (CPR) may help reduce the duration of tissue ischemia by prompting earlier return of spontaneous circulation. Quality CPR may be attained by paying close attention to the rate, depth, and site of compression, minimizing the interruptions required to secure the airway, verify rhythm, and deliver shocks. In addition, adequate venous return is essential for hemodynamically effective chest compression, which can be secured by allowing full re-expansion of the chest cavity, avoiding hyperventilation, and creating an intrathoracic vacuum between compressions by using impedance threshold devices.[86] The following sections address the potential detrimental effects of electrical shocks and adrenergic vasopressor agents along with options to minimize such injury.

Electrical defibrillation

Delivery of electrical shocks during the resuscitation effort may contribute to myocardial injury and worsen postresuscitation electrical and mechanical dysfunction.[87–89] Manifestations of such injury include increased postresuscitation ectopic activity, atrioventricular block, and worsened postresuscitation myocardial dysfunction.[90] Key factors that determine injury include the energy level, number of shocks, and defibrillation waveforms.

Energy level

The presence and severity of myocardial injury is influenced by the amount of energy delivered to the myocardium. In an isolated perfused rabbit heart, Koning and coworkers reported minimal injury after epicardial shocks of 0.6 joule/cm^2. Nevertheless, as the energy was increased to up to 4.2 joule/cm^2 additional and more severe injury developed, including impaired systolic function, myocardial stiffness, release of creatine kinase, and cell necrosis.[91] Similarly, Doherty and coworkers found that significant myocardial injury, as evidenced by creatine kinase release, increased technetium-99m pyrophosphate uptake, and decreased thallium-201 and indium-113m uptake, developed only when the energy of shocks delivered directly to beating canine hearts (15- to 26-kg dogs) exceeded 20 joules.[92] The injury was characterized by dehiscence of intercalated disks between damaged myocytes. Kerber and coworkers, also in dogs, reported contractile abnormalities only when the energy of epicardial shocks was 40 Joules or more in 17- to 45-kg dogs.[93] In the cardiac arrest setting, Xie and coworkers using an intact rat model of VF reported that postresuscitation myocardial dysfunction worsened in close relationship to stepwise increases in the energy used for external defibrillation from 2, to 10, and to 20 Joules.[89] It is important to realize, however, that the energy required to reverse VF is typically below the threshold at which significant myocardial cell injury occurs.[94]

The mechanisms of cell injury following electrical shocks relate in part to increased cytosolic Ca^{2+}. In single-isolated, cultured chick-embryo heart cells, exposure to defibrillator-type electrical shocks causes reversible depolarization followed by intensity-independent Ca^{2+} entry, attributed to opening of normal excitation channels, and intensity-dependent Ca^{2+} entry attributed to cell damage.[95] Further evidence that Ca^{2+} may play a role stems from observations in dogs in which prior administration of the Ca^{2+} channel blocker verapamil – but not the beta-blocker propranolol – attenuates the myocardial injury caused by transthoracic countershocks.[96]

Number of shocks

Multiple shocks are often required to terminate VF. Yet, repetitive electrical shocks may cause myocardial injury beyond that which is caused by individual shocks.[88,90,92,97] Injury may manifest by worsened diastolic dysfunction postresuscitation, despite no adverse effects on postresuscitation systolic function.[98] Thus, efforts to limit the number of electrical shocks are warranted. Until recently, delivery of electrical shocks immediately upon recognition of VF was regarded as an essential component of the chain of survival. Observations in a dog model of VF by Niemann and coworkers[99] and studies in victims of out-of-hospital sudden cardiac arrest by Cobb and coworkers[100] and by Wik and coworkers,[101] however, have challenged such an approach, suggesting that a period of chest compression before attempting defibrillation under conditions of prolonged untreated VF may improve the myocardial responsiveness to electrical shocks. The 2005 guidelines for cardiopulmonary resuscitation recommend that CPR be given for approximately 2 minutes before attempting electrical defibrillation when the ambulance response time is prolonged (i.e., >4 minutes). Moreover, the same recommendation states that only a single shock be given and that CPR be resumed without a pulse check. These recommendations recognize that untimely delivery of electrical shocks may be detrimental to the resuscitation efforts, in part because of interruption in chest compression and because the ischemic myocardium seems to tolerate poorly the repetitive delivery of electrical shocks.

A more optimal approach would be to guide the timing of defibrillation based on real-time analysis of the VF waveform. Previous studies have recognized the value of measuring the amplitude and frequency characteristics of VF waveforms to estimate the duration of untreated VF,[102] assess myocardial energy metabolism,[103] and predict the response to defibrillation attempts.[104,105] Waveform analysis that incorporates amplitude and frequency in a single index has been demonstrated experimentally to have better positive and negative predictor power than VF amplitude and frequency alone.[106] Use of these indices in real-time could allow better targeting of individual shocks, thus avoiding the delivery of shocks when the probability of success is low.

Defibrillation waveforms

Until recently, delivery of electrical shocks by external (transthoracic) defibrillators used monophasic exponential waveforms, but the advent of implantable cardioverter-defibrillators introduced into clinical practice the use of biphasic truncated exponential waveforms. Biphasic waveforms have proven to be more effective for terminating VF and less damaging to the myocardium than monophasic waveforms. In a study of 40- to 45-kg pigs subjected to 10 minutes of VF, Tang and coworkers[107] reported comparable defibrillation efficacy by biphasic (fixed 150-joule) and monophasic (escalating 200-, 300-, and 360-joule) shocks. Biphasic waveform defibrillation was associated with significantly less postresuscitation myocardial dysfunction, as evidenced by lesser postresuscitation reductions in stroke volume, cardiac output, and ejection fraction. In contrast, Niemann and coworkers[37] using 26- to 36-kg pigs subjected to 5 minutes of untreated VF reported comparable defibrillation success using biphasic (fixed 150-joule) and monophasic (escalating 200-, 300-, and 360-joule) shocks without differences in postresuscitation myocardial or hemodynamic function. It is possible that the competitive advantage of biphasic waveform defibrillation occurs at lower energy levels than those that were used in this experimental setting.

In a recent clinical trial, fixed 150-joule impedance-compensating, biphasic truncated exponential defibrillation waveforms were compared with monophasic (truncated exponential or damped sine) defibrillation waveforms in 115 victims of out-of-hospital VF.[108] Biphasic waveform defibrillation was associated with significantly higher rates of successful defibrillation (100% vs. 84%, $P = 0.003$) and return of spontaneous circulation (76% vs. 54%, $P = 0.01$), but not hospital admission (61% vs. 51%, NS) or survival (28% vs. 31%, NS). Although a larger sample size would be required to assess effects on survival outcomes, hospital survivors who had received biphasic waveform defibrillation were noted to have better neurological outcomes. This observation was attributed to possible earlier restoration of spontaneous circulation with biphasic waveform defibrillation. Larger clinical trials are awaited to assess impact on hospital survival.

Vasopressor agents

Although a prominent neuroendocrine vasoconstrictive response occurs during cardiac arrest that reduces distal aortic runoff, enabling preferential perfusion of the coronary and cerebral circuits, this response is limited, and exogenous vasopressor agents are typically required to secure increases in the coronary perfusion pressures above critical resuscitability thresholds. For this purpose, the American Heart Association recommends the use of either adrenaline or vasopressin. Studies have shown, however, that adrenaline under these low-flow conditions may not only fail to improve the myocardial energy deficit despite increases in coronary blood flow,[109] but may actually intensify ischemic injury and worsen postresuscitation myocardial dysfunction and survival.[110,111] These adverse effects of epinephrine are attributed to stimulation of β-receptors whereby the myocardial oxygen requirements are disproportionately increased during cardiac arrest[109] and can be minimized experimentally by using β-blocking agents.[112] In a rat model of VF and closed-chest resuscitation,[111] use of the β_1-blocking agent esmolol in conjunction with epinephrine ameliorated the severity of postresuscitation myocardial dysfunction. Similar effects have been documented in larger animal models of cardiac arrest.[112,113] Even administration of the selective β_1-blocker esmolol alone during chest compression has been shown to ameliorate postresuscitation myocardial dysfunction (Fig. 48.4).[114]

Notwithstanding the adverse effect of adrenergic agents under the low blood flow conditions of standard CPR, provocative studies by Angelos and coworkers suggest that epinephrine may be effective and devoid of its adverse effects when used in association with hemodynamically more effective resuscitation techniques.[115]

An alternative approach is the use of non-adrenergic vasopressor agents such as vasopressin. This agent appears to be more potent than epinephrine and to lack adverse effects on myocardial energy metabolism.[116] Nonetheless, vasopressin has a longer half-life and the vasopressor effects persist during the postresuscitation interval, leading to adverse effects on blood flow to various regional tissue beds. The vasopressor effect may also compromise myocardial performance by increasing afterload.[50]

More recently, activation of α_2- receptors has emerged as a promising new experimental approach. These receptors are expressed in pre- and postsynaptic junctions of vascular smooth cells. Activation of presynaptic α_2-receptors inhibits the release of norepinephrine. Activation of postsynaptic α_2-receptors promotes peripheral vasoconstriction. Studies in rat and pig models of VF and closed-chest resuscitation have shown that administration of the α_2-receptor agonist α-methyl-norepinephrine during chest compression is associated with less postresuscitation myocardial dysfunction when compared to epinephrine.[117,118] Activation of these receptors in Purkinje cells has been shown to reduce reperfusion arrhythmias in rats after left anterior descending coronary artery occlusion and reperfusion.[119] These effects have been linked to signaling via G-protein, causing attenuation in intracellular cyclic adenosine monophosphate levels.

Novel experimental therapies

The realization that ischemia and reperfusion activates a myriad of pathogenic pathways has persuaded researchers to investigate whether targeting such pathways may protect the myocardium and minimize postresuscitation myocardial dysfunction. Some of these studies are described below exposing the specific mechanisms of injury targeted.

Sarcolemmal Na^+–H^+ exchange

Increased sarcolemmal Na^+ influx with subsequent intracellular Na^+ overload due to the inability of the Na^+–K^+ pump to extrude Na^+ during myocardial ischemia has been recognized as an important pathogenic mechanism of cell injury during ischemia and reperfusion.[120–122] Na^+ becomes a "substrate" for reperfusion injury[123] and intensifies processes detrimental to cell function primarily by promoting sarcolemmal Ca^{2+} entry through the Na^+–Ca^{2+} exchanger (NCX) acting in its reverse mode.[124]

The conditions that develop during cardiac arrest are uniquely poised to trigger maximal and sustained NHE-1 activity. The intense intracellular acidosis that develops during ischemia is the initial trigger for NHE-1 activation. The subsequent resuscitation attempt, with closed-chest techniques, promotes reperfusion with coronary flows that rarely exceed 20% of normal. These low blood flow levels are not sufficient to reverse ischemia,[125] but are sufficient to supply the coronary circuit with normo-acidic blood, hence washing out the excess of extracellular protons favoring a trans-sarcolemmal proton gradient that maintains

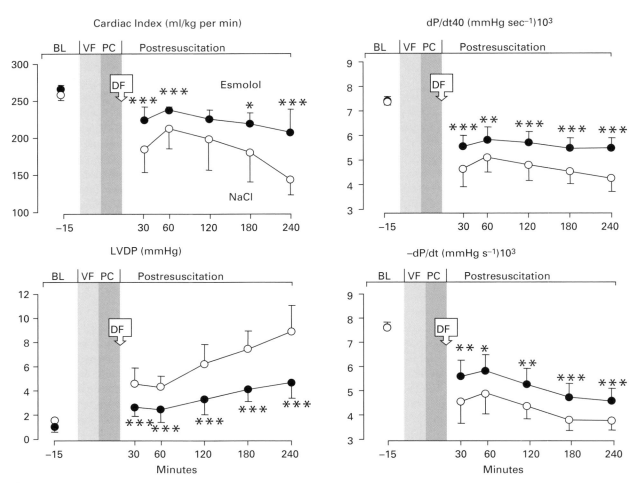

Fig. 48.4. Myocardial effects of β_1-adrenergic blockade during closed-chest resuscitation in a rat model of VF. Esmolol (300 μg/kg, $n = 9$) or NaCl 0.9% ($n = 9$) was given into the right atrium at the second minute of precordial compression (PC) after a 6-minute interval of untreated VF. All esmolol-treated rats but only 5 controls were successfully resuscitated. Closed symbols represent esmolol ($n = 9$); open symbols represent control ($n = 5$). BL = Baseline; LVDP = Left ventricular diastolic pressure. dP/dt_{40} = rate of left ventricular pressure rise at left ventricular pressure of 40 mmHg; – dP/dt = rate of left ventricular pressure decline. Mean ± SD. *$P < 0.05$; **$P \leq 0.03$; *** $P < 0.01$ vs. NaCl. (Adapted from Cammarata G *et al. Crit Care Med* 2004;32:S440.)

NHE-1 activity throughout the resuscitation effort and probably the initial postresuscitation phase.

Administration of selective NHE-1 inhibitors, such as cariporide, has been shown consistently to ameliorate myocardial injury during cardiac resuscitation.[25,27,33,126–129] In an intact pig model, cariporide reduced ischemic contracture during chest compression such that there was less ventricular wall thickening and better preservation of cavity size. This effect enabled chest compression to generate and maintain a coronary perfusion pressure above the threshold for resuscitability and to augment the hemodynamic efficacy of vasopressor agents.[27,128,129] Cariporide also ameliorated postresuscitation ventricular ectopic activity, prevented episodes of recurrent VF, and minimized

postresuscitation myocardial dysfunction (Fig. 48.5).[25,27] Although cariporide inhibits sarcolemmal NHE-1 and ameliorates cytosolic Na$^+$ and Ca^{2+} overload, recent evidence suggests that protection may also involve direct effects on the mitochondria by preserving the inner membrane H$^+$ gradient and delaying ATP depletion.[130]

The potential clinical applicability of NHE-1 inhibitors has been halted for the moment. A recent clinical trial in patients undergoing coronary artery bypass graft surgery demonstrated increased incidence of cerebrovascular occlusive events and higher overall mortality despite a significant reduction in non-fatal postoperative myocardial infarction.[131] Although information on the mechanism of this adverse effect of cariporide is not currently

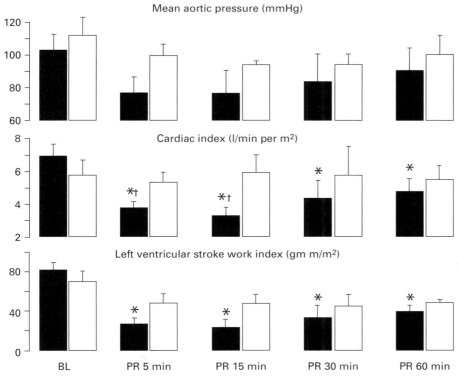

Fig. 48.5. Postresuscitation hemodynamic and left ventricular function in pigs randomized to receive cariporide (3 mg/kg, open bars, $n = 4$) or NaCl 0.9% (closed bars, $n = 4$) immediately before starting chest compression after a 6-minute interval of untreated VF. Each animal was successfully defibrillated after 8 minutes of closed-chest resuscitation and observed for 60 minutes postresuscitation. Mean ± SEM. *$P < 0.05$ vs. baseline (BL) by repeated measures ANOVA; †$P < 0.05$ vs. cariporide by one-way ANOVA. (Adapted from ref. 27.)

available, it appears to be unrelated to the mode of action. Development of newer compounds is anticipated.

K$^+$$_{ATP}$ channel activation

Interventions aimed at activating known mechanisms of preconditioning during cardiac resuscitation may have favorable effects on postresuscitation myocardial dysfunction. One important mechanism of ischemic preconditioning that can be emulated pharmacologically involves opening of mitochondrial K$^+$$_{ATP}$ channels.[132–135] Opening of K$^+$$_{ATP}$ channels leads to increased K$^+$ conductivity of the inner mitochondrial membrane, an effect that is bioenergetically beneficial[136] and limits mitochondrial Ca^{2+} overload.[137] In a rat model of VF and closed chest resuscitation, administration of the K$^+$$_{ATP}$ channel opener cromakalim reduced postresuscitation myocardial function despite a significant reduction in coronary perfusion pressure during chest compression.[138] The favorable effect on postresuscitation myocardial function was comparable to

that of preconditioning and manifested by a higher postresuscitation + dP/dt$_{40}$, -dP/dt$_{max}$, cardiac index, and longer postresuscitation survival.

δ-Opioid receptor activation

Activation of δ-opioid receptors has been shown to play an important role in hibernation, leading to reductions in myocardial oxygen consumption. Activation of δ-opioid receptors, and more specifically δ$_1$- and δ$_2$- receptors, has been shown to ameliorate postischemic myocardial dysfunction and to preserve ultrastructural integrity in chick cardiomyocytes and isolated perfused rabbit hearts.[139,140] Sun and coworkers investigated, in a rat model of VF and closed-chest resuscitation, the effect of administering the δ-opioid receptor agonist pentazocine.[141] Administration of pentazocine was associated with significantly lower postresuscitation arterial lactate and less postresuscitation myocardial dysfunction, evidenced by a higher + dP/dt$_{40}$, -dP/dt$_{max}$, and cardiac index. These effects were abrogated by pretreatment with naloxone.

Lazaroids

Lazaroids are 21-aminosteroid molecules that inhibit lipid peroxidation and scavenge oxygen free radicals.[142–144] Studies in a canine model of cardiac transplantation have shown that the lazaroid compound U-74389G given before reperfusion improves post-transplantation myocardial function.[145] Studies in a rat model of VF and closed chest resuscitation demonstrated that administration of U-74389G before chest compression ameliorates postresuscitation myocardial dysfunction as evidenced by a higher cardiac index and higher $+ dP/dt_{40}$ and a lower left ventricular end diastolic pressure with increased postresuscitation survival time.[146] Administration of the lazaroid was also associated with significantly fewer premature ventricular complexes. These studies suggest that antioxidants may play a role during cardiac resuscitation, further supporting the pivotal role of mitochondria for cardiac resuscitation.[72]

Erythropoietin

Erythropoietin is a 30.4-kDa glycoprotein best known for its action on erythroid progenitor cells and regulation of circulating red cell mass.[147] Within the past few years, however, investigators have reported that erythropoietin also signals survival responses during ischemia and reperfusion in a broad range of tissues including the heart.[148–157] Some of these protective actions are induced immediately upon administration and result in attenuating of ischemia and reperfusion injury even when given after the onset of ischemia and at the time of reperfusion,[154,156,158,159] suggesting that erythropoietin could be beneficial for cardiac resuscitation. Administration of human recombinant erythropoietin in a rat model of prolonged VF (5000 U/kg) at the start of closed-chest resuscitation enabled hemodynamically more effective chest compression and improved postresuscitation hemodynamic function.[160]

Management of postresuscitation myocardial dysfunction

The current approach to cardiac resuscitation emphasizes the prompt reversal of the precipitating cause of cardiac arrest (i.e., terminating VF or correcting hypoxemia) and the generation, by external means, of blood flow across the coronary circuit. This paradigm, however, does not include specific interventions aimed at myocardial protection and prevention of postresuscitation myocardial dysfunction. Yet, as pointed out earlier, opportunities exist to minimize myocardial injury by reducing the time interval for initiating CPR, and by providing quality CPR that can promote higher coronary blood flows. In addition, strategies aimed at more precise timing of shock delivery could minimize injury by avoiding repetitive defibrillation attempts. Regarding vasopressor agents, it is to be hoped that quality CPR might enable more judicious use of vasopressor agents by avoiding excessive dosing, and development of more effective and less toxic vasopressor agents is eagerly awaited. Of increasing interest is the possibility that β-adrenoceptor blocking agents administered during cardiac resuscitation may prevent injury stemming from endogenous and exogenous adrenergic stimulation; clinical studies are awaited to support this concept. The experimental agents shown above to be effective in various animal models of cardiac arrest support the concept that targeting pathways to ischemic injury may be effective. Yet, again, clinical data are awaited.

Recognition and assessment of myocardial dysfunction

Although critical care and emergency medicine physicians are well-trained to recognize and treat acute heart failure, it is not clear that myocardial dysfunction is commonly deemed a diagnostic possibility after an episode of cardiac arrest. Thus, it is important to consider postresuscitation myocardial dysfunction in every patient successfully resuscitated from cardiac arrest. Equally important is to recognize that such dysfunction is potentially reversible, thus justifying efforts to support the failing myocardium until competent pump function resumes. Assessment of postresuscitation myocardial dysfunction follows conventional practice and includes recognition of the classical symptoms and signs of pulmonary vascular congestion and reduced forward blood flow. Accordingly, the assessment should include, at the very least, a focused history and physical examination, a 12-lead electrocardiogram, a chest x-ray, and routine blood tests. Postresuscitation myocardial dysfunction should be suspected in the presence of increased heart rate, decreased arterial blood pressure and cardiac output, and arrhythmias, especially those of ventricular origin. Evaluation of cardiac function and morphology by echocardiography may be critical to establish the presence of and to quantify the severity of myocardial dysfunction. In addition, echocardiography may serve to identify associated conditions such as cardiac tamponade, myocardial infarction, papillary muscle rupture, pulmonary embolism, ruptured aorta, and aortic dissection.[161,162]

Further diagnostic work is dictated by the clinical course and may include the use of a pulmonary artery catheter to assess filling pressures and cardiac output more precisely. As previously discussed, a pattern of myocardial dysfunction found early after successful resuscitation may evolve into a hyperdynamic state as systemic inflammation unfolds (Fig. 48.2). Recognition of this transition is important, because the management is substantially different and large amounts of fluids may be required to ensure hemodynamic stability.

Inotropic interventions

The stunned myocardium is responsive to inotropic stimulation and therefore pump function may be improved by administration of traditional inotropic agents such as β-agonists (i.e., dobutamine) and phosphodiesterase inhibitors (i.e., milrinone). Dobutamine acts primarily on β_1-, β_2-, and α-receptors. Its hemodynamic effects include increases in stroke volume and cardiac output, with decreases in systemic and pulmonary vascular resistance. Studies in animal models of cardiac arrest have demonstrated substantial reversal of postresuscitation

systolic and diastolic dysfunction by using doses ranging between 5 and 10 μg/kg per minute (Fig. 48.6).[163–165] A dose of 5 μg/kg/minute was found in domestic pigs (24 ± 0.4 kg) to provide the best balance, by restoring postresuscitation systolic and diastolic function without adverse effects on myocardial oxygen consumption.[164] Phosphodiesterase inhibitors such as milrinone also exert inotropic and vasodilator effects and have been shown experimentally to improve postresuscitation myocardial dysfunction.[166] Nevertheless, the effectiveness of conventional inotropic agents may be limited by effects on heart rate and the possibility of worsening ischemic injury in settings of critically reduced coronary artery blood flow.

Conventional inotropic agents act by increasing cAMP after stimulation of β-adrenergic receptors or after inhibition of phosphodiesterases. Increased cAMP levels, in turn, signal phosphorylation of several Ca^{2+} regulatory proteins (i.e., L-type Ca^{2+} channels, phospholamban, the ryanodine receptor, TnI, and the myosin binding protein) leading to increased cytosolic Ca^{2+} cycling. Of note, Ca^{2+} cycling consumes energy and may predispose to ventricular arrhythmias. An alternative approach, therefore, is to

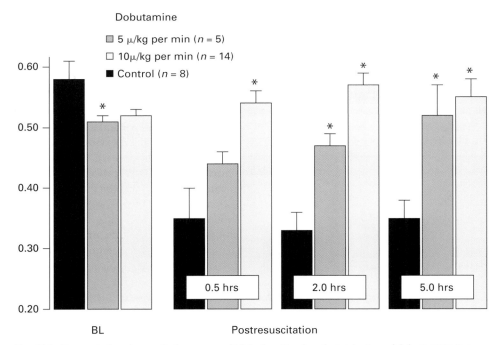

Fig. 48.6. Reversal of postresuscitation myocardial dysfunction by administration of dobutamine in a pig model of VF. VF was untreated for 15 minutes before attempting resuscitation by cardiopulmonary resuscitation including advanced life support and administration of epinephrine. Dobutamine was started at 15 minutes postresuscitation. Mean ± SEM. *$P < 0.05$ control. (Adapted from ref. 163.)

mediate inotropic responses by augmenting the sensitivity of the contractile apparatus to Ca^{2+} acting on TnC and downstream regulatory proteins,[167] so as to exert positive inotropic actions without increasing cAMP or cytosolic Ca^{2+}.

Agents that promote inotropy through these mechanisms are known as Ca^{2+} sensitizers. They are energetically more favorable[168] and are potentially devoid of Ca^{2+}-mediated arrythmogenic effects.[169] One compound, levosimendan, acts by binding to the N-terminal domain of TnC in a Ca^{2+}-dependent manner. Levosimedan was shown by Huang and colleagues in a pig model of VF and closed-chest resuscitation to improve postresuscitation myocardial function, resulting in greater increases in ejection fraction and greater reductions in pulmonary artery occlusive pressure when compared to dobutamine.[170] Further work, however, is required to define dose-response relationships, interactions with underlying coronary and myocardial disease, and the conditions under which inotropic stimulation may help manage postresuscitation myocardial dysfunction and improve outcome.

REFERENCES

1. Zheng, Z.J., Croft, J.B., Giles, W.H. & Mensah, G.A. Sudden cardiac death in the United States, 1989 to 1998. *Circulation* 2001; **104**: 2158–2163.

2. Nichol, G., Stiell, I.G., Laupacis, A. *et al.* A cumulative meta-analysis of the effectiveness of defibrillator-capable emergency medical services for victims of out-of-hospital cardiac arrest. *Ann. Emerg. Med.* 1999; **34**: 517–525.

3. Fredriksson, M., Herlitz, J. & Nichol, G. Variation in outcome in studies of out-of-hospital cardiac arrest: a review of studies conforming to the Utstein guidelines. *Am. J. Emerg. Med.* 2003; **21**: 276–281.

4. Rea, T.D., Eisenberg, M.S., Sinibaldi, G. & White, R.D. Incidence of EMS-treated out-of-hospital cardiac arrest in the United States. *Resuscitation* 2004; **63**: 17–24.

5. Brown, C.G., Martin, D.R., Pepe, P.E. *et al.* and the Multicenter High-Dose Epinephrine Study Group. A comparison of standard-dose and high-dose epinephrine in cardiac arrest outside the hospital. *N. Engl. J. Med.* 1992; **327**: 1051–1055.

6. Kellermann, A.L., Hackman, B.B. & Somes, G. Predicting the outcome of unsuccessful prehospital advanced cardiac life support. *J. Am. Med. Assoc.* 1993; **270**: 1433–1436.

7. Lombardi, G., Gallagher, J. & Gennis, P. Outcome of out-of-hospital cardiac arrest in New York City. The pre-hospital arrest survival evaluation (PHASE) study. *J. Am. Med. Assoc.* 1994; **271**: 678–683.

8. Laurent, I., Monchi, M., Chiche, J.D. *et al.* Reversible myocardial dysfunction in survivors of out-of-hospital cardiac arrest. *J. Am. Coll. Cardiol.* 2002; **40**: 2110–2116.

9. Schoenenberger, R.A., von Planta, M. & von Planta, I. Survival after failed out-of-hospital resuscitation. Are further therapeutic efforts in the emergency department futile? *Arch. Intern. Med.* 1994; **154**: 2433–2437.

10. Laver, S., Farrow, C., Turner, D. & Nolan, J. Mode of death after admission to an intensive care unit following cardiac arrest. *Intens. Care Med.* 2004; **30**: 2126–2128.

11. Klocke, F.J. & Ellis, A.K. Control of coronary blood flow. *Annu. Rev. Med.* 1980; **31**: 489–508.

12. Hoffman, J.I.E. Maximal coronary flow and the concept of coronary vascular reserve. *Circulation* 1984; **70**: 153–159.

13. Yaku, H., Goto, Y., Ohgoshi, Y. *et al.* Determinant of myocardial oxygen consumption in fibrillating dog hearts: Comparison between normothermia and hypothermia. *J. Thorac. Cardiovasc. Surg.* 1993; **105**: 679–688.

14. Gazmuri, R.J., Berkowitz, M. & Cajigas, H. Myocardial effects of ventricular fibrillation in the isolated rat heart. *Crit. Care Med.* 1999; **27**: 1542–1550.

15. Kamohara, T., Weil, M.H., Tang, W. *et al.* A comparison of myocardial function after primary cardiac and primary asphyxial cardiac arrest. *Am. J. Respir. Crit. Care Med.* 2001; **164**: 1221–1224.

16. Neumar, R.W., Brown, C.G., Van Ligten, P., Hoekstra, J., Altschuld, R.A. & Baker, P. Estimation of myocardial ischemic injury during ventricular fibrillation with total circulatory arrest using high-energy phosphates and lactate as metabolic markers. *Ann. Emerg. Med.* 1991; **20**: 222–229.

17. Kern, K.B., Garewal, H.S., Sanders, A.B. *et al.* Depletion of myocardial adenosine triphosphate during prolonged untreated ventricular fibrillation: effect on defibrillation success. *Resuscitation* 1990; **20**: 221–229.

18. Noc, M., Weil, M.H., Gazmuri, R.J., Sun, S., Bisera, J. & Tang, W. Ventricular fibrillation voltage as a monitor of the effectiveness of cardiopulmonary resuscitation. *J. Lab. Clin. Med.* 1994; **124**: 421–426.

19. Kolarova, J.D., Radhakrishnan, J., Sufen, W., Gopalakrishnan, P., Ayoub, I.M. & Gazmuri, R.J. Effects of cariporide on myocardial energy metabolism during resuscitation from VF. *Circulation* 2004; **110**: III-532 (abstract).

20. Johnson, B.A., Weil, M.H., Tang, W., Noc, M., McKee, D. & McCandless, D. Mechanisms of myocardial hypercarbic acidosis during cardiac arrest. *J. Appl. Physiol.* 1995; **78**: 1579–1584.

21. Duggal, C., Weil, M.H., Gazmuri, R.J. *et al.* Regional blood flow during closed-chest cardiac resuscitation in rats. *J. Appl. Physiol.* 1993; **74**: 147–152.

22. Cooley, D.A., Reul, G.J. & Wukasch, D.C. Ischemic contracture of the heart: "Stone Heart". *Am. J. Cardiol.* 1972; **29**: 575–577.

23. Katz, A.M. & Tada, M. The "Stone Heart": A challenge to the biochemist. *Am. J. Cardiol.* 1972; **29**: 578–580.

24. Koretsune, Y. & Marban, E. Mechanism of ischemic contracture in ferret hearts: relative roles of $[Ca^{2+}]_i$ elevation and ATP depletion. *Am. J. Physiol.* 1990; **258**: H9–H16.

25. Gazmuri, R.J., Ayoub, I.M., Hoffner, E. & Kolarova, J.D. Successful ventricular defibrillation by the selective sodium-hydrogen exchanger isoform-1 inhibitor cariporide. *Circulation* 2001; **104**: 234–239.

26. Klouche, K., Weil, M.H., Sun, S. *et al.* Evolution of the stone heart after prolonged cardiac arrest. *Chest* 2002; **122**: 1006–1011.

27. Ayoub, I.M., Kolarova, J.D., Yi, Z. *et al.* Sodium-hydrogen exchange inhibition during ventricular fibrillation: beneficial effects on ischemic contracture, action potential duration, reperfusion arrhythmias, myocardial function, and resuscitability. *Circulation* 2003; **107**: 1804–1809.

28. Berg, R.A., Sorrell, V.L., Kern, K.B. *et al.* Magnetic resonance imaging during untreated ventricular fibrillation reveals prompt right ventricular overdistention without left ventricular volume loss. *Circulation* 2005; **111**: 1136–1140.

29. Sorrell, V.L., Altbach, M.I., Kern, K.B. *et al.* Images in cardiovascular medicine. Continuous cardiac magnetic resonance imaging during untreated ventricular fibrillation. *Circulation* 2005; **111**: e294.

30. Klouche, K., Weil, M.H., Sun, S., Tang, W., Povoas, H. & Bisera, J. Stroke volumes generated by precordial compression during cardiac resuscitation. *Crit. Care Med.* 2002; **30**: 2626–2631.

31. Sharff, J.A., Pantley, G. & Noel, E. Effect of time on regional organ perfusion during two methods of cardiopulmonary resuscitation. *Ann. Emerg. Med.* 1984; **13**: 649–656.

32. Takino, M. & Okada, Y. Firm myocardium in cardiopulmonary resuscitation. *Resuscitation* 1996; **33**: 101–106.

33. Kolarova, J.D., Ayoub, I.M. & Gazmuri, R.J. Cariporide enables hemodynamically more effective chest compression by leftward shift of its flow-depth relationship. *Am. J. Physiol. Heart Circ. Physiol.* 2005; **288**: H2904–H2911.

34. Downey, J.M. Chagrasulis, R.W. & Hemphill, V. Quantitative study of intramyocardial compression in the fibrillating heart. *Am. J. Physiol.* 1979; **237**: H191–H196.

35. Ayoub, I.M., Kolarova, J.D., Radhakrishnan, J., Wang, S. & Gazmuri, R.J. Zoniporide ameliorates post-resuscitation myocardial dysfunction by flow independent mechanisms. *Crit. Care Med.* 2004; **32**: A57 (abstract).

36. Valenzuela, T.D., Roe, D.J., Nichol, G., Clark, L.L., Spaite, D.W. & Hardman, R.G. Outcomes of rapid defibrillation by security officers after cardiac arrest in casinos. *N. Engl. J. Med.* 2000; **343**: 1206–1209.

37. Niemann, J.T., Burian, D., Garner, D. & Lewis, R.J. Monophasic versus biphasic transthoracic countershock after prolonged ventricular fibrillation in a swine model. *J. Am. Coll. Cardiol.* 2000; **36**: 932–938.

38. Kolarova, J., Ayoub, I.M., Yi, Z. & Gazmuri, R.J. Optimal timing for electrical defibrillation after prolonged untreated ventricular fibrillation. *Crit. Care Med.* 2003; **31**: 2022–2028.

39. Tang, W., Weil, M.H., Sun, S. *et al.* The effects of biphasic waveform design on post-resuscitation myocardial function. *J. Am. Coll. Cardiol.* 2004; **43**: 1228–1235.

40. van Alem, A.P., Post, J. & Koster, R.W. VF recurrence: characteristics and patient outcome in out-of-hospital cardiac arrest. *Resuscitation* 2003; **59**: 181–188.

41. Koretsune, Y. & Marban, E. Cell calcium in the pathophysiology of ventricular fibrillation and in the pathogenesis of postarrhythmic contractile dysfunction. *Circulation* 1989; **80**: 369–379.

42. Franz, M.R. Monophasic action potentials recorded by contact electrode method. Genesis, measurement, and interpretations. In Franz, M.R., ed. *Monophasic Action Potentials. Bridging Cell and Bedside.* Armonk, New York: Futura Publishing Company, Inc., 2000: 19–45.

43. Wirth, K.J., Uhde, J., Rosenstein, B. *et al.* K(ATP) channel blocker HMR 1883 reduces monophasic action potential shortening during coronary ischemia in anesthetised pigs. *Naunyn Schmiedebergs Arch. Pharmacol.* 2000; **361**: 155–160.

44. Wirth, K.J., Maier, T. & Busch, A.E. NHE1-inhibitor cariporide prevents the transient reperfusion-induced shortening of the monophasic action potential after coronary ischemia in pigs. *Basic Res. Cardiol.* 2001; **96**: 192–197.

45. Deantonio, H.J., Kaul, S. & Lerman, B.B. Reversible myocardial depression in survivors of cardiac arrest. *PACE* 1990; **13**: 982–985.

46. Gazmuri, R.J., Weil, M.H., Bisera, J., Tang, W., Fukui, M. & McKee, D. Myocardial dysfunction after successful resuscitation from cardiac arrest. *Crit. Care Med.* 1996; **24**: 992–1000.

47. Kern, K.B., Hilwig, R.W., Rhee, K.H. & Berg, R.A. Myocardial dysfunction after resuscitation from cardiac arrest: an example of global myocardial stunning. *J. Am. Coll. Cardiol.* 1996; **28**: 232–240.

48. Kern, K.B. Postresuscitation myocardial dysfunction. *Cardiol. Clin.* 2002; **20**: 89–101.

49. Mullner, M., Domanovits, H., Sterz, F. *et al.* Measurement of myocardial contractility following successful resuscitation: quantitated left ventricular systolic function utilising non-invasive wall stress analysis. *Resuscitation* 1998; **39**: 51–59.

50. Kern, K.B., Heidenreich, J.H., Higdon, T.A. *et al.* Effect of vasopressin on postresuscitation ventricular function: unknown consequences of the recent Guidelines 2000 for Cardiopulmonary Resuscitation and Emergency Cardiovascular Care. *Crit. Care Med.* 2004; **32**: S393–S397.

51. Gazmuri, R.J. Effects of repetitive electrical shocks on postresuscitation myocardial function. *Crit. Care Med.* 2000; **28**: N228–N232.

52. Ruiz-Bailen, M., Aguayo, d.H., Ruiz-Navarro, S. *et al.* Reversible myocardial dysfunction after cardiopulmonary resuscitation. *Resuscitation* 2005; **66**: 175–181.

53. Shyu, K.G., Chang, H., Lin, C.C., Huang, F.Y. & Hung, C.R. Concentrations of serum interleukin-8 after successful cardiopulmonary resuscitation in patients with cardiopulmonary arrest. *Am. Heart J.* 1997; **134**: 551–556.

54. Ito, T., Saitoh, D., Fukuzuka, K. *et al.* Significance of elevated serum interleukin-8 in patients resuscitated after cardiopulmonary arrest. *Resuscitation* 2001; **51**: 47–53.

55. Adrie, C., Adib-Conquy, M., Laurent, I. *et al.* Successful cardiopulmonary resuscitation after cardiac arrest as a "sepsis-like" syndrome. *Circulation* 2002; **106**: 562–568.

56. Kluck, R.M., Bossy-Wetzel, E., Green, D.R. & Newmeyer, D.D. The release of cytochrome c from mitochondria: a primary site for Bcl-2 regulation of apoptosis. *Science* 1997; **275**: 1132–1136.

57. Li, P., Nijhawan, D., Budihardjo, I. *et al.* Cytochrome c and dATP-dependent formation of Apaf-1/caspase-9 complex initiates an apoptotic protease cascade. *Cell* 1997; **91**: 479–489.

58. Green, D.R. & Reed, J.C. Mitochondria and apoptosis. *Science* 1998; **281**: 1309–1312.

59. Crompton, M. The mitochondrial permeability transition pore and its role in cell death. *Biochem. J.* 1999; **341**: 233–249.

60. Weiss, J.N., Korge, P., Honda, H.M. & Ping, P. Role of the mitochondrial permeability transition in myocardial disease. *Circ. Res.* 2003; **93**: 292–301.

61. Halestrap, A.P., Clarke, S.J. & Javadov, S.A. Mitochondrial permeability transition pore opening during myocardial reperfusion – a target for cardioprotection. *Cardiovasc. Res.* 2004; **61**: 372–385.

62. Juhaszova, M., Zorov, D.B., Kim, S.H. *et al.* Glycogen synthase kinase-3beta mediates convergence of protection signaling to inhibit the mitochondrial permeability transition pore. *J. Clin. Invest.* 2004; **113**: 1535–1549.

63. Murphy, E. Primary and secondary signaling pathways in early preconditioning that converge on the mitochondria to produce cardioprotection. *Circ. Res.* 2004; **94**: 7–16.

64. Pan, G., Humke, E.W. & Dixit, V.M. Activation of caspases triggered by cytochrome c in vitro. *FEBS Lett.* 1998; **426**: 151–154.

65. Iwai, T., Tanonaka, K., Inoue, R., Kasahara, S., Kamo, N. & Takeo, S. Mitochondrial damage during ischemia determines post-ischemic contractile dysfunction in perfused rat heart. *J. Mol. Cell. Cardiol.* 2002; **34**: 725–738.

66. Vanden Hoek, T.L., Qin, Y., Wojcik, K. *et al.* Reperfusion, not simulated ischemia, initiates intrinsic apoptosis injury in chick cardiomyocytes. *Am. J. Physiol. Heart Circ. Physiol.* 2003; **284**: H141–H150.

67. Earnshaw, W.C., Martins, L.M. & Kaufmann, S.H. Mammalian caspases: structure, activation, substrates, and functions during apoptosis. *Annu. Rev. Biochem.* 1999; **68**: 383–424.

68. Zou, H., Li, Y., Liu, X. & Wang, X. An APAF-1.cytochrome c multimeric complex is a functional apoptosome that activates procaspase-9. *J. Biol. Chem.* 1999; **274**: 11549–11556.

69. Schlesinger, P.H., Gross, A., Yin, X.M. *et al.* Comparison of the ion channel characteristics of proapoptotic BAX and anti-apoptotic BCL-2. *Proc. Natl Acad. Sci. USA* 1997; **94**: 11357–11362.

70. Niquet, J. & Wasterlain, C.G. Bim, Bad, and Bax: a deadly combination in epileptic seizures. *J. Clin. Invest.* 2004; **113**: 960–962.

71. Ott, M., Robertson, J.D., Gogvadze, V., Zhivotovsky, B. & Orrenius, S. Cytochrome c release from mitochondria proceeds by a two-step process. *Proc. Natl Acad. Sci. USA* 2002; **99**: 1259–1263.

72. Petrosillo, G., Ruggiero, F.M., Pistolese, M. & Paradies, G. Ca^{2+}-induced reactive oxygen species production promotes cytochrome c release from rat liver mitochondria via mitochondrial permeability transition (MPT)-dependent and MPT-independent mechanisms: role of cardiolipin. *J. Biol. Chem.* 2004; **279**: 53103–53108.

73. Van Eyk, J.E., Powers, F., Law, W., Larue, C., Hodges, R.S. & Solaro, R.J. Breakdown and release of myofilament proteins during ischemia and ischemia/reperfusion in rat hearts: identification of degradation products and effects on the pCa-force relation. *Circ. Res.* 1998; **82**: 261–271.

74. Bolli, R. & Marban, E. Molecular and cellular mechanisms of myocardial stunning. *Physiol. Rev.* 1999; **79**: 609–634.

75. Marban, E., Kitakaze, M., Koretsune, Y., Yue, D.T., Chacko, V.P. & Pike, M.M. Quantification of $[Ca^{2+}]_i$ in perfused hearts. Critical evaluation of the 5F-BAPTA and nuclear magnetic resonance method as applied to the study of ischemia and reperfusion. *Circ. Res.* 1990; **66**: 1255–1267.

76. Carrozza, J.P., Jr., Bentivegna, L.A., Williams, C.P., Kuntz, R.E., Grossman, W. & Morgan, J.P. Decreased myofilament responsiveness in myocardial stunning follows transient calcium overload during ischemia and reperfusion. *Circ. Res.* 1992; **71**: 1334–1340.

77. Communal, C., Sumandea, M., de Tombe, P., Narula, J., Solaro, R.J. & Hajjar, R.J. Functional consequences of caspase activation in cardiac myocytes. *Proc. Natl Acad. Sci. USA* 2002; **99**: 6252–6256.

78. Barta, J., Toth, A., Edes, I. *et al.* Calpain-1-sensitive myofibrillar proteins of the human myocardium. *Mol. Cell. Biochem.* 2005; **278**: 1–8.

79. Radhakrishnan, J., Wang, S., Ayoub, I.M., Kolarova, J.D. & Gazmuri, R.J. Myocardial caspase-3 activation after resuscitation from ventricular fibrillation. *Circulation* 2005; **112**:II-324 (abstract).

80. Miller, W.P., McDonald, K.S. & Moss, R.L. Onset of reduced Ca^{2+} sensitivity of tension during stunning in porcine myocardium. *J. Mol. Cell. Cardiol.* 1996; **28**: 689–697.

81. Burkart, E.M., Sumandea, M.P., Kobayashi, T. *et al.* Phosphorylation or glutamic acid substitution at protein kinase C sites on cardiac troponin I differentially depress myofilament tension and shortening velocity. *J. Biol. Chem.* 2003; **278**: 11265–11272.

82. Zaugg, C.E., Ziegler, A., Lee, R.J., Barbosa, V. & Buser, P.T. Postresuscitation stunning: postfibrillatory myocardial dysfunction caused by reduced myofilament Ca^{2+} responsiveness after ventricular fibrillation-induced myocyte Ca^{2+} overload. *J. Cardiovasc. Electrophysiol.* 2002; **13**: 1017–1024.

83. Matsumura, Y., Kusuoka, H., Inoue, M., Hori, M. & Kamada, T. Protective effect of the protease inhibitor leupeptin against myocardial stunning. *J. Cardiovasc. Pharmacol.* 1993; **22**: 135–142.

84. Matsumura, Y., Saeki, E., Inoue, M., Hori, M., Kamada, T. & Kusuoka, H. Inhomogeneous disappearance of myofilament-related cytoskeletal proteins in stunned myocardium of guinea pig. *Circ. Res.* 1996; **79**: 447–454.

85. Rudzinski, T., Mussur, M., Gwiazda, Z. & Mussur, M. Protease inhibitor leupeptin attenuates myocardial stunning in rat heart. *Med. Sci. Monit.* 2004; **10**: BR4–BR10.

86. Aufderheide, T.P., Pirrallo, R.G., Provo, T.A. & Lurie, K.G. Clinical evaluation of an inspiratory impedance threshold device during standard cardiopulmonary resuscitation in patients with out-of-hospital cardiac arrest. *Crit. Care Med.* 2005; **33**: 734–740.

87. Warner, E.D., Dahl, C. & Ewy, G.A. Myocardial injury from transthoracic defibrillator countershock. *Arch. Pathol.* 1975; **99**: 55–59.

88. Mehta, J., Runge, W., Cohn, J.N. & Carlyle, P. Myocardial damage after repetitive direct current shock in the dog: correlation between left ventricular end-diastolic pressure and extent of myocardial necrosis. *J. Lab. Clin. Med.* 1978; **91**: 272–289.

89. Xie, J., Weil, M.H., Sun, S. *et al.* High-energy defibrillation increases the severity of postresuscitation myocardial dysfunction. *Circulation* 1997; **96**: 683–688.

90. Ehsani, A., Ewy, G.A. & Sobel, B.E. Effects of electrical countershock on serum creatine phosphokinase (CPK) isoenzyme activity. *Am. J. Cardiol.* 1976; **37**: 12–18.

91. Koning, G., Veefkind, A.H. & Schneider, H. Cardiac damage caused by direct application of defibrillator shocks to isolated Langendorff-perfused rabbit heart. *Am. Heart J.* 1980; **100**: 473–482.

92. Doherty, P.W., McLaughlin, P.R., Billingham, M., Kernoff, R., Goris, M.L. & Harrison, D.C. Cardiac damage produced by direct current countershock applied to the heart. *Am. J. Cardiol.* 1979; **43**: 225–232.

93. Kerber, R.E., Martins, J.B., Gascho, J.A., Marcus, M.L. & Grayzel, J. Effect of direct-current countershocks on regional myocardial contractility and perfusion. Experimental studies. *Circulation* 1981; **63**: 323–332.

94. Geddes, L.A., Tacker, W.A., Rosborough, J. *et al.* The electrical dose for ventricular defibrillation with electrodes applied directly to the heart. *J. Thorac. Cardiovasc. Surg.* 1974; **68**: 593–602.

95. Krauthamer, V. & Jones, J.L. Calcium dynamics in cultured heart cells exposed to defibrillator-type electric shocks. *Life Sci.* 1997; **60**: 1977–1985.

96. Patton, J.N., Allen, J.D. & Pantridge, J.F. The effects of shock energy, propranolol, and verapamil on cardiac damage caused by transthoracic countershock. *Circulation* 1984; **69**: 357–368.

97. Gazmuri, R.J., Deshmukh, S. & Shah, P.R. Myocardial effects of repeated electrical defibrillations in the isolated fibrillating rat heart. *Crit. Care Med.* 2000; **28**: 2690–2696.

98. Runsio, M., Bergfeldt, L., Brodin, L.A., *et al.* Left ventricular function after repeated episodes of ventricular fibrillation and defibrillation assessed by transoesophageal echocardiography. *Eur. Heart J.* 1997; **18**: 124–131.

99. Niemann, J.T., Cairns, C.B., Sharma, J. & Lewis, R.J. Treatment of prolonged ventricular fibrillation. Immediate countershock versus high-dose epinephrine and CPR preceding countershock. *Circulation* 1992; **85**: 281–287.

100. Cobb, L.A., Fahrenbruch, C.E., Walsh, T.R. *et al.* Influence of cardiopulmonary resuscitation prior to defibrillation in patients with out-of-hospital ventricular fibrillation. *J. Am. Med. Assoc.* 1999; **281**: 1182–1188.

101. Wik, L., Hansen, T.B., Fylling, F. *et al.* Delaying defibrillation to give basic cardiopulmonary resuscitation to patients with out-of-hospital ventricular fibrillation: a randomized trial. *J. Am. Med. Assoc.* 2003; **289**: 1389–1395.

102. Brown, C.G., Dzwonczyk, R. & Martin, D.R. Physiologic measurement of the ventricular fibrillation ECG signal: estimating the duration of ventricular fibrillation. *Ann. Emerg. Med.* 1993; **22**: 70–74.

103. Noc, M., Weil, M.H., Gazmuri, R.J., Sun, S., Biscera, J. & Tang, W. Ventricular fibrillation voltage as a monitor of the effectiveness of cardiopulmonary resuscitation. *J. Lab. Clin. Med.* 1994; **124**: 421–426.

104. Brown, C.G., Griffith, R.F., Van Ligten, P. *et al.* Median frequency – a new parameter for predicting defibrillation success rate. *Ann. Emerg. Med.* 1991; **20**: 787–789.

105. Strohmenger, H.U., Lindner, K.H. & Brown, C.G. Analysis of the ventricular fibrillation ECG signal amplitude and frequency parameters as predictors of countershock success in humans. *Chest* 1997; **111**: 584–589.

106. Povoas, H.P., Weil, M.H., Tang, W., Bisera, J., Klouche, K. & Barbatsis, A. Predicting the success of defibrillation by electrocardiographic analysis. *Resuscitation* 2002; **53**: 77–82.

107. Tang, W., Weil, M.H., Sun, S. *et al.* A comparison of biphasic and monophasic waveform defibrillation after prolonged ventricular fibrillation. *Chest* 2001; **120**: 948–954.

108. Schneider, T., Martens, P.R., Paschen, H. *et al.* Multicenter, randomized, controlled trial of 150-J biphasic shocks compared with 200- to 360-J monophasic shocks in the resuscitation of out-of-hospital cardiac arrest victims. Optimized Response to Cardiac Arrest (ORCA) Investigators. *Circulation* 2000; **102**: 1780–1787.

109. Ditchey, R.V. & Lindenfeld, J. Failure of epinephrine to improve the balance between myocardial oxygen supply and demand during closed-chest resuscitation in dogs. *Circulation* 1988; **78**: 382–389.

110. Berg, R.A., Otto, C.W., Kern, K.B. *et al.* High-dose epinephrine results in greater early mortality after resuscitation from prolonged cardiac arrest in pigs: a prospective, randomized study. *Crit. Care Med.* 1994; **22**: 282–290.

111. Tang, W., Weil, M.H., Sun, S., Noc, M., Yang, L. & Gazmuri, R.J. Epinephrine increases the severity of postresuscitation myocardial dysfunction. *Circulation* 1995; **92**: 3089–3093.

112. Ditchey, R.V., Rubio-Perez, A., Slinker, B.K. Beta-adrenergic blockade reduces myocardial injury during experimental cardiopulmonary resuscitation. *J. Am. Coll. Cardiol.* 1994; **24**: 804–812.

113. Killingsworth, C.R., Wei, C.C., Dell'Italia, L.J. *et al.* Short-acting beta-adrenergic antagonist esmolol given at reperfusion improves survival after prolonged ventricular fibrillation. *Circulation* 2004; **109**: 2469–2474.

114. Cammarata, G., Weil, M.H., Sun, S., Tang, W., Wang, J. & Huang, L. Beta1-adrenergic blockade during cardiopulmonary resuscitation improves survival. *Crit. Care Med.* 2004; **32**: S440–S443.

115. Angelos, M.G., Torres, C.A.A., Waite, D.W. *et al.* Left ventricular myocardial ATP changes during reperfusion of ventricular fibrillation: The influence of flow and epinephrine. *Crit. Care Med.* 2000; **28**: 1503–1508.

116. Wenzel, V. & Lindner, K.H. Arginine vasopressin during cardiopulmonary resuscitation: laboratory evidence, clinical experience and recommendations, and a view to the future. *Crit. Care Med.* 2002; **30**: S157–S161.

117. Sun, S., Weil, M.H., Tang, W., Kamohara, T. & Klouche, K. alpha-Methylnorepinephrine, a selective alpha2-adrenergic agonist for cardiac resuscitation. *J. Am. Coll. Cardiol.* 2001; **37**: 951–956.

118. Klouche, K., Weil, M.H., Tang, W., Povoas, H., Kamohara, T. & Bisera, J. A selective alpha(2)-adrenergic agonist for cardiac resuscitation. *J. Lab. Clin. Med.* 2002; **140**: 27–34.

119. Cai, J.J., Morgan, D.A., Haynes, W.G., Martins, J.B. & Lee, H.C. Alpha 2-Adrenergic stimulation is protective against ischemia-reperfusion-induced ventricular arrhythmias in vivo. *Am. J. Physiol. Heart Circ. Physiol.* 2002; **283**: H2606–H2611.

120. Karmazyn, M. Amiloride enhances postischemic ventricular recovery: possible role of Na^+/H^+ exchange. *Am. J. Physiol.* 1988; **255**: H608–H615.

121. Lazdunski, M., Frelin, C. & Vigne, P. The sodium/hydrogen exchange system in cardiac cells: its biochemical and pharmacological properties and its role in regulating internal concentrations of sodium and internal pH. *J. Mol. Cell. Cardiol.* 1985; **17**: 1029–1042.

122. Avkiran, M. Rational basis for use of sodium–hydrogen exchange inhibitors in myocardial ischemia. *Am. J. Cardiol.* 1999; **83**: 10G–17G.

123. Imahashi, K., Kusuoka, H., Hashimoto, K., Yoshioka, J., Yamaguchi, H. & Nishimura, T. Intracellular sodium accumulation during ischemia as the substrate for reperfusion injury. *Circ. Res.* 1999; **84**: 1401–1406.

124. Mosca, S.M. & Cingolani, H.E. [The Na^+/Ca^{2+} exchanger as responsible for myocardial stunning]. *Medicina (B Aires)* 2001; **61**: 167–173.

125. Ditchey, R.V. & Horwitz, L.D. Metabolic evidence of inadequate coronary blood flow during closed-chest resuscitation in dogs. *Cardiovasc. Res.* 1985; **19**: 419–425.

126. Gazmuri, R.J., Hoffner, E., Kalcheim, J. *et al.* Myocardial protection during ventricular fibrillation by reduction of proton-driven sarcolemmal sodium influx. *J. Lab. Clin. Med.* 2001; **137**: 43–55.

127. Wann, S.R., Weil, M.H., Sun, S., Tang, W. & Yu, T. Cariporide for pharmacologic defibrillation after prolonged cardiac arrest. *J. Cardiovasc. Pharmacol. Ther.* 2002; **7**: 161–169.

128. Kolarova, J., Yi, Z., Ayoub, I.M. & Gazmuri, R.J. Cariporide potentiates the effects of epinephrine and vasopressin by nonvascular mechanisms during closed-chest resuscitation. *Chest* 2005; **127**: 1327–1334.

129. Ayoub, I.M., Kolarova, J., Kantola, R.L., Sanders, R. & Gazmuri, R.J. Cariporide minimizes adverse myocardial effects of epinephrine during resuscitation from ventricular fibrillation. *Crit. Care Med.* 2005; **33**: 2599–2605.

130. Ruiz-Meana, M., Garcia-Dorado, D., Pina, P., Inserte, J., Agullo, L. & Soler-Soler, J. Cariporide preserves mitochondrial proton gradient and delays ATP depletion in cardiomyocytes during ischemic conditions. *Am. J. Physiol. Heart Circ. Physiol.* 2003; **285**: H999–H1006.

131. Mentzer, R.J. Effects of Na^+/H^+ exchange inhibition by cariporide on death and nonfatal myocardial infarction in patients undergoing coronary artery bypass graft surgery: The EXPEDITION study. *Circulation* 2003; **108**: 3M (abstract).

132. Liu, Y. & O'Rourke, B. Opening of mitochondrial K(ATP) channels triggers cardioprotection. Are reactive oxygen species involved? *Circ. Res.* 2001; **88**: 750–752.

133. Kevelaitis, E., Oubenaissa, A., Mouas, C., Peynet, J. & Menasche, P. Ischemic preconditioning with opening of mitochondrial adenosine triphosphate-sensitive potassium channels or Na/H exchange inhibition: which is the best protective strategy for heart transplants? *J. Thorac. Cardiovasc. Surg.* 2001; **121**: 155–162.

134. Nakai, Y., Horimoto, H., Mieno, S. & Sasaki, S. Mitochondrial ATP-sensitive potassium channel plays a dominant role in ischemic preconditioning of rabbit heart. *Eur. Surg. Res.* 2001; **33**: 57–63.

135. O'Rourke, B. Evidence for mitochondrial K^+ channels and their role in cardioprotection. *Circ. Res.* 2004; **94**: 420–432.

136. Ozcan, C., Holmuhamedov, E.L., Jahangir, A. & Terzic, A. Diazoxide protects mitochondria from anoxic injury: implications for myopreservation. *J. Thorac. Cardiovasc. Surg.* 2001; **121**: 298–306.

137. Ishida, H., Hirota, Y., Genka, C., Nakazawa, H., Nakaya, H. & Sato, T. Opening of mitochondrial K(ATP) channels attenuates the ouabain-induced calcium overload in mitochondria. *Circ. Res.* 2001; **89**: 856–858.

138. Tang, W., Weil, M.H., Sun, S., Pernat, A. & Mason, E. K(ATP) channel activation reduces the severity of postresuscitation myocardial dysfunction. *Am. J. Physiol. Heart Circ. Physiol.* 2000; **279**: H1609–H1615.

139. Benedict, P.E., Benedict, M.B., Su, T.P. & Bolling, S.F. Opiate drugs and delta-receptor-mediated myocardial protection. *Circulation* 1999; **100**: II357–II360.

140. McPherson, B.C. & Yao, Z. Signal transduction of opioid-induced cardioprotection in ischemia-reperfusion. *Anesthesiology* 2001; **94**: 1082–1088.

141. Sun, S., Weil, M.H., Tang, W., Kamohara, T. & Klouche, K. Delta-opioid receptor agonist reduces severity of postresuscitation myocardial dysfunction. *Am. J. Physiol. Heart Circ. Physiol.* 2004; **287**: H969–H974.

142. Monyer, H., Hartley, D.M. & Choi, D.W. 21-Aminosteroids attenuate excitotoxic neuronal injury in cortical cell cultures. *Neuron* 1990; **5**: 121–126.

143. Perna, A.M., Liguori, P., Bonacchi, M. *et al.* Protection of rat heart from ischaemia-reperfusion injury by the 21-aminosteroid U-74389G. *Pharmacol. Res.* 1996; **34**: 25–31.

144. Tseng, M.T., Chan, S.A., Reid, K. & Lyer, V. Post-ischemic treatment with a lazaroid (U74389G) prevents transient global ischemic damage in rat hippocampus. *Neurol. Res.* 1997; **19**: 431–434.

145. Takahashi, T., Takeyoshi, I., Hasegawa, Y. *et al.* Cardioprotective effects of Lazaroid U-74389G on ischemia-reperfusion injury in canine hearts. *J. Heart Lung Transpl.* 1999; **18**: 285–291.

146. Wang, J., Weil, M.H., Kamohara, T. *et al.* A lazaroid mitigates postresuscitation myocardial dysfunction. *Crit. Care Med.* 2004; **32**: 553–558.

147. Fisher, J.W. Erythropoietin: physiology and pharmacology update. *Exp. Biol. Med. (Maywood)* 2003; **228**: 1–14.

148. Cai, Z., Manalo, D.J., Wei, G. *et al.* Hearts from rodents exposed to intermittent hypoxia or erythropoietin are protected against ischemia-reperfusion injury. *Circulation* 2003; **108**: 79–85.

149. Calvillo, L., Latini, R., Kajstura, J. *et al.* Recombinant human erythropoietin protects the myocardium from ischemia-reperfusion injury and promotes beneficial remodeling. *Proc. Natl Acad. Sci. USA* 2003; **100**: 4802–4806.

150. Moon, C., Krawczyk, M., Ahn, D. *et al.* Erythropoietin reduces myocardial infarction and left ventricular functional decline after coronary artery ligation in rats. *Proc. Natl Acad. Sci. USA* 2003; **100**: 11612–11617.

151. Parsa, C.J., Matsumoto, A., Kim, J. *et al.* A novel protective effect of erythropoietin in the infarcted heart. *J. Clin. Invest.* 2003; **112**: 999–1007.

152. Tramontano, A.F., Muniyappa, R., Black, A.D. *et al.* Erythropoietin protects cardiac myocytes from hypoxia-induced apoptosis through an Akt-dependent pathway. *Biochem. Biophys. Res. Commun.* 2003; **308**: 990–994.

153. Cai, Z. & Semenza, G.L. Phosphatidylinositol-3-kinase signaling is required for erythropoietin-mediated acute protection against myocardial ischemia/reperfusion injury. *Circulation* 2004; **109**: 2050–2053.

154. Lipsic, E., van der, M.P., Henning, R.H. *et al.* Timing of erythropoietin treatment for cardioprotection in ischemia/reperfusion. *J. Cardiovasc. Pharmacol.* 2004; **44**: 473–479.

155. Parsa, C.J., Kim, J., Riel, R.U. *et al.* Cardioprotective effects of erythropoietin in the reperfused ischemic heart: a potential role for cardiac fibroblasts. *J. Biol. Chem.* 2004; **279**: 20655–20662.

156. Wright, G.L., Hanlon, P., Amin, K., Steenbergen, C., Murphy, E. & Arcasoy, M.O. Erythropoietin receptor expression in adult rat cardiomyocytes is associated with an acute cardioprotective effect for recombinant erythropoietin during ischemia-reperfusion injury. *FASEB J.* 2004; **18**: 1031–1033.

157. Namiuchi, S., Kagaya, Y., Ohta, J. *et al.* High serum erythropoietin level is associated with smaller infarct size in patients with acute myocardial infarction who undergo successful primary percutaneous coronary intervention. *J. Am. Coll. Cardiol.* 2005; **45**: 1406–1412.

158. Hirata, A., Minamino, T., Asanuma, H. *et al.* Erythropoietin just before reperfusion reduces both lethal arrhythmias and infarct size via the phosphatidylinositol-3 kinase-dependent pathway in canine hearts. *Cardiovasc Drugs Ther.* 2005; **19**: 33–40.

159. Hanlon, P.R., Fu, P., Wright, G.L., Steenbergen, C., Arcasoy, M.O. & Murphy, E. Mechanisms of erythropoietin-mediated cardioprotection during ischemia-reperfusion injury: role of protein kinase C and phosphatidylinositol 3-kinase signaling. *FASEB J.* 2005; **19**: 1323–1325.

160. Singh, D., Ayoub, I.M., Kolarova, J.D., Havalad, S. & Gazmuri, R.J. Cardioprotection by erythropoietin during resuscitation from ventricular fibrillation. *Crit. Care Med.* 2005; **33**: A24 (abstract).

161. van der Wouw, P.A., Koster, R.W., Delemarre, B.J., de Vos, R., Lampe-Schoenmaeckers, A.J. & Lie, K.I. Diagnostic accuracy of transesophageal echocardiography during cardiopulmonary resuscitation. *J. Am. Coll. Cardiol.* 1997; **30**: 780–783.

162. Varriale, P. & Maldonado, J.M. Echocardiographic observations during in hospital cardiopulmonary resuscitation. *Crit. Care Med.* 1997; **25**: 1717–1720.

163. Kern, K.B., Hilwig, R.W., Berg, R.A. *et al.* Postresuscitation left ventricular systolic and diastolic dysfunction. Treatment with dobutamine. *Circulation* 1997; **95**: 2610–2613.

164. Vasquez, A., Kern, K.B., Hilwig, R.W., Heidenreich, J., Berg, R.A. & Ewy, G.A. Optimal dosing of dobutamine for treating post-resuscitation left ventricular dysfunction. *Resuscitation* 2004; **61**: 199–207.

165. Studer, W., Wu, X., Siegemund, M., Marsch, S., Seeberger, M. & Filipovic, M. Influence of dobutamine on the variables of systemic haemodynamics, metabolism, and intestinal perfusion after cardiopulmonary resuscitation in the rat. *Resuscitation* 2005; **64**: 227–232.

166. Niemann, J.T., Garner, D., Khaleeli, E. & Lewis, R.J. Milrinone facilitates resuscitation from cardiac arrest and attenuates postresuscitation myocardial dysfunction. *Circulation* 2003; **108**: 3031–3035.

167. Endoh, M. Mechanism of action of Ca^{2+} sensitizers – update 2001. *Cardiovasc. Drugs Ther.* 2001; **15**: 397–403.

168. Kaheinen, P., Pollesello, P., Levijoki, J. & Haikala, H. Effects of levosimendan and milrinone on oxygen consumption in isolated guinea-pig heart. *J. Cardiovasc. Pharmacol.* 2004; **43**: 555–561.

169. Lilleberg, J., Ylonen, V., Lehtonen, L. & Toivonen, L. The calcium sensitizer levosimendan and cardiac arrhythmias: an analysis of the safety database of heart failure treatment studies. *Scand. Cardiovasc. J.* 2004; **38**: 80–84.

170. Huang, L., Weil, M.H., Tang, W., Sun, S. & Wang, J. Comparison between dobutamine and levosimendan for management of postresuscitation myocardial dysfunction. *Crit. Care Med.* 2005; **33**: 487–491.

49

Prevention of postresuscitation neurologic dysfunction and injury by the use of therapeutic mild hypothermia

Wilhelm Behringer[1], Stephen Bernard[2], Michael Holzer[3], Kees Polderman[4], Marjaana Tiainen[5] and Risto O. Roine[6]

[1] University AKH, Vienna, Austria, [2] Department of Epidemiology and Preventive Medicine, Monash University, Australia, [3] University Klinik fur Notfallmedizin, Vienna, Austria, [4] Department of Intensive Care, VU University Medical Center, Amsterdam, The Netherlands, [5] Department of Neurology, Helsinki University Hospital, Finland, [6] Department of Neurology, Turku University Hospital, Finland

This book chapter is dedicated to Peter Safar, the father of modern resuscitation, and world leading pioneer in the field of therapeutic hypothermia.

Introduction

The history of induced hypothermia began in the 1950s with elective moderate hypothermia of the brain, introduced under anesthesia, for the protection–preservation during brain ischemia needed for surgery on heart or brain.[1,2] In the early 1960s, Peter Safar recommended the use of therapeutic resuscitative hypothermia for humans after cardiac arrest in his cardiopulmonary–cerebral resuscitation algorithm.[3] At this time, it was thought that moderate hypothermia (28–32 °C) was required for brain protection. Resuscitative hypothermia research was then given up for 25 years, as experimental and clinical trials had been complicated by the injurious systemic effects of total body cooling, such as shivering, vasospasm, increased plasma viscosity, increased hematocrit, hypocoagulation, arrhythmias, and ventricular fibrillation, when temperatures dropped below 30 °C, and lowered resistance to infection during prolonged moderate hypothermia.[4–7] Moderate hypothermia was too difficult to induce and to maintain.

Peter Safar deserves most of the credit that mild therapeutic hypothermia was re-discovered in the mid 1980s. When he considered the reasons for various outcomes with the same durations of cardiac arrest in his dog experiments, he observed that relatively small differences in brain temperature in the range of mild hypothermia (33–36 °C) at the start of the experiments had a major influence on neurologic outcome. He and his research group then confirmed these observations in systematic studies of mild hypothermia before, during, and after cardiac arrest in dogs.[8–12]

Fritz Sterz, who was research fellow in Safar's laboratory at this time, initiated after his return to Vienna the Hypothermia After Cardiac Arrest (HACA) European multicenter trial in the mid 1990s.[13] This landmark study, together with the Australian study by Bernard,[14] led to the recommendation to use mild hypothermia in patients resuscitated from cardiac arrest by the European Resuscitation Council[15] and the American Heart Association[16] in 2005, more than 40 years after the first recommendation by Peter Safar.

This chapter reviews the current status of therapeutic mild hypothermia in cardiac arrest. Laboratory and clinical studies are described, potential mechanisms and side effects of hypothermia, and cooling methods to induce mild hypothermia. The influence of mild hypothermia on the prediction of neurologic outcome after cardiac arrest is presented. In the conclusion, recommendations for the current use of hypothermia and recommendations for future laboratory and clinical research are given.

Therapeutic mild hypothermia

Animal outcome studies (Behringer)

This section documents the background of therapeutic hypothermia with regard to animal models with cardiac arrest or vessel occlusion that led to the recent trials of therapeutic hypothermia after cardiac arrest in humans.[13,14,17–21]

Cardiac Arrest: The Science and Practice of Resuscitation Medicine. 2nd edn., ed. Norman Paradis, Henry Halperin, Karl Kern, Volker Wenzel, Douglas Chamberlain. Published by Cambridge University Press. © Cambridge University Press, 2007.

Protective hypothermia, induced before cardiac arrest, is differentiated from *preservative* hypothermia, induced during cardiac arrest, and from *resuscitative* hypothermia, induced after resuscitation from cardiac arrest. The first animal studies of *resuscitative* hypothermia after cardiac arrest were reported in the 1950s.[22,23]

Protective-preservative hypothermia

Therapeutic hypothermia was rediscovered in the mid-1980s, when Hossmann reported the beneficial effect of mild hypothermia, unintentionally induced before the experiment, on EEG recovery in cats subjected to 1 hour of global brain ischemia, followed by blood recirculation for 3 hours or longer.[24] At the same time, Safar analysed the outcome data of several cardiac arrest dog studies, and found that dogs that were mildly hypothermic at the beginning of the experiment showed better neurologic outcome than dogs that were normothermic at the beginning of the experiment.[25] These observations were followed by controlled randomized animal studies in various laboratories. In dogs, ventricular fibrillation cardiac arrest of 12.5-minute no-flow was accompanied by head immersion in ice water (which reduced brain temperature by only 1 °C) and followed by reperfusion cooling with brief cardiopulmonary bypass to 34 °C for 1 hour; functional and morphologic brain outcome variables were significantly improved in the hypothermic groups 4 days after the insult.[8] Busto and colleagues found in a 20-minute four-vessel occlusion rat model that small increments of intra-ischemic brain temperature (33°, 34°, 36°, or 39 °C) markedly accentuated histopathological changes following 3-day survival, despite severe depletion of brain energy metabolites during ischemia at all temperatures.[26] Siesjö and colleagues confirmed the beneficial effects of intra-ischemic hypothermia in a two-vessel occlusion rat model with various durations of ischemia by showing that intentional lowering of brain temperature from 37° to 35 °C markedly reduced and to 33 °C virtually prevented neuronal necrosis.[27]

Importantly, the benefit of intra-ischemic mild to moderate hypothermia on neuronal death is regarded as longlasting. Green and colleagues found in a 12.5-minute four-vessel occlusion rat model that intra-ischemic hypothermia to 30 °C protected from behavioral deficits and neuronal injury for up to 2 months.[28] This longlasting effect of intra-ischemic hypothermia was confirmed by the same group in a 10-minute two-vessel occlusion rat model,[29] and by Corbett and colleagues in a 5-minute global ischemia gerbil model with brain temperature to 32 °C.[30]

Resuscitative hypothermia

The rediscovery of protective-preservative mild to moderate hypothermia in brain ischemia led to widespread research of *resuscitative* mild to moderate hypothermia in several animal models in the 1990s. Safar and colleagues conducted a systematic series of outcome studies in dogs of prolonged normothermic cardiac arrest followed by mild resuscitative cerebral hypothermia (34 °C), induced immediately after reperfusion and maintained for 2–3 hours[9,10,12] or 12 hours.[11] Controlled ventilation was maintained for 24 hours, and intensive care was provided for 3 to 4 days, with final evaluation of neurologic outcome and histologic damage in various brain regions. In one study,[9] ventricular fibrillation cardiac arrest after 10-minute no-flow was reversed by standard external cardiopulmonary resuscitation; cooling to 34 °C for 2 hours with a combination of head-neck-trunk surface cooling, plus cold fluid loads administered intravenously, intragastrically, and nasopharyngeally, was induced in one group at the beginning of resuscitation, and in another group after restoration of spontaneous circulation. In both groups, neurologic recovery in terms of histologic damage and functional outcome was improved compared to that in control animals. Next,[10] ventricular fibrillation cardiac arrest of 12.5-minutes no-flow was reversed by brief cardiopulmonary bypass; immediate mild (34 °C) or moderate (30 °C) hypothermia, induced with bypass, for 1 hour improved functional and morphologic brain outcome, but deep postarrest hypothermia (15 °C) did not improve function and worsened brain histology. In the next study,[12] ventricular fibrillation cardiac arrest of 12.5-minute no-flow was reversed by brief cardiopulmonary bypass; delaying cooling (to 34 °C for 1 hour) until 15 minutes after normothermic reperfusion did not improve functional outcome but histologic damage. Finally,[11] ventricular fibrillation cardiac arrest of 11-minute no-flow was reversed by brief cardiopulmonary bypass; a combination treatment of mild hypothermia by head-neck-surface cooling plus peritoneal instillation of cold Ringer's solution to keep brain temperature at 34 °C from reperfusion for 12 hours, plus cerebral blood flow promotion by induced moderate hypertension for 4 hours, plus colloid-induced hemodilution for 12 hours, led to the best outcome yet encountered in dogs, with lowest histologic damage ever achieved. Mild cooling in all dog studies caused no cardiovascular or other side effects.

At the same time, resuscitative hypothermia was also studied in rodent ischemia models. First, Busto and colleagues reduced hippocampal CA1 injury with 3 hours of immediate, but not 30-minute delayed postischemic hypothermia to 30 °C in a two-vessel occlusion rat model with 10 minutes of ischemia and survival to 3 days.[26] Buchan and colleagues reduced hippocampal CA1 injury with 8 hours of immediate hypothermia to 34.5 °C in gerbils with 5 minutes of ischemia and survival to 5 days.[31] Coimbra and colleagues reduced hippocampal CA1 injury with 5 hours of immediate hypothermia to 29 °C in gerbils with 5 minutes of ischemia and survival to 7 days.[32] Chopp and colleagues reduced hippocampal CA1 injury with 2 hours of immediate hypothermia to 34 °C in a two-vessel occlusion rat model with 8 but not 12 minutes of ischemia, and survival to 7 days.[33] Carroll and colleagues progressively reduced hippocampal CA1 injury with immediate hypothermia to 28–32 °C for 1/2, 1, 2, 4, and 6 hours in gerbils after 5 minutes of ischemia, and survival to 4 days; 6 hours of hypothermia delayed for 1 hour after reperfusion also resulted in protection, but 6 hours of hypothermia delayed for 3 hours after reperfusion was not effective. In another study by Coimbra and colleagues hippocampal CA1 injury was reduced with 5 hours of hypothermia to 33 °C, delayed for 2 hours after reperfusion, in a two-vessel occlusion rat model with 10-minutes of ischemia, and survival to 7 days.[34] The same group reduced hippocampal CA1 injury with 5 hours of hypothermia to 33 °C, delayed for 2, 6, and 12 hours, but not for 24 and 36 hours, after reperfusion in a two-vessel occlusion rat model with 10-minutes of ischemia, and survival to 7 days; 3.5 hours of hypothermia delayed for 2 hours after reperfusion was less effective, and 30 minutes of hypothermia delayed for 2 hours after reperfusion was ineffective in the same model.[35]

Although the benefit of intra-ischemic hypothermia on neuronal death is regarded as longlasting,[28,30] results on longlasting effects of postischemic hypothermia are more controversial. Dietrich and colleagues found hippocampal CA1 protection in a two-vessel occlusion rat model with 10-minutes of ischemia and postarrest immediate hypothermia to 30 °C for 4 hours, when histologic evaluation was at 3 days after the insult; this protection significantly declined by 7 days, and was completely absent by 60 days after the insult.[29]

Colbourne and colleagues systematically explored factors affecting neuroprotection of hypothermia in gerbils.[36–38] In the first study,[36] Experiment 1 found that 12 hours of hypothermia (3 °C) delayed for 1 hour after reperfusion attenuated the early (<10-day) ischemia-induced open-field habituation impairments, and substantially reduced CA1 necrosis against 3 minutes of ischemia when assessed at 10 and 30 days, but was only partially effective against a 5-minute occlusion; in Experiment 2, prolonged hypothermia (32 °C) for 24 hours delayed for 1 hour after reperfusion resulted in near total preservation of CA1 neurons at 30 days even after 5 minutes of ischemia. In the

second study with ischemia of 5 minutes.[37] The observation period was extended to 6 months; hypothermia (32 °C) for 24 hours delayed for 1 hour after reperfusion provided substantial CA1 protection at 6 months, but there was less protection than at 1 month. Delaying hypothermia (32 °C, 24 hours) to 4 hours after reperfusion also provided significant protection at 6 months survival, but significantly less than delaying hypothermia for only 1 hour. In the third study with ischemia of 5 minutes,[38] increasing the duration of hypothermia to 48 hours resulted in longlasting protection of neurons at 1 month, even when hypothermia was delayed to 6 hours after reperfusion.

The longlasting effect of delayed (6 hours), prolonged (48 hours) hypothermia (32°–34 °C) on functional and histologic outcome at 1 month was confirmed in rats with 10 minutes of severe four-vessel occlusion ischemia.[39]

The studies described above suggest that minimal delay and longer durations of hypothermia are of critical importance to extend the therapeutic window and to provide permanent protection of resuscitative hypothermia.

Clinical outcome studies (Holzer)

Historic use of therapeutic hypothermia after cardiac arrest

The first experiences of hypothermia after cardiac arrest were obtained in the 1950s by Benson *et al.*[40] who presented four cases of hypothermic therapy after cardiac arrest (temperature 30° to 34 °C) and Williams and Spencer[41] who compared treatment with hypothermia (31°–32 °C) in 12 patients with 7 normothermic controls. In this controlled pioneer case study, patients treated with hypothermia had a favorable neurological recovery in 50% compared to 14% in the control group. Nonetheless, because of hemodynamic and respiratory problems in these early hypothermia protocols, hypothermia was not used clinically for this indication until the late 1990s.

Clinical pilot trials of hypothermia

In 1997 Bernard *et al.*[17] found improved neurologic outcome in survivors of out-of-hospital cardiac arrest with postarrest mild hypothermia (33 °C) by surface cooling with ice packs over 12 hours compared to a historic normothermic control group (11 of 22 vs. 3 of 22 patients).

Yanagawa *et al.*[19] used water-filled cooling blankets in combination with alcohol to cool cardiac arrest survivors to a core temperature between 33 °C and 34 °C over 48 hours. Three of 13 patients in the hypothermia group survived without disabilities as compared to 1 of 15 patients in the historical control group. The long duration of cooling in this study led to a higher rate of pneumonia, but it was stated that in none of these cases the pulmonary infection was a direct cause of death.

In a different approach, Nagao et al.,[42] resuscitated patients in cardiac arrest on arrival at the emergency department with emergency cardiopulmonary bypass and intra-aortic balloon pumping. After successful resuscitation, hypothermia was attained by direct blood cooling to 34 °C via a dialysis coil for a minimum of 48 (71 ± 49) hours. Fifty-two percent of these patients survived with good neurologic recovery and no major side effects were reported.

The pilot study for the HACA trial[20] included 27 comatose patients after ventricular fibrillation cardiac arrest. Cooling blankets (Blanketrol II Hypothermia System, Cincinnati Sub-Zero Products, Inc) were placed within a special mattress consisting of air cushions (TheraKair, Kinetic Concepts, Inc), which allowed cold air to flow around the patient; head and body were cooled with a cooling blanket with constant cold air flow (Polar Bair, Augustin Medical, Inc). Patients were cooled to a target temperature of 33 ±1 °C, which was maintained for 24 hours, after which period the patients were passively rewarmed. After 6 months, good neurological recovery was achieved by 14 (52%) patients, 2 (7%) had poor neurological recovery and 11 (41%) died before discharge. Compared to historic controls this was a twofold improvement of outcome and no major complications were directly related to treatment with mild hypothermia.

For a safety and feasibility trial of therapeutic hypothermia after cardiac arrest, Felberg et al.[43] used external cooling blankets in nine patients with persistent coma and lack of acute myocardial infarction or unstable dysrhythmia. Hypothermia to 33 °C was maintained for 24 hours followed by passive rewarming. Three of the nine patients (33%) recovered completely, and one patient developed unstable cardiac dysrhythmia. Figure 49.1 summarizes outcome data of the pilot trials.

Randomized trials and meta-analysis of therapeutic hypothermia after cardiac arrest

The first randomized trial took place in one of the centers also participating in the European multicenter study.[18] In contrast to the multicenter trial the author included only patients with asystole and pulseless electrical activity and therefore no patient was included in more than one trial. A helmet device (Frigicap®) containing a solution of aqueous glycerol placed around the head and neck induced mild hypothermia in 30 patients. Once a bladder temperature of 34 °C was reached, or if cooling took longer than 4 hours, the patient was allowed to rewarm spontaneously over the next 8 hours. Two of 16 patients in the hypothermia group and none of 14 patients in the normothermia group had a favorable neurologic recovery ($P = 0.49$). Three patients in the hypothermia group survived vs. 1 patient in the normothermia group ($P = 0.60$). Oliguria occurred in 4 hypothermic and in five normothermic patients. There were no further complications reported.

In 2002 two randomized studies on hypothermia after cardiac arrest were published. In the Australian trial, 77 patients with return of spontaneous circulation after cardiac arrest of cardiac origin (ventricular fibrillation or pulseless ventricular tachycardia) were randomly treated with therapeutic hypothermia (33 °C, core temperature over 12 hours, cooled with ice packs) or normothermia.[14]

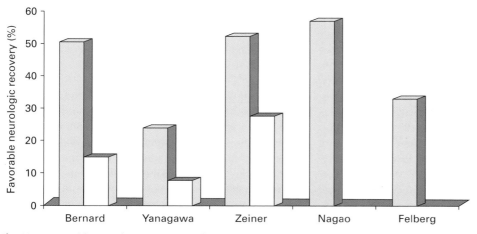

Fig. 49.1. Favorable neurologic recovery in clinical pilot trials of therapeutic hypothermia after cardiac arrest. Therapeutic hypothermia, shaded columns; historic control group, white columns.

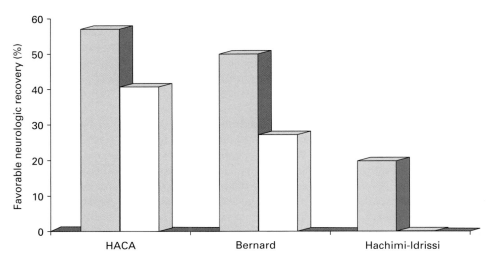

Fig. 49.2. Favorable neurologic recovery in randomized clinical trials of therapeutic hypothermia after cardiac arrest. Therapeutic hypothermia, shaded columns; normothermic control group, white columns.

The primary outcome measure was survival to hospital discharge, with neurologic function appropriate for discharge to home or a rehabilitation facility. Twenty-one of the 43 patients treated with hypothermia (49%) survived with a good neurologic function at hospital discharge as compared with 9 of the 34 treated with normothermia (26%, $P =$ 0.046). After multivariate adjustment for baseline differences, the odds ratio for a good outcome with hypothermia therapy as compared with standard treatment was 5.25 (95% CI, 1.47 to 18.76; $P =$ 0.011). There was no difference in the frequency of adverse events, but hypothermia was associated with a lower cardiac index, higher systemic vascular resistance, and hyperglycemia.

In the European multicenter trial[13] patients resuscitated after ventricular fibrillation or pulseless ventricular tachycardia cardiac arrest were randomly treated with therapeutic hypothermia (32°–34 °C bladder temperature, cooled with cold air) over 24 hours or with normothermia. All patients received standard intensive care according to a detailed protocol including the use of sedation (midazolam, initially 0.125 mg/kg per hour), analgesia (fentanyl, initially 0.002 mg/kg per hour), and relaxation (pancuronium, initially 1 mg/kg every 2 hours, then as needed to prevent shivering). Mechanical ventilation was mandatory for at least 32 hours. The primary end point was a favorable neurologic recovery within 6 months after cardiac arrest; secondary end points were mortality within 6 months and the rate of complications within 7 days. Seventy-five of the 136 patients in the hypothermia group (55%) had a favorable neurologic recovery (defined as cerebral performance category 1 or 2). In the normothermia group 54 of 137 (39%) had favorable neurologic recovery (risk ratio, 1.40; 95% CI 1.08 to 1.81). Mortality at 6 months was 41% in the hypothermia group (56 of 137 patients died), as compared with 55% in the normothermia group (76 of 138 patients; risk ratio, 0.74; 95% CI 0.58 to 0.95). The proportion of patients with any complication was not significantly different between the two groups (93 of 132 patients in the normothermia group (70%) and 98 of 135 in the hypothermia group (73%), $P =$ 0.70). Sepsis was more likely to occur in the hypothermia group, however, this difference was not statistically significant. As inclusion and exclusion criteria were very strict only 8% of patients assessed for eligibility were included in this trial.

In all randomized trials only outcome assessment was blinded and therefore it was possible that some aspects of care differed between the groups. Figure 49.2 shows a summary of the neurologic outcome of the randomized trials.

In a meta-analysis,[44] which included individual patient data of all three randomized trials of therapeutic hypothermia after cardiac arrest it was shown that more patients in the hypothermia group were discharged with favorable neurologic recovery (risk ratio, 1.68; 95% CI 1.29–2.07). Furthermore, the 95% CI of the number-needed-to-treat to allow one additional patient to leave the hospital with favorable neurologic recovery was 4–13. Additionally, patients were more likely to be alive at 6 months with favorable functional neurologic recovery if they were treated with hypothermia (risk ratio, 1.44; 95% CI 1.11–1.76).

Neurologic outcome in recent clinical studies of different cooling methods

In a study of rapid infusion of large volume (30 ml/kg), ice-cold (4 °C) intravenous lactated Ringer's solution, Bernard et al.[45] included 22 patients who were comatose following resuscitation from out-of-hospital cardiac arrest. Eight of these patients had primary rhythms other than ventricular fibrillation. The rapid cold infusion resulted in a significant decrease in median core temperature from 35.5° to 33.8 °C and improvement of the hemodynamic situation. Of the 22 patients 10 (45%) survived to hospital discharge (2 of 8 patients with non-ventricular fibrillation rhythm).

A case series of three patients described the effect of therapeutic hypothermia after cardiac arrest from non-cardiac causes:[46] one patient had cardiac arrest from electrocution (rhythm ventricular fibrillation), one from drowning (rhythm asystole) and one from pulmonary embolism (rhythm pulseless electrical activity). All patients were treated with hypothermia (33 °C) over 24 hours and survived to hospital discharge with favorable neurologic recovery.

In a study evaluating the safety and feasibility of endovascular cooling in comatose patients who had been successfully resuscitated after cardiac arrest, Al-Senani et al.[47] cooled 13 patients to a target bladder temperature of 33 °C for 24 hours, followed by slow controlled rewarming over 18.3 ± 5.9 hours. Five patients (38%) had 30-day favorable neurologic recovery. No unanticipated or procedure-related adverse events occurred.

A pilot study was performed by Friberg et al.[48] using cold intravenous fluids and surface cooling with a cold helmet and a cold-water blanket (Thermowrap® and Allon® control unit, MTRE, Or Akiva, Israel) in five unconscious patients after cardiac arrest; three survived with good recovery to 6-month follow-up (60%). No adverse events were reported during treatment.

Virkkunen et al.[49] cooled 13 adult patients in the prehospital setting with ice-cold Ringer's solution after successful resuscitation from non-traumatic cardiac arrest. After hemodynamic stabilization, 30 ml/kg of Ringer's solution was infused at a rate of 100 ml/min into the antecubital vein. Four of these 13 patients (31%) survived to hospital discharge with favorable neurologic recovery.

Summary

Sufficient clinical evidence supports the use of therapeutic hypothermia after cardiac arrest in unconscious survivors of cardiac arrest, particularly if the primary rhythm was ventricular fibrillation and the arrest occurred outside the hospital; such hypothermia may also be beneficial in patients with other rhythms and in-hospital cardiac arrest.

Initial patient evaluation

The optimal timing and technique for induction of hypothermia after cardiac arrest are uncertain, and this is now the major focus of current research. The induction of hypothermia after cardiac arrest should be an integral component of the initial evaluation and stabilization of the patient. The steps are described below.

Airway/breathing

All patients who have been resuscitated from prolonged cardiac arrest remain comatose and will require endotracheal intubation for airway protection, oxygenation and control of ventilation. Mechanical ventilation with supplemental oxygen at a tidal volume of 10 ml/kg and a rate of 8–10 breaths per minute should ensure adequate oxygenation and normocapnea. Notably, production of CO_2 is decreased by 30% when core temperature is 33 °C, and therefore the minute ventilatory volume will need to be decreased to avoid hypocapnea, as guided by end-carbon dioxide readings and/or arterial blood gas analysis.

To facilitate both mechanical ventilation and assist in the rapid induction of hypothermia, a large dose of a non-depolarizing muscle relaxant should be administered immediately after initial neurological assessment, as well as an infusion of a sedative agent such as midazolam; these medications will abolish shivering.

Circulation

Evidence from laboratory studies indicates that hypertension after cardiac arrest is associated with improved neurological outcome.[11] One treatment that both induces mild hypothermia and improves blood pressure is rapid infusion of large volume (40 ml/kg), ice-cold (4 °C) intravenous fluid (see later). If hypotension (MAP < 90 mmHg) persists despite this fluid therapy, then an inotropic drug may be infused. In our studies of induced hypothermia (IH),[45] adrenaline was the vasoactive drug of first choice as it has a low incidence of adverse cardiac effect. But if it does cause adverse side effects, noradrenaline would be a reasonable alternative.

If the patient is initially hypertensive, additional sedation may be administered (such as propofol) and consideration given to vasodilator therapy with glyceryl trinitrate considered.

Initial procedures

After initial "ABC" resuscitation measures described above, the following procedures and investigations should be undertaken. An orogastric tube should be inserted, since bystander expired air ventilation commonly results in air inflation of the stomach. Insertion of an intra-arterial line facilitates continuous blood pressure monitoring and blood drawing for laboratory tests. A 12-lead electrocardiogram is required to diagnose acute coronary syndromes. A chest X-ray should be obtained during initial evaluation to exclude right main bronchus intubation and to evaluate any pulmonary complications of cardiac arrest such as aspiration pneumonitis and/ or pulmonary edema.

Central venous access may be required for central venous pressure monitoring and/or vasoactive drug infusion. A femoral venous line may be safer in this setting compared with subclavian or internal jugular puncture if thrombolysis is planned.[50]

Core temperature measurement

Core temperature must be monitored continuously and accurately when induction of hypothermia is planned. There is minimal temperature gradient among brain, bladder and rectal temperature[51,52] and it is usually most convenient to monitor bladder temperature after arrival at hospital. Tympanic temperature monitoring may be used pre-hospital, but is less accurate, particularly when the head is surrounded by ice-packs during surface cooling (see below).

Induction of hypothermia

Rapid lowering of core temperature in an adult patient after cardiac arrest requires that shivering be suppressed by administration of sedation and/or muscle relaxants, while heat is concurrently lowered. A range of techniques for rapid cooling may be applicable in this setting, depending on availability of resources and physician expertise (see Table 49.1).

Surface cooling

The simplest technique for cooling after cardiac arrest is extensive application of ice packs to the head, neck, and torso of the patient. In preliminary hypothermia studies,[45] this technique was effective but provided relatively slow core cooling (approximately 0.9 °C per hour). It was also very time-consuming and inconvenient for attending medical and nursing staff.

The European (HACA) study of hypothermia after cardiac arrest used surface cooling with a refrigerated air blanket to induce hypothermia.[13] This was also found to be very slow, however, with a decrease in core temperature of only 0.3 ºC/hour.

Increased conductive heat loss may be achieved using water blankets rather than cold-air blankets. These were compared by Theard *et al.* in surgical patients.[53] Both of these techniques (water and cold-air blankets) were relatively slow and there was no significant difference between

Table 49.1. Techniques for induction of hypothermia after cardiac arrest

- Surface cooling
- Large volume ice cold intravenous fluid
- Intravascular catheter cooling
- Extracorporeal cooling
- Partial liquid ventilation with cold fluorocarbons
- Pharmacological approaches
- Isolated brain cooling
- Body cavity lavage

the groups in the time taken for core temperature to drop from 35 °C to less than 34 °C (mean 178 minutes vs. 142 minutes). Nevertheless, cooling blankets are a feasible and safe for induction of mild hypothermia.[43]

More recently, developments in cooling technology have made surface cooling much more efficient. The most promising commercially available system uses large adhesive pads that are cooled by water at a controlled temperature applied around the trunk and limbs (Arctic Sun, Medivance, Colarado, USA). The water is circulated with a feedback control system, allowing very accurate control of patient core temperature. Although published data on patients after cardiac arrest are limited, this system has provided improved temperature control compared with traditional surface cooling blankets in febrile patients in a neurological intensive care unit.[54] Moreover, this system is non-invasive and can be readily applied by nursing staff.

Surface heat loss can also be attained with evaporative techniques by using fans and alcohol baths, but these are time consuming and impractical in most emergency and critical care units.

The fastest rate of surface cooling has been achieved with complete patient immersion in an ice-water bath.[55] This results in a rapid decrease in core temperature of 9.7 °C/hour, but is impractical for critically ill patients.

Since the skin of the torso and limbs may be poorly perfused in the early post-cardiac arrest period, while brain blood flow is preserved, it was proposed that cooling helmets may be more efficient than cooling blankets, and two studies have investigated this issue. First Wang *et al.* assigned 14 patients with neurological injury to either a cooling helmet or no cooling.[56] Brain temperature was measured directly (just below the surface of the brain) and compared with the patients' core temperatures. Brain surface temperature was reduced by 1.8 °C (range 0.9–2.4 °C) within 1 hour of helmet application, but a mean of 3.4 hours was required to achieve a brain temperature lower than 34 °C and over 6 hours before systemic hypothermia (< 36 °C) occurred. Second, the tympanic temperatures of 16 patients who were cooled after cardiac arrest were compared to those of 14 normothermic controls.[18] The median tympanic temperature on admission to hospital in both groups was 35.5 °C. In the cooling helmet group, the core target temperature of 34 °C was reached after a median time of 180 minutes after resuscitation. The two studies indicate that cooling helmets are relatively slow to provide systemic hypothermia in adults and probably have no advantage over surface cooling with ice packs and/or cooling blankets.

Nevertheless, helmet cooling may be more efficient in neonatal patients, because of the relative size of the head compared with the torso and the presence of open cranial fontanelles. Animal studies have confirmed that moderate cerebral hypothermia can be induced while the body can be maintained at relative normothermia. In one study, Tooley et al. subjected piglets to 45 minutes of global hypoxic-ischaemic insult,[57] after which each piglet was cooled for 7 hours by using a cap wrapped around the head with circulating cold water (median 8.9 °C). Radiant overhead heating was used to warm the body during cerebral cooling. The mean deep brain temperature during the 7-hour cooling period was 31.1 °C, while rectal temperature remained stable at 38.8 °C.

This technique was then used in a clinical trial of hypothermia in neonates with hypoxic-ischemic encephalopathy[58] in which the cooling cap (Olympic Medical Cool Care System, Olympic Medical, Seattle, WA, USA) was placed around the head of the neonate for 72 hours. The system consists of a thermostatically controlled cooling unit and a pump that circulates water between 8 °C and 12 °C through the cap. The infants were also nursed under a radiant overhead heater, which was servo-controlled to the infant's abdominal skin temperature and adjusted to maintain the rectal temperature at 34 °–35 °C. Improved outcomes in neonates with moderate, but not severe, hypoxic-ischemic encephalopathy were shown, and no cardiac arrest complications resulted from the cold cap.

Large-volume ice-cold intravenous fluid
A simple inexpensive technique for induction of mild hypothermia is rapid infusion of a large volume (40 ml/kg) of ice-cold (4 °C) intravenous fluid (LVICF). To date lactated Ringer's solution and normal saline have been used.

This technique was initially tested in volunteers and found to be safe and effective at lowering core temperature, particularly in older patients.[59,60] More recent studies have examined this technique in postcardiac arrest patients. In a study of 22 patients in an Emergency Department by

Bernard et al., 30 ml/kg of LVICF (lactated Ringer's solution) was rapidly infused intravenously, together with a large dose of a long acting neuromuscular blocker to prevent shivering.[45] This infusion decreased core temperature by 1.6 °C and blood pressure was increased and no patient developed pulmonary edema. In addition, there were improvements in acid–base and renal function. Fluid was infused into a peripheral i.v. cannula by using a pressure bag to ensure a high flow rate (100 ml/min) through a standard i.v. giving set.

In a study by Kliegel et al., cardiac arrest patients received 200 ml of LVICF via peripheral venous catheters to initiate IH prior to endovascular catheter insertion.[61] Following 24 ± 7 ml/kg cold fluid, the core temperature decreased from 35.6 °C ± 1.3 °C on admission to 33.8 °C ± 1.1 °C. The target temperature (<34 °C) was reached a mean of 185 minutes after return of spontaneous circulation and 135 minutes after start of infusion. Two patients had radiographic signs of mild pulmonary edema, but no other complications that could be attributed to the LVICF infusion.

Although myocardial dysfunction is common after resuscitation from prolonged cardiac arrest,[62] there is evidence that rapid infusion of LVICF does not result in pulmonary edema in most patients. Kim et al. examined the cardiac effects of LVICF in cardiac arrest patients following hospital admission,[63] by using transthoracic echocardiography to assess cardiac function just before and 1 hour after infusion of LVICF. The infusion resulted in a mean core temperature drop of 1.4 °C without significant changes in vital signs, electrolytes, arterial blood gases, or coagulation indices. The initial mean cardiac ejection fraction was 34%, and the fluid infusion did not effect ejection fraction, central venous pressure, pulmonary pressures, or left atrial filling pressures.

The LVICF has been used for the prehospital induction of hypothermia. In one study of 13 adult patients who were resuscitated from cardiac arrest, 30 ml/kg of lactated Ringer's solution was infused at a rate of 100 ml/minute into an antecubital vein.[49] The mean core temperature decreased from 35.8° ± 0.9 °C at the start of infusion to 34.0° ± 1.2 °C on arrival at hospital (P < 0.0001), with no serious adverse hemodynamic effects.

Although this study was supervised by physicians, it has also been shown that paramedics can administer LVICF after cardiac arrest. In a pre-hospital study, 20 adult patients with return of stable spontaneous circulation following out-of-hospital cardiac arrest were enrolled (Bernard SA, unpublished data). All patients were unconscious after return of spontaneous circulation and were intubated and ventilated. The patients received pancuronium followed by 2000 ml of ice-cold lactated Ringer's solution IV over 20 minutes. Data on vital signs were collected before and after the fluid infusion, before arrival at the emergency department. Core temperature decreased by 1.8 °C. Transient oxygen desaturation in one patient was treated with furosemide without adverse effect.

Since there is evidence that hypothermia may be of maximal benefit when induced during CPR,[9,12] LVICF may be the most feasible technique for cooling during CPR in the field. Although human studies have not been published, this approach was tested in a laboratory study by Nordmark *et al.*[64] In this study, 20 piglets were subjected to 8 minutes of ventricular fibrillation, followed by CPR: they were then randomized into two groups, one given a 30 ml/kg infusion of 4 °C Ringer's solution at 1.33 ml/kg per minute, starting after 1 minute of CPR and the other received the same infusion volume at room temperature. After 9 minutes, cardioversion was used to achieve a return of spontaneous circulation. The mean temperatures in the LVICF animals were significantly reduced by a mean of 1.6 °C compared with 1.1 °C in the control group; there was no difference in cortical cerebral blood flow or hemodynamic variables and no adverse effects of the infusion.

On the other hand, there may be some concern that hypothermia induced during cardiac arrest decreases the effectiveness of defibrillation. This has been studied by Boddicker *et al.* in a swine model of cardiac arrest.[65] The animals were divided into four groups each with eight animals: normothermia; mild hypothermia (35 °C), moderate hypothermia (33 °C); and severe hypothermia (30 °C). Hypothermia was induced by surface cooling before the induction of ventricular fibrillation (VF). After 8 minutes of unsupported VF, without CPR, the animals were defibrillated with successive shocks as needed and then underwent CPR until either resumption of spontaneous circulation or no response at 10 minutes. First-shock defibrillation success was higher in the moderate hypothermia group (6 of 8 hypothermic animals vs. 1 of 8 normothermic animals; $P = 0.04$). Fewer shocks were needed for late defibrillation (≥ 1 minute after initial shock) in all three hypothermia groups compared with the normothermia group (all $P < 0.05$). None of the 8 animals in the normothermia group achieved return of spontaneous circulation, compared with 3 of 8 mild hypothermia ($P = NS$), 7 of 8 moderate hypothermia ($P = 0.001$), and 5 of 8 severe hypothermia ($P = 0.03$) animals. These data suggest that mild hypothermia actually facilitated defibrillation.

Possible contraindications to LVICF include the presence of fulminating pulmonary edema and/or the patient with chronic renal failure (on dialysis) who may be unable to excrete a large fluid load. In these patients, intravenous infusion of a small volume of a much colder liquid might be useful. Recently, an ice "slurry," comprising smoothed 100-micrometre ice particles at subzero temperature, has been developed. Vanden Hoek *et al.* studied the effects of a rapid infusion of this slurry in swine,[66] in which a central catheter infusion of ice slurry (50 ml/kg) was compared to an equal volume of chilled saline. The study included normothermic controls, and compared with these control animals, brain temperatures of the slurry and saline groups dropped by means of 5.3 °C and 3.4 °C ($P = .009$), respectively.

At this time, the use of LVICF appears to be the most feasible and effective approach to rapid core cooling, and it should be administered as soon as possible after resuscitation. On the basis of the promising animal data above, future clinical studies could test this therapy in the prehospital setting and during CPR.

To avoid a rebound increase in temperature as the cold fluid moves into the extra-vascular compartment at the end of the infusion, additional cooling techniques such as surface cooling (as above) or endovascular cooling (see below) may be required for the maintenance of IH.

Endovascular cooling

Several types of endovascular cooling catheters are currently available for induction and maintenance of hypothermia. Although there are minor differences in design, the principles of each catheter type are similar. The catheter is placed in the venous circulation (usually into the inferior vena cava via the femoral vein) and contains circulating saline at a controlled temperature. The fluid is pumped from a bedside heat exchanger that accurately controls fluid and therefore patient core temperature.

Preliminary clinical studies examined the use of this device in febrile neurological patients. Diringer *et al.* compared conventional treatment of fever (acetaminophen and cooling blankets) with this treatment plus an endovascular cooling catheter (Alsius, Irvine, CA) in patients with neurological injury and fever.[67] The "fever burden" (defined as the area under the temperature chart) was 7.92 °C-hours in the conventional group compared with 2.87 °C-hours in the catheter group, which represented a 64% reduction in fever ($P < 0.01$). Rates of infection and use of sedatives, narcotics, and antibiotics were similar in both groups.

The endovascular cooling catheter has also been used for core cooling patients undergoing interventional cardiac procedures. In the "Cool-MI" study, Dixon *et al.* studied the use of a cooling catheter during primary percutaneous coronary intervention (PCI) for acute myocardial infarction.[68] Patients were randomized to primary PCI with either normothermia or cooling by using an endovascular cooling catheter, with a target core temperature of 33 °C. Sedation was administered for patient comfort and to prevent shivering. Cooling was then maintained for 3 hours after reperfusion, and was well tolerated, with no hemodynamic instability or increase in the incidence of arrhythmia. Although the median infarct size was not significantly smaller in patients who received cooling compared with that in the control group, the study established the safety and efficacy of the cooling technology.

The endovascular cooling device has also been used successfully for the induction of mild hypothermia in conscious patients with severe stroke[69] and in the operating room for patients undergoing elective craniotomy for repair of an unruptured cerebral aneurysm.[70]

Endovascular cooling has been used in patients with neurological injury after cardiac arrest by Al-Senani et al.[47] Core temperature was reduced to a target of 33 °C for 24 hours using a closed loop endovascular system placed in the inferior vena cava, followed by controlled rewarming. Thirteen patients (mean age, 60 years) were enrolled. The time from cardiac arrest to ROSC was 14.3 minutes (range 5–32.5). It took a mean of 3 hours and 39 minutes to reach 33 °C (average). The rate of cooling 0.8 °C/hour, range, 0.22 °–1.12 °C/hour). Temperature was tightly maintained for all patients averaging 32.7 ° ± 0.5 °C. Rewarming lasted 18.3 ± 5.9 hours. No procedure-related adverse events occurred.

However, the use of an endovascular cooling catheter is limited to the hospital setting. Moreover, the heat exchanger and catheters are expensive and catheters require insertion by a physician with additional training, which delays induction of hypothermia for some time after hospital arrival. Nevertheless, these devices appear to provide excellent temperature control during maintenance and rewarming from hypothermia.

Extracoporeal circuits

Extracorporeal circulation consists of large intravascular (usually intravenous) catheters, a blood pump, and an in-line heat exchanger. These circuits allow very accurate and rapid control of core temperature, but again this technology is very expensive, and requires specialized physician training for catheter insertion as well as time to prime. Also, the patient usually requires full anticoagulation. Therefore, this approach is unlikely to become commonly used in most emergency and critical care units.

The rapid rate of cooling has been demonstrated by Holzer et al.[71] In large swine, extracorporeal venovenous cooling reduced brain temperature from 38.0 ° to 33.0 °C in a mean of 41 minutes compared with endovascular cooling which took a mean of 126 minutes (P = 0.001). None of the

swine developed significant hemolysis, arrhythmias, or bleeding.

Clinical experience with extracorporeal circuits to induce hypothermia has been limited to a few centers,[72] and only one report in patients with cardiac arrest. Nagas et al. treated 50 patients with out-of-hospital cardiac arrest with standard CPR and, if there was no response, with emergency cardiopulmonary bypass plus intra-aortic balloon pumping.[42] Subsequently, patients with systolic blood pressure above 90 mmHg and Glasgow coma cardiac arrest score of 3 to 5 received mild hypothermia (34 °C for 2 days), induced by extracorporeal coil cooling. Mild hypothermia was induced in 23 patients, and 12 (52%) of them showed good recovery.

Pharmacological techniques

In most patients, the induction of hypothermia requires some therapy assistance to suppress shivering. In conscious patients, sedation alone is used; however, the optimal combination of pharmacological agents is uncertain, but meperidine and buspiridone are widely used to suppress shivering. In general, comatose, ventilated patients are treated with a muscle-relaxant as well as sedative drugs.

Recently, use of magnesium bolus and infusion has been evoked to facilitate induction of hypothermia. In a study of patients with stroke in whom hypothermia (34.5 °C) was induced by surface cooling,[73] patients received meperidine alone, meperidine plus buspirone, meperidine plus ondansetron, or meperidine, ondansetron, and magnesium sulfate 4- to 6-g i.v. bolus of magnesium sulfate was followed by 1 to 3 g per hour infusion. Patients who received magnesium sulfate had a slightly decreased time to achieve a tympanic temperature of 35 °C and also had significantly higher mean comfort scores.

In a similar study, Wadhwa studied 9 healthy volunteers who were assigned to either placebo or magnesium (80 mg/kg) followed by infusion at 2 g/hour.[74] Lactated Ringer's solution (4 °C) was infused via a central venous catheter to decrease tympanic membrane temperature by about 1.5 °C/hour. Magnesium reduced the shivering threshold from a mean of 36.6° to 36.3 °C (P = 0.04). Although this change is statistically significant, this very small drop in the temperature of shivering threshold is unlikely to be clinically important.

Another pharmacological agent that may be useful in the future in induction of hypothermia is a neurotensin analogue. Specific receptors for neurotensin, an endogenous tridecapeptide, are found throughout the central nervous system of mammals, including rats and humans. Neurotensin is elevated in mammals during hibernation, and is thought to induce hypothermia by activation of neurotensin receptors in the brain.

Recently, a neurotensin analog has been developed that can be administered intravenously, which may provide a practical method for rapidly inducing hypothermia within minutes without sedation or general anesthesia. In addition, when neurotensin degrades over 24 hours, the core temperature returns to normal without external application of heat. This has been studied in a rat model of asphyxial cardiac arrest by Katz *et al.*,[75] in which the animals were randomized to normothermia, brief external cooling (6 hours), prolonged external cooling (24 hours), or neurotensin administration 30 minutes after cardiac arrest. The animals with neurotensin-induced hypothermia had improved neurological outcome comparable to prolonged external cooling and improved outcome compared with the brief external cooling, but the feasibility and safety of this drug in humans is currently unknown.

Partial liquid ventilation with cold perflurocarbon

It has been known for many years that mammals can survive prolonged immersion in oxygenated perfluorocarbon (PFC) liquids. The principle of ventilation with oxygen-carrying fluids was subsequently developed to allow partial liquid ventilation in patients with respiratory failure, where it was proposed that the lung/fluid interface would be superior to the lung/gas interface. A clinical trial, however, did not demonstrate patient benefit by this approach.[76]

Nevertheless, instillation into the lungs of a large volume of ice-cold PFC would be expected to provide rapid core cooling, while still allowing adequate oxygenation and ventilation. This has only been studied in animal models at this time.[77]

Body cavity lavage

A number of studies have examined the effects of lavage of various body cavities with ice-cold fluid: these include gastric lavage with cold water, and bladder and peritoneal lavage with cold sterile saline.

Plattner *et al.* compared several of these cooling techniques with surface cooling in volunteers.[55] In addition to surface cooling techniques (ice water immersion) described previously, Plattner also studied gastric lavage (500 ml of ice water every 10 minutes) and bladder lavage (300 ml of iced Ringer's solution every 10 minutes). The first volunteer developed abdominal cramping and diarrhea after gastric lavage and this technique was not used again. Bladder lavage, however, decreased core temperature by 0.8 °C /hour, consequently this technique may be a useful adjunct to cooling, but it requires considerable additional nursing time to maintain the fluid exchanges.

Peritoneal lavage has been studied by Xiao *et al.* in a dog model:[78] 2 litres of Ringer's solution at 10 °C were instilled into the peritoneal cavity, left for 5 minutes, and then drained. Tympanic membrane temperature decreased by a mean of 0.3 °C/min. In addition, pulmonary artery temperature decreased by a mean of 0.8 °C/min. Although insertion of a peritoneal catheter and core rewarming in the Emergency Department has been described for patients with accidental hypothermia, peritoneal cooling has not been studied in postcardiac arrest patients.

Selective brain cooling

To avoid possible complications of systemic hypothermia, isolated brain cooling would be preferable, if this were technically possible. Cannulation of the carotid vessels and the infusion of cooled blood into the cerebral circulation was studied by Mori *et al.*[79] In a swine model of cardiac arrest, VF was induced and cardiac arrest (without CPR) was allowed for 20 minutes. Extracorporeal bypass was then instituted to restore coronary and cerebral perfusion, followed by restoration of cardiac rhythm. Some animals received selective brain hypothermia (32 °C) for 12 hours by use of femoral/carotid bypass. There was significant improvement in the neurohistology scores in the selective brain-cooled animals as compared with those of the normothermic cohort. Nevertheless, given the modest side effects of systemic hypothermia, and the potential complications of cannulating the carotid arteries under emergency conditions, this approach is unlikely to be used in the near future.

Maintenance of hypothermia

The optimal duration of IH after cardiac arrest resuscitation is uncertain. The Australian studies used 12 hours,[17] whereas the European study used 24 hours.[13] Whichever period is chosen, careful control of core temperature during this period is required.

Once a core temperature of 33 °C is reached by one of the techniques described above, adult patients usually become poikilothermic and shivering is largely abolished. The judicious use of sedation rather than pharmacological paralysis may be all that is required to maintain this core temperature. If the core temperature starts to rise (>33.5 °C), additional sedation and/or a muscle relaxant may be administered and ice packs applied to the head, neck, and torso of the patient. If available, a surface or core cooling technology (as described above) would be useful. If temperature decreases (<32.5 °C), ice-packs should be removed and paralyzing drugs withheld while a heated-air blanket is applied. The use of either surface cooling or endovascular cooling (as described above) with feedback controls considerably simplifies the maintenance of IH in the critical care unit.

Rewarming from hypothermia

Active rewarming after a period of IH requires the use of either external heating or endovascular warming to increase core temperature. Some animal data suggests that rewarming from hypothermia should be undertaken slowly.[80] During this time, any shivering must be completely suppressed with sedation. In addition, rewarming may result in peripheral vasodilatation, and (warmed) i.v. fluid therapy may be needed to maintain blood pressure.

Summary

After resuscitation from prolonged out-of-hospital cardiac arrest, current evidence suggests that the comatose patient should be treated with mild hypothermia to improve neurological and overall outcome. Induction of hypothermia requires administration of a large dose of a long-acting muscle relaxant followed by the rapid infusion (>100 ml/min) of ice-cold i.v. crystalloid fluid (i.e., normal saline or lactated Ringer's solution) to a total volume of 40 ml/kg. Current evidence suggests that this is only rarely associated with development of pulmonary edema.

To prevent rewarming, surface cooling should be initiated and core temperature monitored using a bladder temperature probe. Hypothermia should then be maintained for 12–24 hours, and rewarming undertaken over 6–12 hours. Maintenance of hypothermia and later rewarming are most accurately achieved with endovascular or surface cooling devices that have feedback control.

At this time, the use of extracorporeal circuits and/or selective cerebral cooling is expensive and usually not feasible in most hospitals. It is unlikely that such advanced technologies will be shown to be superior to simpler techniques.

Mechanisms and potential side effects of therapeutic mild hypothermia (Poldermann)

Introduction

To apply hypothermia effectively in a clinical setting, it is important to be aware of the mechanisms underlying this treatment, as well as the potential side effects of the treatment. Insufficient understanding of these mechanisms and side effects can decrease their effectiveness, or at worst even lead to treatment failure, as illustrated by early experiences with induced hypothermia in treatment of cardiac

arrest, traumatic brain injury, and for other indications in the 1950s and 1960s.[81–83] At that time hypothermia was presumed to exert its effects exclusively through temperature-dependent reductions in metabolism, leading to a decreased demand for oxygen and glucose in the brain. It is now known that there are multiple effects on the body, as discussed in previous sections, and that the failure of treatment was largely due to the use of temperatures that were too low, lack of understanding of the underlying mechanisms, and failure to treat harmful side effects.

The most important breakthrough in treatment was the realization that neurological outcome could be improved by mild-to-moderate hypothermia (31 °–35 °C) rather than deep hypothermia (≤30 °C), with far fewer and less severe side effects. This new insight stemmed from the observation that the protective effects of hypothermia were not exclusively due to a decrease in oxygen and glucose consumption in the brain. Rather the mechanisms involved were far more complicated.

Numerous destructive processes (collectively termed "postresuscitation disease") begin minutes to hours after an initial (ischemic or traumatic) injury, can continue for hours to several days after initial injury, and can be re-triggered by new episodes of ischemia. Importantly, all of these processes are temperature dependent; thus, they are all stimulated by fever, and can all be mitigated or blocked by mild to moderate hypothermia. The wide-ranging effect of hypothermia on all of these mechanisms may explain why it has proved to be clinically effective, whereas studies with agents that affect just one of the destructive processes have been far less successful.[85,86]

The second important development was the advent of intensive care units to care for critically ill patients. The side effects of hypothermia are far more easily managed in this setting, and the methods for inducing and maintaining hypothermia at a specified level (discussed earlier) have improved significantly since the 1950s.

From studies on mechanisms underlying hypothermia's protective effects, it is clear that the key factors determining the success or failure of hypothermia treatment are speed of induction of hypothermia, duration of cooling, speed of rewarming, and prevention of side effects. Since relative contributions of different destructive mechanisms to the ongoing postresuscitation injury may differ, available "windows of opportunity" for therapeutic interventions such as hypothermia may vary, as well as the required duration of hypothermia. Better understanding of the underlying mechanisms may help us to target our treatments more specifically and help improve outcome.

With respect to side effects of hypothermia, some are intrinsically linked to the protective effects. For example, hypothermia-associated immunosuppression which leads to the suppression of harmful inflammatory processes in the brain and heart, but also to increased risk of wound infections and pneumonia, as observed in various clinical studies.[84]

As discussed above, animal models can be roughly divided into global and focal injury models, to study global anoxia (cardiac arrest model) as well as traumatic brain injury, ischemic stroke, and subarachnoid hemorrhage. Hypothermia has been shown to improve neurological outcome in all of these models and in the overwhelming majority of animal experiments, provided that hypothermia was applied quickly enough. Nonetheless, reproducing these results in clinical trials has proved difficult, because the relative importance of different injury mechanisms may differ between humans and animals, and also among different animal species. Thus, a specific treatment that decreases histological brain damage in rats may also be effective in humans, but the effect may be too small to be clinically significant.[97,98] In addition, specific treatments may modify or inhibit a specific destructive mechanism that plays a central role in the development of injury in a particular animal model, but is far less important in humans.[87,88] The potentially positive effects of hypothermia may be overestimated on the basis of animal experiments; the brains of some animals, especially small animals such as rodents, appear to be more responsive to neuroprotection than is the human brain. But the protective effects may also be *under*estimated if only one mechanism and/or one animal model is examined. For example, many animal studies have focused on the influence of hypothermia on the so-called neuroexitotoxic cardiac arrest, which involves a severe disturbance of intracellular ion homeostasis following an ischemic event.[87–89] This destructive mechanism is a central feature of postischemic injury, and any potential neuroprotective effect depends on the ability of a treatment to influence this particular mechanism. Moreover, various studies in different animal models have shown that the time window to influence this neuroexcitatory cardiac arrest may be limited, ranging from an upper limit of about 120 minutes to as low as 10 minutes.[90] Thus if the benefits of hypothermia were linked to its influence on the neuroexitatory cardiac arrest alone, a "window of opportunity" of about 2 hours, would be expected. Clinical studies have shown improved neurological outcome in patients who remain comatose after cardiac arrest even when induction of hypothermia was delayed for up to 8 hours,[13] strongly suggesting that different mechanisms are probably affected simultaneously when hypothermia is induced.

Potential mechanisms underlying the protective effects of hypothermia

The mechanisms described in more detail below are summarized in Fig. 49.3.

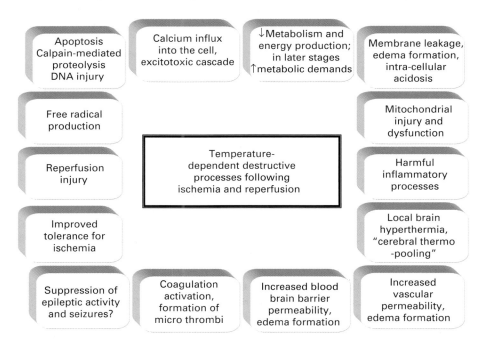

Fig. 49.3. Destructive mechanisms following ischemia and reperfusion.

Decrease in cerebral metabolism

When first applied in a clinical setting, hypothermia was presumed to exert protective effects due to a slowing of cerebral metabolism, leading to a decrease in glucose consumption and oxygen demand. Indeed, cerebral metabolism is reduced by between 5% and 8% for each °C reduction in body temperature during induction of hypothermia.[91] Therefore, these early trials attempted to decrease metabolic rates as much as possible, by lowering body temperature as far as possible. But it was found not only that protective effects could be achieved with mild hypothermia (31°–34 °C); but that the protective effects of cooling appeared to be much greater than could be explained by changes in metabolism alone.[92] Thus, although a decrease in metabolism and oxygen demand is one of the mechanisms underlying hypothermia's protective effects, other mechanisms are equally or more important.

Apoptosis, calpain-mediated proteolysis, and mitochondrial dysfunction

After a period of ischemia and reperfusion, cells can become necrotic, fully or partially recover, or enter a path leading to apoptosis or programmed cell death. Whether a cell will become apoptotic is determined by a number of cellular processes, including mitochondrial dysfunction and disorders in cellular energy metabolism and the release of various enzymes, the caspases. Numerous studies have shown that hypothermia can interrupt the apoptotic pathway and prevent cell injury from leading to apoptosis.[93] Hypothermia probably acts at the early stages of the apoptotic process[94] by influencing mechanisms involved in apoptosis initiation, including inhibition of caspase enzyme activation,[93,94] prevention of mitochondrial dysfunction,[95] decreased overload of excitatory neurotransmitters, and modification of intracellular ion concentrations. Apoptosis is one of the destructive processes that begins relatively late in the postperfusion phase and continues for 48–72 hours or even longer.[96] Thus, prevention or mitigation of apoptosis can be influenced for some time after injury, which in theory provides a wide window of opportunity for therapeutic interventions such as hypothermia. Thus, influencing apoptotic pathways could play an important role in human neuroprotection and reducing postresuscitation injury.

Ion pumps and neuroexcitatory cardiac arrest

A large body of evidence suggests that hypothermia inhibits harmful excitatory processes occurring in brain cells during ischemia and reperfusion. Levels of high-energy metabolites such as adenosine triphosphate (ATP) and phosphocreatine in brain cells decrease within seconds when oxygen supply to the brain is interrupted.[91] The breakdown of ATP and the switch of intracellular metabolism to anaerobic glycolysis leads to an increase in intracellular levels of inorganic phosphate, lactate, and H^+, resulting in both intra- and extracellular acidosis and an influx of calcium (Ca^{2+}) into the cell. Loss of ATP and acidosis also inhibit mechanisms that normally deal with excessive intracellular Ca^{2+} by sequestration of Ca^{2+} from the cell, further aggravating intracellular Ca^{2+} overload. These problems are compounded by failure of ATP-dependent Na^+–K^+ pumps and K^+, Na^+, and Ca^{2+} channels, leading to an additional influx of Ca^{2+}.[89] Excess Ca^{2+} can induce mitochondrial dysfunction (increasing intracellular calcium influx further, in a vicious cycle) and activate numerous intracellular enzyme systems (kinases and proteases). In addition, immediate early genes are activated and depolarization of neuronal cell membranes occurs, with release of large amounts of the excitatory neurotransmitter glutamate into the extracellular space.[89] This leads to prolonged and excessive activation of membrane glutamate receptors, further stimulating Ca^{2+} influx through activation of Ca^{2+} channels again in a vicious cycle. Under normal circumstances, neurons are exposed to only very brief pulses of glutamate; when exposed to glutamate for prolonged periods of time, the neurons remain in a permanent state of hyperexcitability (the "excitotoxic cardiac arrest"), which can lead to additional injury and cell death. Moreover, high levels of glutamate can be neurotoxic, especially in energy-deprived cells. Activation of glutamate receptors can persist for some time after reperfusion, even when glutamate levels have returned to normal, which may also mediate brain cell death. Together, ischemia and reperfusion interrupt a delicate balance between calcium influx and sequestration at the cellular level.

Numerous animal experiments have clearly demonstrated that key destructive processes of the neuroexitatory cardiac arrest (such as calcium influx, accumulation of glutamate, and the release of its co-agonist glycine) can be prevented, interrupted, or mitigated by hypothermia.[26,89,97,98] Even a relatively small decrease in temperature can significantly improve ion homeostasis, whereas the occurrence of fever can trigger and/or stimulate these destructive processes.

The "window of opportunity" available to interrupt the problems described above remain unclear. Disruptions in Ca^{2+} homeostasis begin in the first minutes after injury, but continue in the hours or even days following ischemia, and can be retriggered by each new episode of ischemia. Although, in theory, this would again provide a significant time window for therapeutic interventions such as hypothermia, some animal experiments suggest that the process can be blocked or reversed only if the treatment is initiated in the early phases of the neuroexitatory cardiac arrest.[12,29,87,90,91] Other studies have reported time frames possibly due to different types of injuries and ranging from 30 minutes to up to 6 hours in different species.[8–11,34,35,99–103] Some authors have suggested that the therapeutic window for hypothermia could be extended by combining it with other treatments, such as caspase use of inhibitors or other experimental compounds.[87,104,105]

Immune response and inflammation

In most types of brain injury a significant and protracted inflammatory response begins about 1 hour after a period of ischemia and reperfusion: pro-inflammatory mediators such as tumor necrosis factor-alpha (TNFα) and interleukin-1 (IL-1) are released in large quantities by astrocytes, microglia, and endothelial cells, and levels begin to rise ±1 hour after reperfusion and remain elevated for up to 5 days.[91,106] This stimulates the chemotaxis of activated leukocytes across the blood–brain barrier and leads to an accumulation of inflammatory cells in the injured brain, as well as the appearance of adhesion molecules on leukocytes and endothelial cells. Simultaneously, there is an activation of the complement system, beginning in the very early stages after brain injury further stimulating the passage of neutrophils and (in later stages) monocytes/macrophages.[106] These inflammatory and immunological responses occur predominantly during reperfusion and are accompanied by production of free radicals (see below). Such responses can cause significant (additional) injury through the phagocytic actions of macrophages, synthesis of toxic products, and further stimulation of immune reactions in a vicious cycle.

Notably, however, this inflammatory response is in part physiological, and may have a "dual role" in that some inflammatory mediators have neuroprotective properties, while others are neurotoxic.[106] Nevertheless, there is strong evidence indicating that a disproportionate and persistent production of cytokines and leukocyte infiltration can significantly increase the risk and extent of brain cell injury and infarction;[106] the interleukin-1 family appears to be particularly important in this regard.[107] Of note, this effect is partly time-dependent, with the destructive aspects of inflammation outweighing the potential benefits, especially in the later stages of injury.[106]

Numerous animal experiments and also some clinical studies have shown that hypothermia suppresses ischemia-induced inflammatory reactions and release of pro-inflammatory cytokines in animal and clinical studies.[108,109] Apart from its effect on cytokine levels, hypothermia also prevents or reduces reperfusion-related DNA injury, lipid peroxidation, and leukotriene production,[26,110,111] as well as decreasing production of nitric oxide, a key agent in development of postischemic brain injury.[89] In animal experiments the extent of brain injury and infarct size can be significantly reduced if *any* of these processes is mitigated or interrupted;[89] thus because hypothermia can affect *all* of these steps there is (at least in theory) a huge potential for improving neurological outcome. Moreover, as the inflammatory response begins relatively late (>1 hour) following ischemia and reperfusion, and as the destructive processes require time to develop fully and then continue for prolonged periods of time, they provide a clear therapeutic window for application of hypothermia to reduce the inflammatory response.

Free radical production

A destructive process that is closely linked to, but distinct from the mechanisms discussed above is the release of oxygen free radicals following ischemia and reperfusion. Mediators such as superoxide (O_2^-), peroxynitrite (NO_2^-), hydrogen peroxide (H_2O_2), and hydroxyl radicals (OH^-) play important roles in determining whether injured cells will recover or die.[97,110] Free radicals can oxidize and impair numerous cellular components, and although brain cells have enzymatic and non-enzymatic antioxidant mechanisms to prevent this type of injury, the levels of free radical production following ischemia/reperfusion are so high that these defensive mechanisms are probably overwhelmed, resulting in peroxidation of lipids, proteins, and nucleic acids. Whereas hypothermia does not inhibit free radical production completely, it significantly decreases the amounts of free radicals that are produced[97,110] allowing the endogenous protective (antioxidant) mechanisms to cope better with the free radicals that are released, and thereby preventing or significantly mitigating the peroxidation of lipids, proteins, and nucleic acids. If free radical production is sufficiently reduced, the cell can recover. The degree of inhibition of free radical production parallels the degree of hypothermia, i.e., the lower the temperature, the lower the amount of free radicals.

Vascular permeability, blood–brain barrier disruption, and edema formation

Ischemia/reperfusion leads to disruptions in the blood–brain barrier (BBB), which can significantly increase subsequent development of brain edema.[112–114] Therapeutic interventions such as mannitol administration in traumatic brain injury or stroke can add to the BBB disruption,[113] whereas mild hypothermia significantly reduces the disruptions in the BBB;[112–114] in addition, vascular permeability after ischemia-reperfusion injury is also decreased, which further decreases edema formation.[115] Moreover, in support of this concept, induction of hypothermia decreases the extravasation of hemoglobin after traumatic brain injury.[116] Ischemia and reperfusion can also affect the integrity of the blood–brain barrier in other ways, including decrease in fluidity and integrity of cell membranes and increase in vascular permeability of microvascular endothelial cells in the brain mediated by vascular endothelial growth factor (VEGF) via the release of nitric oxide.[117] These processes of membrane disintegration and hypoxia-induced permeability changes can be relieved or reversed by hypothermia.[117]

In the clinical setting, the development of brain edema is usually assessed by measuring the intracranial pressure (ICP), which can be regarded as a "final common pathway" for all the destructive processes leading to brain edema.[118] Intracranial hypertension and brain edema can also cause development of additional neurological injuries in patients with TBI and stroke as well as causing additional injuries and critically determining outcome in encephalitis and meningitis. Some evidence suggests that brain edema can also affect posthypoxic injury after cardiac arrest.[119]

Since ICH appears to be both a marker for ongoing neurological injury and a cause of additional injury,[118] it seems reasonable that treatments that decrease ICP can also help improve neurological outcome. For example, in patients with traumatic brain injury, ICP is frequently used as a key index to guide treatments and to judge treatment effectiveness.[120]

Notably, although hypothermia has been shown to decrease ICP in many clinical studies, the results in improving survival and neurological outcome have been more mixed,[84,118] with some large trials failing to show any benefits of induced hypothermia.[121] These variable results may be related in part to the management of the side effects of hypothermia;[84,118] see next section below. Speed of induction and the depth and duration of hypothermia may also be important, as evidence suggests that whether or not a lasting protective effect is achieved is critically dependent on these factors.[36,84]

Intra- and extracellular acidosis and cerebral metabolism

The diminished integrity of cell membranes, the failure of various ion pumps, development of mitochondrial dysfunction, inappropriate activation of numerous enzyme systems with cellular hyperactivity, and the disruption of various other intracellular processes all contribute to the development of intracellular acidosis, a factor that powerfully stimulates many of the abovementioned destructive

processes.[122,123] Ischemia/reperfusion also leads to significant rises in cerebral lactate levels, which can be effectively attenuated by hypothermia.[122,123] In addition, utilization of brain glucose is affected by ischemia/reperfusion, and some evidence suggests that hypothermia can improve brain glucose metabolism.[124] Both short- and long-term changes in cerebral metabolism may also develop following TBI, where various animal experiments and some clinical observations have reported initial increases in cerebral glucose metabolism (lasting for several hours) followed by a persistent decrease in metabolic rate, with depression of mitochondrial oxidative phosphorylation and glucose utilization lasting for several weeks.[125] Various studies have shown that hypothermia induced during and after reperfusion increases the speed of metabolic recovery, with better preservation of high-energy phosphates and reduced accumulation of toxic metabolites.[125]

Brain temperature and cerebral thermo-pooling

Even in healthy individuals the temperature of the brain may be somewhat higher than the measured core temperature. This difference can increase significantly in some patients after neurological injury, with differences ranging from 0.1 °C to more than 2 °C.[51,126,127] Moreover, even in healthy subjects there may be small differences in temperature between different areas of the brain, which can increase significantly when brain injury occurs, with injured areas becoming more hyperthermic than non-injured ones[128] because of the destructive "hyperactivity" of injured cells caused by the mechanisms outlined above.

Strong evidence from animal studies establishes that (external) induction of hyperthermia significantly increases the risk and extent of neurological injury,[129–131] because hyperthermia may promote necrosis and apoptosis in ischemic areas, even when fever develops (or is externally induced) some time after the initial injury. For example, Baena et al. demonstrated that moderate, transient whole-body warming to 39 °C–40 °C for 3 hours, induced 24 hours after a brief episode of forebrain ischemia in rats, induced a 2.6-fold increased neuronal injury in the hippocampus,[129] suggesting that fever even of short duration can be detrimental on the day after injury. Moreover, these effects become more pronounced when hyperthermia coincides with cerebral ischemia, suggesting that ischemic brain cells become even more susceptible to the harmful effects of hyperthermia than do reperfused ones.[132]

Numerous clinical studies have confirmed that fever is indeed an independent predictor of adverse neurological outcome and mortality in stroke, TBI and post-anoxic injury.[133–136] Azzimondi and associates prospectively observed stroke patients and noted that developing fever was associated with a 3.4-fold increase in the risk for adverse outcome, with a 95% CI of 1.2 to 9.5.[134] Castillo and associates reported that fever developing within 24 hours after stroke onset was independently related to larger infarct volumes (OR 3.23, 95% CI 1.63 to 6.43) and higher neurological deficits (OR 3.06, 95% CI 1.70 to 5.53) at 3 months.[135] Kammersgaard *et al.* reported that each 1 °C increase of body temperature on admission independently predicted a 30% relative increase in long-term mortality risk, with a 95% CI of 4% to 57%.[136]

Although it has not yet been conclusively proven that fever itself increases neurological injury rather than just being a marker for it, the temporal relationship and the results from animal studies[129–131] strongly suggest that it is. This is in accord with observations from other animal studies that induction of mild hypothermia can prevent fever-related neurological injuries and improves tissue tolerance for ischemia.[84,137–139]

Coagulation activation and formation of micro-thrombi

Various studies have shown that cardiopulmonary arrest and resuscitation are accompanied by a marked activation of coagulation, which can lead to intravascular fibrin formation with blockage of the microcirculation in the brain and heart.[140,141] Administration of anticoagulants such as heparin and rt-PA has been shown to improve microcirculatory reperfusion and survival in various animal experiments;[141,142] in addition, thrombolysis can improve cerebral tolerance to ischemia.[143] Preliminary clinical observations suggest that administering thrombolytic agents to cardiac arrest patients during the very early stages of CPR can indeed improve neurological outcome and survival.[144]

Thus it appears that relatively mild ones, anticoagulants (e.g., low-dose heparin) or more powerful ones (e.g., rt-PA) can improve neurological and cardiac outcome in the early stages of ischemia/reperfusion, by enhancing the microcirculation and removing micro-thrombi. Hypothermia also induces a mild bleeding diathesis, through combined effects on platelet count, platelet function, and the coagulation cascade.[145–150] The anticoagulation effect of hypothermia could provide yet another mechanism for its neuroprotective and cardioprotective effects. But although this hypothesis seems plausible, as outlined above[140–144,151] the concept remains speculative, as there are no studies directly addressing this issue.

Vasoactive mediators

Some evidence suggests that hypothermia can influence the local secretion of vasoactive substances by the endothelium, such as endothelin, thromboxane A2 (TxA2) and prostaglandin I_2, in the brain and at other sites.

Endothelin and TxA2 are both powerful vasoconstrictive agents, while prostaglandin I_2 is a vasodilator; thromboxane can also induce platelet aggregation.[152] These two agents play an important role in regulating local cerebral blood flow, and a balance between the two is required to maintain homeostasis.[152] There is also some evidence suggesting that this local homeostasis may be disrupted after an ischemic and/or traumatic event, with a relative increase in the production of thromboxane.[153] Such disruptions in equilibrium could lead to vasoconstriction and therefore to hypoperfusion and/or thrombogenesis in injured areas of the brain.

This local imbalance in vasoactive mediator production with a relative predominance of vasoconstrictors can be corrected or modified by hypothermia.[111,154,155] Thus, Aibiki *et al.* reported that induction of moderate hypothermia (32 °–33 °C) led to a reduction in prostanoid production and attenuation of the imbalance between thromboxane A2 and prostaglandin I_2 in patients with traumatic brain injury.[154] Chen *et al.* observed decreased production of the vasoconstrictor endothelin-1 associated with hypothermia.[155] Although such preliminary evidence suggests that hypothermia may favorably affect secretion of vasoactive mediators, regulation of cerebral perfusion especially in the injured brain is highly complex, and the impact of hypothermia should be studied in greater detail. Apart from the temperature, local cerebral circulation can be influenced by numerous and highly diverse factors, including the presence or absence of normal cerebral autoregulation, ventilator settings and blood gas management, and concomitantly administered treatments such as mannitol and hypertonic saline, among others.

Improved tolerance for ischemia

Hypothermia has been shown to improve the tolerance for ischemia in various animal models.[156–158] For this reason, it is widely used in the perioperative setting, especially in major vascular surgery, cardiothoracic surgery and neurosurgical interventions. An ability to withstand periods of ischemia more effectively would be an important potential protective mechanism, because patients with different types of neurological injury may develop periods of ischemia for many days following their initial injury. In patients with subarachnoid hemorrhage the development of vasospasm every week after the initial bleeding episode can lead to significant additional ischemic injury. The risk of ischemia long after admission also applies to patients after CPR, where evidence suggests that cerebral ischemia may persist for several hours following successful resuscitation even when saturation and arterial oxygen levels are normal.[159] Thus an increased tolerance for ischemia could be yet another mechanism for beneficial effects of hypothermia.

Role of epileptic activity and other mechanisms
Non-convulsive status epilepticus, i.e., epileptic activity without obvious clinical signs and symptoms, occurs frequently in patients with various types of brain injury (including subarachnoid hemorrhage, stroke, TBI and postanoxic encephalopathy).[160–164] Whether non-convulsive status epilepticus by itself causes permanent (additional) brain injury remains somewhat controversial; however, there is mounting evidence that brain injury can be significantly increased when non-convulsive status occurs in the acute phases of brain injury, i.e., while the destructive processes outlined above are ongoing.[160,161] Thus, although the role of non-convulsive status epilepticus by itself has not been fully clarified, when it occurs in combination with acute brain injury the two are synergistically detrimental, and can markedly increase brain injury.[160,161]

Evidence from various sources suggests that hypothermia can suppress epileptic activity. Various case reports and case series have reported successful use of hypothermia in the treatment of grand mal seizures.[165,166] Animal studies have shown that induction of hyperthermia increases the extent of epilepsy-induced brain injury, while prevention or prompt treatment of hyperthermia reduces these injuries,[167–169] and induction of hypothermia decreases epilepsy-induced brain injury.[169,170] Thus the anti-epileptic effect of hypothermia may also explain its neuroprotective effect.

In addition, an enhanced expression of various so-called *immediate early genes* which are a part of the cellular stress response to injury, and the induction of various *cold shock proteins* that can protect the cell from different types of injury including ischemia and trauma may also be added to protection by hypothermia.[171] There is evidence that hypothermia can suppress so-called *spreading depression-like depolarizations*, which can augment neuronal damage in various types of brain injury.[172] These mechanisms have been studied mainly in TBI and stroke; their role in the transient ischemic brain injury that characterizes cardiac arrest, and the precise influence of induced hypothermia on these processes, remain to be determined.

In summary, there are numerous mechanisms that may underlie the protective effects of hypothermia in various types of brain injury, and perhaps myocardial injury. That hypothermia can influence so many of the destructive mechanisms following ischemia and reperfusion may explain why it has proved effective in a clinical setting, at least in some situations, where other treatments have failed or proved far less successful.

Different destructive mechanism may play a more or less important role in different types of brain injury; in addition, their relative mechanisms may vary among patients, and even over time within the same patient. A more detailed understanding of these processes will help us to apply hypothermia treatment more effectively. The other key element of a successful use of this treatment will be avoiding side effects of hypothermia, as discussed below.

Side effects of induced hypothermia
Hypothermia induces physiological changes in virtually every tract and every organ in the body. The kinetic properties of most enzyme systems are temperature-dependent; thus the speed of various enzyme-mediated reactions (including drug metabolism) is significantly influenced by hypothermia, as well as circulatory, respiratory, and coagulation systems. The physiological changes induced by hypothermia, as well as the implications that this has for methods for inducing hypothermia, are discussed in a separate section above. Here we focus on the most important side effects, those that require detailed attention and management in a clinical setting. Of note that this some changes induced by hypothermia, although physiological, are nevertheless undesirable in critically ill, neurointensive care patients and therefore require preventive measures and/or treatment. In contrast, other consequences of hypothermia are side effects, but pose no great risk to the patient and thus usually do not require active treatment. For example, mild hypothermia frequently induces bradycardia and a decrease in cardiac output, which rarely requires treatment. In contrast, hypothermia induces insulin resistance and a decrease in insulin secretion in many patients, which can lead to hyperglycemia. This physiological consequence of hypothermia requires aggressive treatment because hyperglycemia has been shown to affect outcome adversely in critically ill patients,[173] and to have negative effects on neurological outcome, by increasing brain injury during episodes of ischemia.[87,170]

To discuss risks of side effects, hypothermic treatment is considered in three phases: the induction, maintenance, and rewarming. Each of these phases is associated with different problems and risks, and thus requires a different management approach.

In general, the induction phase of hypothermia, before the target temperature has been reached is where the risk of short-term side effects, (e.g., electrolyte disorders and severe disturbances of glucose metabolism), is greatest. Patients tend to be most "unstable" during this phase, and management is most difficult because many short-term changes occur. For example, ventilator settings and dosage of vasoactive drugs usually require frequent changes, and various metabolic measures should be carefully monitored by frequent blood serum analysis. The risk of side effects of cooling can be minimized by cooling patients rapidly to reach the maintenance phase as quickly as possible. This can be accomplished by using combinations of different cooling methods, such as a combination of large-volume infusion of cold fluids and surface cooling.[174] Once the core temperature decreases below ± 33.5 °C, the patient tends to become more stable, with less risk for fluid loss or intracellular shifts, cessation or significant reduction of shivering, and no further major changes in hemodynamic parameters.[84,175,176]

Once the maintenance phase commences, the risk of acute side effects such as electrolyte disorders diminishes (although some risk still remains). In this phase attention should shift towards the prevention of longer-term side effects such as pneumonia, wound infections, and bed sores (see below).

The rewarming phase is also associated with electrolyte disorders caused by shifts from the intracellular to the extracellular compartment; this can be largely prevented by slow and controlled rewarming, to preserve the neuroprotective effects, rapid rewarming may reactivate the destructive processes outlined above.

The most important side effects of induced hypothermia are discussed below.

Arrhythmias, hemodynamic changes, and cardiovascular effects

Mild hypothermia (32 °–34 °C) induces significant changes in various hemodynamic parameters: cardiac output decreases by about 25% through decreased contractility and reduced heart rate. Central venous pressure usually rises, as well as an increase in arterial resistance. A slight rise in blood pressure, by ± 10 mmHg, is caused by hypothermia-induced vasoconstriction of peripheral arteries and arterioles. This effect is absent or less pronounced in cerebral arteries, where the balance between cerebral blood flow and cerebral metabolism (as measured by oxygen and glucose utilization) is maintained or improved.[177,178] Under normal circumstances hypothermia also induces a small increase in central venous pressure. These observations have been confirmed in clinical trials in adults and in children.[5,179]

Hypothermia also induces electrocardiographic changes and alterations in the heart rhythm. When hypothermic treatment is first started and body temperature begins to decrease from normothermia, patients will develop sinus tachycardia, caused in part by a shift in circulatory volume from the peripheral compartment, especially the skin, to the core compartment. This leads to a relative increase in the venous return to the heart, which can induce a concomitant increase in heart rate. As temperature decreases further, below 35.5 °C sinus bradycardia ensues, with a progressive decrease in heart rate as temperature decreases further. Typically, at core temperatures of 32° the heart rate can decrease to around 40 beats per minute or even lower, although there is a wide inter- and intra-individual variability. This decrease is caused by a decrease in the rate of diastolic depolarization in the cells of the sinus node, and is accompanied by EKG changes, including prolonged PR-interval, widening of the QRS-complex, increased QT-interval, and sometimes so-called Osborne waves. Diastolic and systolic dysfunction may develop with decreased myocardial contractility. Lower heart rate combined with diminished myocardial contractility leads to a decrease in cardiac output of ± 25% at temperatures of 33 °–34 °C. In general, however, the decrease in metabolic rate is equal to or greater than the decrease in cardiac output caused by the bradycardia and decreased myocardial contractility. Mixed venous saturation, which can be measured to determine tissue oxygen extraction, usually remain unchanged or increase reflecting an unchanged or improved circulatory state. Thus hypothermia-associated bradycardia usually does not require treatment. If treatment is considered necessary, because of the mechanism underlying this form of bradycardia, atropine will not be effective. Therefore, stimulation of heart rate can be accomplished by administering isoprenaline, by rewarming the patient to slightly higher temperatures, or (in extreme cases) by inserting a pacing wire, although the last-mentioned is very rarely necessary.

The risk of developing clinically significant arrhythmias is very low as long as the patient's core temperature remains above 30 °C. The risk of severe arrhythmia increases significantly if core temperature drops below 28 °–30 °C, especially if electrolyte disorders have also developed. When arrhythmias do develop, they usually begin with atrial fibrillation (AF), which can be followed by more severe arrhythmias including ventricular tachycardia (VT) and ventricular fibrillation (VF) if temperature decreases further. Importantly, mechanical manipulations can trigger this transition from AF to VF, because the myocardium becomes highly sensitive to mechanical manipulations during hypothermia.[180] Thus, performing chest compressions because of extreme bradycardia this can easily lead to a conversion of sinus rhythm to VF, or AF to VF. A major problem is that once arrhythmias develop in hypothermic patients, they are much more difficult to treat than at normothermia, because the myocardium becomes less responsive to many cardiac and anti-arrhythmic drugs during hypothermia. As these problems are extremely rare at temperatures above 28°–30°C, great care should be taken to keep core temperatures above this limit. In our center we routinely cool some patients to temperatures very close to this limit (between 30.5 and 32°C for refractory intracranial hypertension) without encountering severe arrhythmias, provided that electrolyte levels are carefully monitored and promptly corrected.

The relative increase in venous return induced by hypothermia can lead to an activation of atrial natriuretic peptide and a decrease in the levels of antidiuretic hormone (ADH). This (in combination with other mechanisms such as tubular dysfunction, see below) can lead to a marked increase in diuresis ("cold diuresis"), which if uncorrected can lead to hypovolemia, renal electrolyte loss, and hemoconcentration with increased blood viscosity.[181–183] The risk of hypovolemia is greater when the patient is also treated with agents that can increase diuresis, such as mannitol in patients with traumatic brain injury. The increased blood viscosity (of ± 2% per °C decrease in core temperature) can lead to problems in the microcirculation; the abovementioned mechanisms combined with tubular dysfunction can lead to severe electrolyte disorders (see below) and to a rise in serum sodium levels and osmolarity. Thus, careful attention should be paid to intravascular volume and fluid balance in patients treated with hypothermia, and hypovolemia should be avoided or promptly corrected.

Coronary perfusion and ischemia

From various studies in postoperative patients the presence of hypothermia is associated with increased risk of myocardial infarction, and it is widely believed that hypothermia can lead to coronary vasoconstriction and myocardial ischemia. In addition, various studies have shown that accidental hypothermia in the perioperative setting is associated with an increased risk for morbid cardiac events.[184,185] The actual situation is more complex, in particular because the result probably depends on the pre-existing condition of the patient's coronary arteries and on local factors: in healthy subjects, mild hypothermia (around 35°C) actually increases coronary perfusion,[186] whereas in patients with coronary artery disease hypothermia can induce vasoconstriction in severely atherosclerotic coronary arteries.[187]

Various animal experiments[188–195] and preliminary clinical studies have shown that hypothermia may actually decrease myocardial injury after cardiac arrest, provided it is initiated early enough.[68,196,197] Thus, the question whether hypothermia mitigates myocardial injury should be addressed in further larger studies, available evidence does not suggest that hypothermia *increases* this injury, which might be the case if hypothermia caused vasoconstriction in these patients.

Electrolyte disorders

Patients treated with induced hypothermia are at high risk for developing electrolyte disorders, because of a combination of increased renal excretion of electrolytes and intracellular shift.[182] The mechanisms underlying the increased renal excretion are altered volume regulation and cardiac preload (see above) and tubular dysfunction.[182] This is important because electrolyte disorders, especially hypomagnesemia, may be associated with an increased risk for adverse neurological outcome. In experimental settings depletion of magnesium (Mg) leads to significantly worse neurological outcomes after traumatic injury, whereas administration of Mg during or some time after the event substantially mitigates secondary injury and reduces loss of cortical cells.[198–201] Magnesium may also play a role in prevention of reperfusion injury.[202,203] In addition, loss of Mg is associated with vasoconstriction of cerebral and coronary arteries.[204] Animal studies have shown that administration of magnesium following myocardial infarction is associated with reduced infarct size and improved preservation of myocardial function.[205] In clinical studies, hypomagnesemia has also been linked to atrial and ventricular arrhythmias, neuromuscular abnormalities with muscle weakness (including cardiac insufficiency), bronchospasm, seizures, and metabolic effects including decreased insulin sensitivity.[204] Hypomagnesemia can also induce other electrolyte disorders including hypokalemia, hypocalcemia, hyponatremia, and hypophosphatemia.

In clinical studies, hypomagnesemia is an independent predictor of adverse outcome both in critically ill ICU patients and in less severely ill patients in the general ward.[206,207] It is specifically associated with adverse outcome in patients with unstable angina or myocardial infarction,[208] and administering magnesium has been shown to reduce mortality and infarct size in these patients.[209]

With respect to other electrolyte disorders, hypokalemia and hypophosphatemia can also have highly undesirable effects, including arrhythmias, muscle weakness and neuromuscular abnormalities. Hypophosphatemia can induce weakness of the diaphragm and respiratory muscles leading to an increased risk of respiratory infections and failure to wean, in infants as well as impaired myocardial function and a decrease in cardiac output.[204,210,211]

The clinical consequences of hypokalemia (cardiac arrhythmias, muscle weakness, rhabdomyolysis, renal failure, and hyperglycemia) are usually well recognized, and in most ERs and ICUs, potassium levels are measured promptly and frequently. The potential risks of disorders in sodium metabolism in neurological injury are also usually appreciated, as both hypo- and hypernatremia can significantly increase the severity of brain injury. Magnesium and phosphate usually receive far less attention from ER and ICU physicians, however. The list of potential complications of electrolyte disorders shows that preventing hypothermia-associated electrolyte disorders should be an important goal of therapy in patients treated with induced hypothermia.

Levels of Mg, P, and K should be maintained in the high or high-normal range in all patients with neurological injuries. Of note, serum Mg levels do not always accurately reflect true Mg status; intracellular Mg stores may be significantly depleted while serum Mg levels remain normal.[204] This also applies to levels of ionized Mg, although this better reflects the levels of "active" magnesium.

Hyperglycemia

As already discussed above, hypothermia can simultaneously decrease insulin sensitivity and reduce insulin secretion by pancreatic islet cells. Thus, patients treated with induced hypothermia will be at high risk for developing hyperglycemia, which is associated with increased morbidity and mortality in critically ill patients. Strict control of glucose levels with intensive insulin therapy can reduce morbidity and mortality.[173,212] Hyperglycemia is associated with increased rates of infection, critical illness neuropathy and renal failure.[173] This strongly suggests tight control of glucose levels when hypothermia is induced in critically ill patients.

Other metabolic effects and blood gas analysis

Hypothermia leads to an increase in the synthesis of glycerol, free fatty acids, ketonic acids, and lactate, this will cause a mild metabolic acidosis in most patients, which is a physiological consequence of hypothermia and does not require treatment. In contrast to the pH levels measured extracellularly, *intracellular* pH levels usually increase slightly during hypothermia.

The decrease in metabolic rate (5%–8% per °C drop in core temperature) also decreases oxygen requirements and the synthesis of carbon dioxide (CO_2). Thus the ventilator settings should be adjusted during induction of hypothermia, and blood gases should be monitored frequently especially during the induction phase of cooling.

Of note, the measurement of blood gases is influenced by the temperature of the blood. In blood gas analyzers, samples are warmed to 37 °C, so that when the actual temperature differs significantly from 37 °C, these measurements will not be correct. If blood samples from hypothermic patients are rewarmed under vacuum-sealed conditions, PO_2 and PCO_2 will be overestimated, and pH underestimated. For example, in a patient with an uncorrected core temperature of 30 °C and PCO_2 of 40 mmHg the actual (corrected) PCO_2 value would be 29 mmHg.[213] In the same patient with an uncorrected PO_2 of 100 mmHg, the value corrected for temperature will be 73 mmHg. True pH is also underestimated, with hypothermia leading to a more alkalotic status compared to normothermia (pH increase ± 0.011 pH unit/°C). In the example cited above, the measured pH would be 7.40, whereas the true pH would be 7.50. The concept of CO_2 management in which the PCO_2 obtained by measurement at 37 °C is kept constant (for example, at 40 mmHg) regardless of the actual body temperature is called *alpha-stat*. If the PCO_2 value is corrected for the actual body temperature, and is held constant at the same level as during normothermia, this implies that the "true" amount of CO_2 will increase during hypothermia. This concept of CO_2 management is called *pH-stat*. In other words, when alpha-stat CO_2 management is applied, pH that is not corrected for current body temperature remains constant, while true pH increases because the actual $PaCO_2$ has decreased. When pH-stat CO_2 management is used true pH remains constant, while pH that is not corrected for temperature decreases.

Which method is superior in managing hypothermic patients has not been settled. There is evidence to support both methods.[171,213] Supporters of the pH-stat method argue that it leads to hyperventilation, hypocapnia and hypocapnia-induced cerebral vasoconstriction, while pH-stat management induces a degree of hypercapnia leading to cerebral vasodilatation (provided cerebral autoregulation is intact). The latter would be a more attractive option. However, hypercapnia can impair or abolish cerebral autoregulation, presumably because CO_2-induced vasodilatation limits the vessels' capacity to dilate further.[171,214] This may mean that the body's capacity to divert blood to injured areas is impaired. In addition, some animal studies suggest that respiratory alkalosis is physiologically appropriate during hypothermia to preserve normal physiological conditions.[171]

Regardless of which method of blood gas management is chosen, physicians using mild hypothermia in their patients should be aware of the effects of temperature on blood gas analysis and on other laboratory measurements. In addition, the effect of temperature on PO_2 should be taken into account in all cases, and the measured PaO_2 should always be corrected for current body temperature in hypothermic patients to maintain true PaO_2 in the normal range, regardless of the pCO_2 management method chosen.[213]

Coagulation measures

Hypothermia induces a mild bleeding diathesis, with increased bleeding time due to effects on platelet count, platelet function, the kinetics of clotting enzymes and plasminogen activator inhibitors, and other steps in the coagulation cascade.[145,147–149] Standard coagulation tests will not show abnormalities unless they are performed at the patient's actual core temperature; similar to blood gas analyses, the samples are usually warmed to 37 °C before the clotting tests are performed. Even though the coagulation defects can be caused by hypothermia, the risk of clinically significant bleeding induced by hypothermia in patients who are not already actively bleeding is very low. None of the large clinical trials in patients with TBI, SAH, stroke, or postanoxic coma reported significantly increased risks of intracranial bleeding associated with hypothermia. In patients who are already actively bleeding, for example in multi-traumatized patients, the sites of bleeding should be controlled before hypothermic therapy is initiated.

Infections

Hypothermia impairs immune functions and inhibits various inflammatory responses. This side effect may be advantageous in that impairment of harmful inflammatory reactions in the brain may be one of the mechanisms through which hypothermia can be protective. Nevertheless, hypothermia inhibits secretion of proinflammatory cytokines and suppresses leukocyte migration and phagocytosis. Hypothermia-induced insulin resistance and hyperglycemia may further increase infection risks. Many of the clinical studies that induce hypothermia for various indications have reported a slightly, moderately or in some cases severely increased incidence of pneumonia when hypothermia was used for periods longer than 24 hours,[212,214–216] but if hypothermia is used for 24 hours or less no or only small increases in the rates of infection were reported. Various studies suggest that use of antibiotic prophylaxis in the form of selective decontamination of the digestive tract can decrease ICU mortality and colonization with resistant gram-negative bacteria,[217] and some evidence suggests that selective decontamination can prevent infections during prolonged use of hypothermia.[118,218] Thus antibiotic prophylaxis may be considered in patients treated with induced hypothermia.

An increased risk of wound infections associated with hypothermia has also been reported,[219,220] which may be related both to diminished leukocyte function and to hypothermia-induced vasoconstriction in the skin. Thus extra care should be taken in cooled patients to prevent bed sores, which are more likely to progress and/or show impaired healing. Extra attention should also be paid to catheter insertion sites and to any surgical wounds.

Shivering

When hypothermia is induced, the body will employ various mechanisms to generate heat and decrease heat loss. The latter is accomplished mainly through increasing sympathetic tone and through vasoconstriction in the skin, while heat generation may be accomplished by shivering. Shivering can increase oxygen consumption by between 40% and 100%,[221] an undesirable effect in patients with neurological and/or posthypoxic injury. This is less problematic in mechanically ventilated patients, as the work of breathing will not be increased by shivering. Nevertheless shivering can also present a technical problem by decreasing cooling rates; this problem is discussed more extensively elsewhere.

Shivering can be controlled by administration of sedatives, anesthetics, opiates and/or paralyzing drugs. In most patients shivering can be significantly attenuated by relatively small doses of opiates. When use of paralyzing agents and/or opiates is deemed undesirable, alternatives include administration of clonidine, neostigmine and ketanserine. Care should be taken to avoid adverse effects, however; for example, clonidine may worsen hypothermia-induced bradycardia.

Other side effects

As already stated, hypothermia can significantly influence drug metabolism and pharmacokinetics, because the enzymes that metabolize most drugs are highly temperature-sensitive. For many drugs commonly used in the ER and ICU, the effect of (lower) temperatures is unknown, because drug metabolism and clearance have not been studied at different temperatures. Nonetheless, it seems likely that the clearance of many drugs will be significantly decreased during hypothermia, as has been demonstrated in clinical studies for propofol, fentanyl, muscle paralysers and barbiturates.

Hypothermia can also lead to various changes in laboratory measurements. The most frequently occurring changes are shown in Table 49.2.

Finally, it is clear that most of the side effects of hypothermia can be prevented or well controlled in an appropriate intensive care setting. Patient management problems will vary according to the depth and the duration of hypothermia, and the underlying disease of the patient. In general the use of hypothermia in patients with TBI and stroke will present more problems than the use of hypothermia in patients following cardiac arrest and CPR.[84] It is important that the medical and nursing staff

Table 49.2. Most frequently occurring hypothermia-induced changes in laboratory measurements

Increase in serum amylase levels

Mild-to-moderate thrombocytopenia (platelet count 30×10^{12} -100×10^{12})

Increase in serum lactate levels (2.5–5 mmol/l)

Hyperglycemia

Electrolyte disorders (low Mg, K, P, Ca)

Increase in liver enzymes (SGOT and SGTP)

Mild metabolic acidosis

Mild coagulation disorders

Changes in blood gases

members using induced hypothermia be aware of the physiological and pathophysiological changes that can be expected, and that they can determine which changes require treatment and which do not (Fig. 49.3).

Prediction of neurologic outcome after cardiac arrest in patients treated with therapeutic mild hypothermia (Roine and Tiainen)

Global cerebral ischemia after cardiac arrest is a common cause of extensive brain damage by multiple pathophysiological mechanisms. The clinical syndrome related to global cerebral ischemia is called hypoxic-ischemic encephalopathy (HIE), the severity of which usually determines the outcome of cardiac arrest patients with restored spontaneous circulation. Most patients resuscitated from cardiac arrest are initially comatose. Early prediction of neurological outcome in patients resuscitated from cardiac arrest is a major ethical, medical and economical challenge. To avoid falsely pessimistic prognosis, the prognostic tests used in critical care are usually required to have high specificity and a narrow confidence interval for poor outcome, with less emphasis on sensitivity. When evaluating the prognosis of a comatose patient resuscitated from cardiac arrest, a false prognosis of poor outcome can lead to early withdrawal of care and thus carries a risk of a self-fulfilling prophecy. On the other hand, a falsely optimistic prediction may lead to unnecessary prolongation of intensive care therapy and might prevent admission of other patients who could benefit more.

Clinical status

The times from collapse to the start of basic and advanced life support and especially to defibrillation correlate with survival rate.[222,223] The prognosis declines with increasing duration of coma. No clinical findings on admission have been proven to reliably predict poor outcome and no attempt should be made to assess the neurologic prognosis on admission on clinical grounds. In a recent review article, Booth *et al.* examined all 11 studies between years 1979 and 2000 that addressed clinical signs in outcome prediction after cardiac arrest. They concluded that prognostic assessment of outcome on clinical grounds is not possible before 24 hours have elapsed, and motor signs are not meaningful before 72 hours.[224] This meta-analysis included 1914 comatose survivors of cardiac arrest. Patients sedated or anesthetized during the clinical examination were not included in the analysis. The most useful signs predicting poor outcome were absent corneal and pupillary reflexes, absent motor response at 24 hours, and absent withdrawal to pain at 72 hours after cardiac arrest.[224] Heavy sedation and opiate analgesia are, however, used much more frequently and in higher doses than they were a few decades ago. Old prediction rules based solely on clinical signs and the duration of coma are therefore often outdated or should be revalidated.

Generalized myoclonus status has been reported to be a terminal finding after cardiac arrest and to be incompatible with recovery.[225] Nevertheless, early myoclonic status is not necessarily an agonal event.[226] Therapeutic hypothermia usually requires muscle relaxation to prevent shivering, and this masks myoclonic jerking as well as seizures.

Assessment of clinical status is also masked to some extent by the use of therapeutic hypothermia. Induced hypothermia requires muscle relaxation, sedation and mechanical ventilation, which may complicate the clinical assessment. Hypothermia may also induce changes in drug metabolism and increase the duration of sedative drug effects.[220] The possible effect of individual medications to a patient's clinical status should always be carefully considered. Our own experience is that the sedative effect of both midazolam and propofol can be significantly prolonged in hypothermia-treated patients. Some of our patients did not recover consciousness until day five after cardiac arrest, but made a good recovery thereafter.

Serum markers

Neuron-specific enolase (NSE) is the neuronal form of the intracytoplasmic glycolytic enzyme enolase. NSE is located in neurons and in neuroectodermal cells. It is a dimeric enzyme composed of two γ subunits, with a molecular weight of 78 000 Dalton and biologic half-life of about 24 hours. Neuronal damage and impairment of blood–brain barrier integrity can be detected by release of

NSE into cerebrospinal fluid and eventually to the blood. Increased levels of NSE in cerebrospinal fluid and serum have been reported after ischemic stroke, intracerebral hemorrhage, brain injury, and cardiac arrest. Several studies have found high levels of serum NSE to be associated with poor outcome in patients resuscitated from cardiac arrest.[227-233]

The S-100B protein is an acidic Ca^{2+} binding protein with a molecular weight of approximately 21 000 Dalton and biologic half-life of 0.5 hour. The protein has two subtypes: $\alpha\beta$-heterodimer and $\beta\beta$-homodimer; the $\alpha\beta$-form is found in astroglial cells; and the $\beta\beta$-form is found predominantly in astroglial and Schwann cells, but it has also been demonstrated in tumors such as melanoma, schwannoma, and highly differentiated neuroblastoma. Increased serum levels of protein S-100B have been reported after traumatic brain injury, stroke, cardiac arrest, and cardiopulmonary surgery. High levels of serum S-100B after cardiac arrest have been reported to correlate with unfavorable neurologic outcome.[230,232,234-237]

We studied the time-course of serum NSE and S-100B in hypothermia-treated cardiac arrest patients. The levels of serum NSE were lower in hypothermia- than in normothermia-treated patients during the first 48 hours after cardiac arrest. NSE values decreased between 24 and 48 hours in 30 of 34 patients (88%) in the hypothermia group and in 16 of 32 patients (50%) in the normothermia group ($P<0.001$). Furthermore, the decrease in NSE values was associated with good outcome, and increase with poor outcome at 6 months after cardiac arrest. The results suggest that the time-course of serum NSE between 24 and 48 hours after cardiac arrest may aid in clinical decision-making. Decreasing levels of serum NSE over time may indicate selective attenuation of delayed neuronal death by therapeutic hypothermia.[238] In the same study the levels of serum S-100B did not differ between the two treatment arms. The serum S-100B levels decreased between 24 and 48 hours in 17 of 34 (50%) patients in the hypothermia group and in 15 of 33 (45%) patients in the normothermia group, but the decrease in the levels of serum S-100B during this time period was not related to the outcome. However, in another study by Hachimi-Idrissi et al., the serum S-100B levels decreased significantly between admission and 24 hours after cardiac arrest in the hypothermia-treated group.[239] In our study the ROC-analysis of serum NSE and S-100B at different time-points revealed that cut-off values predicting unfavorable outcome with a specificity of at least 95% were higher in the hypothermia group. Unfortunately, the sensitivity of these tests was remarkably poor in the hypothermia group.[238] The use of hypothermia seems to reduce the prognostic value of both serum NSE and S-100B in outcome prediction, which may be explained by the neuroprotective effect of hypothermia, in preventing the continuing injury and release of these ischemia markers in the blood stream. Hypothermia is also known to maintain the integrity of blood–brain barrier after ischemic damage.[240,241]

Clinical neurophysiology

The short-latency median nerve somatosensory evoked potentials (SSEP) have been found to predict accurately permanent coma after cardiac arrest.[242,243] A bilaterally absent early cortical N20 response (first cortical response occurring approximately 20 ms after stimulation to median nerve at wrist) predicts permanent coma with a specificity of 100% (95% confidence interval 99–100%) and thus the median nerve SSEPs are the method of choice for predicting outcome after cardiac arrest. Significant improvement in SEP have been reported within 24 hours after ROSC,[244] and allowing at least 24 hours after cardiac arrest is recommended for obtaining a reliable prognosis based on SEP. Moreover, normal cortical SEP responses do not guarantee awakening from coma.

Short-latency SEP recording is a non-invasive, reproducible technique that can be easily performed at the bedside in the ICU. Short-latency SEPs are also quite resistant to anesthetic agents. Induced hypothermia requires muscle relaxation, which prevents the adjustment of SEP stimuli intensity based on thumb twitch. The intensity of the stimuli must be sufficient to evoke an ipsilateral supraclavicular response in patients with clinical muscle relaxation. Hypothermia of 33 °C reduces nerve conduction velocity and delays early cortical N20 response. In a study examining 30 still-hypothermic, comatose cardiac arrest survivors at 24–28 hours after resuscitation, the cortical N20 response appeared approximately 24 milliseconds after the stimulus. Bilateral absence of short-latency cortical potentials predicted permanent coma reliably also in these patients.[245]

Long-latency SEPs (N70 response) have been found useful in identifying patients with favourable outcome.[246] Madl et al. also reported that the N70 long-latency sensory evoked potential was more accurate in predicting individual outcome than a panel of three experienced emergency physicians review clinical data 24 hours after cardiac arrest.[247] Because of the slowing of neural transmission with hypothermia, the N70 cut-off values determined on normothermic patients cannot be applied to hypothermic patients. Recording of long-latency SEPs is more demanding than recording of short-latency SEPs, since long-latency SEPs are often less reproducible and more prone to artifacts than short-latency SSEPs, this may be an issue, especially in the ICU environment. So far no studies examining long-latency SEPs in hypothermic cardiac arrest survivors have been published.

The prognostic ability of electroencephalography (EEG) has also been studied in cardiac arrest survivors. EEG is quite sensitive to drug effects and metabolic disturbances, which limits its prognostic usefulness. Only EEG with essentially complete generalized suppression after the first day of the arrest in the absence of sedative or anesthetizing drug effects is associated with invariably poor outcome. Suppression of EEG, periodic complexes, epileptiform activity, burst-suppression or alpha coma pattern does not preclude the possibility of neurologic recovery, although it usually indicates poor outcome.[248] Serial EEGs may offer supplemental information about the evolution of the patient's status. Mild hypothermia produces small changes in the EEG,[249] but no studies evaluating the prognostic value of EEG findings in cardiac arrest patients treated with hypothermia have been published.

Neuroradiological imaging

In the acute stage, conventional MRI or CT may be useful for differential diagnosis. In hypoxic–ischemic encephalopathy, later neuroradiological imaging may reveal bilateral watershed infarcts, laminar cortical necrosis, and cerebellar, white matter, and basal ganglia lesions. Neuroradiological imaging findings apparently have limited prognostic value, except for absent intracranial circulation or increased intracranial pressure. A normal conventional MRI or CT does not exclude the diagnosis of hypoxic-ischemic encephalopathy.[250] FLAIR (fluid-attenuated inversion recovery) and DW (diffusion weighted) imaging may help detect extensive ischemic damage in comatose survivors of cardiac arrest.[251,252] The difficulty of performing MR imaging in critically ill patients often limits the use of this examination.

Limitations of outcome prediction methods

Currently the methods used in assessing the neurologic prognosis are targeted to predict poor outcome (death or persisting coma). Despite all normal examination results some survivors of cardiac arrest never regain consciousness. So far, there are no methods to predict good outcome accurately in the early phase of treatment. Reliable prediction methods are required not just to direct intensive care for the patients benefiting from it, but also in order to alleviate the emotional distress of the patient's family suffering from prolonged uncertainty of their loved one's outcome.

The use of therapeutic hypothermia may complicate the evaluation of outcome. The prediction methods developed on normothermic patients cannot be applied directly to patients treated with hypothermia without validation studies. Therapeutic hypothermia also seems to postpone the first feasible prognostic evaluation, which should not be undertaken during hypothermia or shortly after rewarming the patient. As the amount of evidence and the number of studies concerning prediction of outcome in hypothermia-treated patients are still limited, caution and discretion should be exercised in assessing the neurological prognosis of victims of cardiac arrest and particularly regarding the end-of-life decisions.

Future of preservative hypothermia, suspended animation (Behringer)

Suspended animation

In sudden cardiac death, cooling can be started *before* ischemia (protection), *during* ischemia (preservation), and *after* ischemia (resuscitation). Cerebral protection has been used since the 1950s to protect the brain against global ischemia during cardiac surgery, but is logistically not feasible in sudden cardiac arrest patients. Cerebral resuscitation with mild therapeutic hypothermia after successfully restoring the circulation is described above. The following paragraphs will describe cerebral preservation, which might be feasible during no-flow and low-flow cardiac arrest. The concept of suspended animation, that is: "preservation of the organism during transport and surgical hemostasis, under prolonged controlled clinical death, followed by delayed resuscitation to survival without brain damage"[253] was introduced for trauma victims, who rapidly bleed to death. In these patients, conventional resuscitation attempts are futile, and currently mortality is near 100%. We believe that, if the concept of suspended animation is suitable for normovolemic cardiac arrest, it should be investigated.

Suspended animation in exsanguination cardiac arrest

Protective hypothermia for cardiac surgery is induced slowly and reversed with cardiopulmonary bypass. In the field, cardiopulmonary bypass is not yet available, and in trauma victims who exsanguinate to cardiac arrest, hypothermia must be induced before the brain loses its viability, i.e., within the first minutes of no-flow. Therefore, the use of an aortic cold flush was introduced to induce preservative hypothermia rapidly first in the most sensitive organs, the heart and brain, and cardiopulmonary bypass was used only for resuscitation and rewarming[254,255]. Dogs were exsanguinated over 5 minutes to cardiac arrest no-flow of 15 to 120 minutes.[256–259] At 2 minutes of cardiac arrest, the dogs received the aortic flush via a balloon-tipped catheter, advanced via the femoral artery. Cardiac arrest of 15–120 minutes was reversed with cardiopulmonary bypass, followed by restoration of spontaneous circulation, assisted circulation (with cardiopulmonary bypass) for 2 hours, mild hypothermia for 12 hours, controlled ventilation for 24 hours, and intensive care to 72 hours. Final outcome evaluation at 72 hours was evaluated in terms of overall performance category (OPC), neurologic deficit score (NDS), and total and regional histologic damage scores (HDS) in 19 different brain regions. Results depended on flush volume and flush temperature.

For cardiac arrest of 15 minutes[256] and 20 minutes,[257] aortic arch flush at the start of cardiac arrest with 25 ml/kg saline at 24 °C, decreased tympanic temperature to 36 °C, resulted in poor outcome, while the same flush at 2 °C, decreased tympanic temperature to 34 °C, resulted in good neurologic outcome and only mild histologic damage. For cardiac arrest of 30 minutes,[258] aortic flush at the start of the arrest with 25 ml/kg saline at 2 °C, decreased tympanic temperature to 34 °C resulted in all dogs in coma or brain death, while aortic flush with 100 ml/kg saline at 2 °C, decreased tympanic temperature to 28 °C, resulted in all dogs with good neurologic outcome and zero or only minimal brain HDS. For cardiac arrest of 60 minutes,[259] aortic flush at the start of the arrest with around 3 litres of saline at 2 °C to tympanic temperature 20 °C, resulted in good cerebral outcome, but some disabilities in the hindlegs; aortic flush with around 6 litres of saline at 2 °C to tympanic temperature 15 °C resulted in all dogs with normal outcome and only mild or zero histologic damage, as did flush with around 2 °C saline to tympanic temperature 10 °C. For cardiac arrest of 90 minutes,[259] aortic flush at the start of the arrest with around 10 litres of saline at 2 °C, decreased tympanic temperature to 10 °C, resulted in normal outcome and only zero or minimal brain HDS. For cardiac arrest of 120 minutes,[259] flush to tympanic temperature 10 °C resulted in mixed outcome, and had to include the abdominal viscera; achieving OPC 1 proved feasible but not consistently as observed after 90 minutes of cardiac arrest. With no-flow durations of 30 minutes or longer, the flush had to include the spinal cord to avoid paralysis of the hind legs.

Suspended animation was also explored in a clinically relevant pig model.[260,261] By using readily available equipment, profound hypothermia was induced via a thoracotomy and direct aortic cannulation. A total arrest time of up to 40 minutes at 10 °C core temperature, or a low-flow perfusion of up to 60 minutes at 10 °C core temperature, was survived with normal neurologic recovery. Another group explored the effect of 3 hours of asanguinous low-flow perfusion in dogs with cardiopulmonary bypass with special solutions under ultraprofound hypothermia (< 5 °C), and survival with normal neurologic function to develop a method for protecting the brain during otherwise unfeasible neurosurgical procedures.[262]

Suspended animation in normovolemic cardiac arrest

Sudden normovolemic cardiac arrest accounts for far more deaths than exsanguination cardiac arrest. In Europe, the incidence of normovolemic cardiac arrest is 750 000 patients per year, and good neurologic outcome is achieved in only 6%–23% of them.[263] Therefore, we investigated whether the concept of suspended animation could be adopted for normovolemic cardiac arrest.

One possible approach to suspended animation was shown by Nozari et al. in dogs.[338] In this study, induction of hypothermia was with blood cooled by veno-venous shunt. After cardiac arrest no-flow of 3 minutes, and simulated unsuccessful advanced life support of 17 minutes, dogs were cooled via veno-venous extracorporeal shunt to tympanic temperature 27 °C or 34 °C with ongoing chest compressions for another 20 minutes. Two control groups were kept normothermic, with and without veno-venous blood flow. After 40 minutes of ventricular fibrillation, reperfusion was obtained by cardiopulmonary bypass for 4 hours, including defibrillation to achieve spontaneous circulation. All dogs were maintained at mild hypothermia to 12 hours, and intensive care to 96 hours. In the normothermic groups, all dogs achieved spontaneous circulation, but remained comatose and (except one) died within 58 hours with multiple organ failure. In hypothermia groups, all dogs survived to 96 hours without gross extracerebral organ damage.

Another approach to suspended animation tried in our laboratory was induction of hypothermia with cold aortic saline flush. In exsanguination cardiac arrest, the aortic flush balloon catheter could be inserted by the paramedic or ambulance physician in the field during bleeding, before arrest occurs, whereas in normovolemic cardiac arrest it is clinically unrealistic to think that the aortic flush catheter in place before at least 10 minutes of no-flow, because of the response time of the emergency system and the time required to place the aortic balloon catheter.

Studies in cell cultures and rodents support the concept of suspended animation for normovolemic cardiac arrest. It was shown in myocytes that injury to ischemic cells takes place after reperfusion by initiating several cascades leading to cell death, but not during ischemia itself.[265–267] When ischemic myocytes were made hypothermic before reperfusion, there was less injury to the cells, even when the duration of ischemia was prolonged as compared to cells with normothermic reperfusion.[268] In a cardiac arrest mouse model, induction of moderate hypothermia to 30 °C just before attempted resuscitation resulted in better 72-hour survival compared to mice in which induction of hypothermia was delayed to 30 minutes after the start of resuscitation.[269]

The main challenge in bringing suspended animation to clinical practice consists of the rapid induction of cerebral hypothermia. In one study of exsanguination cardiac arrest in dogs, the aortic flush with 100 ml/kg of saline at 2 °C, decreased tympanic temperature to approximately 28 °C within 4 minutes[258] with a corresponding brain temperature of 18 °C (unpublished data). When the aortic flush as used in the exsanguination cardiac arrest model in dogs[258] was applied in 30-kg swine after 10 minutes of cardiac arrest no-flow, brain temperature remained above 35 °C (unpublished data). One explanation for the difference in brain temperature might be the difference in no-flow time between the two models. In the exsanguination cardiac arrest model, no-flow time before the flush was 2 minutes, whereas in normovolemic cardiac arrest model the no-flow time was prolonged to 10 minutes. Analyzing the pressure curves during the aortic flush with cold saline in normovolemic cardiac arrest, we found no pressure difference between arterial pressure in the descending aorta and venous pressure in the right atrium. Adding vasopressin to the aortic saline flush increased the arterio-venous pressure gradient, which resulted in a rapid decrease of brain temperature to 16 °C during the flush.[270]

After evaluating the feasibility of rapid induction of deep hypothermia after prolonged normovolemic cardiac arrest,[270] the concept of suspended animation was evaluated in a long-term outcome cardiac arrest model in swine.[271] After 15 minutes of ventricular fibrillation, deep hypothermia (about 17 °C) was induced with aortic flush, followed by 20 minutes of hypothermic stasis. At 35 minutes after cardiac arrest, cardiopulmonary bypass was initiated to facilitate restoration of spontaneous circulation and rewarming. Five out of six animals achieved restoration of spontaneous circulation and survived to 9 days, two animals with good neurologic outcome. In the control group, with conventional resuscitation attempts for 20 minutes and jump-start cardiopulmonary bypass, four animals achieved restoration of spontaneous circulation, but only one pig survived to 9 days, with poor neurologic outcome.

How could the results in cell cultures,[265–267] small animals,[269] and our studies[270,271] be translated into daily practice for resuscitating sudden cardiac arrest victims? A futuristic suspended animation scenario might be: when a patient is found in cardiac arrest, resuscitation should not be started by chest compressions, which would result in trickle flow, and thus induce reperfusion injury in a normothermic organism. Instead, once in the field, the emergency physician should insert the flush catheter, and rapidly cool the patient with aortic flush, and only after hypothermia is achieved, start with resuscitation efforts. Before applying suspended animation to humans, many questions must be answered in large animal outcome studies with long-term intensive care and evaluation of neurological outcome: first, it has to be proven that induction of hypothermia after prolonged cardiac arrest no-flow, preceding reperfusion, will improve neurological outcome; secondly, the limit of normothermic no-flow duration has to be determined, i.e., how long can no-flow duration be tolerated so that the animal has normal neurological recovery with induction of hypothermia before reperfusion; third, once cerebral hypothermia is achieved, hypothermic no-flow without chest compression has to be compared to hypothermic trickle-flow with chest compression to bridge the time until initiation of cardiopulmonary bypass for restarting the heart; fourth, the exact level of hypothermia that allows both mitigation of reperfusion injury and protection during hypothermic no-flow, has to be determined; fifth, it has to be proven that a sudden volume load of 100 ml/kg or more by the aortic flush is tolerated by the organism, once restoration of spontaneous circulation is achieved.

Conclusions and recommendations

Hypothermia research has developed enormously since the 1950s. We have learned that hypothermia does much more than simply reduce oxygen metabolism. It took more then 40 years for mild hypothermia after cardiac arrest to be recommended by the European Resuscitation Council and the American Heart Association. There it is stated: *"Unconscious adult patients with spontaneous circulation after out-of-hospital VF cardiac arrest should be cooled to 32 °–34 °C. Cooling should be started as soon as possible and continued for at least 12–24 h. Induced hypothermia might also benefit unconscious adult patients with spontaneous circulation after out-of-hospital cardiac arrest from a non-shockable rhythm, or cardiac arrest in hospital".*[15,16] At the time this chapter was finished in January 2006, the following inclusion criteria for the use of mild hypothermia after cardiac arrest are applied at the Emergency Department at the Medical University of Vienna.

- All patients receiving external chest compressions for any duration due to cardiac arrest, even under sedation.
- Patients not obeying any verbal command at any time after restoration of spontaneous circulation and prior to initiation of cooling.

And only few exclusion criteria are applied.

- Cardiac arrest due to trauma and/or severe bleeding.
- Terminal disease e.g., no further intensive care enhancement/intensification.
- Pregnancy
- Known coagulopathy (except: therapeutic induced)
- Time from sustained restoration of spontaneous circulation until initiation of cooling <240 minutes. An invasive procedure or transport (e.g., CT, PTCA, etc.) is no exclusion for cooling the patient, and cooling should be initiated as soon as possible.

Most of the side effects of hypothermia can be prevented or well controlled in an appropriate intensive care setting, by including sedation and paralysis. Patient management problems will vary according to the depth and the duration of hypothermia, and the underlying disease of the patient. It is important that the medical and nursing staff members using induced hypothermia be aware of the physiological and pathophysiological changes that can be expected, and that they are able to determine which changes require treatment and which do not. Most importantly, hypothermia should be regarded as a drug, and rigorous monitoring of the temperature is mandatory. If the temperature reaches 33 °C, all cooling efforts have to be stopped, and if the temperature drops below 32 °C, the patient has to be rewarmed with heating blankets or warm infusion to avoid further cooling below 32 °C, which might harm the patients. As faster cooling techniques are developed, esophageal temperature is preferred over bladder temperature for temperature monitoring, because bladder temperature lags behind esophageal temperature during fast cooling.

Clinicians should be aware that the use of therapeutic hypothermia might complicate the evaluation of neurologic outcome after cardiac arrest. The prediction methods developed on normothermic patients cannot be applied directly to patients treated with hypothermia without validation studies. The use of therapeutic hypothermia postpones the first feasible prognostic evaluation, to after hypothermia and shortly after rewarming the patient. As the evidence and the number of studies concerning outcome prediction in hypothermia-treated patients are still limited, caution and discretion should be exercised in assessing the neurological prognosis of victims of cardiac arrest and particularly regarding end-of-life decisions.

Despite all the knowledge about hypothermia acquired at this time, additional studies are needed for better definition of the optimal depth and duration of hypothermia, and the optimal rewarming rate after cooling, and to improve the techniques for inducing hypothermia. More laboratory studies in higher non-human primates are needed to investigate the role of hypothermia during cardiac arrest and even before start of resuscita-tion, e.g., suspended animation. In cardiac arrest, mild hypothermia is well established, but mild hypothermia might also benefit patients after stroke, traumatic brain injury, myocardial infarction, hemorrhagic shock, liver failure, pulmonary failure, or sepsis. These fields are all wide open for future research, and should be further pursued in laboratory and clinical studies.

REFERENCES

1. Bigelow, W.G., Linsay, W.K. & Greenwood, W.F. Hypothermia: Its possible role in cardiac surgery. *Ann. Surg.* 1950; **132**: 849–866.
2. Rosomoff, H.L. & Holaday, A. Cerebral blood flow and cerebral oxygen consumption during hypothermia. *Am. J. Physiol.* 1954; **179**: 85–88.
3. Safar, P. Community-wide cardiopulmonary resuscitation. (The CPCR system). *J. Iowa Med. Soc.* 1964; **54**: 629.
4. Friedman, E.W., Davidoff, D. & Fine, J. Effect of hypothermia on tolerance to hemorrhagic shock. In Dripps, R.D., ed. *The Physiology of Induced Hypothermia*. Washington, DC: National Academy of Science Publication, 1956: 369–380.
5. Reuler, J.B. Hypothermia: pathophysiology, clinical settings, and management. *Ann. Intern. Med.* 1978; **89**: 519–527.
6. Steen, P.A., Soule, E.H. & Michenfelder, J.D. Deterimental effect of prolonged hypothermia in cats and monkeys with and without regional cerebral ischemia. *Stroke* 1979; **10**(5): 522–529.
7. Steen, P.A., Milde, J.H. & Michenfelder, J.D. The detrimental effects of prolonged hypothermia and rewarming in the dog. *Anesthesiology* 1980; **52**(3): 224–230.
8. Leonov, Y., Sterz, F., Safar, P. *et al.* Mild cerebral hypothermia during and after cardiac arrest improves neurologic outcome in dogs. *J. Cereb. Blood Flow Metab.* 1990; **10**: 57–70.
9. Sterz, F., Safar, P., Tisherman, S. *et al.* Mild hypothermic cardiopulmonary resuscitation improves outcome after prolonged cardiac arrest in dogs. *Crit. Care Med.* 1991; **19**: 379–389.
10. Weinrauch, V., Safar, P., Tisherman, S., Kuboyama, K. & Radovsky, A. Beneficial effect of mild hypothermia and detrimental effect of deep hypothermia after cardiac arrest in. *Stroke* 1992; **23**: 1454–1462.
11. Safar, P., Xiao, F., Radovsky, A. *et al.* Improved cerebral resuscitation from cardiac arrest in dogs with mild hypothermia plus blood flow. *Stroke* 1996; **27**: 105–113.

12. Kuboyama, K., Safar, P., Radovsky, A., Tisherman, S.A., Stezoski, S.W. & Alexander, H. Delay in cooling negates the beneficial effect of mild resuscitative cerebral hypothermia after cardiac arrest. *Crit. Care Med.* 1993; **21**: 1348–1358.

13. Mild therapeutic hypothermia to improve the neurologic outcome after cardiac arrest. *N. Engl. J. Med.* 2002; **346**(8): 549–556.

14. Bernard, S.A., Gray, T.W., Buist, M.D. *et al.* Treatment of comatose survivors of out-of-hospital cardiac arrest with induced hypothermia. *N. Engl. J. Med.* 2002; **346**(8): 557–563.

15. Nolan, J.P., Deakin, C.D., Soar, J., Bottiger, B.W. & Smith, G. European Resuscitation Council Guidelines for Resuscitation 2005 Section 4. Adult advanced life support. *Resuscitation* 2005; **67** (Suppl 1): S39–S86.

16. Part 4: Advanced Life Support. *Circulation* 2005; **112**(22_Suppl):III-25.

17. Bernard, S.A., Jones, B.M. & Horne, M.K. Clinical trial of induced hypothermia in comatose survivors of out-of-hospital cardiac arrest. *Ann. Emerg. Med.* 1997; **30**(2): 146–153.

18. Hachimi-Idrissi, S., Corne, L., Ebinger, G., Michotte, Y. & Huyghens, L. Mild hypothermia induced by a helmet device: a clinical feasibility study. *Resuscitation* 2001; **51**(3): 275–281.

19. Yanagawa, Y., Ishihara, S., Norio, H. *et al.* Preliminary clinical outcome study of mild resuscitative hypothermia after out-of-hospital cardiopulmonary arrest. *Resuscitation* 1998; 39(1–2):61–66.

20. Zeiner, A., Holzer, M., Sterz, F. *et al.* Mild resuscitative hypothermia to improve neurological outcome after cardiac arrest. A clinical feasibility trial. Hypothermia After Cardiac Arrest (HACA) Study Group. *Stroke* 2000; **31**(1): 86–94.

21. Nolan, J.P., Morley, P.T., Hoek, T.L. & Hickey, R.W. Therapeutic hypothermia after cardiac arrest. An advisory statement by the Advancement Life support Task Force of the International Liaison Committee on Resuscitation. *Resuscitation* 2003; **57**(3): 231–235.

22. Zimmermann, J.M. & Spencer, F.C. The influence of hypothermia on cerebral injury resulting from circulatory occlusion. *Surg. Forum* 1959; **9**: 216.

23. Wolfe, K.B. Effect of hypothermia on cerebral damage resulting from cardiac arrest. *Am. J. Cardiol.* 1960; **6**: 809.

24. Hossmann, K.A. Resuscitation potentials after prolonged global cerebral ischemia in cats. *Crit.l Care Med.* 1988; **16**(10): 964–971.

25. Safar, P. Resuscitation from clinical death: pathophysiologic limits and therapeutic potentials. *Crit. Care Med.* 1988; **16**(10): 923–941.

26. Busto, R., Dietrich, W.D., Globus, M.Y., Valdes, I., Scheinberg, P. & Ginsberg, M.D. Small differences in intraischemic brain temperature critically determine the extent of ischemic neuronal. *J. Cereb. Blood Flow Metab.* 1987; **7**: 729–738.

27. Minamisawa, H., Smith. M.-L. & Siesjö, B.K. The effect of mild hyperthermia and hypothermia on brain damage following 5, 10, and 15 minutes of. *Ann. Neurol.* 1990; **28**: 26–33.

28. Green, E.J., Dietrich, W.D., van Dijk, F. *et al.* Protective effects of brain hypothermia on behavior and histopathology following global cerebral ischemia in rats. *Brain Res.* 1992; **580**(1–2):197–204.

29. Dietrich, W.D., Busto, R., Alonso, O., Globus, M.Y. & Ginsberg, M.D. Intra-ischemic but not post-ischemic brain hypothermia protects chronically following global forebrain. *J. Cereb. Blood Flow Metab.* 1993; **13**: 541–549.

30. Corbett, D., Nurse, S., Colbourne, F. Hypothermic neuroprotection. A global ischemia study using 18- to 20-month-old gerbils. *Stroke* 1997; **28**(11): 2238–2242.

31. Buchan, A. & Pulsinelli, W.A. Hypothermia but not the N-methyl-D-aspartate antagonist, MK-801, attenuates neuronal damage in gerbils subjected to transient global ischemia. *J. Neurosci.* 1990; **10**(1): 311–316.

32. Coimbra, C.G. & Cavalheiro, E.A. Protective effect of short-term post-ischemic hypothermia on the gerbil brain. *Brazilian J. Med. Biol. Res.* 1990; **23**(6–7): 605–611.

33. Chopp, M., Chen, H., Dereski, M.O. & Garcia, J.H. Mild hypothermic intervention after graded ischemic stress in rats. *Stroke* 1991; **22**(1): 37–43.

34. Coimbra, C. & Wieloch, T. Hypothermia ameliorates neuronal survival when induced 2 hours after ischaemia in the rat. *Acta Physiol. Scand.* 1992; **146**: 543–544.

35. Coimbra, C. & Wieloch, T. Moderate hypothermia mitigates neuronal damage in the rat brain when initiated several hours following. *Acta Neuropathol.* 1994; **87**: 325–333.

36. Colbourne, F. & Corbett, D. Delayed and prolonged post-ischemic hypothermia is neuroprotective in the gerbil. *Brain Res.* 1994; **654**(2): 265–272.

37. Colbourne, F. & Corbett, D. Delayed postischemic hypothermia: a six month survival study using behavioral and histological assessments of neuroprotection. *J. Neurosci.* 1995; **15**(11): 7250–7260.

38. Colbourne, F., Auer, R.N. & Sutherland, G.R. Behavioral testing does not exacerbate ischemic CA1 damage in gerbils. *Stroke* 1998; **29**(9): 1967–1970.

39. Kaibara, T., Sutherland, G.R., Colbourne, F. & Tyson, R.L. Hypothermia: depression of tricarboxylic acid cycle flux and evidence for pentose phosphate shunt. *J. Neurosurg.* 1999; **90**: 339–347.

40. Benson, D.W., Williams, G.R., Spencer, F.C. & Yates, A.J. The use of hypothermia after cardiac arrest. *Anesth. Analg.* 1959; **38**: 423–428.

41. Williams, G.R., Spencer, F.C. Clinical use of hypothermia after cardiac arrest. *Ann. Surg.* 1958; **148**: 462–468.

42. Nagao, K., Hayashi, N., Kanmatsuse, K. *et al.* Cardiopulmonary cerebral resuscitation using emergency cardiopulmonary bypass, coronary reperfusion therapy and mild hypothermia in patients with cardiac arrest outside the hospital. *J. Am. Coll. Cardiol.* 2000; **36**(3): 776–783.

43. Felberg, R.A., Krieger, D.W., Chuang, R. *et al.* Hypothermia after cardiac arrest: feasibility and safety of an external cooling protocol. *Circulation* 2001; **104**(15): 1799–1804.

44. Holzer, M., Bernard, S.A., Hachimi-Idrissi, S., Roine, R.O., Sterz, F. & Mullner, M. Hypothermia for neuroprotection after cardiac arrest: systematic review and individual

patient data meta-analysis. *Crit. Care Med.* 2005; **33**(2): 414–418.

45. Bernard, S., Buist, M., Monteiro, O. & Smith, K. Induced hypothermia using large volume, ice-cold intravenous fluid in comatose survivors of out-of-hospital cardiac arrest: a preliminary report. *Resuscitation* 2003; **56**(1): 9–13.

46. Silfvast, T., Tiainen, M., Poutiainen, E. & Roine, R.O. Therapeutic hypothermia after prolonged cardiac arrest due to non-coronary causes. *Resuscitation* 2003; **57**(1): 109–112.

47. Al-Senani, F.M., Graffagnino, C., Grotta, J.C. *et al.* A prospective, multicenter pilot study to evaluate the feasibility and safety of using the CoolGard System and Icy catheter following cardiac arrest. *Resuscitation* 2004; **62**(2): 143–150.

48. Friberg, H., Nielsen, N., Karlsson, T. *et al.* Terapeutisk hypotermi efter hjärtstopp. Kall intravenös vätska, mössa och drakt sänker kroppstemperaturen effektivt. *Läkartidningen* 2004; **101**(30–31):2408–2411.

49. Virkkunen, I., Yli-Hankala, A. & Silfvast, T. Induction of therapeutic hypothermia after cardiac arrest in prehospital patients using ice-cold Ringer's solution: a pilot study. *Resuscitation* 2004; **62**(3): 299–302.

50. Desmond, J. & Megahed, M. Is the central venous pressure reading equally reliable if the central line is inserted via the femoral vein. *Emerg. Med. J.* 2003; **20**(5): 467–469.

51. Henker, R.A., Brown, S.D. & Marion, D.W. Comparison of brain temperature with bladder and rectal temperatures in adults with severe head injury. *Neurosurgery* 1998; **42**: 1071–1075.

52. Crowder, C.M., Tempelhoff, R., Theard, M.A., Cheng, M.A., Todorov, A., Dacey, R.G., Jr. Jugular bulb temperature: comparison with brain surface and core temperatures in neurosurgical patients during mild hypothermia. *J. Neurosurg.* 1996; **85**(1): 98–103.

53. Theard, M.A., Tempelhoff, R., Crowder, C.M., Cheng, M.A., Todorov, A., Dacey, R.G.J. Convection versus conduction cooling for induction of mild hypothermia during neurovascular procedures in adults. *J. Neurosurg. Anesthesiol.* 1997; **9**(3): 250–255.

54. Mayer, S.A., Kowalski, R.G., Presciutti, M. *et al.* Clinical trial of a novel surface cooling system for fever control in neurocritical care patients. *Crit. Care Med.* 2004; **32**(12): 2508–2515.

55. Plattner, O., Kurz, A., Sessler, D.I. *et al.* Efficacy of intraoperative cooling methods. *Anesthesiology* 1997; **87**(5): 1089–1095.

56. Wang, H., Olivero, W., Lanzino, G. *et al.* Rapid and selective cerebral hypothermia achieved using a cooling helmet. *J. Neurosurg.* 2004; **100**(2): 272–277.

57. Tooley, J.R., Eagle, R.C., Satas, S., & Thoresen, M. Significant head cooling can be achieved while maintaining normothermia in the newborn piglet. *Arch. Dis. Child Fetal Neonatal. Ed.* 2005; **90**(3): F262–F266.

58. Gluckman, P.D., Wyatt, J.S., Azzopardi, D. *et al.* Selective head cooling with mild systemic hypothermia after neonatal encephalopathy: multicentre randomised trial. *Lancet* 2005; **365**(9460): 663–670.

59. Rajek, A., Greif, R., Sessler, D.I., Baumgardner, J., Laciny, S. & Bastanmehr, H. Core cooling by central venous infusion of ice-cold (4 degrees C and 20 degrees C) fluid: isolation of core and peripheral thermal compartments. *Anesthesiology* 2000; **93**(3): 629–637.

60. Frank, S.M., Raja, S.N., Bulcao, C. & Goldstein, D.S. Age-related thermoregulatory differences during core cooling in humans. *Am. J. Physiol. Regul. Integr. Comp. Physiol.* 2000; **279**(1): R349–R354.

61. Kliegel, A., Losert, H., Sterz, F. *et al.* Cold simple intravenous infusions preceding special endovascular cooling for faster induction of mild hypothermia after cardiac arrest – a feasibility study. *Resuscitation* 2005; **64**(3): 347–351.

62. Laurent, I., Monchi, M., Chiche, J.D. *et al.* Reversible myocardial dysfunction in survivors of out-of-hospital cardiac arrest. *J. Am. Coll. Cardiol.* 2002; **40**(12): 2110–2116.

63. Kim, F., Olsufka, M., Carlbom, D. *et al.* Pilot study of rapid infusion of 2 L of 4 degrees C normal saline for induction of mild hypothermia in hospitalized, comatose survivors of out-of-hospital cardiac arrest. *Circulation* 2005; **112**(5): 715–719.

64. Nordmark, J. & Rubertsson, S. Induction of mild hypothermia with infusion of cold (4 degrees C) fluid during ongoing experimental CPR. *Resuscitation* 2005; **66**(3): 357–365.

65. Boddicker, K.A., Zhang, Y., Zimmerman, M.B., Davies, L.R. & Kerber, R.E. Hypothermia improves defibrillation success and resuscitation outcomes from ventricular fibrillation. *Circulation* 2005; **111**(24): 3195–3201.

66. Vanden Hoek, T.L., Kasza, K.E., Beiser, D.G. *et al.* Induced hypothermia by central venous infusion: saline ice slurry versus chilled saline. *Crit. Care Med.* 2004; **32**(9 Suppl.): S425–S431.

67. Diringer, M.N. Treatment of fever in the neurologic intensive care unit with a catheter-based heat exchange system. *Crit. Care Med.* 2004; **32**(2): 559–564.

68. Dixon, S.R., Whitbourn, R.J., Dae, M.W. *et al.* Induction of mild systemic hypothermia with endovascular cooling during primary percutaneous coronary intervention for acute myocardial infarction. *J. Am. Coll. Cardiol.* 2002; **40**(11): 1928–1934.

69. Georgiadis, D., Schwarz, S., Kollmar, R. & Schwab, S. Endovascular cooling for moderate hypothermia in patients with acute stroke: first results of a novel approach. *Stroke* 2001; **32**(11): 2550–2553.

70. Steinberg, G.K., Ogilvy, C.S., Shuer, L.M. *et al.* Comparison of endovascular and surface cooling during unruptured cerebral aneurysm repair. *Neurosurgery* 2004; **55**(2): 307–314.

71. Holzer, M., Behringer, W., Janata, A. *et al.* Extracorporeal venovenous cooling for induction of mild hypothermia in human-sized swine. *Crit. Care Med.* 2005; **33**(6): 1346–1350.

72. Piepgras, A., Roth, H., Schurer, L. *et al.* Rapid active internal core cooling for induction of moderate hypothermia in head injury by use of an extracorporeal heat exchanger. *Neurosurgery* 1998; **42**(2): 311–317.

73. Zweifler, R.M., Voorhees, M.E., Mahmood, M.A. & Parnell, M. Magnesium sulfate increases the rate of hypothermia via surface cooling and improves comfort. *Stroke* 2004; **35**(10): 2331–2334.

74. Wadhwa, A., Sengupta, P., Durrani, J. *et al*. Magnesium sulphate only slightly reduces the shivering threshold in humans. *Br. J. Anaesth*. 2005; **94**(6): 756–762.

75. Katz, L.M., Young, A., Frank, J.E., Wang, Y. & Park, K. Neurotensin-induced hypothermia improves neurologic outcome after hypoxic–ischemia. *Crit. Care Med*. 2004; **32**(3): 806–810.

76. Hirschl, R.B., Croce, M., Gore, D. *et al*. Prospective, randomized, controlled pilot study of partial liquid ventilation in adult acute respiratory distress syndrome. *Am. J. Respir. Crit. Care Med*. 2002; **165**(6): 781–787.

77. Hong, S.B., Koh, Y., Shim, T.S. *et al*. Physiologic characteristics of cold perfluorocarbon-induced hypothermia during partial liquid ventilation in normal rabbits. *Anesth. Analg*. 2002; **94**(1): 157–162, table.

78. Xiao, F., Safar, P. & Alexander, H. Peritoneal cooling for mild cerebral hypothermia after cardiac arrest in dogs. *Resuscitation* 1995; **30**(1): 51–59.

79. Mori, K., Saito, J., Kurata, Y. *et al*. Rapid development of brain hypothermia using femoral-carotid bypass. *Acad. Emerg. Med*. 2001; **8**(4): 303–308.

80. Nakamura, T., Miyamoto, O., Sumitani, K., Negi, T., Itano, T. & Nagao, S. Do rapid systemic changes of brain temperature have an influence on the brain? *Acta Neurochir. (Wien)* 2003; **145**(4): 301–307.

81. Bigelow, W.G., Callaghan, J.C. & Hopps, J.A. General hypothermia for experimental intracardiac surgery. *Ann. Surg*. 1950; **132**: 531–537.

82. Rosomoff, H.L. Protective effects of hypothermia against pathologic processes of the nervous system. *Ann. N Y Acad. Sci*. 1959; **80**: 475–486.

83. Hamby, W.B. Intracranial surgery for aneurysm: Effect of hypothermia upon survival. *J. Neurosurg*. 1963; **20**: 41–4510.

84. Polderman, K.H. Application of therapeutic hypothermia in the intensive care unit: Opportunities and pitfalls of a promising. *Intens. Care Med*. 2004; **30**: 757–769.

85. Brain Resuscitation, C.T., I. Randomized clinical study of thiopental loading in comatose survivors of cardiac arrest. *N. Engl. J. Med*. 1986; **314**: 397–403.

86. Brain Resuscitation Clinical Trial II Study Group. A randomized clinical study of a calcium-entry blocker (lidoflazine) in the treatment. *N. Engl. J. Med*. 1991; **324**: 1225–1231.

87. Auer, R.N. Non-pharmacologic (physiologic) neuroprotection in the treatment of brain ischemia. *Ann. N Y Acad. Sci*. 2001; **939**: 271–282.

88. Corbett, D. & Nurse, S. The problem of assessing effective neuroprotection in experimental cerebral ischemia. *Prog. Neurobiol*. 1998; **54**: 531–548.

89. Siesjo, B.K., Bengtsson, F., Grampp, W. & Theander, S. Calcium, excitotoxins, and neuronal death in brain. *Ann. NY Acad. Sci*. 1989; **568**: 234–251.

90. Takata, K., Takeda, Y. & Morita, K. Effects of hypothermia for a short period on histological outcome and extracellular glutamate concentration. *Crit. Care Med*. 2005; **33**: 1340–1345.

91. Small, D.L., Morley, P. & Buchan, A.M. Biology of ischemic cerebral cell death. *Prog. Cardiovasc. Dis*. 1999; **42**: 185–207.

92. Milde, L.N. Clinical use of mild hypothermia for brain protection: a dream revisited. *J. Neurosurg. Anesthesiol*. 1992; **4**: 211–215.

93. Povlishock, J.T., Buki, A., Koiziumi, H., Stone, J. & Okonkwo, D.O. Initiating mechanisms involved in the pathobiology of traumatically induced axonal injury and. *Acta Neurochir*. Suppl 1999; **73**: 15–20.

94. Xu, L., Yenari, M.A., Steinberg, G.K. & Giffard, R.G. Mild hypothermia reduces apoptosis of mouse neurons in vitro early in the cascade. *J. Cereb. Blood Flow Metab*. 2002; **22**: 21–28.

95. Ning, X.H., Chen, S.H., Xu, C.S. *et al*. Hypothermic protection of the ischemic heart via alterations in apoptotic pathways as assessed by gene. *J. Appl. Physiol*. 2002; **92**: 2200–2207.

96. Liou, A.K., Clark, R.S., Henshall, D.C., Yin, X.M. & Chen, J. To die or not to die for neurons in ischemia, traumatic brain injury and epilepsy: a review on the stress-. *Prog. Neurobiol*. 2003; **69**: 103–142.

97. Globus, M.Y., Alonso, O., Dietrich, W.D., Busto, R. & Ginsberg, M.D. Glutamate release and free radical production following brain injury: effects of post-traumatic hypothermia. *J Neurochem* 1995; **65**: 1704–1711.

98. Busto, R., Globus, M.Y., Dietrich, W.D., Martinez, E., Valdés, I. & Ginsberg, M.D. Effect of mild hypothermia on ischemia-induced release of neurotransmitters and free fatty acids in rat. *Stroke* 1989; **20**: 904–910.

99. Hickey, R.W., Ferimer, H., Alexander, H.L. *et al*. Delayed, spontaneous hypothermia reduces neuronal damage after asphyxial cardiac arrest in rats. *Crit. Care Med*. 2000; **28**: 3511–3516.

100. Colbourne, F., Li, H. & Buchan, A.M. Indefatigable CA1 sector neuroprotection with mild hypothermia induced 6 hours after severe forebrain. *J. Cereb. Blood Flow Metab*. 1999; **19**: 742–749.

101. Leonov, Y., Sterz, F., Safar, P. & Radovsky, A. Moderate hypothermia after cardiac arrest of 17 minutes in dogs: effect on cerebral and cardiac outcome: A. *Stroke* 1990; **21**: 1600–1606.

102. Kollmar, R., Schabitz, W.R., Heiland, S. *et al*. Neuroprotective effect of delayed moderate hypothermia after focal cerebral ischemia: an MRI study. *Stroke* 2002; **33**: 1899–1904.

103. Gisvold, S.E., Safar, P., Rao, G., Moossy, J., Kelsey, S. & Alexander, H. Multifaceted therapy after global brain ischemia in monkeys. *Stroke* 1984; **15**: 803–812.

104. Adachi, M., Sohma, O., Tsuneishi, S., Takada, S. & Nakamura, H. Combination effect of systemic hypothermia and caspase inhibitor administration against hypoxic-ischemic. *Pediatr. Res*. 2001; **50**: 590–595.

105. Dietrich, W.D., Busto, R., Globus, M.Y. & Ginsberg, M.D. Brain damage and temperature: cellular and molecular mechanisms. *Adv. Neurol*. 1996; **71**: 177–194.

106. Schmidt, O.I., Heyde, C.E., Ertel, W. & Stahel, P.F. Closed head injury – an inflammatory disease? *Brain Res. Rev*. 2005; **48**: 388–399.

107. Patel, H.C., Boutin, H. & Allan, S.M. Interleukin-1 in the brain: mechanisms of action in acute neurodegeneration. *Ann. NY Acad. Sci.* 2003; **992**: 39–47.

108. Aibiki, M., Maekawa, S., Ogura, S., Kinoshita, Y., Kawai, N. & Yokono, S. Effect of moderate hypothermia on systemic and internal jugular plasma IL-6 levels after traumatic brain. *J. Neurotrauma* 1999; **16**: 225–232.

109. Dietrich, W.D., Chatzipanteli, K., Vitarbo, E., Wada, K. & Kinoshita, K. The role of inflammatory processes in the pathophysiology and treatment of brain and spinal cord trauma. *Acta Neurochir. Suppl* 2004; **89**: 69–74.

110. Globus, M.Y.T., Busto, R., Lin, B., Schnippering, H. & Ginsberg, M.D. Detection of free radical activity during transient global ischemia and recirculation: effects of intra-. *J. Neurochem.* 1995; **65**: 1250–1256.

111. Dempsey, R.J., Combs, D.J., Maley, M.E., Cowen, D.E., Roy, M.M. & Donaldson, D.L. Moderate hypothermia reduces postischemic edema development and leukotriene production. *Neurosurgery* 1987; **21**: 177–181.

112. Huang, Z.G., Xue, D., Preston, E., Karbalai, H. & Buchan, A.M. Biphasic opening of the blood-brain barrier following transient focal ischemia: effects of hypothermia. *Can. J. Neurol. Sci.* 1999; **26**: 298–304.

113. Chi, O.Z., Liu, X. & Weiss, H.R. Effects of mild hypothermia on blood-brain barrier disruption during isoflurane or pentobarbital anesthesia. *Anesthesiology* 2001; **95**: 933–938.

114. Smith, S.L. & Hall, E.D. Mild pre- and posttraumatic hypothermia attenuates blood-brain barrier damage following controlled. *J. Neurotrauma* 1996; **13**: 1–9.

115. Jurkovich, G.J., Pitt, R.M., Curreri, P.W. & Granger, D.N. hypothermia prevents increased capillary permeability following ischemia-reperfusion injury. *J. Surg. Res.* 1988; **44**: 514–521.

116. Kinoshita, K., Chatzipanteli, K., Alonso, O.F., Howard, M. & Dietrich, W.D. The effect of brain temperature on hemoglobin extravasation after traumatic brain injury. *J. Neurosurg.* 2002; **97**: 945–953.

117. Fischer, S., Renz, D., Wiesnet, M., Schaper, W. & Karliczek, G.F. Hypothermia abolishes hypoxia-induced hyperpermeability in brain microvessel endothelial cells. *Brain Res. Mol. Brain Res.* 1999; **74**: 135–144.

118. Polderman, K.H., Ely, E.W., Badr, A.E. & Girbes, A.R. Induced hypothermia in traumatic brain injury: considering the conflicting results of meta-analyses and. *Intens. Care Med.* 2004; **30**: 1860–1864.

119. Guidelines for the management of severe traumatic brain injury. http://www braintrauma org 2005.

120. Ghajar, J. Traumatic brain injury. *Lancet* 2000; **356**: 923–929.

121. Clifton, G.L., Miller, E.R., Choi, S.C. *et al.* Lack of Effect of Induction of Hypothermia after Acute Brain Injury. *N. Engl. J. Med.* 2001; **344**: 556–563.

122. Ding, D., Moskowitz, S.I., Li, R. *et al.* Acidosis induces necrosis and apoptosis of cultured hippocampal neurons. *Exp. Neurol.* 2000; **162**: 1–12.

123. Natale, J.A. & D'Alecy, L.G. Protection from cerebral ischemia by brain cooling without reduced lactate accumulation in dogs. *Stroke*, 1989; **20**: 770–777.

124. Vaquero, J. & Blei, A.T. Mild hypothermia for acute liver failure: a review of mechanisms of action. *J. Clin. Gastroenterol.* 2005; **39**: S147–S157.

125. Lanier, W.L. Cerebral metabolic rate and hypothermia: their relationship with ischemic neurologic injury. *J. Neurosurg. Anesthesiol* 1995; **7**: 216–221.

126. Schwab, S., Spranger, M., Aschhoff, A., Steiner, T. & Hacke, W. Brain temperature monitoring and modulation in patients with severe MCA infarction. *Neurology* 1997; **48**: 762–767.

127. Childs, C., Vail, A., Protheroe, R., King, A.T. & Dark, P.M. Differences between brain and rectal temperatures during routine critical care of patients with severe. *Anaesthesia* 2005; **60**: 759–765.

128. Hayashi, N., Hirayama, T., Udagawa, A., Daimon, W. & Ohata, M. Systemic management of cerebral edema based on a new concept in severe head injury patients. *Acta Neurochir.* Suppl 1994; **60**: 541–543.

129. Baena, R.C., Busto, R., Dietrich, W.D., Globus, M.Y. & Ginsberg, M.D. Hyperthermia delayed by 24 hours aggravates neuronal damage in rat hippocampus following global. *Neurology* 1997; **48**: 768–773.

130. Kim, Y., Busto, R., Dietrich, W.D., Kraydieh, S. & Ginsberg, M.D. Delayed postischemic hyperthermia in awake rats worsens the histopathological outcome of transient focal. *Stroke* 1996; **27**: 2274–2281.

131. Hickey, R.W., Kochanek, P.M., Ferimer, H., Alexander, H.L., Garman, R.H. & Graham, S.H. Induced hyperthermia exacerbates neurologic neuronal histologic damage after asphyxial cardiac arrest in. *Crit. Care Med.* 2003; **31**: 531–535.

132. Ginsberg, M.D., Sternau, L.L., Globus MYT, Dietrich, W.D. & Busto, R. Therapeutic modulation of brain temperature: relevance to ischemic brain injury. *Cerebrovasc. Brain Metab. Rev.* 1992; **4**: 189–225.

133. Schwarz, S., Hafner, K., Aschoff, A. & Schwab, S. Incidence and prognostic significance of fever following intracerebral hemorrhage. *Neurology* 2000; **54**: 354–361.

134. Azzimondi, G., Bassein, L., Nonino, F. *et al.* Fever in acute stroke worsens prognosis. A prospective study. *Stroke* 1995; **26**: 2040–2043.

135. Castillo, J., Davalos, A., Marrugat, J. & Noya, M. Timing for fever-related brain damage in acute ischemic stroke. *Stroke* 1998; **29**: 2455–2460.

136. Kammersgaard, L.P., Jorgensen, H.S., Rungby, J.A., *et al.* Admission body temperature predicts long-term mortality after acute stroke: the Copenhagen Stroke Study. *Stroke* 2002; **33**: 1759–1762.

137. Coimbra, C., Boris-Moller, F., Drake, M. & Wieloch, T. Diminished neuronal damage in the rat brain by late treatment with the antipyretic drug dipyrone or cooling. *Acta Neuropathol.* 1996; **92**: 447–453.

138. Coimbra, C., Drake, M., Boris-Moller, F. & Wieloch, T. Long-lasting neuroprotective effect of postischemic hypothermia and treatment. *Stroke* 1996; **27**: 1578–1585.

139. Piepgras, A., Elste, V., Frietsch, T., Schmiedek, P., Reith, W. & Schilling, L. Effect of moderate hypothermia on experimental severe subarachnoid hemorrhage, as evaluated by apparent. *Neurosurgery* 2001; **48**: 1128–1135.

140. Bottiger, B.W. & Martin, E. Thrombolytic therapy during cardiopulmonary resuscitation and the role of coagulation activation after. *Curr. Opin. Crit. Care* 2001; **7**: 176–183.

141. Fischer, M., Bottiger, B.W., Popov-Cenic, S. & Hossmann, K.A. Thrombolysis using plasminogen activator and heparin reduces cerebral no-reflow after resuscitation from. *Intens. Care Med.* 1996; **22**: 1214–1223.

142. Darius, H., Yanagisawa, A., Brezinski, M.E., Hock, C.E. & Lefer, A.M. Beneficial effects of tissue-type plasminogen activator in acute myocardial ischemia in cats. *J. Am. Coll. Cardiol.* 1986; **8**: 125–131.

143. Kim, Y.H., Park, J.H., Hong, S.H. & Koh, J.Y. Nonproteolytic neuroprotection by human recombinant tissue plasminogen activator. *Science* 1999; **284**: 647–650.

144. Bottiger, B.W., Bode, C., Kern, S. *et al.* Efficacy and safety of thrombolytic therapy after initially unsuccessful cardiopulmonary resuscitation. *Lancet* 2001; **357**: 1583–1585.

145. Michelson, A.D., MacGregor, H., Barnard, M.R., Kestin, A.S., Rohrer, M.J. & Valeri, C.R. Hypothermia-induced reversible platelet dysfunction. *Thromb. Haemost.* 1994; **71**: 633–640.

146. Watts, D.D., Trask, A., Soeken, K., Perdue, P., Dols, S. & Kaufmann, C. Hypothermic coagulopathy in trauma: effect of varying levels of hypothermia on enzyme speed, platelet. *J. Trauma* 1998; **44**: 846–854.

147. Valeri, C.R., MacGregor, H., Cassidy, G., Tinney, R. & Pompei, F. Effects of temperature on bleeding time and clotting time in normal male and female volunteers. *Crit. Care Med.* 1995; **23**: 698–704.

148. Patt, A., McCroskey, B. & Moore, E. Hypothermia-induced coagulopathies in trauma. *Surg. Clin. North Am.* 1988; **68**: 775–785.

149. Ferrara, A., MacArthur, J.D., Wright, H.K., Modlin, I.M. & McMillen, M.A. Hypothermia and acidosis worsen coagulopathy in the patients requiring massive transfusion. *Am. J. Surg.* 1990; **160**: 515–518.

150. Reed, R.L., Bracey, A.W., Hudson, J.D., Miller, T.A. & Fischer, R.P. Hypothermia and blood coagulation: dissociation between enzyme activity and clotting factor levels. *Circ. Shock.* 1990; **32**: 141–152.

151. Gando, S., Kameue, T., Nanzaki, S. & Nakanishi, Y. Massive fibrin formation with consecutive impairment of fibrinolysis in patients with out-of-hospital. *Thromb. Haemost.* 1997; **77**: 278–282.

152. Leffer, C.W. Prostanoids: Intrinsic modulation of cerebral circulation. *News Physiol. Sci.* 1997; **12**: 72–77.

153. Westcott, J.Y., Murphy, R.C. & Stenmark, K. Eicosanoids in human ventricular cerebrospinal fluid following severe brain injury. *Prostaglandins* 1987; **34**: 877–887.

154. Aibiki, M., Maekawa, S. & Yokono, S. Moderate hypothermia improves imbalances of thromboxane A2 and prostaglandin 12 production after. *Cric. Care Med.* 2000; **28**: 3902–3906.

155. Chen, L., Piao, Y., Zeng, F., Lu, M., Kuang, Y. & Ki, X. Moderate hypothermia therapy for patients with severe head injury. *Chin. J. Traumatol.* 2001; **4**: 164–167.

156. Yuan, H.B., Huang, Y., Zheng, S. & Zuo, Z. Hypothermic preconditioning increases survival of purkinje neurons in rat cerebellar slices after an in vitro. *Anesthesiology* 2004; **100**: 331–337.

157. Yunoki, M., Nishio, S., Ukita, N., Anzivino, M.J. & Lee, K.S. Hypothermic preconditioning induces rapid tolerance to focal ischemic injury in the rat. *Exp. Neurol.* 2003; **181**: 291–300.

158. Strauch, J.T., Lauten, A., Spielvogel, D. *et al.* Mild hypothermia protects the spinal cord from ischemic injury in a chronic porcine model. *Eur. J. Cardiothorac. Surg.* 2004; **25**: 708–715.

159. Oku, K., Kuboyama, K., Safar, P. *et al.* Cerebral and systemic arteriovenous oxygen monitoring after cardiac arrest: inadequate cerebral oxygen. *Resuscitation* 1994; **27**: 141–152.

160. Jordan, K.G. Nonconvulsive status epilepticus in acute brain injury. *J. Clin. Neurophysiol.* 1999; **16**: 332–340.

161. Krumholz, A. Epidemiology and evidence for morbidity of nonconvulsive status epilepticus. *J. Clin. Neurophysiol.* 1999; **16**: 314–322.

162. Vespa, P.M., Nuwer, M.R., Nenov, V. *et al.* Increased incidence and impact of nonconvulsive and convulsive seizures after traumatic brain injury. *J. Neurosurg.* 1999; **91**: 750–760.

163. Towne, A.R., Waterhouse, E.J., Boggs, J.G. *et al.* Prevalence of nonconvulsive status epilepticus in comatose patients. *Neurology* 2000; **54**: 340–345.

164. Dennis, L.J., Claassen, J., Hirsch, L.J., Emerson, R.G., Connolly, E.S. & Mayer, S.A. Nonconvulsive status epilepticus after subarachnoid hemorrhage. *Neurosurgery* 2002; **51**: 1136–1143.

165. Maeda, T., Hashizume, K. & Tanaka, T. Effect of hypothermia on kainic acid-induced limbic seizures: an electroencephalographic and 14C-. *Brain Res.* 1999; **818**: 228–235.

166. Karkar, K.M., Garcia, P.A., Bateman, L.M., Smyth, M.D., Barbaro, N.M. & Berger, M. Focal cooling suppresses spontaneous epileptiform activity without changing the cortical motor threshold. *Epilepsia* 2002; **43**: 932–935.

167. Lundgren, J., Smith, M.L., Blennow, G. & Siesjo, B.K. Hyperthermia aggravates and hypothermia ameliorates epileptic brain damage. *Exp. Brain Res.* 1994; **99**: 43–55.

168. Yager, J.Y., Armstrong, E.A., Jaharus, C., Saucier, D.M. & Wirrell, E.C. Preventing hyperthermia decreases brain damage following neonatal hypoxic-ischemic seizures. *Brain Res.* 2004; **1011**: 48–57.

169. Liu, Z., Gatt, A., Mikati, M. & Holmes, G.L. Effect of temperature on kainic acid-induced seizures. *Brain Res.* 1993; **631**: 51–58.

170. Lundgren, J., Smith, M.L. & Siesjo, B.K. Influence of moderate hypothermia on ischemic brain damage incurred under hyperglycemic conditions. *Exp. Brain Res.* 1991; **84**: 91–101.

171. Schaller, B. & Graf, M.L. & Siesjo, B.K. Influence of moderate hypothermia on ischemic brain damage incurred under hyperglycemic conditions. *Exp. Brain Res.* 1991; **84**: 91–101.

172. Busch, E., Gyngell, M.L., Eis, M., Hoehn-Berlage, M. & Hossmann, K.A. Potassium-induced cortical spreading depressions during focal cerebral ischemia in rats: contribution to. *J. Cereb. Blood Flow Metab.* 1996; **16**: 1090–1099.

173. van den, B.G., Wouters, P., Weekers, F. *et al.* Intensive insulin therapy in the critically ill patients. *N. Engl. J. Med.* 2001; **345**: 1359–1367.

174. Polderman, K.H., Rijnsburger, E.R., Peerdeman, S.M., Girbes ARJ. Induction of hypothermia using large volumes of ice-cold intravenous fluid. *Crit. Care Med.* 2005; **33**: in press.

175. Van Zanten, A.R.H. & Polderman, K.H. Early induction of hypothermia: will sooner be better? *Crit. Care Med.* 2005; **33**: 1449–1452.

176. Polderman, K.H. Keeping a cool head: how to induce and maintain hypothermia. *Crit. Care. Med.* 2004; **32**: 2558–2560.

177. Erecinska, M., Thoresen, M. & Silver, I.A. Effects of hypothermia on energy metabolism in Mammalian central nervous system. *J. Cereb. Blood Flow Metab.* 2003; **23**: 513–530.

178. Hagerdal, M., Harp, J., Nilsson, L. & Siesjo, B.K. The effect of induced hypothermia upon oxygen consumption in the rat brain. *J. Neurochem.* 1975; **24**: 311–316.

179. Thoresen, M. & Whitelaw, A. Cardiovascular changes during mild therapeutic hypothermia and rewarming in infants with hypoxic-. *Pediatrics* 2000; **106**: 92–99.

180. Nessmann, M.E., Busch, H.M. & Gundersen, A.L. Asystolic cardiac arrest in hypothermia. *Wis. Med. J.* 1983; **82**: 19–20.

181. Pozos, R.S. & Danzl, D. Human physiological responses to cold stress and hypothermia. In Pandolf, K.B., Burr, R.E., eds. *Medical Aspects of Harsh Environments*. Washington, DC: Borden Institute, Office of the Surgeon General, US Army Medical Department, 2001: 351–382.

182. Polderman, K.H., Peerdeman, S.M. & Girbes, A.R.J. Hypophosphatemia and hypomagnesemia induced by cooling in patients with severe head injury. *J. Neurosurg.* 2001; **94**: 697–705.

183. Polderman, K.H., Tjong Tjin, J.R., Peerdeman, S.M., Vandertop, W.P. & Girbes, A.R.J. Effects of artificially induced hypothermia on intracranial pressure and outcome in patients with severe. *Intens. Care Med.* 2002; **28**: 1563–1567.

184. Frank, S.M., Beattie, C., Christopherson, R. *et al.* Unintentional hypothermia is associated with postoperative myocardial ischemia. The Perioperative. *Anesthesiology* 1993; **78**: 468–476.

185. Mangano, D.T., Browner, W.S., Hollenberg, M., Li, J. & Tateo, I.M. Association of perioperative myocardial ischemia with cardiac morbidity and mortality in men undergoing. *N. Engl. J. Med.* 1990; **323**: 1781–1788.

186. Frank, S.M., Satitpunwaycha, P., Bruce, S.R., Herscovitch, P. & Goldstein, D.S. Increased myocardial perfusion and sympathoadrenal activation during mild core hypothermia in awake. *Clin. Sci.* 2003; **104**: 503–508.

187. Nabel, E.G., Ganz, P., Gordon, J.B., Alexander, R.W. & Selwyn, A.P. Dilation of normal and constriction of atherosclerotic coronary arteries caused by the cold pressor test. *Circulation* 1988; **77**: 43–52.

188. Hale, S.L.and Kloner, R.A. Myocardial temperature in acute myocardial infarction: protection with mild regional hypothermia. *Am. J. Physiol.* 1997; **273**: H220–H227.

189. Hale, S.L., Dae, M.W. & Kloner, R.A. Hypothermia during reperfusion limits 'no-reflow' injury in a rabbit model of acute myocardial infarction. *Cardiovasc. Res.* 2003; **59**: 715–722.

190. Hale, S.L. & Kloner, R.A. Elevated body temperature during myocardial ischemia/reperfusion exacerbates necrosis and worsens no-. *Coron. Artery Dis.* 2002; **13**: 177–181.

191. Hale, S.L. & Kloner, R.A. Myocardial temperature reduction attenuates necrosis after prolonged ischemia in rabbits. *Cardiovasc. Res.* 1998; **40**: 502–507.

192. Hale, S.L., Dae, M.W. & Kloner, R.A. Marked reduction in no-reflow with late initiation of hypothermia in a rabbit myocardial infarct model. *J. Am. Coll. Cardiol.* 2003; **41**: 381–382.

193. Miki, T., Liu, G.S., Cohen, M.V. & Downey, J.M. Mild hypothermia reduces infarct size in the beating rabbit heart: a practical intervention for acute. *Basic Res Cardiol.* 1998; **93**: 372–383.

194. Hale, S.L., Dave, R.H. & Kloner, R.A. Regional hypothermia reduces myocardial necrosis even when instituted after the onset of ischemia. *Basic Res Cardiol.* 1997; **92**: 351–357.

195. Dae, M.W., Gao, D.W., Sessler, D.I., Chair, K. & Stillson, C.A. Effect of endovascular cooling on myocardial temperature, infarct size, and cardiac output in human-sized. *Am. J. Physiol. Heart Circ Physiol.* 2002; **282**: H1584–H1591.

196. Kandzari, D.E., Chu, A., Brodie, B.R., Stuckey, T.A., Hermiller, J.B., Vetrovec GW *et al.* Feasibility of endovascular cooling as an adjunct to primary percutaneous coronary intervention (results of. *Am. J. Cardiol.* 2004; **93**: 636–639.

197. Dixon, S.R., Griffin, J.J., Rizik, D. *et al.* Mild hypothermia during primary percutaneous coronary intervention for acute myocardial infarction: a. *Am. J. Cardiol.* 2005; in press.

198. McIntosh, T.K., V, Yamakami, I. & Faden, A.I. Magnesium protects against neurological deficit after brain injury. *Brain Res.* 1989; **482**: 252–260.

199. Vink, R. Decline in intracellular free $Mg2+$ is associated with irreversible tissue injury after brain trauma. *J. Biol. Chem.* 1988; **263**: 757–761.

200. Vink, R. & Cernak, I. Regulation of intracellular free magnesium in central nervous system injury. *Front Biosc.* 2000; **5**: D656–D665.

201. Polderman, K.H., Zanten, A.V. & Girbes, A.R.J. The importance of magnesium in critically ill patients: a role in mitigating neurological injury and in the. *Intens. Care Med.* 2003; **29**: 1202–1203.

202. Garcia, L.A., Dejong, S.C., Martin, S.M., Smith, R.S., Buettner, G.R. & Kerber, R.E. Magnesium reduces free radicals in an vivo coronary occlusion-reperfusion model. *J. Am. Coll. Cardiol.* 1998; **32**: 536–539.

203. Zhang, Y., Davies, L.R., Martin, S.M., Bawaney, I.M., Buettner, G.R. & Kerber, R.E. Magnesium reduces free radical concentration and preserves left ventricular function after direct current. *Resuscitation* 2003; **56**: 199–206.

204. Weisinger, J.R. & Bellorín-Font, E. Magnesium and phosphorus. *Lancet* 1998; **352**: 391–396.

205. Feliciano, L. & Mass, H.J. Intravenous magnesium sulphate and reperfused myocardium: preservation of function and reduction of. *Magnes. Res.* 1996; **9**: 109–118.

206. Soliman, H.M., Mercan, D., Lobo, S.S., Melot, C. & Vincent, J.L. Development of ionized hypomagnesemia is associated with higher mortality rates. *Crit. Care Med.* 2003; **31**: 1082–1087.

207. Chernow, B., Bamberger, S., Stoiko, M. *et al.* Hypomagnesemia in patients in postoperative intensive care. *Chest* 1989; **95**: 391–397.

208. Abraham, A.S., Rosenman, D., Meshulam, Z., Zion, M. & Eylath, U. Serum, lymphocyte and erythrocyte potassium, magnesium and calcium concentrations and their relation. *Am. J. Med.* 1986; **81**: 983–988.

209. Woods, K.L., Fletcher, S. & Roffe, C. Intravenous magnesium sulphate in suspected acute myocardial infarction: results of the second Leichester. *Lancet* 1992; **339**: 1553–1558.

210. Fisher, J., Magid, N., Kallman, C. *et al.* Respiratory illness and hypophosphatemia. *Chest* 1983; **83**: 504–508.

211. Gravelyn, T.R., Brophy, N., Siegert, C. & Peters-Golden, M. Hypophosphatemia-associated respiratory muscle weakness in a general inpatient population. *Am. J. Med.* 1988; **84**: 870–876.

212. Finney, S.J., Zekveld, C., Elia, A. & Evans, T.W. Glucose control and mortality in critically ill patients. *J. Am. Med. Assoc.* 2003; **290**: 2041–2047.

213. Bacher, A. Effects of body temperature on blood gases. *Intens. Care Med.* 2005; **31**: 24–27.

214. Shiozaki, T., Hayakata, T., Taneda, M. *et al.* A multicenter prospective randomized controlled trial of the efficacy of mild hypothermia for severely head. *J. Neurosurg.* 2001; **94**: 50–54.

215. Schwab, S., Georgiadis, D., Berrouschot, J., Schellinger, P.D., Graffagnino, C. & Mayer, S.A. Feasibility and safety of moderate hypothermia after massive hemispheric infarction. *Stroke* 2001; **32**: 2033–2035.

216. Marion, D.W., Penrod, L.E., Kelsey, S.F. *et al.* Treatment of traumatic brain injury with moderate hypothermia. *N. Engl. J. Med.* 1997; **336**: 540–546.

217. de Jonge, E., Schultz, M.J., Spanjaard, L. *et al.* Effects of selective decontamination of digestive tract on mortality and acquisition of resistant bacteria in. *Lancet* 2003; **362**: 1011–1016.

218. Suehiro, E., Fujisawa, H., Akimura, T. *et al.* Increased matrix metalloproteinase-9 in blood in association with activation of interleukin-6 after traumatic. *J. Neurotrauma* 2004; **21**: 1706–1711.

219. Kurz, A., Sessler, D.I. & Lenhardt, R., and the Study of Wound Infection and Temperature Group. Perioperative normothermia to reduce the incidence of surgical-wound infection and shorten hospitalization. *N. Engl. J. Med.* 1996; **334**: 1209–1215.

220. Sessler, D.I. Complications and treatment of mild hypothermia. *Anesthesiology* 2001; **95**: 531–543.

221. Matsukawa, T., Sessler, D.I., Sessler, A.M. *et al.* Heat flow and distribution during induction of general anesthesia. *Anesthesiology* 1995; **82**: 662–673.

222. Weaver, W.D., Cobb, L.A., Hallstrom, A.P., Fahrenbruch, C., Copass, M.K. & Ray, R. Factors influencing survival after out-of-hospital cardiac arrest. *J. Am. Coll. Cardiol.* 1986; **7**(4): 752–757.

223. Roine, R.O. *Neurological Outcome of Out-of-hospital Cardiac Arrest.* Helsinki: Yliopistopaino, 1993.

224. Booth, C.M., Boone, R.H., Tomlinson, G. & Detsky, A.S. Is this patient dead, vegetative, or severely neurologically impaired? Assessing outcome for comatose survivors of cardiac arrest. *J. Am. Med. Assoc.* 2004; **291**(7): 870–879.

225. Wijdicks, E.F., Parisi, J.E. & Sharbrough, F.W. Prognostic value of myoclonus status in comatose survivors of cardiac arrest. *Ann. Neurol.* 1994; **35**(2): 239–243.

226. Morris, H.R., Howard, R.S. & Brown, P. Early myoclonic status and outcome after cardiorespiratory arrest. *J. Neurol. Neurosurg. Psychiatry* 1998; **64**(2): 267–268.

227. Stelzl, T., von Bose, M.J., Hogl, B., Fuchs, H.H. & Flugel, K.A. A comparison of the prognostic value of neuron-specific enolase serum levels and somatosensory evoked potentials in 13 reanimated patients. *Eur. J. Emerg. Med.* 1995; **2**(1): 24–27.

228. Martens, P. Serum neuron-specific enolase as a prognostic marker for irreversible brain damage in comatose cardiac arrest survivors. *Acad. Emerg. Med.* 1996; **3**(2): 126–131.

229. Fogel, W., Krieger, D., Veith, M. *et al.* Serum neuron-specific enolase as early predictor of outcome after cardiac arrest. *Crit. Care Med.* 1997; **25**(7): 1133–1138.

230. Martens, P., Raabe, A. & Johnsson, P. Serum S-100 and neuron-specific enolase for prediction of regaining consciousness after global cerebral ischemia. *Stroke* 1998; **29**(11): 2363–2366.

231. Schoerkhuber, W., Kittler, H., Sterz, F. *et al.* Time course of serum neuron-specific enolase. A predictor of neurological outcome in patients resuscitated from cardiac arrest. *Stroke* 1999; **30**(8): 1598–1603.

232. Rosen, H., Sunnerhagen, K.S., Herlitz, J., Blomstrand, C. & Rosengren, L. Serum levels of the brain-derived proteins S-100 and NSE predict long-term outcome after cardiac arrest. *Resuscitation* 2001; **49**(2): 183–191.

233. Meynaar, I.A., Oudemans-van Straaten, H.M., van der Wetering, J. *et al.* Serum neuron-specific enolase predicts outcome in post-anoxic coma: a prospective cohort study. *Intens. Care Med.* 2003; **29**(2): 189–195.

234. Rosen, H., Rosengren, L., Herlitz, J. & Blomstrand, C. Increased serum levels of the S-100 protein are associated with hypoxic brain damage after cardiac arrest. *Stroke* 1998; **29**(2): 473–477.

235. Bottiger, B.W., Mobes, S., Glatzer, R. *et al.* Astroglial protein S-100 is an early and sensitive marker of hypoxic brain

damage and outcome after cardiac arrest in humans. *Circulation* 2001; **103**(22): 2694–2698.

236. Mussack, T., Biberthaler, P., Kanz, K.G. *et al.* Serum S-100B and interleukin-8 as predictive markers for comparative neurologic outcome analysis of patients after cardiac arrest and severe traumatic brain injury. *Crit. Care Med.* 2002; **30**(12): 2669–2674.

237. Hachimi-Idrissi, S., Van der Auwera M., Schiettecatte, J., Ebinger, G., Michotte, Y. & Huyghens, L. S-100 protein as early predictor of regaining consciousness after out of hospital cardiac arrest. *Resuscitation* 2002; **53**(3): 251–257.

238. Tiainen, M., Roine, R.O., Pettila, V. & Takkunen, O. Serum neuron-specific enolase and S-100B protein in cardiac arrest patients treated with hypothermia. *Stroke* 2003; **34**(12): 2881–2886.

239. Hachimi-Idrissi, S., Zizi, M., Nguyen, D.N. *et al.* The evolution of serum astroglial S-100 beta protein in patients with cardiac arrest treated with mild hypothermia. *Resuscitation* 2005; **64**(2): 187–192.

240. Wagner, S., Nagel, S., Kluge, B. *et al.* Topographically graded postischemic presence of metalloproteinases is inhibited by hypothermia. *Brain Res.* 2003; **984**(1–2): 63–75.

241. Preston, E. & Webster, J. A two-hour window for hypothermic modulation of early events that impact delayed opening of the rat blood-brain barrier after ischemia. *Acta Neuropathol.* (Berl.) 2004; **108**(5): 406–412.

242. Zandbergen, E.G., de Haan, R.J., Stoutenbeek, C.P., Koelman, J.H. & Hijdra, A. Systematic review of early prediction of poor outcome in anoxic-ischaemic coma. *Lancet* 1998; **352**(9143): 1808–1812.

243. Robinson, L.R., Micklesen, P.J., Tirschwell, D.L. & Lew, H.L. Predictive value of somatosensory evoked potentials for awakening from coma. *Crit. Care Med.* 2003; **31**(3): 960–967.

244. Gendo, A., Kramer, L., Hafner, M. *et al.* Time-dependency of sensory evoked potentials in comatose cardiac arrest survivors. *Intens. Care Med.* 2001; **27**(8): 1305–1311.

245. Tiainen, M., Kovala, T.T., Takkunen, O.S. & Roine, R.O. Somatosensory and brainstem auditory evoked potentials in cardiac arrest patients treated with hypothermia. *Crit. Care Med.* 2005; **33**(8): 1736–1740.

246. Madl, C., Grimm, G., Kramer, L. *et al.* Early prediction of individual outcome after cardiopulmonary resuscitation. *Lancet* 1993; **341**(8849): 855–858.

247. Madl, C., Kramer, L., Domanovits, H. *et al.* Improved outcome prediction in unconscious cardiac arrest survivors with sensory evoked potentials compared with clinical assessment. *Crit. Care Med.* 2000; **28**(3): 721–726.

248. Young, G.B. The EEG in coma. *J. Clin. Neurophysiol.* 2000; **17**(5): 473–485.

249. Kochs, E. Electrophysiological monitoring and mild hypothermia. *J. Neurosurg. Anesthesiol.* 1995; **7**(3): 222–228.

250. Roine, R.O., Raininko, R., Erkinjuntti, T., Ylikoski, A. & Kaste, M. Magnetic resonance imaging findings associated with cardiac arrest. *Stroke* 1993; **24**(7): 1005–1014.

251. Arbelaez, A., Castillo, M. & Mukherji, S.K. Diffusion-weighted MR imaging of global cerebral anoxia. *Am. J. Neuroradiol.* 1999; **20**(6): 999–1007.

252. Wijdicks, E.F., Campeau, N.G. & Miller, G.M. MR imaging in comatose survivors of cardiac resuscitation. *Am. J. Neuroradiol.* 2001; **22**(8): 1561–1565.

253. Bellamy, R., Safar, P., Tisherman, S.A. *et al.* Suspended animation for delayed resuscitation. [Review] [137 refs]. *Crit. Care Med.* 1996; **24**(2 Suppl): S24–S47.

254. Safar, P., Tisherman, S.A., Behringer, W. *et al.* Suspended animation for delayed resuscitation from prolonged cardiac arrest that is unresuscitable by standard cardiopulmonary–cerebral resuscitation [In Process Citation]. *Crit. Care Med.* 2000; **28**(11 Suppl): N214–N218.

255. Tisherman, S.A. Suspended animation for resuscitation from exsanguinating hemorrhage. *Crit. Care Med.* 2004; **32**(2 Suppl): S46–S50.

256. Woods, R.J., Prueckner, S., Safar, P. *et al.* Hypothermic aortic arch flush for preservation during exsanguination cardiac arrest of 15 minutes in dogs. *J. Trauma-Injury Infect. Crit. Care* 1999; **47**(6): 1028–1036.

257. Behringer, W., Prueckner, S., Safar, P. *et al.* Rapid induction of mild cerebral hypothermia by cold aortic flush achieves normal recovery in a dog outcome model with 20-minute exsanguination cardiac arrest. *Acad. Emerg. Med.* 2000; **7**(12): 1341–1348.

258. Behringer, W., Prueckner, S., Kentner, R. *et al.* Rapid hypothermic aortic flush can achieve survival without brain damage after 30 minutes cardiac arrest in dogs.[In Process Citation]. *Anesthesiology* 2000; **93**(6): 1491–1499.

259. Behringer, W., Safar, P., Wu, X. *et al.* Survival without brain damage after clinical death of 60–120 mins in dogs using suspended animation by profound hypothermia. *Crit. Care Med.* 2003; **31**(5): 1523–1531.

260. Rhee, P., Talon, E., Eifert, S. *et al.* Induced hypothermia during emergency department thoracotomy: an animal model. *J. Trauma* 2000; **48**(3): 439–447.

261. Alam, H.B., Bowyer, M.W., Koustova, E. *et al.* Learning and memory is preserved after induced asanguineous hyperkalemic hypothermic arrest in a swine model of traumatic exsanguination. *Surgery* 2002; **132**(2): 278–288.

262. Taylor, M.J., Bailes, J.E., Elrifai, A.M. *et al.* A new solution for life without blood. Asanguineous low-flow perfusion of a whole-body perfusate during 3 hours of cardiac arrest and profound hypothermia. *Circulation* 1995; **91**(2): 431–444.

263. Herlitz, J., Bahr, J., Fischer, M., Kuisma, M., Lexow, K. & Thorgeirsson, G. Resuscitation in Europe: a tale of five European regions. *Resuscitation* 1999; **41**(2): 121–131.

264. Nozari, A., Safar, P., Stezoski, S.W. *et al.* Mild hypothermia during prolonged cardiopulmonary cerebral resuscitation increases conscious survival in dogs. *Crit. Care Med.* 2004; **32**(10): 2110–2116.

265. Vanden Hoek, T.L. & Li, C., Shao, Z., Schumacker, P.T. & Becker, L.B. Significant levels of oxidants are generated by

isolated cardiomyocytes during ischemia prior to reperfusion. *J. Mol. Cell. Cardiol.* 1997; **29**(9): 2571–2583.

266. Vanden Hoek, T.L., Shao, Z., Li, C., Zak, R., Schumacker, P.T. & Becker, L.B. Reperfusion injury on cardiac myocytes after simulated ischemia. *Am. J. Physiol.* 1996; **270**(4 Pt 2): H1334–H1341.

267. Vanden Hoek, T.L., Qin, Y., Wojcik, K. *et al.* Reperfusion, not simulated ischemia, initiates intrinsic apoptosis injury in chick cardiomyocytes. *Am. J. Physiol. Heart Circ. Physiol.* 2003; **284**(1): H141–H150.

268. Vanden Hoek, T.L., Shao, Z., Li, S.Q., Idris, A.H. & Becker, L.B. Do we reperfuse or cool down first to resuscitate ischemic tissue? *Circulation* 2000; **102**[18 (Suppl.)]: 570.

269. Abella, B.S., Zhao, D., Alvarado, J., Hamann, K., Vanden Hoek, T.L. & Becker, L.B. Intra-arrest cooling improves outcomes in a murine cardiac arrest model. *Circulation* 2004; **109**(22): 2786–2791.

270. Janata, A., Holzer, M., Bayegan, K. *et al.* Aortic flush for rapid induction of cerebral hypothremia during normovolemic cardiac arrest in swine. *Resuscitation* 2004; **62**(3): 342.

271. Janata, A., Weihs, W., Bayegan, K. *et al.* Suspended animation after prolonged normovolemic cardiac arrest in swine. *Circulation* 2005; **112**: U378.

50

Postresuscitation neurologic prognostication and declaration of brain death

Romergryko G. Geocadin, Daniel F. Hanley, Scott M. Eleff

Department of Neurology, Neurosurgery and Anesthesiology-Critical Care Medicine, Johns Hopkins University School of Medicine, Baltimore, MD and Department of Anesthesiology, University of Illinois, Chicago, IL, USA

Introduction

The ability to prognosticate or predict accurately the eventual neurologic outcome following successful restoration of native cardiac function has profound clinical, ethical, and financial consequences. Although this chapter focuses on the overall prognosis of the patient who has successfully returned to spontaneous circulation after cardiac arrest, most of the recommendations based on existing data focus on poor or unfavorable outcome. Salient points of recent important studies, focused review, meta-analyses of the existing literature on this topic are included. This chapter provides a sequential approach to evaluating the neurologic status of patients resuscitated from cardiac arrest leading to the ability to predict early trends, especially during the first 72 hours postarrest. The key concepts and discussion of neurologic prognostication are based on intra-arrest factors, clinical examination, and laboratory tests such as electroencephalography (EEG), evoked potentials, analysis of cerebrospinal fluid (CSF) brain enzymes, and brain imaging. A detailed description of how to perform bedside neurologic examination and brain death clinical examinations is provided. A more comprehensive review on brain injury after cardiac arrest, including an expanded discussion of prognostication was recently published.[1]

Consideration in prognostication of neurologic outcomes

Study design

Since the last edition of this book, several new studies, structured reviews, and rigorous meta-analyses have been

undertaken specifically to clarify prognostication of neurologic outcome after cardiac arrest. We focus on the quality of study design of data collection, length of follow-up, methods of analysis, and an understanding of the power of the statistical analysis.[1] Despite guidelines for uniform reporting of data and the follow-up period from out-of-hospital cardiac arrest [2] and in-hospital cardiac arrest[3], significant research problems persist, such as considerable variability in outcome and less than 60% compliance to guidelines[4,5]. The use of the Glasgow–Pittsburgh cerebral performance and overall performance categories as outcome measures has received some degree of acceptance, but many studies still vary significantly in their use of other outcome measures. Therefore, a collective definition for poor outcome encompasses any of the following states: death, persistent vegetative state, or a severe neurological disability requiring full nursing care.

The studies on prognostication in comatose patients after cardiac arrest are obviously, biased towards patients who will have a poor outcome. For this reason, most of the observations relating to the neurologic examination of postcardiac arrest victims and the prognostication of outcome for comatose cardiac arrest victims are skewed toward patients with longer arrest times. Moreover, in studies designed to predict poor outcome there is a tendency to provide less than optimal care to patients thought to have a poor prognosis.

Prognostication and extracerebral complications

The cause of death in the majority of patients after resuscitation is largely extracerebral, which is an important consideration in attempting to assess prognostication of outcome. From the Brain Resuscitation Clinical Trial

Cardiac Arrest: The Science and Practice of Resuscitation Medicine. 2nd edn., ed. Norman Paradis, Henry Halperin, Karl Kern, Volker Wenzel, Douglas Chamberlain. Published by Cambridge University Press. © Cambridge University Press, 2007.

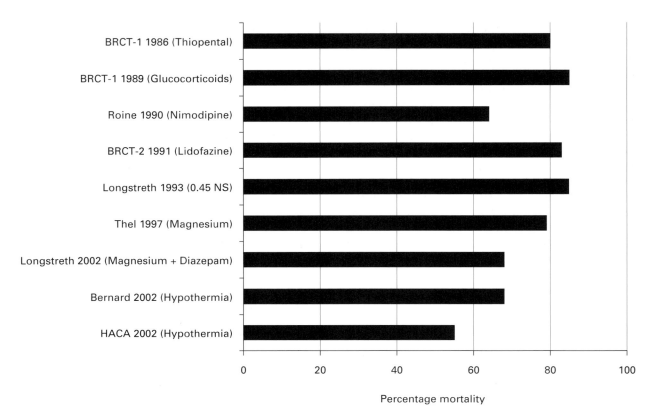

Fig. 50.1. Percentage mortality in the placebo groups of clinical trials for brain injury after cardiac arrest (1986–2002).

(BRCT) 1 study, non-neurologic causes of death accounted for 63.6%, while cerebral causes accounted for 36.4%.[6] A similar proportion was observed in BRCT 2, with extracerebral causes noted in 72.2% of patients and cerebral cause of death in 27.8%.[7] Consequently, a significant number of patients with excellent initial neurologic examination may not have a good outcome, because the patient died of a second cardiac arrest. Management during the postresuscitation period is provided in chapter 47; management of extracerebral or systemic complications in these patients, particularly cardiac injury, is essential for survival and the functional outcome of these patients. We thus examined the placebo arm of controlled human clinical trials over the last three decades. There has been a general overall trend towards a reduction in the percentage mortality of the placebo-treated patients in 8 clinical trials (see Fig. 50.1). With the exception of Roine *et al.* in 1990,[8] who reported a percentage mortality of less than 80%, three of the BRCT from 1986 to 1991[6,7,9] and Longstreth *et al.* in 1993 reported a percentage mortality of 80% or greater. Whereas the BRCT and the Longstreth studies represented a wider spectrum of cardiac arrest severity, the study by Roine *et al.* selected patients with lesser injury by limiting the duration of

cardiac arrest time and resuscitation time.[8] The succeeding trials starting with Thel *et al.* in 1997[10] reported a declining trend, with percentage mortality of those treated with placebo below 80%. An even lower percentage mortality was reported by Longstreth *et al.* in 2002[11] and two recent studies on therapeutic hyothermia.[12,13] Whereas the wide variability in trial design does not allow the precise determination of the factors that lead to the reduction in mortality, two key factors may have changed in the clinical practice during the time these trials were undertaken. First, inclusion of a focused population that will have higher chances of survival after cardiac arrest and thus allow the assessment of functional outcome. Second is the continued improvement in overall standard critical care in patients treated with placebo. As we attempt to define the neurologic injury and its relation to functional outcome, we must also recognize the potential impact of the continued development in critical care therapies provided to these patients.

Prognostication in the era of therapeutic hypothermia

The recent introduction of therapeutic hypothermia,[12,13] which has improved survival and functional outcome, may well alter the current practice of prognostication. Almost all of the data and analysis presented in this chapter were derived from studies conducted in patients before the introduction of therapeutic hypothermia. As the use of therapeutic hypothermia becomes more widespread, factors determining prognostication will need to be redefined. Furthermore, for the first time, a therapy actually shows that brain injury after cardiac arrest can be ameliorated and therefore outcome can be influenced by therapy. In the absence of effective therapies, the detection of irreversible loss of a specific brain function led to prediction of an unfavorable outcome, which often led to the cessation or de-escalation of care. We suggest considering two periods: the early period where the injury can still be ameliorated and effective therapies can be provided, and development of novel markers to assess and perhaps treat patients, and a late period where the significant injury is irreversible and unfavorable outcome almost certain.

The ideal study

As indicated in the first edition, the ideal study should also be prospective and focused on neurologic outcome, both normothermia- and hypothermia-treated patients. To avoid unpredictable biases, all levels of neurologic injury must be included and standardized management is required. The optimal study should have strict intensive care protocols over a long period of time to prevent a model from becoming self-fulfilling. Finally, no study can ever guarantee that the proposed model is definitive in stating that a patient who is not brain-dead will never recover. Therefore, except for the diagnosis of brain death, it is not possible to predict outcome in an individual patient with 100% accuracy. This uncertainty has profound ethical consequences, as well as implications concerning the large financial and personal emotional investment in what, in all likelihood, may be a futile situation. Nonetheless, it is clear that many neurologic findings are highly predictive of outcome and are useful in family counseling and for suggesting ways of assessing the success of therapy.

Prognostication of neurologic outcome

Intracardiac arrest factors

The duration of cardiac arrest as the clinical marker of global ischemia has been correlated with brain injury.[14–17] Several studies have associated some variables relating cardiac arrest and resuscitation to poor outcome, such as increased time[14–15] between collapse and initiation of CPR[14–15] (anoxia time) and the increased duration of CPR. The impact of other characteristics of cardiac arrest (i.e., cardiac rhythm, etiology) and resuscitation (in-hospital and out-of-hospital) are discussed in detail in other chapters of this book.

The BRCT indicated that a cardiac arrest duration of 6 minutes or longer and a resuscitation time to achieve ROSC of 28 minutes or longer predicted poor neurologic recovery[15] whereas shorter cardiac arrest times and resuscitation times, indicating lesser injury were associated with favorable outcome. A similar observation in a European study reported that patients had unfavorable outcome with cardiac arrest time longer than 6 minutes and with resuscitation time longer than 21 minutes.[14]

While most of these variables are associated with poor outcome, the correlations are not sufficient reliably to discriminate patients with poor prognosis from those with a good outcome. The reliability of the CPR as a factor to predict outcome was further placed in doubt after some studies were conducted on the ability of care givers to adhere to resuscitation protocols. In a prospective study of in-hospital CPR quality and compliance with published American Heart Association and international guidelines, it was found that multiple characteristics of CPR were inconsistent and often did not meet published guideline recommendations, even when performed by well-trained hospital staff. These included inadequate chest compression rates, shallow compression depth, and high ventilation rates.[18–19] In an out-of-hospital cardiac arrest resuscitation study in Europe, significant deviations from international CPR guidelines were noted in that chest compressions were not delivered half of the time, and most compressions were too shallow.[20]

Postcardiac arrest factors

Evaluation of the postresuscitation comatose patient
The clinical findings derived from the bedside neurologic evaluation of patients resuscitated from cardiac arrest remain one of the most reliable means of establishing prognosis.[21–22] Therefore, a detailed approach to the bedside neurologic examination is provided below.

Neurologic evaluation is separated into two distinct tasks: first, assessment of the level of consciousness; and second, determination of the integrity of the brain stem and cerebral hemispheres. The overall approach is based on the conventional structure of the neurologic examination which comprises evaluation of mental status, cranial nerve function, and sensorimotor and other reflexes.

Several methods have been developed to standardize the assessment of neurologic function in these patients.

The most widely accepted scale is the Glasgow Coma Scale,[23] which is universally accepted and has been validated for both physicians and nurses. It can be replicated with little interobserver error, performed rapidly, and is easy to learn. This scale is divided into three major components: eye-opening, motor response, and verbal response. Eye-opening is scored as follows: spontaneous to verbal command (3), spontaneous to pain (2), or no opening (1). Motor response is scored as follows: obeys verbal command (6), localizes to pain (5), withdraws to pain (4), flexes to pain (3), extension to pain (2), or no response (1). Verbal response is scored as follows: oriented (5), appropriate words (4), disoriented (3), incomprehensible sounds (2), and no response (1). The addition of the three component scores results in a scale value from 3 to 15. Patients with a GCS score of 3 to 9 have significant impairment of consciousness; 10 to 13 is moderate impairment; and above 13 is mild impairment. Although multiple attempts have been made to define level of consciousness in a stratified manner, there is no uniform agreement on how to describe differences among coma, obtundation, stupor, and such states as delirium or confusion. Significant prognostic value has, however, been attached to the GCS and to the neurologic examination of the brainstem.

A recent method developed to evaluate a comatose patient is the FOUR (Full Outline of UnResponsiveness) score.[24] This consists of four components (eye, motor, brainstem, and respiration), and each component has a maximal score of 4. The Four score provides assessment of critical variables that are important in coma assessment and excludes the verbal response, which has been a major limiting factor in the GCS. Although this is a promising development in coma assessment, the application of this scoring system needs to be established in the postcardiac arrest patient population.

Bedside neurological examination

Level of arousal

To determine the patient's level of arousal, it is necessary to know the patient's best response to specific stimuli. If possible the patient should be informed verbally of the procedure or examination. If noxious stimulation is necessary to get the best response, the least noxious stimulation should be used at the start and the intensity increased until the best response is elicited. Start by calling the patient's name and asking the patient to follow simple commands. If no response is noted, the patient can be tapped or shaken gently, and finally painful pressure such as rubbing the sternum or pinching the trapezius should be applied. Record the specific stimulus that causes a specific response (i.e., eye-opening with voice or extensor posturing of the right side with sternal rub).

If the patient is arousable, he or she should be assessed for ability to follow commands and answer questions. First, have the patient follow simple commands such as "open and close your eyes" or "stick out your tongue", followed by commands involving the extremities, such as "show me two fingers". Next ask questions about orientation: "What's your name? Where are you? What's the date? How did you get here?"

Rapid fluctuation in the level of consciousness, associated with changes in cognition and impaired attention span, should alert the examiner to metabolic dysfunction or even seizures. Serial evaluations must be performed, the trend in level of consciousness is more significant than any specific level of consciousness. Moreover, the findings must be taken in the context of the other significant findings on examination. Intervention must be undertaken to address a rapid or persistent decline in the level of consciousness.

Brainstem evaluation

For the unresponsive patient, the brainstem examination is crucial in assessing the degree of brain injury and the findings are key in prognostication, especially within the first 3 days after cardiac arrest. With the absence of voluntary response in the comatose patient, cranial nerves may be tested by eliciting cranial nerve-based reflexes, such as pupillary light reflex, corneal reflex, grimace, oculovestibular response, caloric response, gag reflex, and cough reflex. By assessing these responses to specified cranial nerves, the pertinent brainstem structures can be evaluated, especially the central portion of the brainstem including the tegmental area, which contains the reticular activating system. An intact reticular activating system is important for neurophysiologic arousal or recovery.

Pupillary response (cranial nerves 2 and 3)

Evaluation of cranial nerves 2 and 3 requires assessment of both responses to light and conjugate eye movements. Reaction of each eye to light is the function of afferent pathways from the retina to the Edinger–Westphal nucleus at the level of the midbrain via the optic nerve. Parasympathetic efferents exit this nucleus via the third nerve. Monocular activation of this reflex with light produces bilateral pupillary constriction. The normal resting pupil size is 4 to 6 mm. Most pupils will constrict to about 2 mm with illumination from a bright flashlight. Normal resting pupillary size is altered by drugs, surgery, and aging. The ability of the pupils to dilate is mediated by sympathetic neurons that travel from the hypothalamus in a longitudinal manner to the cervical cord where they exit and pass rostrally along the carotid vascular system to the eye. Dilation occurs when ambient light is excluded from the patient's retina. The motor aspects of these cranial nerves are assessed with the vestibular system.

Blink reflex (cranial nerves 5 and 7)
The corneal response is a blink reflex when the corneal is touched with a wisp of cotton. This response is activated by sensory afferents of the face that travel via cranial nerve 5 from the face to the trigeminal ganglia and then to the fifth nerve nucleus in the pons. These neurons form synapses with the seventh nerve nucleus in the pons. The seventh nerve nucleus projections innervate the facial muscula-ture, including the orbicularus oculi. Activation of this reflex leads to constriction of the orbicularis oculi and closure of the eye or a blink. In severely obtunded patients, this reflex may be slightly depressed. The most vigorous stimulus is one of direct corneal pressure, which is applied with a clean cotton swab. Gentle pressure on the cornea produces at least a trace constriction of the orbicularis oculi and in many individuals a brisk blink. This reflex is lost with deep general anesthesia but tends to be preserved with moderate sedation. To study the lower facial muscu-lature in a variant of this response, the nasal tickle or grimace reflex is used. This reflex is elicited by either light or deep pressure to the nares and nasal septum area. Pressure here produces a facial grimace often slightly greater on the side of the stimulus. Comparison of the right and left responses allows evaluation of the nasolabial fold and symmetry of lower facial musculature.

Vestibulo-ocular response (cranial nerves 3, 4, 6, and 8)
Cranial nerves 3, 4, 6, and 8 are grouped together, and their evaluation represents oculomotor reflex testing. This reflex involves vestibular afferents that can be activated by either head-turning (doll's eyes) or thermal inputs (caloric response). These stimuli travel to the ponto-medullary junction via cranial nerve 8. Inputs from synapses with the oculomotor system produce coordinated eye movement via brainstem gaze centers, including the parapontine reticular formation and the medial longitudinal fasciculus. These synapses allow coordinated conjugate eye movement. During normal conscious behavior, this system allows sta-bilization of visual fixation with head movement. In an unconsciousness person, volitional eye movements are lost. Such eye movements tend to be rapid in comparison to those evoked by the vestibulo-ocular response. Thus, in the unconsciousness individual, head-turning provokes a slow eye deviation in the direction opposite to head motion. Similarly, cold water irrigation in one ear provokes a slow tonic deviation of eyes in the opposite direction. The pres-ence of both a slow and a fast phase of eye movement after cold water irrigation suggest a conscious state with active visual perception at the cortical level, and is thus associated with behavioral rather than structural etiologies of coma. In a manner similar to the corneal response, sedative drugs will depress this reflex. During low level sedation, however, a vestibulo-ocular response can usually be elicited. If it cannot be elicited, caloric testing, which represents a stronger stimulus to this system, should be used. The caloric test is suppressed by deep general anesthesia. When doll's eyes or caloric testing provokes a response, it is nor-mally the conjugate or equal motion of both eyes in one direction. If individual eyes have either a horizontal or ver-tical asymmetry to their fixation point, damage to an indi-vidual oculomotor nerve should be considered. This is best evaluated by repeating the doll's eye maneuver for both hor-izontal and vertical planes. Each eye should be evaluated individually; if a full range of motion is noted for each eye, the absence of conjugate eye movement is clinically diag-nosed as strabismus rather than as oculomotor palsy.

Gag response (cranial nerves 9 and 10)
The gag response is best tested with both a tongue depres-sor and a cotton swab. While the tongue is depressed, the right and left retropharyngeal areas are stimulated with the cotton swab. This reflex involves the sensory afferents of cranial nerve 9 and a diverse set of motor efferents, includ-ing those of cranial nerves 9 and 10. A normal response includes symmetric elevation of the soft palate and closure of the pharyngeal space from the nasal space. This pha-ryngeal reflex is often lost in individuals who have had pro-longed oral tracheal or nasotracheal intubation. A variant of this reflex is the cough response to deep tracheal suction. Cough reflex involves cranial nerve 10 sensory afferents and abdominal, chest wall, and cranial nerve 10 efferents. The reflex is best produced in individuals with endotracheal intubation, whereby a suction catheter is inserted via this endotracheal route into the carina. Rapid to-and-fro motion produces a gasp and then one to three rapid coughs. A positive response suggests that medullary afferent and efferent centers are intact.

An intact brainstem evaluation suggests the potential for normal arousal. An intact brainstem may be found in comatose patients after cardiac arrest, drug overdose, or closed head injury. An examination demonstrating incom-plete function or asymmetric cranial nerve dysfunction is most often associated with cerebrovascular disease in the vertebrobasilar arterial system or a posterior fossa mass. An alternative explanation for incomplete or asymmetric cranial nerve function is a herniation syndrome secondary to a supratentorial mass. The evaluation of conscious motor behavior is important in cardiac arrest patients because of the high frequency of diffuse cortical injury. Another system that is closely associated with the brainstem is the autonomic system, which may be affected in cardiac arrest. Autonomic manifestations such as an abnormal pattern of breathing, erratic and extreme temperature, arrhythmia and blood pressure lability may be a manifestation of brainstem injury.

Response to pain (motor evaluation)
Conscious behavior requires both an intact reticular activating system and bilateral hemispheric function; therefore, it is important to access hemispheric function as well as brainstem function. The most reproducible assessments of hemispheric functions in unresponsive patients are the motor responses to pain. These responses are elicited individually in each limb, and although they vary with level of consciousness, they should be symmetric. For the unconscious patient, strength cannot be graded objectively so a qualitative description and whether it is reproducible must be provided. The GCS provides a standardized and universal classification system defining five levels of motor response. A conscious individual will obey commands with a defined motor performance. Stuporous or unconsciousness individuals without hemispheric dysfunction will demonstrate purposeful pain avoidance behavior, characterized by rapid attempted withdrawal of the limb from painful stimuli, usually with abducting movements. This is particularly true if painful stimuli are elicited with pinch or deep pressure to the medial aspects of limbs, such as the upper arm triceps area or the adductor region of the thigh, or deep pressure to the medial malleolus at the ankle. A second common behavior is the use of the contralateral limb to remove the noxious stimulus. Deeply comatose individuals do not show this behavior, but rather show simple flexion to painful stimuli. Similarly, individuals with hemispheric lesions may demonstrate brisk and monotonously replicable upper extremity flexion at the shoulder, elbow, wrist, and fingers. When this flexion is asymmetric, a contralateral hemispheric injury or mass is likely. Bihemispheric lesions may demonstrate bilateral flexion. The extension response is present when an injury impairs both cortical and deep basal ganglia and thalamic function. This response is a characteristic extension at the elbow and internal rotation of the forearm with flexion of the fingers. Simultaneous lower extremity extension and adduction are noted. The response represents the unopposed activation of postural extensor muscles by the vestibulospinal system. This response may be asymmetric, suggesting severe cortical and deep hemispheric dysfunction, or bilateral with bilat-

eral hemispheric dysfunction. A final pattern of response to pain is one of no response or minimal flicker of muscles without movement. These findings occur with deep general anesthesia or with bilateral cervical medullary lesions. Taken together, evaluation of the brain stem and the motor response assess the integrity of both sites necessary for conscious behavior, namely, the reticular activating system and the cerebral hemispheres. When the examination suggests that the hemispheres and the reticular activating system are intact, awakening from coma is possible and most likely depends on the underlying disease causing coma. This chapter does not attempt to address the issue of differential diagnosis of coma. With the detailed medical history, laboratory testing, and imaging, a diagnosis is usually possible. Current data provide support that the clinical evaluation of the nervous system and data on the duration of global ischemia are of value in predicting the eventual outcome. Because many cardiac arrests are unwitnessed, the exact duration of ischemia is unknown. For this reason, significant clinical emphasis is placed on the repeated evaluation of the patient at the bedside.

Bedside neurologic examination and prognostication
Numerous studies have reported the importance of specific components of the bedside neurologic examination to functional outcome after in-patient resuscitation from cardiac arrest without therapeutic hypothermia. Studies by Levy and colleagues[25] in 1985 followed by the studies by Rogove and colleagues,[15] and Edgren and colleagues[21] from the Brain Resuscitation Clinical Trials (BRCT) have been largely responsible for defining the key factors in the neurologic examination that are clearly associated with poor functional outcome. Many other studies provide additional support for use of these clinical characteristics in prognostication.[26–30] In 2006, the American Academy of Neurology published an evidence-based review on the predictors of outcome in comatose patients after resuscitation from cardiac arrest.[98] It is important to emphasize that almost all these studies indicate the absence rather than the presence of a specific clinical finding that is best associated with unfavorable outcome after cardiac arrest. This highlights the need for research to provide an early clinical finding that has the ability to determine which patients will have a good recovery postresuscitation.

Of all the clinical findings in the neurologic assessment, a meta-analysis found two clinical findings had 100% specificity at 3 days: absence of pupillary light reflexes (positive likelihood ratio = 10.5 (95% CI 2.1–52.4), and absent motor response to pain (positive likelihood ratio = 16.8 (95% CI 3.4–84.1)).[22] A recent study by Booth and

Table 50.1. Clinical, electrophysiological, and laboratory markers of poor outcome (death or persistent vegetative state, severe disability requiring full nursing care) after cardiac arrest[a]

Based on the current literature, the predictive markers are summarized as follows:

Markers of poor outcome

1. **Clinical markers**

   The absence of pupillary light responses and absence of motor responses to pain in medically stable comatose survivors 3 days after CPR are the most studied and reliable markers.

2. **Electrophysiological markers**

   Bilateral absent cortical responses (N20) on Somatosensory Evoked Potentials recorded > 24 hours is most objective, but expertise and availability limits its widespread use.

   Persisting burst suppression pattern on electroencephalogram recorded > 24 hours after CPR is useful, but less specific than SSEP.

3. **Biochemical markers**

   Serum and cerebrospinal fluid (neuron-specific enolase, S100, creatinine kinase isoenzyme BB) are very useful in prognostication, but variability in cut-off and inability of test in many hospital laboratories limits application.

4. **Neuroimaging markers**

   MR imaging and CT scanning are promising, but data are still insufficient to support or refute use for prognostication.

5. **Multimodality markers**

   The combination of several prognostic markers, such as clinical, electrophysiologic, and biochemical markers, promises to improve the ability predict both poor and good outcome. More studies are needed to validate the used of multimodality markers.

[a] *Prognostic markers may not be reliable in patients receiving sedatives or neuromuscular blocking agents, in patients with severe metabolic derangement, or medically unstable or cardiogenic shock. These prognostic markers were not studied in patients who received therapeutic hypothermia.*

colleagues suggested that similar clinical findings as early as 24 hours can adequately predict poor neurologic outcome: absent response to pain (positive likelihood ratio 4.9 (95% CI 1.6–13.0)), absent pupillary light reflexes (positive likelihood ratio = 10.2 (95% CI 1.8–48.6)), and absent corneal reflexes (positive likelihood ratio = 12.9 (95% CI 2.0–68.7)). With the findings, Booth *et al.* suggest that cessation of life-sustaining therapies may be justifiable. While the 24-hour period may be encouraging in some cases, several studies have reported 18%–36% false positive rates for the absence of pupillary light responses during the first 24 hours after resuscitation.[25,31,32]

The Glasgow Coma Scale which provides a more objective framework for neurologic prognostication, and shows a total aggregate and low component score (especially in the motor response). In a study by Mullie *et al.* of patients who died or were still comatose at 2 weeks, 98% had a GCS score of 4 or less, while only 18% had a GCS-score ≥ 10.[30] Other studies have also used the GCS as a predictive tool[27,33] or as a predominant factor that determines outcome in a more comprehensive score such as the Acute Physiology and Chronic Health Evaluation Score (APACHE) II (Table 50.1).[26,34]

As two of the strongest findings of poor outcome in comatose patients untreated with hypothermia, the absence of pupillary light reflex and absence of motor responses 72 hours after resuscitation may be used to guide the decisions made by clinicians about the intensity and duration of care provided after cardiac arrest. As indicators for poor outcome at 72 hours, these findings have little direct impact on the decision to provide therapies that are currently focused on the first 24 hours. Therefore, there is still a need for research to identify early (within minutes or few hours of injury) neurological markers of brain injury and recovery. Such clinical markers may aid in the development of more effective therapies.

Neuroimaging

Neuroimaging has been used to define brain injury related to cardiac arrest. No large prospective studies have been performed to date. With some limitations, retrospective studies described the brain injury and attempted to define its relation to poor outcome after cardiac arrest. Non-contrast head computerized tomography (CT) is one of the most common screening tools that can rule out a structural abnormality in patients with neurologic dysfunction. An abnormality on CT scan is generally associated with worse outcomes when compared to patients with no CT abnormalities. As global ischemia to the brain leads to cerebral edema, non-contrast head CT will be able to show that edema that leads to effacement of sulci and cisterns also causes a decrease in gray matter density, leading to loss of the gray matter to white matter differentiation. This is pronounced in the basal ganglia and watershed areas.[35]

Quantitatively, the loss of the distinction between gray and white matter on CT, even when normal to the naked eye, has been shown to correspond to neuronal necrosis, watershed infarcts, and periventricular leukomalacia. Torbey and colleagues used CT Housefield units to quantify the loss of gray and white matter (GM/WM) demarcation in association with global cerebral ischemia and found that a lower GM/WM ratio of <1.18 is associated with poor outcome or death after cardiac arrest.[36] The loss of the GM/WM demarcation in a CT scan performed at 48 hours, when combined with the clinical status of the patients such as the GCS and the duration of cardiac arrest, increased the ability of the measure to predict poor functional outcome.[37]

Many retrospective studies on the use of MRI in prognostication have been reported. As an imaging technique, the use of MRI is limited in critically ill patients because of patient safety and possibly lack of compatibility of supportive equipment. A retrospective study defined the role of MRI in prognostication and noted poor prognosis in patients with diffuse cortical signal changes on diffusion-weighted imaging (DWI) or fluid-attenuated inversion recovery (FLAIR).[38] In this study of 10 patients, 8 who remained comatose with no indicator of poor prognosis, such as myoclonic status epilepticus, fixed dilated pupils, absence of SSEP, and burst suppression on EEG, were found to have diffuse and extensive abnormalities in the cortex, thalamus, and cerebellum. The two remaining patients who awoke had normal or localized MRI findings. The study also noted that the DWI abnormalities eventually improved, but the FLAIR abnormalities persisted on follow-up.

Several studies with functional neuroimaging have documented brain injury, but the limited number of patients hamper its reliable application to prognostication. The use of Positron Emission Tomography (PET) has been undertaken in defining the brain injury and prognostication. As in cases of ischemia, changes in lactate and NAA are associated with a specific outcome. However, one study with 8 patients and the other with 7 patients[40] did not find any significant PET index that differentiated between survivors and non-survivors.

Evoked potentials

Somatosensory evoked potentials (SSEP) is a neurophysiological test that measures the integrity of the neuronal pathways from a peripheral nerve, spinal cord, brain stem, and cerebral cortex.[41,42] In the evaluation of brain injury after cardiac arrest, disruption of the neural pathways manifested as slowing or absence of waveforms that are generated by the brain stem and cortex are most important in prognostication. The absence of early cortical SSEPs

(N20/P25) after stimulation of the median nerve has been shown to be a reliable predictor of poor outcome (with persistent coma or death) in several studies of patient series in coma after cardiac arrest.[42–45] The absence of N20 during the first week after cardiac arrest and poor neurologic outcome showed a positive likelihood ratio of 12 (95% CI 5.3–27.6).[22] This ability of SSEP to prognosticate a poor neurologic outcome was also supported by other reviews and large patient series.[42,46] Although the absence of the N20 signal is strongly associated with poor outcome, a normal N20 is only associated with about 60% of those who awake from coma, and a delayed N20 is associated with arousal in only 20% of subjects. (See Fig. 50.2).[42]

Most of these studies report the use of SSEP from several hours to a few days after resuscitation from cardiac arrest, most commonly within 3–4 days. But no studies have established its use earlier than 24 hours. With no reported return of a previous absent N20 in a comatose patient, the absence of the N20 is one of the most significant predictors of poor outcome. Repeated testing must be considered, however, when the N20 responses are present early in the course of postcardiac arrest coma, especially in patients who remain unresponsive. The use of SSEPs in determining a poor prognosis is preferred over other tests, such as EEG and other types of evoked responses, because it is less susceptible to the effect of drugs, metabolic derangements, and temperature. Nevertheless, it may be susceptible to muscle artifact and occasionally the use of muscle relaxants may improve the test quality.

Other evoked response tests, such as brain stem auditory and visual and event-related potential tests, have been used for prognostication but their definitive use still needs to be established. The use of brainstem auditory response is limited by the reversible dysfunction of the cochlear which may lead to the initial absence of brainstem auditory signals that may return over subsequent days.[47] In some studies normal brainstem auditory evoked potential (BAEP) have been seen in patients with poor outcome, including PVS.[48,49] The presence of the late component of the SSEP waveform such as the N70 response was reported to be associated with favorable outcome,[48] but more studies are needed to validate its prognostic ability in these patients.

Electroencephalography (EEG)

EEG is useful for evaluating depth of coma and extent of damage after cardiac arrest. EEG is widely available, easy to perform even in unstable patients, and non-invasive.[41] The widespread application of EEG in prognostication is hampered by several factors, including lack of a unified classification system, which is confounded by the variability of the

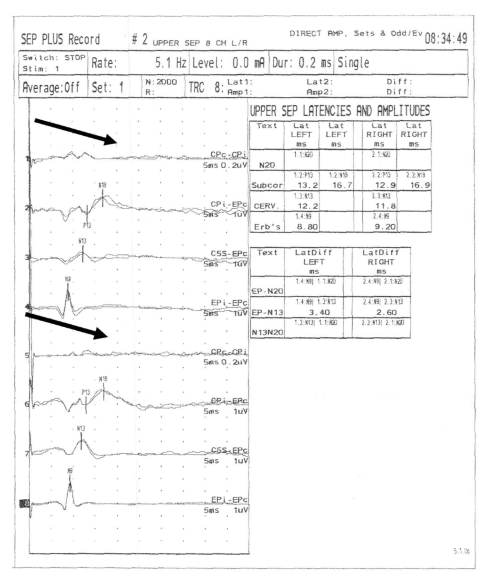

Fig. 50.2. Median nerve SSEP after cardiac arrest demonstrating bilateral absence of the cortical N20 peak (arrows). (From Koenig, M.A., Kaplan, P.W. and Thakor, N.V., Clinical Neurophysiologic Monitoring and Brain Injury from Cardiac Arrest. In Brain Injury after Cardiac Arrest, Neurologic Clinics vol 24 issue 1, Editor: Geocadin, R.G, Publisher – Elsevier 2006, with permission.)

types of EEG patterns in a given category, lack of consistency in the intervals of EEG after resuscitation, and bias toward evaluation of severely injured patients. The numerous EEG studies reviewed for this chapter[41,43,50–54] showed significant variability in the time intervals from CPR to EEG, but the majority seem to be performed around 3 days or later. The key patterns of EEG that provide the basic classification include: presence or absence of EEG activity; reactivity of EEG to specific stimuli; different EEG frequencies (i.e.,

alpha, theta, and delta); certain specific patterns, such as burst suppression or low voltage or isoelectric EEG. These patterns were grouped into five grades in an older classification, which has been consolidated by more recent classifications into three categories for prognostication: malignant, uncertain, and benign. Many classifications of "malignant" EEGs include a combination of suppression, burst-suppression, non-reactive alpha and theta pattern, and generalized periodic complexes.[43,51,52,55,56] The patterns most often associated with poor outcome are generalized suppression to 20 μV, burst-suppression pattern with generalized epileptiform activity, or generalized periodic complexes on a flat background.[57] In a meta-analysis of several relevant studies, EEG recordings with an isoelectric or burst-suppression pattern had a specificity of 100% for poor outcome with a pooled positive-likelihood ratio = 9.0 (95% CI 2.5–33.1) (see Fig. 50.3).

As an early indicator of brain recovery after resuscitation, the early return of continuous and reactive EEG activity may predict good outcomes.[41,58,59] Novel EEG analyses and applications are still being actively investigated as potential objective markers for brain injury, with the ability to track recovery, such as quantitative EEG analysis focusing on real-time changes of EEG, or limited channel recording in order to follow general trends to track recov-

ery or injury processes or development of anoxic encephalopathy, or in detecting sudden changes (such as seizures). EEG may provide potential monitoring for brain recovery during therapeutic hypothermia after cardiac arrest. EEG changes have been described during hypothermia in a limited clinical study.[60] With the exception of a case report detecting seizure activity[61] to date no clinical studies have described a postcardiac arrest population in terms of relating therapeutic hypothermia and EEG.

Biochemical markers

Biochemical markers that can reflect neurologic injury can be measured both in the serum and the CSF. Ideally, a chosen marker should be shown to be released from neurons or glial cells as a result of damage to that cell, and should be easy to obtain.[62] A meta-analysis of published

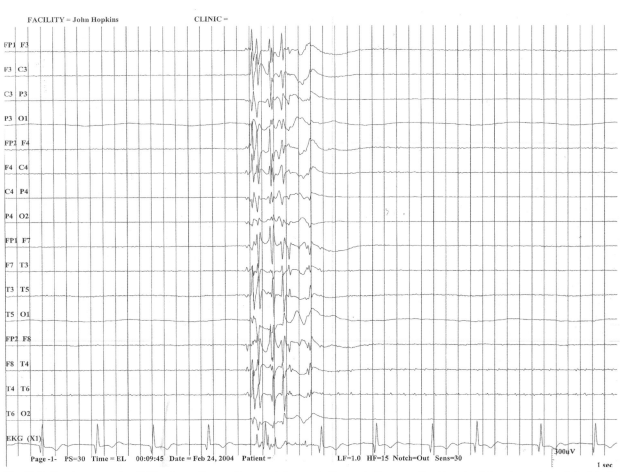

Fig. 50.3. Burst-suppression EEG pattern after cardiac arrest demonstrating periodic generalized bursts of sharply contoured electrical activity separated by periods of EEG suppression (from Koenig, M.A., Kaplan, P.W. and Thaker, N.V., Clinical Neurophysiologic Monitering and Brain Injury from Cardiac Arrest. In Brain Injury after Cardiac Arrest, Neurologic clinics vol 24 issue 1, Editor: Geocadin, R.G., Publisher – Elsevier 2006, with permission).

biochemical tests used to prognosticate outcome after cardiac arrest has been published,[45] as well as several other studies on biochemical tests in serum and CSF.[62–65] While specific cut-off levels are associated with poor outcome, these values vary considerably between studies, even for the same biochemical test (Table 50.1). This significant variability limits the universal translation of these tests into widespread clinical practice. While biochemical markers can detect brain injury and provide prognostication, more controlled clinical studies are required to define precisely their role in prognosticating functional outcome after cardiac arrest.

CSF creatine kinase BB (CKBB)
When the brain is injured, the CKBB in the brain will leak from the cytoplasm of the destroyed cells into the extracellular fluid.[66] CKBB levels in the CSF reach a peak between 48 and 72 hours after cardiac arrest.[67] Several studies investigated the prognostic value of CSF CKBB. The cut-off value higher than 204 units/l predicted poor outcome in these studies.[63,66] In a meta-analysis of 28 studies that included 802 patients,[45] CKBB >204 U/l showed no false-positives for poor outcome. Nevertheless, because of the small numbers of patients studied and methodological limitations, no reliable recommendation can be made for non-treatment decisions. Some concerns have been raised about the safety of CSF sampling as well as the risk of cerebral herniation.

Neuron specific enolase (NSE)
NSE is the neuronal form of the intracytoplasmic glycolytic enzyme enolase, which was first found in extracts of brain tissue (neuronal bodies and axons) and later in neuroendocrine cells (APUD) and neuroendocrine tumors (including small cell lung cancer).[68] It has a relatively high molecular weight, and is therefore unlikely to cross cell membranes unless the cell is damaged. It reaches a peak in the serum and CSF at 72 hours following the ischemic insult.[69] Many studies have investigated the value of increased serum and CSF NSE in patients who remained comatose after cardiac arrest. There is significant variability in the cutoff points for 100% positive predictive value for poor outcome. Some of the larger studies such as that performed by Fogel et al. in 50 patients used a cutoff value of serum NSE of 33 ng/ml and found 80% sensitivity and 100% specificity. Importantly, almost all of these studies were done in normothermic patients.

S-100
This is a dimeric acidic calcium-binding protein present in high concentrations in glial and Schwann cells.[68] It is eliminated by the kidneys, and is also found in certain tumors (including glioma, melanoma, schwannoma, and highly differentiated neuroblastoma).[68] It has a lower molecular weight than NSE and is highly soluble, and therefore more likely to cross the cell membrane.[68] S-100 is a sensitive marker for glial cell damage. The highest levels are usually observed during the first 24 hours after the anoxic insult, and usually decline over the next 48 hours, probably due to ease of permeability.[69] Several studies have used S-100 for prognostication: one used a cutoff value of 0.2 mcg/L, and found a positive predictive value of 79% of S100 2 hours after cardiac arrest, 87% of S-100 24 hours after cardiac arrest, and 75% at 48 hours after cardiac arrest.[70]

NSE, S-100 and hypothermia
Since the positive findings related to therapeutic hypothermia after cardiac arrest, a study by Tiainen et al. of 70 patients to evaluate the effect of therapeutic hypothermia on levels of serum NSE and S-100B protein found that the levels of NSE ($P=0.007$), but not S-100B, were lower in hypothermia-treated patients than in normothermia-treated patients.[64] A decrease in NSE values between 24 and 48 hours was observed in 88% of the hypothermia group and only 50% in the normothermia group ($P<0.001$). This decrease in NSE values was associated with good outcome at 6 months after cardiac arrest ($P=0.005$), recovery of consciousness ($P<0.001$), and survival >6 months after cardiac arrest ($P=0.012$).[64]

Associated manifestations

Elevation of intracranial pressure
Cellular injury and neuronal death from global brain ischemia may lead to cerebral edema. Commonly, increased intracranial pressure is attributed to significant cerebral edema. A study of head CT 3 days after cardiac arrest showed that brain edema was more common in patients who had cardiac arrest due to respiratory distress, and of those patients diagnosed with brain edema, more developed brain death compared to those without brain edema.[71] A study with 10 patients suggests that intracranial pressure elevation (ICP) following CPR does not necessarily increase in the absence of primary intracranial pathology or seizures,[72] but when ICP is elevated, the presence of ICP > 20 mmHg in comatose patients has been associated with poor outcome.[39,73] Although this is a promising indicator of brain injury after cardiac arrest, more studies are needed to establish the usefulness of elevated ICP for prognostication.

Myoclonus status epilepticus
As many as one-third of comatose CPR survivors experience seizure activity at some time during the hospital course,

most commonly within the first 24 hours.[74,75] A detailed discussion of seizures, diagnosis, and management, and impact on outcome after cardiac arrest is provided in a comprehensive review by Koenig and Geocadin.[76]

The prognostic significance of seizure needs to be clarified. Although studies focus on the occurrence of myoclonus status epilepticus as a predictor of poor outcome in selected patients with severe injury,[77,78] other types of seizures may be less ominous, as shown in a general population study by Levy et al.[25] which failed to demonstrate poorer outcomes in the subpopulation with seizures of any type.

Episodic jerking in postcardiac arrest patients must be carefully characterized prior to proposing prognosis. The classical syndrome of postanoxic myoclonus (also known as the Lance–Adams syndrome), which occurs more frequently after respiratory arrest, was previously regarded as a predictor of poor outcome. But a recent report of survivors with postanoxic myoclonus indicates that the myoclonus may improve as neurologic status improves.[79] Nevertheless, myoclonic status epilepticus which presents as repetitive, unrelenting, generalized multifocal myoclonus in the face, limbs, and axial musculature,[74] which is often associated with burst suppression on EEG, is considered to be an indicator of extremely poor prognosis, and it does not respond to anticonvulsants.[74,78]

Multimodality prognostication

Most of the studies on the prognostic markers in cardiac arrest have been made by considering single variables. Few studies have looked at combining the values of the above tests to increase the reliability of predicting outcomes.[43,53,66] Bassetti et al. assessed the value of combining clinical examination, EEG, SSEP, and two serum biochemical markers (ionized calcium and neuron-specific enolase). Individually, clinical examination correctly predicted outcome in 58%, SSEP in 59%, EEG in 41%, and in combination, all three factors (clinical exam, SSEP, and EEG) improved the predictions to 82%. No false poor prediction was observed using the combination.

To improve further the ability of SSEP in predicting poor outcome, Sherman et al. added CSF creatine kinase BB isoenzyme activity (CKBB). As individual tests, they found that poor outcome was predicted with a CKBB ≥ 205 U/l with a sensitivity of 49% and a specificity of 100%, whereas the bilateral absence of the N1 peak had a sensitivity of 53% and a specificity of 100%. The combined presence of CKBB ≥ 205 U/l and bilaterally absent SEP N1 peaks, improved the sensitivity to 69%, while the specificity remained at

100% in predicting a poor outcome.

While novel injury and recovery parameters for prognostication and real-time tracking and application are being developed through research,[80,81] multimodality prognostication provides an opportunity for further enhancement of the ability of clinicians to predict the outcome after cardiac arrest. Although this is a very promising direction, better designed prospective studies with adequate statistical power are needed for real advances in this area.

Withdrawal of life-sustaining therapies

Advances in resuscitation and critical care have allowed the prolongation of life in resuscitated patients, but the desired quality of life is not attained in most of these cases. The practice of withdrawal of life-sustaining therapies is currently widespread in ICUs. Several major organizations, including the American Medical Association,[82–84] the American Academy of Neurology,[85] and the Society of Critical Care Medicine-American College of Chest Physicians,[86] have recognized the right of patients in specific situations to forgo treatment, even if refusal may lead to death. Indeed, research demonstrates widespread support among critical care physicians and nurses for withdrawal of life-sustaining therapies in cases of devastating injury and expected poor outcome.[87–89] The clinical findings in patients with persisting coma presented above, such as the absence of pupillary light flex and motor response on day 3, with or without the SSEP test showing the absence of the N20 wave during the first week, may be used to define the high likelihood of poor outcome.

The actual process leading to the decision to withdraw life-sustaining therapies has not been studied in detail. This is a clinical decision that is based on the clinical condition of the patients in conjunction with treatment and outcome preference of the patients, and clinical expertise of the treating team.[90] A study found that advanced ICU care is provided to treat morbidity and delay mortality, and at the same time to orchestrate the dying process.[91] They also found that the decisions to withhold, provide, continue, or withdraw life support were "socially" negotiated leading to a common decision among family members and clinicians.[91] A survey study showed that 73% of the general public respondents and 70% of nurse respondents advocated a joint decision made by the family and the physician.

A recent report of patients withdrawn from life-sustaining therapies after resuscitation from cardiac arrest indicated that patients with absence of bilateral N20 on SSEP and poor neurologic examination had a shorter period of observation before withdrawal of life support compared to those with poor neurologic examination and indeterminate or present N20 on SSEP.[93] The ICU team and the families decided sooner if the poor neurological examination result was supported by an objective measure like the SSEP.[93] More studies are needed to understand this process and how to apply the information to improve the experience of patients' families and physicians. While the process of withdrawal of life support is widely practiced and discussed, it is still not well known how the clinicians and the families actually process the clinical characteristics used in neurologic prognostication to reach a specific decision.

Evaluation of brain death

Despite the advances in resuscitation techniques and therapies for patients after cardiac arrest, the progression of injury to death is very common. The progression of brain injury after resuscitation from cardiac arrest leading to the irreversible loss of function of the brain and the brain stem underlies the condition of brain death.[94] The practice of declaring brain death has defined criteria that were first established by an ad hoc committee of Harvard Medical School in 1968;[95] the criteria were further developed to be more relevant to clinical practice through a set of guidelines published by the Quality Standards Subcommittee of the American Academy of Neurology (AAN) in 1995.[94] These guidelines are presented below with some additional suggestions pertinent to a patient suspected of brain death following cardiac arrest. It is also strongly advised that the physician performing the brain death examination consults and applies the practice guidelines of the hospital, as well as any established laws of the state or country where the test is performed.

The AAN prerequisites for the declaration of brain death include a known proximate cause for the irreversible absence of brain function;[94] this may be demonstrated by neuroimaging. In patients with global brain ischemia from cardiac arrest, neuroimaging may not be necessary unless other complicating etiologies are considered. For example, medical conditions that may mimic clinical manifestations of brain death or confound the clinical assessment of brain death should be ruled out. These include a severe electrolyte, acid-base, or endocrine disturbance, drug intoxication, use of paralytic and sedative agents, and poisoning. Additionally, significant hypotension must to be corrected, and the patient's core temperature must be greater than or equal to 32 °C (90 °F). In efforts to demonstrate irreversibility and consistency of findings, the determination of brain death requires that two neurological examinations be performed at least more than 6 hours apart. Once all these prerequisites are met, the examination can proceed to establish the presence of the three cardinal findings in brain death: (1) coma or unresponsiveness; (2) absence of brainstem function; and (3) apnea.[94]

Determination of coma

After resuscitation from cardiac arrest, a comatose patient will display no purposeful or spontaneous movements, or response to stimuli of any kind. The depth of the patient's coma may be assessed by the neurological examination. A detailed approach to the determination of the depth of coma was presented above in the section on neurologic assessment. In unresponsive patients, significant noxious stimulation must be used to avoid an erroneous coma diagnosis. If noxious stimulation is to be used, it must be applied first in the midline areas (sternum), and then in the limbs, and in the facial areas as supraorbital ridge pressure. Responses generated by noxious stimulation should not elicit any activity that can be attributable to the brain or brainstem. Not infrequently, reflexive movements generated from the level of the spine may suggest brain or brainstem function.[96] Some of these movements include a minor reflexive flexion in the limb with the application of a noxious stimulant, a slow flexion at the waist, arms raised independently or together, stepping movements, slow turning of the head, movement of toes, facial twitching, or the Babinski reflex.[96] If all the clinical prerequisites are met and the reflexive activity is localized to the spine, the diagnosis of brain death persists.

Examination of brainstem reflexes

Together with the determination of coma, the absence of all clinical functions of the brainstem must also be established. Again, a detailed approach to specific cranial nerves was provided above; the key findings included total absence of the pupillary light reflex (cranial nerve 2) and the persistence of a midpositioned (4 mm) to dilated pupils (9 mm). The absence any ocular response (cranial nerves 3, 4, and 6) with oculocephalic maneuver is consistent with brain death. For patients with known or suspected cervical spine injury, head-turning should not be attempted. All patients undergoing brain death determination should receive cold caloric testing (cranial nerve 8).[94,96,97] During this test, eyes should not deviate while each ear is irrigated with 50 ml of cold water. The patient should be observed for a response for 1 minute following injection, and a period of 5 minutes should be maintained before testing in the patient's other ear. The absence of the cranial nerve 5 and 7 functions can be documented with the absence of the corneal reflex and facial grimace to pain. Finally, pharyngeal and tracheal reflexes (cranial nerve 9 and 10) should be evaluated. The absence of the gag reflex can be documented by the lack of response to tongue depressor placed in the posterior pharynx and the absence of the tracheal cough when tracheal suctioning is applied in intubated patients. The absence of spontaneous respirations or the need for a full ventilatory support also strengthens the diagnosis of brainstem injury in brain death.

The apnea test

The apnea test is performed to determine if the patient's brainstem can trigger a spontaneous breath given an adequate stimulation of carbon dioxide. To perform the test adequately, some prerequisites must be met: a core temperature of 36.5 °C or higher; systolic blood pressure greater than or equal to 90 mmHg; euvolemia; normal pCO_2 (> 40 mmHg), and normal arterial PO_2 with the option to pre-oxygenate to $pO_2 > 200$ mmHg.[94] Close hemodynamic and respiratory monitoring is required because the procedure is closely associated with hypotension and cardiac arrhythmias,[94] especially with the occurrence of systolic blood pressure ≤ 90 mmHg, and significant O_2 desaturation.

The apnea test should begin with a baseline arterial blood gas measurement with the patient connected to a pulse oximeter. The ventilator may then be disconnected, and 100% O_2 should be delivered into the trachea at 6 liters/minute. Oxygen should be delivered using a cannula placed at the level of the carina. The patient should be observed for respiratory movements. Respiration-like movements or abdominal movements may be observed, but a spirometer may be used to confirm the absence of tidal volumes. Arterial PO_2, PCO_2, and pH should be measured every 3–4 minutes.

The test is positive if respiratory movements are absent and PCO_2 reaches a critical level (i.e., ≥ 60 mm Hg, or increase is ≥ 20 mmHg over baseline).[94] The test is negative if respiratory movements are observed. The test may be repeated if negative.[19] The test result is indeterminate if PCO_2 is < 60 mmHg, or increase is < 20 mm Hg over baseline normal level,[94] after which an additional confirmatory test may be considered.

Confirmatory tests

If the determination of brain death cannot be made with certainty on clinical grounds, such as in cases of severe facial trauma, pre-existing pupillary abnormality, toxic drug levels, and severe chronic CO_2 retention, confirmatory testing may be necessary. Confirmatory laboratory testing findings that may help establish the diagnosis of brain death include: (1) absence of cerebral filling at the level of the carotid bifurcation or circle of Willis on conventional angiography; (2) no uptake of isotope in brain parenchyma with technetium-99m hexamethylpropyleneamineoxime brain scan; (3) no electrical activity for at least 30 minutes on the EEG Brain Death protocol by the American Electroencephalographic Society; (4) absence of blood flow on adequate studies with transcranial Doppler; and (5) absence of bilateral N20–P22 response with median nerve stimulation on SSEP based on the protocol adopted by the American Electroencephalographic Society. A detailed discussion of these tests and procedures is provided in AAN guidelines.[94]

Acknowledgments

Dr. Geocadin is supported by R01 HL-071568, R44-HD042872, R44 NS045407; Dr. Hanley is supported by R01 HL-071568.

REFERENCES

1. Geocadin, R.G. (ed.) Brain injury after cardiac arrest. *Neurol. Clinics* 2006; **24** (1): 1–179.
2. Cummins, R.O., Chamberlain, D.A., Abramson, N.S. *et al.* Recommended guidelines for uniform reporting of data from out-of-hospital cardiac arrest: the Utstein Style. Task Force of the American Heart Association, the European Resuscitation Council, the Heart and Stroke Foundation of Canada, and the Australian Resuscitation Council. *Ann. Emerg. Med.* 1991; **20**: 861–874.
3. Cummins, R.O., Chamberlain, D., Haziriski, M.F. *et al.* Recommended guidelines for reviewing, reporting, and conducting research on in-hospital resuscitation: the in-hospital "Utstein style." American Heart Association. *Ann. Emerg. Med.* 1997; **29**: 650–679.
4. Cone, D.C., Jaslow, D.S. & Brabson, T.A. Now that we have the Utstein style, are we using it? *Acad. Emerg. Med.* 1999; **6**: 923–928.
5. Cummins, R.O. Why are researchers and emergency medical services managers not using the Utstein guidelines? *Acad. Emerg. Med.* 1999; **6**: 871–875.
6. Randomized clinical study of thiopental loading in comatose survivors of cardiac arrest. Brain Resuscitation Clinical Trial I Study Group. *N. Engl. J. Med.* 1986; **314**: 397–403.
7. Brain Resuscitation Clinical Trial II Study Group [see comments]. A randomized clinical study of a calcium-entry

blocker (lidoflazine) in the treatment of comatose survivors of cardiac arrest. *N. Engl. J. Med.* 1991; **324**: 1225–1231.

8. Roine, R.O., Kaste, M., Kinnunen, A., Nikki, P., Sama, S. & Kajaste, S. Nimodipine after resuscitation from out-of-hospital ventricular fibrillation. A placebo-controlled, double-blind, randomized trial. *J. Am. Med. Assoc.* 1990; **264**: 3171–3177.

9. Brain Resuscitation Clinical Trial I Study Group. Glucocorticoid treatment does not improve neurological recovery following cardiac arrest. *J. Am. Med. Assoc.* 1989; **262**: 3427–3430.

10. Thel, M.C., Armstrong, A.L., McNulty, S.E., Califf, R.M. & O'Connor, C.M. Randomised trial of magnesium in in-hospital cardiac arrest. Duke Internal Medicine Housestaff. *Lancet* 1997; **350**: 1272–1276.

11. Longstreth, W.T. Jr., Fahrenbruch, C.E., Olsufka, M. *et al.* Randomized clinical trial of magnesium, diazepam, or both after out-of-hospital cardiac arrest. *Neurology* 2002; **59**: 506–514.

12. Hypothermia after Cardiac Asset Study Group. Mild therapeutic hypothermia to improve the neurologic outcome after cardiac arrest. *N. Engl. J. Med.* 2002; **346**: 549–556.

13. Bernard, S.A., Gray, T.W., Buist, M.D. *et al.* Treatment of comatose survivors of out-of-hospital cardiac arrest with induced hypothermia. *N. Engl. J. Med.* 2002; **346**: 557–563.

14. Berek, K., Lechleitner, P., Luef, G. *et al.* Early determination of neurological outcome after prehospital cardiopulmonary resuscitation. *Stroke* 1995; **26**: 543–549.

15. Rogove, H.J., Safar, P., Sutton-Tyrrell, K. & Abramson, N.S. Old age does not negate good cerebral outcome after cardiopulmonary resuscitation: analyses from the brain resuscitation clinical trials. The Brain Resuscitation Clinical Trial I and II Study Groups. *Crit. Care Med.* 1995; **23**: 18–25.

16. Brain Resuscitation Clinical Trial I Study Group. Neurologic recovery after cardiac arrest: effect of duration of ischemia. *Crit. Care Med.* 1985; **13**: 930–931.

17. Rogove, H., Safar, P., Sutton-Tyrrell, K. & Abrahamson, N. Old age does not negate good cerebral outcome from cardiopulmonary arrest: analyses from the brain resuscitation clinical trials. *Crit. Care Med.* 1995; **23**: 18–25.

18. Abella, B.S., Sandbo, N., Vassilatos, P. *et al.* Chest compression rates during cardiopulmonary resuscitation are suboptimal: a prospective study during in-hospital cardiac arrest. *Circulation* 2005; **111**: 428–434.

19. Abella, B.S., Alvarado, J.P., Myklebust, H. *et al.* Quality of cardiopulmonary resuscitation during in-hospital cardiac arrest. *J. Am. Med. Assoc.* 2005; **293**: 305–310.

20. Wik, L., Kramer-Johansen, J., Myklebust, H. *et al.* Quality of cardiopulmonary resuscitation during out-of-hospital cardiac arrest. *J. Am. Med. Assoc.* 2005; **293**: 299–304.

21. Edgren, E., Hedstrand, U., Kelsey, S., Sutton-Tyrrell, K. & Safar, P. Assessment of neurological prognosis in comatose survivors of cardiac arrest. BRCT I Study Group. *Lancet* 1994; **343**: 1055–1059.

22. Zandbergen, E.G., de Haan, R.J., Stoutenbeek, C.P., Koelman, J.H. & Hijdra, A. Systematic review of early prediction of poor outcome in anoxic–ischaemic coma. *Lancet* 1998; **352**: 1808–1812.

23. Teasdale, G. & Jennett, B. Assessment of coma and impaired consciousness. A practical scale. *Lancet* 1974; **2**: 81–84.

24. Wijdicks, E.F., Bamlet, W.R., Maramattom, B.V., Manno, E.M. & McClelland, R.L. Validation of a new coma scale: The FOUR score. *Ann. Neurol.* 2005; **58**: 585–593.

25. Levy, D.E., Caronna, J.J., Singer, B.H. *et al.* Predicting outcome from hypoxic–ischemic coma. *J. Am. Med. Assoc.* 1985; **253**: 1420–1426.

26. Niskanen, M. *et al.* Acute physiology and chronic health evaluation (APACHE II) and Glasgow coma scores as predictors of outcome from intensive care after cardiac arrest. *Crit. Care Med.* 1991; **19**: 1465–1473.

27. Urban, P. & Cereda, J.M. Glasgow coma score 1 hour after cardiac arrest. *Lancet* 1985; **2**: 1012.

28. Berek, K., Jeschow, M. & Aichner, F. The prognostication of cerebral hypoxia after out of hospital cardiac arrest in adults. *Eur. Neurol.* 1997; **37**: 135–145.

29. Bertini, G. *et al.* Prognostic significance of early clinical manifestations in postanoxic coma: a retrospective study of 58 patients resuscitated after prehospital cardiac arrest. *Crit. Care Med.* 1989; **17**: 627–633.

30. Mullie, A. *et al.* Predictive value of Glasgow coma score for awakening after out-of-hospital cardiac arrest. Cerebral Resuscitation Study Group of the Belgian Society for Intensive Care. *Lancet* 1988; **1**: 137–140.

31. Longstreth, W.T., Jr., Inui, T.S., Cobb, L.A. & Copass, M.K. Neurologic recovery after out-of-hospital cardiac arrest. *Ann. Intern. Med.* 1983; **98**: 588–592.

32. Longstreth, W.T., Jr., Diehr, P. & Inui, T.S. Prediction of awakening after out-of-hospital cardiac arrest. *N. Engl. J. Med.* 1983; **308**: 1378–1382.

33. Sacco, R.L., VanGool, R., Mohr, J.P. & Hauser, W.A. Nontraumatic coma. Glasgow coma score and coma etiology as predictors of 2-week outcome. *Arch. Neurol.* 1990; **47**: 1181–1184.

34. Knaus, W.A., Draper, E.A., Wagner, D.P. & Zimmerman, J.E. APACHE II: a severity of disease classification system. *Crit. Care Med.* 1985; **13**: 818–829.

35. Kjos, B., BranZawadski, M. & Young, R. Early CT findings of globl central nervous system hypoperfusion. *Am. J. Radiol.* 1983; **141**: 1277–1232.

36. Torbey, M.T., Selim, M., Knorr, J., Bigelow, C. & Recht, L. Quantitative analysis of the loss of distinction between gray and white matter in comatose patients after cardiac arrest. *Stroke* 2000; **31**: 2163–2167.

37. Torbey, M.T., Geocadin, R. & Bhardwaj, A. Brain arrest neurological outcome scale (BrANOS): predicting mortality and severe disability following cardiac arrest. *Resuscitation* 2004; **63**: 55–63.

38. Wijdicks, E.F., Campeau, N.G. & Miller, G.M. MR imaging in comatose survivors of cardiac resuscitation. *Am. J. Neuroradiol.* 2001; **22**: 1561–1565.

39. Schaafsma, A., de Jong, B.M., Bams, J.L. *et al.* Cerebral perfusion and metabolism in resuscitated patients with severe

post-hypoxic encephalopathy. *J. Neurol. Sci.* 2003; **210**: 23–30.

40. Edgren, E., Enblad, P., Grenvik, A. *et al.* Cerebral blood flow and metabolism after cardiopulmonary resuscitation. A pathophysiologic and prognostic positron emission tomography pilot study. *Resuscitation* 2003; **57**: 161–170.

41. Young, G.B. The EEG in coma. *J. Clin. Neurophysiol.* 2000; **17**: 473–485.

42. Rothstein, T.L. The role of evoked potentials in anoxic-ischemic coma and severe brain trauma. *J. Clin. Neurophysiol.* 2000; **17**: 486–497.

43. Bassetti, C., Bomio, F., Mathis, J. & Hess, C.W. Early prognosis in coma after cardiac arrest: a prospective clinical, electrophysiological, and biochemical study of 60 patients. *J. Neurol. Neurosurg. Psychiatry* 1996; **61**: 610–615.

44. Zandbergen, E.G., de Haan, R.J., Koelman, J.H. & Hijdra, A. Prediction of poor outcome in anoxic-ischemic coma. *J. Clin. Neurophysiol.* 2000; **17**: 498–501.

45. Zandbergen, E.G., de Haan, R.J. & Hijdra, A. Systematic review of prediction of poor outcome in anoxic–ischaemic coma with biochemical markers of brain damage. *Intens. Care Med.* 2001; **27**: 1661–1667.

46. Carter, B.G. & Butt, W. Review of the use of somatosensory evoked potentials in the prediction of outcome after severe brain injury. *Crit. Care Med.* 2001; **29**: 178–186.

47. Sohmer, H., Freeman, S., Gafni, M. & Goitein, K. The depression of the auditory nerve-brain-stem evoked response in hypoxaemia – mechanism and site of effect. *Electroencephalogr. Clin. Neurophysiol.* 1986; **64**: 334–338.

48. Madl, C., Griman, E., Kramer, L. *et al.* Early prediction of individual outcome after cardiopulmonary resuscitation. *Lancet* 1993; **341**: 855–858.

49. Facco, E. & Giron, G.P. Multimodality evoked potentials in coma and brain death. *Minerva Anesthesiol.* 1994; **60**: 593–599.

50. Chen, R., Bolton, C. & Young, G. Prediction of outcome in patients with anoxic coma: A clinical and electrophysiologic study. *Crit. Care Med.* 1996; **24**: 672–678.

51. Scollio-Lavizzari, G. & Bassetti, C. Prognostic value of EEG in post-anoxic coma after cardiac arrest. *Eur. Neurol.* 1987; **26**: 161–170.

52. Synek, V. Value of a revised EEG coma scale for prognosis after cerebral anoxia and diffuse head injury. *Clin. Electroencephalogr.* 1990; **21**: 25–30.

53. Rothstein, T., Thomas, E. & Sumi, S. Predicting outcome in hypoxic-ischemic coma. A prospective clinical and electrophysiological study. *Electroencephalogr. Clin. Neurophysiol.* 1991; **79**: 101–107.

54. Edgren, E., Hedstrand, U., Nordin, M., Rydin, E. & Ronquist, G. Prediction of outcome after cardiac arrest. *Crit. Care Med.* 1987; **15**: 820–825.

55. Young, G.B., McLachlan, R.S., Kreeft, J.H. & Demelo, J.D. An electroencephalographic classification for coma. *Can. J. Neurol. Sci.* 1997; **24**: 320–325.

56. Kaplan, P.W., Genoud, D., Ho, T.W. & Jallon, P. Etiology, neurologic correlations, and prognosis in alpha coma. *Clin. Neurophysiol.* 1999; **110**: 205–213.

57. Young, G.B., Kreeft, J.H., McLachlan, R.S. & Demelo, J. EEG and clinical associations with mortality in comatose patients in a general intensive care unit. *J. Clin. Neurophysiol.* 1999; **16**: 354–360.

58. Jorgensen, E.O. & Malchow-Moller, A. Natural history of global and critical brain ischaemia. Part I: EEG and neurological signs during the first year after cardiopulmonary resuscitation in patients subsequently regaining consciousness. *Resuscitation* 1981; **9**: 133–153.

59. Jorgensen, E.O. & Malchow-Moller, A. Natural history of global and critical brain ischaemia. Part II: EEG and n-eurological signs in patients remaining unconscious after cardiopulmonary resuscitation. *Resuscitation* 1981; **9**: 155–174.

60. Stecker, M.M., Escherich, A., Patterson, T., Bavaria, J.E. & Cheung, A.T. Effects of acute hypoxemia/ischemia on EEG and evoked responses at normothermia and hypothermia in humans. *Med. Sci. Monit.* 2002; **8**: CR223–8.

61. Hovland, A., Nielsen, E.W., Kluver, J. & Salvesen, R. EEG should be performed during induced hypothermia. *Resuscitation* 2006; **68**: 143–146.

62. Mussack, T., Biberthaler, P., Kanz, K.E. *et al.* S-100b, sE-selectin, and sP-selectin for evaluation of hypoxic brain damage in patients after cardiopulmonary resuscitation: pilot study. *World J. Surg.* 2001; **25**: 539–543; discussion 544.

63. Tirschwell, D.L., Longstreth, W.T., Rauch-Matthews, M.E. *et al.* Cerebrospinal fluid creatine kinase BB isoenzyme activity and neurologic prognosis after cardiac arrest. *Neurology* 1997; **48**: 352–357.

64. Tiainen, M., Roine, R.O., Pettila, V. & Takkunen, O. Serum neuron-specific enolase and S-100B protein in cardiac arrest patients treated with hypothermia. *Stroke* 2003; **34**: 2881–2886.

65. Meynaar, I.A., Oudemans-van Straaten, H.M., van den Wetering, J. *et al.* Serum neuron-specific enolase predicts outcome in post-anoxic coma: a prospective cohort study. *Intens. Care Med.* 2003; **29**: 189–195.

66. Sherman, A.L., Tirschwell, D.L., Micklesen, P.J., Longstreth, W.T., Jr. & Robinson, L.R. Somatosensory potentials, CSF creatine kinase BB activity, and awakening after cardiac arrest. *Neurology* 2000; **54**: 889–894.

67. Kjekshus, J.K., Vaagenes, P. & Hetland, O. Assessment of cerebral injury with spinal fluid creatine kinase (CSF-CK) in patients after cardiac resuscitation. *Scand. J. Clin. Lab. Invest.* 1980; **40**: 437–444.

68. Martens, P., Raabe, A. & Johnsson, P. Serum S-100 and neuron-specific enolase for prediction of regaining consciousness after global cerebral ischemia. *Stroke* 1998; **29**: 2363–2366.

69. Rosen, H., Sunnerhagen, K.S., Herlitz, J., Blomstrand, C. & Rosengren, L. Serum levels of the brain-derived proteins S-100 and NSE predict long-term outcome after cardiac arrest. *Resuscitation* 2001; **49**: 183–191.

70. Bottiger, B.W. *et al.* Astroglial protein S-100 is an early and sensitive marker of hypoxic brain damage and outcome after cardiac arrest in humans. *Circulation* 2001; **103**: 2694–2698.

71. Morimoto, Y., Kemmotsu, O., Kitami, K., Matsubara, I. & Tedo, I. Acute brain swelling after out-of-hospital cardiac arrest: pathogenesis and outcome. *Crit. Care Med.* 1993; **21**: 104–110.

72. Sakabe, T., Tateishi, A., Miyauchi, Y. *et al.* Intracranial pressure following cardiopulmonary resuscitation. *Intens. Care Med.* 1987; **13**: 256–259.

73. Gueugniaud, P.Y., Mols, P., Goldstein, P. *et al.* Prognostic significance of early intracranial and cerebral perfusion pressures in post-cardiac arrest anoxic coma. *Intens. Care Med.* 1991; **17**: 392–398.

74. Krumholz, A., Stern, B.J. & Weiss, H.D. Outcome from coma after cardiopulmonary resuscitation: relation to seizures and myoclonus. *Neurology* 1988; **38**: 401–405.

75. Snyder, B.D., Hauser, W.A., Loewenson, R.B. *et al.* Neurologic prognosis after cardiopulmonary arrest: III. Seizure activity. *Neurology* 1980; **30**: 1292–1297.

76. Koenig, M. & Geocadin, R. In *Seizures in Critical Care,* ed. Varelas, P. Totowa, N.J.: Humana Press, 2005

77. Young, G.B., Gilbert, J.J. & Zochodne, D.W. The significance of myoclonic status epilepticus in postanoxic coma. *Neurology* 1990; **40**: 1843–1848.

78. Wijdicks, E., Parisi, J. & Sharbrough, F. Prognostic value of myoclonus status in comatose survivors of cardiac arrest. *Ann. Neurol.* 1994; **35**: 239–243.

79. Werhahn, K.J., Brown, P., Thompson, P.D. & Marsden, C.D. The clinical features and prognosis of chronic posthypoxic myoclonus. *Mov. Disord.* 1997; **12**: 216–220.

80. Geocadin, R.G., Ghodadra, R., Kimura, T. *et al.* A novel quantitative EEG injury measure of global cerebral ischemia. *Clin. Neurophysiol.* 2000; **111**: 1779–1787.

81. Geocadin, R.G., Muthuswamy, J., Sherman, D.L., Thakor, N.V. & Hanley, D.F. Early electrophysiological and histologic changes after global cerebral ischemia in rats. *Mov. Disord.* 2000; **15 Suppl 1**: 14–21.

82. Weir, R.F. & Gostin, L. Decisions to abate life-sustaining treatment for nonautonomous patients. Ethical standards and legal liability for physicians after Cruzan. *J. Am. Med. Assoc.* 1990; **264**: 1846–1853.

83. Council on Scientific Affairs and Council on Ethical and Judicial Affairs. Persistent vegetative state and the decision to withdraw or withhold life support. *J. Am. Med. Assoc.* 1990; **263**: 426–430.

84. Council on Ethical and Judicial Affairs. Medical futility in end-of-life care: report. *J. Am. Med. Assoc.* 1999; **281**: 937–941.

85. American Academy of Neurology. Position of the American Academy of Neurology on certain aspects of the care and management of the persistent vegetative state patient. Adopted by the Executive Board, April 21, 1988, Cincinnati, Ohio. *Neurology* 1989; **39**: 125–126.

86. American College of Chest Physicians/ Society of Critical Care Medicine Consensus Panel. Ethical and moral guidelines for the initiation, continuation, and withdrawal of intensive care. *Chest* 1990; **97**: 949–958.

87. The Society of Critical Care Medicine Ethics Committee. Attitudes of critical care medicine professionals concerning forgoing life-sustaining treatments. *Crit. Care Med.* 1992; **20**: 320–326.

88. Asch, D.A., Hansen-Flaschen, J. & Lanken, P.N. Decisions to limit or continue life-sustaining treatment by critical care physicians in the United States: conflicts between physicians' practices and patients' wishes. *Am. J. Respir. Crit. Care Med.* 1995; **151**: 288–292.

89. Marik, P.E., Varon, J., Lisbon, A. & Reich, H.S. Physicians' own preferences to the limitation and withdrawal of life-sustaining therapy. *Resuscitation* 1999; **42**: 197–201.

90. Haynes, R.B., Devereaux, P.J. & Guyatt, G.H. Physicians' and patients' choices in evidence based practice. *Br. Med. J.* 2002; **324**: 1350.

91. Cook, D.J., Giacomini, M., Johnson, N. & Willms, D. Life support in the intensive care unit: a qualitative investigation of technological purposes. Canadian Critical Care Trials Group. *Cmaj* 1999; **161**: 1109–1113.

92. Sjokvist, P., Nilstun, T., Svantesson, M. & Berggren, L. Withdrawal of life support – who should decide? Differences in attitudes among the general public, nurses and physicians. *Intens. Care Med.* 1999; **25**: 949–954.

93. Geocadin, R.G., Buitrago, M.M., Torbey, M.T. *et al.* The impact of neurological prognostication by clinical examination, EEG and cortical evoked potentials on the withdrawal of life sustaining therapies in patients resuscitated from cardiac arrest. *Neurology* 2003; **60**: A362–A363.

94. The Quality Standards Subcommittee of the American Academy of Neurology. Practice parameters for determining brain death in adults (summary statement). *Neurology* 1995; **45**: 1012–1014.

95. Ad Hoc Committee of the Harvard Medical School. A definition of irreversible coma. Report to Examine the Definition of Brain Death. *J. Am. Med. Assoc.* 1968; **205**: 337–340.

96. Wijdicks, E.F. The diagnosis of brain death. *N. Engl. J. Med.* 2001; **344**: 1215–1221.

97. Wijdicks, E.F. Determining brain death in adults. *Neurology* 1995; **45**: 1003–1011.

98. Wijdicks, E.F., Hijdra, A., Young, G.B., Bassetti, C.L. & Wiebe, S. Practice parameter: prediction of outcome in comatose survivors after cardiopulmonary resuscitation (an evidence-based review), report of the Quality Standards Subcommittee of the American Academy of Neurology. *Neurology* 2006; **67**(2): 203–10.

51

Bringing it all together: brain-oriented postresuscitation critical care

Uwe Ebmeyer[1], Laurence M. Katz[2], Kevin R. Ward[3], and Robert W. Neumar[4]

[1] Clinic for Anaesthesiology and Intensive Therapy, Otto-von-Guericke
[2] Department of Emergency Medicine and University, Magdeburg, Germany
[3] University of North Carolina Department of Emergency Medicine, Virginia Commonwealth University, Detroit, MI, USA
[4] Department of Emergency Medicine, University of Pennsylvania School of Medicine, Philadelphia, PA, USA

Multiple brain-damaging processes occur both during cardiac arrest and after return of spontaneous circulation (ROSC). The first aspect, the actual arrest, is best treated by rapid institution of artificial circulation/ventilation and early ROSC. The details and physiologic background for these procedures are discussed in previous chapters. This chapter will focus on the early period after restoration of spontaneous circulation and treatment aimed to prevent or minimize postischemic brain damage after restoration of spontaneous circulation. The ultimate importance of the postreperfusion (after ROSC) phase for long-term outcome is often underestimated. Currently it is believed that the majority of brain-injuring processes occur not during the no-flow state (cardiac arrest) but during resuscitative reperfusion. This latter stage includes a trickle-, a low-, and a temporary high-flow period. Since significant injury occurs during the resuscitation period, there is a window of opportunity to intervene and affect outcome. Nevertheless, the development of treatments for the multifactorial postresuscitation syndrome is complex and time-consuming and has thus far led to disappointing results. Numerous treatments effective in the laboratory have failed or been shown to have an almost undetectable benefit in clinical studies. Large multicenter studies – the only way to detect small(er) benefits – are extremely expensive and time-consuming and require an enormous administrative and financial investment. Sometimes ethical concerns about obtaining informed consent make clinical resuscitation research increasingly difficult. Nevertheless, definitive clinical studies are the only way to prove the effectiveness of resuscitation and postresuscitation treatment; clinically relevant laboratory studies may only help to select those that are most promising.

Reperfusion

The regulation of cerebral perfusion is complex and only partially understood. Loss of perfusion or insufficient perfusion also results in loss of regulation. Reperfusion but not autoregulation is regained with the initiation of cardiopulmonary resuscitation (CPR). Safar and Bircher have summarized three steps that occur in the failure of early post-ROSC perfusion: (a) immediate multifocal no-flow; (b) transient global "reactive" hyperemia; and (c) delayed, prolonged global, and multifocal hypoperfusion. Later, blood flow either normalizes or hypoperfusion continues, depending on the progress of recovery. Many treatments after ROSC aim to optimize reperfusion and restore autoregulation.[1]

Animal studies have demonstrated that cerebral perfusion early after ROSC is marked by an initial transient period of hyperemia.[2] Although overall cerebral blood flow at this time is greater than normal, however, it is unevenly distributed and the needs of the microcirculation are probably not satisfied. After 15 to 30 minutes of reperfusion, global cerebral blood flow decreases and generalized hypoperfusion develops. This inability to sustain cerebral blood flow after a significant period of flow interruption is part of the no-reflow phenomenon.[3–5] Postischemic blood flow may be impaired for 18 to 24 hours, after which regional cerebral blood flow may either improve, correlating with functional recovery, or decline, correlating with progressive ischemic damage and cell death.[3,4,6] Physiologic mechanisms proposed to explain persistent postischemic hypoperfusion include vasoconstriction,[7,8] decreased red blood cell deformability,[7,9] increased platelet aggregation,[4,6,10] pericapillary cellular edema,[11] and abnormal calcium ion fluxes.[12,13] Intracranial pressure generally does not increase immediately after ROSC and therefore is not a major influence on early cerebral perfusion pressure and consequent cerebral blood flow.[14–18]

Maintenance of adequate cerebral perfusion pressure (dependent on the individual patient's baseline blood pressure before arrest) is a mainstay of postresuscitation care. In normal circumstances, cerebral blood flow is autoregulated such that it is independent of perfusion pressure over a wide range of blood pressures (between approximately 50 and 150 torr mean arterial pressure (MAP)).[19] After global brain ischemia, however, autoregulation is lost, and perfusion becomes dependent on arterial pressure.[20–23] Consequently, the occurrence of postischemic hypotension can severely compromise cerebral blood flow and may result in additional brain damage.[24] Therefore, after restoration of spontaneous circulation, arterial pressure should at least be rapidly normalized, based on prearrest blood pressure levels, by administering intravascular fluids and vasopressors as needed.[8,25]

Experimental evidence indicates that, after a prolonged insult, a transient period of moderate hypertension (MAP at 130 mm Hg) improves postischemic brain reperfusion and neurologic recovery.[8,26–28] Such transient hypertensive reperfusion may occur after resuscitation because of epinephrine loading during resuscitation, or may be induced by administration of vasopressors after ROSC. In dogs an induced brief period of hypertension (MAP 150 to 200 mm Hg for 1 to 5 minutes), followed by controlled normotensive blood pressure levels, abolished evidence of the immediate no-flow state[29,30] and correlated with improved outcome.[8,26,27] Nevertheless, there are potential risks to such an aggressive therapeutic approach: pharmacologically induced hypertension may not be tolerated by the ischemic heart,[11,31] and volume replacement therapy should optimally be guided by monitoring central venous pressure and pulmonary artery pressure. In animal studies, mildly elevated blood pressure (MAP 130 mm Hg) prolonged over the first 4 hours after resuscitation was well tolerated.[27] Although induced hypertension has not been tested in a formal clinical trial, early postarrest hypertension was found to correlate with good cerebral outcome in patients, whereas hypotension correlated with poor cerebral outcome.[32]

For control of early postresuscitation blood pressure, a titrated intravenous infusion of adrenaline or noradrenaline may be more effective than phenylephrine or dopamine. There is also some evidence that noradrenaline may be less arrhythmogenic.[1] Dobutamine may be preferred later for improvement of cardiac output and indirect blood pressure support.[1,33,34] Further, mechanical approaches can also support reperfusion. A spectrum of experimental possibilities, including assisted circulation with cardiopulmonary bypass or aortic balloon pumping, is under development and available for trial.

Emergency cardiopulmonary bypass seems to be a promising approach to accomplish all of the previously described blood flow-promoting treatments. Animal experiment work strongly suggests a beneficial effect of cardiopulmonary bypass after prolonged cardiac arrest.[35–38] Increased ability to resuscitate the heart and improved postresuscitation cardiac and neurologic function have been demonstrated in dogs when cardiopulmonary bypass was instituted after prolonged ischemic insults.[39,40] Use of this technique on an emergency basis via access to femoral vessels may allow restoration of spontaneous circulation in patients refractory to standard CPR and advanced cardiac life support, especially in cardiac arrest secondary to intoxication with central nervous system (CNS) depressant drugs. It may also improve reperfusion of the brain, thereby significantly ameliorating postischemic brain damage. Further, it may assist in the delivery of cerebral resuscitative medications that have cardiodepressant properties. Cardiopulmonary bypass appears to be one of the most effective techniques for rapid induction of therapeutic hypothermia (see discussion of hypothermia). Taken together, the beneficial effects of cardiopulmonary bypass are: (a) to help establish ROSC by optimizing coronary reperfusion; (b) to reduce cardiac work during the early period after ROSC; (c) to reduce the use of catecholamines and in turn reduce myocardial oxygen demand; (d) to allow safe delivery of treatments after ROSC; and (e) to be a potential bridge to heart surgery and heart transplant, if needed. Unfortunately, the practicality of initiating cardiopulmonary bypass during CPR has thus far been limited by the time required for vessel cannulation. Clinical feasibility studies have had limited success in improving outcome.[41] Nevertheless, selective clinical use of this technique may hold promise for future cardiac and cerebral resuscitation.[1,38,41–43]

During the last 10 years several other invasive flow-promoting resuscitation techniques were reevaluated. These include a cup-like direct mechanical ventricular assist device,[44] which requires a relatively large thoracotomy for placement, and a mini-plunger MID-CPR (minimally invasive CPR) placed directly on the pericardium inserted via a small thoracic incision.[45–47] This latter device was developed for actual resuscitation and not for promotion of postresuscitative blood flow. For several reasons, none of these modified CPR techniques has reached clinical acceptance or has been proven to be sufficiently effective in general use. Techniques to improve postischemic organ perfusion by modifying the rheologic characteristics of blood have also been studied.[48] Therapies tested in experimental models include hemodilution with crystalloids, colloids, and fluorocarbons;[49] anticoagulation and/or fibrinolysis with heparin and/or streptokinase;[49–51] blocking of platelet aggregation with prostaglandin inhibitors, such as indomethacin;[52] and the use of calcium entry-blocking drugs to improve deformability[7,9] of red blood cells and microcirculatory flow. The potential benefit of thrombolytic agents remains speculative. In a study of VF in pigs, however, application of hypertonic saline as well as hypertonic HES saline during CPR improved myocardial blood flow, ROSC rate, and survival rate significantly;[53] further studies are planned. New stroma-free hemoglobin (SFH) solutions, currently under development, have so far failed to improve outcome.[54,55] Nonetheless, diaspirin cross-linked hemoglobin (DCLHb) treatment in a 5-min VF, 10 min-CPR pig study increased the ROSC rate, and provided better myocardial O_2 delivery, venous blood O_2 content, and myocardial and cerebral perfusion pressure.[56] The author concluded that this effect was most likely related to improved coronary perfusion and myocardial oxygen delivery. The problem of maximizing blood flow by decreasing viscosity with hemodilution while avoiding a compromise of blood oxygen-carrying capacity has not been resolved. At present, none of these experimental therapies are ready for clinical trials.

Tissue oxygenation

Adequate oxygenation and ventilation of tissues are necessary to preserve cellular function and to allow postischemic reparative processes to occur. Normal arterial PO_2 levels should be maintained by using the lowest FIO_2 possible. Some controversy currently exists concerning the possible role of high arterial oxygen levels in the generation of postischemic, reperfusion-induced free radicals. In recent dog studies,[57] prolonged maximal O_2 administration (before and after arrest) worsened outcome. This was thought to be caused by a triggering of reoxygenation injury cascades induced by free radicals.[57–60] Nevertheless, hippocampal damage in rats resuscitated from cardiac arrest either with hyperoxia (FiO_2 1.0) or normoxia (FiO_2 0.21) did not differ.[61] Therefore, at this time no changes in current clinical practice are recommended.

Ventilation and acid–base balance

Although hyperventilation is still practiced, controversy as to its benefit has developed.[62,63] In pigs hyperventilated during resuscitation, coronary perfusion pressure and postresuscitative survival dropped significantly with higher ventilation rates.[64,65] It has been hypothesized that after prolonged cardiac arrest, early hyperventilation may create a reverse-steal phenomenon that would improve blood flow to the most severely insulted areas of the brain. In these areas, blood vessels lose CO_2-mediated vasomotor responsiveness, whereas vessels in less injured areas may maintain the ability to constrict as CO_2 is lowered. Thus, with hyperventilation, blood may be shunted to the worst areas. Although this modulation of blood flow has been shown to occur, improved outcome has not.[66] Data from patients with head injury suggest that hypocapnia, induced by hyperventilation, may decrease cerebral blood flow and increase differences in cerebral arteriovenous oxygen content, which may worsen neurologic outcome.[67] In brain trauma patients with Glasgow Coma Scale scores below 8, neurologic outcome was worse when $PaCO_2$ was controlled to 24 mm Hg compared to normocapnia (35 mm Hg).[68] With prolonged hyperventilation, cerebrospinal fluid and renal transport mechanisms attempt to compensate by retaining HCO_3.[69] After approximately 4 hours, the effectiveness of hyperventilation may gradually decline.[70] Currently, evidence is insufficient to recommend an optimal $PaCO_2$ level to be maintained.[71–75]

During the early postresuscitation period, washout of elevated tissue PCO_2 into the systemic circulation occurs. In this phase, hyperventilation may help correct postischemic tissue acidosis by enhancing excretion of the CO_2 load generated during ischemia and by the administration of CO_2-generating buffers during CPR.

If hypoperfusion is prolonged after ROSC, the increased tissue CO_2 and the associated acidemia may require pharmacologic treatment. Several buffer solutions are currently in clinical use and are under investigation. Sodium bicarbonate, used during CPR since the early 1960s, is now subjected to critical investigation because CO_2 is produced during a reaction with hydrogen ions. Beside other potential side effects, this additional hypercarbic load may theoretically depress myocardial resuscitability, although animal studies of HCO_3 administration after 5 or 10 minutes of ventricular fibrillation found no harm to the heart and possible benefit to the brain.[76–78] Bicarbonate may only be advantageous when combined with epinephrine; this possibility may not have received enough attention in past studies.[76,78] Other potential buffer agents, such as Tribonate ($NaHCO_3$ + THAM + phosphate acetate) and

Carbicarb ($Na_2CO_3 + NaHCO_3$), are available. In animal studies, low dose Carbicarb (3 ml/kg) administered during resuscitation from asphyxial cardiac arrest attenuated acidosis, improved resuscitation, and reduced neurologic deficits and the number of dead hippocampal neurons.[79] Currently, clinical data are insufficient to support the effectiveness of the use of these drugs during CPR.

In general, buffer solutions should be withheld as an initial intervention during CPR, especially after short arrest periods. When arrest or CPR duration is prolonged, buffer administration may be useful and should be tested in a clinical trial.

After restoration of spontaneous circulation, buffer therapy may be beneficial. Bicarbonate deficit can be estimated by the following formula:

$$\text{bicarbonate deficit} = 0.3 \times \text{body weight (kg)} \times \text{base deficit}$$

Moderate acidemia should be treated initially with an amount of bicarbonate that is only half of the calculated deficit, after which the acid–base status should be corrected over the next few hours. Profound metabolic acidemias should be treated with a bicarbonate bolus of about 1 meq/kg (50 to 150 meq) followed by closely controlled titration. Outcome studies testing the benefit of postresuscitation buffer treatment are needed.

Immobilization and sedation

In the comatose patient the brain responds to external stimuli such as physical examination or airway suctioning with increases in cerebral metabolism and intracranial pressure. This elevated regional brain metabolism requires increased regional cerebral blood flow at a time when oxygen supply and demand may be precariously balanced. Protection from afferent sensory stimuli with administration of titrated doses of sedative-anesthetic drugs and (carefully titrated) muscle relaxants may protect this balance and improve the chance for neuronal recovery, although clinical trials are needed to support this hypothesis.

Anticonvulsant therapy

Seizure activity can increase brain metabolism 300 to 400%.[80–82] This extreme increase in metabolic demand may tip the tissue oxygen supply : demand balance, causing unfavorable neurologic consequences. Clinical evidence confirms this effect after cardiac arrest (Brain Resuscitation

Clinical Trial I, unpublished data). Outcome is worse if convulsions occur at any time within the first 3 days after resuscitation. Not surprisingly, the number of seizures correlates with poor outcome. Although controversy exists about the prophylactic use of anticonvulsant drugs, it is generally agreed that after any signs of seizure activity, anticonvulsive therapy should be administered immediately. Commonly used drugs include barbiturates, phenytoin, and benzodiazepines. Phenytoin has been reported to improve neurologic recovery after experimental global brain ischemia through postulated mechanisms independent of its anticonvulsant effect, such as membrane stabilization.[83,84] Potential beneficial effects of barbiturates are discussed later in this chapter.[55]

Other metabolic factors

Hyperglycemia (observed or experimentally induced) before cardiac arrest has detrimental effects on neurologic outcome.[85] The higher glucose supply available during ischemia and low-flow states serves as a reservoir for continued anaerobic metabolism and results in increased lactate production.[86] Although control of hyperglycemia before arrest is not feasible, blood glucose levels after ROSC can be controlled. In experimental models of forebrain ischemia, hyperglycemia after insult was shown to exacerbate ischemic brain dysfunction.[87–89] In a rat study of asphyxial cardiac arrest, however, administration of glucose during reperfusion did not worsen neurological outcome, most likely because glucose is required for recovery of cellular metabolism after ROSC.[90] Frequently, blood glucose levels observed immediately after resuscitation are elevated, probably because of severe stress and catecholamine release. Reports of detrimental neurologic outcomes in patients with hyperglycemia after ROSC probably reflect the correlation with prolonged resuscitation time rather than a primary effect of the hyperglycemia.[91] Although human studies have not clearly demonstrated a correlation between elevated glucose levels and the effect on neurologic outcome, some clinicians now recommend that at least highly elevated blood glucose levels should be treated aggressively with insulin.

Interestingly, experiments in rats have shown that postischemic high dose insulin treatment may reduce neurologic damage[89,92,93] independent of its glucose-lowering effect. Insulin may also be beneficial for normalization of cerebral blood flow, metabolism, and cardiac function, as well as postulated reparative effects. It seems rational to combine glucose (metabolic substrate for tissue repair) with insulin, to support transport mechanisms and to avoid hypoglycemic side effects. Recently, it has been demonstrated in rats that postresuscitation treatment with a combination of glucose, 1 g/kg, and insulin, 1.2 µg/kg, improved outcome significantly as compared to treatment with placebo, low dose insulin only, or glucose only.[90]

In contrast to the uncertainty concerning the effect of elevated blood glucose levels after cardiac arrest, prolonged hypoglycemia is detrimental.[90,94,95] Hypoglycemia interrupts the autoregulation of cerebral blood flow, disturbs cerebral metabolism, and compromises membrane stability. Thus hypoglycemia after resuscitation must be avoided.

Neurologic protection, preservation, and resuscitation barbiturates

Among the first potential neuroprotective agents to be tested, barbiturates appeared promising because of their ability to reduce cerebral metabolism,[96] edema,[97] intracranial pressure,[26] seizure activity,[98] and damage induced by focal and incomplete ischemia.[99–101] Barbiturates also seemed to improve postischemic brain oxygen supply:demand ratios,[102] cell energy charge,[103] and cyclic adenosine monophosphate (AMP) stores,[104,105] and to lower accumulation of free fatty acids.[106,107] The most influential experimental work indicating that barbiturate administration after complete global brain ischemia ameliorated neurologic damage was performed on rhesus monkeys in the mid 1970s. Even though these studies had methodological problems with blood pressure control, they stimulated studies of clinical feasibility[108] and pilot trials of thiopental loading in comatose CPR survivors,[109] which indicated that high doses of this drug might be administered safely, and also suggested a beneficial effect. A randomized clinical trial of thiopental loading (with up to 30 mg/kg[5,110–112]) between 1979 and 1983 did not show statistically significant differences in neurologic outcome between control and treatment groups.[113–115] On the basis of these data, high-dose thiopental loading has not been recommended for routine clinical use after cardiac arrest. The story may not be completely closed, however, because several studies in dogs have shown a significant improvement in histological outcome with high-dose barbiturate loading (90 mg/kg) after cardiac arrest.[55,116]

Steroids

Commonly administered to patients with intracranial pathologic conditions, steroids may stabilize lysosomal membranes and prevent release of lytic enzymes,[48,117] stabilize mitochondria and preserve adenosine triphosphate (ATP) synthesis,[8,118] inhibit release of free fatty acids from cell membranes,[119,120] and scavenge free radicals generated during postischemic reperfusion.[120] All of these proposed mechanisms contribute to the rationale supporting the use of steroids. Although there is evidence that steroids are beneficial for patients with intracranial tumor-related cerebral edema,[119,121] no clinical evidence documents their efficacy for treatment of brain ischemia.[121]

Methylprednisolone, one of the most widely used steroids, has been shown potentially to improve functional and histological outcome after blunt spinal injuries,[122–127] and when used in dogs after cardiac arrest (as part of a multicomponent treatment) it improved outcome slightly (see discussion of combination treatment).

The effectiveness of 21-aminosteroids ("lazaroids") after global ischemia is still under investigation. Animal models of trauma and focal brain ischemia treated with aminosteroids showed improved outcome.[128–130] After cardiac arrest, however, 21-aminosteroids improved neurologic outcome only when given as a pretreatment.[131,132] New 21-aminosteroids are currently under investigation, but sufficient data are not yet available.[133,134]

Calcium channel-blocking drugs

The potential beneficial effect of calcium channel blockers after cardiac arrest has been demonstrated in (at least) four organ systems:

1. Blood: decreased platelet aggregation, increased red blood cell (RBC) deformability, and decreased blood viscosity[7,9,90]
2. Vessels: decreased vasoconstriction[135,136]
3. Neurons: decreased calcium entry resulting in improved ATP production and decreased production of cytotoxic chemicals[12,137–140]
4. Systemic circulation: improved oxygen supply:demand ratio in myocardium and other tissues.[141]

Postischemic cerebral blood flow may be improved through amelioration of cerebral vasospasm and redistribution of regional flow.[142] It appears that certain calcium channel blockers have a greater effect on cerebral vessels than on peripheral vessels because cerebral vascular muscle tone is more dependent on the entry of extra-cellular calcium.[143] In controlled, blinded animal studies, lidoflazine improved neurologic recovery in dogs when administered after cardiac arrest.[18,144] Nimodipine had the same result in monkeys after cerebral ischemia caused by hypotension and neck tourniquet compression.[135]

Nevertheless, well-conducted clinical trials did not confirm these promising animal experimental findings. No difference was found between patients treated with lidoflazine or standard therapy after cardiac arrest.[145] The reason for these disparities in clinical trials is uncertain, but the beneficial neuroresuscitative properties of these drugs may be neutralized by their deleterious cardiovascular effects. Clinical trials of nimodipine and flunarizine, two other experimental calcium channel blockers, also failed to show evidence of improvement.[96,146]

Temperature control

It is well established that brain temperature before, during, and after cerebral ischemia has a major influence on cerebral outcome.[147–149] Extensive animal experimentation, as well as clinical case reports (especially of drowning victims) as early as the 1970s have shown that hypothermia improves neurological functional outcome after cardiac arrest. The effectiveness and safety of hypothermia after cardiac arrest seems to be maximal between 32 and 34°C, a level termed mild hypothermia.[22,148,150] Temperatures below 32 °C do not seem to increase neuroprotection, but are known to increase the side effects of hypothermia, including increased blood viscosity, decreased cardiac output, and increased susceptibility to infection. The beneficial laboratory data on mild hypothermia was so impressive that a push to have mild hypothermia used as a treatment for cardiac arrest has been advocated for years.[151] Two well-controlled, prospective clinical trials demonstrated that mild (32–34 °C) hypothermia induced as early as possible during cardiac arrest and resuscitation improved neurological outcome.[152–154] Although hypothermia is an effective method of suppressing cerebral metabolic activity, its beneficial effects on cerebral ischemia are believed to differ from CNS depressant drugs. Mild hypothermia not only attenuates the deleterious effects of reperfusion disease,[155–157] but it may have an active role in improving cerebral blood flow and increasing expression and production of brain-derived neurotrophic factor (BDNF).[158,159]

Unfortunately, the beneficial effect of hypothermia on eurological outcome after cardiac arrest is time-dependent. The earlier that hypothermia is induced during cardiac arrest, the more effective it will be in improving neurological outcome.[160] Interestingly, patients early after cardiac arrest have a slight decrease in body temperature, so the magnitude of temperature decrease to reach therapeutic mild hypothermia is relatively small.[161] Normal counter-regulatory mechanisms, such as shivering, however, can slow the process of reaching a therapeutic level.[162] Recent research suggests that the brain's thermostat can be pharmacologically reset to a lower control temperature to speed the rate of attaining therapeutic hypothermia.[163,164] In addition, current therapies are available to overwhelm these counter-regulatory mechanisms and achieve therapeutic hypothermia.[165,166] The precise duration of hypothermia necessary to attain its maximal benefit on neurological outcome has not been established; however, it appears that a minimum of 24 hours of forced mild hypothermia is required to assure that the benefit of therapy is long lasting.[167,168] The optimal method and rate of rewarming after hypothermia has also not been well studied; it is apparent, however, that rapid rewarming (greater than 0.5 °C/hour) may be deleterious to neurological outcome.[169,170] Rewarming is a critical component of therapeutic hypothermia, as several animal studies have documented that even modest hyperthermia worsens histological outcome after an ischemic insult and may negate many of its beneficial properties.[149] Since cerebral metabolic rate changes by about 8% per degree Celsius change in body temperature,[171–173] and regional cerebral metabolic rate determines regional blood flow requirements, elevation of temperature above normal creates the possibility for a significant imbalance between oxygen supply and demand. In addition, the denaturing effect of hyperthermia on proteins may exacerbate structural and biochemical damage. In general, hyperthermia in the postischemic period must be treated aggressively to reduce secondary brain injury.

Cerebral regeneration

The focus of cardiac arrest research has been on reducing brain injury during reperfusion, a field of study referred to as cerebral resuscitation.[174,175] Nevertheless, until recently there has been no research on developing therapies once brain damage has occurred, a phenomenon referred to as cerebral regeneration. The potential to utilize stem cells to repair or replace an injured region of the brain is an area of intense research. Stem cells are broadly categorized as being either embryonic or organ-specific in origin. Oncological research on cell differentiation led to the consideration that embryonic tissue may have therapeutic value for organ repair.[176] The brain is a particularly attractive organ for transplant experiments, because it is historically and clinically considered to have minimal regenerative capabilities after structural damage.[177,178] Experiments with fetal tissue have contributed immensely to the understanding of embryonic stem cell physiology and the potential for tissue repair, especially in the

Table 51.1. Experimental postresuscitation combination treatments with clinical orientation taken from an animal laboratory protocol of the International Resuscitation Research Center (University of Pittsburgh, PA)

		Normothermic	Hypothermic	Comb. 1	Comb. 2	Comb. 3	Comb. 4	Comb. 5	Comb. 6
Temperature	°C	37.5	34	34	34	34	34	34	34
Hematocrit	%	40	40	40	40	30	12	40	35
p_aCO_2	mmHg	30	30	30	30	40	30	30	35
Blood pressure (MAP)	mmHg	100	100	130	130	100	130	130	130
Barbiturate	mg/kg	–	–	90	30	30	–	30	30
Phenytoin	mg/kg	–	–	–	15	15	–	15	15
Methylprednisolone	mg/kg	–	–	–	130	130	–	130	130
Deferoxamine	mg/kg	–	–	–	–	–	–	–	185
$MgSO_4$	mg/kg	–	–	–	–	–	–	290	160
Vitamin C	mg/kg	–	–	–	–	–	–	200	200
Stroma-free hemoglobin	ml/kg	–	–	–	–	–	12.5	–	–

Source: From Ebmeyer, U, Safar, P, Radovsky, A. *et al*. Exploratory studies of effective combination treatments for cerebral resuscitation from cardiac arrest in dogs [partially unpublished].[55]

brain.[179,180] However, in addition to ethical concerns and mechanical limitations of transplantation, fetal tissue is composed of heterogeneous embryonic stem cells, making interpretation of transplant experiments complex. Identification of neural stem cells and neurogenesis in the adult brain has allowed for detailed in vitro analysis of neuronal stem cell development and differentiation as well as in vivo transplant experiments.[181] The advances resulting from studying neurogenesis have brought stem cell transplantation closer to reality as a therapy for tissue repair in the brain. The recognized multipotential of adult stem cells has raised enthusiasm for the notion that stem cells from adult organs aside from the brain may provide unique mechanistic information and therapies for a variety of disease processes, including brain injury.[182–185]

Combination therapies

All novel treatments described in this chapter have shown promise of improvement in outcome in laboratory studies but, except for mild hypothermia, have failed to bring a breakthrough in clinical practice. The complexity of pathologic mechanisms before and after cardiac arrest makes it unreasonable to believe that the treatment of an isolated mechanism could bring a therapeutic breakthrough. Perhaps future research on clinical treatment approaches should simultaneously target at least several of the mechanisms in the postresuscitation syndrome by combining the most promising and clinically relevant results from mechanism-oriented research. Intensive animal research – preferably with outcome models in

large animals – should be performed before initiating clinical trials. An example of this is the research strategy at the International Resuscitation Research Center. In a recently performed series of dog outcome studies[54,55,186] the effects of various combination treatments aimed at treating numerous physical and pharmacologic components of the postresuscitation syndrome were tested by using an established intensive care model (Table 51.1). All components included were previously reported as significantly beneficial for improving outcome in other models. A stepwise combination of physical (hemodilution, hypothermia, normocapnia, initial hypertension) as well as pharmacologic (steroid, barbiturate, anticonvulsive, antimetabolic) interventions was used. Combining these treatments improved outcome only to a limited extent. Drug interactions and combination side effects may be the reason for the plateau in improvement and partially worsened outcome in these highly complex treatment groups.

Hemodynamic support

The eventual outcome of cardiac arrest has only recently been shown to be influenced by complex postresuscitation hemodynamic derangements.[187,188] Several issues may explain why promising therapies from animal studies have not translated into significant improvement in neurologic outcome in humans. First, downtimes in humans may be underestimated so that the total ischemia time, including the low-flow state of CPR, may be outside the effective window for neuronal recovery. This can only be solved by increasing access to and response by emergency medical services. Second, in contrast to laboratory studies of cardiac arrest where animals receive immediate and aggressive postresuscitation care, hemodynamic support for initial survivors of cardiac arrest is often much more variable and less aggressive. Because of the historically poor neurologic prognosis of patients resuscitated from cardiac arrest, many clinicians do not provide these individuals with aggressive care. Nevertheless, because it is not possible immediately after resuscitation to predict definitively what the ultimate neurologic outcome will be, patients should initially be subjected to aggressive postresuscitation management for at least 24 hours. This should include attention to management in global terms; that is, to consider effects on other organ systems that may ultimately affect the heart and brain.

As already stated, the heterogeneous underlying causes of cardiac arrest in humans present a tremendous challenge: their treatment clearly influences the outcome of this insult. Since cardiac arrest is a symptom rather than a disorder *per se*, it is essential to identify and treat any underlying disease (e.g., respiratory diseases, pulmonary embolus, myocardial ischemia, toxic agents, and metabolic abnormalities) after ROSC in order to prevent rearrest.

In terms of oxygen delivery (DO_2), oxygen consumption (VO_2), and oxygen debt, most patients are in a state of shock after ROSC.[187–190] Postresuscitation shock differs from primary cardiogenic shock, however, because of two important events: (a) it is preceded by a period of systemic no-flow and/or extremely low flow during cardiac arrest and CPR; and (b) large doses of catecholamines are usually administered during CPR, which, together with increased output of endogenous catecholamines, may result in further global oxygen debt, impaired myocardial function, and impaired ability to extract oxygen.[187,188] To what extent these abnormalities are reversible is apparently related to the events just described. In studies of other forms of shock, survival and degree of multiorgan failure are found to be related to the cumulative oxygen debt.[190] For a 70-kg man, an oxygen debt of less than $4100 \, ml/m^2$ is rarely if ever fatal; 50% mortality occurs at an oxygen debt of $4900 \, ml/m^2$; and mortality reaches 95% when oxygen debt exceeds $5800 \, ml/m^2$. Oxygen debt is difficult to calculate in humans after cardiac arrest since baseline VO_2 is unknown and the duration of cardiac arrest and prearrest events is also often not known. Assuming a baseline VO_2 of $120 \, ml/min/m^2$, however, a 30-minute cardiac arrest will result in an oxygen debt of $3600 \, ml/m^2$, which is not likely to present a serious problem with dysfunction of many extracerebral organs. Nevertheless, Rivers *et al.* have shown that additional oxygen debt accumulates during the postresuscitation period, which may lead to multiorgan dysfunction.[187,188] Some problems may be due to inappropriate use of catecholamines and reliance on inadequate monitoring (i.e., blood pressure and pulse rate) to guide therapy, as well as insufficient attention to ensuring adequate oxygen transport to the rest of the body.

After ROSC, it is important to determine whether the patient is evolving a myocardial infarction. Standard 12-lead and right-sided electrocardiograms (ECGs) should be obtained as soon as possible to search for ongoing ischemia. Without an appropriate history, it may be difficult to determine whether ischemia showing on the ECG is the cause or result of the cardiac arrest. Treatment for the post-arrest patient evolving a myocardial infarction is obviously optimized if a well-thought out multidisciplinary approach is in place. Patients who have had less than 10 minutes of CPR without evidence of CPR-induced trauma and who are not in vasopressor cardiogenic shock should be considered for thrombolytic therapy.[191] Patients who have had more than 10 minutes of CPR or significant CPR trauma should be considered for immediate angioplasty. Without effective revascularization strategies, myocardial dysfunction is likely to worsen and lead to hypoperfusion of many organs, including the brain. If ischemia is continuing, use of vasopressors to maintain perfusion pressures may increase myocardial oxygen demand above supply, which might result in extension of the infarct or promote dysrhythmias and lead to rearrest. Other hemodynamic supporting measures, such as intraaortic balloon pumping or percutaneous cardiopulmonary bypass, should be considered to increase oxygen delivery and utilization without placing a further burden on the ischemic heart. Heparin and aspirin may be given if there is no evidence of hemorrhage or profound prolonged hypertension. Nitrates and β-blockers as adjunctive therapy are best used when guided by invasive hemodynamic monitoring.

Defects in oxygen utilization, which are observed to various degrees after ROSC, will alter the relationship between VO_2 and DO_2.[187,188] Many patients have venous hyperoxia at lower ranges of DO_2, indicating impaired extraction.[187] Thus, mixed venous oxygen saturation (S_VO_2) will be higher and VO_2 will be lower than values predicted at any given DO_2 under normal conditions. This state indicates ongoing ischemia, shown by continued production of lactic acid, and decreased survival. Notably, these abnormalities cannot be predicted by simple measurements of blood pressure, heart rate, central venous pressure, or initial lactate levels.[187–189,192]

Even though oxygen debt after ROSC cannot be calculated accurately, the debt can be repaid with variable success if the abnormalities described above are taken into consideration. Because of possible decreases in metabolic demand after resuscitation, the debt may be repaid at VO_2 values that are lower than those at baseline. VO_2 values below 90 ml/min/m² are associated with 100% mortality at 24 hours after arrest.[187,188] Inadequate VO_2 during the postresuscitation period may be due largely to insufficient DO_2 and to microcirculatory defects. Critically ill patients with DO_2 below 330 ml/min/m² show progressive lactic acidosis.[189,193] In a specific study of initial survivors of cardiac arrest, those who did not survive to hospital discharge had a maximal DO_2 of 165 ml/min/m², whereas survivors had a DO_2 of 495 ml/min/m².[187,188]

Derangements in oxygen transport are best detected and treated by appropriate hemodynamic monitoring. Pulmonary artery catheter monitoring, particularly with oximetric capabilities, provides the most useful information, including calculations of DO_2, VO_2, and oxygen extraction ratios. If this technique is not available, central venous pressure (CVP) monitoring at the level of the right atrium with continuous or intermittent monitoring of central venous oxygen saturation ($S_{cv}O_2$) is appropriate, even though cardiac output cannot be measured directly. Changes in output may be estimated from changes in S_VO_2, blood pressure, heart rate, CVP, and lactic acid. In the future, non-invasive bioimpedance equipment[194] and gastric tonometry to monitor DO_2 to the visceral organs[195] may aid recognition of decompensation or inadequate resuscitation.

$S_{cv}O_2$ and S_VO_2 have been helpful in monitoring patients, because patients may show normal vital signs even with diminished tissue oxygenation.[196–199] Many of these patients will show abnormally low S_VO_2, which is correlated with increasing lactic acidosis and continuing shock.[192] S_VO_2 decreases when DO_2 has been compromised by declines in hemoglobin, cardiac output, or oxygen saturation or if VO_2 has exceeded supply. As already stated, however, S_VO_2 and $S_{cv}O_2$ alone should not be the sole therapeutic guide, because patients with normal or elevated values may have optimal or suboptimal DO_2 with a low VO_2 because of gross impairments of oxygen extraction. Sequential monitoring of lactate is helpful, with a goal of clearance of 2.5%/hour, which has been associated with improved survival.[193,200]

In postresuscitation cardiogenic shock, it may be difficult to increase DO_2 levels to above normal values (greater than 600 ml O_2/min per m²) as suggested in other shock states.[201,202] Nevertheless, in studies in acute myocardial infarction with cardiogenic shock, carefully monitored aggressive dobutamine and fluid administration can increase DO_2 to about 400 ml/min per m², which increases VO_2 above 100 ml/min/m² and improves survival.[189] When

delivery-independent VO_2 is reached in this manner, further increases in DO_2 will not result in further significant changes in VO_2. Large increases in S_VO_2 will be seen, however, indicating improved oxygen availability.

Increasing catecholamines in patients with limited cardiac reserve may be problematic because they may adversely affect myocardial oxygen demand and exacerbate defects in oxygen utilization. When catecholamines are the only option, volume status should be optimized with a combination of crystalloids and colloids, guided by pulmonary artery or central venous pressures. With volume status optimized, dobutamine and/or noradrenaline may be more effective than dopamine in enhancing oxygen delivery and utilization.[189,203] Supplemental cortisol may also be beneficial and decrease the need for vasopressors, given the significant impairment of adrenal function found in the postresuscitation period.[204,205]

Vasodilators may be required in the postresuscitation state to control hypertension or improve flow by reducing afterload. Since hypertension may occur when volume is depleted, preload should be optimized before vasodilator therapy is instituted.[206,207] Figure 51.1 provides a postresuscitation hemodynamic algorithm based on goal-directed therapy, taking into account that pulmonary artery monitoring may not be available. Until routine monitoring of cerebral arteriovenous oxygen and lactate gradients can be made via such methods as jugular venous bulb catheterization, this goal-directed therapy may be the best readily available alternative to promote adequate cerebral oxygen delivery.[208] Therefore, the algorithm may be viewed as a neuronal salvaging strategy and should help provide adequate oxygen delivery to both cerebral and extracerebral organs and repay oxygen debt, thus potentially preventing development of systemic inflammatory response syndrome and multiorgan dysfunction and failure. The effect of any additional salvaging agents or strategies on these hemodynamic goals should be taken into account. Notably, no therapy will be successful if it is administered outside the effective window.

Summary

For more than 40 years the multifactorial cerebral postresuscitation syndrome has been intensely investigated experimentally and clinically; nevertheless, the mechanisms and interactions underlying this syndrome remain poorly understood. Treatment trials have focused on only one or a few components of the complex of reactions. Hemodynamic resuscitation guided by oxygen transport measures has been largely neglected, although attention to

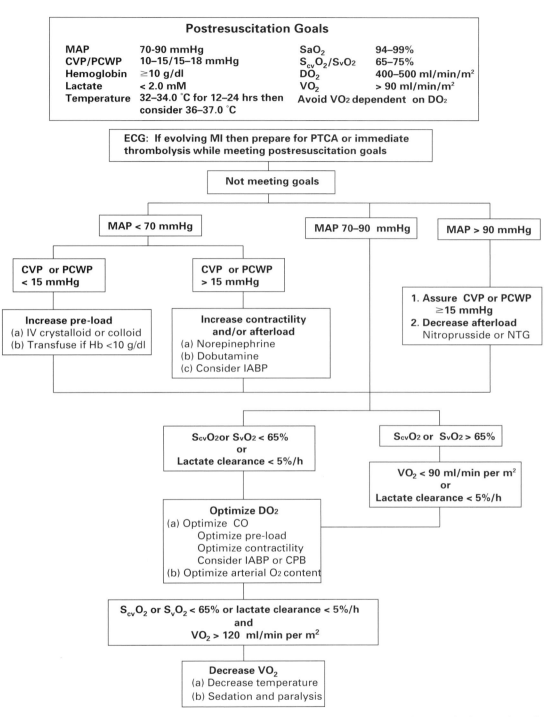

Fig. 51.1. Postresuscitation goal-directed treatment algorithm. These suggested targets and means of achieving them should begin to be instituted as soon as possible after ROSC to prevent further oxygen debt and the development of multiorgan system dysfunction and failure. This should be viewed as a neuronal salvaging strategy in itself. All other neuronal salvaging agents or strategies should take into account how they will affect oxygen transport and utilization characteristics of the body as a whole. PCWP, pulmonary capillary wedge pressure; PTCA, percutaneous transluminal coronary angioplasty; NTG, nitroglycerin; IABP, intraaortic balloon pumping; CPB, cardiopulmonary bypass.[25,209] (From ref. 25 and 209.)

these variables alone might reduce the number of deaths in the immediate postresuscitation period and the frequency of multiorgan dysfunction later in the course, and also improve neurologic outcome in some individuals. For fully effective neuronal salvaging, early attention to the consequence of treatment on oxygen transport to all other organ systems is critical. In addition, mild induced hypothermia should become the standard of care for the neurological treatment of patients who remain comatose after resuscitation from cardiac arrest as long as cardiovascular function is stabilized. Since it is unlikely that a single pharmacologic "magic bullet" will ever be found to relieve this complex syndrome, current research focuses on combination treatments. With the combination of treatments reviewed in this chapter, improvement in neurologic outcome may be possible (Table 51.1).

REFERENCES

1. Safar, P. & Bircher, N.G. Cardiopulmonary Cerebral Resuscitation. 3rd edn. London: W.B. Saunders Company Ltd, 1988.
2. Pulsinelli, W.A., Levy, D.E. & Duffy, T.E. Regional cerebral blood flow and glucose metabolism following transient forebrain ischemia. *Ann. Neurol.* 1982; **11**(5): 499–502.
3. Ames, A., III, Wright, R.L., Kowada, M., Thurston, J.M. & Majno, G. Cerebral ischemia. II. The no-reflow phenomenon. *Am. J. Pathol.* 1968; **52**(2): 437–453.
4. Obrenovitch, T.P. & Hallenbeck, J.M. Platelet accumulation in regions of low blood flow during the postischemic period. *Stroke* 1985; **16**(2): 224–234.
5. Rogers, M.C. & Kirsch, J.R. Current concepts in brain resuscitation. *J. Am. Med. Assoc.* 1989; **261**(21): 3143–3147.
6. Hossmann, V., Hossmann, K.A. & Takagi, S. Effect of intravascular platelet aggregation on blood recirculation following prolonged ischemia of the cat brain. *J. Neurol.* 1980; **222**(3): 159–170.
7. Van Nueten, J.M. & Vanhoutte, P.M. Improvement of tissue perfusion with inhibitors of calcium ion influx. *Biochem. Pharmacol.* 1980; **29**(4): 479–481.
8. White, B.C., Aust, S.D., Arfors, K.E. & Aronson, L.D. Brain injury by ischemic anoxia: hypothesis extension – a tale of two ions? *Ann. Emerg. Med.* 1984; **13**(9 Pt 2):862–867.
9. De Cree, J., De Cock, W., Geukens, H., De Clerck, F., Beerens, M. & Verhaegen, H. The rheological effects of cinnarizine and flunarizine in normal and pathologic conditions. *Angiology* 1979; **30**(8): 505–515.
10. Kleihues, P., Hossmann, K.A., Pegg, A.E., Kobayashi, K. & Zimmermann, V. Resuscitation of the monkey brain after one hour complete ischemia. III. Indications of metabolic recovery. *Brain Res.* 1975; **95**(1): 61–73.
11. Klatzo, I. Brain oedema following brain ischaemia and the influence of therapy. *Br. J. Anaesth.* 1985; **57**(1): 18–22.
12. Siesjo, B.K. Cell damage in the brain: a speculative synthesis. *J. Cereb. Blood Flow Metab.* 1981; **1**(2): 155–185.
13. Siesjo, B.K. Mechanisms of ischemic brain damage. *Crit. Care Med.* 1988; **16**(10): 954–963.
14. Graham, D.I. The pathology of brain ischaemia and possibilities for therapeutic intervention. *Br. J. Anaesth.* 1985; **57**(1): 3–17.
15. Jackson, D.L. & Dole, W.P. Total cerebral ischemia: a new model system for the study of post-cardiac arrest brain damage. *Stroke* 1979; **10**(1): 38–43.
16. Miller, C.L., Alexander, K., Lampard, D.G., Brown, W.A. & Griffiths, R. Local cerebral blood flow following transient cerebral ischemia. II. Effect of arterial PCO_2 on reperfusion following global ischemia. *Stroke* 1980; **11**(5): 542–548.
17. Snyder, J.V., Nemoto, E.M., Carroll, R.G. & Safar, P. Global ischemia in dogs: intracranial pressures, brain blood flow and metabolism. *Stroke* 1975; **6**(1): 21–27.
18. Vaagenes, P., Cantadore, R., Safar, P. *et al.* Amelioration of brain damage by lidoflazine after prolonged ventricular fibrillation cardiac arrest in dogs. *Crit. Care Med.* 1984; **12**(10): 846–855.
19. Shapiro, H.M. Intracranial hypertension: therapeutic and anesthetic considerations. *Anesthesiology* 1975; **43**(4): 445–471.
20. Safar, P. & Kochanek, P. Cerebral blood flow promotion after prolonged cardiac arrest. *Crit. Care Med.* 2000; **28** (8): 3104–3106.
21. Safar, P. Cerebral resuscitation. *Ann. Emerg. Med.* 1993; **22**(4): 759.
22. Safar, P. Resuscitation of the ischemic brain. In Albin, M.S., edn. *Textbook of Neuroanesthesia with Neurosurgical and Neuroscience Prospectives.* New York: McGraw-Hill, 1997: 557–593.
23. Stocchetti, N., Maas, A.I., Chieregato, A. & van der Plas, A.A. Hyperventilation in head injury: a review. *Chest* 2005; **127**(5): 1812–1827.
24. Cantu, R.C., Ames, A., III, Di Giacinto, G. & Dixon, J. Hypotension: a major factor limiting recovery from cerebral ischemia. *J. Surg. Res.* 1969; **9**(9): 525–529.
25. Neumar, R.W. & Ward, K.R. Adult resuscitation. In: Walls, R.N., Marx, J.A., Hockberger, R.S., eds. *Rosen's Emergency Medicine: Concepts and Clinical Practice.* St. Louis: Elsevier Science, 2002: 64–82.
26. Nemoto, E.M., Erdmann, W., Strong, E., Rao, G.R. & Moossy, J. Regional brain PO_2 after global ischemia in monkeys: evidence for regional differences in critical perfusion pressures. *Stroke* 1979; **10**(1): 44–52.
27. Sterz, F., Leonov, Y., Safar, P., Radovsky, A., Tisherman, S.A. & Oku, K. Hypertension with or without hemodilution after cardiac arrest in dogs. *Stroke* 1990; **21**(8): 1178–1184.
28. Wise, G., Sutter, R. & Burkholder, J. The treatment of brain ischemia with vasopressor drugs. *Stroke* 1972; **3**(2): 135–140.
29. Leonov, Y., Sterz, F., Safar, P., Johnson, D.W., Tisherman, S.A. & Oku, K. Hypertension with hemodilution prevents multifocal cerebral hypoperfusion after cardiac arrest in dogs. *Stroke* 1992; **23**(1): 45–53.

30. Sterz, F., Leonov, Y., Safar, P. *et al.* Multifocal cerebral blood flow by Xe-CT and global cerebral metabolism after prolonged cardiac arrest in dogs. Reperfusion with open-chest CPR or cardiopulmonary bypass. *Resuscitation* 1992; **24**(1): 27–47.

31. Bleyaert, A.L., Sands, P.A., Safar, P. *et al.* Augmentation of postischemic brain damage by severe intermittent hypertension. *Crit. Care Med.* 1980; **8**(1): 41–47.

32. Spivey, W.H., Abramson, N.S. & Safar, P. Correlation of blood pressure with mortality and neurologic recovery in comatose postresuscitation patients. *Ann. Emerg. Med.* 1991; **20**: 453.

33. Brillman, J.A., Sanders, A.B., Otto, C.W., Fahmy, H., Bragg, S. & Ewy, G.A. Outcome of resuscitation from fibrillatory arrest using epinephrine and phenylephrine in dogs. *Crit. Care Med.* 1985; **13**(11): 912–913.

34. Otto, C.W., Yakaitis, R.W., Redding, J.S. & Blitt, C.D. Comparison of dopamine, dobutamine, and epinephrine in CPR. *Crit. Care Med.* 1981; **9**(5): 366.

35. Cantadore, R., Vaagenes, P. & Safar, P. Cardiopulmonary bypass for resuscitation after prolonged cardiac arrest in dogs [Abstract]. *Ann. Emerg. Med.* 1984; **13**: 398.

36. Safar, P., Abramson, N.S., Angelos, M. *et al.* Emergency cardiopulmonary bypass for resuscitation from prolonged cardiac arrest. *Am. J. Emerg. Med.* 1990; **8**(1): 55–67.

37. Tisherman, S., Chabal, C., Safar, P. & Stezoski, W. Resuscitation of dogs from cold-water submersion using cardiopulmonary bypass. *Ann. Emerg. Med.* 1985; **14**(5): 389–396.

38. Tisherman, S.A., Grenvik, A. & Safar, P. Cardiopulmonary-cerebral resuscitation: advanced and prolonged life support with emergency cardiopulmonary bypass. *Acta Anaesthesiol. Scand. Suppl.* 1990; **94**: 63–72.

39. Levine, R., Gorayeb, M., Safar, P., Abramson, N., Stezoski, W. & Kelsey, S. Cardiopulmonary bypass after cardiac arrest and prolonged closed-chest CPR in dogs. *Ann. Emerg. Med.* 1987; **16**(6): 620–627.

40. Colwell, C.S., Altemus, K.L., Cepeda, C. & Levine, M.S. Regulation of N-methyl-D-aspartate-induced toxicity in the neostriatum: A role for metabotropic glutamate receptors? *Proc. Natl Acad. Sci. USA* **93**: 1200–1204.

41. Tisherman, S., Safar, P. & Abramson, N.S. Clinical feasibility of emergency cardiopulmonary bypass for resuscitation from CPR-resistant cardiac arrest – a preliminary report [Abstract]. *Ann. Emerg. Med.* 1991; **20**: 491.

42. Tisherman, S.A., Vandevelde, K., Safar, P. *et al.* Future directions for resuscitation research. V. Ultra-advanced life support. *Resuscitation* 1997; **34**(3): 281–293.

43. Wollenek, G., Honarwar, N., Golej, J. & Marx, M. Cold water submersion and cardiac arrest in treatment of severe hypothermia with cardiopulmonary bypass. *Resuscitation* 2002; **52**(3): 255–263.

44. Anstadt, M.P., Bartlett, R.L., Malone, J.P. *et al.* Direct mechanical ventricular actuation for cardiac arrest in humans. A clinical feasibility trial. *Chest* 1991; **100**(1): 86–92.

45. Buckman, R.F., Jr., Badellino, M.M., Mauro, L.H. *et al.* Direct cardiac massage without major thoracotomy: feasibility and systemic blood flow. *Resuscitation* 1995; **29**(3): 237–248.

46. Buckman, R.F., Jr., Badellino, M.M., Eynon, C.A. *et al.* Open-chest cardiac massage without major thoracotomy: metabolic indicators of coronary and cerebral perfusion. *Resuscitation* 1997; **34**(3): 247–253.

47. Paiva, E.F., Kern, K.B., Hilwig, R.W., Scalabrini, A. & Ewy, G.A. Minimally invasive direct cardiac massage versus closed-chest cardiopulmonary resuscitation in a porcine model of prolonged ventricular fibrillation cardiac arrest. *Resuscitation* 2000; **47**(3): 287–299.

48. Gisvold, S.E. & Steen, P.A. Drug therapy in brain ischaemia. *Br. J. Anaesth.* 1985; **57**(1): 96–109.

49. Lin, S.R., O'Connor, M.J., Fischer, H.W. & King, A. The effect of combined dextran and streptokinase on cerebral function and blood flow after cardiac arrest: and experimental study on the dog. *Invest. Radiol.* 1978; **13**(6): 490–498.

50. Safar, P., Stezoski, W. & Nemoto, E.M. Amelioration of brain damage after 12 minutes' cardiac arrest in dogs. *Arch. Neurol.* 1976; **33**(2): 91–95.

51. Stullken, E.H., Jr. & Sokoll, M.D. The effects of heparin on recovery from ischemic brain injuries in cats. *Anesth. Analg.* 1976; **55**(5): 683–687.

52. Hallenbeck, J.M., Leitch, D.R., Dutka, A.J., Greenbaum, L.J., Jr. & McKee, A.E. Prostaglandin I2, indomethacin, and heparin promote postischemic neuronal recovery in dogs. *Ann. Neurol.* 1982; **12**(2): 145–156.

53. Breil, M., Krep, H., Sinn, D. *et al.* Hypertonic saline improves myocardial blood flow during CPR, but is not enhanced further by the addition of hydroxy ethyl starch. *Resuscitation* 2003; **56**(3): 307–317.

54. Ebmeyer, U., Abramson, N. & Katz, L.M. Current research directions in cerebral resuscitation after cardiac arrest. *Curr. Opin. Criti. Care* 1995; **1**: 182–188.

55. Ebmeyer, U., Safar, P. & Radovsky, A. Exploratory studies of effective combination treatments for cerebral resuscitation from cardiac arrest in dogs. (in press) 2006.

56. Chow, M.S., Fan, C., Tran, H., Zhao, H. & Zhou, L. Effects of diaspirin cross-linked hemoglobin (DCLHb) during and post-CPR in swine. *J. Pharmacol. Exp. Ther.* 2001; **297**(1): 224–229.

57. Cerchiari, E.L., Sclabassi, R.J., Safar, P. & Hoel, T.M. Effects of combined superoxide dismutase and deferoxamine on recovery of brainstem auditory evoked potentials and EEG after asphyxial cardiac arrest in dogs. *Resuscitation* 1990; **19**(1): 25–40.

58. Liu, Y., Rosenthal, R.E., Haywood, Y., Miljkovic-Lolic, M., Vanderhoek, J.Y. & Fiskum, G. Normoxic ventilation after cardiac arrest reduces oxidation of brain lipids and improves neurological outcome. *Stroke* 1998; **29**(8): 1679–1686.

59. Rosenthal, R.E., Silbergleit, R., Hof, P.R., Haywood, Y. & Fiskum, G. Hyperbaric oxygen reduces neuronal death and improves neurological outcome after canine cardiac arrest. *Stroke* 2003; **34**(5): 1311–1316.

60. Zwemer, C.F., Whitesall, S.E. & D'Alecy, L.G. Cardiopulmonary–cerebral resuscitation with 100% oxygen exacerbates neurological dysfunction following nine minutes

of normothermic cardiac arrest in dogs. *Resuscitation* 1994; **27**(2): 159–170.

61. Lipinski, C.A., Hicks, S.D. & Callaway, C.W. Normoxic ventilation during resuscitation and outcome from asphyxial cardiac arrest in rats. *Resuscitation* 1999; **42**(3): 221–229.

62. Mickel, H.S., Vaishnav, Y.N., Kempski, O., von Lubitz, D., Weiss, J.F. & Feuerstein, G. Breathing 100% oxygen after global brain ischemia in Mongolian Gerbils results in increased lipid peroxidation and increased mortality. *Stroke* 1987; **18**(2): 426–430.

63. Muizelaar, J.P., Marmarou, A., Ward, J.D. *et al.* Adverse effects of prolonged hyperventilation in patients with severe head injury: a randomized clinical trial. *J. Neurosurg.* 1991; **75**(5): 731–739.

64. Aufderheide, T.P. & Lurie, K.G. Death by hyperventilation: a common and life-threatening problem during cardiopulmonary resuscitation. *Crit. Care Med.* 2004; **32**(9 Suppl): S345–S351.

65. Aufderheide, T.P., Sigurdsson, G., Pirrallo, R.G. *et al.* Hyperventilation-induced hypotension during cardiopulmonary resuscitation. *Circulation* 2004; **109**(16): 1960–1965.

66. Lassen, N.A. & Astrup, J. Cerebral blood flow: normal regulation and ischemic thresholds. In Weinstein, P.R. & Faden, A.I., eds. *Protection of the Brain from Ischemia*. Baltimore: Williams & Wilkins, 1990: 7.

67. Rosner, M.J. & Daughton, S. Cerebral perfusion pressure management in head injury. *J. Trauma* 1990; **30**(8): 933–940.

68. Ward, J.D., Choi, S. & Marmaran, A. Effect of prophylactic hyperventilation on outcome in patients with severe head injury. In: Hoff, J.T. & Betz, A.L., eds. *Intracranial Pressure*. Berlin: Springer Verlag, 1989: 630.

69. Plum, F. & Siesjo, B.K. Recent advances in CSF physiology. *Anesthesiology* 1975; **42**(6): 708–730.

70. Shapiro, H.M. Barbiturates in brain ischaemia. *Br. J. Anaesth.* 1985; **57**(1): 82–95.

71. Berenyi, K.J., Wolk, M. & Killip, T. Cerebrospinal fluid acidosis complicating therapy of experimental cardiopulmonary arrest. *Circulation* 1975; **52**(2): 319–324.

72. Gotoh, F., Meyer, J.S. & Takagi, Y. Cerebral effects of hyperventilation in man. *Arch. Neurol.* 1965; **12**: 410–423.

73. Stewart, J. Management of cardiac arrest, with special reference to metabolic acidosis. *Br. Med. J.* 1964; **5381**: 476–479.

74. von Planta, M., Bar-Joseph, G., Wiklund, L., Bircher, N.G., Falk, J.L. & Abramson, N.S. Pathophysiologic and therapeutic implications of acid–base changes during CPR. *Ann. Emerg. Med.* 1993; **22**(2 Pt 2): 404–410.

75. Wiklund, L., Oquist, L., Skoog, G., Tyden, H. & Jorfeldt, L. Clinical buffering of metabolic acidosis: problems and a solution. *Resuscitation* 1985; **12**(4): 279–293.

76. Bircher, N. Sodium bicarbonate improves cardiac resuscitability, 24 hour survival and neurological outcome after ten minutes of cardiac arrest in dogs [Abstract]. *Anesthesiology* 1991; **75**: A246.

77. Vukmir, R.B., Bircher, N.G., Radovsky, A. & Safar, P. Sodium bicarbonate may improve outcome in dogs with brief or

prolonged cardiac arrest. *Crit. Care Med.* 1995; **23**(3): 515–522.

78. Vukmir, R.B., Bircher, N. & Safar, P. Sodium bicarbonate in cardiac arrest: a reappraisal. *Am. J. Emerg. Med.* 1996; **14**(2): 192–206.

79. Katz, L.M., Wang, Y., Rockoff, S. & Bouldin, T.W. Low-dose Carbicarb improves cerebral outcome after asphyxial cardiac arrest in rats. *Ann. Emerg. Med.* 2002; **39**(4): 359–365.

80. Siesjo, B.K. *Brain Energy Metabolism*. New York: John Wiley & Sons, 1978.

81. Siesjo, B.K. & Siesjo, P. Mechanisms of secondary brain injury. *Eur. J. Anaesthesiol.* 1996; **13**(3): 247–268.

82. Katsura, K., Kristian, T. & Siesjo, B.K. Energy metabolism, ion homeostasis, and cell damage in the brain. *Biochem. Soc. Trans.* 1994; **22**(4): 991–996.

83. Aldrete, J.A., Romo-Salas, F., Jankovsky, L. & Franatovic, Y. Effect of pretreatment with thiopental and phenytoin on postischemic brain damage in rabbits. *Crit. Care Med.* 1979; **7**(10): 466–470.

84. Greenberg, D.A., Cooper, E.C. & Carpenter, C.L. Phenytoin interacts with calcium channels in brain membranes. *Ann. Neurol.* 1984; **16**(5): 616–617.

85. Myers, R.E. & Yamaguchi, S. Nervous system effects of cardiac arrest in monkeys. Preservation of vision. *Arch. Neurol.* 1977; **34**(2): 65–74.

86. Pulsinelli, W.A., Waldman, S., Rawlinson, D. & Plum, F. Moderate hyperglycemia augments ischemic brain damage: a neuropathologic study in the rat. *Neurology* 1982; **32**(11): 1239–1246.

87. D'Alecy, L.G., Lundy, E.F., Barton, K.J. & Zelenock, G.B. Dextrose containing intravenous fluid impairs outcome and increases death after eight minutes of cardiac arrest and resuscitation in dogs. *Surgery* 1986; **100**(3): 505–511.

88. Warner, D.S., Smith, M.L. & Siesjo, B.K. Ischemia in normo- and hyperglycemic rats: effects on brain water and electrolytes. *Stroke* 1987; **18**(2): 464–471.

89. Voll, C.L. & Auer, R.N. Insulin attenuates ischemic brain damage independent of its hypoglycemic effect. *J. Cereb. Blood Flow Metab.* 1991; **11**(6): 1006–1014.

90. Katz, L.M., Wang, Y., Ebmeyer, U., Radovsky, A. & Safar, P. Glucose plus insulin infusion improves cerebral outcome after asphyxial cardiac arrest. *Neuroreport* 1998; **9**(15): 3363–3367.

91. Longstreth, W.T., Jr. & Inui, T.S. High blood glucose level on hospital admission and poor neurological recovery after cardiac arrest. *Ann. Neurol.* 1984; **15**(1): 59–63.

92. Sieber, F.E. & Traystman, R.J. Special issues: glucose and the brain. *Crit. Care Med.* 1992; **20**(1): 104–114.

93. Voll, C.L. & Auer, R.N. The effect of postischemic blood glucose levels on ischemic brain damage in the rat. *Ann. Neurol.* 1988; **24**(5): 638–646.

94. Agardh, C.D., Chapman, A.G., Nilsson, B. & Siesjo, B.K. Endogenous substrates utilized by rat brain in severe insulin-induced hypoglycemia. *J. Neurochem.* 1981; **36**(2): 490–500.

95. Sieber, F.E., Koehler, R.C., Derrer, S.A., Saudek, C.D. & Traystman, R.J. Hypoglycemia and cerebral autoregulation in

anesthetized dogs. *Am. J. Physiol.* 1990; **258**(6 Pt 2): H1714–H1721.

96. Wechsler, L.R., Dripps, R.D. & Kety, S.S. Blood flow and oxygen consumption of the human brain during anesthesia produced by thiopental. *Anesthesiology* 1951; **12**: 308–314.

97. Smith, A.L. & Marque, J.J. Anesthetics and cerebral edema. *Anesthesiology* 1976; **45**(1): 64–72.

98. Todd, M.M., Chadwick, H.S., Shapiro, H.M., Dunlop, B.J., Marshall, L.F. & Dueck, R. The neurologic effects of thiopental therapy following experimental cardiac arrest in cats. *Anesthesiology* 1982; **57**(2): 76–86.

99. Michenfelder, J.D., Milde, J.H. & Sundt, T.M., Jr. Cerebral protection by barbiturate anesthesia. Use after middle cerebral artery occlusion in Java monkeys. *Arch. Neurol.* 1976; **33**(5): 345–350.

100. Smith, A.L., Hoff, J.T., Nielsen, S.L. & Larson, C.P. Barbiturate protection in acute focal cerebral ischemia. *Stroke* 1974; **5**(1): 1–7.

101. Yatsu, F.M., Diamond, I., Graziano, C. & Lindquist, P. Experimental brain ischemia: protection from irreversible damage with a rapid-acting barbiturate (methohexital). *Stroke* 1972; **3**(6): 726–732.

102. Kofke, W.A., Nemoto, E.M., Hossmann, K.A., Taylor, F., Kessler, P.D. & Stezoski, S.W. Brain blood flow and metabolism after global ischemia and post-insult thiopental therapy in monkeys. *Stroke* 1979; **10**(5): 554–560.

103. Nordstrom, C.H., Calderini, G., Rehncrona, S. & Siesjo, B.K. Effects of phenobarbital anaesthesia on postischemic cerebral blood flow and oxygen consumption in the rat. *Acta Neurol. Scand. Suppl.* 1977; **64**: 146–147.

104. MacMurdo, S.D., Nemoto, E.M., Nikki, P. & Frankenberry, M.J. Brain cyclic-AMP and possible mechanisms of cerebrovascular dilation by anesthetics in rats. *Anesthesiology* 1981; **55**(4): 435–438.

105. Nemoto, E.M. Studies on the pathogenisis of ischemic brain damage and its amelioration by barbiturate therapy. *Brain and Heart Infarct.* Berlin: Springer Verlag, 1979.

106. Nemoto, E.M., Shiu, G.K., Nemmer, J.P. & Bleyaert, A.L. Free fatty acid accumulation in the pathogenesis and therapy of ischemic-anoxic brain injury. *Am. J. Emerg. Med.* 1983; **1**(2): 175–179.

107. Shiu, G.K., Nemmer, J.P. & Nemoto, E.M. Reassessment of brain free fatty acid liberation during global ischemia and its attenuation by barbiturate anesthesia. *J. Neurochem.* 1983; **40**(3): 880–884.

108. Breivik, H., Safar, P., Sands, P. *et al.* Clinical feasibility trials of barbiturate therapy after cardiac arrest. *Crit. Care Med.* 1978; **6**(4): 228–244.

109. Mullie, A., Abramson, N. & Safar, P. Clinical pilot studies of thiopental loading after cardiac arrest. *Crit. Care Med.* 1981; **9**: 184.

110. Abramson, N.S., Detre, K., Bradley, K. *et al.* Impact evaluation in resuscitation research: discussion of clinical trials. *Crit. Care Med.* 1988; **16**(10): 1053–1058.

111. Abramson, N.S., Kelsey, S.F., Safar, P. & Sutton-Tyrrell, K. Simpson's paradox and clinical trials: what you find is not necessarily what you prove. *Ann. Emerg. Med.* 1992; **21**(12): 1480–1482.

112. Abramson, N.S. Cerebral resuscitation: let the clinician be wary. *Br. J. Hosp. Med.* 1987; **38**(4): 277.

113. A randomized clinical study of cardiopulmonary–cerebral resuscitation: design, methods, and patient characteristics. Brain Resuscitation Clinical Trial I Study Group. *Am. J. Emerg. Med.* 1986; **4**(1): 72–86.

114. Randomized clinical study of thiopental loading in comatose survivors of cardiac arrest. Brain Resuscitation Clinical Trial I Study Group. *N. Engl. J. Med.* 1986; **314**(7): 397–403.

115. Safar, P. Resuscitation medicine research: quo vadis. *Ann. Emerg. Med.* 1996; **27**(5): 542–552.

116. Ebmeyer, U., Safar, P., Radovsky, A. *et al.* Thiopental combination treatments for cerebral resuscitation after prolonged cardiac arrest in dogs. Exploratory outcome study. *Resuscitation* 2000; **45**(2): 119–131.

117. Katz, L., Vaagenes, P., Safar, P. & Diven, W. Brain enzyme changes as markers of brain damage in rat cardiac arrest model. Effects of corticosteroid therapy. *Resuscitation* 1989; **17**(1): 39–53.

118. Marcy, V.R., O'Connor, M.J. & Welsh, F.A. Permanent energy failure following cerebral ischemia. III. Amelioration by post-ischemic treatment with dead.on. *J. Cereb. Blood Flow Metab.* 1981; Suppl I: 206.

119. Fishman, R.A. Steroids in the treatment of brain edema. *N. Engl. J. Med.* 1982; **306**(6): 359–360.

120. Suzuki, J., Imaizumi, S., Kayama, T. & Yoshimoto, T. Chemiluminescence in hypoxic brain – the second report: cerebral protective effect of mannitol, vitamin E and glucocorticoid. *Stroke* 1985; **16**(4): 695–700.

121. Galicich, J.H. & French, L.A. Use of dexamethasone in the treatment of cerebral edema resulting from brain tumors and brain surgery. *Am. Pract. Dig. Treat.* 1961; **12**: 169–174.

122. Young, W.F., Gopez, J.J. & Legos, J.J. Non-surgical management of spinal cord injury. *Expert Opin. Investig. Drugs* 2002; **11**(4): 469–482.

123. Green, B.A., Kahn, T. & Klose, K.J. A comparative study of steroid therapy in acute experimental spinal cord injury. *Surg. Neurol.* 1980; **13**(2): 91–97.

124. Hoerlein, B.F., Redding, R.W. & Hoff, E.J. Evaluation of naloxone, crocetin, thyrotropin releasing hormone, methylprednisolon, partial myelotomy, and hemi-laminectomy in the treatment of acute spinal cord trauma. *J. Am. Animal Hosp. Assoc.* 1984; **21**: 67.

125. Holtz, A., Nystrom, B. & Gerdin, B. Effect of methylprednisolone on motor function and spinal cord blood flow after spinal cord compression in rats. *Acta Neurol. Scand.* 1990; **82**(1): 68–73.

126. Iizuka, H., Iwasaki, Y., Yamamoto, T. & Kadoya, S. Morphometric assessment of drug effects in experimental spinal cord injury. *J. Neurosurg.* 1986; **65**(1): 92–98.

127. Young, W., DeCrescito, V., Flamm, E.S., Blight, A.R. & Gruner, J.A. Pharmacological therapy of acute spinal cord injury: studies of high dose methylprednisolone and naloxone. *Clin. Neurosurg.* 1988; **34**: 675–697.

128. Braughler, J.M. & Hall, E.D. Involvement of lipid peroxidation in CNS injury. *J. Neurotrauma* 1992; **9** Suppl 1: S1–S7.

129. Hall, E.D., Braughler, J.M. & McCall, J.M. Antioxidant effects in brain and spinal cord injury. *J. Neurotrauma* 1992; **9** Suppl 1: S165–S172.

130. Hall, E.D. Lipid antioxidants in acute central nervous system injury. *Ann. Emerg. Med.* 1993; **22**(6): 1022–1027.

131. Perkins, W.J., Milde, L.N., Milde, J.H. & Michenfelder, J.D. Pretreatment with U74006F improves neurologic outcome following complete cerebral ischemia in dogs. *Stroke* 1991; **22**(7): 902–909.

132. Natale, J.E., Schott, R.J., Hall, E.D., Braughler, J.M. & D'Alecy, L.G. Effect of the aminosteroid U74006F after cardiopulmonary arrest in dogs. *Stroke* 1988; **19**(11): 1371–1378.

133. Wang, J., Weil, M.H., Kamohara, T. *et al.* A lazaroid mitigates postresuscitation myocardial dysfunction. *Crit. Care Med.* 2004; **32**(2): 553–558.

134. Kavanagh, R.J. & Kam, P.C. Lazaroids: efficacy and mechanism of action of the 21-aminosteroids in neuroprotection. *Br. J. Anaesth.* 2001; **86**(1): 110–119.

135. Steen, P.A., Newberg, L.A., Milde, J.H. & Michenfelder, J.D. Nimodipine improves cerebral blood flow and neurologic recovery after complete cerebral ischemia in the dog. *J. Cereb. Blood Flow Metab.* 1983; **3**(1): 38–43.

136. Steen, P.A., Newberg, L.A., Milde, J.H. & Michenfelder, J.D. Cerebral blood flow and neurologic outcome when nimodipine is given after complete cerebral ischemia in the dog. *J. Cereb. Blood Flow Metab.* 1984; **4**(1): 82–87.

137. Hossmann, K.A. Ischemia-mediated neuronal injury. *Resuscitation* 1993; **26**(3): 225–235.

138. White, B.C., Sullivan, J.M., DeGracia, D.J. *et al.* Brain ischemia and reperfusion: molecular mechanisms of neuronal injury. *J. Neurol. Sci.* 2000; **179**(1–2): 1–33.

139. Hossmann, K.A. Treatment of experimental cerebral ischemia. *J. Cereb. Blood Flow Metab.* 1982; **2**(3): 275–297.

140. White, B.C., Winegar, C.D., Wilson, R.F., Hoehner, P.J. & Trombley, J.H., Jr. Possible role of calcium blockers in cerebral resuscitation: a review of the literature and synthesis for future studies. *Crit. Care Med.* 1983; **11**(3): 202–207.

141. Braunwald, E. Mechanism of action of calcium-channel-blocking agents. *N. Engl. J. Med.* 1982; **307**(26): 1618–1627.

142. Ort, E. & Lechner, N. Influence of nimodipine on cerebral blood flow in patients with subacute cerebral infarction. Symposium of the 28th International Congress on Physiologic Sciences. 1980.

143. Allen, G.S. & Banghart, S.B. Cerebral arterial spasm: part 9. In vitro effects of nifedipine on serotonin-, phenylephrine-, and potassium-induced contractions of canine basilar and femoral arteries. *Neurosurgery* 1979; **4**(1): 37–42.

144. Mohamed, A.A., Mendelow, A.D., Teasdale, G.M., Harper, A.M. & McCulloch, J. Effect of the calcium antagonist nimodipine on local cerebral blood flow and metabolic coupling. *J. Cereb. Blood Flow Metab.* 1985; **5**(1): 26–33.

145. A randomized clinical study of a calcium-entry blocker (lidoflazine) in the treatment of comatose survivors of cardiac arrest. Brain Resuscitation Clinical Trial II Study Group. *N. Engl. J. Med.* 1991; **324**(18): 1225–1231.

146. Flunarizine i.v. after cardiac arrest (Fluna-study): study design and organisational aspects of a double-blind, placebo-controlled randomized study. FLUNA Study Group Berlin [corrected]. *Resuscitation* 1989; **17** Suppl: S121–S127.

147. Safar, P. On the future of reanimatology. *Acad. Emerg. Med.* 2000; **7**(1): 75–89.

148. Safar, P.J. & Kochanek, P.M. Therapeutic hypothermia after cardiac arrest. *N. Engl. J. Med.* 2002; **346**(8): 612–613.

149. Minamisawa, H., Smith, M.L. & Siesjo, B.K. The effect of mild hyperthermia and hypothermia on brain damage following 5, 10, and 15 minutes of forebrain ischemia. *Ann. Neurol.* 1990; **28**(1): 26–33.

150. Safar, P. Cerebral resuscitation after cardiac arrest: research initiatives and future directions. *Ann. Emerg. Med.* 1993; **22**(2 Pt 2):324–349.

151. Marion, D.W., Leonov, Y., Ginsberg, M. *et al.* Resuscitative hypothermia. *Crit. Care Med.* 1996; **24**(2 Suppl): S81–S89.

152. Bernard, S.A., Jones, B.M. & Horne, M.K. Clinical trial of induced hypothermia in comatose survivors of out-of-hospital cardiac arrest. *Ann. Emerg. Med.* 1997; **30**(2): 146–153.

153. Bernard, S.A., Gray, T.W., Buist, M.D. *et al.* Treatment of comatose survivors of out-of-hospital cardiac arrest with induced hypothermia. *N. Engl. J. Med.* 2002; **346**(8): 557–563.

154. Mild therapeutic hypothermia to improve the neurologic outcome after cardiac arrest. *N. Engl. J. Med.* 2002; **346**(8): 549–556.

155. Eisenburger, P., Sterz, F., Holzer, M. *et al.* Therapeutic hypothermia after cardiac arrest. *Curr. Opin. Crit. Care* 2001; **7**(3): 184–188.

156. Lei, B., Tan, X., Cai, H., Xu, Q. & Guo, Q. Effect of moderate hypothermia on lipid peroxidation in canine brain tissue after cardiac arrest and resuscitation. *Stroke* 1994; **25**(1): 147–152.

157. Yenari, M.A., Zhao, H., Giffard, R.G., Sobel, R.A., Sapolsky, R.M. & Steinberg, G.K. Gene therapy and hypothermia for stroke treatment. *Ann. N Y Acad. Sci.* 2003; **993**: 54–68.

158. Shaffner, D.H., Eleff, S.M., Koehler, R.C. & Traystman, R.J. Effect of the no-flow interval and hypothermia on cerebral blood flow and metabolism during cardiopulmonary resuscitation in dogs. *Stroke* 1998; **29**(12): 2607–2615.

159. D'Cruz, B.J., Fertig, K.C., Filiano, A.J., Hicks, S.D., DeFranco, D.B. & Callaway, C.W. Hypothermic reperfusion after cardiac arrest augments brain-derived neurotrophic factor activation. *J. Cereb. Blood Flow Metab.* 2002; **22**(7): 843–851.

160. Kuboyama, K., Safar, P., Radovsky, A., Tisherman, S.A., Stezoski, S.W. & Alexander, H. Delay in cooling negates the beneficial effect of mild resuscitative cerebral hypothermia after cardiac arrest in dogs: a prospective, randomized study. *Crit. Care Med.* 1993; **21**(9): 1348–1358.

161. Callaway, C.W., Tadler, S.C., Katz, L.M., Lipinski, C.L. & Brader, E. Feasibility of external cranial cooling during out-of-hospital cardiac arrest. *Resuscitation* 2002; **52**(2): 159–165.

162. Gordon, C.J. The therapeutic potential of regulated hypothermia. *Emerg. Med. J.* 2001; **18**(2): 81–89.

163. Katz, L.M., Wang, Y., McMahon, B. & Richelson, E. Neurotensin analog NT69L induces rapid and prolonged hypothermia after hypoxic ischemia. *Acad. Emerg. Med.* 2001; **8**(12): 1115–1121.

164. Katz, L.M., Young, A., Frank, J.E., Wang, Y. & Park, K. Neurotensin-induced hypothermia improves neurologic outcome after hypoxic-ischemia. *Crit. Care Med.* 2004; **32**(3): 806–810.

165. Al Senani, F.M., Graffagnino, C., Grotta, J.C. *et al.* A prospective, multicenter pilot study to evaluate the feasibility and safety of using the CoolGard System and Icy catheter following cardiac arrest. *Resuscitation* 2004; **62**(2): 143–150.

166. Bernard, S. Hypothermia after cardiac arrest: how to cool and for how long? *Crit. Care Med.* 2004; **32**(3): 897–899.

167. Colbourne, F. & Corbett, D. Delayed postischemic hypothermia: a six month survival study using behavioral and histological assessments of neuroprotection. *J. Neurosci.* 1995; **15**(11): 7250–7260.

168. Krieger, D.W. Therapeutic hypothermia may enhance reperfusion in acute ischemic stroke. *Cleve. Clin. J. Med.* 2004; **71** (Suppl 1): S39.

169. Suehiro, E., Ueda, Y., Wei, E.P., Kontos, H.A. & Povlishock, J.T. Posttraumatic hypothermia followed by slow rewarming protects the cerebral microcirculation. *J. Neurotrauma* 2003; **20**(4): 381–390.

170. Ueda, Y., Suehiro, E., Wei, E.P., Kontos, H.A. & Povlishock, J.T. Uncomplicated rapid posthypothermic rewarming alters cerebrovascular responsiveness. *Stroke* 2004; **35**(2): 601–606.

171. Andjus, R.K., Dzakula, Z., Markley, J.L. & Macura, S. Brain energetics and tolerance to anoxia in deep hypothermia. *Ann. N Y Acad. Sci.* 2005; **1048**: 10–35.

172. Novack, T.A., Dillon, M.C. & Jackson, W.T. Neurochemical mechanisms in brain injury and treatment: a review. *J. Clin. Exp. Neuropsychol.* 1996; **18**(5): 685–706.

173. Robertson, C.S. & Cormio, M. Cerebral metabolic management. *New Horiz.* 1995; **3**(3): 410–422.

174. Safar, P. Reanimatology – the science of resuscitation. *Crit. Care Med.* 1982; **10**(2): 134–136.

175. Safar, P. Cerebral resuscitation: current state of the art. *Ann. Emerg. Med.* 1982; **11**(3): 162–165.

176. Uriel, J. Cancer, retrodifferentiation, and the myth of Faust. *Cancer Res.* 1976; **36**(11 Pt.2): 4269–4275.

177. Cajal, R.Y. *Degeneration and Regeneration of the Nervous System.* New York: Hafner, 1928.

178. Kaufman, S.R. Hidden places, uncommon persons. *Soc. Sci. Med.* 2003; **56**(11): 2249–2261.

179. Aguayo, A.J., David, S. & Bray, G.M. Influences of the glial environment on the elongation of axons after injury: transplantation studies in adult rodents. *J. Exp. Biol.* 1981; **95**: 231–240.

180. Bjorklund, A., Stenevi, U., Dunnett, S.B. & Gage, F.H. Cross-species neural grafting in a rat model of Parkinson's disease. *Nature* 1982; **298**(5875): 652–654.

181. Gage, F.H., Ray, J. & Fisher, L.J. Isolation, characterization, and use of stem cells from the CNS. *Annu. Rev. Neurosci.* 1995; **18**: 159–192.

182. Anderson, D.J., Gage, F.H. & Weissman, I.L. Can stem cells cross lineage boundaries? *Nat. Med.* 2001; **7**(4): 393–395.

183. Chen, J., Li, Y. & Chopp, M. Intracerebral transplantation of bone marrow with BDNF after MCAo in rat. *Neuropharmacology* 2000; **39**(5): 711–716.

184. Shafritz, D.A. & Dabeva, M.D. Liver stem cells and model systems for liver repopulation. *J. Hepatol.* 2002; **36**(4): 552–564.

185. Zhao, L.R., Duan, W.M., Reyes, M., Keene, C.D., Verfaillie, C.M. & Low, W.C. Human bone marrow stem cells exhibit neural phenotypes and ameliorate neurological deficits after grafting into the ischemic brain of rats. *Exp. Neurol.* 2002; **174**(1): 11–20.

186. Ebmeyer, U., Katz, L.M., Safar, P. *et al.* Concluding comments and suggestions for young resuscitation researchers. *Crit. Care Med.* 1996; **24**(2 Suppl): S95–S99.

187. Rivers, E.P., Rady, M.Y., Martin, G.B. *et al.* Venous hyperoxia after cardiac arrest. Characterization of a defect in systemic oxygen utilization. *Chest* 1992; **102**(6): 1787–1793.

188. Rivers, E.P., Wortsman, J., Rady, M.Y., Blake, H.C., McGeorge, F.T. & Buderer, N.M. The effect of the total cumulative epinephrine dose administered during human CPR on hemodynamic, oxygen transport, and utilization variables in the postresuscitation period. *Chest* 1994; **106**(5): 1499–1507.

189. Creamer, J.E., Edwards, J.D. & Nightingale, P. Hemodynamic and oxygen transport variables in cardiogenic shock secondary to acute myocardial infarction, and response to treatment. *Am. J. Cardiol.* 1990; **65**(20): 1297–1300.

190. Shoemaker, W.C., Appel, P.L. & Kram, H.B. Tissue oxygen debt as a determinant of lethal and nonlethal postoperative organ failure. *Crit. Care Med.* 1988; **16**(11): 1117–1120.

191. Gunnar, R.M., Bourdillon, P.D., Dixon, D.W. *et al.* ACC/AHA guidelines for the early management of patients with acute myocardial infarction. A report of the American College of Cardiology/American Heart Association Task Force on Assessment of Diagnostic and Therapeutic Cardiovascular Procedures (subcommittee to develop guidelines for the early management of patients with acute myocardial infarction). *Circulation* 1990; **82**(2): 664–707.

192. Rady, M.Y., Rivers, E.P., Martin, G.B., Smithline, H., Appelton, T. & Nowak, R.M. Continuous central venous oximetry and shock index in the emergency department: use in the evaluation of clinical shock. *Am. J. Emerg. Med.* 1992; **10**(6): 538–541.

193. Rashkin, M.C., Bosken, C. & Baughman, R.P. Oxygen delivery in critically ill patients. Relationship to blood lactate and survival. *Chest* 1985; **87**(5): 580–584.

194. Bishop, M.H., Shoemaker, W.C., Shuleshko, J. & Wo, C.C. Noninvasive cardiac index monitoring in gunshot wound victims. *Acad. Emerg. Med.* 1996; **3**(7): 682–688.

195. Maynard, N., Bihari, D., Beale, R. *et al.* Assessment of splanchnic oxygenation by gastric tonometry in patients with acute circulatory failure. *J. Am. Med. Assoc.* 1993; **270**(10): 1203–1210.

196. Waller, J.L., Kaplan, J.A., Bauman, D.I. & Craver, J.M. Clinical evaluation of a new fiberoptic catheter oximeter during cardiac surgery. *Anesth. Analg.* 1982; **61**(8): 676–679.

197. Krauss, X.H., Verdouw, P.D., Hughenholtz, P.G. & Nauta, J. On-line monitoring of mixed venous oxygen saturation after cardiothoracic surgery. *Thorax* 1975; **30**(6): 636–643.

198. Kasnitz, P., Druger, G.L., Yorra, F. & Simmons, D.H. Mixed venous oxygen tension and hyperlactatemia. Survival in severe cardiopulmonary disease. *J. Am. Med. Assoc.* 1976; **236**(6): 570–574.

199. Birman, H., Haq, A., Hew, E. & Aberman, A. Continuous monitoring of mixed venous oxygen saturation in hemodynamically unstable patients. *Chest* 1984; **86**(5): 753–756.

200. Vincent, J.L., Dufaye, P., Berre, J., Leeman, M., Degaute, J.P. & Kahn, R.J. Serial lactate determinations during circulatory shock. *Crit. Care Med.* 1983; **11**(6): 449–451.

201. Bishop, M.H., Shoemaker, W.C., Appel, P.L. *et al.* Relationship between supranormal circulatory values, time delays, and outcome in severely traumatized patients. *Crit. Care Med.* 1993; **21**(1): 56–63.

202. Shoemaker, W.C., Appel, P.L., Kram, H.B., Waxman, K. & Lee, T.S. Prospective trial of supranormal values of survivors as therapeutic goals in high-risk surgical patients. *Chest* 1988; **94**(6): 1176–1186.

203. Marik, P.E. & Mohedin, M. The contrasting effects of dopamine and norepinephrine on systemic and splanchnic oxygen utilization in hyperdynamic sepsis. *J. Am. Med. Assoc.* 1994; **272**(17): 1354–1357.

204. Schultz, C.H., Rivers, E.P., Feldkamp, C.S. *et al.* A characterization of hypothalamic–pituitary–adrenal axis function during and after human cardiac arrest. *Crit. Care Med.* 1993; **21**(9): 1339–1347.

205. Smithline, H., Rivers, E., Appleton, T. & Nowak, R. Corticosteroid supplementation during cardiac arrest in rats. *Resuscitation* 1993; **25**(3): 257–264.

206. Leach, R.M. & Treacher, D.F. The relationship between oxygen delivery and consumption. *Dis. Mon.* 1994; **40**(7): 301–368.

207. Leier, C.V. Regional blood flow responses to vasodilators and inotropes in congestive heart failure. *Am. J. Cardiol.* 1988; **62**(8): 86E–93E.

208. Oku, K., Kuboyama, K., Safar, P. *et al.* Cerebral and systemic arteriovenous oxygen monitoring after cardiac arrest. Inadequate cerebral oxygen delivery. *Resuscitation* 1994; **27**(2): 141–152.

209. Abramson, N.S., Ebmeyer, U., Ward, K.R. & Neumar, R.W. Bringing it all together: brain-oriented postresuscitation critical care. In Paradis, N.A., Halperin, H.R. & Nowak, R.M., eds. *Cardiac Arrest: The Science and Practice of Resuscitation Medicine.* Baltimore: Williams & Wilkins, 1996: 923–934.

Part VI

Special resuscitation circumstances

52

Prevention of sudden death in patients at risk: channelopathies and arrhythmic syndromes in the structurally normal heart

Alan Cheng, Gordon F. Tomaselli, and Ronald D. Berger

Johns Hopkins University, Baltimore, MD, USA

Introduction

Despite an overall reduction in death caused by cardiovascular diseases, the percentage of death due to arrhythmia-related sudden cardiac death (SCD) has remained high (Fig. 52.1) and is largely accounted for by an increase of death in women over 65 years old (described in detail in Chapter 23).[1] Due in part to its unpredictability and the logistical limitations of immediate access to medical care, the likelihood of surviving an SCD event is estimated between 1% and 5% both in the United States and abroad. Commonly, these events occur in individuals with known cardiac disease (Table 52.1) and can be the initial manifestation of an underlying structural abnormality in 33%–50% of all SCD cases. Although the two most important risk factors for SCD are left ventricular systolic dysfunction[2] and the presence of decompensated heart failure,[3] SCD has also occurred in otherwise healthy individuals with structurally normal hearts and accounts for the bimodal distribution of its incidence with age, particularly in those less than 45 years old.[4] This chapter highlights the syndromes with increased risk of sudden death due to ventricular tachyarrhythmias in the otherwise structurally normal heart. Classic conditions such as right ventricular outflow tract tachycardia and idiopathic ventricular tachycardia are beyond the scope of this chapter because of their low propensity toward sudden death.

Electrophysiologic processes underlying sudden cardiac death

Electrical impulses conducted through myocardial tissue can be fundamentally described by the cardiac action

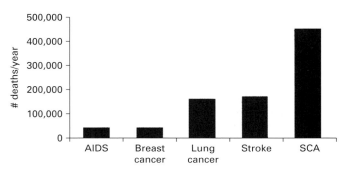

Fig. 52.1 Magnitude of SCA in the USA.[1] SCA claims more lives each year than these other diseases combined.
Source: [1] U.S. Census Bureau, *Statistical Abstract of the United States* 2001. [2] American Cancer Society, Inc., Surveillance Research, Cancer Facts and Figures 2001. [3] 2002 *Heart and Stroke Statistical Update*, American Heart Association. [4] *Circulation*, 2001;104:2158–2163.

potential, which is composed of four different phases of activity (Fig. 52.2). Cardiac action potentials are typically longer than those of other excitable tissues such as neural or striated skeletal muscle cells and range between 200 and 400 msec (in contrast to the latter type of tissue in which the range is between 1 and 5 ms). The action potential profile is governed by the orchestrated activity of multiple ionic currents, each with distinctive time- and voltage-dependent amplitudes as a result of several ion-specific transmembrane channels and transporters. Some are involved with passive flow of ions along electrical and concentration gradients, whereas others are energy-dependent processes that drive ion movements against electrochemical gradients. Depending on the type (e.g., sodium, potassium, calcium)

Cardiac Arrest: The Science and Practice of Resuscitation Medicine. 2nd edn., ed. Norman Paradis, Henry Halperin, Karl Kern, Volker Wenzel, Douglas Chamberlain. Published by Cambridge University Press. © Cambridge University Press, 2007.

Table 52.1. Abnormalities associated with sudden cardiac death

Coronary artery abnormalities
  Atherosclerotic
  Non-atherosclerotic (arteritis, embolism, dissection, congenital malformations, anomalous origin of left coronary artery from
  pulmonary artery or right or non-coronary aortic sinus of Valsalva [artery passing between the aortic and pulmonary artery roots])
Myocardial abnormalities
  Hypertrophic cardiomyopathy
  Idiopathic dilated cardiomyopathy
  Arrhythmogenic right ventricular dysplasia (congenital right ventricular cardiomyopathy)
  Myocarditis
  Sarcoidosis or other infiltrative diseases
  Left ventricular hypertrophy
  Valvular and congenital heart disease
Other conditions
  Aortic dissection
  Acute cardiac tamponade
  Rapid exsanguination
  Pheochromocytoma
  Subarachnoid hemorrhage
  Café coronary (acute glottis obstruction by food)
  Holiday heart syndrome
  Acute alcoholic states
  Massive pulmonary embolism
  Severe asthmatic attacks
  Peripartum air or amnionic fluid embolism
Proarrhythmic effects[a]
  Antiarrhythmic drugs
  Psychotropic agents, phenothiazines, antihistamines, antibiotics, gastrointestinal drugs
  Anorexia nervosa
  Toxic substances
  Electrolyte abnormalities

[a] Often (but not always) associated with QT prolongation (acquired long QT). Classic proarrhythmia usually occurs within days after
initiation of treatment but may extend over one year of exposure.[4]

and number of specific ion channels, regional disparities in the action potential profile can be seen within the heart. The activity of these ion channels (and therefore the action potential) can be affected by a number of factors including electrolyte abnormalities, medications, profound bradycardia, and even mutations or variants in the channel gene. In the proper milieu, arrhythmic triggers such as ventricular extrasystoles and afterdepolarizations can develop, resulting in the initiation of sustained, life-threatening arrhythmias.

Long QT syndrome

The long QT syndrome (LQTS) is an inherited entity, originally described in 1957,[5] that encompasses individuals with a high propensity for sudden cardiac death in the setting of an abnormally prolonged QT interval. All individuals are described to have structurally normal hearts, although early echocardiographic observations have been made suggesting the presence of small ventricular wall motion abnormalities.[6] Initially, two clinical variants were recognized, one of which is associated with congenital deafness and autosomal recessive inheritance (Jervell and Lange–Nielsen syndrome) and the other is dominantly inherited without hearing deficits (Romano–Ward syndrome).[7,8] LQTS is genetically heterogeneous with mutations described in six different genes. Andersen and Timothy syndromes are multisystem inherited diseases associated with deficient ventricular repolarization and QT interval prolongation produced by mutations in *KCNJ2* and *CANC2*, respectively. *KCNJ2* and *CANC2* encode the inward

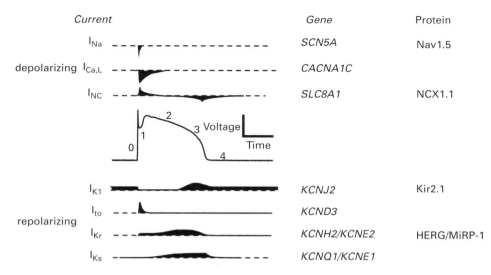

Fig. 52.2 Cardiac action potential: various phases of the cardiac action potential and their respective ionic currents involved in depolarization and repolarization.[96]

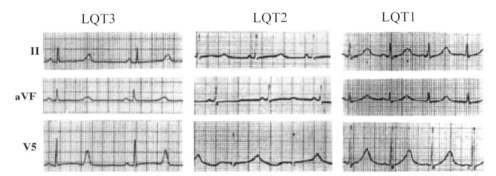

Fig. 52.3 T wave morphologic abnormalities seen in long QT syndrome.[11]

Table 52.2. Different LQT syndromes and their respective genetic abnormalities[97]

Disease	Gene (alternative names)	Protein
LQT-1	*KVLQTI (KCNQ1)*	I_{Ks} K$^+$ channel α subunit
LQT-2	*HERG (KCNH2)*	I_{Kr} K$^+$ channel α subunit
LQT-3	SCN5A	I_{Na} K$^+$ channel α subunit
LQT-4	ANKB	ANKRIN-β
LQT-5	*minK (KCNE1)*	I_{Ks} K$^+$ channel β subunit
LQT-6	*MiRP1 (KCNE2)*	I_{Kr} K$^+$ channel β subunit
LQT-7	KCNJ2	I_{Kr} K$^+$ channel α subunit

rectifier potassium channel (I_{K1}) and dihydropyridine-sensitive calcium channels (Ca$_V$1.2), respectively (Table 52.2). To date, approximately 300 mutations in 6 different ion channels have been associated with this syndrome.[9,10]

The QT interval is a summative representation of myocardial ventricular repolarization, a process that is governed by the interplay of a number of different ion channels. Hence, phenotypic characteristics of the T wave morphology exist based on the specific channel mutated. Although LQT1 patients tend to have considerable variation in their T wave morphologies, LQT2 T waves present with the classic bifid pattern, while LQT3 T waves tend to have late peaks (Fig. 52.3).[11,12] Some variation exists in these observations due in part to variable degrees of penetrance, variations in the genetic background even among

	Points
ECG findings *	
A. QT_o†	
≥ 480 ms	3
460–470 ms	2
450 ms (in males)	1
B. Torsade de pointes‡	2
C. T-Waves alternans	1
D. Notched T wave in three leads	1
E. Low heart rate for age§	0.5
Clinical history	
A. Syncope‡	
With stress	2
Without stress	1
B. Congenital deafness	0.5
Family history‖	
A. Family members with definite LQTS#	1
B. Unexplained sudden cardiac death below age 30 among immediate family members	0.5

LQTS, long QT syndrome.

* In the absence of medications or disorders known to affect these electrocardiographic features.

† QT_o calculated by Bazett's formula, where $QT_c = QT/\sqrt{RR}$.

‡ Mutually exclusive

§ Resting heart rate below the second percentile for age.

‖ The same family member cannot be counted in A and B.

Definite LQTS is defined by an LQTS score ≥ 4. Scoring: ≤ 1 point, low probability of LQTS; 2 to 3 points, intermediate probability of LQTS; ≥4 points, high probability of LQTS.[98]

Table 52.3. Risk factors for torsades de pointes in individuals with acquired long QT syndrome.[99]

Table 2. Risk Factors for Drug-Induced Torsade de Pointes[a]

Female sex
Hypokalemia
Bradycardia
Recent conversion from atrial fibrillation, especially with a
   QT-prolonging drug
Congestive heart failure
Digitalis therapy
High drug concentrations (with the exception of quinidine)
Rapid rate of intravenous infusion with a QT-prolonging drug[17]
Base-line QT prolongation
Subclinical long-QT syndrome
Ion-channel polymorphisms
Severe hypomagnesemia

[a] Studies providing evidence of the effects are cited in the table.

members of the same affected families, environmental factors, or even the severity of the specific mutation.

Since the absolute QT interval measured on the ECG can vary by changes in heart rate, many have employed the Bazett's correction formula to standardize the QT interval (QTc). Classically, QTc intervals in excess of 440 ms and 460 ms are considered prolonged in males and females, respectively. Although extremely prolonged QTc intervals (>600 ms) predict a higher risk for sudden death, it is unclear whether the *degree* of QTc interval prolongation predicts an individual's risk for episodes of ventricular tachyarrhythmias. In normal individuals, QTc intervals vary to some degree with age and gender. Women tend to have slightly longer QTc intervals after puberty when compared to age-matched men,[13] an observation suggesting a hormonal effect on ventricular repolarization. This may explain in part the propensity of this syndrome to affect more women than men, unlike most other diseases

of the cardiovascular system. One fascinating feature of this syndrome is the marked variability in phenotypic penetrance.[14] The variability has been described in members within the same family and even among those carrying the same genetic mutation.[15] This is thought to be due in part to the interplay between genetics and environmental factors, as well as the presence of multiple polymorphisms occurring in related genes.[16]

Diagnostics

Most individuals with LQTS have abnormally prolonged QTc intervals at baseline, but approximately 6%–10% of these patients do not.[17,18] Because of this finding and the variability in phenotypic penetrance, the diagnosis of LQTS may need to be made based on the presence of major and minor diagnostic criteria and a point-scoring system (Fig. 52.4)[19]. There have also been reports of individuals who have normal QTc intervals at baseline, but who have an exaggerated prolongation of the QTc interval in the presence of certain pharmacologic agents or environmental stressors (Table 52.3). The underlying mechanisms of this form of long QT syndrome, also known as "acquired long QT syndrome," may be due in part to several genetic polymorphisms resulting in a reduction of what has been described as "repolarization reserve."[20] On the basis of this concept, individuals with acquired long QT syndrome have no evidence of QT abnormalities at baseline, but in the presence of a stressor (e.g., drugs, heart block, hypokalemia, ischemia), they lack the physiologic mechanisms to accommodate for these insults. Acquired long QT syndrome is not a milder form of congenital long QT syndrome, as evidenced by the observation that the former group of individuals also have an increased risk for torsades de pointes.[21] Identifying individuals at risk for acquired long QT syndrome can often be difficult and many have suggested a number of clinical characteristics that should alert the clinician to the possibility of this risk.[22]

Classically, patients with LQTS are young and present with tachyarrhythmia-associated syncope in the setting of emotional stress, physical exertion, sudden awakening, or menses.[23] Earlier reports have demonstrated ventricular arrhythmias occurring during sleep primarily in individuals with LQT3 with documented mutations in SCN5A.[24] The risk of ventricular arrhythmias also appears to depend on the ion channel mutated. LQT1 and LQT2 patients have the highest risk for ventricular arrhythmias compared to those with LQT3. Although the frequency of events is lower for LQT3 patients, the events occurring in this group are more often fatal. In the end, the cumulative mortality of these three variants is approximately the same.[25]

The surface ECG typically exhibits abnormalities of T wave morphology (as described above) and a prolonged QTc. It is not uncommon for individuals to describe a history of repeated episodes of syncope. The syncopal episodes are invariably due to torsades de pointes that typically terminate spontaneously but may degenerate into ventricular fibrillation. Imaging modalities to assess cardiac function do not help in the diagnosis, as most individuals display grossly normal ventricular systolic function. Diagnosis is based largely on a detailed personal and family history and the ECG.

Risk stratification for sudden cardiac death

The QTc interval on a surface ECG in excess of 500 msec is generally regarded as high risk for sudden cardiac death; however, daily variations in the QTc interval occur even within the same individual. Hence, relying solely on the surface ECG is limited in its scope. Signal-averaged ECGs have been utilized in a number of different conditions for risk assessment of sudden death. Their role in LQTS is limited and not described well enough to warrant routine use.[26] Graded exercise stress testing and other non-invasive tests have been assessed for their ability to aid in risk stratification.[27,28] These early observations suggest that individuals who display prolongation of the QTc at peak exercise are at particularly high risk of arrhythmic events when compared to their age-matched counterparts.[29] The role of invasive electrophysiologic testing has been limited by its lack of robust sensitivity and specificity[30] and is generally

not recommended in these individuals, despite isolated reports of a higher incidence of resting bradycardia[31] or inducibility of ventricular tachyarrhythmias with ventricular burst pacing[32] in this patient population. Universal recommendations for genetic testing in familial cases of long QT syndrome remain equivocal, although a recent article demonstrated that this may be both feasible and cost-effective in certain individuals.[33,34]

Because of the limitations in objective measures for sudden death, a patient's symptoms play a significant role in risk stratification. Individuals with a prior history of syncope (often mistaken for seizure events) or sudden death are naturally at higher risk of a future fatal event, whereas those who are asymptomatic tend to be at lesser risk. Nevertheless, exceptions exist in this observation, especially in asymptomatic individuals with a strong family history of sudden death. Priori *et al.* suggested a method of risk stratification based on gender and genotype analysis and suggest that individuals with LQT1 have a lower risk of arrhythmic events when compared to those with LQT2 and LQT3.[35] Current efforts are underway to make this method widely accessible to the general public.[36]

Preventative strategies

In all patients with LQTS, a careful review of both prescription and non-prescription medications is paramount to identifying agents that may increase the QT interval. Identifying other reversible causes such as ischemia or electrolyte abnormalities is also critical. LQTS patients deemed at high risk for sudden death (e.g., markedly prolonged QTc intervals, history of sudden cardiac death, or recurrent episodes of syncope) are typically managed with β-adrenergic blockers and are recommended to undergo implantation of an ICD. Pharmacotherapy alone does not provide a degree of protection similar to that of an ICD, but may be appropriate in individuals with low–moderate risk for SCD. Since prolongation of the QTc interval in these individuals can result from a number of different ion channelopathies, no single drug should be expected to reduce risk in everyone with LQTS. Beta-blockers are thought to be more effective in LQT1 patients, whereas sodium channel blockers may be more effective in individuals with LQT2 and LQT3.[37] Nevertheless, beta-blockers are recommended in all individuals with LQTS when the genotype is unknown, because a majority of arrhythmic events occur in the setting of heightened adrenergic tone.[38]

Recommendations on physical exertion in patients with LQTS have been addressed by an international panel of experts appointed by the American Heart Association.[39] In this treatise, the type of exercise is graded on the basis of intensity and specific recommendations are made. The reader is referred to this article for specific recommendations on patient management.

Acute management strategies

Tachyarrhythmic syndromes in patients with LQTS are often due to torsades de pointes, polymorphic ventricular tachycardia occurring in the setting of a prolonged QT interval. The acute management of these episodes is heavily based on the degree of hemodynamic instability associated with these arrhythmias. Individuals with asymptomatic episodes of unsustained ventricular tachycardia seen on a cardiac monitor seldom require emergent intervention beyond a careful review of reversible causes of QT prolongation and observation. Individuals presenting acutely with syncope or sudden cardiac death should be promptly managed by the recently revised cardiopulmonary resuscitation treatment recommendations.[40] Once sinus rhythm has been restored, acute secondary preventative measures should be considered. These include infusion of 2–4 g of magnesium intravenously, regardless of the current serum magnesium levels.[41] Magnesium is primarily excreted by the kidneys so individuals with renal insufficiency should be treated cautiously, but this is rarely an absolute contraindication to use. If magnesium proves ineffective in preventing subsequent episodes of sustained ventricular tachyarrhythmias, lidocaine has been demonstrated to be effective in some animal models by blocking sodium channels responsible for rapid depolarizing currents initiated by early afterdepolarizations.[42] Its efficacy in clinical practice has been mixed. Individuals who continue to have episodes of tachyarrhythmias and who fail these initial measures can often be treated with temporary pacing.

In cases of acquired LQTS, temporary rapid atrial pacing should be initiated. This can effectively suppress subsequent episodes of ventricular tachyarrhythmia by reducing the time of myocardial repolarization based on the properties of electrical restitution. If transvenous pacing is unavailable, isoproterenol can be used to increase the heart rate since this agent has a greater chronotropic effect per microgram than other adrenergic agents. Use of isoproterenol is contraindicated in individuals with uncontrolled hypertension, acute coronary syndromes, or a documented history of congenital long QT syndrome.

Short QT syndrome

Recognized as a distinct clinical entity since its discovery in 1999, the short QT syndrome (SQTS) encompasses individuals with QTc intervals <300 ms and clinically presenting with syncope, palpitations, and an increased propensity toward atrial fibrillation, sudden death, or both.[43] Although rare, the true prevalence of this condition is unknown since the brevity of the QT interval is often only recognized with heart rates below 80 bpm. Thus far, mutations in two ion channel genes (HERG and KvLQTI) have been linked to this clinical syndrome, both of which result in a gain of function and increased repolarizing current, presumably I_{Kr} and I_{Ks}, respectively, in the ventricle. On a cellular level, these mutations are thought to contribute to an increase in the heterogeneous dispersion of repolarization between the ventricular M cells and the epicardial cells. Clinically, most individuals have easily inducible ventricular tachycardia during electrophysiologic testing. To date, only 22 confirmed cases of short QT syndrome have been described.[44] Hence, recommendations on management are less well defined. Acute management of these individuals presenting with cardiac arrest should be guided by standard advanced cardiopulmonary life support (ACLS) recommendations; longer term management for those with the most severe presentations should include ICD implantation. The role of drugs that prolong the AP and QT interval in SQTS is not yet defined.

Brugada syndrome

The Brugada syndrome, also referred to as Sudden Unexplained Nocturnal Death syndrome,[45] was described in 1992 after a series of otherwise healthy individuals with structurally normal hearts presented with a high propensity for sudden cardiac death.[46] Classically, this entity is marked by characteristic ECG abnormalities, including the presence of a right bundle branch block pattern and ST segment elevations along V1-V3 (Fig. 52.5). The ECG abnormalities are not pathognomonic for this condition and may be caused by other factors, such as well-conditioned athletic hearts or a variety of drugs (Table 52.4). Although the syndrome has been diagnosed in individuals between 2 and 84 years of age, the mean age of sudden death is 41 ± 15 years and it appears to have an 8:1 predilection for males.[47] Many of the ECG abnormalities seen with this entity are dynamic and occasionally can be accentuated by a febrile state, ischemia, hypotension, or the administration of beta-blockers or sodium channel blockers (e.g., procainamide, flecainide). Often, exercise or adrenergic agents such as isoproterenol can make the ST-segment abnormalities disappear.[48] Hence, the true prevalence of this condition is unknown, although it is estimated to be 5 in 10 000 individuals worldwide. It is

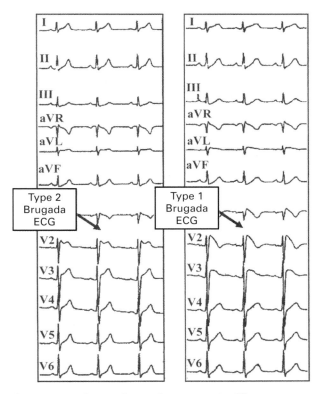

Fig. 52.5 Brugada ECG abnormalities (Type I–III).[100]

generally recognized that individuals from Europe and the United States[49] are less commonly affected while those from Japan[50] and Southeast Asia have higher rates of prevalence for this syndrome. Current estimates (based in large part on epidemiological experiences in Asian populations) report that the Brugada syndrome accounts for 4% of all sudden cardiac deaths and 20% of all sudden cardiac deaths occurring in individuals with structurally normal hearts.[51] In addition to the increased risk for sudden death, 20% of individuals with the Brugada syndrome have recently been described to develop atrial fibrillation as well.[52]

Early work in understanding the molecular pathogenesis of this condition identified loss-of-function mutations in the SCN5A gene,[53] the alpha subunit of the voltage-gated sodium channel originally cloned in 1992.[54] This has also been implicated in a number of other clinical syndromes including progressive familial heart block syndrome[55] and chromosome 3-linked long QT syndrome.[56] More than 80 different mutations[57] in SCN5A have been associated with this condition. Interestingly, only 18%–42% of subjects carrying a clinical diagnosis of Brugada syndrome harbor these mutations;[58] the remaining subjects are thought to

carry mutations in the non-coding portions (e.g., introns) of the gene. How loss-of-function mutations in SCN5A result in the classic ECG abnormalities has been a subject of experimental investigation. It has long been recognized that ventricular myocardium is composed of three functionally distinct layers, the epicardium, the M cell layer, and the endocardium. Normally during Phase I of myocardial repolarization, a gradient exists between the epicardial and endocardial cells that results from a difference in I_{to} current. In the presence of a loss of function mutation such as the Brugada syndrome, this difference is further accentuated whereby an abnormally steep voltage gradient is generated that causes exaggerated J point and ST-segment elevations. The same steep voltage gradient predisposes the myocardium to reentry during the plateau phase of the action potential, thereby initiating rapid ventricular tachycardia.

Diagnostics

The diagnosis of Brugada syndrome is suggested by the presence of distinct repolarization abnormalities noted on the surface ECG marked by the presence of an incomplete right bundle branch block pattern of conduction with coved ST-segment elevations (>2 mm) followed by inverted T waves primarily in leads V1-V3 (Type I pattern). The diagnosis of Brugada is made with Type I ECG abnormalities in addition to one or more clinical features suggestive of an increased propensity toward sudden cardiac death (Table 52.5). Often these abnormalities may be intermittent and are concealed except in the presence of a sodium channel-blocking agent. The absence of these abnormalities by no means excludes this diagnosis. Variations in ECG abnormalities have also been recognized. Type II ECG abnormalities are characterized by the presence of an incomplete right bundle branch block pattern of conduction with "saddleback-like" ST segment elevations (>2 mm) in leads V1-V3. Type III abnormalities are characterized as any Type I or Type II abnormality with minimal ST segment elevation (<2 mm). Type II and Type III abnormalities (in the presence of a clinical feature from Table 52.5) are not diagnostic of Brugada syndrome unless there is conversion of either pattern type to a Type I abnormality in the presence of a sodium channel-blocking agent.

Risk stratification for sudden cardiac death

Not all individuals with Brugada syndrome share the same risk for sudden cardiac death. Hence, developing a strategy to identify those at highest risk permits an economically sound approach to provide aggressive treatment to

Table 52.4. Drug-induced Brugada-like ECG patterns

I. Antiarrhythmic drugs
1. Na$^+$ channel blockers
    Class IC drugs (flecainide, pilsicainide, propafenone)
    Class IA drugs (ajmaline, procainamide, disopyramide, cibenzoline)
2. Ca^{2+} channel blockers
    Verapamil
3. β-Blockers
    Propranolol, etc.
II. Antianginal drugs
1. Ca^{2+} channel blockers
    Nifedipine, diltiazem
2. Nitrate
    Isosorbide dinitrate, nitroglycerine
3. K$^+$ channel openers
    Nicorandil
III. Psychotropic drugs
1. Tricyclic antidepressants
    Amitriptyline, nortriptyline, desipramine, clomipramine
2. Tetracyclic antidepressants
    Maprotiline
3. Phenothiazine
    Perphenazine, cyamemazine
4. Selective serotonin reuptake inhibitors
    Fluoxetine
IV. Other drugs
1. Dimenhydrinate
2. Cocaine intoxication
3. Alcohol intoxication

It is not clear whether individuals who exhibit ECG changes in the setting of these medications have a subclinical form of Brugada syndrome. Drugs listed here do not imply that other drugs of the same class will result in the same ECG changes.[100]

Table 52.5. Brugada syndrome features

Documented ventricular fibrillation or polymorphic ventricular tachycardia
Family history of sudden cardiac death in <45 years old
Coved-type ECG abnormalities in family members
Inducibility of VT with ventricular programmed stimulation
Syncope
Nocturnal agonal respirations

those who need it the most. Much of the early work in identifying sudden cardiac death markers relied on the surface ECG. On the basis of studies of Japanese patients with Brugada syndrome, individuals with a prior episode of ventricular fibrillation arrest had ECGs with widened S waves in V_1 and more pronounced ST segment elevation in V_2 when compared to those without a prior history of cardiac arrest.[59] Other studies have found predictive power in the presence of signal-averaged ECG late potentials or an increase in the body surface area of right precordial ST segments.[60] Despite these reports, no one marker has been found to be particularly more predictive for development of sudden cardiac death than others. Extensive work has also been done regarding the role of electrophysiologic testing in predicting future events.[61–63] Currently, evidence is inconclusive with respect to the role of programmed stimulation in determining whether inducibility of ventricular tachyarrhythmias provides useful prognostic information.

Recent data based on a large cohort of individuals with Brugada syndrome suggest that the risk for sudden death depends on the degree of symptomatology.[64] Eckardt *et al.* followed 212 patients with Type I ECG abnormalities for an average of 3.3 years. Individuals with the highest risk for sudden cardiac death were those who had a history of syncope or a prior history of resuscitation due to ventricular tachyarrhythmias. Asymptomatic individuals had the lowest risk for sudden death. Indeed, only 0.8% of the asymptomatic individuals developed an arrhythmic event (Fig. 52.6). It was also suggested that individuals with spontaneous Type I ECG pattern abnormalities were more likely to develop syncope or sustained ventricular tachyarrhythmias when compared to those whose ECG abnormalities were only noted in the presence of a sodium channel-blocking agent. Genetic testing in Brugada syndrome remains an area of intense research and is currently not recommended for screening of asymptomatic individuals.[65]

Preventative strategies

The classic ECG findings in patients with Brugada syndrome stem from an imbalance of currents, specifically I_{to} and I_{Ca}, during Phase I and Phase II of the action potential (Fig. 52.2).[66,67] Hence, factors affecting these currents can alter the degree of ST-segment elevation seen. Vagal maneuvers (via suppression of I_{Ca} and/or augmentation of potassium currents) and administration of Class IC sodium channel blockers (via its effects on I_{to}) enhance the ST-segment abnormalities seen on the ECG, while beta-adrenergic agonists, through their effects in augmenting I_{Ca}, normalize them. These observations suggest that pharmacologic agents that can augment I_{Ca} or inhibit I_{to} may be pivotal in mitigating the arrhythmogenicity of this condition. Examples include quinidine and 4-aminopyridine, both of which inhibit I_{to}. Commonly used agents, such as tricyclic antidepressants, phenothiazine, selective serotonin reuptake inhibitors, calcium channel blockers, β-blockers, and histaminic H$_1$ receptor antagonists can all accentuate the ST-segment abnormalities seen in patients with Brugada syndrome.[68] It is not clear whether patients with Brugada syndrome are more susceptible to ventricular tachyarrhythmias with the use of these medications, but avoidance of these drugs seems generally prudent in patients with suspected Brugada syndrome, except as noted in the management of acute manifestations of the syndrome.

Current practice guidelines recommend implantation of an ICD in patients with Brugada syndrome with a history of sudden cardiac arrest or syncope. The indications for implanting an ICD in asymptomatic patients remain controversial. Although pharmacologic therapy is less effective than ICDs in preventing SCD, a number of case reports have described the efficacy of quinidine in preventing ventricular fibrillation (VF).[69] Other agents have also been described, including cilostazol, sotalol, and mexiletine.[70] These agents,[71] however, should only be considered as an adjunct to an ICD.

Acute management strategies

Individuals who present with ventricular fibrillatory storm should be treated with β-adrenergic agonists such as isoproterenol and titrated to achieve a 20% increase in the baseline heart rate. Atropine may also be considered, although the effects are ephemeral. Both of these agents act by augmenting I$_{Ca}$. The use of quinidine in ventricular fibrillatory storm has also been described.[70] Additional acute management strategies for this condition should follow current ACLS guidelines.

Catecholamine-induced polymorphic ventricular tachycardia

Catecholamine-induced polymorphic ventricular tachycardia (CPVT) is a rare autosomal disorder originally reported in 1975 to describe children without a history of structural heart disease who were at increased risk for syncope, seizures, or sudden cardiac death.[72] Often these individuals present in the prepubescent period with arrhythmic episodes of bidirectional or polymorphic ventricular tachycardia occurring almost exclusively during physical activity or extreme emotional states. Approximately 72% of these episodes are self-limiting; however, up to 7% may degenerate to ventricular fibrillation.[73] Baseline ECGs, echocardiograms, and histologic cardiac examination of affected individuals are all normal.[74] Estimated risks of sudden death

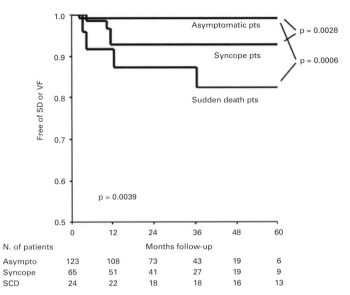

Fig. 52.6 Outcomes of patients with Brugada syndrome risk stratified based on history of syncope or resuscitated sudden death.[64]

range between 30% and 50% in untreated individuals in their second and third decades of life,[75] with approximately 30% of cases having a family history of childhood syncope or sudden death. In a series of 21 children with this condition, Leenhardt *et al.* described the natural history of this condition over a 7-year follow-up period.[76] Most children experienced their first episode of syncope by age 7. In severe cases, these arrhythmia-associated episodes would often be misdiagnosed as manifestations of epilepsy since they were usually associated with a period of hypertonia marked by convulsions and loss of bladder or bowel control. A useful distinction between epilepsy and CPVT is the observation that arrhythmic episodes of CPVT almost always occur in the setting of increased physical or emotional states.

Genetic analyses aimed at elucidating the mechanisms behind this disorder have identified two inherited forms, an autosomal dominant variant and a less common autosomal recessive type. Autosomal dominant CPVT is caused by mutations in the type 2 ryanodine receptor (RyR2), a major transmembrane protein responsible for intracellular calcium transport.[77] Autosomal recessive CPVT is due to mutations in calsequestrin.[78] As such, the initiation of many arrhythmic episodes is due to the development of delayed afterdepolarizations.

Diagnostics and risk stratification for sudden cardiac death

Information obtained from baseline electrocardiograms typically demonstrates sinus bradycardia without evidence of intraventricular conduction delays or prolongation of the QTc interval. Priori *et al.* evaluated 118 individuals with CPVT and assessed current diagnostic modalities in predicting their risk for sudden death.[79] Electrophysiologic testing has little role in risk stratification, with a majority of individuals displaying no inducible arrhythmias during programmed stimulation. Exercise stress testing and ambulatory cardiac monitoring during periods of exercise have often helped in the diagnosis of this condition. During exercise, individuals with this condition elicit a normal increase in the sinus rate. When the rate reaches approximately 120 beats per minute, frequent premature ventricular complexes are seen. With continued exercise, these degenerate into runs of polymorphic ventricular tachycardia.[80] Although these observations appear readily reproducible with physical activity, the role of exercise testing in risk stratification has not been validated. The strongest risk factor for sudden death in this condition appears to be gender, with an increased risk for arrhythmic syncope in males. The presence or absence of symptoms does not appear to predict future risk for sudden death.

Preventative strategies

If left untreated, an individual's risk for sudden death reaches 30%–50% by early adulthood. Hence, proper diagnosis and screening of family members with an affected proband is essential. The use of long-acting beta-blockers without sympathomimetic activity has previously been shown to be highly effective in preventing future episodes of syncope.[73] Recent data from Priori *et al.*,[79] however, demonstrate that beta-blockers are only effective in approximately 50% of individuals. In subjects who underwent ICD implantation, 50% of these patients experienced appropriate ICD firings for ventricular tachyarrhythmias, despite the concomitant use of beta-blockers. The use of calcium channel blockers has limited utility, but recent evidence supports their use in individuals intolerant of beta-blocker therapy.[81] Current recommendations include the use of beta-blockers at the time of diagnosis. The indications for ICD implantation are less clearly defined, but as with any heritable arrhythmia syndrome with a life-threatening presentation, it is prudent in any individual with a history of syncope or resuscitated sudden cardiac death.

Acute management strategies

Individuals presenting with ventricular tachycardia should be treated by currently accepted ACLS guidelines. Since many of these arrhythmias occur in the setting of increased adrenergic tone, the use of intravenous propranolol has been advocated.[82]

Wolff–Parkinson–White syndrome

Wolff, Parkinson, and White (WPW) are credited with describing this syndrome based on their initial experiences of 12 individuals with recurrent episodes of tachycardia and a baseline ECG displaying bundle branch block-like patterns of conduction and a short PR interval.[83] Individuals with these "pre-excited" ECG abnormalities (Fig. 52.7) are diagnosed with the WPW *syndrome* in the presence of paroxysms of tachycardia. Often the tachycardia is regular with a narrow QRS complex (orthodromic reciprocating tachycardia), but it may occasionally present with irregular wide QRS complexes as a result of pre-excited atrial arrhythmias (e.g., atrial fibrillation, atrial tachycardia) or antidromic reciprocating tachycardia. The mechanism for the pre-excitation is a result of a congenital accessory pathway supporting atrioventricular conduction that can manifest in a number of different variations (Fig. 52.8). Normally, the atrioventricular (AV) node serves as the sole means of electrical conduction from the atrium to the ventricles. In patients with WPW, an additional pathway exists composed of working myocardial tissue that allows for activation of the ventricles without the need for the AV node. Unlike the AV node, which has the ability to limit the rate at which impulses are conducted from the atrium to the ventricle, the accessory pathway can often sustain very rapid electrical conduction. Therefore, individuals are at increased risk for sudden death in the setting of pre-excited atrial arrhythmias, such as atrial fibrillation that can rapidly degenerate into ventricular fibrillation.[84] The degree of pre-excitation (i.e., prominence of the delta wave) on a baseline ECG is dependent on the conduction velocity of the AV node and the location of the accessory pathway. Hence, the presence and orientation of the delta wave can provide clues to the location of the pathway (Fig. 52.9).

Clinically, the incidence of WPW syndrome is 1.5 per 1000 persons, with a small predilection toward males.[85] Although most individuals with WPW syndrome have structurally normal hearts, an association with Ebstein's anomaly has been described.[86] Interestingly, patients with Ebstein's anomaly often have multiple accessory pathways. Despite the presence of an accessory pathway,

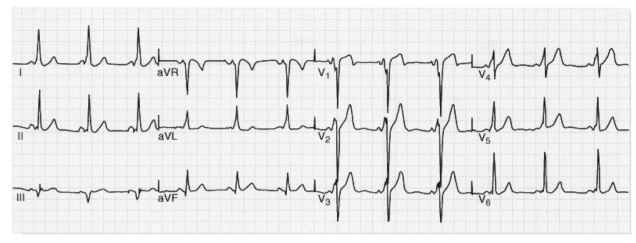

Fig. 52.7 WPW ECG with delta wave and the three classic features (1) short PR<120 ms, (2) QRS >120 ms, (3) ST–T wave changes directed in an opposite direction of the delta and QRS vectors.[87]

episodes of tachyarrhythmias do not occur in all affected individuals. Current estimates of the frequency of paroxysms of tachycardia range between 10% and 36% of patients with a WPW ECG depending on the individual's age.[87] A vast majority (80%) of these tachycardias are atrioventricular reciprocating tachycardias, while the remaining 20% include atrial arrhythmias such as atrial tachycardia, atrial flutter, or atrial fibrillation. The risk of sudden death is small and is estimated to be 0.02%–0.1%.[88]

The natural history of patients with WPW syndrome suggests that the frequency of tachyarrhythmias and the risk of sudden death decreases with age, based on age-related changes in the accessory pathway's conduction velocities.[89] Patients with WPW ECG features but who are otherwise asymptomatic do very well with a low arrhythmic event rate of approximately 1.7 per 100 patient-years.[90]

Diagnostics and risk stratification for sudden cardiac death

The diagnosis of WPW can often be made by the presence of a delta wave on a baseline ECG especially if the pathway is located on the right side of the heart. The absence of a delta wave, however, does not exclude the presence of an accessory pathway, but in these individuals there is no increased risk of sudden death. Individuals with WPW syndrome are often referred for additional testing, including exercise stress testing and/or electrophysiologic testing with ablation. Although the predictive value of ST-T wave changes during exercise testing is poor,[91] the conduction

properties of the accessory pathway can be elucidated in an effort to risk-stratify patients for the development of sudden death. In the presence of pre-excitation at baseline, sudden loss of the delta wave during peak exercise suggests that conduction via the accessory pathway has been blocked and that the patient's risk for sudden death is low.[92] Electrophysiologic testing remains an integral part of the assessment and management of patients with WPW syndrome and should be considered in the absence of known contraindications. Individuals with WPW ECG who are otherwise asymptomatic, however, may not benefit from electrophysiologic testing in light of their low risk for sudden death or tachyarrhythmias. Controversy remains on the optimal management of individuals with asymptomatic WPW ECG patterns.[93,94]

Acute management strategies

Individuals with WPW can present to the emergency department with a variety of tachyarrhythmias. Management of individuals presenting with narrow complex tachycardias should be focused on use of pharmacologic agents that impair AV node conduction, such as adenosine, beta-blockers, or calcium-channel blockers. Individuals presenting with irregular wide complex tachycardias, however, do not rely on the AV node for antegrade conduction. Hence, targeting the AV node will have little effect on the arrhythmia. Antiarrhythmic agents such as procainamide remain the first choice in the acute management of these arrhythmias. Other agents such as disopyramide, dofetilide, and amiodarone have also been described with

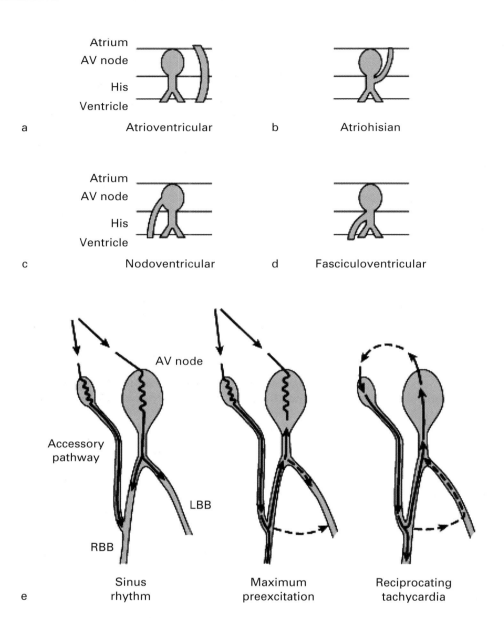

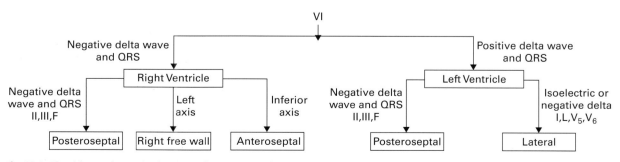

Fig. 52.8 Various types of accessory pathways.[87]

Fig. 52.9 Algorithm to determine location of accessory pathway based on the surface ECG.[87]

moderate degrees of efficacy.[95] Individuals with any degree of hemodynamic compromise should be considered for urgent electrical cardioversion to restore sinus rhythm as described in the ACLS guidelines.

Summary

Sudden cardiac death is typically associated with individuals having structural heart disease. Nevertheless, a number of individuals without structural heart disease but with an increased risk for sudden death have been identified in recent years. Through a series of experimental investigations in both animal models and humans, we have gained a greater understanding of the pathophysiologic mechanisms underlying each of these conditions and consequently realize that pharmacologic therapy is limited in its efficacy. Hence, the ICD remains the standard of care in the primary prevention of SCD for those at increased risk. What is less clear now is determining who is at increased risk. Current efforts aimed at better defining this cohort are now under way and will significantly improve our ability to deliver better care.

REFERENCES

1. Josephson, M. & Wellens, H.J.J. Implantable defibrillators and sudden cardiac death. *Circulation* 2004; **109**: 2685–2691.
2. *Bardy, G.H., Lee, K.L., Mark, D.B. et al.* Amiodarone or an implantable cardioverter–defibrillator for congestive heart failure. *N. Engl. J. Med.* 2005; **352**: 225–237.
3. Kang, S. & Cannom, D.S. Current role of device therapy to reduce sudden cardiac death in heart failure. *Curr. Heart Fail. Rep.* 2004; **1**: 104–110.
4. Wever, E.F. & *Robles de Medina, E.O.* Sudden death in patients without structural heart disease. *J. Am. Coll. Cardiol.* 2004; **43**: 1137–1144.
5. Jervell, A. & Lange-Nielsen, F. Congenital deaf-mutism, functional heart disease with prolongation of the Q-T interval, and sudden death. *Am. Heart J.* 1957; **54**: 59–68.
6. Nador, F., Beria, G., De Ferrari, G.M. *et al.* Unsuspected echocardiographic abnormality in the long QT syndrome: diagnostic, prognostic and pathogenetic implications. 1991; **84**: 1530–1542.
7. Romano, C., Gemme, G. & Pongiglione, R. Aritmie cardiache rare dell'eta pediatrica. *Clin. Pediatr.* 1963; **45**: 656–683.
8. Ward, O.C. A new familial cardiac syndrome in children. *J. Irish Med. Assoc.* 1964; **54**: 103–106.
9. Splawski, I., Shen, J., Timothy, K.W. *et al.* Spectrum of mutations in long-QT syndrome genes. KVLQT1, HERG, SCN5A, KCNE1, and KCNE2. *Circulation* 2000; **102**: 1178–1185.

10. Moss, A.J. T-wave patterns associated with the hereditary long Q-T syndrome. *CEPR* 2002; **6**: 311–315.
11. Moss, A.J., Zareba, W., Benhorin, J. *et al.* ECG T-wave patterns in genetically distinct forms of the hereditary long QT syndrome. *Circulation* 1995; **92**: 2929–2934.
12. Zhang, L., Timothy, K.W., Vincent, G.M. *et al.* Spectrum of ST-T-wave patterns and repolarization parameters in congenital long-QT syndrome: ECG findings identify genotypes. *Circulation* 2000; **102**: 2849–2855.
13. Stramba-Badiale, M., Spagnolo, D., Bosi, G. *et al.* Are gender differences in QTc present at birth? *Am. J. Cardiol.* 1995; **75**: 1277–1278.
14. Vincent, G.M., Timothy, K.W., Leppert, M. & Keating, M. The spectrum of symptoms and QT intervals in carriers of the gene for the long-QT syndrome. *N. Engl. J. Med.* 1992; **327**: 846–852.
15. Kaufman, E.S., Priori, S.G., Napolitano, C. *et al.* Electrocardiographic prediction of abnormal genotype in congenital long QT syndrome: experience in 101 related family members. *J. Cardiovasc. Electrophysiol.* 2001; **12**: 455–461.
16. Tan, B.-H., Valdivia, C.R., Rock, B.A. *et al.* Common human SCN5A polymorphisms have altered electrophysiology when expressed in Q1077 splice variants. *Heart Rhythm* 2005; **2**: 741–747.
17. Priori, S.G., Napolitano, C. & Schwartz, P.J. Low penetrance in the long QT syndrome. Clinical impact. *Circulation* 1999; **33**: 523–533.
18. Garson, A. Jr, Dick, M., Fournier, A. *et al.* The long QT syndrome in children. An international study of 287 patients. *Circulation* 1993; **87**: 1866–1872
19. Schwartz, P.J., Moss, A.J., Vincent, G.M. & Crampton, R.S. Diagnostic criteria for the long QT syndrome. An update. *Circulation* 1993; **88**: 782–784
20. Roden, D.M. Taking the "idio" out of "idiosyncratic": predicting torsades de pointes. *Pacing Clin. Electrophysiol.* 1998; **21**: 1029–1034.
21. Roden, D.M. & Viswanathan, P.C. Genetics of acquired long QT syndrome. *J. Clin. Invest.* 2005; **115**: 2025–2032.
22. Zeltser, D., Justo, D., Halkin, A. *et al.* Torsade de pointes due to noncardiac drugs: most patients have easily identifiable risk factors. *Medicine (Baltimore)* 2003; **82**: 282–290.
23. Schwartz, P.J., Zaza, A., Locati, E. & Moss, A.J. Stress and sudden death. The case of the long QT syndrome. *Circulation* 1991; **83**(Suppl): II71–II80.
24. Schwartz, P.J., Priori, S.G., Locati, E.H. *et al.* Long QT syndrome patients with mutations on the SCN5A and HERG genes have differential responses to Na$^+$ channel blockade and to increases in heart rate. Implications for gene-specific therapy. *Circulation* 1995; **92**: 3381–3386.
25. Zareba, W., Moss, A.J., Schwartz, P.J. *et al.* Influences of genotype on the clinical course of the long QT syndrome. International Long QT syndrome registry research group. *N. Engl. J. Med.* 1998; **339**: 960–965.
26. Tobe, T.J., de Langen, C.D., Bink-Boelkens, M.T. *et al.* Late potentials in a bradycardia-dependent long QT syndrome

associated with sudden death during sleep. *J. Am. Coll. Cardiol.* 1992; **19**: 541–549.

27. Lollgen, H., Wollschlager, H., Schonrich, G. *et al.* Ventricular arrhythmias and Q-Tc interval during stress-ECG. *Herz* 1986; **11**: 303–308.

28. Eggeling, T., Hoeher, M., Osterhues, H.H. *et al.* Significance of noninvasive diagnostic techniques in patients with long QT syndrome. *Am. J. Cardiol.* 1992; **70**: 1421–1426.

29. Dillenburg, R.F. & Hamilton, R.M. Is exercise testing useful in identifying congenital long QT syndrome? *Am. J. Cardiol.* 2002; **89**: 233–236.

30. Bhandari, A.K., Shapiro, W.A., Morady, F. *et al.* Electrophysiologic testing in patients with the long QT syndrome. *Circulation* 1985; **71**: 63–71.

31. Kugler, J.D. Sinus nodal dysfunction in young patients with long QT syndrome. *Am. Heart J.* 1991; **121**: 1132–6.

32. Kirchhof, P., Zellerhoff, S., Monnig, G. & Schulze-Bahr, E. Pauses after burst pacing provoke afterdepolarizations and torsades de pointes in a patient with long QT syndrome. *Heart Rhythm* 2004; **1**: 720–723.

33. *Napolitano, C., Priori, S.G., Schwartz, P.J. et al.* Genetic testing in the long QT syndrome: development and validation of an efficient approach to genotyping in clinical practice. *J. Am. Med. Assoc.* 2005; **294**: 2975–2980.

34. Phillips, K.A., Ackerman, M.J., Sakowski, J. *et al.* Cost-effective analysis of genetic testing for familial long QT syndrome in symptomatic index cases. *Heart Rhythm* 2005; **2**: 1294–1300.

35. Priori, S., Schwartz, P.J., Napolitano, C. *et al.* Risk stratification in the long QT syndrome. *N. Engl. J. Med.* 2003; **348**: 1866–1874.

36. Napolitano, C., Priori, S.G., Schwartz, P.J. *et al.* Genetic testing in the long QT syndrome: development and validation of an efficient approach to genotyping in clinical practice. *J. Am. Med. Assoc.* 2005; **294**: 2975–2980.

37. Shimizu, W., Aiba, T. & Antzelevitch, C. Specific therapy based on the genotype and cellular mechanism in inherited cardiac arrhythmias. Long QT syndrome and Brugada syndrome. *Curr. Pharm. Design* 2005; **11**: 1561–1572.

38. Moss, A.J., Zareba, W., Hall, W.J. *et al.* Effectiveness and limitations of beta-blocker therapy in congenital long-QT syndrome. *Circulation* 2000; **101**: 616–623.

39. Maron, B.J., Chaitman, B.R., Ackerman, M.J. *et al.* Recommendations for physical activity and recreational sports participation for young patients with genetic cardiovascular diseases. *Circulation* 2004; **109**: 2807–2816.

40. 2005 International Consensus Conference on Cardiopulmonary Resuscitation and Emergency Cardiovascular Care Science With Treatment Recommendations. *Circulation* 2005; **112**: III-25–III-54.

41. Bando, S., Yamamoto, H., Nishikado, A. *et al.* Effect of magnesium sulfate on ventricular refractoriness and its efficacy for torsade de pointes. *Tokushima J. Exp. Med.* 1990; **37**: 69–73.

42. Passman, R. & Kadish, A. Polymorphic ventricular tachycardia, Long Q-T syndrome, and torsades de pointes. *Med. Clin. N. Am.* 2001; **85**:

43. Gaita, F., Guistetto, C., Bianchi, F. *et al.* Short QT syndrome. A familial cause of sudden death. *Circulation* 2003; **108**: 965–970.

44. Bjerregaard, P. & Gussak, I. Short QT syndrome: mechanisms, diagnosis and treatment. *Natl Clin. Pract. Cardiovasc. Med.* 2005; **2**: 84–87.

45. Vatta, M., Dumaine, R., Varghese, G. *et al.* Genetic and biophysical basis of sudden unexplained nocturnal death syndrome (SUNDS), a disease allelic to Brugada syndrome. *Hum. Mol. Genet.* 2002; **11**: 337–345.

46. Brugada, P. & Brugada, J. Right bundle branch block, persistent ST segment elevation and sudden cardiac death: a distinct clinic and electrocardiographic syndrome. A multicenter report. *J. Am. Coll. Cardiol.* 1992; **20**: 1391–1396.

47. Alings, M., Wilde, A. "Brugada" syndrome: clinical data and suggested pathphysiological mechanism. *Circulation* 1999; **99**: 666–673.

48. Kasanuki, H., Ohnishi, S., Ohtuka, M. *et al.* Idiopathic ventricular fibrillation induced with vagal activity in patients without obvious heart disease. *Circulation* 1997; **95**: 2277–2285.

49. Hermida, J.S., Lemoine, J.L., Aoun, F.B. *et al.* Prevalence of the Brugada syndrome in an apparently healthy population. *Am. J. Cardiol.* 2000; **86**: 91–104.

50. Miyasaka, Y., Tsuji, H., Yamada, K. *et al.* Prevalence and mortality of the Brugada-type electrocardiogram in one city in Japan. *J. Am. Coll. Cardiol.* 2001; **38**: 771–774.

51. Juang, J.M. & Huang, S.K.S. Brugada syndrome – an underrecognized electrical disease in patients with sudden cardiac death. *Cardiology* 2004; **101**: 157–169.

52. Morita, H., Kusano-Fukushima, K. Nagase, S. *et al.* Atrial fibrillation and atrial vulnerability in patients with Brugada syndrome. *J. Am. Coll. Cardiol.* 2002; **40**: 1437–1444.

53. Chen, Q., Kirsch, G.E., Zhang, D. *et al.* Genetic basis and molecular mechanism for idiopathic ventricular fibrillation. *Nature* 1998; **392**: 293–295.

54. Gellens, M.E., George, A.L., Chen, L. *et al.* Primary structure and functional expression of the human cardiac tetrodotoxin-insensitive voltage-dependent sodium channel. *Proc Natl Acad. Sci. USA* 1992; **89**: 554–558.

55. Schott, J.J., Alshinawi, C., Kyndt, F. *et al.* Cardiac conduction defects associate with mutations in SCN5A. *Nat. Genet.* 1999; **23**: 20–21.

56. Wang, Q., Shen, J., Splawski, I. *et al.* SCN5A mutations associated with an inherited cardiac arrhythmia, long QT syndrome. *Cell* 1995; **80**: 805–811.

57. Antzelevitch, C. The Brugada syndrome: ionic basis and arrhythmia mechanisms. *J. Cardiovasc. Electrophysiol.* 2001; **21**: 268–272.

58. Schulze-Bahr, E., Eckardt, L. *et al.* Sodium channel gene (SCN5A) mutations in 44 index patients with Brugada syndrome: different incidences in familial and sporadic disease. *Hum. Mutat.* 2003; **21**: 651–652.

59. Atarashi, H. & Ogawa, S. New ECG criteria for high-risk Brugada syndrome. *Circ. J.* 2003; **67**: 8–10.

60. Eckardt, L., Bruns, H.J., Paul, M. *et al*. Body surface area of ST elevation and the presence of late potentials correlate to the inducibility of ventricular tachyarrhythmias in Brugada syndrome. *J. Cardiovasc. Electrophysiol.* 2002; **13**: 742–749.

61. Brugada, J., Brugada, R., Antzelevitch, C. *et al*. Long-term follow-up of individuals with the electrocardiographic pattern of right bundle-branch block and ST-segment elevation in precordial leads V1 to V3. *Circulation* 2002; **105**: 73–78.

62. Priori, S., Napolitano, C., Gasparini, M. *et al*. Natural history of Brugada syndrome: insights for risk stratification and management. *Circulation* 2002; **105**: 1342–1347.

63. Kanda, M., Shimizu, W., Matsuo, K. *et al*. Electrophysiologic characteristics and implication of induced ventricular fibrillation in symptomatic patients with Brugada syndrome. *J. Am. Coll. Cardiol.* 2002; **39**: 1799–1805.

64. Eckardt, L., Probst, V., Smits, J.P.P. *et al*. Long-term prognosis of individuals with right precordial ST-segment–elevation Brugada syndrome. *Circulation* 2005; **111**: 257–263.

65. *Ackerman, M.J., Splawski, I., Makielski, J.C. et al*. Spectrum and prevalence of cardiac sodium channel variants among black, white, Asian, and Hispanic individuals: implications for arrhythmogenic susceptibility and Brugada/long QT syndrome genetic testing. *Heart Rhythm* 2004; **1**: 600–607.

66. Yan, G.X. & Antzelevitch, C. Cellular basis for the electrocardiographic J wave. *Circulation* 1996; **93**: 372–379.

67. Yan, G.X. & Antzelevitch, C. Cellular basis for the Brugada syndrome and other mechanisms of arrhythmogenesis associated with ST segment elevation. *Circulation* 1999; **100**: 1660–1666.

68. Shimizu, W., Aiba, T. & Antzelevitch, C. Specific therapy based on the genotype and cellular mechanism in inherited cardiac arrhythmias. Long QT syndrome and Brugada syndrome. *Curr. Pharm. Design* 2005; **11**: 1561–1572.

69. Marquez, M.F., Rivera, J., Hermosillo, A.G. *et al*. Arrhythmic storm responsive to quinidine in a patient with Brugada syndrome and vasovagal Syncope. *PACE* 2005; **28**: 870–873.

70. Marquez, M.F., Salica, G., Hermosillo, A.G. *et al*. Drug Therapy in Brugada Syndrome. *Curr. Drug Targets Cardiovasc. Haematol. Disord.* 2005; **5**: 409–417.

71. Belhassen, B., Viskin, S., Fish, R., Glick, A., Setbon, I. & Eldar, M. Effects of electrophysiologic-guided therapy with Class IA antiarrhythmic drugs on the long-term outcome of patients with idiopathic ventricular fibrillation with or without the Brugada syndrome. *J. Cardiovasc. Electrophysiol.* 1999; **10**: 1301–1312.

72. Reid, D.S., Tynan, M., Braidwood, L. & Fitzgerald, G.R. Bidirectional tachycardia in a child: a study using His bundle electrography. *Br. Heart J.* 1975; **37**: 339–344.

73. Sumitomo, N., Harada, K., Nagashima, M. *et al*. Catecholaminergic polymorphic ventricular tachycardia: electrocardiographic characteristics and optimal therapeutic strategies to prevent sudden death. *Heart* 2003; **89**: 66–70.

74. Swan, H., Piippo, K., Viitasalo, M. *et al*. Arrhythmic disorder mapped to chromosome 1q42-q43 causes malignant poly-

morphic ventricular tachycardia in structurally normal hearts. *J. Am. Coll. Cardiol.* 1999; **34**: 2035–2042.

75. Leenhardt, A., Glaser, E., Burguera, M. *et al*. Short-coupled variant of torsade de pointes: a new electrocardiographic entity in the spectrum of idiopathic ventricular tachyarrhythmias. *Circulation* 1994; **89**: 206 –215.

76. Leenhardt, A., Lucet, V., Denjoy, I. *et al*. Catecholaminergic polymorphic ventricular tachycardia in children: a 7-year follow-up of 21 patients. *Circulation* 1995; **91**: 1512–1519.

77. Laitinen, P.J., Brown, K.M., Piippo, K. *et al*. Mutations of the cardiac ryanodine receptor (RyR2) gene in familial polymorphic ventricular tachycardia. *Circulation* 2001; **103**: 485–490.

78. Lahat, H., Pras, E., Olender, T. *et al*. A missense mutation in a highly conserved region of CASQ2 is associated with autosomal recessive catecholamine-induced polymorphic ventricular tachycardia in Bedouin families from Israel. *Am. J. Hum. Genet.* 2001; **69**: 1378–1384.

79. Priori, S.G., Napolitano, C., Memmi, M. *et al*. Clinical and molecular characterization of patients with catecholaminergic polymorphic ventricular tachycardia. *Circulation* 2002; **106**: 69–74.

80. *Scheinman, M.M. & Lam, J*. Exercise-induced ventricular arrhythmias in patients with no structural cardiac disease. *Annu. Rev. Med.* 2006; **57**: 473–484.

81. Swan, H., Laitinen, R., Kontula, K. *et al*. Calcium channel antagonism reduces exercise-induced ventricular arrhythmias in catecholaminergic polymorphic ventricular tachycardia patients with RyR2 mutations. *J. Cardiovasc. Electrophysiol.* 2005; **16**: 162–166.

82. De Rosa, G., Delogu, A.B., Piastra, M. *et al*. Catecholaminergic polymorphic ventricular tachycardia: successful emergency treatment with intravenous propranolol. *Pediatr. Emerg. Care* 2004; **20**: 175–177.

83. Wolff, L., Parkinson, J., White, P. *et al*. Bundle branch block with short PR interval in healthy young people prone to paroxysmal tachycardia. *Am. Heart J.* 1930; **5**: 685-

84. Klein, G.J., Bashore, T.M., Sellers, T.D. *et al*. Ventricular fibrillation in the Wolff–Parkinson–White syndrome. *N. Engl. J. Med.* 1979; **301**: 1080–1085.

85. Topol, E.J. *Textbook of Cardiovascular Medicine*. 1998; Baltimore: Williams & Wilkins.

86. van Hare, G.F. Radiofrequency ablation of accessory pathways associated with congenital heart disease. *Pacing Clin. Electrophysiol.* 1997; **20**: 2077–2081.

87. Zipes, D.P., Libby, P., Bonow, R.O., & Braunwald, E. *Braunwald's Heart Disease: A Textbook of Cardiovascular Medicine*. 2005; Philadelphia: Elsevier.

88. Fitzsimmons, P.J., McWhirter, P.D., Peterson, D.W. & Kruyer, W.B. The natural history of Wolff–Parkinson–White syndrome in 228 military aviators: a long-term follow-up of 22 years. *Am. Heart J.* 2001; **142**: 530–536.

89. Fan, W., Peter, C.T., Gang, E.S. & Mandel, W. Age-related changes in the clinical and electrophysiologic characteristics of patients with Wolff–Parkinson–White syndrome: compar-

ative study between young and elderly patients. *Am. Heart J.* 1991; **122**: 741–747.

90. Leitch, J.W., Kelin, G.J. & Yee, R. Prognostic value of electrophysiology testing in asymptomatic patients with Wolff–Parkinson–White syndrome. *Circulation* 1990; **82**: 1718.

91. Poyatos, M.E., Suarez, L., Lerman, J. *et al.* Exercise testing and thallium-201 myocardial perfusion scintigraphy in the clinical evaluation of patients with Wolff–Parkinson–White syndrome. *J. Electrocardiol.* 1986; **19**: 319–326.

92. Sharma, A.D., Yee, R., Guiraudon, G. *et al.* Sensitivity and specificity of invasive and noninvasive testing for risk of sudden death in Wolff–Parkinson–White syndrome. *J. Am. Coll. Cardiol.* 1987; **10**: 373–381.

93. Pappone, C., Manguso, F., Santinelli, R. *et al.* Radiofrequency ablation in children with asymptomatic Wolff–Parkinson–White syndrome. *N. Engl. J. Med.* 2004; **351**: 1197–1205.

94. Triedman, J., Perry, J., Van Hare, G. *et al.* Risk Stratification for prophylactic ablation in asymptomatic Wolff–Parkinson–White Syndrome. *N. Engl. J. Med.* 2005; **352**: 92–93.

95. *Redfearn, D.P., Krahn, A.D., Skanes, A.C., Yee, R. & Klein, G.J.* Use of medications in Wolff–Parkinson–White syndrome. *Expert Opin. Pharmacother.* 2005; **6**: 955–963.

96. Shah, M., Akar, F.G. & Tomaselli, G.F. Molecular basis of arrhythmias. *Circulation* 2005; **112**: 2517–2529.

97. Kass, R.S. & Moss, A.J. Long QT syndrome: novel insights into the mechanisms of cardiac arrhythmias. *J. Clin. Invest.* 2003; **112**: 810–815.

98. Schwartz, P.J., Moss, A.J., Vincent, G.M. & Crampton, R.S. Diagnostic criteria for the long QT syndrome: an update. *Circulation* 1993; **88**: 782–784.

99. Roden, D.M. Drug-induced prolongation of the QT interval. *N. Engl. J. Med.* 2004; **350**: 1013–1022.

100. Brugada Syndrome: Report of the Second Consensus Conference. *Heart Rhythm* 2005; **2**: 429.

53

Pediatric cardiopulmonary resuscitation

Robert A. Berg and Vinay M. Nadkarni

Department of Pediatrics, The University of Arizona College of Medicine
Departments of Anesthesia and Pediatrics
University of Pennsylvania School of Medicine
Department of Anesthesia and Critical Care Medicine
The Children's Hospital of Philadelphia, PA, USA

Appropriate pediatric CPR differs from that in adults, because children are anatomically and physiologically different from adults. In addition, the pathogenesis of the cardiac arrests and the most common rhythm disturbances are different in children. In contrast to adults, children rarely suffer sudden ventricular fibrillation (VF) cardiac arrest from coronary artery disease. The causes of pediatric arrests are more diverse and are usually secondary to profound hypoxia or asphyxia due to respiratory failure or circulatory shock. Prolonged hypoxia and acidosis impair cardiac function and ultimately lead to cardiac arrest. By the time the arrest occurs, all organs of the body have generally suffered significant hypoxic-ischemic insults.

Importantly, children of various ages exhibit developmental changes that affect cardiac and respiratory physiology before, during, and after cardiac arrest. For example, newborns undergoing transitional physiological changes during emergence from an environment of amniotic fluid to a gaseous environment certainly differ from adolescents. Similarly, newborns and infants have much less cardiac and respiratory reserve, and higher pulmonary vascular resistance than do older children. Moreover, many children who experience in-hospital cardiac arrest have pre-existing developmental challenges and other organ dysfunction. Finally, pediatrics is developmental medicine, and pediatric neurological tools that are appropriate at one age may not be accurate or valid at another age.

Perhaps the most profound difference between child and adult cardiac arrest is the devastating effect of the death of a child on a family. Coping with a sudden unexpected death is always difficult. When the victim is a child, the loss tends to be even more oppressive. We do not expect children to die before their parents and thus are not prepared for it. Therefore, families and friends are typically overwhelmed. Even "hardened" healthcare providers often become very emotional, and occasionally dysfunctional, when faced with a dying child.

Epidemiology

Our knowledge of the epidemiology and appropriate treatment of pediatric cardiac arrest has been limited, in part, because investigators have categorized diverse diseases and pathophysiologies into general categories. Pediatric studies tend to include all pediatric cardiac arrests, such as those secondary to sudden respiratory failure (e.g., drowning, foreign body aspiration), progressive respiratory failure from infections and/or neuromuscular diseases, trauma, Sudden Infant Death Syndrome (SIDS), septic shock, hypovolemic shock, anaphylaxis, primary cardiomyopathy, primary arrhythmia (e.g., VF or VT), drug intoxications, and others. Some pediatric studies have not clearly differentiated respiratory arrests from cardiac arrests, or CPR episodes from pulseless cardiac arrests, and many have included both pre-hospital and in-hospital cardiac arrests in their data. Moreover, many of the cardiac arrest victims in these studies had been dead for a prolonged period of time (e.g., those with Sudden Infant Death Syndrome) and, therefore, data such as initial cardiac rhythm of asystole and lack of response to therapy are not helpful in terms of understanding the etiology, pathophysiology, or appropriate therapy. The quality of CPR is generally poor, and this is not generally taken into account in most of these studies. Finally, most pediatric arrest studies have inadequate and non-uniform data collection.

Cardiac Arrest: The Science and Practice of Resuscitation Medicine. 2nd edn., ed. Norman Paradis, Henry Halperin, Karl Kern, Volker Wenzel, Douglas Chamberlain. Published by Cambridge University Press. © Cambridge University Press, 2007.

Table 53.1. Summary of representative studies of outcome following in-hospital pediatric cardiac arrest

Author, year	Setting[a]	# of patients	ROSC	Survival to discharge	Good neurological survival
Nadkarni 2005 NRCPR[b]	In-hospital CA	880	459 (52%)	236 (27%)	154 (18%)
Reis 2002	In-hospital CA	129	83 (64%)	21 (16%)	19 (15%)
Extracorporeal Life Support Organization, 2002	In-hospital CA resuscitation by ECMO	232	N/A All needed ECMO	88 (38%)	not reported
Suominen 2000	In-hospital CA	118	74 (63%)	1-year survival 21 (18%)	not reported
Parra 2000	Ped CICU CA	32	24 (63%)	14 (44%)	8 (25%)
Chamnanvanakij 2000	In-hospital intubated NICU pts with chest compressions for bradycardia	39	33 (85%)	CPR 20 (51%) CA 10%	CPR 5 (13%) (6 lost to follow-up)
Slonim 1997	In-hospital PICU CA	205	not reported	28 (14%)	not reported
Torres 1997	In-hospital CA	92	not reported	1-year survival 9 (10%)	7 (8%)
Zaritsky A 1987	In-hospital CA	CA 53	not reported	CA 5 (9%)	not reported
Young 1999	Meta-analysis In-hospital CA	544	not reported	129 (24%)	not reported
Lopez-Herce 2005	Mixed in-hospital and OOH CA	213	110 (52%)	45 (21%)	34 (16%)
Tunstall-Pedoe 1992	Mixed in-hospital and OOH CA	3765	1411 (38%)	706 (19%)	not reported

[a] CA=cardiac arrest.
[b] NRCPR=National Registry of CPR.

Characterization of the process of care and outcomes following pediatric cardiac arrest events has been limited by this lack of consistent data collection and analysis. In particular, pediatric reports often have not clearly differentiated between respiratory arrest, near-arrests (bradycardia with pulses) treated with CPR, and pulseless cardiac arrest. In the early 1990s, international experts developed guidelines for uniform data reporting of out-of-hospital cardiac arrests and in-hospital resuscitation, the so-called Utstein style. Nevertheless, epidemiological information about pediatric cardiac arrests is dominated by retrospective chart reviews with small numbers and inconsistent definitions of cardiac arrest and cardiopulmonary resuscitation, and a few small prospective single-center studies.

Pediatric in-hospital arrests

The true incidence of pediatric pulseless arrest is difficult to estimate because of inconsistent terminology in the literature and difficulty in assessing pulselessness in children. Cardiac arrests were reported in 3% of children admitted to one children's hospital, in 1.8% of all children admitted to pediatric intensive care units in the USA, in 6% of children admitted to one PICU in Finland, and in 4% of children admitted to a pediatric cardiac intensive care unit.

Several well-designed in-hospital pediatric CPR investigations with long-term follow-up have established that pediatric CPR and advanced life support can be remarkably effective (Table 53.1). Typically, one-half to two thirds of these patients were initially successfully resuscitated (i.e., attained sustained ROSC). Survival progressively decreased with time, in large part due to the underlying disease processes. Indeed, most of these arrests/events occurred in pediatric intensive care units because of progressive life-threatening illnesses that had not responded to treatment despite critical care monitoring and supportive care. The 1-year survival rates of 10%–44% are superior to outcomes from out-of-hospital pediatric CPR, and substantially superior to the certain 0% survival rate if CPR and advanced life support were not provided.

Only a few studies have used the more rigorous Utstein-style reporting for exclusively in-hospital pediatric cardiac arrests and CPR. Two describe all CPR events at children's hospitals in Brazil and Finland. The most common causes of the events were progressive respiratory failure and progressive shock: approximately two thirds of the children attained sustained ROSC, and 1-year survival was 15% and 18%, respectively.

A recently published Utstein-style report of in-hospital pediatric cardiac arrests is derived from the American Heart Association's multi-center National Registry of Cardiopulmonary Resuscitation (NRCPR). The NRCPR is a prospective, multicenter observational registry of in-hospital cardiac arrests and resuscitations. The first description of children (<18 years old) from this registry included 880 patients whose arrests occurred between January 1, 2000 and March 30, 2004 in 10 pediatric facilities and 136 mixed pediatric–adult facilities. Because of the size and scope of the NRPCR, and the rigorous data collection, these data are further highlighted in Tables 53.2 and 53.3.

In the NRCPR, a cardiac arrest was defined as cessation of cardiac mechanical activity, determined by the absence of a palpable central pulse, unresponsiveness, and apnea. Events were excluded if the cardiac arrest began out-of-hospital, involved a newborn in a delivery room or neonatal intensive care unit, or was limited to a shock by an implanted cardioverter-defibrillator. Most of these arrests occurred in children with progressive respiratory insufficiency and/or progressive circulatory shock. These children were often succumbing to their critical illnesses despite aggressive critical care monitoring and therapy. Therefore, 95% of these arrests were witnessed and/or monitored, and only 14% occurred on a general pediatric ward. Before the arrest, 57% of these children were mechanically ventilated, 38% had continuous vasoactive infusions, and 29% had continuous direct arterial blood pressure monitoring.

Despite the dire clinical circumstances leading to their arrests, 52% attained sustained ROSC, 36% survived for 24 hours, and 27% survived to hospital discharge. Outcomes for these children were substantially superior to outcomes for adults in this registry (27% survival to discharge versus 18%, respectively; adjusted odds ratio, 2.3 [95%CI, 2.0–2.7]). Importantly, 65% of these children had relatively good neurological outcome, defined as: (1) Pediatric Cerebral Performance Category of 1, 2 or 3; or (2) no change from baseline Pediatric Cerebral Performance Category.

Table 53.2. Characteristics of pediatric in-hospital cardiac arrests

Characteristic	Pediatric cardiac arrest ($N = 880$)
Age, y	
Mean (SD)	5.6 (6.4)
Median (range)	1.8 (0-17.0)
Sex	
Male	473 (54)
Female	407 (46)
Race/ethnicity	
White	447 (51)
Black	226 (26)
Hispanic	105 (12)
Other/unknown	102 (12)
Patient type	
In-patient	750 (85)
Emergency department	121 (14)
Other (outpatient, visitor, or employee)	9 (1)
Illness category	
Medical, cardiac	158 (18)
Medical, non-cardiac	402 (46)
Surgical, cardiac	150 (17)
Surgical, non-cardiac	62 (7)
Trauma	91 (10)
Other	17 (2)
Pre-existing conditions	
Respiratory insufficiency	511 (58)
Hypotension/hypoperfusion	319 (36)
Congestive heart failure	273 (31)
Pneumonia/septicemia/other infection	259 (29)
Arrhythmia	182 (21)
Renal insufficiency	104 (12)
Diabetes mellitus	11 (1)
Metabolic/electrolyte abnormality	178 (20)
Baseline depression in CNS function	151 (17)
Metastatic or hematologic malignancy	43 (5)
Myocardial infarction	21 (2)
None	69 (8)
Hepatic insufficiency	55 (6)
Acute CNS non-stroke event	94 (11)
Acute stroke	5 (1)
Major trauma	97 (11)
Toxicological problem	12 (1)

Interestingly, 200 children who received chest compressions for any reason during this time period were excluded from the NRPCR cardiac arrest analysis because they initially had bradycardia with pulses and did not lose their pulse during the event. Similar to the two previous Utstein-style pediatric in-hospital studies, only 82% of children who received chest compressions fit the definition of

Table 53.3. Event characteristics of pediatric in-hospital cardiac arrests*

Characteristic	Pediatric cardiac arrest ($N=880$)
Event location	
Intensive care unit	570 (65)
Emergency department	116 (13)
General inpatient	123 (14)
Diagnostic area	21 (2)
Outpatient, other, or unknown	20 (2)
Operating department or postanesthetic care	30 (3)
First-documented pulseless rhythm	
Asystole	350 (40)
VF and pulseless VT	120 (14)
VF	71 (8)
Pulseless VT	49 (6)
PEA	213 (24)
Unknown by documentation	197 (22)
Discovery status at time of event	
Witnessed and/or monitored	834 (95)
Witnessed and monitored	727 (83)
Witnessed and not monitored	73 (8)
Monitored and not witnessed	34 (4)
Not monitored and not witnessed	46 (5)
Immediate cause(s) of event	
Arrhythmia	392 (49)
Acute respiratory insufficiency	455 (57)
Hypotension	483 (61)
Acute myocardial infarction or ischemia	12 (2)
Metabolic/electrolyte disturbance	95 (12)
Acute pulmonary edema	33 (4)
Acute pulmonary embolism	6 (1)
Airway obstruction	41 (5)
Toxicological problem	9 (1)

Abbreviations: PEA, pulseless electrical activity; VF, ventricular fibrillation; VT, ventricular tachycardia.

* Data are expressed as No. (%). Because of rounding, percentages may not all total 100.

pulseless cardiac arrest. Of note, and as expected, children who received chest compressions for bradycardia with pulses had a much higher survival to hospital discharge rate (60%) than did those with pulseless cardiac arrest (27%, $P<0.001$).

Are outcomes from in-hospital cardiac arrest improving? The rate of survival to discharge following pulseless cardiac arrest in the NRCPR database, 27%, is substantially higher compared with the two previous studies that used Utstein-style reporting, 15% and 18%, even though

the rate of sustained ROSC was not higher (52% versus 63% and 64%). The better postresuscitation outcomes are especially impressive because these two previous single-center studies reported on all children who received CPR, including many for bradycardia with palpable pulses. It is not clear whether the superior longer term survival after initially successful resuscitation in the present study is due to differences in patient population characteristics, resuscitation performance, reporting bias, or improvements in patient care during the postresuscitation phase (e.g., superior hemodynamic support). The authors believe that better postresuscitation care is probably a major contributor to the apparent improvements in outcome.

Pediatric out-of-hospital arrests

Outcomes following pediatric out-of-hospital arrests appear to be much worse than those from in-hospital arrests (Table 53.4). In particular, the neurological outcomes appear to be much worse among children surviving out-of-hospital arrests. Two diseases have especially poor outcomes: traumatic arrests and SIDS. Traumatic cardiac arrests are typically due to exsanguination resulting in profound circulatory shock; not surprisingly, chest compressions with an empty heart are not likely to provide adequate coronary and cerebral perfusion. SIDS patients have typically been dead for quite a long time before resuscitation is attempted. In most series of out-of-hospital pediatric cardiac arrests, 1/3–1/2 of the children have the diagnosis of SIDS. For other pediatric cardiac arrests in the pre-hospital setting, CPR and advanced life support from EMS providers may be too little, too late (see below). As might be expected, these poor outcomes after pediatric out-of-hospital cardiac arrests are similar to the poor outcomes after adult non-VF out-of-hospital cardiac arrests.

Is CPR in the pre-hospital setting effective for children?

As noted above, the outcomes from pediatric pre-hospital cardiac arrests are frequently dismal. In contrast, outcomes from in-hospital pediatric asphyxial cardiac arrests are much better. For example, in the seminal report from Kouwenhoven and colleagues of successful resuscitation with closed chest cardiac massage, the initial patients were asphyxiated children in the operating room who received immediate effective resuscitation and attained excellent outcomes. Furthermore, our clinical experience suggests

Table 53.4. Summary of representative studies of outcome following out-of-hospital pediatric cardiac arrest

Author, year	Setting	# of patients	ROSC	Survival to discharge	Good neurological survival
Young 1999	Meta-analysis OOH CA	1568	not reported	132 (8%)	not reported
Sirbaugh 1999	OOH CA	300	33 (11%)	6 (2%)	1 (<1%)
Suominen 1998	OOH CA After trauma	41	10 (24%)	3 (7%)	2 (5%)
Suominen 1997	OOH CA	50	13 (26%)	8 (16%)	6 (12%)
Schindler 1996	OOH CA	80	43 (54%)	6 (8%)	0 (0%)
Kuisma 1995	OOH CA	34	10 (29%)	5 (15%)	4 (12%)
Dieckmann 1995	OOH CA	65	3 (5%)	2 (3%)	1 (1.5%)
Lopez-Herce 2005	Mixed in-hospital & OOH CA	213	110 (52%)	45 (21%)	34 (16%)
Tunstall-Pedoe 1992	Mixed in-hospital & OOH CA	3765	1411 (38%)	706 (19%)	not reported

CA = cardiac arrest; OOH = out of hospital.

that excellent outcomes can occur after various types of bystander CPR, including mouth-to-mouth rescue breathing alone (MTM), chest compressions alone (CC), or standard chest compressions and mouth-to-mouth rescue breathing (CC + MTM). Nevertheless, some reports question the effectiveness and advisability of pre-hospital pediatric CPR.

In order to characterize these issues further, pre-hospital pediatric asphyxial arrests were simulated in animal models. In the first study, asphyxia was induced by clamping the tracheal tubes of piglets until cardiac arrest occurred, defined by loss of aortic pulsation. The mean time until loss of aortic pulsations was 8.9 ± 0.4 minutes. After loss of aortic pulsations, animals were randomized to simulated bystander CPR (MTM, CC, or MTM + CC) or no CPR until simulated EMS arrival 8 minutes later. A similar study was performed with intervention at a slightly earlier point in the asphyxial process, when the pulse was "no longer palpable," as defined by systolic pressure <50 mmHg. The mean tracheal tube clamp time to induce this severe hypotension was 6.8 ± 0.3 minutes, clearly a severe asphyxial insult. Not surprisingly, after a complete cardiac arrest, 24-hour survival was clearly superior in the CC + MTM group compared to the other groups (Fig. 53.1). When intervention was provided earlier in the process (i.e., after severe hypotension but before complete loss of aortic pulsation), even though cardiac arrest would have been the clinical diagnosis, 24-hour survival was best with MTM + CC, but was better with MTM or CC than no "bystander CPR" (Fig. 53.2) Interestingly, most of the animals with 24-hour survival had return of spontaneous

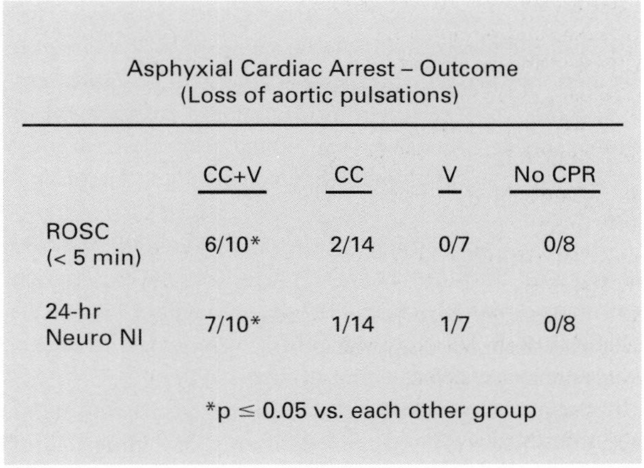

Asphyxial Cardiac Arrest – Outcome (Loss of aortic pulsations)

	CC+V	CC	V	No CPR
ROSC (< 5 min)	6/10*	2/14	0/7	0/8
24-hr Neuro NI	7/10*	1/14	1/7	0/8

*p ≤ 0.05 vs. each other group

Fig. 53.1. Asphyxial Cardiac Arrest – Outcome (Loss of aortic pulsations)

circulation (ROSC) before the simulated EMS arrival. CPR was not futile in these models of pre-hospital pediatric cardiac arrest; excellent CPR was remarkably effective when provided early enough.

In a large prospective study in Houston over 3½ years, Sirbaugh and colleagues found that the outcomes from pediatric pre-hospital cardiac arrests were dismal. Only 6 of the 300 children (2%) survived to hospital discharge, and only 1 of the 300 survived without significant neurological deficits. As in most such studies, the diagnosis of cardiac arrest was determined by EMS providers when they arrived at the scene. Of note, children in cardiac arrest who attained ROSC after bystander CPR before EMS arrival

"Pulseless" Arrest – Outcome (Syst BP <50 mmHg)				
	CC+V	CC	V	No CPR
ROSC (<2 min)	10/10*φ	4/10	6/10*	0/10
24-hr Survival	8/10*	4/10	6/10*	0/10

*p ≤ 0.05 vs. no CPR
φp ≤ 0.01 vs. CC and V combined

Fig. 53.2. "Pulseless" Arrest – Outcome (Syst BP<50 mmHg)

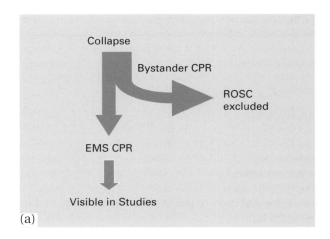

(a)

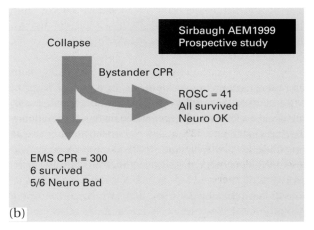

(b)

Fig. 53.3. (a), (b)

were excluded from analysis (Fig. 53.3(a)). Importantly, 41 children who had received bystander CPR were not in cardiac arrest at the time of EMS arrival; all 41 presumably had drowning-related cardiac arrests, and all survived with good neurological outcomes (Fig. 53.3(b)). Most were quite ill when they arrived at a hospital emergency department. In contrast, none of the other 24 children with drowning-related cardiac arrests who were still in cardiac arrest when the EMS personnel arrived survived with a good neurological outcome.

These data and similar data from Hickey *et al.* are consistent with the animal data, reported clinical experience, and in-hospital pediatric CPR data: that is, CPR can be quite effective for asphyxial cardiac arrests, but timing of interventions is critically important.

Recent prospective evaluation of a decade-long, population-based study of pediatric drowning-related events in Houston found 421 children with drowning events in a population of ~2 million total and ~400 000 children (annual incidence of 10.0 per 100 000 children), and 234 required resuscitation. Of these resuscitated children, 193 (82%) received bystander CPR and 72% of these children were long-term survivors. Moreover, 99% of the long-term survivors were neurologically intact. If the child was still apneic and pulseless when EMS personnel arrived, however, less than 5% were revived, and none of these subsequent survivors were ultimately neurologically intact. These data are further evidence that pre-hospital CPR can be quite effective for drowning-associated acute asphyxial cardiac arrests, if provided promptly.

In summary, animal and human data both indicate that CPR for children can be quite effective. In addition, these data support the notion that BLS early is more important than ALS late. Contrary to popular opinion, prompt action

by a citizen bystander in the pre-hospital setting or a provider in the in-hospital setting is generally more effective than late heroic efforts in our intensive care units.

Pediatric ventricular fibrillation

Ventricular fibrillation (VF) is an uncommon, but not rare, electrocardiographic rhythm during out-of-hospital pediatric cardiac arrests. Two studies reported VF as the initial rhythm in 19%–24% of out-of-hospital pediatric cardiac arrests after SIDS deaths were excluded. In studies that include SIDS victims, however, the frequency drops to the range of 6%–10%. The exclusion of SIDS patients can be justified by the rationale that most SIDS patients have been "long dead" by the time emergency medical personnel arrive; therefore, the ECG rhythms when the children were potentially salvageable are not known. Of note, ECG rhythms are often not attained as promptly in children as in adults and VF converts into asystole over time. Therefore, the frequency of VF may have been higher among the children in these studies, but some of the VF may have been undocumented.

The incidence of VF varies by setting and age. In special circumstances, such as tricyclic antidepressant overdose, cardiomyopathy, postcardiac surgery, and prolonged QT syndromes, VF is a more likely rhythm during cardiac arrest. Another special circumstance is commotio cordis, or mechanically initiated VF due to relatively low-energy chest wall impact during a narrow window of repolarization (10–30 ms before the T wave peak in swine models). These tragic events predominantly occur in children, 4 to 16 years old.

VF during an out-of-hospital cardiac arrest is uncommon in infants, but occurs more frequently in children and adolescents. The variance of VF by age was highlighted in a study documenting VF/VT in only 3% of children in cardiac arrest 0–8 years old versus 17% of children 8–19 years old.

Although VF is often associated with underlying heart disease and generally considered the "immediate cause" of cardiac arrest, VF can also occur secondary to asphyxia. In two studies of VF among asphyxiated piglets, the incidence of VF was 28% and 33% at some time during the cardiac arrest. This phenomenon, asphyxia-associated VF, is also well documented among pediatric near-drowning patients. Furthermore, as noted below, VF occurs commonly during in-hospital cardiac arrests, often during resuscitation.

In-hospital pediatric cardiac arrests are uncommon, but not rare. Cardiac arrests occur in ~2% of PICU patients. Although the rhythms during most in-hospital cardiac arrests (both in children and adults) are asystole and pulseless electrical activity (PEA), in a considerable number of arrests the rhythms are VF or pulseless VT. Among the first 1,005 pediatric in-hospital cardiac arrests in the American Heart Association's National Registry of CPR, 10% had an initial rhythm of VF/VT, an additional 15% had subsequent VF/VT (i.e., some time later during the resuscitation efforts), and another 2% had VF/VT but the timing of the arrhythmia was not clear. Therefore, 27% of children with in-hospital cardiac arrests had VF/VT.

In this NRCPR cohort of pediatric in-hospital arrests, survival to discharge was much more common among children with an arrhythmogenic arrest (i.e., initial VF/VT) than among children with VF/VT occurring later during the resuscitation (i.e., subsequent VF/VT): 35% with initial VF/VT vs. 11% subsequent VF/VT (adjusted odds ratio 2.9 [95% CI, 1.2–5.8]). This novel observation is not surprising because children with subsequent VF/VT had hypoxic-ischemic processes before the arrest (i.e., the arrests were generally precipitated by progressive respiratory failure or shock). In addition, the children with subsequent VF/VT had further hypoxic-ischemic insults during resuscitation for asystole or PEA before VF/VT occurred. This is supported by the observation that only 14% of the subsequent VF/VT group had CPR for <15 minutes compared with 44% of the initial VF/VT group.

Surprisingly, the subsequent VF/VT group had worse outcomes than did children with asystole/PEA who never developed VF/VT during the resuscitation: 11% with subsequent VF/VT during resuscitation from asystole/PEA vs. 27% with asystole/PEA alone. Why was the outcome so poor in the subsequent VF/VT group? Rescuers may have been led astray by the initial non-shockable rhythm, so that recognition of VF/VT and defibrillation were delayed. If so, consideration of subsequent VF/VT could have led to earlier recognition, earlier defibrillation, and better outcomes. Another possibility is that subsequent VF/VT was a marker of more severe myocardial pathology. For example, patients with non-shockable rhythms who were most likely to respond promptly to CPR may have attained ROSC before they could develop subsequent VF/VT. Alternatively, resuscitators may have induced VF/VT in some patients by their interventions during the more prolonged CPR for the subsequent VF/VT group (e.g., greater amounts of epinephrine administration).

Traditionally, VF and VT have been considered "good" cardiac arrest rhythms, resulting in better outcomes than asystole and PEA. These NRCPR pediatric VF/VT data suggest a new paradigm: outcomes after *initial* VF/VT are "good," but outcomes after *subsequent* VF/VT are substantially worse than after asystole/PEA without subsequent VF/VT.

Finally, these NRCPR data emphasize the importance of early and repeated electrocardiographic monitoring during resuscitation, because the shockable rhythms of VF/VT occurred in >25% of these children. Even in the setting of progressive respiratory failure and shock with an initial ECG of asystole or PEA, a substantial number of these children developed subsequent shockable VF/VT during CPR.

Treatment of choice: defibrillation

Defibrillation, termination of VF, is necessary for successful resuscitation from VF cardiac arrest. When prompt defibrillation is provided soon after the onset of VF in a cardiac catheterization laboratory, the rates of successful defibrillation and survival approach 100%. When automated external defibrillators are used within 3 minutes of witnessed VF in casinos, long-term survival occurs in ~75%. In general, the mortality increases by 7%–10% per minute of delay to defibrillation. Provision of CPR can improve outcome (i.e., shift the mortality curve).

Because pediatric cardiac arrests are commonly due to progressive asphyxia and/or shock, the treatment of choice is prompt CPR. Therefore, rhythm recognition is relatively less emphasized compared with adult cardiac arrests. Nevertheless, successful resuscitation from VF requires defibrillation. First, we must consider VF, and then diagnose it before we can treat it successfully.

Determinants of defibrillation (termination of VF)

Defibrillation is achieved by attaining current flow adequate to depolarize a critical mass of myocardium. Current flow (amperes) is primarily determined by the shock energy (joules), which is selected by the operator, and the patient's transthoracic impedance (ohms).

Animal studies in the 1970s established that adequate electrical current flow through the myocardium led to successful defibrillation, and too much current flow resulted in postresuscitation myocardial damage (including histopathological evidence of myocardial necrosis). In addition, various extraneous sources of impedance were determined, including paddle size, thoracic gas volume, electrode/paddle contact, and conducting paste. Small paddle size increases resistance, and thereby decreases current through the myocardium. On the other hand, paddles/pads larger than the heart result in current flow through extramyocardial pathways, and thereby less current through the heart (consequently less flow for effective defibrillation). These studies established that current density, i.e., current flow through the myocardium, determines both effectiveness of the shock and myocardial damage.

Further studies established that both poor electrode paddle contact and increased thoracic gas resulted in greater impedance, whereas both conducting paste and increased pressure with the paddle against the skin decreased impedance. Moreover, transthoracic impedance decreased with subsequent shocks, partly due to increased skin blood flow after electrical shocks.

Pediatric defibrillation doses

In the mid-1970s authoritative sources recommended initial defibrillation doses as high as 200 joules for all children. Despite clinical experience indicating that such doses were effective, providing an adult dose to infants seemed potentially dangerous. Because of animal data demonstrating histopathological myocardial damage

with dosages >10 J/kg and further animal data suggesting that 0.5–10 J/kg were generally adequate for defibrillation in a variety of species, some experts recommended a pediatric dose of 2 J/kg.

Gutgesell and colleagues retrospectively evaluated the efficacy of the 2 J/kg pediatric defibrillation strategy. Seventy-one transthoracic defibrillation attempts on 27 children were evaluated. These children were 3 days to 15 years old, and weighed from 2.1 to 50 kg. Fifty-seven of 71 shocks were within 10 joules of the 2 J/kg pediatric dose. Ninety-one percent (52/57) of these shocks effectively terminated VF. The authors did not report any other outcome measures (e.g., successful resuscitation to a perfusing rhythm, 24-hour survival, survival to discharge). Subsequent clinical usage suggests that the 2 J/kg dose is effective for short duration in-hospital defibrillation, although this conclusion has not been rigorously evaluated.

As noted above, current density determines the effectiveness and harm of the shock. Moreover, differences in paddle size, defibrillation energy dose, and the individual's transthoracic impedance are the main determinants of current density. Therefore, Atkins and colleagues investigated the effects of paddle size, age, and weight on transthoracic impedance in children (Fig. 53.4). As expected, transthoracic impedance increased substantially with pediatric paddles. On the basis of those data, the AHA recommends that "pediatric" paddles only be used in infants.

More important, they established that the relationship between transthoracic impedance and weight is not linear. The mean transthoracic impedance in their children was ~50 Ω with 83 cm^2 adult paddles, and varied three-fold among children. With "pediatric" pads (44 cm^2), the mean impedance was ~70 Ω in 3.8–36 kg children. The impedances of their infants were slightly lower than those of their older children, but the range of each was wide and the overlap substantial. Interestingly, the mean transthoracic impedance in adults is typically ~60–80 Ω and it also varies by more than three-fold, yet we shock all adults with the same doses. These data suggest that the pediatric dosage should not vary in a linear manner based on weight. Nevertheless, the pediatric 2 J/kg dose has apparently withstood the test of time over the last 30 years.

Pediatric defibrillation doses for prolonged VF

As noted above, ~16 000 American children suffer a cardiac arrest each year, ~10%–20% with VF as the initial rhythm. There are minimal published data on pediatric defibrillation doses for prolonged VF. Therefore, the approach to pediatric prolonged VF is extrapolated from adult recommendations. For adults, the same defibrillation dose is rec-

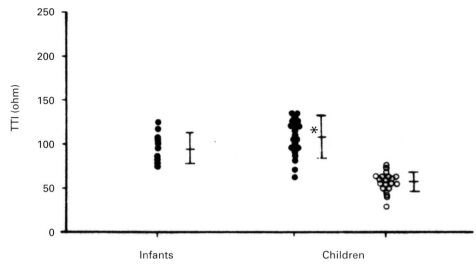

Fig. 53.4. Effect of paddle electrode size on transthoracic impedance (TTI). •, pediatric paddles; ○, adult paddles; *$P<.001$ $v.$ adult paddles; bar indicates standard deviation.

ommended after brief duration or prolonged duration VF, even though the monophasic 200-J dose is often ineffective at terminating prolonged VF (~60% termination of prolonged VF compared with >90% for short duration VF). Adult defibrillation differs from pediatric defibrillation in many ways. First, the adult defibrillation dose is much higher in absolute joules or joules/kg. For example, a 70-kg man would receive 200 J (~3 J/kg), whereas a 70-kg 11-year-old boy may be treated with a pediatric dose of 140 J. Secondly, adult defibrillation from prolonged VF is now typically performed with biphasic defibrillators, and the 150 J or 200 J biphasic AED dosage is nearly 90% successful at terminating prolonged VF (much better than the ~60% effectiveness with 200 J monophasic defibrillation).

Is the currently recommended pediatric VF dose of 2 J/kg by monophasic waveform safe and effective for prolonged VF? A recently published animal study of defibrillation after 7 minutes of untreated VF in 4 to 24 kg piglets suggests that 2 J/kg may be an inadequate dose. Twenty-four piglets were shocked with 2 J/kg, followed by 4 J/kg. The pediatric dose of 2 J/kg monophasic shocks was uniformly unsuccessful at terminating fibrillation in all 24 piglets. This should not be overinterpreted; there could be interspecies differences in defibrillation thresholds.

A small clinical study of pediatric defibrillation attempts, however, also suggests that the 2 J/kg defibrillation dose is often inadequate. Eleven children received 14 pediatric dose shocks of brief duration for VF in the Tucson EMS over a 5-year period, by using the criteria described by Gutgesell in his pediatric in-hospital defibrillation study (2 J/kg ±

10 J). Only 7/14 shocks (50%) terminated out-of-hospital (prolonged) VF vs. 52/57 shocks (91%) in their 27 in-hospital patients ($P<0.01$). Although this small series does not determine what dose we should use, it raises doubts about the efficacy of 2 J/kg monophasic shocks for prolonged VF.

Because standard weight-based dosing strategy for pediatric defibrillation is not easily implemented in automated external defibrillators (AEDs), manufacturers developed an alternative pediatric AED dose of 50–86 J biphasic shocks by attenuating the adult defibrillation dose with pediatric pads/cable systems, thereby delivering 50–86 J rather than 150–360 J. This dose is safe and effective in piglets after either brief or prolonged VF. In addition, the 50 J/75 J/86 J shocks were more effective than the 2 J/kg dose at initial termination of fibrillation after prolonged VF. In another piglet study modelling prolonged out-of-hospital pediatric VF (7 minutes of untreated VF), adult biphasic shocks of 200 J/300 J/360 J were compared with a "pediatric" biphasic AED dose of 50 J/75 J/86 J. Pediatric dosing resulted in fewer elevations of cardiac troponin T levels, less postresuscitation myocardial dysfunction (i.e., smaller decreases in left ventricular ejection fraction 1–4 hours postresuscitation), and superior 24-hour survival with good neurological outcome. These data suggest that adult defibrillation dosing may be harmful to pediatric patients with prolonged VF and support the use of attenuating electrodes with adult automated external defibrillators for pediatric defibrillation. Although human data are certainly needed, these animal data support the

AHA/ILCOR pediatric AED guidelines: "Ideally, the device should deliver a pediatric dose."

It is important to remember that the pediatric defibrillation LD_{100} is 0 joules. The patient uniformly dies if defibrillation is not attempted. Therefore, adult defibrillation doses are preferable to no defibrillation. A single case report in the literature demonstrated that an adult AED dose saved the life of a 3-year-old boy in VF. That child was defibrillated with a biphasic shock of 150 J (9 J/kg) and survived without any apparent adverse effects. In particular, neither serum creatine kinase nor cardiac troponin was elevated, and postresuscitation ventricular function was normal on echocardiogram.

Pediatric AEDs

VF is prolonged in nearly all children with out-of-hospital VF by the time EMS personnel and defibrillators arrive. Until recently, AEDs were not recommended for children <8 years old. Therefore, young children in VF had to wait for a trained operator with a manual defibrillator. Too often, this delay precluded survival. Current international guidelines recommend AED usage for children 1–8 years old. Two issues had to be considered before such recommendations: (1) the safety and efficacy of the AED diagnostic rhythm analysis program in children; and (2) the safety and efficacy of the AED shock dosage.

An important concern was that babies and small children with sinus tachycardia or supraventricular tachycardia can have very high heart rates that might be misinterpreted as "shockable" by AEDs with diagnostic programs developed for adult arrhythmias. Fortunately, published studies of rhythm analysis programs from two leading manufacturers (Philips and Medtronics) have established that they are quite sensitive and specific in detecting the shockable rhythm of VF. Both algorithms were less sensitive at detecting the very uncommon shockable rhythm of VT, but were quite specific (i.e., the algorithm did not misinterpret other rhythms as VT, and therefore did not recommend shocking a "non-shockable" rhythm). On the basis of these two rhythm analysis program studies and the defibrillation dose information noted above, the AHA/ILCOR PALS Task Force recommended that "AEDs may be used for children 1 to 8 years of age with no signs of circulation. Ideally the device should demonstrate high specificity for pediatric shockable rhythms, i.e., the device will not recommend a shock for non-shockable rhythms." Because of the relative rarity of out-of-hospital VF in infants and the limited rhythm analysis program information in infants with VF, the Task Force concluded that "Currently the evidence is insufficient to support a recommendation for or against the use of AEDs in children >1 year of age."

Finally, pediatric AEDs with shock doses are now available. Technological developments have enabled these AEDs to deliver a pediatric dose by attenuating the adult biphasic defibrillation dose with pediatric pads/cable system, thereby delivering 1/4 to 1/3 (50–86 J) of the standard adult energy. As noted above, animal studies and extrapolations from adult defibrillation studies suggest that this pediatric biphasic AED dosage is at least as safe and effective as the 2 J/kg monophasic dose. Although there are theoretical concerns and animal data suggesting that adult AED doses may be less safe than pediatric AED doses, an adult AED dose can terminate VF and save a child's life.

The four phases of cardiac arrest and CPR

There are at least four phases of cardiac arrest: (1) **pre-arrest**, (2) **no-flow** (untreated cardiac arrest), (3) **low-flow** (CPR), and (4) **postresuscitation**. Interventions to improve outcome from pediatric cardiac arrest should optimize therapies targeted to the phase of resuscitation as suggested in Table 53.5. The pre-arrest phase provides the opportunity to have the largest impact on patient survival by preventing cardiopulmonary arrest. Interventions during the pre-arrest phase focus on prevention. Infant safety seats and safe driving to prevent traumatic arrests, water safety programs to prevent drowning arrests, medication safety caps to prevent drug poisoning arrests are well known highly effective efforts to prevent cardiac arrests. Because many pediatric cardiac arrests are due to progressive respiratory failure and shock, the main focus of the Pediatric Advanced Life Support (PALS) is the early recognition and treatment of respiratory failure and shock in children (i.e., prevention of cardiac arrest in the pre-arrest phase). This issue has been popularized as the main focus of medical emergency response teams or rapid response teams.

Interventions during the **no-flow** phase of untreated cardiac arrest focus on early recognition of cardiac arrest and rapid initiation of basic and advanced life support. When there is insufficient oxygen delivery to the brain or heart, CPR should be started. The goal of effective CPR is to optimize coronary perfusion pressure and blood flow to critical organs during the **low-flow** phase. Basic life support with continuous effective chest compressions (i.e., push hard, push fast, allow full chest recoil, minimize interruptions, and do not overventilate) is the emphasis in this phase.

The **postresuscitation** phase is a high-risk period for continuing brain injury, ventricular arrhythmias, and other reperfusion injuries. Injured cells can hibernate, die,

Table 53.5. Phases of cardiac arrest and resuscitation

Phase	Interventions
Pre-arrest phase (**protect**)	• Optimize community education regarding child safety • Optimize patient monitoring and rapid emergency response • Recognize and treat respiratory failure and/or shock to prevent cardiac arrest
Arrest (no-flow) phase (**preserve**)	• Minimize interval to BLS and ACLS (organized response) • Minimize interval to defibrillation, when indicated
Low-flow (CPR) phase (**resuscitate**)	• Push Hard, Push Fast • Allow full chest recoil • Minimize interruptions in compressions • Avoid overventilation • Titrate CPR to optimize myocardial blood flow (coronary perfusion pressures and exhaled CO_2) • Consider adjuncts to improve vital organ perfusion during CPR • Consider ECMO if standard CPR/ALS not promptly successful
Postresuscitation phase: short-term	• Optimize cardiac output and cerebral perfusion • Treat arrhythmias, if indicated • Avoid hyperglycemia, hyperthermia, hyperventilation • Consider mild postresuscitation systemic hypothermia • Debrief to improve future responses to emergencies
Postresuscitation phase: longer-term rehabilitation (**regenerate**)	• Early intervention with occupational and physical therapy • Bioengineering and technology interface • Possible future role for stem cell transplantation

or partially or fully recover function. Interventions such as systemic hypothermia during the immediate postresuscitation phase strive to minimize reperfusion injury and support cellular recovery. Overventilation is frequent and can have adverse effects during and after CPR. The postarrest phase may have the most potential for innovative advances in the understanding of cell injury and death, inflammation, apoptosis, and hibernation, ultimately leading to novel interventions. Thoughtful attention to management of temperature, glucose, blood pressures, coagulation, and optimal ventilation may be particularly important in this phase. The rehabilitation stage of postresuscitation concentrates on salvage of injured cells, recruitment of hibernating cells, and re-engineering of reflex and voluntary communications of these cell and organ systems to improve functional outcome.

The specific phase of resuscitation should dictate the timing, intensity, duration, and focus of interventions. Emerging data suggest that interventions that can improve short-term outcome during one phase may be deleterious during another. For instance, intense vasoconstriction during the low flow phase of cardiac arrest may improve coronary perfusion pressure and probability of ROSC.[2] The same intense vasoconstriction during the postresuscitation phase may increase left ventricular afterload and

worsen myocardial strain and dysfunction. Current understanding of the physiology of cardiac arrest and recovery only enables the crude titration of blood pressure, global oxygen delivery and consumption, body temperature, inflammation, coagulation, and other physiologic parameters to attempt to optimize outcome. Future strategies will likely take advantage of emerging discoveries and knowledge of cellular inflammation, thrombosis, reperfusion, mediator cascades, cellular markers of injury and recovery, and transplantation technology.

Definition of pulseless cardiac arrest

Pulseless cardiac arrest is typically defined as the documented cessation of cardiac mechanical activity, determined by the absence of a palpable central pulse, unresponsiveness, and apnea. As simple as this definition appears, separation of severe hypoxic–ischemic shock from the non-pulsatile state of cardiac arrest can be challenging at any age. This separation can be especially difficult in babies because of their anatomic and physiologic differences.

A rescuer's ability to determine cardiac arrest by a pulse check is neither sensitive nor specific in adults. Not surprisingly, the pulse check is even more problematic in children. In adults, pulses can typically be palpated until the systolic pressure is <50 mmHg. Because the systolic blood pressure in neonates is generally in the 60s, a decrease in blood pressure to "non-palpable pulse" may occur earlier in the continuum from hypoxic–ischemic shock to non-pulsatile cardiac standstill. Furthermore, the best arterial pulse to palpate in an adult is the carotid pulse; however, the short, chunky neck of a baby limits the effectiveness of carotid pulse palpation in babies. Moreover, attempts to palpate the carotid pulse can compress the airway and impede respiration. Therefore, the recommended sites for palpation of pulses in an infant are the brachial, axillary and/or femoral pulses.

Interventions during the low flow phase: CPR

Airway and breathing

As noted above, one of the most common precipitating events for cardiac arrests in children is respiratory insufficiency. Therefore, providing adequate ventilation and oxygenation must remain a high priority. Effective ventilation does not necessarily require a tracheal tube. In one randomized, controlled study of children with out-of-hospital respiratory arrest, those who were treated with bag-mask ventilation did as well as children treated with pre-hospital endotracheal intubation. Effective bag-mask ventilation skills remain the cornerstone of providing effective emergency ventilation. Emergency airway techniques such as transtracheal jet ventilation and emergency cricothyroidotomy are rarely, if ever, required during CPR.

Provision of adequate oxygen delivery to meet metabolic demand and removal of carbon dioxide is the goal of initial assisted ventilation. During CPR, cardiac output and pulmonary blood flow are about 10%–25% of that during normal sinus rhythm. Consequently, much less ventilation is necessary for adequate gas exchange from the blood traversing the pulmonary circulation during CPR. Animal and adult data indicate that rapid rate assisted ventilation (overexuberant rescue breathing) during CPR is common and can substantially compromise venous return and cardiac output. Of most concern, these adverse hemodynamic effects during CPR plus interruptions in chest compressions typically necessary for airway management and rescue breathing can be a lethal combination.

Although **A**irway and **B**reathing hold places of honor in the **ABC** algorithm, that priority has been challenged in certain circumstances. In animal models of sudden VF cardiac arrest, acceptable PaO_2 and $PaCO_2$ persist for 4 to 8 minutes during chest compressions without rescue breathing. Moreover, many animal studies indicate that outcomes from sudden VF cardiac arrests are at least as good with chest compressions alone as with chest compressions plus rescue breathing. In addition, several retrospective studies of adults also suggest that outcomes are similar after bystander-initiated CPR with either chest compressions alone or chest compressions plus rescue breathing. A randomized, controlled study of dispatcher-assisted bystander CPR in adults found a trend toward improved survival in the patients who received chest compressions alone compared to those who received dispatcher-instructed ventilation and chest compressions. In contrast, animal studies of asphyxia-precipitated cardiac arrests have established that rescue breathing is a critical component of successful CPR.

Since oxygenation and ventilation are clearly important for survival from any cardiac arrest, why is rescue breathing not initially necessary for VF, yet quite important in asphyxia? Immediately after an acute fibrillatory cardiac arrest, aortic oxygen and carbon dioxide concentrations do not vary from the pre-arrest state because there is no blood flow and aortic oxygen consumption is minimal. Therefore, when chest compressions are initiated, the blood flowing from the aorta to the coronary and cerebral circulations provides adequate oxygenation at an acceptable pH. At that time, myocardial oxygen delivery is limited more by blood flow than oxygen content. Adequate oxygenation and ventilation can continue without rescue breathing because the lungs serve as a relatively high oxygen/low carbon dioxide reservoir during the low-flow state of CPR. In addition, ventilation can occur due to chest compression-induced gas exchange and spontaneous gasping during CPR in victims of sudden cardiac arrest. Therefore, arterial oxygenation and pH can be adequate with chest compressions alone for VF arrests.

Forgoing ventilation in the pediatric patient is not prudent, because respiratory arrest and asphyxia generally precede pediatric cardiac arrest. During asphyxia, blood continues to flow to tissues; therefore, arterial and venous oxygen saturations decrease while carbon dioxide and lactate continue to increase for many minutes before progression to cardiac arrest. Furthermore, continued pulmonary blood flow before the cardiac arrest depletes the pulmonary oxygen reservoir. Therefore, in contrast to VF, asphyxia results in significant arterial hypoxemia and acidemia prior to resuscitation. In this circumstance, rescue breathing can be life-saving.

Circulation

Basic life support with continuous effective chest compressions is generally the best way to provide circulation during cardiac arrest. As noted in previous chapters of this book, basic life support is often provided poorly or not provided at all. The most critical elements are to Push Hard and Push Fast. Because there is no flow without chest compressions, it is important to minimize interruptions in chest compressions. To allow good venous return in the decompression phase of external cardiac massage, it is important to allow full chest recoil, and to avoid overventilation. The latter can prevent venous return because of increased intrathoracic pressure.

The use of closed-chest cardiac massage to provide adequate circulation during cardiac arrest was initially demonstrated in small dogs with compliant chest walls. Based on reasonable extrapolation, these investigators thought that closed chest cardiac massage would be effective with children, but might not be effective with adults. Therefore, the first patients successfully treated with closed-chest cardiac massage were children. The presumed mechanism of blood flow was direct compression of the heart between the sternum and the spine in these children with compliant chest walls. Later investigations indicated that blood can also be circulated during CPR by the thoracic pump mechanism. That is, increases in intrathoracic pressure induced by chest compression can generate a gradient for blood to flow from the pulmonary vasculature, through the heart, and into the peripheral circulation. Regardless of mechanism, cardiac output during CPR seems to be greater in children (and immature animals) with compliant chest walls than in adults with less compliant chest walls.

Circumferential vs. focal sternal compressions

In adults and animal models of cardiac arrest, circumferential (Vest) CPR improves CPR hemodynamics dramatically. In smaller infants, it is often possible to encircle the chest with both hands and depress the sternum with the thumbs, while compressing the thorax circumferentially. In an infant model of CPR, this "two-thumb" method of compression resulted in higher systolic and diastolic blood pressures and a higher pulse pressure than did traditional two-finger compression of the sternum.

Duty cycle

Duty cycle is the ratio of time of compression phase to the entire compression-relaxation cycle. In a model of human adult cardiac arrest, cardiac output and coronary blood flow are optimized when chest compressions last for 30% of the total cycle time. As the duration of CPR increases, the optimal duty cycle may increase to 50%. In a juvenile swine model, a relaxation period of 250–300 ms (a duty cycle of 40%–50% if 120 compressions are delivered per minute) correlates with improved cerebral perfusion pressure when compared to shorter duty cycles of 30%.

Open chest CPR

Excellent standard closed chest CPR generates a cerebral blood flow that is approximately 50% of normal. By contrast, open chest CPR can generate a cerebral blood flow that approaches normal. While open chest massage improves coronary perfusion pressure and increases the chance of successful defibrillation in animals and humans, performing a thoracotomy to allow open chest CPR is impractical in many situations. A retrospective review of 27 cases of CPR following pediatric blunt trauma (15 with open chest CPR and 12 with closed chest CPR) demonstrated that open chest CPR increased hospital cost without altering rates of ROSC or survival to discharge[4][10a]. No patient in either group survived, however, indicating that the population may have been too severely injured or were treated too late in the process to benefit from this aggressive therapy. Open chest CPR is often provided to children after open heart cardiac surgery status-post sternotomy. Earlier institution of open chest CPR may warrant reconsideration in selected special resuscitation circumstances.

Ratio of compressions to ventilation

Ideal compression–ventilation ratios for pediatric patients are unknown. Current compression–ventilation ratios and tidal volumes recommended during CPR are based upon rational conjecture, tradition, and educational retention theory. Recent physiologic estimates suggest that the amount of ventilation needed during CPR is much less than the amount needed during a normal perfusing rhythm, because the cardiac output during CPR is only 10%–25% of that during normal sinus rhythm. The benefits of positive pressure ventilation (increased arterial content of oxygen and carbon dioxide elimination) must be balanced against the adverse consequence of decreased circulation.

Maximizing systemic oxygen delivery during single rescuer CPR requires a trade-off between time spent doing chest compressions and time spent doing mouth-to-mouth ventilations. Theoretically, neither compression-only nor ventilation-only CPR can sustain systemic oxygen delivery. Some intermediate value of the compression to ventilation ratio is probably optimal. The best intermediate value depends upon many factors including the compression rate, the tidal volume, the blood flow generated by compressions,

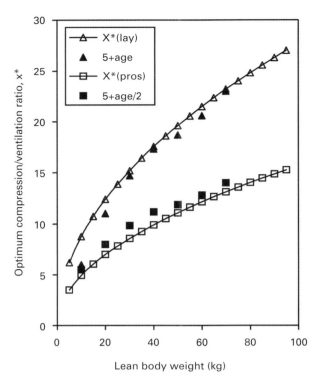

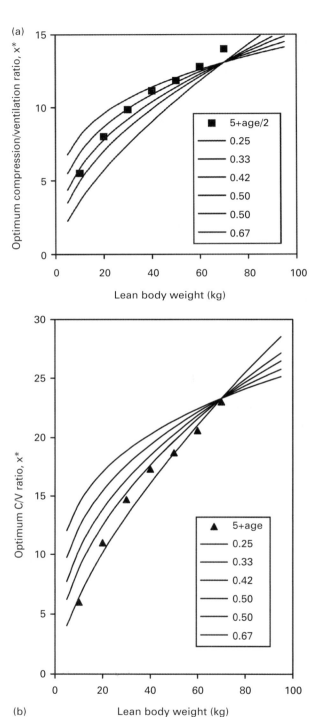

Fig. 53.5. Scaling rules for optimum C/V ratios in pediatric basic life support. Open symbols represent theoretical compression–ventilation ratios for optimal oxygen delivery, scaled for persons having a wide range of body weight. Lay rescuers (lay) are assumed to take 8 seconds to deliver one rescue breath in an adult size individual, in keeping with the observations of Chamberlain and coworkers. Professional rescuers (pros) are assumed to take 2.5 seconds to deliver one rescue breath. Solid symbols indicate approximations to the theoretical curves, based upon average body weights of children ages 1 to 18, according to the rules "5 + patient age in years" for lay rescuers and "5 + one-half patient age in years" for professional rescuers.

and the time that compressions are interrupted to perform ventilations. A chest compression to ventilation ratio of 15:2 delivered the same minute ventilation as CPR with a chest compression to ventilation ratio of 5:1 in a mannequin model of pediatric CPR, but the number of chest compressions delivered was 48% higher with the 15:2 ratio.

In adults, mathematical models of oxygen delivery during CPR performed with variable ratios of healthcare provider chest compressions to ventilations suggest that the optimal compression to ventilation ratio is approximately 30:2 in adults. When the model is adjusted to simulate lay rescuer ability to provide chest compressions and ventilations, the optimal compression to ventilation ratio ranges from 50 to 100:2. Mathematical models of

Fig. 53.6. Sensitivity analysis for scaling rules for optimal C/V ratios in pediatric basic life support. The general effect of body size upon the optimal C/V ratio is insensitive to changes in the exponent of body weight. (A) calculations for professional rescuers, (B) calculations for lay rescuers.

compression–ventilation ratios suggest that matching of the amount of ventilation to the amount of reduced pulmonary blood flow during closed chest cardiac compressions should favor high compression to ventilation ratios. Babbs and Kern suggest that the best way to determine optimal compression to ventilation ratios by using simulation is to choose ratios that maximize oxygen delivery to peripheral tissues. Maximizing oxygen delivery to peripheral tissues during single rescuer CPR requires a trade-off between the time required to compress the chest and time required to provide rescue breathing. If one ignores the relatively small amount of ventilation provided by chest compressions alone, neither compression-only nor ventilation-only CPR can sustain oxygen delivery to the periphery for prolonged periods of CPR. The best ratio depends upon many factors including the compression rate, the tidal volume, the blood flow generated by compressions, and the time that compressions are interrupted to perform ventilations. These factors can be related in a simple mathematical formula based upon classical physiology. These variables necessarily change as a function of the size of the patient. Such considerations may help to refine the amount of ventilation recommended for both adults and children. The ratio of chest compressions to ventilations during "no-flow" and "low-flow" phases of cardiopulmonary-cerebral resuscitation remains an area of high interest, controversy, and future research. These formulas adjusted to the known physiologic variables in children have suggested the potential to simplify the compression: ventilation ratio to 15 chest compressions and 2 ventilations in all children.

Intraosseous vascular access

In infants and children requiring emergent access for resuscitation from cardiac arrest, intraosseous vascular access should be established if reliable venous access cannot be achieved rapidly. Because of the difficulty in establishing vascular access in pediatric cardiac arrest victims, it may be preferable to attempt intraosseous (IO) access immediately. A practical approach is to pursue IO and peripheral or central venous access simultaneously.

Intraosseous vascular access provides access to a non-collapsible marrow venous plexus, which serves as a rapid, safe, and reliable route for administration of drugs, crystalloids, colloids, and blood during resuscitation. Intraosseous vascular access often can be achieved in 30 to 60 seconds. Although a specially designed intraosseous or Jamshidi-type bone marrow stylet needle is preferred to prevent obstruction of the needle with cortical bone, butterfly needles and standard hypodermic needles have been used successfully. The intraosseous needle is typically inserted into the anterior tibial bone marrow; alternative sites include the distal femur, medial malleolus or the anterior superior iliac spine, and the distal tibia. In adults and older children, the medial malleolus, distal radius, and distal ulna are other options.

This intraosseous vascular access technique can be used in all age groups, from pre-term neonates through adulthood. The needle should be twisted into, rather than shoved through, the bone marrow. Evidence for successful entry into the bone marrow includes: (1) the sudden decrease in resistance after the needle passes through the bony cortex, (2) the needle remains upright without support, (3) aspiration of the bone marrow into a syringe (this is not consistently achieved), and (4) the fluid infuses freely without evidence of subcutaneous infiltration.

Resuscitation drugs, fluids, and blood products can be safely administered by the intraosseous route, as well as continuous catecholamine infusions. Onset of action and drug levels following intraosseous infusion during CPR are comparable to those achieved following vascular administration, including central venous administration. Intraosseous vascular access may also be used to obtain blood specimens for chemistry, blood gas analysis, and type and crossmatch, although administration of sodium bicarbonate through the intraosseous cannula eliminates the close correlation with mixed venous blood gases.

Complications have been reported in less than 1% of patients following intraosseous infusion. Such complications include tibial fracture, lower extremity compartment syndrome, severe extravasation of drugs, and osteomyelitis. Most of these complications may be avoided by careful technique. Although microscopic pulmonary fat and bone marrow emboli have been demonstrated in animal models, they have never been reported clinically and appear to occur just as frequently during cardiac arrest without intraosseous drug administration. Animal data and one human follow-up study indicate that local effects of intraosseous infusion on the bone marrow and bone growth are minimal.

Endotracheal drug administration

Before the intraosseous route became commonly used for vascular access during CPR, endotracheal intubation was often easier to attain than vascular access during pediatric CPR. Important lipid-soluble drugs could be administered via the endotracheal tube before vascular access was achieved. In particular, lidocaine, atropine, naloxone, and epinephrine were commonly administered via the endotracheal route. Sodium bicarbonate and calcium are not lipid-soluble, however, and may be very irritating to the airways and lung parenchyma, so they were not recommended for endotracheal administration.

Absorption of drugs into the circulation after endotracheal administration depends on dispersion over the respiratory mucosa, pulmonary blood flow, and matching of the ventilation (drug dispersal) to perfusion. The small volumes of drug that remain as droplets in the tracheal tube are obviously not effective. Inadequate chest compressions resulting in poor pulmonary blood flow will also limit absorption of the drug and prevent its delivery to the heart and systemic circulation. Pre-existing pathophysiologic conditions such as pulmonary edema, pneumonitis, and airway disease also affect the pharmacokinetics of endotracheally administered drugs. Another confounding factor is that the vasoconstrictive effects of epinephrine may limit local pulmonary blood flow, thereby diminishing drug uptake and delivery. It is therefore not surprising that drug absorption varies greatly and that optimal drug doses have not been determined (and probably never can be).

Case reports and our personal experiences suggest that endotracheal epinephrine can be effective and life-saving. Animal studies, however, reveal a wide variability in plasma epinephrine levels and physiological effects after endotracheal administration. On average, 10 times as much endotracheal epinephrine is needed to attain peak plasma levels comparable to intravenous administration. Moreover, a prolonged depot effect typically occurs after endotracheal administration of epinephrine, which can lead to postresuscitation hypertension, tachycardia, and ventricular arrhythmias.

Quinton and associates randomly treated five asystolic adults with 1 mg of endotracheal epinephrine versus seven patients with 1 mg of intravenous epinephrine. Arterial epinephrine levels only increased in the group treated intravenously. They concluded that health care providers should not rely on the endotracheal route.

Endotracheal epinephrine has been considered more important for infants and children than for adults because of vascular access issues. Nevertheless, intraosseous drug administration is more reliable than endotracheal administration because of the inherent problems with the pharmacokinetics of endotracheally administered drugs.

Medication use during cardiac arrest

Although animal studies indicate that epinephrine can improve initial resuscitation success after both asphyxial and VF cardiac arrests, no medication has been shown to improve survival outcome from pediatric cardiac arrest. Because of the dearth of pediatric CPR medication studies, this fact should not be overinterpreted.

Vasopressors

During CPR, the α-adrenergic effect of epinephrine on vascular tone is most important. The α-adrenergic action increases systemic vascular resistance, increasing diastolic blood pressure which, in turn, increases coronary perfusion pressure and blood flow, and improves the likelihood of ROSC. Epinephrine also increases cerebral blood flow during CPR because peripheral vasoconstriction directs a greater proportion of flow to the cerebral circulation. The β-adrenergic effect increases myocardial contractility and heart rate and relaxes smooth muscle in the skeletal muscle vascular bed and bronchi, although this effect of less important. Epinephrine also increases the vigor and intensity of ventricular fibrillation, enhancing the likelihood of successful defibrillation.

High-dose epinephrine (0.05–0.2 mg/kg) improves myocardial and cerebral blood flow during CPR more than does standard-dose epinephrine (0.01–0.02 mg/kg), and may increase the incidence of initial ROSC. Administration of high-dose epinephrine, however, can worsen a patient's postresuscitation hemodynamic condition, with increased myocardial oxygen demand, ventricular ectopy, hypertension, and myocardial necrosis. Retrospective studies indicate that use of high-dose epinephrine in adults or children does not improve survival and may be associated with a worse neurological outcome.

A randomized, controlled trial of rescue high-dose epinephrine vs. standard-dose epinephrine after failed initial standard-dose epinephrine for pediatric in-hospital cardiac arrest indicated a worse 24-hour survival in the high-dose epinephrine group (1/27 vs. 6/23, $P < 0.05$). In particular, high-dose epinephrine seemed to worsen the outcome of patients with asphyxia-precipitated cardiac arrest. High-dose epinephrine cannot be recommended routinely for initial therapy or rescue therapy.

Wide variability in catecholamine pharmacokinetics and pharmacodynamics dictates individual titration of therapy in non-cardiac arrest situations. Therefore, it is likely that a life-saving dose during CPR for one patient may be life-threatening to another. Therefore, high-dose epinephrine should perhaps be considered as an alternative to standard-dose epinephrine in special circumstances of refractory pediatric cardiac arrest (e.g., for a patient on high-dose epinephrine infusion before cardiac arrest) and/or when continuous direct arterial blood pressure monitoring allows titration of the epinephrine dosage to diastolic (relaxation phase) arterial pressure during CPR. Nevertheless, high-dose epinephrine has not been shown to improve outcome and should only be used with caution.

Vasopressin is a long-acting endogenous hormone that acts at specific receptors to mediate systemic vasoconstriction (V_1 receptor) and reabsorption of water in the renal tubule (V_2 receptor). In experimental models of cardiac arrest, vasopressin increases blood flow to the heart and brain and improves long-term survival compared to epinephrine. Vasopressin may decrease splanchnic blood flow during and after CPR. In randomized controlled trials of in-hospital and out-of-hospital arrests in adults, vasopressin had comparable efficacy to epinephrine. Vasopressin did not improve outcome compared with epinephrine.

In a pediatric porcine model of prolonged *ventricular fibrillation*, the use of vasopressin and epinephrine in combination resulted in higher left ventricular blood flow than either pressor alone, and both vasopressin alone and vasopressin plus epinephrine resulted in superior cerebral blood flow than epinephrine alone.[7] By contrast, in a pediatric porcine model of *asphyxial* cardiac arrest, return of spontaneous circulation was more likely in piglets treated with epinephrine than in those treated with vasopressin. A case series of four children who received vasopressin during six prolonged cardiac arrest events suggests that the use of bolus vasopressin may result in return of spontaneous circulation when standard medications have failed. Vasopressin has also been reported to be useful in low cardiac output states associated with sepsis syndrome and organ recovery in children. While vasopressin will not likely replace epinephrine as a first-line agent in pediatric cardiac arrest, there are preliminary data to suggest that its use in conjunction with epinephrine in pediatric cardiac arrest deserves further investigation.

Calcium

For in-hospital pediatric cardiac arrests, hypocalcemia is not uncommon. Although calcium administration is only recommended during cardiac arrest for hypocalcemia, hyperkalemia, hypermagnesemia, and overdose of calcium channel blockers, it is commonly used for in-hospital pediatric cardiac arrests, especially those occurring after cardiac surgery. Administration of calcium has not been found to improve outcome in cardiac arrest. Animal studies suggest that calcium administration may worsen reperfusion injury.

Buffer solutions

Cardiac arrest results in lactic acidosis from inadequate organ blood flow and poor oxygenation. Acidosis depresses myocardial function, reduces systemic vascular resistance, and inhibits defibrillation. Nevertheless, the routine use of sodium bicarbonate for a child in cardiac arrest is not recommended. Clinical trials involving critically ill adults with severe metabolic acidosis did not disclose a beneficial effect of sodium bicarbonate. The presence of acidosis may depress the action of catecholamines, however, so that the use of sodium bicarbonate seems rational in an acidemic child who is refractory to catecholamine administration. The administration of sodium bicarbonate is more clearly indicated in the patient with a tricyclic antidepressant overdose, hyperkalemia, hypermagnesemia, or sodium channel blocker poisoning.

The buffering action of bicarbonate occurs when a hydrogen cation and a bicarbonate anion combine to form carbon dioxide and water. If carbon dioxide is not effectively cleared through ventilation, its build-up will counterbalance the buffering effect of bicarbonate. Other side effects with sodium bicarbonate include hypernatremia, hyperosmolarity, and metabolic alkalosis. Excessive alkalosis decreases calcium and potassium concentration and shifts the oxyhemoglobin dissociation curve to the left.

Antiarrhythmic medications: lidocaine and amiodarone

Administration of antiarrhythmic medications should not delay administration of a shock for a patient with ventricular fibrillation. After unsuccessful attempts at electrical defibrillation, however, medications to increase the effectiveness of defibrillation should be considered. In both pediatric and adult patients, the current first line medication in ventricular fibrillation is epinephrine for improved myocardial readiness, because of improved myocardial blood flow. If epinephrine with or without vasopressin and a subsequent repeat attempt to defibrillate are unsuccessful, the antiarrhythmic agents amiodarone or lidocaine should be considered.

Lidocaine has been recommended traditionally for shock-resistant VF in adults and children. Nonetheless, amiodarone is the only antiarrhythmic agent that has been prospectively determined to improve survival to hospital admission in the setting of shock-resistant VF when compared to placebo. Furthermore, patients who received amiodarone for shock-resistant out-of-hospital ventricular fibrillation had a higher rate of survival to hospital admission than those patients who received lidocaine alone. Neither of these randomized controlled trials included children. Although there are no published comparisons of antiarrhythmic medications for pediatric refractory ventricular fibrillation, extrapolation of the adult studies has led to the recommendation of amiodarone as the preferred antiarrhythmic agent for children.

Postresuscitation interventions

Temperature management

Mild induced hypothermia is the most celebrated goal-directed postresuscitation therapy for adults. Two articles published in the *New England Journal of Medicine* on February 21, 2002 established that mild induced hypothermia could improve outcome for comatose adults after resuscitation from ventricular fibrillation cardiac arrest. In both randomized controlled trials, the inclusion criteria were patients older than 18 years who were persistently comatose after successful resuscitation from nontraumatic ventricular fibrillation. The multicenter European study led by Fritz Sterz and Michel Holzer had a goal of 32–34°C for the first 24 hours post-arrest. The mean time until attainment of this temperature goal was ~8 hours. Six-month survival with good neurological outcome was superior in the hypothermic group (75/136 vs. 54/137 with RR of 1.40 [CI,1.08–1.81]). Similarly, death at 6 months after the event occurred less often in the hypothermic group (56/137 vs. 76/138; RR of 0.74 [CI, 0.58–0.95]). In the same issue of *NEJM*, Bernard reported good outcomes in 21/43(49%) of the hypothermic group vs. 9/34 (26%) of the control group, $P = 0.046$, OR 5.25 (CI, 1.47–18.76).

Importantly, hypotension occurred among over half of the patients in both groups and was aggressively treated with vasoactive infusion in the European study. Similarly, more than half of Bernard's patients received epinephrine infusions during the first 24 hours post-resuscitation.

How should these data affect postresuscitation treatment after pediatric arrests? Fever following cardiac arrest is associated with poor neurological outcome. Hyperthermia following cardiac arrest is common in children. Although it is reasonable to believe that mild induced systemic hypothermia may benefit children resuscitated from cardiac arrest, benefit from this treatment has not been rigorously studied and reported in children or in any patients with non-VF arrests. At a minimum, it is advisable to avoid even mild hyperthermia in children following CPR. Scheduled administration of antipyretic medications *and* use of external cooling devices are often necessary to avoid hyperthermia in this population.

Postresuscitation myocardial support

Postarrest myocardial stunning occurs commonly after successful resuscitation in animals, adults, and children. Moreover, most adults who survive to hospital admission after an out-of-hospital cardiac arrest die in the postresuscitation phase, many due to progressive myocardial dysfunction. Animal studies have demonstrated that postarrest myocardial stunning is a global phenomenon with biventricular systolic and diastolic dysfunction, that typically resolves after 1 or 2 days. This postarrest myocardial stunning is pathophysiologically and physiologically similar to sepsis-related myocardial dysfunction and postcardiopulmonary bypass myocardial dysfunction, including increases in inflammatory mediator and nitric oxide production. Postarrest myocardial stunning is worse after a more prolonged untreated cardiac arrest, after more prolonged CPR, after defibrillation with higher energy shocks and after a larger number of shocks.

In 1998, Mullner and colleagues demonstrated poor LV function in all 20 adults surviving to ICU admission after out-of-hospital cardiac arrest. Similar to the data from the induced hypothermia studies noted above, 17 of these 20 adults were treated with vasoactive infusions (epinephrine, dopamine, and/or dobutamine) during the first 24 hours after resuscitation.

Optimal treatment of postarrest myocardial dysfunction has not been established. As noted above, such myocardial dysfunction has been treated with various continuous inotropic/vasoactive agents, including dopamine, dobutamine, and epinephrine, in both children and adults. Prospective, controlled animal studies have documented amelioration of myocardial dysfunction with post-resuscitation intravenous dobutamine infusions. In addition, milrinone improves the hemodynamic status of children with postcardiopulmonary bypass myocardial dysfunction and septic shock. Milrinone has also improved postarrest myocardial function in a swine investigation. Finally, the new inotropic agent levosimenden has also been effective in animal models of postresuscitation myocardial dysfunction.

Although prospective controlled trials in animals have demonstrated that the myocardial dysfunction can be effectively treated with vasoactive agents, there are no data demonstrating improvements in outcome. Nevertheless, because myocardial dysfunction is common and can lead to secondary ischemic injuries to other organ systems or even cardiovascular collapse, treatment with vasoactive medications is a rational therapeutic choice that may improve outcome. The hemodynamic benefits in animal studies of postarrest myocardial dysfunction, pediatric studies of postcardiopulmonary bypass myocardial dysfunction, and pediatric sepsis-related myocardial dysfunction support the use of inotropic/vasoactive agents in this setting. Furthermore, adult studies document the common occurrence of postarrest hypotension and/or poor myocardial function "requiring" inotropic/vasoactive agents. In summary, because treatment of postarrest myocardial dysfunction with inotropic/vasoactive infusions can improve the patient's hemodynamic status, such treatment should be considered routinely.

Assuming treatment of postresuscitation myocardial dysfunction is appropriate, what should be our therapeutic goal? Should we aim for a normal echocardiographic ejection fraction? Normal cardiac output? Normal blood pressure? Normal mixed venous oxygen saturation? The answers to these questions are not currently available. This is a potentially rich area for further investigation.

Blood pressure management

As noted above, postresuscitation myocardial dysfunction is common and has many similarities to sepsis-associated myocardial dysfunction. Therefore, it should not be surprising that Laurent and colleagues (2002) found that 55% of adults surviving out-of-hospital cardiac arrests required in-hospital vasoactive infusions for hypotension unresponsive to volume boluses.

Compared to healthy volunteers, adults resuscitated from cardiac arrest have impaired autoregulation of cerebral blood flow. Hence, they may not maintain cerebral perfusion pressure when systemic hypotension is present and likewise may not be able to protect the brain from acutely increased blood flow due to systemic hypertension. It is reasonable to presume that blood pressure variability should be minimized as much as possible following resuscitation from cardiac arrest.

Nonetheless, a brief period of hypertension following resuscitation from cardiac arrest may diminish the no-reflow phenomenon. In animal models, brief induced hypertension following resuscitation results in improved neurological outcome compared to normotension. In a retrospective human study, postresuscitative hypertension was associated with a better neurological outcome after controlling for age, gender, duration of cardiac arrest, duration of CPR, and pre-existing diseases.

Given these limited data, what should be our postresuscitation blood pressure goals for children? It seems reasonable to treat aggressively and prevent hypotension, Moreover, it seems unlikely that severe hypertension is desirable. Any further assertions are difficult to support.

Glucose control

Hyperglycemia following adult cardiac arrest is associated with worse neurological outcome, after controlling for duration of arrest and presence of cardiogenic shock. In an animal model of asphyxial cardiac arrest, administration of insulin and glucose, but not administration of glucose alone, improved neurological outcome compared to administration of normal saline. Data are not available to clarify whether clinicians should target tight glucose control to avoid hyperglycemia and hypoglycemia following pediatric cardiac arrests.

Extracorporeal membrane oxygenation CPR

Perhaps the ultimate technology to control postresuscitation temperature and hemodynamic parameters is extracorporeal membrane oxygenation (ECMO). In addition, the concomitant administration of heparin may optimize microcirculatory flow.

The use of veno-arterial ECMO to re-establish circulation and provide controlled reperfusion following cardiac arrest has been published, but prospective, controlled studies are lacking. Nevertheless, these series have reported extraordinary results with the use of ECMO as a rescue therapy for pediatric cardiac arrests, especially from potentially reversible acute postoperative myocardial dysfunction or arrhythmias. In one study, 11 children who suffered cardiac arrest in the PICU after cardiac surgery were placed on ECMO during CPR after 20–110 minutes of CPR. Prolonged CPR was continued until ECMO cannulae, circuits, and personnel were available. Six of these 11 children were long-term survivors without apparent neurological sequelae. More recently, two centers have reported an additional remarkable 8 pediatric cardiac patients provided with mechanical cardiopulmonary support during CPR within 20 minutes of the initiation of CPR. All 8 survived to hospital discharge. Nevertheless, CPR and ECMO are not curative treatments; they are simply cardiopulmonary supportive measures that may allow tissue perfusion and viability until recovery from the precipitating disease process. As such, they can be powerful tools.

Most remarkably, Morris and Nadkarni reported 66 children who were placed on ECMO during CPR at the Children's Hospital of Philadelphia over 7 years. The median duration of CPR before establishment of ECMO was 50 minutes, and 35% (23/66) of these children survived to hospital discharge. We emphasize that these children had brief periods of "no-flow," excellent CPR during the "low-flow" period, and a well-controlled post-resuscitation phase.

What does this ECMO-CPR experience mean? Potential advantages of ECMO come from its ability to maintain tight control of physiologic parameters after resuscitation. For example, blood flow rates, oxygenation, ventilation, and body temperature can be manipulated precisely through the ECMO circuit. As we learn more about the processes of secondary injury after cardiac arrest, ECMO might enable controlled perfusion and temperature management to minimize reperfusion injury and maximize cell recovery.

Conversely, perhaps we should imitate ECMO goals for children successfully resuscitated from cardiac arrest (e.g., maintain adequate SvO_2).

Neuropsychological issues

Information about neurological outcomes and predictors of neurological outcome after both adult and pediatric cardiac arrests is quite limited. Two other pediatric issues create barriers in assessing neurological outcomes of children after cardiac arrests. First, pediatrics is developmental medicine. Prediction of future neuro-psychological status is a complex task for any child, especially babies. This issue is particularly complex after an acute neurological insult like a cardiac arrest. In addition, the need to consider the prearrest neurological potential of a child adds another dimension/barrier to the assessment and prediction of postarrest neurological status. Second, many children who suffer a cardiac arrest have substantial pre-existing neurological problems. For example, 17% of the children with in-hospital cardiac arrests from the NRCPR were neurologically abnormal before the arrest.

Our present knowledge about factors predicting neurological outcome from pediatric cardiac arrest is quite limited. There is little information about the predictive value of clinical neurological examinations, neurophysiological diagnostic studies (e.g., EEG, or somatosensory evoked potentials), biomarkers, or imaging (CT , MRI, or PET) on eventual outcome following cardiac arrest or other global hypoxic–ischemic insults in children.

There are some data indicating that burst-suppression pattern on postarrest EEG is sensitive and specific for poor neurological outcome. One study showed somatosensory evoked potential (SSEP) was highly sensitive and specific in pediatric patients after cardiac arrest. Nevertheless, SSEP is not standardized in the pediatric population and is difficult to interpret.

Biomarkers are emerging tools to predict neurological outcome. In an adult study, serum level of neuron-specific enolase (NSE) and S100b protein showed prognostic value. NSE >33 mcg/liter and S100b >0.7 mcg/liter were highly sensitive and specific for poor neurological outcome (death or persisting unconsciousness). The validation of those biomarkers in pediatric postarrest patients requires further study.

CT scans are not sensitive in detecting early neurological injury. The value of MRI studies following pediatric cardiac arrest is not yet clear. MRI with diffusion weighting, however, should provide valuable information about hypoxic–ischemic injury in the subacute and recovery phases.

Most outcome studies of pediatric cardiac arrest have not included neurological outcomes. Investigations that include neurological outcomes have generally used the Pediatric Cerebral Performance Category, a gross outcome scale. Many neuropsychological tests can detect more subtle, clinically important neuropsychological sequelae from neurological insults. Neuropsychological outcomes are important issues for future studies of outcome after pediatric cardiac arrest.

Conclusions

Outcomes from pediatric cardiac arrest and CPR appear to be improving. It seems likely that the evolving understanding of pathophysiologic events during and after pediatric cardiac arrest and the developing fields of pediatric critical care and pediatric emergency medicine have contributed to these apparent improvements. In addition, there are exciting breakthroughs in basic and applied science laboratories that are on the immediate horizon for study in specific subpopulations of cardiac arrest victims. By strategically focusing therapies to specific phases of cardiac arrest and resuscitation and to evolving pathophysiology, there is great promise that critical care interventions will lead the way to more successful cardiopulmonary and cerebral resuscitation in children.

To shed the "therapeutic orphan" status of treatment for pediatric sudden cardiac arrest and improve outcome for children, the following are necessary: a large pediatric sudden death registry; more and better pediatric sudden arrest and asphyxial arrest animal studies; and multicenter therapeutic trials in pediatric sudden arrest populations. Treatment of sudden death in children in the future needs to be more evidence-based and less anecdotal. Timing of therapeutic interventions to prevent arrest, and protect, preserve, and promote restoration of intact neurological survival is of high priority.

FURTHER READING

2005 American Heart Association (AHA) guidelines for cardiopulmonary resuscitation (CPR) and emergency cardiovascular care (ECC) of pediatric and neonatal patients: pediatric advanced life support. Pediatrics, 2006. **117**(5): p. e1005–28.

2005 American Heart Association (AHA) guidelines for cardiopulmonary resuscitation (CPR) and emergency cardiovascular care (ECC) of pediatric and neonatal patients: pediatric basic life support. Pediatrics, 2006. **117**(5): p. e989–1004.

Abdallah, I. and H. Shawky, *A randomised controlled trial comparing milrinone and epinephrine as inotropes in paediatric patients undergoing total correction of Tetralogy of Fallot.* Egyptian Journal of Anaesthesia, 2003. **19**(4): p. 323–329.

Appleton, G.O., et al., *CPR and the single rescuer: at what age should you "call first" rather than "call fast"?* Ann Emerg Med, 1995. **25**(4): p. 492–4

Atkins, D.L., et al., *Pediatric defibrillation: importance of paddle size in determining transthoracic impedance.* Pediatrics, 1988. **82**(6): p. 914–8.

Atkinson, E., et al., *Specificity and sensitivity of automated external defibrillator rhythm analysis in infants and children.* Ann Emerg Med, 2003. **42**(2): p. 185–96.

Babbs, C.F. and K.B. Kern, *Optimum compression to ventilation ratios in CPR under realistic, practical conditions: a physiological and mathematical analysis.* Resuscitation, 2002. **54**(2): p. 147–157.

Babbs, C.F. and V. Nadkarni, *Optimizing chest compression to rescue ventilation ratios during one-rescuer CPR by professionals and lay persons: children are not just little adults.* Resuscitation, 2004. **61**(2): p. 173–181.

Behringer, W., et al., *Cumulative epinephrine dose during cardiopulmonary resuscitation and neurologic outcome.* Ann Intern Med, 1998. **129**(6): p. 450–6.

Berg, M.D., et al., *Pediatric defibrillation doses often fail to terminate prolonged out-of-hospital ventricular fibrillation in children.* Resuscitation, 2005. **67**(1): p. 63–7.

Berg, R.A., et al., *High-dose epinephrine results in greater early mortality after resuscitation from prolonged cardiac arrest in pigs: a prospective, randomized study.* Crit Care Med, 1994. **22**(2): p. 282–290.

Berg, R.A., et al., *"Bystander" chest compressions and assisted ventilation independently improve outcome from piglet asphyxial pulseless "cardiac arrest".* Circulation, 2000. **101**(14): p. 1743–8.

Berg, R.A., et al., *Attenuated adult biphasic shocks compared with weight-based monophasic shocks in a swine model of prolonged pediatric ventricular fibrillation.* Resuscitation, 2004. **61**(2): p. 189–97.

Berg, R.A., et al., *Better outcome after pediatric defibrillation dosage than adult dosage in a swine model of pediatric ventricular fibrillation.* J Am Coll Cardiol, 2005. **45**(5): p. 786–9.

Berger, P.B., *A glucose-insulin-potassium infusion did not reduce mortality, cardiac arrest, or cardiogenic shock after acute MI.* ACP J Club, 2005. **143**(1): p. 4–5.

Bernard, S.A., et al., *Treatment of comatose survivors of out-of-hospital cardiac arrest with induced hypothermia.* N Engl J Med, 2002. **346**(8): p. 557–563.

Brown, C.G., et al., *A comparison of standard-dose and high-dose epinephrine in cardiac arrest outside the hospital. The Multicenter High-Dose Epinephrine Study Group.* N Engl J Med, 1992. **327**(15): p. 1051–1055.

Callaham, M., et al., *A randomized clinical trial of high-dose epinephrine and norepinephrine versus standard-dose epinephrine in prehospital cardiac arrest.* JAMA, 1992. **268**: p. 2667–2672.

Caffrey, S.L., et al., *Public use of automated external defibrillators.* N Engl J Med, 2002. **347**(16): p. 1242–7.

Ceneviva, G., et al., *Hemodynamic support in fluid-refractory pediatric septic shock.* Pediatrics, 1998. **102**(2): p. e19.

Chamnanvanakij, S. and J.M. Perlman, *Outcome following cardiopulmonary resuscitation in the neonate requiring ventilatory assistance.* Resuscitation, 2000. **45**(3): p. 173–80.

Cecchin, F., et al., *Is arrhythmia detection by automatic external defibrillator accurate for children?: sensitivity and specificity of an automatic external defibrillator algorithm in 696 pediatric arrhythmias.* Circulation, 2001. **103**(20): p. 2483–8.

Cecchin, F., et al., *Is arrhythmia detection by automatic external defibrillator accurate for children? Sensitivity and specificity of an automatic external defibrillator algorithm in 696 pediatric arrhythmias.* Circulation, 2001. **103**(20): p. 2483–2488.

de Mos, N., et al., *Pediatric in-intensive-care-unit cardiac arrest: incidence, survival, and predictive factors.* Crit Care Med, 2006. **34**(4): p. 1209–15.

Dean, J.M., et al., *Age-related changes in chest geometry during cardiopulmonary resuscitation.* J Appl Physiol, 1987. **62**(6): p. 2212–9.

Dieckmann, R.A. and R. Vardis, *High-dose epinephrine in pediatric out-of-hospital cardiopulmonary arrest.* Pediatrics, 1995. **95**(6): p. 901–13.

Donoghue, A.J., et al., *Out-of-hospital pediatric cardiac arrest: an epidemiologic review and assessment of current knowledge.* Ann Emerg Med, 2005. **46**(6): p. 512–22.

Dorian, P., et al., *Amiodarone as compared with lidocaine for shock-resistant ventricular fibrillation.* N Engl J Med, 2002. **346**(12): p. 884–890.

Duncan, B.W., et al., *Use of rapid-deployment extracorporeal membrane oxygenation for the resuscitation of pediatric patients with heart disease after cardiac arrest.* J Thorac Cardiovasc Surg, 1998. **116**(2): p. 305–311.

Eberle, B., et al., *Checking the carotid pulse check: diagnostic accuracy of first responders in patients with and without a pulse.* Resuscitation, 1996. **33**(2): p. 107–16.

Edelson, D.P., et al., *Effects of compression depth and pre-shock pauses predict defibrillation failure during cardiac arrest.* Resuscitation, 2006. **71**(2): p. 137–45.

Egan, J.R., et al., *Levosimendan for low cardiac output: a pediatric experience.* J Intensive Care Med, 2006. **21**(3): p. 183–7.

Feneley, M.P., et al., *Influence of compression rate on initial success of resuscitation and 24 hour survival after prolonged manual cardiopulmonary resuscitation in dogs.* Circulation, 1988. **77**(1): p. 240–250.

Garcia Gonzalez, M.J. and A. Dominguez Rodriguez, *Pharmacologic treatment of heart failure due to ventricular dysfunction by myocardial stunning: potential role of levosimendan.* Am J Cardiovasc Drugs, 2006. **6**(2): p. 69–75.

Gausche, M. and R.J. Lewis, *Out-of-hospital endotracheal intubation of children.* Jama, 2000. **283**(21): p. 2790–2.

Gazmuri, R.J., et al., *Myocardial dysfunction after successful resuscitation from cardiac arrest.* Crit Care Med, 1996. **24**(6): p. 992–1000.

Gerein, R.B., et al., *What are the etiology and epidemiology of out-of-hospital pediatric cardiopulmonary arrest in Ontario, Canada?* Acad Emerg Med, 2006. **13**(6): p. 653–8.

Gluckman, P.D., et al., *Selective head cooling with mild systemic hypothermia after neonatal encephalopathy: multicentre randomised trial.* Lancet, 2005. **365**(9460): p. 663–70.

Graf, W.D., et al., *Predicting outcome in pediatric submersion victims.* Ann Emerg Med, 1995. **26**(3): p. 312–9.

Gurnett, C.A. and D.L. Atkins, *Successful use of a biphasic waveform automated external defibrillator in a high-risk child.* Am J Cardiol, 2000. **86**(9): p. 1051–3.

Gutgesell, H.P., et al., *Energy dose for ventricular defibrillation of children.* Pediatrics, 1976. **58**(6): p. 898–901.

Hallstrom, A.P., et al., *Dispatcher assisted CPR: implementation and potential benefit. A 12-year study.* Resuscitation, 2003. **57**(2): p. 123–9.

Halperin, H.R., et al., *Determinants of blood flow to vital organs during cardiopulmonary resuscitation in dogs.* Circulation, 1986. **73**(3): p. 539–550.

Hickey, R.W., et al., *Hypothermia and hyperthermia in children after resuscitation from cardiac arrest.* Pediatrics, 2000. **106**(1 Pt 1): p. 118–22.

Hintz, S.R., et al., *Utilization and outcomes of neonatal cardiac extracorporeal life support: 1996–2000.* Pediatr Crit Care Med, 2005. **6**(1): p. 33–8.

Hoffman, T.M., et al., *Efficacy and safety of milrinone in preventing low cardiac output syndrome in infants and children after corrective surgery for congenital heart disease.* Circulation, 2003. **107**(7): p. 996–1002.

Hornchen, U., et al., *Endobronchial instillation of epinephrine during cardiopulmonary resuscitation.* Crit Care Med, 1987. **15**(11): p. 1037–1039.

Houri, P.K., et al., *A randomized, controlled trial of two-thumb vs two-finger chest compression in a swine infant model of cardiac arrest.* Prehosp Emerg Care, 1997. **1**(2): p. 65–67.

Huang, L., et al., *Levosimendan improves postresuscitation outcomes in a rat model of CPR.* J Lab Clin Med, 2005. **146**(5): p. 256–61.

Hypothermia After Cardiac Arrest Study Group. Mild therapeutic hypothermia to improve the neurologic outcome after cardiac arrest. N Engl J Med, 2002. **346**(8): p. 549–556. Idris, A.H., et al., *Effect of ventilation on acid-base balance and oxygenation in low blood-flow states.* Crit Care Med, 1994. **22**(11): p. 1827–1834.

Innes, P.A., et al., *Comparison of the haemodynamic effects of dobutamine with enoximone after open heart surgery in small children.* Br J Anaesth, 1994. **72**(1): p. 77–81.

Johnson, L., et al., *Use of intraosseous blood to assess blood chemistries and hemoglobin during cardiopulmonary resuscitation with drug infusions.* Crit Care Med, 1999. **27**(6): p. 1147–1152.

Kamohara, T., et al., *A comparison of myocardial function after primary cardiac and primary asphyxial cardiac arrest.* Am J Respir Crit Care Med, 2001. **164**(7): p. 1221–1224.

Katz, A.M. and H. Reuter, *Cellular calcium and cardiac cell death.* Am J Cardiol, 1979. **44**(1): p. 188–90.

Kern, K.B., et al., *Efficacy of chest compression-only BLS CPR in the presence of an occluded airway.* Resuscitation, 1998. **39**(3): p. 179–88.

Kinney, S.B. and J. Tibballs, *An analysis of the efficacy of bag-valve-mask ventilation and chest compression during different compression-ventilation ratios in manikin-simulated paediatric resuscitation.* Resuscitation, 2000. **43**(2): p. 115–20

Kouwenhoven, W.B., J.R. Jude, and G.G. Knickerbocker, *Closed-chest cardiac massage.* Jama, 1960. **173**: p. 1064–7.

Kudenchuk, P.J., et al., *Amiodarone for resuscitation after out-of-hospital cardiac arrest due to ventricular fibrillation.* N Engl J Med, 1999. **341**(12): p. 871–878.

Kuisma, M., P. Suominen, and R. Korpela, *Paediatric out-of-hospital cardiac arrests—epidemiology and outcome.* Resuscitation, 1995. **30**(2): p. 141–50.

Laitinen, P., et al., *Amrinone versus dopamine and nitroglycerin in neonates after arterial switch operation for transposition of the great arteries.* J Cardiothorac Vasc Anesth, 1999. **13**(2): p. 186–190.

Laitinen, P., et al., *Amrinone versus dopamine-nitroglycerin after reconstructive surgery for complete atrioventricular septal defect.* J Cardiothorac Vasc Anesth, 1997. **11**(7): p. 870–874.

Langhelle, A., et al., *In-hospital factors associated with improved outcome after out-of-hospital cardiac arrest. A comparison between four regions in Norway.* Resuscitation, 2003. **56**(3): p. 247–263.

Laurent, I., et al., *Reversible myocardial dysfunction in survivors of out-of-hospital cardiac arrest.* J Am Coll Cardiol, 2002. **40**(12): p. 2110–2116.

Lindner, K.H., F.W. Ahnefeld, and I.M. Bowdler, *Comparison of different doses of epinephrine on myocardial perfusion and resuscitation success during cardiopulmonary resuscitation in a pig model.* Am J Emerg Med, 1991. **9**(1): p. 27–31.

Lopez-Herce, J., et al., *Outcome of out-of-hospital cardiorespiratory arrest in children.* Pediatr Emerg Care, 2005. **21**(12): p. 807–15.

Lurie, K., et al., *Use of an inspiratory impedance threshold valve during cardiopulmonary resuscitation: a progress report.* Resuscitation, 2000. **44**(3): p. 219–230.

Mann, K., R.A. Berg, and V. Nadkarni, *Beneficial effects of vasopressin in prolonged pediatric cardiac arrest: a case series.* Resuscitation, 2002. **52**(2): p. 149–156.

Mann, K., R.A. Berg, and V. Nadkarni, *Beneficial effects of vasopressin in prolonged pediatric cardiac arrest: a case series.* Resuscitation, 2002. **52**(2): p. 149–56.

Meaney, P.A., et al., *Higher survival rates among younger patients after pediatric intensive care unit cardiac arrests.* Pediatrics, 2006. **118**(6): p. 2424–33.

Menegazzi, J.J., et al., *Two-thumb versus two-finger chest compression during CRP in a swine infant model of cardiac arrest.* Ann Emerg Med, 1993. **22**(2): p. 240–243.

Morris, M.C., G. Wernovsky, and V.M. Nadkarni, *Survival outcomes after extracorporeal cardiopulmonary resuscitation instituted during active chest compressions following refractory in-hospital pediatric cardiac arrest.* Pediatr Crit Care Med, 2004. **5**(5): p. 440–446.

Moule, P., *Checking the carotid pulse: diagnostic accuracy in students of the healthcare professions.* Resuscitation, 2000. **44**(3): p. 195–201.

Nadkarni, V.M., et al., *First documented rhythm and clinical outcome from in-hospital cardiac arrest among children and adults.* JAMA, 2006. **295**(1): p. 50–7.

Nishisaki, A., et al., *Retrospective analysis of the prognostic value of electroencephalography patterns obtained in pediatric in-hospital cardiac arrest survivors during three years.* Pediatr Crit Care Med, 2007. **8**(1): p. 10–7.

Orlowski, J.P., et al., *The safety of intraosseous infusions: risks of fat and bone marrow emboli to the lungs.* Ann Emerg Med, 1989. **18**(10): p. 1062–1067.

Parra, D.A., et al., *Outcome of cardiopulmonary resuscitation in a pediatric cardiac intensive care unit.* Crit Care Med, 2000. **28**(9): p. 3296–300.

Pepe, P.E., et al., *Prospective, decade-long, population-based study of pediatric drowning-related incidents.* Acad Emerg Med, 2002. **9**(5): p. 516–517.

Perondi, M.B., et al., *A comparison of high-dose and standard-dose epinephrine in children with cardiac arrest.* N Engl J Med, 2004. **350**(17): p. 1722–30.

Piazza, O., et al., *S100B is a sensitive but not specific prognostic index in comatose patients after cardiac arrest.* Minerva Chir, 2005. **60**(6): p. 477–80.

Reis, A.G., et al., *A prospective investigation into the epidemiology of in-hospital pediatric cardiopulmonary resuscitation using the international Utstein reporting style.* Pediatrics, 2002. **109**(2): p. 200–9.

Samson, R.A., et al., *Outcomes of in-hospital ventricular fibrillation in children.* N Engl J Med, 2006. **354**(22): p. 2328–39.

Samson, R.A., R.A. Berg, and R. Bingham, *Use of automated external defibrillators for children: an update—an advisory statement from the Pediatric Advanced Life Support Task Force, International Liaison Committee on Resuscitation.* Pediatrics, 2003. **112**(1 Pt 1): p. 163–8.

Samson, R.A., et al., *Use of automated external defibrillators for children: an update: an advisory statement from the pediatric advanced life support task force, International Liaison Committee on Resuscitation.* Circulation, 2003. **107**(25): p. 3250–5.

Schellhammer, F., et al., *Somatosensory evoked potentials: a simple neurophysiological monitoring technique in supra-aortal balloon test occlusions.* Eur Radiol, 1998. **8**(9): p. 1586–9.

Schindler, M.B., et al., *Outcome of out-of-hospital cardiac or respiratory arrest in children.* N Engl J Med, 1996. **335**(20): p. 1473–9.

Shankaran, S., et al., *Whole-body hypothermia for neonatal encephalopathy: animal observations as a basis for a randomized, controlled pilot study in term infants.* Pediatrics, 2002. **110**(2 Pt 1): p. 377–385.

Sheikh, A. and T. Brogan, *Outcome and cost of open- and closed-chest cardiopulmonary resuscitation in pediatric cardiac arrests.* Pediatrics, 1994. **93**(3): p. 392–8.

Sirbaugh, P.E., et al., *A prospective, population-based study of the demographics, epidemiology, management, and outcome of out-of-hospital pediatric cardiopulmonary arrest.* Ann Emerg Med, 1999. **33**(2): p. 174–84.

Skrifvars, M.B., et al., *Improved survival after in-hospital cardiac arrest outside critical care areas.* Acta Anaesthesiol Scand, 2005. **49**(10): p. 1534–9.

Slonim, A.D., et al., *Cardiopulmonary resuscitation in pediatric intensive care units.* Crit Care Med, 1997. **25**(12): p. 1951–5.

Smith, B.T., T.D. Rea, and M.S. Eisenberg, *Ventricular fibrillation in pediatric cardiac arrest.* Acad Emerg Med, 2006. **13**(5): p. 525–9.

Srikantan, S.K., et al., *Effect of one-rescuer compression/ventilation ratios on cardiopulmonary resuscitation in infant, pediatric, and adult manikins.* Pediatr Crit Care Med, 2005. **6**(3): p. 293–297.

Sunde, K., et al., *Implementation of a standardised treatment protocol for post resuscitation care after out-of-hospital cardiac arrest.* Resuscitation, 2007.

Stiell, I.G., et al., *Vasopressin versus epinephrine for inhospital cardiac arrest: a randomised controlled trial.* Lancet, 2001. **358**(9276): p. 105–109.

Stueven, H.A., et al., *The effectiveness of calcium chloride in refractory electromechanical dissociation.* Ann Emerg Med, 1985. **14**(7): p. 626–9.

Suominen, P., et al., *Utstein style reporting of in-hospital paediatric cardiopulmonary resuscitation.* Resuscitation, 2000. **45**(1): p. 17–25.

Suominen, P., J. Rasanen, and A. Kivioja, *Efficacy of cardiopulmonary resuscitation in pulseless paediatric trauma patients.* Resuscitation, 1998. **36**(1): p. 9–13.

Suominen, P., et al., *Paediatric cardiac arrest and resuscitation provided by physician-staffed emergency care units.* Acta Anaesthesiol Scand, 1997. **41**(2): p. 260–5.

Torres, A., Jr., et al., *Long-term functional outcome of inpatient pediatric cardiopulmonary resuscitation.* Pediatr Emerg Care, 1997. **13**(6): p. 369–73.

Tunstall-Pedoe, H., et al., *Survey of 3765 cardiopulmonary resuscitations in British hospitals (the BRESUS Study): methods and overall results.* Bmj, 1992. **304**(6838): p. 1347–51.

Valenzuela, T.D., et al., *Outcomes of rapid defibrillation by security officers after cardiac arrest in casinos.* N Engl J Med, 2000. **343**(17): p. 1206–9.

Voelckel, W.G., et al., *Effects of vasopressin and epinephrine on splanchnic blood flow and renal function during and after cardiopulmonary resuscitation in pigs.* Crit Care Med, 2000. **28**(4): p. 1083–1088.

Voelckel, W.G., et al., *Comparison of epinephrine and vasopressin in a pediatric porcine model of asphyxial cardiac arrest.* Circulation, 1999. **36**: p. 1115–1118.

Wenzel, V., et al., *A comparison of vasopressin and epinephrine for out-of-hospital cardiopulmonary resuscitation.* N Engl J Med, 2004. **350**(2): p. 105–113.

Young, K.D. and J.S. Seidel, *Pediatric cardiopulmonary resuscitation: a collective review.* Ann Emerg Med, 1999. **33**(2): p. 195–205.

Zaritsky, A., et al., *CPR in children.* Ann Emerg Med, 1987. **16**(10): p. 1107–11.

54

Resuscitation in elder persons

Arthur B. Sanders

Department of Emergency Medicine, University of Arizona College of Medicine
Tucson, AZ, USA

The percentage of elder persons throughout the developed world is rapidly increasing. In the USA, for example, the percentage of the population 65 years and older has increased from 4% in 1900 to 13% in 1990 and is projected to be 22% by 2030. The fastest growing segment of the elderly population is the oldest persons who are 85 years or older and made up about 1% of the population in 1990 but will increase to more than 5% over the next 30 years.[1–9]

Similarly in developed countries worldwide (including Japan, Australia, New Zealand, and countries in Europe and North America) the elderly segment of the population is increasing significantly. The highest proportion of elderly people in the world is in Sweden, with 18% of the population 65 years or older.[7] This demographic change with increasing numbers of elder persons in the population is expected to continue over the next 30 to 50 years. By the year 2025, 5%–9% of the population in the developed nations will be 80 years or older.[1–9]

This graying of the population in the developed world is largely due to several demographic factors. This includes a decline in the mortality rate especially from cardiovascular diseases and decreased fertility rates in much of the developed world. The post-World War II baby boom generation in the USA consists of 75 million persons born between 1946 and 1964. These people will be entering the geriatric population over the next 20 years.[1–9]

This increased population of elder persons will have a major impact on the delivery of healthcare. The majority of elder patients suffer from chronic medical conditions and many have limitations on daily activities. Persons over 75 years of age require the greatest amount of medical care per capita of any age group. In addition, the social support systems of the elderly are often less than optimal, with many elderly persons living alone.[1–9]

The number of ED visits in the USA has increased by 26% in the past decade. Elder persons are the most frequent users of the emergency healthcare system. Each year, in the USA there are 64 emergency department visits for each 100 persons over 75 years of age. Heart disease is the most frequent ED diagnosis for elder patients.[10] In 1995, approximately 16% of emergency department visits in the USA were made by patients 65 years or older. Of the 100 million emergency department visits in 1995, it is estimated that 15.7 million patients were 65 years or older, with the most common symptoms related to ischemic heart disease or cardiac dysrhythmias. More than 300 000 elderly patients are treated for cardiac arrest in emergency departments in the USA each year.[1,5] Of patients seen in the emergency department, elderly patients are seven times more likely to be admitted to the hospital, five times more likely to be admitted to an intensive care bed and five times more likely to use ambulance transport compared to younger adult patients.[11] Elder patients seen in the ED are generally sicker than younger patients. Approximately 47% of older patients seen in the ED receive comprehensive ED care, 46% are admitted to the hospital and 39% arrive by ambulance.[11] As the number of elder persons increases over the next four decades and medical resources come under scrutiny, it will be a challenge to ensure that the emergency care needs of elder patients are met.

Aging and the cardiovascular system

The functional reserve of the cardiovascular system and the ability to tolerate stresses such as cardiac arrest or

Cardiac Arrest: The Science and Practice of Resuscitation Medicine. 2nd edn., ed. Norman Paradis, Henry Halperin, Karl Kern, Volker Wenzel, Douglas Chamberlain. Published by Cambridge University Press. © Cambridge University Press, 2007.

acute myocardial infarction decline with age. Although elder persons constitute a heterogeneous group, coronary artery disease, valvular heart disease, hypertension, and myocardial infarction all increase with age.[1–7,12–14] It is difficult to sort out whether it is age itself or accompanying cardiovascular diseases that are responsible for cardiac problems in the elderly. As people age, their arteries stiffen, resulting in increased systolic blood pressure.[1–7,12–14] Left ventricular hypertrophy may accompany the rise in arterial systolic pressure. There is no change in resting heart rate. Nevertheless, maximal heart rate and aerobic capacity decrease with age. The lack of heart rate response to exercise or stress means that cardiac output must be maintained by increases in stroke volume and cardiac dilation.[14] As people age there is increased myocardial stiffness which impairs left ventricular filling increasing the risk for heart failure and arrythmias. About 50% of elder patients have abnormalities in their resting electrocardiogram. With advanced age, there is also an attenuation of responsiveness to beta-adrenergic stimulation.[1–9,12–14]

About 60% of acute myocardial infarctions occur in patients 65 years of age or greater. All of the physiologic changes associated with aging, and particularly the lack of cardiovascular reserve, contribute to the high mortality after acute myocardial infarction in elder persons.[1–7,15–20] Patients over 75 years have a much higher mortality from acute myocardial infarction compared to younger patients. In the GUSTO trial patients 75 years and greater had more than a fourfold increase in mortality compared to those under 65 years. This is thought to be due to comorbid diseases, physiologic dysfunction and lack of physiologic reserve.[21]

Older patients also have a higher mortality some time after myocardial infarction compared to younger patients. Rich *et al.* found the 1-year postdischarge mortality following an acute myocardial infarction was 6.8% in patients under 70 years and 19.1% in those 70 years or older. Hospital mortality was 5.6% in patients under 70 years and 16.1% in patients 70 years or older. Even after adjusting for multiple baseline and therapeutic differences in elder persons, age remained a strong predictor of worsened in-hospital and 1-year mortality.[15] Posthospital mortality is also increased three- to fourfold in elder patients.

The presentation of acute myocardial infarction changes with age. Elderly patients present with atypical symptoms such as shortness of breath, syncope, or confusion. This fact may contribute to a delay in treatment and increased mortality of older persons with acute myocardial infarction. Fewer than half of patients 85 years or older with acute myocardial infarction present with chest pain.[1–5,22]

Ironically, elder patients who are at greater risk for death following acute myocardial infarction are less likely to receive aggressive treatment such as emergent reperfusion.[15,19,23] Even though this observation is partially explained by the atypical presentations and contraindications for some treatments, many elderly patients who are eligible for aggressive treatment do not receive them. In a recent study of more than 2000 older patients with acute myocardial infarction, Magid *et al.* found that older patients were less likely to receive standard treatments even when treatments are controlled for contraindications and atypical presentations. Only 81% of eligible elder patients received aspirin, 60% received beta-blockers, and 78% received acute reperfusion therapy.[23] Weaver *et al.* found that only 25% of potential candidates 75 years or older who would have been eligible to receive thrombolytics were given this therapy.[19] Some healthcare professionals are hesitant to administer key treatments to elder patients; this is unfortunate because older patients with acute myocardial infarction are at the highest risk and have the most to gain in mortality and morbidity benefits.

Outcomes of cardiopulmonary resuscitation in elder persons

The outcome of resuscitation attempts for cardiac arrest in elder persons has been a subject of debate and conflicting recommendations in the medical literature. Comparing different studies in the medical literature is often difficult. Many of the studies looked only at specific populations, such as elderly patients in a nursing home or geriatric unit. Other studies do not differentiate the effects of age from those of other factors such as comorbid diseases, which have a profound effect on survival from cardiac arrest. In some studies of out-of-hospital cardiac arrest, resuscitation rates of elderly and non-elderly patients were not compared. This is important because successful resuscitation of all patients depends highly on the efficiency of the emergency medical services (EMS) system (bystander CPR, time to defibrillation, and other factors). Consequently, without studying a broad population including both older and younger patients, it may be unclear whether poor survival is due to age or an inefficient EMS system. Finally, studies define the elderly population differently: ages above 60, 65, 70, 75 or 80 years have all been used to define an elderly population.

One of the issues in dealing with the special needs of elder patients is understanding societal attitudes about aging. Many misperceptions, even among healthcare professionals, result in stereotyping. For example, some people believe that elder persons who are resuscitated have severe neurologic impairments; therefore some healthcare professionals treat elderly patients less aggressively than they treat younger patients with the same disease. Words in the medical literature are indicative of attitudes. For example, the following titles appeared in prestigious journals: "Should the Elderly be Resuscitated Following Out-of-Hospital Cardiac Arrest?" and "Resuscitation of the Elderly: a Blessing or a Curse?"[24,25] Particular care should be taken in distinguishing attitudes from scientific data and policy recommendations.

Murphy et al. studied 503 patients who suffered cardiac arrest in five Boston health care institutions.[26] Only two of the institutions were acute care hospitals, one was a long-term care institution, and two were chronic care hospitals. Of 503 cases reviewed, 112 (22%) had return of spontaneous circulation, but only 19 (3.8%) survived to hospital discharge.[26] Poor outcomes were noted for patients who had unwitnessed or out-of-hospital arrests or arrests associated with an initial rhythm of asystole or pulseless electrical activity. The prognosis was also very poor in patients who had two or more acute diseases or a severe underlying chronic disorder.

This article was accompanied by an editorial in the *Annals of Internal Medicine* by Podrid, who used these data to demonstrate the futility of resuscitating elderly patients in a cost-conscious environment with a shortage of critical care beds.[25] The editorial states:

When a person is an in-patient, resuscitation should not be attempted even in the absence of a "do not resuscitate" order. . . . In view of the findings of this study, it is perhaps time to establish meaningful guidelines for do not resuscitate orders in the elderly hospitalized patient in order to spare them costly, artificial, and uncomfortable measures that only serve to delay death. . . . Is it reasonable or fair to use critical care beds, which are costly and in short supply, to provide intensive care for those patients who are unlikely to recover or even survive the hospitalization? In this cost conscious environment our resources must be more efficiently allocated to those who are most likely to benefit from them.

This editorial is particularly interesting in light of the significant flaws in the study by Murphy et al.[26] Although the data are interesting and provide a basis for discussion, they are far from convincing and are contradicted by subsequent studies. Murphy et al. describe resuscitation success in an elderly population in the Boston area without comparing it to a control group of non-elder persons in the same area. Out-of-hospital resuscitation success depends highly on an effective EMS system. What was the level of EMS provided in the Boston area at the time of the study? Becker et al. had shown that, while some cities have developed highly sophisticated EMS systems that produced significant resuscitation and survival rates, other cities such as Chicago have dismal resuscitation rates for all patients in cardiac arrest.[27] In a more recent study, survival rates for all patients suffering cardiac arrest in Los Angeles were less than 2%.[28] Is the observation of poor survival in the elderly population the result of age or of a poor EMS system? Another concern is that Murphy et al. mixed populations from a number of healthcare institutions including two acute care hospitals, two chronic care hospitals, and one long-term care institution; yet the conclusions and implications do not clearly distinguish these populations. Is it fair to lump these populations together when many patients in the database were in chronic care facilities? Are there enough data to make conclusions about all elderly patients? Patients, especially in chronic care facilities, have significant comorbid diseases, a fact that was demonstrated in the article by Murphy et al. Patients who had two or more acute problems or one chronic disease had a poor prognosis for long-term survival. Were the poor outcomes the result of age itself or the comorbid diseases that may occur at any age?

Out-of-hospital arrest

The Belgian cerebral resuscitation study group analyzed 2776 out-of-hospital cardiac arrests to determine the effect of age on outcome and neurologic deficit.[28] Overall, 23% of patients were admitted to the hospital and 8% were discharged alive. Age had no effect on hospital admission or discharge rates. Seven percent of patients under 40 years survived to discharge, compared to 7% of patients aged 70 to 79 years and 6% of patients older than 80 years. After cardiac arrest, age had no effect on subsequent death from neurologic causes. There was, however, a significant difference in non-neurologic deaths across the age groups. After resuscitation, more elderly patients died in the hospital from non-neurologic causes than did non-elderly patients. The investigators also compared the effect of age on outcome according to prearrest health status. Although elderly patients more frequently had a dependent lifestyle before the arrest, there was no effect of age on outcome adjusted for prearrest health state. Pulseless electrical activity occurred more frequently in patients 70 years or older (12% vs. 9%). The authors concluded that decision making in cardiac arrest should not be based on age and that age was not associated with overall poor survival or neurologic disability.[29]

Longstreth et al. reviewed the relation between age and outcome in patients treated for out-of-hospital cardiac arrest in Seattle over a 5-year period.[30] Outcomes of 1405 patients 70 years and older were compared to 1624 younger patients. There was no difference in elderly vs. non-elderly patients with regard to resuscitation success (27% vs. 29%) or discharge rate from the hospital (10% vs. 14%). Twenty-four percent of elderly patients with ventricular fibrillation were discharged from the hospital alive. The authors concluded that elderly patients can benefit from attempted resuscitation from out-of-hospital cardiac arrest.[30]

In a series of important studies, Tresch *et al.* provided further insight into the etiology of cardiac arrest in elder persons. They studied 1345 adult victims of out-of-hospital cardiac arrest,[31] and found that ventricular fibrillation as the initial rhythm in cardiac arrest decreased as the age of the patient increased, whereas pulseless electrical activity progressively increased (Fig. 54.1). Fifty-eight percent of patients under 70 years of age demonstrated ventricular fibrillation, compared to 44% of patients over 70 years. Overall, 16% of patients under 70 years of age survived to hospital discharge compared with 9% of patients older than 70 years.

In another study, Tresch *et al.* analyzed 381 patients who had out-of-hospital cardiac arrest witnessed by paramedics.[32] Elderly patients were significantly more likely to have a past history of congestive heart failure (25% vs. 10%) and were more commonly taking digoxin (40% vs. 20%) and diuretics (35% vs. 25%). Before the cardiac arrests, elderly patients were more likely to complain of dyspnea

(53% vs. 40%), whereas younger patients were more likely to complain of chest pain (23% vs. 13%). Ventricular fibrillation was more likely to occur as the initial rhythm in cardiac arrest in younger than in older patients (42% vs. 22%). There was no difference in successful resuscitation rate between younger and elderly patients; however, 24% of younger patients survived to hospital discharge compared to 10% of elder patients. Survival to hospital discharge depended on the patient's age, presenting complaint, and initial cardiac rhythm associated with the arrest. In elder patients, 58% survived if their complaint was chest pain and if ventricular fibrillation was their initial arrest rhythm.[32] This study gives us insight into the etiology of cardiac arrest in elderly patients. It reinforces the concept that chest pain is less common in elder patients as a presenting symptom and that in elder patients congestive heart failure and dyspnea are more common symptoms (and possibly etiologies) of their arrest. Even though resuscitation rates are similar in elderly and younger patients, more elderly patients die postresuscitation in the hospital. This is consistent with the concept that elderly patients have less cardiovascular reserve to withstand the insult of a cardiac arrest and postarrest complications.

Herlitz *et al.* reviewed factors associated with resuscitation in more than 8000 patients in Sweden. The proportion of patients with a cardiac etiology of the arrest increased with age. Fewer patients over 75 years presented with ventricular fibrillation as their initial rhythm. Overall, 1-month survival was worse in older patients, 4.5% for those less than 65 years, 3.2% between 65 and 75 years and 2.5% over 75 years of age. The authors noted that they did not control for comorbid diseases and their effect on outcome in older persons.[33]

Swor *et al.* investigated whether age was a factor in the survival to hospital discharge for more than 2500 patients suffering cardiac arrest over a four year period. Patients 80 years or older were more likely to arrest at home and more likely to have a bradyasystolic initial rhythm than younger patients. Ventricular fibrillation was the initial rhythm in 64% of patients age 40–49 years, but found in only 40% of patients 80 years and older. Survival to hospital discharge was significantly decreased in patients 80 years and older. Only 3.3% of patients over 80 years survived compared to 7.1% of patients age 70–79 and 8.1% for age 60–69. Though the prognosis was not dismal for patients over 80 years, age was an independent factor for decreased survival. In this study, comorbid disease was not taken into account as a variable affecting outcome.[34]

Iwami *et al.* reviewed out-of-hospital cardiac arrest in Osaka, Japan over 2 years. They found that the annual

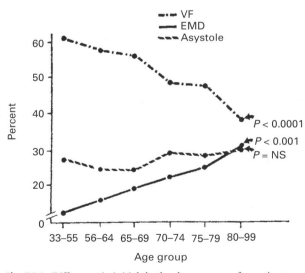

Fig. 54.1. Difference in initial rhythm by age group for patients with out-of-hospital cardiac arrest. Note greater prevalence of electromechanical dissociation (*EMD*) (pulseless electrical activity) and lower prevalence of ventricular fibrillation (*VF*) in older age groups. (From ref. 31. Reprinted with permission from *American Journal of Cardiology*.)

incidence of arrest increased with increasing age. This was due to an increase in cardiac causes of arrest with age, while non-cardiac etiologies of arrest decreased with age. The incidence of witnessed ventricular fibrillation also decreased with age. Overall survival decreased with age. However, some of the decreased survival may have been due to other factors including comorbid diseases.[35]

In summary, the studies on the effect of age on out-of-hospital cardiac arrest show a consistent pattern. Resuscitation of older patients in cardiac arrest is not futile. Many studies show that the overall prognosis for survival is worse for patients age 80 or greater. This observation holds when other emergency medical service factors are accounted for such as bystander CPR, witnessed arrest, time to defibrillation and initial rhythm. Most studies of out-of-hospital arrest, however, do not take into account the important prognostic factors of comorbid diseases and baseline health status. Since older people generally have more comorbid diseases than younger adults, it is unknown whether it is age itself or the comorbid diseases that are responsible for the worse prognosis after age 80. It is also clear from multiple studies that the pattern of cardiac arrest in older persons is different from that in younger adults. Arrests are less frequently witnessed, more frequently of a cardiac etiology and most importantly, less frequently presenting with ventricular fibrillation as an initial rhythm.

In-hospital arrest

Bedell *et al.* studied prognostic factors that determine outcome after in-hospital CPR in 294 patients at a university hospital in Boston.[36] Overall, 14% of patients were discharged alive, with 11% of the 294 patients alive at 6 months. A multivariate analysis showed that pneumonia, hypotension, renal failure, cancer, and a home-bound lifestyle before hospitalization were associated with poor survival. None of the patients in whom the resuscitation attempts took more than 30 minutes survived to hospital discharge. Age did not appear to influence prognosis for survival after CPR or adjustment to illness after discharge from the hospital.[36]

Taffet *et al.* reviewed in-hospital CPR efforts for 77 patients 70 years or older in a Veterans Administration hospital in Houston.[37] Thirty-one percent of patients had return of spontaneous circulation, and 22% were alive after 24 hours, but none survived to hospital discharge. In contrast, 16% of younger patients suffering cardiac arrest were discharged alive. A multivariate analysis indicated that the presence of sepsis, cancer, increased age, number of medications, and absence of witnessed arrest were statistically predictive of a poor outcome.[37] In another study that took place over many years, Gordon and Cheung retrospectively reviewed cardiac arrests in a frail elderly population in a multilevel geriatric care institution.[38] Forty-one patients underwent CPR, and four long-term survivors lived for 60 days or longer. No patient with unwitnessed arrest survived for 60 days. Notably, three of the four survivors were not chronically ill.[38]

Bayer *et al.* reviewed 106 cardiac arrests in a geriatric unit: 39% were successfully resuscitated, 17% were discharged from the hospital, and 15% were alive at 3 months. These survival rates were comparable to those of younger patients. The authors thought that age had no influence on outcome and concluded that resuscitation attempts on geriatric units can benefit a significant minority of patients.[39]

Parish *et al.* assessed the records of more than 2000 patients who suffered in-hospital arrest. The overall survival to hospital discharge was 27%. Geriatric patients had a 24% survival to discharge while other adult patients had a 29% survival rate. Younger age and initial rhythm were correlated with survival. The researchers did not control for comorbid diseases.[40]

De Vos *et al.* reviewed the charts of 553 patients who received in-hospital CPR to determine risk factors for poor survival. Overall, survival to hospital discharge was 22%. Independent risk factors for non-survival were an age of 70 years or older, renal failure before admission and congestive heart failure during hospitalization. Patients with risk factors had a projected survival of less than 10%.[41]

Di Bari *et al.* did a retrospective review of 245 cardiac arrests in a geriatric unit. Overall, long-term survival was 17%. The investigators compared patients above and below 70 years of age. Independent predictors of short-term survival were the initial rhythm in arrest, acute myocardial infarction, heart failure and hypotension. Long-term survival was negatively associated with heart failure. Age was not an independent risk factor when the researchers controlled for comorbid diseases.[42]

Hajbaghery *et al.* reported on factors influencing survival after 206 patients with in-hospital cardiac arrest in Kashan, Iran. Predictors of survival to hospital discharge were CPR duration, time of cardiac arrest, time from cardiac arrest to CPR and defibrillation. Age was not an independent prognostic factor.[43]

Sandroni *et al.* evaluated factors affecting the outcome of 114 patients with in-hospital cardiac arrest over 2 years. The key factor determining survival to hospital discharge was the time to arrival of the cardiac arrest team. Age was not a factor in the survival outcome.[44]

In summary, studies on in-hospital cardiac arrest consistently demonstrate the importance of comorbid diseases and systemic factors in responding to the arrest. In some studies age was an independent factor and in others age was not a factor. It is clear that clinicians should not consider it futile to resuscitate elder patients in cardiac arrest.

Prognosis after return of spontaneous circulation

The hospital course and long-term survival in elderly and younger patients who were successfully resuscitated after out-of-hospital cardiac arrest was also investigated by Tresch *et al.*[24] The investigations were designed to determine whether elderly patients had worse neurologic outcome and utilized more hospital resources than did non-elderly patients. Although hospital deaths were more common in elderly patients resuscitated from cardiac arrest compared to non-elderly patients, the lengths of hospitalization and stay in intensive care units were not significantly different between the age groups. The number of neurologic deaths and residual neurologic impairments were similar in both age groups. Long-term survival curves demonstrated similar survival in both

patient groups after hospital discharge, with approximately 65% of hospital survivors alive at 24 months after discharge (Fig. 54.2).[24] In this important study the authors concluded that resuscitation of elderly patients who suffer out-of-hospital cardiac arrest is appropriate. Although elderly patients are more likely to die during hospitalization, the hospital stay and residual neurologic deficits are no different from those in younger patients.

Studies seem to reinforce the concept that resuscitation of the elderly in cardiac arrest will benefit a significant minority of patients. Elder patients often have more comorbid diseases, and their cardiovascular systems have less reserve. These factors may influence the etiology of the arrest; congestive heart failure and respiratory problems may be more important etiologies in elder persons who suffer cardiac arrest than they are in younger adult patients. We have a similar concept regarding the importance of respiratory compromise as an etiologic factor in children suffering cardiac arrest. Ventricular fibrillation appears to be less common as the initial rhythm, whereas pulseless electrical activity is more common. Since our treatment for the latter condition is much less satisfactory than for ventricular

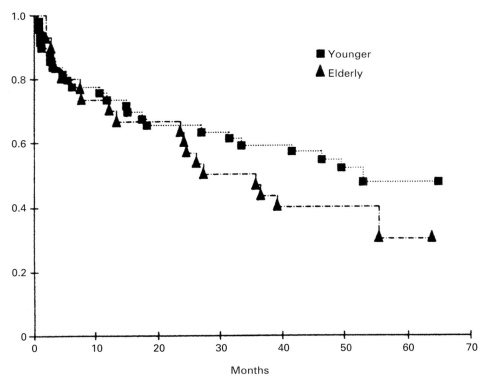

Fig. 54.2. Comparison of long-term survival curves for elderly (70 years and greater) and non-elderly patients. (From ref. 24.)

fibrillation, this may account for some of the observed differences in outcome.

It is also clear that many laypersons as well as healthcare professionals fear that by attempting to resuscitate elderly patients, they risk the possibility of resuscitating patients who are severely neurologically compromised and consume much of society's health care resources. In fact, all the data in the literature indicate that neurologic disability, neurologic deaths, and even hospital resource use are similar for elderly and younger patients following resuscitation from cardiac arrest.

Ethical issues

Ethical issues concerning resuscitation of elder persons are not unique to this population. The same concerns should be relevant to any patient suffering cardiac arrest or in a critical condition. Advance directives have become common in the USA's healthcare system and are particularly relevant where decisions concerning resuscitation must be made immediately. Advance directives convey the wishes of the patient with respect to specific treatment, including resuscitation from cardiac arrest. Written directives in the form of living wills or other recognized documents that specifically direct healthcare providers how to treat patients are particularly useful. Directives that specify "do not attempt resuscitation" (DNAR) are one form of advance directive. These can be portable and used out of the hospital as well as in healthcare institutions. Many EMS systems throughout the USA have standardized portable DNAR forms that a relative can present to the emergency healthcare personnel. Emergency healthcare professionals should respect the wishes of the patient when presented with valid advance directives not to attempt resuscitation.

In effect, advance directives allow patients to make decisions about their healthcare even if they are unconscious or incapacitated. The underlying assumption, however, is that it is the patient who makes the decision about resuscitation. A more thorough discussion of ethical issues in resuscitation can be found in Chapter 66.

Therapeutic considerations

Most studies in the medical literature have focused on the outcome of cardiac arrest in the elderly population. There are few data to modify the existing recommendations for the treatment of older patients in cardiac arrest. Recommendations regarding therapy are therefore based on consideration of the etiology of cardiac arrest. During the cardiac arrest sequence it is important to realize that ventricular fibrillation is less common in elder persons and pulseless electrical activity is more common compared to other adult cardiac arrests. Aggressive anticipation of extracardiac causes of pulseless electrical activity such as hypovolemia from a ruptured aneurysm or dehydration is especially important. Attention to hypoxia is also important, particularly since so many patients present with dyspnea and congestive heart failure.

Recognition that acute myocardial infarction in elder persons can present with atypical symptoms is probably the most important factor preventing cardiac arrest in these patients. Symptoms include dyspnea, dizziness, syncope, and weakness, as well as chest discomfort. Elder persons have a high mortality following an acute myocardial infarction. Therefore, it is most important to treat myocardial infarction in such patients aggressively. Early use of reperfusion strategies as well as other treatments that may limit infarct size is more important in the elderly than in a younger population.

Future directions

In the future it will be important for research to focus on the special etiology and therapeutic needs of the elderly in cardiac arrest. Academicians must do a better job of teaching emergency healthcare personnel about the special needs of elderly patients and the importance of aggressive management of cardiovascular diseases.

REFERENCES

1. Meldon, S.W., Ma, O.J. & Woolard, R. *Geriatric Emergency Medicine.* New York: McGraw-Hill Co., 2004.
2. Kane, R.L., Ouslander, J.G. & Abrass, I.B. *Essentials of Clinical Geriatrics,* 5th edn. New York: McGraw-Hill Co., 2004.
3. Landerfeld, C.S., Palmer, R.M., Johnson, M.A., Johnston, C.B. & Lyons, W.L. *Current Geriatric Diagnosis and Treatment.* New York: McGraw-Hill Co., 2004.
4. Wenger, N.K., ed. *Cardiovascular Disease in the Octogenarian and Beyond.* London: Martin Dunitz Ltd. 1999.
5. *Heart Disease and Stroke Statistics – 2004 Update.* Dallas: American Heart Association. 2004.
6. Evans, J.G. & Williams, T.F., eds. *Oxford Textbook of Geriatric Medicine.* Oxford, UK: Oxford University Press, 1992.
7. American Medical Association Council on Scientific Affairs. American Medical Association white paper on elderly health. *Arch. Intern. Med.* 1990; **150**: 2459–2472.

8. American Medical Association Council on Scientific Affairs. Societal effects and other factors affecting health care for the elderly. *Arch. Intern. Med.* 1990; **150**: 1184–1189.

9. Committee on Leadership for Academic Geriatric Medicine. Report of the Institute of Medicine: academic geriatrics for the year 2000. *J. Am. Geriatr. Soc.* 1987; **35**: 771–773.

10. McGaig, L.F. & Burt, C.W. National Hospital Ambulatory Medical Care Survey: 2003 emergency department summary. Advance data from vital and health statistics; no. 358. Hyattsville, Maryland: National Center for Health Statistics, 2005.

11. Strange, G.R. & Chen, E.H. Use of emergency departments by elder patients: a five-year follow-up study. *Acad. Emerg. Med.* 1998; **5**: 1157–1162.

12. Weisfeldt, M.L., ed. *The Aging Heart.* New York: Raven Press, 1980.

13. Higgenbotham, M.B., Morris, K.G., Williams, R.S., Coleman, R.E. & Cobb, F.R. Physiologic basis for age-related decline in aerobic work capacity. *Am. J. Cardiol.* 1986; **57**: 1374–1379.

14. Rodeheffer, R.J., Gerstenblith, G., Becker, L.C., Fley, J.L., Weisfeldt, M.L., Lakatta, E.G. Exercise cardiac output is maintained with advancing age in healthy human subjects: dilatation and increased stroke volume compensate for a diminished heart rate. *Circulation* 1984; **69**: 203–213.

15. Rich, M.W., Bosner, M.S., Chung, M.K., Shen, J. & McKenzie, J.P. Is age an independent predictor of early and late mortality in patients with acute myocardial infarction? *Am. J. Med.* 1992; **92**: 7–13.

16. Manolio, T.A. & Furberg, C.D. Age as a predictor of outcome: what role does it play? *Am. J. Med.* 1992; **92**: 1–6.

17. Tofler, G.H., Muller, J.E., Stone, P.H. *et al.* Factors leading to shorter survival after acute myocardial infarction in patients ages 65 to 75 years compared with younger patients. *Am. J. Cardiol.* 1988; **62**: 860–867.

18. Udvarhelyi, I.S., Gatsonis, C., Epstein, A.M., Pashos, C.L., Newhouse, J.P. & McNeil, B.J. Acute myocardial infarction in the medicare population. *J. Am. Med. Assoc.* 1992; **268**: 2530–2536.

19. Weaver, W.D., Litwin, P.E., Martin, J.S. *et al.* Effect of age on use of thrombolytic therapy and mortality in acute myocardial infarction. *J. Am. Coll. Cardiol.* 1991; **18**: 657–662.

20. Dooney, A.J., Michelson, E.L. & Topal, E.J. Thrombolytic therapy of acute myocardial infarction. *J. Am. Med. Assoc.* 1992; **268**: 3108–3114.

21. The Gusto Investigators. An international randomized trial comparing four thrombolytic strategies for acute myocardial infarction. *N. Engl. J. Med.* 1993; **329**: 673–682.

22. Bayer, A.J., Chadha, J.S., Farag, R.R. & Pathy, M.S. Changing presentations of myocardial infarction with increasing old age. *J. Am. Geriatr. Soc.* 1986; **34**: 263–266.

23. Magid, D.J., Masoudi, F.A., Vinson, R.D. *et al.* Older emergency department patients with acute myocardial infarction receive lower quality of care than younger patients. *Ann. Emerg. Med.* 2005; **46**: 14–21.

24. Tresch, D.D., Thakur, R.K., Hoffmann, R.G., Olson, D. & Brooks, H.L. Should the elderly be resuscitated following out-of-hospital cardiac arrest? *Am. J. Med.* 1989; **86**: 145–150.

25. Podrid, P.J. Resuscitation in the elderly: a blessing or a curse? *Ann. Intern. Med.* 1989; **111**: 193–195.

26. Murphy, D.J., Murray, A.M., Robinson, B.E. & Campion, E.W. Outcomes of cardiopulmonary resuscitation in the elderly. *Ann. Intern. Med.* 1989; **111**: 199–205.

27. Becker, L.B., Ostrander, M.P., Barrett, J. & Kondos, G.T. Outcome of CPR in a large metropolitan area – where are the survivors? *Ann. Emerg. Med.* 1991; **20**: 355–361.

28. Eckstein, M., Stratton, S. & Chan, L. Cardiac arrest resuscitation evaluation in Los Angeles: CARE-LA. *Ann. Emerg. Med.* 2005; **45**: 504–509.

29. Van Hoeyweghen, R.J., Bossaert, L.L., Mullie, A., *et al.* Survival after out-of-hospital cardiac arrest in elderly patients. *Ann. Emerg. Med.* 1992; **21**: 1179–1184.

30. Longstreth, W.T., Cobb, L.A., Fahrenbruch, C.E. & Copass, M.K. Does age affect outcomes of out-of-hospital cardio-pulmonary resuscitation. *J. Am. Med. Assoc.* 1990; **264**: 2109–2110.

31. Tresch, D.D., Thakur, R., Hoffman, R.G. & Brooks, H.L. Comparison of outcome of resuscitation of out-of-hospital cardiac arrest in persons younger and older than 70 years of age. *Am. J. Cardiol.* 1988; **61**: 1120–1122.

32. Tresch, D.D., Thakur, R.K., Hoffman, R.G., Aufderheide, T.P. & Brooks, H.L. Comparison of outcome of paramedic-witnessed cardiac arrest in patients younger and older than 70 years. *Am. J. Cardiol.* 1990; **65**: 453–457.

33. Herlitz, J., Eek, M., Engdahl, J., Holmberg, M. & Holmberg, S. Factors at resuscitation and outcome among patients suffering from out-of-hospital cardiac arrest in relation to age. *Resuscitation* 2003; **58**: 309–317.

34. Swor, R.A., Jackson, R.E., Tintinalli, J.E. & Pirrallo, R.G. Does advanced age matter in outcomes after out-of-hospital cardiac arrest in community-dwelling adults? *Acad. Emerg. Med.* 2000; &: 762–768.

35. Iwami, T., Hiraide, A., Nakanishi, N. *et al.* Age and sex analysis of out-of-hospital cardiac arrest in Osaka, Japan. *Resuscitation* 2003; **57**: 145–152.

36. Bedell, S.E., Delbanco, T.L., Cook, E.F. & Epstein, F.H. Survival after cardiopulmonary resuscitation in the hospital. *N. Engl. J. Med.* 1983; **309**: 569–576.

37. Taffet, G.E., Teasdale, T.A. & Luchi, R.J. In hospital cardiopulmonary resuscitation. *J. Am. Med. Assoc.* 1988; **260**: 2069–2072.

38. Gordon, M. & Cheung, M. Poor outcome of on-site CPR in a multi-level geriatric facility: three and a half years experience at the Baycrest center for geriatric care. *J. Am. Geriatr. Soc.* 1993; **41**: 163–166.

39. Bayer, A.J., Ang, B.C. & Pathy, M.S. Cardiac arrests in a geriatric unit. *Age Ageing* 1985; **14**: 271–276.

40. Parish, D.C., Dane, F.C., Montgomery, M., Wynn, L.J. & Durham, M.D. Resuscitation in the hospital: Differential relationships between age and survival across rhythms. *Crit. Care Med.* 1999; **27**: 2137–2141.

41. De Vos, R., Koster, R.W., De Haan, R.J., Oosting, H., Van der Wouw, P.A. & Lampe-Schoenmaeckers, A.J. In-hospital

cardiopulmonary resuscitation: Pre-arrest morbidity and outcome. *Arc. Intern. Med.* 1999; **159**: 845–850.

42. Di Bari, M., Chiarlone, M., Fumagalli, L. *et al.* Cardiopulmonary resuscitation of older, inhospital patients: Immediate efficacy and long-term outcome. *Crit. Care Med.* 2000; **28**: 2320–2325.

43. Hajbaghery, M.A., Mousavi, G. & Akbari, H. Factors influencing survival after in-hospital cardiopulmonary resuscitation. *Resuscitation* 2005; **66**: 317–321.

44. Sandroni, C., Ferro, G., Santangelo, S. *et al.* In-hospital cardiac arrest: Survival depends mainly on the effectiveness of the emergency response. *Resuscitation* 2004; **62**: 291–297.

55

Asphyxial cardiac arrest

Peter Safar, Norman A. Paradis[1] and Max Harry Weil[2]

[1]University of Colorado Health Sciences Center
[2]Weil Institute of Critical Care Medicine

There is no malice in this burning coal;
The breath of heaven has blown his spirit out . . .
But with my breath I can revive it, . . .

William Shakespeare

Although asphyxia literally means no pulse (in Greek), it represents an inability to breathe and therefore suffocation. Failure of gas exchange is characterized by hypoxemia and hypercarbia, as originally defined by J.B.S. Haldane.[1] A mechanistic classification of asphyxia (Table 55.1) includes a diversity of pathophysiological processes that preclude movement of gas from the upper airway to the alveoli and ultimately to the tissues, the cells, and then to the mitochondria, thereby sustaining oxidative metabolism in vital organs.

Asphyxia is a cause of sudden death,[1–3] but in contrast to primary cardiac causes, it more often presents with bradycardia and asystole rather than ventricular fibrillation (VF).[4–8] In children, normothermic cardiac arrest is predominantly due to asphyxia. Asphyxia is also the predominant mechanism of cardiac arrest in neonates[9,10] and in infants due to the so-called sudden infant death syndrome,[11,12] Status asthmaticus is an important cause of asphyxia.[13] The most frequent cause is failure of respiratory muscle function.[1–3] Outcomes are worse when VF evolves during asphyxial cardiac arrest than after primary VF in adults.[9–14]

Anoxia or *hypoxia* is defined by critical reductions in arterial oxygen saturation (SaO_2) or arterial oxygen tension (PaO_2). *Hypercarbia* is defined by increases in arterial carbon dioxide tension ($PaCO_2$) in settings of inadequate alveolar ventilation and usually in association with hypoxia.

The more recent and large focus on sudden cardiac death predominantly due to VF followed the introduction and

Table 55.1. Mechanisms of asphyxia

- Impaired alveolar ventilation of neuromuscular cause including impairment of spinal cord, peripheral nerve, in end-plate functions such as myasthenia gravis, neuromuscular blockade
- Obstruction of the airway by foreign particulates, aspiration, blood clots
- Obstruction of the upper airway by soft tissue, especially the tongue, epiglottis
- Mechanical constraints of chest expansion, tension pneumothorax, flail chest
- Tracheobronchial disruption due to trauma, tumor
- Drowning, laryngospasm
- Allergic or inflammatory disease of the airways (tracheitis, asthma, chronic obstructive pulmonary disease)
- Drug-induced apnea caused by sedatives, narcotics, anesthetic agents, neuromuscular blockade
- Generalized seizures (e.g., status epilepticus)
- Cardiogenic and permeability pulmonary edema
- Pulmonary thromboembolism
- Interstitial lung diseases
- Impaired oxygen availability, altitude, confined spaces
- Anemia, including acute hemorrhage, hemodilution
- Hemoglobinopathies, carboxy- and methemoglobinemia, cyanide intoxication
- Neonatal uteroplacental dysfunction, umbilical cord compression
- Sudden infant death syndrome

routine use of defibrillators. Historically, however, resuscitation first focused on patients who had stopped breathing. Indeed, drowning was the first to receive attention and the management of victims of drowning predominated in the

* *This chapter is an update of the late Professor Safar's Chapter in the First Edition of this textbook.*
Cardiac Arrest: The Science and Practice of Resuscitation Medicine. 2nd edn., ed. Norman Paradis, Henry Halperin, Karl Kern, Volker Wenzel, Douglas Chamberlain. Published by Cambridge University Press. © Cambridge University Press, 2007.

evolution of out-of-hospital resuscitation medicine.[1] The "humane societies" of London and Copenhagen were organized for that purpose (see Chapter 1).[1] There is usually opportunity for distinguishing between dysrhythmic cardiac arrest of primary cardiac cause and asphyxia in settings of witnessed cardiac arrest. The time course of asphyxial cardiac arrest is typically prolonged and preceded by overt signs, in contrast to dysrhythmic arrest and sudden death.[3,14–17]

Asphyxia also terminates life either at the beginning or at the end of natural life. Intrauterine asphyxiation and peripartum asphyxiation are major causes of perinatal injury and death.[9,10]

Mouth-to-mouth ventilation was described in the old testament.[18] The earliest implementation of mouth-to-mouth artificial ventilation of asphyxiated newborn infants was by midwives.[1] Before the advent of vaccines and antibiotics, diphtheria- or "croup"-induced laryngeal obstruction or bronchiolitis in the young and pneumonia in the elderly were common causes of fatal asphyxia. Today, increased immune suppression for treatment of autoimmune diseases, chemotherapy for malignancies, and prevention of transplant rejection, as well as the increasing problem of antimicrobial resistance, the incidence of infectious diseases may once again increase. Asphyxia also occurs as a complication of permeability pulmonary edema including the adult respiratory distress syndrome (ARDS). ARDS remains one of the most intractable problems in critical care medicine. Asphyxia therefore remains a major cause of fatalities over the entire age spectrum.

Unlike sudden cardiac arrest, cardiopulmonary dysfunction during asphyxiation is progressive.[19–23] Claude Beck, a famed cardiac surgeon who is credited with electrically defibrillating the heart during surgery,[4,5] observed that the asphyxiated heart became cyanotic. This contrasted with regional ischemia which he described as pink as it advanced to cell death due to myocardial infarction.

Asphyxial cardiac arrest progresses from initial tachycardia to progressive bradycardia terminating in electromechanical dissociation (EMD), now more appropriately described as pulseless rhythm. Cardiac arrest terminates in electrical asystole.[3,20] Prompt reversal of asphyxia minimizes cellular injury and irreversibility.

Complete airway obstruction is typically followed by apnea based on studies in experimental animals (Fig. 55.1).[14–17,19,21–36] Anatomical differences between animal models and patients have been cited by the late Professor Peter Safar as important. Humans and some primates have a kinked upper airway, with greater likelihood of obstruction in comatose patients.[37–43] In contrast, dogs and pigs have a relatively straight upper airway that is more likely to remain open even in the absence of tracheal intubation. Intermittent chest compression may produce adequate tidal volumes in animals without airway obstruction, but not necessarily in comatose human victims and this was ascribed by Professor Safar to differences in anatomy and therefore airway patency.[6,45,48]

Asphyxia has also been documented in patients caused by extravasation of blood during jugular vein cannulation, tracheobronchial thrombus, and esophageal polyps.[41–44]

Pathophysiology

During cardiac arrest, the heart and the brain become the most vulnerable organs.[2,3] This applies to both asphyxial and dysrhythmic cardiac arrest. Current techniques of cardiopulmonary-cerebral resuscitation (CPCR) for reestablishment of spontaneous circulation differ contingent on either asphyxial or dysrhythmic cause. In both instances, however, global brain ischemia is followed by cerebral ischemic injury. Its pathophysiology is more specifically reviewed in Chapters 5 and 13.

Haldane regarded asphyxia as a combination of hypercarbia and hypoxemia in which hypercarbia may make the machine malfunction, but it is hypoxemia that not only stops the machine but also wrecks the machinery.[1] Henderson[9] differentiated among apneic asphyxia, acarbic asphyxia as in carbon monoxide poisoning, and chronic asphyxia as in anemia. Alveolar anoxia alone, without hypercarbia, stops the heart in systole. Hypercarbia without hypoxemia produces hypercarbic acidosis and may impair cardiac function but does not stop the heart beat.[49–56]

Dysrhythmic cardiac arrest represents perfusion failure of the myocardium and therefore failure of oxygen delivery to sustain myocardial metabolism. When patients are maintained on total cardiopulmonary bypass (CPB), no ventilation is required because gas exchange is supplied by the extracorporeal circuit. This contrasts with patients who have supranormal minute ventilation but impaired alveolar ventilation characteristic of respiratory distress syndromes. Accordingly, *processes that critically reduce cellular availability and use of oxygen in the absence of circulatory failure* are appropriately defined under the umbrella of asphyxia (Fig. 55.2).

The asphyxial syndromes are categorized in Table 55.1 and Fig. 55.2. Asphyxia may interfere with energy metabolism at multiple sites between *mouth* and *mitochondria*. Airway obstruction is selectively asphyxial. Impediments to ventilation, such as tension pneumothorax, may impair

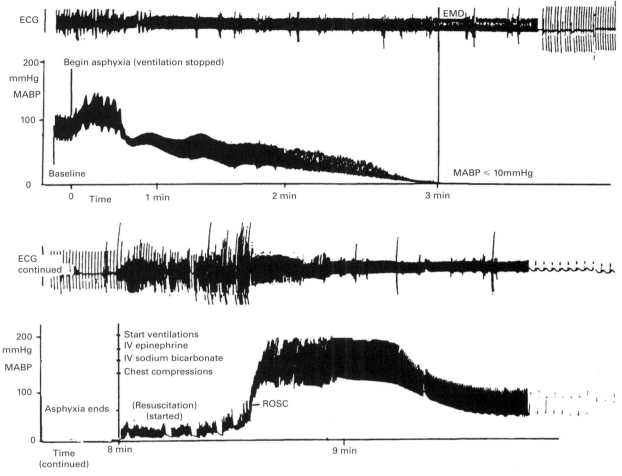

Fig. 55.1. Experimental asphyxiation to cardiac arrest and resuscitation by standard external CPR with intravenous epinephrine and NaHCO3. Electrocardiogram (ECG) and mean and cyclic arterial pressure (MABP) in lightly anesthetized rat before, during, and after apneic asphyxiation. (From Katz L, Ebmeyer U, Safar P, Radovsky A, Neumar R. Outcome model of asphyxial cardiac arrest in rats for functional and morphologic evaluation of cerebral resuscitation. *J Cereb Blood Flow Metab* 1995.

oxygen delivery and therefore organ function through a combination of asphyxial and circulatory mechanisms.

Airway obstruction may produce initial hypoventilation and terminate in apnea after consciousness is reduced.[2,38] Coma, in contradistinction to sleep, is characterized by a loss of muscle function such that the tongue and epiglottis are no longer lifted off the posterior pharyngeal wall.[38] Backward tilt of the head, and in some victims, forward displacement of the mandible lifts the tongue and epiglottis and thereby restores patency of the air passage (Fig. 55.3).[37–43] Approximately one-third of comatose patients require forward displacement of the mandible as part of the so-called triple airway maneuver (Fig. 55.4).[37,38] Intermittent or continuous positive-pressure ventilation

(IPPV, CPPV) minimizes laryngospasm.[57] Nasal obstruction is usually expiratory because of valve-like function of the soft palate.[39,40] If the larynx itself is obstructed, tracheal intubation or cricothyrotomy are life-saving (Fig. 55.5). In settings of asphyxia in a conscious patient, there is a high likelihood of full recovery if ventilation is promptly restored. After cardiac arrest, ventilation and chest compressions have a lesser likelihood of successful outcomes even if spontaneous circulation is restored. Cerebral recovery is likely to be incomplete.[32–34]

Apnea or complete airway obstruction in adult humans breathing air is followed by critical decreases in arterial O_2 saturation to less than 80% within 60 seconds.[37,58] Without alveolar ventilation, arterial PCO_2 increases by 5 to 7 mm

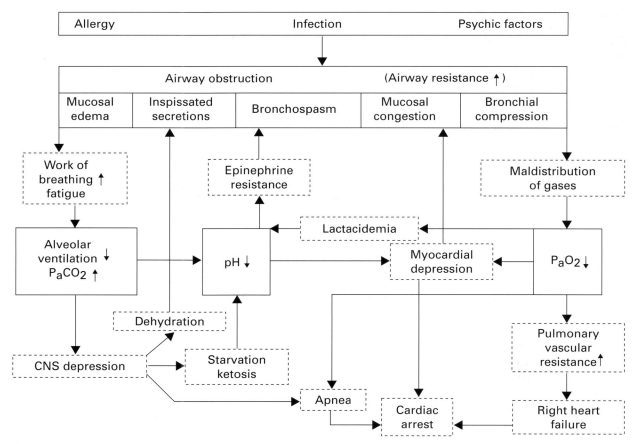

Fig. 55.2. Pathophysiology of asphyxiation in status asthmaticus. Vicious cycle and progression of asphyxiation. Hypoxemia and acidemia (respiratory plus metabolic) are the focal derangements leading to death. (From Safar P. Recognition and management of airway obstruction. *J. Am. Med. Assoc.* 1969; 208: 1008–1011.)

Hg/min. A small number of effective inflations, even with exhaled air, will rapidly normalize blood gas values.[37,58]

Sudden onset of apnea progresses at a slower rate to asphyxial cardiac arrest than does complete airway obstruction during which spontaneous breathing efforts increase oxygen demands.[59] Sudden apnea may result from traumatic or electrical injury, anesthesia, muscle relaxants, narcotics, or hypnotics, or cerebral injury with a sudden increase in intracranial pressure.

In conscious persons, upper airway obstruction provokes coughing, and this represents a spontaneous attempt to relieve obstructions. Powerful ventilatory efforts may clear the airway. Partial obstruction also provokes vigorous ventilatory efforts, which may reduce rather than increase arterial P_{CO_2}. Hypoxemia can be exacerbated by reflex-induced bronchospasm or laryngospasm.

Airway obstruction that provokes increased ventilatory efforts, including exaggerated intercostal and suprasternal retractions, provokes autonomic discharges and in turn, hypertension and tachycardia. A brief interval of hypertension is then followed by hypotension in part due to myocardial impairment. Vagotonus accounts for nodal rhythms followed by ectopic ventricular beats terminating in ventricular asystole or an agonal rhythm or electric asystole.

If the victim is breathing room air, complete airway obstruction is followed by a fall in arterial P_{O_2} of 30 mm Hg and arterial O_2 saturation to 60% or less after approximately 2 minutes. The decline is coincident with loss of consciousness. Between 3 and 10 minutes after complete airway obstruction, apnea and pulselessness supervene. When the arterial P_{O_2} is reduced to approximately 20 mm Hg, apnea begins. The arterial P_{CO_2} is over 70 mm Hg, and the arterial pH is about 6.8 to 7.0. Pulselessness occurs when the arterial P_{O_2} is approximately 10 mm Hg and the arterial pH is 6.3 to 6.8.[17] When arterial pressure decreases below 30 mm Hg, pupillary dilation occurs and progresses

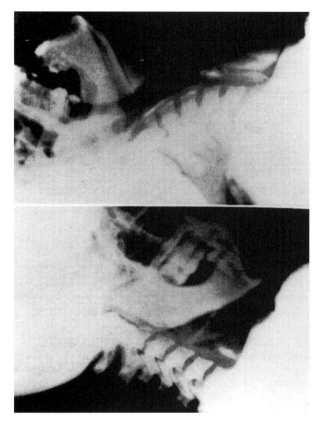

Fig. 55.3. Upper airway (hypopharyngeal) soft tissue obstruction in comatose (anesthetized) adult human. (*Top*) Backward tilt of head stretches anterior neck structures and lifts base of tongue off posterior pharyngeal wall and epiglottis of larynx entrance. (*Bottom*) With head in mid position or flexed, there is hypopharyngeal obstruction by the tongue and laryngeal obstruction by the epiglottis. (From Safar P, Escarraga LA, Chang F. Upper airway obstruction in the unconscious patient. J Appl Physiol 1959; 14: 760–764.)

to an isoelectric electroencephalogram (EEG). With systolic pressure below 25 mm Hg, PEA is apparent.[20–36] Eventually the arterial pressure tracing is almost flat, but ECG complexes may continue, possibly for 5 minutes or longer. Thus complete airway obstruction after air breathing causes clinical death (pulselessness) in 5 to 10 minutes.

After resuscitation from asphyxial cardiac arrest, the circulatory and metabolic abnormalities are similar to those of sudden cardiac arrest due to VF.[3,27,44] Asphyxial arrest is more likely than fibrillatory arrest to cause cerebral ischemic injury.[32–34]

Asphyxia disrupts homeostasis through the interruption of O_2 delivery to the mitochondria. Once the balance between O_2 supply and demand is disturbed, cellular

hypoxia occurs and pyruvate produced by anaerobic glycolysis is converted to lactate. Initial respiratory acidosis becomes combined respiratory and metabolic acidosis (Fig. 55.2). Elevated serum lactate and increases in tissue PCO_2 are among the most sensitive indicators of impaired cellular respiration. It has been suggested that elevated tissue lactate and PCO_2 may of themselves mediate brain injury during asphyxia but the evidence is not persuasive.[60–62]

Effects of hypercarbia

During apnea the increase in arterial PCO_2 is approximately 5 to 7 mm Hg/min. In healthy persons, pre-ventilation with 30% O_2 will maintain arterial PO_2 above 75 mm Hg for at least 5 minutes. Pre-ventilation with 100% O_2 and complete denitrogenation can maintain arterial PO_2 above 75 mm Hg for over 30 minutes if there is no impairment in alveolocapillary diffusion. The arterial PO_2 declines when alveolar O_2 is displaced by CO_2 followed by right-to-left shunting associated with absorption atelectasis of oxygen-filled alveoli. Hypercarbia alone rarely results in death; dogs can tolerate artificial ventilation with up to 70% CO_2 (30% O_2).[53,54] Hypotension begins when the arterial pH decreases to approximately 6.8 and cardiac arrest is likely to occur after arterial pH decreases to 6.5 units. In animals this may require as long as 30 minutes after arterial PCO_2 has risen to about 340 mm Hg provided that arterial PO_2 is maintained above 80 mm Hg. Humans can survive such severe hypercarbia provided that oxygenation is adequately provided so that return to normocarbia is gradual to avoid ventricular arrhythmias attributed to rapid potassium shifts.[50–55]

Neurologic injury and comparison of asphyxia and ventricular fibrillation

VF-induced normothermic cardiac arrest of 3 to 4 minutes' duration can be reversed with complete neurologic recovery and histologically preserved brain. After 5 minutes of VF there may be functional recovery but histological ischemic damage of neurons.[32,63] When the duration of normothermic VF is 7 minutes or longer, some neurologic deficit will be apparent together with permanent histologic brain damage.[44,63,64]

When asphyxiation was reversed just prior to onset of cardiac arrest, complete recovery followed without histologic brain damage. After onset of pulselessness, however, permanent neurologic deficit, with histologic brain damage is observed.[32–34] Neurologic deficit is

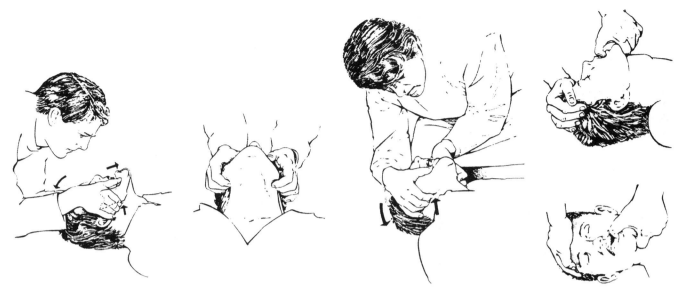

Fig. 55.4. Emergency airway control. Triple airway maneuver (backward tilt of head, lips and teeth separated, forward displacement of mandible [jaw thrust]). A. With operator at patient's vertex, for spontaneously breathing patient. B. With operator at side of patient, for direct mouth-to-mouth ventilation. Seal nose with cheek for mouth-to-mouth breathing. Seal mouth with other cheek for mouth-to-nose breathing. C. Modified triple airway maneuver by thumb–jaw lift method (for relaxed patient only). (From Safar P, Bircher NG, Cardiopulmonary cerebral resuscitation. 3rd ed. World Federation of Societies of Anaesthesiologists. London: Saunders, 1988.)

particularly likely in patients in whom pre-existing illness caused tissue hypoxia prior to asphyxiation.

After asphyxial arrest and resuscitation, ischemic neuronal changes "mature" over 3 days or longer; and injury appears more severe and widespread than after VF of the same duration of circulatory arrest.[32–34] After both insults, injured neurons appear shrunken, with eosinophilic cytoplasm and pyknotic nuclei. Selectively vulnerable are the hippocampus, cerebellum, and neocortex. After asphyxia, however, there are also scattered microinfarcts.[32–34] The severity of injury after asphyxial cardiac arrest is increased when hypotension precedes pulselessness.

In summary, asphyxial cardiac arrest appears more injurious to the brain and less injurious to the heart than does VF cardiac arrest of similar duration. Brain recovery also appears less likely after asphyxial arrest than it does after exsanguination cardiac arrest of equal duration.[65]

Therapeutic considerations

If alveolar ventilation with air or O_2 is restored prior to impairment of blood flow manifested by arterial hypotension, resuscitation is usually prompt and complete. When asphyxiation progresses to profound hypotension or pulselessness, basic life support (BLS) measures *may* still restore spontaneous circulation, but both ventilation and chest compression are needed. After just a brief interval of true cardiac arrest, ROSC may be possible after up to 20 minutes of pulselessness.[16] The brain, however, may not fully recover after as little as 2 minutes of asphyxiation-induced pulselessness.[32–34]

Asphyxial cardiac arrest is the final common pathway for a diverse group of disease processes, and its complete reversal usually requires correction of the underlying disorder. The most important initial interventions are airway control, ventilation, and oxygenation (Table 55.2). The triple airway maneuver, i.e., backward tilt of the head plus forward displacement of the mandible and separation of lips requires no devices (Fig. 55.4). This is often all that is needed to prevent progression of asphyxiation to cardiac arrest. Tracheal intubation or alternate and now less invasive devices are utilized to secure the airway for the longer term. Under immediate life threat, puncture of the cricothyroid membrane may be required (Fig. 55.5).

Asphyxia progressing to pulselessness is often encountered in prehospital settings of cardiac arrest and accounts for PEA and/or asystole.[7] The pathophysiology of asphyxia is fundamentally different from sudden death due to VF. Cardiac arrest is not sudden. Signs of asphyxiation provide opportunities for intervention before the onset of pulselessness. Therapeutic intervention must be rapid, optimally before onset of hypotension.

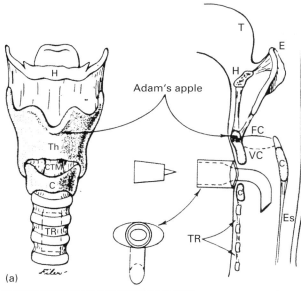

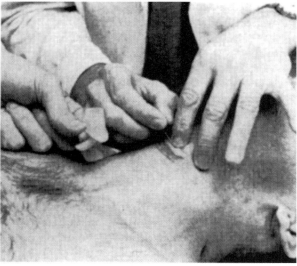

Fig. 55.5. (a). Cricothyroid membrane puncture (cricothyrotomy). Anatomy with cannula in place. *H*, Hyoid bone; *Th*, thyroid cartilage; *C*, cricoid cartilage; *TR*, trachea; *CTM*, cricothyroid membrane; *E*, epiglottis; *T*, tongue; *FC*, false cord; *VC*, vocal chord; *Es*, esophagus. Bevelled, curved cannula with knife blade (with handle rubber stopper, to be carried safely within 15-mm slip joint of cannula) (6-mm diameter cannula for adults, 3-mm diameter for large children). **(b).** Technique of cricothyrotomy via small horizontal skin incision. (From Safar P, Penninckx J. Cricothyroid membrane puncture with special cannula. *Anesthesiology* 1967; 28: 943–948.)

The most common ECG rhythm during asphyxial cardiac arrest is PEA. Defibrillation is indicated only if VF is identified and often follows precordial compression.

The transition from spontaneous circulation to asphyxial cardiac arrest is not easily detected. There are no specific measurements such as blood pressure that would mandate chest compression or alternative circulatory support. Such is also likely to be contingent on the etiology. All patients would best be under the close observation of appropriately skilled clinicians until they are stable and fully awake.

Patients with a potentially reversible etiology of asphyxial arrest who fail to respond to standard BLS-ALS maneuvers may be candidates for open-chest CPR, especially in settings of tension pneumothorax, pericardial tamponade, and other intrathoracic crises.[66,67] Institutions that provide extracorporeal circulation and who have a team prepared to secure the protocol prospectively may utilize extracorporeal circulation.[68]

Airway obstruction

Upper airway soft tissue obstruction during coma of any cause or during general anesthesia is the most common cause of asphyxiation in humans (Fig. 55.3).[2] In an unconscious patient when the head is in the mid or flexed position, the relaxed tongue and epiglottis impinge on the posterior pharyngeal wall and larynx. Such obstruction occurs in diverse body positions: supine, lateral, or prone.[38]

This cause of asphyxia is not only most common but also most easily managed. Simply tilting the head backward or thrusting the jaw forward re-establishes patency of the airway (Fig. 55.3).[37–43] Professor Safar estimated that in 20 to 30% of instances, both techniques are required.[39,40] Airway adjuncts may maintain airway patency (Table 55.2).[2] *Foreign body aspiration* is the second most common cause of life-threatening airway obstruction.

Mouth-to-mouth or mouth-to-nose for BLS advances to mouth-to-adjunct breathing, with or without O_2 and the bag-mask (tube) ventilation with or without O_2.

Airway obstruction may be due to vomitus, blood, or a foreign body or mass lodged in the pharynx or larynx. Obstruction may occur at any level between mouth or nose and bronchioles. In the classic syndrome of sudden solid foreign body obstruction, described as a cafe coronary, food is the obstructing foreign body.[69–75] Altered mental state and especially intoxication by alcohol or drugs and poor dentition are major risk factors. Aspiration, especially in the elderly,[76] may block the airway by direct mechanical obstruction or by triggering laryngospasm and bronchospasm. Laryngospasm reverses after cerebral hypoxia supervenes. Obstruction

Table 55.2. Resuscitation from asphyxial cardiac arrest

1. Establish unresponsiveness
   Activate EMS system
2. Airway control
   (a) Backward tilt of head[a]
   (b) Pharyngeal suctioning
   (c) Supine aligned position[a]
   (d) Pharyngeal airway
   (e) Heimlich maneuver or back   Bronchoscopy
       blows – manual thrusts   Bronchodilation
                                         Pleural drainage
   (f) Side (recovery) position[a]
   (g) Laryngeal mask or esophageal
       obturator airway
3. Lung inflation attempts[a]
4. Triple airway maneuver
   (jaw-thrust, open mouth)[a]
5. Endotracheal intubation
   tracheobronchial suctioning
6. Manual clearing of mouth and throat[a]
7. Cricothyrotomy translaryngeal O_2
   jet insufflation – tracheotomy

[a]Life-supporting first aid.

may also accompany inflammatory, infectious, or neo-plastic diseases.

Complete obstruction of the airway by a "swallowed" foreign body is most commonly due to impaction of the foreign body in the hypopharynx, in the entrance to the larynx, or at the level of the cricoid cartilage.[69] Sudden inability to talk, labored respiratory efforts, and progressive cyanosis constitute the classic signs of foreign body obstruction. The patient may clutch his or her neck. The presence of a high pitched upper airway sound and the capability to vocalize or cough indicate incomplete obstruction. When the obstruction is incomplete and the patient is conscious, the patient should be encouraged to expel the foreign body by himself. Supplementing inspired oxygen is beneficial. Once complete obstruction progresses to unconsciousness, there is impending asphyxial cardiac arrest.

The use of subdiaphragmatic (abdominal) thrusts[70,71] is the primary intervention for relieving the airway obstruction in persons above the age of 1 year and back blows for infants below 1 year. Infants and small children should be placed prone, with the head lowered on the rescuer's hand or knee. Alternatively, back blows may be used in lieu of abdominal thrusts in all age groups. If abdominal thrusts produce only a weak cough-like effect,[73] the chest thrust may be effective and is safer[77] and this is the maneuver

of choice for pregnant women. Abdominal thrusts as described by Heimlich are not without controversy.[2,8,70,72]

Thrusts should best be synchronized with the patient's intrinsic attempts to expel the foreign body. If the victim is conscious, rescuers should be alert to minimize injury to the victim during struggling. Physical attempts to remove the impacted foreign body may result in greater impaction or a human bite to the hand of the rescuer.

Once the patient is unconscious, mouth-to-mouth inflations, digital scooping of the hypopharynx, abdominal or chest thrusts, and back blows are administered and continued until the airway is cleared.[2] When complete obstruction is not relieved, *early* decision to perform cricothyroidotomy is life-saving (Fig. 55.5).

Professional ALS rescuers should be prepared to use airway equipment before unconsciousness occurs. Use of the bag-valve-mask with 100% oxygen is the first option. If the obstruction is complete, the hypopharynx should be visualized with a laryngoscope and attempts made to remove the foreign body with forceps. Blind attempts to remove a foreign body are not advised for they may force the obstructing material to be pushed further in the more distal airway. Endotracheal intubation may be life-saving, yet the risk of advancing the foreign body to the cricothyroid level has grave consequences.

If there is failure to remove the foreign body promptly, cricothyrotomy should not be delayed. One operator should support the triple airway maneuver (Fig. 55.4), with the other person performing cricothyrotomy (Fig. 55.5). Puncture of the trachea or cricothyroid membrane with a catheter needle with insufflation of oxygen distally is another life-saving option.[78–81] Relatively small amounts of oxygen are needed to prevent progression to cardiac arrest. After complete obstruction, care must be taken to prevent overdistending the lungs and causing air trapping. Pressurizing the airway distal to the obstruction in the upper airway may move the foreign body upward, making it easier to remove. If cardiac arrest occurs before patency is established, chest compressions are likely to be futile.

A unique form of sudden and total airway obstruction is hanging,[82–84] but this is not addressed in this chapter.

Stupor and coma

Spontaneous ventilation requires an intact neuraxis and, as stated above, CNS impairment is the most common cause of asphyxial cardiac arrest. Critical loss of innervation between the respiratory center and respiratory muscle fibers impairs ventilation specifically from anesthesia and other drug-induced coma; neurologic diseases, including poliomyelitis or polyneuritis (Guillain–Barré syndrome); head trauma and other causes of increased intracranial pressure; focal cerebral ischemia; intracranial hemorrhage; and seizures.

Metabolic or toxic causes also impair ventilation. Trauma may impair the respiratory center or disrupt transmission through the spinal cord. Polyneuritis can interfere with peripheral transmission of action potentials. The poliomyelitis virus infects and impairs anterior horn motor neurons. Botulism and neuromuscular blocking agents prevent transmission at the neuromuscular end-plates.

A patient who is not fully alert is at risk of asphyxia. Pulse oximetry is likely to forewarn the clinician of progression to asphyxia. Patients presenting with new onset of coma should be routinely intubated and usually provided with supplemental oxygen. Apneic or hypoventilating patients should be mechanically ventilated. Initiation of these measures, including pulse oximetry and optimally, capnometry, should precede evaluation of the underlying etiology prior to cardiac arrest. Measurement of expired CO_2 ($P_{ET}CO_2$) is less reliable to guide interventions during asphyxial cardiac arrest.[85]

Head trauma as the etiology of CNS dysfunction will usually be obvious on presentation. Intoxication by sedatives, narcotics, alcohol, or cocaine have characteristic presentations and are among the most treatable etiologies of asphyxia and these are addressed in Chapter 58. It is important to identify the underlying cause for purposes of specific interventions; nonetheless, BLS-ALS takes precedence. After spontaneous circulation has been restored, attention should then be directed to the underlying cause.

Traumatic brain injury, blunt or penetrating, may cause so-called impact apnea lasting seconds to minutes.[86,87] Immediate ventilation is indicated to prevent hypoxemia with hypercarbia, most especially if the situation is complicated by seizures. Seizures exacerbate ischemic brain injury and BLS may be life-saving. If both apnea and trismus complicate management, mouth-to-nose breathing is indicated. After initial stabilization, care must be taken to avoid secondary failure of spontaneous ventilation due to intracranial hypertension. Comprehensive ICU monitoring of cardiorespiratory function and repetitive neurologic examinations alert the clinician to early intervention.[88,89]

Acute focal brain ischemia follows cerebrovascular accidents, including intracranial hemorrhage and this may be difficult to distinguish from brain ischemia due to transient apnea resulting from airway obstruction.[90] Even if the patient is initially conscious, secondary brain swelling may impair ventilation, especially if there is progression to brain stem herniation. Measures to counter increases in

intracranial pressure and to improve cerebrocortical oxygen delivery are advised.

Generalized convulsions can cause asphyxia from loss of pharyngeal muscle tone, with secondary airway obstruction. The extraordinary increases in metabolic rate and therefore oxygen demands may contribute to the neurologic deterioration that occurs if epilepsy is poorly controlled. Neurologic injury is traced to both hypoxemia during convulsions, and to metabolic failure.

Management of repetitive or prolonged generalized convulsions, so-called status epilepticus, is an indication for mechanical ventilation with oxygen. A muscle relaxant may facilitate external ventilation. A CNS depressant, such as diazepam, or a rapidly acting barbiturate is administered to control the seizures. Seizures themselves lead to death from cardiac causes. Temporal lobe seizures, for example, may cause ventricular arrhythmias and VF by mechanisms that are not fully understood. Electroconvulsive therapy may produce asphyxia due to airway obstruction, apnea, post-ictal coma, or from anesthetics and relaxants administered in conjunction with such treatments. Appropriate airway management and monitoring, including pulse oximetry, has made asphyxia a rare complication of electroconvulsive therapy.

Lightning stroke[91,92] can cause prolonged apnea and cardiac standstill. The heartbeat may return over minutes. Apnea may account for asphyxial cardiac arrest. Household currents may cause cardiac arrest by producing VF.

Traumatic asphyxia

Crushing injury of the thorax is a distinct cause of asphyxia.[93–102] It can occur during stampedes when large crowds panic and attempt to leave a confined area through a restricted exit. Traumatic crush may then be a mass casualty event. Extrication may be delayed and therefore delay restoration of ventilation. If cardiac arrest precedes extrication, it precludes a good outcome. After national disasters such as earthquakes or in military settings, victims may have parts of their body trapped and crushed, and such patients may become unconscious, apneic, and pulseless after release and extrication. This "acute crush release death" of accidental cause following reperfusion must be differentiated from the late postcrush catabolic syndrome caused by myoglobinemia and renal failure.

Sustained thoracic crush injury (squeeze) may result in a distinct syndrome characterized by cephalad cyanosis and edema and facial and conjunctival petechiae.[96–98] Pressure may be transmitted through the venous system into the cranium, increasing intracranial pressure and exacerbating neurologic injury.[99–101] Abdominal structures appear to be relatively protected.[98] After crush injuries, it is likely that if victims do not lose spontaneous circulation and are promptly resuscitated, the outcome is favorable.[95,102] The prognosis worsens considerably after prolonged crushing, when patients progress to hypotension and cardiac arrest. If spontaneous circulation is restored, neurologic impairment is common.

In these settings, there is indication for securing the airway. Cephalad edema may make orotracheal intubation difficult. If shock, and especially cardiac arrest, supervene, a surgical airway is indicated. Crush squeeze injury such as to cause traumatic asphyxia should be distinguished from pulmonary compromise due to multiple rib fractures, flail chest, and pulmonary contusion. These require controlled ventilation.[103–105]

Drowning

Submersion produces asphyxia, usually with water in the lungs.[106–110] Hypoxemia and hypercarbia from submersion without loss of pulse represent "near-drowning." After resuscitation, lung damage usually remains. Progression to cardiac arrest is defined as drowning. If ROSC is achieved, brain damage may be the principal deficit. This subject is specifically addressed in Chapter 61.

Sudden death after submersion is attributed to asphyxia caused by impaired alveolo-capillary exchange of oxygen. Struggling, swallowing, and laryngospasm precede asphyxia,[15] followed by hypoxia-associated relaxation and flooding of the tracheobronchial tree. Alveoli remain damaged after aspiration of either sea water[111] or fresh water.[112] Hypertonic sea water draws fluid from the vascular compartment into the alveoli and causes pulmonary edema. Hypotonic fresh water is less damaging but causes atelectasis after pulmonary surfactant is inactivated. In both instances, asphyxia is potentially reversible with restoration of improved pulmonary gas exchange.[110] Pulmonary damage is typically transient with modern methods of assisted or controlled ventilation.[110] Electrolyte abnormalities are less important than earlier suspected.[110,113,114] Water should be allowed to drain passively from the airways during CPR with the victim horizontal or head slightly lowered; abdominal thrusts[70] are not of proven benefit.[115]

The limiting factor to recovery after *drowning* is postischemic-anoxic encephalopathy. This is contingent on immersion (arrest) time and water temperature. After normothermic drowning, cerebral recovery has been poor, particularly in children.[109,116,117] It comes as no surprise that even brief normothermic pulselessness is predictive of brain damage.[32–34] In cold water drowning, however, cerebral hypothermia is protective and circulatory arrest is delayed.[118] That explains why after 45 or even 60 minutes of ice water submersion, complete recovery has been observed following successful CPR and slow rewarming.[117,119] After cold water drowning, standard external CPR after 45 minutes of submersion[119] and in dogs after 1 hour[120] or even 2 hours of cardiac arrest[121] have allowed restoration of spontaneous circulation and neurological recovery.

Pulmonary failure

Critically ill or injured patients develop hypoxemia in consequence of acute or chronic ventilation-perfusion mismatching, including right-to-left shunting of unoxygenated blood through non-ventilated alveoli.[122] Atelectasis from airway obstruction or failure of surfactant, alveolar edema, and pneumonic exudate are primary causes of such shunts. Etiologies include congenital, infectious, neoplastic, traumatic, toxic, immunologic, and thromboembolic causes. In neonates and children, congenital etiologies are particularly common. As antibiotic resistance and immunologic incompetence have become more prevalent, the incidence of sepsis is increasing together with pulmonary infiltrates characteristic of ARDS.[123–125]

Acute pulmonary insufficiency stimulates hyperventilation, largely driven by peripheral chemoreceptors and by mechanical stimulation of pulmonary stretch receptors. As little as 20% of the total lung tissue suffices to keep arterial PCO_2 within normal limits during spontaneous or artificial hyperventilation. Nevertheless, there is progressive hypoxemia.[126] The clinical features are therefore predominantly those of hypoxemia with varying degrees of hypercarbia. Superimposed lactic acidosis represents circulatory failure. Sudden death from asphyxia of primary pulmonary etiology is traced to acute cardiogenic pulmonary edema, aspiration, near-drowning, inhalation of toxic fumes, and rare cases of fulminating hemorrhagic pneumonitis, including viral causes. The key is to prevent critical decreases in arterial oxygen saturation.[127]

Pulmonary failure alone, without reduced blood flow, causes brain damage or cardiac arrest only when arterial PO_2 falls to <25 mm Hg or less. Severe hypoxemia, however, usually compromises cardiac output and peripheral circulation. When combined with acute circulatory failure and shock, even moderate hypoxemia may damage the brain. In the absence of circulatory failure, hypoxemia is associated with stupor and coma only when the arterial

PO_2 has decreased to <30 mm Hg. In patients with a low-flow state, however, unconsciousness may occur when arterial PO_2 declines to between 40 and 60 mm Hg. The brain suffers irreversible damage only when cerebral blood flow is reduced to <20% of normal in the presence of normal levels of oxygen. The mixed cerebral venous PO_2 values are then 20 mm Hg or less.[128]

Clinicians should consider any patient with pulmonary failure at risk of asphyxia and cardiac arrest. Progression to asphyxia can often be prevented with respiratory management if decompensation is recognized early. Patients with rapidly progressing, potentially reversible pulmonary consolidation, as in fulminant pneumonia, would best have arterial PO_2 maintained above 60 mm Hg. If standard ventilatory techniques cannot maintain adequate oxygenation, extracorporeal circulation (ECMO) has been of value for pediatric patients, especially if instituted early, but ultimate benefit has not been proven for adults.[129,130]

Acute exacerbations of chronic obstructive pulmonary disease (COPD) may progress to asphyxia.[122] Oxygen should not be withheld in these settings. Spontaneous hypoventilation in patients with so-called oxygen-dependent ventilatory drive usually occurs only after an acute event. In patients with longstanding hypercarbia, the brain bicarbonate is greatly increased. Rapid reduction of arterial PCO_2 per se is a cause of coma and convulsions[131] presumably due to cerebral alkalosis and consequent cerebral vasospasm,[132] CO_2 but no bicarbonate crosses the blood–brain barrier rapidly.

Acute asthma

Bronchial asthma, chronic bronchitis, and emphysema represent the triad of clinical COPDs.[122] Asthma affects approximately 5% of the United States population. Its prevalence, morbidity, and mortality have been increasing for unclear reasons.[133,134] In 1990 it was estimated that 1.8 million persons with asthma visited emergency departments for treatment of acute exacerbations of their disease. The general management of asthma is outside the scope of this chapter except for acute and severe episodes representing the so-called "asthmatic crises" and asphyxial cardiac arrest.

Pathophysiology

Asthma is an inflammatory condition. The "hyperreactive lungs" of chronic asthma remain poorly understood, although recent focus on immune derangements promises better insight into mechanisms and improved prevention. The disease is chronic, with episodic exacerbations of bronchial obstruction by thick mucus, bronchial spasm, mucosal edema, and mucosal congestion secondary to variable combinations of allergic, environmental, emotional, and infectious factors.[122] During acute exacerbation, diffuse obstruction of small airways is complicated by dehydration, mucous plugging, exhaustion, arrhythmias, and resistance to sympathomimetic bronchodilators. The morphologic changes seen in patients who died in status asthmaticus include widespread mucous plugging of bronchi and bronchioles, abundance and hypertrophy of goblet cells, infiltration and bronchial exudates with eosinophilic leukocytes, thickening of bronchial musculature, and sometimes interstitial fibrosis.

Clinical presentation

The majority of asthma-related deaths occur outside the hospital and the terminal event is not always understood. A study of near-fatal exacerbations, however, has established that asphyxia, rather than cardiac arrhythmias, is the fatal complication. Therefore undertreatment rather than overtreatment is implicated in most near-fatal or fatal exacerbations.[135–139]

Fatal events have onsets with little warning, and advance to asphyxiation over less than 1 hour. Patients should be prepared to treat themselves first and then only with the help of bystanders. Patients at risk for asthma-related sudden death usually have had a history of multiple emergency department visits, intermittent hospitalizations, and even prior intubations and may have recently withdrawn from corticosteroid therapy, changed locales, or had psychological trauma. Appropriate maintenance therapy with inhaled corticosteroids has allowed more patients to remain crisis-free. This includes especially patients previously treated with oral theophylline or with systemic corticosteroid therapy administered orally. It has allowed lesser use of inhaled β-adrenergic agonists and therefore fewer adverse cardiovascular effects.[139,140]

Patients may have a reduced chemosensitivity to hypoxia and blunted perception of the onset of dyspnea.[141] In cases of sudden onset of fatal asthma, pathologic examination sometimes showed more neutrophils than eosinophils in the airway submucosa,[137,139,141,142] suggesting that a mechanism in addition to allergy, including infection or inflammation, was responsible. Patients with a history of sudden asthmatic crises would best be advised to wear an alert bracelet, and to carry a written treatment plan and injectable epinephrine.[137]

At the onset of an asthmatic crisis, patients are likely to be sitting upright, manifest respiratory distress, and be unable to speak except for a few and often unintelligible words. Tachycardia, pulsus paradoxus, diaphoresis, and overt breathing with accessory muscles will be apparent. The absence of these signs, however, does not rule out the existence of major airflow limitations. In less severely distressed patients, the severity of asthma is best quantified with measurements of forced expiratory volume in 1 second, and/or by the maximal expiratory flow rate (MEFR).

Hypoxemia typically precedes hypercarbia. Patients are likely to be resistant to catecholamine. Progressive dyspnea with diffuse wheezing over the lung fields is followed by altered mental status. Aggressive treatment should be instituted before hypercarbia progresses. Mortality is increased if tension pneumothorax or ventricular arrhythmias supervene.[133]

Management of acute severe asthmatic crisis

Prompt intubation and mechanical ventilation should be instituted. In the still conscious patient, a severe, life-threatening broncho-constriction will be identified if the MEFR declines to 25% or less of the predicted value.

Pharmacologic management[142–152]

Oxygen

Maximal inspired O_2 concentrations are recommended to achieve a PaO_2 of 90 mm Hg or greater. High-flow oxygen by mask with high humidity precedes rapid sequence endotracheal intubation.

β-Agonists

(a) Nebulization of a β-adrenergic agonist, preferably with selective β_2 actions, such as albuterol, for inhalation, is a mainstay of initial therapy. Escalating doses of albuterol are advised with 5.0 mg/70-kg increments at 15- to 20-minute intervals or continuous inhalation in amounts of 15 mg/hour[144,145] with an upper limit of 30 mg/hour. Larger doses can exacerbate tachycardia and may provoke VT and VF.[146] Achieving adequate oxygenation takes precedence. Intravenous administration of a β_2-agonist may not be more effective or less adverse than inhaled drugs with respect to their cardiotoxic actions.[147,148]

(b) Isoproterenol by titrated intravenous infusion has been used, beginning with 0.1 μg/kg/minute and increasing doses up to a maximum of 6.0 μg/kg/minute until arterial PCO_2 is reduced to 50 mm Hg or less. This intervention poses the risk of greater tachycardia and potentially fatal ventricular arrhythmias, however.[147]

(c) The "final" rescue drug is epinephrine by intravenous infusion or injection, but not without risk. Experimentally, epinephrine may increase mortality.[149] The adult intravenous infusion dose is 2 to 10 ml of 1:10 000 administered over an interval of 5 minutes, which may be repeated contingent on response. A continuous infusion of 1 to 20 μg/minute may produce bronchodilation but careful monitoring of the electrocardiogram and blood pressure is important.

Corticosteroids

Corticosteroids reduce the inflammatory mechanisms that accompany acute asthma. Corticosteroid drugs are administered intravenously and may be combined with adrenergic agonists and with increases in inspired oxygen. Methylprednisolone, 2 mg/kg/6 hour, or hydrocortisone, 10 mg/kg/6 hour, are alternatives.

Aminophylline

The use of intravenous aminophylline is no longer routine. Although it may enhance bronchodilation, its adverse effects are significant, including hypotension and cardiac arrhythmias.

Buffer agents

The routine use of buffer agents to reverse acidemia is controversial.[150] Accordingly, normalization of arterial pH with intravenous $NaHCo_3$[151] is of potential but unproven value as an addition to bronchodilation treatment, presumably due to restoring the bronchodilator effects of adrenergic amines. Tris buffer (THAM)[152] has been proposed as a more rational choice, because it is not a CO_2 donor like $NaHCo_3$, but it is also not of proven benefit.

Anticholinergic therapy

This is another option. Nebulized ipratropium bromide may be administered in doses of 0.5 mg/70 kg, and mixed with β-agonist.[150,151]

Magnesium sulfate

Magnesium sulfate has been administered intravenously, but without clear proof of effectiveness, in doses of 2 to 3 g/70 kg, at a rate of 1 g/minute, in conjunction with aggressive β-agonist therapy.[153–155] Excess doses result in hypotension.

Intravenous hydration

This is a priority. Patients are typically dehydrated because of insensible fluid losses. Bronchial mucus is inspissated.

Mechanical ventilation

Mechanical ventilation with 100% oxygen and appropriate prolongation of expiration with the option of pressure and flow assist ventilation is a mainstay of management of potentially fatal bronchoconstriction.[156–158]

Intratracheal artificial ventilation in status asthmaticus

Stupor, coma, and apnea are absolute indications for immediate start of artificial ventilation. Awake intubation after topical anesthesia and intravenous sedation, is preceded by oxygenation by mask. The patient is best managed under light anesthesia and short acting neuromuscular blockade, preferably by an experienced anesthesiologist.[156,157] The almost inevitable "auto-PEEP" is indicative of air trapping and is best managed by maintaining PEEP levels during ventilation that compensate. Typically, there is major benefit when ventilation is adjusted to prolong exhalation, i.e., expiratory retard. Clinical examination, and, specifically lung auscultation, guides adjustments that minimize wheezes, but maintain gas exchange. Complete plugging of bronchi with mucus, however, may account for the absence of wheezes, requiring confirmation that reduced wheezes are accompanied by better gas exchange. Once the patient is intubated and mechanically ventilated, elective hypoventilation may be the only option with which to maintain oxygenation and acceptable inspiratory airway pressure.[158] This results in *permissive hypercarbia*. Although this may lead to relatively high arterial Pco_2 values, there is evidence that it may decrease mortality, but the objective data are not secure, especially in children.[159] Initial ventilator settings may be as follows: FIO_2, 100%; low tidal volumes of 5 to 10 ml/kg, ventilation rate of 10/minute or less to minimize air trapping, PEEP exceeding the measured auto-PEEP, initial inspiratory:expiratory ratio between 1:2 and 1:3, minimize exchange peak inspiratory pressure, and barotraumas. At the time of this writing, the use of high frequency oscillatory ventilation is an option, but without proof of improved survival, including that of newborns.[160]

Volatile anesthetic agents such as halothane, isoflurane, and enflurane, which relax bronchial smooth muscle, have been employed during status asthmaticus unresponsive to initial treatment.[161–164] Nonetheless, technical restraints in delivering these agents in emergency settings to partially "closed" lungs are recognized. The vasodilators and myocardial depressant effects of fluorocarbon anesthetics may be adverse.

Intravenous *ketamine*, in titrated doses, has proven useful for sedation or anesthesia without adverse effects on circulation and with some evidence that it has bron-

chodilation actions.[165–167] It may also have a cerebral protective effect.

During mechanical ventilation when intrathoracic pressure is increased, alveolar distension may lead to deterioration of cardiovascular function and increased risk of barotrauma, including pneumothorax. "Lung massage" has been used for 10 minutes in children with severe asthma undergoing mechanical ventilation. Peak airway pressures decreased and arterial PCO_2 and pH improved. Chest message is applied just after the end of inflation. One operator applies a sustained, firm, bilateral squeeze to the lower chest wall, until the start of the next inflation. There is as yet no proof of survival benefit, however, and it must be regarded as experimental.[168]

If cardiac arrest occurs, the prognosis is very poor. Bilateral tube thoracostomy should be performed simultaneously with other resuscitative measures (Fig. 55.6), because unrecognized *pneumothorax* may contribute to the deterioration.[169] There is no time for confirmation with chest radiography prior to placement of the chest tube. External CPR may be performed after chest tubes are in place. Femorofemoral CPB has been used anecdotally for emergency resuscitation of patients in status asthmaticus, but there is no persuasive proof of better outcomes.

Preload, representing the venous return, may be reduced by the high intrathoracic pressures. Peripherally administered medications may therefore fail to reach the central circulation. Early use of intravascular catheters to monitor blood pressure may aid in differentiating true cardiac arrest from profound hypotension associated with decreased preload.

Pulmonary edema

Pulmonary edema progressing to asphyxia is an extreme form of pulmonary failure. Alveolar spaces are flooded with fluid.[122,170–175] Under normal physiologic conditions, a dynamic equilibrium was described by Starling in his law of capillary–interstitial fluid exchange.[172] The net fluid movement is a function of membrane integrity; capillary, interstitial, and alveolar pressures; plasma and interstitial oncotic pressures; and lymphatic drainage. The net forces change as blood moves through the capillary, and at the venular end of the capillaries, fluid transudes back into the vascular space. Remaining fluid is normally removed via the pulmonary lymphatics.[174]

If the normal forces of fluid movement become deranged by disease, fluid may accumulate in interstitial and alveolar spaces. When interstitial fluid exceeds the capacity of the lymphatic system, it spills into the alveoli, resulting in

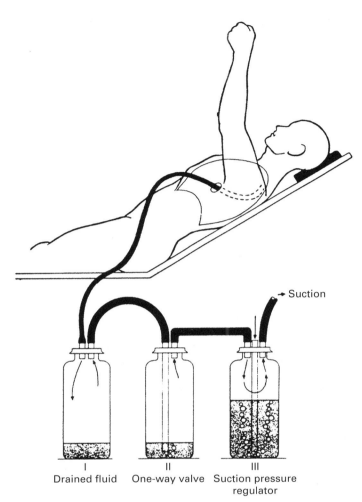

I
Drained fluid

II
One-way valve

III
Suction pressure
regulator

Fig. 55.6. Technique of pleural drainage. The appropriate size chest tube is inserted through a stab incision in the skin and into the pleural cavity, with the open technique (blunt Kelly clamp pierced through the intercostal space and prised open for tube insertion) or the closed technique (using a trocar). The latter technique requires greater skill to avoid complications. One lateral-to-posterior chest tube, with multiple holes, is usually sufficient. The tube is connected to the bottle system consisting of bottle 1 for collection of fluids; bottle 2, a one-way valve; and bottle 3 to keep a constant controllable negative pressure. For transportation a one-way valve instead of the three-bottle system is used. In hospitals the three-bottle system may be replaced by a chest suction device (e.g., Pleurevac) provided it permits control of negative pressure and high flow rate. (From Safar P, Bircher N. Cardiopulmonary cerebral resuscitation. 3rd ed. World Federation of Societies of Anaesthesiologists. London, WB Saunders, 1988.)

pulmonary edema.[175] Alveolar fluid is a barrier to gas exchange. Pulmonary capillary blood then passes through unventilated alveoli, such as to produce pulmonary arterio-venous shunting with hypoxemia and asphyxia.

Any process that alters the osmotic or hydrostatic forces that maintain alveolar-capillary equilibrium may cause pulmonary edema. Increased pulmonary capillary back pressure is most often due to myocardial failure. Decreased plasma oncotic pressure may follow hepatic disease, or extreme losses of plasma albumin as occurs in protein-losing enteropathies.

There are important non-cardiogenic types of pulmonary edemas that may progress to asphyxia. The most common is capillary–alveolar membrane leakage[175] caused by toxic, chemical, bacterial, viral, thermal, or other insults, presenting as ARDS[124,173] with "progressive pulmonary infiltration".[125] When ARDS progresses to cardiac arrest, it is refractory to therapy, because it usually cannot overcome the block to oxygenation caused by the underlying disease state. Non-cardiac pulmonary edema is also caused by membrane damage due to street drugs and especially cocaine. Loss of interstitial negative pressure may be due to pneumothorax, infection, or carcinoma involving pulmonary lymphatics, fibrotic and inflammatory states, or high altitude.[173]

Pulmonary edema should be treated before it progresses to asphyxia and cardiac arrest. During spontaneous circulation, acute pulmonary edema is treated by administration of 100% oxygen delivered with positive pressure.[122,176] The simplest emergency treatment includes spontaneous breathing of 100% oxygen by continuous positive airway pressure, utilizing a mouthpiece or mask.[177–180] If the patient is stuporous or comatose, or has an arterial PO$_2$ of <60 mm Hg, or if the arterial PCO$_2$ increases despite therapy, endotracheal intubation, sedation, paralysis, and 100% oxygen with positive pressure are indicated.[122] Ventilation may be facilitated by administration of a muscle relaxant, but this may delay recovery of spontaneous breathing. Increased airway pressure raises the arterial PO$_2$ by increasing functional residual capacity through recruitment of fluid-filled alveoli with displacement of edema fluid. After oxygenation, fluid should be removed for management of underlying cause.[175] In left-sided heart failure, standard oxygenation may be combined with administration of morphine, a diuretic, and under extreme conditions, phlebotomy. When pulmonary edema has progressed to asphyxial cardiac arrest, the likelihood of ROSC is remote.

Tension pneumothorax

Venting the pleural space, either through the chest wall or through the lung, results in pneumothorax. The cause may be trauma or disease with destruction of lung tissue.[181–184] When the opening is large enough, pressure in one pleural space is increased throughout the respiratory cycle and the ipsilateral lung is compressed. Previously healthy patients then manifest hypoxemia because 40% to 50% of blood flow is shunted through non-ventilated alveoli. If the opening to the pleural space operates as a one-way valve, it causes a tension pneumothorax. Breathing, positive-pressure ventilation, or coughing may further increase the pressure of free gas in the pleural space. Alveoli may rupture, admitting air into the pulmonary interstitial spaces, and thereby producing mediastinal and subcutaneous emphysema. Tension pneumothorax may preclude venous return and therefore preload. Mediastinal shift further impairs venous return. Tension pneumothorax therefore progresses to cardiac arrest by a combination of impaired pulmonary and circulatory mechanisms. The initial event is asphyxial, with impaired delivery of oxygenated blood to the left side of the heart. Subsequently, reduced cardiac filling accounts for decreased cardiac output. Ultimately, circulatory arrest is due to the combined effects of hypoxemia, compression atelectasis, compression of the contralateral lung, and elevated intrathoracic pressures that impede venous return. Compression of major vessels and airways and mediastinal emphysema may contribute to the severity of the insult.

Predisposing causes of tension pneumothorax include lung disease, positive-pressure ventilation, and coughing in the presence of valve-like bronchial obstruction, during asthma and in patients with COPD. Patients with connective tissue disorders, and especially Marfan's syndrome, are at increased risk of pneumothorax as are women with endometriosis.[186,187]

Tension pneumothorax should be suspected when a patient presents with sudden onset of chest discomfort or shortness of breath, especially if predisposing factors are present and are identified. The diagnosis may be made presumptively by diminished or absent breath sounds with hyper-resonance to percussion in one lung, progressive difficulty in ventilation, subcutaneous emphysema, mediastinal and/or tracheal shift. Progressive abdominal distension may accompany tension pneumothorax when pleural gas under pressure breaks through serosal membranes at the openings in the diaphragm.[2]

Confirmation by chest roentgenogram is *not* required in life-threatening settings. A high index of suspicion is needed to diagnose this condition before the hemodynamic crisis occurs.

Needle puncture serves only for confirmation; it is insufficient for relief of gas build-up and has a high false-negative rate.[185] Rapid transformation of the closed pneumothorax into an open pneumothorax is imperative. Thoracostomy with use of a large-bore tube or an intercostal incision to vent the pleural space may be life-saving. Confirmation that the thoracostomy tubes are in the pleural space is made by observation of the characteristic misting with ventilation and subsequent chest radiography. When cardiovascular collapse appears imminent, thoracostomy should proceed without a chest tube tray.[185]

When pulselessness develops, bilateral venting of the pleural space, ventilation, and chest compressions may still restore spontaneous circulation. Open-chest CPR is a final option.

Thromboembolism

Acute pulmonary thromboembolism is among the most common causes of death among old and chronically ill patients.[188,189] It may, however, also occur in persons of seemingly good health. The large list of risk factors includes chronic diseases, especially carcinoma; immobilization, especially in fracture casts; recent surgery; obesity; tobacco abuse; and pregnancy. Deep venous thromboses, predominantly in the veins of the pelvis or a lower extremity, embolize to the pulmonary artery and peripheral pulmonary arteries, impeding pulmonary blood flow.[190] The initial presentation may be circulatory shock or cardiac arrest. Plain chest films in most cases are not helpful but may suggest decreased pulmonary vascularity. If the patient's clinical status permits, a lung scan and arterial blood gas are useful because a normal scan and normal arterial PO_2 virtually rule out significant embolization. If the lung scan is positive and time permits, axial tomography or a pulmonary angiogram confirms the diagnosis.[191,192] The pathogenesis, diagnosis, and management of pulmonary thromboembolism in patients with spontaneous circulation are reviewed elsewhere. The focus of this chapter is on the moribund patient who presents in circulatory shock or cardiac arrest.

The mechanism by which pulmonary thromboembolism progresses to cardiac arrest is a combination of obstructive shock with a low cardiac output together with asphyxia. Acute pulmonary embolism increases not only the physiologic dead space but also right-to-left shunting.[189]

The hypoxemia and a high alveolar–arterial PO_2 gradient are traced to ventilation–perfusion disturbances, including patchy bronchoconstriction and hyperemia, and even scattered pulmonary edema. The severity is contingent on the proportion of the total cross-sectional area of the pulmonary arterial tree that is deprived of blood flow. In patients with previously healthy lungs and heart, more than 30% of the vascular tree is obstructed prior to onset of shock. In patients with cardiopulmonary disease a smaller proportion of the pulmonary vasculature that is suddenly blocked may produce shock and subsequent cardiac arrest.[193] The thrombus in the pulmonary vascular bed has additional local and systemic effects. The primary treatment, however, is to relieve intravascular mechanical obstructions. In the previously fit person with occlusion of one pulmonary artery, bronchial circulation may allow the lung to survive.

A single embolus or multiple small emboli that occlude approximately 50% of the pulmonary vascular bed result in arterial hypotension, tachycardia, pulmonary artery hypertension, and bronchospasm. Prompt anticoagulation and thrombolysis are indicated. More conservative management of the patient with acute pulmonary thromboembolism for whom thrombolysis or mechanical relief is delayed can support vital functions until spontaneous thrombolysis and recanalization of obstructed vessels occurs, at the same time preventing recurrent embolization with anticoagulation.[194–197] Heparinization prevents secondary thrombus formation.[198]

Diagnosis of pulmonary embolism as the cause of cardiac arrest is difficult. If PaO_2 remains markedly reduced when the patient is ventilated with 100% oxygen, and in the absence of gross signs of pulmonary edema, the presumptive diagnosis of pulmonary embolism is supported. ALS is usually ineffective. A central aortic catheter helps to provide better definition of the hemodynamic state[199] and identifies "pseudo-PEA."

Previously healthy patients presenting with probable pulmonary embolism and cardiac arrest represent a special subgroup of patients who may benefit from open-chest CPR or CPB.[200] The decision that standard therapy may not be effective must be made *early*, while a good outcome remains possible. If open-chest CPR is performed, the pulmonary artery should be identified and massaged to break up the thrombus and allow it to move peripherally. If emergency CPB is performed, thoracotomy and embolectomy are appropriate interventions.

Amniotic fluid embolism

Amniotic fluid embolism is an uncommon but tragic cause of sudden death in that two persons, both potentially healthy, may die. It occurs in approximately 1 in 80 000 deliveries.[201,202] Multiparous women are at increased risk, as are those undergoing uterine manipulation. Amniotic fluid embolism causes a distinct pathophysiologic response, indicating that amniotic fluid itself or secondary mediators are biologically active. The pulmonary vascular bed constricts, and at least in part explains progression to cor pulmonale. Oxygen delivery is impaired due to hypoxemia and decreased cardiac output in part as a result of septal shift associated with expansion of right ventricular volume and pressure. Consumptive coagulopathy with hypofibrinogenemia accounts for disseminated intravascular coagulation (DIC).

Amniotic fluid embolism should be suspected when sudden pulmonary or cardiovascular compromise occurs in patients with placenta accreta, cesarean delivery, uterine rupture, retention of the products of conception, or premature separation of the placenta.[203] Sudden collapse with signs of shock is accompanied by dyspnea and cyanosis. More frequently, the event occurs during labor and delivery. Early detection by continuous pulse oximetry has been demonstrated.[204] Therapy includes aggressive respiratory support with 100% oxygen and possibly the addition of pulmonary vasodilator drugs. Aggressive therapy of DIC is recommended.

Management of cardiac arrest is similar to that of pulmonary thromboembolism with the exception that massage of the pulmonary outflow tract is not advised. Early initiation of CPB may be life-saving.[205]

Anaphylaxis

Anaphylaxis is an acute, severe, life-threatening hypersensitivity reaction that may progress to asphyxia and cardiac arrest. Antibodies, principally immunoglobulin E (IgE), that were formed in response to a previous exposure to an antigen, trigger a potentially lethal series of immunologic cascades on re-exposure. Although a very large number of antigens may cause anaphylaxis in sensitized individuals, the most common inciting antigens are β-lactam antibiotics, iodinated contrast media, and Hymenoptera stings.[206] In many cases the etiologic agent may be unclear.

Anaphylaxis is a complex event. The antigen–antibody complex is absorbed by mast cells and basophils. Calcium-dependent degranulation results in the release of bioactive substances. Primary mediators include histamine, serotonin, bradykinin, the slow-reacting substance of anaphylaxis (SRS, now known to be leukotrienes C, D, and E4); the eosinophilic chemotactic factor of anaphylaxis, prostaglandins and leukotrienes, metabolites of arachidonic acid (via the cyclooxygenase and lipoxygenase pathways, respectively); and platelet-activating factor. Secondary mediators include complement and the products of polymorphonuclear leukocytes (prostaglandins [PGs], leukotrienes [LTs], fibrinolysin, plasminogen, elastase); platelets (PGs, LTs, Hageman factor activators, lysosomal enzymes, and serotonin), and eosinophils (collagenase, histaminase, phospholipase D, arylsulfatase D).[207] Most likely, additional mediators will be identified as assays become available.

Anaphylaxis blocks delivery of oxygen in multiple ways. Many of the bioactive substances are smooth muscle and membrane modulators, and their most significant target organs are the airways, lungs, and cardiovascular systems. Pharyngeal and laryngeal edema, bronchospasm, edema of the bronchial mucosa, and vasodilation occur early. Asphyxia is due to upper and lower airway obstructions. Shock develops through a combination of decreased vascular tone and increased capillary permeability. Evidence suggests that the chemical mediators of anaphylaxis may also decrease myocardial function and, together with hypoxemia, exacerbate circulatory shock and cardiac arrest.[208,209] As in all the asphyxial syndromes, aggressive management to prevent progression to cardiac arrest includes airway control, oxygenation, and ventilation. Angioedema and laryngospasm may make orotracheal intubation difficult. Early consideration should be given to transtracheal ventilation or cricothyroidotomy. Early treatment includes relief of bronchospasm.

Epinephrine is life-saving for the treatment of anaphylaxis.[210] Patients known to be at risk should carry an epinephrine auto injector with them and be trained in its use. Epinephrine increases cyclic adenosine monophosphate (cAMP) levels in mast cells and provides inotropic, chronotropic, and pressor support as well as bronchodilation. Anaphylactic shock is treated with intravenous, sublingual, intratracheal, or subcutaneous administration of epinephrine. Intravenous epinephrine is best titrated in 0.1-mg increments. Patients who have received β-blocking drugs may require large doses of epinephrine.

Blood pressure should be closely monitored with an indwelling arterial catheter. Because severe anaphylaxis is associated with hypovolemia,[211,212] fluid challenge is indicated. A corticosteroid may be administered, although its beneficial effect is not immediate. Antihistamines are administered for prophylaxis but are of limited value during resuscitation. In specific situations, antivenoms may be indicated.

Management of anaphylactic shock

Management includes considerations of support for ventilation, circulation, and mitigation of the immunologic response.

Ventilation

1. 100% oxygen by spontaneous breathing or IPPV-CPPV by mask.
2. Endotracheal intubation, transtracheal ventilation, cricothyroidotomy, and IPPV-CPPV.
3. β-Adrenergic agonist, for example, aerosolized albuterol, 0.5 ml in 3 ml saline.
4. Consider neuromuscular blockade (e.g., vecuronium, pancuronium).
5. Consider helium/O_2.
6. Consider general anesthesia (especially intravenous ketamine).

Circulation

1. Crystalloid guided by central venous pressure (fluid challenge).
2. Epinephrine, 5 mg/500 ml ISS, by titrated intravenous infusion. Maintain mean arterial pressure (MAP) at 90 mm Hg or above.

Immunologic support

1. Epinephrine (see above).
2. Antihistamines (diphenhydramine, 50 mg/70 kg); consider cimetidine.
3. Corticosteroid (methylprednisolone, 120 mg/70 kg).
4. Specific antivenom!

A syndrome that combines hypoxemia and hypotension places the patient at high risk for cardiac arrest. Once the pulse is lost, injury to vital organs will occur rapidly. As in all asphyxial syndromes, prevention of cardiac arrest is the primary treatment.[213,214]

Carbon monoxide poisoning

Carbon monoxide (CO) impairs oxygen transport. CO is a colorless, odorless gas that causes more poisoning deaths in the United States than any other single agent.[215] CO has a high affinity for hemoglobin, reversibly displacing oxygen to create carboxyhemoglobin (COHb). Hemoglobin binds carbon monoxide about 200 to 300 times more readily than it binds oxygen. The COHb produced is subsequently not available for oxygen transport. This creates a form of anemic hypoxia without a decrease in plasma hemoglobin.[216] CO toxicity is a more complex process than previously believed. Classically, COHb interferes with O_2 transport. It may also be a cellular poison, interfering with cytochrome function.[217]

CO poisoning does not alter PaO_2 even though available oxygen is reduced. If as little as 0.2% CO is inhaled, COHb will form at a rate of 1.1%/min. If the patient is doing heavy work, the rate will increase to 2.4%/min, and within about 45 minutes CO will saturate 76% of the hemoglobin. Conscious dogs inhaling 1% CO reach 80% CO hemoglobin saturation rapidly followed by sudden death. There is no increase in respiratory drive since the peripheral chemoreceptors sense no decrease in PaO_2.

Most persons who die in fires are asphyxiated. CO intoxication or the effects of other toxic gases are more lethal than decreases in O_2 or increases in CO_2. A key to the early diagnosis is knowledge of the circumstances of intoxication, such as combustion in closed spaces or multiple ill persons within the same family.[218,219]

CO intoxication may manifest itself by headache and variable impairment in mental status and neurologic function. Eventually there is loss of consciousness, followed by hypotension, convulsions, apnea, and cardiac arrest in asystole. IPPV with 100% oxygen delays progression and promotes spontaneous breathing. Permanent cerebral impairment persists even though there is relatively prompt return of spontaneous circulation. Irreversible cerebral damage may occur even in the absence of cardiac arrest.[220]

The initial therapy is to remove the patient from the source of CO. The serum elimination time for COHb is inversely related to the serum partial pressure of oxygen.[218] Administration of 100% oxygen is the primary therapy. Patients with CO poisoning who develop cardiac arrest have a very poor prognosis. Simply intubating these patients and ventilating them with 100% oxygen may not restore an adequate oxygen delivery for favorable neurologic outcomes.

Resuscitation in a hyperbaric chamber has proven effective. Even though the logistics of using such a chamber are daunting, it is the best option.[221]

Cyanide poisoning

Cyanide is the classic cellular asphyxiant; it interrupts the function of oxidative phosphorylation at the mitochondrial level by binding to the ferric (Fe^{3+}) component of cytochrome oxidase. Cells are unable to utilize oxygen as the final electron acceptor, and anaerobic glycolysis results. This is reflected in the early signs of organ dysfunction and increased serum lactate.

Because the block to respiration is at the cellular level, arterial hypoxemia and hypercarbia, the sine qua non of classic asphyxia, will not be present, at least initially. Cyanide asphyxiation presents challenges that are similar to those of CO intoxication. Once cardiac arrest has occurred, the prognosis is bleak. In laboratory studies, amyl nitrite and sodium thiosulfate have not been effective after onset of cardiac arrest.[222,223] The only present option is to prevent progression to arrest.

Conclusions and recommendations

Asphyxial cardiac arrest may be sudden, but it is not immediate. Whatever the cause, the progression from inciting etiology through shock to cardiac arrest provides an opportunity for effective resuscitation before pulselessness sets in. Airway control and artificial ventilation alone are likely to reverse asphyxiation. After cardiac arrest has occurred, return of spontaneous circulation can often be achieved by conventional ALS. Unfortunately, cerebral recovery is less likely after asphyxial cardiac arrest than after primary cardiac arrest due to VF of the same duration. Of the two components in asphyxiation, hypercarbia may cause transient coma and acidosis but is totally reversible, whereas hypoxia–anoxia can cause permanent unresuscitatable damage, particularly to the brain.

REFERENCES

1. Safar, P. History of cardiopulmonary–cerebral resuscitation. In Kaye, W. & Bircher, N., eds. *Cardiopulmonary Resuscitation*. New York: Churchill Livingstone, 1989: 1–53.
2. Safar, P. & Bircher, N.G. World Federation of Societies of Anaesthesiologists. *Cardiopulmonary Cerebral Resuscitation.* 3rd edn. London: Saunders, 1988.
3. Safar, P. & Bircher, N.G. The pathophysiology of dying and reanimation. In Schwartz, G.R., Cayten, C.G., Mangelsen, M.A., Mayer, T.A. & Hanke, B.K., eds. *Principles and Practice of Emergency Medicine*. 3rd edn. Philadelphia: Lea & Febiger, 1992: 3–41.
4. Beck, C. & Rand, H.I. Cardiac arrest during anesthesia and surgery. *J. Am. Med. Assoc.* 1949; **141**: 1230–1233.
5. Beck, C.S. Death after a clean bill of health. *J. Am. Med. Assoc.* 1960; **174**: 133.
6. Redding, J.S. & Pearson, J.W. Resuscitation from ventricular fibrillation. *J. Am. Med. Assoc.* 1968; **203**: 255–260.
7. Eisenberg, M.S., Horwood, B.T., Cummins, R.O., Reynolds-Haertle, R. & Hearne, T.R. Cardiac arrest and resuscitation: a tale of 29 cities. *Ann. Emerg. Med.* 1990; **19**: 179–186.
8. American Heart Association guidelines for cardiopulmonary resuscitation and emergency cardiac care. *Circulation* 2005; **112**(24): IV52–IV57.
9. Henderson, Y. Resuscitation. *J. Am. Med. Assoc.* 1934; **103**: 750.
10. Safar, P. & Holzman, I. Neonatal resuscitation. In Safar, P. & Bircher, N.G., eds. *Cardiopulmonary Cerebral Resuscitation*. London: Saunders, 1988: 286–290.

11. Newton, A.W. & Vandeven, A.M. Unexplained infant and child death: a review of Sudden Infant Death Syndrome, Sudden Unexplained Infant Death, and child maltreatment fatalities including shaken baby syndrome. *Curr. Opin. Pediatr.* 2006; **18**(2): 196–200.

12. Sakai, J., Funayama, M. & Kanetake, J. The relationship between bedding and face-down death in infancy: mathematical analysis of a respiratory simulation system using an infant mannequin to assess gas diffusibility in bedding. *Forens. Sci. Int.* 2006; Apr, In press.

13. Maffei, F.A., van der Jagt, E.W., Powers, K.S. *et al.* Duration of mechanical ventilation in life-threatening pediatric asthma: description of an acute asphyxial subgroup. *Pediatrics* 2004; **114**(3): 762–767.

14. Swann, H.G. & Brucer, M. The cardiorespiratory and biochemical events during rapid anoxic death. *Tex. Rep. Biol. Med.* 1949; **7**: 511.

15. Redding, J., Voigt, C. & Safar, P. Drowning treated with IPPB. *J. Appl. Physiol.* 1960; **15**: 849–854.

16. Redding, J.S. & Pearson, J.W. Resuscitation from asphyxia. *J. Am. Med. Assoc.* 1962; **182**: 283–286.

17. Fenton, T.H. Asphyxia or just hypoxia? *Arch. Dis. Child. Fetal Neonatal. Ed* 2006; **91**(3): F234.

18. II Kings. *Bible King James Version* Chap. 4, Verses 34–35.

19. Toet, M.C., Lemmers, P.M., van Schelven, L.J. & van Bel, F. Cerebral oxygenation and electrical activity after birth asphyxia: their relation to outcome. *Pediatrics* 2006; **117**(2): 333–339.

20. Paradis, N.A., Martin, G.B., Goetting, M.G., Rivers, E.P., Feingold, M. & Nowak, R.M. Aortic pressure during human cardiac arrest: identification of pseudo-electromechanical dissociation. *Chest* 1992; **101**: 123–128.

21. Safar, P., Gisvold, S.E., Vaagenes, P. *et al.* Long-term animal models for the study of global brain ischemia. In Wauquier, A., Borgers, M. & Amery, W.K., eds. *Protection of Tissues Against Hypoxia.* Amsterdam: Elsevier, 1982: 147–170.

22. Vaagenes, P., Safar, P., Moosey, J. *et al.* Asphyxiation versus ventricular fibrillation cardiac arrest in dogs. Differences in cerebral resuscitation effects – a preliminary study. *Resuscitation* 1997; **35**(1): 41–52.

23. Fink, E.L., Alexander, H., Marco, C.D. *et al.* Experimental model of pediatric asphyxial cardiopulmonary arrest in rats. *Pediatr. Crit. Care Med.* 2004; **5**(2): 139–144.

24. Seidl, R., Stockler-Ipsiroglu, S., Rolinski, B. *et al.* Energy metabolism in graded perinatal asphyxia of the rat. *Life Sci* 200; **67**(4): 421–435.

25. Gisvold, S.E., Sterz, F., Abramson, N.S. *et al.* Cerebral resuscitation from cardiac arrest: treatment potentials. *Crit. Care Med.* 1996; **24**(2 Suppl): S69–S80.

26. Smithline, H., Rivers, E., Appleton, T. & Nowak, R. Corticosteroid supplementation during cardiac arrest in rats. *Resuscitation* 1993; **25**(3): 257–264.

27. Katz, L., Young, A., Frank, J.E., Wang, Y. & Park, K. Neurotensin-induced hypothermia improves neurologic outcome after hypoxic–ischemia. *Crit. Care Med.* 2004; **32**(3): 806–810.

28. Song, F.Q., Xie, L. & Chen, M.H. Transoesophageal cardiac pacing is effective for cardiopulmonary resuscitation in a rat of asphyxial model. *Resuscitation* 2006; **69**(2): 263–268.

29. Katz, L.M., Wang, Y., Ebmeyer, U., Radovsky, A. & Safar, P. Glucose plus insulin infusion improves cerebral outcome after asphyxial cardiac arrest. *Neuroreport* 1998; **9**(15): 3363–3367.

30. Fink, E.L., Marco, C.D., Donovan, H.A. *et al.* Brief induced hypothermia improves outcome after asphyxial cardiac arrest in juvenile rats. *Dev. Neurosci.* 2005; **27**: 191–199.

31. Neumar, R.W., Bircher, N.G., Sim, K.M. *et al.* Epinephrine and sodium bicarbonate during CPR following asphyxial cardiac arrest in rats. *Resuscitation* 1995; **29**: 249–263.

32. Huang, L., Weil, M.H., Sun, S., Tang, W. & Fang, X. Carvedilol mitigates adverse effects of epinephrine during cardiopulmonary resuscitation. *J. Cardiovasc. Pharmacol. Ther.* 2005; **10**(2): 113–120.

33. Klouche, K., Weil, M.H., Sun, S., Tang, W. & Zhao, D.H. A comparison of alpha-methylnorepinephrine, vasopressin and epinephrine for cardiac resuscitation. *Resuscitation* 2003; **57**(1): 93–100.

34. Kono, S., Suzuki, A., Obata, Y., Igarashi, H., Bito, H. & Sato, S. Vasopressin with delayed combination of nitroglycerin increases survival rate in asphyxia rat model. *Resuscitation* 2002; **54**(3): 297–301.

35. Kono, S., Bito, H., Suzuki, A., Obata, Y., Igarashi, H. & Sato, S. Vasopressin and epinephrine are equally effective for CPR in a rat asphyxia model. *Resuscitation* 2002; **52**(2): 215–219.

36. Hickey, R.W., Kochanek, P.M., Ferimer, H., Alexander, H.L., Garman, R.H. & Graham, S.H. Induced hyperthermia exacerbates neurologic neuronal histologic damage after asphyxial cardiac arrest in rats. *Crit. Care Med.* 2003; **31**(2): 531–535.

37. Safar, P. Ventilatory efficacy of mouth-to-mouth artificial respiration: airway obstruction during manual and mouth-to-mouth artificial respiration. *J. Am. Med. Assoc.* 1958; **167**: 335–341.

38. Dean, D.E., Schultz, D.L. & Powers, R.H. Asphyxia due to angiotensin converting enzyme (ACE) inhibitor mediated angioedema of the tongue during the treatment of hypertensive heart disease. *J. Forens. Sci.* 2001; **46**(5): 1239–1243.

39. Riesser, T.M. Cardiopulmonary resuscitation. *Clin. Tech. Small Anim. Pract.* 2000; **15**(2): 76–81.

40. Woollard, M., Smith, A., Whitfield, R. *et al.* To blow or not to blow: a randomized controlled trial of compression-only and standard telephone CPR instructions in simulated cardiac arrest. *Resuscitation* 2003; **59**(1): 123–131.

41. Safar, P., Brown, T., Holtey, W.H. & Wilder, R. Ventilation and circulation with closed chest cardiac massage in man. *J. Am. Med. Assoc.* 1961; **176**: 574–576.

42. Morikawa, S., Safar, P. & DeCarlo, J. Influence of head position upon upper airway patency. *Anesthesiology* 1961; **22**: 265–270.

43. Robertsson, S., Grenvik, A. & Wiklund, L. Blood flow and perfusion pressure during open-chest versus closed-chest cardiopulmonary resuscitation in pigs. *Crit. Care Med.* 1995; **23**(5): 715–725.

44. Safar, P. Resuscitation from clinical death: pathophysiologic limits and therapeutic potentials. *Crit. Care Med.* 1988; **16**: 923–941.

45. Kua, J.S. & Tan, I.K. Airway obstruction following internal jugular vein cannulation. *Anesthesia* 1997; **52**(8): 776–780.

46. Lau, H.P., Lin, T.Y., Lee, Y.W., Liou, W.H. & Tsai, S.K. Delayed airway obstruction secondary to inadvertent arterial puncture during percutaneous central venous cannulation. *Acta Anaesthesiol. Sin.* 2001; **39**(2): 93–96.

47. Collins, K.A. & Presnell, S.E. Asphyxia by tracheobronchial thrombus. *Am. J. Forens. Med. Pathol.* 2005; **26**(4): 327–329.

48. Carrick, C., Collins, K.A., Lee, C.J., Prahlow, J.A. & Barnard, J.J. Sudden death due to asphyxia by esophageal polyp: Two case reports and review of asphyxial deaths. *J. Forens. Med. Pathol.* 2005; **26**(3): 275–281.

49. Safar, P. Cerebral resuscitation after cardiac arrest: research initiatives and future directions: a review. *Ann. Emerg. Med.* 1993; **22**(2): 324–349.

50. Schears, G., Creed, J., Zaitseva, T., Schultz, S., Wilson, D.F. & Pastuszko, A. Cerebral oxygenation during repetitive apnea in newborn piglets. *Adv. Exp. Med. Biol.* 2005; **566**: 1–7.

51. Senn, O., Clarenbach, C.F., Kaplan, V., Maggiorini, M. & Bloch, K.E. Monitoring carbon dioxide tension and arterial oxygen saturation by a single earlobe sensor in patients with critical illness or sleep apnea. *Chest* 2005; **128**(3): 1291–1296.

52. Lavie, P. & Hoffstein, V. Sleep apnea syndrome: a possible contributing factor to resistant. *Sleep* 2001; **24**(6): 721–725.

53. Conrad, S.A., Zwischenberger, J.B., Grier, L.R., Alpard, S.K. & Bidani, A. Total extracorporeal arteriovenous carbon dioxide removal in acute respiratory failure: a phase I clinical study. *Intens. Care Med.* 2001; **27**(8): 1340–1351.

54. Nunn, J.F. *Applied Respiratory Physiology: With Special Reference to Anaesthesia.* London: Butterworths, 1975.

55. Rattenborg, C.C. Effect of bicarbonate and THAM on apnea-induced hypercarbia. In Safar, P., ed. *Advances in Cardiopulmonary Resuscitation.* New York: Springer-Verlag, 1977: 128.

56. Zander, R., Mertzlufft, F. Clinical use of oxygen stores: preoxygenation and apneic oxygenation. *Adv. Exp. Med. Biol.* 1992; **317**: 413–420.

57. Ludlow, C.L. Central nervous system control of the laryngeal muscles in humans. *Respir. Physiol. Neurobiol.* 2005; **147**: 205–222.

58. Safar, P. Introduction to respiratory and cardiac resuscitation: a documentary film of human volunteer research. Produced by US Walter Reed Army Institute of Research, Washington, DC, USA. Army film #PMF5349, 1957 and 1961. Available from: University of Pittsburgh Center for Instructional Resources, Pittsburgh, PA 15260, USA.

59. Crile, G.W. & Dolley, D.H. An experimental research into the resuscitation of dogs killed by anesthetics and asphyxia. *J. Exp. Med.* 1906; **8**: 713–724.

60. Siesjo, B.K. Mechanisms of ischemic brain damage. *Crit. Care Med.* 1988; **16**: 954–963.

61. Rehncrona, S., Rosen, I. & Siesjo, B.K. Excessive cellular acidosis: an important mechanism of neuronal damage in the brain. *Acta Physiol. Scand.* 1980; **110**: 435–437.

62. Vukmir, R.B., Bircher, N.G., Radovsky, A. & Safar, P. Sodium bicarbonate may improve outcome in dogs with brief or prolonged cardiac arrest. *Crit. Care Med.* 1995; **23**: 515–522.

63. Radovsky, A., Safar, P., Sterz, F. *et al.* Regional prevalence and distribution of ischemic neurons in dogs' brains 96 hours after cardiac arrest of 0–20 minutes. *Stroke* 1995; **26**(11): 2127–2133.

64. Cerchiari, E.L., Safar, P., Klein, E., Cantadore, R. & Pinsky, M. Cardiovascular function and neurologic outcome after cardiac arrest in dogs. *Resuscitation* 1993; **25**: 9–33.

65. Safar, P., Tisherman, S.A., Behringer, W. *et al.* Suspended animation for delayed resuscitation from prolonged cardiac arrest that is unresuscitable by standard cardiopulmonary–cerebral resuscitation. *Crit. Care Med.* 2000; **28**: N214–N218.

66. Safar, P., Abramson, N.S., Angelos, M. *et al.* Emergency cardiopulmonary bypass for resuscitation from prolonged cardiac arrest. *Am. J. Emerg. Med.* 1990; **8**: 55–67.

67. Tisherman, S.A., Grenvik, A. & Safar, P. Cardiopulmonary-cerebral resuscitation: advanced and prolonged life support with emergency cardiopulmonary bypass. *Acta Anaesthesiol. Scand.* 1990; **94**: 63–72.

68. Martens, P., Mullie, A., Vandekerckhove, Y., Aufiero, T.X. & Chambers, C.E. Case 1 – 1993. Emergency use of cardiopulmonary bypass for resuscitation from CPR-resistant cardiac arrest. *J. Cardiothorac. Vasc. Anesth.* 1993; **7**(2): 227–235.

69. Haugen, R.K. The cafe coronary: sudden death in restaurants. *J. Am. Med. Assoc.* 1963; **186**: 142–144.

70. Heimlich, H.J. A life-saving maneuver to prevent food-choking. *J. Am. Med. Assoc.* 1975; **234**: 398–401.

71. Heimlich, J.H. Death from food-choking prevented by a new life-saving maneuver. *Heart Lung* 1976; **5**: 755–758.

72. Redding, J.S. The choking controversy: critique of evidence on the Heimlich maneuver. *Crit. Care Med.* 1979; **7**: 745.

73. Gordon, A.S., Belton, M.K. & Ridolpho, P.F. Emergency management of foreign body airway obstruction: comparison of artificial cough techniques, manual extrication maneuvers, and simple mechanical devices. In Safar, P., ed. *Advances in CPR.* New York: Springer-Verlag, 1977: 39–50.

74. Mittleman, R.E. & Wetli, C.V. The fatal cafe coronary: foreign-body airway obstruction. *J. Am. Med. Assoc.* 1982; **247**: 1285–1288.

75. Kitay, G. & Shafer, N. Cafe coronary: recognition, treatment and prevention. *Nurse Pract.* 1989; **14**: 35–38, 43, 46.

76. Berzlanovich, A.M., Fazeny-Dorner, B., Waldhoer, T., Fasching, P. & Keil, W. Foreign body asphyxia: a preventable cause of death in the elderly. *Am. J. Prev. Med.* 2005; **28**(1): 65–69.

77. Guildner, C.W., Williams, D. & Subitch, T. Emergency management for airway obstruction by foreign material. In Safar, P., ed. *Advances in CPR.* New York, Springer-Verlag 1977: 51–57.

78. Jacoby, J.J., Hamelberg, W., Ziegler, C.H., Flory, F.A. & Jones, J.R. Transtracheal resuscitation. *J. Am. Med. Assoc.* 1956; **162**: 625–628.

79. Jacobs, H.B. Emergency percutaneous transtracheal catheter and ventilator. *J. Trauma* 1972; **12**: 50–55.

80. Singh, N.P. Transtracheal jet ventilation as a new technique and experiences with ketamine and propandid in India. In Miyazaki, M., ed. *Anesthesiology.* (WFSA Congress Kyoto, 1972). Amsterdam: Excerpta Medica, 1972: 160–161.

81. Klain, M., Keszler, H. & Brader, E. High frequency jet ventilation in CPR. *Crit. Care Med.* 1981; **9**: 421–422.

82. Iserson, K.V. Strangulation: a review of ligature, manual and postural neck compression injuries. *Ann. Emerg. Med.* 1994; **13**: 179–185.

83. Aufderheide, T.P., Aprahamian, C., Mateer, J.R. *et al.* Emergency airway management in hanging victims. *Ann. Emerg. Med.* 1994; **24**: 879–884.

84. Ikeda, N., Harada, A. & Suzuki, T. The course of respiration and circulation in death due to typical hanging. *Int. J. Leg Med.* 1992; **104**: 313–315.

85. Grmec, S., Lah, K. & Tusek-Bunc, K. Difference in end-tidal CO_2 between asphyxia cardiac arrest and ventricular fibrillation/pulseless ventricular tachycardia cardiac arrest in the prehospital setting. *Crit. Care* 2003; **7**(6): R139–R144.

86. Levine, J.E., Becker, D. & Chun, T. Reversal of incipient brain death from head-injury apnea at the scene of accidents [Letter]. *N. Engl. J. Med.* 1979; **301**(2): 109.

87. Levin, H.S., Benton, A.L. & Grossman, R.G. *Neurobehavioral Consequences of Closed Head Injury.* Oxford: Oxford University Press, 1982: 3–48.

88. Fessler, R.D. & Diaz, F.G. The management of cerebral perfusion pressure and intracranial pressure after severe head injury. *Ann. Emerg. Med.* 1993; **22**: 998–1003.

89. Lehman, L.B. Intracranial pressure monitoring and treatment: a contemporary view. *Ann. Emerg. Med.* 1990; **19**: 295–303.

90. Caplan, L.R. Diagnosis and treatment of ischemic stroke. *J. Am. Med. Assoc.* 1991; **266**: 2413–2418.

91. Ravitch, M.M., Lane, R., Safar, P. *et al.* Lightning stroke: recovery following cardiac massage and prolonged artificial respiration. *N. Engl. J. Med.* 1961; **264**: 36–38.

92. Taussig, H.B. Death from lightning and the possibility of living again. *Am. Sci.* 1969; **57**: 306–316.

93. Yeong, E.K., Chen, M.T. & Chu, S.H. Traumatic asphyxia. *Plast. Reconstr. Surg.* 1994; **93**: 739–744.

94. Lee, M.C., Wong, S.S., Chu, J.J. *et al.* Traumatic asphyxia. *Ann. Thorac. Surg.* 1991; **51**: 86–88.

95. Landercasper, J. & Cogbill, T.H. Long-term follow-up after traumatic asphyxia. *J. Trauma* 1985; **25**: 838–841.

96. Loh, F.C. Traumatic asphyxia compounding craniofacial trauma. *J. Craniomaxillofac. Surg.* 1992; **20**: 135–137.

97. Newquist, M.J. & Sobel, R.M. Traumatic asphyxia: an indicator of significant pulmonary injury. *Am. J. Emerg. Med.* 1990; **8**: 212–215.

98. Thompson, A. Jr, Illescas, F.F. & Chiu, R.C. Why is the lower torso protected in traumatic asphyxia? A new hypothesis. *Ann. Thorac. Surg.* 1989; **47**: 247–249.

99. Jongewaard, W.R., Cogbill, T.H. & Landercasper, J. Neurologic consequences of traumatic asphyxia. *J. Trauma* 1992; **32**: 28–31.

100. Purdy, R.H., Cogbill, T.H., Landercasper, J. & Ryan, D.K. Temporary blindness associated with traumatic asphyxia. *J. Emerg. Med.* 1988; **6**: 373–376.

101. Baldwin, G.A., Macnab, A.J. & McCormick, A.Q. Visual loss following traumatic asphyxia in children. *J. Trauma* 1988; **28**: 557–558.

102. Gorenstein, L., Blair, G.K. & Shandling, B. The prognosis of traumatic asphyxia in childhood. *J. Pediatr. Surg.* 1986; **21**: 753–756.

103. Moerch, E.T., Avery, E.E. & Benson, D.W. Hyperventilation in the treatment of crushing injuries of the chest. *Surg. Forum* 1956; **6**: 270.

104. Freedland, M., Wilson, R.F., Bender, J.S. & Levison, M.A. The management of flail chest injury: factors affecting outcome. *J. Trauma* 1990; **30**: 1460–1468.

105. Clark, G.C., Schecter, W.P. & Trunkey, D.D. Variables affecting outcome in blunt chest trauma: flail chest vs. pulmonary contusion. *J. Trauma* 1988; **28**: 298–304.

106. Ornato, J.P. The resuscitation of near-drowning victims. *J. Am. Med. Assoc.* 1986; **256**: 77.

107. Hadley, J.A. & Fowler, D.R. Organa weight effects of drowning and asphyxiation on the lungs, liver, brain, heart, kidneys, and spleen. *Forens. Sci.* 2003; **26**: 239–246.

108. Lunetta, P., Modell, J.H. & Sajantila, A. What is the incidence and significance of "dry-lungs" in bodies found in water? *Am. J. Forens. Med. Pathol.* 2004; **25**(4): 291–301.

109. Quan, L., Gore, E.J., Wentz, K.R. *et al.* Ten-year study of pediatric drownings and near-drownings in King County, WA: lessons in injury prevention. *Pediatrics* 1989; **83**: 1035–1049.

110. Modell, J.H., Graves, S.A. & Ketover, A. Clinical course of 91 consecutive near-drowning victims. *Chest* 1976; **70**: 231–238.

111. Redding, J., Voigt, G. & Safar, P. Treatment of sea water aspiration. *J. Appl. Physiol.* 1960; **15**: 1113–1116.

112. Redding, J. & Cozine, R.A. Restoration of circulation after fresh water drowning. *J. Appl. Physiol.* 1961; **16**: 1071.

113. Yagil, Y., Stalnikowicz, R., Michaeli, J. & Mogle, P. Near drowning in the Dead Sea: electrolyte imbalances and therapeutic implications. *Arch. Intern. Med.* 1985; **145**: 50–53.

114. Orlowski, J.P., Abulleil, M.M. & Phillips, J.M. The hemodynamic and cardiovascular effects of near-drowning in hypotonic, isotonic, or hypertonic solutions. *Ann. Emerg. Med.* 1989; **18**: 1044–1049.

115. Bierens, J.J., Knape, J.T. & Gelissen, H.P. *Drowning Curr. Opin. Crit. Care* 2002; **8**(6): 578–586.

116. Biggart, M.J. & Bohn, D.J. Effect of hypothermia and cardiac arrest on outcome of near-drowning accidents in children. *J. Pediatr.* 1990; **117**: 179–183.

117. Conn, A.W., Miyasaki, K., Katayama, M. *et al.* A canine study of cold water drowning in fresh water versus salt water. *Crit. Care Med.* 1995; **23**(12): 2029–2037.

118. Modell, J.H., Idris, A.H., Pineda, J.A. & Silverstein, J.H. Survival after prolonged submersion in freshwater in Florida. *Chest* 2004; **125**(5): 1948–1951.

119. Siebke, H., Rod, T., Breivik, H. Survival after 40 minutes submersion without cerebral sequelae. *Lancet* 1975; **1**: 1275–1277.

120. Tisherman, S., Chabal, C., Safar, P. & Stezoski, W. Resuscitation of dogs from cold-water submersion using cardiopulmonary bypass. *Ann. Emerg. Med.* 1985; **14**: 389–396.

121. Tisherman, S.A., Safar, P., Radovsky, A. *et al.* Profound hypothermia (<10 °C) compared with deep hypothermia (15 °C) improves neurologic outcome in dogs after two hours' circulatory arrest induced to enable resuscitative surgery. *J. Trauma* 1991; **31**: 1051–1062.

122. Safar, P. & Caroline, N. Acute respiratory insufficiency [Chapter 2]. Respiratory care techniques and strategies [Chapter 11]. In Schwartz, G., Safar, P., Stone, J., Storey, P., Wagner, D., eds. *Principles and Practice of Emergency Medicine.* Philadelphia: Saunders, 1986.

123. Moore, F.D., Lyons, J.H., Pierce, E.C. Post-traumatic pulmonary insufficiency. Philadelphia: Saunders, 1969.

124. Gattinoni, L., Caironi, P., Cressoni, M. *et al.* Lung recruitment in patients with the acute respiratory distress syndrome. *N. Engl. J. Med.* 2006; **354**(17): 1775–1186.

125. Oikonomou, A. & Hansell, D.M. Organizing pneumonia: the many morphological faces. *Eur. Radiol.* 2002; **12**(6): 1486–1496

126. Bendixen, H.H., Egbert, L.D., Hedley-Whyte, J. *et al.* Respiratory Care. St Louis: Mosby, 1965.

127. Safar, P., ed. *Respiratory Therapy.* Philadelphia: Davis, 1965.

128. Symon, L. Flow thresholds in brain ischaemia and the effects of drugs. *Br. J. Anaesth.* 1985; **57**: 34–43.

129. Zapol, W.M., Snider, M.T., Hill, J.D. *et al.* Extracorporeal membrane oxygenation in severe acute respiratory failure: a randomized prospective study. *J. Am. Med. Assoc.* 1979; **242**: 2193–2196.

130. Teresaki, H., Nogami, T., Saito, Y. *et al.* Extracorporeal lung assist without endotracheal intubation and mechanical pulmonary ventilation [Letter]. *Crit. Care Med.* 1987; **15**: 84–85.

131. Rotheram, E.B., Safar, P., Robin, E.D. CNS disorder during mechanical ventilation in chronic pulmonary disease. *J. Am. Med. Assoc.* 1964; **189**: 993–996.

132. Safar, P., Nemoto, E.M. & Severinghaus, J.W. Pathogenesis of central nervous system disorder during artificial hyperventilation in compensated hypercarbia in dogs. *Crit. Care Med.* 1973; **1**: 5–16.

133. McFadden, E.R., Kaiser, R. & DeGroot, W.J. Acute bronchial asthma. *N. Engl. J. Med.* 1973; **288**: 221–225.

134. Nowak, R.M. Adult acute asthma. In Rosen, P., Baker, F., Barkin, R.M., Braen, G.R., Dailey, R.H., Levy, R.C., eds. *Emergency Medicine: Concepts and Clinical Practice.* 3rd edn. St Louis: Mosby, 1992: 1119–1140.

135. Molfino, N.A., Nannini, L.J., Martelli, A.N. & Slutsky, A.S. Respiratory arrest in near fatal asthma. *N. Engl. J. Med.* 1991; **324**: 285–288.

136. Bone, R.C. & Burch, S.G. Management of status asthmaticus. *Ann. Allergy* 1991; **67**: 461–469.

137. Sur, S., Crotty, T.B., Kephart, G.M. *et al.* Sudden-onset fatal asthma: a distinct entity with few eosinophils and relatively more neutrophils in the airway submucosa? *Am. Rev. Respir. Dis.* 1993; **148**: 713–719.

138. ten Brinkle, A., Sterk, P.J., Masclee, A.A. *et al.* Risk factors of frequent exacerbations in difficult-to-treat asthma. *Eur. Respir. J.* 2005; **26**(5): 812–818.

139. Hegde, R.M. & Worthley, L.I. Acute asthma and the life threatening episode. *Crit. Care Resusc.* 1999; **1**(4): 371–387.

140. Woodruff, P.G., Emond, S.D., Singh, A.K. & Camargo, C.A. Jr. Sudden-onset severe acute asthma: clinical features and response to therapy. *Acad. Emerg. Med.* 1998; **5**(7): 695–701.

141. Veen, J.C., Smits, H.H., Ravensberg, A.J., Hiemstra, P.S., Sterk, P.J. & Bel, E.H. Impaired perception of dyspnea in patients with severe asthma. Relation to sputum eosinophils. *Am. J. Respir. Crit. Care Med.* 1998; **158**(4): 1134–1141.

142. Sanders, D.L. & Aronsky, D. Biomedical informatics applications for asthma care: a systematic review. *J. Am. Med. Inform. Assoc.* 2006;Apr, In press.

143. Wasserfallen, J.B., Schaller, M.D. & Perret, C.H. Life-threatening asthma with dramatic resolution. *Chest* 1993; **104**: 616–618.

144. Nowak, R., Emerman, C., Hamrahan, J.P. *et al.*; the XOPENEX Acute Severe Asthma Study Group. A Comparison of levalbuterol with racemic albuterol in the treatment of acute severe asthma exacerbations in adults. *Am. J. Emerg. Med.* 2006; **24**(3): 259–267.

145. Lin, R.Y., Sauter, D., Newman, T., Sirleaf, J., Walters, J. & Tavakol, M. Continuous versus intermittent albuterol nebulization in the treatment of acute asthma. *Ann. Emerg. Med.* 1993; **22**: 1847–1853.

146. Lin, R.Y., Smith, A.J. & Hergenroeder, P. High serum albuterol levels and tachycardia in adult asthmatics treated with high-dose continuously aerosolized albuterol. *Chest* 1993; **103**: 221–225.

147. Crompton, G.K. Nebulized or intravenous beta 2 adrenoceptor agonist therapy in acute asthma? *Eur. Respir. J.* 1990; **3**: 125–126.

148. Salmeron, S., Brochard, L., Mal, H. *et al.* Nebulized versus intravenous albuterol in hypercapnic acute asthma: a multicenter, double-blind, randomized study. *Am. J. Respir. Crit. Care Med.* 1994; **149**: 1466–1470.

149. McCaul, C.L., McNamara, P.J., Engelberts, D. *et al.* Epinephrine increases mortality after brief asphyxial cardiac arrest in an in vivo rat model. *Anesth. Analg.* 2006; **102**(2): 542–548.

150. Bryant, D.H. & Rogers, P. Effects of ipratropium bromide nebulizer solution with and without preservatives in the treatment of acute and stable asthma. *Chest* 1992; **102**: 742–747.

151. Teale, C., Morrison, J.F., Muers, M.F. & Pearson, S.B. Response to nebulized ipratropium bromide and terbutaline in acute severe asthma. *Respir. Med.* 1992; **86**: 215–218.

152. Schiermeyer, R.P. & Finkelstein, J.A. Rapid infusion of magnesium sulfate obviates need for intubation in status asthmaticus. *Am. J. Emerg. Med.* 1994; **12**: 164–166.

153. Rowe, B.H., Camargo, C.A. Jr & Multicenter Airway Research Collaboration (MARC) Investigators. The use of magnesium sulfate in acute asthma: rapid uptake of evidence in North American emergency departments. *J. Allergy Clin. Immunol.* 2006; **117**(1): 53–58.

154. Cheuk, D.K., Chau, T.C. & Lee, S.L. A meta-analysis on intravenous magnesium sulphate for treating acute asthma. *Arch. Dis. Child.* 2005; **90**(1): 74–77.

155. de Abrew, K. Intravenous magnesium sulphate in asthma: current recommendations. *Ceylon Med. J.* 2004: **4**(4): 147.

156. Stevens, T.P., Blennow, M. & Soll, R.F. Early surfactant administration with brief ventilation vs selective surfactant and continued mechanical ventilation for preterm infants with or at risk of RDS. *Cochrane Database Syst. Rev.* 2002; **2**: CD003063.

157. Tan, A., Schulze, A., O'Donnell, C.P. & Davis, P.G. Air versus oxygen for resuscitation of infants at birth. *Cochrane Database Syst. Rev.* 2005; **2**: CD002273.

158. Darioli, R. & Perret, C. Mechanical controlled hypoventilation in status asthmaticus. *Am. Rev. Respir. Dis.* 1985; **129**: 385–387.

159. Woodgate, P.G. & Davies, M.W. Permissive hypercapnia for the prevention of morbidity and mortality in mechanically ventilated newborn infants. *Cochrane Database Syst. Rev.* 2001; **2**: CD002061.

160. Henderson-Smaart, D.J., Bhuta, T., Cools, F. & Offringa, M. Elective high frequency oscillatory ventilation versus conventional ventilation for acute pulmonary dysfunction in preterm infants. *Cochrane Database Syst. Rev.* 2003; **4**: CD00104.

161. Restrepo, R.D., Pettignano, R. & DeMeuse, P. Halothane, an effective infrequently used drug, in the treatment of pediatric status asthmaticus: a case report. *J. Asthma* 2005; **42**(8): 649–651.

162. Revich, L.R., Grinspon, S.G., Parendes, C., Moreno, E., Gene, R. & Jorge, M.A. Respiratory effects of halothane in a patient with refractory status asthmmaticus. *Pulm. Pharmacol. Ther.* 2001; **14**(6): 455–460.

163. Shankar, V., Churchwell, K.B. & Deshpande, J.K. Isoflurane therapy for severe refractory status asthmaticus in children. *Int. Care Med.* 2006; May, In press.

164. Wheeler, D.S., Clapp, C.R., Ponaman, M.L., Bsn, H.M. & Poss, W.B. Isoflurane therapy for status asthmaticus in children. A case series and protocol. *Pediatr. Crit. Care Med.* 2000; **1**(1): 55–59.

165. Petrillo, T.M., Fortenberry, J.D., Linzer, J.F. & Simon, H.K. Emergency department use of ketamine in pediatric status asthmaticus. *J. Asthma* 2001; **38**(8): 657–664.

166. Saulnier, F.F., Durocher, A.V., Deturck, R.A., Lefebvre, M.C. & Wattel, F.E. Respiratory and hemodynamic effects of halothane in status asthmaticus. *Intens. Care Med.* 1990; **16**: 104–107.

167. Hegde, R.M. & Worthy, L.I. Acute asthma and the life threatening episode. *Crit. Care Resusc.* 1999; **1**(4): 371–387.

168. Hondras, M.A., Linde, K. & Jones, A.P. Manual therapy for asthma. *Cochrane Database Syst. Rev.* 2005; **2**: CD001002.

169. Afessa, B., Morales, I. & Cury, J.D. Clinical course and outcome of patients admitted to an ICU for status asthmaticus. *Chest* 2001: **120**(5): 1616–1641.

170. Khan, N., Wazir, M.S., Yasin, M., Mohammad, J. & Javed, A. Etiology, presentation and management outcome of pneumothorax. *J. Ayub Med. Coll. Abbottabad.* 2005; **17**(1): 62–64.

171. Patroniti, N., Bellani, G., Maggioni, E., Manfio, A., Marcora, B. & Pesenti, A. Measurement of pulmonary edema in patients with acute respiratory distress syndrome. *Crit. Care Med.* 2006; **33**(11): 2547–2554.

172. Sibbald, W.J., Anderson, R.R. & Holliday, R.L. Pathogenesis of pulmonary edema associated with the adult respiratory distress syndrome. *Can. Med. Assoc. J.* 1979; **120**: 445–450.

173. Matthay, M.A. & Zimmerman, G.A. Acute lung injury and the acute respiratory distress syndrome four decades of inquiry into pathogenesis and rational management. *Am. J. Respir. Cell Mol. Biol.* 2005; **33**(4): 319–327.

174. Dujon, C., Azarian, R., Mignon, F. & Petitpretz, P. Anomalous pulmonary venous drainage presenting as localized pulmonary oedema. *Rev. Mal. Respir.* 2006; **23**: 89–91.

175. Verheij, J., van Lingen, A., Raijmakers, P.G. *et al.* Effect of fluid loading with saline or colloids on pulmonary permeability, oedema and lung injury score after cardiac and major vascular surgery. *Br. J. Anesth.* 2006; **96**(1): 21–30.

176. Caples, S.M. & Gay, P.C. Noninvasive positive pressure ventilation in the intensive care unit: a concise review. *Crit. Care Med.* 2005; **33**(11): 2651–2658.

177. Villars, P., Koczka, E. & Haynie, C. The use of the laryngeal mask airway with mechanical positive pressure ventilation *AANA J.* 2005; **73**(1): 18.

178. Levine, O.R., Mellins, R.B., Senior, R.M. & Fishman, A.P. The application of Starling's law of capillary exchange to the lungs. *J. Clin. Invest.* 1967; **46**: 934–944.

179. Winck, J.C., Azevedo, L.F., Costa-Pereira, A., Antonelli, M. & Wyatt, J.C. Efficacy and safety of non-invasive ventilation in the treatment of acute cardiogenic pulomonary edema – a systematic review and meta-analysis. *Crit. Care* 2006; **10**(2): R69.

180. Peter, J.V., Moran, J.L., Phillips-Hughes, J., Graham, P. & Bersten, A.D. Effect of non-invasive positive pressure ventilation (NIPPV) on mortality in patients with acute cardiogenic pulmonary oedema: a meta-analysis. *Lancet* 2006; **367**: 1155–1163.

181. McPherson, J.J., Feigin, D.S. & Bellamy, R.F. Prevalence of tension pneumothorax in fatally wounded combat casualties. *J. Trauma* 2006; **60**(3): 573–578.

182. Soundappan, S.V., Holland, A.J., Browne, G. Sports-related pneumothorax in children. *Pediatr. Emerg. Care* 2005; **21**(4): 259–260.

183. Ladurner, R., Qvick, L.M., Hohenbleicher, F., Hallfeldt, K.K., Mutschler, W. & Mussack, T. Pneumopericardium in blunt

chest trauma after high-speed motor vehicle accidents. *Am. J. Emerg. Med.* 2005; **23**(1): 83–86.

184. Leigh-Smith, S. & Christey, G. Tension pneumothorax in asthma. *Resuscitation* 2006; Mar, In press.

185. Aul, A. & Lose, R. Invasive techniques in emergency medicine. II. Preclinical thorax drainage – indications and technique. *Anaesthesist* 2004; **53**(12): 1203–1210.

186. Sakata, K., Murayama, F., Misawa, Y., Sohara, Y., Fukushima, K., Hasegawa, T. Two cases of Marfan syndrome, surgically treated for complicating spontaneous pneumothorax. *Nippon Kyobu Geka Gakkai Zasshi* 1992; **40**(2): 286–289.

187. Peikert, T., Gillespie, D.J. & Cassivi, S.D. Catemenial pneumothorax. *Mayo Clin. Proc.* 2005; **80**(5): 477–680.

188. Pulido, T., Aranda, A., Zevallos, M.A. *et al.* Pulmonary embolism as a cause of death in patients with heart disease: an autopsy study. *Chest* 2006; **129**(5): 1282–1287.

189. Hylands, R. Pulmonary thromboembolism. *Can. Vet. J.* 2006; **47**(4): 385–388.

190. Nathan, S.S., Simmons, K.A., Lin, P.P. *et al.* Proximal deep vein thrombosis after hip replacement for oncologic indications. *J. Bone Joint Surg Am* 2006; **88**(5): 1066–1070.

191. Scatarige, J.C., Weiss, C.R., Diette, G.B., Haponik, E.F., Merriman, B. & Fishman, E.K. Scanning systems and protocols used during imaging for acute pulmonary embolism how much do our clinical colleagues know? *Acad. Radiol.* 2006; **13**(6): 678–685.

192. Nunez-Cambre, I., Argibay-Vazquez, S., Gomez-Buela, J. & Ruibal-Morell, A. Ventilation perfusion scintigraphy and CT: comparative study in the diagnosis of pulmonary thromboembolism. *Med. Clin. (Barc)* 2006; **126**: 357.

193. Bauer, M.P., Vliegen, H.W. & Huissman, M.V. Massive pulmonary embolism with cardiac arrest after an intracardiac electrophysiological study: a strong case for venous thromboprophylaxis. *Blood Coagul. Fibrinolysis* 2006; **17**(10): 57–58.

194. Theron, C. & Laidlow, D.C. Life threatening massive pulmonary embolism treated with reteplase: a case report. *Crit. Care Resusc.* 2000; **2**(4): 214–222.

195. Meneveau, N., Seronde, M.F., Blonde, M.C. *et al.* Management of unsuccessful thrombolysis in acute massive pulmonary embolism. *Chest* 2006; **129**(4): 1043–1050.

196. Aujesky, D., Mazzolai, L. & Perrier, A. The prognosis of pulmonary embolism: are there practical implications for patient management? *Rev. Med. Suisse* 2006; **2**(50): 281–284.

197. Wiles, N. & Hunt, B.J. Anticoagulation via anti-Factor Xa inhibition. *Lupus* 2006; **15**(3): 167–171.

198. Cunningham, R.S. The role of low-molecular-weight heparins as supportive care therapy in cancer-associated thrombosis. *Semin. Oncol.* 2006; **33**: S17–S25.

199. Paradis, N.A., Nowak, R.M. & Martin, G.B. Prospective resuscitation methodologies. *Top. Emerg. Med.* 1989; **11**: 77–86.

200. Benson, D.M., O'Neil, B., Kakish, E. *et al.* Open-chest CPR improves survival and neurologic outcome following cardiac arrest. *Resuscitation* 2005; **64**(2): 209–217.

201. Petrone, P. & Asensio, J.A. Trauma in pregnancy: assessment and treatment. *Scand. J. Surg.* 2006; **95**(1): 4–10.

202. Schoening, A.M. Amniotic fluid embolism: historical perspectives and new possibilities. *Am. J. Matern. Child. Nurs.* 2006; **31**(2): 78–83.

203. Mathelier, A.C. & Krachorlu, K. Placenta previa and accreta complicated by amniotic fluid embolism. *Int. J. Fertil. Wom. Med.* 2006; **51**(1): 28–32.

204. Quance, D. Amniotic fluid embolism: detection by pulse oximetry. *Anesthesiology* 1988; **68**: 951–952.

205. Luciani, N., Gaudino, M. & Possati, G. Surgical treatment of massive pulmonary embolism. *Rays* 1996; **21**(3): 432–438.

206. Tavares, B. Hymenoptera venom allergy. New diagnostic methods. *Acta Med. Port.* 2005; **18**(6): 445–452.

207. Di Lorenzo, G., Pacor, M.L., Mansueto, P. *et al.* Is there a role for antileukotrienes in urticaria? *Clin. Exp. Dermatol.* 2006; **31**(3): 327–334.

208. Marone, G., Bova, M., Detoraki, A., Onorati, A.M., Rossi, F.W. & Spadaro, G. The human heart as a shock organ in anapylaxis. *Novartis Found. Symp.* 2004; **257**: 133–149.

209. Lopez-Abad, R., Rodriguez, F., Garcia-Abujeta, J.L., Martin-Gil, D., Jerez, J. Myocardial ischemia due to severe amoxicillin allergy. *J. Investig. Allergol. Clin. Immunol.* 2004; **14**(2): 162–164.

210. Fitzharris, P., Empson, M., Ameratunga, R. *et al.* Anaphylaxis management: the essential role of adrenaline (epinephrine) auto-injectors. Should PHARMAC fund them in New Zealand? *NZ Med. J.* 2006; **119**: U1965.

211. Brown, S.G. Cardiovascular aspects of analylaxis: Implication fore treatment and diagnosis. *Curr. Opin. Allergy Clin. Immunol.* 2005; **5**(4): 359–364.

212. Morris, R.W., Watterson, L.M., Westhorpe, R.N. & Webb, R.K. Crisis management during anaesthesia: hypotension. *Qual. Saf. Health Care* 2005; **14**(3): e11.

213. Tonnel, A.B. Specific immunotherpay and therapeutic strategies in allergic diseases. What's new? *Bull. Acad. Natl Med.* 2005; **189**(7): 1475–1487.

214. Brown, S.G. Anaphylaxis: Clinical concepts and research priorities. *Emerg. Med. Aust* 2006; **18**(2): 155–169.

215. Bekkedal, M., Sipsma, K., Stremski, E.S., Malecki, K.C. & Anderson, H.A. Evaluation of five data sources for inclusion in a statewide tracking system for accidental carbon monoxide poisonings. *Wisconsin Med. J.* 2006; **105**(2): 36–40.

216. Johnson, C.D. Carbon monoxide toxicity with neurological and cardiac complications. *Bol. Asoc. Med. P. R.* 2005; **97**(4): 315–322.

217. Alonso, J.R., Cardellach, F., Lopez, S., Casademont, J. & Miro, O. Carbon monoxide specifically inhibits cytochrome c oxidase of human mitochondrial respiratory chain. *Pharmcol. Toxicol.* 2003; **93**(3): 142–146.

218. Rosenthal, L.D. Carbon monoxide poisoning. Immediate diagnosis and treatment are crucial to avoid complications. *Am. J. Nurs.* 2006; **3**: 40–46.

219. Sedda, A.F. & Rossi, G. Death scene evaluation in a case of fatal accidental carbon monoxide toxicity. *Forensic Sci. Int.* 2006;Jan, In Press.

220. Weaver, L.K. Carbon monoxide poisoning. *Crit. Care Med.* 1999; **15**(2): 297–317.

221. Hampson, N.B., Dunford, R.G., Ross, D.E. & Wreford-Brown, C.E. A prospective, randomized clinical trial comparing two hyperbolic treatment protocols for carbon monoxide poisoning. *Undersea Hyperb. Med.* 2006; **33**(1): 27–32.

222. Peddy, S.B., Rigby, M.R., Shaffner, D.H. Acute cyanide poisoning. *Pediatr. Crit. Care Med.* 2006; **7**(1): 79–82.

223. Gremion, C., Wicky, R., Niquille, M. Triage and initial treatment of house fire victims. *Rev. Med. Suisse* 2005; **1**(2): 1905–1909.

56

Hemorrhagic shock and hypovolemic cardiac arrest

James L. Atkins, Michael T. Handrigan and David Burris

Uniformed Services University of the Health Sciences, Bethesda, MD, USA

Incidence and current outcomes of post-traumatic cardiopulmonary arrest

Traumatic injury is the leading cause of death among adults under 44 years of age,[1] and it is a worldwide problem. In the year 2000, road traffic injuries were the ninth leading cause of death in the world and this toll is predicted to increase significantly in the next 15 years as road traffic injuries increase in underdeveloped countries.[2] Because traumatic injury has a predilection for the young, it is a major cause of productive life-years lost and it is predicted that by the year 2020, traumatic injury will match or surpass infectious diseases as the leading cause of productive life-years lost world-wide.[3,4] The greatest opportunity to save lives is to improve early care since the majority of traumatic deaths occur within the first few hours after injury.

In the United States as many as 34% of all trauma deaths occur pre-hospital and two major mechanisms predominate as the cause of early death: blood loss and injury to the central nervous system (CNS).[5–7] In a study by Sauaia et al. in 1995,[5] 43% of the overall deaths were due to injury to the central nervous system (CNS), 39% were relegated to exsanguination, and 7% died from multiorgan failure. More recent studies have indicated that the mortality of post-traumatic multi-organ failure is decreasing as a result of improvements in ICU care and now multi-organ failure may account for less than 4% of all traumatic deaths.[8] Multiorgan failure occurs several days after injury while the majority of both CNS and hemorrhage deaths occur within the first 2 hours of injury.[5,9] In the study by Sauaia

et al,[5] exanguination was the most common cause of death among those found dead at the scene and it was the most frequent cause of early hospital deaths. Interventions that may improve early survival include resuscitation after cardiopulmonary arrest (CPR) and therapies aimed at preventing imminent arrest. To date, the results with CPR after trauma (TCPR) have not been encouraging.

Survival rates of pre-hospital closed-chest cardiopulmonary resuscitation after trauma (TCPR) are quite low.[10] Despite an early encouraging report to the contrary by Copass et al.[11] which demonstrated 23% survival in pre-hospital TCPR, numerous subsequent studies have found dismal results with survival rates varying between 0 and 2.6%.[10,12–18] The reason for this discrepancy is not clear, although the study by Copass et al.[11] had a very high prevalence of penetrating injury in the group of survivors. The group of surviving patients included 60% with penetrating injuries and 40% with blunt injuries, while the non-surviving group included 95% with blunt injury and 5% with penetrating injuries. A more favorable outcome of TCPR in patients with penetrating injuries has been seen in some[17] but not all subsequent studies.[12,14,16] There is one subgroup of patients with penetrating injury that may have a clear survival advantage in TCPR, however; that is, patients with isolated penetrating injury to the thorax who can be rapidly transported to the trauma center to receive open-chest CPR and injury repair.[10] More favorable outcome might also be expected in patients with special conditions such as victims of drowning and lightning strike, victims with significant hypothermia, and patients

Disclaimer

The opinions or assertion contained herein are the private views of the authors and are not to be construed as official or reflecting the views of the Department of the Army or the Department of Defense.

in whom the mechanism of injury does not correlate with the clinical condition suggesting a non-traumatic cause of the arrest. The paper by Copass et al.[11] made mention of another special circumstance, the patient with an isolated head injury who is apneic. They proposed that "successful establishment of an endotracheal tube may be lifesaving" in this circumstance. With the increasing frequency of explosive injuries it might be argued that blast-induced apnea[19-22] warrants the same special consideration.

The dire results with TCPR have led several groups to evaluate the risks versus benefits of pre-hospital TCPR. In these considerations the risk-benefit analysis is somewhat unusual, because often the risk evaluated is to the provider while the potential benefit is to the victim. One example of such an evaluation is the consideration of medical care on the battlefield. In a tactical situation when the health care providers are under real risk of receiving fire, the danger to the health care provider administering CPR is quite substantial, and the resources diverted to that likely futile effort might endanger both the security of the team and the ability to provide care to other more salvageable casualties. Under such conditions TCPR is not advised.[23,24] In a peacetime civilian setting the risks to the provider are certainly lower but they may nonetheless be substantial. Recently the National Association of EMS Physicians and the American College of Surgeons Committee on Trauma (NAEMSP/ACSCOTS) have published a position statement proposing guidelines for withholding or terminating resuscitation in prehospital TCPR.[10] In this paper they consider the inherent costs and risks to the community and healthcare providers: (1) "trauma resuscitation consumes significant amounts of ED, operating room, and intensive care unit resources," (2) "there is significant risk for EMS crews and the public associated with emergency transport" and (3) "the chaotic environment of trauma resuscitations may pose a heightened risk of blood-borne pathogen exposure to the involved health care workers." On the basis of these considerations the committee listed specific clinical situations where they believed the likelihood of success is so low that CPR should not be recommended. The debate over these issues is ongoing and recently Pickens et al.[25] have evaluated the guidelines of NAEMO/ACSCOT and concluded that the required clinical assessments could not be obtained reliably in prehospital urban settings. In that study, which had an overall survival to discharge of 7.6%, they concluded that the NAEMO/ACSCOT guidelines might not be applicable to urban systems with rapid transport to a Level 1 Trauma Center. In addition to the consideration that rapid transport to a trauma center may provide improved clinical assessment, rapid transport may also provide the opportunity to have the patient arrive at a Level 1 trauma center before 15 minutes of CPR have elapsed. Both animal[26] and clinical studies indicate a poor outcome is more likely if closed-chest CPR has continued for more than 15 minutes.[14,27] Hence, arrival at a Level 1 center before 15 minutes of closed-chest CPR may provide an opportunity for successful open-chest CPR.

Animal studies have shown that open chest CPR is more effective than closed-chest CPR and produces higher perfusion pressures of the coronaries and brain.[26] Clinical studies seem to confirm better outcomes. A study by Lorenz et al.[28] showed overall 13% survival with open chest CPR, with 2% survival in blunt trauma and 22% survival in penetrating trauma. This confirmed the bias that open chest CPR is more effective in penetrating trauma; however, Fialka et al.[29] have recently found similar survival rates (10%) in open chest CPR in casualties with blunt trauma to the chest or abdomen. In this study all traumatic arrests with severe blunt chest or abdominal trauma isolated or in combination with other injuries were included in the study if the victims were less than 70 years of age and had a documented resuscitation duration of less than 20 minutes. Hachimi-Idrissi et al.[30] studied out-of-hospital open chest CPR and found survival rates of 6%; moreover, they report that the procedure was well accepted by the populace of Belgium.

The NAEMO/ACSCOT guidelines paper emphasizes that their recommendations are based on available research to date and are subject to change as advances are made in the care of the trauma patient.[10] Much of the rest of this chapter will focus on recent research advances that hold promise to improve the treatment of TCPR or to prevent imminent cardiac arrest. We will also explore more basic mechanisms in the body's response to hemorrhage that may account for some of the failures of TCPR and, it is to be hoped, indicate potential new avenues of research.

Research that promises to improve the outcome of TCPR in the future

Emergency preservation and resuscitation (EPR)

Animal studies have examined profound hypothermia as a means to extend the period of time during which surgical repair can be accomplished. Very promising results have been seen in both swine[31-33] and dogs.[34] Following cardiac arrest from hemorrhage, profound hypothermia (core temperature of 10 °C) was induced by rapid cold aortic flush (normal saline at 2 °C at 1.7 l/min in dogs) until core temperature was 10 °C and hypothermia was maintained for 60 minutes. Rewarming was accomplished by cardiopulmonary bypass. After recovery for 72 hours (dogs) or 6 weeks (swine) brain histology and cognitive function were normal. Recently Nozari *et al.*[35] have extended their large series of studies[34,36] to examine the consequence of adding trauma to the hemorrhage model. Splenic injury was induced prior to the hemorrhage. During the profound hypothermia, the spleen was resected and the animals underwent left thoracotomy. Even though there was still 100% survival in all groups, half of the trauma animals (4) had neurologic deficits and three required prolonged mechanical ventilation. The addition of plasma exchange allowed full neurologic recovery even after a 2-hour period of no-flow.[37] This technology may provide sufficient time for repair of even very severe and otherwise unsalvageable vascular injuries in a controlled manner.

Improved ventilation strategies

Hemorrhage sufficient to lower central volume can severely limit venous return and theoretically make it impossible to attain adequate coronary and cerebral perfusion pressure during CPR. The absolute limit to this is total exsanguination after which external chest compressions would essentially squeeze an "empty heart." Cardiac arrest can occur in hemorrhage before there is true exanguination, however, and methods that redistribute the blood to the central core or improve cardiac return have the potential to improve the outcome of TCPR. One such approach is to limit the duration of positive interthoracic pressure during TCPR.

It has been appreciated for some time that positive pressure ventilation can quickly exacerbate a tension pneumothorax and significantly decrease venous return, but recent studies have focused on a much more subtle and more common event that also decreases cardiac return, albeit to a less but still quite significant degree. Positive pressure ventilation decreases cardiac return by raising interthoracic pressure and this effect may be most critical in hypovolemic states.[38] To demonstrate this point, Pepe *et al.*[39,40] recently studied the effect of changes in the rate of positive pressure ventilation in swine with a moderate degree of hemorrhage. Elevated ventilatory rates of 20 and 30 breaths per minute caused a fall in diastolic blood pressure and decreased coronary perfusion pressure as compared to ventilatory rates of 6 breaths per minute. Based on this evidence, the authors raise the concern that rapid ventilatory rates for trauma resuscitation could significantly impair hemodynamics. Krismer *et al.*[41] have examined the use of positive end expiratory pressure (PEEP) after intubation of hemorrhaged swine that had not received fluid

resuscitation. Those treated with PEEP of 5 or 10 cm water had significantly decreased survival compared with those treated with 0 PEEP. Although not directly tested, it might be expected that the same principles apply to animals that arrest as a result of hemorrhage and lower ventilatory rates without PEEP could improve the outcome of TCPR by improving average cardiac return.

A corollary of this concept is that increases in negative interthoracic pressure would improve venous return. It is likely that the body's own compensatory response takes advantage of this concept by the increased ventilatory drive and respiratory alkalosis seen in early hemorrhage and early sepsis. This benefit can be enhanced by the use of a respiratory impedance threshold device (ITD). This valve creates more negative interthoracic pressure during ventilation. It improves blood pressure in hemorrhaged swine with both unassisted ventilation[42] and with ventilation assisted by a phrenic nerve stimulator.[43] In stimulated blood loss in humans accomplished by using lower body negative pressure, the impedance threshold valve improved velocity of cerebral blood flow and preliminary results showed an increase in stroke volume.[44] The ITD coupled to a vacuum source for the generation of controlled – 10 cm water vacuum in the trachea during the decompression phase of CPR, has been shown to improve both cerebral and coronary perfusion pressure during CPR of anesthetized swine in which ventricular fibrillation (VF) cardiac arrest was induced by intracardiac direct electrical current.[45] There was also a remarkable increase in short term survival from 10 to 100% in this group. Hemodynamic parameters were also examined in a group of animals that were subjected to hemorrhage 50% of their estimated blood volume before induction of VF cardiac arrest. These animals also had a significant, but less dramatic, improvement in coronary and cerebral perfusion pressures. Survival was not examined in the hemorrhaged animals.

The results are exciting and provide real hope that changes in pre-hospital ventilatory strategies may prevent arrest in some trauma victims with marginal cardiac return. Moreover, the use of the ITD holds the promise to improve TCPR. Nevertheless, there are still some complexities of CPR after hemorrhage that have not yet been examined with this new methodology. Induction of VF after hemorrhage in propofol-anesthetized animals does not mimic some important features of cardiac arrest after hemorrhage. Cardiac arrest in conscious animals after hemorrhage involves a loss of vasoconstrictor activity and increased vascular compliance. ITD alone may not overcome these additional impediments to venous return and additional therapies may be required to create effective CPR after hemorrhagic arrest. An additive approach to increased venous return may be the use of vasoconstrictors to decrease vascular compliance in non-critical vascular beds.

Hemorrhage-induced vascular collapse

At first glance vasoconstrictors would appear to be an unsuitable adjunctive therapy for the treatment of hemorrhage-associated arrest, because total peripheral resistance is normally increased after hemorrhage, sometimes quite remarkably. In cases of limited fluid resuscitation there are anecdotal stories of alert patients presenting with such severe peripheral vasoconstriction that no peripheral pulses were apparent and there was no bleeding from severed brachial arteries or amputated extremities until fluid resuscitation was initiated. There are animal studies, however, that show specific circumstances when these predominantly vasoconstrictor responses fail. In these circumstances, cardiac arrest ensues in part from an apparently inappropriate vasodilatation or loss of vasoconstrictor action. Two distinct mechanisms have been described that would be expected to occur in two very different circumstances. The literature is somewhat confounded because both of these mechanisms are normally referred to as "irreversible shock" and/or "compensatory failure".[46–49] In order to provide perspective we will first describe the normal sequential responses to continued hemorrhage and then discuss how and when "compensatory failure" may occur.

The body's initial response to hemorrhage is a beautifully orchestrated combination of events involving a delicate balance between an intense increase in vasoconstrictor activity[50] and a large increase in the production of the vasodilator nitric oxide.[51] The net balance of these mediators differs among vascular beds and the systemic effect involves both an increase in total peripheral resistance, which tends to preserve sufficient blood pressure to maintain tissue perfusion, and a redistribution of cardiac output, which tends to preserve blood flow to the coronary and cerebral circulations at the expense of other vascular beds.[50]

In conscious animals, the initial compensatory response to hemorrhage involves a baroreflex-mediated increase in sympathetic activity and a decrease in parasympathetic activity that results in a decrease in vascular conductance and an increase in heart rate. The central pathways involved in this response are quite complex. Numerous neurotransmitters have been implicated in the efferent pathways including classical neurotransmitters, vasopressin,[52,53] histamine,[54] neuropeptides, including CRH, opioids,[49,55] serotonin,[56] neuropeptide Y and galanin, and gaseous mediators like nitric oxide and carbon monoxide.[57] In addition to these complex central pathways, descending autonomic visceromotor cells are activated. The net result of this response is that in awake animals blood pressure is maintained during the initial few minutes of hemorrhage. If rapid hemorrhage continues blood pressure will begin to fall.[58] Somewhat surprisingly this fall in blood pressure is caused in part by a decrease in sympathetic tone and in part by a global vasodilation. Sympathetic tone to most organs will decrease and heart rate will fall in a process referred to as hemorrhage-induced sympathoinhibition (HISI). The fall in blood pressure results in increased production of nitric oxide, which compounds the insult and also contributes to the fall in blood pressure.[59] If the hemorrhage continues at a rapid rate, the combination of these two events results in a further fall in blood pressure to low levels, despite the brisk release of renin, epinephrine and vasopressin. Eventually blood pressure will be too low to preserve perfusion to the coronaries and brain, and ventilatory arrest and death will ensue. The cardiac output threshold for the onset of HISI is influenced by differences in PaO_2[60,61] and various drugs such as α_2-adrenergic antagonists, and perhaps vasopressin and renin.[62] Some controversy exists whether naloxone also influences this threshold.[63–65]

If the initial rate of bleeding was not as fast, the animal may exhibit spontaneous recovery of blood pressure.[66] Angiotensin II and vasopressin are important in this recovery,[67] which appears to be adversely affected by combined brain injury.[68,69] The recovery of blood pressure after severe hemorrhage has also been seen in clinical trials in which little or no fluid resuscitation is given in the initial management of the patient.[70] If blood pressure recovery is adequate then it may tend to remain at the recovery level for some period of time. If the total oxygen debt has already been substantial, however, or if moderate hemorrhage continues, the animals may remain hypotensive or fall back to hypotensive levels where they can remain for some period of time. They can maintain sufficient blood pressure to assure perfusion of critical tissues by a continued rise in total peripheral resistance. During this period of time increased plasma and tissue levels of endothelin have been documented along with increased levels of angiotensin II, but after some time, peripheral resistance will gradually start to fall.

This relatively late fall in peripheral resistance is seen in both awake and anesthetized animals and it occurs at the same time that there is a generalized loss of vascular responsiveness to the vasoconstrictors adrenaline and angiotensin II. This decrease in responsiveness is seen as early as 1 hour after the onset of hypotension in some vascular beds,[71–73] but a systemic decrease in total peripheral resistance can require as long as 2–4 hours of hypotension.[74] The progressive decline in total peripheral resistance likely results from the progressive involvement of more vessels in the phenomenon.

The mechanism of the loss of responsiveness to epinephrine and angiotensin II is not fully explained, but it is associated with increased production of nitric oxide,[71,75] and it may be mediated through an opening of the K-ATP channel in vascular smooth muscle.[74,76] Non-selective nitric oxide synthase inhibition[71,72] and K-ATP channel blockade[76–79] can both return the vascular responsiveness. The continued production of nitric oxide during hemorrhage and the accumulation of nitric oxide adducts like S-nitrosylated proteins[51] may contribute indirectly. It has recently been shown that S-nitrosylation of the RAS/mitogen-activated protein kinase in brain leads to opening of the K-ATP channels.[80] Several other factors in this stage of shock also seem to target this channel, including intercellular acidosis, and decrease in intercellular ATP.[81] The opening of this channel results in hyperpolarization of the vascular smooth muscle, and vasodilation. This process, which also occurs in septic shock, is termed "vasodilatory shock". The net effect may be compounded in hemorrhage by accumulation of extracellular potassium,[82–87] which appears to be mediated in part by loss of transport function of Na-K ATPase.[87] Both uncoupling of the Na-K-ATPase[87] and the presence of an inhibitor[88] have been proposed as the mechanism, but the inhibitor appears to be different from the circulating ouabain-like factor that has recently been shown to be decreased in hemorrhagic shock.[89] The increase in extracellular potassium concentrations to 10–15 mmol[82,84] can contribute to the vasodilation[90] in part by the opening of another related potassium channel, the inward rectified potassium channel (Kir). The importance of these potassium changes has recently been emphasized by the findings of Darlington and Gann who have shown that administration of purine nucleosides[91] especially adenosine[92,93] can increase Na/K ATPase activity, prevent the rise in plasma potassium, and improve survival in hemorrhagic shock. Previous studies have also shown that the protection afforded by modest hypothermia correlates most closely with a slower rise in plasma potassium.[94]

At the late stage of shock there is also a fall in peripheral vasopressin levels perhaps due to depletion of central stores. The hyperpolarization of the vascular smooth muscle and a fall in peripheral vasopressin levels combine to cause a gradual fall in peripheral resistance. At this stage there is also evidence of increased vascular permeability,[95] and although blood pressure can be sustained for some period of time by continued volume replacement, eventually only massive volume infusions[48] are effective in maintaining a life-sustaining blood pressure.

In summary, there are two different mechanisms of vascular collapse following hemorrhage: (1) HISI, which is seen in awake man and animals very early after the start of rapid hemorrhage; and (2) vasodilatory shock, which is seen in both awake and anesthetized animals after a significant oxygen debt. The timing for onset of HISI is minutes after the start of hemorrhage. The timing for onset of vasodilatory shock is variable and will occur as early as half an hour after injury if the hypotension is severe, and as late as several hours if the hypotension is modest. Both mechanisms of vascular collapse can be averted if blood pressure is restored early after hemorrhage by fluid and/or blood resuscitation, but if cardiac arrest intervenes it is possible that the ability to perfuse the brain and coronaries during cardiac compressions is limited by the same mechanisms that initially caused the vascular collapse. Direct evidence for this hypothesis is lacking, but circumstantial evidence implicates HISI in the events surrounding cardiac arrest: (1) HISI is heralded by a fall in heart rate and this biphasic heart rate response to hemorrhage (increased early and then decreased during HISI) may partially account for the finding that heart rate is an unreliable marker of the severity of hemorrhage; (2) HISI may account for the finding that bradycardic rhythms (heart rate below 40 beats per minute) after TCPR are associated with particularly poor outcomes; and (3) HISI is also associated with a marked reduction in oxygen consumption and a fall in core temperature.[96] Hypothermia after severe hemorrhage has also been associated with dismal outcomes. We consider below therapies that may be effective in reversing hemorrhage-induced vascular collapse. Although the two mechanisms may share some common pathways, more targeted therapy may be required that is specific to the mechanism of vascular decompensation.

Therapies to reverse the systemic vasodilation that occurs during rapid hemorrhage

Although HISI is heralded by a fall in heart rate, atropine will not increase blood pressure, even though it does increase the heart rate. Since vasopressin and angiotensin II appear to be involved in spontaneous recovery under normal circumstances, they would be likely as candidates to improve the effectiveness of CPR. Seki *et al.*[97] have shown that low dose hypertonic saline causes sympathetic activation. Two studies evaluated[98,99] vasopressin in model of uncontrolled hemorrhage in pigs. The trigger for vasopressin infusion was a fall in heart rate that occurred surprisingly late at 30 minutes after onset of hemorrhage. Vasopressin increased heart rate and blood pressure without causing further bleeding, and resulted in improved survival. Nevertheless, it is not completely clear if the mechanism of cardiovascular collapse in these studies was HISI or vasodilatory shock. Exciting recent work by Osei-Owusu and Scrogin[100] has shown that Buspirone raises blood pressure after HISI through sympathetic activation and direct activation of α1-adrenergic receptors.

The increased production of nitric oxide as the blood pressure falls in HISI may be more amenable to intervention. Transient non-selective inhibition of nitric oxide synthase (NOS) effectively delays vascular collapse, but this approach to urgent reversal of HISI may be confounded by the finding that there is a significant non-NOS source of nitric oxide during cardiac arrest.[101] Therefore, mechanisms that absorb NO or increase its metabolism may be more effective. Hyperoxia decreases the vasodilatory effect of nitric oxide in two ways, by shortening its half-life (measured in seconds) and by blocking the release of S-nitrosothiols from the red blood cells.[102] Because of increased nitric oxide production and increased formation of S-nitrosothiols,[51] the vasoconstrictor effect of hyperoxia is greatly enhanced early after hemorrhage. Breathing 100% oxygen early after hemorrhage causes a large increase in total peripheral resistance in rats that is associated with an increase in heart rate, cardiac output, plasma norepinephrine, and myocardial contractility(Atkins, unpublished). The sum of these effects results in an increase in mean arterial blood pressure of 60 mmHg, which occurs within 30 seconds of changing the inspired gas to 100% oxygen.[103] PaO_2 averages around 400 mmHg on 100% oxygen, and most of the blood pressure change is seen with inspired oxygen at 60%. The increase in heart rate is prevented by the serotonin blocker ketanserin, but the increase in blood pressure is not prevented by ketanserin, allopurinol, or indomethacin, indicating that this may be a direct effect of decreasing nitric oxide-induced vasodilation. Hyperoxia in early hemorrhage results in a favorable redistribution of cardiac output, causing vasoconstriction in the skeletal muscle[104] and an increase in carotid blood flow.[103] This action may account for the improved survival seen with oxygen inhalation in controlled hemorrhagic shock;[105,106] however, this benefit is not universally seen in uncontrolled hemorrhage,[107,108] presumably because of the increased bleeding caused by the rise in blood pressure. In summary, the results suggest that breathing 100% oxygen may help in reversing HISI.

The desired benefit depends on decreasing levels of nitric oxide rather than meeting tissue oxygen requirements. Nevertheless, high concentrations would be required, and effective delivery during TCPR may be limited by restraints on the use of positive pressure ventilation discussed above. The use of perflurocarbons[109–111] and artificial hemoglobins[112] would also be expected to increase the metabolism of nitric oxide without the same constraints.

The systemic vasodilation resulting from opening of the K-ATP channels in vascular smooth muscle can be reversed by infusion of K-ATP channel blockers glibenclimide and glibizide.[76–79] Vasopressin infusion can also increase blood pressure and prolong survival in very late stage of hemorrhage-induced vasodilatory shock in animals.[113–115,98,116] Evidence suggests that low dose vasopressin may be the most appropriate.[117] On the basis of these promising results in studies of near cardiac arrest it seems reasonable that these same therapies could be useful adjuncts in TCPR, and indeed initial clinical case reports support this conclusion.[118]

Successful TCPR in patients with very rapid hemorrhage and HISI will also certainly require some means to stop the bleeding in the field since effective TCPR with return of spontaneous circulation would likely result in the reinstitution of massive bleeding. Although the relatively selective vasoconstriction of vasopressin may be effective in abdominal bleeding,[114] it is easier to envision success in patients with bleeding in an extremity, in whom the application of a tourniquet before TCPR may prevent a life-threatening rebleed.[119] The population that would likely benefit from glibenclimide or vasopressin are patients with delayed transport to a trauma center.

In summary, recent results make it more likely than ever that the results of TCPR can be dramatically improved in the future by combined strategies of selective vasoconstriction and improved ventilatory techniques. More directed research is needed in this unique cause of cardiac arrest.

Moreover, there may be even more potential to save lives if cardiac arrest can be prevented. In the next sections below, we will discuss therapies and recent advances that may help to prevent cardiac arrest after trauma.

Therapeutic interventions for HS (avenues for the advancement of trauma care)

Clearly, the most effective way of reducing morbidity and mortality related to traumatic arrest is to improve the initial management for the victim of traumatic shock and impending arrest. The approach to resuscitation of the trauma patient follows a very logical and time-honored sequence designed to address life-threatening conditions in a hierarchical and systematic manner: that is to say, the ABC's of trauma treatment. This general approach has provided remarkable improvement and standardization in the prehospital treatment of multiple trauma victims over the last several decades. With this framework of Airway-Breathing-Circulation in mind, we can now consider advanced therapeutic interventions for use during the initial resuscitation that may delay or eliminate the onset of traumatic arrest.

Airway

Airway control remains the first and foremost concern in trauma care. Without adequate airway control all other interventions are destined to fail. Clearly, the importance of simple airway control can not be overstated. Nevertheless, airway manipulation in trauma patients is not without its drawbacks. Positive pressure ventilation results in increased intrathoracic pressure and a concomitant decrease in venous return and diminished cardiac output. This is particularly important in conditions related to volume depletion, such as hemorrhagic shock.[120] Indeed, the application of endotracheal intubation and positive pressure ventilation may exacerbate the already tenuous hemodynamic state and convert impending arrest to full arrest.[121]

Some investigators have begun to explore the reverse effect of this phenomenon as a mode of intervention. That is, to create a relatively negative intrathoracic pressure by way of airway impedance. The result of this maneuver is to create an intrathoracic vacuum effect, thereby improving venous return and cardiac output. Thus, Lurie and coworkers have developed a inspiratory impedance threshold valve for use during active compression–decompression (ACD) cardiopulmonary resuscitation.[122] The device has been shown to improve perfusion of vital organs during resuscitation and has proven to be effective when used during ACD–CPR.[123,124] Investigators have recently demonstrated that such a device may also be effective in preventing circulatory collapse-associated hemorrhagic shock before full arrest in both animal models,[125,126] and in human studies.[127] Use of an impedance device may be a very simple and reliable method for the field stabilization of the trauma victim.

Breathing

Hemorrhagic shock, a low-flow state created by depletion of blood volume, leads to decreased cardiac output, reduced hemoglobin concentration, and alterations in microcirculatory blood flow directly resulting in impaired tissue oxygenation, and thus the accumulation of a cellular oxygen debt.[128] This fundamental precept has led to the nearly universal use of supplemental oxygen in the treatment of traumatic hemorrhage. Although, aside from the very basic goal of improving tissue oxygenation by increasing the available partial pressure of inspired oxygen, supplemental oxygen therapy may have a more subtle benefit for the trauma patient. Sukhotnik and coworkers have demonstrated in several models of hemorrhagic shock that oxygen therapy exerts an independent salutary effect on blood pressure, resulting in redistribution of blood flow from skeletal muscle to the splanchnic and renal vascular beds, which they believe to be a critical component of the beneficial effects of hyperoxia following hemorrhage.[107] Nevertheless, this therapy may increase the risk of bleeding in uncontrolled hemorrhage.[107,108]

As noted above, positive pressure ventilation can have negative hemodynamic effects for the volume-depleted patient. Recently, Pepe and coworkers have proposed an alternative strategy of reduced ventilatory rates aimed at limiting this detrimental effect. Experimental evidence from a swine model of hemorrhagic shock suggests that ventilatory rates as low as 6 breaths per minute can reduce the undesirable intrathoracic pressure changes associated with PPV without adversely affecting oxygenation or acid-base status.[121,129]

Oxygenation is a critical consideration for the patient with traumatic shock. The use of supplemental oxygen may need more careful evaluation because of the potential to increase bleeding. This is a recurrent theme in which inappropriate use of therapeutics that increase blood pressure may result in increased bleeding and prove to be counterproductive. Providing appropriate guidelines for such interventions may prove to be a substantive challenge.

Circulation

Hemorrhage control

The first rule in stabilizing the victim of hemorrhage is to prevent further blood loss. This emphasis has changed very little over time. Whereas, the application of pressure dressings or tourniquets to a wounded extremity remains the mainstay of hemorrhage control in the field, bleeding from non-compressible sites, such as organ injury or proximal vascular injury, continues to represent a significant cause of hemorrhage-related mortality. Approximately 30% of trauma-related deaths result from blood loss alone.[130] To address this problem, considerable attention has been given to the use of both topical and systemic application of procoagulants to stem the tide of blood loss.

Multiple forms of hemostatic wound dressings impregnated with procoagulant compounds have been developed and tested.[131] Active procoagulant compounds used in such hemostatic bandages have included: chitosan, oxidized cellulose, thrombin, fibrinogen, microfibrillar collagen, propyl gallate, aluminum sulfate, and acetylated poly-*N*-acetylglucosamine. A recent direct comparison of several available preparations was conducted in a swine liver injury model. This study demonstrated that a dressing that utilized human fibrinogen, purified human thrombin, factor XIII, and $CaCl_2/cm^2$ freeze dried onto an absorbable polygalactin mesh was most effective,[132] whereas other investigators have shown a chitosan dressing consistently failed within 2 hours after application.[133] In any event, there are sure to be rapid advances in the science of external, emergency hemorrhage control in the near term.

The systemic administration of procoagulants may provide an important advantage to victims of trauma.[134] A retrospective review of in-hospital patients found that 8% of post-traumatic deaths occurred in the operating room. Of these patients, 82% died of uncontrolled hemorrhage and one-quarter of these deaths were attributable to coagulopathy.[135] There are no comparable data on how often coagulopathy contributes to prehospital deaths, but recent data by Brohi *et al.*[136] indicates that a significant number of trauma victims present to the trauma center with a coagulopathy that is not related to the amount of fluid administered, but correlates with the injury severity score. Patients who present with the "fatal triad of death:" acidosis, coagulopathy, and hypothermia, have several independent markers predicting bad outcome.

Although there can be numerous causes of coagulopathy in trauma victims, pharmaceutically enhanced hemostasis has two potential beneficial effects. First, and obviously, it may decrease the amount of initial blood loss, thereby reducing the traumatic insult. Secondly, it may help prevent the hypothermia, acidosis, and dilutional coagulopathy associated with massive transfusions.[137] Interruption of the fatal cycle of worsening hypothermia, coagulopathy, and acidosis may offer a necessary boost needed by these patients. The procoagulant drug that currently appears to be most promising is recombinant factor VIIa (rfVIIa).[138] Boffard and co-workers recently conducted a drug company-sponsored randomized trial of rfVIIa for hemorrhage from both blunt and penetrating trauma.[139] The study demonstrated convincingly that this drug can reduce the overall massive transfusion requirements after blunt trauma, with a similar trend seen in patients with penetrating trauma. While the differences in mortality and reduction in critical complications were less convincing, the drug was shown to be safe in this critically injured population. This may not be a giant leap forward for reduction in trauma mortality, but it is an encouraging advance for the concept of pharmaceutically enhanced hemostasis. A recent review by Ho *et al.*[140] has proposed that the reversal of coagulopathy may be improved with better guidelines for replacement of blood products.

Fluid resuscitation and hemodynamic stabilization

Following adequate airway control, breathing, and the control of hemorrhage, the next step in the standard resuscitation algorithm is to provide fluid resuscitation as needed for hemodynamic stability. The age-old argument of whether to use a crystalloid or colloid fluid for this has evolved into a much more complex and nuanced discussion concerning multiple variables, including volume of resuscitation, blood pressure limits, and an assortment of new fluid choices and additives designed to modulate vascular tone and immune responses. The ideal resuscitative fluid would simulate all of the positive properties of whole blood, be universally acceptable, inhibit further blood loss, abrogate the negative inflammatory consequences of traumatic hemorrhagic shock and subsequent intervention, and provide for hemodynamic stability at low infusion volumes.[141] Consequently, considerable research has been conducted to assess these individual components of resuscitation with the eventual hope of bringing them all together in a simple, easy to use package.

Aggressive fluid resuscitation to normal or even near normal blood pressures has been challenged as a dangerous maneuver likely to lead to exacerbation of blood loss, particularly in patients with non-compressible or uncontrolled hemorrhage.[142,143] This has led to the acceptance of hypotensive resuscitation as a standard of care in some trauma communities.[144,145] The benefit of hypotensive resuscitation for reducing hemorrhage in patients without adequate bleed control is clearly intuitive and has become generally accepted. This approach may also be beneficial in victims with profound blood loss even with adequate hemorrhage control, particularly when there is a delay to definitive care.[66] Currently, hypotensive resuscitation is a concept that is rapidly gaining acceptance in the medical community, but as yet, it is far from a standardized approach ready for insertion into the ACLS guideline. Nonetheless, the benefits of hypotensive resuscitation and the disadvantages of aggressive fluid resuscitation deserve careful consideration. One particular cause of concern is the possibility that hypotensive resuscitation may result in increased incidence of coagulopathy or multiorgan failure.

Late deaths due to multiple organ failure

Multiple organ failure (MOF), or multiple organ dysfunction syndrome (MODS), was previously considered to be the leading cause of death after severe trauma.[146] This became particularly apparent as trauma care improved between the 1970s and 1980s, resulting in more patients surviving their initial injury to develop MOF.[147] Over the last decade, as trauma care has continued to improve, this trend has been reversed, leading to an overall reduction in the mortality risk associated with MOF after traumatic hemorrhage.[148,149] But, despite this encouraging progress, MOF remains an important cause of morbidity after trauma resuscitation and thus continues to be a therapeutic problem for ICU patients.[150]

This may be particularly true for patients surviving an initial arrest and in patients suffering from profound hypovolemic shock. Recent progress concerning the etiology and progression of MOF may offer important insights into possible early therapeutic interventions. The two-hit model proposed by Moore *et al.*[151] continues to play a central role in our understanding of the progress of MOF. Recent work has shown that the development of MOF is likely to be a complex and multifactorial process, with multiple immunologic and molecular events promoting its onset and influencing its severity. MOF is essentially the result of an overexuberant humeral and cellular inflammatory response leading to the expression and release of numerous mediators, such as toxic oxygen species, proteolytic enzymes, adherence molecules, and cytokines.[152]

The initiating events in MOF after shock may occur very early in the course of hemorrhage and mitigation of these events during the initial resuscitation effort may significantly reduce the likelihood of developing MOF following resuscitation. Some of the more important second hit events that may promote the onset of MOF appear to be related to abdominal compartment syndrome,[153] immune activation by postshock mesenteric lymph,[154] red blood cell transfusion,[155] and intravenous fluid infusion itself.[156–159] An early resuscitation strategy designed to mitigate these inflammatory consequences while providing life-saving hemodynamic support may help to decrease further both trauma-related MOF mortality and morbidity. A detailed discussion of the biology of MOF is beyond the scope of this chapter. We will, however, address some of the recent findings concerning the initiation of MOF and possible strategies of early manipulation below.

Immune modulation

Primary immune stimulation in response to trauma, in addition to secondary stimulation due to a subsequent insult such as surgical intervention, infection, and resuscitative interventions, plays an important role in the natural course of trauma. As noted above, the molecular events responsible for the systemic response to traumatic insult may occur very early in the course of injury and treatment. As such, manipulation or modulation of these events during initial resuscitation may offer an effective means of mitigating an exuberant and disruptive inflammatory response. A detailed description of all of the inflammatory consequences of traumatic hemorrhage is beyond the scope of this chapter. Here we will highlight some of the significant contributors to the inflammatory response along with their potential interventions.

The systemic response to traumatic hemorrhage begins with immediate changes in intravascular volume and autonomic discharge intended to redistribute blood flow to critical vascular beds. While these natural responses are intended to prevent irreversible damage to critical organs, the overall cardiovascular effect of significant hemorrhage results in decreased oxygen delivery, decreased tissue perfusion, cellular hypoxia, and organ damage.[160] The resulting stress on vascular endothelium leads to increased platelet aggregation and neutrophil infiltration mediated in part by the release of platelet activating factor (PAF).[161] This microvascular injury is responsible for changes in endothelial integrity that provide a nidus for the inflammatory cascade, which ultimately results in the generalized release of proinflammatory cytokines such as TNF-, IL-1, and IL-6.[162,163] TNF has recently been shown to play a critical upstream role in left ventricular dysfunction after hemorrhage resuscitation.[164] IL-6 is a very consistent marker of injury after hemorrhage resuscitation, so it very surprising that early infusion of IL-6 blunts production of proinflammatory cytokines.[165] The results suggests that IL-6 may be a basic compensatory response to injury rather than a proinflammatory mediator. Recent studies by Tracey and colleagues have identified a pro-inflammatory cytokine that is released late after injury, HMGBI.[166] This may provide a therapeutic target suitable for late interventions.

The early hemodynamic and inflammatory response to hemorrhage also involves the stimulation of nitric oxide (NO) production via constitutively expressed and inducible NO synthases. NO has been shown to exert both local and systemic effects. The immediate local consequence of increased NO concentration is vasodilation, and this along with increased production of carbon monoxide[167] serves to preserve tissue perfusion in the face of the release of potent vasoconstrictors. The appearance of inducible NOS is a relatively late event after hemorrhage,[168] but it has been associated with increased liver,[169,170] gut[171] and lung injury,[172] and the induction of pro-inflammatory cytokines.[173] The interactions of induced heat shock protein, heme oxidase, and inducible NOS, however, are complex and the overall effect on tissue injury or protection is not determined by the expression of a single mediator.[174,175] During resuscitation, increased oxygen tension in the tissues and the production of oxygen radicals can react with nitric oxide from any source and with the nitric oxide adducts accumulated during the period of hypotension to produce reactive nitrogen species, such as NO_3^- and peroxynitrite.[176] Recent work has been designed to interrupt the NO-dependent consequences of these reactive oxygen species. McDonald and coworkers have shown that highly selective inhibitors of iNOS activity may effectively attenuate renal dysfunction as well as liver and pancreatic injury caused by hemorrhage and resuscitation .[177] A membrane-permeable radical scavenger (tempol) has been shown to delay circulatory failure as well as multiple organ injury and dysfunction associated with hemorrhagic shock.[178] Thus a strategy designed to prevent the formation of reactive nitrogen species may represent a novel early therapeutic intervention for hemorrhagic shock.

The gastrointestinal tract may be a particularly important source of posthemorrhage cytokines,[179] and injury to the gut is thought to play a pivotal role in the pathogenesis of MOF after hemorrhage resuscitation.[180] Intestinal injury is seen after resuscitation from hemorrhage and is associated with increased intestinal permeability to hydrophobic solutes,[181,182] appearance of translocated bacteria in mesenteric lymph nodes (of rats),[179,181–183] and the appearance of undefined pro-inflammatory mediators in mesenteric lymph.[184–186] Posthemorrhagic shock mesenteric lymph has been shown to prime neutrophils and cause lung injury.[154] Furthermore, lymphatic diversion can eliminate this injury.[154,187]

Oxidative stress and the formation of peroxynitrite[176] are involved in the intestinal damage and this is apparently exacerbated by a progressive vasoconstriction that begins at the time of resuscitation.[188] Therapeutic interventions have been aimed at minimizing the oxidative injury, reducing the formation of pro-inflammatory mediators, and reversal of the persistent vasoconstriction. Xanthine oxidase is abundant in the intestine and this appears to be a major source of the oxidant injury. Xanthine oxidase inhibitors are protective,[189,189] as are pentoxifyllin and the related compound lisofyllin, both of which may exert their

protection by preventing oxidant injury, although other mechanisms have also been proposed.[190,191] The source of pro-inflammatory mediators in mesenteric lymph is not fully resolved but Schmid-Schonbein and Hugli[186] have proposed a novel theory that postulates that pancreatic enzymes gain access to the intestinal cells after ischemic injury and produce multiple digestion products that are pro-inflammatory. The role of pancreatic enzymes in this process is substantiated by the studies of Cohen et al. showing that ligation of the pancreatic duct prevents distant organ injury after resuscitation from hemorrhage, even though it does not prevent gut injury.[192] Also studies by Doucet et al.[193] have shown that enteral application of pancreatic enzyme inhibitors is also protective. The results clearly indicate that pancreatic enzymes are involved in the formation of pro-inflammatory mediators and potentially provide a real therapeutic option for the prevention of MOF after severe hemorrhagic shock. Therapies that reverse mesenteric vasoconstriction also provide improved survival and are associated with less intestinal pathology. One intriguing approach is that of direct intraperitoneal resuscitation (DPR) proposed by Zakaria et al.[188] The local improvement of blood flow caused by DPR has been attributed to the vasodilatory nature of the dialysis solution. The reason for an increase in lung and muscle blood flow after DPR is less intuitive and remains to be explained. The authors postulate that improved cardiac work, removal of inflammatory mediators from the peritoneal cavity, and reduced leukocyte activation are all likely mediators of this beneficial effect.

In addition to the acute phase inflammatory reaction, profound hemorrhage initiates a molecular response that leads to the promotion and upregulation of genes responsible for heat shock proteins (HSP) and apoptosis. HSP are a family of gene products that likely represent a protective mechanism designed to check possible detrimental effects of physiologic stress. Kiang and coworkers have recently demonstrated specific HSP binding to iNOS and its transcription factor KLF6 after hemorrhage.[175] The result of this binding may lead to inactivation of iNOS and thus to a decrease in NO-related cellular injury. As a result of these findings, it has been postulated that the exogenous stimulation of HSP may be helpful during initial resuscitative efforts.

The stress response to injury concurrently initiates a process of apoptosis, or programmed cell death, designed to limit the extent of inflammation, to clear non-viable cells, and to maintain overall integrity of the organism. As the severity of hemorrhagic shock-related stress increases, the magnitude and extent of apoptosis increases. An exaggerated apoptotic response leads to cell death in multiple cell types and tissues. The subsequent release of inflammatory intracellular components and debris may lead to further local tissue damage as well as detrimental effects at distant organ sites. For example, gastrointestinal apoptosis can result in breakdown in the gut barrier, leading to release of inflammatory intermediates into mesenteric lymph that exacerbate pulmonary apoptosis and the subsequent development of MOF.[194,195]

It has been suggested that regulation of the complex cascade of apoptosis may provide an opportunity for early intervention in the development of organ injury and failure.[196] Therefore, investigators have examined resuscitative strategies designed to limit the negative effects of apoptosis. It has been demonstrated that hemorrhage and resuscitation produce immediate apoptosis and that the magnitude of apoptosis depends, to some extent, on the choice of resuscitative fluid.[197,198] Ongoing work has identified several candidate resuscitative fluids, such as pyruvate Ringer's solution and hypertonic saline, which may help specifically to diminish the magnitude of apoptosis during resuscitation. Additionally, work with pharmacologic adjuncts such as crocetin and glutamine have been shown significantly to improve restoration of cellular energy stores, reduce apoptotic cell death, and improve overall survival.[199]

Cell-mediated immune responses after trauma-hemorrhage are gender-related. Male and female sex steroids produce differing immunomodulatory effects.[200] Proestrus females have been shown to demonstrate beneficial responses following trauma and hemorrhage with respect to splenocyte proliferation, IL-2, IL-3, IFN-gamma release, splenic macrophage IL-6 release, and TNF-alpha.[201] It is likely that this gender-dependent advantage is mediated in part via upregulation of HO-1 expression and activity.[202] These findings support the contention by some authors that the administration of agents such as flutamide, designed to antagonize androgen-receptors and simultaneously upregulate estrogen receptors, may play an important role in improving outcome from shock.

Complement activation has long been recognized to contribute to the inflammatory cascade leading to MODS following hemorrhagic shock.[203] Indeed, inhibition of complement activation before resuscitation has been suggested as a useful adjunct in patients experiencing major hemorrhage for the prevention of the sequelae of gut ischemia.[204] A single bolus treatment of Cl-esterase-inhibitor was shown to abrogate leukocyte adhesion and rolling in the mesenteric microcirculation after hemorrhagic shock.[205]

Recent studies have emphasized the interaction of the neuroendocrine response to hemorrhage and the immune response.[57] Tracey has shown that vagal stimulation blunts the immune response[206] and Guarini *et al.*[207] have shown that vagal stimulation blunts NF-κB activation after hemorrhage and improves short term survival. Moreover, this pathway mediates the protective effect of adrenocorticotropin.[208]

Endothelial dysfunction

A very recent preliminary publication by Mathru and Lang[209] has demonstrated that trauma patients have significant endothelial dysfunction despite adequate resuscitation. Although the authors did not speculate on the presence of nitric oxide inhibitors as a potential cause of this effect, Cooke[210] has postulated that asymmetric dimethyl arginine (ADMA), a naturally occurring inhibitor of nitric oxide synthase, may be an important cause of endothelial dysfunction. This hypothesis is particularly appealing because of the finding by Nijveldt *et al.* that the plasma level of ADMA is an independent risk factor for ICU mortality[211] and a potential cause of multiorgan failure.[212] The link between this and other factors involved in multiorgan failure is yet to be resolved.

New treatment modalities in shock

Hemoglobin-based oxygen carriers (HBOCs)

The hemoglobin-based oxygen carriers, polymerized hemoglobin solutions, represent a potentially significant advance in the treatment of hemorrhagic hypovolemia. The use of HBOCs may meet multiple critical needs of the trauma patient, including volume replacement, oxygen-carrying capacity, and immune modulation. Historically, the treatment of hemorrhagic shock has relied mainly on crystalloid infusion for the immediate stabilization of hemodynamics, followed by surgical intervention and transfusion of stored red blood cells (RBCs). Whereas transfusion with allogenic RBCs remains the gold standard treatment for acute traumatic anemia, human RBC transfusion is not risk-free. Aside from issues of compatibility, disease transmission, and supply limitations, the number of infused RBC units and the age of those units are directly proportional to the risk of subsequent MOF. Resuscitation with an HBOC may offer a means of mitigating these risks. Even though early clinical evaluation of HBOC resuscitation was plagued by increased mortality,[213] current work with newer formulations appears to be quite encouraging.[141,214]

Hemoglobin avidly binds nitric oxide and therefore all the first-generation HBOCs are all vasoconstrictors, as is the hemoglobin within the RBCs. Thus, the question normally posed is whether HBOC absorbs significantly more nitric oxide than the RBCs already present within the circulation. One possible mechanism for an increased vasoconstriction with HBOC is related to the ability of HBOC to extravasate from the vascular compartment and thereby gain access to nitric oxide normally "out of reach" of the RBCs. This is more likely to occur in fenestrated vessels.[112] Persistent hypotension seen with some models of low volume resuscitation may make even a small effect evident.[66] Purification of the HBOC to remove small complexes would tend to minimize this effect.

Recent findings provide another possible explanation for the relative vasoconstrictor effect of HBOCs. Atkins et al.[51] have recently shown in rats that RBCs have an increased content of *S*-nitrosothiols after hemorrhage. Stamler and colleagues[215,216] have proposed that *S*-nitrosothiols may be released from RBCs in vascular beds with low oxygen tension as a result of the conformational change in hemoglobin. The released *S*-nitrosothiols would tend to vasodilate the tissue. Although there is no direct evidence that this "targeted release" occurs in hemorrhage, this "safety valve" mechanism could be functionally important, even if the amount of nitric oxide delivered is small compared to the overall rate of nitric oxide production. If the mechanism is operative in hypoxic vascular beds during hemorrhage, then the endogenous circulating RBCs would tend to vasodilate these beds while transfused RBCs and HBOCs would tend to vasoconstrict them. It remains a very difficult problem to demonstrate this effect *in vivo*, but resolving these questions may help to define the best strategies for the use of HBOCs.

Vasopressin

Return of spontaneous circulation following cardiac arrest due to hemorrhage has historically been considered extremely unlikely. So much so, that interventions, such as CPR and or ED thoracotomy, are discouraged except for the minority of cases involving penetrating torso injury in the patient who has loss of vital signs very close to or in the trauma room. Recently, investigators have begun to explore the use of vasopressin as an adjunct in hemorrhagic shock and cardiac arrest.[217] Administration of vasopressin has been successful in at least one case, albeit temporary, in the treatment of traumatic arrest.[218] The value of this drug may actually be for the hemorrhage victim before frank arrest in helping to stabilize a tenuous hemodynamic state and allowing time for further treatment.[219] Some have argued that in situations of uncontrolled hemorrhage, vasopressin administration along limited fluid infusion may be preferable to standard fluid resuscitation algorithms.[220]

Controlled modest hypothermia

Animal studies have shown a protective effect of modest hypothermia (28 °C to 32 °C) in head trauma and cardiac arrest. Likewise, numerous animal studies have also shown a beneficial effect of modest hypothermia in hemorrhagic shock. Nevertheless, substantial controversy remains about the use of mild (36 °C to 32 °C) or modest hypothermia in trauma, because hypothermia is associated with cardiac arrhythmias, coagulopathies, and increased incidence of infections. Moreover, as previously mentioned, patients who present to the trauma center with hypothermia have a worse outcome. Numerous animal studies have shown that mild or modest hypothermia, however, can improve survival and decrease late organ injury in hemorrhage resuscitation.[94,108,221–225] The controversy may never be resolved, and recently Wu et al.[224,225] have begun a search for the mechanisms that provide the survival benefit from mild hypothermia. Although a daunting task, this may prove to be the most acceptable way to provide this protection to trauma patients.

Conclusions

In developed countries, trauma systems with rapid transport to the hospital continue to make significant improvements in survival and outcome after injury. These advances have been largely based on improved roads and expanded and standardized trauma care systems. Unfortunately, it is unlikely that underdeveloped countries will be able to apply such resource-intensive responses to prevent the predicted increase in deaths from traffic accidents. In this context, improvements in the initial care of trauma patients at the scene could have a very significant impact. Even with the excellent road system and advanced transport systems in the USA, there is still the potential to save many lives through improvements in early care.

REFERENCES

1. *National Safety Council: Injury Facts.* Itasca, IL: National Safety Council; 2000: 13.
2. *Injury: A leading cause of the global burden of disease, 2000.* Geneva: World Health Organization; 2002.
3. *The Global Burden of Disease.* Cambridge, MA: Harvard School of Public Health on behalf of The World Health Organization and the World Bank; 1996: 373–375.
4. Carrico, C.J., Holcomb, J.B. & Chaudry, I.H. Scientific priorities and strategic planning for resuscitation research and life saving therapy following traumatic injury: report of the

PULSE Trauma Work Group. Post Resuscitative and Initial Utility of Life Saving Efforts. *Shock* 2002; **17**: 165–168.

5. Sauaia, A., Moore, F.A., Moore, E.E. *et al.* Epidemiology of trauma deaths: a reassessment. *J. Trauma* 1995; **38**: 185–193.

6. Baker, C.C., Oppenheimer, L., Stephens, B., Lewis, F.R. & Trunkey, D.D. Epidemiology of trauma deaths. *Am. J. Surg.* 1980; **140**: 144–150.

7. Shackford, S.R., Mackersie, R.C., Davis, J.W., Wolf, P.L. & Hoyt, D.B. Epidemiology and pathology of traumatic deaths occurring at a Level I Trauma Center in a regionalized system: the importance of secondary brain injury. *J. Trauma* 1989; **29**: 1392–1397.

8. Demetriades, D., Kimbrell, B., Salim, A. *et al.* Trauma deaths in a mature urban trauma system: is "trimodal" distribution a valid concept? *J. Am. Coll. Surg.* 2005; **201**: 343–348.

9. Trunkey, D.D. Trauma. Accidental and intentional injuries account for more years of life lost in the U.S. than cancer and heart disease. Among the prescribed remedies are improved preventive efforts, speedier surgery and further research. *Sci. Am.* 1983; **249**: 28–35.

10. Hopson, L.R., Hirsh, E., Delgado, J., Domeier, R.M., McSwain, N.E. & Krohmer, J. Guidelines for withholding or termination of resuscitation in prehospital traumatic cardiopulmonary arrest: joint position statement of the National Association of EMS Physicians and the American College of Surgeons Committee on Trauma. *J. Am. Coll. Surg.* 2003; **196**: 106–112.

11. Copass, M.K., Oreskovich, M.R., Bladergroen, M.R. & Carrico, C.J. Prehospital cardiopulmonary resuscitation of the critically injured patient. *Am. J. Surg.* 1984; **148**: 20–26.

12. Shimazu, S. & Shatney, C.H. Outcomes of trauma patients with no vital signs on hospital admission. *J. Trauma* 1983; **23**: 213–216.

13. Rosemurgy, A.S., Norris, P.A., Olson, S.M., Hurst, J.M. & Albrink, M.H. Prehospital traumatic cardiac arrest: the cost of futility. *J. Trauma* 1993; **35**: 468–473.

14. Fulton, R.L., Voigt, W.J. & Hilakos, A.S. Confusion surrounding the treatment of traumatic cardiac arrest. *J. Am. Coll. Surg.* 1995; **181**: 209–214.

15. Pasquale, M.D., Rhodes, M., Cipolle, M.D., Hanley, T. & Wasser, T. Defining "dead on arrival": impact on a level I trauma center. *J. Trauma* 1996; **41**: 726–730.

16. Stratton, S.J., Brickett, K. & Crammer, T. Prehospital pulseless, unconscious penetrating trauma victims: field assessments associated with survival. *J. Trauma* 1998; **45**: 96–100.

17. Battistella, F.D., Nugent, W., Owings, J.T. & Anderson, J.T. Field triage of the pulseless trauma patient. *Arch. Surg.* 1999; **134**: 742–745.

18. Martin, S.K., Shatney, C.H., Sherck, J.P. *et al.* Blunt trauma patients with prehospital pulseless electrical activity (PEA): poor ending assured. *J. Trauma* 2002; **53**: 876–880.

19. Axelsson, H., Hjelmqvist, H., Medin, A., Persson, J.K. & Suneson, A. Physiological changes in pigs exposed to a blast wave from a detonating high-explosive charge. *Mil. Med.* 2000; **165**: 119–126.

20. Guy, R.J., Kirkman, E., Watkins, P.E. & Cooper, G.J. Physiologic responses to primary blast. *J. Trauma* 1998; **45**: 983–987.

21. Ohnishi, M., Kirkman, E., Guy, R.J. & Watkins, P.E. Reflex nature of the cardiorespiratory response to primary thoracic blast injury in the anaesthetised rat. *Exp. Physiol.* 2001; **86**: 357–364.

22. DePalma, R.G., Burris, D.G., Champion, H.R. & Hodgson, M.J. Blast injuries. *N. Engl. J. Med.* 2005; **352**: 1335–1342.

23. Butler, F. Tactical combat casualty care: combining good medicine with good tactics. *J. Trauma* 2003; **54**: S2–S3.

24. Butler, F.K., Jr. Tactical medicine training for SEAL mission commanders. *Mil. Med.* 2001; **166**: 625–631.

25. Pickens, J.J., Copass, M.K. & Bulger, E.M. Trauma patients receiving CPR: predictors of survival. *J. Trauma* 2005; **58**: 951–958.

26. Kern, K.B., Sanders, A.B., Janas, W. *et al.* Limitations of open-chest cardiac massage after prolonged, untreated cardiac arrest in dogs. *Ann. Emerg. Med.* 1991; **20**: 761–767.

27. Mattox, K.L. & Feliciano, D.V. Role of external cardiac compression in truncal trauma. *J. Trauma* 1982; **22**: 934–936.

28. Lorenz, H.P., Steinmetz, B., Lieberman, J., Schecoter, W.P. & Macho, J.R. Emergency thoracotomy: survival correlates with physiologic status. *J. Trauma* 1992; **32**: 780–785.

29. Fialka, C., Sebok, C., Kemetzhofer, P., Kwasny, O., Sterz, F. & Vecsei, V. Open-chest cardiopulmonary resuscitation after cardiac arrest in cases of blunt chest or abdominal trauma: a consecutive series of 38 cases. *J. Trauma* 2004; **57**: 809–814.

30. Hachimi-Idrissi, S., Leeman, J., Hubloue, Y., Huyghens, L. & Corne, L. Open chest cardiopulmonary resuscitation in out-of-hospital cardiac arrest. *Resuscitation* 1997; **35**: 151–156.

31. Alam, H.B., Chen, Z., Ahuja, N. *et al.* Profound hypothermia protects neurons and astrocytes, and preserves cognitive functions in a Swine model of lethal hemorrhage. *J. Surg. Res.* 2005; **126**: 172–181.

32. Alam, H.B., Chen, Z., Honma, K. *et al.* The rate of induction of hypothermic arrest determines the outcome in a Swine model of lethal hemorrhage. *J. Trauma* 2004; **57**: 961–969.

33. Chen, Z., Chen, H., Rhee, P. *et al.* Induction of profound hypothermia modulates the immune/inflammatory response in a swine model of lethal hemorrhage. *Resuscitation* 2005; **66**: 209–216.

34. Tisherman, S.A. Suspended animation for resuscitation from exsanguinating hemorrhage. *Crit. Care Med.* 2004; **32**: S46–S50.

35. Nozari, A., Safar, P., Wu, X. *et al.* Suspended animation can allow survival without brain damage after traumatic exsanguination cardiac arrest of 60 minutes in dogs. *J. Trauma* 2004; **57**: 1266–1275.

36. Carrillo, P., Takasu, A., Safar, P. *et al.* Prolonged severe hemorrhagic shock and resuscitation in rats does not cause subtle brain damage. *J. Trauma* 1998; **45**: 239–248.

37. Nozari, A., Safar, P., Tisherman, S. *et al.* Suspended animation and plasma exchange (SAPEX) enables full neurologic recovery from lethal traumatic exsanguinations, even after 2 h period of no flow. *Crit. Care Med.* **31**[12], A9. 2003. Ref Type: Abstract

38. Pepe, P.E., Roppolo, L.P. & Fowler, R.L. The detrimental effects of ventilation during low-blood-flow states. *Curr. Opin. Crit. Care.* 2005; **11**: 212–218.

39. Pepe, P.E., Lurie, K.G., Wigginton, J.G., Raedler, C. & Idris, A.H. Detrimental hemodynamic effects of assisted ventilation in hemorrhagic states. *Crit. Care Med.* 2004; **32**: S414–S420.

40. Pepe, P.E., Raedler, C., Lurie, K.G. & Wigginton, J.G. Emergency ventilatory management in hemorrhagic states: elemental or detrimental? *J. Trauma* 2003; **54**: 1048–1055.

41. Krismer, A.C., Wenzel, V., Lindner, K.H. *et al.* Influence of positive end-expiratory pressure ventilation on survival during severe hemorrhagic shock. *Ann. Emerg. Med.* 2005; **46**: 337–342.

42. Lurie, K.G., Zielinski, T.M., McKnite, S.H. *et al.* Treatment of hypotension in pigs with an inspiratory impedance threshold device: a feasibility study. *Crit. Care Med.* 2004; **32**: 1555–1562.

43. Samniah, N., Voelckel, W.G., Zielinski, T.M. *et al.* Feasibility and effects of transcutaneous phrenic nerve stimulation combined with an inspiratory impedance threshold in a pig model of hemorrhagic shock. *Crit. Care Med.* 2003; **31**: 1197–1202.

44. Convertino, V.A., Cooke, W.H. & Lurie, K.G. Inspiratory resistance as a potential treatment for orthostatic intolerance and hemorrhagic shock. *Aviat. Space Environ. Med.* 2005; **76**: 319–325.

45. Yannopoulos, D., Nadkarni, V.M., McKnite, S.H. *et al.* Intrathoracic pressure regulator during continuous-chest-compression advanced cardiac resuscitation improves vital organ perfusion pressures in a porcine model of cardiac arrest. *Circulation* 2005; **112**: 803–811.

46. Taylor, J.H., Mulier, K.E., Myers, D.E. & Beilman, G.J. Use of near-infrared spectroscopy in early determination of irreversible hemorrhagic shock. *J. Trauma* 2005; **58**: 1119–1125.

47. Shah, N.S., Kelly, E., Billiar, T.R. *et al.* Utility of clinical parameters of tissue oxygenation in a quantitative model of irreversible hemorrhagic shock. *Shock* 1998; **10**: 343–346.

48. Healey, M.A., Samphire, J., Hoyt, D.B., Liu, F., Davis, R. & Loomis, W.H. Irreversible shock is not irreversible: a new model of massive hemorrhage and resuscitation. *J. Trauma* 2001; **50**: 826–834.

49. Pelaez, N.M., Schreihofer, A.M. & Guyenet, P.G. Decompensated hemorrhage activates serotonergic neurons in the subependymal parapyramidal region of the rat medulla. *Am. J. Physiol. Regul. Integr. Comp. Physiol.* 2002; **283**: R688–R697.

50. Peitzman, A.B., Billiar, T.R., Harbrecht, B.G., Kelly, E., Udekwu, A.O. & Simmons, R.L. Hemorrhagic shock. *Curr. Probl. Surg.* 1995; **32**: 925–1002.

51. Atkins, J., Handrigan, M., Pamnani, M., Zhang, Z., Day, B. & Gorbunov, N. Early formation of nitric oxide adducts in hemorrhagic hypotension. *Shock* 23[S3], 5. 2005. Ref Type: Abstract

52. Jochem, J. Involvement of arginine vasopressin in endogenous central histamine-induced reversal of critical haemorrhagic hypotension in rats. *Inflamm. Res.* 2004; **53**: 269–276.

53. Schadt, J.C. & Hasser, E.M. Interaction of vasopressin and opioids during rapid hemorrhage in conscious rabbits. *Am. J. Physiol.* 1991; **260**: R373–R381.

54. Jochem, J. Involvement of the sympathetic nervous system in the reversal of critical haemorrhagic hypotension by endogenous central histamine in rats. *Naunyn Schmiedebergs Arch. Pharmacol.* 2004; **369**: 418–427.

55. Molina, P.E. Stress-specific opioid modulation of haemodynamic counter-regulation. *Clin. Exp. Pharmacol. Physiol.* 2002; **29**: 248–253.

56. Scrogin, K.E. 5-HT1A receptor agonist 8-OH-DPAT acts in the hindbrain to reverse the sympatholytic response to severe hemorrhage. *Am. J. Physiol. Regul. Integr. Comp. Physiol.* 2003; **284**: R782–R791.

57. Molina, P.E. Neurobiology of the stress response: contribution of the sympathetic nervous system to the neuroimmune axis in traumatic injury. *Shock* 2005; **24**: 3–10.

58. Schadt, J.C. & Ludbrook, J. Hemodynamic and neurohumoral responses to acute hypovolemia in conscious mammals. *Am. J. Physiol.* 1991; **260**: H305–H318.

59. Koch, M.A., Hasser, E.M. & Schadt, J.C. Influence of nitric oxide on the hemodynamic response to hemorrhage in conscious rabbits. *Am. J. Physiol.* 1995; **268**: R171–R182.

60. Blake, D.W., Evans, R.G., Ludbrook, J. & Petring, O.U. Interactions between the circulatory effects of central hypovolaemia and arterial hypoxia in conscious rabbits. *Clin. Exp. Pharmacol. Physiol.* 1994; **21**: 383–396.

61. Eichinger, M.R. & Claybaugh, J.R. Hypoxia attenuates the renin response to hemorrhage. *Am. J. Physiol.* 1992; **263**: R664–R669.

62. Convertino, V.A. & Sather, T.M. Vasoactive neuroendocrine responses associated with tolerance to lower body negative pressure in humans. *Clin. Physiol.* 2000; **20**: 177–184.

63. Schadt, J.C., McKown, M.D., McKown, D.P. & Franklin, D. Hemodynamic effects of hemorrhage and subsequent naloxone treatment in conscious rabbits. *Am. J. Physiol.* 1984; **247**: R497–R505.

64. Lightfoot, J.T., Katz, L. & DeBate, K. Naloxone decreases tolerance to hypotensive, hypovolemic stress healthy humans. *Crit. Care Med.* 2000; **28**: 684–691.

65. Napolitano, L.M. Naloxone therapy in shock: the controversy continues. *Crit. Care Med.* 2000; **28**: 887–888.

66. Handrigan, M.T., Bentley, T.B., Oliver, J.D., Tabaku, L.S., Burge, J.R. & Atkins, J.L. Choice of fluid influences outcome in prolonged hypotensive resuscitation after hemorrhage in awake rats. *Shock* 2005; **23**: 337–343.

67. Schadt, J.C. & Ludbrook, J. Hemodynamic and neurohumoral responses to acute hypovolemia in conscious mammals. *Am. J. Physiol.* 1991; **260**: H305–H318.

68. Law, M.M., Hovda, D.A. & Cryer, H.G. Fluid-percussion brain injury adversely affects control of vascular tone during hemorrhagic shock. *Shock* 1996; **6**: 213–217.

69. Yuan, X.Q., Wade, C.E. & Clifford, C.B. Suppression by traumatic brain injury of spontaneous hemodynamic recovery from hemorrhagic shock in rats. *J. Neurosurg.* 1991; **75**: 408–414.

70. Dutton, R.P., Mackenzie, C.F. & Scalea, T.M. Hypotensive resuscitation during active hemorrhage: impact on in-hospital mortality. *J. Trauma* 2002; **52**: 1141–1146.

71. Thiemermann, C., Szabo, C., Mitchell, J.A. & Vane, J.R. Vascular hyporeactivity to vasoconstrictor agents and hemodynamic decompensation in hemorrhagic shock is mediated by nitric oxide. *Proc. Natl Acad. Sci. U S A* 1993; **90**: 267–271.

72. Liu, L.M., Ward, J.A. & Dubick, M.A. Hemorrhage-induced vascular hyporeactivity to norepinephrine in select vasculatures of rats and the roles of nitric oxide and endothelin. *Shock* 2003; **19**: 208–214.

73. Pieber, D., Horina, G., Sandner-Kiesling, A., Pieber, T.R. & Heinemann, A. Pressor and mesenteric arterial hyporesponsiveness to angiotensin II is an early event in haemorrhagic hypotension in anaesthetised rats. *Cardiovasc. Res.* 1999; **44**: 166–175.

74. Musser, J.B., Bentley, T.B., Griffith, S., Sharma, P., Karaian, J.E. & Mongan, P.D. Hemorrhagic shock in swine: nitric oxide and potassium sensitive adenosine triphosphate channel activation. *Anesthesiology* 2004; **101**: 399–408.

75. Eduardo, dS.-S. & Assreuy, J. Long-lasting changes of rat blood pressure to vasoconstrictors and vasodilators induced by nitric oxide donor infusion: involvement of potassium channels. *J. Pharmacol. Exp. Ther.* 1999; **290**: 380–387.

76. Zhao, K.S., Huang, X., Liu, J. *et al.* New approach to treatment of shock – restitution of vasoreactivity. *Shock* 2002; **18**: 189–192.

77. Evgenov, O.V., Pacher, P., Williams, W. *et al.* Parenteral administration of glipizide sodium salt, an inhibitor of adenosine triphosphate-sensitive potassium channels, prolongs short-term survival after severe controlled hemorrhage in rats. *Crit. Care Med.* 2003; **31**: 2429–2436.

78. Maybauer, D.M., Salsbury, J.R., Westphal, M. *et al.* The ATP-sensitive potassium-channel inhibitor glibenclamide improves outcome in an ovine model of hemorrhagic shock. *Shock* 2004; **22**: 387–391.

79. Salzman, A.L., Vromen, A., Denenberg, A. & Szabo, C. K(ATP)-channel inhibition improves hemodynamics and cellular energetics in hemorrhagic shock. *Am. J. Physiol.* 1997; **272**: H688–H694.

80. Lin, Y.F., Raab-Graham, K, Jan, Y.N., Jan, L.Y. NO stimulation of ATP-sensitive potassium channels: involvement of Ras/mitogen-activated protein kinase pathway and contribution to neuroprotection. *Proc. Natl Acad. Sci. U S A* 2004; **101**: 7799–7804.

81. Landry, D.W. & Oliver, J.A. The pathogenesis of vasodilatory shock. *N. Engl. J. Med.* 2001; **345**: 588–595.

82. Illner, H. & Shires, G.T. The effect of hemorrhagic shock on potassium transport in skeletal muscle. *Surg. Gynecol. Obstet.* 1980; **150**: 17–25.

83. Day, B. & Friedman, S.M. Intracellular sodium and potassium changes in vascular smooth muscle during hemorrhagic shock. *Surg. Gynecol. Obstet.* 1978; **147**: 25–26.

84. Oliver, J.D., Atkins, J.L., Bentley, T.B. & Pamnani, M. Microdialysis measurement of Interstitial Potassium Concentrations during hemorrhagic shock. *FASEB J.* 2002; **16**, A54. Ref Type: Abstract

85. McKinley, B.A., Houtchens, B.A. & Janata, J. Continuous monitoring of interstitial fluid potassium during hemorrhagic shock in dogs. *Crit. Care Med.* 1981; **9**: 845–851.

86. Trump, B.F., Berezesky, I.K., Chang, S.H., Pendergrass, R.E. & Mergner, W.J. The role of ion shifts in cell injury. *Scan Electron Microsc.* 1979; **3**: 1–13.

87. Sayeed, M.M., Adler, R.J., Chaudry, I.H. & Baue, A.E. Effect of hemorrhagic shock on hepatic transmembrane potentials and intracellular electrolytes, in vivo. *Am. J. Physiol.* 1981; **240**: R211–R219.

88. Evans, J.A., Darlington, D.N. & Gann, D.S. A circulating factor(s) mediates cell depolarization in hemorrhagic shock. *Ann. Surg.* 1991; **213**: 549–556.

89. Oliver, J.D., Schooley, J.F, Wang, L., Bentley, T.B., Atkins, J.L. & Pamnani, M.B. Changes in ex vivo Na$^+$, K$^+$-ATPase activity in hemorrhage (H) and resuscitation (R). *Shock* **23**[S3], 28. 2005.

90. Burns, W.R., Cohen, K.D. & Jackson, W.F. K$^+$-induced dilation of hamster cremasteric arterioles involves both the Na$^+$/K$^+$-ATPase and inward-rectifier K$^+$ channels. *Microcirculation* 2004; **11**: 279–293.

91. Darlington, D.N. & Gann, D.S. Purine nucleosides stimulate Na/K ATPase, and prolong survival in hemorrhagic shock. *J. Trauma* 2005; **58**: 1055–1060.

92. Darlington, D.N. & Gann, D.S. Adenosine stimulates NA/K ATPase and prolongs survival in hemorrhagic shock. *J. Trauma* 2005; **58**: 1–6.

93. bdel-Zaher, A.O., bdel-Aal, R.A., Aly, S.A. & Khalifa, M.M. Adenosine for reversal of hemorrhagic shock in rabbits. *Jpn. J. Pharmacol.* 1996; **72**: 247–254.

94. Johnson, K.B., Wiesmann, W.P. & Pearce, F.J. The effect of hypothermia on potassium and glucose changes in isobaric hemorrhagic shock in the rat. *Shock* 1996; **6**: 223–229.

95. Childs, E.W., Udobi, K.F., Hunter, F.A. & Dhevan, V. Evidence of transcellular albumin transport after hemorrhagic shock. *Shock* 2005; **23**: 565–570.

96. Henderson, R.A., Whitehurst, M.E., Morgan, K.R. & Carroll, R.G. Reduced oxygen consumption precedes the drop in body core temperature caused by hemorrhage in rats. *Shock* 2000; **13**: 320–324.

97. Seki, K., Aibiki, M. & Ogura, S. 3.5% hypertonic saline produces sympathetic activation in hemorrhaged rabbits. *J. Auton. Nerv. Syst.* 1997; **64**: 49–56.

98. Voelckel, W.G., Raedler, C., Wenzel, V. *et al.* Arginine vasopressin, but not epinephrine, improves survival in uncontrolled hemorrhagic shock after liver trauma in pigs. *Crit. Care Med.* 2003; **31**: 1160–1165.

99. Stadlbauer, K.H., Wagner-Berger, H.G., Raedler, C. *et al.* Vasopressin, but not fluid resuscitation, enhances survival in

a liver trauma model with uncontrolled and otherwise lethal hemorrhagic shock in pigs. *Anesthesiology.* 2003; **98**: 699–704.

100. Osei-Owusu, P. & Scrogin, K.E. Buspirone raises blood pressure through activation of sympathetic nervous system and by direct activation of alpha1-adrenergic receptors after severe hemorrhage. *J. Pharmacol. Exp. Ther.* 2004; **309**: 1132–1140.

101. Zweier, J.L., Wang, P. & Kuppusamy, P. Direct measurement of nitric oxide generation in the ischemic heart using electron paramagnetic resonance spectroscopy. *J. Biol. Chem.* 1995; **270**: 304–307.

102. McMahon, T.J., Pawloski, J.R., Hess, D.T. *et al.* S-nitrosohemoglobin is distinguished from other nitrosovasodilators by unique oxygen-dependent responses that support an allosteric mechanism of action. *Blood* 2003; **102**: 410–411.

103. Atkins, J., Lee, W., Scott, Z., Johnson, K. & Pearce, F. Oxygen inhalation after hemorrhage increases mean arterial blood pressure (MABP) and carotid blood flow. 1998; *FASEB J.* **11**[3], A286. Ref Type: Abstract

104. Bitterman, H., Brod, V., Weisz, G., Kushnir, D. & Bitterman, N. Effects of oxygen on regional hemodynamics in hemorrhagic shock. *Am. J. Physiol.* 1996; **271**: H203–H211.

105. Crippen, D., Safar, P., Porter, L. & Zona, J. Improved survival of hemorrhagic shock with oxygen and hypothermia in rats. *Resuscitation* 1991; **21**: 271–281.

106. Adir, Y., Bitterman, N., Katz, E., Melamed, Y. & Bitterman, H. Salutary consequences of oxygen therapy on the long-term outcome of hemorrhagic shock in awake, unrestrained rats. *Undersea Hyperb. Med.* 1995; **22**: 23–30.

107. Sukhotnik, I., Krausz, M.M., Brod, V. *et al.* Divergent effects of oxygen therapy in four models of uncontrolled hemorrhagic shock. *Shock* 2002; **18**: 277–284.

108. Kim, S.H., Stezoski, S.W., Safar, P. & Tisherman, S.A. Hypothermia, but not 100% oxygen breathing, prolongs survival time during lethal uncontrolled hemorrhagic shock in rats. *J. Trauma* 1998; **44**: 485–491.

109. Paxian, M., Keller, S.A., Huynh, T.T. & Clemens, M.G. Perflubron emulsion improves hepatic microvascular integrity and mitochondrial redox state after hemorrhagic shock. *Shock* 2003; **20**: 449–457.

110. Lundgren, C.E., Bergoe, G.W. & Tyssebotn, I. The theory and application of intravascular microbubbles as an ultra-effective means of transporting oxygen and other gases. *Undersea Hyperb. Med.* 2004; **31**: 105–106.

111. Kemming, G.I., Meisner, F.G., Wojtczyk, C.J. *et al.* OxygentTtrade mark as a top load to colloid and hyperoxia is more effective in resuscitation from hemorrhagic shock than colloid and hyperoxia alone. *Shock* 2005; **24**: 245–254.

112. Sampei, K., Ulatowski, J.A., Asano, Y., Kwansa, H., Bucci, E. & Koehler, R.C. Role of nitric oxide scavenging in vascular response to cell-free hemoglobin transfusion. *Am. J. Physiol. Heart Circ. Physiol.* 2005; **289**: H1191–H1201.

113. Morales, D., Madigan, J., Cullinane, S. *et al.* Reversal by vasopressin of intractable hypotension in the late phase of hemorrhagic shock. *Circulation* 1999; **100**: 226–229.

114. Stadlbauer, K.H., Wenzel, V., Krismer, A.C., Voelckel, W.G. & Lindner, K.H. Vasopressin during uncontrolled hemorrhagic shock: less bleeding below the diaphragm, more perfusion above. *Anesth. Analg.* 2005; **101**: 830–832.

115. Malay, M.B., Ashton, J.L., Dahl, K. *et al.* Heterogeneity of the vasoconstrictor effect of vasopressin in septic shock. *Crit. Care Med.* 2004; **32**: 1327–1331.

116. Raedler, C., Voelckel, W.G., Wenzel, V. *et al.* Treatment of uncontrolled hemorrhagic shock after liver trauma: fatal effects of fluid resuscitation versus improved outcome after vasopressin. *Anesth. Analg.* 2004; **98**: 1759–1766, table.

117. Holmes, C.L. Vasopressin in septic shock: does dose matter? *Crit. Care Med.* 2004; **32**: 1423–1424.

118. Krismer, A.C., Wenzel, V., Voelckel, W.G. *et al.* Employing vasopressin as an adjunct vasopressor in uncontrolled traumatic hemorrhagic shock. Three cases and a brief analysis of the literature. *Anaesthesist* 2005; **54**: 220–224.

119. Dorlac, W.C., DeBakey, M.E., Holcomb, J.B. *et al.* Mortality from isolated civilian penetrating extremity injury. *J. Trauma* 2005; **59**: 217–222.

120. Morgan, B.C., Crawford, E.W. & Guntheroth, W.G. The hemodynamic effects of changes in blood volume during intermittent positive-pressure ventilation. *Anesthesiology* 1969; **30**: 297–305.

121. Pepe, P.E., Roppolo, L.P. & Fowler, R.L. The detrimental effects of ventilation during low-blood-flow states. *Curr. Opin. Crit Care* 2005; **11**: 212–218.

122. Lurie, K., Voelckel, W., Plaisance, P. *et al.* Use of an inspiratory impedance threshold valve during cardiopulmonary resuscitation: a progress report. [Review] [20 refs]. *Resuscitation* 2000; **44**(3): 219–230.

123. Voelckel, W.G., Lurie, K.G., Zielinski, T. *et al.* The effects of positive end-expiratory pressure during active compression decompression cardiopulmonary resuscitation with the inspiratory threshold valve. *Anesth. Analg.* 2001; **92**(4): 967–974.

124. Plaisance, P., Lurie, K.G., Vicaut, E. *et al.* Evaluation of an impedance threshold device in patients receiving active compression–decompression cardiopulmonary resuscitation for out of hospital cardiac arrest. *Resuscitation* 2004; **61**(3): 265–71.

125. Marino, B.S., Yannopoulos, D., Sigurdsson, G. *et al.* Spontaneous breathing through an inspiratory impedance threshold device augments cardiac index and stroke volume index in a pediatric porcine model of hemorrhagic hypovolemia. *Crit. Care Med.* 2004; **32**: S398–S405.

126. Lurie, K.G, Zielinski, T.M., McKnite, S.H. *et al.* Treatment of hypotension in pigs with an inspiratory impedance threshold device: a feasibility study. *Crit. Care Med.* 2004; **32**: 1555–1562.

127. Convertino, V.A., Cooke, W.H. & Lurie, K.G. Inspiratory resistance as a potential treatment for orthostatic intolerance and hemorrhagic shock. *Aviat. Space Environ. Med.* 2005; **76**: 319–325.

128. Nunn, J.F. & Freeman, J. Problems of oxygenation and oxygen transport during haemorrhage. *Anaesthesia* 1995; **50**: 795–800.

129. Pepe, P.E., Raedler, C., Lurie, K.G. & Wigginton, J.G. Emergency ventilatory management in hemorrhagic states: elemental or detrimental? *J. Trauma* 2003; **54**: 1048–1055.

130. Hoyt, D.B. A clinical review of bleeding dilemmas in trauma. *Semin. Hematol.* 2004; **41**: 40–43.

131. Alam, H.B. Burris, D., DaCorta, J.A. & Rhee, P. Hemorrhage control in the battlefield: role of new hemostatic agents. *Mil. Med.* 2005; **170**: 63–69.

132. Pusateri, A.E.P., Modrow, H.E.P., Harris, R.A.D. *et al.* Advanced hemostatic dressing development program: animal model selection criteria and results of a study of nine hemostatic dressings in a model of severe large venous hemorrhage and hepatic injury in swine. [Article]. *J. Trauma-Injury Infect. Crit. Care* 2003; **55**: 518–526.

133. Kheirabadi, B.S., Acheson, E.M., Deguzman, R. *et al.* Hemostatic efficacy of two advanced dressings in an aortic hemorrhage model in Swine. *J. Trauma* 2005; **59**: 25–34.

134. Dutton, R.P., McCunn, M., Hyder, M. *et al.* Factor VIIa for correction of traumatic coagulopathy. *J. Trauma* 2004; **57**: 709–718.

135. Hoyt, D.B., Bulger, E.M., Knudson, M.M. *et al.* Death in the operating room: an analysis of a multi-center experience. *J. Trauma* 1994; **37**: 426–432.

136. Brohi, K., Singh, J. Heron, M. & Coats, T. Acute traumatic coagulopathy. *J. Trauma* 2003; **54**: 1127–1130.

137. Armand, R. & Hess, J.R. Treating coagulopathy in trauma patients. *Transfus. Med. Rev.* 2003; **17**: 223–231.

138. Holcomb, J.B.M. Use of recombinant activated factor VII to treat the acquired coagulopathy of trauma. [Review]. *J. Trauma-Injury Infect. Crit. Care* 2005; **58**: 1298–1303.

139. Boffard, K.D.M., Riou, B.M., Warren, B.M. *et al.* Recombinant factor VIIa as adjunctive therapy for bleeding control in severely injured trauma patients: two parallel randomized, placebo-controlled, double-blind clinical trials. [Article]. *J. Trauma-Injury Infect. Crit. Care* 2005; **59**: 8–18.

140. Ho, A.M., Karmakar, M.K. & Dion, P.W. Are we giving enough coagulation factors during major trauma resuscitation? *Am. J. Surg.* 2005; **190**: 479–484.

141. Moore, F.A., McKinley, B.A. & Moore, E.E. The next generation in shock resuscitation. *Lancet* 2004; **363**: 1988–1996.

142. Stern, S.A. Low-volume fluid resuscitation for presumed hemorrhagic shock: helpful or harmful? *Curr. Opin. Crit. Care* 2001; **7**: 422–430.

143. Burris, D., Rhee, P., Kaufmann, C. *et al.* Controlled resuscitation for uncontrolled hemorrhagic shock. *J. Trauma* 1999; **46**: 216–223.

144. Dutton, R.P., Mackenzie, C.F. & Scalea, T.M. Hypotensive resuscitation during active hemorrhage: impact on in-hospital mortality. *J. Trauma* 2002; **52**: 1141–1146.

145. Shirley, P.J. & Weaver, A.E. Hypotensive resuscitation in trauma. *J. Trauma* 2002; **53**: 1196.

146. Regel, G., Grotz, M., Weltner, T., Sturm, J.A. & Tscherne, H. Pattern of organ failure following severe trauma. *World J. Surg.* 1996; **20**: 422–429.

147. Regel, G., Lobenhoffer, P., Grotz, M., Pape, H.C., Lehmann, U. & Tscherne, H. Treatment results of patients with multiple trauma: an analysis of 3406 cases treated between 1972 and 1991 at a German Level I Trauma Center. *J. Trauma* 1995; **38**: 70–78.

148. Ciesla, D.J., Moore, E.E., Johnson, J.L., Burch, J.M., Cothren, C.C. & Sauaia, A. A 12-year prospective study of postinjury multiple organ failure: has anything changed? *Arch. Surg.* 2005; **140**: 432–438.

149. Nast-Kolb, D., Aufmkolk, M., Rucholtz, S., Obertacke, U. & Waydhas, C. Multiple organ failure still a major cause of morbidity but not mortality in blunt multiple trauma. *J. Trauma* 2001; **51**: 835–841.

150. Dereeper, E., Ciardelli, R. & Vincent, J.L. Fatal outcome after polytrauma: multiple organ failure or cerebral damage? *Resuscitation* 1998; **36**: 15–18.

151. Moore, E.A., Moore, E.E. & Read, R.A. Postinjury multiple organ failure: role of extrathoracic injury and sepsis in adult respiratory distress syndrome. *New Horiz.* 1993; **1**: 538–549.

152. Yao, Y.M., Redl, H., Bahrami, S. & Schlag, G. The inflammatory basis of trauma/shock-associated multiple organ failure. [Review] [127 refs]. *Inflammation Res.* 1998; **47**(5): 201–10.

153. Balogh, Z., McKinley, B.A., Cox, C.S., Jr. *et al.* Abdominal compartment syndrome: the cause or effect of postinjury multiple organ failure. *Shock* 2003; **20**: 483–492.

154. Gonzalez, R.J., Moore, E.E., Ciesla, D.J., Biffl, W.L., Johnson, J.L. & Silliman, C.C. Mesenteric lymph is responsible for posthemorrhagic shock systemic neutrophil priming. *J. Trauma* 2001; **51**: 1069–1072.

155. Silliman, C.C., Moore, E.E., Johnson, J.L., Gonzalez, R.J. & Biffl, W.L. Transfusion of the injured patient: proceed with caution. *Shock* 2004; **21**: 291–299.

156. Handrigan, M.T., Burns, A.R. & Bowden, R.A. Hydroxyethyl starch inhibits neutrophil adhesion and transendothelial migration. *Shock* 2005; **24**: 434–439.

157. Alam, H.B., Stanton, K., Koustova, E., Burris, D., Rich, N. & Rhee, P. Effect of different resuscitation strategies on neutrophil activation in a swine model of hemorrhagic shock. *Resuscitation* 2004; **60**: 91–99.

158. Alam, H.B., Sun, L., Ruff, P., Austin, B., Burris, D. & Rhee, P. E- and P-selectin expression depends on the resuscitation fluid used in hemorrhaged rats. *J. Surg. Res.* 2000; **94**: 145–152.

159. Rhee, P., Burris, D., Kaufmann, C. *et al.* Lactated Ringer's solution resuscitation causes neutrophil activation after hemorrhagic shock. *J. Trauma* 1998; **44**: 313–319.

160. Wang, P., Ba, Z.F., Burkhardt, J. & Chaudry, I.H. Trauma-hemorrhage and resuscitation in the mouse: effects on cardiac output and organ blood flow. *Am. J. Physiol.* 1993; **264**: H1166–H1173.

161. Childs, E.W., Smalley, D.M., Moncure, M., Miller, J.L. & Cheung, L.Y. Effect of WEB 2086 on leukocyte adherence in response to hemorrhagic shock in rats. *J. Trauma* 2000; **49**: 1102–1107.

162. Roumen, R.M., Hendriks, T., van d, V. *et al.* Cytokine patterns in patients after major vascular surgery, hemorrhagic shock,

and severe blunt trauma. Relation with subsequent adult respiratory distress syndrome and multiple organ failure. *Ann. Surg.* 1993; **218**: 769–776.

163. Yin, W., Hu, X.M., Yuan, J. *et al.* [Potential molecular mechanism of multiple organ dysfunction syndrome induced by hemorrhage and endotoxin]. [Chinese]. *Zhongguo Wei Zhong Bing Ji Jiu Yi Xue /Chin. Crit. Care Med./Zhongguo Weizhongbing Jijiuyixue* 2003; **15**(3): 143–146.

164. Vallejo, J.G., Nemoto, S., Ishiyama, M. *et al.* Functional significance of inflammatory mediators in a murine model of resuscitated hemorrhagic shock. *Am. J. Physiol. Heart Circ. Physiol.* 2005; **288**: H1272–H1277.

165. Brundage, S.I., Zautke, N.A., Holcomb, J.B. *et al.* Interleukin-6 infusion blunts proinflammatory cytokine production without causing systematic toxicity in a swine model of uncontrolled hemorrhagic shock. *J. Trauma* 2004; **57**: 970–977.

166. Yang, H., Wang, H., Czura, C.J. & Tracey, K.J. The cytokine activity of HMGB1. *J Leukoc Biol.* 2005; **78**: 1–8.

167. Rensing, H., Bauer, I., Datene, V., Patau, C., Pannen, B.H. & Bauer, M. Differential expression pattern of heme oxygenase-1/heat shock protein 32 and nitric oxide synthase-II and their impact on liver injury in a rat model of hemorrhage and resuscitation. *Crit. Care Med.* 1999; **27**: 2766–2775.

168. Kiang, J.G. Inducible heat shock protein 70 kD and inducible nitric oxide synthase in hemorrhage/resuscitation-induced injury. *Cell Res.* 2004; **14**: 450–459.

169. Chen, T., Zamora, R., Zuckerbraun, B. & Billiar, T.R. Role of nitric oxide in liver injury. *Curr. Mol. Med.* 2003; **3**: 519–526.

170. Szabo, C. & Billiar, T.R. Novel roles of nitric oxide in hemorrhagic shock. *Shock* 1999; **12**: 1–9.

171. Hierholzer, C., Kalff, J.C., Billiar, T.R., Bauer, A.J., Tweardy, D.J. & Harbrecht, B.G. Induced nitric oxide promotes intestinal inflammation following hemorrhagic shock. *Am. J. Physiol. Gastrointest. Liver Physiol.* 2004; **286**: G225–G233.

172. Menezes, J.M., Hierholzer, C., Watkins, S.C., Billiar, T.R., Peitzman, A.B. & Harbrecht, B.G. The modulation of hepatic injury and heat shock expression by inhibition of inducible nitric oxide synthase after hemorrhagic shock. *Shock* 2002; **17**: 13–18.

173. Hierholzer, C., Harbrecht, B., Menezes, J.M. *et al.* Essential role of induced nitric oxide in the initiation of the inflammatory response after hemorrhagic shock. *J. Exp. Med.* 1998; **187**: 917–928.

174. Billiar, T.R. The diverging roles of carbon monoxide and nitric oxide in resuscitated hemorrhagic shock. *Crit. Care Med.* 1999; **27**: 2842–2843.

175. Kiang, J.G., Bowman, P.D., Wu, B.W. *et al.* Geldanamycin treatment inhibits hemorrhage-induced increases in KLF6 and iNOS expression in unresuscitated mouse organs: role of inducible HSP70. *J. Appl. Physiol.* 2004; **97**: 564–569.

176. Szabo, C. Potential role of the peroxynitrate-poly(ADP-ribose) synthetase pathway in a rat model of severe hemorrhagic shock. *Shock* 1998; **9**: 341–344.

177. McDonald, M.C., Izumi, M., Cuzzocrea, S. & Thiemermann, C. A novel, potent and selective inhibitor of the activity of inducible nitric oxide synthase (GW274150) reduces the organ injury in hemorrhagic shock. *J. Physiol. Pharmacol.* 2002; **53**(4 Pt 1): 555–569.

178. Mota-Filipe, H., McDonald, M.C., Cuzzocrea, S. & Thiemermann, C. A membrane-permeable radical scavenger reduces the organ injury in hemorrhagic shock. *Shock* 1999; **12**: 255–261.

179. Deitch, E.A., Xu, D., Franko, L., Ayala, A. & Chaudry, I.H. Evidence favoring the role of the gut as a cytokine-generating organ in rats subjected to hemorrhagic shock. *Shock* 1994; **1**: 141–145.

180. Hassoun, H.T., Kone, B.C., Mercer, D.W., Moody, F.G., Weisbrodt, N.W. & Moore, F.A. Post-injury multiple organ failure: the role of the gut. *Shock* 2001; **15**: 1–10.

181. Fink, M.P. Gastrointestinal mucosal injury in experimental models of shock, trauma, and sepsis. *Crit. Care Med.* 1991; **19**: 627–641.

182. Yang, R., Gallo, D.J., Baust, J.J., Watkins, S.K., Delude, R.L. & Fink, M.P. Effect of hemorrhagic shock on gut barrier function and expression of stress-related genes in normal and gnotobiotic mice. *Am. J. Physiol. Regul. Integr. Comp. Physiol.* 2002; **283**: R1263–R1274.

183. Fink, M.P. Effect of critical illness on microbial translocation and gastrointestinal mucosa permeability. *Semin. Respir. Infect.* 1994; **9**: 256–260.

184. Deitch, E.A., Forsythe, R., Anjaria, D. *et al.* The role of lymph factors in lung injury, bone marrow suppression, and endothelial cell dysfunction in a primate model of trauma-hemorrhagic shock. *Shock* 2004; **22**: 221–228.

185. Magnotti, L.J., Upperman, J.S., Xu, D.Z., Lu, Q. & Deitch, E.A. Gut-derived mesenteric lymph but not portal blood increases endothelial cell permeability and promotes lung injury after hemorrhagic shock. *Ann. Surg.* 1998; **228**: 518–527.

186. Schmid-Schonbein, G.W. & Hugli, T.E. A new hypothesis for microvascular inflammation in shock and multiorgan failure: self-digestion by pancreatic enzymes. *Microcirculation* 2005; **12**: 71–82.

187. Zallen, G., Moore, E.E., Johnson, J.L., Tamura, D.Y., Ciesla, D.J. & Silliman, C.C. Posthemorrhagic shock mesenteric lymph primes circulating neutrophils and provokes lung injury. *J. Surg. Res.* 1999; **83**: 83–88.

188. Zakaria, E.R., Garrison, R.N., Spain, D.A., Matheson, P.J., Harris, P.D. & Richardson, J.D. Intraperitoneal resuscitation improves intestinal blood flow following hemorrhagic shock. *Ann. Surg.* 2003; **237**(5): 704–711.

189. Deitch, E.A., Bridges, W., Berg, R., Specian, R.D. & Granger, D.N. Hemorrhagic shock-induced bacterial translocation: the role of neutrophils and hydroxyl radicals. *J. Trauma* 1990; **30**: 942–951.

190. Flynn, W.J., Cryer, H.G. & Garrison, R.N. Pentoxifylline restores intestinal microvascular blood flow during resuscitated hemorrhagic shock. *Surgery* 1991; **110**: 350–356.

191. Wattanasirichaigoon, S., Menconi, M.J. & Fink, M.P. Lisofylline ameliorates intestinal and hepatic injury induced

by hemorrhage and resuscitation in rats. *Crit. Care Med.* 2000; **28**: 1540–1549.

192. Cohen, D.B., Magnotti, L.J., Lu, Q. *et al.* Pancreatic duct ligation reduces lung injury following trauma and hemorrhagic shock. *Ann. Surg.* 2004; **240**: 885–891.

193. Doucet, J.J., Hoyt, D.B., Coimbra, R. *et al.* Inhibition of enteral enzymes by enteroclysis with nafamostat mesilate reduces neutrophil activation and transfusion requirements after hemorrhagic shock. *J. Trauma* 2004; **56**: 501–510.

194. Jernigan, T.W., Croce, M.A. & Fabian, T.C. Apoptosis and necrosis in the development of acute lung injury after hemorrhagic shock. *Am. Surg.* 2004; **70**: 1094–1098.

195. Davidson, M.T., Deitch, E.A., Lu, Q. *et al.* Trauma-hemorrhagic shock mesenteric lymph induces endothelial apoptosis that involves both caspase-dependent and caspase-independent mechanisms. *Ann. Surg.* 2004; **240**: 123–131.

196. Sutherland, L.M., Edwards, Y.S. & Murray, A.W. Alveolar type II cell apoptosis. *Comp. Biochem. Physiol. A Mol. Integr. Physiol.* 2001; **129**: 267–285.

197. Deb, S., Martin, B., Sun, L. *et al.* Resuscitation with lactated Ringer's solution in rats with hemorrhagic shock induces immediate apoptosis. *J. Trauma* 1999; **46**: 582–588.

198. Shires, G.T., Browder, L.K., Steljes, T.P., Williams, S.J., Browder, T.D. & Barber, A.E. The effect of shock resuscitation fluids on apoptosis. *Am. J. Surg.* 2005; **189**: 85–91.

199. Van, W.C., III, Dhar, A. & Morrison, D. Hemorrahagic shock: a new look at an old problem. *Mo. Med.* 2003; **100**: 518–523.

200. Angele, M.K., Knoferl, M.W., Schwacha, M.G. *et al.* Sex steroids regulate pro- and anti-inflammatory cytokine release by macrophages after trauma-hemorrhage. *Am. J. Physiol.* 1999; **277** (1 Pt 1): C35–C42.

201. Knoferl, M.W., Angele, M.K., Schwacha, M.G., nantha Samy, T.S., Bland, K.I. & Chaudry, I.H. Immunoprotection in proestrus females following trauma-hemorrhage: the pivotal role of estrogen receptors. *Cell. Immunol.* 2003; **222**(1): 27–34

202. Szalay, L., Shimizu, T., Schwacha, M.G. *et al.* Mechanism of salutary effects of estradiol on organ function after trauma-hemorrhage: upregulation of heme oxygenase. *Am. J. Physiol. – Heart Circ. Physiol.* 2005; **289**(1): H92–H98.

203. Szebeni, J., Baranyi, L., Savay, S. *et al.* Complement activation during hemorrhagic shock and resuscitation in swine. *Shock* 2003; **20**: 347–55.

204. Fruchterman, T.M., Spain, D.A., Wilson, M.A., Harris, P.D. & Garrison, R.N. Complement inhibition prevents gut ischemia and endothelial cell dysfunction after hemorrhage/resuscitation. *Surgery* 1998; **124**(4): 782–791.

205. Horstick, G., Kempf, T., Lauterbach, M. *et al.* Cl-esterase-inhibitor treatment at early reperfusion of hemorrhagic shock reduces mesentry leukocyte adhesion and rolling. *Microcirculation* 2001; **8**: 427–433.

206. Tracey, K.J. The inflammatory reflex. *Nature* 2002; **420**: 853–859.

207. Guarini, S., Altavilla, D., Cainazzo, M.M. *et al.* Efferent vagal fibre stimulation blunts nuclear factor-kappaB activation

and protects against hypovolemic hemorrhagic shock. *Circulation* 2003; **107**: 1189–1194.

208. Guarini, S., Cainazzo, M.M., Giuliani, D. *et al.* Adrenocorticotropin reverses hemorrhagic shock in anesthetized rats through the rapid activation of a vagal anti-inflammatory pathway. *Cardiovasc. Res.* 2004; **63**: 357–365.

209. Mathru, M. & Lang, J.D. Endothelial dysfunction in trauma patients: a preliminary communication. *Shock* 2005; **24**: 210–213.

210. Cooke, J.P. Does ADMA cause endothelial dysfunction? *Arterioscler. Thromb. Vasc. Biol.* 2000; **20**: 2032–2037.

211. Nijveldt, R.J., Teerlink, T., van der, H.B. *et al.* Asymmetrical dimethylarginine (ADMA) in critically ill patients: high plasma ADMA concentration is an independent risk factor of ICU mortality. *Clin. Nutr.* 2003; **22**: 23–30.

212. Nijveldt, R.J., Siroen, M.P., Teerlink, T. & van Leeuwen, P.A. Elimination of asymmetric dimethylarginine by the kidney and the liver: a link to the development of multiple organ failure? *J. Nutr.* 2004; **134**: 2848S–2852S.

213. Sloan, E.P., Koenigsberg, M., Gens, D. *et al.* Diaspirin cross-linked hemoglobin (DCLHb) in the treatment of severe traumatic hemorrhagic shock: a randomized controlled efficacy trial. *J. Am. Med. Assoc.* 1999; **282**: 1857–1864.

214. Gurney, J., Philbin, N., Rice, J. *et al.* A hemoglobin based oxygen carrier, bovine polymerized hemoglobin (HBOC-201) versus Hetastarch (HEX) in an uncontrolled liver injury hemorrhagic shock swine model with delayed evacuation. *J. Trauma* 2004; **57**: 726–738.

215. Pawloski, J.R., Hess, D.T. & Stamler, J.S. Export by red blood cells of nitric oxide bioactivity. *Nature* 2001; **409**: 622–626.

216. Foster, M.W., McMahon, T.J. & Stamler, J.S. S-nitrosylation in health and disease. *Trends Mol. Med.* 2003; **9**: 160–168.

217. Voelckel, W.G., Lurie, K.G., Lindner, K.H. *et al.* Vasopressin improves survival after cardiac arrest in hypovolemic shock. *Anesth. Analg.* 2000; **91** (3): 627–634.

218. Haas, T., Voelckel, W.G. Wiedermann, F., Wenzel, V. & Lindner, K.H. Successful resuscitation of a traumatic cardiac arrest victim in hemorrhagic shock with vasopressin: a case report and brief review of the literature. [Review] [29 refs]. *J. Trauma-Injury Infect. Crit. Care* 2004; **57** (1): 177–179.

219. Krismer, A.C., Wenzel, V., Voelckel, W.G. *et al.* Employing vasopressin as an adjunct vasopressor in uncontrolled traumatic hemorrhagic shock. Three cases and a brief analysis of the literature. *Anaesthesist* 2005; **54** (3): 220–224.

220. Stadlbauer, K.H., Wagner-Berger, H.G., Raedler, C. *et al.* Vasopressin, but not fluid resuscitation, enhances survival in a liver trauma model with uncontrolled and otherwise lethal hemorrhagic shock in pigs. *Anesthesiology* 2003; **98** (3): 699–704.

221. Kentner, R., Rollwagen, F.M., Prueckner, S. *et al.* Effects of mild hypothermia on survival and serum cytokines in uncontrolled hemorrhagic shock in rats. *Shock* 2002; **17**: 521–526.

222. Prueckner, S., Safar, P., Kentner, R., Stezoski, J. & Tisherman, S.A. Mild hypothermia increases survival from severe

pressure-controlled hemorrhagic shock in rats. *J. Trauma.* 2001; **50**: 253–262.

223. Takasu, A., Stezoski, S.W., Stezoski, J., Safar, P. & Tisherman, S.A. Mild or moderate hypothermia, but not increased oxygen breathing, increases long-term survival after uncontrolled hemorrhagic shock in rats. *Crit. Care Med.* 2000; **28**: 2465–2474.

224. Wu, X., Stezoski, J., Safar, P. *et al.* Mild hypothermia during hemorrhagic shock in rats improves survival without significant effects on inflammatory responses. *Crit. Care Med.* 2003; **31**: 195–202.

225. Wu, X., Stezoski, J., Safar, P. *et al.* Systemic hypothermia, but not regional gut hypothermia, improves survival from prolonged hemorrhagic shock in rats. *J. Trauma* 2002; **53**: 654–662.

57

Cardiopulmonary resuscitation in hypothermic patients

P. Mair, B. Schwarz[1], B. Walpoth[2] and T. Silfvast[3]

[1] Department of Anaesthesia and Intensive Care Medicine, Innsbruck Medical University, A-6020 Innsbruck, Austria
[2] Cardiovascular Research Service of Cardiovascular Surgery, University Hospital, CH-1211 Geneva, Switzerland
[3] Department of Anaesthesia and Intensive Care Medicine, Meilhati Hospital of Helsinki, University Central Hospital, FIN-00029 Helsinki, Finland

Introduction

The pathophysiological changes associated with hypothermia make cardiopulmonary resuscitation a unique challenge in patients with severe accidental hypothermia.[1–5] Hypothermia offers protection from ischemic tissue injury. Therefore, hypothermic patients have survived prolonged periods of untreated cardiac arrest and resuscitation efforts lasting for hours.[2,6,7] The arrested hypothermic heart often does not respond to electrical or pharmacological therapy unless rewarmed.[3,8,9] Therefore, diagnosis of irreversible cardiorespiratory arrest is difficult during hypothermia and is often defined as "the failure to revive with rewarming".[3] It is widely accepted that "nobody is dead unless warm and dead."[1] In addition to basic and advanced cardiac life support adopted to the particular needs of hypothermia, rapid core rewarming is an essential cornerstone of any resuscitation effort. Extracorporeal circulation is considered the method of choice to accomplish core rewarming in arrested hypothermic patients while offering optimal circulatory support.[10,11]

Pathophysiology of hypothermic cardiac arrest

Hypothermic cardiac arrest may occur in clinically distinct groups of patients. Cardiac arrest may affect otherwise healthy individuals trapped in cold environments, with cardiac arrest being the sole consequence of the deleterious effects of hypothermia on the cardiovascular system.[12,13] Cardiac arrest may occur in individuals submerged in ice water or snow, who suffer from asphyxia while rapidly cooling.[14,15] In these patients cardiorespiratory arrest is, at least partly, a consequence of asphyxia, and hypothermia may offer protection from irreversible ischemic injury when substantial hypothermia has developed before cardiac arrest. The healthy human body responds to cold stress in a rather uniform way, resulting in a predictable pattern of clinical symptoms and organ dysfunctions depending on the degree of hypothermia (Table 57.1). The two single most important responses to cold stress are an increase in endogenous heat production (e.g., shivering) and an intense sympathetic stimulation.[4,9,16] This results in a central pooling of blood, a marked temperature gradient between the core and the shell of the body of up to 20 °C, cold diuresis, an increase in hematocrit, volume depletion, and depletion of glucose stores.[4,9,17] The response to cold depends on the rate of cooling.[9] The overwhelming cold stress during submersion in ice water will result in a different cardiovascular and metabolic response compared to the prolonged cooling process in an exhausted mountaineer. Sometimes accidental hypothermia affects patients suffering from co-morbidities that alter thermoregulation per se and thus the response to cold stress. Extremes of age, traumatic shock, cerebrovascular accidents, spinal cord injuries, and endocrine disorders (myxedema, hypoglycemia) are the most important among these conditions.[4,9] Mortality of hypothermic patients with disorders of their thermoregulatory system is often determined by their underlying disease rather than by hypothermia.[9,18] Alcohol and drugs like sedatives and opiates also significantly alter the physiological response to cold stress.[19,20] It is important to consider the individual pre-arrest pathophysiology in a hypothermic patient and to adopt treatment protocols to the specific needs of the individual patient.

Cardiac Arrest: The Science and Practice of Resuscitation Medicine. 2nd edn., ed. Norman Paradis, Henry Halperin, Karl Kern, Volker Wenzel, Douglas Chamberlain. Published by Cambridge University Press. © Cambridge University Press, 2007.

Table 57.1. Symptoms of accidental hypothermia

	Mild hypothermia 35°C–32°C	Moderate hypothermia 32°C–28°C	Severe hypothermia < 28°C
Motor function	Involuntary shivering	Shivering gradually disappears	Muscles and joints rigid
Cerebral function	Intellectual impairment	Consciousness	Deep coma[a]
	Agitated, feels intensely cold	increasingly depressed	Pupils may be fixed, dilated
Respiratory function	Hyperventilation	Increasing respiratory depression	Hypoventilation[b]
			Increased bronchial secretion
Cardiocirculatory function	Hypertension, tachycardia	Supraventricular tachyarrhythmias	Bradycardia[b]
	Strong central pulses	Only central pulses palpable	Danger of ventricular fibrillation
			Pulses may be undetectable

[a]Electroencephalogram becomes isoelectric at a core temperature of 20°C; [b]asystole and respiratory arrest occur at a core temperature around 23°C.

Metabolism, oxygen demand, and protection from ischemic tissue injury

The capacity of hypothermia to protect tissue from ischemic injury has been well known for decades and is routinely used in cardiac surgery. After controlled induction of hypothermia (core temperature below 20°C), circulatory arrest is tolerated without obvious neurological injury for periods of up to 45 minutes in adults and up to 60 minutes in infants.[21] In short-term profound hypothermia, the reduction in metabolic rate is the principal component responsible for maintaining tissue viability in cases of ischemic injury. Basically, a reduction in oxygen demand of 5 to 9% of baseline value can be expected with each degree of reduction in body core temperature.[17,22,23] Nonetheless, the impact of hypothermia on metabolism varies significantly among different organs, different cells in a particular organ, and even for different enzymatic reactions within an individual cell.[24] It has been stated repeatedly that during spontaneous circulation the hypothermic myocardium is more susceptible to ischemic injury than is the brain.[25,26] Experimental data suggest that the effect of hypothermia is not linear for various degrees of hypothermia. The temperature coefficient for myocardial protection, which describes the relation between temperature and myocardial preservation for every 10°C change in temperature, is 2.2 for a change from 35°C to 25°C, but 1.6 for a change from 15°C to 5°C.[27] Experimental and human clinical experience suggests that decreasing core temperature below 15°C to 10°C results in a decline in resuscitability rather than further enhanced protection from ischemic injury.[28,29] It is widely accepted that myocardial preservation is optimal during cardioplegic cardiac

arrest in open heart surgery within the temperature range between 10 and 20°C.[24,28] With a core temperature around 10°C, local organ cooling (e.g., brain) is better tolerated than total body hypothermia.[30] Obviously, with such low core temperatures total body hypothermia itself becomes deleterious. One possible explanation for these deleterious effects is the marked difference in the temperature dependence of biological processes. The phenomenon of tissue swelling in response to profound hypothermia, for example, has been attributed to the more pronounced inhibition of the active ion pumps in comparison to passive diffusion among electrochemical gradients.[24] Although extreme hypothermia per se is detrimental, it is not possible to define a borderline temperature below which hypothermia-induced tissue injury is irreversible. Most likely this borderline is different for various organs and depends on the type of cooling (e.g., rapid, controlled cooling with extracorporeal circulation versus slow, uncontrolled cooling during accidental hypothermia). Most of our knowledge about the protective as well as detrimental effects of hypothermia is derived from experimental and clinical data during controlled cooling with use of extracorporeal circulation. It is unclear whether and how these data can be extrapolated to patients with severe accidental hypothermia.

Effects of hypothermia on the myocardium

Hypothermia alters myocardial conduction and results in ECG abnormalities like progressive bradycardia, Q–T prolongation, QRS prolongation, and the "J" wave.[31] Cooling of the heart increases the risk for arrhythmias. Atrial fibrillation is common early during cooling;[16,17] when body core temperature falls below 30 °C, the likelihood for ventricular arrhythmias and ventricular fibrillation is also markedly increased.[2,3,16,17] Possible explanations for the increased irritability of the myocardium during hypothermia are the alterations in the membrane potential secondary to defects of membrane ion channels.[32,33] Consequently, in experimental studies antiarrhythmic drugs like bretylium increase the threshold for ventricular fibrillation in the hypothermic heart.[34-36] Hypoxia, acid–base disturbances, high levels of endogenous catecholamine, myocardial temperature gradients, and rapid endocardial cooling caused by a sudden return of cold blood from the shell of the body (afterdrop) may be additional mechanisms contributing to myocardial irritability during clinical hypothermia.[2,4,9]

Acid–base balance during hypothermia

A unique problem in patients with severe accidental hypothermia is the management of their acid–base balance.[37] Electromechanical neutrality is temperature-dependent and to maintain electromechanical neutrality, pH must increase when temperature decreases. In an electromechanically neutral cell, pH will be 7.40 at 37 °C, but 7.80 at 20 °C. When temperature decreases, the solubility of gases in blood will increase. Consequently, when keeping total CO_2 content in blood constant, the increased solubility will result in a reduction in PCO_2. For example, a given blood CO_2 content corresponds to a PCO_2 of 40 mmHg measured at 37 °C, but only to a PCO_2 of 16 mmHg when measured at a blood temperature of 20 °C. Taken together, this causes a situation where electromechanical neutrality is maintained with temperature changes. Electromechanical neutrality is thought to be essential for the preservation of many cellular processes, e.g., the optimal function of the imidazole buffering system.[21,37]

In clinical practice, blood samples are heated to 37 °C before measuring the acid–base status (temperature uncorrected values). With use of the software of the blood gas analyzer, the values for a given blood temperature can be calculated with the help of nomograms (temperature corrected values). For patient management either corrected or uncorrected PCO_2 values can be taken. Choosing uncorrected values will keep the CO_2 content constant and maintain electromechanical neutrality (alpha-stat acid–base management), whereas choosing the temperature-corrected values will increase total CO_2 content and keep pH constant (pH-stat acid–base management).[21,37] Whether an alpha- or pH-stat regimen should be used during severe hypothermia is a matter of debate. Some experimental animal and clinical data from pediatric cardiac surgical patients indicate that using a pH-stat regimen may improve neurological outcome after cardiocirculatory arrest, reduce myocardial irritability, and increase tissue oxygen delivery.[21] Results are inconsistent, however, and are limited to short-term controlled hypothermia. Therefore, most clinicians use an alpha-stat approach, not only because the preponderance of evidence supports the use of uncorrected blood gas values at least in adult patients,[16] but also because CO_2 to be added to the inspired gas is rarely available in emergency departments or intensive care units. To reach a sufficient CO_2 accumulation for pH-stat management solely by hypoventilation necessitates a degree of hypoventilation that will result in alveolar collapse and hypoxia.[16,38]

Experimental models of hypothermic cardiac arrest

Several experimental studies in animal models of hypothermic cardiopulmonary resuscitation have been published during the last few years. These studies have improved our knowledge and understanding of therapeutic interventions for hypothermic cardiac arrest. Experimental animal data may be of particular interest for evidence-based decision-making, as so far no prospective clinical studies of hypothermic CPR have been published.

External chest compression

Little was known about the efficacy of external chest compression during hypothermia before Maningas studied organ blood flow produced by conventional closed-chest CPR in a swine model in 1986.[39] Maningas demonstrated that, when compared to normothermia, blood flow during hypothermic CPR was lower when comparable forces of chest compression were used, but that it did not decrease over time. The reduced organ blood flow with standard compression forces may be caused by changes in the viscoelastic properties of the thorax during hypothermia. That blood flow is maintained during prolonged external chest compression can be explained by the profound vasoconstriction potency of deep hypothermia. These experimental data suggest that increasing the force of chest compression may improve blood flow, although it is not known whether this increases the risk for CPR-associated injuries.

Drug administration and defibrillation

Several recent experimental studies have focused on the effects of drug administration on coronary perfusion pressure and success of defibrillation. Drug administration is controversial when the core temperature is below 30 °C.[40,41] Vasopressor drugs may not be necessary because of the vasoconstrictor potency of severe hypothermia. Furthermore, antiarrhythmic drugs may not be effective during hypothermia and any drug administered repeatedly may accumulate to toxic levels owing to decreased metabolism.[5]

Experimental studies demonstrated that coronary perfusion pressure during hypothermic CPR increases to a level necessary for restoration of spontaneous circulation only after administration of epinephrine or vasopressin, clearly questioning the assumption that vasopressor drug administration is neither necessary nor effective during hypothermic CPR.[40,41] In accordance with these experimental data, restoration of spontaneous circulation after vasopressor drug administration has been described in case reports of hypothermic clinical CPR.[42–45] Vasopressor drugs, however, may be necessary only after prolonged periods of cardiac arrest. After a short 4-minute period of hypothermic cardiac arrest, coronary perfusion pressure has also been maintained around the threshold associated with restoration of spontaneous circulation without drug administration.[46] The increase in coronary perfusion pressure associated with administration of vasopressor drugs facilitates transient restoration of spontaneous circulation.[40] Without concomitant rewarming efforts, however, no positive effects on long-term survival rates were observed. By contrast, when combined with warm fluid thoracic lavage at 40 °C, 0.4 U/kg of vasopressin significantly improved 1-hour survival rate.[41] Kornberger et al. demonstrated a significantly enhanced mixed venous hypercarbic acidosis and a deteriorated CPR outcome after treatment with epinephrine.[46] This is most likely due to the beta-mimetic side effects of epinephrine and, at least in this pig model of hypothermic CPR, vasopressin may be the vasopressor drug of choice. Two further animal studies demonstrated no positive effects of the antiarrhythmic drug amiodarone alone or in combination with vasopressin on success of defibrillation during hypothermic CPR.[47,48]

A recent experimental animal study evaluated the energy requirements for defibrillation during normothermia and hypothermia.[49] Interestingly, severe hypothermia (30 °C) decreased energy requirements for defibrillation after ventricular fibrillation of short duration. At energies of 20 Joule (J), 30 J, and 50 J the percent success of defibrillation was higher in severe hypothermic conditions. Moderate hypothermia (33 °C) did not affect energy requirements. These findings cannot be explained by a change in transthoracic impedance and transthoracic current, because transthoracic impedance rose and transthoracic current fell. The mechanism for the reduced energy requirements during hypothermia is unknown, but it may be due to altered electrophysiologic or mechanical properties of the hypothermic myocardium.

Clinical management of the hypothermic patient with cardiac arrest

Hypothermic cardiac arrest in the prehospital setting

Because accidental hypothermia may be associated with a multitude of clinical conditions, there is a real risk of overlooking it.[50] Recognition in the prehospital environment is nevertheless important, because of the increased risk for lethal arrhythmias and the good prognosis even during prolonged cardiopulmonary arrest.[2,51] Basically, the possibility of accidental hypothermia should be kept in mind in any patient with a decreased level of consciousness. Depending on the degree of hypothermia, the clinical condition may vary from obtundation to deep coma.[9,16] Sometimes external causes for hypothermia may be obvious, e.g., immersion of the victim in cold water. The potential for significant hypothermia is often less evident, e.g., indoors if subjects are immobile, there is insufficient heating, and drug or alcohol intoxication ("urban hypothermia"). In particular, elderly people seem to be at a increased risk.[9] Profoundly hypothermic patients found outdoors may be considered dead by inexperienced care providers despite a perfusing rhythm, because of the absence of a palpable pulse, shallow and slow breathing, the paleness of the skin, and the stiffness of the limbs.[4,5] In the prehospital setting, resuscitation should be withheld only if the patient has obvious lethal injuries, hypothermia clearly followed normothermic cardiac arrest, or the body is completely frozen, making CPR impossible.[5]

Temperature monitoring

Reliable diagnosis of accidental hypothermia necessitates prehospital determination of body core temperature. Although various sites and different methods to determine body core temperature in the prehospital environment have been described.[2,51,52] The optimal method is controversial. Theoretically, without the possibility of measuring body temperature, a rough estimate can be obtained by feeling the warmth of a central part of the body that has not been in direct contact with the cold environment (e.g., abdomen in a person lying on the back). According to clinical experience, if the skin feels cold to the examiner's hand, hypothermia should be suspected.

Measurements of tympanic membrane temperature are widely used in European emergency medical systems. These measurements are simple and fast to obtain, but may be inaccurate if the victim has been submerged and the ears are wet or full of snow.[51,52] Prehospital measurements are best done with an electrical thermistor probe, as the reliability of infrared emission thermometers in the prehospital environment has been questioned.[53] Other sites accessible for prehospital measurements are the nasopharynx, the esophagus, and the rectum, but appropriate probes and monitors are rarely available in the prehospital environment. Conventional thermometers generally lack a scale that displays temperatures below 32–33 °C. Rectal temperature measurements require undressing of the patient and the thermometer must be inserted deep enough to give accurate readings. Insertion of an esophageal temperature probe may induce arrhythmias.[2,8] Nasopharyngeal temperature measurements often do not give a reasonable estimate of core temperature in the prehospital environment.

General assessment

The most feared complication in the prehospital management of patients with severe accidental hypothermia is a sudden cardiocirculatory collapse during rescue or evacuation ("hypothermic sudden cardiac death," "circum-rescue collapse," "sheltering death").[2–4,51] "Circum-rescue collapse" occurs almost exclusively at a core temperature below 30 °C, and cardiac arrest is usually due to ventricular fibrillation.[3,8] Although there is no solid scientific evidence that ventricular fibrillation is provoked by patient movements, clinical experience suggests that a perfusing rhythm often turns into ventricular fibrillation during rescue or initial patient assessment.[4,16,51] Therefore, if hypothermia is suspected, the operator should avoid any brisk maneuver and unnecessary movements and evacuate and assess the patient as smoothly as possible. It has been argued that movements of the patient mobilize and transfer cold blood from the shell to the center of the body, causing a sudden further decrease in core temperature of 1 °C–2 °C ("afterdrop").[8,9] This may induce ventricular fibrillation, but solid scientific evidence is missing. After prolonged cold water immersion a different explanation for sudden unexpected cardiocirculatory collapse ("post-immersion collapse") has been suggested.[54,55] Rescue from water is associated with a sudden loss of the hydrostatic pressure acting on the human body during submersion, which may cause a marked decrease in myocardial preload and arterial pressure. The phenomenon is further enhanced by evacuating immersed victims vertically.[55] Consequently, evacuating immersed hypothermic

subjects horizontally is a recommended standard procedure for most sea rescue crews.[55]

Diagnosis of cardiopulmonary arrest in the prehospital setting

Signs of life are often hard to detect in patients with severe hypothermia as there is a marked reduction in heart rate, respiratory rate, and cardiac output. Diagnosis of hypothermic cardiopulmonary arrest is therefore often difficult for the lay rescuer or emergency medical personnel not equipped with an ECG.[5] Consequently, the determination of the patient's cardiac rhythm with the help of an ECG in the prehospital environment has a high priority in a suspected cardiac arrest situation. In an obviously lifeless person, besides VF or asystole, an organized bradycardic rhythm without a detectable pulse may be found. In the case of severe hypothermia, slow, weak myocardial contractions may generate a cardiac output sufficient temporarily to meet the reduced demands of the hypothermic brain. Starting external chest compression will often convert this organized rhythm into ventricular fibrillation.[2,4] In extreme bradycardia, it is difficult to decide whether external chest compression should be started or the patient should be transported to hospital without CPR. Although controversial, it may be reasonable to start external chest compression as long as CPR can be maintained without any major interruptions until hospital admission.

Basic and advanced cardiac life support in the prehospital setting

Alterations in the technique of basic life support have been suggested for patients with severe hypothermia.[4,8] Nevertheless, standard ventilation and external chest compression are performed by most clinicians. There is little scientific evidence supporting suggestions to increase the force of chest compression or to reduce the rate to half of normal. The hearts of hypothermic patients undergoing internal cardiac massage were described as "frozen stiff" and "hard as stone".[12] Therefore, the efficiency of external chest compression has been questioned as the myocardium is obviously not compressible.[12] Considering the large number of hypothermic patients successfully resuscitated after prolonged periods of external chest compression, however, conventional external chest compression obviously provides sufficient blood flow to sustain life. The efficiency of external chest compression is best explained by blood flow generated by a general increase in intrathoracic pressure (thoracic pump mechanism) rather than by direct compression of the heart.[56] This is supported by findings from an echocardiographic study that showed blood flow generated by the thoracic pump mechanism in hypothermic patients with a non-compressible myocardium.[57]

In the hypothermic patient, ventricular fibrillation often persists despite defibrillation or recurs immediately after defibrillation.[2,3] Nevertheless, up to three attempts at defibrillation to terminate ventricular fibrillation are generally recommended.[5] If VF continues or recurs, immediate transfer to an appropriate hospital during ongoing CPR is recommended. Because there is no evidence that prehospital drug administration will increase the success of further attempts at defibrillation,[40,48] transfer to hospital should not be delayed by any time-consuming attempts to obtain intravenous access for drug administration. Asystole often indicates prolonged arrest times, concomitant asphyxia, or hypothermia developing after normothermic cardiorespiratory arrest. If standard CPR efforts fail, the prognosis of each patient has to be assessed individually on the basis of history and clinical presentation. If the patient is considered to be potentially salvageable, immediate transfer to an appropriate hospital for rewarming should occur without further delay. There seems to be no reliable correlation between initial cardiac rhythm and outcome as long as cardiac arrest is primarily due to hypothermia.[58]

Whenever possible, an arrested hypothermic patient should be transferred to a hospital with cardiopulmonary bypass capability.[59] Patients tolerate much longer periods of conventional CPR during hypothermia.[6,7] Therefore, the closest hospital is not necessarily the best choice if a center with cardiopulmonary bypass is within reasonable range. Excellent outcome has been reported even after hours of external chest compression before institution of cardiopulmonary bypass.[10,11] Advance notification of the incoming patient is essential to cut treatment delays, and where possible CPR should be continued without major interruptions during patient transfer. Prevention of further heat loss in hypothermic patients in cardiac arrest is recommended,[5] but efforts to rewarm these patients should be withheld until hospital admission.[59]

In-hospital treatment of patients with hypothermic cardiac arrest

Decision to rewarm and resuscitate

The first decision to be made is whether prolonged resuscitation and rewarming efforts should be started in a patient admitted with hypothermic cardiopulmonary arrest. Considering the protective effects of hypothermia, basically the term "nobody is dead unless warm and dead" should be applied. Lifesaving procedures should never be withheld on the basis of clinical presentation alone.[1,5] On the other hand, mortality of hypothermic cardiac arrest is high in many case series despite aggressive resuscitation efforts.[13,60,61,62] Risk factors associated with poor outcome have been identified and may help to determine when to stop resuscitation (Fig. 57.1). Asystole often indicates concomitant asphyxia or hypothermia following normothermic cardiac arrest. In a hypothermic patient, asystole occurs at a core temperature below 23 °C.[4,16,17] Asystole with a higher core temperature typically indicates that factors apart from hypothermia have contributed to cardiopulmonary arrest. Ventricular fibrillation occurs in patients suffering from hypothermic sudden cardiac death and prolonged resuscitation is normally justified as it is in all patients with witnessed cardiocirculatory collapse.[2,3,10] Patients with a history of exposure to cold have a markedly better prognosis when compared to victims with a history of near drowning or snow burial after avalanche accidents.[10,13,58,62] Hypothermia after near drowning normally indicates prolonged submersion, significant tissue hypoxia, and an extremely poor prognosis.[63,64] Only in case of documented very rapid cooling in ice water protection from ischemic injury can be expected. Survivors of ice water-drowning normally have submersion times of less than 40 minutes with a documented maximal submersion time of 66 minutes.[4,14] Most avalanche victims die from asphyxia and only become hypothermic thereafter. Hypothermia should be considered as underlying reason for cardiac arrest in those few avalanche victims with a history of prolonged snow burial and a documented air pocket at extrication.[65] Body core temperature per se does not seem to determine outcome, except that a significant protective effect should be expected only in patients with a core temperature below 30 °C. The lowest body core temperature documented for a survivor of accidental hypothermia is 13.7 °C, and for a survivor of intentional hypothermia the temperature is 9 °C.[66,67] A plasma potassium level exceeding 10 mmol/l may be used to support the diagnosis of irreversible cardiopulmonary arrest.[13,61,62] Survival may be possible despite extraordinarily high plasma potassium concentrations in patients with extensive local freezing injuries.[68,69] On the other hand, plasma potassium levels exceeding 10 mmol/l are a recommended, clinically useful triage criterion in avalanche victims.[65] Taken together, there is no single factor that reliably predicts irreversible cardiopulmonary arrest in the individual hypothermic patient. Common sense and good clinical judgement often allow identification of those hypothermic arrest victims without a reasonable hope of survival. Determining the prognosis of an individual patient is particularly important when several hypothermic arrest victims are admitted simultaneously in avalanche or climbing accidents.

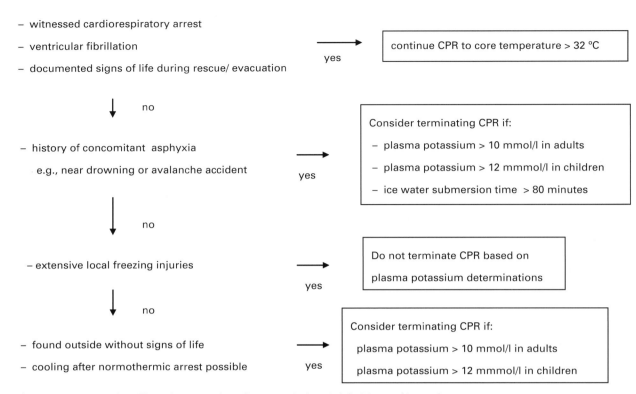

Fig. 57.1. Severe accidental hypothermia with cardiac arrest: in-hospital decision-making and management.

Prevention of cardiocirculatory collapse during in-hospital treatment

Sudden unexpected ventricular fibrillation (hypothermic sudden cardiac death) is not unusual during in-hospital treatment of patients with a core temperature below 28 °C.[2,3,10] Precautions to avoid sudden cardiac death are therefore important in the treatment of severe accidental hypothermia. Although there are no formal studies, it is widely recommended that any direct irritation of the heart (Swan-Ganz catheter, invasive pacing) be avoided and to reduce active and passive movements to a minimum.[2,3,9,16] Insertion of an esophageal temperature probe or of a gastric tube, bladder catheterization, and placement of a thoracostomy tube[2,4,44,70,71] have all been proposed as triggers inducing ventricular fibrillation. The clinician may be well advised to reduce stressful or painful interventions to a minimum. Endotracheal intubation can provoke ventricular fibrillation in profoundly hypothermic patients,[72,73] although this is a very rare event, and it is widely accepted that the advantages of a secure airway and adequate oxygenation outweigh the potential risk of provoking life-threatening arrhythmias.[2,5,16] Rapidly rewarming patients with a core temperature below 28 °C by using an invasive method of active internal rewarming should keep the risk interval for ventricular fibrillation short.[5,16] The efficiency of invasive active internal rewarming techniques such as hemodialysis or body cavity lavage is variable, however, and often there is a significant discrepancy between experimental and clinical efficiency.[16,74–77] Studies demonstrated that forced air rewarming may be a non-invasive, effective and safe alternative for treatment in smaller hospitals.[78–80] Bretylium increases the threshold for ventricular fibrillation during hypothermia and chemical defibrillation after bretylium administration has been reported in a hypothermic patient.[35,81] Amiodarone has no documented antiarrhythmic effects during hypothermia.[47,48] Prophylactic administration of antiarrhythmic drugs to avoid hypothermic sudden cardiac death is neither recommended nor widely used.[5]

Assessment of vital organ perfusion during profound hypothermia

Diagnosis of cardiocirculatory arrest is straightforward in hypothermic patients with asystole or ventricular fibrillation. Diagnosis of inadequate vital organ perfusion, however, may be a problem in patients presenting with extreme bradycardia or unrecordable blood pressure. Extreme bradycardia and weak myocardial contractions may generate a blood flow adequate for the reduced demands during profound hypothermia.[5] The use of Doppler ultrasound probes to detect minimal cardiac output and peripheral blood flow has been suggested.[5] The lowest level of blood pressure that can be tolerated, together with a certain degree of hypothermia, is unknown. Experimental animal data suggest that blood pressure is physiologically reduced to about 50% of baseline at a core temperature of 25 °C.[82] Autoregulation of cerebral blood flow is maintained to a mean arterial pressure as low as 30 mmHg in previously healthy individuals.[83,84] On the other hand, clinical experience demonstrates that many hypothermic patients present with normal arterial pressure despite severe hypothermia, and in some clinical studies low systolic blood pressure was a marker of poor prognosis.[4,85] Interpretation of hemodynamic findings is further obscured by pre-existing cardiovascular diseases, concomitant trauma, or hypovolemia. Sometimes, an obvious discrepancy between the degree of hypothermia and the severity of the hemodynamic compromise may raise doubts that hypotension is solely associated with hypothermia. Furthermore, the therapeutic options to correct bradycardia or hypotension are limited and often controversial. Whether catecholamines, volume load, or vasopressor drugs increase cardiac output and blood pressure or if they can be used safely during hypothermia is controversial and not well studied.[85–88] The efficiency of beta-adrenergic drugs like isoprotenerol in increasing heart rate during hypothermia is controversial.[86,87] Pacing may improve hemodynamics during hypothermia,[89] but invasive transvenous pacing is normally not used as it may induce ventricular fibrillation. The safety and efficiency of transcutaneous pacing has been documented only in a single animal study.[89] Most clinicians would agree to start external chest compression in the in-hospital environment in all hypothermic patients without palpable central pulses or with unrecordable blood pressure, despite the presence of an organized activity in the ECG.

Advanced cardiac life support after hospital admission

Conventional approaches to CPR are often not effective in hypothermic patients with a core temperature below 28 °C.[3,5,9] Repeated administration of epinephrine often proves futile and may damage the heart and result in drug accumulation and delayed toxicity.[5] More than three attempts at defibrillation are considered to be a waste of time without previous rewarming of the myocardium.[5] On the other hand, restoration of spontaneous circulation has been reported in hypothermic patients with a core temperature below 28 °C.[80,90] Electromechanical cardiac activity can be reestablished in patients with a rectal tem-

perature below 20 °C.[80,91] In several case reports, restoration of spontaneous circulation has been reported in close timely association of administration with epinephrine or vasopressin.[8,42,80] In addition, experimental animal data demonstrate that vasopressor drugs increase coronary perfusion pressure during hypothermic CPR (experimental models of hypothermic cardiac arrest). The increase in coronary perfusion pressure may result in an improved CPR outcome when combined with rewarming or after prolonged cardiopulmonary arrest.[41,42] Thus, a pragmatic approach may be to administer at least a single dose of epinephrine or vasopressin. Experimental data available do not support the use of antiarrhythmic drugs during hypothermic CPR.[47,48] It is difficult to perform good quality manual CPR for prolonged periods, because chest compression causes operator fatigue after a few minutes. Use of portable mechanical chest compression devices may achieve an improved and more consistent blood flow.[92] Open chest CPR is an option during prolonged in-hospital resuscitation. Based on his experience in 11 hypothermic patients, Brunette suggested that early emergency room thoracotomy and internal cardiac massage may improve outcome.[71] Nevertheless, in most institutions external chest compression is the preferred method during prolonged CPR efforts. It is perhaps of minor importance how advanced cardiac life support is performed in a hypothermic patient as long as measures do not delay rapid core rewarming in patients without immediate restoration of spontaneous circulation (Table 57.2).

Rewarming options

For hypothermic patients with prolonged cardiac arrest the most important cornerstone of in-hospital resuscitation is initiation of rapid core rewarming.[5] Despite the lack of prospective randomized studies, it is widely accepted that extracorporeal circulation is the method of choice to rewarm arrested hypothermic patients.[3,5,10] When extracorporeal circulation is not available within a reasonable time, successful resuscitation is possible by use of alternative methods of core rewarming during ongoing CPR.[5,71,77,80] Successful resuscitation has been described using non-invasive methods of active rewarming;[80,93,94] nevertheless, invasive methods of active internal rewarming are the recommended therapeutic approach.[5] Experience with peritoneal dialysis, hemodialysis, or warmed fluid thoracic lavage has been reported.[5,74,75,77] The combination of closed chest thoracic lavage with external chest compression seems to be a reasonable, minimal invasive choice suitable for most hospitals (Table 57.3).[77,95–97] Spontaneous circulation was restored in the majority of patients within 2 hours in a

Table 57.2. Key points for the in-hospital treatment of hypothermic cardiac arrest

- Defibrillate three times in case of ventricular fibrillation
  - Consider further attempts after a single dose of epinephrine or vasopressin
- Consider epinephrine or vasopressin in case of asystole
- Check whether blood flow is sufficient to sustain life despite extreme bradycardia
  - Thoroughly check for weak central pulses
  - Consider use of a Doppler ultrasound probe to detect cardiac output
- Decide whether prolonged resuscitation and rewarming is justified
- Check for availability of cardiopulmonary bypass rewarming
  - Advance notification will cut treatment delays
  - Consider an alternative rewarming technique when transfer time to cardiopulmonary bypass exceeds 3 hours
- If prolonged periods of external chest compression are anticipated
  - Check for the availability of a mechanical chest compression device
  - Change resuscitator to avoid poor CPR performance due to fatigue
- Check for alternative rewarming strategies if cardiopulmonary bypass is not an option
  - Closed chest thoracic lavage is a minimal invasive, widely available option

Table 57.3. Suggestion for a minimal invasive treatment protocol for hypothermic cardiac arrest using closed chest thoracic lavage

- Continue external chest compression and consider use of a mechanical compression device
- In case of previous thoracic surgery or thoracic trauma, consider an alternative approach
  - Surface for heat exchange may be limited due to pleural adhesions
- Insert two large bore chest tubes into the left hemithorax
  - One in the mid clavicular line into the second to fourth intercostal space
  - One in the mid axillary line into the fifth to sixth intercostal space
- Infuse 40 °C warmed fluid into the mid clavicular chest tube
  - Actively inject with commercially available pressure-driven fluid warmers
  - Infusion by gravity may be sufficient
  - Use sterile saline if available (use of tap water has been reported)
- Connect standard thoracostomy drainage container to mid axillary chest tube
  - Monitor effluent output to avoid intrathoracic hypertension
- Defibrillate every 15 to 20 minutes of rewarming at least three times
  - Consider application of vasopressin or epinephrine before defibrillation
  - Preferential rewarming of the heart enables defibrillation at low core temperature
- Consider two additional chest tubes in the right hemithorax in case of slow rewarming
  - Rewarming rates of 3 °C to 4 °C/hour should be achieved
- Rewarm to a core temperature > 32 °C before terminating CPR efforts
- Consider use of prophylactic antibiotics after restoration of spontaneous circulation

recently published review on the use of thoracic lavage in arrested hypothermic patients.[77] It is possible that preferential rewarming of the heart during thoracic lavage re-establishes electromechanical activity of the heart more rapidly.[77,95] Experimental animal data suggest that supporting coronary perfusion pressure with vasopressin during rewarming may enhance restoration of spontaneous circulation.[41]

Cardiopulmonary bypass rewarming for hypothermic cardiac arrest

Historical notes

Cardiopulmonary bypass was introduced by Gibbons more than 50 years ago.[98] This technique enables perfusion of the body with oxygenated blood while the heart is arrested. Barratt-Boyes and Kirklin introduced hypothermic circulatory arrest for correction of complex congenital defects and operations involving the aortic arch.[98,99] On the basis of these two techniques, Althaus *et al.* successfully applied cardiopulmonary bypass rewarming to patients with accidental hypothermia and cardiac arrest.[12] Cardiopulmonary bypass rewarming spread rapidly and

has been used worldwide, with mixed results. Reasons for poor outcome are mainly related to indications involving asphyxiated or multitraumatized patients who are either brain-dead due to anoxia, or who develop severe cerebral hemorrhage due to heparinization.[10,100,101]

Indications for cardiopulmonary bypass rewarming

Patients in hypothermic cardiac arrest, without signs of asphyxia or severe brain trauma, are optimal candidates for cardiopulmonary bypass rewarming. Severe hypothermia with impaired cardiorespiratory function can also indicate the need for cardiopulmonary bypass rewarming if the patient is admitted to a hospital with a cardiac surgery unit.[62,102,103] Hypothermic patients without cardio-respiratory arrest can be rewarmed with less invasive or non-invasive methods, such as forced air warming.[5,43,78,79] The latter method is increasingly used in even severely hypothermic patients with good results and is applicable also in small hospitals and for multitraumatized patients.[43,78,79] Possible contraindications to cardiopulmonary bypass rewarming are multisystem-trauma, especially with brain injury since normally a certain level of heparinization is required during cardiopulmonary bypass rewarming.[104] Anticoagulation is necessary even though most hypothermic patients suffer from a severe coagulation disorder. This coagulation disorder may correct itself partly during rewarming, leading to thrombus formation in the cardiopulmonary bypass circuit. Recently, fully heparin-coated cardiopulmonary bypass circuits have permitted the use of lower doses of heparin and, in one published case, the avoidance of any heparinization during cardiopulmonary bypass rewarming.[69]

Advantages and limitations of cardiopulmonary bypass rewarming

The advantages of cardiopulmonary bypass rewarming certainly outweigh the limitations: rapid preferential core rewarming, immediate adequate perfusion and oxygenation of vital organs such as the brain, improved blood rheology, and rapid correction of homeostasis (e.g., acid–base balance). Insertion of a hemofilter into the bypass system allows elimination of noxious substances in cases of intoxication.[10] Nonetheless, some limitations of cardiopulmonary bypass rewarming should be considered. The rate of rewarming with cardiopulmonary bypass is around 8 °C per hour.[10,11] It is not clear whether such rapid rewarming is necessary or could even prove harmful.[105,106] During cardiac surgery fast cooling and rewarming rates are used routinely, but patients with induced hypothermia cannot be compared to patients with accidental, uncontrolled hypothermia. Furthermore, cardiac surgeons try to keep the cardiopulmonary bypass time as short as possible to prevent complications related to the time on an artificial circuit.[107,108] Considering reports of the efficiency of mild hypothermia in preventing brain injury, it may be beneficial to stop rewarming at a core temperature of 33–34 °C and keep the patient mildly hypothermic for 12 to 24 hours.[109] Edema formation is another common problem observed after cardiopulmonary bypass rewarming. Most patients in the study by Walpoth *et al.* developed pulmonary edema already during rewarming,[10] which probably represents a reperfusion injury and there is no reason why a similar phenomenon does not exist in other organs, such as the brain.

Technical aspects of cardiopulmonary bypass rewarming

Technically, cardiopulmonary bypass rewarming is a minor intervention for experienced centers. In the adult patient, peripheral femoral cannulation is preferred and a standard cardiopulmonary bypass circuit or an extracorporeal membrane oxygenation system may be used.[110,111] Extracorporeal membrane oxygenation systems allow cardiopulmonary bypass rewarming outside the operating theatre, e.g., in the emergency department or in an outside hospital.[111–113] Cannulation may be performed percutaneously, allowing rapid cannulation during ongoing CPR.[110,111] In children and infants sternotomy and central cannulation is preferred. In some centers initially low flow perfusion is used,[10] for a few minutes, after which flow rates and temperature are increased step-wise, keeping in mind never to exceed a temperature gradient of 10 °C between the perfusate and the patient's core temperature. With rising temperature, the flow will be increased to calculated full flow values.[10] Defibrillation will occur spontaneously in about 50% of the cases when the temperature rises above 30 °C; defibrillation attempts below 27 °C are rarely successful.[5,10] After weaning from cardiopulmonary bypass care should be taken rigorously to correct the bleeding disorder since there is a synergy of heparin and hypothermia-induced coagulopathy.

Outcome of cardiopulmonary bypass rewarming

The outcome of patients with hypothermic cardiac arrest without asphyxia or brain trauma was excellent in a long-term follow-up study after cardiopulmonary bypass rewarming.[10] Nearly all patients had severe transient pulmonary, brain, or kidney dysfunction immediately after rewarming. Interestingly, cardiovascular complications were rare, probably because of the longer ischemic tolerance of the heart compared to other organs.[10] Outcome after cardiopulmonary bypass rewarming has been described predominantly in case reports or small case series. As most patients not successfully resuscitated will not be reported, it is difficult to determine the exact morbidity and mortality of cardiopulmonary bypass rewarming as long as no international registries that include failed patients have been formed.

Summary

Hypothermic patients have survived prolonged periods of untreated cardiac arrest and resuscitation efforts lasting for hours owing to the protective effects of low body core temperature. Standard protocols for advanced cardiac life support often prove futile in profoundly hypothermic patients and aggressive core rewarming is therefore a cornerstone of any resuscitation effort. Cardiopulmonary bypass rewarming is state-of-the-art for hypothermic patients with cardiac arrest, providing that the technology is available on an immediate basis.

REFERENCES

1. Gregory, R.T., Patton, J.F., Whithey, J.D., Berkley, J.S. & Hilman, H. Treatment after exposure to cold. *Lancet* 1972; **1**: 377–378.

2. Danzl, D.F. & Pozos, R.S. Multicenter hypothermia survey. *Ann. Emerg. Med.* 1987; **16**: 1042–1055.

3. Larach, M.G. Accidental hypothermia. *Lancet* 1995; **345**: 49–498.

4. Lonning, P.E., Skulberg, A. & Abyholm, F. Accidental hypothermia. A review of the literature. *Acta Anaesthesiol. Scand.* 1986; **30**: 601–613.

5. Soar, J., Deakin, C.D., Nolan, J.P. *et al.* European Resuscitation Council Guidelines for resuscitation 2005. Section 7. Cardiac arrest in special circumstances. *Resuscitation* 2005; **67** Suppl I: S135–S170.

6. Roggero, E., Stricker, H. & Biegger, P. Severe accidental hypothermia with cardiopulmonary arrest. Prolonged resuscitation without extracorporeal circulation. *Schweiz Med. Wochenschr.* 1992; **122**: 161–164.

7. Lexow, K. Severe accidental hypothermia: survival after 6 hours 30 minutes of cardiopulmonary resuscitation. *Arctic. Med. Res.* 1991; **50** (Suppl 6): 112–114.

8. Mair, P. & Kornberger, E. Cardiopulmonary resuscitation in accidental hypothermia. *Curr. Opin. Crit. Care* 1999; **5**: 216–222.

9. Lloyd, E.L. Accidental hypthermia. *Resuscitation* 1996; **32**: 111–124.

10. Walpoth, B.H., Walpoth-Aslan, B.N., Mattle, H.P. *et al.* Outcome of survivors of accidental deep hypothermia and circulatory arrest treated with extracorporeal blood warming. *N. Engl. J. Med.* 1997; **337**: 1500–1505.

11. Vretenar, D.F., Urschel, J.D., Parrot, J.C.W. & Unruh, H.W. Cardiopulmonary bypass resuscitation for accidental hypothermia. *Ann. Thorac. Surg.* 1994; **58**: 895–898.

12. Althaus, U., Aeberhard, B., Schuepbach, B., Nachbur, B.H. & Muehlemann, W. Management of profound accidental hypothermia with cardiorespiratory arrest. *Ann. Surg.* 1982; **195**: 492–495.

13. Mair, P., Kornberger, E., Furtwaengler, W., Antretter, H. & Balogh, D. Prognostic markers in patients with severe accidental hypothermia and cardiocirculatory arrest. *Resuscitation* 1994; **27**: 47–54.

14. Bolte, R.G., Black, P.G. & Bowers, S. The use of extracorporeal rewarming in a child submerged for 66 minutes. *J. Am. Med. Assoc.* 1988; **260**: 377–379.

15. Siebke, H., Breivik, H. & Rod, T. Survival after 40 minute submersion without cerebral sequela. *Lancet* 1975, **i**: 1275–1277.

16. Kempainen, R.R., Brunette, D.D. The evaluation and management of accidental hypothermia. *Respir. Care* 2004; **49**: 192–205.

17. Wong, K.C. Physiology and pharmacology of hypothermia *West. J. Med.* 1983; **138**: 227–232.

18. Gentilello, L.M. Advances in the management of hypothermia. *Surg. Clin. North Am.* 1995; **75**: 243–256.

19. Risbo, A., Hagelsten, J.O. & Jesser, K. Human body temperature and controlled cold exposure during moderate and severe experimental alcohol-intoxication. *Acta Anaesth. Scand.* 1981; **25**: 215–218.

20. Kalant, H. & Le, A.D. Effects of ethanol on thermoregulation. *Pharmacol. Ther.* 1984; **23**: 313–314.

21. DiNardo, J.A. Profound hypothermia and circulatory arrest. In Lake, C.L. & Booker, P.D., eds. *Pediatric Cardiac Anaesthesia.* Philadelphia: Lippincott, Williams & Wilkins; **2005**: 253–266.

22. Hegnauer, A.H. & D'Amato, H.E. Oxygen consumption and cardiac output in the hypothermic dog. *Am. J. Physiol.* 1954; **178**: 138–142.

23. Michenfelder, J.D. & Milde, J.H. The relation-ship among canine brain temperature, metabolism, and function during hypothermia. *Anesthesiology* 1991; **75**: 130–136.

24. Rebeyka, I. Hypothermia. In Jonas, J.A. & Elliott, M.J., eds. *Cardiopulmonary Bypass in Neonates, Infants and Young Children.* Oxford, London, Boston: Butterworth-Heinemann, 1994: 54–66.

25. Aoki, M., Nomura, F. & Kawata, H. The effect of calcium and preischemic hypothermia on recovery of myocardial function after cardioplegic ischemia in neonatal lambs. *J. Thorac. Cardiovasc. Surg.* 1993; **104**: 207–213.

26. Frank, S.M., Beatti, C. & Christophersen, R. Unintenional hypothermia is associated with postoperative myocardial ischemia. *Anesthesiology* 1993; **78**: 468–476.

27. Bretschneider, H. Myocardial protection. *Thorac. Cardiovasc. Surg.* 1980; **28**: 295–302.

28. Baldermann, S.C., Binette, J.P. & Chan, A.W. The optimal temperature for preservation of the myocardium during global ischemia. *Ann. Thorac. Surg.* 1983; **35**: 605–614.

29. Keon, W.J., Hendry, P.J. & Taichman, G.C. Cardiac transplantation: the ideal myocardial temperature for graft transport. *Ann. Thorac. Surg.* 1988; **46**: 337–341.

30. Tishermann, S.A., Safar, P. & Radovsky, A. Profound hypothermia ($<$10C) compared with deep hypothermia (15C) improves neurological outcome in dogs after 2 hours circulatory arrest induced to enable resuscitative surgery. *J. Trauma* 1991; **31**: 1051–1062.

31. Trevino, A., Razi, B. & Beller, B.M. The characteristic electrocardiogramm of accidental hypothermia. *Arch. Intern. Med.* 1971; **127**: 470–472.

32. Jacobs, H.K. & South, F.E. Effects of temperature on cardiac transmembrane potentials in hibernation. *Am. J. Physiol.* 1976; **230**: 403–409.

33. Bjornstad, H., Pal, M. Cardiac electrophysiology during hypothermia: implications for medical treatment. *Arct. Med. Res.* 1991; **50** (suppl. 6): 71–75.

34. Bjornstad, H., Mortensen, E., Sager, G. & Refsum, H. Effect of bretylium tosylate on ventricular fibrillation threshold during hypothermia in dogs. *Am. J. Emerg. Med.* 1994; **12**: 407–412.

35. Murphy, K., Novak, R.M. & Tomlanovich, M.C. Use of bretylium tosylate as prophylaxis and treatment in hypothermic ventricular fibrillation in the canine model. *Ann. Emerg. Med.* 1986; **15**: 1160–1166.

36. Orts, A., Alcaraz, C., Delaney, K.A., Goldfrank, L.R., Turndorf, H. & Puig, M.M. Bretylium tosylate and electrically induced cardiac arrhythmias during hypothermia in dogs. *Am. J. Emerg. Med.* 1992; **10**: 311–316.

37. Swan, J.A. Hypothermia and blood pH: a review. *Arch. Intern. Med.* 1988; **148**: 164–1646.

38. Kornberger, E., Mair, P., Hoermann, C., Braun, U. & Bucchardi, H. Hemodynamics and oxygen metabolism in the pig during long term hypothermia: comparison of two pH strategies. *Resuscitation* 1995; **30**: 43–50.

39. Maningas, P.A., DeGuzman, L.R., Hollenbach, S.J., Volk, K.A. & Bellamy, R.F. Regional blood flow during hypothermic arrest. *Ann. Emerg. Med.* 1986; **15**: 390–396.

40. Krismer, A.C., Lindner, K.H., Kornberger, E. *et al.* Cardiopulmonary resuscitation during severe hypothermia in pigs: does epinephrine or vasopressin increase coronary perfision pressure. *Anesth. Analg.* 2000; **90**: 69–73.

41. Schwarz, B., Mair, P., Raedler, C., Deckert, D., Wenzel, V. & Lindner, K.H. Vasopressin improves survival in a pig model of hypothermic cardiopulmonary resuscitation. *Crit. Care Med.* 2002; **30**(6): 1311–1314.

42. Sumann, G., Krismer, A.C., Wenzel, V. *et al.* Cardiopulmonary resuscitation after near drowning and hypothermia: restoration of spontaneous circulation after vasopressin. *Acta Anaesthesiol. Scand.* 2003; **47**: 1–3.

43. Koller, R., Schnider, T.W. & Neidhart, P. Deep accidental hypothermia and cardiac arrest-rewarming with forced air. *Acta Anaesthesiol. Scand.* 1997; **41**: 1359–1364.

44. Irone, M., Mazzaro, E., Zamperetti, N., Dan, M., Fabbri, A. & Mazzuco, A. Extracorporeal membrane oxygenation in emergency resuscitation from deep hypothermia. *Perfusion* 1998; **13**: 211–214.

45. Dominguez, E., Barat, G., Peral, P., Juffe, A., Fernandez, J.M., Avello, F. Recovery from profound hypothermia with cardiac arrest after immersion. *Br. Med. J.* 1973; **289**: 394–395.

46. Kornberger, E., Lindner, K.H., Mayr, V.D. *et al.* Effects of epinephrine in a pig model of hypothermic cardiac arrest and closed-chest cardiopulmonary resuscitation combined with active rewarming. *Resuscitation* 2001; **50**: 301–308.

47. Stoner, J., Martin, G., O'Mara, K., Ehlers, J. & Tomlanovich, M. Amiodarone and bretylium in the treatment of hypothermic ventricular fibrillation in a canine model. *Acad. Emerg. Med.* 2003; **10**(3): 187–191.

48. Schwarz, B., Mair, P., Wagner-Berger, H. Neither vasopressin nor amiodarone improve CPR outcome in an animal model of hypothermic cardiac arrest. *Acta Anaesthesiol. Scand.* 2003; **47**(9): 1114–1118.

49. Rhee, B.J., Zhang, Y., Boddicker, K.A., Davies, L.R. & Kerber, R.E. Effect of hypothermia on transthoracic defibrillation in a swine model. *Resuscitation* 2005; **65**: 79–85.

50. Centre for Disease Control and Prevention. Hypothermia related death-Virginia, November 1996-April 1997. *J. Am. Med. Assoc.* 1998; **279**: 102–104.

51. Giesbrecht, G.G. Prehospital treatment of hypothermia. *Wilderness Environ. Med.* 2001; **12**: 24–31.

52. Morley, A.P. Prehospital monitoring of trauma patients: experience of a helicopter emergency medical service. *Br. J. Anaesth.* 1996; **76**: 726–730.

53. Rogers, J.R., O'Brien, D.L., Wee, C., Smith, A. & Lopez, D. Infrared emission tympanic thermometers cannot be relied upon in a wilderness setting. *Wilderness. Environ. Med.* 1999; **10**: 201–203.

54. Smith, D.E., Kaye, A.D., Mubarek, S.K. *et al.* Cardiac effects of water immersion in healthy volunteers. *Echocardiography* 1998; **15**: 35–42.

55. Stoneham, M.D. & Squires, S.J. Pathogenesis of postimmersion collapse. *Anaesthesia* 1993; **48**: 271–272.

56. Babbs, C.F. New versus old theories of blood flow during CPR. *Crit. Care Med.* 1980; **8**: 191–196.

57. Mair, P., Kornberger, E., Schwarz, B., Baubin, M. & Hoermann, C. Forward blood flow during cardiopulmonary resuscitation in patients with severe accidental hypothermia. An echocardiographic study. *Acta Anaesthesiolog. Scand.* 1998; **42**: 1139–1144.

58. Silfvast, T. & Pettilae, V. Outcome from severe accidental hypothermia in Southern Finland: a 10-year review. *Resuscitation* 2003; **59**: 285–290.

59. Durrer, B., Brugger, H. & Syme, D. International Commission for Mountain Emergency Medicine. The medical on-site treatment of hypothermia. ICAR MedCom recommendations. *High Alt. Med. Biol.* 2003; **4**: 99–103.

60. Auerbach, P.S. Some people are dead when they are cold and dead. *J. Am. Med. Assoc.* 1990; **264**: 1856–1857.

61. Hauty, M.G., Esrig, B.C., Hill, J.G. & Long, W.B. Prognostic factors in severe accidental hypothermia:experience with the Mt. Hood tragedy. *J. Trauma* 1987; **27**: 1107–1112.

62. Schaller, M.D., Fisher, A.D. & Perret, C.H. Hyperkalemia: a prognostic factor during severe acute hypothermia. *J. Am. Med. Assoc.* 1990; **264**: 1842–1845.

63. Suominen, P., Baillie, C., Korpela, R., Rautanen, S., Ranta, S. & Olkkola, K.T. Impact of age, submersion time and water temperature on outcome in near drowning. *Resuscitation* 2002; **52**: 247–254.

64. Quan, L., Wentz, K.R., Gore, E.J. &Copass, M.K. Outcome and predictors of outcome in pediatric submersion victims receiving prehospital care in King County, Washington. *Pediatrics* 1990; **86**: 586–593.

65. Brugger, H., Durrer, B. & Adler-Kastner, L. On-site triage of avalanche victims with asystole by the emergency doctor. *Resuscitation* 1996; **31**: 11–16.

66. Gilbert, M., Busund, R., Skagseth, A., Nilsen, P.A. & Solbo, J.P. Resuscitation from accidental hypothermia of 13.7°C with circulatory arrest. *Lancet* 2000; **355**: 375–376.

67. Niazi, S.A. & Lewis, F.J. Profound hypothermia in man. *Ann. Surg.* 1958; **147**: 264–266.

68. Dobson, J.A.R. & Burgess, J.J. Resuscitation of severe hypothermia by extracorporeal rewarming in a child. *J. Trauma* **40**: 483–485.

69. VonSegesser, L.K., Garcia, E. & Turina, M. Perfusion without systemic heparinization for rewarming in accidental hypothermia. *Ann. Thorac. Surg.* 1991; **52**: 560–561.

70. Kornberger, E. & Mair, P. Important aspects in the treatment of severe accidental hypothermia: the Innsbruck experience. *J. Neurosurg. Anesthesiol.* 1996; **8**: 83–87.

71. Brunette, D.D., Biros, M., Mlinek, E.J., Erlandson, C. & Ruiz, E. Internal cardiac massage and mediastinal irrigation in hypothermic cardiac arrest. *Am. J. Emerg. Med.* 1992; **10**: 32–34.

72. Osborne, L., Kamel El-Din, A.S. & Smith, J.E. Survival after prolonged cardiac arrest and accidental hypothermia. *Br. Med. J.* 1984; **289**: 881–882.

73. Baumgartner, F.J., Janusz, M.T., Jamieson, W.E.R., Winkler, T., Burr, L.H. & Vestrup, J.A. Cardiopulmonary bypass for resuscitation of patients with accidental hypothermia and cardiac arrest. *CJS* 1992; **35**: 184–187.

74. Davis, F.M. & Judson, J.A. Warm peritoneal dialysis in the management of accidental hypothermia.: a report of five cases. *N Z Med. J.* 1981; **94**: 207–209.

75. Jessen, K. & Hagelsten, J.O. Peritoneal dialysis in the treatment of profound accidental hypothermia. *Aviat. Space Environ. Med.* 1978; **49**: 426–429.

76. Lee, H.A. & Ames, A.C. Haemodialysis in severe barbiturate poisioning. *Br. Med. J.* 1965; **231**: 1217–1219.

77. Plaisier, B.R. Thoracic lavage in accidental hypothermia with cardiac arrest – report of a case and review of the literature. *Resuscitation* 2005; **66**: 99–104.

78. Kornberger, E., Schwarz, B., Lindner, K.H. & Mair, P. Forced air surface rewarming in patients with severe accidental hypothermia. *Resuscitation* 1999; **41**: 105–111.

79. Roggla, M., Frossard, M., Wagner, A., Holzer, M., Bur, A. & Roggla, G. Severe accidental hypothermia with and without haemodynamic instability: rewarming without the use of extracorporeal circulation. *Wien Klin. Wochenschr.* 2002; **114**: 315–320.

80. DeCaen, A. Management of profound hypothermia in children without the use of extracorporeal life support therapy. *Lancet* 2002; **360**: 1394–1395.

81. Elenbaas, R.M., Mattson, K., Cole, H., Steele, M., Ryan, J. & Robinson, W. Bretylium in hypothermic-induced ventricular fibrillation in dogs. *Ann. Emerg. Med.* 1984; **13**: 994–999.

82. Tveita, T., Mortensen, E., Hevroy, O., Refsum, H. & Ytrehus, K. Experimental hypothermia: effects of core cooling and rewarming on haemodynamics, coronary blood flow, and myocardial metabolism in dogs. *Anesth. Analg.* 1994; **79**: 212–218.

83. Kern, F.H., Ungerleider, R.M. & Quill, T.J. Cerebral blood flow response to changes in arterial carbon dioxide tension during hypothermic cardiopulmonary bypass in children. *J. Thorac. Cardiovasc. Surg.* 1991; **101**: 618–622.

84. Govier, A.V., Reves, J.G. & McKay, R.D. Factors and their influence on regional cerebral blood flow during nonpulsatile cardiopulmonary bypass. *Ann. Thorac. Surg.* 1984; **38**: 592–600.

85. Vassal, T., Benott-Gonin, B., Carrat, F., Guidet, B., Maury, E. & Offenstadt, G. Severe accidental hypothermia treated in an ICU. *Chest* 2001; **120**: 1998–2003.

86. Hariri, A., Regnier, B., Rapin, M., Lemaire, F. & Le Gall, J.R. Haemodynamic study of prolonged deep accidental hypothermia. *Eur. J. Intens. Care Med.* 1975; **1**: 65–70.

87. Lauri, T. Cardiovascular response to beta-stimulation with isoprotenerol in deep hypothermia. *J. Appl. Physiol.* 1996; **81**: 573–577.

88. Lauri, T. Cardiovascular responses to an acute volume load in deep hypothermia. *Eur. Heart J.* 1996; **17**: 606–611.

89. Dixon, R.G., Dougherty, J.M., White, L.J., Lombino, D. & Rusnak, R.R. Transcutaneous pacing in a hypothermic-dog model. *Ann. Emerg. Med.* 1997; **29**: 602–606.

90. Thomas, R. & Cahill, C.J. Successful defibrillation in profound hypothermia (core temperature 25.6 °C). *Resuscitation* 2000; **47**: 317–320.

91. DaVee, T.S. & Reineberg, E.J. Extreme hypothermia and ventricular fibrillation. *Ann. Emerg. Med.* 1980; **9**: 100–102.

92. Wik, L. & Steinar, K. Use of an automatic mechanical chest compression device as a bridge to establishing cardiopulmonary bypass for a patient with hypothermic cardiac arrest. *Resuscitation* 2005; **66**: 391–394.

93. Bristow, G., Smith, R., Lee, J., Auty, A. & Tweed, W.A. Resuscitation from cardiopulmonary arrest during accidental hypothermia due to exhaustion and exposure. *Can. Med. Assoc. J.* 1977; **117**: 247–249.

94. Wolfe, C.S. Severe hypothermia associated with prolonged cardiorespiratory arrest and full recovery. *J. Am. Board Am. Pract.* 1993; **6**: 594–596.

95. Winegard, C. Successful treatment of severe hypothermia and prolonged cardiac arrest with closed thoracic cavity lavage. *J. Emerg. Med.* 1997; **15**: 629–632.

96. Hall, K.N. & Syverud, S.A. Closed thoracic cavity lavage in the treatment of severe hypothermia in human beings. *Ann. Emerg. Med.* 1990; **19**: 204–206.

97. Iversen, R.J., Atkin, S.H., Jaker, M.A., Quadrel, M.A., Tortella, B.J. & Odom, J.W. Successful CPR in a severely hypothermic patient using continuous thoracostomy lavage. *Ann. Emerg. Med.* 1990; **19**: 1335–1337.

98. Hypothermia, circulatory arrest, and cardiopulmonary bypass. In Kirklin, J.W. & Barratt-Boyes, B.G., eds. *Cardiac Surgery: Morphology, Diagnostic Criteria, Natural History, Techniques, Results and Indications.* 2nd edn. Vol. 1. New York: Churchill Livingstone, 1993; 61–127.

99. Barratt-Boyes, B.G., Neutze, J.M., Clarkson, P.M., Shardey, G.C. &Brandt, P.W.T. Repair of ventricular septal defect in the

first two years of life using profound hypothermia-circulatory arrest techniques. *Ann. Surg.* 1976; **184**: 376–390.

100. Paton, B.C. Accidental hypothermia. *Pharmacol. Ther.* 1983; **22:** 331–337.

101. Davies, D.M., Millar, E.J. & Miller, I.A. Accidental hypothermia treated by extracorporeal blood warming. *Lancet* 1967; **1**: 1036–1037.

102. Bierens, J.J., Knape, J.T. & Gelissen, H.P. Drowning. *Curr. Opin. Crit. Care* 2002; **8**(6): 578–586.

103. Biggart, M.J. & Bohn, D.J. Effect of hypothermia and cardiac arrest on outcome of near-drowning accidents in children. *J. Pediatr.* 1990; **117**: 179–183.

104. Walpoth, B.H., Locher, T., Leupi, F. *et al.* Accidental deep hypothermia with cardiopulmonary arrest. extracorporeal blood rewarming in 11 patients. *Eur. J. Cardiothorac. Surg.* 1990; **4**: 390–393.

105. Rekand, T., Sulg, I.A., Bjaertnes, L. & Jolin, A. Neuro-momitoring in hypothermia and hypothermic hypoxia. *Arct. Med. Res.* 1991; **50** (Suppl. 6): 32–36.

106. Enomoto, S., Hindman, B.J., Dexter, F., Smith, T. & Cutkomp, J. Rapid rewarming causes an increase in the cerebral metabolic rate for oxygen that is temporarily unmatched by cerebral blood flow. *Anesthesiology* 1996; **84**: 1392–1400.

107. Birnbaum, D. & Betz, P. Extracorporeal circulation as a risk factor in heart surgery. *Z. Kardiol.* 1990; **79** (Suppl. 4): 87–93.

108. Okamoto, S., Hashimoto, S., Takei, Y., Yamamoto, H., Tsumori, Y. Influence of prolonged cardiopulmonary bypass on organ function and postoperative complications. *Kyobu Geka.* 1972 Nov; **25**(11): 761–769.

109. Hypothermia after Cardiac Arrest Study Group. Mild therapeutic hypothermia to improve neurological outcome after cardiac arrest. *N. Engl. J. Med.* 2002; **346**: 549–556.

110. Mair, P., Schwarz, B., Kornberger, E. & Balogh, D. Case 5 – 1997. successful resuscitation of a patient with severe accidental hypothermia and prolonged cardiocirculatory arrest using cardiopulmonary bypass. *J. Cardiothorac. Vasc. Anaesth.* 1997; **11**: 901–904.

111. Schwarz, B., Mair, P., Margreiter, J. Experience with percutaneous venoarterial cardiopulmonary bypass for emergency circulatory support. *Crit. Care Med.* 2003; **31**: 758–764.

112. Kumle, B., Doring, B., Mertes, H. & Posival, H. Resuscitation of a near drowning patient by the use of a portable extracorporeal circulation device. *Anaesthesiol. Intensivmed. Notfallmed. Schmerzther.* 1997; **32**: 754–756.

113. Waters, D.J., Belz, M., Lawse, D. & Ulstad, D. Portable cardiopulmonary bypass: resuscitation from prolonged ice water submersion and asystole. *Ann. Thorac. Surg.* 1994; **57**: 1018–1019.

58

Cardiac arrest due to poisoning

Kenneth Heard and Norman A. Paradis

University of Colorado Health Sciences Center, CO, USA

Introduction

Cardiac arrest from poisoning results from direct effects on the cardiovascular or the central nervous system (CNS). Cardiac effects may be caused by perturbation of the autonomic system, antagonism of ion channels, or interference with myocardial metabolism. CNS active poisons cause cardiac arrest through either respiratory suppression (leading to asphyxial arrest) or CNS stimulation with seizures or severe agitation (and the resultant metabolic abnormalities). Restoration of hemodynamics often requires addressing the effects of the poisoning in addition to standard treatment of cardiac arrest.

There are very few studies of specific treatment for cardiac arrest from poisoning. The utility of some interventions, such as ensuring ventilation and oxygenation for patients with cardiac arrest due to CNS depressants, is self-evident. The last two ACLS updates include a section on the treatment of cardiac arrest from poisoning.[1,2] This section was a major advance in that it recognized that cardiac arrest from poisoning is a unique situation, but it also highlighted the lack of quality data in this area. If studies of naloxone are excluded, the recommendations are based on fewer than 500 patients, and most of these data are anecdotal.[3] A few interventions have been studied systematically in animal models of severe poisoning, but there are no systematic animal studies of therapy for cardiac arrest. Given the lack of systematic data, the treatment of cardiac arrest remains more art than science, and the standard of care is poorly defined except for initial supportive care. The recommendations in this chapter are a guide to clinicians, but they should not be considered as standard of care.

Special considerations in the management of cardiac arrest from poisoning

Although many different poisons cause cardiac arrest, the initial treatment must start with standard life-support measures. There are only a handful of specific antidotes that require special consideration during cardiac arrest. Table 58.1 includes the clinical manifestations and treatment of several poisonings that commonly cause cardiac arrest. Although these antidotes may reverse the cardiotoxic effects, they are unlikely to restore perfusion, and must be considered as adjuncts to standard cardiopulmonary resuscitation. Antidotal therapies may help reverse the cardiotoxic effects once perfusion has been restored.

Cardiac arrest from poisoning often occurs in otherwise healthy patients. If the patient's hemodynamics can be supported, there is a potential for recovery. When medications fail, extracorporeal support should be considered.[4–14] For example, one animal study suggested that cardiopulmonary bypass was superior to medical treatment for amitriptyline poisoning.[15] There is also a potential for neuroprotection if the patient is poisoned with barbiturates or calcium channel blockers.[16]

Another consideration is that the optimal doses of commonly used vasoactive medications have not been determined for poisoned patients. In many common overdoses, there is competitive or non-competitive antagonism of the adrenergic receptors. Thus, for example, it is reasonable to exceed the commonly recommended dose range for adrenergic vasopressors.[1,17] Details of treatment for specific poisons are considered below.

Cardiac Arrest: The Science and Practice of Resuscitation Medicine. 2nd edn., ed. Norman Paradis, Henry Halperin, Karl Kern, Volker Wenzel, Douglas Chamberlain. Published by Cambridge University Press. © Cambridge University Press, 2007.

Table 58.1. Presenting symptoms of poisons that commonly cause cardiac arrest and require specific antidotal therapy. These treatments should be used as an adjunct to standard resuscitation measures

Presentation/symptoms	Possible poisoning	Treatment
Bradycardia,heartblock,ventricular or atrial ectopy, hyperkalemia	Acute cardioactive steroid	Digoxin Fab, magnesium, lidocaine, ventricular pacing, amiodarone
Bradycardia, refractory hypotension	Calcium channel antagonists, beta-blocker	Calcium, high dose adrenergic agonists, glucagon
Bradycardia, vasodilatory shock, coma, profound acidosis	Cyanide	Cyanide antidote kit, hydroxocobalamine
Wide complex dysrhythmia, coma, seizures	Tricyclic antidepressants, chloroquine, cocaine	Hypertonic sodium bicarbonate, high dose adrenergic agonists, high dose benzodiazepines
Ventricular fibrillation, shock, profound hypocalcemia	Hydrofluoric acid	High dose calcium chloride
Seizures, pulmonary edema, vomiting/diarrhea, small pupils	Acetylcholinesterase inhibitor (insecticide or chemical weapon)	High dose atropine, high dose benzodiazepines
Marked tachycardia, seizures, vomiting, hypokalemia	Theophylline	Vasopressin, alpha-adrenergic agonists, high dose benzodiazepines
Wide complex dysrhythmias, hypotension	Sodium channel blocking drugs[a]	Hypertonic sodium bicarbonate, adrenergic agonists

[a] See thext for list of drugs reported to block sodium channels.

Calcium channel blockers and beta-adrenergic blockers

Although calcium channel blockers (CCB) and beta-adrenergic blockers have very different mechanisms of action, they produce very similar clinical manifestations when taken in overdose. These medications account for more poisoning deaths than any other cardiovascular drugs and are the second and third most common causes of death from non-narcotic prescription drug poisons.[18]

Pathophysiology

Calcium channel blockers, also known as calcium channel antagonists, bind to and decrease the opening of L-type cardiac and vascular calcium channels. At high doses, these drugs may occupy the channel and completely block entry of calcium, thus preventing the influx of calcium into the cell that is required to activate contraction (or conduction) in these organs. Patients will develop hypotension due to a combination of vasodilatation, bradycardia, and decreased myocardial contraction. Other effects include blocking insulin release, with resultant hyperglycemia and ketosis.[19]

Beta-adrenergic receptor blockers, more commonly known as beta-blockers, are competitive antagonists.

Bradycardia and hypotension are the major manifestations of toxicity from these drugs, which are categorized by their selectivity for beta-1 or beta-2 receptor subtypes. Propranolol also blocks cardiac sodium channels and may produce toxicity similar to quinidine. A few beta-blockers, such as pindolol, have partial beta-adrenergic agonist activity,[19] but it is not clear how these effects alter toxicity following overdose.

Presentation and diagnosis

Calcium channel blocker or beta-blocker poisoning should be suspected when a patient has hypotension, heartblock, and profound bradycardia. Although the hypotension is well tolerated initially, patients often deteriorate rapidly.

Treatment

There are several case reports of successful resuscitation of patients in cardiac arrest after overdose from both CCB and beta-blockers. These reports suggest that multiple therapies, including high-dose calcium, adrenergic agents, and glucagon are often required (see below). Extracorporeal support, including cardiopulmonary bypass and intra-aortic balloon pump, has also been used to treat hemodynamically unstable patients.

Calcium, which has a rapid onset of effect, has been used as first line treatment of hypotension and cardiac arrest from CCB and beta-blocker overdose.[20-24] There are also reported failures of calcium therapy, however, possibly because of inadequate dosing.[25,26] One to 3 grams of calcium chloride may be given as repeated boluses; indeed, one patient required more than 30 g over 12 hours.[27,28]

Adrenergic vasopressors are of rapid onset, and should be considered first line therapies for patients with hemodynamic instability or cardiac arrest. Epinephrine is most commonly used for treatment of cardiac arrest, but norepinephrine and isoproterenol have been used successfully to treat hypotension from CCB poisoning. Phenylephrine is less effective than other vasopressors in animal models.[29,30] Very high doses of vasopressors may be effective when standard doses are inadequate.

Glucagon is considered the "antidote" for both beta-blocker and CCB toxicity. Several animal studies suggest that glucagon may reverse hypotension from these agents, but human case reports are mixed.[31-34] In animals and humans the effects may not be noted for 15–30 minutes after administration,[30] suggesting that glucagon is at best an adjunct to more rapidly acting drugs for patients in cardiac arrest. The normal dose is 5–15 mg as a bolus, followed by an infusion of 1–10 mg/hr.[19]

The most recent advance in the treatment of CCB toxicity is utilization of high-dose insulin therapy. Several well designed animal trials have shown improved survival and metabolic indices compared to standard therapies.[36-40] and this therapy has also been used in several human cases. The effects of insulin are not immediate, and patients may not improve for 30 minutes or more.[41] Therefore, insulin should be considered as a post-resuscitation supportive treatment. The usual dose is 1 unit/kg as a bolus followed by a 1 unit/kg/hour infusion. A glucose infusion is also started to maintain euglycemia.

Non-adrenergic vasopressors are of uncertain efficacy. Vasopressin increased mortality in an animal study of verapamil poisoning.[42] There are no compelling human reports suggesting that vasopressin is effective for hypotension or cardiac arrest in the setting of verapamil poisoning. Animal studies of phosphodiesterase inhibitors gave mixed results.[43,44] In several case reports amrinone was used as an adjunct to other vasopressors, and phosphodiesterase inhibitors are a reasonable adjunctive therapy for patients with refractory hypotension.[34,45,46]

Stimulants

Cocaine and amphetamine derivatives are the most commonly encountered CNS stimulants. As most patients are not taking these drugs with self-harm intent, cardiac arrest is a rare complication of their use. Nevertheless, stimulants still account for several thousand deaths each year. Most intensivists and emergency physicians will have to care for critically ill patients intoxicated with these drugs.

Pathophysiology

Stimulants act directly on the brain to cause agitation and seizures.[47] Activation of the sympathetic nervous system can also cause vasospasm. In addition, cocaine blocks cardiac sodium channels, and patients may require specific treatment to reverse sodium channel antagonism (see sodium channel blocking drugs below).[47]

Presentation and diagnosis

Most patients with stimulant intoxication present with restlessness, anxiety, hypertension, tachycardia, and other signs of sympathetic nervous system activation. Ventricular tachycardia may be due to ischemia from increased oxygen demand or vasospasm. Cocaine may produce a wide complex tachycardia from direct antagonism of sodium channels; these channels are pH-dependent, so that the binding wide tachycardia most commonly occurs after a seizure.[48] Cocaine use can also cause subarachnoid hemorrhage, which may present as cardiac arrest.[49]

Treatment

There are several reports of successful treatment of cardiac arrest from cocaine toxicity.[48] These patients had severe agitation and seizures followed by hemodynamic collapse. Patients should be treated with benzodiazepines (diazepam 5–20 mg i.v.) to control the seizures, sodium bicarbonate (1–2 meq/kg i.v.) to reverse the myocardial sodium channel antagonism, and epinephrine (1 mg i.v.) to restore perfusion.[48]

Cocaine use is also associated with accelerated atherosclerosis, vasospasm, and is prothrombotic.[50-52] Thus, patients may present with sudden cardiac death from an acute coronary occlusion precipitated by cocaine use.[53] In general, management of these patients is similar to the management of other myocardial infarction patients. Once perfusion has been restored, patients with appropriate electrocardiographic criteria should be considered for early revascularization. Patients with CNS symptoms of sympathomimetic intoxication should be sedated with benzodiazepines as described above?[54,55] Beta-blockers are contraindicated in the setting of acute cocaine poisoning.[1]

Asphyxiants/CNS depressants

These two types of poisons are considered together because they both kill patients by producing systemic hypoxia. Asphyxiants are gases that displace oxygen in the atmosphere, producing a hypoxic environment. Common asphyxiant gases include methane, propane, carbon dioxide, and nitrogen, but any gas can become an asphyxiant at high concentrations. Common CNS depressants include ethanol, benzodiazepines, opioids, barbiturates, and many other therapeutic and abused drugs. Although some of these drugs may have effects beyond CNS depression (e.g., cardiodepression from high doses of barbiturates, sodium channel antagonism from norpropoxyphene, or cardiac sensitization from chloral hydrate), most cases of cardiac arrest are due to respiratory depression and hypoxia.

Pathophysiology

The importance of oxygen for cellular function has been described in detail in several previous chapters. As described above, simple asphyxiants cause hypoxemia by decreasing the concentration of oxygen in the environment. This hypoxemia produces an initial increase in respiratory drive, and ventilation will increase until the respiratory centers become depressed from hypoxia. CNS depressant drugs inhibit respiratory centers and cause hypoxia through hypoventilation.

Presentation and diagnosis

Patients exposed to asphyxiants usually develop signs of hypoxia before losing consciousness. Upon removal from the hypoxic environment, they often improve dramatically. Persistent symptoms suggest that there is hypoxic brain injury. Patients with a brief period of asphyxia may respond rapidly to resuscitation once the heart is oxygenated. Patients who suffer cardiac arrest due to hypoxia and hypoventilation from CNS depressant toxicity may also have a rapid return of circulation once myocardial oxygen delivery is restored. Nevertheless, they do not usually have a rapid return of consciousness, as the effects of the CNS depressant remain.

Treatment

The key to treatment for cardiac arrest from exposure to either asphyxiants or CNS depressants is to provide adequate oxygenation as soon as possible. One study of prehospital cardiac arrest from these poisons found that many patients recovered pulses with CPR alone.[56] There are no specific animal studies of cardiac arrest due to poisoning by CNS depressants, but high dose epinephrine or vasopressin plus epinephrine is more effective at restoring circulation than vasopressin, and improves survival in an animal models of asphyxiated cardiac arrest.[57] Whereas there is no evidence that prolonged resuscitative attempts are warranted, many of the CNS depressant medications have been shown to have neuroprotective effects in animal models of cardiac arrest and this clinical scenario is similar to the pretreatment design of animal studies.[16] This has led to the recommendation that prolonged resuscitative attempts may be warranted in these patients. There are no controlled data, however, and this author was unable to find any quality case reports to support this assertion.

Theophylline

Theophylline use has decreased dramatically over the past 10 years, with only 10 theophylline poisoning deaths reported to US poison centers in 2003.[18] Theophylline and caffeine are both methylxanthines that occur naturally in coffee and tea; more concentrated sources include energy supplements and diet pills. Caffeine toxicity rarely results in cardiovascular or neurologic effects, but when serious toxicity occurs, the effects and management are similar to those of theophylline.

Pathophysiology

Theophylline is an indirect activator of the adrenergic system and this increases plasma catecholamines and causes increased sympathetic activity.[58] The methylxanthines do not cause severe peripheral vasoconstriction and therefore patients are not usually hypertensive. Theophylline is also a potent adenosine receptor antagonist, and this effect may be the primary mechanism of therapeutic action. Adenosine antagonism is responsible for the seizures that are the hallmark of severe theophylline intoxication.[59]

Presentation and diagnosis

The diagnosis of theophylline toxicity should be considered when patients present with marked tachycardia, vomiting, and seizures.[60] Most patients have a history of pulmonary disease. Laboratory findings that suggest theophylline poisoning include hypokalemia, metabolic acidosis, and hyperglycemia.[58]

Treatment

The most common cause of cardiac arrest following theophylline poisoning is ventricular dysrhythmias.[60] A patient with recurrent episodes of ventricular fibrillation and prolonged hypotension survived with repeated defibrillation, lidocaine (a total of 240 mg/h), metoprolol (10 mg), benzodiazepines (20 mg diazepam followed by a midazolam infusion of 5 mg/hour), electrolyte replacement, and hemoperfusion once hemodynamics were restored.[61] Another report of a patient with chronic theophylline intoxication who developed cardiac arrest also was readily defibrillated.[62] In a series of 38 theophylline overdoses, there were three cases of ventricular fibrillation and two responded "promptly" to defibrillation.[63] Finally, there is one well documented case of a patient who developed hypotension refractory to 160 mcg/min of epinephrine and 250 mcg/min of phenylephrine. This patient survived for 48 hours but was treated with several different combinations of vasopressors (including norepinephrine), and ultimately developed ventricular dysrhythmias and hypotension that were refractory to treatment.[64]

On the basis of these case reports, patients with ventricular fibrillation in the setting of theophylline poisoning should be treated with prompt defibrillation and lidocaine. There are no reports of the use of amiodarone, but it is a rational choice. Patients may require high doses of adrenergic agents to maintain adequate blood flow. There are no data on the use of vasopressin as a vasopressor for theophylline overdose, but, given the role of endogenous catecholamines in the adverse cardiovascular effects of theophylline poisoning, it is a reasonable choice. Vasopressin has been used to treat refractory hypotension from caffeine poisoning.[65] Beta-blockers have been used successfully to treat the cardiovascular effects of theophylline,[66,67] and they should be considered for patients who recover hemodynamics after cardiac arrest. Esmolol should be administered to patients with persistent ectopy or dysrhythmias and an adequate mean arterial pressure. Low doses should be administered initially, after which the dose should be titrated to control ventricular rate and prevent ectopy.

Adenosine is an intriguing potential antidote for theophylline poisoning. A 1-mg bolus of adenosine reversed the hemodynamic effects of 50 mg/kg of theophylline in a rat model;[68] this would translate into very high doses (approximately 200–400 mg) for a human. One theoretical treatment that might be reasonable in severe cases is administration of dipyramidole, which is an adenosine uptake inhibitor, and may therefore prolong the activity of adenosine. The dose used in cardiac stress testing is 0.56 mg/kg i.v. over 4 minutes.[69]

Hydrocarbon inhalation

Deliberate inhalation of hydrocarbon products ("huffing", "glue," or "paint sniffing") is a growing problem among US adolescents.[70] Death from hydrocarbon abuse may be from dysrhythmias ("sudden sniffing death") or from asphyxia.

Inhalation of hydrocarbons must be differentiated from aspiration of hydrocarbons. Inhalation does not cause acute pulmonary symptoms. The hydrocarbon is volatilized, allowing the gaseous form to pass through the alveoli and into the blood. Aspiration occurs when the liquid hydrocarbon enters the lung, usually when the product is swallowed or vomited. In liquid form, the hydrocarbon can interact with lung structure causing atelectasis and non-cardiogenic pulmonary edema.

Pathophysiology

Butane and toluene are commonly found in abused products in the USA and benzene is used in many industrial types of glue; it is frequently abused in other countries. These drugs are abused for their effects on the CNS. They have general anesthetic properties, and inhalation is associated with euphoria, followed by CNS depression. There are several techniques for inhaling these products: the most common is to pour the substance on a cloth and then inhale the vapors from the rag. Over time, the patient develops tolerance, and requires higher doses of the vapor to achieve the desired effect. Tolerant subjects may increase their dose by inhaling the vapors in a bag rather than on a cloth. Sometimes subjects will place a bag over their head or use other elaborate delivery systems to increase the concentration of the hydrocarbon. These techniques not only increase the concentration of hydrocarbon in the inhaled vapor, but also decrease the amount of oxygen that is inhaled. The combination of hypoventilation and hypoxic environment leads to asphyxial cardiac arrest.

In addition to asphyxia, inhaled hydrocarbons also may precipitate cardiac dysrhythmias.[71] Acute exposure to hydrocarbons sensitizes the myocardium to epinephrine.[72–74] This is the proposed mechanism of "sudden sniffing death"; a hydrocarbon abuser is startled and has an acute release of adrenaline, which precipitates ventricular dysrhythmias.

Presentation and diagnosis

Symptoms of hydrocarbon intoxication include slurred speech, ataxia, confusion, and somnolence; chronic use leads to tremor and encephalopathy. The diagnosis can often be confirmed by the presence of paint on the patient's face or hands and a strong odor of hydrocarbons. Patients who present with these symptoms are unlikely to develop complications. Hydrocarbon abusers may also present with ventricular dysrhythmias. Premature ventricular contractions and non-sustained ventricular tachycardia suggest myocardial sensitization. Patients may also present in cardiac arrest from ventricular fibrillation. Finally, toluene may cause a renal tubular acidosis and profound hypokalemia that may lead to paralysis and respiratory arrest.

Treatment

Patients who present with only CNS symptoms can be observed and discharged when their mental status has returned to baseline. Patients who present with ventricular ectopy or dysrhythmias may benefit from beta-blockade (metoprolol 5 mg i.v.); however, most cases will resolve without therapy. It is reasonable to check electrolytes, including magnesium, in patients with ventricular ectopy. Two patients with ventricular fibrillation following butane abuse were successfully resuscitated with amiodarone.[75,76] Other cases have also responded to standard ACLS treatments.[77,78]

Some authors have advocated avoiding adrenergic vasopressors (i.e., epinephrine) when treating cardiac arrest in the setting of hydrocarbon intoxication,[76] arguing that the dysrhythmia is precipitated by myocardial sensitization to epinephrine, and that additional epinephrine should be avoided. Vasopressin offers a reasonable alternative with no beta-adrenergic effects, but there are no experimental data to support this position. Patients who have hemodynamically significant cardiac ectopy after return of a perfusing rhythm should be treated with beta-blockade.[76]

As toluene abuse causes renal wasting of cations, toluene abusers who develop polymorphic ventricular tachycardia should be treated with magnesium (2 g i.v.). Overdrive pacing is a reasonable therapy, but medical treatments to increase heart rate (e.g., isoproterenol) should be avoided as they may worsen myocardial irritability. As hydrocarbons appear to have a mechanism of action similar to the inhaled anesthetics, it is possible that they will provide some neuroprotection during cardiac arrest. Therefore it is reasonable to prolong resuscitative therapy.

Tricyclic antidepressants, chloroquine, and other sodium channel blocking agents

Deaths from tricyclic antidepressant (TCA) poisoning have decreased over the past decade, yet these drugs remain an important cause of mortality from poisoning. Most emergency physicians and intensivists will have to care for a critically ill TCA-poisoned patient during their careers. Other poisons share some of the toxic properties of TCAs (sodium channel blockade), but not all of these poisons produce the seizures and cardiovascular collapse that are the hallmark of TCA poisoning.

Pathophysiology

Sodium channel blockade is responsible for the major cardiac effects of TCA toxicity and for the dysrhythmias observed in many other poisonings. By decreasing inward sodium currents, intracardiac conduction of electrical impulses is slowed. These effects are first detected on the ECG as prolongation of the terminal depolarization of the heart, which can then progress to prolongation of the QRS, and eventually the patient develops a wide complex rhythm.[79] The effect of these drugs on the cardiac conduction system is pH-dependent,[80] and systemic acidosis increases the chance of dysrhythmias.[48]

Although large overdoses of many medications can produce cardiac dysrhythmias, TCA and chloroquine-poisoned patients appear to be more likely to result in cardiovascular collapse and death than patients poisoned with other medications that cause sodium channel blockade. TCAs are potent alpha-adrenergic antagonists and cause vasodilatation;[81] they also directly impair myocardial contractility.[82] Furthermore, TCAs frequently cause seizures, and the resultant lactic acidosis increases sodium channel antagonism. TCA-mediated altered mental status and seizures have been attributed to antagonism of muscarinic cholinergic, histamine, and GABA receptors.[83,84]

Presentation and diagnosis

TCA intoxication should be suspected in any patient who develops seizures and cardiac dysrhythmias after self-poisoning.[85] Patients who present with a complaint of TCA ingestion require intensive monitoring as abrupt deterioration is common. The electrocardiogram is the diagnostic test of choice; the risk of dysrhythmias is correlated with the duration of the QRS interval. One prospective study suggests that a QRS duration of more than 160 ms indicates that the patient is at risk for cardiac dysrhythmia,[86] but others have disputed this cutoff.[87]

Overdoses of chloroquine, quinine, hydroxychloroquine, flecanide, and propafenone cause severe cardiovascular effects from sodium channel blockade. Many other drugs cause QRS widening due to sodium channel antagonists, but do not cause cardiovascular collapse. The treating physician should not expect that these cases will develop cardiovascular effects, but he should be prepared to treat them if they do occur.

Treatment

There are multiple reports of survival following cardiac arrest from TCA poisoning,[88–90] but patients presenting with acute severe TCA poisoning require several simultaneous interventions. Airway management allows hyperventilation (to help raise serum pH) and ensures adequate oxygenation.[91,92] Seizures, which often precede cardiovascular collapse,[93] should be treated with high-dose benzodiazepines (lorezepam 4–6 mg repeated as needed). Paralysis will stop the neuromuscular activity associated with the seizures that produces the metabolic acidosis. Dysrhythmias should be treated with sodium bicarbonate boluses.[94,95] An initial dose of 2 meq/kg should be administered, and this dose should be repeated at least every 5 minutes or until a perfusing rhythm has been restored. Magnesium has been used in animal models and a single case report, but human experience is insufficient to recommend its routine use.[95,96] High-dose vasopressors may be required. Animal data suggest that epinephrine is more effective than norepinephrine.[97] A reasonable initial dose is 1 mcg/kg per minute as an infusion, but the dose should be rapidly increased if perfusion is not improved. The only available human data suggest that norepinephrine is more effective than dopamine; however, this study was uncontrolled and the dosing was at the discretion of the treating physician.[98] Glucagon has also been used as a vasopressor for patients with refractory shock, but there are no controlled data.[99,100] Phenytoin and beta-blockers are not recommended for treatment of TCA overdose.

There are also several reports of survival following cardiac arrest from chloroquine poisoning.[87,101–104] These patients are treated with an epinephrine infusion, high-dose benzodiazepines (diazepam 1–2 mg/kg), and early intubation. Animal data suggest that sodium bicarbonate may also be useful.[105]

Fluoride and hydrofluoric acid

Fluoride and hydrofluoric acid account for several deaths each year in the USA.[18] Exposure to fluoride-containing dental products rarely produces serious symptoms,[106] and most cases are due to exposure to hydrofluoric acid or other industrial fluoride products (ammonium fluoride). Indeed, severe fluoride toxicity may occur after exposure to as little as an ounce of a household rust remover.[107]

Pathophysiology

Fluoride is the most electronegative element and therefore it binds avidly to divalent cations, producing profound hypocalcemia and hypomagnesemia. These abnormalities are thought to cause the cardiac effects observed in fluoride-poisoned patients. Fluoride also interferes with the function of several enzyme pathways, however, including the Krebs cycle.[108] In animal models, cardiac arrest is temporally associated with a profound hyperkalemia, which is thought to be due to release of intracellular potassium from erythrocytes.[109] Nonetheless, hyperkalemic animals did not respond to standard treatment, suggesting that hyperkalemia is not the only cause of arrest.[110] Ultimately, fluoride-poisoned patients develop cardiovascular collapse from dysrhythmias, vasodilatation, and myocardial dysfunction.

Presentation and diagnosis

Severe fluoride toxicity may occur after ingestion of products, after dermal exposures, or after inhalation of fluoride-containing vapors. Patients with ingestion of HF products may develop life-threatening effects without significant gastrointestinal complaints. Dermal exposures to low concentration products (<10%) are unlikely to produce toxicity unless they are extensive. Nevertheless, severe toxicity may occur with only a 1% BSA exposure to a 50% HF preparation.[111,112] Patients who develop fluoride toxicity after inhalational exposure present with severe respiratory complaints and acute lung injury before developing effects from the fluoride exposure.[113]

Diagnosis of fluoride poisoning is based on history of exposure, clinical presentation, and laboratory findings. Severe effects should be anticipated for patients who present after deliberate oral exposures. Clinical effects may be minimal initially, and the patient may progress to cardiovascular collapse without other significant symptoms.[107] Serum fluoride levels are not routinely available and are not considered useful in the acute management of patients. Serum calcium levels are markedly low in patients who develop serious fluoride toxicity.

Management

No systematic human studies have evaluated treatment of cardiac arrest due to fluoride poisoning, but several reported cases of cardiac arrest have responded to large doses of calcium (5–10 g of calcium chloride).[114–117] Animal studies suggest that early administration of calcium salts may attenuate fluoride toxicity and increase the dose of fluoride required to produce cardiac arrest.[118,119] Systemic alkalosis has also been reported to prolong survival in animal models.[120]

As there are very few adverse effects from acute hypercalcemia, patients who have deliberately ingested HF products should receive empiric treatment with calcium salts (1–3 g i.v. over 30 minutes) while awaiting results.[108] The goal of calcium therapy is to maintain serum levels in the high–normal range. Low serum calcium levels are an ominous sign and these patients should receive 1–3 g of calcium chloride iv bolus. Patients who have dysrhythmias or hypotension should receive a minimum of 3 g of calcium as an iv bolus and be treated with systemic alkalinization to a serum pH of 7.5. Patients with cardiac arrest in the setting of fluoride poisoning should be treated with 3–5 g of calcium chloride and sodium bicarbonate (1–2 meq/kg) in addition to vasopressors and defibrillation. Resuscitation after prolonged cardiac arrest has been reported.[114–117]

Cardioactive steroids

The most commonly encountered cardioactive steroids are the medications digitialis and digitoxin. Plant sources of cardioactive steroids include foxglove (the source of digitalis), oleander, and red squill. Animal sources of cardioactive steroids include bufotoxin, which is produced by the boreal toad. There have been several cases of severe toxicity and even deaths reported following ingestion of aphrodisiacs made from bufo toad skin.[121] These toads also produce a hallucinogenic toxin, so there have been reports of mild intoxication following "toad licking."

Pathophysiology

Cardiac glycosides have two main effects on the cardiovascular system. They have potent negative chronotrophic effects, partially mediated through the vagal system, slowing the rate of sinus node firing and slowing conduction through the AV node. Cardioactive steroids also alter transcellular ion

gradients, causing atrial and ventricular ectopy. The overall effect is the classic finding of digoxin toxicity: increased ectopy (atrial or ventricular) with heartblock.[122]

Presentation and diagnosis

The presentation of cardiac arrest may differ in acute and chronic cardioactive steroid poisoning. Acute poisoning frequently causes refractory heartblock and bradycardia, leading to bradyasystolic arrest. Patients with chronic cardioactive steroid poisoning usually have bradycardia, and many also have intracardiac conduction abnormalities. These patients usually die from refractory ventricular dysrhythmias. Non-cardiac symptoms include vomiting, confusion, and changes in vision. After acute ingestion of any cardioactive steroid, the serum potassium is the most important marker of toxicity. In a large series of poisoned patients (before the development of digoxin Fab), the mortality for patients with a serum potassium level above 5.5 meq/ml was 100%, whereas no patients with a serum potassium level below 5.0 meq/ml died.[123] Interestingly, low serum potassium exacerbates dysrhythmias observed in the setting of chronic digoxin toxicity.[124,125] Serum digoxin levels do not accurately discriminate toxic from non-toxic patients.[125,126]

Treatment

The treatment of cardiac glycoside poisoning was revolutionized by antidigoxin antibody fragments (Fab). Before Fab was available, the mortality of cardiac arrest from acute digoxin poisoning approached 100%. In the initial trial of Fab, almost half of cardiac arrest patients treated with digoxin Fab survived.[127] The recommended dose for cardiac arrest is 20 vials as an intravenous bolus.[127] If possible, higher doses are recommended for non-digoxin cardioactive steroids.

The treatment of cardioactive steroid poisoning when digoxin Fab is not available is obviously more complicated. Most hospitals do not stock sufficient Fab to treat critically poisoned patients.[128] The treatment of cardiac arrest depends on the manifestation: thus, bradydysrhythmias may respond to atropine,[129–131] but pacing is considered the treatment of choice.[132] Ideally, the pacer should be placed before severe dysrhythmias develop. The rate should be increased until the ventricular ectopy is suppressed. Ventricular dysrhythmias have been treated with phenytoin, magnesium, and lidocaine. Phenytoin is administered as an i.v. bolus in doses of 100–350 mg.[123,133] Magnesium has also been used to treat ventricular ectopy[134–137] and, in one case report, intracardiac magnesium administration was associated with restoration of circulation.[138] Lidocaine was used frequently to treat ventricular dysrhythmias from digoxin, but there is very little published experience, and at least one death was temporally associated with lidocaine administration.[139,140] There are two case reports of successful use of amiodarone to treat patients in cardiac arrest, although in one case digoxin Fab was also administered.[125,141–143] Finally, there is a report of successful use of extracorporeal support to treat a severely poisoned child.[9]

Acetylcholinesterase inhibitors (insecticides and nerve agents)

The organophosphate insecticides are an uncommon cause of poisoning death. The nerve agent chemical weapons are also organophosphates, however, so there is a potential that a mass exposure could result in multiple casualties.

Pathophysiology

Organophosphates act by inhibiting acetylcholinesterase in plasma and in synapses. This results in an excess of cholinergic stimulation and produces the classic DUMBELS (Defecation, Urination, Miosis, Bradycardia+ Bronchorrhea, Emesis, Lacrimation, Seizures) presentation. These effects are primarily due to excess stimulation of muscarinic cholinergic receptors. Acetylcholine excess at the neuromuscular junction causes fasciculations and weakness that may progress to respiratory paralysis. Although deaths can occur from the combination of weakness and pulmonary secretions, animal studies suggest that early deaths are due to the effects of excess acetylcholine in the CNS.[144]

Presentation and diagnosis

The effects of organophosphate poisoning range from non-specific malaise and gastrointestinal effects to seizures, coma, and cardiovascular collapse. The diagnosis will usually be made clinically, on the basis of the presentation of a patient with profound vomiting and diarrhea, seizures, muscle fasciculations, and small pupils. In the event of a chemical attack, multiple patients may present with similar symptoms. Exposure to an organophosphate can be confirmed by measurement of cholinesterase levels, serum and red blood cells, but this test is not available rapidly. Clinicians should also realize that government identification of a chemical agent during an attack may be misleading. For example, the poison in the sarin attacks on the Tokyo subway was initially identified as cyanide.

Treatment

Patients must be decontaminated before treatment. Many victims in the Tokyo subway attack were healthcare workers exposed while treating patients who had sarin vapors trapped in their clothing.[145] After decontamination, patients should have ventilation established, ACLS implemented, and treatment with atropine and benzodiazepines initiated. As noted above, CNS effects play a significant role in severely poisoned patients. Therefore, critically ill patients should be treated with very high doses of benzodiazepines (20 mg of diazepam or the equivalent; this should be repeated rapidly if seizures do not cease). Atropine should be administered in 1-mg boluses and titrated until it results in drying of pulmonary secretions. If patients do not respond rapidly, the bolus dose should be doubled. In a series of patients reported after the Tokyo attack, four patients were successfully resuscitated by using these therapies.[146]

Cyanide

Cyanide and hydrogen sulfide are both mitochondrial poisons that can produce rapid onset of coma and cardiovascular collapse. Cyanide is commonly used in industry and hydrogen cyanide could be used as a chemical weapon. The most common forms are salts such as sodium or potassium cyanide and these may cause toxicity following ingestion. When these salts are exposed to an acid, hydrogen cyanide gas is released. Hydrogen sulfide is a strong smelling gas often released with methane. Occupational exposures may occur when workers enter an enclosed space such as a storage tank or sewer. Unfortunately, the characteristic smell disappears at high levels.

Pathophysiology

Cyanide and hydrogen sulfide bind to cytochrome proteins in the electron transport chain and prevent ATP formation. This results in rapid loss of function in organs with a high metabolic rate (such as the brain and heart). As aerobic metabolism is not possible, all ATP production will occur through anaerobic metabolism.

Presentation and diagnosis

The main CNS effects include headache and nausea at low levels, but loss of consciousness and seizures occur very rapidly with high level exposures. The initial cardiovascular effects are tachycardia and hypertension, followed by a vasodilatation hypotension,[147] myocardial suppression, and cardiovascular collapse.[148] Wide complex bradydys-rhythmias are a pre-terminal rhythm. Common metabolic abnormalities include lactic acidosis and hyperkalemia. Patients who survive may have permanent injury to the basal ganglia.[149,150] Whereas most cases of cardiac arrest from cyanide occur soon after exposure, acetonitrile (found in some artificial fingernail products) is metabolized to cyanide and there is a report of cardiac arrest 24 hours after exposure.[151] Hydrogen sulfide causes a rapid onset of coma, but cardiovascular effects are less common. The effects generally resolve quickly if the patient is removed from the exposure.

Acute cyanide poisoning is primarily a clinical diagnosis. It should be considered in patients with a history of poisoning, altered mental status, and cardiovascular collapse. Laboratory studies such as hyperkalemia, profound metabolic acidosis, and high serum lactate are supporting data, but treatment should not be delayed while waiting for results. A whole blood cyanide level will confirm the exposure, but this test is not available on an emergent basis.

Treatment

Secondary exposure of healthcare workers while treating a cyanide-poisoned patient is unlikely, although it is possible that the vomitus of a patient who ingests cyanide salts could release cyanide gas. Therefore, workers should protect themselves from exposure to vomitus, and the patient should be treated in a well ventilated area. Several cases of cardiovascular collapse and recovery after cyanide poisoning have been reported, as have cases of resuscitation from cardiac arrest.[133,148,152,153] Standard ACLS should be initiated. Patients may have an initial response to vasopressor therapy, but this response may be short-lived if antidotal treatment is not administered. Several antidotes are available for treatment of cyanide poisoning; all work by binding the cyanide. In the United States, a three-part kit is used. Amyl and sodium nitrite are administered to induce formation of methemoglobin, which can bind cyanide. Amyl nitrite is provided as a ampule that can be broken allowing the vapors to be inhaled. Once intravenous access is established, sodium nitrite can be administered. The third component of the kit is sodium thiosulfate, which provides substrate to allow the formation of thiocyanate in the liver; the thiocyanate is then excreted in the urine. The usual dose of sodium nitrite is 300 mg and the dose of sodium thiosulfate is 12.5 g. Hydroxocobalamin is another antidote that is used commonly in Europe; it binds cyanide to form

cyanocobalamin (vitamin B_{12}). This drug has an excellent safety profile and is used routinely in France to treat smoke inhalation victims with suspected cyanide poisoning. It causes peripheral vasoconstriction in animal models of cyanide poisoning,[154,155] and this may improve coronary perfusion during cardiac arrest . The usual dose of hydroxocobalamin is 5 g, which should effectively neutralize a serum level of 40 mcg/ml in an adult.[156]

REFERENCES

1. Albertson, T.E., Dawson, A., de Latorre, F. et al. TOX-ACLS: toxicologic-oriented advanced cardiac life support. *Ann. Emerg. Med.* 2001; **37**: S78–S90.
2. Anonymous Part 10.2: Toxicology in ECC. *Circulation* 2005; **112**: IV126–IV132.
3. Heard, K., Paradis, N.A. & Dart, R.C. American Heart Association guidelines for resuscitation of the poisoned patient. *Internet J. Med. Toxicol.* 2001; **4**: 24.
4. Massetti, M., Bruno, P., Babatasi, G., Neri, E. & Khayat, A. Cardiopulmonary bypass and severe drug intoxication. *J. Thorac. Cardiovasc. Surg.* 2000; **120**: 424–425.
5. Ohuchi, S., Izumoto, H., Kamata, J. et al. A case of aconitine poisoning saved with cardiopulmonary bypass. *Kyobu Geka* 2000; **53**: 541–544.
6. Pasic, M., Potapov, E., Kuppe, H. & Hetzer, R. Prolonged cardiopulmonary bypass for severe drug intoxication. *J. Thorac. Cardiovasc. Surg.* 2000; **119**: 379–380.
7. Holzer, M., Sterz, F., Schoerkhuber, W. et al. Successful resuscitation of a verapamil-intoxicated patient with percutaneous cardiopulmonary bypass. *Crit. Care Med.* 1999; **27**: 2818–2823.
8. Corkeron, M.A., van Heerden, P.V., Newman, S.M. & Dusci, L. Extracorporeal circulatory support in near-fatal flecainide overdose. *Anaesth. Intens. Care* 1999; **27**: 405–408.
9. Behringer, W., Sterz, F., Domanovits, H. et al. Percutaneous cardiopulmonary bypass for therapy resistant cardiac arrest from digoxin overdose. *Resuscitation* 1998; **37**: 47–50.
10. Schmidt, W., Reissig, M. & Neuhaus, K.L. Percutaneous extracorporeal circulation in cardiogenic shock caused by combined poisoning with methyldigoxin, nifedipine and indapamide. *Dtsch. Med. Wochenschr.* 1995; **120**: 996–1002.
11. Fitzpatrick, A.J., Crawford, M., Allan, R.M. & Wolfenden, H. Aconite poisoning managed with a ventricular assist device. *Anaesth. Intens. Care* 1994; **22**: 714–717.
12. McVey, F.K. & Corke, C.F. Extracorporeal circulation in the management of massive propranolol overdose. *Anaesthesia* 1991; **46**: 744–746.
13. Hendren, W.G., Schieber, R.S. & Garrettson, L.K. Extracorporeal bypass for the treatment of verapamil poisoning. *Ann. Emerg. Med.* 1989; **18**: 984–987.
14. Noble, J., Kennedy, D.J., Latimer, R.D. et al. Massive lignocaine overdose during cardiopulmonary bypass. Successful

treatment with cardiac pacing. *Br. J. Anaesth.* 1984; **56**: 1439–1441.

15. Larkin, G.L., Graeber, G.M. & Hollingsed, M.J. Experimental amitriptyline poisoning: treatment of severe cardiovascular toxicity with cardiopulmonary bypass. *Ann. Emerg. Med.* 1994; **23**: 480–486.

16. Safar, P. Cerebral resuscitation after cardiac arrest: a review. *Circulation* 1986; **74**: IV138–153.

17. Kalman, S., Berg, S. & Lisander, B. Combined overdose with verapamil and atenolol: treatment with high doses of adrenergic agonists. *Acta Anaesthesiol. Scand.* 1998; **42**: 379–382.

18. Watson, W.A., Litovitz, T.L., Klein-Schwartz, W. *et al.* 2003 annual report of the American Association of Poison Control Centers Toxic Exposure Surveillance System. *Am. J. Emerg. Med.* 2004; **22**: 335–404.

19. DeWitt, C.R. & Waksman, J.C. Pharmacology, pathophysiology and management of calcium channel blocker and beta-blocker toxicity. *Toxicol. Rev.* 2004; **23**: 223–238.

20. Isbister, G.K. Delayed asystolic cardiac arrest after diltiazem overdose; resuscitation with high dose intravenous calcium. *Emerg. Med. J.* 2002; **19**: 355–357.

21. Haddad, L.M. Resuscitation after nifedipine overdose exclusively with intravenous calcium chloride. *Am. J. Emerg. Med.* 1996; **14**: 602–603.

22. Lam, Y.M., Tse, H.F. & Lau, C.P. Continuous calcium chloride infusion for massive nifedipine overdose. *Chest* 2001; **119**: 1280–1282.

23. Brimacombe, J.R., Scully, M. & Swainston, R. Propranolol overdose – a dramatic response to calcium chloride. *Med. J. Aust.* 1991; **155**: 267–268.

24. Pertoldi, F., D'Orlando, L. & Mercante, W.P. Electro-mechanical dissociation 48 hours after atenolol overdose: usefulness of calcium chloride. *Ann. Emerg. Med.* 1998; **31**: 777–781.

25. Crump, B.J., Holt, D.W. & Vale, J.A. Lack of response to intravenous calcium in severe verapamil poisoning. *Lancet* 1982; **2**: 939–940.

26. Ramoska, E.A., Spiller, H.A. & Myers, A. Calcium channel blocker toxicity. *Emerg. Med.* 1990; **19**: 649–653.

27. Buckley, N.A., Whyte, I.M. & Dawson, A.H. Overdose with calcium channel blockers. *B. Med. J.* 1994; **308**: 1639.

28. Buckley, N., Dawson, A.H., Howarth, D. & Whyte, I.M. Slow-release verapamil poisoning. Use of polyethylene glycol whole-bowel lavage and high-dose calcium. *Med. J. Aust.* 1993; **158**: 202–204.

29. Gay, R., Algeo, S., Lee, R., Olajos, M., Morkin, E. & Goldman, S. Treatment of verapamil toxicity in intact dogs. *J. Clin. Invest.* 1986; **77** (6): 1805–1811.

30. Stone, C.K., May, W.A. & Carroll, R. Treatment of verapamil overdose with glucagon in dogs. *Ann. Emerg. Med.* 1995; **25**: 369–374.

31. Doyon, S. & Roberts, J.R. The use of glucagon in a case of calcium channel blocker overdose. *Ann. Emerg. Med.* 1993; **22**: 1229–1233.

32. Zaritsky, A.I., Horowitz, M. & Chernow, B. Glucagon antagonism of calcium channel blocker induced myocardial dysfunction. *Crit. Care Med.* 1988; **16**: 246–254.

33. Walter, F.G., Frye, F., Mullen, G.T. *et al.* Amelioration of nifedipine poisoning associated with glucagon therapy. *Ann. Emerg. Med.* 1993; **22**: 1234–1237.

34. Wolf, L.R., Spadafora, M.P. & Otten, E.J. Use of amrinone and glucagon in a case of calcium channel blocker overdose. *Ann. Emerg. Med.* 1993; **22**: 1225–1228.

35. Stone, C.K., May, W.A. & Carroll, R. Treatment of verapamil overdose with glucagon in dogs. *Ann. Emerg. Med.* 1995; **25**: 369–374.

36. Kline, J.A., Tomaszewski, C.A., Schroeder, J.D. & Raymond, R.M. Insulin is a superior antidote for cardiovascular toxicity induced by verapamil in the anesthetized canine. *J. Pharmacol. Exp. Therap.* 1993; **267**(2): 744–750.

37. Kline, J.A., Raymond, R.M., Schroeder, J.D. & Watts, J.A. The diabetogenic effects of acute verapamil poisoning. *Toxicol. App. Pharmacol.* 1997; **145**(2): 357–362.

38. Kline, J.A., Raymond, R.M., Leonova, E.D., Williams, T.C. & Watts, J.A. Insulin improves heart function and metabolism during non-ischemic cardiogenic shock in awake canines. *Cardiovasc. Res.* 1997; **34**(2): 289–298.

39. Kline, J.A., Leonova, E., Williams, T.C., Schroeder, J.D. & Watts, J.A. Myocardial metabolism during graded intraportal verapamil infusion in awake dogs. *J. Cardiovasc. Pharmacol.* 1996; **27**(5): 719–726.

40. Kline, J.A., Leonova, E. & Raymond, R.M. Beneficial myocardial metabolic effects of insulin during verapamil toxicity in the anesthetized canine. *Crit. Care Med.* 1995; **23**(7): 1251–1263.

41. Yuan, T.H., Kerns, W.P., Tomaszewski, C.A., Ford, M.D. & Kline, J.A. Insulin-glucose as adjunctive therapy for severe calcium channel antagonist poisoning. *Clin. Toxicol.* 1999; **37**: 463–474.

42. Sztajnkrycer, M.D., Bond, G.R., Johnson, S.B. & Weaver, A.L. Use of vasopressin in a canine model of severe verapamil poisoning: a preliminary descriptive study. *Acad. Emerg. Med.* 2004; **11**: 1253–1261.

43. Koury, S.I., Stone, C.K. & Thomas, S.H. Amrinone as an antidote in experimental verapamil overdose. *Acad. Emerg. Med.* 1996; **3**: 762–767.

44. Tuncok, Y., Apaydin, S., Kalkan, S., Ates, M. & Guven, H. The effects of amrinone and glucagon on verapamil-induced cardiovascular toxicity in anaesthetized rats. *Int. J. Exp. Pathol.* 1996; **77**: 207–212.

45. Goenen, M., Col, J., Compere, A. & Bonte, J. Treatment of severe verapamil poisoning with combined amrinone-isoproterenol therapy. *Am. J. Cardiol.* 1986; **58**: 1142–1143.

46. Hantson, P., Ronveau, J.L., De Coninck, B., Horn, J.L., Mahieu, P. & Hassoun, A. Amrinone for refractory cardiogenic shock following chloroquine poisoning. *Intens. Care Med.* 1991; **17**: 430–431.

47. Goldfrank, L.R. & Hoffman, R.S. The cardiovascular effects of cocaine. *Ann. Emerg. Med.* 1991; **20**: 165–175.

48. Wang, R.Y. pH-dependent cocaine-induced cardiotoxicity. *Am. J. Emerg. Med.* 1999; **17**(4): 364–349.

49. Broderick, J.P., Viscoli, C.M., Brott, T. *et al.* Major risk factors for aneurysmal subarachnoid hemorrhage in the young are modifiable. *Stroke* 2003; **34**: 1375–1381.

50. Lange, R.A. & Hillis, L.D. Cardiovascular complications of cocaine use. *N. Engl. J. Med.* 2001; **345**: 351–358.

51. Moliterno, D.J., Willard, J.E., Lange, R.A. *et al.* Coronary-artery vasoconstriction induced by cocaine, cigarette smoking, or both. *N. Engl. J. Med.* 1994; **330**: 454–459.

52. Lange, R.A., Cigarroa, R.G., Yancy, C.W. Jr. *et al.* Cocaine-induced coronary-artery vasoconstriction. *N. Engl. J. Med.* 1989; **321**: 1557–1562.

53. Ascher, E.K., Stauffer, J.C. & Gaasch, W.H. Coronary artery spasm, cardiac arrest, transient electrocardiographic Q waves and stunned myocardium in cocaine-associated acute myocardial infarction. *Am. J. Cardiol.* 1988; **61**(11): 939–941.

54. Honderick, T., Williams, D., Seaberg, D. & Wears, R. A prospective, randomized, controlled trial of benzodiazepines and nitroglycerine or nitroglycerine alone in the treatment of cocaine-associated acute coronary syndromes. *Am. J. Emerg. Med.* 2003; **21**: 39–42.

55. Baumann, B.M., Perrone, J., Hornig, S.E., Shofer, F.S. & Hollander, J.E. Randomized, double-blind, placebo-controlled trial of diazepam, nitroglycerin, or both for treatment of patients with potential cocaine-associated acute coronary syndromes. *Acad. Emerg. Med.* 2000; **7**: 878–885.

56. Paredes, V.L., Rea, T.D., Eisenberg, M.S. *et al.* Out-of-hospital care of critical drug overdoses involving cardiac arrest.[see comment]. *Acad. Emerg. Med.* 2004; **11**(1): 71–74.

57. Mayr, V.D., Wenzel, V., Voelckel, W.G. *et al.* Developing a vasopressor combination in a pig model of adult asphyxial cardiac arrest. *Circulation* 2001; **104**: 1651–1656.

58. Shannon, M. Hypokalemia, hyperglycemia and plasma catecholamine activity after severe theophylline intoxication. *J. Toxicol. Clin. Toxicol.* 1994; **32**: 41–47.

59. Shannon, M. & Maher, T. Anticonvulsant effects of intracerebroventricular adenocard in theophylline-induced seizures. *Ann. Emerg. Med.* 1995; **26**: 65–68.

60. Shannon, M. Life-threatening events after theophylline overdose: a 10-year prospective analysis. *Arch. Intern. Med.* 1999; **159**: 989–994.

61. Filejski, W., Kurowski, V., Batge, B., Mentzel, H. & Djonlagic, H. The clinical course and therapy of massive theophylline poisoning. *Dtsch. Med. Wochenschr.* 1993; **118**: 1641–1646.

62. Aderka, D., Shavit, G., Garfinkel, D., Santo, M., Gitter, S. & Pinkhas, J. Life-threatening theophylline intoxication in a hypothyroid patient. *Respiration* 1983; **44**: 77–80.

63. Henderson, A., Wright, D.M. & Pond, S.M. Management of theophylline overdose patients in the intensive care unit. *Anaesth. Intens. Care* 1992; **20**: 56–62.

64. Dettloff, R.W., Touchette, M.A. & Zarowitz, B.J. Vasopressor-resistant hypotension following a massive ingestion of theophylline. *Ann. Pharmacother.* 1993; **27**: 781–784.

65. Holstege, C.P., Hunter, Y., Baer, A.B., Savory, J., Bruns, D.E. & Boyd, J.C. Massive caffeine overdose requiring vasopressin infusion and hemodialysis. *J. Toxicol. Clin. Toxicol.* 2003; **41**: 1003–1007.

66. Biberstein, M.P., Ziegler, M.G. & Ward, D.M. Use of beta-blockade and hemoperfusion for acute theophylline poisoning. *West. J. Med.* 1984; **141**: 485–490.

67. Kempf, J., Rusterholtz, T., Ber, C., Gayol, S. & Jaeger, A. Haemodynamic study as guideline for the use of beta blockers in acute theophylline poisoning. *Intens. Care Med.* 1996; **22**: 585–587.

68. Ujhelyi, M.R., Hulula, G. & Skau, K.A. Role of exogenous adenosine as a modulator of theophylline toxicity. *Crit. Care Med.* 1994; **22**: 1639–1646.

69. Rossen, J.D., Simonetti, I., Marcus, M.L. & Winniford, M.D. Coronary dilation with standard dose dipyridamole and dipyridamole combined with handgrip. *Circulation* 1989; **79**: 566–572.

70. Neumark, Y.D., Delva, J. & Anthony, J.C. The epidemiology of adolescent inhalant drug involvement. *Arch. Pediatr. Adolesc. Med.* 1998; **152**: 781–786.

71. Shepherd, R.T. Mechanism of sudden death associated with volatile substance abuse. *Hum. Toxicol.* 1989; **8**: 287–291.

72. Ikeda, N., Takahashi, H., Umetsu, K. & Suzuki, T. The course of respiration and circulation in "toluene-sniffing". *Forensic. Sci. Int.* 1990; **44**: 151–158.

73. Reinhardt, C.F., Mullin, L.S. & Maxfield, M.E. Epinephrine-induced cardiac arrhythmia potential of some common industrial solvents. *J. Occup. Med.* 1973; **15**: 953–955.

74. Reinhardt, C.F., Azar, A., Maxfield, M.E., Smith, P.E. Jr. & Mullin, L.S. Cardiac arrhythmias and aerosol "sniffing". *Arch. Environ. Health.* 1971; **22**: 265–279.

75. Edwards, K.E. & Wenstone, R. Successful resuscitation from recurrent ventricular fibrillation secondary to butane inhalation. *Br. J. Anaesth.* 2000; **84** (6): 803–805.

76. Adgey, A.A., Johnston, P.W. & McMechan, S. Sudden cardiac death and substance abuse. *Resuscitation* 1995; **29**: 219–221.

77. Cunningham, S.R., Dalzell, G.W., McGirr, P. & Khan, M.M. Myocardial infarction and primary ventricular fibrillation after glue sniffing. *Br. Med. J. (Clin. Res. Ed.)* 1987; **294**: 739–740.

78. Roberts, M.J., McIvor, R.A. & Adgey, A.A. Asystole following butane gas inhalation. *Br. J. Hosp. Med.* 1990; **44**: 294

79. Hoffman, J.R., Votey, S.R., Bayer, M. & Silver, L. Effect of hypertonic sodium bicarbonate in the treatment of moderate-to-severe cyclic antidepressant overdose. *Am. J. Emerg. Med.* 1993; **11**: 336–341.

80. Sasyniuk, B.I. & Jhamandas, V. Mechanism of reversal of toxic effects of amitriptyline on cardiac Purkinje fibers by sodium bicarbonate. *J. Pharmacol. Exp. Ther.* 1984; **231**: 387–394.

81. Auguet, M., Clostre, F. & DeFeudis, F.V. Effects of antidepressants on receptor-activated and Ca^{2+}-activated contractions of rabbit isolated aorta. *Gen. Pharmacol.* 1986; **17**: 607–610.

82. Heard, K., Cain, B.S., Dart, R.C. & Cairns, C.B. Tricyclic antidepressants directly depress human myocardial mechanical

function independent of effects on the conduction system. *Acad. Emerg. Med.* 2001; **8**: 1122–1127.

83. Malatynska, E., Knapp, R.J., Ikeda, M. & Yamamura, H.I. Antidepressants and seizure-interactions at the GABA-receptor chloride-ionophore complex. *Life Sci.* 1988; **43**: 303–307.

84. Squires, R.F. & Saederup, E. Antidepressants and metabolites that block GABAA receptors coupled to 35S-t-butylbicy-clophosphorothionate binding sites in rat brain. *Brain Res.* 1988; **441**: 15–22.

85. DeWitt, C. & Heard, K. Cardiovascular toxicology. In Markovchick, V.J. & Pons, P.T., eds. *Emergency Medicine Secrets*, 3rd edn. pp. 431–444. Philadelphia PA: Hanely and Belfus

86. Boehnert, M.T. & Lovejoy, F.H. Value of the QRS duration versus the serum drug levels in predicting seizures and ventricular arrhythmias after an acute overdose of tricyclic antidepressants. *N. Engl. J. Med.* 1985; **313**: 474–479.

87. Buckley, N.A., Chevalier, S., Leditschke, I.A., O'Connell, D.L., Leitch, J. & Pond, S.M. The limited utility of electrocardiography variables used to predict arrhythmia in psychotropic drug overdose. *Crit. Care* 2003; **7**: R101–R107.

88. Sandeman, D.J., Alahakoon, T.I. & Bentley, S.C. Tricyclic poisoning–successful management of ventricular fibrillation following massive overdose of imipramine. *Anaesth. Intens. Care* 1997; **25**: 542–545.

89. Citak, A., Soysal, D.D., Ucsel, R., Karabocuoglu, M. & Uzel, N. Efficacy of long duration resuscitation and magnesium sulphate treatment in amitriptyline poisoning. *Eur. J. Emerg. Med.* 2002; **9**: 63–66.

90. Christiaens, F., Lessire, H., Dellers, I., Denis, B., Vankeerberghen, L. & Verborgh, C. Successful prolonged cardiopulmonary resuscitation after a combined intoxication with a tricyclic antidepressant, a benzodiazepine and a neuroleptic. *Eur. J. Emerg. Med.* 2000; **7**: 229–236.

91. Kingston, M.E. Hyperventilation in tricyclic antidepressant poisoning. *Crit. Care Med.* 1979; **7**: 550–551.

92. Bessen, H.A. & Niemann, J.T. Improvement of cardiac conduction after hyperventilation in tricyclic antidepressant overdose. *J. Toxicol. Clin. Toxicol.* 1985–1986; **23**: 537–546.

93. Taboulet, P., Michard, F., Muszynski, J., Galliot-Guilley, M. & Bismuth, C. Cardiovascular repercussions of seizures during cyclic antidepressant poisoning. *J. Toxicol. Clin. Toxicol.* 1995; **33**: 205–211.

94. Knudsen, K. & Abrahamsson, J. Effects of epinephrine, norepinephrine, magnesium sulfate, and milrinone on survival and the occurrence of arrhythmias in amitriptyline poisoning in the rat. *Crit. Care Med.* 1994; **22**: 1851–1855.

95. Knudsen, K. & Abrahamsson, J. Effects of magnesium sulfate and lidocaine in the treatment of ventricular arrhythmias in experimental amitriptyline poisoning in the rat. *Crit. Care Med.* 1994; **22**: 494–498.

96. Knudsen, K. & Abrahamsson, J. Magnesium sulphate in the treatment of ventricular fibrillation in amitriptyline poisoning. *Eur. Heart J.* 1997; **18**: 881–882.

97. Knudsen, K. & Abrahamsson, J. Effects of epinephrine and norepinephrine on hemodynamic parameters and arrhythmias during a continuous infusion of amitriptyline in rats. *J. Toxicol. Clin. Toxicol.* 1993; **31**: 461–471.

98. Tran, T.P., Panacek, E.A., Rhee, K.J. & Foulke, G.E. Response to dopamine vs norepinephrine in tricyclic antidepressant-induced hypotension. *Acad. Emerg. Med.* 1997; **4**: 864–868.

99. Sensky, P.R. & Olczak, S.A. High-dose intravenous glucagon in severe tricyclic poisoning. *Postgrad. Med. J.* 1999; **75**: 611–612.

100. Sener, E.K., Gabe, S. & Henry, J.A. Response to glucagon in imipramine overdose. *J. Toxicol. Clin. Toxicol.* 1995; **33**: 51–53.

101. McKenzie, A.G. Intensive therapy for chloroquine poisoning. A review of 29 cases. *S. Afr. Med. J.* 1996; **86**: 597–599.

102. Boereboom, F.T., Ververs, F.F., Meulenbelt, J. & van Dijk, A. Hemoperfusion is ineffectual in severe chloroquine poisoning. *Crit. Care Med.* 2000; **28**: 3346–3350.

103. Bauer, P., Maire, B., Weber, M., Bollaert, P.E., Larcan, A. & Lambert, H. Full recovery after a chloroquine suicide attempt. *J. Toxicol. Clin. Toxicol.* 1991; **29**: 23–30.

104. Collee, G.G., Samra, G.S. & Hanson, G.C. Chloroquine poisoning: ventricular fibrillation following 'trivial' overdose in a child. *Intens. Care Med.* 1992; **18**: 170–171.

105. Curry, S.C., Connor, D.A., Clark, R.F., Holland, D., Carrol, L. & Raschke, R. The effect of hypertonic sodium bicarbonate on QRS duration in rats poisoned with chloroquine. *J. Toxicol. Clin. Toxicol.* 1996; **34**: 73–76.

106. Augenstein, W.L., Spoerke, D.G., Kulig, K.W. *et al.* Fluoride ingestion in children: a review of 87 cases. *Pediatrics* 1991; **88**: 907–912.

107. Kao, W.F., Deng, J.F., Chiang, S.C. *et al.* A simple, safe, and efficient way to treat severe fluoride poisoning–oral calcium or magnesium. *J. Toxicol. Clin. Toxicol.* 2004; **42**: 33–40.

108. McIvor, M.E. Acute fluoride toxicity: Pathophysiology and management. *Drug Safety* 1990; **5**: 79–85.

109. McIlvor, M.E., Cummings, C.C., Mover, M.M. *et al.* The manipulation of potassium efflux during fluoride intoxication: implications for therapy. *Toxicology* 1985; **37**: 233–239.

110. McIlvor, M.E., Cummings, C.E., Mower, M.M. *et al.* Sudden cardiac death from acute fluoride intoxication: The role of potassium. *Ann. Emerg. Med.* 1987; **16**: 777–781.

111. Kirkpatrick, J.J. & Burd, D.A. An algorithmic approach to the treatment of hydrofluoric acid burns. *Burns* 1995; **21**(7): 495–499.

112. Muriale, L., Lee, E., Genovese, J. & Trend, S. Fatality due to acute fluoride poisoning following dermal contact with hydrofluoric acid in a palynology laboratory. *Ann. Occup. Hyg.* 1996; **40**(6): 705–710.

113. Watson, A.A., Oliver, J.S. & Thorpe, J.W. Accidental death due to inhalation of hydrofluoric acid. *Med. Sci. Law* 1973; **13**(4): 277–279.

114. Stremski, E.S., Grande, G.A. & Ling, L.J. Survival following hydrofluoric acid ingestion. *Ann. Emerg. Med.* 1992; **21**: 1396–1399.

115. Greco, R.J., Hartford, C.E., Haith, L.R. & Patton, M.L. Hydrofluoric acid-induced hypocalcemia. *J. Trauma.* 1988; **28**: 1593–1596.

116. Klasner, A.E., Scalzo, A.J., Blume, C., Johnson, P. & Thompson, M.W. Marked hypocalcemia and ventricular fibrillation in two pediatric patients exposed to a fluoride-containing wheel cleaner. *Ann. Emerg. Med.* 1996; **28**: 713–718.

117. Mullins, M.E., Warden, C.R. & Barnum, D.W. Anonymous 1998.

118. Strubelt, O., Iven, H. & Younes, M. The pathophysiological profile of the acute cardiovascular toxicity of sodium fluoride. *Toxicology* 1982; **24**: 313–323.

119. Heard, K., Hill, R.E., Cairns, C.B. & Dart, R.C. Calcium neutralizes fluoride bioavailability in a lethal model of fluoride poisoning. *J. Toxicol. Clin. Toxicol.* 2001; **39**: 349–353.

120. Reynolds, K.E., Whitford, G.M. & Pashley, D.H. Acute fluoride toxicity: The influence of acid-base status. *Toxicol. Appl. Pharmacol.* 1978; **45**: 415–427.

121. Bismuth, C., Motte, G., Conso, F., Chauvin, M. & Gaultier, M. Acute digitoxin intoxication treated by intracardiac pacemaker: experience in sixty-eight patients. *Clin. Toxicol.* 1977; **10**: 443–456.

122. Chung, E.K. Digitalis-induced cardiac arrhythmias: a report of 180 cases. *Jpn. Heart J.* 1969; **10**(5):409–427.

123. Lang, T.W., Bernstein, H., Barbieri, F., Gold, H. & Corday, E. Digitalis toxicity. Treatment with diphenylhydantoin. *Arch. Intern. Med.* 1965; **116**(4): 573–580.

124. Sonnenblick, M., Abraham, A.S., Meshulam, Z. & Eylath, U. Correlation between manifestations of digoxin toxicity and serum digoxin, calcium, potassium, and magnesium concentrations and arterial ph. *Br. Med. J. Clin. Res. Ed.* 1983; **286** (6371):1089–1091.

125. Gomez-Arnau, J., Maseda, J., Burgos, R. *et al.* Cardiac arrest due to digitalis intoxication with normal serum digoxin levels: effects of hypokalemia. *Drug. Intell. Clin. Pharm.* 1982; **16**(2): 160–161.

126. Shapiro, W. Correlative studies of serum digitalis levels and the arrhythmias of digitalis intoxication. *Am. J. Cardiol.* 1978; **41**(5):852–859.

127. Antman, E.M., Wenger, T.L. & Butler, V.P. Treatment of 150 cases of life threatening digitalis intoxication with digoxin specific Fab antibody fragments: Final report of a multicenter study. *Circulation* 1990; **81**: 1744–1752.

128. Dart, R.C., Stark, Y., Fulton, B., Koziol-McLain, J. & Lowenstein, S.R. Insufficient stocking of poisoning antidotes in hospital pharmacies. *J. Am. Med. Assoc.* 1996; **276**: 1508–1510.

129. Duke, M. Atrioventricular block due to accidental digoxin ingestion treated with atropine. *Am. J. Dis. Child.* 1972; **124** (5): 754–756.

130. Smith, T.W. & Willerson, J.T. Suicidal and accidental digoxin ingestion. Report of five cases with serum digoxin level correlations. *Circulation* 1971; **44**(1): 29–36.

131. Navab, F. & Honey, M. Self-poisoning with digoxin: successful treatment with atropine. *Br. Med. J.* 1967; **3**(566): 660–661.

132. Bismuth, C., Motte, G., Conso, F., Chauvin, M. & Gaultier, M. Acute digitoxin intoxication treated by intracardiac pacemaker: experience in sixty-eight patients. *Clin. Toxicol.* 1977; **10**: 443–456.

133. Yen, D., Tsai, J., Wang, L.M. *et al.* The clinical experience of acute cyanide poisoning. *Am. J. Emerg. Med.* 1995; **13**: 524–528.

134. Green, S.M. & Naftel, J. Antiarrhythmic efficacy of magnesium in the setting of life-threatening digoxin toxicity [letter]. *Am. J. Emerg. Med.* 1989; **7**(3): 347–348.

135. French, J.H., Thomas, R.G., Siskind, A.P., Brodsky, M. & Iseri, L.T. Magnesium therapy in massive digoxin intoxication. *Ann. Emerg. Med.* 1984; **13**(7): 562–566.

136. Kinlay, S. & Buckley, N.A. Magnesium sulfate in the treatment of ventricular arrhythmias due to digoxin toxicity. *Clin. Toxicol.* 1995; **33**: 55–59.

137. Eisenberg, C.D., Simmons, H.G. & Mintz, A.A. The effects of magnesium upon cardiac arrhythmias. *Am. Heart J.* 1950; **39**: 703–712.

138. Zwilliger, L. Uber die magnesiumwirkung auf das herz. *Klin. Wochenschr.* 1935; **14**: 1429–1433.

139. Castellanos, A., Ferreiro, J., Pefkaros, K., Rozanski, J.J., Moleiro, F. & Myerburg, R.J. Effects of lignocaine on bidirectional tachycardia and on digitalis-induced atrial tachycardia with block. *Br. Heart J.* 1982; **48**(1): 27–32.

140. Agrawal, B.V., Singh, R.B., Vaish, S.K. & Edin, H. Cardiac asystole due to lignocaine in a patient with digitalis toxicity. *Acta. Cardiol.* 1974; **29**(4): 341–347.

141. Siegers, A. & Board, P.N. Amiodarone used in successful resuscitation after near-fatal flecainide overdose. *Resuscitation* 2002; **53**: 105–108.

142. Nicholls, D.P., Murtagh, J.G. & Holt, D.W. Use of amiodarone and digoxin specific fab antibodies in digoxin overdosage. *Br. Heart J.* 1985; **53**(4): 462–464.

143. Maheswaran, R., Bramble, M.G. & Hardisty, C.A. Massive digoxin overdose: successful treatment with intravenous amiodarone. *British Medical Journal Clinical Res. Ed.* 1983; **287**(6389): 392–393.

144. Bird, S.B., Gaspari, R.J. & Dickson, E.W. Early death due to severe organophosphate poisoning is a centrally mediated process. *Acad. Emerg. Med.* 2003; **10**: 295–298.

145. Okumura, T., Takasu, N., Ishimatsu, S. *et al.* Report on 640 victims of the Tokyo subway sarin attack. *Ann. Emerg. Med.* 1996; **28**: 129–135.

146. Ohbu, S., Yamashina, A., Takasu, N., Yamaguchi, T. *et al.* Sarin poisoning on Tokyo subway. *South. Med. J.* 1997; **90**: 587–593.

147. Feihl, F., Domenighetti, G. & Perret, C. Massive poisoning with cyanide with favorable outcome. Hemodynamic study. *Schweiz. Med. Wochenschr.* 1982; **112**: 1280–1282.

148. Chen, K.K. & Rose, C.L. Treatment of acute cyanide poisoning. *J. Am. Med. Assoc.* 1956; **162**: 1154–1155.

149. Feldman, J.M. & Feldman, M.D. Sequelae of attempted suicide by cyanide ingestion: a case report. *Int. J. Psychiatry Med.* 1990; **20**: 173–179.

150. Carella, F., Grassi, M.P., Savoiardo, M., Contri, P., Rapuzzi, B. & Mangoni, A. Dystonic-Parkinsonian syndrome after cyanide poisoning: clinical and MRI findings. *J. Neurol. Neurosurg. Psychiatry* 1988; **51**: 1345–1348.

151. Boggild, M.D., Peck, R.W. & Tomson, C.R. Acetonitrile ingestion: delayed onset of cyanide poisoning due to concurrent ingestion of acetone. *Postgrad. Med. J.* 1999; **66**(771): 40–41.

152. Stewart, R. Cyanide poisoning. *Clin. Toxicol.* 1974; **7**: 561–564.

153. Mutlu, G.M., Leikin, J.B., Oh, K. & Factor, P. An unresponsive biochemistry professor in the bathtub. *Chest* 2002; **122**(3): 1073–1076.

154. Riou, B., Berdeaux, A., Pussard, E. & Giudicelli, J.F. Comparison of the hemodynamic effects of hydroxocobalamin and cobalt edetate at equipotent cyanide antidotal doses in conscious dogs. *Intens. Care Med.* 1993; **19**: 26–32.

155. Riou, B., Gerard, J.L., La Rochelle, C.D., Bourdon, R., Berdeaux, A. & Giudicelli, J.F. Hemodynamic effects of hydroxocobalamin in conscious dogs. *Anesthesiology* 1991; **74**: 552–555.

156. Sauer, S.W. & Keim, M.E. Hydroxocobalamin: improved public health readiness for cyanide disasters. *Ann. Emerg. Med.* 2001; **37**: 635–641.

59

Cardiac arrest during anesthesia

Wolfgang Ummenhofer[1], Andrea Gabrielli[2], Quinn Hogan[3], Eldar Soreide[4] and Mathias Zuercher[5]

[1] Department of Anesthesia, University Hospital, Basle, Switzerland
[2] Division of Critical Care Medicine, University of Florida, Gainesville, FL, USA
[3] Department of Anesthesiology, Medical College of Wisconsin, Milwaukee, WI, USA
[4] Intensive Care Unit, Stavanger University Hospital, Stavanger, Norway
[5] Department of Anesthesia, University Hospital, Basle, Switzerland

Introduction

Without the inherent risk of cardiac arrest (CA), anesthesia might not have developed as an acknowledged medical specialty in its own right. Only a year after painless surgery was made possible in 1846 by W.T.G. Morton's use of ether as an anesthetic, cases of death under inhalation anesthesia occurred in England. In 1848, Hannah Green, a young healthy patient undergoing a trivial procedure for removal of an infected toenail, became the first reported fatality from chloroform anesthesia and, even today, her name stands for every anesthesiologist's nightmare.[1]

John Snow, whose work on resuscitation is less well known than his contributions to the scientific foundations of anesthesia for infants,[2] had by 1841 accumulated considerable expertise in the field of resuscitating asphyxiated stillborns.[3] With his monograph *On Chloroform and Other Anaesthetics* published in 1858, John Snow became the world's first scientific anesthesiologist, and with his review of 50 cases of fatal chloroform administration he also became the first researcher on the mechanism of critical incidents and the first promoter of modern resuscitation medicine. Some of his recommended techniques of resuscitation included use of the "tracheal tube," administration of oxygen, mouth-to-mouth or mouth-to-nostril ventilation, compression of the ribs and abdomen, and introduction of galvanic current.[4] Thus, CA strongly influenced the professionalization of anesthetic practice, while at the same time anesthesia offered the hitherto unknown opportunity for investigating and treating a multitude of expected, observed, and, later on, monitored and instrumented cases of CA that have facilitated the successes in modern resuscitation medicine during the last 150 years.

Initially, CA seemed only to be related to the use of general anesthesia (GA), but with the increased use of regional anesthesia (RA) during the first half of the twentieth century, fatal outcome of painless surgery was shown not to be restricted to GA. Neuraxial anesthesia, intravenous RA (Bier-Block), peripheral RA, and local anesthesia were associated with risks specific for CA because of the loss of sympathetic reflexes, drug toxicity, convulsions, and early or delayed hypoxia.

For many years, efforts to decrease fatal adverse events concentrated on the technical, pharmacological, equipment, and monitoring aspects of anesthetic care; more recently human factors involved in anesthesia management (presence, experience, and carefulness of personnel providing care) have been shown to significantly influence severe morbidity and mortality of patients exposed to anesthesia.[5] Mishaps and human failure to recognize and handle fatal adverse events are among the most frequent bases for all closed-claims' investigations. Litigation rarely considers that personal failings usually reflect organizational or working place deficiencies.

Anesthesiologists tend to feel that proficiency in cardiopulmonary resuscitation is part of their natural area of expertise. Nevertheless, the poor quality of resuscitation skills among medical staff is well documented[6–10] and this, unfortunately, includes anesthesiologists.[11] Educational programs must consider these realities.

This chapter focuses on creating care and vigilance in the multicausal etiology of fatal outcome in perioperative states and contributing to preventive measures for major adverse events.

Epidemiology

Incidence, definitions

CA in association with anesthesia is rare and, in contrast to the out-of-hospital area, is associated with an excellent outcome with good recovery in over 80% of cases. Several recent studies report similar rates between 0.5 and 1 case per 10 000 anesthetics for adults[12–15] and up to 1.4 cases per 10 000 anesthetics for children.[16] There are major problems in comparing reports in the literature, however, because of lack of uniformly accepted definitions and reporting methods. These include:

(a) Considerable variation in keywords used as trial inclusion criteria: pulselessness, circulatory collapse, CA requiring external chest compression, indication for electric defibrillation, asystole, ventricular fibrillation, electromechanical dissociation, death in association with anesthesia.

(b) Different time-periods studied: preoperative (from drug intake for premedication) to the induction of anesthesia, during stay in the operating room (OR) emergence from anesthesia, postoperative transport, recovery room, intensive care unit (ICU), ward (up to 6 hours after anesthesia, up to 24 hours after anesthesia with a maximal postoperative time of up to 30 days).

(c) Use of different reporting systems: most information is based on case series, closed-claim analysis, computer record systems, and voluntary critical incident and national anesthetic record systems. CAs managed without postoperative consequences were probably not uniformly recorded and therefore underestimated. The quality of data depends on the accuracy and honesty of those reporting them, so that use of defined terms by all participants would aid obtaining uniform results.

(d) Assessment of the heterogeneity of the investigated patients: no uniformly used grading system is available to quantify age-mix, comorbidities, and complexity of surgery performed.

(e) Use of retrospective data records, which cannot provide first-hand information about the case.

Beecher and Todd in 1954 reported on the first prospective cohort study on mortality and morbidity of anesthesia and identified 384 deaths out of 599 548 anesthetics administered between 1948 and 1952 in ten large American teaching hospitals as being attributable to anesthesia alone or anesthesia as a major contributing factor. They calculated an incidence of 6.4 deaths per 10 000 anesthetics and concluded that "deaths from anesthesia are certainly a matter for public health concerns."[17]

Six major cohort studies were published between 1980 and 1990 with more than one million anesthetics administered (Table 59.1). Incidence of CA was between 1.3 and 6 per 10 000 anesthetics with a mortality rate between 0.3 and 3 per 10 000 anesthetics. These six studies are not comparable, as they report on different observation time periods, that is: 1 year;[18] 17 years;[19] time periods from 1967 to 1987, age-mixed cohorts[20] or just children and infants,[21] nationwide cohort studies[20] or individual hospital surveys.[22,23] Nevertheless, these reports do offer rough figures for incidences of that time period and investigated patient populations.

The 10 years between 1995 and 2005 included nine large investigations from the United States,[14,16] Australia, New Zealand,[24,25] Japan,[13,26] and Europe,[12] reflecting more than 4.5 million anesthetics and over 5200 reported claims. Incidence of CA in the perioperative period varied between 0.15 and 1.1 per 10 000 anesthetics in adults and up to 1.4 per 10 000 in children, with a mortality rate between 0.1 and 0.9 per 10 000 for adults and 0.4 for children.

The incidence of anesthesia-related CA is believed to have decreased over the last decades (Fig. 59.1). Comparing the periods from 1980 to 90 and 1995 to 2005 and that the published studies were not performed in a similar manner, the reported incidence declines from a range of 1.3 to 6 per 10 000 anesthetics (1989–90) to a range of 0.5 to 2.8 per 10 000 (1995–2005). There is no clear trend with regard to anesthetic-related deaths resulting from CA with a rather stable incidence between 0.1 and 0.9 per 10 000. Nevertheless, after an extensive literature search, Lagasse *et al.*[27] argue that the anesthetic-related mortality rate has been stable over time since 1992 and that, because of lack of a worldwide standardization in definitions and methodology, no scientific evidence demonstrates an increased safety in anesthesia in the last decade.

In contrast, a dramatic change in the characteristics of the surgical population over the last 20 years is well documented. Today, patients are older and sicker, and more complex surgical procedures are being performed. A large French survey of over 7 937 000 anesthetic procedures in 1996 compared these data with data from 1980 and concluded that the number of anesthetic procedures increased by 120% over the 16 years, which corresponds to an increase in the population-corrected rate from 6.6 to 13.5 per 100 population. Elderly patients and those with high American Society of Anesthesiologists (ASA) physical status classifications (Table 59.2) had the greatest increase: ASA class 1: + 30%, ASA class 3: + 268%.[28]

Several studies comparing early with more recent observation periods provide insight into the development of CA

Table 59.1. Studies of anesthesia-related cardiac arrest and mortality

Author	Pub Year	Study Type	Study Period	Country	Follow up	Anesthesia-related CA per 10,000 Anesthetics	Anesthesia-related Death per 10,000 Anesthetics	Anesthesia-related CA (n)	Anesthesia-related Deaths/Veg State (n)	Anesthesia-related Deaths/Veg State (%)	Population/claims (n)	Remarks
Beecher(17)	1954	CH	1948–52	USA	to discharge	–	6.4	–	–	–	355 548	
Hovi-Viander (18)	1980	CI	1975	Finland	to discharge	2.6	1.9	89	12	13	338 934	
Pottecher (20)	1984	CH	1978–82	France	24 hours	6.0	3.4	119	67	56	198 103	
Keenan (23)	1985	CR	1969–83	USA	24 hours	1.7	0.9	27	14	52	163 240	
Olsson (19)	1988	CH	1967–84	Sweden	OR	4.5	0.3	115	9	8	250 543	
Tiret (21)	1988	CR	1978–82	France	24 hours	3.0	0.25	12	1	8	40 240[a]	
Chopra (22)	1990	CI	1978–87	Netherlands	OR	1.3	0.6	13	6	46	97 496	
Aubas (48)	1991	CR	1983–87	France	OR, RR	2.8	1.1	29	11	38	102 468	
Morray (33)	1993	CI	1985–91	USA	–	–	–	–	1185	–	2 400	
Tikkanen (29)	1995	CI	1986	Finland	3 days	–	0.15	–	20	–	325 585	
Warden (25)	1996	CI	1984–90	Australia	24 hours	–	0.5	–	48	–	3 500 000	
Auroy (41)	1997	CI	1994	France	–	3.1	0.67	32	7	22	103 730[b]	
Morray (16)	2000	CI	1994–98	USA	OR, RR	1.4	0.36	150	39	26	1 089 200[a]	
Biboulet (12)	2001	CH	1989–95	France	12 hours	1.1	0.6	11	6	55	101 769[c]	
Auroy (38)	2002	CI	1998–99	France	–	0.6	0.25	10	4	40	158 083[b]	
Newland (14)	2002	CH	1989–99	USA	48 hours	2.1	0.9	15	7	47	72 959	
Kawashima (13)	2003	CH	1994–98	Japan	7 days	1.0	0.13	237	37	16	2 363 038	
Sprung (15)	2003	CH	1990–2000	USA	discharge	0.5	0.1	24	5	21	518 294	
Lee (163)	2004	CI	1980–90	USA	–	–	–	81	73	90	1 005[b]	
Mason (34)	2004	CI	1994–98	France	OR, RR	1.4	0.36	150	39	26	1 089 200[d]	
Kopp (39)	2005	CH	1983–2002	USA	OR	1.7	0.5	26	8	31	150 370[b]	
Runciman (24)	2005	CI	1996 ongoing	Australia	–	–	–	129	25	19	4 000	

CH: cohort study   CI: critical incidence report/closed claim   CR: case series, case reports.

OR: operating room   RR: recovery room   Veg: vegetative.

[a] only pediatric   [b] only RA   [c] ASA class 5 excluded   [d] identical population a Morray 16, 2000.

n number of patients.

Table 59.2. American Society of Anesthesiologists (ASA) Patient Classification

ASA class 1:	Healthy individual
ASA class 2:	Mild systemic disease without functional limitations
ASA class 3:	Severe systemic disease with functional limitations
ASA class 4:	Severe systemic disease that poses a daily threat to life
ASA class 5:	Moribund patient not expected to survive 24 hr with or without surgery

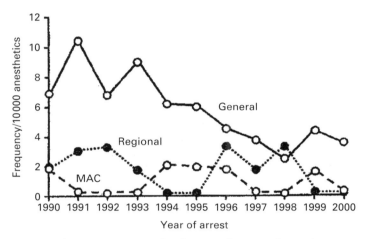

Fig. 59.1. Frequency of cardiac arrest by year and type of anesthesia.[15] Reproduced with permission.

over time with less methodological bias. A computer-based anesthetic record system at Karolinska Hospital, Stockholm, Sweden was used to analyze 170 CAs out of 250 543 anesthetic record files between 1967 and 1984. There was a nearly 10-fold decrease in incidence of CA during anesthesia between 1967 and 1984, most prominent between 1967 and 1974.[19] In the non-cardiac surgical patient collective study at the Mayo Clinic, Rochester, MN between the years 1990 and 2000, of 518 294 patients, 223 experienced CA between the start of anesthesia and discharge from the recovery room.[15] Incidence for patients receiving GA decreased over the 11 years from a rate of 7.8 per 10 000 anesthetics (1990–92) to 3.2 per 10 000 (1998–2000). But only 24 of these 223 CAs were attributed to anesthesia. Analysis of the Finnish Mortality Associated with Anesthesia and Surgery Survey 1986 (325 585 procedures)[29] compared these results with a similar study of the Finnish collective in 1975 (338 934 procedures).[18] Tikkanen

et al. identified 5 cases in the 1986 survey compared with 67 cases in the 1975 survey and calculated a more than 10-fold reduction in the incidence of death related to anesthesia (from 1.9 to 0.15 per 10 000 anesthetics) over this 20-year period.[29]

The debate continues as to whether the safety of anesthesia has improved over time. The reported rates of anesthesia-related mortality vary widely among published studies. No uniform methods, definitions, observation periods, and/or markers are used for normalizing patient age-mix, comorbidities, and complexity of surgical procedures, thus making comparisons of published data extremely difficult. Nevertheless, as highlighted by Cooper and Gaba,[30] the truth will end up somewhere between major progress as declared by the Committee on Quality of Health Care in America in 1999[31] and no progress in the improvement of safety in anesthesia over the last 25 years, as concluded in the literature review published by Lagasse *et al.* in 2002.[32]

Risk factors

CA during anesthesia is predominantly multifactorial in origin: poor preoperative patient conditions associated with inadequate preoperative risk estimation, inappropriate or delayed anesthesia management, and human error or misjudgement.[12,15] The incidence of anesthetic-related CA or death is so low that no statistical single variables are identifiable as being independent and solely responsible risk factors leading to CA and consequent mortality. Moreover, without uniform definitions, CA in acute coronary syndrome or severe kidney failure would not be attributed by most authors as anesthetic-related, but rather as an underlying patient disease. Thus, we have only discussed studies where the categories of risk factors were identified by univariate or multivariate analysis.

Infants and children

Compared with adults, the incidence for perioperative CAs in infants and children is increased. In 1985, Keenan and Boyan reported a threefold increased risk for the pediatric group.[23] A French survey of over 40 240 anesthetics in patients younger than 15 years reported an incidence of CA in infants of 19 per 10 000 and in children of 2.1 per 10 000.[21] Respiratory failure was predominant in infants, whereas respiratory and circulatory events were equally distributed in children. The most comprehensive survey on the pediatric patient collective reported 289 cases

Table 59.3. Incidence of cardiac arrest and mortality as a function of the America Society of Anesthesiologists (ASA) Physical Status Classification

	Biboulet et al.[12]		Sprung et al.[15]		Newland et al.[14]		Olsson et al.[19]		Kopp et al.[39]	
	CA	Fatal	CA	Fatal	CA	Fatal	CA	Fatal	CA	Fatal
I	1	0	1	0	1	0	11		3	1
II	2	1	5	0	2	0	53		9	1
III	6	3	16	5	8	6	39		12	4
IV	2	2	2	0	3	1	17		2	2
V					1	0			0	0
Unknown/missing							5			
Total	11	6	24	5	15	7	115	9	26	8
Elective	9	5	22	5	11	6	101		25	7
Emergency	2	1	2	0	4	1	14		1	1

recorded in the Pediatric Perioperative CA (POCA) Registry:[16] 150 cases (52%) were related to anesthesia: 83 of these (55%) occurred in infants (less than 12 months), and 47 (31%) in children aged 12 months to 5 years; the remaining 20 cases were in older children. Distribution for ASA classifications were 33% in ASA physical status classes 1 and 2, and 67% in ASA classes 3 to 5. Causes were categorized as 37% medication-related, 32% cardiovascular, and 20% respiratory events. The medication-related cause significantly predominated in ASA classes 1 and 2 patient groups, and cardiovascular causes in the ASA classes 3 and 4 patient groups. In 68% of all reported cases, the patients recovered without long-term injury. Higher ASA classifications and emergency procedures were most often associated with poor outcome.

Compared to the Pediatric Closed Malpractice Study[33] in 1993, where respiratory events (43%) were the most common, the distribution of causes in the POCA registry represents a major change in reported causes. Nonetheless, that study could be biased, because chest compression was mandatory as an inclusion criterion for the POCA registry. Mason emphasizes that use of pulse oximetry and capnography in the POCA registry was 98% and 86%, respectively, compared with only 7% for pulse oximetry in 1993, and she concluded that increased use of these monitoring devices was probably effective in preventing adverse respiratory events.[34] Newland et al. reported 22 CAs out of 16,051 cases in patients younger than 20 years with an incidence of 13.7 per 10 000 anesthetics.[14] Eighteen of these patients were preoperatively classified as very ill (ASA class 4 or 5), and therefore do not represent the typical pediatric patient population.

Age

In 2001, a consecutive cohort analysis of over 101 769 anesthetics identified 24 CAs including 13 not related to anesthesia.[12] Age above 80 years was identified in a univariate analysis as a risk factor. This corresponds with the results of Olsson and Hallen that indicated[19] a four times higher risk for patients aged over 80 years compared with patients aged 30–39 years, but age was not an independent risk factor in the recent survey of Sprung et al.[15]

ASA physical status classification

The ASA physical status classification was introduced as a marker for estimated perioperative risk. It assigns the preoperatively assessed comorbidities of a patient to a score between 1 and 5. ASA class 1 indicates a "healthy patient" without increased anesthetic risk and ASA class 5 indicates a "moribund patient not expected to survive 24 hours with or without surgery." Coexisting diseases such as acute or chronic coronary syndrome, acute renal failure or diabetes, and patient factors such as morbid obesity that increased risk were summarized and normalized by the ASA physical status classification.

It is not surprising that a higher ASA physical status classification is associated with an elevated risk of CA and death (Table 59.3). The risk of perioperative CA for patients with an ASA class 5 is 300 times that of class 1 or 2, and patients with class 3 have a higher risk than ASA class 1 or 2.[14] Similar distributions of ASA classifications were found by Biboulet et al.[12] (8 of 11 anesthetic-related CAs and 5 of 6 mortalities, ASA physical status class over 2), and by Sprung *et al.*[15] (44% of all CAs, ASA class of 4 or 5, and 18 of 24 of the anesthetic-related CAs (75%) occurred in patients with an ASA class of 3 or 4).

Obstetric anesthesia

Anesthesia for cesarean section and other emergency peripartum procedures has been associated with a relatively high risk of death among otherwise young and healthy women. Failed airway management due to the anatomical changes during pregnancy, increased risk of gastric acid aspiration during airway management, and acute respiratory distress syndrome have been identified as major risk factors for perioperative death. The 2005 published report on 50 years of the "Confidential Enquiries into Maternal Death" in Great Britain concludes that anesthesia for cesarean section is now 30 times safer than it was 50 years ago,[35] with a major contributing factor being the change in anesthetic technique (avoidance of GA whenever possible and use of neuraxial anesthesia). Rates of direct death attributable to anesthesia were 36 per 10 000 cesarean sections in 1964–66 and 1 per 10 000 in 2000–02.[36] Pregnancy is apparently not associated with an increased risk of fatal outcome from neuraxial anesthesia. There were no deaths directly attributed to RA in the 2000–02 report and only one case in the 1997–1999 report.[36,37]

Regional anesthesia

Although CA might actually be less likely to occur under RA compared with GA, our review of the literature over the last 20 years shows an incidence between 0.04 and 1.8 per 10 000 major regional blocks[12,38–40] which is the same order of magnitude reported for GA, but it appears to have declined over the last 20 years. Neuraxial anesthesia techniques are associated with a higher risk of CA compared with peripheral plexus or nerve blocks, and the highest risk is associated with spinal anesthesia.[38,39,41] This result has to be interpreted with caution, however, as there is no correction for the large increase in spinal anesthesia compared with epidural anesthesia over the last years.[28] Furthermore, the analyses of Critical Incidence Reporting Systems may represent only the worst outcome associated with a particular technique, rather than all results from a broad population. Also, patients receiving GA and those receiving RA were not similar with regard to ASA physical status classifications, comorbidities, types of surgery, and ratios of elective to emergency surgery.

A comprehensive report representing 20 years of RA at the Mayo Clinic, Rochester, MN analyzed over 70 000 neuraxial anesthesias.[39] CA was defined as hemodynamic instability (severe hypotension and/or bradycardia) that resulted in loss of consciousness requiring defibrillation, chest compression, and/or vasopressors. They included only the period after initiation of regional anesthesia and before discharge to the recovery room or ICU. Twenty-six patients in the last 15 years who had a CA were described in detail. The overall incidence of CA was 1.8 per 10 000 neuraxial procedures with a predominance for spinal compared with epidural anesthesia (2.9 vs. 0.9 per 10 000). The ratio of patients who survived CA to discharge did not differ between spinal and epidural anesthesia (14 of 20 vs. 3 of 6, p = 0.29). The incidence declined between the first 5 years (1988–92) from 3.3 to 1.0 per 10 000 in the last 5 years (1998–2002). In particular, in the spinal anesthesia group, incidence declined from 5.6 per 10 000 in the first 5 years of the study to 1.4 per 10 000 in the last 5 years (1998–2002). Table 1 from Kopp *et al.* shows 40 CAs, 28 of them in the period after 1988 where the number of anesthetics was known and the corresponding incidence was calculated. Two patients from the original 28 were apparently lost and were not included in his results.

Auroy *et al.* performed two large French surveys on complications of RA.[38,41] In the 2002 report, 487 anesthesiologists voluntarily reported 56 serious complications related to RA (overall, 150 083 regional blocks were performed in adults (74%), children (3%), or for obstetric purposes (23%)). CA occurred in 10 patients during spinal anesthesia and in 1 patient during a posterior lumbar plexus block, with an incidence of 0.83 vs. 0.08 per 10 000. In a 1997 French report of 103 730 regional blocks there were 89 serious complications related to anesthesia: CA in 32 cases (spinal: 26, epidural: 3, peripheral nerve block: 3), and fatal outcome in 7 cases (spinal: 6 of 26, epidural: 0, peripheral nerve block: 1 of 3). Bradycardia was the main precursor in all CAs during spinal anesthesia, and more elderly than younger patients were involved.

Liu and McDonald emphasize that risk factors for bradycardia are baseline heart rate lower than 60 beats/ min, ASA physical status class 1, use of β-blockers, prolonged PR interval on the electrocardiogram, and spinal block higher than T5.[40] The closed-claim analysis identified administration of sedation and lack of early treatment with epinephrine as typical patterns of management in cases of CA.[42] Pollard argues that the evidence for a respiratory etiology for CA during neuraxial anesthesia is sparse and that CAs occur with oxygen saturation readings of 95%–100%.[43] Bradyarrhythmia is commonly found before CA and could be related to blockade of sympathetic activity and/or cardiovascular reflexes[44] related to a relative hypovolemia induced by vasodilatation. Unfortunately, some CAs that occurred during spinal anesthesia have fatal outcomes even in young and otherwise healthy patients.[43,45]

Causes of cardiac arrest

The vast majority of CAs are ascribed to concomitant disease or surgical factors. Fatal outcome associated with anesthetic and surgical procedures in Finland was about the same in 1986 as in 1975. But the role of surgery had decreased to about one-third and of anesthesia to less than one-tenth as the main contributing cause of the death;[29] similar progress in anesthetic safety has been reported for the same time period.[46,47] A large Japanese survey divided etiologies of fatal accidents into four categories, those resulting from: preoperative complications (65%); surgical procedures (24%); intraoperative pathological events (9%); and those attributable to anesthetic management (2%).[26] The major cause of preoperative complication-related deaths was pre-existing hemorrhagic shock, followed by cardiovascular diseases, such as myocardial ischemia and congestive heart failure. Excessive surgical bleeding comprised 70% of surgical procedure-related deaths. The major causes of intraoperative pathological events were myocardial ischemia, pulmonary embolism, and severe arrhythmias. Half the anesthetic management-related deaths were caused by airway or ventilatory problems, followed by medication accidents, and infusion/transfusion mishaps.

Principal causes of CA and other critical incidents due to etiologies during anesthesia and surgery are listed in Table 59.4.

Several epidemiological studies have analyzed the possible causes for intraoperative CA.[12–15,19,21,23,25,29,48,49] Identifying the causes of CA that are primarily attributable to anesthetic management would allow for institution of preventive measures. From the very beginning, as has been shown for incidences, the classification of deaths and causes of CA during surgery and anesthesia has varied considerably.[50–54] In addition, it is often impossible to retrieve sufficient information retrospectively in order to reliably identify the causative factors. Moreover, adverse events are generally multifactorial in origin, and CA in particular is often the culmination of different reasons,[14,27,30] one of which might well include anesthetic interventions or, rather, the lack thereof.[15]

Thus, in an Australian study, 129 cases of CA were grouped into five categories reflecting monofactorial and multifactorial origins: (a) anesthetic technique (11 cases with this category alone; 32 with this and one or more of the other categories, representing 25% of all 129 CA); (b) drug-related (16; 32, 25%); (c) associated with surgical procedure (9; 29, 22%); (d) associated with pre-existing medical or surgical disease (30; 82, 64%); (e) unknown (8; 14, 11%).[24]

Patients

Hypoxemia

For all anesthesiologists, hypoxia as a main cause of CA is always worrisome, especially in a "cannot intubate – cannot ventilate" scenario. Hypoxia during anesthesia occurs in failure of airway management; misplacement of the endotracheal tube (esophageal or endobronchial; accidental tracheal extubation in the prone position);[14,15,19] aspiration of gastric contents;[14] laryngospasm mainly due to mechanical irritation during inadequate depth of anesthesia;[19] severe bronchospasm because of anaphylactic or intrinsic reactions; and/or errors in oxygen supply.

During the first 100 years of anesthesia, hypoventilation in spontaneously breathing patients resulting from deep inhalation anesthesia and accompanying cardiovascular compromise was a major source of fatal outcome. In their 1985 study of incidence and causes of CA due to anesthesia, Keenan and Boyan found failure of adequate ventilation in 50% and overdose inhalation in 33% of the cases.[23] In a contemporary Scandinavian survey, ventilatory problems were the most frequent causative factors of "anesthetic CA."[19] More recently, Irita et al. similarly attributed half of anesthesia-related deaths to airway and ventilatory management.[26] Sprung et al. classify 46% of CA that are attributable to anesthesia as associated with airway/ventilation problems:[15] CA due to a loss of airway patency had a poor outcome. Of note, none of the patients who experienced CA from anesthesia and had resuscitation for longer than 20 minutes survived; all of these patients had lost airway patency.

With the introduction of endotracheal intubation and controlled mechanical ventilation, the inability to establish a secure protected airway became more common. In a survey of patients whose lungs could not be ventilated and whose tracheas could not be intubated, Nagaro et al. identified 26 out of 151 300 cases of GA in university hospitals in Japan.[55] Newland et al. attributed only 20% of CA to problems of airway management.[14] Respiratory depression due to narcotics or benzodiazopines and inadequate reversal of muscle relaxation contribute to hypoventilation during the emergence from anesthesia.[19] Monitoring the intensity of muscle relaxation at the end of surgery and introduction of

Table 59.4. Causes of cardiac arrest

I   *Respiratory events*

   A.   Failure to ventilate
- Airway management failure: cannot intubate – cannot ventilate; misplacement of the endotracheal tube; aspiration of gastric contents; laryngospasm
- Inability to ventilate despite secure airway: bronchospasm; tension pneumothorax; tracheal disruption; tube dysfunction / occlusion; mediastinal collapse (mediastinal mass)

   B.   Apnea/Hypoventilation
- Respiratory depression in spontaneously breathing patients
- Failure in ventilator setting
- Loss of gas supply; breathing circuit disconnection
- Apnea in neuraxial blockade
- Pneumoperitoneum

   C.   Lack of oxygen carrier
- Severe anemia
- Carboxyhemoglobinemia; Methemoglobinemia (Prilocaine)

   D.   Ventilation/Perfusion-Mismatch
- Pulmonary embolism
- Pulmonary hypertension / vasoconstriction

II.   *Circulatory events*

   A.   Vascular failure
- Hypovolemia: hypovolemic shock; surgical bleeding
- Failure in systemic resistance: anaphylaxis; sepsis; neurogenic shock; neuraxial sympathetic block; pheochromocytoma; monoamino oxidase inhibitors; eclampsia; thyroid storm; Addison crisis
- Tension pneumothorax
- Mediastinal collapse (mediastinal mass)
- Embolism: thrombus (surgical sources: hip replacement); air (sitting position and neurosurgery); amniotic fluid

   B.   Pump failure
- Arrhythmia: coronary artery disease; conduction abnormalities (Wolff–Parkinson–White syndrome; high-degree conduction block; sick sinus syndrome); mechanical stimulation (inadequate depth of anesthesia and sympathetic stimulation; central venous or pulmonary artery catheterization); vagal reflexes; local anesthetics; hypokalemia; hyperkalemia (succinylcholine); hypocalcemia; hypomagnesemia; interference of pacemakers/AIDs; hypothermia
- Ischemia: hypoxia; anemia; increased oxygen demand (tachycardia); thrombus (myocardial infarction); end-stage congestive heart failure
- Myocardial depressant factors: volatile anesthetics; induction agents; endotoxins
- Valvular/congenital heart disease: neuraxial anesthesia and aortic stenosis

III. *Environmental causes*

   A.   Equipment failure
- Loss of gas supply
- Tube disconnection
- Failure of anesthetic machine; breathing circuit; laryngoscope; airway device
- Laser/electrocautery mishaps (airway fire)
- Monitor malfunction

   B.   Human factors
- Inadequate vigilance
- Monitoring negligence
- Drug overdose (induction agents, inhalational anesthetics, muscle relaxants)
- Drug selection error
- Blood transfusion error
- Line misconnection (venous – arterial – epidural)
- Gas flow/ventilator setting error
- Gas misconnection (N_2O instead of O_2)
- Inappropriate airway management
- Inadequate fluid management (hypovolemia; fluid overload)
- Organizational deficiencies: lack of educated and trained personnel; lack of support; workload; fatigue; communication problems; lack of checklists; missing standard operating procedures

short-acting muscle-relaxing drugs probably reduced complications during recovery. In addition, the availability of postanesthesia care units was a great advantage in preventing perioperative ventilatory disasters. More recently, use of monitored anesthesia care as the technique of choice for a variety of invasive or non-invasive procedures is increasing.[56] In a closed-claims analysis, severity of monitored anesthesia care claims was comparable to GA claims, with 41% of the claims being for death or permanent brain damage. Respiratory depression as a result of oversedation was the most common mechanism of injury.[57]

During neuraxial anesthesia, cardiovascular collapse can develop secondarily after the unrecognized development of apnea. A spinal anesthetic followed by excessive patient movement or coughing might promote arrival of the local anesthetic (LA) at cervical levels that are high enough to produce blockade of motor fibers to both the diaphragm and inspiratory muscles of the chest and neck (e.g., C3). In contrast with spinal anesthesia, epidural anesthesia usually does not compromise ventilation, unless the injection is performed cervically. Nonetheless, accidental subarachnoid injection of an anesthetic intended for the epidural space could produce apnea because the dose is 6- to 8-fold higher than that intended for subarachnoid injection, resulting in a high level of blockade and compromise of ventilatory muscles. Apnea might similarly result from an unintended subarachnoid injection of LA during retro-orbital, interscalene, or greater occipital nerve blocks.

Tension pneumothorax

During controlled mechanical ventilation, tension pneumothorax is a potentially fatal problem.[13] Awareness of its possibility, especially following central venous catheterization, and the decreasing use of nitrous oxide have reduced incidence of this complication.

Anemia

There are few data regarding CA secondary to normovolemic anemia. Anesthesiologists currently tolerate lower levels of hemoglobin than formerly, but in patients with pre-existing coronary artery disease, myocardial ischemia can occur. If hemoglobin levels in healthy patients are allowed to fall below 8 g/dl, intensified monitoring such as mixed venous saturation and/or control of serum lactate is required to prevent inadequate oxygen delivery and acidosis.[1]

Pulmonary embolism

A sudden decrease in oxygen saturation along with an additional decrease in end-tidal CO_2 measurement are strong indicators for pulmonary embolism. After a brief evaluation of ventilator settings and ruling out mechanical obstruction of tubing and other ventilation-perfusion mismatches, immediate diagnosis, as for example, with trans-esophageal echocardiography, is mandatory.

Allergic reactions

Allergic reactions are relatively common during anesthesia (frequencies range from 2.2 per 10 000 to 22.4 per 10 000), but only 3–4% of them are lethal or otherwise serious.[29,58] Anaphylaxis can occur as a result of drug administration (e.g., antibiotics, thiopental, muscle relaxants) or repeated exposure to latex. Intravenous administration of drug boluses in short sequences is characteristic of GA. It has been suggested that many unexplained deaths during GA can be retrospectively attributed to anaphylactic reactions.[59] In a Scandinavian study, 5 CAs that occurred during 200 543 anesthetic procedures were related to anaphylaxis;[19] and in a Japanese survey, 4 CAs occurred out of a total of 2.3 million.[13] With dextran as a prophylaxis against thrombosis, anaphylactic CA occurred more often,[19,29] and a case report described a fatal intraoperative event related to aprotinin after local application of fibrin glue.[60] Severe anaphylactic shock due to antibiotic wound cleaning occurred after tourniquet release at the end of minor orthopedic surgery of the limbs under RA.[61] Muscle relaxant allergies have accounted for 60 to 80% of the cases of anaphylactic shock during anesthesia.[62] Unfortunately, during GA, signs and symptoms of allergic reactions are often hidden, and hypotension, tachycardia, and bronchospasm are misinterpreted as, for example, inadequate depth of anesthesia or ventilator problems.

Allergy to LA drugs

Allergy to LA drugs is a rare cause of hypotension and circulatory arrest, particularly for amide anesthetics, but this may occur with amino-ester drugs because of their metabolites related to p-aminobenzoate. Skin testing is of uncertain utility. Allergies can also exist for methylparaben and metabisulfite used as preservatives. Many events attributed to allergy can also be the result of absorption of the coinjected epinephrine.

Cardiovascular events

Serious arrhythmias, myocardial infarction, ischemia, coronary spasm as well as pulmonary embolism account for the third to fifth ranked principal causes of total CA during surgery in Japan.[13] CA patients who had coronary ischemia preoperatively had the worst prognosis: 47% of these patients died.[63]

Neuraxial block and aortic stenosis

Hypotension from extensive neuraxial block can be especially problematic in the presence of aortic stenosis.

Although coronary perfusion pressure falls with development of systemic sympathetic block, left ventricular systolic pressures may remain high because of the stenotic valve, resulting in high oxygen demand. Development of myocardial ischemia and contractile dysfunction further compromises coronary perfusion pressure, and a vicious cycle is initiated that could result in CA.

Vagal reflexes

Vagal reflexes due to mechanical stimulation of parasympathetic nerves are associated with CA.[14] Olsson and Hallen found that succinylcholine administration resulted in 23 cases of CA;[19] notably, only 3 cases were elicited by the first administration of the drug; additional doses were given up to seven times! The authors note that succinylcholine-induced CA became rare after routine use of a small dose of non-depolarizing muscle relaxant before administration of succinylcholine although it still occurred. Sprung *et al.* describe many asystolic CAs after application of neuromuscular reversal agents.[15] In all of these cases, prognosis for successful resuscitation was very good.[15,19]

Postinduction hypotension

Hypotension is a common precursor of anesthesia-related CA.[12,14,15,19] In one of these studies, 50% of CA patients had received more than 5 mg/kg of thiopental.[19] Data from all studies suggest that CA after postinduction hypotension can be regarded as a relative overdose of narcotic and/or hypnotic induction dose (see below).

Hypovolemia

Hypovolemia and/or impaired venous return is another important cause of intraoperative CA.[12,14,19] This group includes misguided fluid replacement of expected or hidden hemorrhage, as well as other fluid losses, such as sudden evacuation of ascites. Mediastinal compression by tumor or lymphatic masses is dangerous, reducing venous return especially if combined with positive pressure ventilation.[19,64–68] Intraoperative mobilization of a hypovolemic patient can also trigger CA.[12] Prone position reinforces relative hypovolemia resulting from impaired venous return and can induce circulatory collapse together with a reduced compensatory ability.[19]

Acid–base and electrolyte imbalances

Acid–base and electrolyte imbalance are other major sources of CA.[13,19,69] Dehydration and hypokalemia are possible contributors, but the effect of hypokalemia has been studied only in small randomized trials.[70] Nevertheless, hypokalemia might contribute to a worse outcome in patients with myocardial infarction.[71,72] Most commonly,

hyperkalemia triggers CA. Inadvertent administration of potassium and calcium can affect myocardial activity and could result in cardiovascular standstill during diastole or systole. The ratio of potassium-to-calcium in blood is important; hyperkalemia is more dangerous in the presence of less ionized calcium. Evaluation of serum potassium must consider effects of changes in serum pH. When serum pH decreases, serum potassium increases because potassium shifts from the cellular to the vascular space. Likewise, when serum pH increases, serum potassium shifts intracellularly. Elevated levels of serum potassium should be anticipated before use of succinylcholine in abnormal muscle states like paraplegia or tetraplegia, inactiveness, tissue breakdown (ischemia of bowels or limbs, rhabdomyolysis, tumor lysis, hemolysis, and burn injuries), specific drugs (angiotensin-converting enzyme inhibitors, angiotensin II receptor blockers, potassium-sparing diuretics, non-steroidal anti-inflammatory drugs, β-blockers, and trimethoprim), metabolic acidosis, and endocrine disorders (Addison's disease, or hyperkalemic periodic paralysis).[73] Hyperkalemia causing anesthesia-related CA in pediatric patients has been observed after massive transfusion, reperfusion following liver transplantation, and in renal insufficiency.[16] Renal failure is the most common reason for increasing of total body potassium. Acute exacerbation of hyperkalemia occurs if acidemia develops secondary to hypoventilation or hypoperfusion. Typically, during emergence from GA, patients with acute or chronic renal failure become acidotic because of hypoventilation, and are at risk of an additional and potentially fatal shift of intracellular potassium into the intravascular compartment.[74] For treatment of hyperkalemic CA, aggressive reduction of extracellular potassium is mandatory. Hyperventilation, calcium chloride, sodium bicarbonate, and glucose plus insulin drive potassium back into the intracellular compartment and support return of the cellular membrane potential towards normal.

Environment

Anesthesia is an area in which environmental effects influence the margin of patient safety. Lagasse defined and distinguished different types of error.[27] Table 59.5 summarizes categories for system error and human error, with common examples of each.[32,75]

CA during anesthesia is not always regarded as caused by error. But if the definition of error is "an act that through ignorance, deficiency, or accident departs from or fails to achieve a desired outcome," all adverse outcomes, especially ultimately serious ones like CA, are errors.[27] Lagasse's

Table 59.5. Types of error

	Error	Example
System error	Technical accident	Postdural puncture headache follows a properly performed spinal anesthetic
	Equipment failure	Equipment malfunction results in death despite proper maintenance and checks
	Communication error	Medical consultant's report is delayed when following the usual channels of communication
	Limitation of therapeutic standards	Appropriate resuscitative efforts result in death of a multiple trauma victim
	Limitation of diagnostic standards	Preoperative assessment fails to predict difficult airway management
	Limitation of available resources	Lack of available blood products results in death due to massive bleeding
	Limitation of supervision	Attending anesthesiologist is unable to prevent a resident anesthesiologist from committing a human error because of multiple supervisory responsibilities
Human error	Improper technique	A short catheter placed in an internal jugular vein dislodges and results in hematoma formation
	Misuse of equipment	Neglecting to perform the prescribed equipment check results in equipment failure that contributes to patient death
	Disregard of available data	Failure to avoid known drug allergen results in unplanned hospital admission
	Failure to seek appropriate data	Failure to check appropriate extubation criteria results in premature extubation, subsequent respiratory failure and need for reintubation
	Inadequate knowledge	Incorrect interpretation of hemodynamic variables results in pulmonary edema

(From Ref. 27, reproduced with permission.)

definition is consistent with the definition from the Committee on Quality of Health Care in America: "Failure of a planned action to be completed as intended" or "use of a wrong plan to achieve an aim"; the accumulation of errors results in accidents.[31]

Kawashima *et al.* identified detailed causes of CA due to equipment failure including gas supplies or sources, anesthetic machine, breathing circuit, airway device, laser machine, and other sources.[13] Disconnection or misconnection of breathing circuit, arterial/venous lines and loss of gas (oxygen) supplies have been described.[19] Equipment complications following central venous or pulmonary artery catheterization such as arrhythmia that progresses to ventricular fibrillation, tamponade, hemothorax, or pneumothorax are well known. Complications associated with central venous access caused 20% of CAs in one study;[14] in pediatric anesthesia-related CA, complications of anesthesiologist-placed central lines are the most common equipment-related problems.[16] CA from pulmonary outflow-tract obstruction due to a double-lumen tube has been described.[76]

CA during anesthesia is traditionally considered to occur generally in the OR. In the Australian Incident Monitoring Study, 129 reported CA occurred in the OR (70%), recovery room (11%), introduction room (7%), ICU (5%), general

ward (4%), imaging room (1.5%), and in transit (1.5%).[24] In contrast, induction room CA is considerably higher, and CA during the course of anesthesia is significantly lower (20%) in two American surveys (Fig. 59.2).[14,15] For neuraxial anesthesia, the CA occurred at: time of block placement (4%), between block placement and surgical incision (19%), during the surgical procedure (62%), and after surgical closure (15%).[39] Proper recovery room care is very important in reducing anesthetic complications,[58] because as many as 60% of patients need special attention in the postanesthesia care unit.[77] The limiting factor to appropriate postoperative care seemed to be lack of personnel.[29]

Monitoring negligence, malfunction, or available but not used monitors relate to human error (Table 59.5): inadequate vigilance, overdose of drug or inhaled agent, selection error, and inappropriate airway management are among the most frequent causes of so called "human factors."[13] Selection error refers to mistaking one drug for another,[78] as well as to application mishaps, such as CA resulting from an inadvertent overdose of lidocaine through an arterial pressure line.[79] Errors in drug administration occur during anesthesia; "syringe swap" (selection of the wrong syringe and the erroneous administration of its contents) is the most frequent error,[80,81] occurring in 0.11%–0.75% of cases.[82,83]

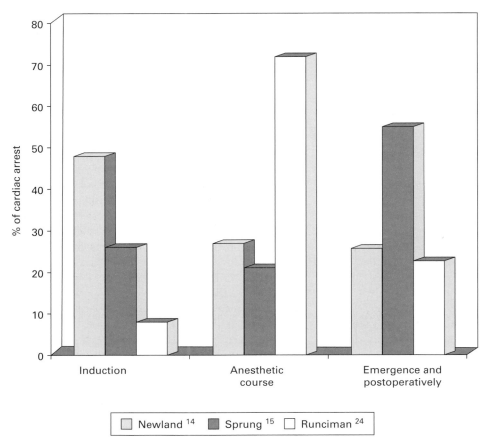

Fig. 59.2. Locations and phases of anesthesia-related cardiac arrest in three studies.

The impact of emergency procedures compared with elective anesthesia remains controversial. Earlier studies found higher overall mortality during emergency operations,[20,84–86] which was also observed in a study of intraoperative CA in the tropics: 75% of CA occurred during emergency procedures as opposed to 25% for elective cases.[87] Keenan and Boyan found a 6-fold higher incidence of CA in emergency cases, but, surprisingly, only a very small difference in incidence between ordinary hospital working hours and other times of the day.[23] Similarly, newer studies do not suggest a higher incidence of CA during non-regular hospital working hours.[14,15,39] Newland *et al.* showed that although 60% of CAs were emergencies, none of the CA cases attributable to anesthesia were emergencies.[14] In the survey by Sprung *et al.*, 168 (75%) CAs occurred during standard working hours and only 53 (25%) occurred during the night or on weekends.[15] Notably, if not the incidence of CA, then at least the likelihood of survival was better for patients who had CA during standard versus non-standard working hours.[15]

This finding might be partly explained by poorer performance induced by fatigue. For example, sleep loss and circadian disruption result in reduced attention vigilance, impaired memory and decision-making, prolonged reaction time, and disrupted communications. These create a situation where there is increased risk of the occurrence of errors, critical incidents, and accidents.[88] On the other hand, worse outcome for CA during non-regular working hours might also be explained by delayed access to surgical resources and fewer available personnel; Sprung *et al.* calculated the overall CA outcome and not that related to the anesthesia.[15]

Arbous *et al.* performed a seminal case-control study on the importance of the "human environment" for anesthesia patient safety.[5] Simple anesthetic management principles appear to have a major effect on perioperative mortality: direct availability of an additional anesthesiologist to help or troubleshoot when needed, the use of full-time compared with part-time anesthetic team members, and the presence of two persons from the anesthetic team during emergence from anesthesia had dramatically positive effects that were associated with reduced perioperative mortality within 48 hours after surgery and anesthesia.

General anesthesia

As discussed above, CA during anesthesia occurs under GA, RA, or monitored anesthesia care. The higher incidence observed during GA reflects the higher percentage of more complex interventions in more complex surroundings for sicker patients rather than the technique itself. Nevertheless, there are inherent risks during GA related to drugs and techniques.

Inhalation anesthetics

The type of anesthesia affects hemodynamic variables before and during the onset of CA. In animals the effect of induced CA differs widely based on the anesthetic protocol adopted before CA, a variable that is unfortunately not always controlled.[89] In general, anesthetic drugs can significantly affect the cardiovascular system in various ways: direct myocardial depression, parasympathetic stimulation, sympathetic stimulation, increased excitability of ventricular muscle, hypotension (especially in patients who are unable to increase cardiac output by increasing heart rate, such as those with severe valvular stenosis), heart block, constrictive pericarditis, or anaphylactic reaction.[90] Inhalation anesthetics can exacerbate and slow atrioventricular conduction and also have an added negative inotropic effect. GA can also sensitize the myocardium to the antiarrhythmic effect of catecholamines.[91] In animal models, where a critical constriction has been created, of inhalation agents reduces coronary flow autoregulation and transient episodes of sympathetic overactivity can be associated with myocardial ischemia. The presence of coronary artery disease is often found postmortem in patients who die from CA during anesthesia and whose resuscitation was ineffective.[92] Although the ischemia resolves at the end of the anesthetic, mild reductions in the ejection fraction might persist and contribute to postoperative cardiovascular complications that can be exacerbated by the use of large doses of α-blockers and β-blockers.[93]

Muscle relaxants

CA related to loss of airway has an extremely poor outcome; essentially no patients survive without neurological deficits after resuscitation requiring more than a few minutes after the loss of airway. The use of neuromuscular blocking agents accounts for the largest category of hypoxic CA[14,19,23,94]. In general, the adverse effects of non-depolarizing muscle relaxants are related to the inability to ventilate or intubate a patient who does not have spontaneous ventilation after induction or after extubation. Irreversible hypoxic brain damage is the most apparent consequence of this type of CA during GA, while hypoxic brain damage can also be an unexpected finding following dysrhythmic CA.[95]

Succinylcholine continues to be the drug of choice for urgent tracheal intubation in the perioperative period, in the emergency room, in the ICU, and even outside the hospital during emergency transportation of patients.[96–98] Because succinylcholine has a rapid onset of effect even when administered intramuscularly, it is also used to treat laryngospasm, especially when there is associated desaturation with no intravenous access. In some instances, however, adverse hemodynamic consequences, including death may occur. One of the most deleterious side effects is the acute onset of hyperkalemia and cardiovascular instability associated with its administration in susceptible patients.[99] In particular, depolarizing muscle relaxants are associated with bradycardia and asystole, especially in children[100] and in adults after repeated doses.[19,101] Bradycardia and asystole probably arise from direct stimulation of the carotid baroreceptors producing reflex bradycardia and accumulation of acetylcholine, because of competition for available cholinesterase by the paralytic agent.[101] Patients with congenital muscular dystrophies are susceptible to hyperkalemia and rhabdomyolysis following administration of succinylcholine.[102] This also occurs with acquired pathological states such as upper or lower motor denervation, immobilization, infection, direct muscle trauma, muscle tumor or inflammation, and burn injury.[99]

The electrophysiological effects of CA during hypoxemia elicited by misuse of muscle relaxants are dramatic and unique.[103] An initial sympathetic stimulation is followed by severe bradycardia and asystole. Increased serum potassium and acute metabolic and respiratory acidosis potentiate the cardiovascular depressant effect of the anesthetic. Hypercapnia from hypoventilation results in increased circulating catecholamines, but increased serum potassium levels will eventually enhance the asystole induced by vagal stimulations.

Intravenous anesthetics and sedatives

Several intravenous anesthetic agents can contribute to the onset of asystole, including etomidate, with or without depolarizing relaxants,[104,105] and propofol, the putative mechanism being increased vagal activity.[106–108] Several surgical stimuli can enhance or initiate the dysrhythmia through a vagal reflex mechanism that can lead to bradycardia or asystole. These surgical areas include: rectum, uterus and cervix, larynx, bronchial tree, bladder and urethra, mesentery, carotid sinus, heart, biliary tract, extraocular muscles, and testicles. In addition, long-term propofol infusion has been shown to be associated with metabolic acidosis, rhabdomyolysis, and cardiac failure in adults,[109,110] as well as in children.[111]

Dexmedetomidine, a recently introduced α_2-adrenergic receptor agonist with sedative, analgesic, and anxiolytic properties has been associated with CA.[112] This agent, a full agonist of the α_2-adrenergic receptor that decreases the requirement of GA with relevant respiratory depression, is associated with severe bradycardia and hemodynamic instability. The effects of dexmedetomidine can be increased by an epidural block, and dexmedetomidine itself can potentiate other negative chronotropic drugs such as digoxin and pyridostigmine. The asystole is usually brief and responds to parasympatholytic agents. In patients undergoing GA with dexmedetomidine, the potential for asystolic CA should be kept in mind.

Medication associated with prolonged Q–T interval

Sudden episodes of unexplained CA during surgery have been attributed to Q–T prolongation. In general, CA is unexpected in this patient population and very difficult to reverse.[113] High adrenergic state, intrinsic myocardial disease, electrolyte abnormalities such as hypokalemia, hypocalcemia, and anti-arrhythmic agents like quinidine, procainamide, imipramine, amiodarone, and phenothiazines can all promote acquired Q–T prolongation. This latter group of patients often has a normal preoperative baseline electrocardiogram. If the diagnosis is suspected or confirmed, preoperative aggressive electrolyte correction of calcium, potassium, and magnesium as well as mild β-blockade and perioperative cardiac pacing should be considered.

Malignant hyperthermia (MH)

Malignant hyperthermia (MH) is a rare but well-described cause of CA during GA.[114] Although there are no stereotypically clinical features of MH, conditions such as masseter spasm by exaggerated response to succinylcholine could indicate the syndrome. Hypermetabolic state follows with increased lactate levels, body temperature, and CO_2 production; muscle rigidity with evidence of massive rhabdomyolysis is seen in both urine and serum. The ultimate cause of death is usually asystole

from hyperkalemia secondary to massive rhabdomyolysis and extrusion of potassium from damaged cells that is exacerbated by sympathetic stimulation and severe metabolic acidosis. The pathophysiological trigger of this disease is an increased sensitivity to halogenated anesthetic drugs such as halothane, isoflurane, sevoflurane, and desflurane, or depolarizing neuromuscular blocking agents, e.g., succinylcholine. The triggering agent causes an imbalance of ionized calcium homeostasis within skeletal muscle cells. Increased intracellular calcium increases glycolysis demand for ATP and metabolism. The massive activity of ATPase becomes important in lack of myofilament relaxation and calcium sequestration of the sarcoplasmic reticulum and sarcolemma. Increased body temperature and CO_2 production (end-tidal CO_2) are usually indicators that the hypermetabolic response has already started. More than 50% of MH families have mutations in the ryanodine receptor, the calcium channel of the sarcoplasmic reticulum.[114] This pharmacogenetic disease is inherited as an autosomal dominant trait, and penetrance is variable. In MH families with known MH causative mutations, molecular genetic diagnosis of MH susceptibility is an established procedure.[115,116] Because of the heterogeneity of the MH trait, an MH-negative diagnosis must not be concluded without the halothane and caffeine *in vitro* muscle contraction test. Clinical findings that raise suspicion of MH are: family history, masseter rigidity, respiratory acidosis, hypoxemia, rhabdomyolysis with increased creatine kinase and myoglobin urea, increasing temperature (usually a late sign), and cardiac dysrhythmias.

Awareness of the problem and introduction of sodium dantrolene have decreased the mortality of MH during GA from 80% in the 1960s to less than 10% today.[117] If MH is thought to be the cause of CA in the OR, the triggering agent must be immediately discontinued and the patient should be ventilated with 100% oxygen at high flow. Use of calcium as an add-on to the resuscitation protocol should be an immediate consideration; a solution of dextrose 50% in water and IV insulin 1 unit for each 10 g of glucose should also be given. Early administration of bicarbonate and hyperventilation might be necessary to decrease extravasation of potassium. The patient should also be cooled as soon as feasible. The main therapy is immediate administration of sodium dantrolene. Ideally, the therapy is started with a dantrolene bolus of 2.5 mg/kg and repeated every 5 minutes to a total dose of 10 mg/kg. A proven MH should trigger rapid and comprehensive communication with the patient and the family to take appropriate steps to protect themselves from an MH crisis if they undergo GA.[118]

Regional anesthesia

Introduction

RA is often chosen over GA because of the belief that disastrous complications will be less likely. Although this is certainly true for peripheral nerve blocks with a small volume of LA, such as a digital block, evidence indicating a lower CA rate for RA is weak. In part, this is due to the overall low rates of catastrophic circulatory complications during both RA and GA. There are, however, factors unique to RA that are inherently risky. Sudden loss of sympathetic activity in an extensive portion of the body is unique to neuraxial (spinal and epidural) anesthesia. Also, RA is the only routine medical treatment in which the intended target for injection might be only a few millimeters from a locale that would result in a massive toxic response, such as intravascular injection of LA solution during brachial plexus blockade, or intrathecal injection during epidural blockade.

Systemic LA toxicity

The desired effect of LAs when used for RA is temporary interruption of axonal conduction in peripheral nerves, thereby suspending sensation and motor activity of the distal body part. LA toxicity/neurotoxicity at the injection site is a rare clinical problem that could produce cauda equina syndrome after lidocaine spinal anesthesia or delayed recovery of function after peripheral nerve blockade. Much more serious systemic consequences may follow unintended intravascular injection of large doses of LA solution intended for nerve plexus blockade or epidural blockade.

Presentation

The earliest signs of systemic LA toxicity are due to subtle cerebral dysfunction, including tinnitus, odd metallic taste, or confusion and dysphasia, which may be followed by generalized seizure activity. Higher serum levels may be tolerated if levels rise slowly, whereas abrupt increases in circulating levels, such as from unintended intravascular delivery of a large LA bolus, are more likely to cause complications. The predominant circulatory manifestations in the deeply sedated patient or in one in whom RA is combined with concurrent GA are low cardiac output and blood pressure. Alternatively, dysrhythmias are often the initial circulatory manifestation in awake patients. A less common mechanism for systemic LA toxicity is rapid uptake from the injection site in the absence of direct injection into a vessel, such as when a large volume of agent is administered throughout a large area of tissue so that a large surface is involved in uptake. This occurs with multiple intercostal blocks or extensive subcutaneous infiltration for liposuction.

Etiology

Peripheral circulatory effects of LAs

Studies of direct effects of LAs on vessels show highly variable responses, from constriction to dilatation, depending on dose.[119,120] Toxic levels of bupivacaine in intact animals raise systemic vascular resistance, and when systemic toxicity leads to seizures, increased sympathetic tone causes vasoconstriction. Thus, the principal mechanism by which LAs depress the circulation is through actions on the heart.

Depression of myocardial contractility

LAs produce a dose-dependent decrease in myocardial contractile force. Whereas the clinical efficacy of LAs is through blockade of neuronal voltage-gated Na^+ channels, myocardial depression probably results from other mechanisms.[121] LAs, especially bupivacaine, block cardiac Ca^{2+} channels,[122] which in turn, reduces the Ca^{2+} available for triggering its release from intracellular Ca^{2+} stores. Release from this sarcoplasmic Ca^{2+} pool is also inhibited by the action of LAs on the Ca^{2+} release channel of the sarcoplasmic reticulum.[123,124] The final result is a lower level of cytoplasmic Ca^{2+} and therefore weakened contraction.

Additional evidence points to disruption of cellular energy metabolism by LAs at various sites in the production and use of ATP.[125,126] Two processes have been identified as targets for inhibition by LA. In isolated mitochondria, LAs uncouple mitochondrial oxidative phosphorylation and increase metabolic rate. Additionally, inhibition of complex I of the respiratory chain reduces energy production.[127] The relative contribution of lowered intracellular Ca^{2+} and inhibition of energy metabolism to myocardial depression is not clear, but the high LA concentrations necessary to inhibit Ca^{2+} entry indicate that altered energy metabolism might predominate at usual concentrations. LA inhibition of cyclic AMP production (particularly by bupivacaine) might also contribute to myocardial depression and interfere with the therapeutic effects of epinephrine,[128] probably by inhibiting binding of β-adrenergic receptor agonists.[129] At equipotent doses, bupivacaine depresses contractility somewhat more strongly than lidocaine, as demonstrated by injections into the coronary arteries, which avoids other systemic effects.

Altered cardiac electrophysiology

The pattern of dysrhythmia caused by toxic doses of long acting agents such as bupivacaine and etidocaine differ from that of other LAs. Whereas lidocaine in progressive doses eventually leads to circulatory failure and hypotension with only sinus bradycardia or atrioventricular block, the typical pattern with bupivacaine is widening of the QRS complex, malignant ventricular dysrhythmias, electromechanical dissociation, and refractory asystole. Cardiovascular collapse occurs at doses only 3.7 times the dose that causes seizures. This "safety ratio" for lidocaine is 7.1 and etidocaine is intermediate at 4.4. In many clinical and laboratory reports, resuscitation is especially difficult with bupivacaine.

These unique features of bupivacaine are due to the kinetics of its binding to cardiac Na^+ channels. LAs bind channels during their open configuration. Bupivacaine dissociates from the inactivated channel with a time constant of 1.5 seconds, unlike the 0.15 second for lidocaine. Even with normal heart rates, bupivacaine does not completely leave the channel during diastole, so that the next depolarization and channel opening binds more bupivacaine, producing an accumulation in the heart.[130] Lidocaine has time to leave the inactivated channels during diastole, so accumulation and intensification of blockade do not occur. At death, the heart:blood concentration ratio for bupivacaine is 3.5 compared with 2.0 for lidocaine.

Automaticity is somewhat depressed by LAs in most studies. Phase 4 depolarization of pacemaker cells during diastole is slowed, due to Ca^{2+} channel blockade. In isolated hearts, pacemaker rates are slowed more by bupivacaine than by lidocaine and the effect is amplified by hypoxia and acidosis. Both effects are greater in neonatal hearts.[131] Conduction alterations occur at concentrations of LA lower than are necessary for changes in automaticity, and are responsible for the most troublesome electrophysiological complications, namely ventricular tachydysrhythmias for the long-acting amides and heart block for the other agents. Cardiac impulse conduction is slowed by LAs,[132–134] because diminished inward Na^+ current depolarizes adjacent membrane more slowly, which produces a prolonged PR interval, a widened QRS complex, and atrioventricular block. Slowed conduction also leads to unidirectional block and reentry, which in turn can produce ventricular tachycardia and fibrillation. Intracoronary doses necessary to produce these dysrhythmic arrests are 16 times greater for lidocaine than for bupivacaine.[135] A central nervous mechanism might contribute to bupivacaine cardiotoxicity. Direct intracranial bupivacaine administration is followed by ventricular dysrhythmias,[136] probably via activation of the sympathetic nervous system,[137] but this has been disputed.[138]

Contributory factors

Hypoxia and acidosis have consistently been observed to increase the cardiac toxicity of LAs, especially bupivacaine. Hyperkalemia decreases the dose of lidocaine and, especially, bupivacaine necessary for cardiovascular collapse in ventilated dogs, whereas it has no effect on seizure threshold.[139] Pregnancy probably does not increase bupivacaine cardiotoxicity.[140]

New LA drugs

Levobupivacaine, the S(-) enantiomer (one of a pair of mirror image isomers) of bupivacaine, has been known for some time to be less toxic than the R(+) enantiomer or the racemic mixture.[141] Ropivacaine is similar in structure to bupivacaine and mepivacaine, but is prepared as a pure S(-) enantiomer. Ropivacaine exits the Na^+ channel more rapidly than bupivacaine does, but still much more slowly than lidocaine.[142] Myocardial depression produced by circulating ropivacaine, bupivacaine, and lidocaine is proportional to their nerve-blocking potency.[143] With the more serious complication of conduction disturbance, in vitro studies show ropivacaine and levobupivacaine are much less potent than bupivacaine in depressing cardiac excitation and conduction.[144–146] The diminished dysrhythmogenesis from levobupivacaine is supported by studies with intact animals,[147–149] whereas results for ropivacaine are less clear.[140,150] Like bupivacaine, demise from ropivacaine is most often accompanied by ventricular dysrhythmias.[150] Higher circulating levels of ropivacaine after equal doses compromise its increased cardiac safety. Comparisons of ropivacaine and levobupivacaine toxicity in vivo have not demonstrated a difference in dysrhythmogenesis.[151,152]

Sympathetic block-related bradycardic arrest

Presentation

Bradycardia or nausea may be the first indications of circulatory compromise from extensive blockade.[153] Factors that increase the risk of hypotension after spinal anesthesia include age (greater in adults than in children and in adults over 40 years of age), extensive block, low initial blood pressure (systolic less than 120 mmHg), in combination with GA, higher puncture site for injection, and inclusion of phenylephrine in the anesthetic solution.[154–156] Additional factors may include female gender, cementing a prosthesis, and deflation of a leg tourniquet.[157,158]

Whereas hypotension during neuraxial anesthesia is common and easily treated, a combination of profound bradycardia, asystole, and circulatory collapse can occasionally develop without any obvious precipitating cause during spinal or epidural anesthesia, often with poor outcome.[42,159] The patient may be conscious and talking right up to the moment of arrest. The typical bradycardic event occurs well after injection of the anesthetic and is not clearly related to unintended levels of blockade,[45] unlike the incidence of hypotensive events.[160] The timing of the onset is a mystery, but it may be due to a situation of diminished stimulation of the patient. The initial presentation might be apnea or bradycardia. Prodromal slowing of the heart rate is not a uniform feature, nor is hypoxia or excessive sedation,[42,43,161] although these can contribute. In one study, however, use of sedation decreased the incidence of hemodynamic side effects of spinal anesthesia,[160] conceivably due to avoidance of emotional stress that may also trigger severe bradycardia during sympathetic blockade.[162] Epinephrine infusion is not preventive.[42] It appears that bradycardic CA during neuraxial anesthesia is increasing.[163]

Factors predisposing to the common form of bradycardia without arrest are more easily determined than are those leading to reflex bradycardic arrest, which is rare. These risk factors include low baseline heart rate, use of β-adrenergic blockers, prolonged PR interval, extensive anesthetic block, young age, and low ASA status (i.e., healthy subjects).[154,158,164] It is not certain that these factors also put a patient at risk for full arrest, but they require extra attention. It is possible that obesity and the prone position are also risk factors.

Etiology

Neuraxial anesthesia substantially limits sympathetic activity to the areas of the body affected by sensory blockade. Whereas a block limited to the lower extremities rarely produces serious hemodynamic problems, more extensive blockade can produce hypotension and diminished cardiac output. Blockage of sympathetic innervation to the heart (T1–T5) minimally affects myocardial contractility, and chronotropic responses to isolated cardiac denervation are mild. Unlike narrow segmental block, however, extensive spinal or epidural block with significant vasodilatation typically produces bradycardia and a depressed baroreceptor response, so that low systemic blood pressure fails to induce accelerated heart rates. This change in baroreceptor performance does not require blocking of T1–T5, indicating that the heart rate response to neuraxial

anesthesia is not due to blockade of cardiac accelerator fibers. Indeed, heart rate changes and increased baroreceptor reflex sensitivity due to blockage of T7 and below can be reversed by compression of the legs and abdomen by inflation of MAST trousers.[165] The reflex changes following neuraxial block are probably due to unloading of low-pressure receptors in the heart and great veins. Endogenous opiate mechanisms in the central nervous system contribute to abrupt vasodilatation that accompanies substantial hypovolemia, so naloxone therapy could be considered.[166]

The mechanism behind these phenomena originates with sensory events in the heart.[167–169] Inhibitory depressor reflexes can be initiated by vigorous contraction around an almost empty ventricular chamber, which produces wall deformation.[170] The combination of an increased inotropic state of the heart and decreased left ventricular volume is the most potent stimulus for this response.[171] The Bezold–Jarisch reflex is a similar depressor phenomenon originating in the heart in response to chemical stimuli.[44]

As noted above, the sympathectomy state is unique with regard to regulation of heart rate. Low systemic blood pressures are not accompanied by high heart rates. This creates an unstable system with positive feedback: venodilation, especially of the splanchnic circulation,[172,173] decreases cardiac filling and leads to further sympathetic withdrawal and vagal hyperactivity. Increased cardiac contractility from elevated sympathetic activity in unblocked segments may amplify the cardiac wall deformation that stimulates the depressor reflex. There is evidence that neuraxial anesthesia may trigger such a reflex sequence.[174] Overall, these events resemble typical fainting from other causes in upright subjects. Like fainting, this hemodynamic sequence is not found in patients receiving sedation or GA. Patients who develop hypotension and bradycardia display a sudden increase in the baroreceptor sensitivity and frequency domain, which is evidence of elevated sympathetic activity.[175] Sympathetic block prevents an effective baroreceptor-driven compensation. A downward spiral is further encouraged by cerebral hypoperfusion and an obtunded response to hypoxia from epidural block.[176]

Prevention

Although there are no data to guide strategies to avoid sudden bradycardic arrest during neuraxial anesthesia, development of substantial hypovolemia should be avoided in patients with extensive neuraxial blocks, especially if they are young and fit, and hypovolemia should be corrected before initiating neuraxial anesthesia. Treatment of heart rates lower than 50 beats/minute should be considered, in order to anticipate and prevent the potential development of more severe bradycardia and arrest.[43,177]

Anesthesia outside the operating room (non-OR anesthesia)

Overview

Anesthesia outside the operating room (non-OR) has the same inherent risk factors and causes of CA as described above, but with certain specific problems. Most are linked to anesthetic drugs, techniques, and equipment being used in unfamiliar and less controlled surroundings, often by less trained personnel. Consequently, risks of CA as a fatal complication to anesthetic practice may be higher than in the more controlled OR environment.[178]

GA is frequently used for emergency airway management. Anesthetic drugs are used for procedural sedation in the emergency department with the inherent risk of complications such as CA, especially in children.[179]

Office-based anesthesia and anesthesia in remote areas

Office-based anesthesia has become increasingly popular. It can be viewed as an extension of ambulatory (day case) anesthesia taking place in free standing (solo) physicians' and dentists' offices.[180] Most procedures involve a combination of LA and sedation or GA with drugs like propofol and sevoflurane.

In the day-surgery clinics, in both private and academic practices, overdosages of either inhalation or intravenous anesthetics have been described as associated with CA,[181,182] in particular in dental practices. Indeed, in a disproportionate number of patients CA occurs in oral/dental maxillofacial office practices, which suggests that the anesthetic risk might be significantly increased in this patient population even though the event is still relatively rare.[183] In the early 1990s, a questionnaire was sent to all dentists practicing in the United States and follow-up letters describing 43 cases of CA were reported with a total mortality of 81.4% of the cases.[184] Remarkably, pre-existing diseases were not statistically associated with mortality, but multiple pharmacological agents and limited monitoring and resuscitative efforts were statistically associated with mortality. Basic and advanced cardiac life support was used in fewer than 50% of the cases.

Both GA and monitored anesthesia care were responsible for CA although the data were limited. The greater the number of pharmacological sedative agents used, the higher the risk of CA, indicating the need for a more widespread knowledge of anesthetic agents and their adverse effects, and of resuscitation skills for health professionals involved in dental practices.[185,186] The danger of CA with office-based anesthesia was brought to public attention when a review in the United Kingdom showed several cases of anesthetic deaths in dental offices.[187] This resulted in specific recommendations on who should provide anesthesia and what resuscitation equipment and emergency drugs should be available. With an ever increasing demand for anesthesia in this context, there are obvious medicolegal aspects as to who provides the anesthetic service.[188]

There are scant data on the epidemiology of CA during office-based anesthesia. The overall mortality and risk of severe morbidity appears to be very low,[180] particularly when solo practitioners report their own data,[189,190] whereas state or national audits report less favorable safety records.[187,191]

Office-based anesthesia aims to reduce overhead costs of ambulatory surgery. This can conflict with the obvious need to provide national practice guidelines for anesthetic personnel, anesthetic equipment, monitoring, recovery areas, availability of emergency equipment, and resuscitation drugs. Patients should demand the same standards of care for both solo ambulatory surgical and diagnostic units.[180]

Other non-OR anesthetic locations are classified as "remote areas":[178,180] psychiatric hospitals for electroconvulsive therapy, gastroenterology laboratories for endoscopy, the radiology department for diagnostic procedures such as computed tomography and magnetic resonance imaging or interventional neuroradiology, and, increasingly, the cardiology laboratory for acute percutaneous coronary angiography and/or percutaneous coronary intervention. Sprung *et al.* studied the outcome of CA in patients undergoing invasive cardiology procedures over an 11-year period (1990–2000).[192] The overall incidence of CA was 21.9 per 10 000 procedures; this rate decreased from 33.9 per 10 000 before 1995 to 13.1 per 10 000 after 1995. Overall survival to hospital discharge after CA was 56.1%.

In all "remote" locations anesthesia providers may not be accustomed to the special machines and monitors, and have limited access to both the patient and an experienced assistant. Although the risk of anesthesia complications resulting from technical and human failures in remote areas might be expected to be higher than in a hospital setting, this has not been frequently studied[178] and problems tend to be illustrated by case reports.[193]

Anesthesia and sedation in the ICU and emergency department

In the ICU and emergency department (ED) anesthesia is mainly used to facilitate emergency airway management in critically ill and injured patients. Rapid sequence endotracheal intubation in these patients carries the risk of CA linked to patient factors, to the use of cardiodepressive drugs in patients with circulatory failure with different etiologies, and to hypoxia and bradycardia following difficult or failed intubation. Assistance during the procedure and back-up help from more experienced personnel might not be available to the same extent and adequate monitoring and alternative airway devices might also not be present. Hence, the use of anesthesia in these circumstances carries a higher risk of complications than in the more controlled environment of the OR.

Anesthetic drugs like propofol, etomidate, ketamine, or fentanyl are generally used alone to provide procedural sedation and analgesia, but they can also be used in combination, and although descriptions like "sedoanalgesia," "controlled sedation," and "awake sedation" are used, this practice carries the same risks (overdosing patients, losing control of the airways, and other side-effects) for CA as with giving "full anesthesia".[179,194,195] In most hospitals, doctors (anesthesiologists, intensivists, emergency physicians) provide this care, although elsewhere, it may be provided by nurse anesthetists. Independent of care provider training, both quality and safety aspects of airway management must be considered in deciding who should provide anesthetic and sedative service in the ICU and emergency department, and how such service is provided.

Prehospital anesthesia and analgesia

The same concerns also apply to prehospital anesthesia and analgesia. Again, anesthetic drugs are mainly used to facilitate endotracheal intubation.[196] One difference compared with hospital care is that in many emergency medical service systems non-physicians (paramedics, flight nurses) are allowed to use rapid sequence endotracheal intubation.[197] Further, the prehospital working environment is variable, not secure, and uncontrolled. Hence, the legal, quality, and safety aspects of prehospital anesthesia are of major concern. Although in many studies, self-reporting of data has concluded that the prehospital use of anesthetic drugs and techniques by non-anesthesiologists is both safe and improves outcome, recent studies[198,199] and editorials[197] have cast doubt on the benefits and safety of this practice. Importantly, even in prehospital EMS staffed with anesthesiologists, the incidence of critical incidents with the potential for CA is reported to be almost 10%.[196] Hence, both training and experience of personnel, adequate monitoring and equipment, as well as documentation are important to ensure high quality prehospital anesthesia and analgesia. Patient safety is the key word. The potential benefits of inducing anesthesia must always be weighed against its risks, whether the goal is to ensure ETI in critically ill patients or to provide adequate pain relief in trauma patients.

Prevention

Perioperative CA is rare and has a better outcome than either in-hospital or out-of-hospital CA.[94,200] A substantial percentage of anesthetic-related CAs are caused by human error (inadequate vigilance, inappropriate airway management, drug overdose) and are considered to have been preventable (53% Kawashima et al.;[13] 91% Biboulet et al.[12]). We describe below some key elements that can contribute to effective crisis management.

Monitoring requirements

Large closed-claim analyses have identified associations and causes leading to CA.[13,15,42,201,202] Adequate monitoring is mandatory for real-time assessment of a patient's condition, especially as adverse outcomes occur as a result of unexpected reactions. Thus, monitoring devices that provide sufficient real-time information to manage unexpected adverse events should be available whenever patients are exposed to increased risk due to iatrogenic intervention. The minimal recommended monitoring consists of: a two-lead electrocardiogram monitor, non-invasive blood measuring device, and pulse oximetry. Capnography is mandatory whenever endotracheal intubation is performed. Nasal side stream capnography is more sensitive than pulse oximetry in detecting hypoventilation during conscious sedation. Whenever artificial ventilation is used, oximetry of the inspired gas and a disconnecting alarm system should be available. Invasive arterial blood pressure monitoring is very helpful in patients with a higher risk for cardiovascular collapse during induction or maintenance of anesthesia. Bispectral index monitoring is a new device used as a marker for the patient's hypnotic state. Several case reports indicate a potential benefit for its use during resuscitation in the perioperative setting.[203–206] There should be continuous monitoring from the start of anesthesia until the patient is in the recovery room or intensive care unit, including the transfer between the different suites.

While monitoring requirements have been defined for areas where anesthesia is normally administered, remote areas such as obstetric wards have less equipment. Notably, in an RA closed-claims analysis, most of the CA cases that were not monitored occurred outside the OR.[163] Discordance between different monitoring devices or between clinical signs and the results from monitoring equipment must be carefully checked and reassessed,[207] to avoid likely medical errors.

Minimal safety standards

Because these are only a few major causes for the majority of all adverse events, and most of these adverse events are considered to be preventable and are associated more often with human error than with technical or equipment failure, practice standards (rules or requirements representing generally accepted principles of sound patient management) and guidelines (systematically developed recommendations that have a higher degree of adherence) have been developed.[201,202,208] They describe a range of broadly accepted basic management strategies judged to be feasible by experts and based on the best available evidence from the literature;[209,210] nevertheless, they can be modified depending on circumstances. Many national societies of anesthesiologists have promulgated collections of practice standards, recommendations, and/or guidelines that contain minimal safety standards.[211]

Minimal safety standards for anesthesia require the following:

- A sedated or anesthetized patient is never without surveillance by an anesthesiologist or a nurse anesthetist.
- During induction and emergence, the person in charge of the anesthesia has to be supported by another qualified person trained to assist with anesthesia.
- A staff anesthesiologist has to be immediately available.
- The minimal equipment (including prepared drugs for management of potential side effects) and monitoring devices must be available and checked for function before the anesthesia is started.
- Each patient has an intravenous line inserted as soon as possible and checked for correct infusion.
- Emergency materials such as defibrillator, difficult airway management tools, and ventilation bag with transportable oxygen are easily available.
- Standard operation protocols for RA and GA techniques including rapid sequence induction have to be defined and implemented.

Checklists for control of equipment and material before the start of a procedure as well as for defined emergencies (i.e., CA, toxicity of LA or MH) offer clear-cut guidance during complex and stressful crisis management. In contrast to the aviation industry, acceptance and daily use of checklists are still not yet established in medicine.

Treatment principles

If minimal safety standards[211] are followed, CA during anesthesia will always be witnessed and immediately diagnosed. Indeed, CA during anesthesia has clear advantages compared with other in-hospital or out-of-hospital locations: pre-established intravenous access, emergency drugs, oxygen, airway management devices, monitoring equipment, and a defibrillator are immediately available. Furthermore, anesthesiologists and nurse anesthetists should be familiar with resuscitation guidelines and should also be regularly retrained. Additional personnel should be close by or at least on call and quickly available. These advantages may explain the far better outcome of patients who have CA during anesthesia compared with CA in other situations. Guidelines and all the specific technical and pharmacological aspects of resuscitation are discussed in detail in Chapters 25–42.

Some features of CA specific to perioperative conditions are addressed briefly: the major cardiac rhythm at the onset of CA from anesthesia is bradycardia or asystole (45%); other pathological cardiac rhythms are tachycardia, ventricular tachycardia, or ventricular fibrillation (14%), pulseless electrical activity (7%), and not assessed rhythms (33%) (Table 59.6).[24] Treating CA during anesthesia must take these different circumstances into account and the published CPR guidelines, which were developed for the non-anesthesia-related CA patient population, must be adapted to the situation.

The basic goal is to restore cardiac pump function without hypoxic side effects to the brain and heart. Today, the use of pulse oximetry and capnography is mandatory and CA as the first sign of hypoxemia should be the exception. Nevertheless, inadequate alveolar oxygen supply must be ruled out: 100% oxygen should be administered in all cases of CA. If supplemental oxygen administration is a standard operating procedure (SOP) for all patients experiencing GA or neuraxial RA, a supranormal alveolar oxygen tension at the beginning of CA can be expected.

Maintenance of perfusion pressure and blood flow in coronary arteries and cerebral circulation is the other most important goal to ensure oxygenation and drug transport to the target organs and improve the chances for successful restoration of cardiac pump function. In witnessed CA with tachydysrhythmia, immediate defibrillation is the therapy of choice.[212] If a defibrillator is not instantly available or if the cardiac rhythm at the time of arrest is not shockable, chest compression must be started immediately and rigorously,[213,214] despite the risks of compromised asepsis and/or mechanical tissue damage at the surgical field as well as at the cardiopulmonary site. Epinephrine

Table 59.6. ECG rhythm at time of cardiac arrest (%)

	Runciman[24]	Spring[15]
Asystole/Bradycardia	46	83
Tachycardia/VF/VF	14	13
Normal	7	4
Not Indicated	33	

and atropine, if indicated, should be administered aggressively. The side effects of the recommended dosages have to be balanced against the potentially harmful blood pressure elevations during ongoing surgery. There is evidence that management of CA in association with anesthesia tends to be less aggressive than recommended,[24,163] but the impact of these defensive reactions on outcome is unknown.

Identifiable causes of CA during anesthesia have to be treated aggressively during ongoing CPR. Hypovolemia must be prevented and, if present, aggressively corrected. Tension pneumothorax must always be kept in mind during mechanical ventilation. Opioids, muscle relaxant drugs, and sedative or anesthetic drugs influence physiological respiratory regulation. Hypoventilation during mechanical and spontaneous ventilation leads to acute respiratory acidosis and could cause harmful electrolyte disorders with the risk of CA, especially in susceptible patients. Thus, during emergence from anesthesia and immediately thereafter (transfer to and early recovery room period) patients must be carefully checked.

CA and RA

Effective management of CA during RA must be aware of the toxicity of LAs, relative or absolute hypovolemia, and/or imbalanced vegetative nervous system reactions caused by neuraxial RA.

Toxicity from LAs: Early and aggressive treatment of seizures and cardiovascular collapse, including repeated large doses of epinephrine, might reduce mortality from massive intravenous doses of bupivacaine.[215] Although both epinephrine and bupivacaine are dysrhythmogenic drugs, epinephrine is less likely to cause dysrhythmia after bupivacaine than without.[216] Amiodarone can prevent cardiovascular collapse.[217] Magnesium sulfate suppresses bupivacaine-induced dysrhythmias.[218] Unfortunately, there is no magic cure for CA that results from LA toxicity. Aggressive standard resuscitation techniques should be sustained for a prolonged period and electrolyte as well as acid–base imbalances should be normalized.

CA during neuraxial anesthesia: CA is typically associated with extensive blocks reaching to sensory levels T4–T5. With a sensory block of T4, the cardiac accelerator fibers originating from T1–T4 may be completely blocked. Effects of direct blockade of cardiac sympathetic outflow and indirect mechanisms via cardiac reflexes cause severe bradycardia.[44,219] The relative hypovolemia induced by vasodilatation also results in reduced venous return. Basic treatment must increase cardiac frequency (β-mimetic effect of epinephrine and atropine blocking the increased vagal tone) and restore the intravasal volume (fluid resuscitation, supported by vasoconstricting agents). Successful resuscitation aims for efficient coronary perfusion pressure. Epinephrine is recommended at doses of 0.01 to 0.1 mg/kg for profound bradycardia, whereas 1 mg of epinephrine is recommended for CA.[42,43,220,221] Vasopressin might be advantageous for CA during RA compared with epinephrine.[222]

Instant call for help, communication, organization, and delegation of tasks are crucial for managing CA successfully. Resuscitation requires a team leader who coordinates and gives clear directions. CA is always stressful for the team involved. Checklists should help participating personnel to proceed in a well organized fashion and without missing key points even when managing CA caused by rare events. Debriefing should be part of the procedure, irrespective of the outcome.

Educational aspects

"To Err is Human: Building a Safer Health System" was published in 1999 by the Institute of Medicine.[31] This report stated that as many as 98 000 people die annually as the result of medical errors, which initiated a worldwide expression of concern about patient safety. Although progress since then has been slow, the Institute of Medicine report truly "changed the conversation" to a focus on changing systems, stimulated a broad array of stakeholders to engage in patient safety, and motivated hospitals to adopt new safety practices (Table 59.7). The pace of change is likely to accelerate, particularly in the implementation of electronic health records, diffusion of safe practices, team training, and full disclosure to patients following injury.[223] The concept that bad systems, not bad people, lead to the majority of errors and injuries, will become one of the mainstays in healthcare education.

Impact of human factors

Most of the anesthesia-related CAs are considered to be preventable and to have involved human error or

Table 59.7. Clinical effectiveness of safe practices

Intervention	Results
Perioperative antibiotic protocol	Surgical site infections decreased by 93%[a]
Physician computer order entry	81% Reduction of medication errors
Pharmacist rounding with team	66% Reduction of preventable adverse drug events 78% Reduction of preventable adverse drug events
Protocol enforcement	95% Reduction in central venous line infections[b] 92% Reduction in central venous line infections[c]
Rapid response teams	Cardiac arrests decreased by 15%
Reconciling medication practices	90% Reduction in medication errors
Reconciling and standardizing medication practices	60% Reduction in adverse drug events over 12 mo (from 7.6 per 1000 doses to 3.1 per 1000 doses) 64% Reduction in adverse drug events in 20 mo (from 3.8 per 1000 doses to 1.39 per 1000 doses)
Standardized insulin dosing	Hypoglycemic episodes decreased 63% (from 2.95% of patients to 1.1%) 90% Reduction in cardiac surgical wound infections (from 3.9% of patients to 0.4%)[d]
Standardized warfarin dosing	Out-of-range international normalized ratio decreased by 60% (from 25% of tests to 10%)
Team training in labor and delivery	50% Reduction in adverse outcomes in preterm delivery[e]
Trigger tool and automation	Adverse drug events reduced 75% between 2001 and 2003
Ventilator bundle protocol	Ventilator-associated pneumonias decreased by 62%[a]

Table 59.7. (*notes*)

[a] J. Whittington, written communication, March 2005.
[b] P. Pronovost, Johns Hopkins Hospital, written communication, January 2005.
[c] R. Shannon, written communication, January 2005.
[d] K. McKinley, Geisinger Clinic, written communication, April 2005.
[e] B. Sachs, Beth Israel Deaconess Medical Center, written communicion. October 2004.
From Ref. 223 (reproduced with permission.)

inadequate human resources.[13,24] The incidence of CA coincides with the number of qualified anesthesiologists in a department (Fig. 59.3),[19] and organizational factors such as intraoperative presence of trained anesthetic personnel are associated with decreased mortality after surgery.[5] The mortality rate and failure to rescue from CA were lower when anesthesiologists directed anesthetic care and when a board-certified anesthesiologist was in charge.[224,225] A higher nurse-to-patient ratio and higher level of education of the nurses decreases postoperative mortality and failure to rescue.[226,227] It is suggested that the best outcomes take place when anesthesia is provided by a professional care team.[228,229] Such care teams cannot rely merely on new scientific developments or technology, but they must also incorporate non-technical information. This has recently been introduced,[230] because a profound deficit of core skills still remains, such as: team performance, behavior, learning from and with others, and increasing sensitivity to the pitfalls and human factors influencing interactive and interdisciplinary procedures. In a recent editorial, Gaba addresses the important question, "What makes a "good" anesthesiologist?".[231] Although good clinical care in anesthesia has many components, the ability to diagnose and treat acute, life-threatening perioperative abnormalities is near the top of most anesthesiologists' lists.[232]

Individual behavior and team

Medical education must include information that considers "human factors." Disciplines and companies traditionally involved in risk management procedures originally focused on improving safety and usability at the interface between humans and machines through improved design. The term "human factors" relates to a much broader interdisciplinary study of the working environment. Human factors draw on the fields of sociology and psychology (emphasizing cognitive, industrial,

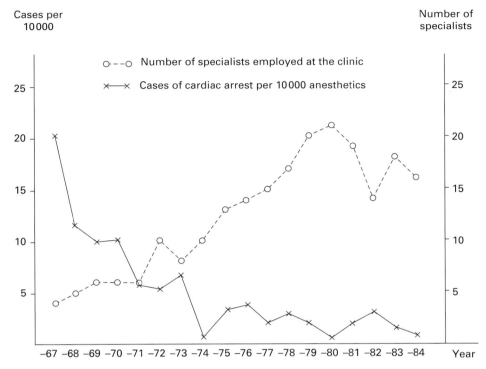

Fig. 59.3. Incidence of anesthesia-related cardiac arrest and numbers of departmental specialists. (From Ref. 19, reproduced with permission.)

organizational, personality, and social psychology) as well as engineering. Research in human factors includes the discovery and application of knowledge about individual and team interactions with technology. An important aspect is the use of a system perspective that considers both the influence of individual as well as group characteristics and the contribution of organizational and national cultures.[233] With regard to "error culture," the aviation industry's experience has shown that the majority of accidents in technical professions are caused by human error and this is undoubtedly true for anesthesia-related fatal accidents in the OR.[30,208] These errors tend to involve interpersonal issues: communication, conflicts, leadership, and/or flawed decision-making. The aviation community responded by initiating formal instruction in the interpersonal aspects of human factors through programs that are known as "Crew Resource Management."[234] Interestingly, hazardous industries such as aviation have succeeded in becoming relatively safe. Unfortunately, modern health-care technology is certainly more complex than that of most other industries, and a busy OR is a perfect model of complexity. Different types of medical specialties and subspecialties interact with each other and with an equally large array of

allied health professions with different hierarchies such as nursing staff and technicians. Separate procedures during anesthesia on different patients occur simultaneously; for instance, induction of anesthesia is done in one area, while emergence from anesthesia is cared for in another, with the same personnel involved and responsible for both. Sadly, the more complex a system, the more possibilities it has to fail. There is considerable evidence that team communication and information-sharing is one of the most important team behaviors for developing common situation assessment, overcoming "groupthink," stimulating creative problem-solving, learning from experiential feedback, encouraging full participation, and achieving enhanced performance.[235–237]

Another challenge is medicine's tenacious commitment to individual professional autonomy. Creating cultures of safety requires major changes in behavior that professionals easily perceive as threats to their personal authority.[238] Comprehensive anesthesia simulation is considered to be a useful tool in studying the "chain of accident evolution".[210,239] Simulation studies involving residents, faculty, and community anesthesiologists challenged the ubiquitous perception that "experience" itself is a guarantee of success in all tasks:[240–242] some highly experienced personnel failed catastrophically in managing certain acute events, whereas some juniors performed exceptionally well.[241] Acute care skills simulation can be used to study complex task-solving capabilities in near-fatal anesthetic complications.[243]

With surgical factors responsible for sizeable numbers of intraoperative CAs, changes in the climate of surgical education have been considered.[244] Whereas formerly the OR was regarded as the best classroom for surgical education, this point of view has recently been challenged. In the OR, a teaching session cannot be well designed or predicted; steps cannot be repeated, and the patient cannot be reassembled to start over if failure occurs. Furthermore, the greatest learning and performance potential occurs in an environment of moderate stress.[244] High-end simulation is an ideal tool to create such an environment. Strategic management simulations accurately assess the performance of surgical residents,[245] and team factors that determine resuscitation success have been identified.[246] For the specific circumstances of perioperative CA, suitable case scenarios should be included within simulation-based education that reflects the different features caused by GA or RA.

Algorithms

As mentioned above, autonomy in the medical profession is a very strong attitude favoring working procedures that depend on personal experiences, circumstances, temporary mood, or time of the day. What might be a reasonable approach under controlled conditions, however, may become hazardous in the face of potentially escalating complications. This is why SOP have been defined for management of critical incidents in risk-prone enterprises. These SOPs should be clear to every team member especially for team organization, course of action, priorities, aims of intervention, task distribution, and rescue strategies, so that the group functions along a well-structured and predictable pathway. Algorithms have been established to deliver evidence-based standards of care for management of otherwise fatal or near-fatal complications. For SOP to work within stress-burdened and uncontrolled escalating emergencies, they have to be integrated far ahead of the emergency and become part of our professional armamentarium. SOPs should be integrated into formal medical education, and medical staff should be trained and periodically retrained in SOPs to guarantee that SOPs become instinctive when needed. Algorithms for the immediate management of life-threatening conditions have become a cornerstone in the treatment of serious complications and the knowledge and skills required are, therefore, a mandatory prerequisite for competent professional performance.

For anesthesiologists, management of difficult airways is a core competence that is best accomplished by relying on algorithm-based sequence of action. Benumof described the advantage of a well-structured approach in expected or unforeseen difficult circumstances in which the patient's lungs could not be ventilated or the trachea could not be intubated.[247] Several recommendations[248–250] have established practice guidelines for management of the difficult airway, which is of an overwhelming importance for all anesthetic care providers. Circumstances in which the lungs cannot be ventilated and the trachea cannot be intubated continue to occur after the induction of anesthesia with any induction method, after repeated attempts at tracheal intubation with any intubation method, and after malplacement of a tracheal tube in patients with anatomical abnormalities of the face and/or neck.[55]

Algorithms can also be helpful to indicate potentially dangerous circumstances during the different phases of anesthesia. Post-induction hypotension triggers substantial episodes of CA. SOP should therefore include close monitoring of hemodynamic stability following induction of GA and neuraxial anesthesia, and the decreased blood-pressure measurement interval during this critical period will enable an immediate response should hemodynamic compromise occur.

Unfortunately, established management-guidelines and algorithms[212] do not reflect the peculiar features of intraoperative CA. The pattern of etiological factors is different, as are the prevailing cardiac rhythms, with bradycardia and asystole predominating. Thus, the statement in the American Heart Association's guidelines, "although the algorithms provide a good cookbook, the patient always requires a thinking cook",[251] accurately describes the peculiar circumstances of perioperative CA. Two factors significantly influence diagnosis and treatment of anesthesia-related CA: first, there is a continuous reduction of cardiac output that makes it difficult to determine at which point it becomes significant; second, an arbitrary decision has to be made about what constitutes a serious duration of arrest. For example, should a vaso-vagal arrest of 30 seconds with prompt recovery be counted? When to react and by which degree of invasiveness? Consequently, management of CA related to anesthesia tends to be less aggressive than is recommended in the respective guidelines. In their Australian study, Runciman et al. suggest that chest compression was not performed in 28% of CA patients.[24] On the other hand, the efficacy of early and aggressive intervention for anesthesia-related CA has been confirmed clinically and in animal models.[39,252]

Checklists

Formal education should also include and support use of checklists to control material, equipment, ventilator and monitor settings, identification of drugs, patient identification, intended procedures, available preoperative information, and patient's consent. Most anesthesiologists theoretically support the importance of checking anesthetic equipment before use, but do not follow the guidelines because they perceive checklists as too time-consuming.[253,254] A further disadvantage of routine checking might be that routine measures have an inherent risk of reducing awareness. Nevertheless, machine checks detected significant percentages of defaults, of which 11% to 18% were deemed serious.[255,256] Investigators of critical incidents identified failure to perform an equipment check as a frequent risk factor.[22,208,257–261] Equipment checks, performed with a checklist and protocol, are associated with a decreased risk of perioperative morbidity and mortality, as well as documentation of the check.[5] Using an airline pilot's checklist to investigate errors and omissions in anesthesia, a simulation study by Hart and Owen found that important checks were often forgotten when memory alone was relied upon and that the use of a checklist improved performance.[262]

Critical incidents reporting systems

A critical incident is a human error or equipment failure that could have led (if not discovered or corrected in time) or did lead to an undesirable outcome, ranging from increased length of hospital stay to death.[208] The theory of organizational safety stresses that "safety" is a never-ending process whose success cannot be measured strictly by epidemiological methods.[263] The willingness and readiness to communicate critical incidents can be another method to improve safety. Equipment failure is often reported because it shifts responsibility from the person to the technical or manufacturer's side. As the development of more and more sophisticated electronics in anesthetic machines and monitoring devices continues to create an increasingly complex environment, reporting technical failures becomes even more important. Prompt reporting of critical incidents of technical failure allows rapid investigation and implementation of design improvements to this equipment.[264]

Physicians and nurses have considerable difficulty in dealing with human error when it occurs. The culture of medical practice continues to involve its members in striving for error-free practice.[238] Therefore, medical schools and clinical institutions have to fight to change attitudes.

Introduction of reporting systems should be accompanied with serious efforts to maintain anonymity, confidentiality, and privacy of the participating individuals. Nevertheless, adverse events have to be collated, analyzed, and regularly discussed among those responsible for the department or unit; gradually, consistent reporting activities should result in improved safety behavior. Without a strong commitment to such tasks from unit or departmental leaders, most systems will fail.[265]

Reporting systems can successfully identify specific features of CA in association with anesthesia,[24] as the diagnosis is made earlier and with greater precision compared with resuscitation situations encountered elsewhere. But, at the same time, SOPs are used less frequently and to a lesser degree. If CA is encountered and treatment is initiated, alleviation of specific anesthetic or surgical causes is often possible and the outcome is generally good, with the majority of patients leaving the hospital alive and apparently well.

Conclusions

Undergoing anesthesia is intrinsically hazardous for the patient. Anesthesiologists have struggled for years to determine the incidence of catastrophic adverse outcomes.[30] Anesthetic risk has continued to be the subject of numerous investigations, editorials, and journal correspondence since the first anesthetic death was reported in 1848.[266] Undoubtedly, anesthesia for healthy patients is now much safer than it once was. But even though patients are increasingly older and enter the OR with serious pre-existing diseases, the perioperative rate of mortality for surgical patients is still too high. Ascribing CA to preoperative conditions may transfer responsibility from the individual who provides the anesthesia and shift it towards patient's factors, but, whatever the cause, CA and/or death following surgery remains devastating. CA during anesthesia has some unique features that are beyond the scope of current guidelines, and anesthesiologists have to develop and maintain awareness and competence to handle the situation. Without constant effort to improve, anesthesiologists will lose their leadership role in addressing organizational safety culture in all of health care.[30] Nearly 60 years ago, Macintosh stated that no patient should be harmed *by* anesthesia.[267] Today, we, as anesthesiologists, should go beyond this statement and increase our responsibilities beyond the causative aspects and consider pre-existing disease, preoperative conditions, and surgical factors. For the future, our aim should be that fewer and fewer patients are harmed during or following anesthesia.

REFERENCES

1. Rosenberg, J. & Wahr, J. Cardiac arrest during anesthesia. In Paradis, N., Halperin, H. & Nowak, R., eds. *Cardiac Arrest: The Science and Practice of Resuscitation Medicine.* 1st edn Baltimore: Williams and Wilkins, 1996: 783–811.
2. Shephard, D.A. & Baskett, T.F. John Snow and resuscitation. *Resuscitation* 2001; **49**: 3–7.
3. Snow, J. On asphyxia and on the resuscitation of stillborn children. *Lond. Med. Gaz.* 1841; **29**: 222–227.
4. Snow, J. *On Chloroform and other Anaesthetics: Their Action and Administration.* London: John Churchill, 1858.
5. Arbous, M.S., Meursing, A.E., van Kleef J.W. *et al.* Impact of anesthesia management characteristics on severe morbidity and mortality. *Anesthesiology* 2005; **102**: 257–268; quiz 491–492.
6. Abella, B.S., Alvarado, J.P., Myklebust, H. *et al.* Quality of cardiopulmonary resuscitation during in-hospital cardiac arrest. *J. Am. Med. Assoc.* 2005; **293**: 305–310.
7. Casey, W.F. Cardiopulmonary resuscitation: a survey of standards among junior hospital doctors. *J. Roy. Soc. Med.* 1984; **77**: 921–924.
8. Lowenstein, S.R., Hansbrough, J.F., Libby L.S. *et al.* Cardiopulmonary resuscitation by medical and surgical house-officers. *Lancet.* 1981; **2**: 679–681.
9. Skinner, D.V., Camm, A.J. & Miles, S. Cardiopulmonary resuscitation skills of preregistration house officers. *Br. Med. J. (Clin. Res. Ed.)* 1985; **290**: 1549–1550.
10. Wik, L., Kramer-Johansen, J., Myklebust, H. *et al.* Quality of cardiopulmonary resuscitation during out-of-hospital cardiac arrest. *J. Am. Med. Assoc.* 2005; **293**: 299–304.
11. Semeraro, F., Signore, L. & Cerchiari, E.L. Retention of CPR performance in anaesthetists. *Resuscitation* 2006; **68**: 101–108.
12. Biboulet, P., Aubas, P., Dubourdieu, J. *et al.* Fatal and non fatal cardiac arrests related to anesthesia. *Can. J. Anaesth.* 2001; **48**: 326–332.
13. Kawashima, Y., Takahashi, S., Suzuki, M. *et al.* Anesthesia-related mortality and morbidity over a 5-year period in 2,363,038 patients in Japan. *Acta Anaesthesiol. Scand.* 2003; **47**: 809–817.
14. Newland, M.C., Ellis, S.J., Lydiatt, C.A. *et al.* Anesthetic-related cardiac arrest and its mortality: a report covering 72,959 anesthetics over 10 years from a US teaching hospital. *Anesthesiology* 2002; **97**: 108–115.
15. Sprung, J., Warner, M.E., Contreras, M.G. *et al.* Predictors of survival following cardiac arrest in patients undergoing non-cardiac surgery: a study of 518 294 patients at a tertiary referral center. *Anesthesiology* 2003; **99**: 259–269.
16. Morray, J.P., Geiduschek, J.M., Ramamoorthy, C. *et al.* Anesthesia-related cardiac arrest in children: initial findings of the Pediatric Perioperative Cardiac Arrest (POCA) Registry. *Anesthesiology* 2000; **93**: 6–14.
17. Beecher, H.K. & Todd, D.P. A study of the deaths associated with anesthesia and surgery: based on a study of 599, 548 anesthesias in ten institutions 1948–1952, inclusive. *Ann. Surg.* 1954; **140**: 2–35.
18. Hovi-Viander, M. Death associated with anaesthesia in Finland. *Br. J. Anaesth.* 1980; **52**: 483–489.
19. Olsson, G.L. & Hallen, B. Cardiac arrest during anaesthesia. A computer-aided study in 250,543 anaesthetics. *Acta Anaesthesiol. Scand.* 1988; **32**: 653–664.
20. Pottecher, T., Tiret, L., Desmonts, J.M. *et al.* Cardiac arrest related to anaesthesia: a prospective survey in France (1978–1982). *Eur. J. Anaesthesiol.* 1984; **1**: 305–318.
21. Tiret, L., Nivoche, Y., Hatton, F. *et al.* Complications related to anaesthesia in infants and children. A prospective survey of 40240 anaesthetics. *Br. J. Anaesth.* 1988; **61**: 263–269.
22. Chopra, V., Bovill, J.G. & Spierdijk, J. Accidents, near accidents and complications during anaesthesia. A retrospective analysis of a 10-year period in a teaching hospital. *Anaesthesia* 1990; **45**: 3–6.
23. Keenan, R.L. and Boyan, C.P. Cardiac arrest due to anesthesia. A study of incidence and causes. *J. Am. Med. Assoc.* 1985; **253**: 2373–2377.
24. Runciman, W.B., Morris, R.W., Watterson, L.M. *et al.* Crisis management during anaesthesia: cardiac arrest. *Qual. Saf. Health Care* 2005; **14**: e14.
25. Warden, J.C., Horan, B.F. Deaths attributed to anaesthesia in New South Wales, 1984–1990. *Anaesth. Intens. Care* 1996; **24**: 66–73.
26. Irita, K., Kawashima, Y., Iwao, Y. *et al.* Annual mortality and morbidity in operating rooms during 2002 and summary of morbidity and mortality between 1999 and 2002 in Japan: a brief review. *Masui* 2004; **53**: 320–335.
27. Lagasse, R.S. Anesthesia safety: model or myth? A review of the published literature and analysis of current original data. *Anesthesiology* 2002; **97**: 1609–1617.
28. Clergue, F., Auroy, Y., Pequignot, F. *et al.* French survey of anesthesia in 1996. *Anesthesiology* 1999; **91**: 1509–1520.
29. Tikkanen, J. & Hovi-Vianer, M. Death associated with anaesthesia and surgery in Finland in 1986 compared to 1975. *Acta Anaesthesiol. Scand.* 1995; **39**: 262–267.
30. Cooper, J.B. & Gaba, D. No myth: anesthesia is a model for addressing patient safety. *Anesthesiology* 2002; **97**: 1335–1337.
31. Kohn, L., Corrigan, J., Donaldson, M. *To Err is Human: Building a Safer Health System.* Washington, DC: National Academy Press, 1999.
32. Lagasse, R.S., Steinberg, E.S., Katz, R.I. & Saubermann, A.J. Defining quality of perioperative care by statistical process control of adverse outcomes. *Anesthesiology* 1995; **82**: 1181–1188.
33. Morray, J.P., Geiduschek, J.M., Caplan, R.A. *et al.* A comparison of pediatric and adult anesthesia closed malpractice claims. *Anesthesiology* 1993; **78**: 461–467.
34. Mason, L.J. An update on the etiology and prevention of anesthesia-related cardiac arrest in children. *Paediatr. Anaesth.* 2004; **14**: 412–416.
35. Ngan Kee, W.D. Confidential enquiries into maternal deaths: 50 years of closing the loop. *Br. J. Anaesth.* 2005; **94**: 413–416.

36. Cooper, G.M. & McClure, J.H. Maternal deaths from anaesthesia. An extract from *Why Mothers Die 2000–2002, the Confidential Enquiries into Maternal Deaths in the United Kingdom*: Chapter **9**: Anaesthesia. *Br. J. Anaesth.* 2005; **94**: 417–423.

37. Thomas, T.A. & Cooper, G.M. Maternal deaths from anaesthesia. An extract from *Why mothers die 1997–1999, the Confidential Enquiries into Maternal Deaths in the United Kingdom*. *Br. J. Anaesth.* 2002; **89**: 499–508.

38. Auroy, Y., Benhamou, D., Bargues, L. *et al.* Major complications of regional anesthesia in France: The SOS Regional Anesthesia Hotline Service. *Anesthesiology* 2002; **97**: 1274–1280.

39. Kopp, S.L., Horlocker, T.T., Warner, M.E. *et al.* Cardiac arrest during neuraxial anesthesia: frequency and predisposing factors associated with survival. *Anesth. Analg.* 2005; **100**: 855–865, table of contents.

40. Liu, S.S. & McDonald, S.B. Current issues in spinal anesthesia. *Anesthesiology* 2001; **94**: 888–906.

41. Auroy, Y., Narchi, P., Messiah, A. *et al.* Serious complications related to regional anesthesia: results of a prospective survey in France. *Anesthesiology* 1997; **87**: 479–486.

42. Caplan, R.A., Ward, R.J., Posner, K. & Cheney, F.W. Unexpected cardiac arrest during spinal anesthesia: a closed claims analysis of predisposing factors. *Anesthesiology* 1988; **68**: 5–11.

43. Pollard, J.B. Cardiac arrest during spinal anesthesia: common mechanisms and strategies for prevention. *Anesth. Analg.* 2001; **92**: 252–256.

44. Campagna, J.A. & Carter, C. Clinical relevance of the Bezold–Jarisch reflex. *Anesthesiology* 2003; **98**: 1250–1260.

45. Lovstad, R.Z., Granhus, G. & Hetland, S. Bradycardia and asystolic cardiac arrest during spinal anaesthesia: a report of five cases. *Acta Anaesthesiol. Scand.* 2000; **44**: 48–52.

46. Harrison, G.G. Death due to anaesthesia at Groote Schuur Hospital, Cape Town—1956–1987. Part, I. Incidence. *S. Afr. Med. J.* 1990; **77**: 412–415.

47. Zeitlin, G.L. Possible decrease in mortality associated with anaesthesia. A comparison of two time periods in Massachusetts, USA. Closed Claims Study Committee. *Anaesthesia* 1989; **44**: 432–433.

48. Aubas, S., Biboulet, P., Daures, J.P. & du Cailar, J. Incidence and etiology of cardiac arrest occurring during the perioperative period and in the recovery room. Apropos of 102,468 anesthesia cases. *Ann. Fr. Anesth. Reanim.* 1991; **10**: 436–442.

49. Lunn, J.N. & Devlin, H.B. Lessons from the confidential enquiry into perioperative deaths in three NHS regions. *Lancet* 1987; **2**: 1384–1386.

50. Dripps, R.D., Lamont, A. & Eckenhoff, J.E. The role of anesthesia in surgical mortality. *J. Am. Med. Assoc.* 1961; **178**: 261–266.

51. Edwards, G., Morton, H.J., Pask, E.A. & Wylie, W.D. Deaths associated with anaesthesia. A report on 1,000 cases. 1956. *Anaesthesia* 1995; **50**: 440–453; discussion 39.

52. Harrison, G.G. Anaesthetic contributory death — its incidence and causes. II. Causes. *S. Afr. Med. J.* 1968; **42**: 544–549.

53. Harrison, G.G. Anaesthetic-associated mortality. *S. Afr. Med. J.* 1974; **48**: 550–554.

54. Lauwers, P. Anesthetic death. *Acta Anaesthesiol. Belg.* 1978; **29**: 19–28.

55. Nagaro, T., Yorozuya, T., Sotani M. *et al.* Survey of patients whose lungs could not be ventilated and whose trachea could not be intubated in university hospitals in Japan. *J. Anesth.* 2003; **17**: 232–240.

56. Sa Rego, M.M., Watcha, M.F. & White, P.F. The changing role of monitored anesthesia care in the ambulatory setting. *Anesth. Analg.* 1997; **85**: 1020–1036.

57. Bhananker, S.M., Posner, K.L., Cheney, F.W. *et al.* Injury and liability associated with monitored anesthesia care: a closed claims analysis. *Anesthesiology* 2006; **104**: 228–234.

58. Tiret, L., Desmonts, J.M., Hatton, F. & Vourc'h G. Complications associated with anaesthesia – a prospective survey in France. *Can. Anaesth. Soc. J.* 1986; **33**: 336–344.

59. Watkins, J. Investigation of allergic and hypersensitivity reactions to anaesthetic agents. *Br. J. Anaesth.* 1987; **59**: 104–111.

60. Oswald, A.M., Joly, L.M., Gury, C. *et al.* Fatal intraoperative anaphylaxis related to aprotinin after local application of fibrin glue. *Anesthesiology* 2003; **99**: 762–763.

61. Laxenaire, M.C., Mouton, C., Frederic, A. *et al.* Anaphylactic shock after tourniquet removal in orthopedic surgery. *Ann. Fr. Anesth. Reanim.* 1996; **15**: 179–184.

62. Laxenaire, M.C. Substances responsible for peranesthetic anaphylactic shock. A third French multicenter study (1992–94). *Ann. Fr. Anesth. Reanim.* 1996; **15**: 1211–1218.

63. Irita, K., Kawashima, Y., Morita, K. *et al.* Life-threatening coronary ischemia in the operating room: analysis of annual survey from 1999 to 2001 conducted by Japanese Society of Anesthesiologists. *Masui* 2003; **52**: 304–319.

64. Flaherty, S. & Grishkin, B.A. Airway obstruction by anterior mediastinal mass. Successful management by percutaneous aspiration. *Chest* 1994; **106**: 947–948.

65. Goh, M.H., Liu, X.Y. & Goh, Y.S. Anterior mediastinal masses: an anaesthetic challenge. *Anaesthesia* 1999; **54**: 670–674.

66. Keon, T.P. Death on induction of anesthesia for cervical node biopsy. *Anesthesiology* 1981; **55**: 471–472.

67. Levin, H., Bursztein, S. & Heifetz, M. Cardiac arrest in a child with an anterior mediastinal mass. *Anesth. Analg.* 1985; **64**: 1129–1130.

68. Pullerits, J. & Holzman, R. Anaesthesia for patients with mediastinal masses. *Can. J. Anaesth.* 1989; **36**: 681–688.

69. Wong, K.C., Schafer, P.G. & Schultz, J.R. Hypokalemia and anesthetic implications. *Anesth. Analg.* 1993; **77**: 1238–1260.

70. Vitez, T.S., Soper, L.E., Wong, K.C. & Soper, P. Chronic hypokalemia and intraoperative dysrhythmias. *Anesthesiology* 1985; **63**: 130–133.

71. Glaser, R. Chronic hypokalemia and intraoperative dysrhythmias. *Anesthesiology* 1986; **64**: 408–409.

72. Hulting, J. In-hospital ventricular fibrillation and its relation to serum potassium. *Acta Med. Scand.* Suppl 1981; **647**: 109–116.

73. Soar, J., Deakin, C.D., Nolan, J.P. *et al.* European Resuscitation Council guidelines for resuscitation 2005. Section 7. Cardiac

arrest in special circumstances. *Resuscitation* 2005; **67** (Suppl 1): S135–S170.

74. Otto, C.W., Yakaitis, R.W., Redding, J.S. & Blitt, C.D. Comparison of dopamine, dobutamine, and epinephrine in CPR. *Crit. Care Med.* 1981; **9**: 640–643.

75. Edbril, S.D. & Lagasse, R.S. Relationship between malpractice litigation and human errors. *Anesthesiology* 1999; **91**: 848–855.

76. Wells, D.G., Zelcer, J., Podolakin, W. *et al.* Cardiac arrest from pulmonary outflow tract obstruction due to a double-lumen tube. *Anesthesiology* 1987; **66**: 422–423.

77. Zelcer, J. & Wells, D.G. Anaesthetic-related recovery room complications. *Anaesth. Intens. Care* 1987; **15**: 168–174.

78. Irita, K., Tsuzaki, K., Sawa, T. *et al.* Critical incidents due to drug administration error in the operating room: an analysis of 4,291,925 anesthetics over a 4 year period. *Masui* 2004; **53**: 577–584.

79. Gilbert, T.B. Cardiac arrest from inadvertent overdose of lidocaine hydrochloride through an arterial pressure line flush apparatus. *Anesth. Analg.* 2001; **93**: 1534–1536, table of contents.

80. Currie, M., Mackay, P., Morgan, C. *et al.* The Australian Incident Monitoring Study. The "wrong drug" problem in anaesthesia: an analysis of 2000 incident reports. *Anaesth. Intens. Care* 1993; **21**: 596–601.

81. Haslam, G.M., Sims, C., McIndoe, A.K. *et al.* High latent drug administration error rates associated with the introduction of the international colour coding syringe labelling system. *Eur. J. Anaesthesiol.* 2006; **23**: 165–168.

82. Fasting, S. & Gisvold, S.E. Adverse drug errors in anesthesia, and the impact of coloured syringe labels. *Can. J. Anaesth.* 2000; **47**: 1060–1067.

83. Webster, C.S., Merry, A.F., Larsson, L. *et al.* The frequency and nature of drug administration error during anaesthesia. *Anaesth. Intens. Care* 2001; **29**: 494–500.

84. Fowkes, F.G., Lunn, J.N., Farrow, S.C. *et al.* Epidemiology in anaesthesia. III: Mortality risk in patients with coexisting physical disease. *Br. J. Anaesth.* 1982; **54**: 819–825.

85. Marx, G.F., Mateo, C.V. & Orkin, L.R. Computer analysis of postanesthetic deaths. *Anesthesiology* 1973; **39**: 54–58.

86. Vacanti, C.J., VanHouten, R.J. & Hill, R.C. A statistical analysis of the relationship of physical status to postoperative mortality in 68,388 cases. *Anesth. Analg.* 1970; **49**: 564–566.

87. Ugwu, B.T., Isamade, E.S. & Isamade, E.I. Intra-operative cardiac arrest–a tropical experience. *West. Afr. J. Med.* 2000; **19**: 277–280.

88. Howard, S.K., Rosekind, M.R., Katz, J.D. & Berry, A.J. Fatigue in anesthesia: implications and strategies for patient and provider safety. *Anesthesiology* 2002; **97**: 1281–1294.

89. Wenzel, V., Padosch, S.A., Voelckel, W.G. *et al.* Survey of effects of anesthesia protocols on hemodynamic variables in porcine cardiopulmonary resuscitation laboratory models before induction of cardiac arrest. *Comp. Med.* 2000; **50**: 644–648.

90. Rajgor, M.B. & Multani, S.T. Management of cardiac arrest in operation theatre. *J. Indian Med. Assoc.* 1998; **96**: 341–344.

91. Foex, P. Cardiac arrest during anesthesia. *Am. J. Emerg. Med.* 1984; **2**: 241–245.

92. Mueller, R.N., Uretsky, B.F., Hao, L. *et al.* Cardiac arrest on induction of anesthesia due to triple vessel coronary artery disease despite a "Negative" angiogram. *Anesthesiology* 2002; **97**: 745–749.

93. Hunter, J.M. Synergism between halothane and labetalol. *Anaesthesia* 1979; **34**: 257–259.

94. Dumot, J.A., Burval, D.J., Sprung, J. *et al.* Outcome of adult cardiopulmonary resuscitations at a tertiary referral center including results of "limited" resuscitations. *Arch. Intern. Med.* 2001; **161**: 1751–1758.

95. Adams, J.H. Hypoxic brain damage. *Br. J. Anaesth.* 1975; **47**: 121–129.

96. Bulger, E.M., Copass, M.K., Sabath, D.R. *et al.* The use of neuromuscular blocking agents to facilitate prehospital intubation does not impair outcome after traumatic brain injury. *J. Trauma* 2005; **58**: 718–723; discussion 23–24.

97. Sakles, J.C., Laurin, E.G., Rantapaa, A.A. & Panacek, E.A. Airway management in the emergency department: a one-year study of 610 tracheal intubations. *Ann. Emerg. Med.* 1998; **31**: 325–332.

98. Schwartz, D.E., Matthay, M.A. & Cohen, N.H. Death and other complications of emergency airway management in critically ill adults. A prospective investigation of 297 tracheal intubations. *Anesthesiology* 1995; **82**: 367–376.

99. Martyn, J.A. & Richtsfeld, M. Succinylcholine-induced hyperkalemia in acquired pathologic states: etiologic factors and molecular Mechanisms. *Anesthesiology* 2006; **104**: 158–169.

100. Robinson, A.L., Jerwood, D.C. & Stokes, M.A. Routine suxamethonium in children. A regional survey of current usage. *Anaesthesia* 1996; **51**: 874–878.

101. McLeskey, C.H., McLeod, D.S., Hough, T.L. & Stallworth, J.M. Prolonged asystole after succinylcholine administration. *Anesthesiology* 1978; **49**: 208–210.

102. Gronert, G.A. Cardiac arrest after succinylcholine: mortality greater with rhabdomyolysis than receptor upregulation. *Anesthesiology* 2001; **94**: 523–529.

103. Sachs, B.P., Oriol, N.E., Ostheimer, G.W. *et al.* Anesthetic-related maternal mortality, 1954 to 1985. *J. Clin. Anesth.* 1989; **1**: 333–338.

104. Inoue, K. & Reichelt, W. Asystole and bradycardia in adult patients after a single dose of suxamethonium. *Acta Anaesthesiol. Scand.* 1986; **30**: 571–573.

105. Van den Hurk, A.W. & Teijen, H.J. Cardiac complications during use of etomidate. *Anaesthesia* 1983; **38**: 1183–1184.

106. Baraka, A. Severe bradycardia following propofol-suxamethonium sequence. *Br. J. Anaesth.* 1988; **61**: 482–483.

107. Guise, P.A. Asystole following propofol and fentanyl in an anxious patient. *Anaesth. Intens. Care* 1991; **19**: 116–118.

108. Tramer, M.R., Moore, R.A. & McQuay, H.J. Propofol and bradycardia: causation, frequency and severity. *Br. J. Anaesth.* 1997; **78**: 642–651.

109. Cremer, O.L., Moons, K.G., Bouman, E.A. *et al.* Long-term propofol infusion and cardiac failure in adult head-injured patients. *Lancet* 2001; **357**: 117–118.

110. Eriksen, J. & Povey, H.M. A case of suspected non-neurosurgical adult fatal propofol infusion syndrome. *Acta Anaesthesiol. Scand.* 2006; **50**: 117–119.

111. Kumar, M.A., Urrutia, V.C., Thomas, C.E. *et al.* The syndrome of irreversible acidosis after prolonged propofol infusion. *Neurocrit. Care.* 2005; **3**: 257–259.

112. Ingersoll-Weng, E., Manecke, G.R., Jr. & Thistlethwaite, P.A. Dexmedetomidine and cardiac arrest. *Anesthesiology* 2004; **100**: 738–739.

113. Wig, J., Bali, I.M., Singh, R.G. *et al.* Prolonged Q-T interval syndrome. Sudden cardiac arrest during anaesthesia. *Anaesthesia* 1979; **34**: 37–40.

114. Hopkins, P.M. Malignant hyperthermia: advances in clinical management and diagnosis. *Br. J. Anaesth.* 2000; **85**: 118–128.

115. Girard, T., Treves, S., Voronkov, E. *et al.* Molecular genetic testing for malignant hyperthermia susceptibility. *Anesthesiology* 2004; **100**: 1076–1080.

116. Urwyler, A., Deufel, T., McCarthy, T. & West, S. Guidelines for molecular genetic detection of susceptibility to malignant hyperthermia. *Br. J. Anaesth.* 2001; **86**: 283–287.

117. Krause, T., Gerbershagen, M.U., Fiege, M. *et al.* Dantrolene – a review of its pharmacology, therapeutic use and new developments. *Anaesthesia.* 2004; **59**: 364–373.

118. Christiansen, L.R. & Collins, K.A. Pathologic findings in malignant hyperthermia: a case report and review of literature. *Am. J. Forens. Med. Pathol.* 2004; **25**: 327–333.

119. Johns, R.A., DiFazio, C.A. & Longnecker, D.E. Lidocaine constricts or dilates rat arterioles in a dose-dependent manner. *Anesthesiology* 1985; **62**: 141–144.

120. Nakamura, K., Toda, H., Kakuyama, M. *et al.* Direct vascular effect of ropivacaine in femoral artery and vein of the dog. *Acta Anaesthesiol. Scand.* 1993; **37**: 269–273.

121. Clarkson, C.W. & Hondeghem, L.M. Evidence for a specific receptor site for lidocaine, quinidine, and bupivacaine associated with cardiac sodium channels in guinea pig ventricular myocardium. *Circ. Res.* 1985; **56**: 496–506.

122. Coyle, D.E. & Sperelakis, N. Bupivacaine and lidocaine blockade of calcium-mediated slow action potentials in guinea pig ventricular muscle. *J. Pharmacol. Exp. Ther.* 1987; **242**: 1001–1005.

123. Lynch, C., 3rd. Depression of myocardial contractility in vitro by bupivacaine, etidocaine, and lidocaine. *Anesth. Analg.* 1986; **65**: 551–559.

124. Nieman, C.J. & Eisner, D.A. Effects of caffeine, tetracaine, and ryanodine on calcium-dependent oscillations in sheep cardiac Purkinje fibers. *J. Gen. Physiol.* 1985; **86**: 877–889.

125. Eledjam, J.J., de La Coussaye, J.E., Brugada. J. *et al.* In vitro study on mechanisms of bupivacaine-induced depression of myocardial contractility. *Anesth. Analg.* 1989; **69**: 732–735.

126. Sztark, F., Tueux, O., Erny, P. *et al.* Effects of bupivacaine on cellular oxygen consumption and adenine nucleotide metabolism. *Anesth. Analg.* 1994; **78**: 335–339.

127. Sztark, F., Malgat, M., Dabadie, P. & Mazat, J.P. Comparison of the effects of bupivacaine and ropivacaine on heart cell mitochondrial bioenergetics. *Anesthesiology* 1998; **88**: 1340–1349.

128. Butterworth J.Ft., Brownlow, R.C., Leith, J.P. *et al.* Bupivacaine inhibits cyclic-3',5'-adenosine monophosphate production. A possible contributing factor to cardiovascular toxicity. *Anesthesiology.* 1993; **79**: 88–95.

129. Voeikov, V.L. & Lefkowitz, R.J. Effects of local anesthetics on guanyl nucleotide modulation of the catecholamine-sensitive adenylate cyclase system and on beta-adrenergic receptors. *Biochim. Biophys. Acta* 1980; **629**: 266–281.

130. Clarkson, C.W. & Hondeghem, L.M. Mechanism for bupivacaine depression of cardiac conduction: fast block of sodium channels during the action potential with slow recovery from block during diastole. *Anesthesiology* 1985; **62**: 396–405.

131. Bosnjak, Z.J., Stowe, D.F. & Kampine, J.P. Comparison of lidocaine and bupivacaine depression of sinoatrial nodal activity during hypoxia and acidosis in adult and neonatal guinea pigs. *Anesth. Analg.* 1986; **65**: 911–917.

132. Hotvedt, R., Refsum, H. & Helgesen, K.G. Cardiac electrophysiologic and hemodynamic effects related to plasma levels of bupivacaine in the dog. *Anesth. Analg.* 1985; **64**: 388–394.

133. Komai, H. & Rusy, B.F. Effects of bupivacaine and lidocaine on AV conduction in the isolated rat heart: modification by hyperkalemia. *Anesthesiology* 1981; **55**: 281–285.

134. Moller, R.A. & Covino, B.G. Cardiac electrophysiologic effects of lidocaine and bupivacaine. *Anesth. Analg.* 1988; **67**: 107–114.

135. Nath, S., Haggmark, S., Johansson, G. & Reiz, S. Differential depressant and electrophysiologic cardiotoxicity of local anesthetics: an experimental study with special reference to lidocaine and bupivacaine. *Anesth. Analg.* 1986; **65**: 1263–1270.

136. Heavner, J.E. Cardiac dysrhythmias induced by infusion of local anesthetics into the lateral cerebral ventricle of cats. *Anesth. Analg.* 1986; **65**: 133–138.

137. Bernards, C.M. & Artu, A.A. Hexamethonium and midazolam terminate dysrhythmias and hypertension caused by intracerebroventricular bupivacaine in rabbits. *Anesthesiology* 1991; **74**: 89–96.

138. de La Coussaye, J.E., Eledjam, J.J., Bruelle, P. *et al.* Mechanisms of the putative cardioprotective effect of hexamethonium in anesthetized dogs given a large dose of bupivacaine. *Anesthesiology* 1994; **80**: 595–605.

139. Avery, P., Redon, D., Schaenzer, G. & Rusy, B. The influence of serum potassium on the cerebral and cardiac toxicity of bupivacaine and lidocaine. *Anesthesiology* 1984; **61**: 134–138.

140. Santos, A.C., Arthur, G.R., Wlody, D. *et al.* Comparative systemic toxicity of ropivacaine and bupivacaine in nonpregnant and pregnant ewes. *Anesthesiology* 1995; **82**: 734–740; discussion 27A.

141. Aberg, G. Toxicological and local anaesthetic effects of optically active isomers of two local anaesthetic compounds. *Acta Pharmacol. Toxicol. (Copenh.)* 1972; **31**: 273–286.

142. Arlock, P. Actions of three local anaesthetics: lidocaine, bupivacaine and ropivacaine on guinea pig papillary muscle sodium channels (V_{max}). *Pharmacol. Toxicol.* 1988; **63**: 96–104.

143. Reiz, S., Haggmark, S., Johansson, G. & Nath, S. Cardiotoxicity of ropivacaine — a new amide local anaesthetic agent. *Acta Anaesthesiol. Scand.* 1989; **33**: 93–98.

144. Mazoit, J.X., Boico, O. & Samii, K. Myocardial uptake of bupivacaine: II. Pharmacokinetics and pharmacodynamics of bupivacaine enantiomers in the isolated perfused rabbit heart. *Anesth. Analg.* 1993; **77**: 477–482.

145. Moller, R. & Covino, B.G. Cardiac electrophysiologic properties of bupivacaine and lidocaine compared with those of ropivacaine, a new amide local anesthetic. *Anesthesiology* 1990; **72**: 322–329.

146. Pitkanen, M., Feldman, H.S., Arthur, G.R. & Covino, B.G. Chronotropic and inotropic effects of ropivacaine, bupivacaine, and lidocaine in the spontaneously beating and electrically paced isolated, perfused rabbit heart. *Reg. Anesth.* 1992; **17**: 183–192.

147. Chang, D.H., Ladd, L.A., Wilson, K.A. *et al.* Tolerability of large-dose intravenous levobupivacaine in sheep. *Anesth. Analg.* 2000; **91**: 671–679.

148. Denson, D.D., Behbehani, M.M. & Gregg, R.V. Enantiomer-specific effects of an intravenously administered arrhythmogenic dose of bupivacaine on neurons of the nucleus tractus solitarius and the cardiovascular system in the anesthetized rat. *Reg. Anesth.* 1992; **17**: 311–316.

149. Huang, Y.F., Pryor, M.E., Mather, L.E. & Veering, B.T. Cardiovascular and central nervous system effects of intravenous levobupivacaine and bupivacaine in sheep. *Anesth. Analg.* 1998; **86**: 797–804.

150. Nancarrow, C., Rutten, A.J., Runciman, W.B. *et al.* Myocardial and cerebral drug concentrations and the mechanisms of death after fatal intravenous doses of lidocaine, bupivacaine, and ropivacaine in the sheep. *Anesth. Analg.* 1989; **69**: 276–283.

151. Groban, L., Deal, D.D., Vernon, J.C. *et al.* Ventricular arrhythmias with or without programmed electrical stimulation after incremental overdosage with lidocaine, bupivacaine, levobupivacaine, and ropivacaine. *Anesth. Analg.* 2000; **91**: 1103–1111.

152. Groban, L., Deal, D.D., Vernon, J.C. *et al.* Cardiac resuscitation after incremental overdosage with lidocaine, bupivacaine, levobupivacaine, and ropivacaine in anesthetized dogs. *Anesth. Analg.* 2001; **92**: 37–43.

153. Ratra, C.K., Badola, R.P., Bhargava, K.P. A study of factors concerned in emesis during spinal anaesthesia. *Br. J. Anaesth.* 1972; **44**: 1208–1211.

154. Carpenter, R.L., Caplan, R.A., Brown, D.L. *et al.* Incidence and risk factors for side effects of spinal anesthesia. *Anesthesiology* 1992; **76**: 906–916.

155. Curatolo, M., Scaramozzino, P., Venuti, F.S. *et al.* Factors associated with hypotension and bradycardia after epidural blockade. *Anesth. Analg.* 1996; **83**: 1033–1040.

156. Dohi, S., Naito, H. & Takahashi, T. Age-related changes in blood pressure and duration of motor block in spinal anesthesia. *Anesthesiology* 1979; **50**: 319–323.

157. Kahn, R.L., Marino, V., Urquhart, B. & Sharrock, N.E. Hemodynamic changes associated with tourniquet use under epidural anesthesia for total knee arthroplasty. *Reg. Anesth.* 1992; **17**: 228–232.

158. Tarkkila, P.J. and Kaukinen, S. Complications during spinal anesthesia: a prospective study. *Reg. Anesth.* 1991; **16**: 101–106.

159. Liguori, G.A. & Sharrock, N.E. Asystole and severe bradycardia during epidural anesthesia in orthopedic patients. *Anesthesiology* 1997; **86**: 250–257.

160. Arndt, J.O., Bomer, W., Krauth, J. & Marquardt, B. Incidence and time course of cardiovascular side effects during spinal anesthesia after prophylactic administration of intravenous fluids or vasoconstrictors. *Anesth. Analg.* 1998; **87**: 347–354.

161. Mackey, D.C., Carpenter, R.L., Thompson, G.E. *et al.* Bradycardia and asystole during spinal anesthesia: a report of three cases without morbidity. *Anesthesiology* 1989; **70**: 866–868.

162. Frerichs, R.L., Campbell, J. & Bassell, G.M. Psychogenic cardiac arrest during extensive sympathetic blockade. *Anesthesiology* 1988; **68**: 943–944.

163. Lee, L.A., Posner, K.L., Domino KB. *et al.* Injuries associated with regional anesthesia in the 1980s and 1990s: a closed claims analysis. *Anesthesiology* 2004; **101**: 143–152.

164. Liu, S., Paul, G.E., Carpenter RL. *et al.* Prolonged PR interval is a risk factor for bradycardia during spinal anesthesia. *Reg. Anesth.* 1995; **20**: 41–44.

165. Baron, J.F., Decaux-Jacolot, A., Edouard, A. *et al.* Influence of venous return on baroreflex control of heart rate during lumbar epidural anesthesia in humans. *Anesthesiology* 1986; **64**: 188–193.

166. Ludbrook, J. & Rutter, P.C. Effect of naloxone on haemodynamic responses to acute blood loss in unanaesthetized rabbits. *J. Physiol.* 1988; **400**: 1–14.

167. Abboud, F.M. Ventricular syncope: is the heart a sensory organ? *N. Engl. J. Med.* 1989; **320**: 390–392.

168. Mark, A.L. The Bezold–Jarisch reflex revisited: clinical implications of inhibitory reflexes originating in the heart. *J. Am. Coll. Cardiol.* 1983; **1**: 90–102.

169. Zucker, I.H. & Cornish, K.G. The Bezold–Jarisch in the conscious dog. *Circ. Res.* 1981; **49**: 940–948.

170. Oberg, B. & Thoren, P. Increased activity in left ventricular receptors during hemorrhage or occlusion of caval veins in the cat. A possible cause of the vaso-vagal reaction. *Acta Physiol. Scand.* 1972; **85**: 164–173.

171. van Lieshout, J.J., Wieling, W., Karemaker, J.M. & Eckberg, D.L. The vasovagal response. *Clin. Sci. (Lond.)* 1991; **81**: 575–586.

172. Arndt, J.O., Hock, A., Stanton-Hicks, M. & Stuhmeier, K.D. Peridural anesthesia and the distribution of blood in supine humans. *Anesthesiology* 1985; **63**: 616–623.

173. Hogan, Q.H., Stadnicka, A., Stekiel, T.A. *et al.* Effects of epidural and systemic lidocaine on sympathetic activity and

mesenteric circulation in rabbits. *Anesthesiology* 1993; **79**: 1250–1260.

174. Jacobsen, J., Sofelt, S., Brocks, V. *et al.* Reduced left ventricular diameters at onset of bradycardia during epidural anaesthesia. *Acta Anaesthesiol. Scand.* 1992; **36**: 831–836.

175. Gratadour, P., Viale, J.P., Parlow, J. *et al.* Sympathovagal effects of spinal anesthesia assessed by the spontaneous cardiac baroreflex. *Anesthesiology* 1997; **87**: 1359–1367.

176. Hogan, Q.H., Amuzu, J., Clifford, P.S. *et al.* Hypoxia causes apnea during epidural anesthesia in rabbits. *Anesthesiology* 1998; **88**: 761–767.

177. Stienstra, R. Mechanisms behind and treatment of sudden, unexpected circulatory collapse during central neuraxis blockade. *Acta Anaesthesiol. Scand.* 2000; **44**: 965–971.

178. Melloni, C. Morbidity and mortality related to anesthesia outside the operating room. *Minerva Anestesiol* 2005; **71**: 325–334.

179. Cote, C.J., Notterman, D.A., Karl, H.W. *et al.* Adverse sedation events in pediatrics: a critical incident analysis of contributing factors. *Pediatrics* 2000; **105**: 805–814.

180. White, P.F. & Freire, A.R. Ambulatory (outpatient) anesthesia. In Miller, R.D. ed. *Anesthesia*, Philadelphia: Elsevier Churchill Livingstone, **2005**: 2589–2635.

181. Memery, H.N. Anesthesia mortality in private practice. A ten-year study. *J. Am. Med. Assoc.* 1965; **194**: 1185–1188.

182. White, P.F. & Roizen, M.F. Cardiac arrest in a day surgery patient. *Anesthesiology* 1990; **72**: 771–772.

183. Brahams, D. Death in the dentist's chair. *Lancet* 1989; **2**: 991–992.

184. Krippaehne, J.A. & Montgomery, M.T. Morbidity and mortality from pharmacosedation and general anesthesia in the dental office. *J. Oral Maxillofac. Surg.* 1992; **50**: 691–698; discussion 8–9.

185. Holden, C.G., Monaghan, D. & Cassidy, M. Retention of cardiopulmonary resuscitation skills of dental nurses. *SAAD Dig* 1996; **13**: 3–7.

186. Luyk, N.H. & Ferguson, J.W. The safe practice of intravenous sedation in dentistry. *N Z Dent. J.* 1993; **89**: 45–49.

187. James, D.W. General anaesthesia, sedation and resuscitation in dentistry. *Br. Dent. J.* 1991; **171**: 345–347.

188. Whitmire, H.C., Jr. Medicolegal considerations for office-based anesthesia in dentistry. *Dent. Clin. North Am.* 1999; **43**: 361–372, vii, 73–77.

189. Bitar, G., Mullis, W., Jacobs, W. *et al.* Safety and efficacy of office-based surgery with monitored anesthesia care/sedation in 4778 consecutive plastic surgery procedures. *Plast. Reconstr. Surg.* 2003; **111**: 150–156; discussion 7–8.

190. Perrott, D.H., Yuen, J.P., Andresen, R.V. & Dodson, T.B. Office-based ambulatory anesthesia: outcomes of clinical practice of oral and maxillofacial surgeons. *J. Oral Maxillofac. Surg.* 2003; **61**: 983–995; discussion 95–96.

191. Coldiron, B., Shreve, E. & Balkrishnan, R. Patient injuries from surgical procedures performed in medical offices: three years of Florida data. *Dermatol. Surg.* 2004; **30**: 1435–1443; discussion 43.

192. Sprung, J., Ritter, M.J., Rihal, C.S. *et al.* Outcomes of cardiopulmonary resuscitation and predictors of survival in patients undergoing coronary angiography including percutaneous coronary interventions. *Anesth. Analg.* 2006; **102**: 217–224.

193. Russ, M.J. & Bailine, S.H. Asystole and bradycardia related to anesthetic induction during ECT: a case report. *J. Ect.* 2004; **20**: 195–197.

194. Brown, T.B., Lovato, L.M. & Parker, D. Procedural sedation in the acute care setting. *Am. Fam. Physician.* 2005; **71**: 85–90.

195. Pershad, J. & Godambe, S.A. Propofol for procedural sedation in the pediatric emergency department. *J. Emerg. Med.* 2004; **27**: 11–14.

196. Thierbach, A., Piepho, T., Wolcke, B. *et al.* [Prehospital emergency airway management procedures. Success rates and complications]. *Anaesthesist* 2004; **53**: 543–550.

197. Spaite, D.W. & Criss, E.A. Out-of-hospital rapid sequence intubation: are we helping or hurting our patients? Ann. Emerg. Med. 2003; **42**: 729–730.

198. Bochicchio, G.V., Ilahi, O., Joshi M. *et al.* Endotracheal intubation in the field does not improve outcome in trauma patients who present without an acutely lethal traumatic brain injury. *J. Trauma* 2003; **54**: 307–311.

199. Dunford, J.V., Davis, D.P., Ochs, M. *et al.* Incidence of transient hypoxia and pulse rate reactivity during paramedic rapid sequence intubation. *Ann. Emerg. Med.* 2003; **42**: 721–728.

200. Hazinski, M.F., Nadkarni, V.M., Hickey, R.W. *et al.* Major changes in the 2005 AHA Guidelines for CPR and ECC: reaching the tipping point for change. *Circulation* 2005; **112**:IV206–211.

201. Caplan, R.A., Posner, K.L., Ward, R.J. & Cheney, F.W. Adverse respiratory events in anesthesia: a closed claims analysis. *Anesthesiology* 1990; **72**: 828–833.

202. Cheney, F.W., Posner, K.L. & Caplan, R.A. Adverse respiratory events infrequently leading to malpractice suits. A closed claims analysis. *Anesthesiology* 1991; **75**: 932–939.

203. Azim, N. & Wang, C.Y. The use of bispectral index during a cardiopulmonary arrest: a potential predictor of cerebral perfusion. *Anaesthesia* 2004; **59**: 610–612.

204. England, M.R. The changes in bispectral index during a hypovolemic cardiac arrest. *Anesthesiology* 1999; **91**: 1947–1949.

205. Kluger, M.T. The bispectral index during an anaphylactic circulatory arrest. *Anaesth. Intens. Care* 2001; **29**: 544–547.

206. Szekely, B., Saint-Marc, T., Degremont, A.C. *et al.* Value of bispectral index monitoring during cardiopulmonary resuscitation. *Br. J. Anaesth.* 2002; **88**: 443–444.

207. Kuroda, M., Kawamoto, M. & Yuge, O. Undisrupted pulse wave on pulse oximeter display monitor at cardiac arrest in a surgical patient. *J. Anesth.* 2005; **19**: 164–166.

208. Cooper, J.B., Newbower, R.S. & Kitz, R.J. An analysis of major errors and equipment failures in anesthesia management: considerations for prevention and detection. *Anesthesiology* 1984; **60**: 34–42.

209. Eichhorn, J.H., Cooper, J.B., Cullen, D.J. *et al.* Standards for patient monitoring during anesthesia at Harvard Medical School. *J. Am. Med. Assoc.* 1986; **256**: 1017–1020.

210. Gaba, D.M. Anaesthesiology as a model for patient safety in health care. *Br. Med. J.* 2000; **320**: 785–788.

211. ASA. http://www.asahq.org/publicationsServices.htm.

212. 2005 American Heart Association Guidelines for Cardiopulmonary Resuscitation and Emergency Cardiovascular Care. *Circulation* 2005; **112**:IV1–203.

213. Berg, R.A., Hilwig, R.W., Ewy, G.A. & Kern, K.B. Precountershock cardiopulmonary resuscitation improves initial response to defibrillation from prolonged ventricular fibrillation: a randomized, controlled swine study. *Crit. Care Med.* 2004; **32**: 1352–1357.

214. Ewy, G.A., Kern, K.B., Sanders, A.B. *et al.* Cardiocerebral resuscitation for cardiac arrest. *Am. J. Med.* 2006; **119**: 6–9.

215. Feldman, H.S., Arthur, G.R., Pitkanen, M. *et al.* Treatment of acute systemic toxicity after the rapid intravenous injection of ropivacaine and bupivacaine in the conscious dog. *Anesth. Analg.* 1991; **73**: 373–384.

216. Kulier, A.H., Woehlck, H.J., Hogan, Q.H. *et al.* Epinephrine dysrhythmogenicity is not enhanced by subtoxic bupivacaine in dogs. *Anesth. Analg.* 1996; **83**: 62–67.

217. Haasio, J., Pitkanen, M.T., Kytta, J. & Rosenberg, P.H. Treatment of bupivacaine-induced cardiac arrhythmias in hypoxic and hypercarbic pigs with amiodarone or bretylium. *Reg. Anesth.* 1990; **15**: 174–179.

218. Solomon, D., Bunegin, L. & Albin, M. The effect of magnesium sulfate administration on cerebral and cardiac toxicity of bupivacaine in dogs. *Anesthesiology* 1990; **72**: 341–346.

219. Rosenberg, J.M., Wortsman, J., Wahr, J.A. *et al.* Impaired neuroendocrine response mediates refractoriness to cardiopulmonary resuscitation in spinal anesthesia. *Crit. Care Med.* 1998; **26**: 533–537.

220. Brown, D.L., Carpenter, R.L. & Moore, D.C. Cardiac arrest during spinal anesthesia III (letter). *Anesthesiology* 1988; **68**: 971–972.

221. Rosenberg, J.M., Wahr, J.A., Sung, C.H. *et al.* Coronary perfusion pressure during cardiopulmonary resuscitation after spinal anesthesia in dogs. *Anesth. Analg.* 1996; **82**: 84–87.

222. Krismer, A.C., Hogan, Q.H., Wenzel, V. *et al.* The efficacy of epinephrine or vasopressin for resuscitation during epidural anesthesia. *Anesth. Analg.* 2001; **93**: 734–742.

223. Leape, L.L. & Berwick, D.M. Five years after To Err Is Human: what have we learned? *J. Am. Med. Assoc.* 2005; **293**: 2384–2390.

224. Silber, J.H., Kennedy, S.K., Even-Shoshan O. *et al.* Anesthesiologist direction and patient outcomes. *Anesthesiology* 2000; **93**: 152–163.

225. Silber, J.H., Kennedy, S.K., Even-Shoshan, O. *et al.* Anesthesiologist board certification and patient outcomes. *Anesthesiology* 2002; **96**: 1044–1052.

226. Aiken, L.H., Clarke, S.P., Cheung, R.B. *et al.* Educational levels of hospital nurses and surgical patient mortality. *J. Am. Med. Assoc.* 2003; **290**: 1617–1623.

227. Aiken, L.H., Clarke, S.P., Sloane, D.M. *et al.* Hospital nurse staffing and patient mortality, nurse burnout, and job dissatisfaction. *J. Am. Med. Assoc.* 2002; **288**: 1987–1993.

228. Abenstein, J.P. & Warner, M.A. Anesthesia providers, patient outcomes, and costs. *Anesth. Analg.* 1996; **82**: 1273–1283.

229. Needleman, J., Buerhaus, P., Mattke S. *et al.* Nurse-staffing levels and the quality of care in hospitals. *N. Engl. J. Med.* 2002; **346**: 1715–1722.

230. Fletcher, G., Flin, R., McGeorge P. *et al.* Anaesthetists' Non-Technical Skills (ANTS): evaluation of a behavioural marker system. *Br. J. Anaesth.* 2003; **90**: 580–588.

231. Gaba, D.M. What makes a "good" anesthesiologist? *Anesthesiology* 2004; **101**: 1061–1063.

232. Anesthesiology Residency Review Committee. *Program Requirements for Graduate Medical Education in Anesthesiology (Document 040pr703)* Accreditation Council for Graduate Medical Education. Chicago, 2004.

233. Helmreich, R. & Davies, J. *Human Factors in the Operating Room: Interpersonal Determinants of Safety, Efficiency, and Morale.* London: Balliere Tindall, 1996.

234. Helmreich, R.L. On error management: lessons from aviation. *Br. Med. J.* 2000; **320**: 781–785.

235. Blum, R.H., Raemer, D.B., Carroll, J.S. *et al.* A method for measuring the effectiveness of simulation-based team training for improving communication skills. *Anesth. Analg.* 2005; **100**: 1375–1380, table of contents.

236. Bohmer, R.M. & Edmondson, A.C. Organizational learning in health care. *Health Forum J.* 2001; **44**: 32–35.

237. Morey, J.C., Simon, R., Jay, G.D. *et al.* Error reduction and performance improvement in the emergency department through formal teamwork training: evaluation results of the MedTeams project. *Health Serv. Res.* 2002; **37**: 1553–1581.

238. Leape, L.L. Error in medicine. *J. Am. Med. Assoc.* 1994; **272**: 1851–1857.

239. DeAnda, A. & Gaba, D.M. Unplanned incidents during comprehensive anesthesia simulation. *Anesth. Analg.* 1990; **71**: 77–82.

240. DeAnda, A. & Gaba, D.M. Role of experience in the response to simulated critical incidents. *Anesth. Analg.* 1991; **72**: 308–315.

241. Gaba, D.M., Howard, S.K., Flanagan B. *et al.* Assessment of clinical performance during simulated crises using both technical and behavioral ratings. *Anesthesiology* 1998; **89**: 8–18.

242. Schwid, H.A. & O'Donnell, D. Anesthesiologists' management of simulated critical incidents. *Anesthesiology* 1992; **76**: 495–501.

243. Murray, D.J., Boulet, J.R., Kras, J.F. *et al.* Acute care skills in anesthesia practice: a simulation-based resident performance assessment. *Anesthesiology* 2004; **101**: 1084–1095.

244. Haluck, R.S. & Krummel, T.M. Computers and virtual reality for surgical education in the 21st century. *Arch. Surg.* 2000; **135**: 786–792.

245. Satish, U., Streufert, S., Marshall, R. *et al.* Strategic management simulations is a novel way to measure resident competencies. *Am. J. Surg.* 2001; **181**: 557–561.

246. Marsch, S.C., Muller, C., Marquardt, K. *et al.* Human factors affect the quality of cardiopulmonary resuscitation in simulated cardiac arrests. *Resuscitation* 2004; **60**: 51–56.

247. Benumof, J.L. Management of the difficult adult airway. With special emphasis on awake tracheal intubation. *Anesthesiology* 1991; **75**: 1087–1110.

248. Practice guidelines for management of the difficult airway. A report by the American Society of Anesthesiologists Task Force on Management of the Difficult Airway. *Anesthesiology* 1993; **78**: 597–602.

249. Practice guidelines for management of the difficult airway: an updated report by the American Society of Anesthesiologists Task Force on Management of the Difficult Airway. *Anesthesiology* 2003; **98**: 1269–1277.

250. Crosby, E.T., Cooper, R.M., Douglas, M.J. *et al.* The unanticipated difficult airway with recommendations for management. *Can. J. Anaesth.* 1998; **45**: 757–776.

251. Guidelines for cardiopulmonary resuscitation and emergency cardiac care. Emergency Cardiac Care Committee and Subcommittees, American Heart Association. Part III. Adult advanced cardiac life support. *J. Am. Med. Assoc.* 1992; **268**: 2199–2241.

252. Cheney, F.W. The American Society of Anesthesiologists Closed Claims Project: what have we learned, how has it affected practice, and how will it affect practice in the future? *Anesthesiology* 1999; **91**: 552–556.

253. Mayor, A.H., Eaton, J.M. Anaesthetic machine checking practices. A survey. *Anaesthesia* 1992; **47**: 866–868.

254. Zorab, J.S. Anaesthetic machine checking practices. *Anaesthesia* 1993; **48**: 267.

255. Barthram, C. & McClymont, W. The use of a checklist for anaesthetic machines. *Anaesthesia* 1992; **47**: 1066–1069.

256. Kendell, J. & Barthram, C. Revised checklist for anaesthetic machines. *Anaesthesia* 1998; **53**: 887–890.

257. Cooper, J.B., Newbower, R.S., Long, C.D. & McPeek, B. Preventable anesthesia mishaps: a study of human factors. *Anesthesiology* 1978; **49**: 399–406.

258. Craig, J. & Wilson, M.E. A survey of anaesthetic misadventures. *Anaesthesia* 1981; **36**: 933–936.

259. Kumar, V., Barcellos, W.A., Mehta, M.P. & Carter, J.G. An analysis of critical incidents in a teaching department for quality assurance. A survey of mishaps during anaesthesia. *Anaesthesia* 1988; **43**: 879–883.

260. Short, T.G., O'Regan, A., Jayasuriya, J.P. *et al.* Improvements in anaesthetic care resulting from a critical incident reporting programme. *Anaesthesia* 1996; **51**: 615–621.

261. Webb, R.K., Russell, W.J., Klepper, I. & Runciman, W.B. The Australian Incident Monitoring Study. Equipment failure: an analysis of 2000 incident reports. *Anaesth. Intens. Care* 1993; **21**: 673–677.

262. Hart, E.M. & Owen, H. Errors and omissions in anesthesia: a pilot study using a pilot's checklist. *Anesth. Analg.* 2005; **101**: 246–250, table of contents.

263. Reason, J. *Managing the Risks of Organizational Accidents.* Aldershot, UK: Ashgate Publishing Limited, 1997.

264. Usher, A.G., Cave, D.A. & Finegan, B.A. Critical incident with Narkomed 6000 Anesthesia System. *Anesthesiology* 2003; **99**: 762; discussion.

265. Flaatten, H. How to learn from adverse events? *Acta Anaesthesiol. Scand.* 2005; **49**: 889–890.

266. Beecher, H.K. The first anesthesia death with some remarks suggested by it on the fields of the laboratory and the clinic in the appraisal of new anesthetic agents. *Anesthesiology* 1941; **2**: 443–449.

267. Macintosh, R. Deaths under anaesthetics. *Br. J. Anaesth.* 1948; **21**: 107–136.

60

Resuscitation of the pregnant patient suffering sudden cardiac death

Mark Stacey and Stephen Morris

Anaesthetic Department, Llandough Hospital, Cardiff, UK

Clinical scenario: A 20-year-old pregnant woman is admitted to the emergency room having had a cardiac arrest at home. Cardiac massage and intubation had been performed at home with the patient in the left lateral position. An emergency Cesarean section takes place on the emergency room trolley in "not particularly aseptic conditions", and a live infant is born. The mother's cardiovascular system now responds to resuscitative measures. Three weeks later, after a stormy period in the intensive care unit, she is discharged to the ward with a left hemiparesis. Eighteen years later she sees her son get a place at university.

Introduction

Pregnancy places considerable stress on the cardiorespiratory system. Despite this, cardiac arrest is uncommon – Willis and Rees estimated it to occur once in approximately 30 000 late deliveries,[1] but survival from such an event is exceptional. The United Kingdom's Confidential Enquiry into Maternal and Child Health (CEMACH), formerly known as the Confidential Enquiry into Maternal Deaths, reports that most maternal deaths are from acute causes, with many mothers receiving some form of resuscitation. Nevertheless, the number of indirect deaths (deaths from medical conditions exacerbated by pregnancy) is greater than that of deaths from conditions that arise from pregnancy itself. These indirect deaths seem to be increasing as a result of both social trends and medical progress. The advance of surgical procedures and medical treatments has meant that women who previously would not have survived to adulthood may now reach pregnancy. Those who

have had corrective surgery for congenital cardiac lesions provide a good example. Causes of cardiac arrest during pregnancy include those found in the normal population (arrhythmias, congenital and acquired heart disease, pulmonary emboli, trauma) and those specific to pregnancy (amniotic fluid embolism, hemorrhage, and iatrogenic causes such as magnesium overdose, intravenous bupivacaine, syntocinon-induced pulmonary edema) (See Table 60.1). The dramatic cardiovascular and respiratory changes that occur in pregnancy mandate that several aspects of resuscitation have to be modified if they are to have any prospect of success in a very different clinical situation.

The following recommendations are based on summaries of relevant case reports and knowledge of maternal physiology. In terms of the strength of evidence, because of the obvious difficulties in carrying out research into maternal cardiac arrest, they are at best the opinions of respected authorities, based on clinical evidence, descriptive studies, or reports of expert committees.

Physiological changes in pregnancy

Cardiovascular system

In normal parturients, plasma volume increases throughout pregnancy to approximately 150% of prepregnancy values at 32 weeks' gestation. About half the increase occurs by 10 weeks' gestation and 80% at 20 weeks. Increased erythropoiesis causes an increase in the red cell mass in a more linear fashion by about 25%. The discrepancy between these changes in plasma volume and red

Table 60.1. Examples of pathology that has caused cardiac arrest in pregnancy

Causes	Ref
Pregnancy-related	
Peripartum cardiomyopathy	58, 59
Amniotic fluid embolus	60, 61
Pre-eclampsia/eclampsia	62
Laryngeal edema	
Magnesium overdose	63
Anesthetic-related	
General anesthesia	
Airway problems	22, 64
Local anesthesia	
Intravenous drug toxicity	65
Local anesthetics	66, 67
Spinal anesthesia	66, 68
Fetal injection of potassium	69
Non-pregnant causes	
Trauma	70
Pulmonary embolus	71, 72
Air embolus	73
Myocardial sarcoid	74
Aortic dissection	55
Adenocarcinoma	75

cell mass account for the fall in hemoglobin throughout pregnancy.[1-3]

Pulse rate also rises throughout pregnancy, ultimately reaching 10 to 20 beats per minute higher at term, with most changes occurring by 8 weeks' gestation. Stroke volume has been shown either to increase or decrease, but usually shows little change.[4] The increased oxygen consumption in pregnancy causes cardiac output to increase throughout pregnancy, reaching a peak at 32 weeks. It remains at this level only to increase further during labor.

It was previously believed that cardiac output decreases in the latter stages of pregnancy. This decrease in cardiac output, however, is due to aortocaval compression. In ten maternal volunteers, who had pulmonary artery flow catheters inserted to measure cardiac output, it was found that there was a decrease in cardiac output in the supine position. This fall could be reversed by using the left or right lateral positions.[5] This study showed no difference between the two positions, but the left tilt is used preferentially, as the inferior vena cava lies on the right side of the vertebral column. Significant rises in systemic and pulmonary vascular resistance occurred to maintain arterial pressure when cardiac output fell with the subject in the supine position.

The gravid uterus, by virtue of its weight and size, compresses not only the inferior vena cava but also the aorta. This compression is responsible for an additional fall in cardiac output of 10%–25% when the mother is supine, and exacerbates the reduction in venous return that already exists during cardiopulmonary resuscitation. Utero-placental blood flow is also further compromised by compression of the abdominal aorta by the uterus. Placing the mother in the left lateral position or displacing the uterus to the left is essential to minimize aortocaval compression.

Systemic vascular resistance in pregnancy is usually low, thereby minimizing the rise in blood pressure associated with the increase in circulating volume. The central venous and pulmonary capillary wedge pressures seem to remain at prepregnancy values.

During labor there are further dramatic changes in cardiac output. Basal cardiac output increases by 13% in the first stage of labor between contractions and by 34% during contractions. Each contraction displaces a further 300 ml of blood back into the central circulation.[6] Within 24 hours of delivery, all hemodynamic values return to normal.[7]

Respiratory system

Appreciable changes in the respiratory system also occur during pregnancy. Unfortunately, they make the mother less able to tolerate a cardiac arrest. Pregnant women hyperventilate to excrete the excess waste products produced by the feto-placental unit. This hyperventilation leads to a respiratory alkalosis, which is partly compensated for by a decrease in serum HCO_3^- levels that reduces the mother's buffering capacity during circulatory hypoperfusion or cardiac arrest.

Functional residual capacity decreases by as much as 25%, because of upward displacement of the diaphragm.[8] This is further decreased with the patient in the supine position and the dependent airway may close during tidal breathing.[9] Normal oxygen consumption in non-pregnant women is about $3\,ml\,kg^{-1}min^{-1}$, but in pregnancy it increases by up to 16% due to the metabolic demands of the feto-placental unit and the enlarging uterus. Both these factors markedly reduce the tolerance of gravid women to apnea: they rapidly become hypoxemic.

Generalized vasodilatation occurs in the skin and mucous membranes during pregnancy.[9a] Progesterone-induced engorgement of the mucosal membranes can lead to nasal stuffiness and epistaxis.[10] Pregnancy-induced hypertension or upper respiratory tract infection may lead to further edema, exacerbating upper airway problems that add to the difficulty of securing the airway.

Gastrointestinal tract

Progesterone also causes decreased motility of the gastrointestinal tract. Moreover, the position of the stomach is altered by the enlarging uterus, which pushes its long axis – which is usually parallel to the spine – into a more horizontal position.[11] This may hinder gastric emptying and increase the risk of aspiration. The concern over aspiration adds to the importance of securing the airway rapidly during cardiac arrest.

Fetal physiology and outcome

The outcome of resuscitation of the mother determines fetal outcome. The more rapidly the mother is resuscitated (which may include immediate delivery), the more likely the fetus will recover with intact neurological and cardiovascular function. Primate research and human case reports show successful fetal resuscitation if delivery occurs between 5 and 20 minutes after arrest.[12,13]

The fetus has several physiological responses to hypoxia. Shunting and other compensatory mechanisms are known to occur, which may help the infant tolerate hypoxia for slightly longer than adults. Peeters *et al.* showed in sheep that as PO_2 drops, blood is shunted to the heart, brain, and adrenals.[14] Windle found that in rhesus monkeys brain damage occurred after as little as 6 minutes of asphyxia.[15] Clinically there is likely to be additional time taken to deliver and reoxygenate the neonate. Despite these tight timetables, there have been at least two successful resuscitations of a baby after 45 minutes of unsuccessful resuscitation, both in previously healthy mothers who suffered traumatic death.[16,17] It is possible that maternal cardiac arrest may occur after a period of impaired placental perfusion such that fetal adaptive mechanisms may already have been exhausted. For this reason, results from animal models of acute cardiac arrest may not be directly applicable to humans. It is therefore in the interests of both mother and fetus for delivery to occur in as short a time as possible, preferably within 5 minutes of arrest.

Cardiopulmonary resuscitation in pregnancy

Although there is very little research on cardiac arrest in pregnancy, it is generally accepted that conventional protocols recommended by the Resuscitation Councils should be followed, with the modifications listed below. The most recent guidelines can be found on www.resus.org.uk and www.americanheart.org.

Basic life support

Airway

A clear airway must be rapidly established with a head tilt-jaw thrust or head tilt-chin lift maneuvre which must be maintained. Suction should be used to aspirate vomit. Badly fitting dentures and other foreign bodies should be removed and an oral airway inserted. When inserting the airway it is important to place fingers behind the posterior ramus of the mandible in order for the airway to sit behind the tongue. Four-hand ventilation involves using two hands to provide the jaw thrust and another two hands to provide the bag squeezing.[18] These procedures should be performed with the patient inclined laterally or supine with the uterus displaced laterally (see lateral displacement of uterus below).

Breathing

In the presence of apnea, positive pressure ventilation should be started once the airway is cleared; mouth to mouth, mouth to nose, or mouth to airway ventilation should be carried out until a self-inflating bag and mask are available. Ventilation should then be continued with 100% oxygen and reservoir bag. Because of the increased risk of pulmonary aspiration of gastric contents in late pregnancy, cricoid pressure may protect the airway until it is secured by a cuffed tracheal tube. In practice, cricoid pressure may be difficult to apply during the course of resuscitation, particularly in a patient in the lateral position. In addition, when applied by personnel not trained in its regular use, cricoid pressure may cause or worsen airway obstruction and make tracheal intubation more difficult.

Ventilation of the lungs is made more difficult by reduced chest compliance caused by rib flaring and splinting of the diaphragm by the abdominal contents. Because of the increased oxygen requirements of pregnancy, effective pulmonary ventilation is especially important. Observing the rise and fall of the chest in pregnant patients is also more difficult.

Circulation

Circulatory arrest is diagnosed by the absence of a palpable pulse in a large artery (carotid or femoral). Chest compressions are performed at a rate of 100 per minute in a ratio of 15 compressions to 2 breaths. Chest compression is made more difficult by large breasts, obesity, flared ribs, raised diaphragm, and reduced chest compliance. Although no current guidelines exist, it is possible that the hand position for cardiac massage should be moved up the sternum as the diaphragm, and hence the heart, are pushed upwards by the abdominal contents.

The complicating factor of aortocaval compression by the gravid uterus has already been mentioned. Some authorities believe that all attempts at resuscitation will be futile unless the compression is relieved by either placing the patient in an inclined lateral position, using a wedge, or by displacing the uterus manually. Raising the patient's legs will also improve the venous return. Nevertheless, even optimal chest compression with adrenaline in the supine non-pregnant victim produces at best 30% of normal cardiac output, 30%–50% of cerebral blood flow, and only 5%–20% of coronary blood flow.[19] It is not known whether the output from chest compressions with the pregnant patient in the lateral position is adequate for maternal or utero-placental circulation.[20] As early Cesarean section is recommended in such resuscitation situations, open cardiac compression has been advocated because the simple equipment required is already at hand.

In cases of pre-eclampsia or acute fatty liver of pregnancy, the enlarged liver may be more prone to damage during chest compression. If the cause of arrest is thought to be pulmonary embolus, the use of thrombolysis or surgical embolectomy may be life-saving.

According to the 2002 CEMACH report, 34% of mothers were classified as overweight and 23% as obese, an increase from 16% in 1993. Obesity is known to increase the risk of almost every complication of pregnancy and delivery, and the exaggeration of all the physiological difficulties described will make resuscitation more difficult.

Lateral displacement of the uterus

Effective forces for chest compression can be generated with patients inclined at angles of up to 30 degrees, but pregnant women tend to roll into a full lateral position at angles greater than this, making chest compression difficult. Different methods of tilting the mother for cardiac massage include the Cardiff resuscitation wedge[1], the human wedge, or the upturned chair (see Figs. 60.1–60.3). These offer a firm base for chest compressions, at an angle sufficient to displace the uterus. In the human wedge technique, the patient is tilted on to a rescuer's knees to provide a stable position for basic life support, although with an obese parturient this may be uncomfortable for the rescuer. Alternatively, a pillow or foam wedge may be used[21] to wedge the patient into the left inclined position. An assistant should move the uterus further off the inferior vena cava by lifting it with two hands to the left and towards the patient's head. The important principle is to relieve aortocaval compression while allowing adequate chest compression to be performed.

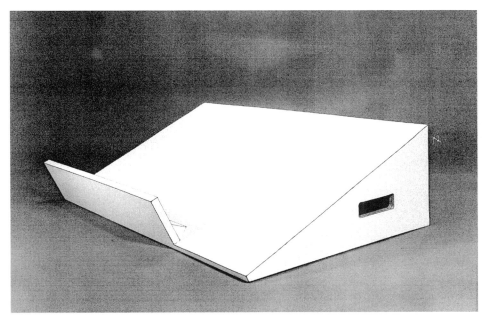

Fig. 60.1. The Cardiff wedge consists of a board with a 30 degree tilt allowing cardiac massage to be performed with the uterus displaced to prevent aorto-caval compression.

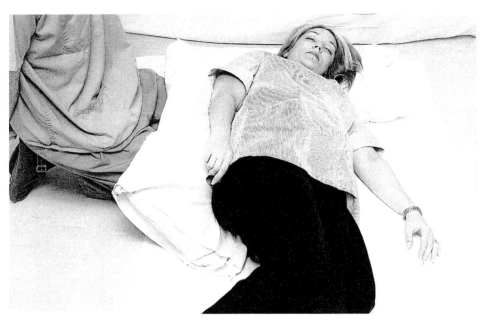

Fig. 60.2. The human wedge: the rescuer uses their knees in order to tilt the patient.

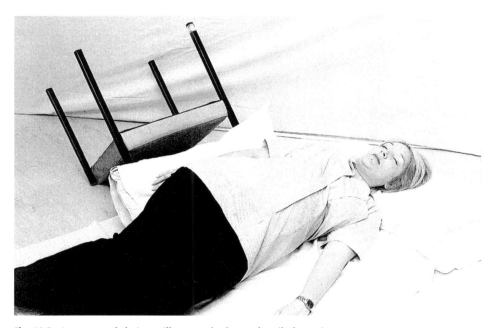

Fig. 60.3. An upturned chair or pillow can also be used to tilt the patient.

Advanced life support

Intubation

Three deaths cited in the anesthetic section of the most recent CEMACH report[22] were directly associated with the failure of airway skills – highlighting the importance of the technique and training of basic airway skills, the use of four-hand ventilation, the right molar approach (see below), and ensuring the correct position of the endotracheal tube after intubation.

Tracheal intubation should be carried out as soon as facilities and skill are available. Difficulty in tracheal intubation is encountered up to 10 times more frequently in women who are pregnant compared with those who are not.[23] Specialized equipment for advanced airway management may be required. A short obese neck and full breasts due to pregnancy may make it difficult to insert the laryngoscope into the mouth. The use of a short-handled laryngoscope or one with its blade mounted at more than 90 degrees (polio/adjustable blade) or demounting the blade from the handle during insertion into the mouth may help. Use of the right molar approach may improve the laryngeal view and increase the likelihood of successful intubation – the laryngoscope is passed down the right molar teeth to access the epiglottis.[24] Furthermore, it is useful to have a gum elastic bougie at hand to aid intubation.

Mouth-to-mouth or bag and mask ventilation is best done without pillows under the head so that the head and neck are fully extended. The position for intubation, however, requires at least one pillow to flex the neck and extend the head. Any pillow removed at initial ventilation must therefore be kept at hand for intubation.

In the event of failure to intubate the trachea or ventilate the patient's lungs with a bag and mask, insertion of a laryngeal mask airway (LMA) should be attempted. Cricoid pressure must be removed temporarily in order to place the LMA successfully.[25] Once the LMA is in place, cricoid pressure should be reapplied. In the non-pregnant population, ventilation through the laryngeal mask is associated with a lower incidence of regurgitation than bag and mask ventilation, suggesting it might have a role as a first-line airway device[26] If the patient has pre-eclampsia, a smaller cuffed endotracheal tube (6.0 mm) should be used for intubation, as there is the potential for laryngeal edema.

Confirmation of correct tube positioning in the trachea ideally would include using capnography to measure end-tidal carbon dioxide levels, but reliance on clinical methods – seeing the endotracheal tube pass through the cords – or use of an esophageal detector[27] may be necessary, depending on the location of the arrest and available equipment.

Defibrillation and drugs

Defibrillation and drug administration should follow advanced life support recommendations. It is difficult to apply an apical defibrillator paddle with the patient inclined laterally, and great care must be taken to ensure the dependent breast does not come into contact with the hand holding the paddle. It is easiest to avoid this problem if adhesive electrodes are used, although defibrillation in an anteroposterior direction is an option. Case reports indicate that shocks of up to 300J have not led to adverse effects in the fetus.[28] Furthermore, elective cardioversion

suggests that the fetal heart is not compromised by the external shock applied to the mother's chest.[29]

Drug delivery

Ideally, all drugs should be injected *via* the intravenous route, preferably by using a central vein. The action of drugs given into the femoral or saphenous veins may be delayed in the presence of aortocaval compression. The administration of drugs by the transtracheal route is probably ineffective[30] because of erratic absorption and unpredictable pharmacokinetics. It is limited to drugs such as adrenaline (epinephrine), atropine, and lidocaine and probably requires doses at least 2–3 times more than the intravenous dose. In the absence of venous access, the intraosseous route is probably a more reliable method of injecting drugs, but its use has not been reported in the resuscitation of pregnant patients.

Intravenous fluids

If the arrest is due to hypovolemia it is appropriate to transfuse intravenous fluids: crystalloid, colloid, or blood may be given. It is always advisable to give resuscitation drugs into a fast running intravenous infusion. If a coagulopathy develops, for example following amniotic fluid embolus, appropriate blood products should be used (fresh frozen plasma, platelets, cryoprecipitate) in consultation with a hematologist. In a resuscitation involving massive blood loss, all fluids should be given via a rapid infusor capable of reliably warming fluids at high flow rates. Such devices should be available in every labor ward and emergency department.

Drug therapy

Standard drug therapy should be used without modification in pregnancy as the primary goal is resuscitation of the mother.[31] Adrenaline should be used, even though vasopressors induce uteroplacental vasoconstriction. Neither calcium nor bicarbonate is recommended in the current resuscitation algorithms. Magnesium, recommended for the treatment of eclampsia, is also often used in the management of pre-eclampsia, and in overdose can cause cardiorespiratory arrest. It is therefore important that volumetric infusion pumps be used, with careful monitoring of plasma concentrations to prevent any inadvertent overdose. If cardiopulmonary arrest is thought to be due to a magnesium overdose, the infusion must be stopped at once, calcium chloride or gluconate should be administered, and immediate delivery should be considered.

The use of sodium bicarbonate to treat maternal acidosis is contentious, as its use will lead to fetal hypercarbia and acidosis.[20] Nonetheless, maternal metabolic acidosis increases the reactivity of the uteroplacental vasculature to alpha-adrenergic agents so that it may be useful to administer bicarbonate post-arrest to correct acidosis if maternal PO_2 and PCO_2 are normal.

Local anesthetic toxicity

Bupivacaine is the commonest long-acting local anesthetic used in obstetric practice, but can produce profound cardiovascular depression after intravenous injection. Bupivacaine rapidly blocks sodium channels by entering intracellular spaces during systole, but its dissociation from sodium channels during diastole is slow, leading to an increase in sodium channel blockade and reduction in traffic through the conducting system.[32] It has been recognized for many years that resuscitation from overdose may be difficult,[33] and this has spurred much animal research into the most effective method of resuscitation. Amrinone,[34–36] vasopressin,[37] insulin and glucose,[38] noradrenaline, isoprenaline, dopamine,[39] magnesium,[40] and lipid emulsion[41] have all been tried with varying degrees of success. Appreciable species differences have been reported in experimental animals.[34,36,42] For this reason and because of the various study methodologies, extrapolation of results to humans requires caution. Some reports do, however, deserve consideration. Adrenaline may worsen ventricular arrhythmias associated with bupivacaine toxicity,[36,39,43] whereas amiodarone may have a role as a relatively safe antiarrhythmic[44] after the discontinuation of bretylium, which was considered the drug of choice for treatment of ventricular arrhythmias.[45–47] Lidocaine should not be used because it lowers the threshold to ventricular tachycardia.[45,48] Weinberg and colleagues[41] found that after a 10 ml/kg bolus of 10% lipid emulsion, normal rhythm was established within 5 minutes, with no electrical countershock, in all of nine experimental dogs even when the administration of the lipid was delayed for 10 minutes to simulate a more realistic arrest scenario. The potential human applications of these findings have been discussed in an editorial (Picard & Meek, 2006). Either the lipid provides a fat-rich compartment into which the local anesthetic becomes partitioned, or the inhibition of carnitine acylcarnitine translocase by the local anaesthetic is overwhelmed. An example of Weinberg's dose regimen for humans is described. (See below). The use of propofol as a source of lipid is not recommended, however. Magnesium is now the treatment of choice for torsades de pointes[49] and should be considered in cases of refractory VF, particularly as patients in late pregnancy may have hypomagnesemia. Its usefulness in cardiac arrest may be limited in that the 2 g

loading dose has to be given over 15 minutes. It is contraindicated if women have received magnesium for the treatment of pre-eclampsia or eclampsia.

Despite these concerns over the toxicity of bupivacaine, it does have a very good safety record in obstetric practice, with **no** reports of maternal death in CEMACH. Furthermore, with the advent of the newer, less toxic, amide local anesthetics ropivacaine and levobupivacaine, the risk of cardiac arrest should be reduced even further.

Weinberg's dose regimen for use in humans (Weinberg, 2004). In cardiac arrest secondary to local anaesthetic toxicity which is unresponsive to standard therapy, intravenous administration of a lipid such as Intralipid® 20% is recommended in the following regimen:

1. give 1 ml kg.$^{-1}$ over 1 min;
2. repeat twice more at 3–5 min intervals;
3. then (or sooner if stability restored), convert to an infusion at a rate of 0.25 ml kg^{-1} per min, continuing until haemodynamic stability is restored;
4. increasing dose beyond 8 ml kg^{-1} is unlikely to be useful;
5. in practice, in resuscitating an adult weighing 70 kg:
   - take a 500 ml bag of Intralipid® 20% and a 50 ml syringe;
   - draw up 50 ml and give it *stat* intravenously, then draw up and give another 20 ml;
   - do exactly the same thing up to twice more as you give epinephrine – if necessary or appropriate;
   - then attach the Intralipid® bag to a giving set and run it intravenously over the next 15 min.

Cesarean section

In 715 BC, the Roman senate decreed that no woman in advanced pregnancy should be placed in the sepulchre until the child was removed from the parent body.[50] Cesarean section was practiced in Egyptian, Persian, Hindu, Finnish, and North American Indian culture.[13,51] Even Shakespeare refers to the practice in "the Scottish play."[52] Because delivery of the fetus is essential to improve maternal and fetal survival, it is advisable to have a simple Cesarean section pack on the maternity unit cardiac arrest cart. Maternal and fetal outcome is determined by a number of factors including: gestational age of fetus, time from maternal arrest to delivery, cause of the arrest, and previous maternal health. Prognosis after cardiac arrest in pregnancy is improved if Cesarean section can be performed within 5 minutes of maternal arrest; after 20 minutes the prognosis is poor.[13,16,53] Once a decision has been made to perform a perimortem Cesarean section, cardiopulmonary resuscitation must be continued throughout and after delivery.

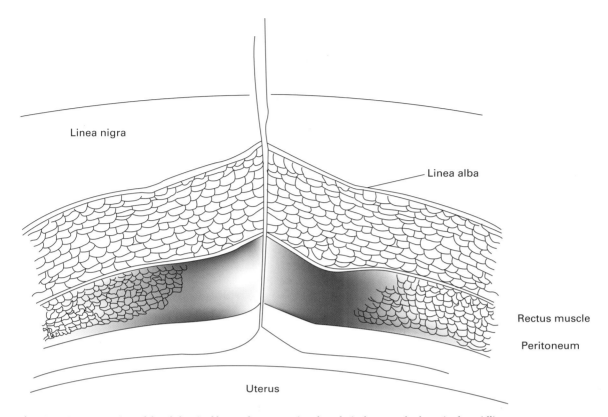

Fig. 60.4. A cross-section of the abdominal layers demonstrating the relatively avascular layer in the midline.

Performing the perimortem Cesarean section

As discussed above, a perimortem Cesarean section is indicated on a pregnant patient in cardiac arrest who has failed to respond to initial resuscitation attempts. The procedure should begin as soon as it is accepted that the mother has little chance of recovery. Resuscitative measures are continued during the surgical procedure in order to maximize uteroplacental perfusion. A few moments are allowed for sterile abdominal preparation, while the bladder is catheterized to decompress it.

A surgeon who is an experienced obstetrician may wish to use a conventional Pfannenstiel incision, but a vertical incision using a scalpel offers the most rapid access into the peritoneal cavity and is probably through one of the more anatomically uncomplicated areas of the abdomen.[54,55] The incision should run from pubis to umbilicus along the linea nigra, between the usually divaricated recti. Ideally the incision should be through the fascial and peritoneal layers, avoiding bowel, bladder, or uterine vessel injury (Fig. 60.4).

Once the peritoneal cavity is entered, the bladder is retracted caudally, away from the uterus. The uterus is entered in the lower segment, just above the bladder, and

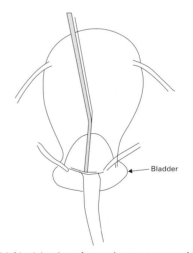

Fig. 60.5. Initial incision into the uterine segment avoiding the bladder.

the vertical incision is extended cranially using scissors. The other hand is placed inside the uterus to protect the fetus from the scissors as the incision continues towards the fundus of the uterus (Figs 60.5 and 60.6). A sufficiently long incision is the key to a rapid delivery.

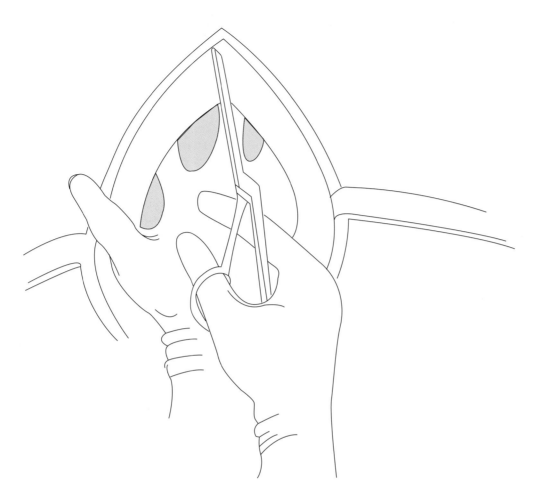

Fig. 60.6. Extension of the uterine incision using the fingers to protect the fetus.

If the placenta lies anteriorly, it must be incised rapidly to deliver the baby.

After completing the uterine incision, all retractors are removed in order to avoid injury to the fetus on delivery. If the fetus is in a vertex position, a hand is inserted between the fetal head and the pubic symphysis; the head is then lifted gently out of the incision. Delivery of the head and shoulders is followed by spontaneous delivery of the body. If the fetus is in breech or transverse position, a feet-first delivery is easiest. Traction to the feet is applied in a gentle progressive manner. In order to minimise damage to the fetus, pressure on the abdomen or lower back should be avoided, with the fetal neck kept in flexion to avoid injury to the cervical spine. Upon delivery of the infant, gentle suction should be applied to nose and pharynx, and clamps applied to the umbilical cord and the placenta.

The child should then be resuscitated as necessary. The open abdomen permits the use of internal cardiac massage. The inside of the uterus must be palpated to exclude the possibility of twins and remove the placenta. After successful delivery, both mother and infant should be transferred to their appropriate intensive care units as soon as clinical conditions permit.

Medicolegal considerations

A perimortem lower segment Caesarean section has the potential for major ethical and consent issues. Operating without consent may be considered as assault on the woman. The doctrine of an "emergency exception" to consent would be applied in most countries, however, allowing for legally acceptable implied consent when a delay in treatment may cause harm or injury.[13] In an emergency situation, where consent cannot be obtained, then doctors may under common law (in some countries), provide treatment to anyone who needs it, provided the treatment is limited to what is immediately necessary to save life or prevent significant deterioration (unless they are aware of a valid advance refusal).

In reality, in view of the 5-minutes time frame, the responsible physician will have to act rapidly and decisively to maximize the chance of a successful resuscitation.

Training

Because cardiac arrest in pregnancy is so rare, it is difficult for groups such as obstetricians and midwives to maintain their skills. There are a number of resuscitation courses available. Some, such as MOET used in the UK,[56] are specifically designed for staff working on delivery suites. Nevertheless, regular update sessions and "fire drills" are essential for the teams to practice their response to life-threatening emergencies.

Ideally, members of the public and healthcare professionals in the emergency service should be aware of the additional problems associated with resuscitation in late pregnancy, because they may have to act as the first responders in the crucial first few minutes after collapse.

Summary

Cardiac arrest in pregnancy is rare, but, if it occurs, requires decisive and rapid treatment. Modification to normal CPR protocols include left tilt, early intubation, and early delivery of the fetus. The key factors for successful resuscitation are that all midwifery, nursery, and medical staff concerned with obstetrics should be trained in cardiopulmonary resuscitation.[57]

REFERENCES

1. Rees, G.A.D. & Willis, B.A. Resuscitation in late pregnancy. *Anaesthesia* 1988; **43**: 347–349.
2. Mable, W.C., Disessa, T.G., Crocker, L.E., Sibai, B.M. & Arheart, K.L. A longitudinal study of cardiac output in normal human pregnancy. *Am. J. Obstet Gynecol* 1994; **170**(3): 849–856.
3. Sadaniantz, A., Kocheril, A.G., Emaus, S.P., Garber, C.E. & Parisi, A.F. (1992). Cardiovascular changes in pregnancy evaluated by two-dimensional and Doppler echocardiography. *J. Am. Soc. Echocardiogr.*1992; **5**(3): 253–258.

4. Mashini, I.S., A.S., Fadel, H.E., Abdulla, A.M. *et al.* Serial non-invasive evaluation of cardiovascular hemodynamics during pregnancy. *Am. J. Obstet. Gynecol.* 1987; **156**(5): 1208–1213.
5. Clark, S.L., Cotton, C.D., Pivarnik, J.M., *et al.* Position change and central hemodynamic profile during normal third-trimester pregnancy and post partum. *Am. J. Obstet. Gynecol.* 1991; **164**(3): 883–887.
6. Hendricks, C.H. The hemodynamics of a uterine contraction. *Am. J. Obstet. Gynecol.* 1958; **76**: 969–982.
7. Robson, S.C., D.W., Boys, R.J. & Hunter, S. Cardiac output during labour. *Br. Med. J. (Clin. Res. Ed.).* 1987; **295**(6607): 1169–1172.
8. Novy, M.J., E.M. Respiratory problems in pregnancy. *Am. J. Obstet. Gynecol.* 1967; **99**(7): 1024–1045.
9. Russell, I.F. & Chambers, W.A. Closing volume in normal pregnancy. *Br. J. Anaesth.* 1981; **53**(10): 1043–1047.
9a Wong, R.C., Ellis, E.C. Physiologic skin changes in pregnancy. *Semin. Dermatol.* 1989 **8**(1): 7–11.
10. Cooley, S.M., Geary, M., O'Connell, M.P. & Keane, D.P. Hypovolaemic Shock Secondary to epitaxis in pregnancy. *J.Obst. Gynaecol.* 2002; **22**(2), 229–230.
11. Williams, N.H. Variable significance of heartburn. *Am. J. Obstet. Gynecol.* 1941; **42**: 814–819.
12. Lanoix, R., Akkapeddi, V. & Goldfeder, B. Perimortem cesarean section: case reports and recommendations. *Acad. Emerg. Med.* 1995; **2**(12): 1063–1067.
13. Katz, V.L., Dotters, D.J. & Droegemueller, W. Perimortem cesarean delivery. *Obstet. Gynecol.* 1986; **68**(4): 571–576.
14. Peeters, L.L., Sheldon, R.E. Jones, M.D. Jr., Makowski, E.L. & Meschia, G. Blood flow to fetal organs as a function of arterial oxygen content. *Am. J. Obstet. Gynecol.* 1979; **135**(5): 637–646.
15. Windle, W. F. Brain damage at birth. Functional and structural modifications with time. *J. Am. Med. Assoc.* 1968; **206**(9): 1967–1972.
16. Lopez-Zeno, J.A., Carlo, W.A. O'Grady, J.P. & Fanaroff, A.A. Infant survival following delayed postmortem cesarean delivery. *Obstet. Gynecol.* 1990; **76**(5 Pt 2): 991–992.
17. Yildirim, C., Goksu, S. Kocoglu, H. Gocmen, A. Akdogan, M. & Gunay, N. Perimortem cesarean delivery following severe maternal penetrating injury. *Yonsei. Med. J.* 2004; **45**(3): 561–563.
18. Stacey, M. Failed intubation in obstetrics. *Anaesth. intens. Care Med.* 2004; **5**(6): 266–268.
19. Lindner, K.H. Cardiopulmonary resuscitation, *Curr. Opin. anaesthesiol.* 1997; **10**: 114–118.
20. Ornato, J.P., Paradis, N. Bircher, N. *et al.* Future directions for resuscitation research. III. External cardiopulmonary resuscitation advanced life support. *Resuscitation* 1996; **32**(2): 139–158.
21. Goodwin, A.P. & Pearce, A.J. The human wedge. A manoeuvre to relieve aortocaval compression during resuscitation in late pregnancy. *Anaesthesia* 1992; **47**(5): 433–434.
22. Cooper, G.M. & McClure, J.H. Maternal deaths from anaesthesia. An extract from *Why Mothers Die 2000–2002, the*

Confidential Enquiries into Maternal Deaths in the United Kingdom: Chapter 9: *Anaesthesia. Br. J. Anaesth.* 2005; **94**(4): 417–423.

23. Barnardo, P.D. & Jenkins, J.G. Failed tracheal intubation in obstetrics: a 6-year review in a UK region. *Anaesthesia* 2000; **55**(7): 690–694.

24. Yamamoto, K., Tsubokawa, T. Ohmura, S., Itoh, H. & Kobayashi, T. Left-molar approach improves the laryngeal view in patients with difficult laryngoscopy. *Anesthesiology* 2000; **92**(1): 70–74.

25. Asai, T., Barclay, K. Power, I. & and Vaughan, R.S. Cricoid pressure impedes placement of the laryngeal mask airway. *Br. J. Anaesth.* 1995; **74**(5): 521–525.

26. Stone, B.J., Chantler, P.J. & Baskett, P.J. The incidence of regurgitation during cardiopulmonary resuscitation: a comparison between the bag valve mask and laryngeal mask airway. *Resuscitation.* 1998; **38**(1): 3–6.

27. Wee, M.Y. The oesophageal detector device. Assessment of a new method to distinguish oesophageal from tracheal intubation. *Anaesthesia* 1988; **43**(1): 27–29.

28. Curry, J.J. & Quintana, F.J. Myocardial infarction with ventricular fibrillation during pregnancy treated by direct current defibrillation with fetal survival. *Chest* 1970; **58**(1): 82–84.

29. Cullhed, I. Cardioversion during pregnancy. A case report. *Acta Med. Scand.* 1983; **214**(2): 169–172.

30. Quinton, D.N., O'Byrne, G. & Aitkenhead, A.R. Comparison of endotracheal and peripheral intravenous adrenaline in cardiac arrest. Is the endotracheal route reliable? *Lancet* 1987; **1**(8537): 828–829.

31. Dildy, G.A. & Clark, S.L. Cardiac arrest during pregnancy. *Obstet. Gynecol. Clin. North Am.* 1995; **22**(2): 303–314.

32. Reiz, S., Nath, S. Cardiotoxicity of local anaesthetic agents. *Br. J. Anaesth.* 1986; **58**: 736–46.

33. Albright, G.A. Cardiac arrest following regional anesthesia with etidocaine and bupivacaine. *Anesthesiology*, 1979; **51**: 285–87.

34. Saitoh, K., Hirabashi, Y., Shimizu, R. & Fukuda, H. Amrinone is superior to epinephrine in reversing bupivacaine-induced cardiovascular depression in sevoflurane anesthetized dogs. *Anesthesiology* 1995; **83**: 127–133.

35. Lindgren, L., Randell, T., Suzuki, N., Kytta, J., Yli-Hankala, A. & Rosenberg, P.H. The effect of amrinone on recovery from severe bupivacaine intoxication in pigs. *Anesthesiology* 1992; 77: 309–315.

36. Heavner, J.E., Mather, L.E., Pitkanen, M. & Shi, B. Should epinephrine be used to treat local anesthetic-induced cardiotoxicity? *Anesthesiology* 1994; **80**: 1179.

37. Mayr, V.D., Raedler, C., Wenzel, V., Lindner, K.H. & Strohmenger, H.U. A comparison of epinephrine and vasopressin in a porcine model of cardiac arrest after rapid intravenous injection of bupivacaine. *Anesth. Analg.* 2004; **99**: 1875–1876.

38. Cho, H.S., Lee, J.J., Chung, I.S., Shin, B.S., Kim, J.A. & Lee, K.H. Insulin reverses bupivacaine-induced cardiac depression in dogs. *Anesth. Analg.* 2000; **91**: 1096–1102.

39. Heavner, J.E., Pitkanen, M.T., Shi, B. & Rosenberg, P.H. Resuscitation from bupivacaine-induced asystole in rats:

comparison of different cardioactive drugs. *Anesth. Analg.* 1995; **80**: 1134–1139.

40. Solomon, D., Bunegin, L. & Albin, M. The effect of magnesium sulphate administration on cerebral and cardiac toxicity of bupivacaine in dogs. *Anesthesiology* 1990; **72**: 341–346.

41. Weinberg, G., Ripper, R., Feinstein, D.L. & Hoffman, W. Lipid emulsion rescues dogs from bupivacaine-induced cardiac toxicity. *Reg. Anesth. Pain Med.* 2003; **28**: 198–202.

42. Kasten, G.W. & Martin, S.T. Comparison of resuscitation of sheep and dogs after bupivacaine-induced cardiovascular collapse. *Anesth. Analg.* 1986; **65**: 1029–1032.

43. Groban, L., Deal, D.D., Vernon, J.C., James, R.L. & Butterworth, J. Cardiac resuscitation after incremental overdosage with lidocaine, bupivacaine, levobupivacaine and ropivacaine in anaesthetized dogs. *Anesth. Analg.* 2001; **92**: 37–43.

44. Kudenchuk, P.J. Intravenous antiarrythmic drug therapy in the resuscitation from refractory ventricular arrythmias. *Am. J. Cardiol.* 1999; **84**: 52–55.

45. Kasten, G.W. & Martin, S.T. Bupivacaine cardiovascular toxicity: comparison of treatment with bretylium and lidocaine. *Anesth. Analg.* 1985; **64**: 911–916.

46. Feldman, H.S., Arthur, G.R., Pitkanen, M., Hurley, R., Doucette, A.M. & Covino, B.G. Treatment of acute systemic toxicity after the rapid intravenous injection of ropivacaine in the conscious dog. *Anesth. Analg.* 1991; **73**: 373–384.

47. Haasio, J., Pitkanen, M.T., Kytta, J. & Rosenberg, P.H. Treatment of bupivacaine-induced cardiac arrythmias in hypoxic and hypercarbic pigs with amiodarone or bretylium. *Reg. Anesth.* 1990; **15**: 174–179.

47a. Picard, J. & Meek, T. Lipid emulsion to treat overdose of local anaesthetic: the gift of the glob. *Anaesthesia* 2006; **61**:107–109.

47b. Weinberg, G. Reply to Drs. Goor, Groban and Butterworth – Lipid rescue: Caveats and recommendations for the "silver bullet" (letter). *Reg. Anesth. Pain Med.* 2004; **29**: 74.

48. Simon, L., Kariya, N., Pelle-Lancien, E. & Mazoit, J.X. Bupivacaine-induced QRS prolongation is enhanced by lidocaine and by phenytoin in rabbit hearts. *Anesth. Analg.* 2002; **94**: 203–207.

49. Tzivoni, D., Keren, A., Cohen, A.M. *et al.* Magnesium therapy for Torsade de Pointes. *Am. J. of Cardiol.* 1984; **53**: 528–530.

50. Lattuada, H.P. Postmortem cesarean section; surgical and legal aspects. *Am. J. Surg.* 1952; **84**(2): 212–214.

51. Weber, C. E. Postmortem cesarean section: review of the literature and case reports. *Am. J. Obstet. Gynecol.* 1971; **110**(2): 158–165.

52. Shakespeare, W. Macbeth.Act, V., scene viii. *William Shakespeare: the Complete Works.* Hamlyn Publishing Group Ltd., 1968.

53. Marx, G.F. Cardiopulmonary resuscitation of late-pregnant women. *Anesthesiology* 1982; **56**(2): 156.

54. Whitten, M. & Irvine, L.M. Postmortem and perimortem caesarean section: what are the indications? *J. R. Soc. Med.* 2000; **93**(1): 6–9.

55. Dezarnaulds, G. & Nada, W. Perimortem Caesarean section: a case report. *Aust. N Z J. Obstet. Gynaecol.* 2004; **44**(4): 354–355.

56. Johanson, R., Cox, C., Grady, K., Howell, C., eds. *Managing Obstet. Emerge. Trauma.* London: RCOG Press; 2003.

57. Morris, S. & Stacey, M. Resuscitation in pregnancy. *Br. Med. J.* 2003; **327**(7426): 1277–1279.

58. O'Connor, R.L. & Sevarino, F.B. Cardiopulmonary arrest in the pregnant patient: a report of a successful resuscitation. *J. Clin. Anesth.* 1994; **6**(1): 66–68.

59. McIndoe, A.K., Hammond, E.J. & Babington, P.C. Peripartum cardiomyopathy presenting as a cardiac arrest at induction of anaesthesia for emergency caesarean section. *Br. J. Anaesth.* 1995; **75**(1): 97–101.

60. Fletcher, S.J. & Parr, M.J. Amniotic fluid embolism: a case report and review. *Resuscitation* 2000; **43**(2): 141–146.

61. Nagar, M.P., Gratrix, A.P., O'Beirne, H.A. & Enright, S.M. Survival following amniotic fluid embolism and cardiac arrest complicated by sub-capsular liver haematoma. *Int. J. Obstet. Anesth.* 2005; **14**(1): 62–65.

62. Milne, S.E. A pregnancy complicated by haemorrhage, cardiac arrest and eclampsia. *Int. J. Obstet. Anesth.* 1998; 7(2): 140–141.

63. Swartjes, J.M., Schutte, M.F. & Bleker, O.P. Management of eclampsia: cardiopulmonary arrest resulting from magnesium sulfate overdose. *Eur. J. Obstet. Gynecol. Reprod. Biol.* 1992; **47**(1): 73–75.

64. Singh, S. & Loeb, R.G.. Fatal connection: death caused by direct connection of oxygen tubing into a tracheal tube connector. *Anesth. Analg.* 2004; **99**(4): 1164–1165.

65. Marx, G.F. Obstetric anesthesia: advances in the 1980s. *Clin. Perinatol.* 1982; **9**(1): 3–12.

66. Eldridge, A.J., Popat, M.T. & Carrie, L.E. Cardiorespiratory arrest and combined spinal/epidural anaesthesia for caesarean section. *Anaesthesia* 1994; **49**(1): 84–85.

67. Parker, J., Balis, N. Chester, S. & Adey, D. Cardiopulmonary arrest in pregnancy: successful resuscitation of mother and infant following immediate caesarean section in labour ward. *Aust. N Z J. Obstet. Gynaecol.* 1996; **36**(2): 207–210.

68. Scull, T.J. & Carli, F. Cardiac arrest after Caesarean section under subarachnoid block. *Br. J. Anaesth.* 1996; **77**(2): 274–276.

69. Coke, G.A., Baschat, A.A., Mighty, H.E. & Malinow, A.M. Maternal cardiac arrest associated with attempted fetal injection of potassium chloride. *Int. J. Obstet. Anesth.* 2004; **13**(4): 287–290.

70. Bowers, W. & Wagner, C. Field perimortem cesarean section. *Air. Med. J.* 2001; **20**(4): 10–11.

71. Ilsaas, C., Husby, P., Koller, M.E., Segadal, L. & Holst-Larsen, H. Cardiac arrest due to massive pulmonary embolism following caesarean section. Successful resuscitation and pulmonary embolectomy. *Acta Anaesthesiol. Scand.* 1998; **42**(2): 264–266.

72. Cardosi, R.J. & Porter, K.B. Cesarean delivery of twins during maternal cardiopulmonary arrest. *Obstet. Gynecol.* 1998; **92**(4 Pt 2): 695–697.

73. Kaiser, R.T. Air embolism death of a pregnant woman secondary to orogenital sex. *Acad. Emerg. Med.* 1994; **1**(6): 555–558.

74. Reuhl, J., Schneider, M., Sievert, H., Lutz, F.U. & Zieger, G. Myocardial sarcoidosis as a rare cause of sudden cardiac death. *Forensic Sci. Int.* 1997; **89**(3): 145–153.

75. Gourley, C., Monaghan, H., Beattie, G., Court, S., Love, C. & Gabra, H. Intra-uterine death resulting from placental metastases in adenocarcinoma of unknown primary. Clin. Oncol. (R. Coll. Radiol.) 2002; **14**(3): 213–216.

61

Drowning

Joost Bierens[1], Robert Berg[2], Peter Morley[3], David Szpilman[4] and David Warner[5]

[1] Department of Anesthesiology, VU University Medical Centre, Amsterdam, the Netherlands
[2] The University of Arizona College of Medicine, Tucson, AZ, 85718, USA
[3] Intensive Care Unit, Royal Melbourne Hospital, Victoria, Australia
[4] Intensive Care Unit, Hospital Miguel Couto, Sociedade Brasileira de Salvamento Aquatico, Rio de Janeiro, Brasil
[5] Departments of Anesthesiology, Neurobiology, and Surgery, Duke University Medical Center, Durham, NC, USA

Drowning refers to submersion and immersion. This chapter focuses on submersion and reviews the epidemiology, pathophysiology, and treatment of this mainly respiratory problem. Hypothermia-related immersion issues are described in Chapter 49.[1]

Epidemiology

Circumstances of drowning vary around the world; from healthy toddlers to desperate boat refugees, and from beach to bathtub. According to the WHO report, each year between 350 000 and 450 000 persons die from drowning. In addition, in some years, over 500 000 persons have drowned in floods and tsunamis. Most drowned victims are children, and the potential years of life lost are immense. Within this global perspective, 97% of all drowning occurs in South East Asia, the Pacific, and Africa. In some areas, the drowning rate is as high as 400 persons per 100 000 inhabitants. The leading cause of drowning in these areas is multifactorial. Leisure, work, transport, and collecting water for household purposes occur in the surroundings of water. Swimming skills are lacking, as is the knowledge on how to perform rescue, first aid, or basic life support (BLS). Also, prevention efforts, rescue resources, or communication equipment are poor.[2–4]

In the Western world, a combination of socioeconomic factors, legislation, multifaceted prevention programs, improved rescue techniques, and up-to-date medical systems have resulted in a 10- to 20-fold decrease in drowning rates during the last 50 years. The death rate is between 0.1 and 2.5 per 100 000 inhabitants. High risk groups are children (because of their exploratory behavior), ethnic minorities (because they have poorer swimming skills and are unfamiliar with water hazards), car occupants (because of blocked escape routes from cars with maximum active safety protection), and water recreationers (because of inadequate preparation and alcohol use). Certain countries or areas have specific, and sometimes unique, risk groups: Alaska and Iceland (commercial fisherman),[5,6] Japan (hot tub drowning),[7] and Australia and the southern areas of the USA (private swimming pool drowning).[8,9] Recent data from the Netherlands suggest another new trend: scoot-mobiles and walker-related drowning in the elder generation.[10] An important cause of drowning in the Western world is suicide, and in some countries the incidence of suicidal drowning is three times larger than that of accidental drowning.[11] Homicide has been suggested to be underreported in pediatric bathtub drowning.[12] For most types of drowning, males have an approximately 4-fold greater incidence of drowning than do females, except for suicide.[12,13]

Prevention remains the most powerful therapeutic intervention and can be effective in more than 85% of drownings. Many predisposing and etiological factors have been identified that can be influenced by improved understanding and training on prevention.[14]

Definition of drowning and data collection

During the 2002 World Congress on Drowning, a consensus was reached on a new definition of drowning: Drowning is the process of experiencing respiratory impairment from submersion or immersion in liquid. This definition is

Cardiac Arrest: The Science and Practice of Resuscitation Medicine. 2nd edn., ed. Norman Paradis, Henry Halperin, Karl Kern, Volker Wenzel, Douglas Chamberlain. Published by Cambridge University Press. © Cambridge University Press, 2007.

accepted by the World Health Organization but needs further classification of causes, morbidity, and mortality.[15,16] Also during this congress, a standard nomenclature on drowning incidents and a standardized reporting mechanism for these data were proposed.[17]

In the definition, two different drowning mechanisms are included. During submersion the head of the victim remains under water and the primary problems are related to hypoxic injuries. During immersion, the head of the victim initially remains above water and the life-threatening dangers are related to the immediate or late consequences of hypothermia. During immersion, splashes of water in the face can result in aspiration, hyponia and unconsciousness with submersion as a result. So both mechanisms can occur simultaneously.

Recognition of a drowned person

A drowning victim usually does not wave or call for help, but remains with the mouth just above the water level and with the arms extended laterally, slapping the water. The victim may submerge and surface several times during 10 to 60 seconds before final submersion occurs. Because all efforts are desperately needed to inhale air, the victim is usually unable to cry out for help.[18] Individuals close by may therefore not recognize that a person is drowning. Children and toddlers typically disappear instantaneously under water without any sign or call of distress.

Pathophysiology of drowning

In spite of the wide variety of drowning circumstances, the pathophysiology of drowning has common characteristics. Some characteristics are distinct from cardiac arrest (for example, gradual onset of circulatory arrest in drowning vs. immediate onset in cardiac arrest) or from trauma (for example: no energy impact in drowning vs. massive energy impact in trauma). Cardiac arrest due to drowning occurs as a result of prolonged anoxia, in a time frame between a few minutes and an hour, or as a result of cold-induced cardiac arrest in a time frame of hours or even days, and is the result of the mechanical impairment of the hypothermic heart and conduction disorders, typically ventricular fibrillation. The most important pathophysiological mechanisms, hypoxia and hypothermia, may be complicated by other factors, such as the diving reflex, aspiration, and trauma.

Submersion

Hypoxia and the circulatory consequences of submersion

When a victim submerges (disappears under water) the most likely immediate response to hypoxia is a short period of tachycardia. As the vagal response of the diving reflex blunts the tachycardia, the victim becomes progressively bradycardic, which is sometimes associated with ventricular ectopy.[19–21] Hypoxia will lead to hypotension and a narrow pulse. This may progress to profound cardiac dysfunction and then cardiac arrest with pulseless electric activity (PEA) or non-perfusing ventricular fibrillation (VF) or ventricular tachycardia (VT). The extreme hypoxic–ischemic insult will ultimately result in asystole.

The circulatory consequences of submersion are in contrast to an arrhythmogenic VF cardiac arrest, where the cardiopulmonary system initially has abundant oxygen. In a submersion cardiac arrest the cardiopulmonary system has profound depletion of oxygen which is clinically obvious by a profound metabolic and respiratory acidosis.[22,23]

Hypoxia and the neurological consequences of submersion

The brain is exquisitely sensitive to interrupted delivery of oxygen and glucose, even if for only a few minutes. Energy failure causes unregulated neurotransmitter release and failure of neurotransmitter reuptake. This leads to excitotoxic stimulation of postsynaptic neurons and breakdown of transmembrane ionic gradients critical for neuronal function. Abrupt cessation of energy supply also causes global shutdown of protein synthesis and failure of proteins to be folded into functional tertiary structures. This creates a toxic state in the endoplasmic reticulum that must be reversed before protein synthesis can recover. In selectively vulnerable structures, this latter process may not be reversible.[24,25]

At the same time, hypoxia impairs mitochondrial function and leads to formation of reactive oxygen and nitrogen species (ROS-RNS) during the early phase of recirculation. Oxidative stress stimulates cellular mechanisms designed to eliminate injured cells by apoptosis and also upregulation of inflammatory mediators. The reaction of ROS-RNS with cell membranes, DNA, and proteins disrupts functions and stimulates futile efforts to repair molecular damage, but at the same time consumes large quantities of energy, thus contributing to further hypoxic damage. The inflammatory responses activate microglia and recruit neutrophils, which in turn further promote oxidative stress. Selective neurological vulnerability is demonstrated in survivors of cardiac arrest. Hippocampal damage may be prominent, while other parts of the brain are unaffected. As a result, survivors who recover consciousness still may have sustained permanent impairment of new memory formation.[26] More severe anoxic insults cause tissue damage in the basal ganglia, cortex, and cerebellum, resulting in motor deficits or permanent impairment of consciousness and cognition. Virtually no study of cerebral pathology has been performed in drowning models. Hence, our understanding of brain damage resulting from drowning is extrapolated from the knowledge of other brain injuries.[27]

Hypoxia and the double role of hypothermia in submersion

Water has a heat conductance capacity that is 25 times greater than air and the body temperature of a person in water drops five times faster than it does in air. As a result, depending on water temperature, body temperature can drop to a lethal level within minutes to hours. This is attributable to hypothermia-induced cardiac arrest. In some drowning cases, however, hypothermia can provide a protective mechanism that allows victims to survive prolonged submersion episodes, in exceptional cases longer than 60 minutes.[28] An important underlying mechanism is reduction of energy consumption by the brain. Reduced oxygen consumption prolongs the interval until cellular anoxia and ATP depletion occur. Hypothermia also stabilizes cellular integrity and slows pathologic processes. Through these mechanisms, hypothermic cells can retain viability until circulation is restored. There is less acidosis and neurotransmitter release, mitochondrial functions are less impaired, and there are fewer signs of oxidative stress and disrupted protein synthesis. These factors are in contrast to non-hypothermic cardiac arrest where deranged brain metabolism has its onset within seconds of interrupted circulation. Hypothermia reduces the electrical and metabolic activity of the brain in a temperature-dependent fashion. The rate of cerebral oxygen consumption is reduced by approximately 5% per °C reduction in temperature within the range of 37–20 °C.[29–33] Thus, reduction of brain temperature by 10 °C reduces the rate of ATP consumption by approximately 50%, doubling the duration of time the brain can survive absence of blood flow. Colder temperatures provide even more profound preservation of energy stores, such that reduction of temperature to 16–18 °C can allow intervals of no-flow of more than 60 minutes in humans.[22]

Table 61.1. Circumstances that facilitate hypothermia and allow the protective effects of low body temperature to become effective

Water colder than 5 °C
Young age
No insulating clothing or body fat
Aspiration of large quantities of water
No survival struggle
Immersion followed by submersion

The conditions that permit miraculous outcomes with cerebral preservation are summarized in Table 61.1. Hypothermia, if present, may prolong the window of opportunity for successful resuscitation, allowing victims of a cardiac arrest secondary to submersion in cold water potentially to have a much better outcome than would otherwise be expected.[34]

The diving reflex and submersion

Some experts on drowning speculate that the diving reflex provides a protective mechanism against drowning pathophysiology. The diving reflex is a well-known reflex in aquatic mammals, such as whales and dolphins, and occurs when the animal submerges under water.[19,21] The diving reflex has also been studied in humans during diving into very deep water,[20] in studies on the diabetes-related autonomic dysfunction of the sympathetic and parasympathetic nervous systems, and in other diseases.[35,36]

Selective vasoconstriction is the mechanism of protection in the diving reflex. When the head, and specifically the sensory distribution of the trigeminal nerve, is in sudden contact with water, blood flow is preferentially directed to the heart and brain, the organs most vulnerable to hypoxia. Cold water enhances the occurrence of the reflex. Because oxygen consumption in these two organs is less than total body oxygen consumption, oxygenation of the brain and heart is better sustained. The reduced total body oxygen consumption delays the time interval until a hypoxia-induced cardiac arrest occurs. It is hypothesized that the diving reflex buys time until the organ-protective effects of hypothermia come into action. Bradycardia is the clinically observed consequence of the diving reflex, with a heart rate often below 40 beats per minute.[20,21]

Aspiration and submersion

A still less understood pathophysiological factor in submersion is aspiration. Although drowning victims, by definition, have signs of respiratory impairment, not all drowning victims have signs of aspiration, and respiratory impairments often resolve spontaneously. Signs of aspiration are found in 80–90% of the autopsies of fatal submersion incidents.[37] The percentage of patients who are admitted with signs of aspiration varies among countries and health systems. Clinical signs of aspiration occur only in 10%–20% of submerged victims admitted to hospitals in The Netherlands,[38,39] while this is almost 100% in hospitals in Brazil.[40]

In many drowning victims, laryngospasm occurs instantaneously when inhaled water contacts the vocal cords and this laryngospasm will temporarily prevent aspiration. Many victims will be saved before laryngospasm has ceased. In other victims the dying process will have advanced to a stage where efforts to breathe occur after laryngospasm has ceased. For this reason, but possibly also due to other yet unknown factors, massive aspiration is seldom present and most drowned victims will have aspirated limited amounts of water.

Small amounts of aspirated water may have serious clinical consequences. Water in the alveoli causes wash-out of surfactant (mostly in fresh water) or destruction of surfactant (mostly in salt water), or both. Differences in osmotic gradients can pull water from the lungs to the circulation with fresh-water drowning. In contrast, more water can be drawn into the lungs from the circulation with salt-water drowning. In either situation, the effect of the osmotic gradient on the very delicate alveolar-capillary membrane can disrupt the integrity of the membrane, increase its permeability and exacerbate fluid, plasma, and electrolyte shifts.[41,47]

The clinical picture of the damage caused to the alveolar–capillary membrane is a massive, often red stained, pulmonary edema. The combined effects of fluids in the lungs, loss of surfactant, and increased capillary–alveolar permeability can result in decreased lung compliance, increased right-to-left shunting in the lungs (up to 80%), atelectasis, and bronchospasm. Although the clinical picture resembles the classical adult respiratory distress syndrome (ARDS), the underlying mechanism in drowning is due to local damage rather than systemic inflammatory reactions. This is probably the main reason why ARDS after drowning resolves within 48 hours, unless an underlying pulmonary infection, chemically induced pneumonia, or massive aspiration of gastric contents is present.[38]

Electrolyte disorders during submersion

In the 1970s, electrolyte disorders were considered to be the most relevant pathophysiological threat in drowning.[42–44]

It has now been confirmed that electrolyte disorders play a minor role in the initial cardiovascular events after submersion. These disorders, if they occur at all, can be corrected by common regulatory mechanisms when the victim reaches a hospital. The salinity of the water in which the victim has been submerged generally has limited impact on the pathophysiology and outcome, except in extreme conditions such as drowning in the Dead Sea or drowning in unusual industrial environments.[45–47] No evidence exists for any therapeutic benefit of administration of hypertonic solutions after fresh water submersion or hypotonic solutions after salt-water submersion.[48]

Treatment

Very few emergency medical system (EMS) personnel and clinicians have had sufficient clinical experience with the treatment of drowned victims. Those who have this experience often have a specific geographically determined focus on the treatment of these victims, such as drowning on the beaches of Rio de Janeiro (most of which are in warm water) or drowning in the cold North Sea (most of which are in cold water). Since the body's response to drowning is related to the environment in which drowning occurs, local circumstances should be taken into consideration in deciding treatment strategies and protocols.[49]

Rescue and in-water basic life support

Rescue and in-water BLS is a typical link in the management of drowning victims (Fig. 61.1). All persons who attempt a rescue from the water should be aware of the risks of the sometimes hostile environment.[50]

Rescuers should avoid becoming second victims by advising the victim on how to get out of the dangerous situation, by reassuring that assistance is coming, or by using a "throw or reach rescue technique." When entering water is unavoidable, this should be done cautiously. The victim should be transported to shore immediately without further treatment, and removed from the water, when possible with the head above body level to avoid vomiting and aspiration. The victim should then be placed parallel to the waterline, and, when the accident occurs on a seashore, far enough from incoming waves.

Trained rescuers have learned how to avoid unnecessary risks, to calm the victim, to reach out in a safe way, and to bring the victim to land.[50,51] In some countries rescuers have learned in-water ventilation (Perkins, 2005). Although this may seem futile, in-water ventilation applied by two or three professional lifesavers in Rio de Janeiro

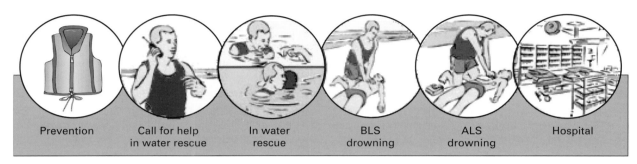

| Prevention | Call for help in water rescue | In water rescue | BLS drowning | ALS drowning | Hospital |

Fig. 61.1. Basic life support (BLS) is a typical link in the management of drowning victims.

(Brazil) can increase survival sevenfold.[52] In most other situations, ventilation is initiated after the victim is removed from the water, when the physical support of ground, boat, or surfboard is available. Even for trained rescuers a pulse check in water is unreliable and thoracic compressions in water are impossible.[50]

There has been some concern about cervical spine injuries, especially from high energy impact, such as occurs with kite-surfers, water skiers, and occupants of motorized water craft.[54,55] Yet in several large studies of water-related episodes, the incidence of cervical spine injuries among submersion victims is less than 0.5%.[11,51] The possibility of a spinal injury causes conflicting priorities with respect to whether resuscitation or spinal stabilization should take precedence. If there are no signs of cervical spinal injury (history of trauma or a bruised forehead), no time should be spent to immobilize the cervical spine. BLS measures always have priority above spine stabilization. Indeed, if the victim is not breathing spontaneously, resuscitation should start without any special attention to the cervical spine. When spinal cord injury is suspected, however, rescuers should float the victim horizontally supine with an open airway well out of the water. If there is spontaneous breathing, the hands of the rescuers can stabilize the neck in a neutral position. If immediately available, a floating back support device can be used to facilitate alignment of the victim's head, neck, chest, and body before moving the victim.[53]

Basic life support (BLS) on land

Cardiopulmonary or respiratory arrest occurs only in 0.5% of all rescued victims, but most drowning victims have some level, albeit temporary, of respiratory, circulatory, or neurological impairment (Szpilman 1997). Immediate bystander BLS on land is crucial in all these situations, but is most important in victims of cardiac arrest. Chance of

survival dramatically decreases if BLS is delayed.[56] For this reason, policemen, firefighters, and EMS personnel should know how to perform a water rescue, and those who work or live close to water should know how to perform BLS on a drowning victim.[57]

The first BLS action for an unconscious drowning victim on land is to open the obstructed airway and to place the victim in a recovery position. When the victim is not breathing, mouth-to-mouth ventilation should be started. This can be strenuous because of increased airway resistance, loss of surfactant, and hypothermia-induced tissue rigidity.

After 2 minutes of mouth-to-mouth ventilation, the presence of circulation should be assessed to determine if thoracic compressions should be performed. A pulse check in drowning victims is likely to be unreliable. Vasoconstriction and bradycardia are often present, caused by hypoxia, hypothermia, and the diving reflex, but if there are no signs of circulation, thoracic compressions should be started.

Ventricular fibrillation is rare in drowning patients. The automated external defibrillator (AED) therefore has a limited role in BLS after drowning[58] (www.ilsf.org: position statement). Limiting BLS to thoracic compressions only, as recommended as a good alternative in primarily cardiac arrest, is counterproductive in drowning because the lethal component is hypoxia. Thus, ventilation of the lungs must be restored first.

Prevention of aspiration of vomitus is important. Vomiting occurs in 50% of initially symptom-free victims, in more than 65% of victims who need ventilation, and 85% of victims who need BLS.[8,51] Vomitus in the mouth must be removed. A check for seaweed, sand, or mud in the airway is only performed in rare situations, when effective ventilation cannot be achieved.

Active drainage of the lungs by placing the victim head down, by firmly compressing the thorax, or by abdominal thrust is not recommended, because this increases the risk of vomiting more than fivefold and leads to 19% increase in mortality (www.ilsf.org: position statement).

Advanced Life Support (ALS) on land

The skills and qualifications to provide ALS by EMS providers differ among countries and even within counties.[1,56] The preferred situation is that all ALS measures be provided by the EMS system, but if the EMS is unable to do so, BLS should be continued while the victim is transported as soon as possible to a hospital. When on shore, both the victim and the rescuer should always receive medical attention from the EMS team.

The immediate treatment of the respiratory consequences is essential. Also, when circulation is intact, oxygen is the first-line therapy. Initially, oxygen can be administered by a non-rebreathing mask at 15 liters per minute. Minor cases may require only a nasal cannula with 5 liters of oxygen per minute. With respiratory arrest, artificial bag-mask ventilation is initially performed with 15 liters of oxygen and an estimated tidal volume of 5–8 ml per kg of body weight. If the respiratory situation does not improve, an endotracheal tube should be inserted immediately. Suctioning through the endotracheal tube to enable visualization of the vocal cords when intubating may be necessary when copious pulmonary edema foam drains from the trachea. Once the victim is intubated, oxygenation and ventilation with positive end expiratory pressure (PEEP) can be started. The initial PEEP-level at 5 cm H_2O is increased when hemoglobin oxygen saturation, as measured by pulse oximetry, is below 92%. The initial oxygen inspiration fraction (F_iO_2) is 1 but can be reduced to 0.45 or less when hemoglobin oxygen saturation is above 92%. The quality of the signal of the pulse oximeter in the cold, and thus vasoconstricted, patient should always receive extra attention when interpreting the results, as in this situation readings may be inaccurate.[59,60]

In many life-threatening postrescue situations, the initial rhythm is an extreme bradycardia or PEA. If improvement of oxygenation has not resulted in improved circulation, cardiotonic drugs are started. Because of the cold-induced vasoconstriction and the non-cardiogenic pulmonary edema fluid in the airways, both the peripheral and endotracheal administration of drugs are unreliable. A central venous approach via the external or internal jugular vein is the preferred route.[18]

In a cardiorespiratory arrest situation, cardiac compression should be started as soon as oxygenation and ventilation are secured. High-dose epinephrine can be considered in drowning if 1-mg doses fail, because the pathophysiological mechanisms are different, the cardiac arrest is secondary to hypoxia, the pharmocodynamic effects of hypothermia require a higher initial dose to be effective, and the time elapsed to cardiac arrest can be very long. Many victims have initially marginal cardiac function. If circulation and a regular cardiac rhythm with a mean arterial pressure (MAP) below 90 mmHg is present after rescue, and circulation measures do not improve with oxygenation and lifting of the legs, rapid crystalloid infusion is indicated.[18,61]

Drowning severity and treatment decision scheme

One of the most difficult medical decisions for those who provide BLS or ALS at the rescue site is how to treat victims with less life-threatening conditions appropriately. In these situations, a treatment decision scheme can be used (Table 61.2). The scheme is validated for 41 279 rescues, including 1831 drownings.[40]

Treatment in the emergency department

In situations where the EMS system has established all ALS measures, treatment in the emergency department (ED) focuses on:

– acquisition of information
  ● circumstances of the drowning incident
  ● previous illnesses of the victim
  ● quality of rescue, BLS and ALS
– further optimization of ALS measures and diagnosis
– decision-making
  ● continue or stop resuscitation efforts
  ● admit to an ICU
  ● observation in the ED
  ● discharge

When the EMS system is not able to provide some, or all, ALS measures in the prehospital situation, all remaining ALS measures must be established first.

Additional ALS measures may also be needed in the ED, for example when the clinical condition of the patient worsens after an initially mild clinical course. Notably, in these patients a very aggressive therapeutic approach is needed in order to stay ahead of a rapidly evolving life-threatening complication.

Acquisition of information in the ED

Relevant information includes details on the location, cause, and circumstances of the accident, water and air temperature, water salinity and contamination (bacteria,

Table 61.2. Drowning treatment decision scheme at the rescue site

Grade	Signs and symptoms	Treatment on land (basic and advanced life support)	Mortality on site (%)	Mortality in hospital (%)
Rescue	Conscious, normal auscultation, no coughing, foam or difficulty in breathing	Evaluation and release from the accident site without further medical care	0	0
1	Normal pulmonary auscultation, coughing, no foam in mouth or nose	Rest, warm and calm the victim. No further medical care	0	0
2	Rales in some pulmonary fields, small amount of foam in mouth or nose	5 liters oxygen per minute by nasal cannula; warm and calm the victim; recovery position, hospitalization	0.6	4.0
3	Large amount of foam in mouth or nose, normotension, palpable radial pulse	15 liters oxygen per minute by non-rebreathing mask, intubation when possible; recovery position if unconscious; hospitalization.	5.2	11.5
4	Large amount of foam in mouth or nose, hypotension, no radial pulse but palpable carotid pulse	Grade 3 treatment extended by crystalloid infusion via peripheral vein until restoration of systolic arterial pressure >90 mmHg; hospitalization	19.4	19.4
5	Isolated respiratory arrest	Mouth-to-mouth (when possible with 15 liters of oxygen) until restoration of normal breathing, then treat as grade 4.	44.0	33.3
6	No cardiac activity on ECG, cardiopulmonary arrest	Start CPR; insert tracheal tube, obtain venous access, give epinephrine; defibrillate if necessary. After succesful CPR: follow grade 4.	93.0	43.5
Dead body	Submersion time over 1 hour and no cardiac activity on ECG monitoring; or obvious rigor mortis, putrefaction or dependent lividity	Do not start BLS or ALS; arrange morgue.	100	100

Adapted from ref. 40.

chemical), wave conditions, submersion time, timing and quality of rescue, BLS and ALS.

Causes of the submersion incident should be sought and may include accidents,[54] epilepsy,[62] acute myocardial infarction, stroke, alcohol use, drug use, and psychiatric conditions.[39] History of the victim, but also of family members, may reveal the possibilty of a prolonged QT syndrome.[63–65] Focal neurological signs suggest stroke or trauma. A significant number of submersion victims are foreign to the area and language difficulties may cause problems in acquiring this information.[66]

Further optimizing ALS measures and diagnosis in the ED

The position of an endotracheal tube inserted out-of-hospital should always be checked immediately on admission to the ED, because the wet surface of the skin, transport on rough ground, and high inflation pressures increase the risk of tube dislocation. Airway obstruction due to foreign bodies is rare, but fiberoptic bronchoscopy should always be considered. Bronchoscopy allows therapeutic clearing of sand, gravel, and other solids, which can lead to atelectasis of large lung areas. The extent of airway injury can be determined and cultures obtained to define bacterial infection.

Each drowned patient needs a thorough respiratory check-up. Inspiratory crackles indicate the presence of ARDS or atelectasis as a result of aspiration.[67] Arterial blood gas analysis, with and without oxygen, and a chest radiograph will further confirm the presence of pulmonary problems and provide baseline information. When an endotracheal tube is in place, a nasogastric tube should also be placed. The reduction of gastric distention, resulting from insufflation during BLS, facilitates ventilation and prevents further aspiration.

The respiratory condition of a submersion victim often improves during the first 6 hours. In some patients, however, the condition can seriously deteriorate and continous pulse oximetry as well as regular arterial blood gas analysis and monitoring of respiratory rate and respiratory efforts are needed to identify this category. An altered chest radiograph on admission should not be interpreted as pneumonia, as this is usually the result of pulmonary edema and aspirated water in the alveoli and bronchi. Young victims are often able to compensate for respiratory insufficiency with extra respiratory effort during prolonged periods. These patients are likely to seriously decompensate and it is advised not to wait until the moment of exhaustion to perform endotracheal intubation. In some patients, continuous positive airway pressure (CPAP) or other non-invasive respiratory therapies may be beneficial, provided that this is not contraindicated for the patient and this technique does not cause panic or gastric distension.[68–70]

Ventilation in drowning patients with ARDS can be extremely difficult because of massive pulmonary edema, decreased pulmonary compliance, and bronchospasm. High levels of PEEP improve oxygenation after drowning, but may impair hemodynamics. PEEP may be increased by 2 to 3 cm H_2O increments until arterial blood gases show an intrapulmonary shunt (QS:QT) of 20% or less, or until a PaO_2:FiO_2 ratio of 250 or more is achieved. Optimal PEEP can also be titrated by determining the lower inflection point of the compliance curve of the respiratory system, or by PEEP trials between 5 and 15 cm H_2O PEEP.[71–73] Once the desired oxygenation is achieved, that given level of PEEP should ideally be maintained unchanged for 48 hours before attempting to decrease the PEEP level. This period is needed for adequate surfactant regeneration. Unlike ARDS of a systemic cause, arterial oxygenation often improves dramatically when local lung damage has recovered and PEEP can be progressively decreased. Once weaning from the ventilator commences, it is almost always successful within 48–72 hours

and some 75% of the patients with ARDS after drowning survive.[38]

The Brain Resuscitation Task Force at the World Congress on Drowning 2002 concluded that maintenance of normocapnia is recommended during the ICU period for the best chance of neurological recovery.[27] Because both hypocapnia and permissive hypercapnia have unwanted circulatory and neurological effects,[74] the usual strategy for lung protection by permitting hypercapnia should be avoided.[75]

Low cardiac output is common after severe drowning and is the result of the hypoxic insult, arrhythmias, relative or absolute hypovolemia, and hypothermia.[48] Often, the circulation state improves with better oxygenation, 2–3 liters of crystalloid fluid, and rewarming. Monitoring of urine output and clinical assessment of the peripheral circulation in the extremities provides relevant information on the quality of circulation. Poor response to the therapy requires additional information (e.g., by central venous pressure measurements, echocardiography, or transesophageal echocardiography) for further assessment of cardiac function. Depending on this information, further volume loading with colloids, inotropic support, or use of vasopressors may be indicated. Titration of adrenaline or dobutamine administered through a central venous catheter to a MAP of 90–100 mmHg is reasonable. The sometimes paradoxical hemodynamic effects of these drugs in a hypothermic patient should always be taken into consideration.[76–78] Traumatic blood loss should always be excluded in hemodynamically unstable patients.[79] The pulmonary edema seen in drowning patients is most likely of non-cardiogenic origin and thus furosemide is rarely indicated. The use of prophylactic antiarrhythmics, even after ventricular fibrillation, is controversial. Treatment of arrhythmias that have negative effects on circulation is appropriate. Before starting with antiarrhythmic drugs, oxygenation, circulation, sedation, and pain treatment should be adequate and electrolyte abnormalities (especially K^+ and Mg^{2+}) should be corrected.

The majority of the submerged victims in the ED have a metabolic and respiratory acidosis.[18,22,80–82] This should be corrected with adequate ventilation and circulation. The use of bicarbonate is only indicated when the pH remains below 7.1, or the bicarbonate level remains below 12 mEq/l, despite improved circulation and ventilation.

Extremes of temperature may occur. Hypothermia is often present and can contribute to a reversible loss of consciousness. Hypothermia may have some potential benefit for organ preservation. Attempts at rewarming should be tempered by the potential neurological benefits associated with induced hypothermia after cardiac arrest.[27,83,84] Hypothermia also adds complex management issues with regard to the appropriate timing, speed, and techniques for rewarming. In the case of a hypothermic cardiac arrest, resuscitation should be continued until the temperature reaches 33 °C, because below this temperature many drugs, as well as defibrillation, are less effective. Above 33 °C the cardiac physiology returns to normal.

The several methods of rewarming are included in Chapter 49.

On the other hand, hyperthermia may also occur as an overshooting reaction on rewarming or as a systemic response to pulmonary or systemic damage. Hyperthermia should be prevented or aggressively treated as the increased temperature severely enhances neurological damage.[27]

Important other investigations in the ED include measurement of electrolytes, blood urea nitrogen, creatinine, and hemoglobin. Free hemoglobin measures hint at aspiration of fresh water.[85] Additional investigations should be guided by the presentation and likelihood of abnormalities.

If cervical spine injuries are suspected, appropriate radiological procedures should be undertaken to guide further management.[86] High-speed impact injuries should be treated as if caused by trauma and films of cervical spine and pelvis are needed. Focal neurological signs suggest a need for a head computerized tomogram (CT).

Decision where to go after the ED

Hospitalization can be avoided in drowning victims who have a normal pulmonary examination, a normal chest radiograph, normal room air oxygen saturation after 6–8 hours of observation, and who have no significant comorbid disease.[38,40,87] Prediction of the likelihood of successful resuscitation is very difficult and survivors have been reported after particularly severe physiological conditions. In hypothermic pediatric patients, prognosis is even more difficult.[1,22,23,82,88,8,9] In general, a submersion period of 10 minutes is associated with good survival when rescue, BLS, and ALS are performed adequately and no other factors interfere (such as previous illnesses or trauma). Often the submersion duration is unknown. Most normothermic adult and pediatric patients are neurologically intact if restoration of spontaneous circulation occurs within 25 minutes of the initiation of ALS techniques or within 1 hour of the initiating submersion event.[39,90,91]

Given reports of asystolic drowning victims who were eventually resuscitated after several hours of ALS, it is appropriate to continue cardiopulmonary resuscitation efforts until adequate rewarming has occurred. The decision to proceed with time, material, and manpower measures that are so time-consuming must be based on clinical experience, availability of resources, and the patient's premorbid state. Information on a slow speed and low quality of rescue, the delayed start of bystander resuscitation, injuries, co-morbidities, and complications is relevant to the decision to discontinue resuscitation. In deep hypothermic cardiac arrest, cardiopulmonary bypass (CPB) is the most effective therapy to improve circulatory, ventilatory, and biochemical indices.[92] The transfer of a hypothermic cardiac arrest child to a center with CPB facilities has been life-saving on several occasions.

Complications in the ICU

In the Intensive Care Unit (ICU), the treatment that started in the prehospital setting and ED must be continued. Most complications that occur in the ICU are common for intensive care patients, but some additional considerations are needed.

Respiratory complications at the ICU

Usually, the water from pools and beaches have too few bacterial colonies to result in pneumonia just after the incident. If the victim needs mechanical respiratory assistance, the incidence of secondary pneumonia increases to 52% on the third or fourth day of hospitalization, a time when pulmonary edema caused by drowning has usually resolved.[38] As a general rule, prophylactic antibiotics should be avoided in the ICU as they tend to select out resistant organisms. This should be limited to scenarios where obviously contaminated water has been involved. The choice of antibiotic agents is complex, but beta-lactam agents (e.g., penicillins or cephalosporins) are reasonable first-line agents for prophylaxis.

In all cases, daily monitoring of tracheal aspirates with Gram stain, culture, and sensitivity is recommended. A large variety of common and uncommon endogenous and exogenous micro-organisms can be detected. The first signs of pulmonary infection usually occur after the first 48 to 72 hours: prolonged fever, sustained leukocytosis, persistent or new pulmonary infiltrates, and presence of leukocytes in the tracheal aspirate. Antibiotic therapy is selected on the basis of the predominant organism in cultures in the ICU and their sensitivities. Some pulmonary infections are very severe. Irreversible multiple organ failure and other septic complications have been reported in the first 24 hours after successful resuscitation.

Artificial exogenous or endogenous surfactant has been used successfully in these very serious ARDS cases as rescue treatment, although insufficient data exist about the appropriate delivery techniques, quantities, and timing of administration.[93,94] Also extracorporeal membrane oxygenation[95,96] and the use of the prone position have been reported to be successful.[97] Treatment of pulmonary edema with corticosteroids has no benefit,[98] although corticosteroids may be useful together with bronchodilators to treat bronchospasm.

Apart from ventilation-related infections, the intensivist must be constantly vigilant for volutrauma and barotrauma. Spontaneous pneumothoraces, secondary to positive pressure ventilation, and local areas of hyperinflation occur in some 10% of ventilated drowning patients admitted to the ICU. Sudden hemodynamic instability during the first hour of mechanical ventilation should be considered to be due to volume depletion, after which a tension pneumothorax (or other barotrauma) should be excluded as a cause.

Circulatory complications

Hypotension may initially be attributed to a period of severe hypoxia, hypovolemia, or hypothermia. When hypotension persists after adequate treatment, pre-drowning myocardial disease, hypoxic myocardial dysfunction, or a profound inflammatory response (that develops over the subsequent hours) should be considered. Information from echocardiography and a pulmonary artery catheter about preload and contractility may be required to facilitate diagnosis and optimal management. A protocol with routine use of central venous catheter and SVO_2 in the early resuscitative phase of patients with sepsis appeared to improve outcome,[99] but the use of invasive monitoring (including a pulmonary artery catheter) still remains controversial.[100,101] The role of these or newer methods of monitoring the circulation, such as PICCCO®, has yet to be studied in drowning.

Neurological complications

Among survivors of a drowning accident, success will be measured in terms of the quality of neurologic recovery.[102] Despite this, there is little information derived from either patients or from animal models that specifically addresses appropriate cerebral resuscitation. This is most likely attributable to the sporadic presentation of drowning victims to any one center and the considerable variability of severity of insult with respect to duration of circulatory arrest, body temperature, and efforts by first responders to provide BLS. Thus, current practice to treat neurological complications is largely extrapolated from the study of anoxic encephalopathy, traumatic brain injury, and stroke.

Restoration of oxygenated blood flow to the brain is the highest priority in drowning victims to restore lack of oxygen, the principal cause of cellular demise in the brain. Immediate cardiopulmonary resuscitation remains the most effective response to drowning.

When circulation and ventilation are established, additional therapies are of limited benefit. Tissue plasminogen activator (t-PA) has been effective for treating some forms of ischemic brain injury. t-PA serves to lyse clots in stroke victims however, and thus has little or no role in drowning patients. Although the anachronistic practice of treating brain injury patients with steroids persists in some environments, both experimental and human evidence indicates that steroids are most likely to increase mortality and worsen neurological outcome, either by promoting hyperglycemia or increasing the frequency of systemic complications.[103] Thus, pharmacological therapy for drowning victims is currently limited to management of seizures, which, at least in cardiac arrest are a common complication of anoxic encephalopathy.

Physiologic factors can play a major role in achieving an optimal neurological outcome from acute brain injury. Although none of these factors has been studied specifically in human or experimental drowning scenarios, sufficient evidence is available from study of other forms of acute brain injury to suggest recommendations for the management of temperature, blood glucose concentration, and blood gas characteristics.

Of these, temperature management seems most promising. In most animal models, brain temperature causes profound effects on the extent of ischemic brain injury. Mild hypothermia (32–34 °C) is highly protective, even if started after circulation has been restored, but postresuscitation-induced hypothermia must be sustained for intervals of 12–24 hours to provide persistent benefit. With use of this strategy, benefit from induced mild hypothermia in comatose survivors of out-of-hospital ventricular fibrillation cardiac arrest has been demonstrated.[78,104,105]

In many drowning victims, resuscitation is started in a mild or severe hypothermic patient. Therefore, the Brain Resuscitation Task Force assembled at the World Congress of Drowning 2002 recommended that hypothermic drowning victims who remain comatose after restoration of spontaneous circulation be maintained at 32 °C –34 °C or be treated with deliberate mild hypothermia initiated as soon as possible,[27] and sustained for 12–24 hours. Patients treated with mild hypothermia should be endotracheally intubated, mechanically ventilated, with shivering prevented. Hypnotics, analgesics, and neuromuscular blockade may be used as required to maintain hypothermia. Electroencephalographic monitoring should be considered to detect seizures. At completion of induced hypothermia, passive rewarming is recommended at a rate no greater than 0.5–1.0 °C per hour.

Hyperthermia is a common sequel to acute brain injury in humans, with the incidence in cardiac arrest survivors approaching 70%[106] is also common in drowning victims in the ICU. Hyperthermia has been shown repeatedly profoundly to exacerbate brain injury in experimental animals, even when onset of hyperthermia occurs many hours after the primary insult.[107] It is therefore recommended that hyperthermia in drowning survivors be treated aggressively.

Hyperglycemia exacerbates most forms of experimental brain injury. This has been attributed to enhanced anaerobic glycolysis resulting in intracellular acidosis and increased corticosterone concentration.[105,108] Although hyperglycemia is most damaging when present during the insult, there is accumulating evidence that ongoing strict regulation of blood glucose reduces mortality and complications.[109–111] Based on this evidence, blood glucose concentration in the drowning patient with a neurologic deficit should be monitored frequently and it appears reasonable to aim for normoglycemic values (80–110 mg/dl; 4.4–6.1 mM).

There is an increasing capability to monitor both the physiology and neurophysiology of brain-injured humans. Although monitoring of evoked potentials, intracerebral microdialysates (neurotransmitters and lactate concentrations), jugular venous oxygen saturation, and intracranial pressure (ICP) have been utilized in traumatic brain injury, there is little evidence that use of these monitors alters outcome from anoxic encephalopathy (but see ref.112). ICP monitoring may be considered, however, if permissive hypercapnia is required for oxygenation in drowning victims with ARDS.

In cardiac arrest studies, repeated assessment of S-100B and neuron specific enolase has been shown to have value in predicting neurologic outcome,[113,114] but although promising, there is insufficient evidence at this time to recommend routine use of these neurochemical markers in guiding management of drowning encephalopathy.

Other complications

Hypoxia and hypothermia result in pathophysiological injuries at a celluluar level in all organs. The brain and the heart are the most vulnerable, but all other organs can also

be affected. Many drowning victims suffer from a wide range of complications that can extensively prolong the ICU stay, ranging from the induction of otherwise asymptomatic conditions (Yoshinaga *et al.* 1999), to various acute stresses on the respiratory and cardiovascular systems, including myocardial infarction, stroke, renal failure, and rhabdomyolysis.

Specific pediatric aspects

Drowning is a leading cause of morbidity and mortality in the pediatric population of most countries.[2–4] There is less information concerning morbidity, but it is estimated that, for each drowning death, there are 1 to 4 non-fatal submersions requiring hospitalization. Such submersion injuries are often severe, requiring prolonged care and considerable monetary and emotional costs.[3,11,90,91] Childhood drowning generally occurs in two groups: toddlers and adolescents. Toddlers often enter water unintentionally and during brief lapses in supervision. Once immersed in even small amounts of water, toddlers are unable to rescue themselves because of their cognitive and physical immaturity. Both males and females have a peak in drowning rates during toddler years.

The pathophysiology of childhood drowning is similar to that for adults except that children have a relatively larger ratio of surface area to body mass. Therefore, children can become hypothermic during icy water drownings much more readily than adults, perhaps resulting in better protection of the brain and heart. Also the diving reflex is more likely to occur in children. At the same time, toddlers rarely show panic when drowning, but remain calm while under water. Both aspects keep the oxygen consumption low. This may explain the great preponderance of children in reports of impressively good saves, notably from prolonged icy water drownings.

Most will agree that childhood deaths have a greater impact on society than do adult deaths. For each child drowning death, more years of productive life are lost compared with an adult drowning death. Furthermore, there is a devastating impact on multiple persons associated with the victim. Childhood death from drowning leads to far-reaching impacts on public health[3,91,115]

Coping with a sudden unexpected death is always difficult. When the victim is a child, the loss is generally even more devastating. In modern developed countries, childhood death is unusual and many people have a strong belief that children are not supposed to die. Consequently, the death of a child is often difficult to accept. Children are an integral part of a family unit and their death has a deep and lasting impact for those close to them. The death of their child is frequently inconceivable to parents. In addition to immediate family, the profound and long-lasting impact often affects large numbers of people who have relationships with the child and family.

Childhood death is also stressful for health care providers. They may feel an additional burden in caring for the family as well as for the victim, while concurrently attempting to deal with their own emotions regarding childhood death. Many prehospital and emergency personnel are inexperienced in caring for children and feelings of inadequacy may provoke additional stress after an unsuccessful pediatric resuscitation. Decision-making is different when the victim is a child and some health care providers are uncomfortable with a process that involves an extended family unit. Others may appreciate the support system that families typically provide for their children.

Support for families of childhood drowning victims and for healthcare providers involved in the unsuccessful resuscitation deserves great emphasis.

Summary

In low and middle income countries, drowning is an important but neglected issue. In high income countries the incidence of drowning is low and attracts limited clinical and research attention. It is important to realize that drowning is primarily a process of acute respiratory impairment. The drowning patient is most of all a challenge for those involved in preventive medicine, rescue, BLS, and ALS. Diagnostic flaws and therapeutic obstacles have to be dealt with in the prehospital situation. In the hospital, rapidly presenting ARDS, optimal usage of hypothermic protection, providing cardiovascular stability, and optimal neurological outcome are therapeutic challenges.

REFERENCES

1. Bierens, J.J.L.M., Knape, J.T.A. & Gelissen, H.P.M.M. Drowning. *Curr. Opin. Crit. Care* 2002; 8: 578–586.

2. Krug, R. *Injury. A Leading Cause of the Global Burden of Disease.* WHO: Geneva, 1999.

3. WHO. *Facts about Injuries: Drowning.* WHO, Geneva, 2003. www.who.int/violence_injury_prevention/

4. UNICEF/TASC. Towards a world safe for children. Bangkok 2004. www.tasc-gcipf.org

5. Rafnsson, V. & Gunnarsdottir, H. Risk of fatal accidents occurring other than at sea among Icelandic seamen. *Br. Med. J.* 1993; **306**: 1379–1381.

6. Lincoln, J.M. & Conway, G.A. Preventing commercial fishing deaths in Alaska. *Occup. Env. Med.* 1999; **56**: 691–695.

7. Yoshioka, N., Chiba, T., Yamauchi, M., Monma, T. & Yoshizaki, K. Foresic considerations of death in the bath tub. *Legal Med.* 2003; **5**: S375–S381.

8. Manolios, N. & Mackie, I. Drowning and near-drowning on Australian beaches patrolled by life-savers: a 10-year study, 1973–1983. *Med. J. Aust.* 1988; **148**: 165–167 and 170–171.

9. Scott, I. Prevention of drowning in home pools-lessons from Australia. *Inj. Control Saf. Promot.* 2003; **10**: 227–236.

10. Maatschappij tot Redding van Drenkelingen (MRD). Recommendations World Congress on Drowning. Amsterdam 2003. www.drowning.nl.

11. Bierens, J.J.L.M. Drowning in The Netherlands. Pathophysiology, epidemiology and clinical studies. Ph.D. thesis. University Utrecht; 1996.

12. Kemp, A.M., Mott, A.M. & Sibert, J.R Accidents and child abuse in bathtub submersions. *Arch. Dis. Child* 1994; **70**: 435–438.

13. Howland, J., Hingson, R., Mangione, T.W., Bell, N. & Bak, S. Why are most drowning victims men? Sex differences in aquatic skills and behaviors. *Am. J. Public Health* 1996; **86**: 93–96.

14. Bennett, E. National and community campaigns. In Bierens, J.J.L.M. (ed.) *Handbook on Drowning. Prevention, Rescue, Treatment.* Springer Verlag 2005: 117–132.

15. Beeck, F. van, Branche, C., Szpilman, D., Modell, J. & Bierens, J.J.L.M. A new definition of drowning: towards documentation and prevention of a global public health problem. *Bull. World Health Org.* 2005; **83**: 1–4

16. Papa, L., Hoelle, R. & Idris, A. Systematic review of definitions for drowning incidents. *Resuscitation* 2005; **65**: 255–264.

17. Idris, A.H., Berg, R.A., Bierens, J. *et al.* Recommended guidelines for uniform reporting of data from drowning: The Utstein Style. *Circulation* 2003; **108**: 2565–2574.

18. Orlowski, J.P. & Szpilman, D. Drowning. Rescue, resuscitation, and reanimation. *Pediatr. Clin. N. Am.* 2001; **48**: 627–646.

19. Hochachka, P.W., Gunga, H.C. & Kirsch, K. Our ancestral physiological phenotypes: an adaptation for hypoxia tolerance and for endurance performance ? *Proc. Natl Acad. Sci. USA* 1998; **95**: 1915–1920.

20. Lemaitre, F., Bernier, F., Petit, I., Renard, N., Gardette, B. & Joulia, F. Heart rate responses during a breath-holding competition in well-trained divers. *Int. J. Sports Med.* 2005; **26**: 409–413.

21. Foster, G.E. & Sheel, A.W. The human diving response, its function, and its control. *Scand. J. Med. Sci. Sports* 2005; **15**: 3–12.

22. Gilbert, M., Busund, R., Skagseth, A., Nilsen, P.Å. & Solbø, J.P. Resuscitation from accidental hypothermia of 13.7 °C with cardiac arrest. *Lancet* 2000; **355**: 375–376.

23. Wollenek, G., Honawar, N., Golej, J. & Marx, M. Cold water submersion and cardiac arrest in treatment of severe

hypothermia with cardiopulmonary bypass. *Resuscitation* 2002; **52**: 255–263.

24. Petito, C.K., Feldman, E., Pulsinelli, W.A. & Plum, F. Delayed hippocampal damage in humans following cardiorespiratory arrest. *Neurology* 1987; **37**: 1281–1286.

25. Zola-Morgan, S., Squire, L.R., Rempel, N.L., Clower, R.P. & Amaral, D.G. Enduring memory impairment in monkeys after ischemic damage to the hippocampus. *J. Neurosci.* 1992; **12**: 2573–2581.

26. Grubb, N.R., O'Carroll, R., Cobbe, S.M., Sirel, J. & Fox, K.A.A. Chronic memory impairment after cardiac arrest outside hospital. *B. Med. J.* 1996; **313**: 143–146.

27. Warner, D. & Knape, J. Recommendations and consensus brain resuscitation in the drowning victim. In Bierens, J.J.L.M (ed). *Handbook on Drowning. Prevention, Rescue, Treatment.* Springer Verlag, 2005: 436–439.

28. Bolte, R.G., Black, P.G., Powers, R.G., Kent-Thorne, J. & Cornell, H.M. The use of extracorporeal rewarming in a child submerged for 66 minutes. *J. Am. Med. Assoc.* 1988; **260**: 377–379.

29. Silverberg, G.D., Reitz, B.A. & Ream, A.K. Hypothermia and cardiac arrest in the treatment of giant aneurysms of the cerebral circulation and hemangioblastoma of the medulla. *J. Neurosurg.* 1981; **55**: 337–346.

30. Michenfelder, J.D. & Milde, J.H. The relationship among canine brain temperature, metabolism, and function during hypothermia. *Anesthesiology* 1991; **75**: 130–136.

31. Milde, L.N. Clinical use of mild hypothermia for brain protection: a dream revisited. *J. Neurosurg. Anesthesiol.* 1992; **4**: 211–215.

32. Wass, C.T., Lanier, W.L., Hofer, R.E., Scheithauer, B.W. & Andrews, A.G. Temperature changes of $>1\,^{\circ}C$ alter functional neurologic outcome and histopathology in a canine model of complete cerebral ischemia. *Anesthesiology* 1995; **83**: 325–335.

33. Polderman, K.H. Application of therapeutic hypothermiua in the ICU: opportunities and pitfalls of a promising treatment modality. Part 1: indications and evidence. *Intens. Care Med.* 2004; **30**: 556–575.

34. Kuisma, M. & Jaara, K. Unwitnessed out-of-hospital cardiac arrest: is resuscitation worthwhile? *Ann. Emerg. Med.* 1997; **30**: 69–75.

35. Oei-Reyners, A.K.L. Cardiovascular autonomic function tests: methodological considerations and clinical application. PhD thesis University Groningen. Groningen 2002

36. Paton, J.F., Boscan, P., Pickering, A.E. & Nalivaiko, E.The yin and yang of cardiac autonomic control: vago-sympathetic interactions revisited. *Brain Res. Rev.* 2005; **49**: 555–565.

37. Modell, J.H. Aspiration. In Bierens J.J.L.M. (ed.) *Handbook on Drowning. Prevention, Rescue, Treatment.* Springer Verlag 2005: 407–410.

38. Berkel, M. van, Bierens, J.J.L.M., Lie, R.L.K. *et al.* Pulmonary oedema, pneumonia and mortality in submersion victims. A retrospective study in 125 patients. *Int. Care Med.* 1996; **22**: 101–107.

39. Bierens, J.J.L.M., Velde, E.A., van der, Berkel, M. van & Zanten, J.J. van. Submersion in the Netherlands: prognostic indicators and results of resuscitation. *Ann. Emerg. Med.* 1990; **19**: 1390–1395.

40. Szpilman, D. Near-drowning and drowning classification: a proposal to stratify mortality based on the analysis of 1,831 cases. *Chest* 1997; **112**: 660–665.

41. Modell, J.H., Moya, F. & Newby, E.J. The effects of fluid volume in sea water drowning. *Ann. Int. Med.* 1967; **67**: 68–80.

42. Giammona, S.T. & Modell, J.H. Drowning by total immersion: effects on pulmonary surfactant of distilled water, isotonic saline and sea water. *Am. J. Dis Child.* 1967; **114**: 612–616.

43. Modell, J.H., Calderwood, H.W. *et al.* Effects of ventilatory patterns on arterial oxygenation after near-drowning in sea water. *Anesthesiology* 1974; **40**: 376–384.

44. Modell, J.H., Graves, S.A. & Ketover, A. Clinical course of 91 consecutive near-drowning victims. *Chest* 1976; **70**: 231–238.

45. Hussain, I.R., Edenborough, F.P., Wilson, R.S. & Stableforth, D.E. Severe lipoid pneumonia following attempted suicide by mineral oil immersion. *Thorax* 1996; **51**: 652–853; discussion 656–657.

46. Segev, D., Szold, O., Fireman, E., Kluger, Y. & Sorkine, P. Kerosene-induced severe acute respiratory failure in near drowning: reports on four cases and review of the literature. *Crit. Care Med.* 1999; **27**: 1437–1440.

47. Saidel-Odes, L.R. & Almog, Y. Near-drowning in the Dead Sea: a retrospective observational analysis of 69 patients. *Isr. Med. Assoc. J.* 2003; **5**: 856–858.

48. Orlowski, J.P., Abulleil, M.M. & Phillips, J.M. The hemodynamic and cardiovascular effects of near-drowning in hypotonic, isotonic, or hypertonic solutions. *Ann. Emerg. Med.* 1989; **18**: 1044–1049.

49. Soar, J., Deakin, C.D., Nolan, J.P. *et al.* European Resuscitation Council guidelines for resuscitation 2005. Section 7. Cardiac arrest in special situations. *Resuscitation* 2005; **6751**: S135-S170.

50. Szpilman, D., Morizot-Leite, L., Vries, W. *et al.* First aid courses for the aquatic environment. In Bierens, J.J.L.M. (ed.) *Handbook on Drowning: Prevention, Rescue,Treatment.* Springer Verlag, 2005.

51. Szpilman, D., Idris, A. & Cruz-Filho, F.E.S. Position of drowning resuscitation victim on sloping beaches; World Congress on Drowning, Amsterdam 2002, *Book of Abstracts*:168.

52. Szpilman, D. & Soares, M. In-water resuscitation: is it worthwhile? *Resuscitation* 2004; **63**: 25–31.

53. Wernicki, P., Fenner, P. & Szpilman, D. Immobilisation and extraction of spinal injuries. In: Bierens, J.J.L.M. (ed.) *Handbook on Drowning. Prevention, Rescue, Treatment.* Springer Verlag, 2005: 291–295.

54. Shatz, D.V., Kirton, O.C., McKenney, M.G. *et al.* Personal watercraft crash injuries: an emerging problem. *J. Trauma* 1998; **44**: 198–201.

55. Watson, R.S., Cummings, P., Quan, L., Bratton, J. & Weiss, N.S. Cervical spine Injuries among submersion victims. *J. Trauma* 2001; **51**: 658–662.

56. Pepe, P. & Wenzel, V. Advanced life support: In Bierens, J.J.L.M. *Handbook on Drowning: Prevention*, Rescue Treatment. Springer Verlag, 2005: 348–351.

57. American Heart Association in collaboration with International Liaison Committee on Resuscitation. Guidelines 2000 for Cardiopulmonary Resuscitation and Emergency Cardiovascular Care: International Consensus on Science,. Part 8: advanced challenges in resuscitation. Section 3: special challenges in ECC. 3B: submersion or near-drowning. *Resuscitation* 2000 ;**46**: 1–3, 273–277.

58. Beerman, S. & Løfgren, B. Automated external defibrillators in the aquatic environment. In Bierens, J.J.L.M. (ed.) *Handbook on Drowning. Prevention, Rescue Treatment.* Springer Verlag, 2005: 331–336.

59. MacLeod, D.B., Cortinez, L.I., Keifer, J.C. *et al*. The desaturation response time of finger pulse oximeters during mild hypothermia. *Anesthesia* 2005; **60**: 65–71.

60. Kober, A., Scheck, T., Lieba, F. *et al*. The influence of active rewarming on signal quality of pulse oximetry in prehospital trauma care. *Anesth. Analg.* 2002; **95: 961–966.**

61. Farstad, M. & Husby, P. Fluid management during treatment of immersion hypothermia. In Bierens, J.J.L.M. (ed.) *Handbook on Drowning. Prevention, Rescue, Treatment.* Springer Verlag, 2005: 514–519.

62. Diekema, D.S., Quan, L. & Holt, V. Epilepsy as a risk factor for submersion injury in children. *Pediatrics* 1993; **9**: 612–616.

63. Ackerman, M.J., Tester, D.J. & Porter, C.J. Swimming, a gene-specific arrhythmogenic trigger for inherited long QT syndrome. *Mayo Clin. Proc.* 1999; **74**: 1088–1094.

64. Ott, P., Marcus, F.I. & Moss, A.I. Ventricular fibrillation during swimming in a patient with long QT syndrome. *Circulation* 2002; **106**: 521–522.

65. Bove, A., & Rienks, R. Long Q.T. Syndrome and drowning: In Bierens J.J.L.M. *Handbook on Drowning; Prevention, Rescue Treatment.* Springer Verlag, 2005: 352–356.

66. Leahy, S.J., Fenner, P.J., Harrison, S.L. & Tebb, N. Olympic visitors need to be told about the dangers of the Australian surf. Australian and New Zealand *J. Public Health* 1999; **4**: 442.

67. Simcock, A.D. Near drowning. In Grieves, I. & Porter, K. (eds.). *Pre-hospital Medicine.* London: Arnold 1999.

68. Hore, C.T. Non-invasive positive pressure ventilation in patients with acute respiratory failure. *Emerg. Med.* 2002; **14**: 281–295.

69. Truwit, J.D. & Bernard, G.R., Noninvasive ventilation: Don't push too hard. *N. Engl. J. Med.* 2004; **350**: 2512–2515.

70. Caples, S.M. & Gay, P.C. Noninvasive positive pressure ventilation in the intensive care unit : a concise review. *Crit. Care Med.* 2005; **33**: 2651–2658.

71. Barbes, C.S., Matos de, G.F., Okamoto, V., Borges, J.B., Amato, M.B. & Carvalho, C.R. Lung recruitment maneuvers in acute respiratory distress syndrome. *Respir. Care Clin. N. Am.* 2003; **9**: 401–418.

72. Albaiceta, G.M., Luyando, L.H., Parra, D. *et al*. Inspiratory vs expiratory pressure-volume curves to set end-expiratory pressure in acute lung injury. *Int. Care Med.* 2005; **31**: 1370–1378.

73. Pestana, D., Hermandez-Gancedo, C., Royo, C., Perez-Chrzanowska, H. & Criado, A. Pressure–volume curve variations after recruitment manoeuvre in acute lung injury/ARDS patients: implications for the understanding of the inflection points of the curve. *Eur. J. Anesthesiol.* 2005; **22**: 175–180.

74. Aufderheide, T.P., Sigurdsson, G., Pirrallo, R.G. *et al*. Hyperventilation-induced hypotension during cardiopulmonary resuscitation. *Circulation* 2004; **109**: 1960–1965.

75. The Adult Respiratory Distress Syndrome Network. Ventilation with lower tidal volumes as compared to traditional tidal volumes for acute lung injury and the acute respiratory distress syndrome. *N. Engl. J. Med.* 2000; **342**: 1301–1308.

76. Weiss, S.J., Muniz, A., Ernt, A.A., Lippton, H.L. & Nick, T.G. The effect of prior hypothermia on the physiological response to norepinephrine. *Resuscitation* 2000; **45**: 201–207.

77. Kornberger, E., Lindner, K.H., Mayer, V.D.P. *et al*. Effects of epinephrine in a pig model of hypothermic cardiac arrest and close-chest cardiolpulmonary resuscitation combined with active rewarming. *Resuscitation* 2001; **50**: 301–308.

78. Bernard, S.A., Gray, T.W., Buist, M.D. *et al*. Treatment of comatose survivors of out-of-hospital cardiac arrest with induced hypothermia. *N. Engl. J. Med.* 2002; **346**: 557–563.

79. Pepe, P.E., Raedler, C., Lurie, K. & Wigginton, J.G. Emergency ventilatory management in hemorrhagic states: elemental or detrimental. *J. Trauma* 2003; **54**: 1048–1057.

80. Opdahl, H. Survival put to the acid test: extreme arterial blood acidosis (pH 6.33) after near drowning. *Crit. Care Med.* 1997; **25**: 1431–1436.

81. Schummer, W. & Schummer, C. Survival put to the acid test: extreme arterial blood acidosis (pH 6.33) after near drowning. *Crit. Care Med.* 1999; **27**: 2071–2073.

82. Suominen, P., Baillie, C., Korpela, R., Rautanen, S., Ranta, S. & Olkkola, K.T. Impact of age, submersion time and water temperature on outcome in near-drowning. *Resuscitation* 2002; **52**: 247–254.

83. Bernard, S.A. & Buist, M.Induced hypothermia in critical care medicine: a review. *Crit. Care Med.* 2003; **31**: 2041–2051.

84. Nolan, J.P., Morley, P.T., Vanden Hoek, T.L. & Hickey, R.W. Therapeutic hypothermia after cardiac arrest: an advisory statement by the advanced life support task force of the International Liaison Committee on Resuscitation. *Circulation* 2003; **108**: 118–121.

85. Conn, A.W., Miyasaka, K., Katayama, M. *et al*. A canine study of cold water drowning in fresh versus salt water. *Crit. Care Med.* 1995; **23**: 2092–2037.

86. Morris, C.G., McCoy, E.P. & Lavery, G.G. Spinal immobilisation for unconscious patients with multiple injuries. *Br. Med. J.* 2004; 329; 495–499.

87. Causey, A.L., Tilelli, J.A. & Swanson, M.E. Predicting discharge in uncomplicated near-drowning. *Am. J. Emerg. Med.* 2000; **18**: 9–11.

88. Lavelle, J. & Shaw, K. Near-drowning: Is emergency department cardiopulmonary resuscitation or intensive care unit

cerebral resuscitation indicated? *Crit. Care Med.* 1993; **21**: 368–373.

89. Salomez, F. & Vincent, J.-L. Drowning: a review of epidemiology, pathophysiology, treatment and prevention. *Resuscitation* 2004; **63**: 261–268.

90. Quan, L. & Kinder, D. Pediatric submersions: prehospital predictors of outcome. *Pediatrics* 1992; **90**: 909–913.

91. Ellis, A.A. & Trent, R.B. Hospitalizations for near drowning in California: incidence and costs. *Am. J. Public Health* 1995; **85**: 1115–1118.

92. Walpoth, B.H., Walpoth-Aslan, B.N., Mattle, H.P. *et al.* Outcome of survivors of accidental deep hypothermia and circulatory arrest treated with extracorporeal blood warming. *N. Engl. J. Med.* 1997; **20**: 1500–1505.

93. Anker, A.L., Santora, T. & Spivey, W. Artificial surfactant administration in an animal model of near drowning. *Acad. Emerg. Med.* 1995; **2**: 204–210.

94. Haitsma & Lachmann, B. Surfactant therapy. In Bierens, J.J.L.M. (ed.). *Handbook on Drowning. Prevention, Rescue, Treatment.* Springer Verlag, 2005: 419–423.

95. Eich, C., Brauer, A. & Kettler, D. Recovery of a hypothermic drowned child after resuscitation with cardiopulmonary bypass followed by prolonged axtracorporeal membrane oxygenation. *Resuscitation* 2005; **67**: 145–148.

96. Peralta, R., Ryan, D.P., Iribrane, A. & Fitzsimons, M.G. Extracorporeal membrane oxygenation and CO_2 removal in an adult after near drowning. *J. Extra Corpor. Technol.* 2005; **37**: 71–74.

97. Tulleken, J.E., Werf, T.S. van der, Ligtenberg, J.J., Fijen, J.W. & Zijlstra, J.G. Prone position in a spontaneously breathing near-drowning patient. *Int. Care Med.* 1999; **25**: 1469–1470.

98. Foex, B.A. Corticosteroids in the management of near-drowning. *Emerg. Med. J.* 2001; **18**: 465–466.

99. Rivers, E., Nguyen, B., Havstad, S. *et al.* Early goal-directed therapy in the treatment of severe sepsis and septic shock. *N. Engl. J. Med.* 2001; **345**: 1368–1377.

100. Kern, J.W. & Shoemaker, W.C. Meta-analysis of hemodynamic optimization in high-risk patients. *Crit. Care Med.* 2002; **30**: 1686–1692.

101. Richard, C., Warszawski, J. Anguel, N. *et al.* Early use of the pulmonary artery catheter and outcomes in patients with and acute respirtory distress syndrome A randomised controlled trial. *J. Am. Med. Assoc.* 2003;**290**:2713–2720.

102. Bohn, D.J., Biggar, W.D., Smith, C.R., Conn, A.W. & Barker, G.A. Influence of hypothermia, barbiturate therapy, and intra-cranial pressure monitoring on morbidity and mortality after near-drowning. *Crit. Care Med.* 1986; **14**: 529–534.

103. Roberts, I., Yates, D., Sandercock, P. *et al.* Effect of intravenous corticosteriods on death within 14 days in 10008 adults with clinically significant head injury (MRC CRASH trial): randomised placebo-controlled trial. *Lancet* 2004; **364**: 1321–1328.

104. Colbourne, F. & Corbett, D. Delayed postischemic hypothermia: a six month survival study using behavioral and histologic assessments of neuroprotection. *J. Neurosci.* 1995; **15**: 7250–7260.

105. Hypothermia After Cardiac Arrest Study (HACAS) Group. Mild therapeutic hypothermia to improve the neurologic outcome after cardiac arrest. *N. Engl. J. Med.* 2002; **346**: 549–556.

106. Albrecht, R.F., Wass, C.T. & Lanier, W.L. Occurrence of potentially detrimental temperature alterations in hospitalized patients at risk for brain injury. *Mayo Clin. Proc.* 1998; **73**: 629–635.

107. Baena, R.C., Busto, R., Dietrich, W.D., Globus, M.Y. & Ginsberg, M.D. Hyperthermia delayed by 24 hours aggravates neuronal damage in rat hippocampus following global ischemia. *Neurology* 1997; **48**: 768–773.

108. Payne, R.S., Tseng, M.T. & Schurr, A. The glucose paradox of cerebral ischemia: evidence for corticosterone involvement. *Brain Res.* 2003; **97**: 9–17.

109. Li, P.A. & Siesjo, B.K. Role of hyperglycaemia-related acidosis in ischaemic brain damage. *Acta Physiol. Scand.* 1997; **161**: 567–580.

110. Van den Bergh, G., Wouters, P., Weekers, F. *et al.* Intensive insulin therapy in critically ill patients. *N. Engl. J. Med.* 2001; **345**: 1359–1367.

111. Krinsley, J.S. Effect of an intensive glucose management protocol on the mortality of critically ill adult patients. *Mayo Clin. Proc.* 2004; **79**: 992–1000.

112. Hermon, M.M., Golej, J., Burda, G. & Trittenwein, G. Monitoring of cerebral oxygen saturation with a jugular bulb catheter after near-drowning and respiratory failure. *Wien. Klin. Wochenschr.* 2003; **115**: 128–131.

113. Rosen, H., Rosengren, L., Herlitz, J. & Blomstrand, C. Increased serum levels of the S-100 protein are associated with hypoxic brain damage after cardiac arrest. *Stroke* 1998; **29**: 473–427.

114. Schoerkhuber, W., Kittler, H., Sterz, F. *et al.* Time course of serum neuron-specific enolase. A predictor of neurological outcome in patients resuscitated from cardiac arrest. *Stroke* 1999; **30**: 1598–1603.

115. Christensen, D.W., Jansen, P. & Perkin, R.M. Outcome and acute care hospital costs after warm water near drowning in children. *Pediatrics* 1997; **99**: 715–721.

62

Anaphylactic shock

Richard Pumphrey

Department of Immunology, Manchester Royal Infirmary, Manchester M13 9WL, UK

The discovery of anaphylaxis

In 1902, Richet and Portier were attempting to immunize dogs with venom extracted from sea anemones (Actinia). To their surprise, instead of being protected, some dogs had apparently become more sensitive to the effect of the venom: they became acutely ill and died within minutes of the second injection. They had expected protection (prophylaxis) but had, they thought, achieved the opposite, which they termed anaphylaxis.[1] It soon became clear that this was not enhanced toxicity of the venom, but rather a dangerously severe acute allergic reaction that could equally be triggered by non-toxic proteins. Prausnitz demonstrated in 1921[2] that this hypersensitivity could be transferred by a heat-labile component of the serum, but it was not until 1966 that the Ishizakas identified this component as immunoglobulin E (IgE).[3]

Hypersensitivity reactions take many forms and these were classified in 1968 by Gell and Coombes;[4] IgE-mediated hypersensitivity was labelled type I. More recently, the nomenclature committee of the European Academy of Allergy and Clinical Immunology (EAACI) has recommended it should simply be called "IgE-mediated hypersensitivity."[5]

Definitions of anaphylaxis

The term "anaphylaxis" has been used for all types of acute life-threatening illness triggered by abnormal sensitivity to a trigger agent, and for apparently spontaneous attacks with similar features (idiopathic anaphylaxis). This has made it difficult to define. The EAACI Nomenclature Committee proposed the following broad definition:[5]

Anaphylaxis is a severe, life-threatening, generalized or systemic hypersensitivity reaction.

The term allergic anaphylaxis should be used when the reaction is mediated by an immunological mechanism such as IgE, IgG, or complement activation by immune complexes. An anaphylactic reaction mediated by IgE antibodies, such as peanut-induced food anaphylaxis, may be referred to as IgE-mediated allergic anaphylaxis. The term "anaphylactoid" reaction had been introduced for anaphylactic reactions not mediated by IgE,[6] but the EAACI committee has recommended that this term should no longer be used. These proposals were updated in 2003.[7]

This proposal has not been universally accepted. An authoritative recent American practice parameter[8] states: "Anaphylaxis is defined . . . as a condition caused by an IgE-mediated reaction. Anaphylactoid reactions are defined as those reactions that produce the same clinical picture as anaphylaxis but are not IgE mediated."

Diagnosis

In practical terms, **anaphylaxis is a variable acute illness, characteristically evolving over minutes. It may cause fatal shock or asphyxia, but otherwise resolves spontaneously within hours** (Table 62.1).

Although anaphylaxis commonly involves respiratory, cutaneous, and circulatory changes, variations such as shock with gastrointestinal disturbance or shock alone are possible. Alternatively, reactions may be fatal without

Cardiac Arrest: The Science and Practice of Resuscitation Medicine. 2nd edn., ed. Norman Paradis, Henry Halperin, Karl Kern, Volker Wenzel, Douglas Chamberlain. Published by Cambridge University Press. © Cambridge University Press, 2007.

Table 62.1. Mode of death in 188 cases of fatal anaphylaxis recorded in the UK fatal anaphylaxis register

	Age (years)	0–9	10–19	20–29	30–39	40–49	50–59	60–69	70–79	≥ 80
Foods	shock		1	2	2					
	larynx			5	1	4		1		1
	d.i.b		3	10	4		1			
	asthma	4	18	6	4	2	1	1		
	inhaled vomit		2			1				
Stings	shock			1	3	7	3	4	3	2
	larynx					2	3	1	3	1
	d.i.b					1	1	2		
	asthma			1			1		1	
Drugs	shock	2	1	3	5	5	9	14	13	3
	larynx			1	1	1	3		2	
	d.i.b			1		1		2		1
	asthma		1		3		1	3	2	1

"d.i.b" signifies difficulty breathing due to a combination of upper and lower airways obstruction or cases where the location of the obstruction was uncertain; "larynx" includes laryngeal and other upper airway angioedema.

significant shock except as the terminal event following respiratory arrest.[9] Because of its variability, certain other conditions have commonly proved difficult to distinguish from anaphylaxis.

1. There is a continuous spectrum between anaphylaxis, from anaphylaxis with predominantly asthmatic features, to a pure acute asthma attack with no other features of anaphylaxis. Even life-threatening asthma with no features of anaphylaxis may be triggered by food allergy,[10] in which case it should be classified as an acute severe generalized or systemic hypersensitivity reaction – in other words, anaphylaxis.

2. Similarly, there is a continuous spectrum between angioedema and anaphylaxis, and between various forms of urticaria and anaphylaxis, with shock and/or difficulty breathing in the most severe reactions. Particular care must be taken to recognize cases where asphyxia due to upper airway angioedema has been caused by ACE inhibitors or C1 esterase inhibitor deficiency, as this often does not respond to adrenaline, may need tracheostomy, and may respond to infusion of normal fresh frozen plasma[11] or C1 esterase concentrate.

3. Panic is usual in anaphylaxis, which is often accompanied by a characteristic sense of impending doom. Panic without anaphylaxis may cause a sensation of difficulty swallowing, of difficulty breathing leading to hyperventilation, or may cause uncontrollable coughing and difficulty with inspiration. Patients presenting with these features may be anywhere along the spectrum between panic and anaphylaxis.

4. Vasovagal attacks are commoner than anaphylaxis after injections for immunization and also may occur after stings, particularly around the mouth. This has led to confusion with anaphylaxis.

5. Anaphylactic shock may occur without other visible features of anaphylaxis and will cause myocardial ischemia:[12] it may therefore be difficult to distinguish from myocardial infarction due to coronary artery disease.

In distinction to the endless variability of features caused by anaphylaxis, the time course is characteristic and reactions evolving over a longer time period or resolving too quickly are more likely to have a different diagnosis. The time course may be more rapid (as short as a minute to cardiorespiratory arrest after intravenous injection) or slower (but rarely more than 6 hours to reach a peak) depending on the cause(s), severity, general health and make-up of the patient, and any medication taken daily by the patient or given to treat the reaction. In most cases when the onset of severe symptoms was as slow as 5–6 hours, antihistamines or adrenaline taken for early symptoms may have delayed the reaction.

Anaphylactic shock may be cardiogenic (typically older patients in hospital with pre-existing cardiac pathology) or due to volume redistribution (typically younger patients, slower reactions, outside hospital). Myocardial ischemia with ECG changes is expected within minutes of anaphylactic shock becoming severe (Fig. 62.1).

Asphyxia may be due to upper airway occlusion caused by angioedema, or bronchospasm with mucus plugging of the lower airways; the latter most commonly occurs in patients taking daily treatment for asthma. Both these processes may occur simultaneously in patients reacting to foods, latex, beta-lactam antibiotics, or aspirin.

Anaphylaxis usually resolves in 2–8 hours but secondary pathology arising from the reaction or its treatment may prolong the condition. In a few cases of food anaphylaxis, the reaction itself may be prolonged, possibly because the causative agent is still being absorbed from the gut. Resolution is complete except when cerebral anoxia at the peak of the reaction has caused significant brain damage, or when disordered clotting leads to bleeding, or when panic during the reaction leads to a lasting phobia of the cause. A third of fatal cases are resuscitated after the reaction, but die from complications a variable time later (median 60 hours) without regaining consciousness.

Causes and epidemiology of anaphylaxis

Foods

Acute allergic reactions have been triggered by almost every food, but some cause reactions more commonly than others.[13] Eight food groups have been singled out as high risk in the USA:[14] cereals containing gluten, crustaceans, eggs, fish, peanuts & soybeans, tree nuts, milk (lactose included), and sulphite in concentrations of 10 mg/kg or more. Three additional foods are regarded as high risk in Europe (celery, mustard, sesame);[15] these potently allergenic foods and all their products are subject to additional regulatory control during manufacture of packaged foods and must be identified in ingredient lists to help those with food allergy to avoid reactions. Which foods are most allergenic depends on geographic and ethnic factors: for example, celery (or more precisely, celeriac) allergy predominantly affects German Switzerland;[16] in Japan the list of potently allergenic foods includes buckwheat (*Fagopyrum esculentum*).[17] Allergy to cow's milk most commonly affects infants, and resolves within 1–3 years except in a small proportion.[18] In the UK deaths from milk anaphylaxis have mostly occurred in patients aged from 5 months to 16 years, reaching a peak around age 8 years;[19] all these were predominantly asthmatic reactions. Although allergy to hen's eggs is also commonest in infancy, the only recent UK death from egg allergy was in a 43-year-old. The prevalence of peanut and tree nut allergy is increasing and currently affects around 1% of UK[20] and US[21] children, with lower prevalence in most other countries; deaths from this cause occur predominantly in teenagers and young adults.[22]

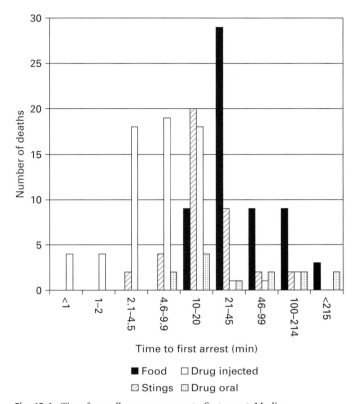

Fig. 62.1. Time from allergen exposure to first arrest. Median times were 5 minutes for injected drugs, 15 minutes for stings, 25 minutes for oral drugs and 30 minutes for food.

Animal dander and secretions

Allergy to domestic animals is common. The dominant allergen in cats is a protein present in the sebum and saliva,[23] whereas for horses the dominant allergen is in the dander,[24] and in rats, the urine.[25] The allergy most commonly manifests as rhinitis, asthma, or contact urticaria but anaphylaxis may occur, for example, following bites from rats in laboratory workers or domestic animals such as horses[26] or hamsters.[27]

Pollens, spores and dust

Microscopic airborne particles contain a wide variety of bacterial, fungal, plant, and animal allergens that cause reactions on mucosal surfaces. Occasionally reactions may become systemic, particularly if there is contact with a larger amount of allergen; for example, pollen accumulated on the surface of late snow and inoculated into the skin by grazing contact during winter sports caused anaphylaxis.[28] Allergen-specific immunotherapy (repeated injection of increasing quantities of allergen in the hope of inducing tolerance) has repeatedly led to anaphylaxis when an inappropriately large dose has been given.[29] The digestive proteins of a variety of common mites (including *Dermatophagoides pteronyssinus*) are particularly potent allergens, affecting 15–20% of population in temperate climates where these mites abound.[30] Although respiratory and conjunctival symptoms are very common, anaphylaxis is rare and there has only been one report of a fatal reaction to natural exposure.[31]

Latex

Natural rubber latex is the sap of the rubber tree *Hevea braziliensis*. More than a dozen allergenic proteins have been identified in the sap and on rubber goods made from latex.[32] Some of these proteins cross-react with proteins found in pollens, fruit, and other plant products: thus around half of those allergic to latex will also react to one or more of banana, avocado, sweet chestnut, kiwi fruit, and, less commonly, a range of other foods. There is genetic[33] and geographical variation in the foods most commonly cross-reactive with latex. IgE-mediated reactions to latex are mostly limited to contact urticaria or asthma from inhaling latex protein-impregnated starch particles from powdered gloves. A small fraction of those with latex allergy suffer severe generalized reactions and latex anaphylaxis has occasionally been fatal.[34,35] The National Patient Safety Agency recently issued an alert which requires NHS Trusts to have policies and procedures in place to reduce the risk to patients who have allergies associated with latex. As well as surgical gloves and catheters, latex is widely used for manufacture of bathing caps, condoms, hot water bottles, and adhesives; one fatal anaphylactic reaction followed the use of a latex-based adhesive designed to attach hair pieces during coiffure.[36]

Stings

Venom in the stings of bees, wasps, and related insects such as fire ants contains highly allergenic proteins and peptides.[37] IgE antibodies are commonly formed following stings, reaching a peak 3–8 weeks after a sting and sometimes persisting for many years;[38] a second sting from the same or cross-reactive venom will then cause an allergic reaction. Sting allergy may be specific for a particular family or genus; less commonly it is broadly cross-reactive, so that some people will react to stings from both bees and wasps.[39,40] Severe reactions to stings cause shock or upper airway blockage;[41] asthmatic reactions are uncommon and largely restricted to those taking daily treatment for asthma.[19] Anaphylaxis is not the only cause of death from stings: some were caused by local angioedema around the upper airway due to the direct toxic effect of the sting,[41] and high numbers of stings when a large nest had been disturbed have caused death through the systemic toxic effects of the venom.[42] There may be other manifestations of acute illness following stings: serum sickness-like illness[43] or other unusual symptoms may occur.[44] The geographical distribution of sting anaphylaxis is obviously dependent on the habitats of the stinging insects: these have already changed due to global warming and further changes are to be expected.

The venom in scorpion stings triggers maximal release of endogenous adrenaline:[45] it is therefore interesting that whereas other stings commonly cause anaphylaxis, there are no reports of anaphylaxis to scorpion stings.

Other plant, animal, or human products

Rare cases of anaphylaxis have been caused by coelenterate (jellyfish) stings,[46] bites by hemiptera (bugs),[47] diptera (flies)[48] and other insects, animal[49] and human seminal fluid,[50] extracts of plants and animals used as food coloring such as annatto,[51] cochineal[52] and so on. No clear pattern has yet emerged that reliably predicts which proteins will be allergenic and which will not.

Parasites including hydatid disease

IgE antibodies are thought to have evolved principally to protect against infestation by parasites[53] and many helminthic parasites are very effective at inducing this class of antibodies. Sudden exposure to antigens from these parasites can trigger anaphylaxis: this has been most commonly observed when an echinococcal cyst has been ruptured during surgery,[54] but there are cases of anaphylaxis following spontaneous rupture of hydatid cysts; some have been fatal.[9] Anaphylaxis has also been triggered by fish nematodes (*Anisakis*) when these have been accidentally eaten in a fish meal.[55]

Drugs

During the early years of its use, penicillin became famous as a potent cause of anaphylaxis.[56] Reactions to penicillin V or G are now rare, but aminopenicillins such as ampicillin and amoxicillin, and similar cephalosporins such as cefaclor are now the commonest causes of fatal antibiotic anaphylaxis.[57] Interpretation of the literature on cross-reactivity between penicillins and cephalosporins is complicated by the variety of mechanisms for these adverse reactions and the low frequency of reactions on challenge among those claiming "penicillin allergy:" nevertheless, significant cross-reactivity between aminopenicillins and aminocephalosporins is common for IgE-mediated anaphylaxis.[58,59]

By far the commonest situation for iatrogenic anaphylaxis is at induction of anesthesia, when an opioid, an intravenous anesthetic, and a muscle relaxant are injected within seconds of each other. There is compelling evidence that these reactions are IgE-mediated and that there may be cross-reactivity between opiates and relaxants,[60] giving scope for synergism between these drugs when they are injected together. Recent observations by a Norwegian group suggest a curious possibility for how patients become sensitized to relaxants. The first observation was that anaphylaxis to relaxants such as rocuronium was far more common in Norway than in Sweden. Because previous theories for sensitization to relaxants focused on environmental quaternary ammonium compounds such as those found in cosmetics and detergents, Florvaag et al. investigated the differences in exposure and found that pholcodine cough syrup was a likely candidate:[61] this medicine is widely used in Norway but is not available in Sweden. A dramatic rise in IgE reactive with pholcodine, morphine, and relaxants followed exposure of individuals sensitized to pholcodine.[62]

Aspirin and other non-selective cyclooxygenase (COX) inhibitors will trigger attacks of asthma or urticaria/angioedema in susceptible individuals.[63] The mechanism is widely thought to be due to diversion of the arachidonic acid pathway away from prostaglandin towards leukotriene production,[64] combined with susceptibility to the effects of the leukotrienes. High levels of mast cell tryptase found in some of these reactions, however,[65] suggest the possibility of more complex interactions including mast cell activation. This is non-IgE-mediated, at least in the majority of cases.

Epoxylated castor oil (cremophore) is used as a solvent for several water-insoluble drugs such as althesin, vitamin K, and taxol. After repeated use, it may cause non-IgE-mediated anaphylaxis. Complement activation occurs, but the mechanism for this is not known.[66] Excipients such as Povidone (polyvinyl pyrrholidone) can cause IgE-mediated anaphylaxis. As they are used in many different medicines, the pattern of reactions to the solvents may be confusing and the cause difficult to establish if this possibility is not considered.[67]

Immunization

Passive immunization with antisera or antitoxins raised in horses carries a high risk of anaphylaxis. In those who have previously received horse antiserum, this is likely to be due to high levels of IgG anti-horse antibodies, leading to immune complex formation and rapid complement activation. Patients with pre-existing IgE-mediated allergy arising from contact with horses may suffer IgE-mediated anaphylaxis on their first injection of horse serum.[68]

Active immunization carries a much lower risk of anaphylaxis and fatalities are exceptionally rare. In addition to the antigen for immunization, the allergenic agent may be contaminant proteins or antibiotics left over from production, such as avian egg or chick proteins,[69] an excipient such as gelatine,[70,71] a preservative such as a mercury-containing compound,[72] or an adjuvant such as alum. Acute adverse events following immunization, however, are more commonly due to vasovagal attacks or panic; these have resulted in medical emergencies when inappropriate treatment was given, such as intravenous adrenaline or even intramuscular adrenaline during a panic attack when the endogenous adrenaline is already high.

Infusions and transfusions

Of all the types of transfusion reaction, anaphylaxis must be among the rarest; a variety of allergens have been described and both non-IgE-[73] and IgE-dependent mechanisms have been postulated.[74]

Contrast media

Large volume bolus injections have obvious potential for triggering adverse effects, so it is perhaps surprising that more reactions to contrast media do not occur. The mechanism of most non-IgE-mediated reactions is still unclear[75] but they are more common when ionic media of high osmotic strength are used.[76] Fatal reactions have usually been associated with grossly raised mast cell tryptase, occur mainly in males[9,77] (whereas non-fatal reactions have a strong female predominance),[78] and may be associated with IgE antibodies. Occasionally individuals are identified with positive skin prick tests (SPT) to contrast media,[79] although this may not necessarily indicate IgE-mediated allergy to the contrast medium.[80]

Disinfectants, sterilizing agents, and fixatives

Chlorhexidine is widely used as a disinfectant and has emerged recently as a cause of anaphylaxis both in the operating theatre and at home.[81]

Orthophthaldehyde is used to sterilize instruments and endoscopes; these may then cause anaphylaxis in susceptible individuals. These reactions may take an hour or more to become severe and thus often occur after the patient has left the operating theater.[82] Formaldehyde can also cause anaphylaxis: this has been reported in a variety of circumstances, including, for example, root canal treatment in dentistry.[83] Positive skin prick tests have been reported following reactions to chlorhexidine, orthophthalaldehyde and formaldehyde and standard commercial tests are available to detect IgE antibodies to formaldehyde.

Physical causes

Urticaria may be triggered in many ways, including heat and cold. In some cases it is possible to block heat-induced urticaria by anticholinergic drugs[84] – its original classification as "cholinergic" followed speculation that acetylcholine caused release of histamine:[85] some of these patients have positive SPT to their own sweat,[86] providing an explanation of how anticholinergic drugs might block the reaction. Occasionally cholinergic urticaria is severe enough to be classified as anaphylaxis. Other mechanisms must exist whereby exercise can lead to anaphylaxis – some are dependent on food allergy, some on aspirin, and some when both are present.[87]

It seems likely a variety of processes can lead to cold-induced urticaria, but the precise explanation remains obscure.[88] Cold-induced urticaria may lead to anaphylaxis – for example, after immersion in cold water.[89]

Amniotic fluid embolus

This has been termed the anaphylactoid syndrome of pregnancy and has many features of anaphylaxis, including the time course and mast cell degranulation[90] with raised tryptase levels;[91] it is fatal in 30%–86% of cases.[92] Estimates of incidence range from 1:8000 to 1:120000 pregnancies, attacks typically occurring during vigorous labor but also following termination or blunt injury during pregnancy. The mechanism leading to mast cell activation is not known but speculation includes IgE antibodies reactive with amniotic fluid,[96] non-IgE-mediated allergy and non-immune anaphylaxis.

Rare causes

Occasionally unusual causes are identified for anaphylaxis that do not fall into any of the categories already described. For example, although reactions to hair dye (reaction products of hydrogen peroxide with p-phenylenediamine or p-toluidinediamine)[94] usually result from contact sensitization, rarely reactions are IgE-mediated and lead to anaphylaxis; this has been fatal.[19,95]

Idiopathic

If no external cause of anaphylaxis can be identified, the reaction may be labelled as idiopathic. This is not simply a failure to identify the cause; these reactions commonly have characteristics that set them apart from the reactions described above. In one subgroup, the reaction typically starts with itching of the palms and/or soles (not common in allergen-mediated anaphylaxis), followed by abdominal cramps with diarrhea, and then severe tremor affecting all muscle groups. There may be loss of consciousness due to hypotension during the later phases of this acute illness. Mast cell tryptase is grossly raised in some cases, but not in others.

Another type of idiopathic anaphylaxis is at the severe end of idiopathic urticaria/angioedema; in these reactions there may be difficulty in breathing due to bronchospasm. The difference between these attacks and reactions to recognizable allergens lies in the timing of the reaction; they often have a more insidious onset and frequently recur several times over the course of a few days. Reports of "biphasic reactions" may arise from failure to identify these attacks as idiopathic anaphylaxis.[92] There may be a single attack, or there may be recurrences at intervals varying from a few days up to months or even years; generally the first or second attack is the worst, and subsequent attacks decrease in severity. Various epidemiological studies report the fraction of anaphylaxis that is idiopathic as 5–37%.[96–107]

Conditioned anaphylaxis

Neurological processes may possibly trigger repeat reactions in the absence of the original cause.[108,109]

Pathophysiology of anaphylaxis and factors increasing the probability of cardiorespiratory arrest

Because anaphylaxis in its broad sense comprises a heterogeneous collection of acute severe transitory illnesses, it has proved difficult to study in humans, and experimental animal models may not accurately portray the human conditions. Mouse models suggest that mast cell activation is only one of the pathways – macrophage triggering by IgG antibodies leads to a platelet activating factor-dependent, histamine-independent pathway.[110] They also suggest that cytokines such as IL-4 and IL-13 can alter the sensitivity of mice, increasing the tendency for anaphylaxis. There is no doubt that human susceptibility for severe reactions varies from time to time as a result of infection or stress, consistent with the idea that we too may respond to cytokines in this way.

In human anaphylaxis, IgE-mediated reactions are generally regarded as the most typical, such as might be triggered by a sting, peanuts, or amoxicillin. At some time prior to the reaction the subject must have become sensitized, leading to the production of antibodies of the IgE class.[111] After their synthesis and release by plasma cells, these bind to the high affinity IgE receptor (Fc$_\varepsilon$RI) on cytoplasmic membranes of mast cells and basophils. Triggering of these cells requires that the mobility of at least two receptor molecular complexes is limited by bridging between them – usually when the IgE antibodies bind to allergen;[112] large rafts of cross-linked receptors

lead to more rapid triggering, causing a sequence of changes within the mast cell or basophil.[113] Redistribution of calcium within the cell then leads to release of granules containing histamine and a variety of proteins including mast cell tryptase, chymase, and carboxypeptidase, and proteoglycans including heparin and chondroitin sulphate.[114] Other synthetic pathways are initiated, leading to release of arachidonic acid from phospholipids in the nuclear membrane and its conversion to prostaglandins such as PGD2 and leukotrienes such as LTC4; platelet activating factor (PAF) is also formed (Fig. 62.2).

PAF may be the key to the difference between mild allergic reactions and anaphylaxis: it comprises a variety of related phospholipid derivatives with an ether linkage at the sn-1 position of the glycerol backbone, a short acyl chain, usually an acetyl residue, at the sn-2 position, and the polar head group of choline or ethanolamine at the sn-3 position. The length of the alkyl chain at the sn-1 position and the number of double bonds also affect its

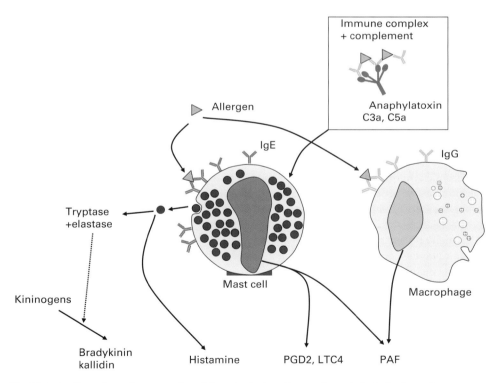

Fig. 62.2. Outline scheme for generation of the principal mediators of anaphylaxis. Preformed mediators including histamine are released from mast cell granules. PAF, leukotrienes and prostaglandins are synthesized from membrane lipids. Kinins are split from kininogens, possibly by proteases released from mast cell granules. There is evidence from mouse models that some types of anaphylaxis are caused by PAF release from macrophages: similar processes may play a part in human reactions.

biological activity. PAF has potent effects on the heart, blood vessels, and the airways, all of which cause changes typical of severe anaphylaxis.[115] PAF acetyl hydrolase comprises a family of enzymes that inactivate PAF; genetic variants with reduced or absent activity have been associated with increased severity of asthma and anaphylaxis.[116]

The kinin system is also activated in anaphylaxis.[117] Mast cell peptidases detach bradykinin from its precursor, the high molecular weight kininogen,[118] and kallidin from the low molecular weight kininogen. There may be other routes of activation such as the more usual activation of factors XII and XI of the blood clotting cascade and of kallikrein.[119] These kinins have potent effects on blood vessels, similar in many ways to those of histamine but with a slower time course.[120] Because angiotensin converting enzyme (ACE) is one of the main brakes on the kinin system (it acts as a carboxypeptidase, inactivating the kinins), ACE inhibitors potentiate anaphylaxis, increasing the tendency to both shock[121] and swelling, both because they increase the bradykinin activity and because they lower angiotensin activity; angiotensin is a natural antagonist of anaphylaxis.[122] Genetic deficiency of aminopeptidase P (another enzyme like ACE that inactivates bradykinin) is another cause of angioedema when ACE inhibitors are administered.[123]

Anaphylatoxin (split products of complement activation) was one of the earliest recognized mediators of anaphylaxis.[124] It is produced in vitro during complement activation and if injected, leads to anaphylaxis. Plasma carboxypeptidases quickly inactivate anaphylatoxin,[125] however, and it is less certain what effect this has in vivo. Complement activation occurs in dextran reactions,[126] where IgG antibodies form immune complexes with the dextran. The resulting anaphylaxis may well be due to anaphylatoxin but multiple other pathological changes occur.[127] Dextran anaphylaxis may be fatal.[128]

As might be expected with so many potent mediators, there are rapid effects on many tissues and organs. Arterioles relax and dilate, increasing the pressure in capillaries and venules. The postcapillary venular endothelium leaks fluid into the tissue resulting in angioedema and augmenting the decrease in vascular return caused by the increase in intravascular volume. In other cases, direct action of mediators on the myocardium[115,129] may reduce cardiac output by decreasing contractility or causing arrhythmia of any kind; when this happens there may be insufficient pressure to cause urticaria or angioedema, resulting in anaphylactic shock with no other manifestation of an allergic reaction.

Shock is affected by posture and there is a remarkable association between upright posture and irreversible cardiac arrest from anaphylaxis, to the extent that in all fatalities from anaphylaxis outside hospital where the postural history was known, there had either been a change to a more upright posture or an upright posture had been maintained after loss of consciousness.[12] A possible mechanism for this is that although the blood pressure is low, there is some venous return while the posture is horizontal, but on assuming a more upright posture insufficient blood returns to the vena cava and it rapidly empties. Within a few beats, the heart becomes empty and as there is no cardiac output, the vena cava remains empty and resuscitation by external cardiac massage is impossible. As with all severe shock, the decreased cardiac output leads to myocardial ischemia with typical ECG changes. When there are no other manifestations of anaphylaxis, this has been mistaken for primary myocardial infarction.

Simultaneously, mediators may lead to respiratory difficulty, either through angioedema in the pharynx, larynx, or trachea, or through bronchospasm. In asthmatics with remodelling of the airways this will be more severe and is accompanied by secretion of viscid mucus which contributes to the airways occlusion. Asthma, particularly when it is not optimally treated, is a risk factor for fatal anaphylaxis, particularly to foods and NSAIDs.[9,22]

There may also be rhinitis with sneezing, irritation of airways with coughing, and panic because of a feeling of loss of control over what is happening in the body. A sense of impending doom is characteristic of panic and is frequently reported by those with anaphylaxis.[130] Nevertheless, panic with hyperventilation (which may lead to wheezing, particularly if the subject has exercise-induced asthma), coughing with panic and paradoxical vocal chord movement or laryngospasm with stridor, have all been mistaken for anaphylaxis and vice versa. Both the increased sympathetic tone and the rise in circulating adrenaline that occur in panic protect against progression to anaphylaxis; this may explain why exhaustion may promote severe reactions, because of depletion of sympathetic reserves.

The formation of PAF during anaphylaxis in mice[110] causes disordered clotting with intravascular coagulation.[131] Clotting is also disturbed in human anaphylaxis and the ensuing bleeding may be difficult to manage, particularly when there are other sequelae such as cerebral ischemia or adult respiratory distress syndrome.

Biphasic reactions have been reported to occur commonly by some authors.[132,136] and to be unusual by others.[9] Possible explanations include undertreatment leading to recurrence of symptoms (particularly omission of steroids from the initial treatment, predisposing to late-phase asthmatic symptoms), or inclusion in the series of idiopathic anaphylaxis, where there may be one or more cycles of partial resolution and recrudescence over days or even weeks. Mouse models suggest the late phase may be related to PAF activation.[133]

Management of anaphylaxis

There is more to the management of anaphylaxis than simply giving the correct treatment to anyone who has a reaction. The first problem is recognizing that the acute illness (or if the patient is already ill, the acute deterioration) is due to anaphylaxis.

Strategies for optimal management of anaphylaxis depend on the likely mode of death, and this in turn depends on the cause of the attack. Once the patient has been rescued from this danger, the cause for the reaction must be found and the patient advised about how to prevent a recurrence, both by preventing reexposure and by minimizing the severity of a reaction if accidental reexposure occurs.

Diagnosis

Anaphylaxis is surprisingly difficult to diagnose. It is usually unexpected; and even in situations when it might be expected, experience shows that the correct diagnosis is frequently not achieved in time to give treatment that will stop progression to anaphylaxis. The main confusions have been listed above.

Treatment of the acute reaction

Even patients with severe untreated reactions recover with much the same time course as those of similar severity who are treated. The primary objective of treatment is to prevent the incipient illness turning into anaphylaxis; once cardiac arrest is established it should be treated according to standard protocols.

Recommendations for management of anaphylaxis vary according to the situation. What is appropriate for a paramedic is not what will be needed by an anesthetist. Separate UK guidelines have been published for first responders,[134] paramedics, anesthetists, and radiologists; the guidance for immunization reactions has now been brought in line with that for first responders. Other countries have published consensus guidance (e.g., USA).[8] In every situation, however, the first drug to be given is adrenaline. Although there has never been a randomized controlled trial, there are good theoretical grounds to suppose this is a logical treatment[135] and there is sufficient anecdotal evidence supporting its use to ease breathing difficulty and restore adequate cardiac output. Both alpha and beta activity are needed, centrally increasing the force of the myocardial contractions and, paradoxically, slowing the rhythm by increasing peripheral resistance, which in turn helps reduce peripheral leakage from the postcapillary venules by a combination of increased arteriolar tone and reduced venular permeability. In the lungs, the beta-2 activity relaxes the bronchiolar smooth muscle, easing bronchospasm. In some cases, upper airways angioedema may respond dramatically to adrenaline, whereas in others there may be little benefit and tracheostomy may occasionally be needed.

The earlier adrenaline is given, the higher the probability it will prevent anaphylaxis from developing.[136] In addition to the actions listed above, there are beta-2 adrenergic receptors on mast cells[137] that inhibit activation[138] and consequently early adrenaline administration attenuates the severity of IgE-mediated allergic reactions. Because of this, beta-blockers enhance the severity of anaphylaxis.[139]

There has been argument about the optimal route for administration of adrenaline.[140] Absorption of adrenaline from muscle depends on the blood flow. Blood flow through subcutaneous tissues (predominantly alpha-adrenergic receptors) is restricted by even very low concentrations of adrenaline[141] and adrenaline is poorly absorbed from this site, which should not be used when treating anaphylaxis. Beta-adrenergic activity at physiological concentrations causes vasodilatation:[142] absorption therefore depends on the ratio of beta- to alpha-adrenergic receptors. Beta receptors are induced in muscle blood vessels by exercise;[143] possibly because of this, absorption is better from the extensor muscles of the thigh than from the arm.[144] The preferred site for intramuscular injection of adrenaline is therefore the midpoint of the thigh, on the anterolateral aspect. If an autoinjector is used, it is important to ascertain that the needle is long enough to deliver the injection into the muscle [see below].[145]

Once shock is established, however, adrenaline loses its effectiveness[146,147] and repeated bolus injection may have only transient effect on the blood pressure.[148] In this case, infusion has proved more effective in experimental models[149] and anecdotally in humans. In cases where adrenaline fails to restore the blood pressure, selective alpha-agonists may be tried[150] but it may be more logical to use vasopressin.[151] There is some evidence that glucagon may be helpful for those who are unresponsive to adrenaline because they are on beta-blockers.[152] Rapid fluid infusion is essential if the pressure is so low that the central venous return is threatened; in this situation posture can be critical and raising the legs may assist venous return as much as 0.5–1.0 l of fluid.[153]

While 1.0 mg of adrenaline i.v. is recommended in the treatment of cardiac arrest, it is crucial to realize that intravenous adrenaline is dangerous in the conscious patient. Bolus injection of as little as 0.5 mg leads to dangerous elevation of the blood pressure with a range of harmful, sometimes lethal effects. Pulmonary edema is a regular effect (intravenous adrenaline is the basis for experimental models of pulmonary edema):[154] if the resulting difficulty in breathing is mistaken as a worsening of the anaphylaxis and more adrenaline is given, a vicious spiral may result, ending with the death of the patient. Alternatively, the rapid extreme increase in blood pressure may lead to dissection of arterial intima – typically in the vertebral arteries, with subsequent thrombosis which may detach and lodge at the bifurcation of the basilar arteries, causing infarction of the thalamus and optic cortex. In other cases there has been arterial bleeding into the brain. Persistent memory, cognitive, and intellectual impairment has regularly followed intravenous bolus injection of adrenaline. There may also be myocardial ischemia.[155] It is therefore strongly recommended that intravenous adrenaline is only used in monitored patients and the dose titrated against the effect.[134] Even so, vomiting is common following slower i.v. adrenaline use. This is particularly dangerous if the patient's stomach is loaded with allergen: inhalation of vomit has been a regular cause of death in such cases.

Although adrenaline will relieve bronchospasm, it is usual in addition to treat wheezing by nebulized salbutamol. Bronchospasm resistant to both adrenaline and salbutamol may be a result of excessive daily use of salbutamol.[156] In this case a bronchodilator acting through a different mechanism will be needed, such as aminophylline or magnesium sulphate.[157,158]

After adrenaline, an antihistamine should be used such as chlorphenamine 10 mg by intramuscular or slow intravenous injection and steroids are recommended to prevent late phase recrudescence of the reaction: these are commonly given as hydrocortisone 100–400 mg i.v., but this may cause very unpleasant side effects with intense paresthesia and sometimes shock.[159] This has been mistaken as a sudden worsening of the reaction and has led to inappropriate injection of adrenaline.

Various other strategies have been suggested. Military antishock trousers may reverse some of the volume redistribution.[160] Methylene blue antagonizes the effects of NO on the vessels.[161]

Investigation of causes and mechanisms

A recurrence of anaphylaxis is common[162] and has been fatal. It is therefore essential that anyone with anaphylaxis is referred to an appropriate specialist for investigation of the cause and advice about management.

Minimizing chance of reexposure

The cause of the reaction may seem obvious, but mistakes are common. Proper investigation is important because, however careful the avoidance is, it will be ineffective if the patient avoids the wrong thing. Effective allergen avoidance may demand a lifestyle change and is likely to affect the quality of life.[163] The patient needs to know more after penicillin anaphylaxis than simply that they should avoid penicillin, or after reacting to food, that it may have contained nuts and they must avoid nuts in future. Patients are more likely to get good advice from an appropriately trained specialist and should therefore be referred accordingly.

Minimizing danger from effects of reexposure

Allergen avoidance can never guarantee safety from accidental exposure[164] but the effect on the patient of such an accident can be minimized in a variety of ways. Allergen-specific immunotherapy (desensitization) is available for bee and wasp sting anaphylaxis and will greatly reduce the risk of a recurrence. Gradually increasing doses of pure venom are injected, followed by maintenance treatment at 4–6 week intervals for 3–5 years: this leads to long-lasting protection.[165] This therapy has proved too dangerous for routine use with food allergy,[166] but as most food-induced anaphylactic deaths have been dominantly asthmatic reactions in those taking suboptimal daily treatment for their asthma,[9,22] improved daily asthma management will be at least partially protective.

Patients with anaphylaxis to food or stings may be advised to carry self-injectible adrenaline.[167] Devices are available that deliver one or two doses of 0.3 mg or, suitable for those under 30 kg body mass, 0.15 mg of adrenaline. This equipment will only be effective if the patient carries the adrenaline at all times there is a risk of exposure, knows how and when to use the injection, and has an autoinjector that can deliver an intramuscular injection. One or more of these conditions are commonly not met.[145,168] Needle length depends on the make and varies from 9 to 16 mm. It is important to confirm that the skin-to-muscle thickness is less than this in the target area (anterolateral aspect of the mid-section of the thigh).[145] Skin-fold thickness may give an estimate in some patients; others will need an ultrasound or MR scan. Patients with autoinjectors need to have regular reviews to ensure that their device is still appropriate, that they remember how and when to use it, that it is in date, that they have not been prescribed drugs that have adverse interactions with adrenaline and so on.[169]

REFERENCES

1. Richet, C.R. L'Anaphylaxie. Paris, 1909; Chapter 1. English translation: Murray Bligh, J. Anaphylaxis. Liverpool-London: Constable & Co Ltd, The University Press, 1913; 1.

2. Prausnitz, C. & Küstner, H. Studien über die Überempfindlichkeit. Zentralbl Bakt Parasits Infect I Abt Orig 1921; **86**: 160–169.

3. Ishizaka, K., Ishizaka, T. & Hornbrook, M.M. Physicochemical properties of reaginic antibody. V. Correlation of reaginic activity with cE-globulin antibody. *J. Immunol.* 1966; **97**: 840.

4. Gell, P.G.H. & Coombes, R.R.A.(eds.) *Clinical Aspects of Immunology.* Oxford: Blackwell, 1962.

5. Johansson, S.G.O., Hourihane, J.O'B., Bousquet, J. *et al.* A revised nomenclature for allergy [An EAACI position statement from the EAACI nomenclature task force] *Allergy* 2001: **56**: 813–824.

6. Hanzlik, P.J. & Karsner, H.A.T. Anaphylactoid phenomena from the intravenous administration of various colloids, arsenicals and other agents. *J. Pharmacol. Exp. Ther.* 1920; **14**: 379.

7. Johansson, S.G.O., Bieber, T., Dahl, R. *et al.* Revised nomenclature for allergy for global use: Report of the Nomenclature Review Committee of the World Allergy Organization, October 2003. *J. Allergy Clin. Immunol.* 2004; **113**: 832–836.

8. Joint Task Force on Practice Parameters. The diagnosis and management of anaphylaxis: an updated practice parameter. *J. Allergy Clin. Immunol.* 2005; **115**: S483–S523.

9. Pumphrey, R.S.H. Lessons for management of anaphylaxis from a study of fatal reactions. *Clin. Exp. Allergy* 2000; **30**: 1144–1150.

10. Roberts, G., Patel, N., Levi-Schaffer, F., Habibi, P. & Lack, G. Food allergy as a risk factor for life-threatening asthma in childhood: a case-controlled study. *J. Allergy Clin. Immunol.* 2003; **112**: 168–174.

11. Warrier, M.R., Copilevitz, C.A., Dykewicz, M.S. & Slavin, R.G. Fresh frozen plasma in the treatment of resistant angiotensin-converting enzyme inhibitor angioedema. *Ann. Allergy Asthma Immunol.* 2004; **92**: 573–575.

12. Pumphrey, R.S.H. Fatal posture in anaphylactic shock. *J. Allergy Clin. Immunol.* 2003; **112**: 451–452.

13. Mills, E.N. & Breiteneder, H. Food allergy and its relevance to industrial food proteins. *Biotechnol. Adv.* 2005; **23**: 409–414.

14. Taylor, S.L. Emerging problems with food allergens. *Food, Nutri. Agric.* 2000; **26**: 14–23.

15. Directive 2000/13/EC.

16. Ballmer-Weber, B.K., Vieths, S., Luttkopf, D., Heuschmann, P. & Wuthrich, B. Celery allergy confirmed by double-blind, placebo-controlled food challenge: a clinical study in 32 subjects with a history of adverse reactions to celery root. *J. Allergy Clin. Immunol.* 2000; **106**: 373–378.

17. Hamamoto, T. Food and agricultural import regulations and standards: revised allergen labeling requirements. Global Agriculture Information Network: 2005; report JA5037.

18. Sampson, H.A. Food allergy. Part 1: immunopathogenesis and clinical disorders. *J. Allergy Clin. Immunol.* 1999; **103**: 717–728.

19. Pumphrey, R.S. Fatal anaphylaxis in the UK, 1992–2001. *Novartis Found. Symp.* 2004; **257**: 116–128.

20. Grundy, J., Bateman, B.J., Gant, C., Matthews, S.M., Dean T.P. & Arshad, S. Peanut allergy in three year old children – a population based study [abstract]. *J. Allergy Clin. Immunol.* 2001; **107**: S231.

21. Sicherer, S.H., Munoz-Furlong, A. & Sampson, H.A. Prevalence of peanut and tree nut allergy in the United States determined by means of a random digit dial telephone survey: a 5-year follow-up study. *J. Allergy Clin. Immunol.* 2003; **112**: 1203–1207.

22. Bock, S.A., Muñoz-Furlong, A. & Sampson, H.A. Fatalities due to anaphylactic reactions to foods. *J. Allergy Clin. Immunol.* 2001; **107**: 191–193.

23. Mata, P., Charpin, D., Charpin, C., Lucciani, P. & Vervloet, D. Fel d I allergen: skin and or saliva? *Ann. Allergy* 1992; **69**: 321–322.

24. Erwin, E.A., Woodfolk, J.A., Custis, N. & Platts-Mills, T.A. Animal danders. Immunol Allergy *Clin. North Am.* 2003; **23**: 469–481.

25. Nieuwenhuijsen, M.J., Putcha, V., Gordon, S. *et al.* Exposure-response relations among laboratory animal workers exposed to rats. *Occup. Environ. Med.* 2003; **60**: 104–108.

26. Guida, G., Nebiolo, F., Heffler, E., Bergia, R. & Rolla, G. Anaphylaxis after a horse bite. Allergy. 2005; **60**: 1088–1089.

27. Lim, D.L., Chan, R.M.E., Wen, H., van Bever, H.P.S. & Chua, K.Y. Anaphylaxis after hamster bites-identification of a novel allergen. *Clin. Exp. Allergy* 2004; **34**: 1122–1123.

28. Spitalny, K.C., Farnham, J.E., Witherell, L.E. *et al.* Alpine slide anaphylaxis. *N. Engl. J. Med.* 1984; **310**: 1034–1037.

29. Borchers, A.T., Keen, C.L. & Gershwin, M.E. Fatalities following allergen immunotherapy. *Clin. Rev. Allergy Immunol.* 2004; **27**: 147–158.

30. Jarvis, D., Luczynska, C., Chinn, S. *et al.* Change in prevalence of IgE sensitization and mean total IgE with age and cohort. *J. Allergy Clin. Immunol.* 2005; **116**: 675–682.

31. Edston, E. & Hage-Hamsten, M. Death in anaphylaxis in a man with house dust mite allergy, *Int. J. Legal Med.* 2003; **117**: 299–301.

32. Yeang, H.Y. Natural rubber latex allergens: new developments. *Curr. Opin. Allergy Clin. Immunol.* 2004; **4**: 99–104.

33. Blanco, C., Sanchez-Garcia, F., Torres-Galvan, M.J. *et al.* Genetic basis of the latex-fruit syndrome: association with HLA class II alleles in a Spanish population. *J. Allergy Clin. Immunol.* 2004; **114**: 1070–1076.

34. Ownby, D.R., Tomlanovich, M., Sammons, N. & McCullough, J. Anaphylaxis associated with latex allergy during barium enema examinations. *Am. J. Roentgenol.* 1991; **156**: 903–908.

35. Martinez Jabaloyas, J.M., Broseta Rico, E., Ruiz Cerda, J.L., Sanz Chinesta, S., Osca Garcia, J.M. & Jimenez Cruz, J.F. Extracorporeal shockwave lithotripsy in patients with urinary diversion. *Actas Urol. Esp.* 1995; **19**: 143–147.

36. Pumphrey, R.S., Duddridge, M. & Norton, J. Fatal latex allergy. *J. Allergy Clin. Immunol.* 2001; **107**: 558.

37. King, T.P. & Guralnick, M. Hymenoptera allergens. *Clin. Allergy Immunol.* 2004; **18**: 339–453.

38. Bilo, B.M., Rueff, F., Mosbech, H. *et al.* Diagnosis of Hymenoptera venom allergy. *Allergy* 2005; **60**: 1339–1349.

39. Straumann, F., Bucher, C. & Wuthrich, B. Double sensitization to honeybee and wasp venom: immunotherapy with one or with both venoms? Value of FEIA inhibition for the identification of the cross-reacting ige antibodies in double-sensitized patients to honeybee and wasp venom. *Int. Arch. Allergy Immunol.* 2000; **123**: 268–274.

40. Egner, W., Ward, C., Brown, D.L. & Ewan, P.W. The frequency and clinical significance of specific IgE to both wasp (Vespula) and honey-bee (Apis) venoms in the same patient. *Clin. Exp. Allergy* 1998; **28**: 26–34.

41. Mosbech, H. Death caused by wasp and bee stings in Denmark 1960–1980. *Allergy* 1983; **38**: 195–200.

42. Müller, U.R. *Insect Sting Allergy: Clinical Picture, Diagnosis and Treatment.* Gustav Fischer Verlag / VCH, 1990: 46.

43. Reisman, R.E. & Livingston, A. Late-onset allergic reactions, including serum sickness, after insect stings. *J. Allergy Clin. Immunol.* 1989; **84**: 331–337.

44. Reisman, R.E. Unusual reactions to insect stings. *Curr. Opin. Allergy Clin. Immunol.* 2005; **5**: 355–358.

45. Nouira, S., Elatrous, S., Besbes, L. *et al.* Neurohormonal activation in severe scorpion envenomation: correlation with hemodynamics and circulating toxin. *Toxicol. Appl. Pharmacol.* 2005; **208**: 111–116.

46. Togias, A.G., Burnett, J.W., Kagey-Sobotka, A. & Lichtenstein, L.M. Anaphylaxis after contact with a jellyfish. *J. Allergy Clin. Immunol.* 1985; **75**: 672–675.

47. Moffitt, J.E., Venarske, D., Goddard, J., Yates, A.B. & deShazo, R.D. Allergic reactions to Triatoma bites. *Ann. Allergy Asthma Immunol.* 2003; **91**: 122–128.

48. Hemmer, W., Focke, M., Vieluf, D., Berg-Drewniok, B., Gotz, M. & Jarisch, R. Anaphylaxis induced by horsefly bites: identification of a 69 kd IgE-binding salivary gland protein from *Chrysops* spp. (Diptera, Tabanidae) by western blot analysis. *J. Allergy Clin. Immunol.* 1998; **101**: 134–136.

49. Holden, T.E. & Sherline, D.M. Bestiality, with sensitization and anaphylactic reaction. *Obstet. Gynecol.* 1973; **42**: 138–140.

50. Shah, A. & Panjabi, C. Human seminal plasma allergy: a review of a rare phenomenon. *Clin. Exp. Allergy* 2004; **34**: 827–838.

51. Lucas, C.D., Hallagan, J.B. & Taylor, S.L. The role of natural color additives in food allergy. *Adv. Food Nutr. Res.* 2001; **43**: 195–216.

52. Wuthrich, B., Kagi, M.K. & Stucker, W. Anaphylactic reactions to ingested carmine (E120). *Allergy* 1997; **52**: 1133–1137.

53. Hagel, I., Di Prisco, M.C., Goldblatt, J. & Le Souef, P.N. The role of parasites in genetic susceptibility to allergy: IgE, helminthic infection and allergy, and the evolution of the human immune system. *Clin. Rev. Allergy Immunol.* 2004; **26**: 75–83.

54. Buyuk, Y., Turan, A.A., Uzun, I., Aybar, Y., Cin, O. & Kurnaz, G. Non-ruptured hydatid cyst can lead to death by spread of cyst content into bloodstream: an autopsy case. *Eur. J. Gastroenterol. Hepatol.* 2005; **17**: 671–673.

55. Dominguez-Ortega, J., Alonso-Llamazares, A., Rodriguez, L. *et al.* Anaphylaxis due to hypersensitivity to *Anisakis simplex*. *Int. Arch. Allergy Immunol.* 2001; **125**: 86–88.

56. Welch, H., Lewis, C.N., Weinstein, H.I. & Boeckman, B.B. Severe reactions to antibiotics; a nationwide survey. *Antibiotics Annual* 1957–1958; 296–309.

57. Pumphrey, R.S. & Davis, S. Underreporting of antibiotic anaphylaxis may put patients at risk. *Lancet* 1999; **353**: 1157.

58. Romano, A., Gueant-Rodriguez, R.M., Viola, M., Pettinato, R. & Gueant, J.L. Cross-reactivity and tolerability of cephalosporins in patients with immediate hypersensitivity to penicillins. *Ann. Intern. Med.* 2004; **141**: 16–22.

59. Romano, A., Gueant-Rodriguez, R.M., Viola, M. *et al.* Diagnosing immediate reactions to cephalosporins. *Clin. Exp. Allergy* 2005; **35**: 1234–1242.

60. Baldo, B.A., Pham, N.H. & Zhao, Z. Chemistry of drug allergenicity. *Curr. Opin. Allergy Clin. Immunol.* 2001; **1**: 327–335.

61. Florvaag, E., Johansson, S.G., Oman, H. *et al.* Prevalence of IgE antibodies to morphine. Relation to the high and low incidences of NMBA anaphylaxis in Norway and Sweden, respectively. *Acta Anaesthesiol. Scand.* 2005; **49**: 437–444.

62. Florvaag, E., Johansson, S.G.O., Öman, H., Harboe, T. & Nopp, A. Pholcodine stimulates a dramatic increase of IgE in IgE-sensitized individuals. *Allergy* 2006; **61**: 49.

63. Simon, R.A. Adverse respiratory reactions to aspirin and nonsteroidal anti-inflammatory drugs. *Curr. Allergy Asthma Rep.* 2004; **4**: 17–24.

64. Hamad, A.M., Sutcliffe, A.M. & Knox, A.J. Aspirin-induced asthma: clinical aspects, pathogenesis and management. *Drugs* 2004; **64**: 2417–2432.

65. Bosso, J.V., Schwartz, L.B. & Stevenson, D.D. Tryptase and histamine release during aspirin-induced respiratory reactions. *J. Allergy Clin. Immunol.* 1991; **88**: 830–837.

66. Szebeni, J. Complement activation-related pseudoallergy: a new class of drug-induced acute immune toxicity. *Toxicology* 2005; **216**: 106–121.

67. Ronnau, A.C., Wulferink, M., Gleichmann, E. *et al.* Anaphylaxis to polyvinylpyrrolidone in an analgesic preparation. *Br. J. Dermatol.* 2000; **143**: 1055–1058.

68. Demoly, P., Botros, H.G., Rabillon, J., David, B. & Bousquet, J. Anaphylaxis to antitetanus toxoid serum. *Allergy* 2002: **57**: 860–861.

69. Patja, A., Makinen-Kiljunen, S., Davidkin, I., Paunio, M. & Peltola, H. Allergic reactions to measles–mumps–rubella vaccination. *Pediatrics* 2001; **107**: E27.

70. Pool, V., Braun, M.M., Kelso, J.M. *et al.* Prevalence of anti-gelatin Ig E antibodies in people with anaphylaxis after measles–mumps–rubella vaccine in the United States. *Pediatrics* 2002; **110**(6): e71.

71. Sakaguchi, M., Nakayama, T. & Inouye, S. Food allergy to gelatin in children with systemic immediate-type reactions, including anaphylaxis, to vaccines. *J. Allergy Clin. Immunol.* 1996; **98**: 1058–1061.

72. Lee-Wong, M., Resnick, D. & Chong, K. A generalized reaction to thimerosal from an influenza vaccine. *Ann. Allergy Asthma Immunol.* 2005; **94**: 90–94.

73. Vassallo, R.R. Review: IgA anaphylactic transfusion reactions. Part, I. Laboratory diagnosis, incidence, and supply of IgA-deficient products. *Immunohematology* 2004; **20**: 226–233.

74. Shimada, E., Tadokoro, K., Watanabe, Y. *et al.* Anaphylactic transfusion reactions in haptoglobin-deficient patients with IgE and IgG haptoglobin antibodies. *Transfusion* 2002; **42**: 766–773.

75. Morcos, S.K. Review article: Acute serious and fatal reactions to contrast media: our current understanding. *Br. J. Radiol.* 2005; **78**(932): 686–693.

76. Katayama, H., Yamaguchi, K., Kozuka, T., Takashima, T., Seez, P. & Matsuura, K. Adverse reactions to ionic and nonionic contrast media. *Radiology* 1990; **175**: 621–628.

77. Wang, D.Y., Forslund, C., Persson, U. & Wiholm, B.E. Drug attributed anaphylaxis. *Pharmacoepidemiol. Drug Saf.* 1998; **7**: 269–274.

78. Lang, D.M., Alpern, M.B., Visintainer, P.F. & Smith, S.T. Gender risk for anaphylactoid reaction to radiographic contrast media. *J. Allergy Clin. Immunol.* 1995; **95**: 813–817.

79. Kanny, G., Pichler, W., Morisset, M. *et al.* T cell-mediated reactions to iodinated contrast media: evaluation by skin and lymphocyte activation tests. *J. Allergy Clin. Immunol.* 2005; **115**(1): 179–185.

80. Schwartz, E.E., Glick, S.N., Foggs, M.B. & Silverstein, G.S. Hypersensitivity reactions after barium enema examination. *Am. J. Roentgenol.* 1984; **143**(1): 103–104.

81. Krautheim, A.B., Jermann, T.H. & Bircher, A.J. Chlorhexidine anaphylaxis: case report and review of the literature. *Contact Dermatitis* 2004; **50**: 113–116.

82. Sokol, W.N. Nine episodes of anaphylaxis following cystoscopy caused by Cidex OPA (orthophthalaldehyde) high-level disinfectant in 4 patients after cytoscopy. *J. Allergy Clin. Immunol.* 2004; **114**: 392–397.

83. Kunisada, M., Adachi, A., Asano, H., & Horikawa, T. Anaphylaxis due to formaldehyde released from root-canal disinfectant. *Contact Dermatitis* 2002, **47**, 215–218.

84. Commens, C.A. & Greaves, M.W. Tests to establish the diagnosis in cholinergic urticaria. *Br. J. Dermatol.* 1978; **98**: 47–51.

85. Grant, R.T., Bruce Pearson, R.S. & Comeau, W.J. Observations on urticaria provoked by emotion, by exercise and by warming the body. *Clin. Sci.* 1936; **2**: 253–272.

86. Fukunaga, A., Bito, T., Tsuru, K. *et al.* Responsiveness to autologous sweat and serum in cholinergic urticaria classifies its clinical subtypes. *J. Allergy Clin. Immunol.* 2005; **116**: 397–402.

87. Matsuo, H., Morimoto, K., Akaki, T. *et al.* Exercise and aspirin increase levels of circulating gliadin peptides in patients with wheat-dependent exercise-induced anaphylaxis. *Clin. Exp. Allergy.* 2005; **35**: 461–466.

88. Asero, R., Tedeschi, A. & Lorini, M. Histamine release in idiopathic cold urticaria. *Allergy* 2002; **57**: 1211–1212.

89. Alangari, A.A., Twarog, F.J., Shih, M.C. & Schneider, L.C. Clinical features and anaphylaxis in children with cold urticaria. *Pediatrics* 2004; **113**: e313–e317.

90. Rainio, J. & Penttilä, A. Amniotic fluid embolism as cause of death in a car accident – a case report. *Forens. Sci. Int.* 2003; **137**(2–3): 231–234.

91. Nishio, H., Matsui, K., Miyazaki, T., Tamura, A., Iwata, M. & Suzuki, K. A fatal case of amniotic fluid embolism with elevation of serum mast cell tryptase. *Forens. Sci. Int.* 2002; **126**: 53–56.

92. Tufnell, D.J. United Kingdom amniotic fluid and embolism register. *Br. J. Obstet. Gynecol.* 2005; **112**: 1625–1629.

93. Benson, M.D. Anaphylactoid syndrome of pregnancy. *Am. J. Obstet. Gynecol.* 1996; **175**: 749.

94. Goldberg, B.J., Herman, F.F. & Hirata, I. Systemic anaphylaxis due to an oxidation product of p-phenylenediamine in a hair dye. *Ann. Allergy* 1987; **58**: 205–208.

95. Belton, A.L. & Chira, T. Fatal anaphylactic reaction to hair dye. *Am. J. Forens. Med. Pathol.* 1997; **18**(3): 290–292.

96. Pumphrey, R.S. & Stanworth, S.J. The clinical spectrum of anaphylaxis in north-west England. *Clin. Exp. Allergy* 1996; **26**: 1364–1370.

97. Thong, B.Y., Cheng, Y.K., Leong, K.P., Tang, C.Y. & Chng, H.H. Anaphylaxis in adults referred to a clinical immunology/allergy centre in Singapore. *Singapore Med. J.* 2005; **46**: 529–534.

98. de Bruyne, J.A. & Lee, B.W. Anaphylaxis in the Asia Pacific. *Allergy Clin. Immunol. Int.* 2004; **16**: 137–141.

99. Bohlke, K., Davis, R.L., DeStefano, F. *et al.* Epidemiology of anaphylaxis among children and adolescents enrolled in a health maintenance organization. *J. Allergy Clin. Immunol.* 2004; **113**: 536–542.

100. Helbling, A., Hurni, T., Mueller, U.R. *et al.* Incidence of anaphylaxis with circulatory symptoms: a study over a 3-year period comprising 940 000 inhabitants of the Swiss Canton Bern. *Clin. Exp. Allergy* 2004; **34**: 285–290.

101. Helbling, A., Hurni, T., Mueller, U.R. *et al.* Incidence of anaphylaxis with circulatory symptoms: a study over a 3-year period comprising 940 000 inhabitants of the Swiss Canton Bern. *Clin. Exp. Allergy* 2004; **34**: 285–290.

102. Brown, A.F., McKinnon, D. & Chu, K. Emergency department anaphylaxis: a review of 142 patients in a single year. *J. Allergy Clin. Immunol.* 2001; **108**: 861–866.

103. Cianferoni, A., Novembre, E., Mugnaini, L. *et al.* Clinical features of acute anaphylaxis in patients admitted to a university hospital: an 11-year retrospective review (1985–1996). *Ann. Allergy Asthma Immunol.* 2001; **87**: 27–32.

104. Pastorello, E.A., Rivolta, F., Bianchi, M. *et al.* Incidence of anaphylaxis in the emergency department of a general

hospital in Milan. *J. Chromatogr B. Biomed. Sci.* Appl 2001; **756**: 11–17.

105. Novembre, E., Cianferoni, A., Bernardini, R. *et al.* Anaphylaxis in children: clinical and allergologic features. *Pediatrics* 1998; **101**: E8.

106. Kemp, S.F., Lockey, R.F., Wolf, B.L. *et al.* Anaphylaxis. A review of 266 cases. *Arch. Intern. Med.* 1995; **155**: 1749–1754.

107. Yocum, M.W. & Khan, D.A. Assessment of patients who have experienced anaphylaxis: a 3-year survey. *Mayo Clin. Proc.* 1994; **69**: 16–23.

108. Russell, M., Dark, K.A., Cummins, R.W., Ellman, G., Callaway, E. & Peeke, H.V. Learned histamine release. *Science* 1984; **225**(4663): 733–734.

109. Palermo-Neto, J. & Guimaraes, R.K. Pavlovian conditioning of lung anaphylactic response in rats. *Life Sci.* 2000; **68**: 611–623.

110. Finkelman, F.D., Rothenberg, M.E., Brandt, E.B., Morris, S.C. & Strait, R.T. Molecular mechanisms of anaphylaxis: lessons from studies with murine models. *J. Allergy Clin. Immunol.* 2005; **115**: 449–457.

111. Vercelli, D. Genetic regulation of IgE responses: Achilles and the tortoise. *J. Allergy Clin. Immunol.* 2005; **116**: 60–64.

112. Oliver, J.M., Pfeiffer, J.R., Surviladze, Z. *et al.* Membrane receptor mapping: the membrane topography of Fc(epsilon)RI signaling. *Subcell. Biochem.* 2004; **37**: 3–34.

113. Iwaki, S., Tkaczyk, C., Metcalfe, D.D. & Gilfillan, A.M. Roles of adaptor molecules in mast cell activation. *Chem. Immunol. Allergy* 2005; **87**: 43–58.

114. Metcalfe, D.D., Baram, D. & Mekori, Y.A. Mast cells. *Physiol. Rev.* 1997; **77**: 1033–1079.

115. Montrucchio, G., Alloatti, G. & Camussi, G. Role of platelet-activating factor in cardiovascular pathophysiology. *Physiol. Rev.* 2000; **80**: 1669–1699.

116. Karasawa, K., Harada, A., Satoh, N., Inoue, K. & Setaka, M. Plasma platelet activating factor-acetylhydrolase (PAF-AH). *Prog. Lipid Res.* 2003; **42**: 93–114.

117. Smith, P.L., Sobotka, A., Bleeker, E.R. *et al.* Physiologic manifestations of human anaphylaxis. *J. Clin. Invest.* 1980; **66**: 1072–1080.

118. Kozik, A., Moore, R.B., Potempa, J., Imamura, T., Rapala-Kozik, M. & Travis, J. A novel mechanism for bradykinin production at inflammatory sites. Diverse effects of a mixture of neutrophil elastase and mast cell tryptase versus tissue and plasma kallikreins on native and oxidized kininogens. *J. Biol. Chem.* 1998; **273**: 33224–33229.

119. Kaplan, A.P., Joseph, K. & Silverberg, M. Pathways for bradykinin formation and inflammatory disease. *J. Allergy Clin. Immunol.* 2002; **109**: 195–209.

120. Leeb-Lundberg, L.M., Marceau, F., Muller-Esterl, W., Pettibone, D.J. & Zuraw, B.L. International union of pharmacology. XLV. Classification of the kinin receptor family: from molecular mechanisms to pathophysiological consequences. *Pharmacol. Rev.* 2005; **57**: 27–77.

121. Ober, A.I., MacLean, J.A. & Hannaway, P.J. Life-threatening anaphylaxis to venom immunotherapy in a patient taking an angiotensin-converting enzyme inhibitor. *J. Allergy Clin. Immunol.* 2003; **112**: 1008–1009.

122. Hermann, K. & Ring, J. The renin angiotensin system and hymenoptera venom anaphylaxis. *Clin. Exp. Allergy* 1993; **23**: 762–769.

123. Nikpoor, B., Duan, Q.L. & Rouleau, G.A. Acute adverse reactions associated with angiotensin-converting enzyme inhibitors: genetic factors and therapeutic implications. *Expert Opin. Pharmacother.* 2005; **6**: 1851–1856.

124. De Kruif, P. Anaphylatoxin and anaphylaxis: VIII. Primary toxicity of normal serum. *J. Inf. Dis.* 1917; **20**: 717–775.

125. Campbell, W.D., Lazoura, E., Okada, N. & Okada, H. Inactivation of C3a and C5a octapeptides by carboxypeptidase R and carboxypeptidase N. *Microbiol. Immunol.* 2002; **46**: 131–134.

126. Ring, J. Anaphylactoid reactions to intravenous solutions used for Volume substitution. *Clin. Rev. Allergy* 1991; **9**: 397–414.

127. Ljungström, K.G., Revenäs, B., Smedegård, G., Hedin, H., Richter, W. & Saldeen, T. Histopathological lung changes in immune complex mediated anaphylactic shock in humans elicited by dextran. *Forens. Sci. Int.* 1988; **38**: 251–258.

128. Hernández, D., de Rojas, F., Martínez Escribano, C. *et al.* Fatal dextran-induced allergic anaphylaxis. *Allergy* 2002: **57**: 862–862.

129. Marone, G., de Crescenzo, G., Adt, M., Patella, V., Arbustini, E. & Genovese, A. Immunological characterization and functional importance of human heart mast cells. *Immunopharmacology* 1995; **31**(1): 1–18.

130. Schmidt-Traub, S. & Bamler, K.J. The psychoimmunological association of panic disorder and allergic reaction. *Br. J. Clin. Psychol.* 1997; **36**: 51–62.

131. Choi, I.H., Ha, T.Y., Lee, D.G. *et al.* Occurrence of disseminated intravascular coagulation (DIC) in active systemic anaphylaxis: role of platelet-activating factor. *Clin. Exp. Immunol.* 1995; **100**: 390–394.

132. Brazil, E. & MacNamara, A.F. "Not so immediate" hypersensitivity – the danger of biphasic anaphylactic reactions. *J. Accid. Emerg. Med.* 1998; **15**: 252–253.

133. Choi, I.W., Kim, Y.S., Kim, D.K., *et al.* Platelet-activating factor-mediated NF-kappaB dependency of a late anaphylactic reaction. *J. Exp. Med.* 2003; **198**: 145–151.

134. Project Team of the Resuscitation Council (UK). Update on the emergency medical treatment of anaphylactic reactions for first medical responders and for community nurses. *Emerg. Med. J.* 2001; **18**: 393–395.

135. Brown, S.G. Cardiovascular aspects of anaphylaxis: implications for treatment and diagnosis. *Curr. Opin. Allergy Clin. Immunol.* 2005; **5**: 359–364.

136. Sampson, H.A., Mendelson, L. & Rosen, J.P. Fatal and near-fatal anaphylactic reaction to food in children and adolescents. *N. Engl. J. Med.* 1992; **327**: 380–384.

137. Kay, L.J. & Peachell, P.T. Mast cell beta2-adrenoceptors. *Chem. Immunol. Allergy* 2005; **87**: 145–153.

138. Chong, L.K., Morice, A.H., Yeo, W.W., Schleimer, R.P. & Peachell, P.T. Functional desensitization of beta agonist responses in human lung mast cells. *Am. J. Respir. Cell Mol. Biol.* 1995; **13**: 540–546.

139. Muller, U. & Haeberli, G. Use of beta-blockers during immunotherapy for hymenoptera venom allergy. *J. Allergy Clin. Immunol.* 2005; **115**: 606–609.

140. Sadana, A., O'Donnell, C., Hunt, M.T. & Gavalas, M. Managing acute anaphylaxis. Intravenous adrenaline should be considered because of the urgency of the condition. *Br. Med. J.* 2000; **320**(7239): 937–938.

141. Liu, S., Carpenter, R.L., Chiu, A.A., McGill, T.J. & Mantell, S.A. Epinephrine prolongs duration of subcutaneous infiltration of local anesthesia in a dose-related manner. Correlation with magnitude of vasoconstriction. *Reg. Anesth.* 1995; **20**: 378–384.

142. Hoffman, B.B. & Lefkowitz, R.J. Catecholamines, sympathomimetics drugs and adrenergic receptor antagonists. In Hardman, J.G., Gilman, A.G. & Limbird, L.E. eds. *The Pharmacological Basis of Therapeutics*, 9th edn. New York: McGraw-Hill, 1996: 199–248.

143. Wolfel, E.E., Hiatt, W.R., Brammell, H.L. *et al.* Effects of selective and nonselective beta-adrenergic blockade on mechanisms of exercise conditioning. *Circulation* 1986; **74**: 664–674.

144. Simons, F.E., Gu, X. & Simons, K.J. Epinephrine absorption in adults: intramuscular versus subcutaneous injection. *J. Allergy Clin. Immunol.* 2001; **108**: 871–873.

145. Song, T.T., Nelson, M.R., Chang, J.H., Engler, R.J.M. & Chowdhury, B.A. Adequacy of the epinephrine autoinjector needle length in delivering epinephrine to the intramuscular tissues. *Ann. Allergy Asthma Immunol.* 2005; **94**: 539–542.

146. Tsuda, A., Tanaka, K.A., Huraux, C. *et al.* The in vitro reversal of histamine-induced vasodilation in the human internal mammary artery. *Anesth. Analg.* 2001; **93**: 1453–1459.

147. Bautista, E., Simons, F.E., Simons, K.J. *et al.* Epinephrine fails to hasten hemodynamic recovery in fully developed canine anaphylactic shock. *Int. Arch. Allergy Immunol.* 2002; **128**: 151–164.

148. Smith, P., Kagey-Sobotka, A., Bleecker, E.R. *et al.* Physiologic manifestations of human anaphylaxis. *J. Clin. Invest.* 1980; **66**: 1072–1080.

149. Mink, S.N., Simons, F.E., Simons, K.J., Becker, A.B. & Duke, K. Constant infusion of epinephrine, but not bolus treatment, improves haemodynamic recovery in anaphylactic shock in dogs. *Clin. Exp. Allergy* 2004; **34**: 1776–1783.

150. Heytman, M. & Rainbird, A. Use of alpha-agonists for management of anaphylaxis occurring under anaesthesia: case studies and review. *Anaesthesia* 2004; **59**: 1210–1215.

151. Kill, C., Wranze, E. & Wulf, H. Successful treatment of severe anaphylactic shock with vasopressin. Two case reports. *Int. Arch. Allergy Immunol.* 2004; **134**: 260–261.

152. Thomas, M. & Crawford, I. Best evidence topic report. Glucagon infusion in refractory anaphylactic shock in patients on beta-blockers. *Emerg. Med. J.* 2005; **22**: 272–273.

153. Boulain, T., Achard, J.M., Teboul, J.L., Richard, C., Perrotin, D. & Ginies, G. Changes in BP induced by passive leg raising predict response to fluid loading in critically ill patients. *Chest* 2002; **121**(4):1245–1252.

154. Maron, M.B. Dose–response relationship between plasma epinephrine concentration and alveolar liquid clearance in dogs. *J. Appl. Physiol.* 1998; **85**: 1702–1707.

155. Arfi, A.M., Kouatli, A., Al-Ata, J., Arif, H. & Syed, S. Acute myocardial ischemia following accidental intravenous administration of epinephrine in high concentration. *Indian Heart J.* 2005; **57**: 261–264.

156. Pumphrey, R.S. & Nicholls, J.M. Epinephrine-resistant food anaphylaxis. *Lancet* 2000; **355**: 1099.

157. Cheuk, D.K., Chau, T.C. & Lee, S.L. A meta-analysis on intravenous magnesium sulphate for treating acute asthma. *Arch. Dis. Child.* 2005; **90**: 74–77.

158. Blitz, M., Blitz, S., Beasely, R. *et al.* Inhaled magnesium sulfate in the treatment of acute asthma. *Cochrane Database Syst. Rev.* 2005; **19**: CD003898.

159. Calogiuri, G.F., Muratore, L., Nettis, E., Ventura, M.T., Ferrannini, A. & Tursi, A. Anaphylaxis to hydrocortisone hemisuccinate with cross-sensitivity to related compounds in a paediatric patient. *Br. J. Dermatol.* 2004; **151**: 707–708.

160. Granata, A.V., Halickman, J.F. & Borak, J. Utility of military anti-shock trousers (MAST) in anaphylactic shock – a case report. *J. Emerg. Med.* 1985; **2**: 349–351.

161. Oliveira Neto, A.M., Duarte, N.M., Vicente, W.V., Viaro, F. & Evora, P.R. Methylene blue: an effective treatment for contrast medium-induced anaphylaxis. *Med. Sci. Monit.* 2003; **9**: CS102–CS106.

162. Mullins, R.J. Anaphylaxis: risk factors for recurrence. *Clin. Exp. Allergy* 2003; **33**: 1033–1040.

163. Avery, N.J., King, R.M., Knight, S. & Hourihane, J.O. Assessment of quality of life in children with peanut allergy. *Pediatr. Allergy Immunol.* 2003; **14**: 378–382.

164. Sicherer, S.H., Burks, A.W. & Sampson, H.A. Clinical features of acute allergic reactions to peanut and tree nuts in children. Pediatrics. 1998; **102**: e6 (http://www.pediatrics.org/cgi/content/full/102/1/e6).

165. Golden, D.B. Discontinuing venom immunotherapy. *Curr. Opin. Allergy Clin. Immunol.* 2001; **1**: 353–356.

166. Oppenheimer, J.J., Nelson, H.S., Bock, S.A., Christensen, F. & Leung, D.Y. Treatment of peanut allergy with rush immunotherapy. *J. Allergy Clin. Immunol.* 1992; **90**: 256–262.

167. Sicherer, S.H. & Simons, F.E. Quandaries in prescribing an emergency action plan and self-injectable epinephrine for first-aid management of anaphylaxis in the community. *J. Allergy Clin. Immunol.* 2005; **115**: 575–583.

168. Sicherer, S.H., Forman, J.A. & Noone, S.A. Use assessment of self-administered epinephrine among food-allergic children and pediatricians. *Pediatrics* 2000; **105**: 359–362.

169. Gold, M. & Sainsbury, R. First aid anaphylaxis management in 68 children who were prescribed an epinephrine auto-injector device (EpiPen). *J. Allergy Clin. Imunol.* 2000; **106**: 171–176.

63

High altitude resuscitation

Philip Eisenburger, Benjamin Honigman, Susan Niermeyer, Robert Roach and Wolfgang Voelckel

Universität fur Notfallmedizin, Vienna, Austria

Cardiac arrest in remote areas such as in the wilderness and at high altitude cannot be compared directly with cardiac arrest in the urban setting, and both scenarios merit specific consideration. Given that mountains and, in particular, ski resorts have become increasingly popular with tourists, the occurrence of cardiac arrest in more remote places becomes an epidemiologic problem. Moreover, millions of people worldwide travel by plane, where they are exposed to a high altitude environment that may contribute to cardiocirculatory problems or even cardiac arrest. This chapter focuses on both of these specific settings and their relevant physiologic and epidemiologic characteristics.

Cardiac arrest resulting from high altitude on mountains

Worldwide, it is estimated that approximately 40 million individuals live above 8000 feet, and 25 million live above 10 000 feet.[1] Both travelers who arrive abruptly into an hypoxic environment and residents who live year round at such altitudes have different risks for cardiac arrest. Mountain sports activities and tourism are attracting increasing numbers of participants each year. This, combined with the rapid ascent made possible by air transportation, results in increased members of unacclimatized individuals at risk for high-altitude illness. More than 1 million visitors travel annually to the remote high mountain ranges of Asia, Africa, and South America.[1] Approximately 35 million visitors travel annually to high-altitude recreation areas in the western United States.[1]

The clinical syndrome of high-altitude illness comprises several symptoms that may overlap and share a common pathophysiology. If individuals fail to acclimatize and ignore the clinical signs of the typically benign and usually self-limited acute mountain sickness (AMS), they are at risk of developing high altitude pulmonary (HAPE) or cerebral edema (HACE). Approximately 8% of individuals who develop AMS at 14 000 feet (4000 m) will develop these life-threatening conditions at higher altitudes,[2] and both HAPE and HACE can deteriorate and result in cardiac arrest.

The incidence of AMS varies with altitude and rate of ascent. It increases from 3% at 6000 ft (1829 m) in trekkers in the eastern Alps not staying at this altitude overnight[3] to 9% at 2850 m (9000 ft)[4] to 25% in tourists in the western US at 2400 m (8000 ft),[5] 47% in those who fly into the Khumbu region of Mt Everest at 12 000 ft (3600m)[2] and 67% in hikers on Mount Rainier at 14 000 ft (4000 m).[6] These incidence rates depend on many variables, including the velocity of ascent, highest altitude reached, sleeping altitude, duration of stay at any altitude, and individual susceptibility. Both HAPE and HACE are more common with a longer duration of visit and higher sleeping altitude. Gender does not affect the incidence of AMS; however, women may have less risk of developing HAPE.[2,7]

The number of elderly people visiting mountain resorts is increasing. Six million visitors older than 55 years of age travel annually to the Colorado Rocky Mountains, according to the Colorado Tourism Board. Many of these individuals have underlying health problems, including lung disease (10%), heart disease (25%), and hypertension (30%).[8] Despite these pre-existing risk factors, older adults are less likely to develop AMS when compared with other age groups,[8] yet there are clues that the elderly may not

Cardiac Arrest: The Science and Practice of Resuscitation Medicine. 2nd edn., ed. Norman Paradis, Henry Halperin, Karl Kern, Volker Wenzel, Douglas Chamberlain. Published by Cambridge University Press. © Cambridge University Press, 2007.

react well to acute high-altitude exposure. Pulmonary vital capacity decreases almost one-third in elderly individuals who go from sea level to 14 000 feet (4000 m) for 1 week, producing a significant drop in both oxygen saturation and maximal oxygen uptake during exercise. For elderly individuals residing at moderate elevations, oxygen saturation is approximately 92% at rest.[8]

Epidemiology of AMS-induced cardiac arrest

While AMS may contribute to fatalities of other causes such as trauma, and misjudgment of danger in a proportion of deaths, the disease itself is uncommonly lethal. From 1950 to 2003, among approximately 30 000 mountaineers in the Himalayas, 664 died. Of those, 43 (6.5%) died of AMS/HACE/HAPE and 53 (8%) had AMS as a contributing factor to some other form of death[9] (e.g., "Hammann [. . . had] cerebral edema and froze to death;" Report DHAI-951-02 of the Himalayan Database).

Of 23 people who died on expeditions to summits > 7000 meters, 4 died of worsened AMS.[10] In a period of 3 1/2 years, helicopter rescue flights at moderate altitude in the Himalayas responded to 1 HAPE and 2 HACE patients out of 23 dead and to 38 AMS patients out of 111 live trekkers who were evacuated.[11] The response time for the helicopter to arrive was more than 24 hours. There are no data on the actual number of fatalities. It is estimated that there are about 100–200 deaths world-wide secondary to altitude illness and most of these are in soldiers in Pakistan and India, climbers on Kilimanjaro and Aconcagua, and unknown tourists in Asia and South America. In the United States and Europe, deaths are obviously rare, and no reliable data are available (personal communication, Peter Hackett 2005).

Definitions

Moderate altitude is between 8000 and 12 000 feet (2400–3600 m) of elevation. Although most people do not experience significant arterial oxygen desaturation until they reach higher altitudes, high-altitude illness is common with rapid ascents above 2500 m (8200 ft). Individuals with underlying medical problems may be predisposed to developing altitude illness at these lower levels.

High altitude is between 12 000 and 18 000 feet (3600–5500 m). Most serious altitude illness occurs at these levels. The pathophysiologic effects of high altitude begin when the oxygen saturation of the arterial blood begins to fall below the 90% level. The sigmoidal shape of the oxyhemoglobin dissociation curve prevents a significant fall of

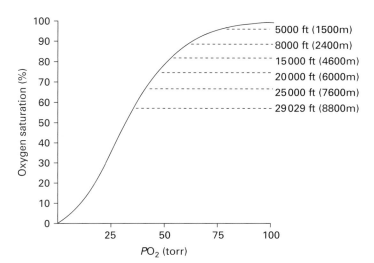

Fig. 63.1. SaO_2 dissociation curve changes with increasing altitude = decreasing partial pressure of oxygen

arterial oxygen saturation (SaO_2) in most individuals up to an altitude of approximately 12 000 feet. At this altitude, the steep portion of the curve is encountered, and rapid desaturation begins, with relatively small increases in altitude (Fig. 63.1). Some predisposed individuals may become desaturated to less than 90% at altitudes as low as 8000 feet (2400 m).

Extreme altitude is above 18 000 feet (5500 m). At this height, the human organism is not able to cope with the environmental conditions, and to adjust physiologic function for long-term survival. Accordingly, prolonged visits above this level will inevitably result in progressive deterioration. Moreover, in cases of life-threatening high-altitude illness, air rescue by helicopter – although proven feasible – is unavailable.

Acclimatization

Acclimatization occurs gradually and involves multiple respiratory, cardiovascular, and hematologic adjustments, allowing a greater ability to survive and perform in the high-altitude environment. It begins at the altitude that causes the oxygen saturation of arterial blood to fall below sea-level values. The ability to acclimatize is different among individuals, in part depending on the so-called hypoxic ventilatory response, the hyperventilation triggered by the carotid bodies, and central mechanisms in the medulla.[1,12]

Respiratory adaptation consisting of an increase in minute ventilation is the most important physiologic change that occurs during acclimatization, causing a decrease in the partial pressure of carbon dioxide in arterial blood ($PaCO_2$). The alveolar gas equation states that, as the alveolar PCO_2 decreases, a corresponding increase in PO_2 occurs, thereby increasing arterial oxygenation. Thus the level of ventilation determines alveolar oxygen for a given inspired oxygen tension.

Pathophysiology

The clinical syndrome of high-altitude illness represents a spectrum of symptoms (Table 63.1) sharing common and interconnected pathophysiologic mechanisms.

For a detailed description of the pathophysiology of altitude illness, the reader is referred to several references.[13–17] Briefly, the initiating factor is believed to be hypobaric hypoxemia which sets into motion a complex pathologic process that involves the circulatory, pulmonary, endocrine, and central nervous systems and leads to the development of the various clinical symptoms.

Hypoxemia alters fluid homeostasis, resulting in a generalized fluid retention, followed by the shift of fluid into the intracellular spaces. This is regulated by an interplay of antidiuretic hormone (ADH), the renin-angiotensin-aldosterone system, and the atrial natriuretic peptide. The inappropriate release of these hormones is thought to be the underlying pathogenic mechanism for the development of high-altitude edema.

Hypoxia is a potent pulmonary vasoconstrictor, and pulmonary vascular resistance is increased. In the lungs, hypoxemia resulting from high-altitude exposure causes pulmonary artery hypertension. Uneven pulmonary vasoconstriction in HAPE-susceptible individuals may result in distention, injury, and increased permeability of the pulmonary vasculature. Pulmonary blood flow is also increased as a result of hypoxia increasing cardiac output. In HAPE victims an uneven distribution of pulmonary vasoconstriction may result in overperfusion, distention, and leakage in the remaining vessels,[18] which may explain the patchy nature of the infiltrate visualized on chest x-ray films of patients with HAPE (Fig. 63.2). Exercise and cold stress on arrival at high altitudes are commonly associated with HAPE, as well as sympathetic nervous system stimulation with catecholamine release.[19]

The manifestations of mild AMS/HACE appear to be the result of central nervous system dysfunction: vasogenic edema resulting from increased permeability of brain capillary endothelial cells may be the primary mechanism.[20] Hypoxemia also produces changes in cerebral blood flow and blood volume, which along with a loss of

Table 63.1. Symptoms of acute altitude-related sickness

- Nausea and vomiting
- Severe headache
- Fatigue
- Tachycardia
- Respiratory distress
- Mental alteration
- Dry coughing
- Vertigo
- Ataxia
- Oliguria ($<$ 500 ml / day)
- Sleeplessness

autoregulation may also play a part in the pathogenesis of AMS/HACE.

Hypoxemia also results in an increase of cerebral blood flow, but this is mitigated at high altitude by the vasoconstrictive effect of hypocapnia secondary to hyperventilation.[21] Cerebral blood flow is thought to increase, despite the hypocapnia, when PaO_2 is less than 60 mm Hg (altitude greater than 12 500 feet). This net increase of blood flow increases intracranial volume and may contribute to changes in intracranial pressure.

High-altitude pulmonary edema

HAPE is the most common fatal manifestation of severe high-altitude illness. Although HAPE is uncommon below 10 000 feet, it can occur, and even be fatal, at altitudes as low as 8000 feet. Episodes occurring between 8000 and 10 000 feet are usually related to heavy exercise or due to malformation of the cardiovascular/pulmonary system, but at higher altitudes pulmonary edema may also occur at rest or with only light activity.[22] The incidence of HAPE varies from 0.01% to 2% in most studies, but has reached 15.5% among soldiers who were flown directly to 14 500 feet without a chance to acclimatize at a lower altitude.[23,24]

Susceptibility for developing HAPE may exist in some individuals who may experience HAPE with each ascent to altitude. Many patients, however, have a single episode of HAPE and subsequently are able to return to high altitude without a recurrence. Conversely, those with previously uneventful high-altitude exposures may develop HAPE in a future ascent.

Individuals who have been residents at high-altitude locations for extended periods, pulmonary edema may develop on re-ascent from a trip to low altitude. This phenomenon, which occurs primarily in children and adolescents, has been termed reentry HAPE.

Clinical presentation

The initial symptoms of HAPE usually begin insidiously 2 to 4 days after arrival at high altitude. Although most cases occur during the second night, HAPE may develop rapidly, with early symptoms apparent after just a few hours at high altitude. Marked dyspnea on exertion, fatigue with minimal to moderate effort, and dry cough are early manifestations of the disease. The symptoms of AMS usually occur concurrently with the development of HAPE.

Physical examination reveals a few rales in mild HAPE, usually in the region of the right middle lobe, progressing to unilateral or bilateral rales, then diffuse bilateral rales and audible rhonchi and gurgles that can be heard without a stethoscope. Central cyanosis, tachypnea, tachycardia, and slightly elevated temperatures are also common. A respiratory tract infection may occasionally be seen. As the condition intensifies, cerebral edema or simply severe hypoxemia causes central nervous system dysfunction, such as ataxia and altered mentation. Coma may follow and precede death in a few hours if oxygen therapy is not instituted, or immediate descent is not possible.

Ancillary tests

Chest radiographs can help elucidate the nature of the illness. The infiltrates seen in HAPE victims are fluffy (alveolar) and patchy in distribution, with areas of clearing between the patches. Unilateral infiltrates may be seen in mild cases. Bilateral infiltrates indicate a severe form of HAPE, and involvement of the right midlung field is a common sign (Fig. 63.2). Pleural effusion is rare but may be present in severe cases. The extent of the edema present on the chest film roughly parallels the clinical severity.[22] The radiographic findings of cardiomegaly, batwing distribution of infiltrates, and Kerley B lines, which are typical of cardiogenic pulmonary edema, are absent in HAPE.

Radiographic evidence for HAPE clears rapidly after initiation of treatment; some mild cases may clear in 4 to 6 hours and most clear by 24 hours. In some cases of severe HAPE, however, infiltrates may persist for as long as 2 weeks even though the clinical symptoms have resolved.

An electrocardiogram (ECG) prior to arrest will usually reveal tachycardia and evidence of right-heart strain, including right axis deviation, P-wave abnormalities, tall R waves in the precordial leads, and S waves in the lateral leads (Fig. 63.3).[22] Invasive hemodynamic monitoring shows increased pulmonary vascular resistance, elevated

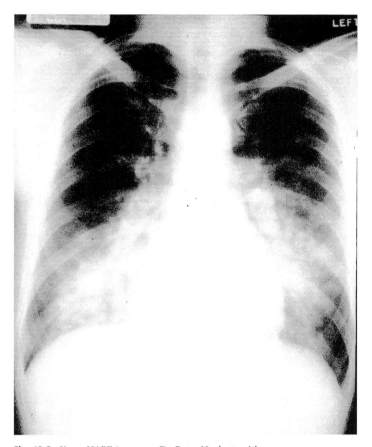

Fig. 63.2. X-ray HAPE (courtesy Dr. Peter Hackett, with permission). Chest X-ray of a patient with high altitude pulmonary edema (HAPE).

pulmonary artery pressures, but normal pulmonary wedge pressures.[25] Likewise, echocardiography studies demonstrate high estimated pulmonary artery pressures, pulmonary vascular resistance, and normal left ventricular function.[26,27]

High-altitude cerebral edema

HACE is the least common yet most severe form of high-altitude illness. The incidence of HACE is lower than that of HAPE, and although it usually occurs together with HAPE, it may be seen as an isolated entity. Death from HACE at as low as 8200 feet has been reported, although most cases occur above 12 000 feet.[28] Mild AMS may progress rapidly to severe HACE with coma within 12 hours.[5] The usual time course is 1 to 3 days for the development of severe symptoms, but in some cases severe symptoms and coma do not develop for 5 to 9 days.[29]

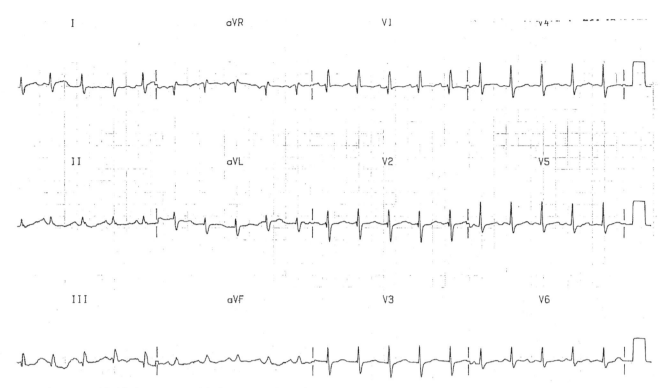

Fig. 63.3. ECG right heart strain. Right heart strain due to hypoxic vasoconstriction in pulmonary arteries in a patient exposed to high altitude

Clinical presentation

HACE is characterized by evidence of global cerebral dysfunction and represents the most severe manifestation of AMS. Symptoms of severe AMS (headache, fatigue, vomiting), as well as those of HAPE (cough and dyspnea), are usually present. HACE-specific signs include ataxia, generalized seizures, slurred speech, rare focal neurologic deficits, and altered mentation. The last mentioned can range from mild emotional lability or confusion to hallucinations, and ultimately decreased levels of consciousness that may proceed to coma and death.[29] MRI scans in patients with HACE reveal white matter changes consistent with vasogenic edema (Fig. 63.4).[30] Ataxia alone is an indication for immediate descent.

Progression to cardiac arrest

Deterioration of AMS, HAPE, and/or HACE will ultimately result in cardiac arrest if adequate therapy is not available in the appropriate time. Once the patient suffers cardiac arrest, successful resuscitation may be considerably less likely than it is in other settings. First, because of the remote location, i.e., wilderness or high altitude, proper performance of CPR will be limited by several factors, such as fatigue of the rescuers, environmental issues, and the availability of advanced life support means. Second, cardiac arrest caused by deteriorated HAPE or HACE is typically the result of prolonged hypoxemia. While central respiratory depression due to cerebral edema can be treated sufficiently by artificial ventilation, it is obvious that the pulmonary pathology of HAPE will not immediately respond to oxygen therapy. In addition, it is well known that asphyxial cardiac arrest is associated with poor outcome. Third, since resuscitation efforts focus on the restoration of cerebral perfusion and re-oxygenation, cerebral edema and elevated intracranial pressures during HACE will further limit the chance for successful CPR.[31]

The key to successful resuscitation is recognizing the patient's deterioration and treating the underlying problems before cardiac arrest develops. In addition, the specific pathophysiology of altitude-related illness deserves a distinct therapeutic approach. Since the cause of a cardiac arrest at high altitude may not necessarily be AMS, but may also include myocardial infarction, stroke, or pulmonary embolism, it is obvious that therapy will be difficult to direct.

Cardiac arrest in children and young adults at high altitude

The etiology of cardiac arrest in infants and children at high altitude is predominantly asphyxial; respiratory failure often precedes cardiac arrest. Especially during infancy, high-altitude hypoxemia may unmask a pre-existing cardiopulmonary condition that may be well compensated at low altitudes. Interruption of the postnatal decline in pulmonary artery pressure. Unusually severe anemia before postnatal erythropoiesis accelerates, and presentation of previously undiagnosed congenital heart malformations are examples of risks unique to altitude exposure in the very young. Coupled with limited ability of the patient to communicate distress clearly, and the non-specific signs of illness in infancy, diagnosis of altitude-related illness may be delayed until a critical point has been reached. Conversely, the vulnerability of young children usually means that parents protect them from exposure to extremes of high altitude. Lack of exposure to the conditions resulting in severe high altitude cerebral edema may account for the absence of reports in the medical literature of fatal cases of HACE in children.[32]

The pathophysiology underlying cardiac arrest may differ substantially between infants and children who stay temporarily at high altitude (sojourners) as compared to those who are long-term residents there.

Sojourners

Children apparently experience an incidence of AMS very similar to that observed in adults.[32] Acute exposure to high altitude can result in an exaggerated hypoxemia that may potentiate other underlying pathophysiologic conditions, such as bronchopulmonary dysplasia following preterm birth and respiratory distress syndrome, congenital heart disease, severe anemia, or pulmonary hypoplasia. High altitude pulmonary edema does occur in children, although the incidence has not been well established.[32] As in adults, risk varies with rapidity of ascent, altitude reached, and previous history of HAPE. In addition, certain risk factors such as antecedent illness,[33] especially viral respiratory tract infections, or as mentioned above, underlying congenital heart disease, and other genetic conditions may uniquely predispose children to HAPE.

A lethal episode of HAPE has been described in an adolescent with unilateral absence of the pulmonary artery.[34] Several case reports of non-lethal occurrences also document such an association.[32]

Children with trisomy 21 (Down syndrome) have multiple medical risk factors that place them at higher risk for HAPE; these factors include chronic pulmonary hypertension,

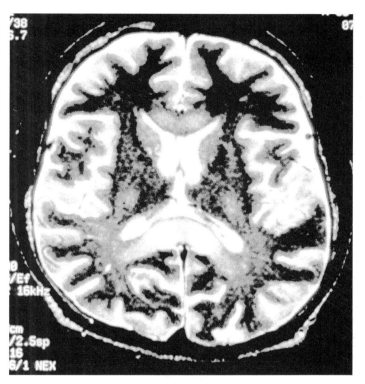

Fig. 63.4. MRI HACE (courtesy Dr. Peter Hackett, with permission). Cranial MRI of a patient with High Altitude Cerebral Edema (HACE).

pulmonary overperfusion from left-to-right shunts (ventricular septal defect (VSD), patent ductus arteriosus (PDA), atrial septal defect (ASD), and more complex congenital heart malformations), and frequent infections. A retrospective review of 52 patients treated for HAPE at The Children's Hospital in Denver, Colorado identified 6 children with trisomy 21.[35] All but one of these children had either chronic pulmonary hypertension or an active or surgically repaired left-to-right shunt; the remaining child had a history of preceding or concurrent illness, as did 4 other children in the series. The rapid onset of pulmonary edema and the relatively low altitudes (1738 m to 3252 m – 5100–10700 ft) suggest the need for heightened awareness when children with Down syndrome travel above sea level.

Sudden death has been reported in the setting of high altitude and extreme exertion among young adults with sickle cell trait.[36] Four young men (ages 19–21 years) experienced sickling crises and sudden death during moderate-to-severe exercise after recent arrival at relatively high altitude (1240 m – 4060 ft). Vaso-occlusive and splenic crises have been well described among patients with sickle cell anemia, sickle/hemoglobin C disease, and sickle/thalassemia who travel to the mountains above 2000 m (6600 ft).[37,38]

Residents

Among children resident at high altitude, pulmonary hypertension and high-altitude pulmonary edema are pathophysiologic mechanisms of great importance. Hypoxemia at high altitude also potentiates mortality from lower respiratory infections and may increase the incidence of sudden infant death syndrome.[39–42]

Symptomatic high-altitude pulmonary hypertension must be recognized as an important, and potentially lethal altitude-associated illness.[43] Typically, subacute pulmonary hypertension at high altitude develops in young children (generally under 18 months) of low-altitude ancestry who are exposed continuously to altitudes above 3000 m for periods longer than 1 month.[44–46] Oxygen administration and descent are often sufficient to bring improvement after timely diagnosis. Nevertheless, cardiac arrest occurs in cases with advanced right ventricular failure and irreversible pulmonary hypertension.[46,47] A well-documented autopsy series revealed severe right ventricular hypertrophy and vascular changes of pulmonary hypertension, with medial hypertrophy of pulmonary arteries and extensive muscularization of small pulmonary arteries and arterioles as a result of chronic hypoxic pulmonary vasoconstriction.[46]

Children with congenital heart disease may be at higher risk for developing complications of pulmonary hypertension at high altitude. An autopsy series of 280 infants (under 1 year of age) who died of congenital heart disease revealed 6 cases of severe pulmonary hypertensive changes (Heath Edwards grade IV) in the pulmonary vasculature.[48] A variety of cardiac lesions were represented in the series, including transposition of the great vessels, coarctation/interruption of the aorta, atrioventricular canal, and double outlet right ventricle; common to most cases was the presence of a ventricular septal defect and/or patent ductus arteriosus. Although this series from 1959–1978 predates modern echocardiographic diagnosis and early surgical intervention, similar pathophysiology and clinical evolution may occur today in many high-altitude areas of the world where diagnostic and treatment facilities are remote and poorly accessible.

The nature and incidence of HAPE differ among children resident at high altitude as compared to those who reside at low altitude and then travel to high altitude. Among children who reside at high-altitude, HAPE commonly occurs as a re-entry phenomenon, that is, upon reascent to the altitude of residence after travel to low altitude. Children resident at high altitude have an apparently higher incidence of re-entry HAPE than do adults.[32,49,50] Symptoms respond to supportive care with rest and oxygen. A variety of empirical pharmacologic therapies have been reported

as well, most commonly diuretics and calcium channel blockers. Children with re-entry HAPE and abnormal cardiac examinations, ECGs, or echocardiograms, however, may have previously unsuspected underlying abnormalities, such as unilateral absence of the pulmonary artery.[51]

Conflicting reports exist regarding the possibility of increased risk of SIDS among children living at high altitude.[39–41] The most rigorous study conducted at moderate high altitude (500–1900 m – 1640–6234 ft) concluded that the risk of SIDS increased gradually with increasing altitude of residence.[41]

Adult cardiac arrest on mountains not related to acute mountain sickness

(for cardiac arrest due to hypothermia see Chapter 57)

Cardiac arrest and sudden non-traumatic death is an epidemiologic problem in areas of alpine mass tourism, such as major ski resorts or high-altitude sightseeing spots. It is not entirely clear whether death in tourists to high elevations occurs because of natural progression of disease, or whether the hypoxic environment triggers sudden cardiac death. The risk of coronary heart disease at high altitude appears to depend mainly on the population and the amount of physical activity undertaken. Populations frequenting ski resorts are different from those trekking in Nepal, with the former more likely to in poorer health, not very physically active, and overweight. Healthy mountaineers´ hearts can tolerate exertion at the utmost hypoxia of extreme altitude (with arterial oxygen saturations below 50% and oxygen extraction rates of over 80%) without any sign of myocardial ischemia by clinical examination, echocardiography, ECG, or Swan-Ganz catheter determinations.[52–54] By contrast, individuals who died suddenly on a mountain in Austria (mostly in areas of mass tourism at altitudes from 1100 to 2100 m), had known coronary heart disease with or without prior myocardial infarction, arterial hypertension, and lack of regular exercise as independent risk factors of sudden death compared to controls.[55] The issue of whether altitude and the hypoxic environment itself (and not physical activity) poses a risk to people with known coronary artery disease has been discussed extensively.[56]

"Going up to the mountains to trek or ski is a safe undertaking for those who believe they are able to do this"[57] and "At high altitude, physical activity is limited by dyspnea and pulmonary gas exchange and not by the circulatory pump or cardiac output. . ." The patient with coronary disease is therefore more likely to die while running at sea level than trekking at high altitude because "trekking does not involve maximal work, but a comfortable pace that can be continued for many hours."[58] Rennie[57] and Hultgren[58] state that in asymptomatic patients, there is no indication that a stress ECG is of any help and is likely to lead to false positive results.

Downhill skiing receives little appreciation by some as being a true sport "where the work is done by the lift, . . . not an impressive aerobic challenge. . .".[57] Halhuber *et al.* observed 434 patients during a period of rehabilitation after myocardial infarction at altitudes of 1700 – 3200 m over 4 weeks and found only one reinfarction[59] and no deaths in this group. They also found a very low incidence of sudden death in alpine vacationers (6 / 151 000) at moderate altitudes (2 by myocardial infarction, 2 unclear, 1 mitral stenosis, and 1 myocardial infarction in the valley).[59]

Others argue that skiing is indeed physical work causing coronary stress. Grover *et al.* used telemetric ST-segment analysis during downhill skiing and found ST-depressions in 5 out of 149 volunteers.[60] Morgan *et al.* compared treadmill performance in nine patients with confirmed coronary heart disease at 1600 and at 3100 meters without acclimatization. They found a significantly shorter time of exercise and a lower workload before onset of ischemia (ST depression or angina) at high altitude.[61] Two out of the nine patients were short of breath after arrival at 3100 meters.

Irrespective of whether altitude is raising or lowering the individual risk of coronary insufficiency, sudden cardiac death does occur in resorts with a large tourist population, but is rarely seen at higher elevations where only trained and experienced mountaineers can (or should) go. Malignant primary arrhythmias also do not appear to play a role in sudden death on mountains.[14,59–62]

Peer-reviewed original publications on the incidence of death on mountains are rare.[11,63,64] Data on sudden death on the mountains originate from various epidemiologic settings, and the overall risk of suffering myocardial ischemia on a mountain is hard to determine. Much of the data presented is from research letters[10,55,65–67] and even articles in yearbooks of mountaineering clubs[68–70] and should be regarded with the necessary scientific caution.

In areas with large tourist populations, i.e., mostly skiing resorts, sudden death accounts for about 30% of all deaths; the other 70% are due to trauma.[55,63,65,67] The totality of cases can only be extrapolated from the different sources, as the included causes of death or populations vary. Cases of pulmonary embolism, intracranial hemorrhage, and dissecting aortic aneurysms, if known, were excluded from some analyses[63] or are incorporated into the "deaths by heart failure."[70] Most of the published data comes from Austria. Here, approximately 8.5 million people engaged in mountain hiking, downhill skiing, or both each year before 1993.[55] In contrast, Lienhart *et al.* cite the presence of

1 million skiers in the year 2004 in one single resort in Austria,[64] with a maximum of 20 000 persons at a time. Burtscher gives different numbers of victims over several overlapping time intervals, depending on the combination of skiing (downhill or cross country), hiking, and climbing. He reports 642 arrests in people who were skiing, hiking, and climbing over 9 years;[66] 416 victims while hiking or downhill skiing over 7 years;[55] and 285 deaths during hiking over 7 years.[65] The Austrian mountain rescue association reported 373 deaths of all causes in 2003[70] encompassing any activity on a mountain, of which 112 were due to non-traumatic sudden death (including pulmonary embolism, stroke, myocardial ischemia, and others). The range of victims between 1984 and 2003 was 205–373, mean 304.[70] The activity before the arrest is depicted in Fig. 63.5.

Usually, alpine cardiac arrest victims appear to be included in reports of regional emergency medical service systems,[71] but this has been debated as being inconclusive.[72] Breitfeld and Voelckel reported all air rescue missions in Austria over 3 years performed by the major air rescue provider in Austria.[68] In total, rescue helicopters responded to 98 cardiac arrests, in which 80 (82%) victims received bystander basic life support. Automated external defibrillators for basic life support were not available to non-physicians at that time. Standard advanced cardiac life support was instituted after 25 ± 5 min. Return of spontaneous circulation was achieved in 6 patients, of whom 3 died before transport. The remaining 3 (3%) reached the hospital alive, but none survived to hospital discharge (unpublished details[68]) The majority of all arrests (62%) were observed during winter and mainly in ski resorts (75%). In summer, at least one-third of all cardiac arrest cases occurred close to lodges or alpine resorts. On the basis of these data, the authors initiated a public access defibrillation programme on a glacier ski resort with 1 million visitors per year and a maximum of 20 000 guests per day. As reported by Lienhart *et al.* four automated external defibrillators were placed at appropriate locations within the resort. Within the following 2 years, 3 cardiac arrest victims received bystander CPR and automated external defibrillation. Two patients survived to hospital admission, and one was discharged in good neurological condition.[64]

In a setting completely different from that described above, the Himalayas, Shlim and Houston[19] report helicopter missions over 31/2 years for trekking (not mountaineering) tourists in Nepal. Among 148 000 persons, 23 died and were evacuated by helicopter, and another 111 were rescued alive. Of the dead victims, none was classified to have died from myocardial ischemia (4 causes were unknown), and among the ones rescued alive, cardiac problems were the chief complaint in only 6 cases. The

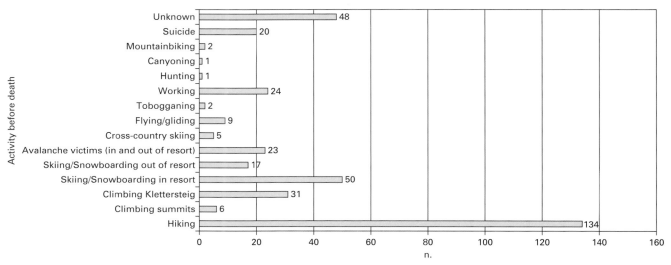

Fig. 63.5. Activity before death on mountains, Austria. (Adapted from ref. 70.)

study was repeated with a different methodology. Shlim and Gallie[73] found that four patients had died from heart attacks during trekking among a total of 275 950 trekkers over 41/2 years (total number of deaths, 40: traumatic cardiac arrest, 12; acute mountain sickness, 10; non-AMS illness, 14, missing, 4).

Trekkers death rates (15/100 000[11]) contrast sharply to deaths in climbers (2900/100 000[74]) in the Himalayas, which are primarily due to trauma, hypothermia, and avalanches. In the Himalayas, among the 165 non-traumatic deaths, cardiac arrest was caused by illness (not acute mountain sickness) in 27 cases[9] (Fig. 63.6), but the total number of autopsies was extremely rare since most victims could not be transported home and were buried on the spot. Therefore, it usually remains unclear why a person suddenly collapses. The large database by Elisabeth Hawley[9] documenting all mountaineering expeditions to Nepalese summits over 40 years relies on interviews with climbers after their return and their description of events. The symptoms of altitude-related illness are well known and are distinguished from those of other illnesses.

Berghold and Schaffert from Austria assume that fulminant pulmonary embolism accounts for most non-traumatic deaths at extreme altitude,[75] although there are no data to support this (personal communication, Franz Berghold, 2004). Their reasoning is that extreme mountaineers have healthy hearts not susceptible to the injury caused by hypoxia.[54] Therefore, a possible explanation for sudden death besides AMS, hypothermia, or trauma may well be pulmonary embolism. It is known that climbers at

extreme altitudes have a high incidence of deep venous thrombosis due to hyperviscosity caused by elevation in hematocrit and dehydration[76,77] and immobility[77–82] when confined in a tent, constrictive clothing, and cold.[14] Hypobaric hypoxia is thought by some[76,83,84] to be an independent risk factor of thrombosis through altered coagulability[76,80–88] while others dispute this claim.[89,90]

Recently, airplane travel thrombosis – where similar pathophysiologic mechanisms apply – has been stated to occur mainly[91] or only[92] in patients with predisposing congenital coagulation abnormalities such as protein-c deficiency.

Irrespective of the mechanism, pulmonary embolism (PE) is found in 0.3%–57% of patients at altitude (table from Dickinson[94])[93–98] supporting Berghold's[75] assumption. The wide range of these data comes from different groups of patients (6 out of 1692 patients seen at hospital after altitude stay[98] and 9 out of 40 patients presenting with HAPE to hospital).[93] In a series of seven altitude-related deaths, pulmonary embolism was at least a contributing factor to death in 4 patients.[94] The signs and symptoms of PE may mimic those of HAPE, but embolic disease tends to have a more rapid onset, and pleuritic chest pain is a more prominent feature (Table 63.2).

Stroke – both ischemic and hemorrhagic – may also be a cause of sudden collapse and death at high and extreme altitude. High altitude death has been found to be associated with intracranial petechiae or hematomas (table from Dickinson[94]). Stroke is a problem at high altitude,[98–102] but as with pulmonary embolism it cannot

Table 63.2. Postmortem findings in seven trekkers who died of mountain sickness

| Case No | Age (y) | Lungs | | | | Brain | | | Deep vein thrombosis |
		Pulmonary thrombosis	Red infarcts	Bronchopneumonia	Edema	Thrombosis	Hemorrhage	Edema	
1	54	+	0	+ +	+	0	0	+ +	0
2	38	+ +	+ +	+	0	Subarachnoid venous with hemorrhage. Petechiae	+	0	0
3	27	+ +	+ +	+	0	Venous with subarachnoid hemorrhage. Posterior dural venous sinuses	+	+	0
4	54	+ +	+	+ +	0	0	0	+	+
5	41	0	0	0	+ +	0	+	+ +	0
6	46	0	0	+	+ +	0	0	+ +	0
7	62	+ +	0	+	+ +	. . .	. . .	. . .	0

From ref. 94. Reproduced with permission.

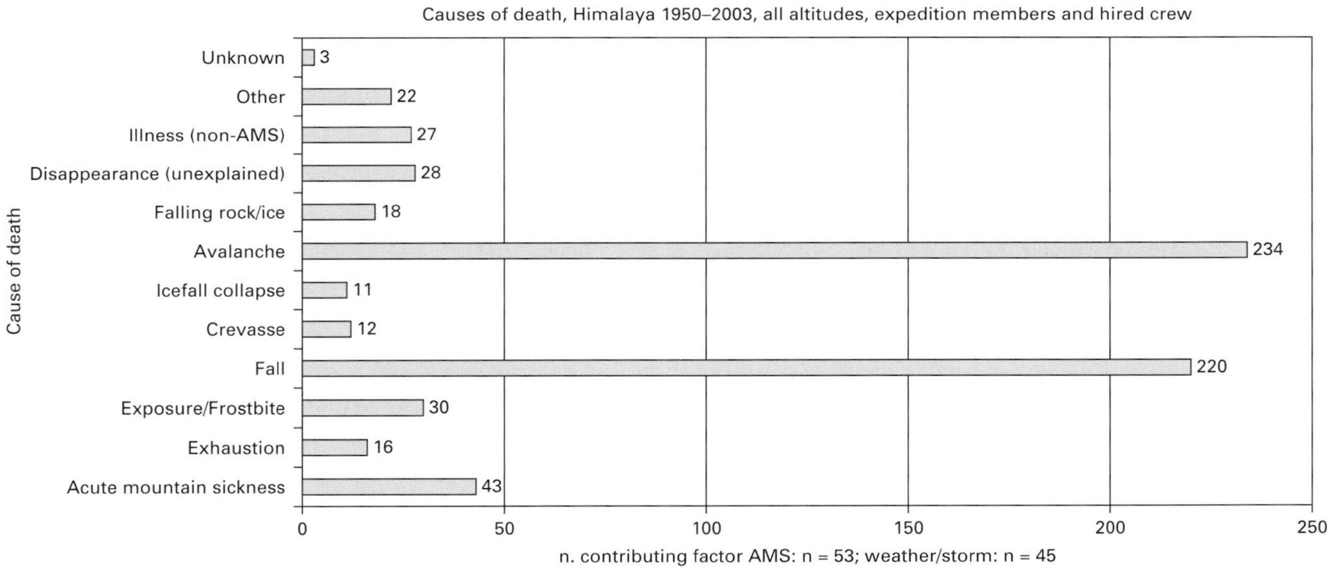

Fig. 63.6. Causes of death in Himalayas 1950–2003. (Adapted from ref. 9.)

clearly be stated whether the incidence is high, relatively low, or can only be put in perspective when considering the selection mechanism of the populations studied where patients with cardiac or pulmonary diseases are excluded a priori.

Cardiac arrest aboard commercial airplanes

In-flight cardiac arrest is uncommon. About 0.31–0.8 death per million passengers are reported[103,104] annually. With passenger numbers increasing exponentially over recent decades,[105] this converts into large variations in absolute numbers. Incidence data also vary if the denominator is a single airline,[106,107,107b] an airport,[103,108–110] data collected at the Federal Aviation Administration,[105,106] or the International Air Transport Association (IATA).[104] Rodenberg describes 90 deaths over 20 years in one large airline,[106] and Lyznicki *et al.* found over 33 deaths on domestic US flights over 2 years.[105] O'Rourke *et al.* report 27 cardiac arrests on international flights in 55 overseas airplanes for a death rate of 4.7 per million passengers on Quantas Airlines;[107] only 59% were witnessed arrests. Six passengers had ventricular fibrillation, and 2 of these (7.4%) survived to hospital discharge. No patient with a non-shockable rhythm survived. Whether long flight diversions on international flights from or to Australia played a role is unclear. Magalhães *et al.*[111] report 3 fatal arrests on 34 of Brazil's 80 VARIG airplanes over 6 months (passenger numbers not provided). Cummins and Schuback report five cardiac arrests out of 14.4 million passengers arriving at Seattle Tacoma International Airport during 1 year. Interestingly, none of them had the arrest during flight.[108] McKim Davis and Schuriet[109] report 11 cardiac arrests among travellers brought to one out of three hospitals from Dallas/Fort Worth Airport within 1 year. Three received basic life support during flight and one survived with neurological deficits. Speizer *et al.*[103] report 6 cardiac arrest (all fatal) out of 8 375 000 passengers during flights inbound to Los Angeles International airport in a 6-month period. In total, 25 patients were hospitalized for various symptoms including cardiac arrest, but none of the patients was diagnosed with pulmonary embolism. The fatal cardiac arrests were assumed to be of myocardial origin. Sarvesvaran[110] describes 104 deaths that were reported to the coroner of Heathrow Airport over 3 years, of whom 61 were in-flight cardiac arrests. Eleven of these were due to pulmonary embolism and 43 were due to cardiac ischemia. Ten out of the 11 pulmonary embolic deaths occurred in flights of more than 12 hours' duration. In the group of 28 "would-be passengers" with an arrest while still on the ground, only one had pulmonary embolism as the cause of arrest. No patient with a cardiac arrest was younger than 40 years, with the exception of five chronically ill patients, whose disease was their reason of final travel. In a 10-year period with many fewer passengers than today (1971–1980), 10-year incidence of medical events on US domestic flights was 7789 and deaths ranged from 21 deaths to 100 per year.[106] Cummins *et al.*[104] depict 577 in-flight deaths reported to the IATA in an 8-year period, with a response rate of approximately 25% of all IATA airlines, which represent approximately 50–60% of all airlines. Extrapolation of these data to worldwide incidences is not appropriate, however,

because of the distribution of long range flights among carriers and the resulting different incidences ranging from zero to 59 arrests in one airline over 8 years.

It is not completely clear to what extent the hypobaric hypoxic environment in an airplane plays a role. Commercial aircraft set their cabin pressure at a level that refers to an altitude of approximately 1900 m (6200 ft), but sometimes pressure values of 2700 m (8915 ft) are reached.[112] This leads to a decrease of the inspired oxygen partial pressure from 159 mmHg at sea level to 113 mmHg at 9000 ft.

Considering the very low relative and absolute death rate aboard airplanes, it appears that flying is a safe mode of travel for the vast majority of the population. Myocardial ischemia, massive pulmonary embolism, and cerebrovascular disasters are causes of death with sudden onset. In contrast, cancer or other chronic diseases may keep people from flying near the end of life, leading to a selection bias in individuals who die suddenly on airplanes.

Interestingly, there are no reports of acute mountain sickness during flights, although this would be expected to happen regularly. The cabin altitude is high enough for this disease.[3] As stated above, acute mountain sickness usually develops within the first 12 hours[5] (or very rarely even sooner[94]), a time range that is often reached on international flights. Whether the lack of physical activity might be a possible explanation for this phenomenon is still to be investigated.

Commercial air travel with infants and children

The possibility of a link between prolonged (intercontinental) flights and subsequent SIDS was raised in a research article published in a major medical journal.[113] Clinically healthy infants were exposed to 15% oxygen to identify the effects on arterial oxygenation and the frequency of apneic pauses. This publication aroused considerable alarm, especially among families with surviving siblings of SIDS victims, but subsequent critique of the study design, methodology and conclusions, resulted in consensus that such an association is unsubstantiated. There are no reports of cardiac arrest in pediatric passengers during flights in commercial airlines. Even with an assumed strong negative publication bias, the problem would not be a large one in absolute numbers.

Air transport of patients

Medical transport of patients may be accomplished by rotor- or fixed-wing aircraft. Although helicopter emergency medical service (HEMS) programs typically focus on primary rescue missions, daily interhospital transfer flights are routine. For long distance or intercontinental flights, patients may be transported either on board major airlines or dedicated charter flights. Such aircraft generally are pressurized only to an atmospheric pressure that approximates an altitude of 1515 m (5000 ft) and the cabin altitude may be as high as 2440 m (8000 ft) at the highest cruising altitudes.[114,115]

Transport by helicopter is done in unpressurized cabins, so that pressure inside the aircraft corresponds directly to the flight altitude. Even in alpine rescue or transfer flights, however, flight level typically does not exceed 3000 m.

Nevertheless, rapid ambient pressure change is a major concern in aero-medical transport. Enclosed collections of gas within the body can expand rapidly during normal ascent or sudden depressurization of the aircraft. While expansion of air in the middle ear can be acutely painful, expansion of a pneumothorax, pneumopericardium, or cystic adenomatoid malformation in pediatric patients can lead to critical reductions in cardiac output and subsequent cardiac arrest if unrelieved. Moreover, volume expansion of intestinal gas (i.e., in patients with acute bowel obstruction) may cause gut distension and subsequently impair respiratory function. Accordingly, detection and adequate treatment of the aforementioned pathologies (i.e., chest tube placement) prior to air transport is crucial. Once the patient is on board the aircraft, auscultation of breath sounds will be significantly compromised by the ambient noise and vibration during flight. Thus, it is important to utilize comprehensive hemodynamic monitoring and to have a high index of suspicion for air leaks in patients who present with sudden onset of respiratory distress, hypoxemia, bradycardia, and/or hypotension during transport. For transfer flights of intubated and mechanically ventilated patients, a regular check of tube position, bilateral ventilation, tube patency, equipment (oxygen supply pressure), and stomach distension is mandatory. The cuff of the tracheal tube should be evaluated at different altitudes, as the air inside the cuff expands when the aircraft or helicopter gains altitude (2000 feet or more) and inadvertent high cuff pressures may cause mucosal damage in the trachea.[116] If the patient is intubated on the mountain and flown to the valley, the cuff is compressed and needs to be refilled. Alternatively, as in the hyperbaric chamber treatment for diving accidents, the cuff may be inflated with water or saline.

When a patient is treated with a transport ventilator, at high altitude with lower barometric ambient pressure, the ventilator delivers more volume per minute to the patient (approximately 15% more minute volume at 2000 m[117] or 3000 m[118] when compared with volumes at sea level).

Monitoring of the given ventilation volume is therefore warranted during all kinds of patient transport.

Prior to air transport, patients with impaired cardiopulmonary function must be stabilized appropriately, and supplemental oxygen should be administered routinely in order to maintain adequate oxygenation during transport. If patients are at risk for malignant arrhythmias, an option for defibrillation during flight is given. Although transthoracic defibrillation with hand-held paddles is not likely to interfere with the helicopter's flight safety, self-adhesive electrodes are advantageous, and these electrodes should be attached prior to flight.

Austrian air rescue responds to 15 000 rescue missions per year, and about 3% are for cardiac arrest patients. Therefore, air rescue crews must be familiar with current CPR guidelines, and even more important, must be able to perform CPR in remote locations, difficult terrain, and during flight. Even though the quality of chest compressions is limited during transport (ground and air), ongoing cardiac massage during flight is justified under certain circumstances such as severe hypothermia. The cabin space of modern EMS helicopter allows performance of prolonged chest compressions even during flight, but air rescue teams must be familiar with the management of cardiac arrest patients during flight. An adjusted in-cabin advanced life support training should be part of ongoing educational programs for the entire air rescue crew.

Treatment of high altitude cardiac arrest

In those areas and altitudes where emergency medical services are available in acceptable time ranges, especially in resorts with large tourist populations, myocardial ischemia can be assumed to be the leading cause of death, although other causes of sudden death, i.e., pulmonary embolism, CNS events, and other cardiac and respiratory conditions should also be considered. Accordingly, standard advanced cardiac life support should be instituted by rescuers. Programmes for public access defibrillation[64] should be encouraged. Use of thrombolytics for specific etiologies should follow standard recommendations (See Chapter 41).

For individuals with cardiac arrests in remote areas (wilderness, airplanes, and others), use of expensive and possibly dangerous regimens must be counterbalanced and should not put rescue crew members at inappropriate risk. On mountains, response intervals will be far too long to make resuscitation success likely.[11] There are reports of response times for helicopter evacuation of 24 hours. Even when response times are moderate in wilderness locations, outcomes are exceedingly poor.[68] Nonetheless, there are a few special circumstances (such as severe altitude illness) in both major tourist resort areas and in remote locations that may require adjustments to usual treatment regimens.

Cardiac arrest management in patients with altitude illness

If a patient is known to be affected by acute mountain sickness and develops cardiac arrest (not suddenly but usually after hours to days), treatment may be different from standard ACLS. Because of the pathophysiologic mechanisms described above, the aim of treatment must be to lower the pulmonary vascular resistance for HAPE patients, as oxygen alone may not be sufficient,[119] and to lower intracranial pressure in HACE patients. No prospective studies have been performed on these rare entities (one death per year in the Himalayas[11]), and there are no case reports with precise descriptions of ACLS except in non-medical mountaineering literature (e.g., J. Krakauer – Into Thin Air). Since literature is limited, it is noteworthy that the following treatment proposal is entirely speculative and is not supported by sound scientific data.

Oxygen is a mainstay of treatment for altitude illness. Rescue personnel should air-drop oxygen supplies if immediate evacuation to lower altitudes will be delayed. High-flow rates of oxygen (10–12 l/min) by mask should be delivered initially to victims with severe HAPE until improvement is seen. Lower flow rates may then be used until recovery or descent is completed. This may take days to weeks, as oxygen alone does not completely solve the problem of pulmonary vasoconstriction.[119] Delivering oxygen with a continuous positive airway pressure mask improves oxygenation in HAPE victims compared with normal oxygen delivery.[120]

Patients with severely altered levels of consciousness require intubation for airway management and hyperventilation to control elevated intracranial pressures, although at moderate and extreme altitude, patients are already spontaneously hyperventilating and hypocapneic.

When a patient is ventilated with supplemental oxygen (via bag valve mask or endotracheal tube), the ventilation volume per minute is not a clear target. Some degree of hyperventilation appears to be desirable in a patient with cardiac arrest from HACE and suspected elevated intracranial pressures. In this regard, the rescuers must be aware that spontaneous hyperventilation and subsequently low arterial PCO_2 values are part of the physiologic adaptation to high altitude (PCO_2 values as low as 7.5 mmHg have been observed on the summit of Mount Everest without any cerebral damage[121]). Accordingly, despite improved

oxygenation after initiation of artificial ventilation, reduction of minute ventilation might be harmful.

Anecdotal reports of the successful treatment of HACE in hyperbaric chambers exist. Coma may persist for several days after descent to lower altitudes, so placement of HACE patients in a hyperbaric device may only delay the more comprehensive care available in the hospital setting. If immediate descent is impossible, portable hyperbaric therapy may be life-saving. Early treatment for HACE generally results in good outcomes, but after coma occurs, mortality exceeds 60%.[122]

Death is usually due to cerebral edema and herniation, and sometimes from antemortem cerebral infarcts from the high intracranial pressure and decreased cerebral blood flow. In addition, the clinician should be careful not to make the patient ischemic secondary to overventilation. If the patient appears to be herniating then hyperventilation appears advisable.

If HAPE is recognized early and treated properly, cardiac arrest and death usually can be avoided. Descent to a lower altitude, bed rest, and supplemental oxygen are the most effective methods of therapy;[22] portable hyperbaric chambers[123,124] generating 103 mmHg (2 psi) above the ambient pressure thereby simulating descent are a valuable substitute if oxygen is not available. Because of the nature and construction of these devices, it is not possible to perform CPR while the patient is in the portable chamber.

Supplemental oxygen administration addresses the primary insult of high-altitude exposure and corrects hypoxemia. Delaying descent while HAPE progresses or waiting for rescue personnel to initiate evacuation has proven fatal. Descents of 1500 to 3000 feet should be adequate to begin the recovery phase.

The evaluation of drug therapy in treating HAPE has been limited. There are no reports of modifications of standard ACLS drugs in patients with HAPE who have cardiac arrest. In addition to standard ACLS drugs, agents that lower pulmonary artery pressure, pulmonary blood volume, and pulmonary vascular resistance would intuitively be useful. Furosemide is beneficial in treating HAPE and, when combined with morphine for the initial dose, results in even greater diuresis and clinical improvement. Some authors caution that deleterious dehydration may result from furosemide therapy and that the potential ventilatory depression caused by morphine can further increase the severity of the hypoxemia that underlies AMS.[22] Others argue that, during the state of antidiuresis found with severe AMS, furosemide may be useful and that no documented reports of deleterious effects from this treatment exist. Furosemide may also be useful in settings where both oxygen therapy and descent are not available;

however, caution must be exercised because of limited experience. Its application in altitude-related cardiac arrest is unclear and without scientific evidence of success.

As used in the treatment of AMS before cardiac arrest, dexamethasone (8 mg parenterally, followed by 4 mg every 6 hours) is likely to result in more benefit than harm.

This is less clear with nifedipine: usually, ACLS aims at raising systemic and coronary blood pressure, and treatment with intravenous boluses of nifedipine can be expected to do the opposite. But, because of its action as a pulmonary vasodilator, nifedipine has been used to treat HAPE prior to cardiac arrest with good results.[26,27,125] Nifedipine does not improve pulmonary hemodynamics as effectively as oxygen and does not have an additive effect when administered with oxygen.[26] Therefore, intuitively it does not appear to be beneficial in a patient during ACLS who is intubated and receiving 100% oxygen.

Cardiac arrest from chronic pulmonary artery hypertension (not related to altitude) has been treated with bolus injections of 50 µg of iloprost, a prostacyclin analogue,[126] but this was not a randomized controlled trial. Of 513 patients with cardiac arrest, 8 survived with no neurological deficit; 7 of these patients had correctable causes of cardiopulmonary arrest, such as vasovagal reactions, digitalis toxicity, or pericardial tamponade. In 3 of the 8 survivors, iloprost had been used, but in many of the unsuccessful attempts it was used it was not reported.

Recent studies have shown the effectiveness of the phosphodiesterase type 5 inhibitors on the pulmonary vasoconstriction associated with HAPE in human and animal studies. Sildenafil has been used successfully for lowering pulmonary vascular resistance when given 100 mg orally in healthy volunteers,[127] or 1 mg/kg in children with congenital heart disease (without altitude-related problems).[128] In a small study of 6 patients it has been shown to lower pulmonary arterial pressure if taken orally (40 mg 3 times per day) beginning several hours after arrival at altitude of 4350 m.[129] As both a preventive and non-preventive treatment strategy, sildenafil lowered pulmonary artery pressure in rats at doses of 25 and 75 mg kg^{-1} per d.[130] Because of its potential to cause severe hypotension, however, it should be used with caution in patients in extremis.

Bosentan, an endothelin antagonist, has been discribed in long-term use for treating children with pulmonary hypertension and HAPE due to congenital heart disease,[51] but not for acute treatment of HAPE. Other treatment options used for pulmonary hypertension[131] have not been studied in HAPE.

Beta-2 agonists such as salmeterol have been applied in the prevention of HAPE with a reduction from 74 to 33% in susceptible persons going to 4559 m within 22 hours,[132] but again, this was not a treatment for acutely decompensating, overt HAPE. If available, in-line beta-agonists may be attempted for the ventilated patient during resuscitation.

With respect to treatment of HACE, anecdotal reports support steroid therapy, which resulted in recovery without neurological deficits in some patients. The initial dose of dexamethasone is 8 mg parenterally, followed by 4 mg every 6 hours.

Diuretics (e.g., furosemide) and hypertonic solutions (e.g., mannitol) have been used to decrease intracranial pressure. Many patients with HACE are already volume-depleted from poor fluid intake and loss of fluid through hyperventilation, and care must be taken to ensure adequate intravascular volumes if a diuretic agent is used. Acetazolamide is a carbonic anhydrase inhibitor that induces a renal bicarbonate diuresis causing a metabolic acidosis, thereby increasing ventilation and arterial oxygenation. This drug also lowers CSF volume and pressure, which may play an additional role in its therapeutic and prophylactic use. The use of acetazolamide parenterally in cardiac arrest has never been reported but with other drugs used for lowering intracerebral pressures, an IV bolus of 250–375 mg, may be beneficial.

Between one-half and two-thirds of arrests on mountains are caused by trauma.[9,11,55,70,73] The prognosis of these patients, which is very serious in urban settings, is disastrous in the wilderness. If patients are found by rescuers without a pulse, resuscitation is virtually futile (see chapter 57 for traumatic arrest).[133] Since trauma represents the largest group, the suggested strategy of preventive anticoagulation treatment anticipating salvageable victims of sudden death by myocardial ischemia or pulmonary embolism does not appear to be of value.[134]

In conclusion, the key to success in AMS-related cardiac arrest lies in prevention, early diagnosis, early therapy with descent and oxygen with positive endexpiratory pressure (PEEP), acetazolamide, and dexamethasone. Once asphyxial cardiac arrest has occurred, treatment is unclear and survival is unlikely.

Acknowledgments

We are indebted to Peter Hackett, MD (USA) and Martin Roeggla, MD (Austria) for their help with this chapter.

REFERENCES

1. Moore, L.G. Altitude-aggravated illness: examples from pregnancy and prenatal life. *Ann. Emerg. Med.* 1987; **16**(9), 965–973.

2. Hackett, P.H., Rennie, I.D. & Levine, H.D. The incidence, importance, and prophylaxis of acute mountain sickness, *Lancet* 1976; **2**: 1149–1154.

3. Roeggla, G., Roeggla, M., Hirschl, M.M., Wagner, A. & Laggner, A.N. Zur Inzidenz der Acute Mountain Sickness (AMS) in mittlerer Höhe in Österreichs Alpen (On the incidence of acute mountain sickness in moderate height in Austrian alps). *Wien. Klin. Wochenschr.* 1992; **104**; Suppl. 194, S7–S10.

4. Maggiorini, M., Buhler, B., Walter, M. & Oelz, O. Prevalence of acute mountain sickness in the Swiss Alps. *Br. Med. J.* 1990; **301** (6756): 853–855.

5. Honigman, B., Theis, M.K., Koziol-McLain, J. *et al.* Acute mountain sickness in a general tourist population at moderate altitudes. *Ann. Intern. Med.* 1993; **118**(8): 587–592. Erratum in: *Ann. Intern. Med.* 1994; **120**(8): 698.

6. Larson, E.B., Roach, R.C., Schoene, R.B. & Hornbein, T.F. Acute mountain sickness and acetazolamide. *J. Am. Med. Assoc.* 1982; **248**: 328–332.

7. Houston, C.S. *Going Higher: The Story of Man at High Altitude*, Boston: Little, Brown, 1987.

8. Roach, R.C., Houston, C.S., Honigman, B. *et al.* How well do older persons tolerate moderate altitude? *West. J. Med.* 1995; **162**: 32–36.

9. Hawley, E. & Salisbury, R. The Himalayan Database – The Expedition Archives of Elizabeth Hawley. The American Alpine Club, Golden, CO, USA 2004.

10. Pollard, A. & Clarke, C. Deaths during mountaineering at extreme altitude. *Lancet* 1988; **1**(8597): 1277. Letter.

11. Shlim, D.R. & Houston, R. Helicopter rescues and deaths among trekkers in Nepal. *J. Am. Med. Assoc.* 1989; **261**(7): 1017–1019.

12. Matsuzawa, Y., Kobayashi, T., Shinozaki, S. *et al.* Low hypoxic ventilatory response and relative hypoventilation in acute mountain sickness, *Jpn J. Mountain Med.* 1990: 10.

13. Basnyat, B. & Murdoch, D.R. High-altitude illness. *Lancet* 2003; **361**(9373): 1967–1974.

14. Hackett, P.H. & Roach, R.C. High altitude medicine. In Auerbach, P. (ed.) *Wilderness Medicine*, 4th edn, St.Louis: Mosby Year Book 2001: 2–43.

15. West, J.B. The physiologic basis of high-altitude diseases. *Ann. Intern. Med.* 2004; **141**: 789–800.

16. Hackett, P.H. & Roach, R.C. High altitude illness. *N. Engl. J. Med.* 2001; **345**: 107–114.

17. Brundrett, G. Sickness at high altitude: a literature review. *J. Roy. Soc. Promot. Health* 2002; **122**: 14–20.

18. Hultgren, H.N., Grover, R.F. & Hartley L.H. Abnormal circulatory responses to high altitude in subjects with a previous history of high altitude pulmonary edema, *Circulation* 1971; **44**: 759–770.

19. Koyama, S., Kobayashi, T., Kubo, K. *et al.* The increased sympathoadrenal activity in patients with high altitude pulmonary edema is centrally mediated. *Jpn J. Med.* 1988; **27**: 10–16.

20. Hackett, P. High altitude cerebral edema and acute mountain sickness: a pathophysiology update. In Roach, R., Wagner, P.

& Hackett, P. (eds.) *Hypoxia: into the Next Millennium*, New York: Kluwer Academic/Plenum, 1999.

21. Huang, S.Y., Sun, S., Droma, T. *et al.* Internal carotid and vertebral arterial flow velocity in men at high altitude, *J. Appl. Physiol.* 1987; **63**: 395–400.

22. Hultgren, H.N. High altitude pulmonary edema. In Staub, N.C. (ed.) *Lung Water and Solute Exchange*, New York: Dekker, 1978.

23. Houston, C.S. Incidence of acute mountain sickness. *Am. Alpine J.* 1985; **27**: 162–165.

24. Singh, I., Kapila, C.C., Khanna, P.K., Nanda, R.B. & Rao, B.D. High altitude pulmonary edema, *Lancet* 1965; **1**: 229–234.

25. Penaloza, D. & Sime, F. Circulatory dynamics during high altitude pulmonary edema, *Am. J. Cardiol.* 1969; **23**: 369–378.

26. Hackett, P.H., Roach, R.C., Hartig, G.S., Greene, E.R. & Levine, B.D. The effect of vasodilators on pulmonary hemodynamics in high altitude pulmonary edema: a comparison. *Int. J. Sports Med.* 1992; **13** Suppl. 1: S68–S71.

27. Oelz, O., Noti, C., Ritter, M., Jenni, R. & Bärtsch, P. Nifedipine for high altitude pulmonary edema, *Lancet* 1989; **2**: 1241–1244.

28. Houston, C.S. High altitude illness: disease with protean manifestations, *J. Am. Med. Assoc.* 1976; **236**: 2193–2195.

29. Houston, C.S. & Dickinson, J.G. Cerebral form of high altitude illness, *Lancet* 1975; **2**: 758–761.

30. Hackett, P.H., Marnett, P.R., Hill, R. *et al.* High-altitude cerebral edema evaluated with magnetic resonance imaging: clinical correlation and pathophysiology, *J. Am. Med. Assoc.* 1998; **280**: 1920–1925.

31. Kurkciyan, I., Meron, G., Sterz, F. *et al.* Spontaneous subarachnoid haemorrhage as a cause of out-of-hospital cardiac arrest. *Resuscitation* 2001; **51**(1): 27–32.

32. Pollard, A.M., Niermeyer, S. & Barry, P. Children at high altitude: an international consensus statement by an ad hoc committee of the International Society for Mountain Medicine, March 12, 2001. *High Altitude Med. Biol.* 2001; **2**: 389–403.

33. Carpenter, T.C., Reeves, J.T. & Durmowicz, A.G. Viral respiratory infection increases the susceptibility of young rats to hypoxia-induced pulmonary edema. *J. Appl. Physiol.* 1998; **84**: 1048–1054.

34. Schoene, R.B. Fatal high altitude pulmonary edema associated with absence of the left pulmonary artery. *High Altitude Med. Biol.* 2001; **2**(3): 405–406.

35. Durmowicz, A.G. Pulmonary edema in 6 children with Down Syndrome during travel to moderate altitudes. *Pediatrics* 2001; **108**(2): 443–447.

36. Jones, S.R., Binder, R.A. & Donowho, E.M.J. Sudden death in sickle-cell trait. *N. Engl. J. Med.* 1970; **282**(6): 323–325.

37. Githens, J.H., Gross, G.P., Eife, R.F. & Wallner, S.F. Splenic sequestration syndrome at mountain altitudes in sickle/hemoglobin C disease. *J. Pediatr.* 1977; **90**(2): 203–206.

38. Mahoney, B.S. & Githens, J.H. Sickling crises and altitude. *Clin. Pediatr.* 1979; **18**(7): 431–438.

39. Barkin, R.M., Hartley, M.R. & Brooks, J.G. Influence of high altitude on sudden infant death syndrome. *Pediatrics* 1981; **68**: 891–892.

40. Getts, A.G. & Hill, H.F. Sudden infant death syndrome: incidence at various altitudes. *Dev. Med. Child Neurol.* 1982; **24**: 61–68.

41. Kohlendorfer, U., Kiechl, S. & Sperl, W. Living at high altitude and risk of sudden infant death syndrome. *Arch. Dis. Child.* 1998; **79**: 506–509.

42. Wisborg, K., Kesmodel, U., Henriksen, T.B., Olsen, S.F. & Secher, N.J. A prospective study of smoking during pregnancy and SIDS. *Arch. Dis. Child.* 2000; **83**(3): 203–206.

43. Niermeyer, S. The cardiopulmonary transition at high altitude during infancy. *High Altitude Med. Biol.* 2003; **4**(2): 225–239.

44. Khoury, G.H. & Hawes, C.R. Primary pulmonary hypertension in children living at high altitude. *J. Pediatr.* 1963; **62**: 177–185.

45. Hurtado Gomez, L., Calderon, R.G. Hipoxia de altura en la insuficiencia cardiaca del lactante. *Bol. Soc. Boliviana Pediatr.* 1965; **IX**(1): 11–23.

46. Sui, G.J., Liu, Y.H., Cheng, X.S. *et al.* Subacute infantile mountain sickness. *J. Pathol.* 1988; **155**: 161–170.

47. Wu, T. & Miao, C. High altitude heart disease in children in Tibet (ltr). *High Altitude Med. Biol.* 2002; **3**(3): 323–325.

48. Alt, B. & Shikes, R.H. Pulmonary hypertension in congenital heart disease: irreversible vascular changes in young infants. *Pediat. Pathol.* 1983; **1**: 423–434.

49. Scoggin, C.H., Hyers, T.M., Reeves, J.T. & Grover, R.F. High-altitude pulmonary edema in the children and young adults of Leadville, Colorado. *New Engl. J. Med.* 1977; **297**: 1269–1272.

50. Fasules, J.W., Wiggins, J.W. & Wolfe, R.R. Increased lung vasoreactivity in children from Leadville, Colorado, after recovery from high-altitude pulmonary edema. *Circulation* 1985; **72**: 957–962.

51. Das, B.B., Wolfe, R.R., Chan, K.C., Larsen, G.L., Reeves, J.T. & Ivy, D. High-altitude pulmonary edema in children with underlying cardiopulmonary disorders and pulmonary hypertension living at altitude. *Arch. Pediatr. Adolesc. Med.* 2004; **158**(12): 1170–1176.

52. Reeves, J.T., Groves, B.M., Sutton, J.R. *et al.* Operation Everest II: preservation of cardiac function at extreme altitude. *J. Appl. Physiol.* 1987; **63**(2): 531–539.

53. Sutton, J.R., Reeves, J.T., Groves, B.M. *et al.* Oxygen transport and cardiovascular function at extreme altitude: lessons from Operation Everest, II. *Int. J. Sports Med.* 1992; **13** (Suppl. 1): S13–S18.

54. Aigner, A., Berghold, F. & Muss, N. Herz-Kreislauf-Untersuchungen im Hochgebirge bis 7800 m Höhe (Investigations on the cardiovascular system at altitudes up to a height of 7,800 meters). *Z. Kardiol.* 1980; **69**(9): 604–610.

55. Burtscher, M., Philadelphy, M. & Likar, R. Sudden cardiac death during mountain hiking and downhill skiing. *N. Engl. J. Med.* 1993; **329**(23): 1738–1739. Letter.

56. Trekking in Nepal: safety after coronary artery bypass. QUESTIONS AND ANSWERS. *J. Am. Med. Assoc.* 1988; **259**: 3184.

57. Rennie, D. Will mountain trekkers have heart attacks? *J. Am. Med. Assoc.* 1989; **261**: 1045–1046. Editorial.

58. Hultgren, H.N. The safety of trekking at high altitude after coronary bypass surgery. *J. Am. Med. Assoc.* 1988; **260**: 2218. Letter.

59. Halhuber, M.J., Humpeler, E., Inama, K. & Jungmann, H. Does altitude cause exhaustion of the heart and circulatory system? In Jokl, E. & Hebbelinck, M., eds. *Medicine and Sport Science. High Altitude Deterioration.* Vol 19. Basel: Karger, S. 1985, 192–202.

60. Grover, R.F., Tucker, C.E., McGroarty, S.R. & Travis, R.R. The coronary stress of skiing at high altitude. *Arch. Intern. Med.* 1990; **150**(6): 1205–1208.

61. Morgan, B.J., Alexander, J.K., Nicoli, S.A. & Brammell, H.L. The patient with coronary heart disease at altitude: observations during acute exposure to 3100 meters. *J. Wilderness Med.* 1990; **1**: 147–153.

62. Alexander, J.K. Age, altitude and arrhythmia. *Texas Heart Ins. J.* 1995; **22**: 308–316.

63. Burtscher, M., Pachinger, O., Mittleman, M.A. & Ulmer, H. Prior myocardial infarction ist the major risk factor associated with sudden cardiac death during downhill skiing. *Int. J. Sports Med.* 2000; **21**: 613–615.

64. Lienhart, H.G., Breitfeld, L. & Voelckel, W. Frühdefibrillation im Gletschergebiet: übertrieben oder Überleben? 3 Fallberichte und eine Standortbestimmung (Public access defibrillation in alpine skiing areas: three case reports and a brief survey of the literature). *Anaesthesiol. Intensivmed. Notfallmed. Schmerzther.* 2005; **40**: 150–155.

65. Burtscher, M. Time-dependent SCD risk during mountain hiking. *Circulation* 1994; **89**(6): 2948–2949. Letter.

66. Burtscher, M. & Mittleman, M.A. Time-dependent SCD risk during mountain sports changes with age. *Circulation* 1995; **92**(10): 3151–3152. Letter.

67. Burtscher, M., Philadelphy, M., Nachbauer, W. & Likar, R. The risk of death to trekkers and hikers in the mountains. *J. Am. Med. Assoc.* 1995; **273**(6): 460. Letter.

68. Breitfeld, L. & Voelckel, W. Der plötzliche Herztod im Gebirge und halbautomatische externe Defibrillatoren – grundsätzliche Überlegungen (Sudden cardiac death on mountains and automatic external defibrillators – general considerations). *Jahrb Österreichischen Gesellsch. Alpin- und Höhenmedi.* 2002: 55–65.

69. Mosimann U. Swiss Alpine Club. Bergnotfälle 2002 (Mountain Emergencies 2002). *Die Alpen* 2003; **6**: 24–29.

70. Sladek, F. Alpinunfallbericht 2003. In *Österreichisches Kuratorium für Alpine Sicherheit, Jahrbuch 2004*, Innsbruck, 2004: 159–169.

71. Eisenburger, P., Czappek, G., Sterz, F. *et al.* Cardiac arrest patients in an alpine area during a six year period. *Resuscitation* 2001; **51**(1): 39–46.

72. Breitfeld, L. & Voelckel, W. Cardiac arrest and the local emergency cardiac care system. *Resuscitation* 2002; **54**(3): 314. Letter.

73. Shlim, D.R. & Gallie, J. The causes of death among trekkers in Nepal. *Int. J. Sports Med.* 1992; **13** Suppl. 1: S74–S76.

74. Hawley, E. Quoted in Shlim, D.R. & Houston, R. Helicopter rescues and deaths among trekkers in Nepal. *J. Am. Med. Assoc.* 1989; **261**(7): 1017–1019.

75. Berghold, F. & Schaffert, W. Höhenakklimatisation und Höhenmedizin. In Lösch, R. (ed.) *Schutzimpfungen und Reisemedizin. Demeter Verlag im Spitta Verlag*, Balingen, 1997.

76. Maher, J.T., Levine, P.H. & Cymerman, A. Human coagulation abnormalities during acute exposure to hypobaric hypoxia. *J. Appl. Physiol.* 1976; **41**(5 Pt. 1): 702–707.

77. Ward, M.P., Milledge, J.S. & West, J.N. *High Altitude Medicine and Physiology*. London: Arnold, 2000.

78. Simpson, K. Shelter deaths from pulmonary embolism. *Lancet* 1940; **ii**, 744.

79. Homans, J. Thrombosis of the deep leg vein due to prolonged sitting. *N. Engl. J. Med.* 1954; **250**; 148–149.

80. Schobersberger, W., Mittermayer, M., Innerhofer, P. *et al.* Coagulation chages and edema formation during long-distance bus travel. *Blood Coagul. Fibrinol.* 2004; **15**: 419–425.

81. Beasley, R., Raymond, N., Hill, S., Nowitz, M. & Hughes, R. Thrombosis: the 21st century variant of venous thromboembolism associated with immobility. *Eur. Respir. J.* 2003; **21**(2): 374–376.

82. Lapostolle, F., Surget, V., Borron, S.W. *et al.* Severe pulmonary embolism associated with air travel. *N. Engl. J. Med.* 2001; **345**(11): 779–783.

83. Bendz, B., Rostrup, M., Sevre, K., Andersen, T.O. & Sandset, P.M. Association between acute hypobaric hypoxia and activation of coagulation in human beings. *Lancet* 2000; **356**(9242): 1657–1658. Research letter.

84. Bendz, B. & Sandset, P.M. Acute hypoxia and activation of coagulation. *Lancet* 2003; **362**(9388): 997–998. Research letter.

85. Singh, I. & Chohan, I.S. Abnormalities of blood coagulation at high altitude. *Int. J. Biometeorol.* 1972; **16**(3): 283–297.

86. Schobersberger, W., Fries, D., Mittermayer, M. *et al.* Changes of biochemical markers and functional tests for clot fomation during long-haul flights. *Thromb. Res.* 2003; **108**: 19–24.

87. Hudson, J.G., Bowen, A.L., Navia, P. *et al.* The effect of high altitude on platelet counts, thrombopoietin and erythropoietin levels in young Bolivian airmen visiting the Andes. *Int. J. Biometeorol.* 1999; **43**(2): 85–90.

88. Le Roux, G., Larmignat, P., Marchal, M. & Richalet, J.P. Haemostasis at high altitude. *Int. J. Sports Med.* 1992; **13** Suppl. 1: S49–S51.

89. Bärtsch, P., Haeberli, A., Franciolli, M., Kruithof, E.K. & Straub, P.W. Coagulation and fibrinolysis in acute mountain sickness and beginning pulmonary edema. *J. Appl. Physiol.* 1989; **66**(5): 2136–2144.

90. Crosby, A., Talbot, N.P., Harrison, P., Keeling, D. & Robbins, P.A. Relation between acute hypoxia and activation of coagulation in human beings. *Lancet* 2003; **361**(9376): 2207–2208. Research letter.

91. Schobersberger, W. Hauer, B., Sumann, G., Gunga, H.C. & Partsch, H. Die Reisethrombose – Häufigkeit, Ursachen, Prävention. *Wien Klin. Wochenschr.* 2002; **114**: 14–20.

92. Schwarz, T., Siegert, G., Oettler, W. *et al.* Venous thrombosis after long-haul flights. *Arch. Intern. Med.* 2003; **163**(22): 2759–2764.

93. Khan, D.A., Hashim, R., Mirza, T.M. & Matloob-ur-Rahman, M. Differentiation of pulmonary embolism from high altitude pulmonary edema. *J. Coll. Phys. Surg. Pak* 2003; **13**: 267–270.

94. Dickinson, J., Heath, D., Gosney, J. & Williams, D. Altitude-related deaths in seven trekkers in the Himalayas. *Thorax* 1983; **38**(9): 646–656.

95. Nakagawa, S., Kubo, K., Koizumi, T., Kobayashi, T. & Sekiguchi, M. High-altitude pulmonary edema with pulmonary thromboembolism. *Chest* 1993; **103**(3): 948–950.

96. Shlim, D.R. & Papenfus, K. Pulmonary embolism presenting as high-altitude pulmonary edema. *Wilderness Environ. Med.* 1995; **6**(2): 220–224.

97. Heffner, J.E. & Sahn, S.A. High-altitude pulmonary infarction. *Arch. Intern. Med.* 1981; **141**(12): 1721.

98. Anand, A.C., Jha, S.K., Saha, A., Sharma, V. & Adya, C.M. Thrombosis as a complication of extended stay at high altitude. *Natl. Med. J. India* 2001; **14**: 197–201.

99. Jha, S.K., Anand, A.C., Sharma, V., Kumar, N. & Adya, C.M. Stroke at high altitude: Indian experience. *High Alt. Med. Biol.* 2002; **3**(1): 21–27.

100. Basnyat, B., Wu, T. & Gertsch, J.H. Neurological conditions at altitude that fall outside the usual definition of altitude sickness. *High Alt. Med. Biol.* 2004; **5**(2): 171–179.

101. Niaz, A. & Nayyar, S. Cerebrovascular stroke at high altitude. *J. Coll. Phys. Surg. Pak.* 2003; **13**(8): 446–448.

102. Jaillard, A.S., Hommel, M. & Mazetti, P. Prevalence of stroke at high altitude (3380 m) in Cuzco, a town of Peru; a population based study. *Stroke* 1995; **26**: 562–568.

103. Speizer, C., Rennie, C.J. III & Breton, H. Prevalence of in-flight medical emergencies on commercial airlines. *Ann. Emerg. Med.* 1989; **18**: 26–29.

104. Cummins, R.O., Chapman, P.J., Chamberlain, D.A., Schubach, J.A. & Litwin, P.E. In-flight deaths during commercial air travel. How big is the problem? *J. Am. Med. Assoc.* 1988; **259**(13): 1983–1988.

105. Lyznicki, J.M., Williams, M.A., Deitchman, S.D. & Howe, J.P. 3rd; Council on Scientific Affairs, American Medical Association. Inflight medical emergencies. *Aviat. Space Environ. Med.* 2000; **71**(8): 832–838.

106. Rodenberg, H. Medical emergencies aboard commercial aircraft. *Ann. Emerg. Med.* 1987; **16**: 1373–1377.

107. O'Rourke, M.F., Donaldson, E. & Geddes, J.S. An airline cardiac arrest program. *Circulation* 1997; **96**(9): 2849–2853.

107b. Page, R.L., Joglar, J.A., Kowal, R.C. *et al.* Use of automated external defibrillators by a U.S. airline. *N. Engl. J. Med.* 2000; **343**(17): 1210–1216.

108. Cummins, R.O. & Schubach, J.A. Frequency and types of medical emergencies among commercial air travelers. *J. Am. Med. Assoc.* 1989; **261**(9): 1295–1299.

109. McKim Davis, M. & Schuriet, W. In-flight deaths. *J. Am. Med. Assoc.* 1989; **262**: 31–32. Letter.

110. Sarvesvaran, R. Sudden natural death associated with commercial air travel. *Med. Sci. Law.* 1986; **26**: 35–38.

111. Magalhães Alves, P., Jensen de Freitas, E.J., Mathias, H.A. *et al.* Use of automated external defibrillators in a Brazilian airline. A 1-year experience. *Arq. Bras. Cardiol.* 2001, **76**: 310–314.

112. Cottrell, J.J. Altitude exposures during aircraft flight. Flying higher. *Chest* 1988; **93**(1): 81–84.

113. Parkins, K.J., Poets, C.F., O'Brien, L.M., Stebbens, V.A. & Southall, D.P. Effect of exposure to 15% oxygen on breathing patterns and oxygen saturation in infants: interventional study. *Br. Med. J.* 1998; **316**: 887–891.

114. American Academy of Pediatrics Committee on Hospital Care. Guidelines for air and ground transport of pediatric patients. *Pediatrics* 1986; **78**(5): 943–950.

115. Samuels, M.P. The effects of flight and altitude. *Arch. Dis. Child.* 2004; **89**: 448–455.

116. Smith, R.P. & McArdle, B.H. Pressure in the cuffs of tracheal tubes at altitude. *Anaesthesia* 2002; **57**(4): 374–378.

117. Thomas, G. & Brimacombe, J. Function of the Drager Oxylog ventilator at high altitude. *Anaesth. Intens. Care* 1994; **22**(3): 276–280.

118. Roeggla, M., Roeggla, G., Wagner, A., Eder, B. & Laggner, A.N. Emergency mechanical ventilation at moderate altitude. *Wilderness Environ. Med.* 1995; **6**(3): 283–287.

119. Groves, B.M., Reeves, J.T., Sutton, J.R. *et al.* Operation Everest II: elevated high-altitude pulmonary resistance unresponsive to oxygen. *J. Appl. Physiol.* 1987; **63**(2): 521–530.

120. Schoene, R.B., Roach, R.C., Hackett, P.H., Harrison, G. & Mills, W.J. Jr. High altitude pulmonary edema and exercise at 4,400 meters on Mount McKinley. Effect of expiratory positive airway pressure. *Chest* 1985; **87**(3): 330–333.

121. West, J.B., Hackett, P.H., Maret, K.H. *et al.* Pulmonary gas exchange on the summit of Mt. Everest. *J. Appl. Physiol.* 1983; **55**: 678–687.

122. Clarke, C. High altitude cerebral oedema, Int. *J. Sports Med.* 1988; **9**: 170–174.

123. Kasic, J.F., Yaron, M., Nicholas, R.A., Lickteig, J.A., and Roach, R. Treatment of acute mountain sickness: hyperbaric versus oxygen therapy, *Ann. Emerg. Med.* 1991; **20**: 1109–1112.

124. Roach, R.C. & Hackett, P.H. Hyperbaria and high altitude illness. In Sutton, J.R., Coates, G. & Houston, C.S., eds. *Hypoxia and Mountain Medicine*, Burlington, VT: Queen City Press, 1992.

125. Oelz, O., Maggiorini, M., Ritter, M. *et al.* Prevention and treatment of high altitude pulmonary edema by a calcium channel blocker. *Int. J. Sports Med.* 1992; **13**: S65–S68.

126. Hoeper, M.M., Galiè, N., Murali, S. *et al.* Outcome after cardiopulmonary resuscitation in patients with pulmonary arterial hypertension. *Am. J. Respir. Crit. Care Med.* 2002; **165**: 341–344.

127. Zhao, L., Mason, N.A., Morrell, N.W. *et al.* Sildenafil inhibits hypoxia-induced pulmonary hypertension. *Circulation* 2001; **104**: 424–428.

128. Schulze-Neick, I., Hartenstein, P., Li, J. *et al.* Intravenous sildenafil is a potent pulmonary vasodilator in children with congenital heart disease. *Circulation* 2003; **108** Suppl. 1: II167–II173.

129. Richalet, J.P., Gratadour, P., Robach, P. *et al.* Sildenafil Inhibits altitude-induced hypoxemia and pulmonary hypertension. *Am. J. Respir. Crit. Care Med.* 2005; **171**: 275–281.

130. Sebkhi, A., Strange, J.W., Phillips, S.C., Wharton, J. & Wilkins, M.R. Phosphodiesterase type 5 as a target for the treatment of hypoxia-induced pulmonary hypertension. *Circulation* 2003; **107**: 3230–3235.

131. Humbert, M., Sitbon, O. & Simonneau, G. Treatment of pulmonary arterial hypertension. *N. Engl. J. Med.* 2004; **351**: 1425–1436. Review.

132. Sartori, C., Allemann, Y., Duplain, H. *et al.* Salmeterol for the prevention of high-altitude pulmonary edema. *N. Engl. J. Med.* 2002; **346**(21): 1631–1636.

133. Falcone, R.E., Herron, H., Johnson, R., Childress, S., Lacey, P. & Scheiderer, G. Air medical transport for the trauma patient requiring cardiopulmonary resuscitation: a 10-year experience. *Air Med. J.* 1995; **14**(4): 197–203.

134. Segler, C.P. Prophylaxis of climbers for prevention of embolic accidents. *Med. Hypotheses* 2001; **57**(4): 472–475.

64

Electrical injuries

Wolfgang Lederer[1], Erga Cerchiari[2] and Norman A. Paradis[3]

[1] Department of Anaesthesiology and Critical Care, Innsbruck Medical University, Austria
[2] Department of Anaesthesiology and Intensive Therapy, Maggiore Hospital, Bologna, Italy
[3] University of Colorado Health Sciences Center

Today, human-made and natural sources together kill about 1100 to 1200 people each year in the United States.[1,2] The number of people injured worldwide by electricity, however, remains unclear, because it is generally under-reported and it is common for survivors to avoid medical care initially. Although scientific investigations of electrical injuries date back to 1884, with current scientific knowledge and the clinical appearance of electrical injuries, we now know that the outcomes of electrical injuries differ substantially, depending on whether technical electricity with low-volt household current, high-volt current, or lightning is the underlying cause.

Injuries after electrocution are often dramatic and potentially fatal. In the majority of victims injuries are caused by the effects of electrical, thermal, and mechanical energy. Secondary trauma may result from falls, explosions, or violent muscle contractions.[3] Cardiac and respiratory arrest may occur immediately or secondary to direct effects of current.[4] Many victims die before advanced life support can be provided, and survivors may suffer permanent disabilities.[5] What is unique about electrical injuries, however, is the potential for good resuscitation outcome even after long arrest times.[4,6] This may be a result of the electrical shock itself or because these accidents tend to occur in younger persons with few or no underlying pathological conditions.

Considering the magnitude of the voltage and current involved, it is amazing that anyone survives an encounter with a bolt of lightning. Lightning can cause harm by electrical energy (e.g., direct hit, side splash, upward streamer, ground strike, conducted current, step voltage) and can cause trauma (e.g., heat, explosion, fall).[7] Circulatory arrest due to asystole or after prolonged respiratory arrest, hypoxia and acidosis can be expected in about one-third of patients.[4] Lightning-associated injuries such as burns, fractures, mechanical injury to internal organs, or hemorrhage are contributing factors.[8,9] Contrary to general opinion, victims of lightning strike have a good prognosis if appropriate cardiopulmonary resuscitation is instituted without delay.[10]

Epidemiology

Technical electricity

Human-generated technical electricity causes about 5000 non-fatal injuries per year and accounts for about 5% of all admissions to burn centers in the United States. Electric shock is associated with a mortality rate of 0.5 to 2.5 per 100 000 persons/year.[2] Because of a lack of reliable reporting services and data recording, the incidence may be much higher and may vary considerably in different countries. There is thus a need for a comprehensive worldwide epidemiological survey of current-induced casualties. Up to 70% of electrical deaths from high-volt current are related to occupation (Table 64.1).[11–13] Electrocution-related deaths predominate in young males, comprising 7.5% of all lethal occupational accidents in the United States.[12] Approximately three-quarters of deaths occur in electrical and construction workers and result from direct contact with power lines. Most cases of high-voltage injury occur in linemen and construction workers, but they also occur in adventurous persons, usually juvenile males, who climb trees or poles near electricity lines.[14] Late mortality in those who survive initial injuries is mostly due to septicemia, pneumonia,

Cardiac Arrest: The Science and Practice of Resuscitation Medicine. 2nd edn., ed. Norman Paradis, Henry Halperin, Karl Kern, Volker Wenzel, Douglas Chamberlain. Published by Cambridge University Press. © Cambridge University Press, 2007.

Table 64.1. Epidemiology of low volt and high volt technical electricity and lightning associated injuries

Characteristic	Technical electricity		Lightning
	Low volt	High volt	
Incidence (/100 000/yr)	Approx. 70		Approx. 0.09–0.12
Fatality rate	Approx 3%	Up to 30%	10% to 30%
Sex preponderance	Male	Male (> 85%)	Male (> 85%)
Age of greatest risk	Children	20 to 29 yr	20–29 yr
Time of day	Daytime	Working hours	4 to 6 PM
Season	Any	Summer	Summer
At occupation		up to 70%	up to 33%
Activity	Playing, household	Linepersons, electricians	Farmers, golfers

and renal failure.[15,16] Electrocution has been reported as a method of suicide and is still practiced as a means of torture and capital punishment in some countries.[17–19]

About 60% to 70% of electrical injuries are due to low-voltage current, which accounts for one-half of deaths from electricity and up to 1% of accidental household deaths.[16] More than 20% of all electrical injuries occur in children.[20] Household low-voltage electrical injuries are more frequently observed in pre-school children and toddlers,[15,21,22] while high-voltage exposures are more common in those over 12 years old.[23]

Electrocution during pregnancy entails high risks for fetal health because the fetus is exquisitely sensitive to electrical shock.[24] Spontaneous abortions after electrical injury and injury from electric-shock weapons have been reported.[25,26] The path of electricity in electrical cardioversion, however, does not include the uterus and this procedure has been applied safely in all trimesters of pregnancy.[27]

Lightning

Although the majority of persons struck by lightning are merely stunned and may have transient difficulty moving, lightning-related injuries account for several thousand deaths worldwide each year.[11,28] The overall yearly incidence rate of reported cases ranges from 0.09 to 0.12 per 100 000, with case fatality rate up to 30%.[29,30] Eighty-five percent of all people killed by lightning in the United States are male, with a median age of 26 years (Table 65.1). One-third of all lightning strike-related deaths occur in relation to the victim's occupation.[2,31] The time of injury reaches a peak from 16:00 to 18:00 hours, and most casualties occur between May and September.[28,29,32] Approximately one-third of victims killed were injured on the job.[33] Three-quarters of survivors sustain significant permanent sequelae. Most of these epidemiological data are represen-

tative for the USA; the incidence in other countries may differ owing to different exposure rates and data recording.

Prevention

Technical electricity

Both natural and technical electrocution are avoidable problems. Better understanding of the epidemiology of electrical cardiac arrest may result in improved education and product safety. The public should be made more aware of risk factors for electrical shocks. Risky behavior and misuse, e.g., climbing of utility poles, tampering with electrical installations and equipment by unqualified persons, lack of residual current breakers, and improper handling of electrical equipment, must be avoided.[5,34]

Household current in the United States is 120 volts, whereas many other countries use 220 volts. Although high-voltage electricity is more lethal than low-voltage electricity, most electrical injuries result from standard household and business appliances and the power lines that supply them. High-voltage current, defined as a voltage exceeding 1000 volts, commonly results in severe burns and deep tissue damage. Depending on humidity and electrical conduction of surrounding air, as well as the magnitude of voltage and amperage, arcing current may occur within a certain proximity to the high-voltage source. To avoid harm by step voltage from ground current, rescuers are advised to keep a minimum distance of 10 meters unless the power line has been switched off by expert personnel and is visibly grounded.

When an electrical appliance catches fire, it should be unplugged or turned off from the current fuse box. Only a class C fire extinguisher is adequate, in no case should water be used to extinguish fires.

Household electrical cords are the major electrocution hazard in children younger than 12 years.[23] Oral contact with electrical cords or placing objects in a cord socket are frequent causes of injury in toddlers.[35] Water may contribute to electrocution in up to half of all fatalities, and electric sources in bathrooms remain a constant problem, in particular when house wiring is faulty.[36] After use, electrical appliances should be unplugged and kept out of the reach of small children. Use of electrical safety switches, plug covers, circuit breakers, and immersion detectors should become standard practice in private homes and elsewhere.[21]

All electrical equipment on a construction site must comply with the prescribed standards and be maintained by trained and qualified personnel only. Safety equipment, including portable residual current protective devices, use of adequate protective clothing, ground-fault protection on construction sites and at work places, and compliance with established procedures are mandatory.[13] Preventive measures taken by professional associations have reported successful reduction of the frequency of electrical arc accidents.[37] Electrical safety training should be compulsory for utility and construction workers, and any employees handling electrical equipment. Training should include salvage and self-rescue by disconnection of the power line or intentionally dropping to the ground. A health safety program to provide guidance for safe practice is mandatory.[12,13]

Lightning

Information on lightning prevention is based on experimental findings and empirical data from single fatalities. With respect to evidence-based medicine, we lack randomized study findings to prove the various precautions related to lightning. As lightning is related to conduction between negative and positive electric charges, it may occur within a 15-kilometer radius of the thunderstorm. Threat of lightning injury may occur before the beginning of the storm and continue even when the storm has passed. Occasionally lighting may even strike out of the blue sky.[38] Therefore, people are urged to pay attention to local weather forecasts before undertaking outdoor activities. Lightning-associated injuries most commonly reported from open fields, at swimming pools, and in tents. Accidents are related to work, e.g., on or near docks and during leisure time activities in the open. On the surface below a thunderhead (cumulonimbus), ground charges accumulate on tall objects including telephone poles, electricity poles, and isolated trees and increase the chance of these being hit by a lightning bolt. Taking shelter close to metal pipes, rails, and other metallic paths that can transmit lightning energy from a nearby strike must be avoided.[2,31,32] People should stop outdoor activities, especially swimming, diving, or boating whenever a thunderstorm appears imminent; if persons are caught outdoors in a lightning storm, and feel as if their hair is standing on end or their skin is prickling, they are advised to keep low, squat down, put their feet together, and cover their ears. This is recommended to counteract injuries caused by ground current and shock wave. Proximity to other people of less than 10 m should be avoided.

Although no place in a thunderstorm is absolutely safe, large enclosed structures such as buildings or fully closed and hard-topped metal vehicles provide good shelter from lightning threat. Indoors, people should stay away from doors and windows and avoid elevated locations such as rooftops. Rooms that have excess plumbing, such as kitchens and bathrooms, should be avoided until the storm has passed. In particular, using the telephone, taking a shower, or any contact with conductive surfaces with exposure to the outside should be avoided.[39] About 10% of lightning injuries occur during transport.[40] Whereas lightning remains a potential risk to aircraft passengers, modern airplanes are well equipped to reduce the dangers from accidents due to lightning. Moreover, lightning detection systems help trace early stages of incipient thunderstorms.

Pathophysiology

Technical electricity

Experimental knowledge about the effects of electricity on humans indicates that current flow is directly proportional to tissue damage and systemic effects. Severity of electrical trauma, however, cannot be concluded solely from an electrophysical point of view, e.g., the amperage, voltage, type, duration, and pathway of the electric current.[3,14,41,42] Tissue damage results from conversion of electric energy to heat, on the one hand, and from the direct effect of current on cell membranes and vascular smooth muscle, on the other hand. After brief exposure to potential gradients it is cell membranes that are mainly impaired. Cellular damage results in increased cell permeability, leading to ion leakage, escape of metabolites, cellular edema, and irreversible cellular damage. Leakage of ions leads to an osmotic imbalance which in turn causes a colloidal hemolysis of the red cells. In addition, electrolysis of the blood may cause embolism by formation of gas bubbles and thrombosis. Permeabilization of cell membranes and direct electroconformational denaturation of proteins contributes to further tissue damage.[43,44] Injured tissue

Table 64.2. Expected physiological response in relation to amperage (A) by direct current (DC) and alternating current (AC)

Grade	Amperage (A)		Physiologic response
	DC	AC	
I	< 0.08	0.001 to 0.004	Unpleasant, tingling sensation
		0.01 to 0.02	Tetanic skeletal muscle contractions
II	0.08 to 0.3	0.03 to 0.05	Thoracic muscle tetany, respiratory arrest
		0.05 to 0.08	Brady/tachyarrhythmia, atrial fibrillation
III	0.3 to 8	0.08 to 8	Ventricular fibrillation
IV	> 8	> 8	Thermal damage, ventricular fibrillation or asystole

may be salvageable as long as membrane permeabilization is the primary pathologic condition. Severity of injury is closely related to the magnitude of current passing through the tissues when current is high and exposure time is long.[34] When contact time is long, secondary damage from joule heating can directly affect the whole cell.

Furthermore, the extent of injury depends on the nature of the tissues. Bone and skin are most resistant to the passage of electric current, whereas muscle, blood vessels, and nerves conduct with least resistance. Resistance to current flow varies according to the tissue fluid and electrolyte content and the duration of exposure. In addition, surface moisture, sweat, and ointments reduce the impediment to current flow. In general, the skin of babies and children offers lower dermal resistance. Fetal skin is approximately 200 times less resistant to current flow than is postnatal skin. Further, the hyperemic pregnant uterus and amniotic fluid are excellent conductors of electricity. Together this explains why up to 70% of fetuses die, even if the mother survives an electrical injury.[24]

The area of the contact point and exposure time are important, because it is the amount of energy per unit tissue that determines the extent of injury. A small area of contact usually concentrates electrical energy and leads to serious damage of the skin and underlying tissue, whereas the same current may not cause any visible external damage if applied over a wide surface area. The low cross-sectional area of extremities increases current density.

Alternating current (AC) at 50 to 60 cycles per second is extremely dangerous at even low amperage levels, particularly with prolonged exposure time. The likelihood of ventricular fibrillation increases once exposure continues for a complete cardiac cycle.[25] The heart and diaphragm are most susceptible to frequencies at 50 to 60 hertz; hence respiratory and cardiac arrest are more likely when the current passes directly through the trunk, compared with a straddle or vertical path.[45,46] There is clinical evidence that hand-to-hand (transthoracic) pathways are the most lethal followed by head-to-foot (vertical) pathways. Leg-to-leg pathways may result from ground charge that induces a potential difference between the victim's legs. In comparison, direct current (DC) is generally tolerated at much higher strengths (Table 64.2). Electrocardiogram (ECG) changes and positive MB fraction of creatine phosphokinase (CK-MB) are attributed to the direct effect of current and coronary spasms, which cause patchy damage throughout the myocardium.[47] Although uncommon, true Q wave infarctions have been reported after electrical injury.[48] Finally, conduction disturbances as well as severe dysrhythmias are common after electrical shock, although more benign rhythm disturbances such as atrial fibrillation and sinus tachycardia have been reported as well.[49] Several mechanisms appear to underlie the ability of technical electricity to precipitate sudden death: (*a*) myocardial cell damage from the overwhelming inotropic stimulus; (*b*) direct electrical alteration of cell membrane potential; (*c*) released catecholamines; and (*d*) tissue hypoxia from concurrent apnea. In general, the rhythm on presentation is the worst rhythm; however, there are some reports of life-threatening ventricular arrhythmias occurring up to 12 hours after technical electrocution.[50] Victims often develop hypovolemia and metabolic acidosis secondary to extensive fluid losses from cutaneous and deep tissue damage.

Lightning

Lightning is a transfer of electrical charge within a cloud, between clouds, or between the ground and clouds. Rising air within a thundercloud carries positive charges to the top and leaves negative charges at the bottom layer of the cloud. The electrical potential forces an invisible conductive path between negative charges from the cloud to the positively charged earth and a return charge from the

Table 64.3. Differences between low-volt and high-volt technical electricity and lightning regarding voltage, amperage, duration, common tissue pathway, and injury type

| Characteristic | Technical electricity | | Lightning |
	Low-volt	High-volt	
Type of current	Alternating (AC)	Alternating (AC)	
	Direct (DC)		Electrical impulse
Voltage (V)	< 1000 V	1000 to 380 000 V	up to 1 billion V
Amperage (A)	10 to 15 A	up to 1000 A	> 200 000 A
Duration (s)	Variable	Variable	0.0001 to 0.001 s
Tissue pathway	Superficial tissue	Deep tissue	Skin flashover
Injury type	Cardiac rhythm	Burn, shock	Trauma: blunt, thermal, explosive

earth to the cloud. Contact of charges is followed by a visible surge of electricity. As air is a poor conductor of electricity even when humidity is high, discharge of electrical energy will not occur until a potential difference of 30 000 volts or higher exceeds the inherent resistance of the air.

Once at the surface, lightning can harm people in various ways. A direct strike is the most dangerous type and occurs when the primary contact point is on the victim's body. A splash strike is the most common and occurs when an object such as a tree or car is struck primarily, before the strike enters a person. A ground strike can harm the victim when the lightning bolt has struck the ground and the spreading current makes contact through the feet. Rapid heating of air and explosive expansion of atmospheric gases of the surrounding air create shock waves with the typical "sledgehammer effect" of lightning.[28,51]

The direct current lightning strike differs from the more common alternating current electrocution in several ways (Table 64.3). A single lightning bolt can transfer up to 1 billion volts with 200 000 amperes of current. Because of the short duration of approximately 0.0001 to 0.003 second, the resistance of the skin is protective and a relatively small amount of energy is delivered.[28] In addition, high current tends to travel along the outside of a conductor. Sweat, rainwater and metallic materials in the victim's dress contribute to increased peripheral conductivity. Burns may occur from heated metal objects close to the skin and clothing. The superficial current pathway often resembles a skin flashover, leaving a typically fern leaf-patterned superficial sign. Internal current flow leading to deep tissue necrosis is uncommon and fluid requirements are usually low.[28] Reported blunt injuries include myocardial, pulmonary, and abdominal visceral contusion, tympanic membrane rupture, and orthopedic injury.

Clinical manifestations

Victims of electrical shock can sustain a wide variety of injuries, ranging from a transient unpleasant sensation to cardiac arrest. Respiratory arrest may be caused by electric current passing through the brain, by tetanic contraction during exposure, and by prolonged paralysis of respiratory muscles. The electrically injured patient often presents with multisystem injury, either directly related to the electrical shock or secondary to concurrent trauma.[9] Such injuries include burns, fractures, dislocations, contusions, hemorrhage, visceral injury and neurological injury. Thus, the clinician who evaluates a victim of electrical injury must be highly suspicious of secondary injuries.

Technical electricity

Clinical signs and symptoms after electrical injury to the heart can be atypical, delayed in onset, or obscured by other trauma.[50] The physiological response varies depending on magnitude of amperage and whether current was direct or alternating (Table 65.2). Alternating current at low voltage is frequently associated with arrhythmias, varying from ectopic beats, atrial fibrillation, sinus tachycardia or bradycardia, to ventricular fibrillation and asystole.[52] The underlying cause of cardiac arrhythmia may be direct damage to the myocardial cell, hypoxia secondary to central respiratory arrest, or extensive catecholamine release. Myocardial damage can be caused directly by the current and the heat it produces and indirectly by decreased perfusion secondary to coronary artery spasm or unstable arrhythmias.[53]

High-voltage electric shocks are prone to provoke asystole, but non-specific changes in ECG, including prolongation of the corrected QT interval, transient ST segment inversion or elevation, are observed in up to half of all patients.[54,55] CK-MB levels may be elevated, but myocardial necrosis is rarely diagnosed.[22,56] In non-survivors, however, histopathologic investigation of the heart may reveal widespread focal necrosis involving the entire myocardium, including the specialized tissue of the sinus and atrioventricular nodes.[57]

Relatively low levels of current across the chest are enough to cause tetanic spasm of the respiratory muscles. Current passing through the brain can directly damage the medullary respiratory center.[43] Consequent respiratory arrest may resolve spontaneously or lead to secondary cardiac arrest due to asphyxia.[54] Cases of pulmonary edema and respiratory distress syndrome have been reported after electrocution.[58]

Transient damage to the nervous system occurs in up to 70% of electrical injuries. Neurological deficits include coma, seizure, blindness, deafness, and aphasia.[59] Delayed and persistent neuropathy is common. High-voltage electrical injury may cause cerebral vein thrombosis with significant early and delayed brain and spinal cord injury. Spinal involvement indicated by ascending paralysis, spastic paraplegia and associated sensory loss has been reported. Patients may suffer from emotional lability, anxiety reactions, loss of appetite and libido, sleep disorders, depression, post-traumatic stress disorder, and psychosis.[10,34,60]

Musculoskeletal and cutaneous injuries dominate the clinical picture. Low-voltage current, especially alternating current, can lead to sustained muscular contractions and subsequent fracture of adjacent bones or dislocation of affected joints. Severe burn injuries are frequently complicated by damaged deep tissues.[61] Extensive myonecrosis, compartment syndrome, thrombosis, may be associated with cyanotic and pulseless limbs. Early radical fasciotomy and debridement may allow better salvage rates of functional limbs and a reduction in systemic effects such as hypotension, infection and sepsis.[5,14,62] Amputation of one or more limbs may be indicated.[63] Massive tissue necrosis leading to rhabdomyolysis and myoglobinuria may cause acute tubular necrosis. Consequent renal shutdown is more likely after volume depletion and prolonged shock.[64]

Lightning

No large series of cases treated by one institution is available to provide sufficient information on the variety of clinical features in lightning victims. There are, however, a few characteristics that appear to be pathognomonic for lightning.[65] Factors that tend to be in the victim's favor are the very short duration of a lightning strike and because the favored pathway for a majority of the current is along the skin on the outside of the body. There are reports of

prolonged, successful cardiopulmonary resuscitation in lightning victims who initially had non-responding cardiac dysrhythmias.[6,10]

Changes in heart rhythm are common, but generally resolve. A direct hit may cause myocardial damage, pericardial effusion, conduction disturbances, or dysrhythmia.[7] The entire myocardium is simultaneously depolarized, and the heart is thrown into a forceful, sustained contraction until current flow ends. In many cases, cardiac automaticity inherent in the myocardium may restore an organized rhythm with spontaneous circulation. Secondary cardiac impairment can occur due to release of catecholamine or autonomic stimulation. ECG may reveal non-specific changes; only direct hits result in a prolonged QT interval or abnormalities revealed by echocardiography. Severely decreased left and right ventricular ejection fraction has been observed, but can be reversible.

Respiratory arrest due to paralysis of the medullary respiratory centers is common. It can outlast the duration of the cardiac arrest and may lead to secondary hypoxic cardiac arrest.[4,30] Contusion of the lungs can occur with pneumothorax or hemothorax. Bronchospasm and pulmonary edema after lightning strike have been reported.[66]

The low resistance of nervous tissue explains its increased vulnerability in lightning strike. Neurological findings vary from short-term loss of consciousness and transient paralysis to coma, seizure, increased intracranial pressure, or even intracranial hemorrhage.[67] Neurological deficits may present as blindness, deafness, and aphasia. Sequelae, e.g., confusion, amnesia, agitation, mood disturbance, sleep disturbance, anxiety attacks, fear, pain syndromes, major depression, and frank psychosis have been reported in victims of lightning strike.[68]

Blunt trauma may be caused by the shock wave produced by lightning. Muscle contractions caused by the current may result in fractures and dislocations.[28,68] Limb paralysis with sensory symptoms, pallor, coolness, and absent pulses may occur from intense vasospasm (keraunoparalysis) due to autonomic nervous system dysfunction. Initially cyanotic and pulseless limbs, however, are prone to revert spontaneously to normal. Delay of fasciotomy for several hours is reasonable.

The gastrointestinal tract can be afflicted with ileus, contusion, or perforation, and the kidneys are susceptible to decreased clearance compounded with a myoglobin load from muscle breakdown.

In victims of lightning strike, burns of any degree can injure the skin, but the extremely short flashover, extensive burns and tissue destruction are uncommon.[69] The external path of the direct current may show an arborizing or fern leaf pattern. Ruptured tympanic membranes from shock

Table 64.4. Distinctions in sequence of resuscitation between low volt, high volt and lightning associated injuries

Characteristic	Technical electricity		Lightning
	Low-volt	High-volt	
Emergency call	Nature and intensity of injury	Nature and intensity of injury Need for expert personnel	Nature and intensity of injury Limit call time by conventional telephone during thunderstorm
Self-protection	Unplugged electrical device Switched-off power line Switched off fuse	Keep minimum distance of 10 m unless power line was switched off by expert personnel and visibly grounded	Avoid locations with high risk of lightning Avoid proximity on site
Triage	Conventional	Conventional	Modified
Spine protection	Immobilization, if indicated	Immobilization mandatory	Immobilization mandatory
External cooling	Not indicated	Cool water on 1° and 2° burn area of less than 30% for up to 10 min Remove smoldering clothes	Not indicated
Airway management	Conventional	Early tracheal intubation and ventilation in orofacial edema	Avoid hypoxic cardiac arrest by early ventilation
IV access	Single peripheral IV access	Multiple large-bore IV lines	Single peripheral IV access
IV fluid administration	IV fluid administration restricted	IV 4–7 ml/kg per day x % burn	IV fluid administration restricted
CPR onset	CPR during extrication	CPR during extrication	Delayed onset after initial ventilation if necessary
CPR termination	Conventional	Conventional	Modified
Referral	Intensive care unit	Trauma/burn center	Trauma center

waves and damage to cornea or retina are common in lightning victims. Cataracts can occur from a few days to several months after the lightning strike.

Clinical case reports suggest that resuscitation may be successful in victims of lightning strike, even when the interval between arrest and therapy is prolonged and refractory rhythms (e.g., asystole) are present.[70] To explain this observation, it was hypothesized that lightning causes cellular metabolism to cease temporarily, thereby delaying the onset of anoxic tissue damage and reducing the potential for irreversible cardiac and cerebral injury. No basic or clinical scientific data are available to validate this assumption.

Resuscitation

Cardiac arrests induced by both natural and technical electricity require special treatment and management of current-induced casualties differs according to whether their injuries are caused by low-voltage, high-voltage, or lightning (Table 65.4). Generally the degree of cardiac and neurological malfunction after primary successful resuscitation correlates with duration of cardiac arrest time.[71] Special treatment recommendations for lightning and electrical injuries have been based on case reports rather than laboratory and clinical investigations. There are reports supporting the thesis that in victims of electrical injury, resuscitation may be effective even after a prolonged interval between the electrical injury and the resuscitative attempt.[4,6] Because the victims are often young and have no co-morbid diseases, reports that good outcomes may occur after long arrest times are compelling reasons to sustain resuscitation efforts.

Emergency call and response

Information about the likely number of victims and the type of injury must be provided immediately to the dispatch center to ensure early EMS arrival on the scene. If expert personnel are needed in the case of high-voltage accidents it must be recognized early. Furthermore, the dispatch center can give CPR instructions. During a thunderstorm calls by conventional telephone should be kept as short as possible, and only wireless calls by cell phone or radio are regarded as safe.[38] The person calling must stay on the line with the dispatch center and must not disconnect the line of communication.

Modified triage

Rapid triage and early emergency medical treatment are mandatory if numerous victims have been severely injured following electrocution. Whenever the number of patients exceeds the capacity of rescue personnel, the lowest priority is given to those without a palpable pulse.[72] In lightning, when two or more victims are struck simultaneously, standard triage principles are reversed: highest priority is given to those without a palpable pulse, rather than to victims who are awake but confused.[4] It is unlikely that those who survived the initial injury will develop delayed life-threatening conditions. If there are many injured patients, triage extends to the use of monitoring equipment as well. While pulsoxygraphy is adequate for initial observation of an unconscious patient, ECG may be applied when the patient is awake.

Discontinuing exposure and evacuation

Unlike the victims of lightning strike, patients experiencing technical electrocution should be assumed still to have current flowing through them. The victim may still be gripping the live wire or object because of tetanic spasm of the flexor muscles. For low-voltage electrical injury, electrical sources must be turned off, unplugged, or carefully removed with rubber or wooden instruments before rescue is attempted. If electrical shock occurs in a location that is not readily accessible, such as while the victim is atop a utility pole or is swimming, effective CPR attempts will not be possible until the victim is extricated.[73] The spine should be immobilized and remain so during out-of-hospital emergency treatment as patients frequently fall, resulting in a high incidence of neck trauma.[3,74]

In high-voltage incidents the rescuers must wait at a distance until expert personnel have turned off and visibly grounded the power supply. Unidentified current is regarded as high-voltage unless expert personnel disagree. The recommended safe distance from the electrical transmission lines is at least twice the distance from the insulator to the utility pole, with a minimum of 10 meters.[75]

During a thunderstorm, rescuers are cautioned to minimize their exposure to lightning as much as possible. Victims of lightning carry no electrical charge and can be touched safely immediately after the strike. On the other hand, the lightning strike indicates that the situation might still be dangerous. If providing CPR takes the rescuer to the highest point in the midst of a severe storm, then addi-

tional casualties may occur. In most cases, however, the risk to rescuers in treating the victims of lightning strike is minimal. If the injury occurs on moist ground or in water, it is acceptable to give a few quick breaths before moving the patient to a safer place and starting CPR. A protective layer between patient and ground may diminish the risk of hypothermia. Spinal protection and immobilization should be maintained during extrication and treatment if head or neck trauma appears to be likely.

Cardiopulmonary resuscitation

When cardiac arrest occurs in remote locations that are far from medical care facilities, response times for professional rescue are prolonged. The principles for management of electrically injured victims[76] and victims of lightning[77,78] include ensuring rescuer safety and providing for CPR to be started immediately by bystanders. The goal is to oxygenate the heart and brain adequately until cardiac activity is restored. The sequence of actions follows the International Guidelines for Basic Life Support (BLS) and Advanced Life Support (ALS) with respect to electric shock and lightning strike.[79,80]

BLS

In victims of high-voltage current with first and second degree burns of less than 30% body surface, further extension of thermal injury should be avoided by applying copious amounts of cool water to the burned area. Cold water should not be used as it induces vasoconstriction and consequently increases the afterburn effect. Application is restricted to 10 minutes to avoid further harm from hyper- or hypothermia. Smoldering shoes, belts, and clothes should be removed unless they are stuck to burn lesions. If the victim is not breathing spontaneously, emergency medical service (EMS) system activation, prompt CPR and, if available, use of automated external defibrillator (AED) are initiated by bystanders. Basic life support by mouth-to-mouth ventilation together with cardiac compression in the ratio 2:30 is started. As soon as circulation returns, ventilation should be continued until sufficient spontaneous breathing is restored.

ALS

When advanced life support can be established, the initial cardiac activity is quickly assessed by using defibrillator paddles or self-adhesive electrode pads. The two defibrillator paddles or electrode pads are placed one below the right clavicle and the other at the opposite lateral chest wall with the heart maintained in the center between the two paddle surfaces. The rhythm on the monitor is determined as being either shockable, e.g., ventricular fibrillation or pulseless ventricular tachycardia, or non-shockable rhythm. With shockable rhythm it has to be ensured that everybody is clear of the patient. A one-shock strategy and immediate resumption of effective chest-compressions after each shock may improve outcome by reducing interruptions of CPR.[80] The total number of countershocks and the power applied should be kept to a minimum because myocardial injury may be cumulative.[81] The chance for successful defibrillation increases when coronary perfusion can be improved prior to defibrillation.[82] When rhythm is non-shockable, CPR is continued and signs of circulation, e.g., palpable carotid pulse, are repeatedly checked for.

Airway management

Patients with insufficient and absent breathing should receive immediate ventilatory support with positive pressure ventilation and a high inspired oxygen concentration, preferably 100%. When administering oxygen on site, a safe distance to burning or hot objects must be maintained. A secure airway is established early, and the gold standard is tracheal intubation. This allows adequate mechanical ventilation and the administration of emergency drugs, with the exception of sodium bicarbonate. A definitive airway is also important in patients with burns of the face, mouth, or neck or whenever inhalation injury is expected. Intubation should be accomplished on an elective basis before signs of airway obstruction become severe. With high-voltage injury, in particular, extensive soft tissue swelling may develop rapidly and compromise the airway and breathing, necessitating emergency cricothyroidotomy or tracheotomy. Airway protection and ventilation are particularly important in lightning victims as the critical factor in mortality from lightning is the duration of respiratory arrest rather than the time of circulatory standstill.[4]

Drug treatment

Drug treatment including vasopressors, inotropic support, and other standard therapies are administered as needed. Close monitoring of patient response is important. Once return of spontaneous circulation has been achieved, further therapies may be started. Dosages and administration schedules do not differ from general recommendations, but it is not clear whether the application of therapies that depend on cardiac electrophysiology, such as antiarrhythmic drugs and cardiac pacing, is altered by the preceding electrical injury.

Venous access

Peripheral venous cannulation, e.g., via the external jugular vein, is usually sufficient to establish vascular access, but central veins are the optimal route for delivering drugs rapidly into the central circulation and for administering infusions. This applies especially to patients with high-voltage injuries, who may have severe burns and significant tissue destruction.

Fluid administration

Vigorous fluid therapy in the early phase of resuscitation with crystalloids (preferably normo-saline solution) is critical to both immediate survival and ultimate outcome. Colloids are not recommended in patients with severe burns unless multiple systems are injured. Colloids potentially increase edema and therefore could add to secondary tissue damage. Fluid requirements are often greater than those estimated by the Parkland formula, because severe burn and extended tissue damage frequently occur together. Infusions should be continued after successful resuscitation at a rate between 4 and 7 ml/kg per % body surface area burned per day.[83]

From emergency medical point of view, this is about 1 l of crystalloids per hour in adults (children: 10 – 15 ml/kg per hour) unless additional injuries other than burns increase the volume demand. Fluid administration should be adequate to maintain diuresis to facilitate excretion of myoglobin, potassium and other by-products of tissue destruction. Lightning victims generally do not require volume expansion, and indeed this can worsen the cerebral edema that commonly accompanies the injury.[4] Once spontaneous circulation is reestablished, intravenous fluid therapy must be restricted.

Prognosis

The various reports of good outcomes even after prolonged arrest times justify early transport and continued CPR en route to the hospital.[6] Heroic therapies such as open chest CPR may be effective in some patients.[84]

Referral and definitive care

Generally, hospitalization is advised for all victims of electrical trauma as the magnitude and severity of internal tissue damage cannot be accurately gauged from external examination alone. Particular attention should be paid to the development of compartment syndrome, hyperkalemia, myoglobinemia and renal injury. Sequelae of internal tissue injury tend to occur along the path of current flow. Furthermore, all victims of electrical injury require a complete neurologic assessment. Delayed neurological injury is common in victims of both lightning and technical electrocution. As soon as the patient's condition has stabilized, smooth and quick transport to the most suitable intensive care center should be arranged. Victims of high-voltage injury are transferred to the trauma and burn center. Patients who have been struck by lightning are regarded as trauma patients and are transferred to the trauma center. Continuous monitoring of vital signs during transport is mandatory.

REFERENCES

1. Cooper, M.A. Electrical and lightning injuries. *Emerg. Med. Clin. North Am.* 1984; **2**(3): 489–501.

2. Duclos, P.J. & Sanderson, L.M. An epidemiological description of lightning-related deaths in the United States. *Int. J. Epidemiol.* 1990; **19**(3): 673–679.

3. Fish, R. Electric shock, Part III: Deliberately applied electric shocks and the treatment of electric injuries. *J. Emerg. Med.* 1993; **11**(4): 599–603.

4. Fontanarosa, P.B. Electrical shock and lightning strike. *Ann. Emerg. Med.* 1993; **22**(2): 378–386.

5. Haberal, M.A. An eleven-year survey of electrical burn injuries. *J. Burn. Care. Rehabil.* 1995; **16**(1): 43–48.

6. Marcus, M.A., Thijs, N. & Meulemans, A.I. A prolonged but successful resuscitation of a patient struck by lightning. *Eur. J. Emerg. Med.* 1994; **1**(4): 199–202.

7. Lichtenberg, R., Dries, D., Ward, K., Marshall, W. & Scanlon, P. Cardiovascular effects of lightning strikes. *J. Am. Coll. Cardiol.* 1993; **21**(2): 531–536.

8. Wetli, C.V. Keraunopathology. An analysis of 45 fatalities. *Am. J. Forensic. Med. Pathol.* 1996; **17**(2): 89–98.

9. Fahmy, F.S., Brinsden, M.D., Smith, J. & Frame, J.D. Lightning: the multisystem group injuries. *J. Trauma* 1999; **46**(5): 937–940.

10. Leibovici, D., Shemer, J. & Shapira, S.C. Electrical injuries: current concepts. *Injury* 1995; **26**(9): 623–627.

11. Taylor, A.J., McGwin, G., Jr., Valent, F. & Rue, L.W. 3rd. Fatal occupational electrocutions in the United States. *Inj. Prev.* 2002; **8**(4): 306–312.

12. Jones, J.E., Armstrong, C.W., Woolard, C.D. & Miller, G.B., Jr. Fatal occupational electrical injuries in Virginia. *J. Occup. Med.* 1991; **33**(1): 57–63.

13. Ore, T. & Casini, V. Electrical fatalities among U.S. construction workers. *J. Occup. Environ. Med.* 1996; **38**(6): 587–592.

14. Arnoldo, B.D., Purdue, G.F., Kowalske, K., Helnn, P.A., Burris, A. & Hunt, J.L. Electrical injuries: a 20-year review. *J. Burn Care Rehabil.* 2004; **25**(6): 479–484.

15. Koumbourlis, A.C. Electrical injuries. *Crit. Care Med.* 2002; **30**(11 Suppl): 424–430.

16. Haberal, M., Ucar, N., Bayraktar, U., Oner, Z. & Bilgin, N. Visceral injuries, wound infection and sepsis following electrical injuries. *Burns* 1996; **22**(2): 158–161.

17. Al-Alousi, L.M. Homicide by electrocution. *Med. Sci. Law* 1990; **30**: 239–246.

18. Fernando, R. Suicide by electrocution. *Med. Sci. Law* 1990; **30**: 219–220.

19. Moreno, A. & Grodin, M.A. Torture and its neurological Sequelae. *Spinal Cord* 2002; **40**(5): 213–223.

20. Baker, M.D. & Chiaviello, C. Household electrical injuries in children. *Am. J. Dis. Child* 1989; **143**(1): 59–62.

21. Nguyen, B.H., MacKay, M., Bailey, B. & Klassen, T.P. Epidemiology of electrical and lightning related deaths and injuries among Canadian children and youth. *Inj. Prev.* 2004; **10**(2): 122–124.

22. Bailey, B., Gaudreault, P., Thivierge, R.L. & Turgeon, J.P. Cardiac monitoring of children with household electrical injuries. *Ann. Emerg. Med.* 1995; **25**(5): 612–617.

23. Rabban, J.T., Blair, J.A., Rosen, C.L., Adler, J.N. & Sheridan, R.L. Mechanisms of pediatric electrical injury. New implications for product safety and injury prevention. *Arch. Pediatr. Adolesc. Med.* 1997; **151**(7): 696–700.

24. Goldman, R.D., Einarson, A. & Koren, G. Electrical shock during pregnancy. *Can. Fam. Physician* 2003; **49**: 297–298.

25. Robinson, M.N., Brooks, C.G. & Renshaw, G.D. Electric shock devices and their effects on the human body. *Med. Sci. Law* 1990; **30**(4): 285–300.

26. Denk, W., Misshwetz, J., Wieser, I. & Tauschitz, C. Electroshock devices as weapon. *Arch. Kriminol.* 1995; **196**(3–4): 78–86.

27. Fatovich, D.M. Electric shock in pregnancy. *J. Emerg. Med.* 1993; **11**: 175–177.

28. Blount, B.W. Lightning injuries. *Am. Fam. Physician.* 1990; **42**(2): 405–414.

29. Cooper, M.A. Lightning injuries: prognostic signs for death. *Ann. Emerg. Med.* 1980; **9**(3): 134–138.

30. Adeloya, N. & Nolte, K.B. Struck-by-lightning deaths in the United States. *J. Environ. Health* 2005; **67**(9): 45–50, 58.

31. Epperly, T.D. & Stewart, J.R. The physical effects of lightning injury. *J. Fam. Pract.* 1989; **29**(3): 267–272.

32. Langley, R.L., Dunn, K.A. & Esinhart, J.D. Lightning fatalities in North Carolina 1972–1988. *N C Med. J.* 1991; **52**(6): 281–284.

33. Cooper, M.A. Lightning injuries. *Emerg. Med. Clin. North Am.* 1983; **1**(3): 639–641.

34. Cooper, M.A. Emergent care of lightning and electrical injuries. *Semin. Neurol.* 1995; **15**(3): 268–278.

35. Palin, W.E., Jr., Sadove, A.M., Jones, J.E., Judson, W.F. & Stambaugh, H.D. Oral electrical burns in a pediatric population. *J. Oral Med.* 1987; **42**(1): 17–21.

36. Budnick, L.D. Bathtub-related electrocutions in the United States 1979 to 1982. *J. Am. Med. Assoc.* 1984; **252**(7): 918–920.

37. Strauch, H. & Wirth, I. Fatal electric arc accidents due to high voltage. *Arch. Kriminol.* 2004; **214**(5–6): 163–172.

38. Dwyer, J.R. A bolt out of the blue. *Sci. Am.* 2005; **292**(5): 64–71.

39. Andrews, C.J. Telephone-related lightning injury. *Med. J. Aust.* 1992; **157**(11–12): 823–826.

40. Cherington, M. Lightning and transportation. *Semin. Neurol.* 1995; **15**(4): 362–366.

41. Lee, R.C. Injury by electrical forces: pathophysiology, manifestations, and therapy. *Curr. Probl. Surg.* 1997; **34**(9): 677–764.

42. Cooper, M.A. A fifth mechanism of lightning injury. *Acad. Emerg. Med.* 2002; **9**(2): 172–174.

43. Clausen, T. & Gissel, H. Role of Na,K pumps in restoring contractility following loss of cell membrane integrity in rat skeletal muscle. *Acta Physiol. Scand.* 2005; **183**(3): 263–271.

44. Lee, R.C., Zhang, D. & Hannig, J. Biophysical injury mechanisms in electrical shock trauma. *Annu. Rev. Biomed. Eng.* 2000; **2**: 477–509.

45. Edlich, R.F., Farinholt, H.M., Winters, K.L., Britt, L.D. & Long, W.B. 3rd. Modern concepts of treatment and prevention of electrical burns. *J. Long Term Eff. Med. Implants.* 2005; **15**(5): 511–532.

46. Chandra, N.C., Siu, C.O. & Munster, A.M. Clinical predictors of myocardial damage after high voltage electrical injury. *Crit. Care Med.* 1990; **18**(3): 293–297.

47. Lewin, R.F., Arditti, A. & Sclarovsky, S. Non-invasive evaluation of electrical cardiac injury. *Br. Heart J.* 1983; **49**(2): 190–192.

48. Kinney, T.J. Myocardial infarction following electrical injury. *Ann. Emerg. Med.* 1982; **11**(11): 622–625.

49. Fineschi, V., D: Donato, S., Mondillo, S. & Turillazzi, E. Electric shock: cardiac effects relative to non-fatal injuries and post-mortem findings in fatal cases. *Int. J. Cardiol* 2005; Oct 26, [Epub ahead of print].

50. Jensen, P.J., Thomsen, P.E., Bagger, J.P., Norgaard, A. & Baandrup, V. Electrical injury causing ventricular arrhythmias. *Br. Heart J.* 1987; **57**(3): 279–283.

51. O'Keefe, Gatewood, M. & Zane, R.D. Lightning injuries. *Emerg. Med. Clin. North Am.* 2004; **22**(2): 369–403.

52. Carleton, S.C. Cardiac problems associated with electrical injury. *Cardiol. Clin.* 1995; **13**(2): 263–266.

53. Xenopoulos, N., Movahed, A., Hudson, P., & Reeves, W.C. Myocardial injury in electrocution. *Am. Heart. J* 1991; **122**(5): 1481–1484.

54. Ku, C.S., Lin, S.I., Hsu, T.L., Wang, S.P. & Chang, M.S. Myocardial damage associated with electrical injury. *Am. Heart J.* 1989; **118**(3): 621–624.

55. Cunningham, P.A. The need for cardiac monitoring after electrical injury. *Med. J. Aust.* 1991; **154**(11): 765–766.

56. Hammond, J.S. & Ward, C.G. Myocardial damage and electrical injuries: significance of early elevation of CPK-MB isoenzymes. *South. Med. J.* 1986; **79**(4): 414–416.

57. Housinger, T.A., Green, L., Shahangian, S., Saffle, J.R. & Warden, G.D. A prospective study of myocardial damage in electrical injuries. *J. Trauma* 1985; **25**(2): 122–124.

58. Schein, R.M., Kett, D.H., De Marchena, E.J. & Sprung, C.L. Pulmonary edema associated with electrical injury. *Chest* 1990; **97**(5): 1248–1250.

59. Grossman, A.R., Tempereau, C.E., Brones, M.F. Kulber, H.S. & Pembrook, L.J. Auditory and neuropsychiatric behaviour after electrical injury. *J. Burn Care Rehabil.* 1993; **14**(2): 169–175.

60. Primeau, M. Neurorehabilitation of behavioral disorders following lightning and electrical trauma. *Neuro Rehabilitation* 2005; **20**(1): 25–33.

61. Selvaggi, G., Montstrey, S., Van Landuyt, K., Hamdi, M. & Blondeel, P. Rehabilitation of burn injured patients following lightning and electrical trauma. *Neuro Rehabilitation* 2005; **20**(1): 35–42.

62. Holliman, C.J., Saffle, J.R., Kravitz, M. & Warden, G.D. Early surgical decompression in the management of electrical injuries. *Am. J. Surg.* 1982; **144**(6): 733–739.

63. Parshley, P.F., Kilgore, J., Pulito, J.F., Smiley, P.W. & Miller, S.H. Aggressive approach to the extremity damaged by electric current. *Am. J. Surg.* 1985; **150**(1): 78–82.

64. Bhatt, D.L., Gaynor, D.C. & Lee, R.C. Rhabdomyolysis due to pulsed electric fields. *Plast. Reconstr. Surg.* 1990; **86**(1): 1–11.

65. Graber, J., Ummenhofer, W. & Herion, H. Lightning accident with eight victims: case report and brief review of the literature. *J. Trauma* 1996; **40**(2): 288–290.

66. Lutalo, S.K., Ummenhofer, W. & Herion, H. Acute pulmonary oedema caused by lightning. *Cent. Afr. J. Med.* 1989; **35**(11): 534–537.

67. Cherington, M. Central nervous system complications of lightning and electrical injuries. *Semin. Neurol.* 1995; **15**(3): 233–240.

68. Cherington, M. Spectrum of neurologic complications of lightning injuries. *Neuro Rehabilitation* 2005; **20**(1): 3–8.

69. Eriksson, A. & Ornehult, L. Death by lightning. *Am. J. Forens. Med. Pathol.* 1988; **9**(4): 295–300.

70. Ghezzi, K.T. Lightning injuries. A unique treatment challenge. *Postgrad. Med.* 1989; **85**(8): 201–208.

71. Cerchiari, E.L., Safar, P., Klein, E., Cantadore, R. & Pinsky, M. Cardiovascular function and neurologic outcome after cardiac arrest in dogs. The cardiovascular post-resuscitation syndrome. *Resuscitation* 1993; **25**(1): 9–33.

72. Ueberle, H.K. & Rose, T.K. Medical policy in the management of a mass casualty situation with special regard to sorting. *Med. Law* 1985; **4**(3): 275–282.

73. Towne, G.E. Pole-top cardiopulmonary resuscitation. *J. Occup. Med.* 1971; **13**(8): 3998–4001.

74. Lammertse, D.P. Neuro rehabilitation of spinal cord injuries following lightning and electrical trauma. *Neuro Rehabilitation* 2005; **20**(1): 9–14.

75. Hauf, R. First aid and therapeutic measures at the place of the accident and in the hospital in electrical accidents. *Zentralbl. Arbeitsmed. Arbeitsschutz Prophyl.* 1978; **28**(11): 305–310.

76. Lederer, W., Wiedermann, F.J., Cerchiari, E. & Baubin, M.A. Electricity-associated injuries I: outdoor management of current-induced casualties. *Resuscitation* 1999; **43**(1): 69–77.

77. Lederer, W., Wiedermann, F.J., Cerchiari, E. & Baubin, M.A. Electricity-associated injuries II: outdoor management of lightning-induced casualties. *Resuscitation* 2000; **43**(2): 89–93.

78. Electric Shock and Lightning Strikes. International Guidelines 2000 for CPR and ECC – A consensus on Science. In Baskett, P., ed. *Resuscitation Official Journal of the European Resuscitation Council.* Amsterdam, Lausanne, New York, Oxford, Shannon, Tokyo: Elsevier, 2000: 297–299.

79. Second and subsequent shocks. International Liaison Committee on Resuscitation (ILCOR), Part 3. Defibrillation. Elsevier Ireland Ltd. 2005; **67**: 203–211.

80. Zafren, K., Durrer, B., Herry, J.P. & Brugger, H. Lightning injuries: prevention and on-site treatment in mountains and

remote areas: Official guidelines of the International Commission for Mountain Emergency Medicine and the Medical Commission of the International Mountaineering and Climbing Federation (ICAR and UIAA MEDCOM). *Resuscitation* 2005; **65**(3): 369–372.

81. Bunai, Y., Tsujinaka, M., Nakazawa, T. *et al.* Myocardial damage by resuscitation methods. *Leg. Med.* 2003; Suppl. 1: S302–S306.

82. Wik, L., Hansen, T.B., Fylling, F. *et al.* Delaying fibrillation to give basic cardiopulmonary resuscitation to patients with out-of-hospital ventricular fibrillation: a randomized trial. *J. Am. Med. Assoc.* 2003; **289**(11): 1389–1395.

83. Bortolani, A., Governa, M. & Barisona, D. Fluid replacement in burned patients. *Acta Chir. Plast.* 1996; **38**(4): 132–136.

84. Paradis, N.A. et al. Use of open chest CPR after failure of standard closed chest CPR: illustrative cases. *Resuscitation* 1992; **24**: 61–71.

65

Rare syndromes, commotio cordis, sudden death in athletes

Tommaso Pellis[1], Mark Link[2], Charles Antzelevitch[3], and Peter Kohl[4]

[1] Cardiac Mechano-Electric Feedback Lab, University Laboratory of Physiology, Oxford, UK
[2] Tufts University School of Medicine, Boston, USA
[3] Masonic Medical Research Laboratory, Utica, USA
[4] The University Laboratory of Physiology, Oxford, UK

Introduction

Athletes deliberately expose themselves to extreme environments (such as high altitude mountaineering and deep-sea diving) and physical challenges (from weight lifting to marathon running), which may give rise to the manifestation of rare cardiac conditions, or cause sudden death (SD). Indeed, the renowned Athenian long distance runner Pheidippides suffered SD in 490 BC after running from the battlefield of Marathon to Athens to announce the great victory of the Greeks over the invaders.

An analysis of the very dissimilar physical and environmental conditions to which athletes are exposed, and related health risks, is beyond the scope of this chapter and will not be conducted. Instead, we will focus on SD from cardiac causes.

Incidence

Sudden cardiac death

It is commonly understood, and substantiated by clinical evidence, that regular moderate physical exercise has beneficial cardiovascular effects.[1] Several prospective epidemiological studies consistently associate exercise with a reduced risk of coronary artery disease (CAD) and sudden cardiac death (SCD).[2,3]

The incidence of SCD in adolescents and young adults (here defined as the age group <35 years) is about 1 in 100 000 per year;[4] this is 100 times less than in the older population (1 in 1000 per year; Fig. 65.1).[5] Predominant causes of SCD in athletes change with age. In those over

35 years of age, the most common etiology is atherosclerotic CAD, often severe and diffuse, even in individuals without known risk factors or symptoms.[6] In contrast, in younger athletes, a variety of cardiac diseases, largely congenital and often rare, account for the majority of SCD.[4,6–8]

Despite the above-mentioned general health benefit of regular exercise, young athletes can have a *higher* incidence of SD than age-matched non-athletes.[10] Thus, Corrado *et al.*[4] found in the Veneto region of Italy that the SCD incidence in athletes was 2.8 times that of non-athletes (all aged 12–35 years), demonstrating that *competitive sports activity* can actually enhance the risk of SD (Fig. 65.2). Young competitive athletes who died suddenly were primarily affected by silent cardiovascular diseases, predominantly cardiomyopathies, premature CAD, and congenital coronary anomalies (Fig. 65.3). Sports activity, in this context, is therefore not *per se* a cause of the increased mortality; rather, it triggers manifestation of underlying cardiovascular diseases, predisposing athletes to life-threatening ventricular arrhythmias during physical exercise.

In keeping with this view, up to 90% of deaths among young athletes occur during training or competition.[4,7] For this reason, unexplained syncope in young athletes in the context of exercise should be taken very seriously indeed (presuming an "aborted SD"), unless proven otherwise.

Furthermore, current evidence suggests a gender difference of SD in athletes, with a striking male predominance (male-to-female ratio 10:1; Table 65.1).[4,7,11] This predominance of fatal events in male athletes was initially explained by the lower number of females participating in competitive sports. Male gender is in itself a risk factor for sports-related SD, however, as demonstrated by Corrado

Cardiac Arrest: The Science and Practice of Resuscitation Medicine. 2nd edn., ed. Norman Paradis, Henry Halperin, Karl Kern, Volker Wenzel, Douglas Chamberlain. Published by Cambridge University Press. © Cambridge University Press, 2007.

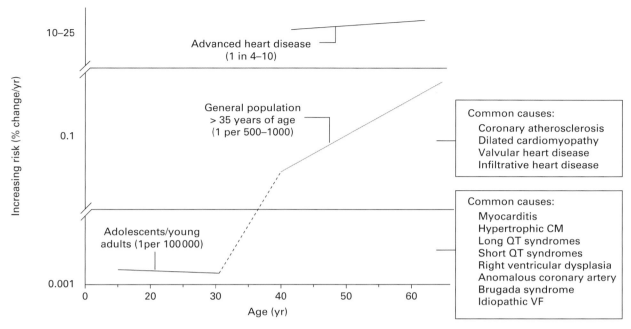

Fig. 65.1. Age-related and disease-specific risk for SCD. For the general population (35 years of age and older) the SCD risk is 0.1 to 0.2% per year (1 per 500 to 1000). In adolescents and adults younger than 30 years, the overall risk of SCD is 1 per 100 000, or 0.001% per year. The risk of SCD increases dramatically beyond the age of 35 years and continues to rise. CM = cardiomyopathy; VF = ventricular fibrillation. (With permission from ref. 9.)

et al.[4] Compared to females, male athletes are generally exposed to more intense training and higher levels of intensity during competition, and they have a greater prevalence and/or phenotypic expression of cardiac diseases with risk of arrhythmic cardiac arrest, such as cardiomyopathies[12] and premature CAD in the given age range.[13] Moreover, there appear to be gender differences in mechanisms underlying cardiac electrophysiology, such as a lower level of the transient outward current in females, which could serve to protect them from arrhythmogenic SD linked, for example, to the Brugada syndrome.[14] A role for sex hormones has been conjectured in this and other ion channelopathies.[15]

Based on the Minneapolis Heart Institute Foundation registry, Maron *et al.*[16] report that a majority of athletes who died suddenly of hypertrophic cardiomyopathy (HCM) were African Americans (55%; Fig. 65.4). This predominance is unlikely to be solely attributable to differences in relative rates or types of sports participation compared to other ethnic communities. It is possible that HCM in African Americans represents a more virulent form of the disease, perhaps due to a malignant genetic substrate when associated with exercise,[17] thereby predisposing to SD on the athletic field. In contrast, arrhythmogenic right ventricular cardiomyopathy (ARVC) and aortic valve

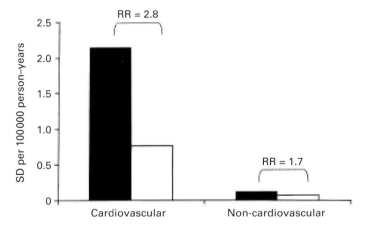

Fig. 65.2. Incidence and relative risk (RR) of sudden death (SD) among athletes (solid columns) and non-athletes (open columns) from cardiovascular and non-cardiovascular causes. Athletes had a 2.8 RR of cardiovascular SD (confidence interval [CI] 1.9 to 3.7; $P < 0.001$) compared to 1.7 RR of non-cardiovascular SD (CI 0.3 to 5.7; $P = 0.39$). (With permission from ref. 4.)

stenosis are both significantly more common in white than in African American athletes (Fig. 65.4).[16]

Despite a number of investigations, the *actual* incidence of SCD in adolescents and young adults in

Table 65.1. Characteristics of sudden death victims

	Athletes ($n = 55$)	Non-athletes ($n = 245$)	*P* value
Mean age (yrs)	23.1 ± 7	23.9 ± 9	1.0
Gender			
Males	50	170	0.002
Females	5	75	
Circumstances of death			
Exercise-related	49 (89%)	22 (9%)	< 0.0001
During effort	40	15	
After effort	9	7	
Unrelated to exercise	6 (11%)	225 (91%)	
Medical history			
Familial history of SD	5 (9%)	27 (11%)	0.8
Previous symptoms	18 (32%)	56 (23%)	0.2
ECG abnormalities/ arrhythmias	22 (40%)	36/63 (57%)	0.1

Data are presented as the mean value ± standard deviation or number (%) of subjects. ECG = electrocardiographic; SD = sudden death.
With permission from ref. 4.

Table 65.2. Causes of sudden death in 387 young athletes in the USA

Cause	Number of athletes	Percent
Hypertrophic cardiomyopathy	102	26.4
Commotio cordis	77	19.9
Coronary-artery anomalies	53	13.7
Left ventricular hypertrophy of indeterminate causation[a]	29	7.5
Myocarditis	20	5.2
Ruptured aortic aneurysm (Marfan's syndrome)	12	3.1
Arrhythmogenic right ventricular cardiomyopathy	11	2.8
Tunneled (bridged) coronary artery[b]	11	2.8
Aortic-valve stenosis	10	2.6
Atherosclerotic coronary artery disease	10	2.6
Dilated cardiomyopathy	9	2.3
Myxomatous mitral-valve degeneration	9	2.3
Asthma (or other pulmonary condition)	8	2.1
Heat stroke	6	1.6
Drug abuse	4	1.0
Other cardiovascular cause	4	1.0
Long-QT syndrome[c]	3	0.8
Cardiac sarcoidosis	3	0.8
Trauma involving structural cardiac injury	3	0.8
Ruptured cerebral artery	3	0.8

Data are from the registry of the Minneapolis Heart Institute Foundation.[16]
[a] Findings at autopsy were suggestive of hypertrophic cardiomyopathy but were insufficient to be diagnostic.
[b] Tunneled coronary artery was deemed the cause in the absence of any other cardiac abnormality.
[c] The long-QT syndrome was documented on clinical evaluation.
With permission from ref. 18.

competitive sports remains controversial. The issue has been addressed primarily in the United States (US) and in Italy, two very different countries with dissimilar racial and genetic backgrounds, scope of popular sports activities, screening regulations, and health care provision. The reported annual prevalence of athletic field deaths ranges from 0.5 in 100,000 in US high-school athletes in Minnesota[11] to 2.3 in 100 000 in Northern Italy.[4]

In the majority of US reports that include autopsy data, HCM is the most common underlying disease linked to these deaths (Table 65.2).[6,7] In contrast, HCM is uncommon in Italian studies of SD on the athletic field. A probable reason for this difference is the compulsory pre-participation screening of young athletes, which leads to early exclusion of HCM sufferers from competitive sports. Instead, diseases that are more difficult to screen, such as ARVC, have become the most common causes of SCD in North-Italian athletes (Table 65.3).[4,8]

It is interesting, however, that in spite of the apparently efficient pre-participation screening program, the overall incidence of SCD is higher in Italy than in the US. Among a number of possible explanations are differences in population background (both biological and social), sports participation (range and type of activities), reporting, and others. In addition, a high prevalence of genetic predisposition to ARVC in Italy, particularly in the Veneto region, may play a role, and this clearly warrants further investigation. Another surprising facet is the observation

that SD rates in young US athletes are apparently lower than in the age-matched general population (the data collected in the respective studies may be affected by ethnic and socioeconomic differences in the population sampled, e.g., athletes in the Minnesota area may not be representative of the general US population). Equally deserving further investigation is the fact that Italian athletes are at such a relatively high risk, compared to age-matched non-athletes, despite efficient pre-screening for HCM and other cardiovascular conditions (ARVC may

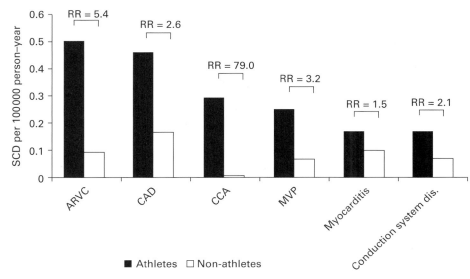

Fig. 65.3. Incidence and relative risk (RR) of sudden cardiac death (SCD) among athletes and non-athletes from: arrhythmogenic right ventricular cardiomyopathy (ARVC), coronary artery disease (CAD), congenital coronary artery anomaly (CCA), mitral valve prolapse (MVP), myocarditis and conduction system disorders. (With permission from ref. 5.)

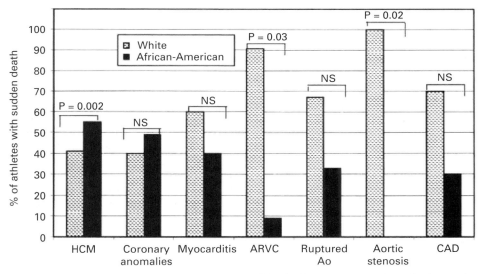

Fig. 65.4. Impact of race on cardiovascular causes of sudden death. Ao = aorta; ARVC = arrhythmogenic right ventricular cardiomyopathy; CAD = coronary artery disease; HCM hypertrophic cardiomyopathy. (With permission from ref. 16.)

present a particular exercise-induced risk that has yet to be identified).

Before speculating on any of the above differences, it is clear that currently available incidence numbers should be interpreted with care. Thus, Maron *et al.*[11] investigated the annual incidence of SD from undiagnosed cardiovascular

disease based on a longstanding insurance program for catastrophic injury or death in Minnesota. The reported incidence of SCD was 1 in 200 000 high-school athletes participating in organized sports. This estimate is based on three episodes of SCD over a 12-year period (with such small case numbers, the actual observation period

Table 65.3. Causes of sudden death in athletes and non-athletes 35 years of age or less in the Veneto region of Italy 1979–1996

Cause	Athletes (N = 49)	Non-athletes (N = 220)	Total (N = 269)
	number (percent)		
Arrhythmogenic right ventricular cardiomyopathy	11 (22.4)	18 (8.2)[a]	29 (10.8)
Atherosclerotic coronary artery disease	9 (18.4)	36 (16.4)	45 (16.7)
Anomalous origin of coronary artery	6 (12.2)	1 (0.5)[b]	7 (2.6)
Disease of conduction system	4 (8.2)	20 (9.1)	24 (8.9)
Mitral-valve prolapse	5 (10.2)	21 (9.5)	26 (9.7)
Hypertrophic cardiomyopathy	1 (2.0)	16 (7.3)	17 (6.3)
Myocarditis	3 (6.1)	19 (8.6)	22 (8.2)
Myocardial bridge	2 (4.1)	5 (2.3)	7 (2.6)
Pulmonary thromboembolism	1 (2.0)	3 (1.4)	4 (1.5)
Dissecting aortic aneurysm	1 (2.0)	11 (5.0)	12 (4.5)
Dilated cardiomyopathy	1 (2.0)	9 (4.1)	10 (3.7)
Other	5 (10.2)	61 (27.7)	66 (24.5)

[a] $P = 0.008$ for the comparison with the athletes.
[b] $P < 0.001$ for the comparison with the athletes.
With permission from ref. 8.

profoundly affects calculated incidence), and all victims were male (so that the incidence in female athletes remains unknown). Another example of how small numbers may hamper interpretation of SD incidence is the attempt to establish such risk in marathon runners.[19] Out of 215 413 runners who completed the Marine Corps Marathon over a period of 19 years (1976 to 1994) and the Twin Cities Marathon (1982 to 1994), only 4 exercise-related SD occurred. Nonetheless, all deaths were clustered in the last 9 years of observation; thus, if reported during the first 10 years (1976 to 1985) the incidence would have been 0, whereas during the last 10 years it would have almost doubled (compared to the 19 years data).

Assessment of the precise SD frequency in young athletes is further complicated because most previous studies were retrospective. This may have resulted in an underestimation of the true prevalence of sports-related SD, because such studies rely on reporting from individual schools and institutions, or media accounts.[7] Moreover,

limited or missing information on pre-participation screening, and on the number of athletes barred from competition on health grounds, influences outcome.

These limitations were largely avoided in the previously mentioned 21-year prospective cohort study of all inhabitants of Veneto, a region in northeast Italy.[4] According to Italian sports medicine guidelines, athletes aged 12 to 35 years who are participating in organized sports requiring regular training and competition *must* undergo annual screening of their medical history, a physical examination with 12-lead electrocardiogram, and limited exercise testing (as mandated by Italian law).[20] This population, for the 21 years of observation, provided 29 118 600 age-specific person-years. In all cases of SD, an autopsy was carried out (Table 65.4). After excluding non-cardiac causes of death, all hearts were fixed and forwarded to the Referral Center of Pathological Anatomy at the University of Padua for detailed morphologic assessment by a single institution. The subject's clinical history, athletic activity, and circumstances surrounding the cardiac arrest were recorded in each case.[4] The reported annual incidence of all-cause SD of 2.3 per 100 000 athletes, and of 2.1 per 100 000 athletes from cardiovascular diseases[4] will be fairly accurate for the given population, but probably should not be extrapolated to either the whole Italian population, or other countries.

Sudden non-cardiac death

Non-cardiac SD in athletes has been reported from extreme hyperthermia (heat stroke);[21] head and spine trauma (football players, pole vaulters); uncontrolled bronchial asthma;[4] ruptured cerebral artery aneurysm;[4] sickle cell trait;[22] or drug abuse.[16] The incidence of non-cardiac SD is 6% in (pre-screened) Italian athletes,[4] and exceeds 33% (198 out of 584) in the US.[16]

Sudden cardiac death involving structural abnormalities

Hypertrophic cardiomyopathy

General

HCM is a complex and relatively common genetic disorder, characterized by an asymmetrically hypertrophied, non-dilated left ventricle, with heterogeneous clinical, morphologic, and genetic expression (Fig. 65.5).[23] The prevalence of phenotypically expressed HCM in the adult general population is about 0.2% (1 in 500).[23] This excludes a probably

Table 65.4. Causes of sudden death by gender and age in athletes and non-athletes

	Total (N = 300)		Athletes (n = 55)			Non-athletes (n = 245)		
	n	Age (yrs)	Males (n = 50)	Females (n = 5)	Age (yrs)	Males (n = 70)	Females (n = 75)	Age (yrs)
Cardiovascular	259	23.8 ± 8	46	5	23.1 ± 7	150	58	23.9 ± 9
Atherosclerotic CAD	58	29.1 ± 5	10	0	28.9 ± 6	43	5	29.2 ± 5
Arrhythmogenic RV cardiomyopathy	37	25.2 ± 7	12	0	22.6 ± 4	17	8	26.9 ± 7
Myocarditis	32	22.3 ± 7	5	0	22.5 ± 7	21	6	22.1 ± 7
Mitral valve prolapse	27	22.7 ± 6	4	2	23.0 ± 3	8	13	22.4 ± 6
Disease of the conduction system	25	21.5 ± 9	3	1	21.2 ± 5	17	4	21.6 ± 5
Hypertrophic cardiomyopathy	23	22.3 ± 7	1	0	15	18	4	22.3 ± 7
Aortic rupture	12	21.2 ± 8	1	0	21	8	3	21.3 ± 9
Dilated cardiomyopathy	11	22.1 ± 7	1	0	14	7	3	22.0 ± 7
Anomalous origin of CAD	8	20.2 ± 6	6	1	21.5 ± 9	0	1	13
Non-atherosclerotic CAD	7	21.4 ± 8	0	0	—	2	5	21.4 ± 8
Myocardial bridge	6	21.7 ± 9	2	0	23.5 ± 4	2	2	20.9 ± 8
Aortic valve stenosis	4	20.7 ± 3	0	0	—	4	0	20.7 ± 3
Postoperative CHD	4	13.2 ± 5	0	0	—	2	2	13.2 ± 5
Pulmonary thromboembolism	4	23.4 ± 2	1	0	24	1	2	23.0 ± 1
Long QT syndrome	1	20	0	1	20	0	0	—
Non-cardiovascular	23	24.1 ± 8	3	0	25.2 ± 6	9	11	22.9 ± 7
Asthma	10	23.2 ± 7	0	0	—	6	4	23.2 ± 3
Cerebral berry aneurysm	6	27.8 ± 8	1	0	28	1	4	27.6 ± 4
Cerebral embolism	5	22.2 ± 6	2	0	23.5 ± 4	1	2	21.3 ± 6
Other	2	24.5 ± 6	0	0	—	1	1	24.5 ± 6
Unexplained	18	23.2 ± 8	1	0	28	11	6	22.9 ± 8

Data are presented as the number of subjects and mean value ± standard deviation.

CAD = coronary artery disease; CHD = congenital heart disease; RV = right ventricular.

With permission from ref. 4.

substantial proportion of individuals harboring a mutant gene for HCM without clinical symptoms.

HCM is a unique cardiovascular disease with the potential for clinical presentation during any phase of life, from infancy to old age. The clinical course is typically variable and may cause disability or death; indeed, patients may remain stable over long periods of time, with up to 25% of HCM sufferers achieving normal longevity (Fig. 65.6).[25] Nevertheless, HCM is also a prominent cause of SCD in the young, including athletes.[7,26] SCD may actually be the first disease presentation in asymptomatic or mildly symptomatic young people.[7,26,27] Death may occur during mild exertion or sedentary activity including sleep, but it is not infrequently triggered by vigorous physical exertion.[7] Indeed, in the US population, HCM is the most common cause of SCD in young people and competitive athletes (Fig. 65.7).[7]

Although the usual diagnostic criterion for HCM is a maximal left ventricular (LV) wall thickness ≥ 15 mm, genotype-phenotype correlations have shown that virtually any wall thickness, including values within the normal range, may be associated with presence of an HCM mutant gene.[17] Not all individuals harboring a genetic defect express clinical symptoms, such as abnormal electrocardiogram (ECG) and echocardiography, or impaired cardiac function.[17,30] Most commonly, substantial LV remodeling with spontaneous appearance of hypertrophy occurs with accelerated body growth during adolescence, and morphologic expression is usually complete at physical maturity.[31] In trained athletes, modest segmental wall thickening (13–15 mm) requires differential diagnosis between extreme manifestations of physiologically based "athlete's heart"[32,33] and mild morphologic expressions of HCM,[33] which can usually be conducted non-invasively.[32]

A distinctive clinical observation in some patients with obstructive HCM is the dynamic pressure gradient in the subaortic area that divides the left ventricle into high-pressure (apical) and a low-pressure (subaortic) regions (Fig. 65.8).[34] This form of dynamic subaortic obstruction is typically produced by mitral valve systolic anterior

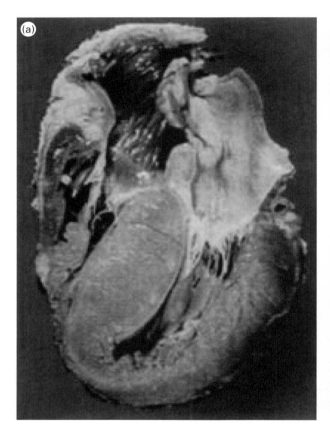
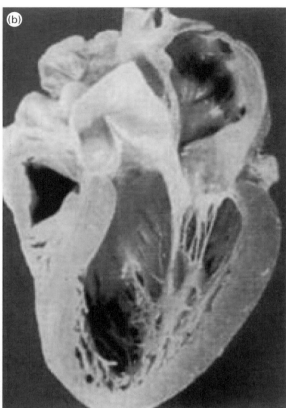

Fig. 65.5. Gross pathological specimens of the cardiomyopathies. (a) Hypertrophic cardiomyopathy, showing a marked increase in myocardial mass and preferential hypertrophy of the interventricular septum. (b) Normal heart, with normal left ventricular dimensions and thickness. (With permission from ref. 24.)

motion and septal contact[35,36] caused by drag effect[36] or possible Venturi phenomenon[35] and is responsible for a loud systolic murmur. Even if this feature attracted much attention, HCM is predominantly expressed as the non-obstructive phenotype (75% of patients show no sizable resting outflow tract gradient).[30,37]

In cases where a subaortic gradient is present, it is now generally accepted that values of ≥30 mm Hg, and associated elevation in LV pressure, reflect a true mechanical impairment to outflow, and are of pathophysiologic and prognostic importance for HCM patients.[28,39] Indeed, outflow obstruction is a strong, independent predictor of disease progression to HCM-related death (relative risk vs. non-obstructed patients: 2.0).[39] Treadmill or bicycle exercise testing in association with Doppler echocardiography has been proposed as the most physiologic and preferred provocative maneuver to identify latent gradients during and/or immediately following exercise for the purpose of major management decisions, given that HCM-related symptoms are typically elicited with exertion.[40]

Genetics

HCM is an inherited, autosomal dominant trait and is caused by a mutation in any of the more than 10 identified genes encoding for components of thick or thin filaments with contractile, structural or regulatory functions (Fig. 65.9).[17] The close functional association of these proteins has resulted in consideration of diverse HCM spectra as a single disease entity and primary sarcomere disorder. Although DNA analysis for mutant genes is the most definitive method for diagnosing HCM, it is not yet a routine clinical strategy.[17] The substantial genetic heterogeneity, low frequency of individual mutations in the general HCM population, and methodological difficulties associated with identifying single mutations, have all hindered the

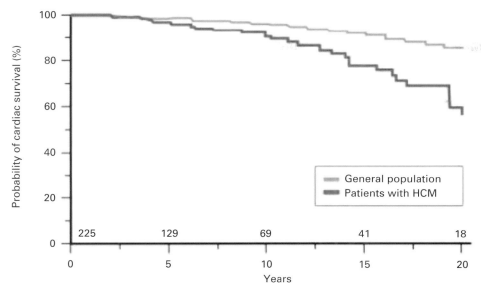

Fig. 65.6. Kaplan–Meier survival curve of 225 community-based patients with hypertrophic cardiomyopathy (HCM) and age-matched control subjects. The numbers above the horizontal axis refer to the number of patients at each follow-up period. The annual total mortality rate of the patients with HCM was 1.3%. (With permission from ref. 28.)

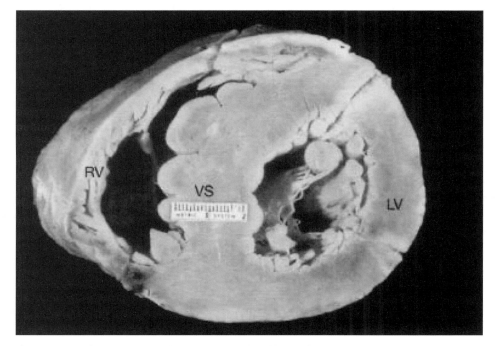

Fig. 65.7. Gross heart specimen of a 13-year-old male athlete with hypertrophic cardiomyopathy, presenting a disproportionate thickening of the interventricular septum (VS) compared with the left ventricular (LV) free wall. RV = right ventricular free wall. (With permission from ref. 29.)

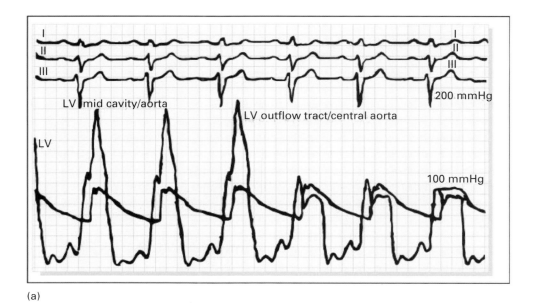

(a)

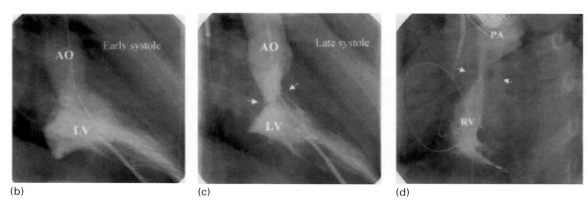

(b)   (c)   (d)

Fig. 65.8. Hemodynamic and angiographic findings in hypertrophic cardiomyopathy with biventricular involvement. (a) Simultaneous pressure recordings from the mid left ventricular (LV) cavity and aorta show a 100 mmHg gradient. The aortic tracing shows a "spike-and-dome" pattern related to systolic anterior movement of the anterior leaflet of the mitral valve. The subaortic location of the gradient is confirmed as the LV catheter is pulled back from the midcavity (left) to the subaortic outflow tract (right). (b) and (c) Left ventriculogram in the right anterior oblique projection. Arrows show systolic anterior mitral valve movement in late systole with attendant obstruction of the outflow tract. (d) Right ventriculogram in the left lateral projection showing massive hypertrophy of the right ventricular (RV) outflow area (arrows) with an "hourglass" configuration. AO = aorta; PA = pulmonary artery. (With permission from ref. 38.)

translation of genetic research into practical applications and routine clinical strategy, leaving mutation analysis confined to a few research-oriented laboratories.[40]

HCM may be initially suspected because of heart murmur,[7] positive family history, and new symptoms, or abnormal ECG patterns,[8] for example during sports pre-participation examinations.[8] Definite clinical diagnosis of HCM is best established with 2-dimensional echocardiography,[17,23,26] imaging the hypertrophied but non-dilated LV chamber in the absence of another cardiac or systemic disease capable of producing the observed magnitude of hypertrophy (Fig. 65.10).[41]

Pathogenesis

Microscopic findings in HCM are distinctive, showing disorganized LV myocardial architecture, comprising hypertrophied myocytes with irregular shapes and multiple intercellular connections, often arranged in a chaotic order

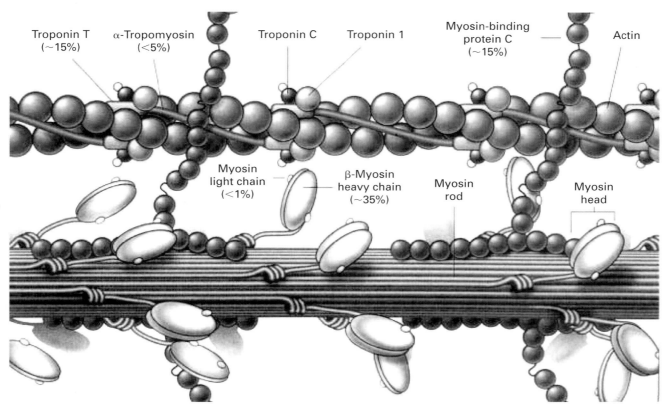

Fig. 65.9. Drawing showing components of the sarcomere and mutations in hypertrophic cardiomyopathy. Mutations may impair protein interactions resulting in ineffectual contraction and thereby producing hypertrophy. Percentages represent the estimated frequency with which a mutation causes hypertrophic cardiomyopathy. (With permission from ref. 37.)

or aligned at oblique and perpendicular angles, culminating in an irregular pattern (Fig. 65.11).[42] Such cellular disarray may be widely distributed and appears to be most extensive in young victims of the disease (Fig. 65.12(a)).[42] Abnormal intramural coronary arteries, characterized by thickened walls with increased intimal and medial collagen and narrowed lumen, may be regarded as a form of small vessel disease (Fig. 65.12(b)).[43] Such architectural alterations of the microvasculature and the expanded interstitial collagen compartment,[44] as well as mismatch between myocardial mass and coronary circulation are probably responsible for impaired coronary vasculature reserve[45] and bursts of myocardial ischemia,[45] leading to myocyte death and tissue remodelling in the form of patchy or transmural replacement scarring.[46]

Disorganized cellular architecture,[42] myocardial scarring,[46] and expanded matrix[44] probably serve as arrhythmogenic substrates, predisposing to life-threatening electrical instability. This substrate may give rise to primary ventricular tachycardia (VT) and ventricular fib-

rillation (VF), which appear to be the predominant mechanisms of SD.[27]

Life-threatening tachyarrhythmias can be provoked in HCM by a number of variables, either secondary to environmental factors, such as intense physical exertion, or alternatively intrinsic to the disease process. Physical exertion, in particular, can trigger a vicious cycle of increasing myocardial ischemia[45] and diastolic dysfunction,[47] possibly affected by outflow obstruction,[39] systemic arterial hypotension,[48] or supraventricular tachyarrhythmias[49] that lead to a decrease in stroke volume and coronary perfusion.

Moreover, HCM is not infrequently associated with cardiovascular congenital abnormalities which may contribute to, or account *per se* for, SCD. As documented by the Minneapolis Heart Institute Foundation registry, out of 102 athletes who died suddenly with documented HCM, 9 had associated abnormalities that may have contributed to death, including tunneled (bridged) left anterior descending coronary artery ($n = 7$) and coronary artery hypoplasia ($n = 2$).[16]

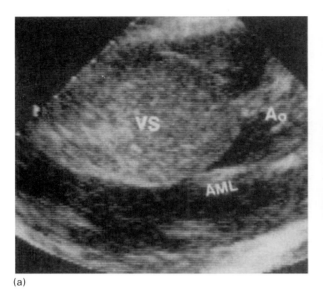
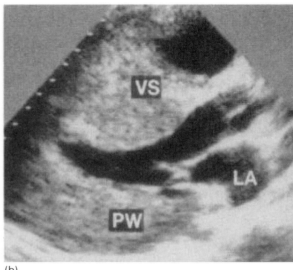

(a)   (b)

Fig. 65.10. Heterogeneity in the pattern and extent of left ventricular wall thickening in hypertrophic cardiomyopathy as shown by echocardiography (long-axis views). (a) Massive hypertrophy of the ventricular septum (VS) with wall thickness greater than 50 mm. (b) Distal VS thickening greater than proximal VS. Ao = aorta; AML = anterior mitral leaflet; LA = left atrium; PW = posterior wall. (With permission from ref. 41.)

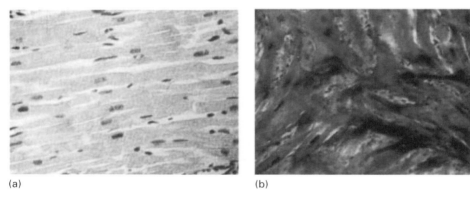

(a)   (b)

Fig. 65.11. Histopathology of hypertrophic and dilated cardiomyopathy. (a) The normal architecture of healthy myocardium shows orderly alignment of myocytes with minimal interstitial fibrosis. (b) Hypertrophic cardiomyopathy, demonstrating marked enlargement and disarray of myocytes (red) with increased interstitial fibrosis (blue). Stains: A, hematoxylin and eosin; B, Masson trichrome. (With permission from ref. 24.)

Risk stratification

The highest risk for SCD has been associated with the following conditions: (1) prior cardiac arrest or spontaneously occurring and sustained VT;[50] (2) family history of premature HCM-related SD;[30] (3) identification of a high-risk mutant gene;[17] (4) unexplained syncope, particularly in young patients or when exertional or recurrent;[37] (5) nonsustained VT (of 3 beats or more and of at least 120 beats/min) evident on ambulatory (Holter) ECG recordings;[51] (6) abnormal blood pressure response during upright exercise which is attenuated or hypotensive, in patients less than 50 years old;[37,38] and (7) extreme LV hypertrophy with maximum wall thickness of 30 mm or more, particularly in adolescents and young adults.[26] The last mentioned risk factor derives from a continuous, direct relationship between maximum LV wall thickness and SD, which supports the magnitude of LV wall thickness as a determinant of the risk of SCD.[26] Impaired consciousness,

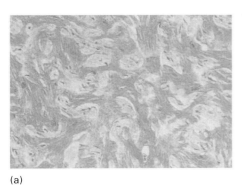 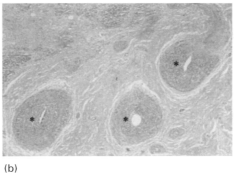

(a) (b)

Fig. 65.12. Histological specimen of hypertrophic cardiomyopathy in a 13-year-old showing (a) marked cellular disarray with hypertrophied cells arranged in a chaotic pattern; (b) several abnormal intramural coronary arteries, with markedly thickened walls and narrowed lumina. Hematoxylin and eosin stain; original magnifications ×50. (With permission from ref. 29.)

such as syncope or near-syncope, is a most striking clinical risk indicator and should never be underestimated.[28]

Finally, variability between ECG leads in measurements of QTc (QTc dispersion) is thought to reflect regional variations in myocardial recovery and excitability.[52] Subjects with HCM have greater QTc dispersion than control subjects,[53] and patients with ventricular arrhythmias have significantly larger QTc dispersion than patients without arrhythmias.[54] Increased QTc dispersion is therefore believed to be an important risk factor for SCD.[53]

Prevention and treatment

Intense physical exertion constitutes a SD trigger in susceptible individuals.[7] Therefore, to reduce risk, disqualification from most competitive sports has been recommended by a number of consensus statements for athletes with unequivocal evidence of HCM.[55,56]

In HCM, treatment strategies to reduce risk for SD have historically relied on drugs such as β-blockers, verapamil, and antiarrhythmic agents (procainamide and amiodarone).[51,57] Nevertheless, there is little evidence[57] that prophylactic pharmacological strategies reduce SD risk. Furthermore, because of its potential toxicity, amiodarone is unlikely to be tolerated throughout the long risk periods of young HCM patients. At present, implantable cardioverter-defibrillators (ICD) appear to be the most effective intervention for high-risk HCM patients.[27] In one multicenter retrospective study, ICD appropriately sensed and automatically aborted potentially lethal ventricular tachyarrhythmias by restoring sinus rhythm in almost 25% of a high-risk cohort, followed for a relatively brief period of 3 years.[27] This is in line with ACC/AHA/NASPE 2002 guidelines that recommend ICD

for primary SCD prevention (class IIb indication), and for secondary prevention after one cardiac arrest (class I indication).[58]

For adults and children with obstructive HCM and severe drug–refractory symptoms, ventricular septal myotomy–myectomy (Morrow procedure) has become an established operation, on the basis of the experience acquired throughout the past 40 years, and is regarded as the standard therapeutic option.[30,37,59] Nevertheless, only a small, though significant, proportion (5%) of the overall HCM population is truly eligible for the procedure.[37]

Arrhythmogenic right-ventricular cardiomyopathy

General

ARVC is a primary myocardial disease, characterized by adipose or fibro-adipose substitution of right ventricular (RV) myocardium. Originally considered a cause of RV failure,[60] ARVC was more recently found to be responsible for severe ventricular arrhythmias in adults[61] and SCD in young persons and athletes (Fig. 65.13(a)).[62] Although initially considered to be strictly confined to the RV, there is growing clinical evidence that, over time, the LV shares RV cardiomyopathic changes;[63] hence the definition of the World Health Organization of a disease "characterized by progressive fibrofatty replacement of RV myocardium, initially with typical regional and later global RV and some LV involvement" (Fig. 65.13).[64]

ARVC is associated with a high incidence of ventricular arrhythmias, including polymorphic non-sustained VT and VF, as well as recurrent sustained VT.[66] In a large proportion of victims (up to 80%), the first manifestation of the disease is "unexplained" syncope or SCD.[67]

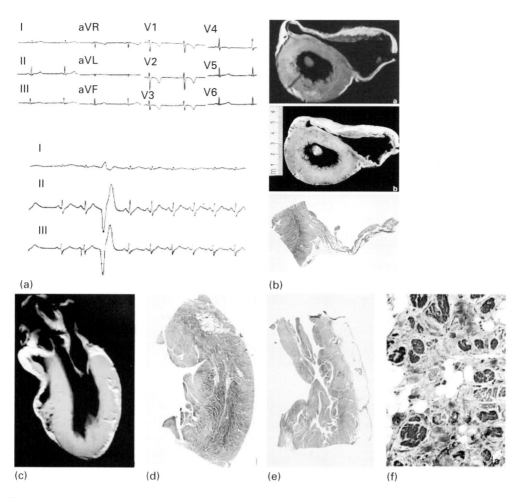

Fig. 65.13. (a) An asymptomatic 17-year-old boy died suddenly during a soccer game. Retrospectively, the only signs of the disease were basal ECG T-wave inversion in right precordial leads up to V4 and an isolated premature ventricular beat of left bundle-branch block morphology during step test. (b) same case, in vitro NMR cross-sectional view showing a uniformly whitish right ventricular free wall with anterior and inferior aneurysms (note a spotty involvement of the posterolateral wall of the left ventricle); also, corresponding cross section of the heart specimen with infundibular and inferior subtricuspidal aneurysms, and panoramic histological view of the inferior aneurysm showing wall thinning with fibrofatty replacement. (c) in vitro NMR scan in the long-axis view showing extensive involvement of the anterior free wall of the right ventricle and patchy involvement of the posterior wall of the left ventricle; the interventricular septum is spared. (d) corresponding panoramic histological view of the left ventricle showing a spot of fibrofatty replacement of the myocardium. (e) control heart from a 20-year-old man who died in a motor vehicle accident. Panoramic histological view of the lateral free wall of the right ventricle: the fatty tissue is limited to the subepicardium and only slightly infiltrates the myocardium. (f) Myocardial atrophy with fibrous and fatty tissue replacement (Azan stains; original magnification B, D, and E ×2.5, F ×240; (With permission from ref. 65.)

The clinical diagnosis is formulated in patients with ventricular arrhythmias with a left bundle branch configuration,[68] abnormal T wave inversion and epsilon waves in the right precordial leads,[69] increased ventricular volume, localized or diffuse trabecular disarrangement with fibrous or fibrofatty replacement of myocardial tissue on endomyocardial biopsy,[70] and dynamic abnormalities of the RV free wall.[71] The characteristic progressive loss of myocardium coincides with the onset of cardiac electrical instability. Clinicopathological data suggest a wide age range, spanning adolescence to adulthood, during which the disease may become symptomatic and fatal.[65,72] ARVC is diagnosed in 90% of cases after the age of 20 (usually before reaching 50 years), probably because it is concealed during earlier life.[72] Several disease stages have been identified, from an early clinically silent phase with or without minor arrhythmias and with myopathic abnormalities localized only to the RV, during which SD may be the first manifestation of the disease;[62] to an "overt electrical instability" with severe arrhythmias and impending cardiac arrest, characterized by segmental or global RV structural changes;[73] finally followed by "pump failure" characterized by biventricular cardiomyopathy mimicking dilated cardiomyopathy (DCM) with cardiomegaly, congestive heart failure requiring transplantation, and the risk of thromboembolic complications.[74]

It has been proposed that in some young people a sudden change from the subclinical to a clinical stage may produce life-threatening arrhythmias as the first symptom, suggesting that the juvenile form of ARVC is not benign.[75] The experience of SD as first clinical manifestation of ARVC in young people and athletes is in accordance with this hypothesis. In the adult, the disease probably reaches a stable phase in which abrupt changes in electrical instability are less common.

A history of cardiac arrest or VT with hemodynamic compromise, young age, and LV involvement have all been identified as independent predictors of VF.[76] SCD is often exercise-related, and in regions of the world where screening for HCM has excluded the affected athletes from competition, ARVC has emerged as the most common cause of sports-related SCD.[8]

In patients with ARVC, VF has been associated with active phases of myocyte death occurring in younger affected patients with progressive disease, whereas hemodynamically well-tolerated monomorphic VT is caused by a re-entry mechanism around a stable myocardial scar as the result of healing and remodeling processes that occur at a later stage of the disease course.[72] This view is reinforced by the finding that younger age is an independent risk factor for VF.[67]

Macroscopic or histologic LV involvement, or both, can be found in 76% of the hearts analyzed, thus confirming that ARVC affects the LV in the majority of cases. LV changes usually affect both the septum and LV free wall, either diffusely or, more often, regionally (Fig. 65.13(b) and (d)).[67] However, patients with isolated RV changes are younger and more often die suddenly without having experienced warning symptoms compared to patients with coexistent LV abnormalities.[67]

Genetics

A genetic basis for ARVC is being explored. A large proportion of cases, up to an estimated 30%–50% appear to have a familial distribution.[67,77] The inheritance pattern is autosomal dominant, except for the geographically clustered *Naxos* disease (chromosome 17).[77] Autosomal dominant ARVC has been mapped to eight chromosomal loci on three putative genes. These genes link ARVC to mutations in the *RYR2*-gene[78] which encodes the sarcoplasmic calcium release channel (aka Ryanodine Receptor [RyR]; the same gene is also implicated in familial catecholaminergic polymorphic ventricular tachycardia [CPVT]), and the *DSP* and *JUP*-genes which encode for the cell adhesion proteins desmoplakin and plakoglobin, respectively.[79]

Risk, prevention and treatment

During the concealed phase, affected young persons involved in sports activities are particularly vulnerable to electrical instability with risk of cardiac arrest; early recognition is thus a medical challenge, and exclusion from all sports is mandatory.[65,67]

A large observational study that addressed the clinical impact of ICD therapy on the natural history of patients with ARVC treated for prevention of SD[76] demonstrated that a history of either cardiac arrest or VT with hemodynamic compromise, young age, and LV involvement are independent predictors of potentially lethal ventricular arrhythmias and can help in identifying those ARVC patients who would benefit most from ICD implantation. The major finding was that nearly half the patients ($n = 64$) had at least one episode of ventricular tachyarrhythmia that required ICD intervention despite antiarrhythmic drug therapy over a mean follow-up period of 3.3 years, and 24% experienced VF that, in all likelihood, would have been fatal without termination by the device (Fig 65.14). This high incidence of ICD interventions is in agreement with data from smaller series of patients with ARVC previously reported.[80] Moreover, the majority of appropriate ICD interventions occurred despite concomitant therapy with sotalol, amiodarone, or β-blockers (alone or in combination).[76]

Coronary artery abnormalities

A variety of congenital coronary artery anomalies represent common causes of exercise-related SD in young athletes.[4,8] Corrado *et al.*[4] report 9 out of 55 SD in athletes

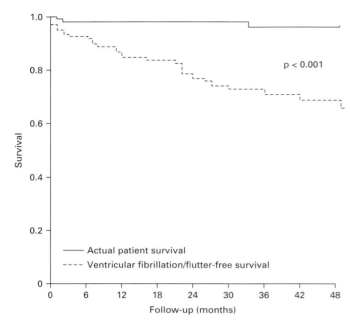

Fig. 65.14. Kaplan–Meier analysis of actual survival of ICD-implanted patients, compared with the predicted survival in the same population if no ICD interventions had occurred (assuming that ventricular fibrillation/flutter would, if untreated, have been lethal). Divergence between lines reflects estimated survival benefit of ICD therapy. (With permission from ref. 76.)

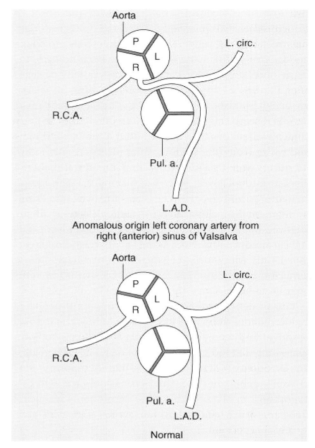

Fig. 65.15. Congenital coronary artery anomaly of wrong aortic sinus origin, which may cause SD in young athletes. **Top,** Anomalous origin of the left main coronary artery arising from right (anterior) sinus of *Valsalva*. Note acute leftward bend of left main coronary artery at its origin and its posterior course between aorta and pulmonary artery trunk (Pul. a.). **Bottom,** Normal coronary artery anatomy is shown for comparison. L.A.D. = left anterior descending; L. circ. = left circumflex; L = left sinus; R = right sinus; P = posterior sinus; R.C.A. = right coronary artery. (With permission from ref. 6.)

to be secondary to coronary abnormalities, with 7 due to wrong coronary sinus origin, and the remaining related to myocardial bridging. The mechanism of SD is believed to be episodic myocardial ischemia.[81,82] Diagnosis represents a serious challenge, but is particularly important as surgical correction is feasible.[83] The possibility of a coronary anomaly should always be considered in a young athlete with a history of chest pain or syncope, particularly if the episodes are triggered by exercise.[84] Transthoracic or transesophageal echocardiography and magnetic resonance imaging can be used to diagnose the anomaly,[83] and diagnostic coronary arteriography can ultimately be performed. Patients usually do *not* have abnormalities on 12-lead or even exercise electrocardiograms,[83,85] because the myocardial ischemia is episodic, thereby limiting the value of random screening.

Acquired coronary abnormalities, particularly premature CAD, account for another major substrate for unexpected death in athletes, despite implementation of pre-participation screening programs.[4,8]

Wrong coronary sinus origin

General

Anomalous origin of coronary arteries is a rare congenital disease, found in approximately 0.6% to 1% of all coronary angiograms, and in 0.3% of all autopsies (Fig. 65.15).[86,87] Although an anomalous origin of coronary arteries may have a completely benign and asymptomatic course, it can be a cause for SD in the young, more commonly in competitive athletes than in non-athletes.[4,8]

Risk

Recognized as an important cardiovascular cause of SD on the athletic field (Tables 65.3 and 65.4),[4,8,83] these anomalies may be more common than previously thought.[85]

Left main coronary artery origin from the right aortic sinus of *Valsalva* represents the most serious anomaly, associated with the highest incidence of symptoms and SD.[87] As reported by Taylor *et al.*,[87] in 242 patients with isolated coronary artery anomalies, SD and exercise-related death were most common with origin of the left main coronary artery from the right coronary sinus (57% and 64% of cases, respectively). Anomalous origin of the right coronary artery from the left coronary sinus was also commonly associated with exercise-related SD (46% of cases). High-risk anatomy further involved abnormalities of the initial coronary artery segment, or the coursing of the anomalous artery between the pulmonary artery and aorta. Younger patients (≤30 years old) were significantly more likely to die suddenly than were older patients (62% vs. 12% overall; 40% vs. 2% during exercise).[87] Although the type of malformation may affect life expectancy, this may be less relevant in the elderly as large vessel stiffening may afford some degree of protection, in particular for coronary vessels routed "between" cardiac outflow branches.

Diagnosis

Coronary origin anomalies are rarely suspected and usually first recognized at autopsy, largely because they are not recognized during routine or pre-participation screening, as the affected subjects are often asymptomatic (Fig. 65.16).[8,88]

The available clinical data suggest that myocardial ischemia in young athletes with aortic sinus coronary artery anomalies probably occurs in infrequent bursts, which may be cumulative with time. This view is supported by normal ECG patterns in patients who had *postmortem* pathologic evidence of acute myocardial ischemic damage and/or chronic ischemic injury with replacement-type fibrosis.[83] Thus, repetitive ischemic episodes may result in patchy myocardial necrosis and fibrosis, which could predispose to lethal ventricular tachyarrhythmias by creating an electrically unstable myocardial substrate with increased structural and functional tissue heterogeneity. Considering that trained athletes perform intense physical exercise many times before any fatal event, it is most likely that critical impairment of coronary flow to the myocardium occurs only sporadically.

Pathogenesis

Although the exact pathophysiology of this decreased blood flow is not fully understood, several potential mechanisms have been proposed to explain exercise-related myocardial ischemia and SD in patients with wrong sinus coronary anomalies: the acute take-off angle and kinking or torsion of the coronary artery as it arises from the aorta and passes between the great vessels (Fig. 65.16(b));[89]

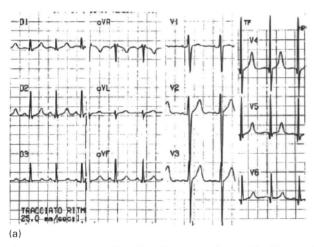
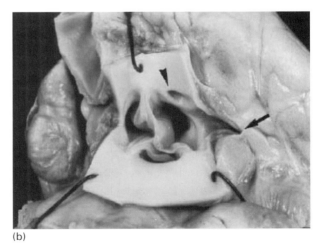

(a)   (b)

Fig. 65.16. A 15-year-old male Italian soccer player with a history of exertional syncope 1 year before death, who died suddenly while running during the second half of a game. (a) A 12-lead ECG performed 10 months before death, as part of routine pre-participation screening, is within normal limits. (b) View of the aortic root; the right coronary artery arises normally from the right aortic sinus (arrow), and the left main coronary artery arises anomalously from the right sinus with an acute angle take-off producing a slit-like lumen (arrowhead). (With permission from ref. 83.)

flap-like closure of the abnormal slit-like coronary orifice;[90] compression of the anomalous coronary artery between the aorta and pulmonary trunk (Fig. 65.15),[87] especially during exercise-induced distention of the sinus of *Valsalva*;[91] and spasm of the anomalous coronary artery, possibly as a result of endothelial injury.[92] The consequent myocardial ischemia, exacerbated by increased myocardial oxygen requirements during exertion, in particular in the presence of tissue heterogeneity caused by previous incidents, may trigger and sustain life-threatening ventricular arrhythmias and SD.[86]

Moreover, in some patients the proximal portion of the anomalous coronary artery is essentially intramural (i.e., within the aortic tunica media), which can further aggravate the coronary obstruction, particularly with expansion of the aorta during exercise.[83]

Prevention

A strategy for clinical identification of wrong sinus coronary artery anomalies in young athletes has been proposed.[83] If the index of suspicion is sufficiently high because of the presence of potential clinical markers such as exertional syncope or chest pain, even in the setting of both a normal 12-lead ECG and maximal exercise test, the anatomy of these malformations should be defined non-invasively by transthoracic or transesophageal echocardiography. Pelliccia *et al.*[93] demonstrated that echocardiographic imaging of left and right coronary arteries is feasible and reliable in a substantial proportion of young athletes (~95%). Consistently, identification of coronary artery origins should be generally included as part of any routine echocardiographic examination.[85] Further anatomic definition, if warranted, may be obtained by coronary angiography or possibly with magnetic resonance imaging[94] or computed tomography.[95]

Myocardial bridging

General

Myocardial bridging (MB) occurs when a band of cardiac muscle overlies a segment of a coronary artery, the 'intramural' segment being referred to as a "tunneled artery." Usually, the coronary vessels course over the epicardial surface of the heart but may dip into the myocardium for varying lengths and then reappear on the heart's surface.[82] The left anterior descending coronary artery is by far the most often bridged vessel; however, diagonal branches are occasionally involved, as well as the posterior descending right coronary artery or marginal branches of the circumflex artery (Fig. 65.17).[82]

Risk

Systolic compression of the left anterior descending coronary artery is a well-recognized angiographic phenomenon.[96] There is, however, a wide discrepancy in pathological data on MB incidence, ranging from 15% to 85% of the population,[97,98] and angiographic observations, from 0.5% to 2.5%.[96,99] This large discordance suggests that only a minor fraction of patients with MB are at risk for clinical symptoms. Moreover, among patients with angiographically documented systolic narrowing of a coronary artery, a substantial percentage (~50%) have

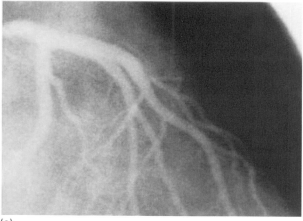
(a)

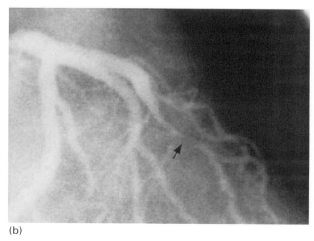
(b)

Fig. 65.17. Coronary angiogram of a patient with myocardial bridging of the left anterior descending coronary artery in the right anterior oblique position. (a) An absence of constriction during diastole is shown. (b) This depicts the redistribution of blood during systole, also referred to as "milking effect" (arrow). (With permission from ref. 82.)

concomitant LV hypertrophy, HCM, atherosclerotic, or valvular heart disease, which independently affect clinical outcome as well as treatment strategy.[100] Finally, among patients with isolated MB documented at angiography, only about two-thirds exhibit a >50% narrowing of the vessel during systole.[100]

Pathogenesis

The progressive increase in LV wall tension, with maturation may explain, at least in part, why MB – even if present from birth – produces symptoms only later in life.[100] Typically, patients are predominantly male, 5 to 10 years younger than patients with symptomatic coronary disease, and they tend to have severe anginal symptoms.[82] When symptom-limited exercise electrocardiograms are performed, a significant ischemic ST segment depression is identified in 28% to 67% of patients.[82] Consequently, such anomalies may have important clinical implications during intense athletic activity (Fig. 65.18).[82] Indeed, tunneled coronary arteries are occasionally the sole abnormality found at autopsy and are within the most frequent 10 abnormalities responsible for SCD in athletes.[7,18]

MB has been associated with other concomitant cardiovascular abnormalities, in particular HCM.[100] In both conditions, myocardial ischemia has been recognized as the predominant arrhythmogenic substrate.[101] MB with compression of an epicardial coronary artery[96] occurs in 30% to 50% of adults who have HCM.[102]

Until recently, visual interpretation of coronary angiograms only revealed systolic narrowing if induced by significant MB of a coronary artery. Coronary flow, however, occurs predominantly during diastole; therefore, it appeared unlikely that this systolic phenomenon would itself cause pronounced myocardial ischemia.

With the advent of quantitative coronary angiography, intravascular ultrasonography, and intracoronary Doppler flow velocity measurements, it has become possible to identify diastolic hemodynamic disturbances in MB patients.[103] There is mounting evidence for a diastolic time-lag during which the previously compressed coronary vessel remains underfilled (30% to 75% of diastole).[81] This prolongation of compression well into diastole is likely to compromise myocardial perfusion, and will have a greater effect in young adults and children, especially during exercise, because their heart rates are faster and diastolic perfusion times are shorter.[81]

Two mechanisms are regarded as responsible for the reduced coronary flow reserve in distal vessels and for

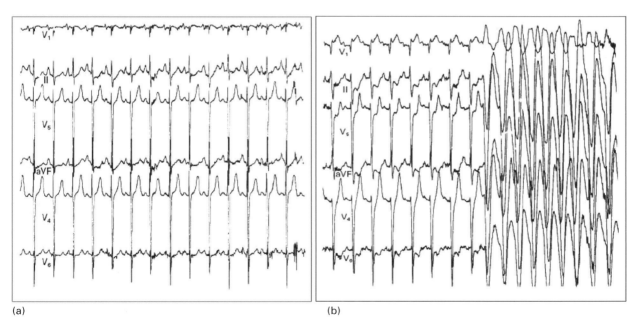

(a) (b)

Fig. 65.18. Electrocardiogram obtained during exercise testing in a patient with myocardial bridging and induced myocardial ischemia and ventricular arrhythmia. After 9 minutes of a treadmill exercise test, ST segments were normal (Panel (a)) and the patient's heart rate was 131 beats per minute. After 9 minutes and 36 seconds, the patient's heart rate was 141 beats per minute and the electrocardiogram showed acute elevation of the ST segment in lead V1 and depression of the ST segment in leads II, aVF, V5, and V6, followed by rapid ventricular tachycardia and ventricular fibrillation (Panel (b)). (With permission from ref. 81.)

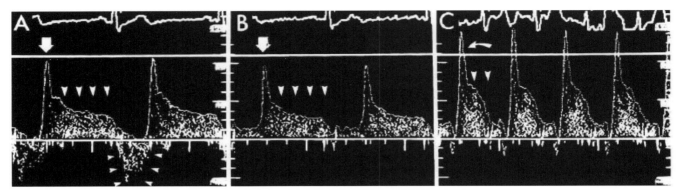

Fig. 65.19. Intracoronary Doppler blood flow velocity profile showing the characteristic "finger-tip"-like flow velocity acceleration during early diastole (single arrow) followed by a plateau phase at mid-to-late diastole (arrows in (a) and (b)). During systole, there is almost no flow within the bridged segment, but a retrograde flow phenomenon occurs at the entry site of the myocardial bridge (horizontal arrows in (a)). During rapid atrial pacing, absolute diastolic flow velocities are increased, and the duration of the plateau phase is reduced owing to shortened diastole (c). (With permission from ref. 104.)

clinical symptoms and signs of myocardial ischemia: (1) a phasic systolic vessel compression with persistent mid-to-late reduction in diameter in diastole and (2) increased intracoronary Doppler flow velocities with abnormal qualitative flow profiles. Qualitative analysis of the Doppler flow profile shows a highly characteristic pattern in approximately 90% of MB patients, with abrupt early diastolic flow acceleration, termed "finger tip" phenomenon (Fig. 65.19).

As an alternative or additional mechanism, vasospastic coronary constriction may be associated with MB.[105] The systolic compression of the vessel may produce endothelial damage, especially at high heart rates, which may stimulate platelet aggregation and enhance coronary vasospasm. These alterations, particularly in association with aggravating factors such as increased heart rate, pressure, and pre-existing coronary vasospasm, may explain the occurrence of symptoms and myocardial ischemia in patients with symptomatic MB.[82]

Myocardial damage resulting from chronic ischemia may cause diffuse fibrosis and increasing disarray of myocardial fibers, which may secondarily create an arrhythmogenic substrate. Yetman *et al.*[81] documented a higher incidence of VT on Holter ambulatory monitoring in MB patients. In addition, ischemic ST segment changes that culminate in VT have been observed in at least one patient with MB (Fig. 65.18). Finally, a greater degree of QTc dispersion is present in patients with MB.[81] These patients have a larger incidence of ischemia, which may lead to an arrhythmogenic substrate in association with abnormal and variable repolarization.

Treatment

Three different treatment strategies are available medical therapy, percutaneous coronary intervention, and direct surgical myotomy or coronary bypass grafting. Medical therapy is the first and principal strategy.[82] It usually includes β-blockers, calcium channel blockers, and antiplatelet agents, with the objective of relieving symptoms and signs of myocardial ischemia and/or protecting against the risk of future coronary events.

Stables *et al.*[106] demonstrated that intracoronary stent implantation can achieve internal stabilization of the coronary artery lumen against external compression by MB. Prior to the availability of coronary stenting, surgical myotomy was regarded as the surgical treatment of choice for patients with persistent symptoms.[82] Alternatively, internal mammary artery anastomosis to the distal vessel segment may be a suitable treatment in patients with unsuccessful coronary stenting or in-stent restenosis.[107]

Atherosclerotic coronary artery disease

General

Several pathological studies have demonstrated that coronary atherosclerotic disease, complicated by thrombosis, is the most common morphological substrate of acute coronary events and SD in adults of the general population.[108,109] In line with this finding, atherosclerotic CAD is the most common cause of SD in athletes >35 years of age.[110,111] In younger subjects, even after stringent pre-participation screening, coronary atherosclerosis is the second most common cause of SCD, accounting for 18% of SD in the athletic population (Table 65.3).[8]

SD due to premature CAD occurs predominantly in the older segment of under 35-year-old athletes, and in non-athletes (29.1 ± 5 years; Table 65.4).[4] Premature CAD is associated with a high risk of sports-related SD (relative risk 2.6; Fig. 65.3).[4]

Pathogenesis

Few studies have addressed the pathological lesions of coronary atherosclerosis and pathophysiological mechanisms of fatal myocardial ischemia in young people.[13] Single-vessel obstructive CAD, mostly affecting the proximal left anterior descending coronary artery, is most commonly observed in young adults and athletes (Fig. 65.20).[4,13] This finding probably reflects early development of CAD, which only later in life will progress and become a more generalized obstructive process. In this context, previous necropsy

studies in adult and elderly victims of sudden coronary death showed a high frequency of multivessel CAD.[108,109]

The increase in myocardial oxygen demand, in the presence of fixed supply, may be the mechanism underlying exercise-induced arrhythmias and SD. The absence of angina pectoris and ECG-documented ischemic changes in the history of the patients suggests that the obstructive coronary plaques, observed at histology, may not be flow-limiting in vivo at rest.[13] The dynamic nature of the pathophysiology of coronary events has led to the recognition that superimposed acute lesions create a setting in which alterations in the metabolic or electrolyte state of the myocardium may lead to disturbed electrical activity.[9] The coexistence of both such factors during, and immediately after, physical exertion could account for the higher incidence of SD in athletes.

A modification in flow dynamics may induce mechanical injury to the vessel wall and explain the propensity for obstructive plaque localization at the proximal tract of the left anterior descending coronary artery, just below the left main coronary artery bifurcation, where flow velocity is critically reduced and wall shear stress is increased.[112] Thus, in subjects from 1 to 20 years of age, the proximal left anterior descending coronary artery is most prone to the formation of fibrocellular intimal thickenings and early non-obstructive coronary plaques,[113] as confirmed by an autopsy study on young trauma victims <35 years old.[114]

In most of the young victims of atherosclerotic CAD-induced SD, obstructive plaques are fibrous, with a stratum of smooth muscle cell hyperplasia occupying up to 46% of the total plaque cross-sectional area (Fig. 65.21).[13] These fibrocellular plaques represent an early stage of mature atheromatous plaques.[115]

Acute thrombosis is present in only 22% of obstructive plaques in athletes and young adult victims of sudden

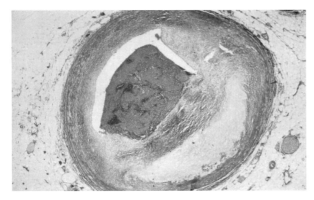

Fig. 65.20. Fresh occlusive thrombosis of the proximal anterior descending coronary artery superimposed by an eccentric atheromatous plaque with a large lipid core in a 33-year-old man who died suddenly. Azan stain, original magnification ×25. (With permission from ref. 13.)

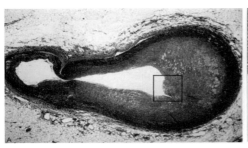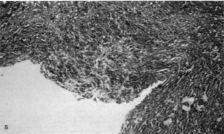

Fig. 65.21. Proximal left anterior descending coronary artery of a 30-year-old man who died suddenly. (a) Histology showing an obstructive eccentric fibrous plaque at the origin of the first diagonal branch. Note the preserved tunica media. Azan stain, original magnification ×25. (b) Close-up of the boxed area showing a layer of intimal cell hyperplasia. Azan stain, original magnification ×200. (With permission from ref. 13.)

coronary death, a much lower frequency than that observed in older adults, where 73% of plaques are complicated by thrombosis.[13] A normal tunica media and a layer of intimal fibrocellular hyperplasia in the absence of thrombosis may represent the potential substrate accounting for coronary hypervasoreactivity.[13] The normally thick tunica media is an anatomic prerequisite for preserved vasomotor reactivity in the atherosclerotic coronary artery. Constrictive coronary hyperreactivity accompanies both experimental[116] and clinical[117] accelerated atherosclerosis, which shows many similarities to the smooth muscle cell hyperplasia overlying the fibrous plaques observed in the young.

Prevention and treatment

CAD is the primary cause of SCD in the adult; therefore, prevention and treatment are discussed in dedicated chapters. It is less common in the young but the mechanism and therefore the therapeutic approach and prevention strategies are the same.

Coronary vasospasm

General

Coronary vasospasm is a potential trigger of transient myocardial ischemia[118] which, in turn, may precipitate VT/VF and cause SCD (Fig. 65.22).[119]

Risk

Coronary vasospasm is a rare cause of SCD in athletes.[18,120]

Pathophysiology

Coronary artery spasm and modulation of coronary collateral flow may be linked to local endothelial dysfunction, which exposes the myocardium to the double hazard of transient ischemia and reperfusion.[121] Smooth muscle cell hyperplasia has been described as a distinctive feature in coronary plaques retrieved by directional atherectomy from patients with unstable angina, and may provide an alternative mechanism to thrombus formation precipitating myocardial ischemia at rest and during competition.[122] Neurogenic influences are also likely to play a role, but do not appear to be a *sine qua non* factor to trigger spasm. Vessel susceptibility and humoral factors, particularly those related to platelet activation, also appear to be important contributors.[9]

Prevention and treatment

As before, this has been extensively discussed elsewhere in the book. Also, the pathophysiology of this entity is largely speculative, and will not be addressed in detail here.

Valvular heart disease

Aortic stenosis

General

The natural history of aortic stenosis is typically characterized by a long asymptomatic period during which the degree of stenosis increases. In 1968 Ross and Braunwald showed that the risk of SCD is low (3–5%) in asymptomatic patients.[123] More recently, a prospective study showed that SCD did not occur in any of 123 asymptomatic patients followed for 2.5 years.[124] Accordingly, in the absence of cardiac symptoms, survival is excellent without valve replacement.

Risk and diagnosis

The prognostic value of hemodynamic and electrophysiological testing is limited. Clinical manifestations of aortic stenosis include syncope, angina pectoris and/or dyspnea. Both syncope and SCD are exertional in many patients but it is not clear if syncope is a necessary and/or reliable predictor of SCD.[125] The difficulty is to predict the natural history of aortic stenosis in an asymptomatic patient since the risk of SCD is low.[125] The degree of stenosis, amount of calcification and severity of LV hypertrophy can be used to predict the speed of progression of stenosis requiring surgical intervention.[126]

Once symptoms develop, the prognosis worsens dramatically and the incidence of SCD among symptomatic patients rises to 8–34%.[123,126,127] Analysis of Holter ECG in seven patients who died suddenly demonstrated the presence of VT in six patients, while only in one patient was death associated with bradyarrhythmia.[128]

Prevention

Restriction of physical activity should be advised in patients with moderate and especially with severe aortic stenosis.[125] Such a policy resulted in the absence of SCD related to aortic stenosis over 20 years of pre-participation screening in northeast Italy, as demonstrated by Corrado *et al.*[4] In the absence of such screening, aortic stenosis accounts for 2.6% of SCD in athletes.[18] In line with this reasoning the following recommendations for athletic participation have been proposed:[129]

1. Athletes with mild aortic stenosis (<20 mmHg) can participate in all competitive sports.
2. Athletes with mild to moderate aortic stenosis (21 to 40 mmHg) should participate in low or moderate intensity sports only.
3. Athletes with severe aortic stenosis (>40 mmHg) or symptoms should not engage in any competitive sports.

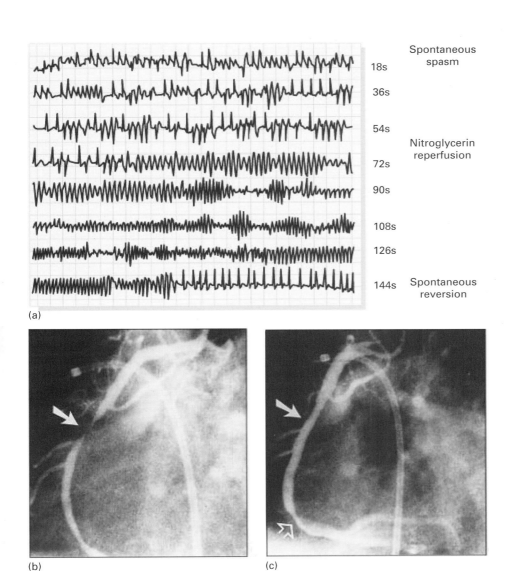

Spontaneous spasm

18s

36s

54s

Nitroglycerin reperfusion

72s

90s

108s

126s

144s Spontaneous reversion

(a)

(b)   (c)

Fig. 65.22. Life-threatening ventricular arrhythmias associated with acute myocardial ischemia related to coronary artery spasm and reperfusion. (a) Continuous lead II electrocardiographic monitor recording during ischemia (time 0 to 55 seconds) caused by spasm of the right coronary artery. There is an abrupt transition (time 56 to 72 seconds) from repetitive ventricular ectopy to a rapid polymorphic, prefibrillatory tachyarrhythmia (time 80 to 130 seconds) associated with nitroglycerin-induced reversal of the spasm. (b) and Closed arrows, site of spasm before and after nitroglycerin; open arrow, lower grade distal lesion. (With permission from ref. 9.)

4. Athletes with bicuspid aortic valve, even without stenosis but with aortic dilatation, can participate in low intensity sports only. Serial 6-monthly echocardiographic monitoring of aortic root and ascending aorta is recommended.

Treatment

Prevention of SCD is one of the goals of surgical treatment of aortic stenosis. If surgery is considered in order to reduce the risk of SCD, however, this risk must outweigh perioperative mortality and known complications of prosthetic valves.[130] On this ground, surgical intervention is usually deferred until clinical symptoms occur.

Mitral valve prolapse

General

Mitral valve prolapse is equally common in men and women, although men seem to have a higher incidence of complications, including infective endocarditis, severe mitral regurgitation, cerebrovascular ischemic events, and SCD.[131,132] Mitral leaflet thickening greater than 5 mm (that is classic prolapse) is associated with a 14-fold higher risk of complications, including SD.[131]

Risk

The risk of SCD is relatively low (40 in 10 000)[133] – twice the incidence expected in the general population – and the causal relation between mitral valve prolapse and SD is not fully resolved. Nonetheless, increased risk of SD is observed in patients with severe mitral regurgitation and/or severe valvular deformation,[131,133] depressed LV function,[134] QT interval prolongation,[135] and a history of syncope and palpitations. The presence of severe mitral regurgitation with a flail segment appears to carry a particularly high risk of SCD (up to 2% per year).[134]

Prevention and treatment

The mechanism of SD in mitral valve prolapse appears to be linked to the presence of VT. Therefore, it is prudent to disqualify from competitive sports athletes with mitral valve prolapse associated with a history of ventricular arrhythmias.[18,136]

Nevertheless, most patients with mitral valve prolapse have an excellent prognosis with an expected survival similar to that of the general population.[131,132] Indeed, most patients do not develop symptoms or significant echocardiographic abnormalities, and most asymptomatic patients with mitral valve prolapse can be followed conservatively.[132] Neither their activity level nor lifestyle need to be restricted; to the contrary, routine exercise may be preferable.[132]

Marfan syndrome

General

This autosomal dominant disorder is relatively frequent (2–3 per 10 000) and occurs in all races and ethnic groups.[137] Marfan syndrome, with its characteristic phenotype resulting from excessive growth of the long bones and joint laxity, may be underdiagnosed, particularly in populations of elite basketball players.[120] SD in Marfan syndrome is commonly due to aortic dissection.[138] Even with the discovery of the genetic and biochemical basis of the condition, the diagnosis of Marfan syndrome outside families with the classic phenotype remains entirely clinical.[120] Athletes with Marfan syndrome can participate successfully in strenuous competitive sports for many years without experiencing a catastrophic event, presumably before aortic dilatation becomes marked and the predisposition to dissection or rupture increases critically. Treatment with β-blockers is thought to reduce the risk of progressive aortic dilation and SD.[139]

Risk

A large cohort of patients with Marfan syndrome, followed by a single institution to assess long-term outcome, demonstrated a significant incidence of ventricular arrhythmias.[140] Patients were started on medical management early in the course of their disease, mainly β-blockers and angiotensin converting enzyme inhibitor. A high prevalence of LV dilation with associated abnormalities of repolarization was documented. Over an average follow-up period of 24 years, few patients required surgical intervention. The mortality rate from presumed arrhythmogenic death was 4%, exceeding by far the rate of aortic rupture.[140] Such repolarization abnormalities may account for the increased risk of ventricular ectopy and possibly SCD.

Prevention and treatment

Patients with Marfan syndrome and ventricular dysrhythmias may be at particularly high risk for SCD. Accordingly, aggressive treatment modalities including amiodarone or ICDs may be warranted in selected patients.

SCD involving functional abnormalities

About 2% of young athletes who die suddenly have normal cardiac structure at autopsy, and no definitive cause of death can be established.[7,141]

Ion channelopathies

The list of congenital and acquired arrhythmias, secondary to mutations or polymorphisms in genes encoding for cardiac ion channels, has expanded impressively in recent years. These ion channel disorders include long QT syndrome (LQTS), short QT syndrome (SQTS), Brugada syndrome and CPVT, atrial fibrillation (AF), and conduction system disease (Table 65.5). Recent studies have suggested that a small proportion (5–10%) of SD in infants is also

Table 65.5. Genetic disorders secondary to ion channelopathies

Ventricular	Rhythm		Inheritance	Locus	Ion Channel	Gene
Long QT	TdP		AD			
syndrome (RW)	LQT1			11p15	I_{Ks}	*KCNQ1, KvLQT1*
	LQT2			7q35	I_{Kr}	*KCNH2, HERG*
	LQT3			3p21	I_{Na}	*Na$_v$1.5 , SCN5A*
	LQT4			4q25		*ANKB, ANK2*
	LQT5			21q22	I_{Ks}	*KCNE1, minK*
	LQT6			21q22	I_{Kr}	*KCNE2, MiRP1*
	LQT7		(Andersen-Tawil syndrome)	17q23	I_{K1}	*KCNJ2, Kir 2.1*
	LQT8		(Timothy syndrome)	6q8A	I_{Ca-L}	Ca$_v$1.2
LQT syndrome (JLN)	TdP		AR	11p15	I_{Ks}	*KCNQ1, KvLQT1*
				21q22	I_{Ks}	*KCNE1, minK*
Brugada syndrome	VT/VF		AD	3p21	I_{Na}	*Na$_v$1.5 , SCN5A*
				3p22–25		
Short QT syndrome	VT/VF		AD	7q35	I_{Kr}	*KCNH2, HERG*
SQT1	SQT2			11p15	I_{Ks}	*KCNQ1, KvLQT1*
	SQT3			17q23.1–24.2	I_{K1}	*KCNJ2, Kir2.1*
Catecholaminergic VT	CPVT1	VT	AD	1q42–43	*RyR2*	
	CPVT2	VT	AR	1p13–21	*CASQ2*	
Supraventricular						
Atrial fibrillation	AF		AD	10q22		
			AD	11p15	I_{Ks}	*KCNQ1*
Atrial standstill	SND, AF		AD	3p21	I_{Na}	*SCN5A*
Cardiac conduction disorders						
Progressive conduction disease	CCD1	AVB	AD	3p21	I_{Na}	*Na$_v$1.5, SCN5A*
				16q23–24		
				19q13.2–13.3		

Abbreviations: AD: autosomal dominant, AF: atrial fibrillation, AR: autosomal recessive, AVB: atrioventricular block, AVRT: atrioventricular re-entrant tachycardia, JLN: Jervell and Lange–Nielsen, LQT: Long QT, RW: Romano-Ward, SND: sinus node dysfunction, TdP: Torsades de Pointes, VF: ventricular fibrillation, VT: ventricular tachycardia, CPVT: catecholaminergic polymorphic ventricular tachycardia.

linked to ion channelopathies, including LQTS, SQTS and Brugada syndrome.[142,143]

Clinical diagnosis is generally made by identification of the disease phenotype on standard 12-lead ECG. Some of these cases have previously been classified as idiopathic VF, a category describing syndromes for which a mechanistic understanding is lacking.

Long QT syndrome

General

LQTS is characterized by the appearance of long QT intervals in the ECG, an atypical polymorphic VT known as Torsades de Pointes, and a relatively high risk for SCD.[144] Congenital LQTS is subdivided into seven genotypes, distinguished by mutations in at least six different ion channel genes and a structural anchoring protein located on chromosomes 3, 4, 7, 11, 17, and 21.[145–147] Timothy syndrome, classified by some as LQT8, is a rare congenital disorder characterized by multiorgan dysfunction, including prolongation of the QT interval, lethal arrhythmias, webbing of fingers and toes, congenital heart disease, immune deficiency, intermittent hypoglycemia, cognitive abnormalities, and autism. Timothy syndrome has been linked to mutations in Ca$_v$1.2, which encodes for a portion of the calcium channel.[148]

The estimated prevalence of this disorder is 1–2:10 000. The ECG diagnosis is based on the presence of prolonged repolarization (QT interval) and abnormal T wave morphology.[149] Cardiac events are often precipitated by physical or emotional stress, but may also occur at rest. The mainstay of therapy is represented by antiadrenergic intervention with β-blockers. For patients unresponsive to this approach, ICD implantation and/or cardiac sympathetic denervation represent the therapeutic alternative.[150]

Genetics

Two patterns of inheritance have been described: 1) a rare autosomal recessive disease associated with deafness (Jervell and Lang-Nielsen), caused by two genes that encode for the slowly activating delayed rectifier potassium channel (*KCNQ1* and *KCNE1*); and 2) the much more common autosomal dominant form known as the Romano Ward syndrome, caused by mutations in eight different genes, including *KCNQ1* (KvLQT1; LQT1); *KCNH2* (HERG;LQT2); *SCN5A* (Na$_v$1.5; LQT3); *ANKB* (LQT4); *KCNE1* (minK; LQT5); *KCNE2* (MiRP1; LQT6); *KCNJ2*; Kir2.1; (LQT7; Andersen's syndrome) and *CACNA1C* (Ca$_v$1.2; LQT8; Timothy syndrome). Six of the eight genes encode for cardiac potassium channels, one for the cardiac sodium channel (SCN5A) and one for a protein called Ankyrin B, which is involved in anchoring of ion channels to the cellular membrane (ANKB).

Acquired LQTS refers to a syndrome similar to the congenital form, but caused by exposure to drugs that prolong the duration of the ventricular action potential (AP)[151] or QT prolongation secondary to cardiomyopathies such as DCM or HCM, as well as to abnormal QT prolongation associated with bradycardia or electrolyte imbalance.[152]

Pathophysiology

A number of studies point to amplification of spatial dispersion of repolarization within the ventricular myocardium as principal arrhythmogenic substrate in both acquired and congenital LQTS. The accentuation of spatial dispersion, typically secondary to an increase of transmural, trans-septal, or apicobasal dispersion of repolarization, and the development of early afterdepolarization-induced triggered activity underlie the substrate and trigger for the development of Torsades de Pointes arrhythmias observed under LQTS conditions.[153] Models of LQT1, LQT2, and LQT3 have been developed by using the canine arterially perfused LV wedge preparation. These models suggest that in these three forms of LQTS, preferential prolongation of the M cell AP duration (APD) leads to an increase in the QT interval as well as an increase in transmural dispersion of repolarization (TDR), which contributes to the development of spontaneous as well as stimulation-induced Torsades de Pointes.[154]

Genotype-phenotype correlation studies point to major differences among patients with the three most common LQTS loci (LQT1, LQT2, LQT3), which account for approximately 95% of all genotyped patients. Genotype-specific ECG patterns have been identified[155]

and the environmental triggers for cardiac events have been shown to be gene-specific: LQT1 patients experience 97% of cardiac events during physical activity, as opposed to LQT3 patients who present the majority of cardiac events at rest. Moreover, auditory stimuli and arousal have been shown to be relatively specific triggers for LQT2 patients, whereas swimming leads to cardiac events in LQT1 patients.[156]

The response to sympathetic activation displays a very different time-course in LQT1 and LQT2, both in experimental models and in the clinic.[153,157] In LQT1, isoproterenol produces an increase in TDR that is most prominent during the first 2 minutes, but which persists, although to a lesser extent, during the steady-state. Incidence of Torsades de Pointes is enhanced during the initial period as well as during the steady-state. In LQT2, isoproterenol produces only a transient increase in TDR that persists for less than 2 minutes, so that Torsades de Pointes incidence is enhanced only briefly. In LQT3, β-adrenergic stimulation abbreviates APD of all cardiac cell types, reducing TDR and suppressing Torsades de Pointes,[158] thus providing an explanation for the prevalence of cardiac events in LQT3 patients at rest. These observations help to explain the important differences in autonomic activity and other gene-specific triggers that contribute to events in patients with different LQTS genotypes as well as the genotype-specific response to treatment with β-blockers.[159,160]

Prevention and treatment

Because of the great heterogeneity in clinical expression of LQTS, individualized patient management is required. Evaluation is geared toward discerning which asymptomatic family members are affected and who among the affected individuals harbors a "ticking time bomb." Prohibition of competitive sports is one of the biggest issues facing families of children and adolescents diagnosed with LQTS, even though physical activity poses no risk to some patients with this disorder. Unfortunately, clinical testing cannot always accurately determine individuals at risk; while LQT1 and LQT2 patients are universally restricted from high-exertion sports, many LQTS experts support participation in "recreational sports with moderate exertion" in properly treated LQTS patients.

Brugada syndrome

General

The Brugada syndrome, first described in 1992, is characterized by an accentuated coved-type ST segment elevation, or J wave, appearing principally in the right precordial leads (V1-V3), often followed by a negative T wave, and a high incidence of SCD secondary to a rapid polymorphic VT or VF.[161] The ECG sign of the Brugada syndrome is dynamic and often concealed, but can be unmasked by potent sodium channel blockers such as ajmaline, flecainide, procainamide, disopyramide, propafenone, and pilsicainide.[162] The syndrome may also be unmasked or precipitated by a febrile state, vagotonic agents, α-adrenergic agonists, β-adrenergic blockers, tricyclic or tetracyclic antidepressants, a combination of glucose and insulin, and hypokalemia, as well as by alcohol and cocaine toxicity.[163]

Clinical manifestations of the disease (syncope or cardiac arrest) generally appear in the third to fourth decade of life, although malignant forms with childhood or neonatal onset have been reported.[164] Cardiac events typically occur during sleep or at rest.[165] The disease is inherited as an autosomal dominant trait but there is a striking male to female ratio of 10:1 in the occurrence of clinical manifestations. These gender differences have been attributed to differences in the intensity of the transient outward current (I_{to}).[14]

Genetics

Familial autosomal dominant and sporadic forms have been linked to mutations in the α-subunit of the cardiac sodium channel gene, SCN5A (the same gene responsible for LQT3) in 20% of patients with the Brugada syndrome. Another locus was reported on the short arm of chromosome 3, but no gene has been identified.

Sudden unexplained nocturnal death syndrome, found predominantly in young Southeast Asian males (i.e., from Thailand, Japan, Philippines, and Cambodia), is a disorder causing SD during sleep due to VT/VF. Sudden unexplained nocturnal death and Brugada syndrome have been shown to be phenotypically, genetically, and functionally the same disorder.

Pathophysiology

The arrhythmogenic substrate responsible for the development of extrasystoles and polymorphic VT in the Brugada syndrome is thought to be secondary to amplification of phase 1 (early AP repolarization)-mediated notch in the RV epicardial AP. Rebalancing of the currents active at the end of phase 1 is thought to underlie the accentuation of the AP notch in RV epicardium, which is responsible for the augmented J wave and ST segment elevation associated with the Brugada syndrome (see ref. 166 for details). The ST segment is normally close to isoelectric due to the absence of major transmural voltage gradients at the level of the AP plateau. Accentuation of the RV AP notch under pathophysiologic conditions leads to exag-

geration of transmural voltage gradients and thus to accentuation of the J wave, or to J point elevation. If the epicardial AP continues to repolarize before that of the endocardium, the T wave remains positive, giving rise to a saddleback configuration of the ST segment elevation. Further accentuation of the notch is accompanied by a prolongation of the epicardial AP causing it to repolarize after the endocardium, thus leading to inversion of the T wave.

The down-sloping ST segment elevation, or accentuated J wave, observed in experimental wedge models, often appears as an R', suggesting that the appearance of a right bundle branch block morphology in Brugada patients may be due in large part to early repolarization of RV epicardium, rather than major delays in impulse conduction in the right bundle.[167] Despite the appearance of a typical Brugada sign, accentuation of the RV epicardial AP notch alone does not give rise to an arrhythmogenic substrate. The arrhythmogenic substrate may develop with a further shift in the balance of currents, leading to loss of the AP dome at some epicardial sites but not others. Marked TDR develops as a consequence, creating a vulnerable window, which when captured by a premature extrasystole can trigger a re-entrant arrhythmia. Because loss of the AP dome in epicardium is generally heterogeneous, epicardial dispersion of repolarization develops as well. Conduction of the AP dome from sites at which it is maintained to sites at which it is lost may cause local re-excitation via phase 2 re-entry, leading to the development of a closely coupled extrasystole capable of capturing the vulnerable window across the ventricular wall, thus triggering a circus movement re-entry in the form of VT/VF.[168] Support for these hypotheses derives from experiments involving the arterially perfused RV wedge preparation[168] and from recent studies in which monophasic AP electrodes were positioned on the epicardial and endocardial surfaces of the RV outflow tract in patients with the Brugada syndrome.[169,170]

Prevention and treatment

An ICD is the most widely accepted approach to therapy. ICD implantation is not an appropriate solution for infants and young children, however, or for patients residing in regions of the world where an ICD is out of reach because of economic factors. Although arrhythmias and SCD generally occur during sleep or at rest, associated with slow heart rates, a potential therapeutic role for cardiac pacing remains largely unexplored. A recent report by Haissaguerre and coworkers[171] points to focal radiofrequency ablation as a potentially valuable tool in controlling arrhythmogenesis by focal ablation of the ventricular premature beats that trigger VT/VF in the Brugada syndrome.

Data relative to a cryosurgical approach or the use of ablation therapy are very limited at this time.

A pharmacologic approach to therapy, based on a rebalancing of currents active during the early phases of the epicardial AP in the right ventricle to reduce the AP notch and/or restore the AP dome, has been a focus of basic and clinical research in recent years. Because the presence of a prominent transient outward current, I_{to}, is central to the mechanism underlying the Brugada syndrome, the most rational approach to therapy, regardless of the ionic or genetic basis for the disease, is partial inhibition of I_{to}. Cardioselective and I_{to}-specific blockers are not currently available. The only agent on the market with significant I_{to}-blocking properties is quinidine. It was therefore suggested as a therapeutic approach for treatment of this syndrome.[172] Experimental studies have shown quinidine to be effective in restoring the epicardial AP dome, thus normalizing the ST segment and preventing phase 2 re-entry and polymorphic VT in experimental models of the Brugada syndrome.[168] Clinical evidence of the effectiveness of quinidine in normalizing ST segment elevation in patients with the Brugada syndrome has been reported.[173,174]

The effects of quinidine in preventing inducible and spontaneous VF were recently reported by Belhassen and coworkers[174] in a prospective study of 25 Brugada syndrome patients. These results are consistent with those reported by the same group in prior years[175] and more recently by other investigators.[176,177] The data highlight the need for randomized clinical trials to assess the effectiveness of quinidine, preferably in patients with frequent events who have already received an ICD.

Agents that boost the calcium current, such as β-adrenergic agents like isoproterenol, are useful as well.[166,168,178] Isoproterenol, sometimes in combination with quinidine, has been shown to normalize ST segment elevation in patients with the Brugada syndrome and in controlling "electrical storms," particularly in children.[173,179] A recent addition to the pharmacological armamentarium is the phosphodiesterase III inhibitor, cilostazol,[178] which normalizes the ST segment, most likely by augmenting calcium currents as well as by reducing I_{to} secondary to an increase in heart rate.

Other than isolated anecdotal reports of exertion-induced VT/VF, no data exist concerning the risk of participation in sports. Accordingly, patients with the Brugada syndrome at present are not excluded or restricted from participating in sports. This fact notwithstanding, because bradycardia and increased vagal activity are both known to predispose to the development of ST segment elevation and arrhythmogenesis in Brugada syndrome patients, a case can be made for avoiding these manifestations of a well-trained athlete. Thus, adaptation of the cardiac autonomic nervous system to training, which results in increased vagal activity and/or withdrawal of sympathetic activity, may enhance the propensity of athletes with Brugada syndrome to die suddenly at rest, during sleep, or immediately after exercise.[180]

Short QT syndrome

General

In 2000, Gussak et al.[181] proposed SQTS as a new clinical entity. Short-QT syndrome is an inherited syndrome characterized by a QTc $\leq$ 300 ms and high incidence of VT/VF in infants, children, and young adults.[182] The familial nature of this syndrome was confirmed by Gaita et al. in 2003.[183]

Genetics

The first genetic defect (SQT1) responsible for the SQTS, reported by Brugada et al. in 2004, involved two different missense mutations (substitution of one amino acid for another) resulting in the same amino acid substitution in HERG (*N588K*), which caused a gain of function in the rapidly activating delayed rectifier channel, I_{Kr}.[184] A second gene (SQT2) was recently reported by Bellocq et al.[185] A missense mutation in *KCNQ1* (KvLQT1) was found to cause a gain of function in the slowly activating delayed rectifier potassium current (I_{Ks}). A third gene (SQT3), involving mutations in *KCNJ2*, the gene that encodes for the inward rectifier channel, was found to cause a gain of function in the inwardly rectifying potassium current (I_{K1}), leading to an abbreviation of QT interval. SQT3 is associated with QTc intervals of <330 ms, not quite as short as SQT1, and SQT2.

Pathophysiology

SQTS is also characterized by the appearance of tall peaked symmetrical T waves in the ECG. The augmented T_{peak}–T_{end} interval associated with this electrocardiographic feature of the syndrome suggests that TDR is increased. Recent data collected using a ventricular wedge model of SQTS has provided evidence to support the hypothesis that an increase in outward repolarizing current can preferentially abbreviate endocardial/M cell APD in the left ventricle and this increases TDR and thus creates the substrate for re-entry.[186] The potassium channel opener pinacidil causes heterogeneous APD abbreviation among the different cell types spanning the ventricular wall, thus creating a substrate for VT under conditions associated with short QT intervals. Polymorphic VT could be readily induced with programmed electrical stimulation. The increase in TDR was further accentuated by isoproterenol, leading to easier induction and more persistent VT/VF. The latter is probably due to the reduction in the wavelength of the re-entrant circuit, which reduces the path-length required for maintenance of re-entry.[186]

Therapy

Because of the recent identification of the short QT syndrome as a new clinical entity, the approach to therapy is still evolving. An ICD is clearly the therapy of choice in patients with syncope and a positive family history of SCD. Nonetheless, ICD therapy in patients with a short QT syndrome has an increased risk for inappropriate shock delivery due to T wave oversensing secondary to the presence of tall peaked T waves. A variety of drugs, including sotalol, ibutilide, flecainide, and quinidine, have been tested in SQT1. Quinidine was the only drug that effectively suppressed the gain-of-function of I_{Kr} leading to a prolongation of the QT interval and rendering VT/VF non-inducible. Quinidine has been proposed as an adjunct to ICD therapy and is a possible alternative treatment, especially for children and newborns.[187] At present there is little evidence on which to base a restriction of activity of patients with SQTS. Events have been reported at rest, during exertion, exercise and during sleep.

Wolff–Parkinson–White syndrome

General

Wolff–Parkinson–White (WPW) syndrome is caused by accessory atrioventricular (AV) connections, bypassing the AV-node and His bundle. WPW is rarely associated with other congenital cardiac anomalies.

Pathophysiology

The short anterograde effective refractory period of the accessory pathway allows extremely rapid ventricular responses during AF, with the risk of deterioration into VF.[188] Anterograde effective refractory periods <250 ms are considered unfavorable in symptomatic patients.[189] Patients with WPW have an SCD risk of less than 1 in 1000 per year of follow-up.[190] Most survivors of SCD have experienced arrhythmias before the event but, in up to 10%, SCD may occur as first manifestation.[191]

Prevention and treatment

For symptomatic patients, catheter ablation is now first-choice therapy with >95% effectiveness.[192] If ineffective, antiarrhythmic drugs prolonging the anterograde effective refractory period of the accessory pathway, or cardiac surgery, are the only alternatives. Consensus remains that in asymptomatic patients catheter ablation is not indicated.[193]

In many cases, the resting ECG shows pre-excitation. The athlete with a WPW pattern on the ECG and no symptoms of palpitations, syncope, or presyncope represents a more difficult problem. It is thought that although these individuals have a lifelong risk of developing arrhythmias, the risk of developing a fatal arrhythmia is quite low; therefore, most experts do not advise routine electrophysiologic testing of these individuals or exclusion from physical activity.[194,195] Electrophysiological testing and ablation therapy is recommended in special circumstances, such as family history of SCD, high risk profession (e.g., pilot), or athletes who may be at higher risk for developing AF.[125]

Catecholaminergic polymorphic ventricular tachycardia

General

In 1975, Coumel *et al.*[196] described four cases of severe ventricular arrhythmias in children with normal QT intervals. VT/VF was reproducibly induced by any form of sympathetic stimulation and termed catecholaminergic polymorphic ventricular tachycardia (CPVT). A remarkable feature of CPVT is its high lethality, demonstrated by the occurrence of 19 juvenile SCD in 10 affected families and by the occurrence of appropriate ICD shocks in 6 of 12 patients implanted with an ICD, over a follow-up period of ~2 years.[197]

Genetics

The recent identification of mutations of the cardiac ryanodine receptor gene (RyR2), underlying CPVT,[198] lends support to the hypothesis that stress-induced life-threatening arrhythmias, occurring in the structurally intact heart, are phenotypical variants of the same disease. Cardiac ryanodine receptor gene mutations have been identified in a similar proportion of patients with bidirectional VT (36%), polymorphic VT (58%), and catecholaminergic VF (50%), suggesting that the diagnosis of CPVT may extend to all patients with polymorphic VT or VF occurring in the structurally intact heart in the absence of a prolonged QT interval (Fig. 65.23).[197] Mutations of RyR2 have been identified in subjects who had unexplained cardiac arrest during physical or emotional stress, without arrhythmias inducible at exercise stress testing or Holter monitoring.[197]

Pathophysiology

A diagnosis of CPVT should be considered in subjects of all ages with idiopathic polymorphic ventricular arrhythmias occurring during exercise or emotional stress in the absence of structural abnormalities or prolonged QT interval.[197] In athletes with structural heart disease and

(a)

(b)

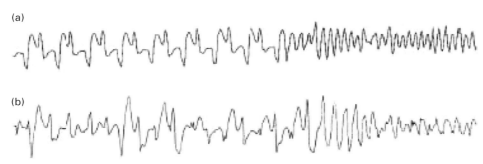

Fig. 65.23. Examples of bidirectional (a) and polymorphic ventricular tachycardia (b) degenerating into ventricular fibrillation in patients with catecholaminergic ventricular tachycardia. (With permission from ref. 197.)

syncope, the cause of the syncope should be presumed to be arrhythmic, and athletes should be treated similarly to those who have experienced resuscitated SD, unless another clear diagnosis explains syncope.[199] In athletes without known structural heart disease, syncope during peak exertion should warrant an extensive work-up.

Interestingly, the age of onset of syncope is significantly lower in patients with RyR2 CPVT than in patients with non-genotyped CPVT; however, the mean age of SD among individuals in families with RyR2 CPVT suggests that, if not identified and treated during childhood, the disease becomes lethal in early adulthood.[197] A strong predominance of symptomatic female subjects has been observed among patients with non-genotyped CPVT, whereas male sex appears to be a strong risk factor (relative risk, 4.2) for syncope in patients with RyR2 CPVT.[197] The morphology of the ventricular arrhythmias is independent of the genetic defect, as demonstrated by the presence of discordant phenotypes in individuals with the same mutation.[197]

Prevention and treatment

Analogies may exist between CPVT and LQTS,[197] and further genetic research is required for clarification. CPVT patients must comply with medical therapy, namely β-blockers. ICD treatment may become part of therapy, although attention should be given to the catecholaminergic effects of ICD shock delivery. As in LQTS, ICD should therefore not be implanted without concomitant administration of β-blockers.

Right ventricular outflow tract tachycardia

General

This VT appears to originate from the RV outflow tract and has the characteristic ECG of a left bundle brunch block contour in V_1 and inferior axis in the frontal plane (Fig. 65.24).

Pathophysiology

Vagal maneuvers, including administration of adenosine, terminate the VT, whereas exercise, stress, isoproterenol infusion, and rapid or premature stimulation can initiate or perpetuate the tachycardia. The mechanism responsible may be cyclic adenosine monophosphate-triggered activity[200] resulting from early or delayed afterdepolarizations. Two types can be distinguished: paroxysmal VT and repetitive monomorphic VT. The paroxysmal type is exercise-induced, whereas the repetitive monomorphic type occurs at rest with sinus beats interposed between runs of non-sustained VT that may be precipitated by transient increases in sympathetic activity unrelated to exertion.

Therapy

Radiofrequency catheter ablation can eliminate tachycardia in 83% to 100% of patients.[201]

Familial atrial fibrillation

AF is the most common sustained arrhythmia encountered in the clinic (in part at least, because in contrast to VF it is compatible with life). AF is usually secondary to ischemic heart disease, hypertension, or congestive heart failure. In a fraction of cases (3–30%) no underlying cardiovascular disease is apparent and in some AF appears to be familial. A locus on chromosome 10, linked to familial AF, was described in 1997, but the specific gene has not yet been identified. More recently, familial AF has been identified as an autosomal dominant trait, linked to mutations in KCNQ1, and associated with LQTS, SQTS, and Brugada syndromes.[203]

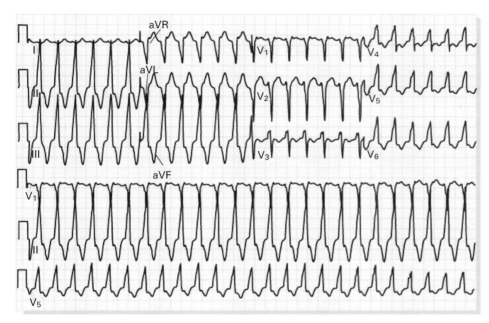

Fig. 65.24. Ventricular tachycardia originating from the right ventricular outflow tract. This tachycardia is characterized by a left bundle branch block contour in V1 and an inferior axis. (With permission from ref. 202.)

Conduction system disease

A progressive cardiac conduction defect, also known as Lev-Lenegre disease, is characterized by escalating impairment of conduction in the His-Purkinje system, leading to widening of the QRS complex. Conduction block can give rise to long pauses and/or bradycardia that may cause syncope. Sick sinus syndrome is a disorder phenotypically similar to progressive cardiac conduction defect. Familial occurrence of both syndromes has been reported, with an autosomal dominant pattern of inheritance. An ionchannelopathy in the form of SCN5A mutations is thought to contribute to these defects.

Idiopathic VF

In some patients, neither underlying disease nor distinct electrophysiologic abnormalities or electrolyte or metabolic derangements may be demonstrable. VF in these conditions is referred to as "idiopathic".[204] Idiopathic VF is a diagnosis by exclusion. Therefore, it can only be made when thorough clinical evaluation does not provide evidence for structural heart disease or other known causes of VT/VF. This does not necessarily imply that a patient's heart is completely free of any structural or functional abnormality, but merely that if an abnormal finding (e.g.,

first-degree AV block or AF) is present, it is not considered responsible for the VF episode.[121]

Because idiopathic VF is unlikely to represent a homogeneous disease, future research may identify specific causes in certain subsets, as was the case for LQTS and CPVT. Current consensus is that some minor abnormalities, unknown to be associated with the occurrence of VF, do not rule out the diagnosis. A combined Task Force of the Unexplained Cardiac Arrest Registry of Europe and Idiopathic Ventricular Fibrillation Registry of the US[121] has summarized a variety of minor abnormalities that may be compatible with a diagnosis of idiopathic VF.

Previously, prognosis was considered excellent.[205] There appeared to be agreement that only symptomatic patients with recurrent arrhythmia should be treated. Initially, no particular efforts were directed toward identification of high-risk subgroups or SCD prevention. Data from several more recent studies, however, suggest recurrence rates of VF, syncope, or cardiac arrest varying from 25% to 43% over longer follow-up.[121,205] In the early 1990s, Wever et al.[205] were the first to report results of a prospective study on patients with primary electrical disease who survived a VF episode. The major finding was the high recurrence rate of life-threatening events during long-term follow-up, often in young patients (<35 years). In a subsequent study on survivors of out-of-hospital cardiac

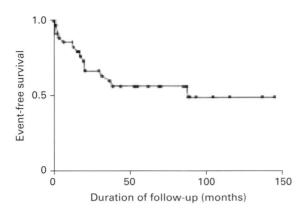

Fig. 65.25. Kaplan–Meier curve showing survival free of major events (sudden death, recurrent episodes of syncope, or documented ventricular tachyarrhythmia) of 37 consecutive patients with idiopathic ventricular fibrillation. (With permission from ref. 204.)

arrest due to idiopathic VF, this finding was confirmed.[204] During an average 77 months of follow-up, 43% of patients had recurrent episodes of syncope, documented ventricular tachyarrhythmia, or SCD (Fig. 65.25). Mean age was 35 years and retrospective analysis showed that 9 of 37 patients (24%) could have been classified as having Brugada syndrome.

SCD involving externally caused pathologies

Myocarditis

General

Myocarditis is an insidious disease that is usually asymptomatic; thus, important clues to its epidemiology come from postmortem studies.[206] Such studies suggest that myocarditis is a major cause of SD, accounting for approximately 20% of cases in adults < 40 years of age,[207] including young athletes.[208] In addition, prospective and retrospective studies have identified myocardial inflammation in 1% – 9% of routine postmortem examinations.[209]

Pathophysiology

Initially, selected viruses were implicated by demonstration of rising antibody titers in the serum of patients during acute myocarditis and convalescence.[210] Recently, however, the enterovirus genome has been identified in the myocardium of patients with myocarditis and patients with DCM.[211] Enterovirus and enterovirus-like RNA sequences have also been identified in endomyo-

cardial biopsy specimens from patients with clinically suspected myocarditis and from those with idiopathic DCM.[212]

Prevention and treatment

Myocarditis is difficult to diagnose clinically and may be suggested in the absence of symptoms on the basis of ECG abnormalities alone, which include heart block and ventricular arrhythmias.[213] Reverse-transcriptase–polymerase-chain-reaction assays allow identification of a viral genome in endomyocardial biopsy specimens.[214] Although myocarditis usually has an infectious origin, it can also be a consequence of drug abuse.[215,216]

Bed rest should be considered during viremia, in contrast with non-inflammatory DCM, although this recommendation is based solely on animal studies, and on the observation that myocarditis is often lethal in young athletes.[213]

Commotio cordis

General

Induction of arrhythmias, including SCD, by non-penetrating chest wall impact in the absence of structural injury to the ribs, sternum, and heart is known as *Commotio cordis* (*CC*). First described in the European medical literature during the 19th century,[217–219] *CC* was initially associated with workplace accidents, involving falls or impacts by tools and animal body parts. Since the twentieth century, the focus of *CC* has shifted almost entirely to sporting activities.[220]

The incidence of lethal *CC* in contemporary sports has traditionally been estimated to be < 5 deaths per annum in the US,[220] but under-reporting and misclassification of deaths is likely to occur, and the true number of deaths due to relatively mild chest wall impacts may be significantly higher. Indeed, in the last 5 years, the number of reported *CC* victims has increased in the US to 20 per annum (probably due to better awareness and reporting), with up to 20% of deaths on the athletic field caused by chest wall impact.[18, 221]

Clinical profile

The US *CC* Registry in Minneapolis, established in 1996, has documented in detail more than 170 cases. *CC* victims have a mean age of 14 years (80% ≤ 18 years),[220] and it is thought that young athletes are at particular risk because of their more pliable chest wall that facilitates the transmission of chest impact energy to the myocardium. With age, the thoracic cage stiffens and the chest wall absorbs more of the impact energy. Males comprise 95% of the victims, a proportion seemingly too high to be accounted for solely by the predominance of males in sports.

In the US, the most common sporting activity causing *CC* is baseball (~50%). Other sports include softball, ice hockey, and lacrosse; in each of these sports the impact object is a solid projectile. *CC* is rarely reported after blows from air-filled balls such as used in European soccer and American football. In these sports, *CC* is mostly caused by chest blows with a body part such as a knee, elbow, head, or fist (as in karate).

While organized competitive sports account for about 60% of all *CC* lethalities, some 20% occur in non-competitive recreational athletic activities, often during play with peers. The remainder of events occur during routine activities, parental disciplining, playful boxing, gang rituals, or blows by plastic projectiles or playground swings.

Pathophysiology

Collapse after impact is either immediate (~50%), or occurs following a brief period of consciousness, often marked by extreme lightheadedness. In the 74 cases from the *CC* Registry in which a postcollapse rhythm was documented, 48 showed VF. After prolonged cardiopulmonary resuscitation, asystole is common.[220] In the few survivors, in whom a 12-lead ECG was available, marked ST segment elevation, especially in the anterior leads, was observed, which resolved over time without development of Q-waves or elevation of myocardial enzymes.

Although CC initially was reported to be almost invariably fatal, survival now appears to approach 15%, including some cases with spontaneous resolution (see Fig. 65.26).[221] The greater likelihood of survival is probably related to at least two factors. The first is a reversal of a bias to report only fatal cases: we are becoming aware of many non-fatal cases with either spontaneous or defibrillated recovery. The most important determinant of increased survival is probably due to the better recognition of *CC* in the community, however, which translates into more timely cardiopulmonary resuscitation and defibrillation. Of 78 Registry events in which resuscitation was initiated within 3 minutes, 25% survived (compared to only 8% in which resuscitation was delayed for > 3 minutes).

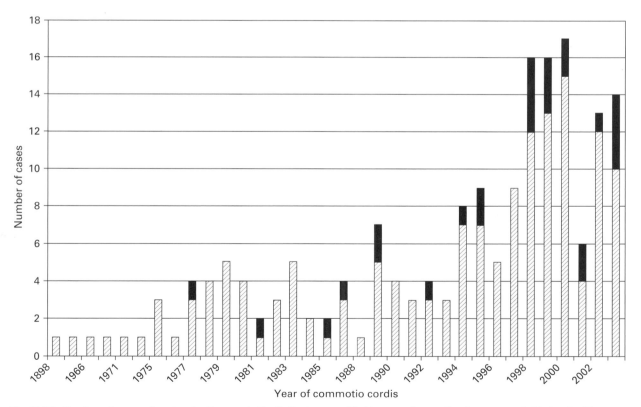

Fig. 65.26. Number of cases referred to the Commotio Cordis Registry stratified by year of event. Deaths are recorded in hatched bars, and survivors are represented by solid bars. Note the increasing number of reported cases and increasing likelihood of survivors in more recent years, both of which are probably caused by increased awareness of this phenomenon. (With permission from ref. 221.)

Experimental insight

Early experimental efforts generally focused on relatively severe chest wall trauma, such as that typically seen with victims of motor vehicle accidents, falls from heights, and bomb blasts.[217,218] In these models, morphologic cardiac damage was typically produced. Riedinger and Kümmell first distinguished between Cardiac Contusion (in which structural cardiac damage is present) and Commotion (where the heart remains intact).[218] The first systematic experimental insight into *CC* came from Schlomka's extensive experimental research[222] which highlighted the intrinsic cardiac nature of heart rhythm responses to precordial impact, and which suggested coronary vasospasms as a cause of arrhythmia in *CC* (reviewed in detail elsewhere).[219]

This concept had to be revised in recent years, largely as a result of the introduction of a new sophisticated porcine model, developed to clarify the mechanism of *CC*.[223] In this model, ventricular arrhythmias, including VF, can be produced by controlled (timing, location, amplitude) chest wall impact with a baseball in the absence of structural damage to the heart.

When impacts caused VF, this was not preceded by ventricular tachycardia, heart block, or ischemic ST changes (Fig. 65.27). One of the most important determinants of VF is the timing of the chest impact in the cardiac cycle. If a 49 km h^{-1} (30 mi h^{-1}) projectile impact occurs during a 20-ms window on the upslope of the T wave, approximately 30% of strikes will initiate VF. Impacts occurring outside of this narrow window, but still on the upslope of the T-wave, trigger VF only in 5% of cases, while blows at all other times of the cardiac cycle (including the down-slope of the T wave) do not result in VF.[224] Also of note, non-sustained bursts of VF are occasionally induced, as well as transient complete heart block. Non-sustained VF always terminated within 10 s (once it persisted >10 s, defibrillation

was required), and heart block was never permanent (usually lasted < 5 beats). These non-sustained arrhythmic episodes may account for cases of *CC* in which collapse after the chest blow is transient, and recovery occurs spontaneously within 10 to 20 s.[220]

Other important variables predisposing to *CC* include the site and velocity of the chest blow. For example, VF will not occur with a chest blow outside of the cardiac silhouette, while impacts at the center of the cardiac silhouette are most likely to provoke VF. Impacts near the base and the apex only occasionally trigger VF; at all other sites on the chest, including the right and left thorax and back, blows will not induce VF.[225] *CC* events occur over a wide range of velocities in humans, ranging from minor blows to impacts from hockey pucks or lacrosse balls, at impact velocities of up to 160 km h^{-1} (100 mi h^{-1}). Of note, in the above porcine model, when the velocity of impacts is increased to 65 km h^{-1} (40 mi h^{-1}), the frequency of VF increases dramatically, up to 70%. On raising impact velocity further to 80–110 km h^{-1} (50–70 mi h^{-1}), however, VF becomes *less* frequent, despite an increased occurrence of cardiac structural damage.[226] The mechanism for decreased vulnerability for *CC* at particularly high impact velocities is unresolved, but it may be related to the requirement for a critical mass of myocardial tissue that is *not* affected by the mechanical stimulus to sustain re-entrant arrhythmias, reduced overall heterogeneity with increasing impact strength, or possibly to critical LV pressure changes produced by the chest wall blow.

Immediately following impact, segmental and transient wall motion abnormalities were observed at the apex, a region distant from the area of precordial impact.[223] Immediate (within 60 s) coronary angiography did not reveal any epicardial coronary artery abnormalities,[223] thereby directly contradicting the "coronary vasospasm" theory of Schlomka.[222]

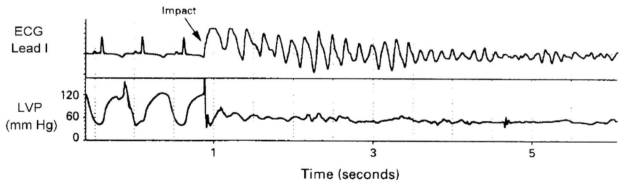

Fig. 65.27. ECG (lead I, top) and left ventricular pressure recording (LVP, bottom), obtained from an anesthetized pig, subjected to a precordial impact that coincided with the upstroke of the T-wave. Note the swiftness of mechanical induction of VF and loss of contractility (within one cardiac cycle). (With permission from ref. 223.)

Cellular mechanisms of *CC*

In humans and in experimental models it appears that VF, initiated by a chest wall blow, may underlie SCD observed in the context of *CC*. Induction of VF by a chest blow in the absence of structural damage to the heart is a primary electrical event, rather than secondary to other factors such as structural heart block, myocardial ischemia, or hemorrhage. Given the swift electrical response to an impact, *CC* is likely to act via effects on cardiac ion channels.

Myocardial stretch is a probable contributor to the VF in *CC*,[227] potentially mediated via an increase in LV pressure,[225,226] as peak probability of VF was seen at LV pressures between 250 and 450 mmHg. The rapid rise in ventricular pressure observed in this setting may mediate ion channel activation via myocardial stretch, compression, membrane deformation, or possibly by direct action on the ion channels themselves.

Because of certain electrical similarities between *CC* and myocardial ischemia, such as ST segment elevation, a possible contributor is the K^+_{ATP} channel. This is particularly plausible since, on the one hand, K^+_{ATP} channels are understood to be primarily responsible for ST segment elevation and to affect the risk of VF in myocardial ischemia,[228] while the same channel population is also mechanosensitive.[229] Indeed, glibenclamide (a blocker of K^+_{ATP} channels), reduces the magnitude of ST segment elevation with QRS strikes, and the incidence of VF following strikes at the upstroke of the T-wave,[230] suggesting that activation of this channel by chest wall impact is critical for the initiation and/or maintenance of VF in *CC*.

Other channels[231] may be activated by myocardial stretch, and in this way underlie the genesis of ventricular arrhythmias following chest blows. Cation non-selective stretch-activated channels (SAC) in particular would seem to be likely candidates for the initiation of VF with chest wall blows[227] since their activation causes depolarization that may trigger AP in resting cardiomyocytes.[232] This theory has recently been addressed in a randomized and blinded study, with streptomycin, a convenient blocker of SAC in isolated myocytes (at 40 μM; at higher concentrations streptomycin also blocks L-type calcium channels and several potassium channels).[233] In whole animal experiments, streptomycin had no significant effect on the frequency of VF induction, yet the magnitude of ST segment elevation was depressed by the drug.

Interestingly, a recent report highlights the ambiguity of streptomycin effects in native tissue, and suggests that SAC (but not L-type calcium channels) may be protected *in situ* from the blocking effect of streptomycin.[235] An alternative drug to dissect the possible role of SAC *in situ* would be GsMTx-4, a peptide isolated from the Chilean tarantula toxin, which has been shown to be highly selective and efficient in blocking mechanically promoted AF in isolated heart.[236] Its limited availability and exceedingly high cost make whole animal experiments with this drug difficult, but with the emergence of isolated heart models of CC,[234] it is to be hoped that this concern will be addressed in the not too distant future (Fig. 65.28).

Illicit substance abuse

Sudden unexpected death, non-fatal stroke, and acute myocardial infarction in trained athletes have been attributed to the abuse of cocaine, anabolic steroids, and dietary and nutritional supplements.[237,238] Dietary supplements such as ma huang (*Ephedra sinica*), a herbal source of ephedrine, which is a potentially arrhythmogenic cardiac stimulant, are also often taken to enhance athletic performance.[238] Ephedra was initially found in a Neolithic grave in the Middle East, which may indicate that Ephedra was used as a medicine more than 60 000 years ago. In China, Ephedra was the first herbal remedy to yield an active

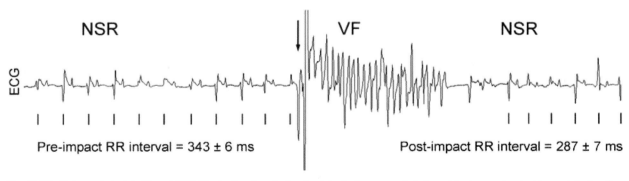

Fig. 65.28. Guinea pig isolated heart ECG, illustrating the electrophysiological response to left ventricular mechanical impact during the T-wave. The stimulus (arrow) causes a short run of ventricular fibrillation (VF), preceded and followed by normal sinus rhythm (NSR). (With permission, ref. 234.)

constituent, in this case ephedrine. Causal linkage between the use of dietary supplements and cardiovascular events is largely inferential, based on a close temporal relation between the ingestion of the compound and adverse events in otherwise healthy people (see also http://www.ncbi.nlm.nih.gov/books/bv.fcgi?rid=hstat1a. section.41090).

Cocaine

With more than 30 million Americans having tried cocaine at least once, and with a reported 5 million regular users,[239] a better understanding of the magnitude of this cardiac risk is important from a public health perspective.

Illicit use of cocaine is often associated with acute cardiovascular events, including stroke, myocardial infarction, coronary thrombosis, arrhythmia, and SD.[237] Cocaine induces an increase in the three major determinants of myocardial oxygen demand: heart rate, systemic arterial pressure, and LV contractility. At the same time, the ingestion of even small amounts of the drug causes vasoconstriction of epicardial coronary arteries.[240] Cocaine also increases endothelial production of endothelin[241] and decreases production of nitric oxide[242] – effects that may cause or enhance vasoconstriction.

In addition to vasoconstriction, cocaine may induce thrombus formation in the coronary arteries.[243] Its use is associated with enhanced platelet activation and aggregability[244] as well as increases in the concentration of plasminogen-activator inhibitor,[245] which may contribute to thrombogenesis. Taken together, these concomitant factors explain why cocaine has been associated with an increased risk of a myocardial infarction (24 times) in the first hour after its use in persons who are otherwise at low risk.[246]

Long-term cocaine abuse has been reported to cause LV hypertrophy[247] and systolic dysfunction. Several reports have described DCM in long-term cocaine users, as well as reversible, profound myocardial depression after binge cocaine use.[248] Moreover, chronic cocaine ingestion presents a clinical and pathological profile similar to myocarditis.[18]

The profound repetitive sympathetic stimulation induced by cocaine bears comparison with that observed in patients with pheochromocytoma; both are associated with cardiomyopathy and characteristic microscopic changes of subendocardial contraction band necrosis.[216] Finally, the concomitant administration of drugs and infectious agents may cause myocarditis or endocarditis, which has been seen on occasion in postmortem studies of intravenous cocaine users.[215,249]

Anabolic steroids, dietary and nutritional supplements (particularly ephedrine-containing compounds)

Several reports link the adverse response of ma huang to concurrent use of caffeine, guarana (a source of caffeine and theophylline) or exercise.[238] Moreover, over the last few years, several studies examining substance use patterns, particularly among student populations, have shown an increase in use of steroids abuse.[250,251]

The real incidence of androgenic anabolic steroids is difficult to evaluate, but it has been suggested that more than 1 million Americans are current or former users.[252] Unfavorable cardiovascular events have been linked to both cocaine and anabolic-androgenic steroid abuse in healthy, physically active individuals. Steroid intake has been associated with vascular complications,[253] cardiomyopathy,[254] coronary atherosclerosis,[255] and cardiac hypertrophy,[256] and in several clinical reports, intake was associated with acute myocardial infarction.[257,258]

Despite the above indications, only 9 SCD cases had been examined and confirmed at autopsy by 2001.[259] The mechanism proposed for SCD in athlete consumers of anabolic-androgenic steroids is related to the adrenergic stress imposed to the heart, which is documented by the extensive early contraction band necrosis, triggered by terminal physical efforts.[260]

Athletes taking anabolic steroids tend to have increased QT intervals and an increase in QT dispersion, contributing to an increased risk of arrhythmic events.[261] Moreover, endomyocardial biopsy specimens have revealed increased fibrous tissue and fat droplets in the myocardium of anabolic steroid abusers.[262]

Even if the cause-effect relationship among anabolic-androgenic steroids, body-building, and myocardial infarction currently lacks solid clinical evidence, the concept of cardiac arrest caused by catecholamine myotoxicity, associated with VF, is supported by an experimental study in which anabolic steroids, administered in combination with exercise training, induced degenerative changes within the intracardiac sympathetic neurons of the mouse.[263] It is not surprising, therefore, that concomitant abuse of anabolic steroids and cocaine greatly enhances the risk of cardiovascular events. Indeed, testosterone at concentrations that have no effect on their own can potentiate the cocaine effect on endothelial and platelet functions.[264]

Healthcare implications

Physical inactivity and a sedentary lifestyle have been recognized as risk factors for the development or progression of coronary heart disease and for adverse cardiovascular and non-cardiovascular events and death.[1,265] Further-more, regular aerobic exercise and fitness have many cardiovascular benefits in both men and women,[266,267] and reduce the risk of fatal or non-fatal myocardial infarction, as well as other coronary events.[1,265] Accordingly, regular exercise is being regarded as a means of primary and secondary prevention of CAD and, consequently, promoted (regardless of age) as a public health goal.[265]

Nonetheless, the consequences of exercise are more complex than they might seem at first, since vigorous physical exertion can be regarded as a two-edged sword.[268] Besides offering protection from coronary events and SCD in those who regularly engage in exercise, it can simultaneously increase the short-term risk of SD or myocardial infarction, particularly in persons who are not accustomed to regular exercise ("weekend warriors").[269,270] Indeed, a case-crossover cohort study confirmed a 17-fold increase in SCD during vigorous exercise, compared to lower levels of activity or inactive states.[268] The absolute risk for events was very low (1 event per 1.5 million exercise sessions), however, and an active lifestyle with habitual vigorous exercise markedly attenuated the risk (probably via blunting the transient risk of SD associated with occasional intense exertion).

A mechanism suggested to underlie the exercise-induced risk is activation of the sympathetic nervous system during physical exertion, which can destabilize vulnerable atherosclerotic plaques or, on the ground of a susceptible myocardium, including exercise-induced rhythm disturbances, trigger fatal arrhythmias.[271]

In contrast, regular modest physical activity enhances myocardial electrical stability by promoting a higher vagal tone, hence raising the threshold of VF (exceptions include Brugada syndrome patients).

Sports participation screening

Recently the European Society of Cardiology (ESC) released a consensus statement[56] recommending systematic cardiovascular pre-participation screening of young competitive athletes for the timely detection of cardiovascular abnormalities predisposing to sport-related cardiac death. Following a previous consensus statement from the American Heart Association,[88] the ESC has promoted a standard for medical evaluation of competitive athletes. The recommended protocol for pre-participation cardiovascular screening includes a 12-lead ECG in addition to medical history and physical examination (Fig. 65.29), which is the only screening modality proven to be effective in identifying athletes with HCM, and preventing SD.[4,8]

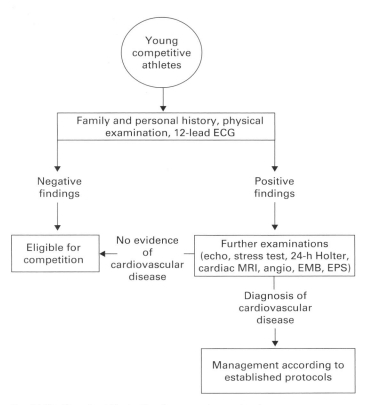

Fig. 65.29. Flowchart illustrating the screening protocol proposed by the European Society of Cardiology. The initial cardiovascular protocol includes family and personal history, physical examination with determination of blood pressure, and basal 12-lead ECG. Additional tests, such as echocardiography, 24-h Holter monitoring, or stress testing and cardiac MRI are requested only for subjects who had positive findings at the initial evaluation. In uncertain cases, invasive tests such as contrast ventriculography (both right and left), coronary angiography, endomyocardial biopsy, and electrophysiological study may be necessary in order to confirm (or rule out) the diagnosis of cardiovascular disease. Athletes diagnosed with clinically relevant cardiovascular abnormalities are managed according to available guidelines for assessing athletic risk. Angio, angiography EMB, endomyocardial biopsy; EPS, electrophysiological study; MRI, magnetic resonance imaging; SAECG, signal-averaged ECG. (With permission from ref. 56.)

The proposed strategy builds on the Italian experience of mandatory and government-sponsored medical evaluations, in which six million athletes participating in organized sports (~10% of the Italian population) are screened *annually* by specially trained and certified sports medicine physicians.[8,20] This initiative has derived numerous benefits for athletes, including recognition of the additive

Table 65.6. Cardiovascular conditions responsible for disqualification from competitive sports in 621 athletes in Padua, 1979 to 1996

Condition	Number (%)
Rhythm and conduction abnormalities	238 (38.3)
Systemic hypertension	168 (27.1)
Valvular diseases (including mitral-valve prolapse)	133 (21.4)
Hypertrophic cardiomyopathy	22 (3.5)
Others	60 (9.7)

With permission from ref. 8.

diagnostic power of the ECG in identifying certain cardiac disease risks, particularly HCM.[8] Similar results have also been observed in large populations of young military recruits in Italy with use of the same protocol (with an ECG).[272]

Corrado *et al*.[8] reported the 17-year experience from the Center for Sports Medicine of Padua. During the period of 1979–1996, a consecutive series of 33 735 young athletes (≤35 years) underwent pre-participation cardiovascular evaluation. Of these, 1058 were disqualified for medical reasons: 621 (1.8%) because of clinically relevant cardiovascular abnormalities. The most frequent disqualifying conditions were rhythm and conduction abnormalities (38.3%); hypertension (27%); valvular diseases (21.4%); and HCM (3.6%; Table 65.6). Less frequent reasons for non-eligibility included DCM, congenital and rheumatic heart diseases, and pericarditis.

Of the 33 735 athletes initially screened, 3016 (8.9%) were referred for echocardiographic evaluation because of their family history, abnormal physical findings, or ECG abnormalities.[8] Twenty-two had definite evidence of HCM on echocardiographic examination. No significant differences in the degree of LV hypertrophy were seen before and after deconditioning. None of the 22 athletes who were disqualified because they had HCM died during the follow-up period.

Studies from the US have consistently identified HCM as the most common cause of cardiac arrest in young competitive athletes (up to 30%),[7,273] whereas in the Italian cohort of athletes HCM caused only one death. At the same time, the prevalence of HCM among young non-athletes who died suddenly was comparable between Italy and the US.[8,274] This provides indirect but strong evidence to suggest that screening reduces SD from HCM by reducing the prevalence of HCM among athletes.

Pre-participation cardiovascular screening has traditionally been performed (in the US) by medical history and physical examination, but without 12-lead ECG or other non-invasive testing, which are requested largely at the discretion of the examining physician.[88,275] This screening method has been recommended by the Sudden Death and Congenital Defects Committee of the American Heart Association on the assumption that 12-lead ECG is not cost-effective for screening a large population of young athletes, because of its low specificity.[88] The above screening strategy, however, may have a limited power to detect potentially lethal cardiovascular abnormalities in young athletes. One retrospective analysis of 134 high school and collegiate athletes who died suddenly showed that cardiovascular abnormalities were suspected by standard history and physical examination screening in only 3% of the examined athletes and, eventually, less than 1% received an accurate diagnosis.[7]

The Italian screening modality has proved more sensitive than the current US protocol. Among the 22 Italian athletes (20 males and 2 females, aged 20 ± 4 years) who were identified and disqualified because they had HCM,[8] 82% had shown ECG changes at pre-participation evaluation, which included repolarization abnormalities (87.5%), elevated QRS precordial voltages (69%), and abnormal Q waves (31%). Moreover, premature ventricular beats were recorded in 5 (23%). It is noteworthy that only 5 of these 22 athletes (23%) had a positive family history, a cardiac murmur, or both, at pre-participation evaluation. These findings indicate that the Italian screening modality, including 12-lead ECG, has 77% greater power for detecting HCM, and it is expected to result in a corresponding additional number of lives saved, compared with the AHA-endorsed protocol. Taking into account this difference in diagnostic power, a three times greater cost-effectiveness has been estimated for the Italian screening strategy (compared to the US) for identification and prevention of SD of athletes with HCM alone.[276,277]

On the basis of currently available data, addition of echocardiography would not seem significantly to improve efficacy of the pre-participation screening in identifying HCM. As reported by Pelliccia *et al*.[278] routine echocardiographic examination did not identify any additional HCM case among 4450 athletes previously cleared by ECG at pre-participation evaluation. There are also several limitations that undermine echocardiographic recognition of ARVC, in particular the technical difficulty in visualizing the right ventricle and in assessing its function along with the existence of a wide age range and pathological features including minor and localized structural abnormalities which may nevertheless act as substrate for lethal arrhythmias.[279]

The 12-lead ECG, in contrast, offers the potential to detect, or raise clinical suspicion of, other lethal conditions, such as ARVC, DCM, LQTS, Brugada syndrome, SQTS, and WPW syndrome. Overall, these conditions, including HCM, account for up to 60% of SD in young competitive athletes.[4,7,8,18]

Tools and targets for pre-participation screening will continue to be developed further over time, and their impact on mortality should be reassessed regularly. For example, the Italian screening for ARVC showed that 82% of athletes who died from this disease had a history of syncope, ECG changes consisting of inverted T waves in the right precordial leads, and/or ventricular arrhythmias with a left bundle-branch block pattern.[8] These athletes were not identified at earlier pre-participation screening, however, since ARVC was discovered relatively recently (two decades ago) and remained underdiagnosed or was regarded with skepticism by cardiologists.[280] The number of athletes with ARVC identified and disqualified from active competition significantly increased throughout 1992 to 2001, compared to the previous decade.[277]

Socioeconomic impact

Screening of large athletic populations may have a significant socioeconomic impact. Strategies for implementing the proposed screening program depend on the specific socioeconomic and cultural background as well as on the medical systems in place in different countries. The Italian experience indicates that a comprehensive screening program that includes 12-lead ECG is feasible, with the side effect of reduced cost of 12-lead ECG in a setting of mass screening. The cost of performing a pre-participation cardiac history/physical examination by qualified physicians has been estimated to be 20 Euros per athlete; this rises to 30 Euros per athlete if the 12-lead ECG is added. In Italy, the screening cost is covered by the athlete or by his team, except for athletes under 18 years of age, for whom the expense is sustained by the National Health System. Costs of infrastructure and training courses for pre-participation screening are not included in this calculation, and introducing a comprehensive coverage will increase cost.

Diagnostic challenges: athlete's heart vs. cardiovascular disease

Structural changes

Regular physical training leads to cardiovascular adaptations including both structural and functional changes, which are referred to as "athlete's heart." Modifications include structural remodeling, an increase in LV cavity size

and wall thickness by 10–20%, and an increase in LV mass by up to 45% with preservation of systolic and diastolic function.[281] The abnormal cardiac dimensions associated with athletic training are normally scaled to body-surface area or lean body mass and are usually less pronounced in female athletes.[281,282]

This physiological form of hypertrophy is regarded as a benign adaptation to systematic athletic training, with no overt adverse cardiovascular consequences.[56,283] Other physiological adaptations to training include a variety of abnormal patterns on 12-lead ECG in about 40% of athletes,[284] some of which resemble cardiac diseases, namely increased voltages, Q waves, and repolarization abnormalities.[284]

The magnitude of physiological remodeling may be such that in some highly trained individuals it may pose a challenge for differential diagnosis from cardiac diseases such as HCM and ARVC (Fig. 65.30).[32,281,285] A distinction between physiological adaptation to exertion and cardiac disease is important since in the attempt to minimize the risk of SD, identification of cardiovascular disease translates into disqualification from further competitive sports participation,[56,136] so that both false-positive and false-negative findings are undesirable.

Several studies have evaluated methods to differentiate between HCM and physiological hypertrophy of the athlete's heart,[32] often non-invasively by assessing the reduction of cardiac mass after short periods of deconditioning (usually 3 months),[286,286] or by echocardiographic measurement of diastolic filling.[32] Further support, in particular to avoid false-negative identification of cardiac disease, may come from evaluation of family history.[287] The absence of HCM in relatives does not exclude the diagnosis, however, since the disease may be the result of a *de novo* mutation responsible for the "sporadic" form.[288]

In general, HCM patients have localized hypertrophy with reduced cavity dimensions and evidence of impaired diastolic function, whereas athletes develop symmetric hypertrophy and have normal or slightly increased LV cavity dimensions (Table 65.7). A small LV cavity dimension, enlarged left atrial diameter, abnormal diastolic filling pattern, pathologic Q waves, and ST–T abnormalities on the ECG are suggestive of HCM, whereas supranormal metabolic exercise indices, such as peak oxygen consumption >50 ml/kg per min or >20%, are most likely secondary to physiological hypertrophy.[289] Metabolic indices of exercise provide a useful tool for differentiating between physiologic hypertrophy and HCM since they are abnormal in most patients affected by HCM regardless of the magnitude of hypertrophy.[289]

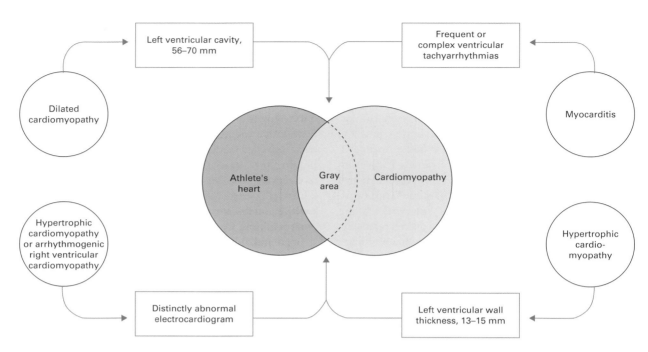

Fig. 65.30. Gray area of overlap between athlete's heart and cardiomyopathies, including myocarditis, hypertrophic cardiomyopathy and arrhythmogenic right ventricular cardiomyopathy. (With permission from ref. 18.)

Functional changes

Physical activity increases vagal tone.[290] This enhanced parasympathetic activity is held responsible for a variety of arrhythmias and conduction alterations observed in elite athletes, which include premature atrial and ventricular beats, supraventricular tachycardia, junctional rhythm, and first-degree AV block (Mobitz type I). Alternatively, intense endurance training has been shown to shift autonomic modulation from parasympathetic to sympathetic predominance,[291] which may predispose to an electrical instability of the ventricles and eventually trigger ventricular tachyarrhythmias.[292] Several ambulatory Holter studies have shown a higher prevalence of ventricular ectopic beats (70%) and frequent and/or complex forms (25% to 63%), such as non-sustained VT and couplets, in athletic populations.[283,293]

Arrhythmias can be a marker of heart disease and therefore generate appropriate concern when observed in athletes. Indeed, the clinical assessment and interpretation of such arrhythmias may be difficult, since this may be the only expression of potentially lethal cardiac diseases (such as ARVC), myocarditis or even substance abuse.[213,237,283] It has been generally accepted that when frequent and/or complex ventricular ectopic beats are detected in apparently healthy persons who are thoroughly examined

non-invasively and are found free of structural heart disease, it is a benign condition with a favorable prognosis.[293] A large study on almost 16 000 athletes seems confirmatory and extends that observation to extensively trained young adults.[283] Of the 355 athletes who had >3 premature ventricular contractions on 12-lead ECG or a history of palpitations, only 7% harbored structural cardiovascular abnormalities. Nonetheless, structural heart disease was 15 times more frequent in athletes with frequent and complex VT than in those with less severe arrhythmias.

Reversibility

The extreme alterations in cardiac dimensions evident in some athletes have inevitably raised the question of whether such exercise-related adaptations are truly physiological and benign. Reverse LV remodeling is evident after long-term detraining (deconditioning), with significant reduction in cavity size and normalization of wall thickness. Regression in cavity dimension and/or wall thickness typically occurs within weeks to months after cessation of competitive activity.[285] A longitudinal echocardiographic study, however, showed incomplete reversal and substantial residual dilatation of the chambers in 20% of retired, deconditioned athletes.[294] Similarly, LV mass remained

Table 65.7. Echocardiographic features of athlete's heart and HCM

	Athlete's heart	HCM
Maximal left ventricular wall thickness (mm)	< 16	≥ 16
LVH pattern	Concentric	ASH/variable
Left ventricular cavity size	Large	Small
Diastolic function	Normal	Impaired
Left atrial size	Normal	Dilated

ASH, Asymmetrical septal hypertrophy; LVH, left ventricular hypertrophy.
With permission from ref. 129.

increased in about half of the former athletes.[294] Although firm evidence is lacking, we cannot exclude the possibility that extreme ventricular remodeling associated with intense exercise-related conditioning may represent an irreversible consequence and may have adverse clinical consequences in the long term.[294,295] Unfortunately, detraining is not usually monitored as efficiently as is active athletic performance, which may contribute to incomplete deconditioning and deficient reverse remodeling.

Reversibility of arrhythmias after deconditioning was observed both in athletes with and without cardiovascular abnormalities.[286] Biffi *et al.*[286] assessed the impact of deconditioning on ventricular arrhythmias in 70 athletes who had ≥2000 premature ventricular contractions per day and/or bursts of non-sustained VT on ambulatory ECG recording. After a deconditioning period of at least 3 months, a second 24-h recording demonstrated a clear reduction in arrhythmias for the group overall. Total premature ventricular contraction frequency decreased by 80%, couplets decreased by 80%, and the number of non-sustained VT episodes decreased by 90%. Reversibility of arrhythmia with deconditioning did not, however, always indicate absence of structural heart disease: 26% of patients who showed a clear decrease in ectopy had heart diseases, including mitral valve prolapse, myocarditis, DCM, and ARVC. In athletes with heart disease, resolution of arrhythmias after detraining could explain the mechanism by which the restriction of these athletes from competition may reduce their risk for SCD. Conversely, in athletes without cardiovascular abnormalities, the reversibility of ventricular tachyarrhythmias and the absence of cardiac events in the follow-up period support the benign clinical nature of these arrhythmias as a functional expression of athlete's heart.[286]

Medicolegal implications

Once a cardiovascular abnormality is diagnosed, the recommendations of the 26th Bethesda Conference offer clear criteria by which athletes should be withdrawn from sports competition.[296] The rationale for guidelines on sports eligibility or disqualification is the evidence that intense training and competition increases the risk of SD in those athletes who harbor cardiovascular diseases and, most importantly, that this risk is reduced after withdrawal from athletic competition.[4,8,88,297]

Given the extreme diversity of conditions to which competitive athletes are exposed and the intrinsic variability of each cardiovascular disease, the precise risk of SD to which a single individual is exposed cannot be identified with certainty. Therefore, elite athletes with heart disease may not appreciate the beneficial implications of medical advice, and rather accept the risks than abandon their professional career.[297,298] Also, disqualification of athletes with cardiovascular disease may be difficult to implement.[297–299]

An already difficult medical decision may be further influenced by pressures exerted on the physician by the athletes, their family members, team coaches, and potential sponsors. Athletes may also solicit multiple medical opinions in attempts to regain eligibility (circumventing diagnosis).[299] At the same time, waivers of responsibility that athletes may be willing to sign may not be recognized as ethically and legally binding.[296,297] A precedent for resolving medicolegal disputes comes from the US where an appellate court[297] ruled that guidelines such as the Bethesda Conference report[296] can be used by physicians to formulate appropriate decisions about an athlete's eligibility.

Recommendations for the eligibility of athletes without cardiovascular abnormalities, but with frequent and/or complex ventricular tachyarrhythmias, currently are not available. It is nevertheless common practice to withdraw such athletes for 3 to 6 months and then re-evaluate with ambulatory Holter ECG monitoring. If the frequency of ventricular tachyarrhythmias is significantly reduced or abolished at the end of the detraining period, then athletes are normally allowed to resume training and competition. Close follow-up of such athletes is warranted for the assessment of new symptoms or worsening of arrhythmias.[300]

Conclusions

Regular moderate physical exercise has beneficial cardiovascular effects. Several prospective epidemiological studies consistently associate exercise with a reduced risk of CAD and SCD. Despite the general health benefit of regular exercise, young athletes can have a higher incidence of SD than age-matched non-athletes. In young athletes, a variety of cardiac diseases, largely congenital and often rare, account for the majority of SCD. Sports activity triggers manifestation of underlying cardiovascular diseases, predisposing athletes to life-threatening ventricular arrhythmias during physical exercise. It is therefore not *per se* a cause of the increased mortality.

In most US reports that include autopsy data, HCM is the most common underlying disease linked to these deaths. In contrast, HCM is uncommon in Italian studies of SD on the athletic field. A probable reason for this difference is the compulsory pre-participation screening of young athletes in Italy, which leads to early exclusion of HCM sufferers from competitive sports. Instead, diseases that are more difficult to screen, such as ARVC, have become most common causes of SCD in North Italian athletes.

About 2% of young athletes who die suddenly have normal cardiac structure at autopsy, and no definitive cause of death can be established. The list of congenital and acquired arrhythmias, secondary to mutations or polymorphisms in genes encoding for cardiac ion channels, has expanded impressively in recent years and may be largely responsible for such unexplained deaths. These ion channel disorders include LQTS, SQTS, Brugada syndrome, CPVT, AF, and conduction system disease. SCD may also be secondary to myocarditis, illicit substance abuse, and direct mechanical insults, i.e., CC.

Provided that efficient health screening is implemented, the impact on recreational and competitive sports can be kept to a minimum. In keeping with this view, the European Society of Cardiology has released a consensus statement recommending systematic cardiovascular pre-participation screening of young competitive athletes. The protocol includes a 12-lead ECG in addition to medical history and physical examination, which is the only screening modality proven to be effective in identifying athletes with HCM, and preventing SD. Given the socioeconomic impact strategies for implementing the proposed screening program, success will depend on the specific socio-economic and cultural background, as well as on the medical systems in place in different countries.

REFERENCES

1. Paffenbarger, R.S., Jr., Hyde, R.T., Wing, A.L. *et al.* The association of changes in physical-activity level and other lifestyle characteristics with mortality among men. *N. Engl. J. Med.* 1993; **328**(8): 538–545.

2. Slattery, M.L., Jacobs, D.R., Jr. & Nichaman, M.Z. Leisure time physical activity and coronary heart disease death. The US Railroad Study. *Circulation* 1989; **79**(2): 304–311.

3. Ekelund, L.G., Haskell, W.L., Johnson, J.L. *et al.* Physical fitness as a predictor of cardiovascular mortality in asymptomatic North American men. The Lipid Research Clinics Mortality Follow-up Study. *N. Engl. J. Med.* 1988; **319**(21): 1379–1384.

4. Corrado, D., Basso, C., Rizzoli, G. *et al.* Does sports activity enhance the risk of sudden death in adolescents and young adults? *J. Am. Coll. Cardiol.* 2003; **42**(11): 1959–1963.

5. Myerburg, R.J. Sudden cardiac death: exploring the limits of our knowledge. *J. Cardiovasc. Electrophysiol.* 2001; **12**(3): 369–381.

6. Maron, B.J., Epstein, S.E. & Roberts, W.C. Causes of sudden death in competitive athletes. *J. Am. Coll. Cardiol.* 1986; **7**(1): 204–214.

7. Maron, B.J., Shirani, J., Poliac, L.C. *et al.* Sudden death in young competitive athletes. Clinical, demographic, and pathological profiles. *J. Am. Med. Assoc.* 1996; **276**(3): 199–204.

8. Corrado, D., Basso, C., Schiavon, M. *et al.* Screening for hypertrophic cardiomyopathy in young athletes. *N. Engl. J. Med.* 1998; **339**(6): 364–369.

9. Myerburg, R. & Castellanos, A. Cardiac arrest and sudden cardiac death. In Zipes, D.P., Libby, P., Bonow, R.O. *et al.*, eds. *Heart Disease.* Philadelphia: Elsevier Saunders; 2005: 865–908.

10. Thiene, G., Basso, C. & Corrado, D. Is prevention of sudden death in young athletes feasible? *Cardiologia* 1999; **44**(6): 497–505.

11. Maron, B.J., Gohman, T.E. & Aeppli, D. Prevalence of sudden cardiac death during competitive sports activities in Minnesota high school athletes. *J. Am. Coll. Cardiol.* 1998; **32**(7): 1881–1884.

12. Nava, A., Bauce, B., Basso, C. *et al.* Clinical profile and long-term follow-up of 37 families with arrhythmogenic right ventricular cardiomyopathy. *J. Am. Coll. Cardiol.* 2000; **36**(7): 2226–2233.

13. Corrado, D., Basso, C., Poletti, A. *et al.* Sudden death in the young. Is acute coronary thrombosis the major precipitating factor? *Circulation* 1994; **90**(5): 2315–2323.

14. Di Diego, J.M., Cordeiro, J.M., Goodrow, R.J. *et al.* Ionic and cellular basis for the predominance of the Brugada syndrome phenotype in males. *Circulation* 2002; **106**(15): 2004–2011.

15. Antzelevitch, C. Androgens and male predominance of the Brugada syndrome phenotype. *Pacing Clin. Electrophysiol.* 2003; **26**(7 Pt 1): 1429–1431.

16. Maron, B.J., Carney, K.P., Lever, H.M. *et al.* Relationship of race to sudden cardiac death in competitive athletes with hypertrophic cardiomyopathy. *J. Am. Coll. Cardiol.* 2003; **41**(6): 974–980.

17. Maron, B.J., Moller, J.H., Seidman, C.E. *et al.* Impact of laboratory molecular diagnosis on contemporary diagnostic criteria for genetically transmitted cardiovascular diseases: hypertrophic cardiomyopathy, long-QT syndrome, and marfan syndrome: a statement for healthcare professionals from the councils on clinical cardiology, cardiovascular disease in the young, and basic science, american heart association. *Circulation* 1998; **98**(14): 1460–1471.

18. Maron, B.J. Sudden death in young athletes. *N. Engl. J. Med.* 2003; **349**(11): 1064–1075.

19. Maron, B.J., Poliac, L.C. & Roberts, W.O. Risk for sudden cardiac death associated with marathon running. *J. Am. Coll. Cardiol.* 1996; **28**(2): 428–431.

20. Decree of the Italian Ministry of Health February 18. Norme per la tutela sanitaria dell'attivita' sportiva agonistica (rules concerning the medical protection of athletic activity). *Gazzetta Ufficiale.* 1982; **63**.

21. Bouchama, A. & Knochel, J.P. Heat stroke. *N. Engl. J. Med.* 2002; **346**(25): 1978–1988.

22. Kark, J.A., Posey, D.M., Schumacher, H.R. *et al.* Sickle-cell trait as a risk factor for sudden death in physical training. *N. Engl. J. Med.* 1987; **317**(13): 781–787.

23. Maron, B.J., Gardin, J.M., Flack, J.M. *et al.* Prevalence of hypertrophic cardiomyopathy in a general population of young adults. Echocardiographic analysis of 4111 subjects in the CARDIA Study. Coronary Artery Risk Development in (Young) Adults. *Circulation* 1995; **92**(4): 785–789.

24. Seidman, J.G. & Seidman, C. The genetic basis for cardiomyopathy: from mutation identification to mechanistic paradigms. *Cell* 2001; **104**(4): 557–567.

25. Maron, B.J., Casey, S.A., Hauser, R.G. *et al.* Clinical course of hypertrophic cardiomyopathy with survival to advanced age. *J. Am. Coll. Cardiol.* 2003; **42**(5): 882–888.

26. Spirito, P., Bellone, P., Harris, K.M. *et al.* Magnitude of left ventricular hypertrophy and risk of sudden death in hypertrophic cardiomyopathy. *N. Engl. J. Med.* 2000; **342**(24): 1778–1785.

27. Maron, B.J., Shen, W.K., Link, M.S. *et al.* Efficacy of implantable cardioverter-defibrillators for the prevention of sudden death in patients with hypertrophic cardiomyopathy. *N. Engl. J. Med.* 2000; **342**(6): 365–373.

28. Kofflard, M.J., Ten Cate, F.J., van der Lee, C. *et al.* Hypertrophic cardiomyopathy in a large community-based population: clinical outcome and identification of risk factors for sudden cardiac death and clinical deterioration. *J. Am. Coll. Cardiol.* 2003; **41**(6): 987–993.

29. Maron, B.J. Hypertrophic cardiomyopathy. *Curr. Probl. Cardiol.* 1993; **18**: 637.

30. Maron, B.J. Hypertrophic cardiomyopathy. *Lancet* 1997; **350**(9071): 127–133.

31. Hagege, A.A., Dubourg, O., Desnos, M. *et al.* Familial hypertrophic cardiomyopathy. Cardiac ultrasonic abnormalities in genetically affected subjects without echocardiographic evidence of left ventricular hypertrophy. *Eur. Heart J.* 1998; **19**(3): 490–499.

32. Maron, B.J., Pelliccia, A. & Spirito, P. Cardiac disease in young trained athletes. Insights into methods for distinguishing athlete's heart from structural heart disease, with particular emphasis on hypertrophic cardiomyopathy. *Circulation* 1995; **91**(5): 1596–1601.

33. Pelliccia, A., Maron, B.J., Spataro, A. *et al.* The upper limit of physiologic cardiac hypertrophy in highly trained elite athletes. *N. Engl. J. Med.* 1991; **324**(5): 295–301.

34. Braunwald, E., Morrow, A.G. & Cornell, W.P. Idiopathic hypertrophic subaortic stenosis: Clinical, hemodynamic and angiographic manifestations. *Am. J. Med.* 1960; **29**: 924–928.

35. Wigle, E.D., Rakowski, H., Kimball, B.P. *et al.* Hypertrophic cardiomyopathy. Clinical spectrum and treatment. *Circulation* 1995; **92**(7): 1680–1692.

36. Sherrid, M.V., Chu, C.K., Delia, E. *et al.* An echocardiographic study of the fluid mechanics of obstruction in hypertrophic cardiomyopathy. *J. Am. Coll. Cardiol.* 1993; **22**(3): 816–825.

37. Spirito, P., Seidman, C.E., McKenna, W.J. *et al.* The management of hypertrophic cardiomyopathy. *N. Engl. J. Med.* 1997; **336**(11): 775–785.

38. Doshi, S.N., Kim, M.C. & Sharma, S.K. Images in cardiovascular medicine. Right and left ventricular outflow tract obstruction in hypertrophic cardiomyopathy. *Circulation* 2002; **106**: e3.

39. Maron, M.S., Olivotto, I., Betocchi, S. *et al.* Effect of left ventricular outflow tract obstruction on clinical outcome in hypertrophic cardiomyopathy. *N. Engl. J. Med.* 2003; **348**(4): 295–303.

40. Maron, B.J., McKenna, W.J., Danielson, G.K. *et al.* American College of Cardiology/European Society of Cardiology Clinical Expert Consensus Document on Hypertrophic Cardiomyopathy. A report of the American College of Cardiology Foundation Task Force on Clinical Expert Consensus Documents and the European Society of Cardiology Committee for Practice Guidelines. *Eur. Heart J.* 2003; **24**(21): 1965–1991.

41. Klues, H.G., Schiffers, A. & Maron, B.J. Phenotypic spectrum and patterns of left ventricular hypertrophy in hypertrophic cardiomyopathy: morphologic observations and significance as assessed by two-dimensional echocardiography in 600 patients. *J. Am. Coll. Cardiol.* 1995; **26**(7): 1699–1708.

42. Maron, B.J., Anan, T.J. & Roberts, W.C. Quantitative analysis of the distribution of cardiac muscle cell disorganization in the left ventricular wall of patients with hypertrophic cardiomyopathy. *Circulation* 1981; **63**(4): 882–894.

43. Tanaka, M., Fujiwara, H., Onodera, T. *et al.* Quantitative analysis of narrowings of intramyocardial small arteries in normal hearts, hypertensive hearts, and hearts with hypertrophic cardiomyopathy. *Circulation* 1987; **75**(6): 1130–1139.

44. Shirani, J., Pick, R., Roberts, W.C. *et al.* Morphology and significance of the left ventricular collagen network in young

patients with hypertrophic cardiomyopathy and sudden cardiac death. *J. Am. Coll. Cardiol.* 2000; **35**(1): 36–44.

45. Krams, R., Kofflard, M.J., Duncker, D.J. *et al.* Decreased coronary flow reserve in hypertrophic cardiomyopathy is related to remodeling of the coronary microcirculation. *Circulation* 1998; **97**(3): 230–233.

46. Basso, C., Thiene, G., Corrado, D. *et al.* Hypertrophic cardiomyopathy and sudden death in the young: pathologic evidence of myocardial ischemia. *Hum. Pathol.* 2000; **31**(8): 988–998.

47. Briguori, C., Betocchi, S., Romano, M. *et al.* Exercise capacity in hypertrophic cardiomyopathy depends on left ventricular diastolic function. *Am. J. Cardiol.* 1999; **84**(3): 309–315.

48. Sadoul, N., Prasad, K., Elliott, P.M. *et al.* Prospective prognostic assessment of blood pressure response during exercise in patients with hypertrophic cardiomyopathy. *Circulation* 1997; **96**(9): 2987–2991.

49. Olivotto, I., Cecchi, F., Casey, S.A. *et al.* Impact of atrial fibrillation on the clinical course of hypertrophic cardiomyopathy. *Circulation* 2001; **104**(21): 2517–2524.

50. Cecchi, F., Maron, B.J. & Epstein, S.E. Long-term outcome of patients with hypertrophic cardiomyopathy successfully resuscitated after cardiac arrest. *J. Am. Coll. Cardiol.* 1989; **13**(6): 1283–1288.

51. Cecchi, F., Olivotto, I., Montereggi, A. *et al.* Prognostic value of non-sustained ventricular tachycardia and the potential role of amiodarone treatment in hypertrophic cardiomyopathy: assessment in an unselected non-referral based patient population. *Heart* 1998; **79**(4): 331–336.

52. Day, C.P., McComb, J.M. & Campbell, R.W. QT dispersion in sinus beats and ventricular extrasystoles in normal hearts. *Br. Heart J.* 1992; **67**(1): 39–41.

53. Miorelli, M., Buja, G., Melacini, P. *et al.* QT-interval variability in hypertrophic cardiomyopathy patients with cardiac arrest. *Int. J. Cardiol.* 1994; **45**(2): 121–127.

54. Buja, G., Miorelli, M., Turrini, P. *et al.* Comparison of QT dispersion in hypertrophic cardiomyopathy between patients with and without ventricular arrhythmias and sudden death. *Am. J. Cardiol.* 1993; **72**(12): 973–976.

55. Maron, B.J., Chaitman, B.R., Ackerman, M.J. *et al.* Recommendations for physical activity and recreational sports participation for young patients with genetic cardiovascular diseases. *Circulation* 2004; **109**(22): 2807–2816.

56. Corrado, D., Pelliccia, A., Bjornstad, H.H. *et al.* Cardiovascular pre-participation screening of young competitive athletes for prevention of sudden death: proposal for a common European protocol: Consensus Statement of the Study Group of Sport Cardiology of the Working Group of Cardiac Rehabilitation and Exercise Physiology and the Working Group of Myocardial and Pericardial Diseases of the European Society of Cardiology. *Eur. Heart J.* 2005.

57. Ostman-Smith, I., Wettrell, G. & Riesenfeld, T. A cohort study of childhood hypertrophic cardiomyopathy: improved survival following high-dose beta-adrenoceptor antagonist treatment. *J. Am. Coll. Cardiol.* 1999; **34**(6): 1813–1822.

58. Gregoratos, G., Abrams, J., Epstein, A.E. *et al.* ACC/AHA/NASPE 2002 Guideline Update for Implantation of Cardiac Pacemakers and Antiarrhythmia Devices – summary article: a report of the American College of Cardiology/American Heart Association Task Force on Practice Guidelines (ACC/AHA/NASPE Committee to Update the 1998 Pacemaker Guidelines). *J. Am. Coll. Cardiol.* 2002; **40**(9): 1703–1719.

59. Morrow, A.G., Reitz, B.A., Epstein, S.E. *et al.* Operative treatment in hypertrophic subaortic stenosis. Techniques, and the results of pre and postoperative assessments in 83 patients. *Circulation* 1975; **52**(1): 88–102.

60. Dalla Volta, S., Battaglia, G. & Zerbini, E. "Auricularization" of right ventricular pressure curve. *Am. Heart J.* 1961; **61**: 25–33.

61. Berder, V., Vauthier, M., Mabo, P. *et al.* Characteristics and outcome in arrhythmogenic right ventricular dysplasia. *Am. J. Cardiol.* 1995; **75**(5): 411–414.

62. Maron, B.J. Right ventricular cardiomyopathy: another cause of sudden death in the young. *N. Engl. J. Med.* 1988; **318**(3): 178–180.

63. Pinamonti, B., Sinagra, G., Salvi, A. *et al.* Left ventricular involvement in right ventricular dysplasia. *Am. Heart J.* 1992; **123**(3): 711–724.

64. Richardson, P., McKenna, W., Bristow, M. *et al.* Report of the 1995 World Health Organization/International Society and Federation of Cardiology Task Force on the Definition and Classification of cardiomyopathies. *Circulation* 1996; **93**(5): 841–842.

65. Basso, C., Thiene, G., Corrado, D. *et al.* Arrhythmogenic right ventricular cardiomyopathy. Dysplasia, dystrophy, or myocarditis? *Circulation* 1996; **94**(5): 983–991.

66. Corrado, D., Basso, C., Nava, A. *et al.* Arrhythmogenic right ventricular cardiomyopathy: Current diagnostic and management strategies. *Cardiol. Rev.* 2001; **9**(5): 259–265.

67. Corrado, D., Basso, C., Thiene, G. *et al.* Spectrum of clinicopathologic manifestations of arrhythmogenic right ventricular cardiomyopathy/dysplasia: a multicenter study. *J. Am. Coll. Cardiol.* 1997; **30**(6): 1512–1520.

68. Nava, A., Martini, B., Thiene, G. *et al.* [Arrhythmogenic right ventricular dysplasia. Study of a selected population]. *G. Ital. Cardiol.* 1988; **18**(1): 2–9.

69. Nava, A., Canciani, B., Buja, G. *et al.* Electrovectorcardiographic study of negative T waves on precordial leads in arrhythmogenic right ventricular dysplasia: relationship with right ventricular volumes. *J. Electrocardiol.* 1988; **21**(3): 239–245.

70. Angelini, A., Thiene, G., Boffa, G.M. *et al.* Endomyocardial biopsy in right ventricular cardiomyopathy. *Int. J. Cardiol.* 1993; **40**(3): 273–282.

71. Daliento, L., Rizzoli, G., Thiene, G. *et al.* Diagnostic accuracy of right ventriculography in arrhythmogenic right ventricular cardiomyopathy. *Am. J. Cardiol.* 1990; **66**(7): 741–745.

72. Daliento, L., Turrini, P., Nava, A. *et al.* Arrhythmogenic right ventricular cardiomyopathy in young versus adult patients: similarities and differences. *J. Am. Coll. Cardiol.* 1995; **25**(3): 655–664.

73. Rossi, P., Massumi, A., Gillette, P. *et al.* Arrhythmogenic right ventricular dysplasia: clinical features, diagnostic techniques, and current management. *Am. Heart J.* 1982; **103**(3): 415–420.

74. Ricci, C., Longo, R., Pagnan, L. *et al.* Magnetic resonance imaging in right ventricular dysplasia. *Am. J. Cardiol.* 1992; **70**(20): 1589–1595.

75. Basso, C., Frescura, C., Corrado, D. *et al.* Congenital heart disease and sudden death in the young. *Hum. Pathol.* 1995; **26**(10): 1065–1072.

76. Corrado, D., Leoni, L., Link, M.S. *et al.* Implantable cardioverter-defibrillator therapy for prevention of sudden death in patients with arrhythmogenic right ventricular cardiomyopathy/dysplasia. *Circulation* 2003; **108**(25): 3084–3091.

77. Priori, S.G., Barhanin, J., Hauer, R.N. *et al.* Genetic and molecular basis of cardiac arrhythmias: impact on clinical management parts I and II. *Circulation* 1999; **99**(4): 518–528.

78. Tiso, N., Stephan, D.A., Nava, A. *et al.* Identification of mutations in the cardiac ryanodine receptor gene in families affected with arrhythmogenic right ventricular cardiomyopathy type 2 (ARVD2). *Hum. Mol. Genet.* 2001; **10**(3): 189–194.

79. Rampazzo, A., Nava, A., Malacrida, S. *et al.* Mutation in human desmoplakin domain binding to plakoglobin causes a dominant form of arrhythmogenic right ventricular cardiomyopathy. *Am. J. Hum. Genet.* 2002; **71**(5): 1200–1206.

80. Tavernier, R., Gevaert, S., De Sutter, J. *et al.* Long term results of cardioverter-defibrillator implantation in patients with right ventricular dysplasia and malignant ventricular tachyarrhythmias. *Heart* 2001; **85**(1): 53–56.

81. Yetman, A.T., McCrindle, B.W., MacDonald, C. *et al.* Myocardial bridging in children with hypertrophic cardiomyopathy – a risk factor for sudden death. *N. Engl. J. Med.* 1999; **339**(17): 1201–1209.

82. Bourassa, M.G., Butnaru, A., Lesperance, J. *et al.* Symptomatic myocardial bridges: overview of ischemic mechanisms and current diagnostic and treatment strategies. *J. Am. Coll. Cardiol.* 2003; **41**(3): 351–359.

83. Basso, C., Maron, B.J., Corrado, D. *et al.* Clinical profile of congenital coronary artery anomalies with origin from the wrong aortic sinus leading to sudden death in young competitive athletes. *J. Am. Coll. Cardiol.* 2000; **35**(6): 1493–1501.

84. Goldschlager, N., Epstein, A.E., Grubb, B.P. *et al.* Etiologic considerations in the patient with syncope and an apparently normal heart. *Arch. Intern. Med.* 2003; **163**(2): 151–162.

85. Davis, J.A., Cecchin, F., Jones, T.K. *et al.* Major coronary artery anomalies in a pediatric population: incidence and clinical importance. *J. Am. Coll. Cardiol.* 2001; **37**(2): 593–597.

86. Roberts, W.C. Major anomalies of coronary arterial origin seen in adulthood. *Am. Heart J.* 1986; **111**(5): 941–963.

87. Taylor, A.J., Rogan, K.M. & Virmani, R. Sudden cardiac death associated with isolated congenital coronary artery anomalies. *J. Am. Coll. Cardiol.* 1992; **20**(3): 640–647.

88. Maron, B.J., Thompson, P.D., Puffer, J.C. *et al.* Cardiovascular preparticipation screening of competitive athletes. A statement for health professionals from the Sudden Death Committee (clinical cardiology) and Congenital Cardiac Defects Committee (cardiovascular disease in the young), American Heart Association. *Circulation* 1996; **94**(4): 850–856.

89. Liberthson, R. Ectopic origin of a coronary artery from the aorta with aberrant proximal course. *Congenital Heart Disease: Diagnosis and Management of Children and Adults.* Boston, Massachusetts: Little Brown; 1989: 209–217.

90. Cheitlin, M.D., De Castro, C.M. & McAllister, H.A. Sudden death as a complication of anomalous left coronary origin from the anterior sinus of Valsalva, a not-so-minor congenital anomaly. *Circulation* 1974; **50**(4): 780–787.

91. Ness, M.J. & McManus, B.M. Anomalous right coronary artery origin in otherwise unexplained infant death. *Arch. Pathol. Lab. Med.* 1988; **112**(6): 626–629.

92. Maddoux, G.L., Goss, J.E., Ramo, B.W. *et al.* Angina and vasospasm at rest in a patient with an anomalous left coronary system. *Cathet. Cardiovasc. Diagn.* 1989; **16**(2): 95–98.

93. Pelliccia, A., Spataro, A. & Maron, B.J. Prospective echocardiographic screening for coronary artery anomalies in 1,360 elite competitive athletes. *Am. J. Cardiol.* 1993; **72**(12): 978–979.

94. McConnell, M.V., Ganz, P., Selwyn, A.P. *et al.* Identification of anomalous coronary arteries and their anatomic course by magnetic resonance coronary angiography. *Circulation* 1995; **92**(11): 3158–3162.

95. Mousseaux, E., Hernigou, A., Sapoval, M. *et al.* Coronary arteries arising from the contralateral aortic sinus: electron beam computed tomographic demonstration of the initial course of the artery with respect to the aorta and the right ventricular outflow tract. *J. Thorac. Cardiovasc. Surg.* 1996; **112**(3): 836–840.

96. Juilliere, Y., Berder, V., Suty-Selton, C. *et al.* Isolated myocardial bridges with angiographic milking of the left anterior descending coronary artery: a long-term follow-up study. *Am. Heart J.* 1995; **129**(4): 663–665.

97. Ishii, T., Hosoda, Y., Osaka, T. *et al.* The significance of myocardial bridge upon atherosclerosis in the left anterior descending coronary artery. *J. Pathol.* 1986; **148**(4): 279–291.

98. Ferreira, A.G., Jr., Trotter, S.E., Konig, B., Jr. *et al.* Myocardial bridges: morphological and functional aspects. *Br. Heart J.* 1991; **66**(5): 364–367.

99. Colleran, J.A., Tierney, J.P., Prokopchak, R. *et al.* Angiographic presence of myocardial bridge after successful percutaneous transluminal coronary angioplasty. *Am. Heart J.* 1996; **131**(1): 196–198.

100. Noble, J., Bourassa, M.G., Petitclerc, R. *et al.* Myocardial bridging and milking effect of the left anterior descending coronary artery: normal variant or obstruction? *Am. J. Cardiol.* 1976; **37**(7): 993–999.

101. Dilsizian, V., Bonow, R.O., Epstein, S.E. *et al.* Myocardial ischemia detected by thallium scintigraphy is frequently related to cardiac arrest and syncope in young patients with hypertrophic cardiomyopathy. *J. Am. Coll. Cardiol.* 1993; **22**(3): 796–804.

102. Pey, J., de Dios, R.M. & Epeldegui, A. Myocardial bridging and hypertrophic cardiomyopathy: relief of ischemia by surgery. *Int. J. Cardiol.* 1985; **8**(3): 327–330.

103. Ge, J., Jeremias, A., Rupp, A. *et al.* New signs characteristic of myocardial bridging demonstrated by intracoronary ultrasound and Doppler. *Eur. Heart J.* 1999; **20**(23): 1707–1716.

104. Schwarz, E.R., Klues, H.G., vom Dahl, J. *et al.* Functional characteristics of myocardial bridging. A combined angiographic and intracoronary Doppler flow study. *Eur. Heart J.* 1997; **18**(3): 434–442.

105. Kuhn, F.E., Reagan, K., Mohler, E.R., 3rd *et al.* Evidence for endothelial dysfunction and enhanced vasoconstriction in myocardial bridges. *Am. Heart J.* 1991; **122**(6): 1764–1766.

106. Stables, R.H., Knight, C.J., McNeill, J.G. *et al.* Coronary stenting in the management of myocardial ischaemia caused by muscle bridging. *Br. Heart J.* 1995; **74**(1): 90–92.

107. Haager, P.K., Schwarz, E.R., vom Dahl, J. *et al.* Long term angiographic and clinical follow up in patients with stent implantation for symptomatic myocardial bridging. *Heart* 2000; **84**(4): 403–408.

108. Liberthson, R.R., Nagel, E.L., Hirschman, J.C. *et al.* Pathophysiologic observations in prehospital ventricular fibrillation and sudden cardiac death. *Circulation* 1974; **49**(5): 790–798.

109. Davies, M.J. & Thomas, A. Thrombosis and acute coronary-artery lesions in sudden cardiac ischemic death. *N. Engl. J. Med.* 1984; **310**(18): 1137–1140.

110. Waller, B.F. & Roberts, W.C. Sudden death while running in conditioned runners aged 40 years or over. *Am. J. Cardiol.* 1980; **45**(6): 1292–1300.

111. Virmani, R., Robinowitz, M. & McAllister, H.A., Jr. Nontraumatic death in joggers. A series of 30 patients at autopsy. *Am. J. Med.* 1982; **72**(6): 874–882.

112. Sabbah, H.N., Khaja, F., Hawkins, E.T. *et al.* Relation of atherosclerosis to arterial wall shear in the left anterior descending coronary artery of man. *Am. Heart J.* 1986; **112**(3): 453–458.

113. Angelini, A., Thiene, G., Frescura, C. *et al.* Coronary arterial wall and atherosclerosis in youth (1–20 years): a histologic study in a northern Italian population. *Int. J. Cardiol.* 1990; **28**(3): 361–370.

114. Joseph, A., Ackerman, D., Talley, J.D. *et al.* Manifestations of coronary atherosclerosis in young trauma victims – an autopsy study. *J. Am. Coll. Cardiol.* 1993; **22**(2): 459–467.

115. Ip, J.H., Fuster, V., Badimon, L. *et al.* Syndromes of accelerated atherosclerosis: role of vascular injury and smooth muscle cell proliferation. *J. Am. Coll. Cardiol.* 1990; **15**(7): 1667–1687.

116. Shimokawa, H., Tomoike, H., Nabeyama, S. *et al.* Coronary artery spasm induced in atherosclerotic miniature swine. *Science* 1983; **221**(4610): 560–562.

117. Bertrand, M.E., Lablanche, J.M., Fourrier, J.L. *et al.* Relation to restenosis after percutaneous transluminal coronary angioplasty to vasomotion of the dilated coronary arterial segment. *Am. J. Cardiol.* 1989; **63**(5): 277–281.

118. Maseri, A. & Chierchia, S. Coronary artery spasm: demonstration, definition, diagnosis, and consequences. *Prog. Cardiovasc. Dis.* 1982; **25**(3): 169–192.

119. Myerburg, R.J., Kessler, K.M., Mallon, S.M. *et al.* Life-threatening ventricular arrhythmias in patients with silent myocardial ischemia due to coronary-artery spasm. *N. Engl. J. Med.* 1992; **326**(22): 1451–1455.

120. Maron, B.J. Cardiovascular diseases in athletes. In Zipes, D.P., Libby, P., Bonow, R.O. *et al.*, eds. *Heart Disease.* Philadelphia: Elsevier Saunders, 2005: 1985–1991.

121. Survivors of out-of-hospital cardiac arrest with apparently normal heart. Need for definition and standardized clinical evaluation. Consensus Statement of the Joint Steering Committees of the Unexplained Cardiac Arrest Registry of Europe and of the Idiopathic Ventricular Fibrillation Registry of the United States. *Circulation* 1997; **95**(1): 265–272.

122. Flugelman, M.Y., Virmani, R., Correa, R. *et al.* Smooth muscle cell abundance and fibroblast growth factors in coronary lesions of patients with nonfatal unstable angina. A clue to the mechanism of transformation from the stable to the unstable clinical state. *Circulation* 1993; **88**(6): 2493–2500.

123. Ross, J., Jr. & Braunwald, E. Aortic stenosis. *Circulation* 1968; **38**(1 Suppl): 61–67.

124. Otto, C.M., Burwash, I.G., Legget, M.E. *et al.* Prospective study of asymptomatic valvular aortic stenosis. Clinical, echocardiographic, and exercise predictors of outcome. *Circulation* 1997; **95**(9): 2262–2270.

125. Priori, S.G., Aliot, E., Blomstrom-Lundqvist, C. *et al.* Task Force on sudden cardiac death of the European Society of Cardiology. *Eur. Heart J.* 2001; **22**(16): 1374–1450.

126. Horstkotte, D. & Loogen, F. The natural history of aortic valve stenosis. *Eur. Heart J.* 1988; **9** Suppl E: 57–64.

127. Lund, O., Nielsen, T.T., Emmertsen, K. *et al.* Mortality and worsening of prognostic profile during waiting time for valve replacement in aortic stenosis. *Thorac. Cardiovasc. Surg.* 1996; **44**(6): 289–295.

128. Olshausen, K.V., Witt, T., Pop, T. *et al.* Sudden cardiac death while wearing a Holter monitor. *Am. J. Cardiol.* 1991; **67**(5): 381–386.

129. Firoozi, S., Sharma, S. & McKenna, W.J. Risk of competitive sport in young athletes with heart disease. *Heart* 2003; **89**(7): 710–714.

130. Pellikka, P.A., Nishimura, R.A., Bailey, K.R. *et al.* The natural history of adults with asymptomatic, hemodynamically significant aortic stenosis. *J. Am. Coll. Cardiol.* 1990; **15**(5): 1012–1017.

131. Nishimura, R.A., McGoon, M.D., Shub, C. *et al.* Echocardiographically documented mitral-valve prolapse. Long-term follow-up of 237 patients. *N. Engl. J. Med.* 1985; **313**(21): 1305–1309.

132. Hayek, E., Gring, C.N. & Griffin, B.P. Mitral valve prolapse. *Lancet* 2005; **365**(9458): 507–518.

133. Kligfield, P., Levy, D., Devereux, R.B. *et al.* Arrhythmias and sudden death in mitral valve prolapse. *Am. Heart J.* 1987; **113**(5): 1298–1307.

134. Grigioni, F., Enriquez-Sarano, M., Ling, L.H. *et al.* Sudden death in mitral regurgitation due to flail leaflet. *J. Am. Coll. Cardiol.* 1999; **34**(7): 2078–2085.

135. Tieleman, R.G., Crijns, H.J., Wiesfeld, A.C. *et al.* Increased dispersion of refractoriness in the absence of QT prolongation in patients with mitral valve prolapse and ventricular arrhythmias. *Br. Heart J.* 1995; **73**(1): 37–40.

136. Maron, B.J. & Mitchell, J.H. Revised eligibility recommendations for competitive athletes with cardiovascular abnormalities. *J. Am. Coll. Cardiol.* 1994; **24**(4): 848–850.

137. Pyeritz, R.E. The Marfan syndrome. *Annu. Rev. Med.* 2000; **51**: 481–510.

138. Devereux, R.B. & Roman, M.J. Aortic disease in Marfan's syndrome. *N. Engl. J. Med.* 1999; **340**(17): 1358–1359.

139. Shores, J., Berger, K.R., Murphy, E.A. *et al.* Progression of aortic dilatation and the benefit of long-term beta-adrenergic blockade in Marfan's syndrome. *N. Engl. J. Med.* 1994; **330**(19): 1335–1341.

140. Yetman, A.T., Bornemeier, R.A. & McCrindle, B.W. Long-term outcome in patients with Marfan syndrome: is aortic dissection the only cause of sudden death? *J. Am. Coll. Cardiol.* 2003; **41**(2): 329–332.

141. Maron, B.J. Cardiovascular risks to young persons on the athletic field. *Ann. Intern. Med.* 1998; **129**(5): 379–386.

142. Antzelevitch, C. Molecular genetics of arrhythmias and cardiovascular conditions associated with arrhythmias. *Heart Rhythm* 2004; **1**(5C): 42C–56C.

143. Priori, S.G. Inherited arrhythmogenic diseases: the complexity beyond monogenic disorders. *Circ. Res.* 2004; **94**(2): 140–145.

144. Moss, A.J., Schwartz, P.J., Crampton, R.S. *et al.* The long QT syndrome. Prospective longitudinal study of 328 families. *Circulation* 1991; **84**(3): 1136–1144.

145. Wang, Q., Shen, J., Splawski, I. *et al.* SCN5A mutations associated with an inherited cardiac arrhythmia, long QT syndrome. *Cell* 1995; **80**(5): 805–811.

146. Mohler, P.J., Schott, J.J., Gramolini, A.O. *et al.* Ankyrin-B mutation causes type 4 long-QT cardiac arrhythmia and sudden cardiac death. *Nature* 2003; **421**(6923): 634–639.

147. Curran, M.E., Splawski, I., Timothy, K.W. *et al.* A molecular basis for cardiac arrhythmia: HERG mutations cause long QT syndrome. *Cell* 1995; **80**(5): 795–803.

148. Splawski, I., Timothy, K.W., Sharpe, L.M. *et al.* Ca(V)1.2 calcium channel dysfunction causes a multisystem disorder including arrhythmia and autism. *Cell* 2004; **119**(1): 19–31.

149. Schwartz, P.J., Priori, S.G. & Napolitano, C. The long QT syndrome. In Zipes, D.P., Jalife, J., eds. *Cardiac Electrophysiology: From Cell to Bedside.* Philadelphia: Saunders, 2000: 597–615.

150. Schwartz, P.J., Priori, S.G., Cerrone, M. *et al.* Left cardiac sympathetic denervation in the management of high-risk patients affected by the long-QT syndrome. *Circulation* 2004; **109**(15): 1826–1833.

151. Bednar, M.M., Harrigan, E.P., Anziano, R.J. *et al.* The QT interval. *Prog. Cardiovasc. Dis.* 2001; **43**(5 Suppl 1): 1–45.

152. Tomaselli, G.F. & Marban, E. Electrophysiological remodeling in hypertrophy and heart failure. *Cardiovasc. Res.* 1999; **42**(2): 270–283.

153. Antzelevitch, C. & Shimizu, W. Cellular mechanisms underlying the long QT syndrome. *Curr. Opin. Cardiol.* 2002; **17**(1): 43–51.

154. Shimizu, W. & Antzelevitch, C. Cellular basis for the ECG features of the LQT1 form of the long-QT syndrome: effects of beta-adrenergic agonists and antagonists and sodium channel blockers on transmural dispersion of repolarization and torsade de pointes. *Circulation* 1998; **98**(21): 2314–2322.

155. Zhang, L., Timothy, K.W., Vincent, G.M. *et al.* Spectrum of ST-T-wave patterns and repolarization parameters in congenital long-QT syndrome: ECG findings identify genotypes. *Circulation* 2000; **102**(23): 2849–2855.

156. Moss, A.J., Robinson, J.L., Gessman, L. *et al.* Comparison of clinical and genetic variables of cardiac events associated with loud noise versus swimming among subjects with the long QT syndrome. *Am. J. Cardiol.* 1999; **84**(8): 876–879.

157. Noda, T., Takaki, H., Kurita, T. *et al.* Gene-specific response of dynamic ventricular repolarization to sympathetic stimulation in LQT1, LQT2 and LQT3 forms of congenital long QT syndrome. *Eur. Heart J.* 2002; **23**(12): 975–983.

158. Shimizu, W. & Antzelevitch, C. Differential response of transmural dispersion of repolarization and Torsade de Pointes to beta-adrenergic agonists and antagonists in LQT1, LQT2 and LQT3 models of the long QT syndrome. *PACE* 1999; **22**(II): 730.

159. Schwartz, P.J., Priori, S.G., Spazzolini, C. *et al.* Genotype-phenotype correlation in the long-QT syndrome: gene-specific triggers for life-threatening arrhythmias. *Circulation* 2001; **103**(1): 89–95.

160. Priori, S.G., Napolitano, C., Schwartz, P.J. *et al.* Association of long QT syndrome loci and cardiac events among patients treated with beta-blockers. *J. Am. Med. Assoc.* 2004; **292**(11): 1341–1344.

161. Brugada, P. & Brugada, J. Right bundle branch block, persistent ST segment elevation and sudden cardiac death: a distinct clinical and electrocardiographic syndrome. A multicenter report. *J. Am. Coll. Cardiol.* 1992; **20**(6): 1391–1396.

162. Priori, S.G., Napolitano, C., Gasparini, M. *et al.* Clinical and genetic heterogeneity of right bundle branch block and ST-segment elevation syndrome: a prospective evaluation of 52 families. *Circulation* 2000; **102**(20): 2509–2515.

163. Antzelevitch, C., Brugada, P., Borggrefe, M. *et al.* Brugada Syndrome. Report of the Second Consensus Conference. Endorsed by the Heart Rhythm Society and the European Heart Rhythm Association. *Circulation* 2005; **111**(5): 659–670.

164. Priori, S.G., Napolitano, C., Giordano, U. *et al.* Brugada syndrome and sudden cardiac death in children. *Lancet* 2000; **355**(9206): 808–809.

165. Brugada, P., Brugada, R. & Brugada, J. Sudden death in patients and relatives with the syndrome of right bundle

branch block, ST segment elevation in the precordial leads V(1)to V(3)and sudden death. *Eur. Heart J.* 2000; **21**(4): 321–326.

166. Antzelevitch, C. The Brugada syndrome: ionic basis and arrhythmia mechanisms. *J. Cardiovasc. Electrophysiol.* 2001; **12**(2): 268–272.

167. Gussak, I., Antzelevitch, C., Bjerregaard, P. *et al.* The Brugada syndrome: clinical, electrophysiologic and genetic aspects. *J. Am. Coll. Cardiol.* 1999; **33**(1): 5–15.

168. Yan, G.X. & Antzelevitch, C. Cellular basis for the Brugada syndrome and other mechanisms of arrhythmogenesis associated with ST-segment elevation. *Circulation* 1999; **100**(15): 1660–1666.

169. Antzelevitch, C., Brugada, P., Brugada, J. *et al.* Brugada syndrome: a decade of progress. *Circ. Res.* 2002; **91**(12): 1114–1118.

170. Kurita, T., Shimizu, W., Inagaki, M. *et al.* The electrophysiologic mechanism of ST-segment elevation in Brugada syndrome. *J. Am. Coll. Cardiol.* 2002; **40**(2): 330–334.

171. Haissaguerre, M., Extramiana, F., Hocini, M. *et al.* Mapping and ablation of ventricular fibrillation associated with long-QT and Brugada syndromes. *Circulation* 2003; **108**(8): 925–928.

172. Antzelevitch, C., Brugada, P., Brugada, J. *et al. Clinical Approaches to Tachyarrhythmias. The Brugada Syndrome.* Armonk, NY: Futura Publishing Company; 1999.

173. Alings, M., Dekker, L., Sadee, A. *et al.* Quinidine induced electrocardiographic normalization in two patients with Brugada syndrome. *Pacing Clin. Electrophysiol.* 2001; **24**(9 Pt 1): 1420–1422.

174. Belhassen, B. & Viskin, S. Pharmacologic approach to therapy of Brugada syndrome: quinidine as an alternative to ICD therapy? In Antzelevitch, C., Brugada, P., Brugada, J. *et al.*, eds. *The Brugada Syndrome: From Bench to Bedside.* Oxford: Blackwell Futura; 2004: 202–211.

175. Belhassen, B., Viskin, S., Fish, R. *et al.* Effects of electrophysiologic-guided therapy with Class IA antiarrhythmic drugs on the long-term outcome of patients with idiopathic ventricular fibrillation with or without the Brugada syndrome. *J. Cardiovasc. Electrophysiol.* 1999; **10**(10): 1301–1312.

176. Hermida, J.S., Denjoy, I., Clerc, J. *et al.* Hydroquinidine therapy in Brugada syndrome. *J. Am. Coll. Cardiol.* 2004; **43**(10): 1853–1860.

177. Mok, N.S., Chan, N.Y. & Chiu, A.C. Successful use of quinidine in treatment of electrical storm in Brugada syndrome. *Pacing Clin. Electrophysiol.* 2004; **27**(6 Pt 1): 821–823.

178. Tsuchiya, T., Ashikaga, K., Honda, T. *et al.* Prevention of ventricular fibrillation by cilostazol, an oral phosphodiesterase inhibitor, in a patient with Brugada syndrome. *J. Cardiovasc. Electrophysiol.* 2002; **13**(7): 698–701.

179. Tanaka, H., Kinoshita, O., Uchikawa, S. *et al.* Successful prevention of recurrent ventricular fibrillation by intravenous isoproterenol in a patient with Brugada syndrome. *Pacing Clin. Electrophysiol.* 2001; **24**(8 Pt 1): 1293–1294.

180. Corrado, D., Pelliccia, A., Antzelevitch, C. *et al.* ST segment elevation and sudden death in the athlete. In Antzelevitch, C., Brugada, P., Brugada, J. *et al.*, eds. *The Brugada Syndrome: From Bench to Bedside.* Oxford: Blackwell Futura; 2004: 119–129.

181. Gussak, I., Brugada, P., Brugada, J. *et al.* Idiopathic short QT interval: a new clinical syndrome? *Cardiology* 2000; **94**(2): 99–102.

182. Gussak, I., Brugada, P., Brugada, J. *et al.* ECG phenomenon of idiopathic and paradoxical short QT intervals. *Cardiol. Electrophysiol. Rev.* 2002; **6**(1–2): 49–53.

183. Gaita, F., Giustetto, C., Bianchi, F. *et al.* Short QT Syndrome: a familial cause of sudden death. *Circulation* 2003; **108**(8): 965–970.

184. Brugada, R., Hong, K., Dumaine, R. *et al.* Sudden death associated with short-QT syndrome linked to mutations in HERG. *Circulation* 2004; **109**(1): 30–35.

185. Bellocq, C., van Ginneken, A.C., Bezzina, C.R. *et al.* Mutation in the KCNQ1 gene leading to the short QT-interval syndrome. *Circulation* 2004; **109**(20): 2394–2397.

186. Extramiana, F. & Antzelevitch, C. Amplified transmural dispersion of repolarization as the basis for arrhythmogenesis in a canine ventricular-wedge model of short-QT syndrome. *Circulation* 2004; **110**(24): 3661–3666.

187. Gaita, F., Giustetto, C., Bianchi, F. *et al.* Short QT syndrome: pharmacological treatment. *J. Am. Coll. Cardiol.* 2004; **43**(8): 1494–1499.

188. Klein, G.J., Bashore, T.M., Sellers, T.D. *et al.* Ventricular fibrillation in the Wolff–Parkinson–White syndrome. *N. Engl. J. Med.* 1979; **301**(20): 1080–1085.

189. Klein, G.J., Ideker, R.E., Smith, W.M. *et al.* Epicardial mapping of the onset of ventricular tachycardia initiated by programmed stimulation in the canine heart with chronic infarction. *Circulation* 1979; **60**(6): 1375–1384.

190. Zipes, D.P. & Wellens, H.J. Sudden cardiac death. *Circulation* 1998; **98**(21): 2334–2351.

191. Bromberg, B.I., Lindsay, B.D., Cain, M.E. *et al.* Impact of clinical history and electrophysiologic characterization of accessory pathways on management strategies to reduce sudden death among children with Wolff–Parkinson–White syndrome. *J. Am. Coll. Cardiol.* 1996; **27**(3): 690–695.

192. Manolis, A.S., Wang, P.J., Estes, N.A., 3rd. Radiofrequency catheter ablation for cardiac tachyarrhythmias. *Ann. Intern. Med.* 1994; **121**(6): 452–461.

193. Morady, F. Radio-frequency ablation as treatment for cardiac arrhythmias. *N. Engl. J. Med.* 1999; **340**(7): 534–544.

194. Zardini, M., Yee, R., Thakur, R.K. *et al.* Risk of sudden arrhythmic death in the Wolff–Parkinson–White syndrome: current perspectives. *Pacing Clin Electrophysiol.* 1994; **17**(5 Pt 1): 966–975.

195. Krahn, A., Klein, G. & Yee, R. The approach to the athlete with Wolff–Parkinson–White syndrome: risk of sudden cardiac death. In Estes, N. III, Salem, D., Wang, P., eds. *Sudden Cardiac Death in the Athlete.* Armonk, NY: Futura Publishing Co.; 1998.

196. Coumel, P., Fidelle, J., Lucet, V. *et al.* Catecholamine-induced

severe ventricula arrhythmias with Adam-Stokes syndrome in children: report of four cases. *Br. Heart J.* 1978; **40** (Suppl): 28–37.

197. Priori, S.G., Napolitano, C., Memmi, M. *et al.* Clinical and molecular characterization of patients with catecholaminergic polymorphic ventricular tachycardia. *Circulation* 2002; **106**(1): 69–74.

198. Priori, S.G., Napolitano, C., Tiso, N. *et al.* Mutations in the cardiac ryanodine receptor gene (hRyR2) underlie catecholaminergic polymorphic ventricular tachycardia. *Circulation* 2001; **103**(2): 196–200.

199. Kramer, M.R., Drori, Y. & Lev, B. Sudden death in young soldiers. High incidence of syncope prior to death. *Chest* 1988; **93**(2): 345–347.

200. Markowitz, S.M., Litvak, B.L., Ramirez de Arellano, E.A. *et al.* Adenosine-sensitive ventricular tachycardia: right ventricular abnormalities delineated by magnetic resonance imaging. *Circulation* 1997; **96**(4): 1192–1200.

201. Flemming, M.A., Oral, H., Kim, M.H. *et al.* Electro-cardiographic predictors of successful ablation of tachycardia or bigeminy arising in the right ventricular outflow tract. *Am. J. Cardiol.* 1999; **84**(10): 1266–1268, A1269.

202. Olgin, J.E. & Zipes, D.P. Specific arrhythmias: diagnosis and treatment. In Zipes, D.P., Libby, P., Bonow, R.O. *et al.*, eds. *Heart Disease*. Philadelphia: Elsevier Saunders; 2005: 803–863.

203. Brugada, R. Is atrial fibrillation a genetic disease? *J. Cardiovasc. Electrophysiol.* 2005; **16**(5): 553–556.

204. Wever, E.F.D. & De Medina, E.O.R. Sudden death in patients without structural heart disease. *J. Am. Coll. Cardiol.* 2004; **43**(7): 1137–1144.

205. Wever, E.F., Hauer, R.N., Oomen, A. *et al.* Unfavorable outcome in patients with primary electrical disease who survived an episode of ventricular fibrillation. *Circulation* 1993; **88**(3): 1021–1029.

206. Coxsackie B5 virus infections during 1965. A report to the Director of the Public Health Laboratory Service from various laboratories in the United Kingdom. *Br. Med. J.* 1967; **4**(579): 575–577.

207. Drory, Y., Turetz, Y., Hiss, Y. *et al.* Sudden unexpected death in persons less than 40 years of age. *Am. J. Cardiol.* 1991; **68**(13): 1388–1392.

208. McCaffrey, F.M., Braden, D.S. & Strong, W.B. Sudden cardiac death in young athletes. A review. *Am. J. Dis. Child.* 1991; **145**(2): 177–183.

209. Gore, I. & Saphir, O. Myocarditis: a classification of 1402 cases. *Am. Heart J.* 1947; **34**: 827–830.

210. Cambridge, G., MacArthur, C.G., Waterson, A.P. *et al.* Antibodies to Coxsackie B viruses in congestive cardiomyopathy. *Br. Heart J.* 1979; **41**(6): 692–696.

211. Bowles, N.E., Richardson, P.J., Olsen, E.G. *et al.* Detection of Coxsackie-B-virus-specific RNA sequences in myocardial biopsy samples from patients with myocarditis and dilated cardiomyopathy. *Lancet* 1986; **1**(8490): 1120–1123.

212. Jin, O., Sole, M.J., Butany, J.W. *et al.* Detection of enterovirus RNA in myocardial biopsies from patients with myocarditis and cardiomyopathy using gene amplification by polymerase chain reaction. *Circulation* 1990; **82**(1): 8–16.

213. Feldman, A.M. & McNamara, D. Myocarditis. *N. Engl. J. Med.* 2000; **343**(19): 1388–1398.

214. Pauschinger, M., Bowles, N.E., Fuentes-Garcia, F.J. *et al.* Detection of adenoviral genome in the myocardium of adult patients with idiopathic left ventricular dysfunction. *Circulation* 1999; **99**(10): 1348–1354.

215. Isner, J.M., Estes, N.Ad., Thompson, P.D. *et al.* Acute cardiac events temporally related to cocaine abuse. *N. Engl. J. Med.* 1986; **315**(23): 1438–1443.

216. Tazelaar, H.D., Karch, S.B., Stephens, B.G. *et al.* Cocaine and the heart. *Hum Pathol.* 1987; **18**(2): 195–199.

217. Meola, F. La commozione toracica. *Gior. Internaz. Sci.* 1879; **1**: 923–937.

218. Riedinger, F. & Kümmell H. Die Verletzungen und Erkrankungen des Thorax und seines Inhaltes. In von Bergman, E. & von Bruns, P., eds. *Handbuch der Praktischen Chirurgie*. Stuttgart: Ferd. Enke, 1903: 373–456.

219. Nesbitt, A.D., Cooper, P.J. & Kohl, P. Rediscovering commotio cordis. *Lancet* 2001; **357**: 1195–1197.

220. Maron, B.J., Link, M.S., Wang, P.J. *et al.* Clinical profile of commotio cordis: an under appreciated cause of sudden death in the young during sports and other activities. *J. Cardiovasc. Electrophysiol.* 1999; **10**(1): 114–120.

221. Link, M.S., Estes N.A.M. III & Maron, B.J. Sudden death caused by chest wall trauma (Commotio cordis). In Kohl, P., Sachs, F. & Franz, M.R., eds. *Cardiac Mechano-electric Feedback and Arrhythmias: From Pipette to Patient*. Philadelphia: Elsevier Saunders; 2005: 270–276.

222. Schlomka, G. Commotio cordis und ihre Folgen. (Die Einwirkung stumpfer Brustwandtraumen auf das Herz.) *Ergebn Inn Med Kinderheilk* 1934; **47**: 1–91.

223. Link, M.S., Wang, P.J., Pandian, N.G. *et al.* An experimental model of sudden death due to low-energy chest-wall impact (commotio cordis). *N. Engl. J. Med.* 1998; **338**(25): 1805–1811.

224. Link, M.S. Mechanically induced sudden death in chest wall impact (commotio cordis). *Prog. Biophys. Mol. Biol.* 2003; **82**(1–3): 175–186.

225. Link, M.S., Maron, B.J., VanderBrink, B.A. *et al.* Impact directly over the cardiac silhouette is necessary to produce ventricular fibrillation in an experimental model of commotio cordis. *J. Am. Coll. Cardiol.* 2001; **37**(2): 649–654.

226. Link, M.S., Maron, B.J., Wang, P.J. *et al.* Upper and lower limits of vulnerability to sudden arrhythmic death with chest-wall impact (commotio cordis). *J. Am. Coll. Cardiol.* 2003; **41**(1): 99–104.

227. Kohl, P., Nesbitt, A.D., Cooper, P.J. *et al.* Sudden cardiac death by commotio cordis: role of mechanico-electrical feedback. *Cardiovasc. Res.* 2001; **50**: 280–289.

228. Kondo, T., Kubota, I., Tachibana, H. *et al.* Glibenclamide attenuates peaked T wave in early phase of myocardial ischemia. *Cardiovasc. Res.* 1996; **31**: 683–687.

229. Van Wagoner, D.R. Mechanosensitive gating of atrial ATP-sensitive potassium channels. *Circ. Res.* 1993; **72**: 973–983.

230. Link, M.S., Wang, P.J., VanderBrink, B.A. *et al.* Selective activation of the K+ ATP channel is a mechanism by which sudden death is produced by low-energy chest-wall impact (commotio cordis). *Circulation* 1999; **100**: 413–418.

231. Kohl, P., Hunter, P. & Noble, D. Stretch-induced changes in heart rate and rhythm: clinical observations, experiments and mathematical models. *Prog. Biophys. Molec. Biol.* 1999; **71**: 91–138.

232. Craelius, W., Chen, V. & El-Sherif, N. Stretch activated ion channels in ventricular myocytes. *BioSci. Rep.* 1988; **8**: 407–414.

233. Belus, A. & White, E. Effects of streptomycin sulphate on ICaL, IKr and IKs in guinea-pig ventricular myocytes. *Eur. J. Pharmacol.* 2002; **445**: 171–178.

234. Cooper, P.J., Epstein, A., MacLeod, I.A. *et al.* Soft tissue impact characterisation kit (STICK) for ex situ investigation of heart rhythm responses to acute mechanical stimulation. *Prog. Biophys. Molec. Biol.* 2005; 2006; **90**: 444–468.

235. Cooper, P. & Kohl, P. Species- and preparation-dependence of stretch effects on sino-atrial node pacemaking. *ANYAS* 2005; **1047**: 324–335.

236. Bode, F., Sachs, F. & Franz, M.R. Tarantula peptide inhibits atrial fibrillation. *Nature* 2001; **409**: 35–36.

237. Lange, R.A. & Hillis, L.D. Cardiovascular complications of cocaine use. *N. Engl. J. Med.* 2001; **345**(5): 351–358.

238. Valli, G. & Giardina, E.G. Benefits, adverse effects and drug interactions of herbal therapies with cardiovascular effects. *J. Am. Coll. Cardiol.* 2002; **39**(7): 1083–1095.

239. *Annual Data 1987. Data from the Drug Abuse Warning Network. Series 1, No. 7 of National Institute on Drug Abuse series.* Rockville, Md: National Institute on Drug Abuse; 1988.

240. Lange, R.A., Cigarroa, R.G., Yancy, C.W.J. *et al.* Cocaine-induced coronary-artery vasoconstriction. *N. Engl. J. Med.* 1989 1989; **321**(23): 1557–1562.

241. Wilbert-Lampen, U., Seliger, C., Zilker, T. *et al.* Cocaine increases the endothelial release of immunoreactive endothelin and its concentrations in human plasma and urine: reversal by coincubation with sigma-receptor antagonists. *Circulation* 1998; **98**(5): 385–390.

242. Mo, W., Singh, A.K., Arruda, J.A. *et al.* Role of nitric oxide in cocaine-induced acute hypertension. *Am. J. Hypertens.* 1998; **11**(6 Pt 1): 708–714.

243. Stenberg, R.G., Winniford, M.D., Hillis, L.D. *et al.* Simultaneous acute thrombosis of two major coronary arteries following intravenous cocaine use. *Arch. Pathol. Lab. Med.* 1989; **113**(5): 521–524.

244. Heesch, C.M., Wilhelm, C.R., Ristich, J. *et al.* Cocaine activates platelets and increases the formation of circulating platelet containing microaggregates in humans. *Heart* 2000; **83**(6): 688–695.

245. Moliterno, D.J., Lange, R.A., Gerard, R.D. *et al.* Influence of intranasal cocaine on plasma constituents associated with endogenous thrombosis and thrombolysis. *Am. J. Med.* 1994; **96**(6): 492–496.

246. Mittleman, M.A., Mintzer, D., Maclure, M. *et al.* Triggering of myocardial infarction by cocaine. *Circulation* 1999; **99**(21): 2737–2741.

247. Brickner, M.E., Willard, J.E., Eichhorn, E.J. *et al.* Left ventricular hypertrophy associated with chronic cocaine abuse. *Circulation* 1991; **84**(3): 1130–1135.

248. Chokshi, S.K., Moore, R., Pandian, N.G. *et al.* Reversible cardiomyopathy associated with cocaine intoxication. *Ann. Intern. Med.* 1989; **111**(12): 1039–1040.

249. Virmani, R., Robinowitz, M., Smialek, J.E. *et al.* Cardiovascular effects of cocaine: an autopsy study of 40 patients. *Am. Heart J.* 1988; **115**(5): 1068–1076.

250. Green, G.A., Uryasz, F.D., Petr, T.A. *et al.* NCAA study of substance use and abuse habits of college student-athletes. *Clin. J. Sport. Med.* 2001; **11**(1): 51–56.

251. Bahrke, M.S., Yesalis, C.E., Kopstein, A.N. *et al.* Risk factors associated with anabolic-androgenic steroid use among adolescents. *Sports Med.* 2000; **29**(6): 397–405.

252. Sturmi, J.E. & Diorio, D.J. Anabolic agents. *Clin. Sports Med.* 1998; **17**(2): 261–282.

253. Akhter, J., Hyder, S. & Ahmed, M. Cerebrovascular accident associated with anabolic steroid use in a young man. *Neurology* 1994; **44**(12): 2405–2406.

254. Ferrera, P.C., Putnam, D.L. & Verdile, V.P. Anabolic steroid use as the possible precipitant of dilated cardiomyopathy. *Cardiology* 1997; **88**(2): 218–220.

255. Sullivan, M.L., Martinez, C.M., Gennis, P. *et al.* The cardiac toxicity of anabolic steroids. *Prog. Cardiovasc Dis.* 1998; **41**(1): 1–15.

256. Melchert, R.B. & Welder, A.A. Cardiovascular effects of androgenic-anabolic steroids. *Med. Sci. Sports Exerc.* 1995; **27**(9): 1252–1262.

257. Crook, D. Testosterone, androgens and the risk of myocardial infarction. *Br. J. Clin. Pract.* 1996; **50**(4): 180–181.

258. Madea, B., Grellner, W., Musshoff, F. *et al.* Medico-legal aspects of doping. *J. Clin. Forens. Med.* 1998; **5**(1): 1–7.

259. Fineschi, V., Baroldi, G., Monciotti, F. *et al.* Anabolic steroid abuse and cardiac sudden death: a pathologic study. *Arch. Pathol. Lab. Med.* 2001; **125**(2): 253–255.

260. Eliot, R.S., Baroldi, G. & Leone, A. Necropsy studies in myocardial infarction with minimal or no coronary luminal reduction due to atherosclerosis. *Circulation* 1974; **49**(6): 1127–1131.

261. Higham, P.D. & Campbell, R.W. QT dispersion. *Br. Heart J.* 1994; **71**(6): 508–510.

262. Nieminen, M.S., Ramo, M.P., Viitasalo, M. *et al.* Serious cardiovascular side effects of large doses of anabolic steroids in weight lifters. *Eur. Heart J.* 1996; **17**(10): 1576–1583.

263. Hartmann, G., Addicks, K., Donike, M. *et al.* Testosterone application influences sympathetic activity of intracardiac nerves in non-trained and trained mice. *J. Auton. Nerv. Syst.* 1986; **17**(2): 85–100.

264. Togna, G.I., Togna, A.R., Graziani, M. *et al.* Testosterone and cocaine: vascular toxicity of their concomitant abuse. *Thromb. Res.* 2003; **109**(4): 195–201.

265. Fletcher, G.F., Balady, G., Blair, S.N. *et al.* Statement on exercise: benefits and recommendations for physical activity programs for all Americans. A statement for health professionals by the Committee on Exercise and Cardiac Rehabilitation of the Council on Clinical Cardiology, American Heart Association. *Circulation* 1996; **94**(4): 857–862.

266. Wannamethee, G., Shaper, A.G., Macfarlane, P.W. *et al.* Risk factors for sudden cardiac death in middle-aged British men. *Circulation* 1995; **91**(6): 1749–1756.

267. Manson, J.E., Hu, F.B., Rich-Edwards, J.W. *et al.* A prospective study of walking as compared with vigorous exercise in the prevention of coronary heart disease in women. *N. Engl. J. Med.* 1999; **341**(9): 650–658.

268. Albert, C.M., Mittleman, M.A., Chae, C.U. *et al.* Triggering of sudden death from cardiac causes by vigorous exertion. *N. Engl. J. Med.* 2000; **343**(19): 1355–1361.

269. Mittleman, M.A., Maclure, M., Tofler, G.H. *et al.* Triggering of acute myocardial infarction by heavy physical exertion. Protection against triggering by regular exertion. Determinants of Myocardial Infarction Onset Study Investigators. *N. Engl. J. Med.* 1993; **329**(23): 1677–1683.

270. Willich, S.N., Lewis, M., Lowel, H. *et al.* Physical exertion as a trigger of acute myocardial infarction. Triggers and Mechanisms of Myocardial Infarction Study Group. *N. Engl. J. Med.* 1993; **329**(23): 1684–1690.

271. Jouven, X., Zureik, M., Desnos, M. *et al.* Long-term outcome in asymptomatic men with exercise-induced premature ventricular depolarizations. *N. Engl. J. Med.* 2000; **343**(12): 826–833.

272. Nistri, S., Thiene, G., Basso, C. *et al.* Screening for hypertrophic cardiomyopathy in a young male military population. *Am. J. Cardiol.* 2003; **91**(8): 1021–1023, A1028.

273. Maron, B.J., Roberts, W.C., McAllister, H.A. *et al.* Sudden death in young athletes. *Circulation* 1980; **62**(2): 218–229.

274. Burke, A.P., Farb, A., Virmani, R. *et al.* Sports-related and non-sports-related sudden cardiac death in young adults. *Am. Heart J.* 1991; **121**(2 Pt 1): 568–575.

275. Maron, B.J., Bodison, S.A., Wesley, Y.E. *et al.* Results of screening a large group of intercollegiate competitive athletes for cardiovascular disease. *J. Am. Coll. Cardiol.* 1987; **10**(6): 1214–1221.

276. Corrado, D., Basso, C., Schiavon, M. *et al.* Identification of athletes with hypertrophic cardiomyopathy at risk of sudden death: cost effectiveness analysis of screening strategies. *Circulation* 2002; **106**: II–701.

277. Corrado, D., Basso, C., Schiavon, M. *et al.* Arrhythmogenic right ventricular dysplasia and hypertrophic cardiomyopathy: identification with the Italian preparticipation athletic screening program. In Maron, B.J., ed. *Diagnosis and Management of Hypertrophic Cardiomyopathy.* Armonk, NY: Blackwell Futura; 2004: 393–403.

278. Pelliccia, A., Di Paolo, F., De Luca, R. *et al.* Efficacy of preparticipation screening for the detection of cardiovascular abnormalities at risk of sudden death in competitive athletes: the Italian experience. *J. Am. Coll. Cardiol.* 2001; **37**: 151A.

279. McKenna, W.J., Thiene, G., Nava, A. *et al.* Diagnosis of arrhythmogenic right ventricular dysplasia/cardiomyopathy. Task Force of the Working Group Myocardial and Pericardial Disease of the European Society of Cardiology and of the Scientific Council on Cardiomyopathies of the International Society and Federation of Cardiology. *Br. Heart J.* 1994; **71**(3): 215–218.

280. Corrado, D., Fontaine, G., Marcus, F.I. *et al.* Arrhythmogenic right ventricular dysplasia/cardiomyopathy: need for an international registry. Study Group on Arrhythmogenic Right Ventricular Dysplasia/Cardiomyopathy of the Working Groups on Myocardial and Pericardial Disease and Arrhythmias of the European Society of Cardiology and of the Scientific Council on Cardiomyopathies of the World Heart Federation. *Circulation* 2000; **101**(11): E101–E106.

281. Pelliccia, A., Culasso, F., Di Paolo, F.M. *et al.* Physiologic left ventricular cavity dilatation in elite athletes. *Ann. Intern. Med.* 1999; **130**(1): 23–31.

282. Pelliccia, A., Maron, B.J., Culasso, F. *et al.* Athlete's heart in women. Echocardiographic characterization of highly trained elite female athletes. *J. Am. Med. Assoc.* 1996; **276**(3): 211–215.

283. Biffi, A., Pelliccia, A., Verdile, L. *et al.* Long-term clinical significance of frequent and complex ventricular tachyarrhythmias in trained athletes. *J. Am. Coll. Cardiol.* 2002; **40**(3): 446–452.

284. Pelliccia, A., Maron, B.J., Culasso, F. *et al.* Clinical significance of abnormal electrocardiographic patterns in trained athletes. *Circulation* 2000; **102**(3): 278–284.

285. Maron, B.J., Pelliccia, A., Spataro, A. *et al.* Reduction in left ventricular wall thickness after deconditioning in highly trained Olympic athletes. *Br. Heart J.* 1993; **69**(2): 125–128.

286. Biffi, A., Maron, B.J., Verdile, L. *et al.* Impact of physical deconditioning on ventricular tachyarrhythmias in trained athletes. *J. Am. Coll. Cardiol.* 2004; **44**(5): 1053–1058.

287. Thierfelder, L., Watkins, H., MacRae, C. *et al.* Alpha-tropomyosin and cardiac troponin T mutations cause familial hypertrophic cardiomyopathy: a disease of the sarcomere. *Cell* 1994; **77**(5): 701–712.

288. Watkins, H., Thierfelder, L., Hwang, D.S. *et al.* Sporadic hypertrophic cardiomyopathy due to de novo myosin mutations. *J. Clin. Invest.* 1992; **90**(5): 1666–1671.

289. Sharma, S., Elliott, P.M., Whyte, G. *et al.* Utility of metabolic exercise testing in distinguishing hypertrophic cardiomyopathy from physiologic left ventricular hypertrophy in athletes. *J. Am. Coll. Cardiol.* 2000; **36**(3): 864–870.

290. Goldsmith, R.L., Bigger, J.T., Jr., Bloomfield, D.M. *et al.* Physical fitness as a determinant of vagal modulation. *Med. Sci. Sports Exerc.* 1997; **29**(6): 812–817.

291. Iellamo, F., Legramante, J.M., Pigozzi, F. *et al.* Conversion from vagal to sympathetic predominance with strenuous training in high-performance world class athletes. *Circulation* 2002; **105**(23): 2719–2724.

292. Grassi, G., Seravalle, G., Bertinieri, G. *et al.* Behaviour of the adrenergic cardiovascular drive in atrial fibrillation and

cardiac arrhythmias. *Acta Physiol. Scand.* 2003; **177**(3): 399–404.

293. Gaita, F., Giustetto, C., Di Donna, P. *et al.* Long-term follow-up of right ventricular monomorphic extrasystoles. *J. Am. Coll. Cardiol.* 2001; **38**(2): 364–370.

294. Pelliccia, A., Maron, B.J., De Luca, R. *et al.* Remodeling of left ventricular hypertrophy in elite athletes after long-term deconditioning. *Circulation* 2002; **105**(8): 944–949.

295. Estes, N.A., 3rd, Link, M.S., Cannom, D. *et al.* Report of the NASPE policy conference on arrhythmias and the athlete. *J. Cardiovasc. Electrophysiol.* 2001; **12**(10): 1208–1219.

296. 26th Bethesda Conference: recommendations for determining eligibility for competition in athletes with cardiovascular abnormalities. January 6–7, 1994. *J. Am. Coll. Cardiol.* 1994; **24**(4): 845–899.

297. Maron, B.J., Mitten, M.J., Quandt, E.F. *et al.* Competitive athletes with cardiovascular disease – the case of Nicholas Knapp. *N. Engl. J. Med.* 1998; **339**(22): 1632–1635.

298. Maron, B.J. Sudden death in young athletes. Lessons from the Hank Gathers affair. *N. Engl. J. Med.* 1993; **329**(1): 55–57.

299. Maron, B.J., Thompson, P.D., Puffer, J.C. *et al.* Cardiovascular preparticipation screening of competitive athletes: addendum: an addendum to a statement for health professionals from the Sudden Death Committee (Council on Clinical Cardiology) and the Congenital Cardiac Defects Committee (Council on Cardiovascular Disease in the Young), American Heart Association. *Circulation* 1998; **97**(22): 2294.

300. Heidbuchel, H., Hoogsteen, J., Fagard, R. *et al.* High prevalence of right ventricular involvement in endurance athletes with ventricular arrhythmias. Role of an electrophysiologic study in risk stratification. *Eur. Heart J.* 2003; **24**(16): 1473–1480.

Special issues in resuscitation

66

The ethics of resuscitation and end of life decisions

Peter Baskett, Arthur B. Sanders and Petter Steen

Stanton St Quentin, Wiltshire, UK, Department of Emergency Medicine, University of Arizona, Tucson, AZ, USA, Oslo, Norway

Introduction

Successful resuscitation attempts have brought extended, useful, and precious life to many, and happiness and relief to their relatives and loved ones. And yet there are occasions when resuscitation attempts have merely prolonged suffering and the process of dying. In a few cases, resuscitation has resulted in the ultimate tragedy – the patient in a persistent vegetative state. It is to be remembered that resuscitation attempts are unsuccessful in 70%–95% of cases and death ultimately is inevitable. All would wish to die with dignity.

A number of ethical decisions are required to ensure that the decisions to attempt or withhold resuscitation are appropriate and the patients and their loved ones are treated with dignity. These decisions may be influenced by individual, international, and local cultural, legal, traditional, religious, social and economic factors.[1–10] Sometimes the decisions can be made in advance, but often they have to be made in a matter of seconds at the time of the emergency. Therefore, it is important that healthcare providers understand the principles involved before they are put in a situation where a resuscitation decision must be made.

This chapter will deal with the following ethical aspects and decisions:

- Advance directives, sometimes known as Living Wills
- When not to start resuscitation attempts
- When to stop resuscitation attempts
- Decision making by non-physicians
- When to withdraw treatment in those in a persistent vegetative state following resuscitation
- Decisions regarding active euthanasia

- Decisions regarding family members or loved ones who wish to be present during resuscitation
- Decisions regarding research and training on the recently dead
- The breaking of bad news to relatives and loved ones
- Staff support.

There are many different schools in medical ethics with emphasis on different principles such as duty (deontology, Kantian ethics), virtue, or the consequences of the decisions (utilitarian). Most common in the Western world today are the four principles of biomedical ethics, first presented by Beauchamp and Childress[11] based upon discussions in a US Presidential commission. The four key principles are *beneficence, non-maleficence, justice, and autonomy*.

Beneficence implies that healthcare attendants must provide benefit while balancing benefit and risks. Commonly, this will involve attempting resuscitation, but on occasion it will mean withholding cardiopulmonary resuscitation. Beneficence may also include responding to the overall needs of the community, such as establishing a program of public access to defibrillation.

Non-maleficence means doing no harm. Resuscitation should not be attempted in futile cases, nor when it is against the patient's wishes (expressed when the individual is in a mentally competent state).

Justice implies a duty to spread benefits and risks equally within a society. If resuscitation is provided, it should be made available to all who will benefit from it within the available resources. Also the needs of others may be compromised if excessive resources are allocated to futile attempts at resuscitation. The ethical principle of justice is independent of legal systems or cultural traditions, but

Cardiac Arrest: The Science and Practice of Resuscitation Medicine. 2nd edn., ed. Norman Paradis, Henry Halperin, Karl Kern, Volker Wenzel, Douglas Chamberlain. Published by Cambridge University Press. © Cambridge University Press, 2007.

these two factors will affect how ethical justice is emphasized within a context.

Autonomy relates to the patients being able to make informed decisions on their own behalf, rather than being subjected to paternalistic decisions being made for them by the medical or nursing professions. This principle was introduced, particularly during the past 30 years, arising from legislature such as the Helsinki Declaration of Human Rights and its subsequent modifications and amendments.[12] Autonomy requires that the patient is adequately informed, competent, free from undue pressure, and that there is consistency in the patient's preferences.

Advance Directives

Advance directives have been introduced in many countries emphasizing the importance of patient autonomy. Advance directives are a method of communicating the patient's wishes concerning future care, particularly towards the end of life, and must be expressed while the patient is mentally competent and not under duress. They are likely to specify limitations concerning terminal care, including the withholding of cardiopulmonary resuscitation (CPR). The term advance directive applies to any expression of patient preferences, including mere dialogue between patient and/or close relatives and loved ones and/or medical or nursing attendants. This may help healthcare attendants to assess the patient's wishes in the event of the patient becoming mentally incompetent. Nevertheless, problems can arise. The relative may misinterpret the wishes of the patient, or indeed may have a vested interest in the death (or continued existence) of the patient. Healthcare providers tend to underestimate sick patients' desire to live.

Written directions by the patient, legally administered living wills, or powers of attorney may eliminate some of these problems, but are not without limitations. The patient should describe the situation envisaged when life support should be withheld or discontinued as precisely as possible. This may be aided by a medical adviser. For instance, many would prefer not to undergo the indignity of futile CPR if there was end-stage multiorgan failure with no reversible cause, but would welcome the attempt at resuscitation should ventricular fibrillation occur in association with a remediable primary cardiac cause.

In sudden out-of-hospital cardiac arrest the attendants usually do not know the patient's situation and wishes, and an advance directive is often not readily available. Some communities have a standard prehospital advance directive form that will be respected when presented to an emergency healthcare professional. Unless there is a clear advance directive requesting no resuscitation, resuscitation is begun immediately and questions addressed later. There is no ethical objection to stopping the resuscitation attempt that has started if the healthcare providers are later presented with an advance directive limiting care. The family doctor can provide an invaluable link in these situations.

There is considerable international variation in the medical attitude to written advance directives.[1] In some countries the written advanced directive is considered to be legally binding and disobedience is considered to be an assault; in others the advance directive is flagrantly ignored if the doctor does not agree with the contents. In recent years, however, there is a growing tendency towards compliance with patient autonomy and a reduction in a patronizing attitude by the medical profession.[1]

When to withhold a resuscitation attempt

Whereas patients have a right to refuse treatment, they do not have an automatic right to demand treatment; they cannot insist that resuscitation must be attempted in any circumstance. A doctor is required only to provide treatment that is likely to benefit the patient and is not required to provide treatment that would be futile, although it would be wise to seek a second opinion in making this momentous decision, for fear that his/her own personal values, or the question of available resources, may influence his/her opinion.[13]

The decision to withhold a resuscitation attempt raises a number of ethical and moral questions. What constitutes futility? What exactly is being withheld? Who should decide? Who should be consulted? Who should be informed? Is informed consent required? When should the decision be reviewed? What religious and cultural factors should be taken into consideration?

What constitutes futility?

Futility exists if resuscitation will be of no benefit in terms of prolonging life of acceptable quality. Futility must be discussed in terms of goals or purpose. Some of the controversy regarding futility revolves around disagreements on the goals of resuscitation – prolongation of life compared with the perceived judgement of meaningful life. It is difficult to evaluate the quality of life of another person and its inclusion can imply value judgements. Futility must also be defined in terms of quantitative aspect – how likely is it that the stated goal can be achieved?[14] What is the threshold of anticipated success for deciding that health care providers will not begin a resuscitation attempt – 10%,

5%, 1%. 0.5%. 0.1%? It is problematic that while predictors for non-survival after attempted resuscitation have been published,[15–18] none has been tested on an independent patient sample with sufficient predictive value, apart from end-stage multiorgan failure with no reversible cause. In addition, studies on resuscitation are particularly dependent on system factors such as time to CPR, time to defibrillation, and others. These may be prolonged in any study, but are not applicable to an individual case. For example, studies may show survival from community cardiac arrest in some large cities is as low as 1%–2%, but does that mean that resuscitation should not be attempted for a patient who arrests outside a hospital with a defibrillator available in a few minutes?

Inevitably, judgements will have to be made, and there will be grey areas where subjective opinions are required in patients with heart failure and severe respiratory compromise, asphyxia, major trauma, head injury, and neurological disease. The age of the patient may feature in the decision but age, itself, is a relatively weak predictor of outcome.[19,20] Nonetheless, age is frequently associated with comorbidity, which has an influence on prognosis. At the other end of the scale, most doctors will err on the side of intervention in children for emotional reasons, even though the overall prognosis is often worse in children than in adults. It is therefore important that clinicians understand the factors that influence success of resuscitation.

What exactly should be withheld?

Do not attempt resuscitation (DNAR) means that in the event of cardiac or respiratory arrest CPR should not be performed – nothing more than that. Other treatment should be continued, especially pain relief and sedation, as required. Ventilation and oxygen therapy, nutrition, antibiotics, fluid and vasopressors, and other interventions should be continued as indicated, if they are considered to be contributing to the quality of life. If not, orders not to continue or initiate any such treatments should be specified independent of DNAR orders.

While DNAR orders for many years in many countries were written by single doctors, often without consulting the patient, relatives, or other health personnel, there are now clear procedural requirements in many countries such as the USA, UK, and Norway.

Who should decide not to attempt resuscitation?

This very grave decision is usually made by the senior doctor in charge of the patient after appropriate consultations. Decisions by committee are impractical and have not been shown to work, and hospital management personnel lack the training and experience on which to base a judgement. Decisions by legal authorities are fraught with delays and uncertainties, especially if there is an adversarial legal system, and should be sought only if there are irreconcilable differences between the parties involved. Such decisions are usually associated with undignified media attention that is not in anyone's interest, especially the patient's. In especially difficult cases, the senior doctor may wish to consult his/her own medical defence society for a legal opinion.

Medical Emergency Teams, acting in response to concern about a patient's condition from ward staff, can assist in initiating the decision-making process concerning DNAR.[21] In addition, some hospitals have Ethics Committees that will provide multidisciplinary consultations and advice to the senior physician before a decision regarding limitation of care is made.

Who should be consulted?

Having stated that the ultimate decision for DNAR should be made by the senior doctor in charge of the patient, he or she would be foolish and arrogant not to consult others in arriving at that decision. Following the principle of patient autonomy, it is prudent, when possible, to ascertain the patient's wishes in regard to a resuscitation attempt. This must be done in advance, when the patient is able to make an informed choice. Opinions vary as to whether such discussions should be a routine matter for every hospital admission (which might cause undue alarm in the majority of cases) or only if the diagnosis of a potentially life-threatening condition is made (when there is a danger that the patient may be too ill to make a balanced judgement). It has been shown that doctors find these discussions difficult and in a review of US institutions only 20%–38% of seriously ill patients had discussed possible resuscitation with their physician.[22] Another report from the UK has indicated that the number of cases designated as DNAR fell significantly when there was a directive that discussion of resuscitation decisions with the patient should be mandatory in all who are compos mentis.[23] In presenting the facts to the patient, the doctor must be as certain as possible of the diagnosis and the prognosis and may seek a second or third medical opinion in this matter. It is vital that the doctor should not allow his/her own life values to distort the discussion – in matters of acceptability of a certain quality of life, the patient's opinion should prevail.

It is considered essential for the doctor to have discussions with close relatives and loved ones if at all possible. Although they may influence the doctor's decision, it should be made clear to them that the ultimate decision will be that of the doctor. It is unfair and unreasonable to place the burden of decision on the relative.

The doctor would also be wise to discuss the matter with the nursing and junior medical personnel, who are often closer to the patient and more likely to be given personal information. The patient's family doctor may have very close and long-term insight into the patient's wishes and the family relationships based on years of knowledge of the particular situation.

Who should be informed?

Once the decision has been made, it must be communicated clearly to all who may be involved, including patient and relatives. The decision and the reasons for it, and a record of who has been involved in the discussions should be written down – ideally on a special DNAR form that should be placed in a prominent place in the patient's notes – and recorded in the nursing records. Sadly, there is evidence of a reluctance to commit such decisions in writing by doctors in some centers in some countries.[24]

When to abandon the resuscitation attempt

The vast majority of resuscitation attempts do not succeed and have to be abandoned. A number of factors will influence the decision to stop the resuscitative effort. These include the medical history and anticipated prognosis, the period between cardiac arrest and start of CPR, the interval to defibrillation, and the period of advanced life support with continuing asystole and no reversible cause.

In many cases, particularly for out-of-hospital cardiac arrest, the underlying cause of arrest may be unknown or merely surmised and the decision is made to start resuscitation while further information is gathered. If it becomes clear that the underlying cause renders the situation futile, then resuscitation should be abandoned. Information, such as an advance directive, can also become available, which makes discontinuation of the resuscitation attempt ethically correct.

In general, resuscitation should be continued as long as ventricular fibrillation persists. It is generally accepted, however, that ongoing asystole for more than 20 minutes in the absence of a reversible cause, and with all advanced life support measures in place, is justification for abandoning the resuscitation attempt.[25] There are reports of exceptional cases that prove the general rule and each case must be assessed individually.

In out-of-hospital cardiac arrest of cardiac origin, if recovery is going to occur, a return of spontaneous circulation usually takes place on-site. Patients with primary cardiac arrest who require ongoing CPR without any return of a pulse during transport to hospital rarely survive neurologically intact.[26]

Many will persist with the resuscitation attempt for longer if the patient is a child. This decision is not generally justified on scientific grounds, for the prognosis after cardiac arrest in children is certainly no better, and probably worse, than in adults. Nevertheless, the decision to persist in the distressing circumstances of the death of a child is quite understandable and the potential enhanced recruitment of cerebral cells in children after an ischemic insult is an unknown factor to be reckoned with. Similar decisions, based purely on emotion, may occur if the patient is a celebrity or well known to the resuscitating team, such as a member of staff, but purely emotional decisions do not stand up to evidence-based scientific scrutiny.

The decision to abandon the resuscitation attempt is made by the team leader, but after consultation with the other team members, who may have valid points to contribute. Ultimately the decision is based on the clinical judgement that the patient's arrest is unresponsive to advanced life support. In the end, the final conclusion should be reached by the team leader taking all facts and views into consideration and dealing sympathetically, but firmly, with any dissenter.

Decision-making by non-physicians

Many cases of out-of-hospital cardiac arrest are dealt with by emergency medical technicians or paramedics, who face similar dilemmas of when resuscitation is futile and when it should be abandoned. Clearly, resuscitation is futile in cases of cardiac arrest with a mortal injury such as decapitation and hemicorporectomy, known prolonged submersion, incineration, rigor mortis, dependent lividity and fetal maceration. In such cases the non-physician is making a diagnosis of death but is not certifying death (which in most countries can be done only by a physician). In some countries emergency medicine technicians operate under the authority of a base station physician or medical director specific protocols. Consultation with the base hospital physician is strongly advised when the decision is being considered regarding medical futility.

But what of the decision to abandon a resuscitation attempt? Should paramedics trained in, and able to provide, advanced life support in terms of cardiac monitoring, ventilation with oxygen through a secure airway, and appropriate drug administration be able to declare death after 20 minutes of asystole in the absence of reversible causes – bearing in mind the very negative results achieved with on-going CPR during transport? Opinions vary from country to country.[27] In some countries it is routine, and it is clearly unreasonable to expect paramedics to continue with resuscitation in the precise circumstances where it would be abandoned by a doctor. In making this recommendation it is essential that times are recorded very accurately and written guidelines are provided.[28] The answer would appear to lie in superior training and thereafter confidence in those who have been trained to make the decision.

Similar decisions and a diagnosis of death may have to be made by nurses in nursing homes for the aged and terminally ill without a resident doctor. It is to be hoped that a decision as to the merits of a resuscitation attempt will have been made previously. DNAR consideration should always be addressed for patients in these establishments.

Mitigating circumstances

Certain circumstances such as hypothermia will enhance the chances of recovery without neurological damage. The phrase "not dead until warm and dead" is often cited as a guiding principle to follow, but this only applies to patients with cardiac arrest secondary to hypothermia, not necessarily to other etiologies.

Sedative and analgesic drugs obscure the assessment of the level of consciousness in the patient who has a return of spontaneous circulation.

Withdrawal of treatment after a resuscitation attempt

Assessment of the overall prognosis of the neurological status after resuscitation with a return of spontaneous circulation, but continuing loss of consciousness, is difficult during the first 3 days. During that time, efforts should be made to ensure that blood chemistry and hematology are restored to normal values. There are no specific clinical signs that can predict outcome in the first few hours after the return of spontaneous circulation. Measurement of cerebral spinal fluid creatinine kinase or serum S-100 levels have been found to have a high specificity for determining a poor neurological outcome, but only after about 3 days, and if combined with absent pupillary responses and an absence of motor response to pain and electrophysiological testing, the specificity rises to almost 100%.[29,30] Of note, however, the introduction of therapeutic hypothermia after cardiac arrest appears to have changed the predictive values, and these should be viewed with caution until new predictive values have been established for these patients.

In a very small number of distressing cases, patients regain spontaneous circulation but remain in a long-term persistent vegetative state. The question may arise as to whether such an existence is in the patient's best interest compared to the alternative of dying. If it is found to be the patient's wish not to continue in this state, the question arises as to whether basic treatment such as food and fluids should be withdrawn to terminate life. Generally there is agreement between relatives and the doctors and nurses as to the path to follow. If that agreement means continuing with basic supportive treatment, then there is usually no problem. Similarly, if there is general agreement that life should be terminated by withdrawing basic treatment this can be done with or without the involvement of legal authorities as required in the country. Difficulties arise if there is a disagreement between the doctors and nurses and the relatives, or between the relatives. The very sad case of Terri Schiavo in the United States in 2005 highlights the extreme protracted legal wrangling and indignity that can be associated with such a situation which attracts the intrusive, and often uninformed, media and internet celebrities and figures to add their gratuitous opinions in a highly charged atmosphere.[31] It is of interest that opinion polls in the US supported the withdrawal of the feeding tube in this case and the majority felt that the wishes of the spouse should be upheld, as opposed to the views expressed by the patient's parents and some politicians, who wished to prolong life regardless.[32] The case has prompted many to make an Advance Directive for the first time. In Europe, although there also may be extreme views supporting either side, it seems that many are content to leave the decision to the family and physicians in private.

Family presence during resuscitation

The question of permitting close family members to be present during a resuscitation attempt, if they so wished, was first raised in the literature during the late 1980s[33] and was a subject of continuing debate during the 1990s.[34] Initial reaction to the suggestion by the medical profession (particularly among internists) was very negative,[35,36] particularly if relatives were uninformed and unsupported and there was a general feeling that the process would be very difficult and stressful for staff.[37] Emergency physicians and pediatricians and the nursing staff were more supportive of this concept. The antagonists cited fears that the procedure would be most distressing for the relative, particularly if defibrillation and very invasive measures were being performed. Others maintained that the distraught relative might interfere with the resuscitation process or put the rescuers off their prime objective of saving the patient's life. It was thought by some that the presence of a relative would make the decision to abandon the resuscitation attempt very difficult. Some were afraid that medicolegal action might be taken if apparent weaknesses or failures were perceived to have occurred. Public expectation of success rates from resuscitation endeavors as shown on fictional medical series on television (70%–80%) is much higher than occurs in reality (20%–30% at best) .In practice there has been no evidence to support these fears.

Indeed, there has been a continuing flow of papers supporting the concept of family members being present during the resuscitation process, if they wish.[38–45] Many relatives would wish to be present during resuscitation attempts, and of those who have had this experience, over 90% would to do it again. Most parents would expect to be with their child at this time and would not take kindly to being excluded.[46]

Relatives have noted a number of benefits from being permitted to be present.

These include:

- help in coming to terms with the reality of death and easing the bereavement process;
- being able to communicate with, and touch, their loved one in their final moments while they were still warm. Many feel that their loved one appreciated their presence at that moment, and this may be quite possible if consciousness returns during effective CPR (as has been recorded on occasion, especially with mechanical CPR);
- feeling that they had been present during the final moments and that they had been a support to their loved one when they needed it;
- feeling that they had been there to see that everything that could be done, was actually done.

Clearly a number of measures are required to ensure that the experience of the relative is the best under the circumstances.

- The resuscitation should be seen to be conducted competently under good team leadership with an open and welcoming attitude to the relative. "Black humour," so often the saviour of staff working in such stressful situations, should be postponed until afterwards at the staff debriefing session.
- The relatives should be briefed, in terms that they can understand, before entering and offered continual support during the event by a member of staff (usually a nurse) trained in this subject. They should be given to understand that the choice to be present is entirely

theirs, and no feelings of guilt should be provoked, whatever their decision.

- They should be made aware of the procedures they are likely to see and the patient's response (e.g., convulsive movements after defibrillation) and the possible invasive techniques such as tracheal intubation and placement of central venous lines that may be required. The importance of not interfering with any procedures should be emphasized and any dangers of doing so should be explained clearly.
- In the majority of cases it will be necessary to explain that the patient has not responded to the resuscitation attempt and that the attempt has to be abandoned. The decision should be made by the team leader involving the members of the team. The relative should not be burdened with this responsibility. It should be explained to the relative that there may be a brief interval while equipment is removed and that then they will be able to return to be with their loved one at their leisure, alone or supported, as they wish. Certain tubes and cannulae may have to be left in place for medicolegal reasons.
- Finally, there should be an opportunity for the relative to reflect and ask questions about the cause and the process and be given advice about the procedure for registering the death and the support services available.

In the event of an out-of-hospital arrest the relatives may already be present, and possibly performing basic life support. They should be offered the option to stay and may appreciate the opportunity to help and travel in the ambulance to hospital. If death is pronounced at the scene, the relatives should be offered the help and support of their family doctor or community nurse and bereavement councillor.

For resuscitation staff, both in- and out-of-hospital, it is worth offering training on the best way to help relatives who wish to be present. The Resuscitation Council (UK) has designed a program for such a study day.[47]

From increasing experience of family presence during resuscitation attempts, it is clear that problems rarely, if ever, arise. In the majority of instances the relative comes in and stays but a few minutes and then leave – satisfied that they have taken the opportunity to be there to support their loved one and say good bye as they would have wished. Ten years ago most would not have countenanced the presence of relatives being present during resuscitation, but a recent survey has shown an increasingly open and less patronizing attitude and appreciation of the autonomy of both patient and relative.[1] International cultural and social variations still exist, and must be understood and appreciated with sensitivity.

Training and research on the recently dead

Another matter that has raised considerable debate is the ethics, and in some cases the legality, of undertaking training and/or research on the recently dead.

Training

The management of resuscitation can be taught using scenarios with manikins and modern simulators, but training in certain skills required during resuscitation is notoriously difficult. External chest compressions and, to an extent, expired air ventilation, insertion of the oropharyngeal and nasopharyngeal airways can be taught using manikins, but many other skills, needed on a regular basis during resuscitation, can be acquired satisfactorily only through practice on a human subject, dead or alive, even though the design of manikins and simulators improves year by year. These other skills include, for example, central and peripheral venous access, arterial puncture and cannulation, venous cutdown, bag/valve/mask ventilation, tracheal intubation, cricothyrotomy, needle thoracostomy, chest drainage, and open chest cardiac massage. Some of these skills may be practiced during routine clinical work, mostly involving anesthesia, and to some lesser degree, surgery, but others such as cricothyrotomy, needle thoracostomy, and open chest cardiac massage cannot, and are needed only in a life-threatening emergency when it is difficult to justify a teaching exercise. In modern day practice, with practitioners being called increasingly to account and patient autonomy prevailing, it is becoming more and more difficult to obtain permission for student practice of skills in the living. Gone are the days when admission to a "teaching hospital" implied automatic consent for students to practice procedures on patients under supervision as they wished. And yet the public expect, and are entitled to, competent practitioners for generation after generation.

So the question arises – is it ethically and morally appropriate to undertake training and practice on the living – or the dead?

There is a wide diversity of opinion on this matter.[48] Many, particularly those in, but not limited to, the Islamic nations, find the concept of any skills training and practice on the recently dead completely abhorrent because of an innate respect for the dead body. Others will accept the practice of non-invasive procedures that do not leave a mark, such as tracheal intubation. And some are open and frank enough to accept that any procedure may be learned on the dead body with the justification that the learning of skills is paramount for the well-being of future patients. One option is to request informed consent for the procedure from the relative of the deceased. Nevertheless, only some will obtain permission[1,48] and many find this very difficult to do, especially in the harrowing context of breaking bad news to the recently bereaved. As a result, only non-invasive procedures may be practiced, on the basis that distress will not be caused by what is not seen. Clearly, the days of undertaking any procedure without consent are rapidly coming to an end. Perhaps it is now becoming increasingly necessary to mount a publicity campaign to exhort the living to give permission for training on their bodies after death through advance directives, in much the same way as permission for transplant of organs may be given. It is possible that an "opt-out" rather than an "opt-in" arrangement may be adopted, but this will require changes in the law in most countries. It is advised that healthcare professionals learn local and hospital policies regarding this issue and follow the established policy.

Research

There are important ethical issues regarding advancing the quality of resuscitation by performing randomized clinical trials for patients in cardiac arrest who cannot give informed consent to participate in research studies. Progress in improving the dismal rates of successful resuscitation will only come through the advancement of science through clinical studies. The utilitarian concept in ethics looks to the greatest good for the greatest number of people. This must be balanced with respect for patient autonomy in which patients should generally not be enrolled in research studies without their informed consent. Over the past decade, legal directives have been introduced into the United States and the European Union[49,50] that place significant barriers to research in patients during resuscitation unless there is informed consent from the patient or immediate relative. Data show that such regulations deter research progress in resuscitation. It is indeed possible that these directives may in themselves conflict with the basic human right to good medical treatment as set down in the Helsinki Agreement.[12] Research in resuscitation emanating from the United States has fallen dramatically in the last decade,[51] and it appears very likely that the European Union will follow suit as the rules are implemented there. The United States authorities have, to a very limited extent, sought to introduce methods of exemption,[49] but these are still associated with problems and almost insurmountable difficulties.[52]

Research on the recently dead is likely to encounter similar restrictions unless prior permission is granted as part of an advance directive by the patient, or permission can be given there and then by the relative who is next of kin. Legal ownership of the recently dead is established only in a few countries, but in many countries it is at least tacitly agreed that the body "belongs" to the relatives (unless there are suspicious circumstances or the cause of death is unknown) and permission for any research must be granted by the next of kin unless there is an advance directive giving consent. Obtaining consent from relatives in the stressful circumstances of immediate bereavement is unenviable and potentially damaging to the relationship between doctor and relative. The introduction of these prohibitive directives, as they apply at present, will prevent research in humans into potentially valuable drugs for resuscitation. Research can still be carried out during postmortem examination, for instance, to study the traumatic damage arising as a result of using specific methods of chest compressions, but all body parts must be returned to the patient unless specific permission is obtained from relatives to do otherwise.

Breaking bad news and bereavement counselling

Breaking news of the death of a patient to a relative is an unenviable task. It is a moment that the relative will remember forever, so it is very important that it be done as correctly and sensitively as possible. It also places a considerable stress on the healthcare provider who has this difficult duty. Both may need support in the ensuing hours and days. It is notable that the breaking of bad news is seldom taught in medical school or at postgraduate level.[1]

Contacting the family in case of death of a relative without the relatives being present

If the relatives are not present when the patient dies, they must be contacted as soon as possible. The caller may not be known to the relative and must take great care to ensure that his or her identity is made quite clear and, in turn, the caller must make sure of the relationship of the call recipient to the deceased. In most cases it is wise not to state on the telephone that the patient has actually died, unless the distance and travel time involved is very long (e.g., the relative is in another country). It may be better to say that the patient is seriously and critically ill or injured and that the relatives should come to hospital immediately. It is wise to ask the relative to ask a friend to drive them to hospital and to state that nothing will be gained by driving at speed. When relatives arrive they should be greeted right away by a competent and knowledgeable member of staff and the situation explained immediately. Delays in being told the facts are agonizing.

Who should break the bad news to the relative?

It is no longer acceptable for the patronizing senior doctor to delegate the breaking of bad news to his junior assistant. Nowadays, it is generally agreed that it is the duty of the senior doctor or the Team Leader to talk to the relatives. Nevertheless, it is wise to be accompanied by an experienced nurse who may be a great comfort for the patient (and indeed the doctor).

Where and how should bad news be given?

The environment where bad news is given is vitally important. There should be a room set aside for relatives of the seriously ill that is tastefully and comfortably furnished, with fresh flowers daily, a television and free access to a telephone. There are some basic principles that should be followed when breaking bad news if grave errors are to be avoided and the relative is not to be discomforted. It is essential to know the facts of the case and to make quite sure that you are talking to the correct relatives.

Body language is vital – always sit at the same level as the patient – do not stand up when they are sitting. Make sure you are cleanly dressed – wearing blood-stained clothing is not good. Do not give the impression that you are busy and in a hurry. Give the news they are anxious to hear immediately using the words "dead" or "has died" – "I am very sorry to have to tell you that your father/husband/son has died." Do not leave any room for doubt by using such phrases as "passed on" or left us" or "gone up above".

Going into the complete medical details at this stage is not helpful – wait until they are asked for. Touching may be appropriate, such as holding hands or placing an arm on the shoulder, but people and customs vary and the doctor needs to be aware of these. Do not be ashamed if you shed a tear yourself. Allow time for the news to be assimilated by the relative. Reactions may vary from relief ("I am so glad his suffering is over" or "He went suddenly – that is what he would have wished"), to anger with the patient (" I told him to stop smoking" or "He was too fat to play squash" or " Look at the mess he has left me in"), to self-guilt ("If only I had not argued with him this morning before he left for work" or "Why did I not tell the doctor he got chest pain"), to anger with the medical system ("Why did the ambulance take so long" or "The doctor was far too young and did not know what he was doing") , to uncontrollable wailing and crying and anguish, to complete expressionless catatonia. It may be useful to reassure the family that they did everything correctly such as calling for help and getting to the hospital; however, in the vast majority of cases health care providers are unable to restart the heart.

Some time may elapse before conversation can resume and at this stage ask the relative if they have any questions about the medical condition and the treatment given. It is wise to be completely open and honest about this, but always say if appropriate "He did not suffer". In the majority of cases the relative will wish to see the body. It is important that the body and bedclothes are clean and all tubes and cannulae are removed, unless these are needed for postmortem examination. The image of the body will leave an impression on the relative that will last forever. A postmortem examination may be required and this should requested with tact and sensitivity by explaining that the procedure will be carried out by a professional pathologist and will help to determine the precise cause of death.

Children

Breaking bad news to children may be perceived to present a special problem but experience seems to indicate that it is better to be quite open and honest with them, so helping to dispel the nightmarish fantasies that children may concoct about death. It is helpful to contact the school so that the teachers and fellow pupils can be prepared to receive the child back into the school environment with support and sensitivity.

Closure

In many cases this will be the relative's first experience of death and help should be offered with the bewildering administration of the official registration of death, funeral arrangements, and socioeconomic support by the hospital or community social worker.

Depending on religious beliefs, the hospital padre or priest may play a vital role. Whenever possible, the family physician should be informed immediately by telephone or e-mail with the essential details of the case so that they can give full support to the relatives. A follow-up telephone call to the relative a day or two later from a member of the hospital staff who was involved, enquiring if they can be of any help, and with an offer to answer any questions that the relative may have forgotten about at the time, is always appreciated.

Staff debrief

Although many members of staff seem, and often are, little affected by death in the course of their work, this should not be assumed. Their sense of accomplishment and job satisfaction may be adversely affected and there may be feelings of guilt, inadequacy, and failure. This may be especially apparent in, but not restricted to, very junior members of staff. A team debrief of the event with positive and constructive critique of techniques should be conducted and personal bereavement counselling offered to those with a particular need. How this is done will vary with the individual and will range from an informal chat in the pub or cafe (which seems to deal effectively with many cases) to professional counselling. It should be explained that distress after a death at work may be a normal reaction to an abnormal situation.

Conclusions

Resuscitation has given many a new lease on life to the delight of patients and their relatives, but has the potential to bring misery to a few. This chapter addresses how that misery can be reduced by not attempting resuscitation in inappropriate circumstances or in patients with a valid advance directive and when to discontinue the resuscitation attempt in cases of futility or persistent vegetative state. Ethical issues such as training and research on the recently dead, and the presence of family members during the resuscitation attempt place further burdens on the medical profession, but must be dealt with sympathetically, and with an appreciation of growing patient autonomy and Human Rights throughout the world. Finally, the breaking of bad news is one of the most difficult tasks to be faced by the medical and nursing professions. It requires time, training, compassion and understanding.

REFERENCES

1. Baskett, P.J.F. & Lim, A. The varying ethical attitudes towards resuscitation in Europe. *Resuscitation* 2004; **62**: 267–273.
2. Sprung, C.L., Cohen, S.L., Sjokvist, P. *et al.* End of life practices in European intensive care units; the Ethicus study. *J. Am. Med. Asoc.* 290: 790–797.
3. Richter, J., Eisemann, M.R., Bauer, B., Kreibeck, H. & Astrom, S. Decision making in the treatment of elderly people: a cross-cultural comparison between Swedish and German physicians and nurses. *Scand. J. Caring Sci.* 2002; **16**: 149–156.
4. daCosta, D.E., Ghazal, H., Al Khusaiby, S. Do Not Resuscitate orders and ethical decisions in a neonatal intensive care unit in a Muslim community. *Arch. Dis. Child Fetal Neonatal. Ed.* 2002; **86**: F115–F119.
5. Ho, N.K. Decision making: initiation and withdrawing life support in the asphyxiated infant in developing countries. *Singapore Med. J.* 2001; **42**: 402–405.
6. Richter, J., Eisemann, M. & Zgonnikova, E. Doctors' authoritarianism in end-of-life treatment decisions. A comparison

between Russia, Sweden and Germany. *J. Med Ethics* 2001; **27**: 186–191.

7. The EURONIC Study group. End-of-life decisions in neonatal intensive care: physicians self reported practice in seven European countries. *Lancet* 2000; **355** (9221): 2112–2118.

8. Konishi, E. nurses attitudes towards developing a do not resuscitate policy in Japan. *Nurs. Ethics.* 1998; **5**: 218–227.

9. Muller, J.H. & Desmond, B. Ethical dilemmas in a cross-cultural context. A Chinese example. *West. J. Med.* 1992; **157**: 323–327.

10. Edgren, E. The ethics of resuscitation; differences between Europe and the USA – Europe should not adopt American guidelines without debate. *Resuscitation.* 1992; **23**: 85–89.

11. Beauchamp, T.L. & Childress, J. *Principles of Biomedical Ethics.* 3rd edn. Oxford: Oxford University Press, 1994.

12. Declaration of Helsinki. Ethical principles for medical research involving human subjects adopted by the 18th WMA General Assembly, Helsinki, Finland, June 1964 and amended at the 29th, 35th, 41st, 48th, and 52nd WMA Assemblies.

13. Aasland, O.G., Forde, R. & Steen, P.A. Medical end-of-life decisions in Norway. *Resuscitation* 2003; **57**: 312–313.

14. Moskop, J. Medical futility. In *Ethics in Emergency Medicine.* 2nd edn. Tucson, Arizona, USA: Galen Press, 1995.

15. Danciu, S.C., Klein, L., Hosseini, M.M., Ibrahim, L., Coyle, B.W. & Kehoe, R.F. A predictive model for survival after in-hospital cardiopulmonary arrest. *Resuscitation* 2004; **64**: 35–42.

16. Duatzenberg, P.L., Broekman, T.C., Hoover, C., Schonwetter, R.S. & Duursma, S.A. Review: patient-related predictors of cardiopulmonary resuscitation of hospitalised patients. *Age Ageing* 1993; **22**: 464–465.

17. Haukoos, J.S., Lewis, R.J. & Niemann, J.T. Prediction rules for estimating neurologic outcome following out-of-hospital cardiac arrest. *Resuscitation* 2004; **63**: 145–155.

18. Herlitz, J., Engdahl, J., Svensson, L., Young, M., Angquist, K.A. & Holmberg, S. Can we define patients with no chance of survival after out of-hospital cardiac arrest? *Heart* 2004; **9**: 1114–1118.

19. Herlitz, J., Engdahl, J., Svensson, L., Angquist, K.A., Young, M. & Holmberg, S. Factors associated with an increased chance of survival among patients suffering from an out-of-hospital cardiac arrest in a national perspective in Sweden. *Am. Heart J.* 2005; **149**: 61–66.

20. Ebell, M.H. Prearrest predictors of survival following in-hospital cardiopulmonary resuscitation: a meta-analysis. *J. Fam. Pract.* 1992; **34**: 551–558.

21. Hillman, K., Parr, M., Flabouris, A., Bishop, G. & Stewart, A. Redefining in-hospital resuscitation – the concept of the Medical Emergency Team. *Resuscitation* 2001; **48**: 102–110.

22. Layson, R.T., Adelman, H.M., Wallach, P.M., Pfeifer, M.P., Johnston, S. & McNutt, R.A. Discussions about the use of life-sustaining treatments: a literature review of physicians' and patients' attitudes and practices. End of life Study group. *J. Clin. Ethics* 1994; **5**: 195–203.

23. Diggory, P., Cauchi, L. & Griffith, D. The influence of new guidelines on cardiopulmonary resuscitation decisions. Five cycles of audit of a clerk proforma which included a resuscitation decision. *Resuscitation* 2003; **56**: 159–165.

24. Sovik, O. & Naess, A.C., Incidence and content of written guidelines for "do not resuscitate" orders. A survey of six different hospitals in Oslo. *Tidsskr Nor Laegeforen* 1997; **117**: 4206–4209.

25. Bonnin, M.J., Pepe, P.E., Kimball, K.T. & Clark, P.S. Jr. Distinct criteria for termination of resuscitation in the out-of-hospital setting. *J. Am. Med. Assoc.* 1993; **270**: 1457–1462.

26. Kellerman, A.L., Hackman, B.B. & Somes, G. Predicting the outcome of unsuccessful prehospital advanced life support. *J. Am. Med. Assoc.* 1993; **270**: 1433–1436.

27. Naess, A.C., Steen, E. & Steen, P.A. Ethics in treatment decisions during out-of-hospital *Resuscitation* Resuscitation. 1997; **33**: 245–256.

28. Joint Royal Colleges Ambulance Liaison Committee. *Newsletter* 1996 and 2001. Royal College of Physicians, London.

29. Edgren, E., Hedstrand, U., Kelsey, S., Sutton Taylor, K. & Safar, P. Assessment of neurological prognosis in comatose survivors of cardiac arrest. BRCT I Study Group. *Lancet* 1994; **343**: 1055–1059.

30. Attia, J. & Cook, D.J. Prognosis in anoxic and traumatic coma. *Crit. Care Clin.* 1998; **14**: 497–511.

31. Eisenberg, D. Lessons of the Schiavo battle. *Time Magazine* April 4th 2005; 20–28.

32. Robinson, S. Europe's way of death. *Time Magazine* April 4th 2005; 32–33.

33. Doyle, C.J. Post, H., Burney, R.E., Maino, J. & Kee, F.E. & Rhee, K.J. Family participation during resuscitation – an option. *Ann. of Emerg. Med.* 1987; **16**: 673–675.

34. Adams, S., Whitlock, M., Higgs, R, Bloomfield, P. & Baskett, P.J.F. Should relatives be allowed to watch resuscitation? *Br. Med. J.* 1994; **308**: 1689.

35. Shilling, R.J. No room for spectators (Letters). *Br. Med. J.* 1994; **309**: 406.

36. Osuwagu, C.C.ED codes: keep the families out. *J. Emerg. Nurs.* 1991; **17**: 363–364.

37. BAEM/RCN Bereavement Care in A and E departments. Report of a Working Group. Published 1995 by The Royal College of Nursing, London.

38. Hanson, C. & Strawser, D. Family presence during cardiopulmonary resuscitation: Foote Hospital emergency department's nine year perspective. *J. Emerg. Nurs.* 1992; **18**: 104–106.

39. Awoonor-Renner, S. I desperately need to see my son. *Br. Med. J.* 1991; **302**: 351.

40. Gregory, C.M. I should have been with Lisa when she died. *Accid. Emerg. Nurs.* 1991; **3**: 136–8.

41. Boie, E.T., Moore, G.P., Brummett, C. & Nelson, D.R. Do parents want to be present during invasive procedures in the emergency department? A survey of 400 patients. *Ann. Emerg. Med.* 1999; **34**: 70–74.

42. Boudreaux, E.D., Francis, J.L. & Loyacano, T. Family presence during invasive procedures and resuscitation in the emergency department: a critical review and suggestions for future research. *Ann. Emerg. Med.* 2002; **40**: 193–205.

43. Martin, J. Rethinking traditional thoughts. *J. Emerg. Nurs.* 1991; **17**: 67–68.

44. Robinson, S.M., Mackenzie-Ross, S., Campbell Hewson, G.L., Egleston, C.V. & Prevost, A.T. Psychological effect of witnessed resuscitation on bereaved relatives. *Lancet* 1998; **352**: 614–617.

45. Baskett, P.J.F. The Ethics of Resuscitation. In Colquohoun, M.C., Handley, A.J. & Evans, T.R., eds. The *ABC of Resuscitation*. 5th edn London: BMJ Publishing Group.

46. Bouchner, H., Vinci, R. & Waring, C. Pediatric procedures: do parents want to watch? *Pediatrics* 1989; **84**: 907–909.

47. Resuscitation Council UK – Project Team. *Should Relatives Witness Resuscitation?* p. 13. 5th Floor, Tavistock House North, Tavistock Square, London WC1H 9HR: The Resuscitation Council (UK), 1996.

48. Morag, R.M., De Sousa, S., Steen, P.A. *et al.* Performing procedures on the newly deceased for teaching purposes: what if we were to ask? *Arch. Intern. Med.* 2005; **165**: 92–96.

49. US Department of Health and Human Services. Protection of Human Subjects: Informed Consent and Waiver of Informed Consent requirements in certain emergency circumstances. In 61 Federal Register 51528 (1996) codified at CFR #50.24 and #46.408.

50. Fontaine, N. & Rosengren, B. Directive/20/EC of the European Parliament and Council of 4th April 2001 on the approximation of the laws, regulations and administrative provisions of the Member States relating to the implementation of good clinical practice in the conduct of trials on medical products for human use. EN. *Offic. J. Eur. Commun.* 2001; **121**: 34–44.

51. Mosesso, V.N., Brown, L.H., Leon Greene, H. *et al.* Conducting research using the emergency exception from informed consent: the Public Access Defibrillation (PAD) Trial experience. *Resuscitation* 2004; **61**: 29–37.

52. Nichol, G., Huszti, E., Rokosh, J., Dumbrell, A., McGowan, J. & Becker, L. Impact of informed consent requirements on cardiac arrest research in the United States: exemption from consent or exemption from research? *Reuscitation* 2004; **62**: 3–23.

67

The economics of treating sudden cardiac arrest

Alastair Fischer and Graham Nichol

St George's University of London.
University of Washington-Harborview Center for Prehospital Emergency Care, University of Washington, USA

Introduction

Each year, about 360 000 of about 2.4 million deaths in the USA are caused by sudden cardiac arrest (SCA). Any other cause of death that gives rise to mortality on such a scale (about 15% of all deaths) has seen huge research funding and effort, and funding devoted to finding the cause and successful treatment of the condition. Although much is now known about the cause of sudden cardiac episodes, efforts to apply successful treatment have not received the funding that could be expected of such a large cause of death.

The two main reasons for this are the speed and near-certainty of death. The speed of onset of the condition requires an exceedingly fast response. Successful treatment is available, but it must be applied quickly. Increasing the speed of response of emergency medical services is expensive, and this dominates in the estimation of cost-effectiveness. A fundamental but unresolved question is the extent to which it is worth providing a swift response, and the circumstances in which a society or a health service provider is willing to divert resources from other disease areas, given the uncertainty surrounding the value of the benefits of adding resources to improve the likelihood of success of the treatment. The second reason for the lack of resources is the near certainty of death when the condition strikes. There are relatively few survivors: in most countries, no more than 5% of patients leave hospital alive. Hence, there are few patient support groups to provide a higher profile and act as a lobby group for more effective treatment. There is also a general belief that survivors do not have long to live, whereas the average length of survival is about 6 years, and somewhat longer for those who arrest at a younger age.[1]

But even though sudden cardiac arrest is a common form of death, it is nevertheless a rare event. If the lifetime incidence is 15%, and average life expectancy is 75 years, then there will still only be one sudden cardiac death event every 500 person-years. Once a sudden cardiac arrest (SCA) arrhythmia has become established, the primary means of avoiding death is by defibrillation. Five hundred years is a long time for a defibrillator, if it were to be dedicated to a single person, to have to wait for a single use. Since defibrillators require maintenance, training and retraining of operators, all requiring ongoing costs, it is easy to see why there is not one in every home and on every street corner.

This chapter examines the economics of defibrillation, and tries to generate some general principles. Among other things, the following types of question will be addressed. What is worthwhile doing and what is not? How does the cost of the technology impinge on the total cost of defibrillation? How can training be made less expensive? The chapter also looks more broadly at where there are gaps in knowledge of the cost-effectiveness of combating sudden cardiac death. In particular, modeling will be required to evaluate systems devoted to the treatment of SCA. How could one establish whether emergency service provision in a region requires more or less resources than other uses of resources to maximize the health gain in that community?

The focus of this chapter is the use of automated external defibrillators (AEDs) out of hospital. Implantable defibrillators are not considered except briefly as an alternative therapy and as a potential downstream cost, nor is in-hospital defibrillation. The role of cardiopulmonary resuscitation (CPR) is considered only in passing, but the

Cardiac Arrest: The Science and Practice of Resuscitation Medicine. 2nd edn., ed. Norman Paradis, Henry Halperin, Karl Kern, Volker Wenzel, Douglas Chamberlain. Published by Cambridge University Press. © Cambridge University Press, 2007.

model could be extended to assess the incremental cost-effectiveness of community training or other methods of achieving bystander CPR.

Given the cost of defibrillators and their infrequent use, they will not be cost-effective under all circumstances (i.e., they will not be cost-effective if placed in every home and on every street corner); thus, the limits to what circumstances are cost-effective must be determined on a case-by-case basis. In what follows, we assume that the objective of the provider of defibrillators is to use resources in such a way as to maximize the number of quality-adjusted life years gained for the community under consideration.

For this purpose, two strategies are considered:

1. To bring the defibrillator to the patient (via the emergency services: ambulance, fire brigade, police)
2. To site defibrillators where there are large gatherings of people (sporting events, large auditoriums, airports, railway stations and large shopping centers): public access defibrillators (PADs). About 16%–17% of SCA episodes occur in public places.[1]

Beyond this, there are special cases, such as long-distance aircraft and trains, where an offsite defibrillator cannot be transported to the patient without considerable delay, but where the number of people served by the PAD is smaller than in 2 above, yet still moderately large. Moreover, in the case of air and rail travel there are trained "carers" of the traveling public (hostesses and stewards) who know the location of defibrillators and can be trained in their use.

To estimate the relative magnitudes involved in these two strategies, consider 100 cases of out-of-hospital SCA. About 50 incidents are witnessed, of which some 33 would be at home or in places not served by a PAD. Some of the 17 patients who could be covered by PADs will be treated by them, while for the remainder, the emergency service will arrive first. So in round figures, some 40 to 45% of people could expect to be covered by emergency service and some 5 to 10% by PADs;[2] only a very small proportion of the remaining 50% will receive defibrillation in time to prevent premature death. Each implementation of defibrillation in the community has costs and effects.

The main issues in cost-effectiveness analysis

In assessing the costs and effects of an intervention, it is important to determine

- the population under consideration,
- the intervention,
- the comparator or comparators,
- the perspective of the study,

- the effects (benefits), and
- the costs.

Analysis and modeling of the underlying processes involved also generally require some knowledge of factors (or covariates) that determine the costs and outcomes of the intervention.

The first three of these points are straightforward: the population consists of people suffering out-of-hospital SCA, the intervention is an external defibrillator (either carried by a specialized team such as emergency service personnel, or placed as a public access device), and the comparison is with not using a defibrillator. The other three points: perspective, costs, and benefits, require some discussion.

Perspective

The importance of the perspective of a cost-effectiveness study is often underestimated. There are perhaps three main perspectives that can be taken: that of society, that of a health service as a whole (equivalently, a third-party payer perspective), and that of part of the health service such as an emergency service.

If we take a societal perspective, we must ask ourselves what are the total costs of treating a person suffering SCA with a defibrillator, and what are the total costs of treating them without a defibrillator. Without a defibrillator, there will be virtually no survivors, so the costs will be limited in time. With a defibrillator, however, there will be a small proportion of survivors. They will accrue health care costs for the rest of their lives, which may stretch on for years and occasionally for decades. These costs are relevant to the analysis. They include those of long-term care for people with poor neurological outcomes, and implantable defibrillators for those who receive them.

The perspective also helps to determine how the cost-effectiveness analysis will be carried out. From a societal perspective, we may be interested in comparing the effect of using additional resources for treating SCA on the one hand, with anything else, such as education, defense or the environment, or allowing individuals to spend their extra earnings as they wish rather than be collected as taxes, on the other hand. To determine the allocation of resources between such competing uses, we must place a monetary value on benefits as well as on costs, leading to a cost-benefit analysis.

Nevertheless, we may also be concerned with the costs and benefits to society as a whole (that is, take a societal perspective) without wishing to make comparisons outside the health sector. In that case, it is not necessary to go as far as having to convert health benefits into monetary equivalents. An accepted common currency to compare the full range of health benefits is a quality-adjusted life year (QALY).

To determine how best to spend money within an emergency service, most comparisons can be made by estimating how many seconds can be subtracted from average response time for a given cost of different innovations. The innovation that gives rise to the greatest reduction in average response time for a given cost will in most circumstances be the innovation that gains the most QALYs for a given cost. It is that innovation that should be the first to be adopted. It is only when there is a need to compare spending of additional money within an emergency service with the same money spent elsewhere on health care that recourse to QALYs is required.

The perspective of an economic analysis refers to the group within society that bears the costs and gains the benefits of health care decisions, but the term is also used when examining costs from either an accounting or an economic perspective. Often these perspectives are the same, but sometimes they can be quite different. The accounting approach attributes the cost of a health care worker to the time spent on a task, multiplied by their hourly wage rate. The economic approach attributes the cost of the labor component of making an innovation operational by determining the value of the time spent by looking at what that person would otherwise be doing with the time. In EMS agencies, some of a provider's time is spent waiting for a call to aid, known as on-call time, or using the jargon of linear programming, slack time. If a provider were to be engaged in an activity in place of what would otherwise be slack time, then the so-called "opportunity cost" of their labor will be zero. In other words, it does not cost anything in economic terms if slack time is used for a productive purpose. Conversely, the opportunity cost of delaying an ambulance on its way to defibrillate an SCA victim will be hundreds if not thousands of dollars per minute.

By considering a scenario, we illustrate some of the difficult distinctions that should be made with respect to perspective. Some of these distinctions overlap with decisions about how to deal with costs, and to some degree, the discussion could easily be carried out in the following section on costs.

Suppose that an emergency service with 20 active ambulances carries 1000 people with SCA per year to hospital, where 60 are discharged alive. If SCA patients comprise (say) 1% of all calls, and if they take the same crew-time as a call of average duration, should the SCA calls be debited with 1% of all costs? It is unclear in terms of economic or accounting costs, as there are no theorems to say how joint costs should be apportioned. The decision to allocate costs

as a proportion of resources used is widely utilized as an accounting approach to costs, but is no more than a pragmatic decision.

From an economic perspective, we can gain some idea of how to allocate these costs by supposing that the ambulance service, after pressure from the community, is given resources that would double the number of ambulances from 20 to 40. The service carries no more SCA patients than before (indeed, no more of any sort of patient). Because there are more ambulances than before, response times decrease, and as a result, we suppose that of the 1000 patients with SCA, the number of survivors increases from 60 to 80. The response times for every other sort of patient will also improve. If the active resources have been doubled in order to deal with life-threatening conditions (and for no other reason), however, then the life-threatening conditions alone should be ascribed the cost of the additional ambulances. These costs should not be spread over the people with non-life-threatening conditions who are carried by ambulance. If, perversely, the only people eligible to be carried by an ambulance were those *without* a life-threatening condition, society would probably not provide resources for ambulances at all, and probably rightly so. Notably also, as a consequence of why the ambulances are being provided, ambulances should give priority to people who have life-threatening conditions over those who do not.

So how much of an emergency service's costs should be attributed to SCA patients? Certainly not only the time taken per call. To this must be apportioned on-call time, as a very minimum. But according to the above logic, almost the whole cost of the service should accrue to life-threatening calls, of which SCA calls will be a large portion.

If the perspective is that of the emergency service, we do not need to estimate the cost of postsurvival care for survivors. Find the increased cost of the 10 ambulances, apportion a large chunk (as described above) of this cost to SCA patients, and note that there are 20 additional survivors. If the average number of life-years saved is 6 per survivor, then there would be 2 additional survivors and 12 additional life-years gained per additional ambulance. The cost per life-year saved is thus the cost of the increased number of ambulances divided by 12 if *all* the costs are attributed to SCA, and less if some of the costs are attributed elsewhere (to other life-threatening conditions, and a little to the non-life-threatening conditions carried by the ambulances).

Since we cannot separate the various uses of an ambulance, the most satisfactory solution to this problem of apportionment is to estimate the number of quality-adjusted life-years gained (QALYs) from all uses in aggregate that would be gained from a given increase in resources. That is, the emergency service has to be evaluated for cost-effectiveness as a whole, and not just for its role in treating/transporting cardiac arrest patients.

Nonetheless, while it might be important within an emergency service to consider only ambulance costs, it is clearly not the case for the health service as a whole. All the costs of treating the survivor, however long he or she may live, and whatever future condition is treated, should be included on a time-discounted basis. (We return later to estimate the cost per life-year saved in an emergency service.) These costs would not accrue if the patient had died of SCA, but would accrue otherwise, so they should be counted. Note that the approach of counting later medical costs of survivors of a condition is not always used in economic evaluation, because it is often too difficult to estimate future costs of what will in many cases be unrelated conditions. Therefore, in the model of an emergency service developed later, we will model scenarios where survivor costs are at first excluded and then included.

From a health service or third-party payer perspective, we do not need to consider the benefit that accrues to people who are able to return to work after an SCA episode. Clearly, however, a societal perspective will include such benefits. What proportion of SCA survivors returns to work? The answer appears to be: 'not many,' as the average age of survivors is typically in the late 60s. Perhaps 20% were working prior to their SCA episode, however, so it is not unreasonable to suggest that perhaps half of these people, or 10% of all SCA survivors, are able to return to work. The gain to society is to be found in the additional product, be it the amount of extra food produced by a farmer-survivor or the amount paid for legal services offered by a lawyer-survivor that would not otherwise be produced. In a society with severe unemployment, the return to work of the survivor may cause a temporary replacement to become unemployed, so no additional product would be forthcoming, and the benefit would be zero. Unemployment on this scale has not been common in industrialized societies since the early 1930s.

The situation with respect to survivors who have retired or who are unable to work after SCA also depends on perspective. In society as a whole, giving a pension paid out of current taxes is merely a transfer payment and is assumed not to involve any change in the amount of work undertaken. Thus from a societal perspective, the payment of a pension is not a cost. It is simply a redistribution of existing resources. From the perspective, not of society, but of a government as a whole, if the budget for the country is of fixed size, then the payment of a pension to a survivor will mean that funds are not available for other purposes, so

the pension payment is a cost. From the perspective of the health service/third-party payer, or the emergency service, which does not pay the pension, a pension payment reverts to not being an economic cost.

Costs

The four main cost components are:
1. cost of device
2. maintenance cost of device
3. training and retraining in the use of CPR and defibrillators
4. costs of subsequent health care for survivors.

The reason costs have been broken into components is to see which costs are important. If costs change in the future due to innovation, what changes in cost effectiveness does this imply? Where should effort be placed to reduce costs? Studies show that the cost of the defibrillator itself is not a major component of total costs. Typical costs of a defibrillator are now about $1000 compared with some $2000–2500 in the early 1990s. Modern defibrillators have relatively low annual maintenance costs, but costs of training (and retraining) in the efficient use of defibrillators are relatively high, because training needs to be given to many people. Typically, therefore, maintenance and training costs of a defibrillator over its lifetime will be several times greater than the initial cost of the device.

The cost per survivor of a defibrillator program depends on whether the defibrillator is a public access device or is carried by an emergency service. For a PAD, relative costs depend on how often the device is used; for an emergency service, relative costs are a trade-off between the number of devices and the speed with which patients can be reached. Subsequent healthcare costs for survivors are also a relatively high proportion of total costs.

Questions must be asked in relation to maintenance and training costs. In settings in which a large proportion of workers' time is on call, the cost of maintaining PADs and of training staff in their use may actually be much lower than costs measured by the time taken to perform them. The real cost of training emergency service officers in the use of defibrillators should be much lower than their accounting cost, apart from instructor time. This is because many such officers have large amounts of slack time. If they were instructed in the use of defibrillators during a time that would otherwise be waiting time, the cost of undertaking the training would be free. If the unit being instructed were called in the middle of training, they would immediately be required to abort the training session to attend the call, and in that case, it would be the time of the instructor that is wasted. If 60% of emergency service officer time were slack, then the instructor is at best likely to complete only 3 out of every 5 training sessions (the proportion of completions would be lower if slack times were continually interspersed with brief bursts of activity). Thus, in this example, a premium of 1.67 or more would be attached to the instructor's productive time.

The costs of treating an SCA episode are generally not very high, because the vast majority of people die within a short time, and treatment is not prolonged. For the survivors, most leave hospital within a few days or occasionally within several weeks. A small minority has high costs of continued care because of brain damage. For the majority of survivors, the largest costs are usually occasioned by illnesses that they suffer subsequently, and for many of them, the illness will not be of cardiac origin.

Benefits

The benefits of using defibrillators out of hospital are easy to state but uncertain in their extent: they are the sum of the years of additional life gained by survivors discounted by disability and the effluxion of time. The years of extra life can be estimated retrospectively by long-term follow-up of the survivors from about 1970 onwards. As therapy for people with heart conditions improves, however, it is likely that survival from SCA will change. On one hand, it will increase to the extent that follow-up after survival from SCA will improve. On the other hand, it will decrease to the extent that the kind of person having an SCA episode may be older and most probably sicker than those of past years, because of improvements in therapy for people with heart conditions.

Although to be considered with caution, the life expectancy of survivors, even if it changes by 20% up or down, will be relatively well estimated, however. In comparison, estimation of survival *differences* between earlier and later use of defibrillators is fraught with potentially enormous errors.

Cost-effectiveness estimates of PADs from the literature

Several studies have assessed the economics of EMS without focusing on the cost-effectiveness of specific prehospital interventions for cardiac arrest.[3–14] Others have focused on EMS interventions for other disorders.[15,16] We focus here on previous economic evaluations of EMS (Table 67.1) and non-EMS interventions for cardiac arrest (Table 67.2). Estimates published in these articles were converted to US dollars and adjusted for inflation. Since

few of these studies evaluated the incremental cost per QALY, outcomes were expressed as cost per life saved.

The range of incremental costs of EMS or other interventions for out-of-hospital cardiac arrest is highly variable. Comparisons of the incremental cost effectiveness of EMS interventions or lay responder defibrillation for out-of-hospital cardiac arrest are difficult, because of the heterogeneity of interventions considered, completeness of costs, perspective, and the degree to which uncertainty or sensitivity analyses were used to assess the robustness of the economic results. Although it is generally recommended that health economic evaluations express effectiveness in quality-adjusted life–years, and some survivors of cardiac arrest can have reduced quality of life, the majority of previous studies evaluated lives saved. Thus, comparison with other health interventions is difficult. Assuming an average life expectancy of 6 years among survivors, the cost per life–year (without discounting for costs and benefits that occur in the future) will be 1/6 of the cost per life saved.

Cost-effectiveness of defibrillation in an emergency service

We shall now return to examine in more detail the estimation of costs and benefits in an emergency service, where the surrogate for benefit is the reduction in ambulance response time. In a very simple scenario, we described above an emergency service that extended two lives per year from SCA for each additional ambulance added to the fleet. By knowing the cost of running an additional ambulance, we can then estimate the cost per life extended, and by estimating the average additional life expectancy, we can estimate the cost per life–year gained. We said nothing about how one might estimate the number of people saved in this way in the real world.

First, however, let us contrast the economic evaluation of the provision of PADs with that of the provision of an emergency service. The problem of optimal provision of PADs is to place them in those public places where they will be used sufficiently often to justify their provision. This can be judged by estimating the cost per QALY of the provision at different sorts of location. Nevertheless, the optimal provision of defibrillators in an emergency service (assuming that each responder is equipped with a defibrillator) depends on the (incremental) costs and the (incremental) benefits of increasing the number of responders. This research has never apparently been carried out satisfactorily. Two studies go some way towards an answer, but in each case, they look only at comparing different innovations

Table 67.1. Previous economic evaluations of EMS interventions for cardiac arrest

Author (year)	Intervention	Comparator	Perspective	Costs Included	Incremental cost-effectiveness $ per life saved
Nichol (1996) (17)	Reduction in response time: In all-ALS system by adding ALS providers	Existing EMS agency	Society	EMS and initial hospital costs only; not ICD or ambulatory costs	2,627, 000
	In BLS+ALS system by adding defibrillator-capable first responders in fire vehicles				383,500
	by adding defibrillator-capable first responders in EMS vehicles				1,134,400
	Change from all-ALS system to BLS+ALS system by adding defibrillator-capable first responders in fire vehicles				286,900
	by adding defibrillator-capable first responders in EMS vehicles				678,200
Jermyn (2000) (18)	Implementation of first responder defibrillation program	Existing EMS agency	EMS	Training and consumables but not capital equipment	
	In urban setting				7,800
	In rural setting				57,400
Ornato (1988) (19)	Treatment by range of emergency medical technicians (EMT)	Existing EMS agency	EMS	Training costs only	
	EMT				12,900
	Defibrillation-capable				3,600
	EMT				3,800
	Advanced cardiac life support				
Urban (1981) (20)	Advanced cardiac life support	Existing EMS agency	Societal	EMS and initial hospital costs only	91,900
Hallstrom (1981) (21)	Rapid defibrillation by EMTs; rapid defibrillation by EMTs with paramedic backup response.	EMTs without defibrillation	EMS	EMS costs assumed	48,100
					80,900
Valenzuela (1990) (22)	Advanced cardiac life support	Existing EMS agency	EMS	Training, equipment and on-time costs	181,000
Jackobsson (1987) (23)	EMTs	Existing EMS agency	Societal	EMS and hospital only	2,800

within an emergency service system. Nichol *et al.*[17] examined the relative merits of adding single responder units or fully-equipped ambulances, but the study was not designed to find out how many additional such units could be added to an EMS fleet for each successive addition to remain cost-effective. Costs per QALY were obtained for each process, but these would pertain only to the margin, and could not tell us how long we should keep adding units to the fleet.

Table 67.2. Lay responder defibrillation interventions for cardiac arrest

Author (year)	Intervention	Comparator	Perspective	Costs included	Incremental cost-effectiveness, $ per life saved
Forrer (2002) (24)	Police automated defibrillation program in coverage area	Existing EMS agency	EMS	Training and equipment but not medical oversight or quality assurance	84,000
Pell (2002) (25)	Lay responder defibrillation program in all airports, railway and bus stations	Existing EMS agency	Society	EMS, hospital and ambulatory but not ICD costs	1,219,300
Nichol (1998) (26)	Defibrillation by police in coverage area	Standard EMS agency	Society	EMS and hospital but not ambulatory or ICD costs	107,000
	Defibrillation by lay responders in coverage area				190,000
Nichol (2003) (27)	Defibrillation by security guards in casinos	Standard EMS agency	Society	EMS, hospital, ICD and ambulatory costs	183,000
van Alem (2004) (28)	Reduction in time to shock by	Standard EMS agency	Society	EMS, hospital and ambulatory costs to six months but not ICD	
	2 min				23,400
	4 min				19,100
	6 min				17,000

Fischer et al.[29] carried out a somewhat different exercise that also compared the cost-effectiveness of a new practice with that of an existing practice. Although this study looked beyond marginal changes in resources, it was carried out from the perspective of an emergency service (in terms of cost per second of a reduction in response time). It did not compare the cost-effectiveness of an emergency service with that of other parts of a health service or use cost per QALY as a unit of measurement. A third study (the OPALS study)[30] claims that average response times should be lower than present response times (because benefits increase exponentially as response times decrease), but says nothing at all about costs, which increase faster than benefits when response times decrease sufficiently.

The model

We now outline a means of estimating the optimal size of an EMS service. This outline is for demonstration and pedagogical purposes and needs to be adapted to local circumstances before being used to guide decision-making in a EMS agency.

The model used is therefore a simple one. Since most of the estimates were derived from studies in England, the analysis is in pounds sterling (£), for which the current exchange rate is £1 = $US1.75. Since costs will vary from one country to another in ways that are not accounted for by either the official exchange rate or a purchasing power parity exchange rate, the model should use country-specific costs if is to be utilized outside the UK.

The objective is to express, in terms of response time, both the total costs and the total benefits of increasing the size of the emergency service within a given geographical area and with given technology and procedures. From there, we find the range of response times for which an emergency service should be provided, and estimate the response time that maximizes the total net benefits (= total benefits − total cost) of the service.

Estimation of total cost

First, we find an expression for annual total cost of an emergency service in terms of response time, as follows.

We define T to be the time from collapse to defibrillation.

T comprises a lag of "a" minutes from collapse to calling the EMS, plus b minutes of activation time from receipt of call to dispatch of responder, plus t minutes of travel time, plus c minutes from arrival to administration of the first shock.

Thus $T = a + b + t + c.$ (67.1)

Response time $R = b + t$ (i.e., activation time + travel time)   (67.2)

Travel time t depends on the distance travelled by a responder, and we assume direct proportionality between time and distance travelled. The distance travelled will depend on the number of responders and whether they are optimally positioned. In the simplest case, assume that the population is uniformly distributed on an infinite plane and that the ambulances (which are uniformly spaced) travel on a rectangular grid. (Think of the ambulances at the centre of each square on a chess board.) The average distance travelled will be half the distance to the top or bottom of the square, plus half the distance to the left or right boundary. The total distance travelled on average will therefore be the distance from the center of the square to the top or bottom. When there are four times as many ambulances, the average distance will halve; when there are nine times as many ambulances, the average distance travelled will be one-third of the original. Thus, for n on-call ambulances, the average distance will be $1/$(the square root of n) compared with the distance for one ambulance. It is likely that as the number of responders increases and average distances fall, average speeds will also fall marginally, and the centralized dispatcher of vehicle placement will place them less optimally, but in the base case of this model, those factors have been ignored.

Thus $T = a + b + d \cdot n^{-1/2} + c$ (67.3)

(If the average speed of responders falls and they become less optimally placed as n increases, this may be modeled by changing the exponent on n in the direction of zero. The exponent on n was estimated by Fischer to be -0.37 for the Surrey Ambulance Service, but the magnitude of this exponent estimated by using a different but plausible functional form was -0.43. A reasonable alternative magnitude for sensitivity analysis would therefore be -0.4.)

Since $R = b + t = b + d \cdot n^{-1/2}$, by rearranging, we obtain

$n = (d/(R - b))^2$ (67.4)

We assume that costs are proportional to the number of ambulance units on duty, which we call $n + n^*$, where n are on-call (and waiting) and n^* are in use.

The total cost of equipping, staffing and operating an ambulance for a year in England is about £300 000 (about $550000). Thus the total cost (TC) of running $(n + n^*)$ ambulances is about £300 000 $(n + n^*)$.

Substituting from (67.4) for n yields
TC = 300 000 $(d/(R - b)^2 + n^*)$ (67.5)

Note that this analysis has been carried out from an emergency service perspective, because the cost of hospitalization and future illness costs for survivors have not been included in Equation 67.5. From a societal perspective, we must add to 5 an average hospital cost H and a cost of future illness of F for each of the $N.S$ survivors, where N is the number of patients annually carried to hospital with SCA and where S is the probability of survival for an individual.

We assume that the survival curve T minutes after collapse, derived from the OPALS study,[30] is given by

$S = \exp(-0.23T)$ (67.6)

Since $T = R + a + c$, then

$S = \exp(-0.23(R + a + c))$ (67.7)

If N people with SCA are carried by the emergency service in a year, the expected number of survivors will be

NS = $N.\exp(-0.23(R + a + c))$.   (67.8)

Thus the total cost of current and future illnesses of survivors is

$(H + F)N.\exp(-0.23(R + a + c))$.   (67.9)

Thus from equations 67.5 and 67.9, total societal cost becomes

TC(soc) = $300000((d/(R - b))^2 + n^*) +$
         $(H + F)N.\exp(-0.23(R + a + c))$ (67.10)

Estimation of total benefits

First, we find the total benefits (TB) for SCA patients in terms of R, from the perspective of the emergency service.

We assume that the NS survivors on average live Y = 6 years at a utility value of 0.7 after an SCA episode, and that the value of a life-year saved (at utility = 0.7) to the health service/third-party payer is £21 000, equivalent to £30 000 ($52 500) per QALY. Clearly, the threshold cost per QALY varies from country to country: for the USA, a figure often used is $100 000; for low-income countries, the figure would be substantially lower.

Thus, using equation (67.8),

$$TB = 21\,000.\,N.Y.\exp(-0.23(R + a + c))$$
$$= 126\,000.\,N.\exp(-0.23(R + a + c)) \qquad (67.11)$$

From a societal perspective, some survivors will be able to return to work. Compared with being on a state pension, society benefits by the additional production that is measured by their earned income. For the sake of this exercise (as we have no data to inform this scenario), we assume that 10% of survivors work at an annual salary of £20 000 for an additional 5 years, giving an additional benefit of an average of £10 000 per survivor. Thus total societal benefit is given by

$$TB\,(soc) = 136\,000.\,N.\exp(-0.23(R + a + c)) \qquad (67.12)$$

Estimation of total net benefit

A ***net*** benefit is defined as the difference between benefit and cost. If the net benefit is positive, the activity will be worth undertaking; if it is negative, then some combination of other activities will be worth doing instead.

Thus the total net benefit from the perspective of the emergency service, using equations (67.5) and (67.11), is given by

$$TNB = TB - TC \qquad (67.13)$$

Societal net benefit (SNB) is given by equations (67.10) and (67.12) as

$$SNB = TB(soc) - TC(soc) \qquad (67.14)$$

The objects of the exercise are to establish, first, the range of values of R for which TNB > 0, and second, the value of R which maximizes TNB, and then to repeat the exercise by using SNB in place of TNB.

We assume that

- $a + c$ = 4.3 minutes (the sum of the time lag between collapse and contact with the emergency service, plus the lag between arrival of the emergency service and the first shock).

    (The magnitude of the first lag, a, will probably never be known accurately, as it relies on people's notoriously poor recollections, but it is probably approaching 2 minutes. The magnitude of the second lag, c, appears to be at least 2 minutes.[30] The figure of 4.3 minutes makes the data consistent with the OPALS predicted survival curve.)

- b = 1.5 minutes (control room activation time, from receipt of call to the departure of a responder).

    (The literature suggests that this is between 1 and 2 minutes.)

- N = 1100 SCA patients carried in any one year.

- n = 20 (average number of ambulances on call (and not in use).

- n^* = 8 (average number of ambulances in use).

- d = 33 (assuming average response time is 8.9 minutes when n = 20, and using equation (67.4)).

    (N, n, n^* and d are derived from Fischer's study of the Surrey Ambulance Service.[29] The average response time was 8 minutes 52 seconds at the time that the Service was studied. Note that as N, n, n^* and d are all inter-related, it would not be appropriate to change one of these variables without changing the others. A different set of these four variables will pertain to each emergency service.)

- F = £40 000 (= $70 000) of future illness costs for each survivor.

- H = £1700 (= $3000) of hospitalization costs.

    (The values for F and H come from the study of Nichol *et al.* (1998) of emergency services in the USA.[26] They have not been adjusted for inflation, because it is likely that the UK costs would have been a little lower in the first instance.)

Thus SNB = $[149\,600\,000.\exp(-0.23(R + 4.3))]$ −
$[300\,000((1095/(R - 1.5))^2 + 8) +$
$41\,700.\exp(-0.23(R + 4.3))]$
$= 107\,900\,000.\exp(-0.23(R + 4.3))$ −
$2\,400\,000 - 328\,500\,000/(R - 1.5)^2$

We show the graphs of total costs and total benefits and the total net benefits from both a societal perspective and an emergency service perspective. The difference between the two results is that the emergency service perspective stops at the hospital door, whereas the societal perspective includes proximate hospital costs and all future health costs of survivors as well as all indirect costs.

According to the assumptions of this model, if the only benefits from operating an emergency service accrue to SCA survivors, and to nobody with other conditions, the service should not be funded, as the net benefits are negative for all response times. This is shown in Fig. 67.1, where the net benefits from an emergency service perspective are maximized at an average response time of 9.2 minutes and a net benefit of −£1.7 million per year. From a societal perspective, the net benefit curve is flat from an average response time of 10 minutes or more, at a value of −£2.8 million per year.

If the benefits of operating an emergency service for other conditions are proportional to those of cardiac arrest for all average response times, and we ascribe a high enough level of benefit to other conditions, then the net benefits of an emergency service become positive for a range of response times. We illustrate this by assuming that all other uses of an emergency service (at each average response time) produce the same net benefits as are gained by people with SCA.

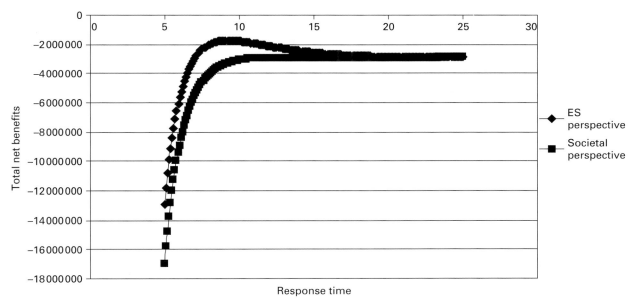

Fig. 67.1. Total net benefits by response time if the only benefits are for SCA.

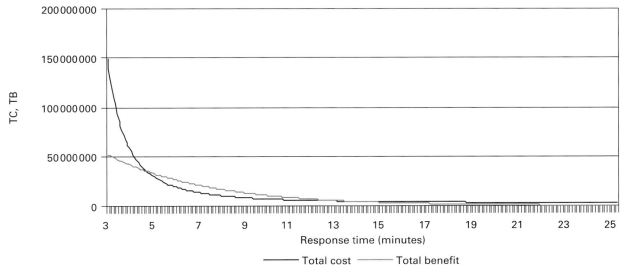

Fig. 67.2. Total costs and benefits by response time when benefits for other treatments are benefits for SCA.

Figure 67.2 shows how both total costs and total benefits change as R changes. As more resources are made available to the service (that is, as R falls) total benefits at first rise faster than total costs. As response times fall sufficiently, however, total costs begin to rise faster than total benefits. The curves cross twice, and at these points, TC equals TB, and net benefits are zero. Between the two crossing points ($R = 4.7$ minutes and $R = 13.4$ minutes), an emergency service is justified. The greatest net benefit of £7.6 million

per year occurs when $R = 6.5$ minutes, as is shown in Fig. 67.3. From a societal perspective, the two crossing points are at 5.8 minutes and 11.1 minutes, the optimal R is at 7.4 minutes and the maximum benefits are estimated to be £2.2 million per year.

The relationship between 75% response time and average response time was estimated by Fischer[29] to be "75Resp" $= 0.136 + 1.163R$, so $R = 6.5$ (the optimum from the emergency service perspective) corresponds to "75Resp" $= 7$ minutes

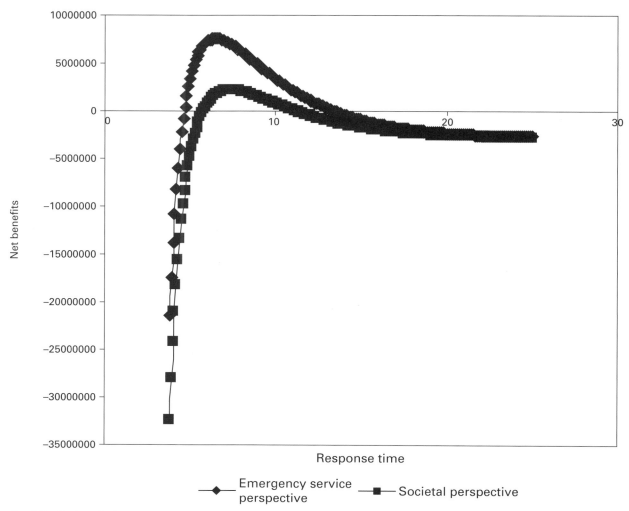

Fig. 67.3. Net benefits by response time if benefits for other treatments equal benefits for SCA.

42 seconds. That is, according to this model, the optimal target for emergency services in urban areas in Britain is approximately correct. From the optimal response time, we calculate that optimal value of n will be $n = (33/(6.5 − 1.5))^2 = 44$ compared with actual 20, and opt $(n + n^*)$ will be $44 + 8 = 52$ instead of $20 + 8 = 28$, a considerable increase. From a societal perspective, opt $R = 7.4$ minutes, and "75Resp" = 8.7 minutes, requiring $n = 31$ ambulances, or $n + n^* = 39$ rather than the actual 28.

The assumption that all calls will have the same average response time is a simplification. To be carried out more realistically, response time should have a distribution and the whole exercise should be done as a Monte Carlo simulation. Since the TC and TB curves are convex to the origin, the optimal response time will be slightly lower than the one calculated in this exercise.

The results would indicate that running an emergency service in a low-income country is probably not a good use of scarce health care resources, because the willingness and/or ability to pay for the service is not likely to be sufficient. In a country that is sufficiently wealthy to afford emergency services, the results depend critically on the extent of benefits from treating and transporting people with conditions other than cardiac arrest.

Discussion

This chapter utilizes some simple economic notions to illustrate how the cost effectiveness of treatments for SCA can be both measured and improved. Among these notions is the idea of opportunity cost applied to otherwise slack time. The opportunity cost of such time is zero, so the idea should be to pack as much new productive work into that time without losing efficiency in the main task of providing a rapid response to emergencies. The extent to which this is possible in practice may be limited. Nevertheless, opportunities to utilize this time will not be sought if a non-zero price is placed on such time by people charged with examining the cost effectiveness of using slack time more productively. But also important are the ideas of marginal/incremental costs and benefits; of perspective; and of the pitfalls in apportioning costs to a single disorder when the same individuals are on call to treat all disorders. It is relatively easy to estimate average costs and benefits; marginal costs and benefits are often much harder to deal with, as the prototype modeling exercise on the optimal level of resource provision indicates. Yet it is the margin that is relevant when changes to the resource base are proposed. Perspective is also important, because it determines which costs and which benefits to include. At the very least, apportioning costs to life-threatening conditions (or more particularly in the context of this discussion, to SCA) is fraught with difficulties. In the context of the appropriate provision of resources for emergency services, the most appropriate approach is to consider the costs of expanding or contracting the emergency service provider as a whole, and to compare these costs with the estimated benefits of doing so.

So where are the boundaries of cost effectiveness with defibrillators?

The first question is whether resources should be put into PADs or emergency services. The cost-effectiveness of PADs has been examined in rather more detail than that of emergency services, probably because the former estimation is much easier to do. For emergency services, it is difficult both to formulate the problem and to estimate the benefits at the margin. We have provided a prototype model that may be modified in many ways, that attempts to discover the optimal level of emergency service provision given current practice.

Currently, in high-income countries, PADs may be justified in cost-effectiveness terms in places where large numbers of people congregate. How many is the lower boundary of "large" in this context? Other things being equal, it will be:

- smaller in the US than in countries that have lower incomes (and therefore a lower ability to provide health care resources),
- larger, the proportion of the at-risk members of the gathering fitted with an ICD
- smaller, the lower the cost of acquiring a PAD
- larger, the greater the extent of vandalism (this makes the average PAD less effective than otherwise)

- smaller, the lower the training and maintenance costs of PADs
- smaller, utilizing the "slack" time of bystanders as training time
- smaller, making the device easy for amateurs to use
- larger, the greater the presence and efficiency of emergency services.

For airlines, it would appear that PADs can be justified for large planes (200+ passengers) in the US, but not for smaller ones. Clearly, this would change if passengers could be trained in defibrillator use in their waiting (slack) time, provided that the device were simple enough to use without prior hands-on experience, and assuming that there is no "learning-by-doing." This conclusion also ignores diversion costs of airliners and the cost of litigation if PADs are not carried.

The appropriate level of funding of emergency services, has probably never been properly estimated. That in this chapter, a crude illustration of how to go about working out the cost-effectiveness of an emergency service, is apparently as good an estimate as has ever been produced, and shows the rudimentary state of the art in this area. Unlike PADs, which have (arguably) probably been provided up to the limit of their cost-effectiveness, it would seem that in many countries, emergency services have been something of a Cinderella service in health care.

Turning to the model proposed in this chapter, changing the values of each parameter in turn could be used to explore the appropriateness of the model in different circumstances. For example, changing the willingness-to-pay variable (assumed to be £30 000 per QALY in the above) would allow a more appropriate analysis for higher-income countries (USA) and lower-income countries. Changing N would act as a surrogate for lower population density. Changing the different assumed time lags would give an indication of their importance and whether it would be worthwhile reducing them. Estimating the benefits for carriage of people with life-threatening conditions other than SCA is very important, as the size of the total benefit of an emergency service determines whether the service should be provided, and if provided, at which level.

The model could also be extended to include single responders as well as fully equipped ambulances. The optimal mix of these two types of responder could be estimated from such a model.

In most situations, decreasing returns mean that the provision of a resource will be limited, because eventually the costs of a further increase of provision will outweigh its benefits. For emergency services, however, we have shown that benefits may increase faster than costs at certain levels of provision, even though the eventual result will be a limit in provision. According to the lower curve in Fig. 67.3, the costs of providing a service with an average response time of over about 12 minutes would generally outweigh the benefits of the service (which is why sufficiently remote areas are not served by emergency services). But as the response time dips below 12 minutes, the benefit (per minute of decrease in response time) increases at an increasing rate, as can be seen from the slope of the curve. Nevertheless, the cost of resources that will allow a decrease of a minute of response time will increase as response time decreases. That is because, if there is a four-fold increase in the number of ambulances, the travel time will not on average be one-quarter of the previous time, but one-half. Thus, at first, the cost-effectiveness of ambulances will actually improve as more resources are added, and in countries where this is so, there is added reason for an increase in those resources.

This analysis has several strengths. First, it provides a framework for decision makers to assess the marginal cost of improving response time by addition of emergency response vehicles to an existing EMS system, whereas most previous analyses have considered the incremental cost of improving the skill level of providers in the field. Second, the framework can be adapted to local circumstances by substituting local effectiveness values. Although the overall survival observed in the OPALS study, the basis of this economic analysis, was low, an EMS system staffed by highly trained, experienced EMS providers who treat a high volume of calls and perform a high volume of procedures each year, with independent medical oversight and quality assurance can achieve survival of 15% to 20%[31] (and unpublished data, Seattle Medic One program, August 28, 2005). In Seattle, WA, survival decreased by 3% with every 1-minute delay in CPR and by 4% with every 1-minute delay in defibrillation.[32] Third, the framework can be adapted to local circumstances by comparison to local thresholds for willingness to pay. The latter is important since a society's willingness to expand EMS can depend on the availability of competing alternatives and adequate resources.

This analysis also has weaknesses. First, it provides a point estimate of the incremental cost of improving response time. Since it relies on several assumptions, there is likely to be large uncertainty in this estimate. Future extensions of this model should use Monte Carlo simulation to evaluate this uncertainty. Second, the model assumes that technology and dispatch protocols are constant through time. Response time can be improved by changes in both technology and protocols, however, or location of vehicles closer to where calls are likely to occur. The costs of these alternate interventions were not considered. Third,

this analysis underestimates the incremental cost-effectiveness by assuming no benefit to use of emergency vehicles for other conditions in one case, and by artificially assuming that cardiac benefits are half of all benefits in the other case. Fourth, the use of OPALS data underestimates survival by assuming zero survival once a VF rhythm has ceased. Despite these limitations, we believe that this analysis represents an important advance over previous analyses of the economics of EMS interventions, and should be validated in a variety of settings.

REFERENCES

1. Engdahl, J. & Herlitz, J. Localization of out-of-hospital cardiac arrest in Goteborg 1994–2002 and implications for public access defibrillation. *Resuscitation* 2005; **64**(2): 171–175.

2. Culley, L.L., Rea, T.D., Murray, J.A. *et al.* Public access defibrillation in out-of-hospital cardiac arrest: a community-based study. *Circulation* 2004; **109**(15): 1859–1863.

3. Riediger, G. & Fleischmann-Sperber, T. Efficiency and cost-effectiveness of advanced EMS in West Germany. *Am. J. Emerg. Med.* 1990; **8**(1): 76–80.

4. Brazier, J., Nicholl, J. & Snooks, H. The cost and effectiveness of the London Helicopter Emergency Medical Service. *J. Health Serv. Res. Policy* 1996; **1**(4): 232–237.

5. Snooks, H.A., Nicholl, J.P., Brazier, J.E. & Lees-Mlanga, S. The Costs and Benefits of Helicopter Emergency Ambulance Services in England and Wales. *J. Public Health Med.* 1996; **18**(1): 67–77.

6. Daberkow, S.G. Location and cost of ambulances serving a rural area. *Health Serv. Res.* 1977; **12**(3): 299–311.

7. Pascarelli, E.F. & Katz, I.B. Planning and developing a prehospital mobile intensive care system in an urban setting. *Am. J. Public Health* 1978; **68**(4): 389–393.

8. Kurola, J., Wangel, M., Uusaro, A. & Ruokonen, E. Paramedic helicopter emergency service in rural Finland – do benefits justify the cost? *Acta Anaesthesiol. Scand.* 2002; **46**(7): 779–784.

9. Gearhart, P.A., Wuerz, R. & Localio, A.R. Cost-effectiveness analysis of helicopter EMS for trauma patients. *Ann. Emerg. Med.* 1997; **30**(4): 500–506.

10. Lechleuthner, A., Koestler, W., Voigt, M. & Laufenberg, P. Helicopters as part of a regional EMS system – a cost-effectiveness analysis for three EMS regions in Germany. *Eur. J. Emerg. Med.* 1994; **1**(4): 159–166.

11. Bruhn, J.D., Williams, K.A. & Aghababian, R. True costs of air medical vs. ground ambulance systems. *Air Med. J.* 1993; **12**(8): 262–268.

12. Nicholl, J.P., Beeby, N.R. & Brazier, J.E. A comparison of the costs and performance of an emergency helicopter and land ambulances in a rural area. *Injury.* 1994; **25**(3): 145–153.

13. Hauswald, M. & Yeoh, E. Designing a Prehospital System for a Developing Country: Estimated Cost and Benefits. *Am. J. Emerg. Med.* 1997; **15**: 600–603.

14. Suchard, J.R., Fenton, F.R. & Powers, R.D. Medicare expenditures on unsuccessful out-of-hospital resuscitations. *J. Emerg. Med.* 1999; **17**(5): 801–805.

15. Cretin, S. Cost/benefit analysis of treatment and prevention of myocardial infarction. *Health Services Research.* 1977; **12**(2): 174–189.

16. Lammers, R.L., Roth, B.A. & Utecht, T. Comparison of ambulance dispatch protocols for nontraumatic abdominal pain. *Ann. Emerg. Med.* 1995; **26**(5): 579–589.

17. Nichol, G., Laupacis, A., Stiell, I. *et al.* A cost-effectiveness analysis of potential improvements to emergency medical services for victims of out-of-hospital cardiac arrest. *Ann. Emerg. Med.* 1996; **27**(6): 711–720.

18. Jermyn, B.D. Cost-effectiveness analysis of a rural/urban first-responder defibrillation program. *Prehosp. Emerg. Care* 2000; **4**(1): 43–47.

19. Ornato, J.P., Craren, E.J., Gonzalez, A., *et al.* Cost-effectiveness of defibrillation by emergency medical technicians. *Am. J. Emerg. Med.* 1988; **6**: 108–112.

20. Urban, N., Bergner, L. & Eisenberg, M.S. The costs of an suburban paramedic program in reducing deaths due to cardiac arrest. *Med. Care* 1981; **19**: 379–392.

21. Hallstrom, A., Eisenberg, M.S. & Bergner, L. Modeling the effectiveness and cost-effectiveness of an emergency service system. *Soc. Sci. Med. [Med. Econ].* 1981; **15**C(1): 13–17.

22. Valenzuela, T., Criss, E.A., Spaite, D. *et al.* Cost-effectiveness analysis of paramedic emergency medical services in the treatment of prehospital cardiopulmonary arrest. *Ann. Emerg. Med.* 1990; **19**: 1407–1411.

23. Jakobsson, J., Nyquist, O., Rehnqvist, N. *et al.* Cost of a life saved following out-of-hospital cardiac arrest resuscitated by specially trained ambulance personnel. *Acta Anesthesiol. Scand.* 1987; **31**: 426–429.

24. Forrer, C.S., Swor, R.A., Jackson, R.E., Pascual, R.G., Compton, S. & McEachin, C. Estimated cost effectiveness of a police automated external defibrillator program in a suburban community: 7 years experience. *Resuscitation* 2002; **52**(1): 23–29.

25. Pell, J.P., Sirel, J.M., Marsden, A.K., Ford, I., Walker, N.L. & Cobbe, S.M. Potential impact of public access defibrillators on survival after out of hospital cardiopulmonary arrest: retrospective cohort study. *Br. Med. J.* 2002; **325**(7363): 515.

26. Nichol, G., Hallstrom, A., Ornato, J.P. *et al.* Potential cost-effectiveness of public access defibrillation in the United States. *Circulation* 1998; **97**(13): 1315–1320.

27. Nichol, G., Valenzuela, T., Roe, D., Clark, L., Huszti, E. & Wells, G.A. Cost effectiveness of defibrillation by targeted responders in public settings. *Circulation* 2003; **108**(6): 697–703.

28. van Alem, A.P., Dijkgraaf, M.G., Tijssen, J.G. & Koster, R.W. Health system costs of out-of-hospital cardiac arrest in relation to time to shock. *Circulation* 2004; **110**(14): 1967–1973.

29. Fischer, A.J., O'Halloran, P., Littlejohns, P., Kennedy, A. & Butson, G. Ambulance Economics *Journal of Public Health Medicine* 2000; **22**,(3): 413–421.

30. De Maio, V.J., Stiell, I.G., Wells, G.A. & Spaite, D.W. Optimal defibrillation response intervals for maximum out-of-hospital cardiac arrest survival rates. *Ann. Emerg. Med.* 2003; **42**(2): 242–250.

31. Fahrenbruch, C.E., Olsufka, M. & Copass, M.K. Changing incidence of out-of-hospital ventricular fibrillation, 1980–2000. *J. Am. Med. Assoc.* 2002; **288**(23): 3008–3113.

32. Weaver, W.D., Cobb, L.A., Hallstrom, A.P. *et al.* Considerations for improving survival from out-of-hospital cardiac arrest. *Ann. Emerg. Med.* 1986; **15**: 1181–1186.

68

Medicolegal aspects

Richard Pawl

Department of Emergency Medicine, Medical College of Georgia, GA, USA

Part 1:   Introduction

Discussing the law in the context of cardiovascular resuscitation would seem to involve a small number of topics. Most commonly, one might consider the malpractice consequences of negligence in the conduct of medical personnel performing cardiopulmonary resuscitation for a dying patient. Certainly, malpractice law is a legal aspect of cardiopulmonary resuscitation (CPR). Yet, because of the nature of the act of CPR, it rarely, alone, becomes the focus of malpractice litigation. Most commonly, malpractice litigation focuses upon the alleged malpractice that leads up to a patient's resuscitation. However, when the resuscitative efforts of medical professionals are the focus of a malpractice suit, the legal theories may be similar to those one may find in other malpractice litigation (e.g., negligent administration of drugs or negligently performing procedures) to more unique causes of action that arise from the resuscitation of a patient with Do-Not-Resuscitate (DNR) orders, such as the wrongful life legal complaint when the patient designated as a "DNR patient" is successfully resuscitated. Indeed, the more one delves into topics related to the law and CPR, the more one finds that to do adequate justice to the topic one must study the bioethics of death and dying and the evolution of advanced directives and how they apply to all patients – competent and incompetent alike. Because the law relating to death and dying is at the cusp of the interface between bioethics and the law, one must also pursue an understanding of the evolution of our laws as they relate to personhood, self-autonomy, and privacy. The "law of privacy" is still controversial in the United States because the concept of privacy as a "right of privacy" largely became a critical issue in legal cases that involved contraception, sexuality, and abortion.[1] Although readers may disagree about the validity of the evolution of the law as it relates to death, dying, and resuscitation, it is the *law of the land* in the United States, and understanding such law enables one to understand the evolution of this law.

In order to see the relationships between the evolution of the law related to death and dying (and thereby, resuscitation) one must begin with the bioethical philosophies that gave rise to some of the legal concepts that have emerged in the course of litigation and legislation. Nevertheless, it would be naïve to consider that an overview of bioethical considerations could ever do justice to the complexities of the topic. Similarly, it would be naïve to consider that any system of thought could adequately address all of the issues that relate to any particular individual's problems in the course of treating each patient in clinical practice. One can only hope to provide ethical and legal information as tools that the clinician may utilize to solve the ethical and legal dilemmas that confront us in the practice of medicine.

Courts have looked to some principles within their common law and precedents that overlap with bioethical principles, such as the concept of patient autonomy. In the present legal climate, for most scenarios, patient autonomy, the right to self-determination, and the right to privacy have emerged as the leading principles that courts will use in medical decision-making cases. As medicine's capability to preserve life became technologically more advanced over the past 35 years, courts have had to face controversies in patient care decision-making that had previously been non-issues. Although it is not always apparent from reading courts' opinions, judges will often look beyond precedents for guidance for their jurisprudence.

Cardiac Arrest: The Science and Practice of Resuscitation Medicine. 2nd edn., ed. Norman Paradis, Henry Halperin, Karl Kern, Volker Wenzel, Douglas Chamberlain. Published by Cambridge University Press. © Cambridge University Press, 2007.

They may delve into bioethical literature, but how judges use that literature may sometimes be in direct conflict with how healthcare providers may apply such literature in treating their patients. In fact, some court decisions regarding issues of patient care and end-of-life decision-making may make sense from a legal point of view, but may seem to be a perverse decision from a healthcare provider's point of view. Nevertheless, parallels between bioethical principles and legal principle may be drawn.

For example, over the last 35 years, medical ethics has been dominated by a body of thought that is often referred to as "principlism" in the bioethics literature. The tenets of principlism may be traced back to *The Belmont Report* that was a product of the National Commission for the Protection of Human Subjects.[2] Created by the National Research Act of 1974 (PL 93-348), the Commission was given the charge to develop ethical guidelines in human research. The four basic principles that were proposed by *The Belmont Report* were autonomy, beneficence, non-maleficence, and justice. Principlism was primarily brought into the mainstream of bioethics by the influence of the authors Tom Beaucamp and James Childress in their publication *Principles of Biomedical Ethics*.[3]

One would think that the legal application of patient autonomy, for example, would merge with the bioethical principles of patient autonomy, and indeed, in some cases they do. The primacy of patient informed consent and informed refusals within medicine arguably were merged from the legal concepts of the same names as they developed within the law. Nevertheless, medicine generally will contend with environments wherein patients and healthcare providers will agree with medical care. That is, patients desire their ability to make autonomous decisions given the appropriate communication with their treating physicians. Courts, on the other hand, must contend with scenarios where providers, their patients, and the patient's surrogates are in conflict. Within those conflicts lies the divergence between principles that seem to be so similar in law and medicine. In some cases, as will be discussed later, a court may actually avoid confronting critically important issues that confront physicians and bioethicists because such issues are far from settled issues for medicine – for example, concepts of futility, ethnocentric issues, and gender issues.

Bioethicists do have the freedom to venture into controversial issues without having to be concerned about the legal concepts with which courts must contend, such as *stare decisis*. Stare decisis represents the legal doctrine of precedent, under which it is necessary for a court to follow earlier judicial decisions within their jurisdiction when the same points arise again within litigation. Additionally, judges must always be aware that their decisions must be respected by other courts within their jurisdictions under the same doctrine of stare decisis. Bioethicists do not have to follow such doctrine, nor do healthcare providers. Hence, bioethicists may freely criticize that the concepts of principlism represent the bioethics of the privileged patient and fail to take into account the inequities of gender and race. Legal scholars have a similar freedom to criticize judicial decisions as decisions that represent value systems applied by largely male, well-insured judges. Nonetheless, judges must be constrained by the accepted principles of law and the future consequences of their decisions. Additionally, although there are valid legal criticisms that some judges have 'legislated from the bench,' judges must deal with conflicts and controversies within a body of law that must be constrained by the will of the people, and leave making new law to the representatives in the legislatures of our system of government. It is because of some of these legal constraints on the courts that parallel concepts in medicine and the law diverge.

To shed light on the differences between decision-making in medicine versus decision-making in the law, it is useful to discuss some cases. It is an accepted biomedical principle throughout the medical community that the concept of patient autonomy includes the right of a patient to be a fully informed participant in every aspect of the medical decision-making process as well as the right to refuse a prescribed treatment, even if such treatment is life-saving treatment. However, patient autonomy does not give rise to the entitlement to receive inappropriate or futile treatment.[4] "No ethical principle or law has ever required physicians to offer or accede to demands for treatments that are futile. Even civil malpractice standards do not require a physician to render useless interventions."[5] But, in 1991, a Minnesota Probate Court Decision rendered an opinion that forced a patient's healthcare providers to render care that many would consider futile.[6]

In December of 1989, an 86-year-old woman by the name of Helga Wenglie broke her hip.[7] After successful treatment at Hennepin County Medical Center (HCMC), she was sent to a nursing home. A month later, however, she developed respiratory failure, returned to HCMC, and had to be supported with mechanical ventilation.[8] Although conscious and aware of her surroundings, attempts to wean Ms. Wanglie from her ventilator repeatedly failed over the ensuing 5 months.[9]

Subsequently, Ms. Wanglie was transferred to a facility that cared for ventilator-dependent patients. While at this facility she had a cardiopulmonary arrest, was resuscitated, and was transferred to an acute care hospital in St. Paul. Because Ms. Wanglie had suffered brain injury from oxygen deprivation after the cardiopulmonary arrest, she remained in a persistent vegetative state. Her health-care providers suggested limiting further life-support treatment and removing her from the ventilator, but her family resisted the suggestion, and had her transferred back to HCMC. However, the healthcare providers at HCMC reached the same conclusion that Ms. Wanglie would remain in a persistent vegetative state and also suggested that Ms. Wanglie be removed from the ventilator. Again, resisting the medical staff's opinion regarding the poor prognosis for Ms. Wanglie, the family believed that only God could take a life, and that allowing the medical staff to remove Ms. Wanglie from her ventilator would be the moral equivalent of playing God.[10]

An HCMC ethics committee reviewed Ms. Wanglie's case and initially advised that the hospital staff should err on the side of continuing treatment while the hospital staff make reasonable attempts to resolve the moral conflicts between the family and the staff. Furthermore, HCMC and the Wanglie family made extensive, unsuccessful efforts to find another provider that would be willing to accept the transfer of Ms. Wanglie to that provider. Ms. Wanglie had become the medical equivalent of a "hot potato."[11]

The hospital turned to the courts to attempt to solve the problem.[12] The hospital first sought the appointment of an independent conservator to decide if the continued use of the mechanical ventilator was beneficial for Ms. Wanglie. Secondarily, if the independent conservator found that the mechanical ventilation was not beneficial, the hospital sought a judgment from the court as to whether the hospital had a duty to continue to provide the ventilator support. Mr. Wanglie filed a motion to be appointed conservator of his wife. After a 4-day trial, Judge Patricia L. Belois found clear and convincing evidence that Mr. Wanglie was the best person to be Mrs. Wanglie's conservator.[13] Judge Belois found that Mr. Wanglie was in the best position "to investigate and act upon Helga Wenglie's conscientious, religious, and moral beliefs" and noted that "[e]xcept with regard to the issue of removing the ventilator, [he] has thoughtfully agreed with the treating physicians about every major decision in his wife's care."[14] Mr. Wanglie then demanded that the hospital continue his wife's death-delaying treatment.[15] After Mr. Wanglie was appointed conservator, the hospital agreed to continue to provide respiratory support to Helga Wanglie, although her physicians deemed such treatment to be non-beneficial because it would not heal her lungs, palliate her suffering, or enable her to experience life.[16] Ironically, Ms. Wanglie died several days after her husband had been appointed her conservator by the court.

Although it was evident in *Wanglie* that the health-care providers were clearly addressing the concept of the futility of Ms. Wanglie's respiratory support, the court successfully ducked the issue of futility. One can speculate that the court appropriately avoided dealing with that issue because to rule on the futility of Ms. Wanglie's care would be the equivalent of forming a definition of futile care in Minnesota. Under the doctrine of stare decisis, such a decision would have lasting consequences on similar controversies heard by other courts in the jurisdiction. However, the court's decision resulted in forcing the providers for Ms. Wanglie to continue "futile" or "non-beneficial" care, an act that bioethical principles would generally not support.

Another case that illustrates the divergence between medical ethics and the law can be found in *In re Baby K*.[17] In October of 1992, Baby K was born with anencephaly.[18] She had suffered from breathing difficulties at birth and required mechanical ventilation.[19] Her initial respiratory support gave her physicians time to explain to her mother that babies with anencephaly usually die within a few days from respiratory failure and other complications.[20] Because aggressive treatment would serve no therapeutic or palliative purpose, Baby K's physicians recommended that she should be provided with only supportive care including nutrition, hydration, and warmth.[21] They also discussed the possibility of a Do-Not-Resuscitate (DNR) order for Baby K.

The mother refused to allow the removal of needed respiratory support and refused to allow the DNR order.[22] As a result of the disagreement between the mother and the caretakers, the hospital sought to transfer Baby K to another hospital, but all the hospitals with pediatric intensive care declined to accept the transfer.[23] Like Mrs. Wanglie, Baby K had become a medical hot potato.[24] But, by November 1992, Baby K was able to survive without mechanical ventilation so the hospital arranged to transfer her to a nearby nursing home.[25]

After being transferred to the nursing home, Baby K required three return visits to the acute care hospital wherein she was given respiratory support, stabilization, and a return to the nursing home.[26] After her second admission, the hospital filed an action in a federal district court in the 4th Circuit Court to resolve the issue as to whether it was obligated to provide emergency medical treatment to Baby K that it deemed medically and ethically inappropriate.[27] Note that this case was heard in a federal court because most of the issues that arose giving the court jurisdiction over this case surrounded the Emergency Medical Treatment and Active Labor Act (EMTALA) rather than the futility of providing Baby K with continued medical treatment.[28] The hospital sought a declaratory judgment that it was not obligated under EMTALA to provide treatment other than warmth, nutrition, and hydration to Baby K.[29] The district federal court held that the hospital was obligated to treat Baby K's breathing difficulty since it qualified as an emergency medical condition, which triggers the hospital's duty under EMTALA to provide stabilizing treatment within their capacity. The hospital appealed to the Fourth Circuit Court of Appeals, which confirmed the district court's decision.

Both courts' decisions hinged on the strict interpretation of EMTALA, which has been the approach the federal courts have generally taken when addressing issues surrounding EMTALA. EMTALA requires a hospital to provide stabilizing treatment within its capabilities to any patient who presents to the hospital with an emergency medical condition.[30] Baby K would present to the hospital filing the appeal from the nursing home with respiratory distress, an emergency medical condition under EMTALA. The hospital argued that (1) the court had previously interpreted EMTALA as only requiring uniform treatment of all patients exhibiting the same condition; (2) that in prohibiting disparate emergency medical treatment Congress did not intend to require physicians to provide treatment outside the prevailing standard of medical care; (3) that an interpretation of EMTALA that requires a hospital to provide respiratory support to an anencephalic infant fails to recognize a physician's ability, under Virginia law, to refuse to provide medical treatment that the physician considers medically or ethically inappropriate; and (4) that EMTALA only applies to patients who are transferred from a hospital in an unstable condition.[31]

The 4th Circuit Court of Appeals rejected all of the hospital's arguments. On the first point, the court determined that the non-discrimination aspect of EMTALA applied to the application of the medical screening exam requirement of EMTALA, pointing out that the statute requires that a hospital must provide stabilizing treatment as required to prevent the material deterioration of a patient's condition.[32] Rejecting the hospital's second argument, the court stated that the plain language of EMTALA included stabilizing treatment to patients with emergency medical conditions and it was outside its "judicial function" to go beyond the statute in considering the issues regarding morally and ethically inappropriate care.[33] The court suggested that the defendants should redress these policy concerns not to the court, but to Congress.[34]

The hospital's third argument was based upon the Virginia Health Care Decisions Act, which recognized that the statute did not expect the doctors in the state to provide treatment they considered to be medically or ethically inappropriate.[35] The Fourth Circuit rejected this argument because of a well-established federal jurisdiction doctrine of pre-emption. The doctrine requires that when state laws are in direct conflict with laws passed by Congress, the state laws are invalid where the states law conflicts directly with a federal law.[36] The hospital's final argument was also rejected by the court based upon the strict interpretation of EMTALA.

Baby K is illustrative of the courts' restrictions in interpreting moral issues that confront medicine. Federal courts have generally interpreted EMTALA as a strict liability statute (with some exceptions that have not withstood the test of time).[37] From a legal point of view, the court followed *stare decisis* by respecting previous decisions of other federal courts addressing EMTALA. Additionally, this court recognized that its duty was to interpret the law, not to legislate it. By refusing to address policy concerns regarding medically and ethically inappropriate care, the court properly suggested that the venue for addressing policy issues in the law is Congress.

From a moral and ethical point of view, however, the decisions in *Baby K* and *Wanglie* are frustrating to many healthcare providers and bioethicists because, in fact, the courts avoided the bioethical concerns that were at the heart of the provider's concerns. It is important to remember during the course of studying decisions made by courts regarding moral issues that confront medicine that easy and clear solutions may not be forthcoming from our courts. Moral and policy issues in medicine are profoundly more complex than those which we may be able to expect the courts to solve. Certainly, our society has made progress in the arena of patient care decision-making over the last 35 years, but we still have a long way to go.

Part 2: Advanced directives and the patient self-determination act

Strictly speaking, advanced directives relate to *any* type of document that either empowers someone to act as a surrogate decision-maker in the event of a person's incapacity or any document that provides some guidance of a person's intents and desires in the event of that person's incapacity. *Black's Law Dictionary* includes both a durable power of attorney document as well as the document often referred to as a living will.[1] In other words, advanced directives are . . . "written instructions . . . recognized under state law, relating to the provision of health care when an individual's condition makes him or her unable to express his or her wishes."[2] Since the beginning of the last decade of the twentieth century, all states and the District of Columbia have enacted some form of advanced directive legislation.[3]

Although the concept of a living will was first proposed in the late 1960s as a response to newly developing medical technology that could prolong a patient's life, the discussion was relegated primarily to the medical and legal literature until the story of Karen Ann Quinlan became a "cause celebre" in the mid-1970s.[4] In fact, inquiring about an opinion regarding Karen Ann Quinlan became a popular interview question in the late 70s for prospective medical students.[5]

Karen Ann Quinlan entered into a persistent vegetative state (PVS) after she had ingested some combination of narcotic-based drugs.[6] Although she did exhibit some basic motor reflexes, it was apparent to her doctors that she was unlikely to awaken from her PVS. At some point, Ms. Quinlan's father sought judicial approval to disconnect his daughter from her mechanical ventilator and allow her to die. However, there were no advanced directives that had been executed by this 21-year-old woman. There existed only indirect evidence that she would not have wanted to continue to live in the condition that she was enduring at the time of her father's petition to the court. Having no precedent, the court accepted her alleged casual oral remarks that she would not have wanted to live in her condition and held that Ms. Quinlan's autonomy should not be discarded merely because she could no longer exercise it on her own.[7]

Subsequently, much public debate ensued regarding life-prolonging treatment, extraordinary measures to prolong life, persistent vegetative states, and methodologies to allow patients to exert their rights to self-determination after such patients became incompetent. Living wills became one answer to dealing with an incompetent patient's right to self-determination. Likewise, documents such as durable power of attorney for health were also advocated.[8] It is beyond the scope of this writing to discuss the details of executing advance directives; however, it is prudent to be aware of the Patient Self-Determination Act and its effects, or lack thereof, on the utilization by patients of advance directives.[9]

Although not without criticisms, advance directives became tools that patients could use to direct their own medical care in the event that these patients became incompetent. In an attempt to buttress the use of advance directives, the US Congress enacted the Patient Self-Determination Act of 1990 (PSDA).[10] Applying to all hospitals, skilled nursing facilities, home health agencies, hospice programs, and managed care organizations receiving Medicaid and/or Medicare funding, the PSDA requires providers to maintain written policies and procedures that will educate patients and the public as to their right to execute advance directives and to direct

their medical care after the time they may lose their decision-making capacity.[11] The providers must also provide materials that inform all adult individuals receiving medical care of that individual's right under state law to make decisions concerning their medical care, including the right to refuse medical or surgical treatments.[12]

Being another unfunded mandate such as EMTALA, the whole thrust of the PSDA was to alert the public about advance directives with the hope that more individuals would begin to use them.[13] Nonetheless, numerous authors have criticized the PSDA as being an abject failure for numerous reasons.[14] One fairly obvious reason is that few patients being admitted to any of the PSDA-mandated institutions are focused on many of the documents that they are routinely given and asked to sign when they enter into these institutions. Additionally, in the absence of any incentives to do so, little time is taken by the personnel providing the written documentation to explain what the documents actually mean. Physicians have no incentives under the PSDA to spend time with their patients discussing advance directives. Merely being *aware* that one has legal rights is not the equivalent of having the requisite understanding in order to execute documents asserting those rights. Furthermore, without adequate knowledge under the *informed consent* doctrine, one could argue that even executed advance directives may not actually allow patients to exercise their rights of self-determination.

In the end, making patients aware of advance directives will not necessarily encourage our patients to take advantage of them. Many laypersons have insufficient information with which to understand the ramifications of such advance directives in the absence of having advisors who can explain what such documents actually mean. Furthermore, being documents that are executed before a person loses decision-making capacity, healthcare providers, surrogates, and courts may find that a patient's advance directives do not address the healthcare issues that an incompetent patient may actually be facing.

Part 3: Evolution of the law of healthcare decision-making

The legal theories and precedents that are now used in the course of litigation involving healthcare decision-making largely evolved from litigation that occurred in the latter part of the twentieth century. Indeed, most of the hallmark decisions that delineated the law of healthcare decision-making largely evolved out of constitutional issues that were evaluated by the United Stated Supreme Court (with some exceptions). We must look to the cases of the Supreme Court to understand the evolution of healthcare decision-making. But first, the constitutional concept of *implied fundamental rights* must be introduced.[1]

The United States Constitution protects a number of individual rights. For example, the right to equal protection under the law is an express right granted by the Fourteenth Amendment of the United States Constitution.[2] The right to free speech is an express right that is provided by the First Amendment of the US Constitution.[3] However, many of the Supreme Court decisions rely upon rights that have been defined by the Court as fundamental rights, yet have not clearly been listed in the Constitution. Over the years, the fundamental rights upon which the Supreme Court relied that are not clearly delineated by the Constitution have come to be known as *implied fundamental rights*. One of the frequently used implied fundamental rights in decisions involving healthcare decision-making is the *right to privacy*.

In common law, one can see that early concepts of one's right to freedom from interference with one's person were already expressed in criminal law, namely the tort of battery. Battery is defined as a harmful or offensive contact with a person, resulting from an act intended to cause the plaintiff or a third person to suffer such a contact.[4] A mere touching of an individual against one's will is enough to cause a battery; however, the act must have been intended rather than accidental. It still holds true that if a physician intentionally performs an unwanted touching of a patient, a battery has been committed by that physician. Yet, battery is not a concept that was sufficiently broad to satisfy the complexities of medicolegal jurisprudence.

American law developed throughout its history with the underlying, carefully guarded concept that every person holds the right to be free from unwanted contact from others as well as unwanted restraints by others. Although, at times, the activities of the population in the United States had double standards with regard to this type of personal freedom (e.g., slavery), even in the nineteenth century there were jurists who were protecting such rights. For example, in 1891, the US Supreme Court asserted that

No right is held more sacred, or is more carefully guarded by the common law, than the right of every individual to the possession and control of his own person, free from all restraint or interference of others, unless by clear and unquestionable authority of law.[5]

An early twentieth-century recognition by a court of a person's right to self-determination was uttered by J. Cardozzo in a 1914 decision in *Schlendorf v. Society of N.Y. Hosp.* wherein he stated that "[e]very human being of adult years and sound mind has the right to determine what shall be done with his body."[6] Another early recognition by a court suggesting that a right to privacy existed was described in a dissent by Justice Brandeis in a case decided in 1928 (during Prohibition). The case involved defendants who were convicted of violating the National Prohibition Act with evidence gathered by the new technique of telephone tapping. In dissenting from the conviction, Justice Brandeis asserted that the protection guaranteed by the Amendments (of the United States Constitution)

[I]s much broader in scope. The Makers of our Constitution undertook to secure conditions favorable to the pursuit of happiness. They recognized the significance of man's spiritual nature, of his feelings, of his intellect. They knew that only a part of the pain, pleasure, and satisfactions of life are to be found in material things. They sought to protect Americans in their beliefs, their thoughts, their emotions and their sensations. They conferred, as against the Government, the *right to be let alone* – the most comprehensive of rights and the right most valued by the individual. (*Emphasis by author*)[7]

Privacy and implied fundamental rights

Over time, the judiciary has evolved the concept of implied fundamental rights largely from the "liberty" protected by the due process clause of the Fifth and Fourteenth Amendments of the United States Constitution.[8] In fact, many writers support the approach of deriving implied fundamental rights from the Constitution by pointing out that the Ninth Amendment of the Constitution avers that there exist other valid rights supported by the Constitution that have not been enumerated in the Constitution.[9] Although there are constitutional scholars who debate the validity of implied fundamental rights under our Constitution, the fact of the matter is that the Supreme Court has based many decisions upon the existence of implied fundamental rights. Hence, the right to privacy is here to stay, for now. The debate regarding whether the US Constitution actually accommodated the concept of implied fundamental rights is beyond the scope of this essay.[10]

The right to privacy may be said to have obtained its stature as an established implied fundamental right in a contraception case in the mid-1960s when the Supreme Court heard *Griswold v. Connecticut*.[11] This case involved a Connecticut statute that prohibited any person from using "any drug, medicinal article, or instrument for the purpose of preventing contraception."[12] Griswold was the Executive Director of the Planned Parenthood League of Connecticut, who was the appellant to the Supreme Court along with Dr. Buxton, who was a licensed physician and a professor at the Yale Medical School who served as the medical director for the League at its Center in New Haven. The appellants had been convicted as accessories to the violation of the Connecticut contraception statute by a married couple whom they advised and who had used contraceptives.

Justice Douglas delivered the opinion of the Court. In the course of his opinion, Justice Douglas evolved the right to privacy in one of the most obscure statements in Supreme Court history. After proceeding past a discussion of various cases involving "rights of assembly," Justice Douglas created the "zone of privacy" right:

The foregoing cases suggest that specific guarantees in the Bill of Rights have penumbras, formed by emanations from those guarantees that help give them life and substance . . . Various guarantees create zones of privacy . . . [t]he present case, then, concerns a relationship lying within the zone of privacy created by several fundamental constitutional guarantees. And it concerns a law which . . . seeks to achieve its goals by means of having a maximum destructive impact upon that relationship. Such a law cannot stand in light of the familiar principle . . . that a governmental purpose to control or prevent activities constitutionally subject to state regulation may not be achieved by means which sweep unnecessarily broadly and thereby invade the area of protected freedoms. NAACP v. Alabama, 377 U.S. 288,307. Would we allow the police to search the sacred precincts of marital bedrooms for telltale signs of the use of contraceptives? The very idea is repulsive to the notions of privacy surrounding the marriage relationship.[13]

Hence, the zone, or the right, of privacy was born from the emanations formed from a penumbra of the Bill of Rights. Many lawyers had to pull out their dictionaries while reading Griswold for the first time.[14] A penumbra is a term that describes the partial shadow in an eclipse or the edge of a sunspot,[15] whereas an emanation is a term for gas created from radioactive decay.[16] Essentially, *Griswold* established the right to privacy for a married couple. In 1972, the Supreme Court considered contraceptives and unmarried couples in *Eisenstadt v. Baird*.[17] Although Justice Brennan, in writing the opinion for the court, did not have to use the marital privacy right discussed in *Griswold* to decide the case, he nevertheless argued for expanding the right to privacy in dicta:

If under *Griswold* the distribution of contraceptives to married persons cannot be prohibited, a ban on distribution to unmarried persons would be equally impermissible. It is true that in *Griswold* the right of privacy in question inherent in the marital relationship. Yet the married couple is not an independent entity with a mind and heart of its own, but an association of two individuals each with a separate intellectual and emotional makeup . . . [i]f the right of privacy means anything, it is the right of the individual, married or single, to be free from unwanted governmental intrusion in to matters so fundamentally affecting a person as the decision whether to bear or beget a child.[18]

Justice Brennan was expanding the right of privacy to apply to begetting and bearing children likely in anticipation of *Roe v. Wade*,[19] which, at the time of *Eisenstadt*, had been argued in front of the Court twice but had not yet been decided.[20] Without going into the controversies involved with the decision in *Roe*, the right to privacy was further delineated by Justice Blackmun in this case:

The Constitution does not explicitly mention any right of privacy. [But], the Court has recognized that a right of personal privacy, or a guarantee of certain areas or zones of privacy, does exist under the Constitution. In varying contexts, the Court or individual Justices have, indeed, found at least the roots of that right in the First Amendment; . . . in the Fourth and Fifth Amendments; in the penumbras of the Bill of Rights, in the Ninth Amendment; or in the concept of liberty guaranteed by the first section of the Fourteenth Amendment. These decisions make it clear that only personal rights that can be deemed "fundamental" or "implicit in the concept of ordered liberty" are included in this guarantee of personal privacy.[21]

Informed consent

As the right to privacy emerged from the basic concept of autonomy in American jurisprudence, so did the doctrines of informed consent and refusal emerge out of American medical malpractice jurisprudence. In the late nineteenth century and early twentieth century, courts were using the general rule that the physician could not treat a patient without his consent.[22] In the late 1950s, however, several courts began to articulate clearly the physician's duty to communicate properly to the patient necessary information with which the patient could make an informed decision about undergoing a proposed course of treatment. In *Salgo v. Leland Stanford Jr. University Board of Trustees*, a California appellate court held that the physician had an affirmative duty to make a "full disclosure of facts necessary to an informed consent."[23] The following year, in *Bang v. Charles T. Miller Hospital*, the Minnesota Supreme Court held a physician liable for failing to disclose information about alternative treatments to the patient undergoing surgery on his prostate wherein the patient's spermatic cords were severed in the course of the operation.[24]

Generally considered to be the beginning of the contemporary period of the informed consent doctrine, two state supreme courts articulated the parameters of what would be considered the informed consent doctrine. In *Natason v. Kline*, after the plaintiff had sustained injuries she did not expect from radiation treatment after mastectomy, the plaintiff claimed the physician "failed to warn [the patient] the course of treatment which he undertook to administer involved great risk of bodily injury or death."[25] Citing *Salgo*, the court held that the doctor was "obligated to make a reasonable disclosure to the [patient] of the nature and probable consequences of the suggested or recommended cobalt irradiation treatment, and he was also obligated to make a reasonable disclosure of the dangers within his knowledge which were incident to, or possible in, the treatment he proposed to administer . . . in language as simple as necessary . . . [the nature of the ailment, the probability of success, and the alternative methods of treatment]."[26]

Several days later in Missouri, the Missouri Supreme Court decided *Mitchell v. Robinson*.[27] The action was against a physician for negligence arising from the performance of insulin shock and electroshock treatment for the patient's schizophrenia. Along with the negligence action, the patient alleged that he had never been informed of the inherent risk that the convulsions experienced during the treatment could fracture bones. The court held that "considering the nature of Mitchell's illness and this rather new and radical procedure with its rather high incidence of serious and permanent injuries not connected with the illness, the doctors owed their patient in possession of his faculties the duty to inform him generally of the possible serious collateral hazards."[28]

Different jurisdictions will have different standards with regard to what is considered to be reasonable and what a physician is obligated to tell the patient in the process of informed consent. Some courts have held that a physician is obligated to tell a patient the information regarding a course of treatment that a reasonable physician would provide in similar circumstances.[29] This is known as the professional standard of informed consent. This standard has been criticized because it requires the plaintiff to establish that there exists a community standard of informed consent by bringing forth expert witnesses to testify to standard. Other jurisdictions use a layperson's standard of informed consent wherein a physician is obligated to provide information considering a course of proposed treatment that a reasonable layperson would wish to have revealed.[30] Criticisms of this approach include that the decision to disclose is a medical professional's decision

and only the medical professional can judge the patient's health and the psychological impact of a disclosure; and that the lay standard for disclosure would waste a doctor's time in disclosing all the risks and limit the doctor's flexibility in caring for the patient's needs.[31]

Traditionally, an action based upon a lack of informed consent would sound in the intentional tort of battery – unless an effective consent is given to the medical practitioner, an unconsented touching or battery has occurred. As the concept evolved under malpractice law, however, courts determined that a physician owes a duty to a patient to disclose fully all information that is pertinent to the proposed treatment and obtain an informed consent. Failure to perform such duty is considered a breach of a physician's duty to the patient and the action sounds in negligence or the tort of medical malpractice. The generally acceptable elements of informed consent would include a physician's duty to inform the patient of his medical condition, the nature of the proposed treatment for that condition, the benefits reasonably expected from the proposed treatment together with the material risks and dangers of that treatment, as well as treatment alternatives and their risks and benefits.[32]

The most commonly invoked exception to informed consent is the emergency exception. Usually fact-specific, the emergency exception to informed consent may be invoked by the healthcare provider where a delay in treatment in order to inform the patient would be life-threatening. The scenario wherein this condition would be most apparent would be in situations where the patient needs an immediate medical intervention, such as cardioversion. Legal authorities will sometimes define this exception as more of a privilege.[33] Requirements of this privilege include "(a) the patient must be unconscious or without capacity to make a decision, while no one legally authorized to act as an agent for the patient is available, (b) time must be of the essence, in the sense that it must reasonably appear that delay until such time as an effective consent could be obtained would subject the patient to a risk of serious bodily injury or death which prompt action would avoid; and (c) under the circumstances, a reasonable person would consent, and the probabilities are that the patient would consent."[34] However, the emergency exception cannot be invoked when it is known by the healthcare providers that the contemplated intervention, regardless of the consequences, had been previously refused by the competent patient who had been properly informed of the needs of such intervention.

Two other exceptions to informed consent are the therapeutic privilege exception and the patient waiver exception. The therapeutic privilege waiver is rarely invoked but it allows physicians to withhold information from a patient when a disclosure of that information would cause the patient emotional or physical harm in the determination of the physician. *Canterbury* upheld a therapeutic exception that allowed physicians to withhold disclosure of certain information to a patient when such information posed a threat to the patient's well-being or in the case of an emergency.[35] The therapeutic privilege exception actually undermines the patient-based standard of informed consent by "allowing physicians to employ their professional discretion to withhold information from their patients."[36]

The patient waiver exception to informed consent allows patients to forgo their right to being fully informed about their medical condition and the proposed treatment.[37] Although rarely invoked by patients, a waiver of informed consent would be appealing to those individuals who prefer to trust the provider's professional judgment or who, because of cultural preferences, would prefer to rest medical decision-making with significant others in their family. Healthcare practitioners would be well-advised to obtain such waivers in writing from patients who are competent to provide consent to treatment in the first place.

Negligence

Negligence emerged in the 19th century in the appearance of liability on behalf of certain persons who professed to be competent in certain "public callings."[38] "A carrier, an innkeeper, a blacksmith, or a surgeon, was regarded as holding oneself out to the public as one in whom confidence might be reposed, and hence as assuming an obligation to give proper service, for the breach of which, by any negligent conduct, he might be liable."[39] Intentional torts became more and more grouped together towards criminal liabilities, and negligence became the more dominant cause of actions for accidental and/or unintentional injuries. Negligence is but one kind of conduct. But a cause of action sounding in negligence requires four distinct elements. First, there must be a duty on the part of a defendant, recognized under the law, to provide a certain standard of conduct, for the protection of others against unreasonable risks. For healthcare practitioners, this duty is usually established by the patient–practitioner relationship. Second, the person owing the duty to the other must have failed to perform his duty in a legally recognizable way. Such failure is otherwise known as a breach of duty. Third, there must exist a reasonably close relationship between the breach of the duty owed and the injury sustained by the

other party – known as proximate cause. Finally, there must be a legally measurable injury to the person alleging the breach of duty.

The healthcare provider's duty arises from the patient/provider relationship. The provider begins the duty to the patient usually by initially rendering treatment to that patient. Although this relationship usually ensues with a "person-to-person" contact, some courts have held that if a physician is "on-call" to an emergency department, and contact is made with that on-call physician for the benefit of a patient being attended to in the emergency department, a physician/patient relationship is established even if the on-call physician has refused to see the patient or is not available to attend to the patient.[40]

Once a duty owed is established by the patient/provider relationship, there must be proof that there was a breach of duty of the provider to the patient for a negligence action to occur. Generally, a breach of duty is characterized as conduct that falls below the standard established by law for the protection of others against unreasonable risk of harm.[41] In the case of physicians, the duty of care is the degree of reasonable care and skill expected of members of the medical profession under the same or similar circumstances.[42] The standard of care for the purposes of a negligence action must be established by the testimony of expert witnesses, i.e., other physicians. States have different requirements for the qualifications of expert witnesses, but it is beyond the scope of this writing to go into the nuances of expert witness qualifications in medical malpractice actions.

It is a necessary element of a negligence action to show that the negligence of the physician is the immediate, proximate cause of the patient's injuries. It must be shown that the alleged negligence was a cause, "which in a natural and continuing sequence produced the event or injury, and without which the event or injury would not have occurred".[43] This is sometimes referred to as the "but for" test – that is, but for the negligence of the defendant, the plaintiff's injuries would not have occurred. The plaintiff must also prove under this element of negligence that the event or injury was foreseeable. "Foreseeability exists when a physician of ordinary skill, knowledge, care, and prudence, in the exercise of ordinary care, would have been able to reasonably anticipate . . . that the event . . . would have occurred as a natural and probably consequence of his conduct."[44]

Finally, the plaintiff must prove damages – that injuries actually were suffered by the patient as a result of the negligence of the defendant. Additionally, the patient may have incurred recurring medical costs, loss of income, pain and suffering damages, loss of consortium damages, and so on, which if quantifiable, could be part of the injuries resulting from the breach of duty of the defendant.

Part 4:   Patient care decision-making at the end of life

The body of law that deals with end-of-life decision-making is hardly settled law. Because the welfare of citizens is largely the concern of individual states, judicial decisions regarding end-of-life issues in healthcare vary among the states.[1] The courts of one state have no legal duty to honor the decisions of any other state although jurists may look to other jurisdictions for non-binding guidance on issues that arise before any court. Over time, parallel, though not identical, trends may be perceived between the courts of different states. However, medical advancements in the last quarter of a century created issues in patient care decision-making that courts had not faced prior to the 1960s. Hence, there has been much less time for development of the body of law dealing with end-of-life decision-making than for many other areas within the law. Therefore, it is difficult to make broad generalizations for every issue that one may encounter in patient care decision-making. The following discussion attempts to identify some clear trends in this area of the law as a guide to understanding and contending with end-of-life decision-making. It is essential to advise the readers always to consult experienced attorneys within their own jurisdictions when faced with critical issues regarding end-of-life decision-making.

The competent adult

Legal scholars tend to agree that there are some general principles that generally apply across all jurisdictions.[2] Probably the most well-established general principle that virtually every jurisdiction will follow is that a competent adult patient will always be given the autonomy to control the medical care he or she accepts or refuses. To state this as a principle . . . "[a]n adult patient with decision-making capacity may refuse any treatment unless the refusal will endanger the public health (or in a small minority of jurisdictions and under very narrow circumstances, a dependent or unborn child). The family has no standing to be involved in the decision-making but may be if the patient wishes".[3]

Competent adults have a broad legal prerogative to decide how to respond to medical conditions that threaten their well-being and even their lives. A competent adult has a privacy right to be free from unwanted interventions even if such interventions are meant to maintain that person's life. Such a scenario occurred in *Farrell*.[4] Kathleen Farrell was suffering from amyotrophic lateral sclerosis and was dependent upon a ventilator to keep her breathing. Even though her physician informed her that removing her from the ventilator would cause her death, Ms. Farrell insisted upon having her ventilator turned off. Her husband filed a complaint with the court seeking his appointment as Special Medical Guardian for his wife with specific authority to disconnect her respirator. Although Ms. Farrell had died while still connected to her ventilator by the time the New Jersey Supreme Court heard the case, the court decided nevertheless to hear the case because of the importance of the issues involved.[5] Citing *Quinlan*, the New Jersey Supreme Court asserted that Ms. Farrell, as a competent adult, could assert her right to privacy to refuse mechanical ventilation because her right to privacy was protected in the common law, the state, and federal constitutions.[6]

Another case illustrative of the principle that competent adults have the right to accept or refuse medical care under common law and constitutional law is useful to review because of the personal and social issues that arose that are not actually reflected in the decision of the court. Elizabeth Bouvia was a 28-year-old quadriplegic woman afflicted with cerebral palsy since birth, who was confined to bed in a public hospital who petitioned the court for a writ of mandate to compel the hospital to stop feeding her through a nasogastric tube.[7] She had previously stated that she wished to starve herself to save her from a life she now considered futile and meaningless.[8] Despite her disabilities, Ms. Bouvia had acquired a college degree and had been married,[9] but her fragile life had become unraveled. Her husband left her and she suffered a miscarriage. Her parents, no longer wishing to provide the care that she needed, turned her out of their home. A search for a place for her to live was unsuccessful, necessitating her living in a public hospital for her care.[10] The court, in granting Ms. Bouvia's request to remove her feeding tube asserted that her motive for the removal was irrelevant because no one's approval was needed for her to exercise her right to refuse medical care.[11] This right to refuse medical care was "basic and fundamental" as "part of the right of privacy protected by both the state and federal constitutions."[12] However, 2 years after her successful court battle, she was interviewed by the L.A. Times, stating that . . . "people should have the right . . . to decide if they want to suffer or not."[13] Professor M. R.

Flick points out in describing Ms. Bovia's plight that perhaps she really had not wanted to die, but had wanted to be wanted.[14] This very poignant observation contains a warning to all clinicians to remember to examine a competent patient's true motives for the refusal of medical care before that patient's options are terminated by death.

There exist some cases where a competent adult was denied the ability to refuse medical care when the well-being of the adult's children was threatened. For example, in *Dubreuil*, a Florida court authorized the administration of life-saving blood transfusion required because of uncontrolled bleeding after delivery of her child, despite her objections to receiving the transfusion on religious grounds.[15] The appellate court invoked the state's *parens patriae* interests in the welfare of Ms. Dubreuil's children necessitating the transfusions against her will, because the court found that the patient was the mother of four minor children and there was no evidence that anyone other than Ms. Dubreuil would be available to care for them in the event of her death from exsanguination.[16]

It is generally true that, except where a state finds that the interests and well-being of minors may be affected by a competent adult's decision for forgo life-saving medical care, a competent adult will always have the right to make decisions regarding the medical care he or she will accept or refuse.

Surrogate decision-making in end-of-life decision-making

Generally, incompetent adults and minors require some sort of surrogate medical decision-making. When it comes to minors, the surrogate decision-makers are typically that minor's parents. Previously competent adults may have a surrogate appointed to make decisions for them either by statutory direction or through an advance directive. Unfortunately, many previously competent adults have no advance directives that provide assistance to providers when such patients need a surrogate. Despite public awareness of living wills, it has been estimated that only 10% to 20% of the adult population in the United States has completed a formal advance directive.[17] Never-competent adults typically will have a public guardian appointed by a court who would be responsible for making medical care decisions for them. Typically, such a guardian would be a close relative, but wards of a state would likely have a public guardian appointed. It is very important for clinicians to keep in mind that there exist limitations to surrogate decision-making, and that such limitations may vary depending on the jurisdiction. Hence, despite generalizations that may

be made below, surrogate decision-making, particularly for end-of-life decisions, will be unique to varying degree in every jurisdiction, so it is prudent for clinicians to be familiar with the laws governing the jurisdiction within which they practice.

Minors

A fairly clear trend in the law is that a . . . "parent, or if there is no parent, the legal guardian, may refuse treatment for a minor who is terminally ill or irreversibly unconscious, so long as the minor agrees."[18] There are some limitations concerning such decisions with regard to infants in some states under federal and state child abuse laws.[19] No parent has the right to refuse beneficial medical treatment provided that the treatment is a generally accepted practice in the medical community and that beneficial outcome is expected. "Parents may be free to become martyrs themselves. But it does not follow [that] they are free, in identical circumstances, to make martyrs of their children before they have reached the age of full and legal discretion when they can make that choice for themselves."[20]

On the other hand, when treatment is "futile" based upon the generally accepted standard of care, and the healthcare providers and parents (or guardian) agree, it is legally acceptable to have life-sustaining treatment withheld or withdrawn.[21] "Futile" life-sustaining care may also be withdrawn upon the agreement of parents and providers if the minor is in a persistent vegetative state.[22] If a minor's parents and healthcare providers disagree upon a course of treatment that is subject to differences of opinion within the medical community, it would be advisable for the providers to seek the advice of experienced attorneys in their jurisdiction before contemplating going to court in such situations. As is usually true, provider communication with the parents often surmounts issues that lead to a decisional impasse. Nevertheless, controversial treatments or treatments with which reasonable clinicians may differ could lead to provider liability.

Importantly Congress enacted the Federal Child Abuse Prevention and Treatment Act in 1984 which provided general standards for the care of infants with defective medical conditions when the infant's life is immediately in danger.[23] The Act generally prohibits withholding or withdrawing treatment for infants when such treatment can be reasonably estimated to correct or stabilize a condition that could be life-threatening. Clinicians caring for infants should also be familiar with their state's child abuse statutes as they may apply to newborns and infants with defective medical conditions.

Adults

Surrogate decision-making law for adults is the most variable and lies at the cutting edge of bioethics and the law in some scenarios. It is beyond the scope of this writing to entertain the wide range of opinions in the bioethics and legal literature on this topic. It is hoped that some useful guidelines may be provided within this area of patient care decision-making, but disagreements between parties involved in the care of incompetent patients will still likely end up in court.

Formerly competent adults

Most laws governing surrogate decision-making will respect a formerly competent patient's autonomy interests by requiring a surrogate to follow the course of treatment the patient would presumably want.[24] Such issues are most clear when the formerly competent patient left explicit instructions in an advance directive. When explicit instructions have been left, the surrogate must follow those instructions if they apply to the medical scenario that the incompetent patient is facing, leaving little independent judgment to the surrogate. There is little controversy when the surrogate must decide *in favor* of recommended medical treatment. Indeed, one may say that the surrogate is merely acceding to the supposed wishes of the patient rather than making a decision on behalf of the patient. Additionally, when an advance directive is clear that a patient would refuse certain treatment if certain conditions are present, there is little argument that such treatment can be refused by the surrogate on behalf of the patient without going to court. Unfortunately, because of the uncertainties of medicine and many ambiguities in advance directives as they exist today, advance directives may sometimes be too vague to assist surrogate decision-making effectively.[25]

If a formerly competent patient made an informed decision to reject certain medical care before becoming incompetent, such decisions will generally be given continuing effect as long as the circumstances have not materially changed.[26] For example, in *Yetter*, the now incompetent Ms. Yetter had refused a breast biopsy for a breast mass when she had been hospitalized for schizophrenia.[27] The patient's caseworker testified that at the time of her hospitalization, Ms. Yetter was "lucid, rational, and appeared to understand that the possible consequences of her refusal included death".[28] Later, Ms. Yetter's mental illness became more profound to the point where she was no longer capable of discussing the matter of the breast biopsy.

Although deemed incompetent at the court hearing, the court gave continuing effect to Ms. Yetter's refusal for the breast biopsy. Citing *Roe v. Wade*, the court stated that "the constitutions right of privacy includes the right of a mature competent adult to refuse to accept medical recommendations that may prolong one's life . . . [and] that the right of privacy includes a right to die with which the State should not interfere where there are no minor or unborn children and no clear and present danger to the public health, welfare, or morals."[29]

Although *Yetter* represents only one jurisdiction, it is likely that, if a formerly competent patient made an informed decision to refuse certain medical treatment when that patient was competent, that patient's autonomy interests would be served by giving continuing effect to that decision. As long as the circumstances have not materially changed, it seems likely that such prior decisions would be respected by the courts.[30] Many of the problems with surrogate decision-making for formerly competent patients arise when there exists little or no information available with which a surrogate can make decisions.

When a formerly competent patient expressed no strong preference or written advance directive regarding the refusal of certain treatment prior to that patient's incompetence, a surrogate decision-maker's choices will be more restricted. It seems possible that, in light of the US Supreme Court's decision in *Cruzan*, state courts that have no clear precedent for surrogate decision-making may impose firm restrictions upon surrogate abilities to withdraw treatment in the absence of an incompetent's clearly articulated preferences.[31] In *Cruzan*, the Supreme Court held that the US Constitution does not forbid a state to require clear and convincing evidence of an incompetent's wishes to withdraw life-sustaining treatment.[32] The "clear and convincing" evidentiary standard represents the strictest civil court evidentiary standard. The only standard more strict is the familiar, "beyond a shadow of a doubt" evidentiary standard that is used in criminal law. The "clear and convincing" evidentiary standard is not a *requirement* of the US Constitution. *Cruzan* merely asserts that a state may set its own standards.

Courts are more likely to allow the discontinuation of life-sustaining treatment when it is clear that the patient in question is in a persistent vegetative state or is terminally ill.[33] Yet, when there is absence of a terminal condition, surrogates may have to surmount evidentiary standards of the courts within their jurisdictions. For example, in *Ragona v. Preate*, the court heard a petition from the guardian and husband of a woman who was in a persistent vegetative state, but was not terminal.[34] The petition requested permission to remove Ms. Ragona's feeding tube. Although the final result of the decision was to allow the removal of the feeding tube the court began its opinion by pointing out that Ms. Ragona's . . . "right to self-determination is [its] guiding principle; the court does not decide whether to withdraw the life-supporting treatment, rather [the court's] role is to determine and effectuate Ruth Ragona's express intent."[35] Citing *Cruzan*, the court stated that Ms. Ragona's intent would have to be proven by clear and convincing evidence and pointed out that . . . "the court must not manage morality or temper theology. Its charge is to examine what law there is and apply it to the facts proven in this cause."[36] The court heard testimony from the treating physician and an independent medical expert to establish that Ms. Ragona was truly in a persistent vegetative state. Subsequently, extensive testimonial evidence was gathered from her husband and her son regarding her previously expressed opinions concerning her wishes. Ms. Ragona had expressed her wishes clearly that she would not wish to live in a vegetative state.[37] The court found the evidence to be "highly persuasive" evidence of Ms. Ragona's intent and granted the husband's petition to remove the feeding tube.[38] One can speculate that if there had been less evidence to support Ms. Ragona's opinions regarding the issues faced by the court that the court would have been disinclined to have her feeding tube removed.

Given the evidentiary requirements that courts may apply, courts will certainly be less inclined to allow a surrogate to refuse medical care when the incompetent patient is not terminal or is in something less than a clearly persistent vegetative state. For example, a New Jersey court ordered that an enterostomy tube be inserted to support the life of a patient who was severely debilitated from a stroke, but who was neither terminally ill nor in a persistent vegetative state.[39] In *Clark*, the patient at issue had not executed a living will or healthcare power of attorney document,[40] nor had he ever expressed any desires regarding medical treatment to any known person. Judging that the court had no basis upon which to base a "substituted" judgment on his behalf, the court used an "objective" test to make "[a] determination of whether certain treatment should be provided or withheld . . . strictly on a weighing of the burdens of life with the treatment versus the benefits of that life to the patient."[41] The court held that the burdens of the surgery to insert the enterostomy tube did not outweigh the benefits that the patient derived from life.

In *Wendland v. Superior Court*, an appellate court required the appointment of an independent counsel when the patient's wife sought appointment as his permanent conservator and to have his feeding tube removed.[42]

Mr. Wendland was a 43-year-old man who had been severely impaired as a result of a motor vehicle accident approximately 2½-years earlier. After being comatose for more than a year, he "awoke" and was found to be substantially brain-injured. He was paralyzed on his right side and was able to follow simple commands.[43] His wife, asserting that Mr. Wendland had made statements that he would not want to live in a state of total dependence, was making arrangements to transfer Mr. Wendland to a convalescent hospital where his feeding tube would be removed and he would be allowed to die.[44] This decision had been supported by Mr. Wendland's physicians and the hospital's ethics committee. Mr. Wendland's mother and sister did not agree with this decision, however, and sought the appointment of an independent counsel for Mr. Wendland in the conservatorship proceedings. The appellate court held that Mr. Wendland was entitled to an independent counsel to represent his interests because "his very life was at stake."[45] Citing *Cruzan*, a concurring opinion went on to say that . . . "this much is clear: a person has a constitutional right to refuse unwanted medical procedures, including artificial hydration and nutrition."[46] "There is little doubt that if [Mr. Wendland] were competent, he could refuse further medical treatment. However, in light of his incompetence . . . [Mr. Wendland's] freedom of choice 'is a legal fiction at best' . . . the court must select a conservator who has a broad authority to make decisions regarding treatment, guided by the patient's best interests."[47]

The evaluation of cases dealing with surrogate decision-making provides some guidance to clinicians, though such guidance is less than ideal. In her treatise on healthcare decision-making the author Claire C. Obade summarized the trends for surrogate decision-making at the present time:

A surrogate may authorize, and perhaps compel, the discontinuation of medical treatment for an adult person without decision-making capacity if the patient is terminally ill, or if the proposed treatment will not be of benefit to the patient. However, the surrogate cannot make a decision contrary to the known preferences of the patient, nor can a surrogate refuse medical care which is reasonably likely to be even of limited benefit. The closest relative is presumably the proper surrogate unless there is a court-appointed guardian or the patient has previously designated another decision-maker. State law should be consulted for priority if there is a disagreement among the guardian, designated surrogate and/or close family members".[48]

Although the evidentiary standards differ amongst the states, the vast majority of jurisdictions in the United States have attempted to ascertain the wishes of the formerly competent patient when evaluating surrogates' requests for or against treatment. The clear and convincing evidentiary standards are applied most vigorously in states such as Missouri and New York.[49] Michigan and Wisconsin apply similar standards for dying patients who still have the capacity to relate to their environment.[50] Fortunately, most states have less rigorous standards for evidentiary proof of a patient's prior intentions.[51] Additionally, courts have the discretion to determine the value of the weight of the evidence they evaluate. Regardless of the evidentiary standards used, the courts will typically attempt to apply a *substituted judgment* on behalf of the previously competent patient. Some courts may use a *best interests* test when previously competent patients have never been found to have expressed their wishes regarding end-of-life issues. The best interests test objective is to treat people the way most people would want to be treated, in other words, evaluating a patient's interests based upon what are believed to be societal standards.

Never-competent adults

Adults who were never competent are considered by the state to be vulnerable constituents whose rights should be carefully guarded. In most scenarios, such incompetent adults should be considered to have the legal status similar to minors. Particularly when such incompetents are wards of the state, regulatory issues must be taken into consideration. The state's mental health statutes may also have a bearing upon the treatment of such individuals. Erring on the side of favoring beneficial treatment is always the preferable rule-of-thumb when providing medical care to these patients. Inevitably, there will arise decision points where it will be necessary to consider the decision to withdraw or withhold treatment for such patients who are in a terminally ill situation or a persistent vegetative state. The prudent clinician should consult with legal counsel familiar with the laws of their jurisdiction whenever considering the withholding or withdrawing of life-saving treatment.

In states where their life-sustaining treatment can only be withdrawn or withheld based upon clear and convincing evidence of the patient's preferences, it is unlikely that a court in such a state would allow the removal or withholding of life-sustaining treatment to a never competent adult. The states that use a "substituted judgment" standard for evaluating the removal of life-sustaining treatment for an incompetent patient may find that the application of this standard to a never-incompetent patient may be stretched and unwieldy.[52] The states that

use a "best interests" test in evaluating an incompetent's rights to refuse or withhold medical treatment would probably be in the best position to contend with these issues in their application to a never-competent patient.[53]

Two authors have proposed a statutory theme that, if enacted, could provide an extra-judicial pathway to forgoing life-sustaining treatments for never-competent patients that would protect the interests of public wards.[54] Although specifically limiting the proposal to developmentally disabled persons who have been adjudicated as incompetent to make their own health care decisions, the authors Deborah K. McKnight and Maureen Bellis provide a solid starting place for dealing with the never-competent patient for end-of-life decision-making. The proposal designates a group of decision-makers for the developmentally disabled public ward who together as a unanimous group could decide to withhold or withdraw life-sustaining treatment without seeking judicial review.[55] The group would comprise an "involved guardian," the patient's attending physician, and either two physicians with relevant experience or the endorsement of a prognosis committee.[56] Patient surrogates acting in good faith and physicians exercising reasonable medical judgment would be immune from civil or criminal liability under this proposal.[57] The proposal outlines four situations in which the decision-makers may choose to forgo life-sustaining treatment: (1) the patient has been in a persistent vegetative state for 12 months, (2) the patient has a terminal illness with uncontrollable pain, (3) the patient is in an advanced stage of a terminal illness with severe and permanent deterioration, and (4) if the patient did not fall under any of the other three conditions a decision for treatment withdrawal only could be made after a conscientious effort that the burdens of continuing treatment outweigh the benefits.[58] The decision-makers would then have to agree that a decision to withhold or withdraw life-sustaining treatment would be in the *patient's* best interest with any disputes between the decision-makers requiring court intervention.[59] Finally, palliative care would always have to be provided.[60]

Without some statutory framework for the purpose of making end-of-life decision-making for never-competent patients, it seems unlikely that such decisions can be made without some court supervision. There have been court decisions that have contended with such issues for patients who have never been competent, but they are few.[61] In light of the struggles that courts have had in dealing with formerly-competent patients, it is similarly unlikely that the courts will be the best venues to solve the problems involved inherent to end-of-life decision-making for never-competent patients.

Medical futility and the courts

The bioethical community and legal scholars have written extensively regarding various definitions of medical futility and their applications to end-of-life decision-making. However, it is not the purpose of this essay to provide an overview of such discussions, but rather to discuss the law that has addressed such issues. Some courts, in cases such as *Wanglie* and *In re Baby K*, that have had the opportunity to address futility issues, have rendered opinions that were clearly frustrating to health care providers as well as bioethicists and some legal scholars.[62] To be sure, few courts have actually had to contend with futility issues. Given the moral and ethical controversies involved with the concept of medical futility in the bioethical and legal literature, it seems clear that the courts will struggle with cases that come before them that force them to contend with the issue. *Wanglie* was one of the few cases in which there was an opportunity to address futile care had the judge decided to appoint a neutral guardian for Mrs. Wanglie who was in a persistent vegetative state. Instead, Ms. Wanglie's husband was appointed the guardian and, as guardian, Mr. Wanglie insisted upon the continued life-support of his wife against the opinion of the hospital and healthcare providers that the continued life-support for her was futile.[63] The Fourth Circuit of Appeals ducked the issue of futility completely when it held that a Virginia hospital was required under EMTALA to provide repeated emergency life-saving respiratory support to an anencephalic infant who had to be repeatedly transferred from a nursing facility to the hospital for recurrent respiratory failure.[64] However, there are a few other cases that have dealt with decisions surrounding the withdrawal or withholding of futile care.

In *Causey v. St. Francis Medical Center*, a physician withdrew life-sustaining care to a 31-year-old quadriplegic woman with end-stage renal failure and stage IV coma over the strong objections of the family.[65] The physician had considered the continued life-supporting treatment morally and ethically inappropriate and was supported by the decision of the hospital's Morals and Ethics Board.[66] The patient's husband and son filed an action against the hospital and the physician as an intentional battery claim. Nonetheless, the trial court dismissed the claim as premature because the doctor and hospital "acted in accordance with professional opinions and professional judgment" and under Louisiana's malpractice act therefore this was required to be submitted to a medical review panel prior to being reviewed by the court.[67] The plaintiffs appealed and the Court of Appeal of Louisiana, Second Circuit, heard the appeal. The appellate court first stated that the Louisiana

state legislature had enacted a statute respecting individual autonomy and the right to self-determination by giving a competent, terminally-ill person the right to *refuse* medical treatment.[68] The court went on to say that . . . "the right or autonomy to refuse treatment is simply a severing of the relationship with the physician . . . [i]n this case, however, the patient (through her surrogate) is not severing a relationship, but demanding treatment the physician believes is inappropriate."[69] Holding that the issue was whether the actions of the physician and the hospital met the standard of care of the medical profession, the court held that the issue fell under the Medical Malpractice Act and must first be submitted to a medical review panel.[70] Although the appellate court did not directly confront the issues of futility, it held that such determinations were in the purview of the standard of care.

A Georgia appellate court found that there were factual issues in dispute that would be required to be submitted to a jury in a case where a physician terminated the life-support treatment of a 9-day-old, critically ill infant.[71] The parents had brought a malpractice suit and an intentional tort suit against a physician for terminating the life-support of their daughter. The infant was born at 24 weeks' gestation on the side of the road on the way to the hospital.[72] The infant had been successfully resuscitated in the emergency room of the hospital, but required life-saving care including blood pressure and respiratory support.[73] The attending physician alleged that he had orally obtained the consent of the parents to stop treatment, which the parents disputed. The malpractice claim was dismissed on procedural grounds, but inconsistencies in the facts were such that the appellate court recognized that the parents could have a valid claim for the wrongful death of the infant based upon the reckless disregard of the consequences of the physician's actions or the heedless indifference to the rights and the safety of others.[74] Coupled with a reasonable foresight that injury would occur, the court suggested that if such allegations were proved, such actions would amount to . . . "criminal negligence equivalent to an intentional tort" and sent the case back down to the trial level.[75]

In sum, a healthcare provider treads on thin ice when walking on the surface of the medical futility issues in contravention of a surrogate's wishes. The results of such conflicts, when they reach the courts, are unpredictable and very fact-specific, dependent upon the jurisdiction. Fortunately, most healthcare providers and surrogates agree with the decisions regarding medically futile care. Unfortunately, when disputes are not resolvable through careful communication, consultations with ethics committees, and alternative dispute resolution techniques, submitting the issues to a court will be fraught with uncertainties. There is no clear line of decision-making upon which a provider can rely when acting on an opinion that certain medical care is futile without the consent of a surrogate. It seems that when a provider has made an effort to act carefully within a reasonable standard of care, and with the independent opinions of other physicians or an ethics committee endorsement, courts will give greater deference to a decision to withhold or withdraw care that is considered futile. That being said, the reader must understand that the preceding statement is merely an observational opinion. Providers should consult with attorneys within their jurisdiction for pertinent legal advice.

NOTES

Part 1: Introduction

1. *E.g Griswold v. Connecticut*, 381 U.S. 485(1965) (*J. Douglas' infamous statement evolved the right of privacy from the U.S. Constitution by deriving the right from the Bill of Right's penumbras, formed by emanationsf from those [specific] guarantees [from the Bill of Rights] that help give them life and substance*'; *Roe v. Wade*, 410 U.S 113 (1973) (*J. Blackman finds the right to privacy in the First, Fourth, Fifth and Ninth Amendments and the precedent set forth in Griswold*).

2. *See generally,* The Belmont Report: Ethical Guidelines for the Protection of Human Subjects of Research (National Commission for the Protection of Human Subjects of Biomedical and Behavioral Research, ed., 1978).

3. Tom L. Beaucamp and James F. Childress, Principles of Biomedical Ethics (4th Ed. 1994). Although the authors are often regarded as champions of principlism, their bioethical philosophy is regarded as more complex that that of principlism. However, because of the influence of their publication, they have become associated with this bioethical philosophy.

4. *See generally,* George P. Smith, II, Utility and the Principle of Medical Futility: Safeguarding Autonomy and the Prohibition Against Cruel and Unusual Punishment, 12 J. Contemp. Health L. & Pol'y, 1 (Fall, 1995).

5. Ibid. *at* 22.

6. *In re Helga Wanglie*, PX-91-283 (Hennepin County, Minn., 4th Dist. Ct., P. Ct. Div. July 1, 1991).

7. *See* Ronald E. Cranford, *Helga Wanglie's Ventillator*, Hastings Center Rep., July-Aug. 1991.

8. Ibid. *at* 23.

9. Ibid.

10. Ibid.

11. *See generally,* Judith F. Daar, A Clash at the Bedside: Patient's Autonomy versus A Physician's Professional Conscience, 44 Hastings L. J. 1241. Many states require medical providers to seek transfer of a patient when disputes regarding the care of a patient arise between the patient's providers, the patient, or the patient's surrogates. When disputes rise to the level of court action, particularly cutting-edge public legal and moral issues, other providers and healthcare facilities become reluctant to accept transfer of these 'problem cases.' As a result, the solution for transferring such a patient to another provider willing to care for the patient as the family wishes (as suggested by

courts and state legislation) essentially become an impossibility. These cases are referred to colloquially by some critics as hot potato cases.

12. *See* Stephen Miles, Informed Demand for 'Non-Beneficial Treatment, 325 New Eng. J. Med. 512 (1991).

13. *Wanglie*, at 13.

14. Ibid.

15. *See* FN. 12 *at* 513.

16. Ibid.

17. *In re Baby K*, 16 F.2d 590 (4th Circ.), Cert. denied, 115 S. Ct. 91 (1994).

18. Ibid. *at* 592.

19. Ibid.

20. Ibid.

21. Ibid.

22. Ibid. *at* 593.

23. Ibid.

24. *See* FN. 11, *supra*.

25. *Baby K at* 593.

26. Ibid.

27. Ibid.

28. EMTALA, 42 U.S.C.A. Sec 1395dd.

29. *In re Baby K, at* 592.

30. 42 U.S.C.A. Sec 1395dd *et. seq.*

31. *In re Baby K, at* 595.

32. Ibid.

33. Ibid.

34. Ibid.

35. Ibid. *at* 597. The hospitals argument was based upon Section 54.1-2990 of the Health Care Decisions Act of Virginia that recognized that "nothing in this article shall be construed to require a physician to prescribe or render medical treatment that the physician determines to be medically or ethically inappropriate." Va. Code Ann. Sec. 54.1-2990.

36. Ibid.

37. A detailed discussion of EMTALA is beyond the scope of this chapter. For more details on EMTALA, *see generally* Robert A. Bitterman, Ed., Providing Emergency Care Under Federal Law: EMTALA, American College of Emergency Physicians, 2000 *and* James Hubler, Ed., EMTALA; The Essential Guide to Compliance, Thomson American Health Consultants, Inc., 2003.

Part 2: Advanced directives and the patient self-determination act

1. Advance directive: 1. A durable power of attorney that takes effect upon one's incompetency and designates a surrogate decision-maker for healthcare matters . . . 2. A legal document explaining one's wishes about medical treatment if one becomes incompetent or unable to communicate-Also termed *medical directive; physician's directive; written directive*. Cf. LIVING WILL, *Black's Law Dictionary, 7th Ed.*, Bryan A Garner, Ed., West Group, 1999.

2. Thaddeus Mason Pope, *The Maladaptation of Miranda to Advanced Directives: A Critique of the Implementation of the Patient Self-Determination Act,* 9 Health Matrix 139, (Winter 1999).

3. In 1992, Pennsylvania became the 50th state to enact advance directives legislation. 20 Pa. Cons. Stat. Ann., Sections 5401–16 (West 1998).

4. *See* Luis Kutner, Due Process of Euthanasia: The Living Will, A Proposal, 44, Ind. L.J. 539 (1969); *In re Quinlan*, 355 A. 2d 647 (N.J. 1976).

5. Author's personal oberservation.

6. *In re Quinlan*, 355 A. 2d at 655-56.
7. Ibid. *at* 663.
8. *See* Bretton J. Hortter, A survey of Living Will and Advance Health Care Directives, 74 N.D. L. Rev. 233 (1998).
9. *See* Patient Self-Determination Act-Providers Offer Information on advance directives but Effectiveness Uncertain, GAO/HEHS Doc. No. 95–135 (1995).
10. Signed into law on November, 5, 1990 by President George Bush as a part of the Omnibus Budget Reconcilliation Act of 1990, the law did not go into effect until December 1, 1991. Omnibus Budget Reconcilliation Act of 1990, Pub. L. No. 101–508 Sec. 4206, 104 Stat. 1388, 1388–115 to 117, 1388204 to –206 (codified as amended in scattered sections of 42 U.S.C. (1990)).
11. *See* 42 U.S.C. Sec. 1395cc(f)(1)(A)(i) and 1395cc(f)(3).
12. Ibid.
13. EMTALA, Emergency Medical Transfer and Active Labor Act, 42 U.S.C. 1395dd *et. seq.*
14. *See generally* FN. 2, *supra; see also* Edward J. Larson and Thomas A. Eaton, The Limits of advance directives: A History and Assessment of the Patient Self-Determination Act, 32 Wake Forest L. R. , 249, 259, 267 (1997).

Part 3: Evolution of the law of healthcare decision-making

1. Implied fundamental rights are sometimes called substantive due process rights, but the author chooses to use the term implied fundamental rights for the sake of clarity. The "substantive due process rights" appellation is a useful moniker when discussing these rights amongst constitutional scholars.
2. "No State shall make or enforce any law which shall . . . deny to any person within its jurisdiction the equal protection of the laws." 14th Amendment, United States Constitution.
3. "Congress shall make no law . . . abridging the freedom of speech", 1st Amendment, United States Constitution.
4. Prosser and Keeton on Torts, 5th Edition, W. Page Keeton, ed, West Publishing Co. (1984).
5. Union and Pac. R. R. Co. v. Botsford, 141 U.S.250, 251. 11 S. Ct. 1000, 351 L. Ed. 734, 735 (1891).
6. Schloendorff v. Society of N.Y. Hospitals, 211 N.Y. 125, 105 N.E. 92 (1914).
7. Olmstead v. United States, 277 US 438, 478 (1928)(dissenting opinion).
8. The Fifth Amendment states that no person shall be . . . 'deprived of life, liberty, or property, without due process of law.' The Fourteenth Amendment states that . . . 'no State [shall] deprive any person of life, liberty, or property, without due process of law.'
9. "The enumeration in the Constitution, of certain rights, shall not be construed to deny or disparage others retained by the people." Ninth Amendment, United States Constitution.
10. The reader who may be interested in the debate regarding implied fundamental rights should consider starting with recognized Constitutional law textbooks, such as American Constitutional Law by Laurence Tribe (published by The Foundation Press, Inc.
11. **Griswold v. Connecticut,** 381 U.S. 479 (1965).
12. **Ibid.** *at* 479.
13. **Ibid.** *at* 484 *et. seq.*
14. *See* Mark R. Levin, Men in Black: How the Supreme Court is Destroying America, Regnery Publishing Co., 2005. For an interesting foray into a description of judicial activism in the Supreme

Court, Mr. Levin describes numerous instances of what he considers to be stretched interpretation of the U.S. Constitution by some justices of the Supreme Court.
15. *Ibid.* *at* 57.
16. *Ibid.*
17. **Eisenstadt v. Baird**, 405 U.S. 438 (1972).
18. Ibid. *at* 453.
19. **Roe v. Wade,** 410 U.S. 113 (1973). It is interesting to note that *Roe* had been.
20. *See* FN 12, at 60.
21. **Ibid.** *at* 151 *et. seq.*
22. *See* Burroughs v. Crichton, 48 App. D.C. 596; Pratt v. Davis 224 Ill. 300, 79 N.E. 562 (1906); State v. Housekeeper, 70 Md. 162, 16 A. 382, 1889); Mohr v. Williams, 95 Minn. 261, 104 N.W. 12 (1905).
23. Salgo v. Leland Stanford Jr. Board of Trustees, 154 Cal. App. 2d 560, 578, 317 P. 2d 170, 181 (1957).
24. Bang v. Charles T. Miller Hospital, 251 Minn. 427, 434, 88 N.W. 2d 190 (1958).
25. Nateson v. Kline, 186 Kan 393, 400, 350 P. 2d 1093, 1099 (1960).
26. Ibid.
27. Mitchell v. Robinson, 334 S.W. 2d 11(M0. 1960).
28. Ibid *at* 19.
29. *E.g.* Govin v. Hunter, 374 P. 2d 421 (Wyo. 1962).
30. *See* Canterbury v. Spence, 464 F. 2d 772 (D.C. Cir.), cert. denied. 409 U.S. 1064 (1972).
31. *See e.g.* Wooley v Hnederson, 418 A. 2d 1123, 1128–21 (Me. 1980); Aiken v. Clary, 396 S.W. 2d 668, 674–75 (mo. 1965); Folger v. Corbett, 118 N.H. 737, 394 A.2d 63 (1978).
32. *See* Susan O. Scheutzow, Patient Care, Fundamentals of Health Law, 3rd Ed., Bernadette M. Broccolo, *et. al.*, Ed., American Health Lawyers Association, July, 2004.
33. *See* FN. 4 *at* 117.
34. Ibid.
35. *See* FN 30 *at* 788–89.
36. Elysa Gordon, Multiculturalism in Medical Decisionmaking: The notion of Informed Waiver, 23 Fordham Urb. L. J. 1321 *at* 1339.
37. Ibid. *at* 1340.
38. *See* FN. 4 *at* 161.
39. Ibid.
40. *See generally*, S.O. Scheutzow, FN 32 *at* 37; *See e.g.* Millard v Cirrado, Miss. Ct. App. ED Dec. 14. 1999, Case No. 75420; Hiser v. ¶andoph, 126 Ariz. 608, 617 P. 2d 774 (Ct. App. AZ. 1980).
41. *See generally*, Terry O. Tottenham, Liability for Patient Care *at* 9–10, *in* Health Law Practice Guide, American Health Lawyers Association, Thomson/West Publishers, 2005.
42. Ibid. *at* 9–11.
43. Ibid. *at* 9–13.
44. Ibid. *at* 9–14.

Part 4: Patient care decision-making at the end of life

1. The Tenth Amendment of the United States Constitution ratified as part of the Bill of Rights in 1791 provides that any powers not constitutionally delegated to the federal government, nor prohibited to the states, are reserved for the states or the people. Also known as the Reserved Power Clause, the Tenth Amendment empowers each state with the interest in the welfare of its constituents, among other powers.
2. For readers who want a comprehensive discussion regarding healthcare decision-making from a legal perspective, *see* Claire C.

Obade, Heathcare Decision-Making, Patient Autonomy, and Professional Responsibility, *in* Health Law Practice Guide, Vol.1, at 8-1 *et. seq.,* A. G. Gosfield, et. al., Ed., American Health Lawyers Assoc., Thompson/West (2005). Obade is a superlative writer in this area of law and covers this topic from the viewpoint of an attorney fairly comprehensively.

3. Ibid. *at* 8–67.
4. *In re Farrell,* 108 N.J. 335, 529 A.2d 404 (1987).
5. Ibid. *at* 410.
6. Ibid.
7. *Bouvia v. Superior Court,* 179 Cal. App. 3d 1127, 225 Cal. Rptr. 297 (1986).
8. Ibid. *at* 297.
9. Ibid. *at* 300.
10. Ibid.
11. Ibid. *at* 306.
12. Ibid.
13. Michael R. Flick, The Due Process of Dying, 79 Calif. L. Rev. 1121, 1143 quoting from L.A. Times, May 23, 1988, Sec. 1 at 14, col. 2.
14. Ibid.
15. *In re Dubreuil,* 603 So. 2d 538 (Fla. App. 1987).
16. Ibid.
17. Thaddeus Mason Pope, The Maladaptation of Miranda to advance directives: A Critique of the Implementation of the Patient Self-Determination Act, 9 Health Matrix 139 (Winter 1999) *at* 154.
18. *See* FN. 2, *at* 8–68.
19. Ibid.
20. Ibid. *at* 8–26, quoting the U.S. Supreme Court in *Prince v. Massachusetts,* 321 U.S. 158, 170, reh'g denied, 321 U. S. 804 (1944).
21. *See* FN. 2 *at* 8–27. *See also, e.g.* C*ustody of a Minor,* 385 Mass. 697, 434 N.E. 2d 601 (1982).
22. Ibid.
23. 42 U.S.C.A. Sec. 5101(a); 45 C.F.R. Sec 11340.15. *See* FN. 2 *at* 8–32.
24. Norman L. Cantor, Twenty-Five Years after Quinlan: A Review of the Jurisprudence of Death and Dying, 29 J. L. Med. & Ethics 182, *at* 182.
25. Ibid. *at* 190.
26. *See* FN. 2 *at* 8–19
27. *In re Yetter,* 62 Pa. D. & C. 2d 619 (C.P. Northampton 1973).
28. Ibid. *at* 621.
29. Ibid. *at* 623.
30. *See* FN. 2 *at* 8–20.
31. Cruzan v. Director, Missouri Dep't of Health, 497 U.S. 261, 110 S. Ct. 2841, 111 L. Ed. 2d 224 (1990).
32. Ibid. *at* 284.
33. *In re Storar,* 52 N.Y. 2d 363, 438 N.Y.S. 2d 266 (1981), court authorized removal of a mechanical ventilator from a vegetative, terminally ill patient where the decision was consistent with medical recommendations and the patient's previously expressed wishes.
34. *Ragona v. Preate,* 6 Pa. D. & C. 4th, 202; 1990 Pa. D. & C. LEXIS 176.
35. Ibid. *at* 203.
36. Ibid.
37. Ibid. *at* 213.
38. Ibid. *at* 219.
39. *In re Clark,* 210 N.J. Super. 548, 510 A. 2d 136 (Ch. Div. 1986); *see generally,* FN. 2 *at* 8–21.
40. Ibid. *at* 560.
41. Ibid. *at* 564–65.
42. *Wendland v. Superior Court,* 56 Cal. Rptr. 2d 595 (Cal. App. 3d Dist. 1996).
43. Ibid. *at* 597.
44. Ibid.
45. Ibid. *at* 600.
46. Ibid. *at* 601, *citing Cruzan v. Director, Missouri Dep't of Health,* 497 U.S. 261, 277 (1990).
47. Ibid.
48. *See* FN. 2, *supra.*
49. *See* Cantor *supra,* FN. 24 *at* 190.
50. Ibid.
51. Ibid.
52. *See Superintendent of Belchertown State School v. Joseph Saikerwicz,* 373 Mass. 728, 370 N.E. 2d 417, 1977 Mass. LEXIS 1129.
53. *See supra,* FN. 2, *at* 8–24.
54. *See generally,* Deborah K. McKnight and Maureen Bellis, *Foregoing Life-Sustaining Treatment for Adult, Developmentally Disabled, Public Wards: A Proposed Statute,* 18 Am. J. L. and Med. 203 (1992).
55. Ibid. *at* 215.
56. Ibid. *at* 216.
57. Ibid.
58. Ibid. *at* 220–23.
59. Ibid. *at* 225.
60. Ibid.
61. *See e.g., Saikewicz,* FN. 52, *supra; In re Moorehouse,* 250 N.J. Super. 307, 593 A 2d 1256, 1991 N.J. Super. LEXIS 280 (1991); *In re Lawrence,* 579 N.E. 2d 32, 1991 Ind. LEXIS 170 (1991).
62. *See discussion, supra.*
63. *See Wanglie, supra.*
64. *See Baby K, supra.*
65. *Causey v. St. Francis Medical Center,* 719 So. 2d 1072 (1998).
66. Ibid. *at* 1074.
67. Ibid. *at* 1073. Louisiana's Medical Malpractice Act, La. R.S. 40:1299.41 *et. seq.,* requires that medical malpractice actions be submitted to a medical review panel established under the act before being submitted to a court. The trial judge considered the action to be a medical malpractice action.
68. Ibid.
69. Ibid. *at* 1074.
70. Ibid. *at* 1075.
71. *Velez v. Bethune,* 219 Ga. App. 679,466 S.E. 2d 627, 1995 Ga. App. LEXIS 1115, 96 Fulton County D. Rep. 49.
72. Ibid. *at* 679.
73. Ibid. *at* 630–31.
74. Ibid. *at* 680.
75. Ibid. *at* 681.

The near-death experience, long-term psychological outcomes and support of survivors

Sam Parnia, K. Spearpoint, and P.B. Fenwick

Consciousness Research Group, University of Southampton, and
Critical Care Department, Hammersmith Hospitals NHS Trust, London, UK

Since the 1950s and 1960s improvements in resuscitation techniques have led to improved survival for patients following cardiac arrest. Although many studies have focused on prevention and acute medical treatment of cardiac arrest, relatively few have studied cognitive functioning during and after this event. Nevertheless, this is one of the most intriguing aspects of cardiopulmonary resuscitation. Much of the work in this area has evolved from the finding that a proportion of cardiac arrest survivors report thought processes, reasoning, and memory formation that are consistent with previously described near-death experiences. These experiences are reported to have occurred at a time during cardiac arrest when consciousness appears to be absent. The first part of this chapter thus focuses on the history and phenomenology of near-death experiences, their relationship to cardiac arrest and current explanations for the experiences. We then review the longer-term psychological outcomes of surviving a cardiac arrest, as well as the impact of having a near-death experience on long-term quality of life. Finally we review the wider potential philosophical implications of research into near-death experiences during cardiac arrest.

History of near-death experiences

Although modern heart and lung resuscitation methods were established in the 1950s and 1960s, there is a long history, going back centuries, of attempts to resuscitate people after they had become 'lifeless'. These involved using warm ash and hot water, whipping, blowing hot smoke in the mouth and rectum, as well as rolling people back and forth on a wine barrel or a horse to help the chest expand and take air in. The outcome of these methods was understandably poor. Nevertheless despite these primitive methods of resuscitation and the generally poor prognosis of anyone coming close to death there have been many anecdotal reports of unusual experiences during a close brush with death.

The earliest recorded reference to an experience during the dying process is in Plato's Republic.[1] A soldier, Er, suffers a near fatal injury on the battlefield, is revived and describes a journey from darkness to light accompanied by guides, a moment of judgement, feelings of peace and joy, and visions of extraordinary beauty and happiness. Historically, events closely resembling NDEs have been described by Bolivian, Argentinean, and North American Indians, as well as in Buddhist texts, Islamic texts and accounts from China, Siberia and Finland.[2] Two of the most interesting cases are a fifteenth-century painting as well as an eighteenth-century near drowning case. The fifteenth-century painting "ascent to empyrean" by Hieronymus Bosch [Fig. 69.1] depicts a tunnel leading to a bright light and has been found very much to resemble modern descriptions of near-death experiences. An NDE account from Admiral Beaufort, a British admiral who narrowly escaped drowning in Portsmouth harbour in 1795 describes a historical case of what would now be recognized as an archetypal life review.[2]

. . . circumstances minutely associated with home, were the first reflections. Then they took a wider range, our last cruise . . . a former voyage and shipwreck, my school and boyish pursuits and adventures. Thus travelling backwards, every past incident of my life seemed to glance across my recollection in retrograde succession; not however in mere outline, as here stated, but the picture filled up with every minute and collateral feature. In short, the

Cardiac Arrest: The Science and Practice of Resuscitation Medicine. 2nd edn., ed. Norman Paradis, Henry Halperin, Karl Kern, Volker Wenzel, Douglas Chamberlain. Published by Cambridge University Press. © Cambridge University Press, 2007.

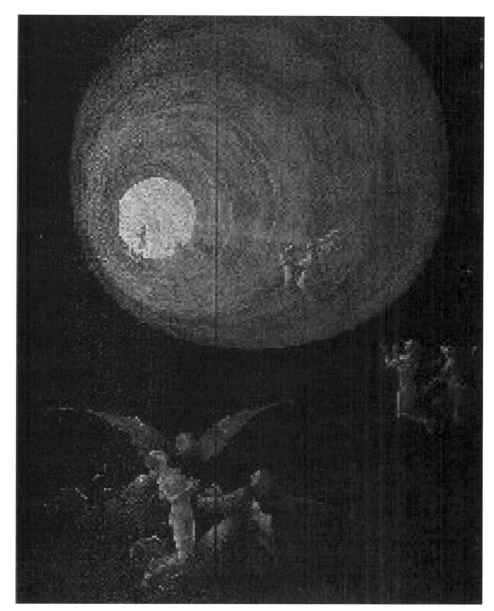

Fig. 69.1. Ascent to Empyrean. Hieronymus Bosch (1450–1516).

whole period of my existence seemed to be placed before me in a kind of panoramic review, and each of it seemed to be accompanied by a consciousness of right or wrong, or by some reflection on its cause or consequences; indeed many trifling events which had been forgotten then crowded into my imagination, and with the character of recent familiarity.

The first systematic collection of accounts from people who had experienced a close encounter with death were reported by a nineteenth-century Swiss geologist and mountaineer, Albert Heim.[3] Heim had survived a near-fatal

mountaineering accident himself and then went on to collect 30 first-hand accounts from other survivors of near-fatal mountaineering accidents, and found that they had had similar experiences.

Modern studies of near-death experiences

Despite these limited reports, it was not really until as late as the 1970s that this subject entered the realms of science, after Raymond Moody, an American psychiatrist with a background in philosophy, published his best selling book, *Life after Life* in which he had collected the accounts given by 150 survivors of near-death encounters.[4] His series of survivors of near-death encounters was not limited to cardiac arrest, but included reported experiences of people who were considered sufficiently ill to have otherwise died without medical intervention. He found that the survivors who had had experiences described similar phenomena including feelings of peace, a tunnel and a bright light, seeing deceased relatives, a life review, a perception of separation from the body (out of body experience) and entering a heavenly domain.[4] The experiences were usually described as happening when the individual was unconscious and often resulted in a more spiritual and socially orientated outlook and a reduced fear of death. Moody termed these experiences "near-death experiences" (NDE).

Since then it has been found that near-death experiences have been described in many different cultures, including India, China, South America and the Middle East.[2,5,6] Although the central features are universally present, the interpretation of the experience reflects personal religious or cultural views.

Following Moody's work, Sabom,[7] Noyes and Kletti,[8] Ring,[9] and Greyson[10] described and classified the experiences in more detail. A number of actual NDE cases collected by the authors that illustrate some of the typical features are described below. One of the most interesting aspects of these cases is that during the cases many have claimed to have been able to recall very specific details about events that had actually taken place during their experience. One woman explained:

. . . during my operation I was floating around the operating theatre. I could see the surgeon and nurses working on my body, . . . the surgeon said he would leave the wound open to let it drain as the appendix had burst. He then visited me on the ward afterwards to explain what he had done and I already knew as I had heard him. He said I couldn't possibly have heard him and suggested that a nurse had been to my bedside and told me . . . I did not tell him I had seen the operation being performed . . .' [Personal communication to the author]

. . . I can remember so vividly being above and to the right of the bed in the delivery room at the head end in a white-like tunnel, but it was white, absolutely brilliant white . . . I looked down and I could see Dr Gallagher, I could see what he was doing and I saw him run round the bottom end of the delivery bed . . . he must have forgotten [a bucket] was there because I saw him kick it in his haste to get round the other side and he kicked this bucket and it knocked into a trolley with all the instruments on, things like bowls, etc., and that trolley whizzed across the room and hit the wall. It didn't tip right up but you could see things falling off it and he then came round to me on my left-hand side and I saw him

thumping on my chest, thumping and thumping. I heard nothing, I could see nothing, no sound whatsoever, I just saw what he was doing . . . It was peace, it was peace, it was absolute peace . . . I just looked down on myself . . . I could possibly say it was a tunnel where you were looking down [from], but all this light was around you, it was a brilliant light . . . and then there was a noise, a terrible noise . . . I just said, "Let me go back, it was beautiful . . ." The next day I spoke to the doctor and I was telling him what he had done and he was furious and wanted to know which nurse had told me!' [Personal communication to the author]

During the 1980s NDEs were also studied in children. Dr. Melvyn Morse, an American pediatrician, and others found that children's NDEs share many of the same features as those of adults – separating from the body, watching events, feeling peaceful, seeing a bright light and beings of light, but they are often described in children's terminology and during the course of play, sometimes over many months.[11–14]

The following is one case of NDE recalled by a small child that was sent to the authors by his grandmother:

John's heart had stopped . . . . . . they were pressing on his chest and he was lifeless and blue . . .They put him in an ambulance and took him to hospital . . .

[After he had been discharged from hospital] one day, during the course of play, he said, "Grandma, when I died I saw a lady." He was not yet three years old. I asked my daughter if anyone had mentioned anything to John about him dying and she said, "No, absolutely not." But over the course of the next few months he continued to talk about his experience. It was all during the course of play and in a child's vocabulary.

He said, "When I was in the doctor's car the belt came undone and I was looking down from above." He also said, "When you die, it is not the end . . . a lady came to take me . . . There were also many others, who were getting new clothes, but not me, because . . . I was going to come back."

John's parents noticed that he kept on drawing the same picture over and over again. As he got older, it got more complex. When asked what the balloon was, he said, "When you die you see a bright lamp and . . . are connected by a cord" (Fig. 69.2(a), (b)).

Long-term effects of having a near-death experience

One of the aspects of NDE that was first described by Moody, was that NDEs have a long-term positive protective psychological effect. This has been shown in other studies also. Fenwick and Fenwick[15] in a questionnaire survey of 358 people who had had NDEs in widely differing circumstances and who had written in after a television programme about

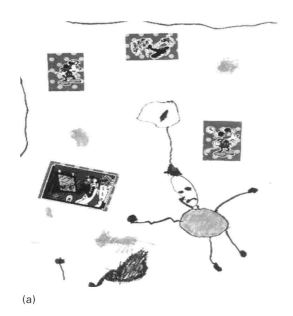 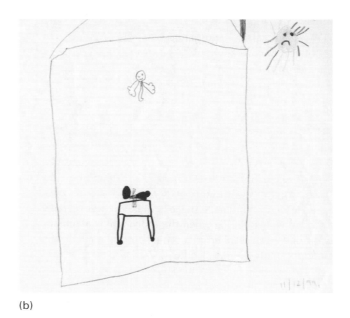

(a)   (b)

Fig. 69.2. Two drawings depicting a NDE experienced by a small child. These are two drawings by John, a child who had a near-death experience when he was less than three years old. His family had at first been concerned because they saw that he kept on drawing the same theme. Here, there is a drawing from when he was younger (a) and one when he had grown a little older (b).

NDEs found that 82% had less fear of death, 42% reported that they were more spiritual, 22% claimed to be a better person and 40% said they were more socially conscious than before. As only 10% of this sample had their NDEs after cardiac arrest, it would appear that simply having an NDE is the positive factor, and the positive changes are not related to the pathology causing the NDE.[15]

Greyson[16] suggested that near-death experiences reportedly foster value transformations and decrease suicidal ideation. Eighty-nine survivors of near-death experiences judged values related to material and social success as less important than did 175 control subjects. The reduction in feelings of personal failures may account for the reported suicide-inhibiting effect.[16] Greyson also studied a group of patients who attempted suicide and found that 26% of them had NDEs.[18] Extending this to other studies on suicide, he found that people who had had an NDE during a suicide attempt were less likely to attempt suicide again.[17,18]

Scientific theories for the causation of NDE

Many theories to account for the occurrence of NDE have been proposed. These include physiological states such as cerebral hypoxia,[19,20] hypercarbia[21] hormone and neurotransmitter release such as endorphins,[22,23] serotonin,[14] and abnormal NMDA receptor activation,[24] abnormal activation of the temporal lobes leading to seizures,[25] or limbic lobe activation.[26-28] Various drugs and, in particular, drugs that are known to cause hallucinations, such as ketamine, which activate the NMDA receptor have been suggested.[24] An alternative view, which is undoubtedly true in a few situations, is that the experience is a psychological response to stress or a form of depersonalization or dissociation in the face of actual or perceived danger or death.[8, 32]

The final moments of the dying process invariably involves a period of hypoxia. Therefore, it has been proposed that hypoxia may lead to overactivity in the visual processing areas of the brain and as there are more cells involved with central vision than peripheral vision, this may therefore create an illusion of seeing a light in the centre that fades out towards the periphery, or in other words a tunnel effect.[19,20] It has also been proposed that hypoxia may induce hyperactivity of the NMDA receptor that may in turn lead to an NDE.[24] Other theories involving other neurotransmitters or hormones such as serotonin and endorphins have also been proposed.[25-27]

More recently some have suggested that out-of-body experiences may be related to a dysfunction at the temporo-parietal junction.[29–31] It is argued that a multi-sensory disintegration at this area may lead to the disruption of several phenomenological and cognitive aspects of self-processing, causing an illusory reduplication, self-location, and perspective of the self that is experienced as an out-of-body experience.[30,31] This theory has followed from a case report of a single patient who was undergoing evaluation for epilepsy treatment in whom an "out-of-body"-like experience was induced following focal electrical stimulation of the brain's right angular gyrus.[29] Unfortunately this explanation does not take into account the observation that people who have had an out-of-body experience report actually being able to recall specific details of events that had taken place at a time when they had been unconscious. If correct, this would make it unlikely that such experiences are simply illusions, even if the trigger for the experience and hence the neurological intermediary pathway for such an experience may lie in the temporoparietal region of the brain.

In general, all the brain-based and psychological theories for the causation of NDE have proposed possible physical or psychological triggers that may either lead to or mediate the NDE. Although none of the above hypotheses can account for the NDE in its entirety, the NDE is undoubtedly mediated by neuronal intermediaries and may be triggered by either a physical or psychological stimulus. Identifying the neurological changes that mediate an experience, however, cannot identify or determine the "reality" of the experience and this includes near-death experiences. Every subjective experience is mediated by neuronal changes, and is triggered by physical or psychological stimuli, including familiar experiences such as maternal love and compassion; however, identifying the detailed neuronal circuitry that mediates these experiences does not define their "reality." In the same way, eventually identifying the neuronal pathways that mediate NDE cannot determine their "reality." Reality, on the other hand, is socially and not neurologically determined.[33] As explained above, they also do not take into account that people who have had an out of body experience report actually being able to recall specific details of events that had taken place at a time when they had been unconscious, so simply identifying the neurological triggers for the experience may not help determine its reality.

Almost all of our understanding of cognitive neuroscience and its representation in brain structure depends on correlates of cognition. The models of cognition that are built from those data are, however, correlative rather than causative models.

The limitation of early studies

Nevertheless, despite the large number of interesting cases and retrospective studies carried out in the 1970s and 1980s, one of the greatest difficulties in studying these so-called near-death experiences had been the difficulty in defining the actual proximity of the individuals to clinical death. Most cases involving such near-death experiences had not been recorded in conjunction with actual medical data demonstrating objective proximity to death. In some cases, such as the ones illustrated in this text, the patients' own accounts appeared to indicate the existence of a period of cardiac arrest. Therefore because near-death experiences can occur in widely varying circumstances, one of the difficulties in studying them has been the problem of defining the actual proximity of the individuals to clinical death.

The cardiac arrest model of the near-death experience

In clinical practice, death is diagnosed when the heart stops beating, the person stops breathing, and the brainstem and hence the rest of the brain have stopped functioning. The ideal model to study the near-death experience, therefore, is one in which these criteria are met, namely a cardiac arrest.[34]

In this condition patients develop two out of the three criteria of clinical death – no heartbeat, no breathing – and also develop the third – fixed dilated pupils of the eyes* – within a few seconds owing to the loss of brain and, in particular, brainstem function. Secondly, cardiac arrest mimics the initial period of the dying process biologically. Finally, irrespective of the cause of death, the last steps in the dying process are the cessation of breathing and heartbeat – in other words a cardiac arrest. What people experience at that time can provide us with a unique window of understanding into the subjective experiences of the dying process.[34]

In the 1970s Sabom had interviewed a group of cardiac arrest survivors and matched their descriptions of the arrest to the medical notes. He had concluded that patients

---

*   In cardiac arrest, drugs may be administered such as epinephrine and atropine that can also make the pupils look fixed and dilated. Other measures of brainstem reflexes such as the gag reflex are also lost, however, indicating that this vital part of the brain does not work.

who had out-of-body experiences were able to describe the resuscitation process as recorded in the medical notes.[35] In 1994, Martens[36] conducted a small retrospective study looking at a group of out-of-hospital cardiac arrest survivors. Since no near-death experiences had been found in this group, it was concluded that this phenomenon must be very rare in cardiac arrest survivors.

The first published prospective study to identify NDE accounts in cardiac arrest survivors was a small 1-year prospective study which showed that 6% of 63 cardiac arrest survivors reported having lucid well-structured thought processes, together with reasoning and memory formation.[34] This study was based upon interviewed accounts obtained within 1 week of the arrest. The experiences recalled were typical of those reported in other studies.

The main features that were recalled were coming to a border of no return, feeling peace, feeling joy, seeing a bright light, losing awareness of the body, and seeing deceased relatives. The authors found no evidence to support a specific role of drugs, hypoxia, hypercarbia, or electrolyte disturbances in the causation of the experiences. This was, however, a small study and therefore the authors concluded that a larger study would be needed. In a larger Dutch study 344 cardiac arrest survivors from 10 hospitals were interviewed over a 2-year period, and 41 (12%) reported experiences similar to those from the British study.[37] Approximately 24% of those who had an NDE also had an out-of-body experience and some reported having been able to watch and recall events from their cardiac arrest.

In one case, a nurse had reported having removed a patient's dentures and placed them in a drawer in a special trolley. Throughout the 1.5 hours of his resuscitation the patient had remained in a coma. One week later he had returned to the same ward where the nurse worked and after seeing her said "Oh, that nurse knows where my dentures are." He went on to describe how she took his dentures out of his mouth and put them into the crash trolley. He added "It had all these bottles on it and there was this sliding drawer underneath and that's where you put my teeth."

The nurse is quoted as saying:

I was especially amazed because I remembered this happening while the man was in a deep coma and in the process of CPR. When asked further, it appeared that the man had seen himself lying in bed and that he had perceived from above how the nurses and doctors had been busy with CPR. He had also been able to describe correctly and in detail the small room in which he had been resuscitated as well as the appearance of those present . . . At the time . . . he had

been very much afraid that we would have to stop CPR and that he would die. And it is true that we had been very negative about his prognosis due to his very poor medical condition when admitted.

The authors found that the occurrence of NDEs was not influenced by the duration of unconsciousness or the type of cardiac arrest, or by medication, but that there were more NDEs in those who had previous CPR, previous NDEs and also in the group of survivors who died shortly after their experience, suggesting that maybe the closer the patients were to death, the more likely they were to get an NDE.

This study also extended and confirmed the findings of the retrospective studies described above that a near-death experience has long-term life-enhancing sequelae. Using a life-change inventory[38] Van Lommel assessed the long-term attitude changes in a subset of his sample. 23 patients with an NDE had a 2- and an 8-year follow-up, and 15 matched patients with no NDE were interviewed at the same time intervals.

The authors found that there were changes in attitude after a cardiac arrest even amongst the people who did not have an NDE, although they were not as marked as those seen in patients who did have such an event. It is clear that a cardiac arrest in itself is a very powerful event and leads to changed attitudes. Both groups became less fearful of death, but interestingly, spirituality decreased in the non-NDE group but increased in the NDE group. They concluded that patients who have an NDE after a cardiac arrest have larger and more positive changes in attitude than those who do not.[37]

Two other studies of NDE in cardiac arrest were published from the USA. One study of 1,595 people who had been admitted to a cardiac unit over a 30-month period, also found that the incidence of NDE increased with the severity of the cardiac disease: only 1% of those admitted with stable cardiac disease reported NDEs; this increased to 10% of those with cardiac arrest. Those who had had an NDE were no different from those who had not in terms of social or demographic variables, cognitive function, or degree of heart disease.[39] Another US study found that 23% of cardiac arrest survivors had an NDE and that again those with NDEs became transformed in a positive manner after 6 months.[40]

It is clear from both retrospective studies and the prospective cardiac arrest studies that having an NDE during a cardiac arrest may have life-enhancing sequelae. In general those with an NDE are happier, more socially orientated, less materialistic, more altruistic and less afraid of death than those who do not have this experience.[4,15,37,40]

Table 69.1. Summary of changes in cardiac arrest survivors at 2-year and 8-year follow-up

Life-change inventory questionnaire	2-year follow-up		8-year follow-up	
	NDE (*n*=23)	no NDE (*n*=15)	NDE (*n*=23)	no NDE (*n*=15)
Social attitude				
Showing own feelings	42	16	78	58
Acceptance of others	42	16	78	41
More loving, empathic	52	25	68	50
Understanding others	36	8	73	75
Involvement in family	47	33	78	58
Religious attitude				
Understand purpose of life	52	33	57	66
Sense inner meaning of life	52	25	57	25
Interest in spirituality	15	−8	42	−41
Attitude to death				
Fear of death	−47	−16	−63	−41
Belief in life after death	36	16	42	16
Others				
Interest in meaning of life	52	33	89	66
Understanding oneself	58	8	63	58
Appreciation of ordinary things	78	41	84	50

NDE = near-death experience. The sums of all individual scores per item are reported in the same 38 patients who had both follow-up interviews.

Participants responded in a five-point scale indicating whether and to what degree they had changed: strongly increased (+2), somewhat increased (+1), no change (0), somewhat decreased (−1), and strongly decreased (−2). Only in the reported 13 (of 34) items in this table were significant differences found in life-change scores in the interview after 2 years.

Consciousness and awareness during cardiac arrest: what can we learn from awareness during anesthesia?

Although the reports of consciousness, thought processes, reasoning and memory formation during cardiac arrest are relatively new, reports of awareness while under general anesthesia have been noted since the introduction of anesthesia in the nineteenth century. In these cases such awareness is usually caused by insufficient anesthesia or by light levels of anesthesia allowed by the use of muscle relaxants. After being aware during general anesthesia, patients report hearing conversations, sensations of paralysis and pain, anxiety, panic, and helplessness.[41] Subsequent psychological sequelae may arise, with sleep disturbances, nightmares, flashbacks and a preoccupation with death.[42] This phenomenon is rare and is thought to arise in less than 1% of patients who undergo general anesthesia, but following its occurrence a longer term post-traumatic stress disorder may also arise.[43]

Four stages of perception during general anesthesia with memory of intraoperative events have been described.[44] At the first stage there is conscious perception with explicit memory. This has been reported in the unfortunate case of those who have been administered a muscular paralytic agent together with inadequate anesthesia and are thus able to feel and perceive events fully but appear completely unconscious. As actual anesthesia is administered and deepened, explicit recall of intraoperative events is lost, but conscious perception remains, such that the apparently anesthetized patient is capable of responding to commands yet appears amnesic of events afterwards. This is the stage of conscious perception without explicit memory (stage 2). There is evidence that with deeper anesthesia there is the possibility of subconscious perception with only implicit memory of intraoperative events (stage 3). A progressive increase in anesthetic concentration leads first to a progressive reduction in working memory, then loss of consciousness and explicit memory, whereas implicit memory of intra-anesthetic events may remain (stage 4). In one study that supports this finding, during anesthesia half of the patients were presented with target words from the category of fruit and colour, whilst the other half had seaside noises played to them through headphones. Postoperatively no patient had explicit recall of the sounds but the experimental group of patients generated more target words when asked to name the first three fruits and colors that came to mind.[44] At deeper levels of anesthesia there is no perception and no memory.

Using what is understood from awareness during anesthesia it may thus be possible to conclude that perhaps during cardiac arrest there are different levels of consciousness depending on the degree of cerebral depression that occurs as a consequence of reduced cerebral blood flow. Nevertheless, as described later in this chapter much of the evidence regarding cerebral function during cardiac arrest indicates that there is a lack of electrical activity in the brain during cardiac arrest. It has thus been proposed to study the phenomenon of consciousness and its relationship to cerebral function during cardiac arrest by using bispectral EEG monitoring.

Long-term psychological and cognitive effects of surviving a cardiac arrest

It is now widely recognized that severe mental reactions may occur in response to a stressful event and that having a cardiac arrest may be emotionally extremely stressful. In addition, as many patients may have suffered from hypoxic brain injury,[41] and moderate to severe neuropsychological sequelae have been found in approximately 50% of cardiac arrest survivors after 1 year,[45] this has highlighted the significance of studying the long-term psychological effects of surviving a cardiac arrest. Relatively few studies have addressed this issue, nevertheless, sufficient work has been done to show that cardiac arrest survivors enjoy a good overall quality of life, but may suffer from cognitive and emotional impairments. It is not clear whether those who have had an NDE during their cardiac arrest are protected against these effects as no comparative studies have yet been carried out.

Quality of life after cardiac arrest

Granja et al.[46] studied the health-related quality of life 6 months after a cardiac arrest using the EQ-5D Generic Quality of Life Instrument, developed by the EuroQol Group. The authors studied all cardiac arrest patients between April 1997 and December 2000 who had been resuscitated after cardiac arrest. These survivors filled in the questionnaire 6 months after discharge. A matched control group consisted of similar aged patients with an approximately equal Apache II score from randomly selected ICU patients without cardiac resuscitation. This was a small study, as although 36 patients were discharged from hospital, 12 of these died before their 6-month evaluation. A further five were not evaluated. Overall, 19 patients completed the questionnaire, of whom only 8 were working at that time. Eleven patients were retired, however, and 7 of these returned to their previous level of activity. Interestingly, there was no difference on the HR-Qol scores between the survivors of cardiac arrest and those from other ICU patients. The authors comment: "These results agree with previous reports stating that CPR is frequently unsuccessful, but if survival is achieved, a fairly good quality of life can be expected."

Further work by Nichol et al.,[47] in a study examining both in-hospital and out-of-hospital cardiac arrest survivors showed that quality of life issues were correlated with clinical parameters. The surviving cohort was followed up for a minimum of 6 months after discharge. From an original group of 126 survivors, 86 patients were interviewed with the Health Utilities Index Mark III used as the quality of life assessment tool. The results indicated that "utilities" were highest in patients with the shortest times to initiation of CPR and that the mean utility scores were lower than those found in the general population or people not limited by chronic disease. Survival was considered to be poor, but most of the survivors retained an acceptable health-related quality of life. With use of the Health Utilities Index Mark III, another study in survivors of out-of-hospital cardiac arrest examined the health-related quality of survival in 268 one-year survivors from an original group of 8091 patients. Scores achieved by these patients compared well with age- and sex-matched members from the general population. Patients aged 80 or more were the most affected and bystander CPR was associated with better health-related quality of life outcomes. The authors concluded, ". . . such survivors have good health-related quality of life and functional status".[48]

Long-term emotional effects and the occurrence of post-traumatic stress disorder after cardiac arrest

Post-traumatic stress disorder (PTSD) is a unique symptom configuration after an extreme event consisting of intrusion re-experiencing (flash-back), avoidance and numbness, and hyperarousal symptoms.[49] Until recently, few studies had examined the occurrence of PTSD in cardiac arrest patients, even though this condition may potentially be one of the most traumatizing conditions for patients.

In a study aiming to examine the long-term prevalence and emotional disability in cardiac arrest survivors. Ladwig *et al.*[50] conducted follow-up analysis in a group of 21 survivors of out-of-hospital cardiac arrest who had sufficient cerebral performance to enable appropriate psychodiagnostic assessment. A cohort was selected from in-hospital patients who had experienced ventricular tachycardia or fibrillation arrest specifically. These were then compared to a "control" group containing cardiac patients with unstable angina, but who did not suffer cardiac arrest. The results were complex; however, the study group did display healthy levels of emotional stability and had a mean anxiety score lower than did the comparative group (using the Hospital Anxiety and Depression scale). When surveyed via self-assessment, the cardiac arrest group indicated no differences from the angina group with respect to mental condition and their somatic condition or illness-related quality of life issues. The only detectable difference between the two groups concerned ability to concentrate which was more impaired in the cardiac arrest group. Over half of the cardiac arrest group patients stated that having had a cardiac arrest had significantly affected their lives. Identification of a subset of the cardiac arrest patients who had PTSD (identified by the use of Impact of Event scores on intrusive thoughts, avoidance states and increased arousal) showed that patients who had PTSD scored higher for depression and anxiety, which was also seen in the self-assessment results. These patients had a more negative outlook about their disease progression, were less able to concentrate, and were more preoccupied with somatic complaints. An important point is that patients who were sedated at the onset of the events they experienced were five times less likely to develop PTSD.

In another study of 143 cardiac arrest survivors who had been followed up on average 45 months after the arrest, it was found that 27% fulfilled criteria for PTSD according to the Davidson Trauma Score. Patients with PTSD had a significantly lower quality of life. The only independent risk factor for the development of PTSD was younger age. Nonetheless, in this study there was no difference between patients with or without PTSD in use of sedation and analgesia during or after cardiac arrest.[51] In a smaller study comparing 27 patients who had survived an in-hospital cardiac arrest with 27 patients who had a myocardial infarction uncomplicated by cardiac arrest, a similar incidence of PTSD was found. 19% of the cardiac arrest survivors and 7% of the MI survivors fulfilled the DSM-IV criteria for PTSD when assessed by structured clinical interview.[52]

Cognitive and behavioral changes after cardiac arrest

Despite the relatively good quality of life, many studies have indicated that cardiac arrest may be associated with long-term memory impairment in approximately 20%–50% of survivors. In particular, studies have indicated impairment of long-term memory and executive function impairment together with focal cognitive deficits.

Grubb *et al.*[53] found that when assessing cognitive function, between 2 months to 1 year after cardiac arrest, up to 40% of survivors from out-of-hospital cardiac arrest have memory impairment of the ability to "recall" rather than "recognition" memory. It was suggested that this may occur as a consequence of hippocampal damage, as "recall" memory is mediated by the hippocampus. In a further study by the same group which aimed to assess longer-term memory effects of surviving cardiac arrest, 10 of the previously identified survivors of out-of-hospital cardiac arrest were followed up to 3 years after the index event and re-examined for cognitive impairments. These patients were age- and sex-matched with control subjects with myocardial infarction without cardiac arrest. Using the "Rivermead Behavioural Memory test" (RBMT), a test of the ability to extract information from short- to long-term memory and hence a test of memory impairment that may affect everyday activities, as well as the "Doors and People" test, which identifies "recall memory", they were able to show that although the RBMT scores declined in both groups, the cardiac arrest patients were significantly more affected. The DPT scores remained poor in the cardiac arrest group, whereas they were normal in the MI group. This study demonstrated that the memory deficits that take place after a cardiac arrest are persistent and focal, and that "cognitive impairment is a serious and underdiagnosed complication of prolonged cardiac arrest" with considerable effects on normal living activities.[54]

Further work by O'Reilly and colleagues[55] regarding memory impairment compared three groups: in-hospital cardiac arrest survivors, out-of-hospital cardiac arrest survivors and patients with myocardial infarction without cardiac arrest. Four tests were applied to each respective cohort, each consisting of 35 subjects. The tests sought to identify the current state of "affect" (Hospital anxiety and depression scale), premorbid intelligence (National adult reading test), short-term memory (digit span test), and long-term episodic memory (Rivermead behavioural memory test). The in-hospital cardiac arrest survivors displayed higher anxiety levels than did the other two groups, and moderate or severe memory loss was identified in 26% of these patients. The memory impairment in these patients was not significantly different for the out-of-hospital survivors; however, 38% of them were categorized as moderately or severely impaired. None of the MI group experienced this level of memory impairment. There were no significant differences between the groups with respect to premorbid intelligence and short-term memory tests, with both groups scoring within the normal range expected for unimpaired adults.

Some cognitive defects have been shown to be present soon after cardiac arrest. In one study 60% of patients were found to have moderate to severe cognitive deficits 3 months after cardiac arrest. At 12 months, almost 50% of survivors still had moderate to severe deficits; 45% had evidence of depression and 24% had severe depression.[45]

Nunes[56] studied the long-term effects of surviving a cardiac arrest. Eleven cardiac arrest survivors from the intensive care unit were examined between 1 and 3 years after cardiac arrest. Patients were classified by using the Cerebral Performance Categories (CPC), neurological examination, detailed cognitive testing and computerized tomography (CT) scan with qualitative and quantitative imaging analysis. Six of the 11 patients had good cerebral performance. The verbal and visuospatial short-term memory scores were associated with CPC, such that all patients with at least moderate cerebral disability were found to have abnormal verbal memory test results compared with only one survivor with good CPC score (CPC 1); visuospatial short-term memory was abnormal in four moderately affected survivors and normal in those with good CPC score (CPC 1). CT scan findings correlated with the verbal memory score and the executive functions score, suggesting involvement of different brain areas in these functions. CT imaging revealed atrophy in both qualitative and quantitative analysis, and correlated with impairment in cognitive testing. This was found in the frontal and temporal areas. Another study with MRI has also suggested that memory impairment in cardiac arrest survivors is associated with global cerebral atrophy and not just selective hippocampal damage,[57] which relates to executive and language dysfunction found in affected patients.

Long-term psychological care of cardiac arrest survivors

Although the study of cognition and consciousness during cardiac arrest as well as the longer term psychological outcomes of surviving a cardiac arrest comprise a relatively new area of study, significant advances have been made in this field in the last decade. It has been demonstrated that many cardiac arrest survivors may have cognitive processes during the time of their arrest and anecdotally some have also been able to describe verified events accurately during their arrest, indicating the presence of consciousness. Near-death experiences appear to have a long-term protective psychological effect, even though many studies have shown that a significant proportion of cardiac arrest survivors may suffer from behavioural, cognitive, and emotional disturbances that may begin soon after the cardiac arrest and persist for many years. More work is needed to identify ways of preventing and treating these impairments in cardiac arrest survivors.

To date, there are no standardized programs for the long-term psychological care of cardiac arrest survivors, but as recent studies have indicated that many patients who undergo a cardiac arrest may have long-term psychological outcomes, care should be focused on identifying and appropriately managing patients after the arrest. The authors suggest the establishment of follow-up procedures for cardiac arrest survivors through trained health care professionals who can identify those who may be suffering depression, post-traumatic stress disorder, and emotional or other cognitive effects.

Implications of the study of cognition and consciousness during cardiac arrest

An interesting point that had been raised as a consensus of opinion by the authors of the four published prospective studies of near-death experiences during cardiac arrest, was that the occurrence of lucid well-structured cognitive processes together with memory formation and recall of detailed accounts of events from the period of resuscitation may be a scientific paradox. It has been proposed that this may, in turn, have profound implications for the scientific discovery of the nature of consciousness and its relation with the brain, which is one of the most profound questions facing science today.[58]

The basic scientific problem of consciousness is simple to describe but difficult to answer: how does our sense of self-awareness together with all our subjective thoughts, feelings, and emotions arise from the brain? Traditionally, in philosophical circles this has been referred to as the mind–body problem, and whereas many well-known philosophers including Plato and Descartes have argued that the mind and brain are separate entities, many modern scientists have proposed that the mind is a product of brain activity. The common views for its occurrence can be broadly divided into conventional and non-conventional neurobiological theories. Those in support of the conventional neurobiological theories have commonly proposed that mind and consciousness are products of neuronal activity and arise as an epiphenomenon from cerebral activity. Conceptually, this is similar to how light arises from a light bulb, but is not the same as the underlying processes within the light bulb. A number of different theories have been proposed to account for this phenomenon, which portray consciousness as an emergent property of neuronal activity in the brain.[59–62] Evidence to support these theories has come from the observation that specific changes in function, such as personality or memory are associated with specific cerebral lesions. In addition, fMRI and PET scanning have also shown a correlation between metabolic activity and different mental states. Although these provide evidence for the role of neuronal networks as an intermediary for the manifestation of thoughts, they do not necessarily imply that those cells also produce the thoughts. Almost all our understanding of cognitive neuroscience and its representation in brain structure depends on correlates of cognition. The models of cognition that are built from these data are correlative rather than causative models. Thus, we proceed with our third-person objective science we cannot get close to subjective experience. This has led to alternative "non-conventional" explanations for consciousness.

It has been proposed that mind and consciousness may arise from quantum processes within neuronal microtubules,[63] or may actually be an irreducible scientific entity in its own right,[64,65] similar to many of the concepts in physics such as mass and gravity, which are also irreducible entities. Consciousness has thus been proposed to be similar to the discovery of electromagnetic phenomena in the nineteenth century, or quantum mechanics in the twentieth century, both of which were inexplicable in terms of previously known principles and were introduced as fundamental entities.[64] Some have argued that this entity is a product of the brain, whereas others, such as the late Nobel laureate Sir John Eccles, have argued that it may be an entirely separate entity not produced by the brain. Furthermore, it has also been proposed that consciousness may be an irreducible scientific entity that is composed of a very subtle type of matter that is still not amenable to measurement by our scientific tools, but is similar in concept to electromagnetic waves, and is governed by precise laws, axioms and theorems.[65]

In spite of obvious interest, no testable, plausible biological mechanism to account for how the brain may give rise to the mind or consciousness has been proposed. Despite a number of theories, progress has been hampered by a lack of experimental models to test such theories. The study of the human mind and consciousness during cardiac arrest has been proposed as a novel and innovative method that has arisen in the last few years for testing any theory of consciousness.[58]

This is because studies have indicated that during cardiac arrest there is little or no cerebral perfusion and hence no measurable EEG function. Although more accurate studies are needed to verify the occurrence of consciousness and thought processes during the actual process of cardiac arrest, evidence gathered so far appears to indicate that, paradoxically, thought processes with accurate recall of events, reasoning and memory formation may occur during cardiac arrest. Evidence from human and animal studies has shown that there is a loss of global brain function during cardiac arrest. Immediately after a cardiac arrest due to the cessation of the heartbeat, the blood pressure drops to unmeasurable levels. During properly performed chest compressions, the systolic values may rise to sufficient levels, but the diastolic values and hence the mean arterial pressure still remain low.[66,67] The use of vasopressors such as epinephrine and vasopressin has been shown to increase blood pressure, as well as cardiac and cerebral perfusion pressures as compared with chest compressions alone.[68,69] Coronary and cerebral perfusion rely on adequate diastolic pressures and therefore the pressures generated during cardiac arrest with chest compressions and the use of epinephrine, although better than no intervention, are still generally too low for adequate perfusion. Cerebral perfusion pressure (CPP) is determined by the difference between the mean arterial pressure and the intracranial pressure (MAP – ICP). It has been shown that the more prolonged a cardiac arrest, the higher the ICP rises and hence a higher MAP is needed to maintain CPP.[70] Relatively low mean arterial blood pressures are maintained until the resumption of cardiac output despite conventional cardiopulmonary resuscitation.[67–69,71]

In clinical practice the EEG is often used to assess cerebral ischemia during procedures such as cardiac and neurosurgery and to assess cerebral function during cardiac arrest in animals and humans. The data from humans are largely limited to those obtained during defibrillation threshold testing at defibrillator implantation, or individual case reports on patients who had suffered a cardiac arrest while connected to an EEG. In patients with early defibrillated arrhythmias, concurrent EEG monitoring during a cardiac arrest has shown an initial slowing of the EEG, which then progresses to an isoelectric (flat) line within approximately 10–20 seconds and remains flat until the resumption of cardiac output.[71] In cases of prolonged cardiac arrest, however, EEG activity may not return for many tens of minutes after cardiac output has returned.[72] Cerebral blood flow is severely impaired, which leads to a lack of electrophysiological activity in the cortex, which worsens with the length of the arrest. Animal studies have shown that an absence of cortical EEG activity correlates with an absence or reduction in activity of the deep brain structures as measured by in-dwelling electrodes.[73,74] As a result, consciousness is rapidly lost during a cardiac arrest.

Although there is minimal blood flow to the brain during a cardiac arrest, it has also been shown that, after a cardiac arrest, local cerebral blood flow and hence cerebral perfusion are also severely impaired, despite the restoration of an adequate blood pressure and gross cerebral blood flow rate. This is due to local increases in vasoconstriction, possibly brought about by an imbalance in the local production of vasoconstrictors and vasodilators, which can also explain the observed lack of electrical activity on EEG after the maintenance of adequate blood pressure during the recovery phase of cardiac arrest. The main factor responsible for this reduced cerebral blood flow after a cardiac arrest is the initial period of ischemia before adequate resuscitation.[70] From a clinical point of view these observations are supported by the continued loss of brainstem reflexes such as the gag reflex and continuing unconsciousness. The unconsciousness is due both to reduced cerebral perfusion and to the absence of brainstem function required to maintain cortical activity.

The occurrence of lucid, well-structured cognitive processes such as attention and memory recall of specific events during a cardiac arrest (NDE) raises a number of interesting and perplexing questions. As described above these experiences are reported to be occurring during unconsciousness at a time when cerebral function is severely impaired or absent. Cerebral localization studies have indicated that cognitive processes are mediated through the activation of a number of different cortical areas. Therefore a globally disordered brain will not support lucid thought processes. It has been shown that even relatively minor reductions in blood flow lead to impaired attention.[76] The experiences reported from cardiac arrest are clearly not confusional and occur at a time when consciousness and memory formation should not be possible.

An alternative explanation is that the experiences may actually be arising at a time when consciousness is either being lost or regained, rather than during the cardiac arrest. Experiments during simple fainting episodes have shown that experiences arising during loss of consciousness occur in conjunction with ongoing mental experiences at the beginning of the episode,[77] which is not classically seen in NDEs. EEG data during fainting show a gradual slowing of the cerebral rhythms with the appearance of delta activity before finally, in a minority of cases, the EEG becomes flat.[78] During cardiac arrest, the process

is accelerated, with the EEG showing changes within a few seconds.[79] Cerebral insult leads to a period of both anterograde and retrograde amnesia.[80,81] Memory is a very sensitive indicator of brain injury and the length of these amnesic periods is a measure of the severity of the injury.[82] Therefore, events that occur just before or just after loss of consciousness would not be expected to be recalled, or if they were, the memory would be confusional.[81,82] As described above, cerebral function as measured by EEG may not return until tens of minutes or even a few hours after successful resuscitation. Despite these observations it can still be argued that some of the recalled features may be occurring during the recovery phase, although the patient believes that they occurred during the arrest. The many anecdotal reports of patients being able to "see" and recall specific details relating to the resuscitation period, however, which have been verified by hospital staff, cannot be simply explained in this way and point away from this conclusion. For memory to take place, consciousness would need to be present during the actual cardiac arrest itself.

Studying cognitive function during cardiac arrest allows examination of the relationship between consciousness and brain function. It is perhaps the only clinical situation in which global brain function temporarily ceases, so if consciousness is indeed present, then it clearly cannot be entirely dependent on brain function. The exciting point that we currently face is that for the first time this can now be tested objectively through large studies. It has been proposed to test the claims of "consciousness" and being able to "see" during cardiac arrest objectively by the use of hidden targets that are only visible from a vantage point above the patient and accurately timing these experiences. If it can be proven that this period of consciousness had indeed taken place during cardiac arrest, rather than before or after it, this will have significant implications for science. The study of consciousness has for many years been a neglected area of science, but has now become a significant point of debate in neuroscience. This new approach may provide an insight into this intriguing, yet largely unexplored area of science.

REFERENCES

1. Dent, Plato, *The Republic*. London, 1937; **10**: 318–325.
2. Roberts, G. & Owen, J. The near-death experience. *Br. J. Psychiatry* 1988; **153**: 607–617.
3. Heim, A. Notizen uber den Tod durch Absturtz. Jahrbuch des schweizer. *Alpenclub* 1892; **27**: 327–337.
4. Moody, R.A. *Life after Life*. Bantam Press, 1975.

5. Pascricha, S. & Sevenson, I. Near death experiences in India. *J. Nerv. Ment. Dis.* 1986; **55**(4): 542–549.

6. Feng, Z., A research on near death experiences of survivors in big earthquake of Tangshan, 1976. *Chung Hua Shen Ching Ching Shen Ko Tsa Chih* 1992; **25**(4): 222–225, 253–254.

7. Sabom, M., *Recollections of Death: A Medical Investigation.* New York: Harper & Row, 1983.

8. Noyes, R. & Kletti, R. Depersonalisation in the face of life threatening danger: a description. *Psychiatry* 1976; **39**: 251–259.

9. Ring, K. *Life at Death.* New York: Coward Mc Cann, 1980.

10. Greyson, B., The near death experience scale construction, reliability, and validity. *J. Nerv. Ment. Dis.* 1983; **171**: 369–375.

11. Morse, M.L. Near death experiences of children. *J. Ped. Onc. Nursing* 1994; **11**(4): 139–144.

12. Serdahely, W.J. Pediatric near death experiences *J. Near Death Studies* 1990; **9**(1).

13. Herzog, D.B. & Herrin, J.T. Near death experiences in the very young. *Crit. Care Med.* **13**(12): 1074–1075.

14. Morse, M., Castillo, P., Venecia, D., Milstein, J. & Tyler, D.C. Childhood near death experiences. *Am. J. Dis. Child.* 1986; **140**: 1110–1114.

15. Fenwick, P. & Fenwick, E. *The Truth in the Light,* London: Hodder Headline, 1995.

16. Greyson, B. Near death experiences and personal values *Am. J. Psychiatry* 1983; **140**(5): 618–620.

17. Greyson, B. Near-death experiences and attempted suicide. *Suicide Life Threat Behav.* 1981; **11**(1): 10–16.

18. Greyson, B. Incidence of NDEs following attempted suicide. *Suicide Life Threat Behav.* 1986; **16**(1): 40–45. 11, 10–16.

19. Blackmore, S.J. & Troscianko, T. The physiology of the tunnel. *J. Near Death Stud.* 1988; **8**: 15–28.

20. Blackmore, S.J. Near death experiences. *J. R. Soc. Med.* 1996; **89**: 73–76.

21. Meduna, L. *Carbon Dioxide Therapy: A Neurophysiological Treatment of Nervous Disorders,* 2nd edn. Springfield, IL: Charles C Thomas Publisher, 1958.

22. Carr, D.B. Endorphins at the approach of death. *Lancet* 1981; **1**: 8216.

23. Sotelo, J., Perez, R., Guevara & Fernandez, A. Changes in brain, plasma and cerebrospinal fluid contents of B-endorphin in dogs at the moment of death. *Neurol. Res.* 1985; **17**: 223.

24. Jansen, K. Near death experience and the NMDA receptor. *Br. Med. J.* 1989; **298**: 1708.

25. Appleton, R.E. Reflex anoxic seizures. *Br. Med. J.* 1993; **307**: 214–215.

26. Lempert, T. Syncope and near death experience. *Lancet* 1994; **344**: 829–830.

27. Carr, D. Pathophysiology of stress induced limbic lobe dysfunction: a hypothesis for NDEs. *J. Near Death Stud.* 1982; **2**: 75–89.

28. Morse, M., Venecia, D. & Milstein, J., Near-death experiences: a neurophysiologic explanatory model. *J. Near Death Stud.* 1989; **8** (1): 45–53.

29. Blanke, O., Ortigue, S., Landis, T. & Seeck, M. Stimulating illusory own-body perceptions. *Nature* 2002; **419**(6904): 269–270.

30. Blanke, O., Out of body experiences and their neural basis. *Br. Med. J.* 2004; **329**(7480): 1414–1415.

31. Blanke, O. & Arzy, S. The out-of-body experience: disturbed self-processing at the temporo-parietal junction. *Neuroscientist* 2005; **11**(1): 16–24.

32. Owens, J.E., Cook, E.W. & Stevenson, I., Features of "near death experience" in relation to whether or not patients were near death: *Lancet* 1990; **336**: 1175–1177.

33. Henslin, J., *Down to Earth Sociology: Introductory Readings* Free Press 13th edn, 2005, 259–268.

34. Parnia, S., Waller, D., Yeates, R. & Fenwick, P. A qualitative and quantitative study of the incidence, features and aetiology of near death experiences in cardiac arrest survivors. *Resuscitation* 2001; **48**: 149–156.

35. Sabom, M. *Recollections of Death: A Medical Perspective.* New York: Harper and Row, 1982.

36. Martens, P.R., Near-death-experiences in out-of-hospital cardiac arrest survivors. Meaningful phenomena or just fantasy of death? *Resuscitation* 1994; **27**(2): 171–175.

37. Van Lommel, P., Wees Van, R., Meyers, V. & Elfferich, I., Near-death experience in survivors of cardiac arrest: a prospective study in the Netherlands. *Lancet.* 2001; **358**(9298): 2039–2045.

38. Ring, K. *Life at Death. A Scientific Investigation of the Near-Death Experience.* New York: Coward McCann and Geoghenan, 1980.

39. Greyson, B. Incidence and correlates of near death experiences in a cardiac care unit. *Gen. Hosp. Psychiatry* 2003; **25**(4): 269–276.

40. Schwaninger, J. A prospective analysis of Near Death Experiences in cardiac arrest patients *J. Near Death Experiences* 2002; **20**(4): 215–232.

41. Moerman, N., Bonke, B. & Oosting, J. Awareness and recall during general anaesthesia: Facts and feelings. *Anaesthesiology* 1993; **79**: 454–464.

42. Blacher, R.S. On awakening paralysed during surgery. *J. Am. Med. Assoc.* 1975; **234**: 67–68.

43. Bailey, A.R. & Jones, J.G. Patients' memories of events during general anaesthesia. *Anaesthesia* 1997; **52**: 460–476.

44. Jelic, M., Bonke, B., De Roode, A. & Boville, J.G. Implicit learning during anaesthesia. In Sebel, P.S., Bonke, B. & Winograd, E., eds. *Memory and Awareness in Anaesthesia,* New Jersey: Prentice Hall, 1993: 81–84.

45. Roine, R.O., Kajaste, S. & Kaste, M. Neuropsychological sequelae of cardiac arrest. *J. Am. Med. Assoc.* 1993; **269**: 237–242.

46. Granja, C., Cabral, G., Pinto, A.T. & Costa-Pereira, A. Quality of life 6-months after cardiac arrest. *Resuscitation* 2002; **55**(1): 37–44.

47. Nichol, G., Stiell, I.G., Hebert, P., Wells, G.A., Vandemheen, K. & Laupacis, A. What is the quality of life for survivors of cardiac arrest? A prospective study. *Acad. Emerg. Med.* 1999; **6**(2): 95–102.

48. Stiell, I., Nichol, G., Wells, G. *et al.* OPALS Study Group. Health-related quality of life is better for cardiac arrest survivors who received citizen cardiopulmonary resuscitation. *Circulation* 2003; **108**(16): 1939–1944. Epub 2003 Oct 6.

49. Bisson, J. Post traumatic stress disorder. *Clin. Evid.* 2004; **11**: 1343–1361.

50. Ladwig, K., Schoenfinius, A., Dammann, G., Danner, R., Gurtler, R. & Herrman, R. Long-acting psychotraumatic properties of a cardiac arrest experience. *Am. J. Psychiatry* 1999; **156**: 912–919.

51. Gamper, G., Willeit, M., Sterz, F. *et al.* Life after death: post-traumatic stress disorder in survivors of cardiac arrest – prevalence, associated factors, and the influence of sedation and analgesia. *Crit. Care Med.* 2004; **32**(2): 378–383.

52. O'Reilly, S.M., Grubb, N. & O'Carroll, R.E. Long-term emotional consequences of in-hospital cardiac arrest and myocardial infarction. *Br. J. Clin. Psychol.* 2004; **43**(1): 83–95.

53. Grubb, N.R., O'Carroll, R., Cobbe, S.M., Sirel, J. & Fox, K.A. Chronic memory impairment after cardiac arrest outside hospital. *Br. Med. J.* 1996; **313**(7050): 143–146.

54. Drysdale, E, Grubb, N., Fox, K. & O'Carroll, R. Chronicity of memory impairment in long-term out-of-hospital cardiac arrest survivors. *Resuscitation* 2000; **47**: 27–32.

55. O'Reilly, S.M., Grubb, N.R. & O'Carroll, R.E. In-hospital cardiac arrest leads to chronic memory impairment. *Resuscitation* 2003; **58**(1): 73–79.

56. Nunes, B., Pais, J., Garcia, R., Magalhaes, Z., Granja, C. & Silva, M.C. Cardiac arrest: long-term cognitive and imaging analysis. *Resuscitation* 2003; **57**(3): 287–297.

57. Grubb, N.R., Fox, K.A., Smith, K. *et al.* Memory impairment in out-of-hospital cardiac arrest survivors is associated with global reduction in brain volume, not focal hippocampal injury *Stroke* 2000; **31**(7): 1509–1514.

58. Parnia, S. & Fenwick, P. Near death experiences in cardiac arrest: visions of a dying brain or visions of a new science of consciousness. *Resuscitation* 2002; **52**(1): 5–11.

59. Greenfield, S. Mind, brain and consciousness, *Br. J. Psychiatry* 2002; **181**: 91–93.

60. Crick, F. & Cock, K. The hidden mind, *Scientific American* (special issue) Aug 2002, 10–17.

61. Dennett, D. *Consciousness Explained.* Penguin, 1991.

62. Tunoni, G. & Edelman, G.M. Consciousness and complexity *Science* 1998; **282**: 1846–1851.

63. Hameroff, S., Nip, A., Porter, M. & Tuszynski, J., Conduction pathways in microtubules, biological quantum computation, and consciousness, *BioSystems* 2002; **64**: 149–168.

64. Chalmers, D.J. The puzzle of conscious experience, mysteries of the mind. *Scientific American* (special issue) 1997: 30–37.

65. Elahi, B. *Foundations of Natural Spirituality.* Element Books, 1997 and *Spirituality is a Science* Cornwall Books, 1999.

66. Paradis, N.A., Martin, G.B. & Goetting, M.G., Simultaneous aortic jugular bulb, and right atrial pressures during cardiopulmonary resuscitation in humans: insights into mechanisms. *Circulation* 1989; **80**: 361–368.

67. Angelos, M., Safar, P. & Reich, H. A comparison of cardiopulmonary resuscitation with cardiopulmonary bypass after prolonged cardiac arrest in dogs. Reperfusion pressures and neurologic recovery. *Resuscitation* 1991; **21**: 121–135.

68. Gonzalez, E.R., Ornato, J.P. & Garnett, A.R. Dose dependent vasopressor response to epinephrine during CPR in human beings. *Ann. Emerg. Med.* 1991; **18**: 920–926.

69. Paradis, N.A., Martin, G.B. & Rosenberg, J. The effect of standard and high dose epinephrine on coronary perfusion pressure during prolonged cardiopulmonary resuscitation. *J. Am. Med. Assoc.* 1991; **265**: 1139–1144.

70. Fischer, M. & Hossman, K.A. Volume expansion during cardiopulmonary resuscitation reduces cerebral no-reflow *Resuscitation* 1996; **32**: 227–240.

71. De Vries, J.W., Bakker, P.F., Visser, G.H., Diephuis, J.C. & van Huffelen, A.C. Changes in cerebral oxygen uptake and cerebral electrical activity during defibrillation threshold testing. *Anesth. Analg.* 1998; **87**: 16–20.

72. Kano, T., Hashiguchi, A. & Sadanaga, M. Cardiopulmonary – cerebral resuscitation by using cardiopulmonary bypass through the femoral vein and artery in dogs. *Resuscitation* 1993; **25**: 265–281.

73. Lavy, S. & Stern, S. Electroencephalographic changes following sudden cessation of artificial pacing in patients with heart block. *Confin. Neurol.* 1967 (Basel); **29**: 47.

74. Mayer, J. & Marx, T. The pathogenesis of EEG changes during cerebral anoxia In J Van Der Drift, ed. *Cardiac and Vascular Diseases Handbook of Electroencephalography and Clinicial Neurophysiology.* Amsterdam, 1972, vol. 14: 5–11.

75. Buunk, G., Van der Hoeven, J.G. & Meinders, A.E. Cerebral blood flow after cardiac arrest. *Netherlands J. Med.* 2000; **57**: 106–112.

76. Marshall, R.S., Lazar, R.M. & Spellman, J.P. Recovery of brain function during induced cerebral hypoperfusion. *Brain* 2001; **124**: 1208–1217.

77. Lishman, A. *Organic Psychiatry* 2nd edn. Oxford: Blackwell, 1987: 257–258.

78. Gastaut, H. & Fischer-Williams, M. Electroenchephalographic study of syncope: its differentiation from epilepsy. *Lancet* 1957; **2**: 1018–1025.

79. Clute, H.L. & Levy, W.J. Electroencephalographic changes during brief cardiac arrest in humans. *Anesthesiology* 1990; **73**: 821–825.

80. Cartlidge, N. Head injury, outcome and prognosis. In Swash, M. & Oxbury, J. eds. *Clinical Neurology.* Churchill Livingstone, 1991: Vol 1, 699–707.

81. Teasdale, G. Head injury – concussion, coma and recovery from altered states of consciousness. In Swash, M. & Oxbury, J. *Clinical Neurology.* Churchill Livingstone, 1991: Vol 1, 684–686.

82. Lishman, W.A. *Organic Psychiatry*, 2nd edn, Chapter 5, Head Injury. London: Blackwell, 1987: 137–150.

70

CPR training

Michael Shuster[1], Walter Kloeck[2], Edward R. Stapleton[3], Ulrik Juul Christensen[4], and Allan Braslow[5]

[1] Mineral Springs Hospital, Box 1050 Banff, Alberta, Canada
[2] Fairland, Johannesburg, South Africa
[3] Health Science Center, State University of NY, Stonybrook, New York
[4] Sophus Medical ApS, Copenhagen, Denmark
[5] Greenwich, CT, USA

The most important factor in survival from sudden cardiac arrest is the presence of a trained rescuer who is equipped to intervene. The most effective tools of the trained rescuer are CPR and defibrillation. CPR has been taught as a formal program to professionals since the late 1960s and to the lay public since the early 1970s. The program has changed markedly in scope and complexity as well as educational format and philosophy since its inception. Resuscitation councils that promote and teach CPR have sprung up around the world. Yet, despite this long history of the availability of CPR programs and their promotion, most victims of cardiac arrest do not receive bystander CPR.[1-6] Moreover, when CPR is performed, the quality of the CPR is often not ideal.[7,8] Although the development of the automated external defibrillator (AED), its increasing affordability, widespread promotion and availability to non-professionals have all contributed to earlier defibrillation, the number of people who are resuscitated is still limited by the low numbers of people who receive bystander CPR before defibrillation and the often poor quality of CPR when it is provided.

This chapter will address the challenge of teaching CPR effectively in various contexts: to the lay public, to laypersons with a duty to respond (such as police, fire, lifeguards, and airline employees), and to healthcare professionals. It will also discuss advanced educational technologies and present a model for new course development.

Teaching CPR

The lay public

Bystander CPR has consistently been shown to more than double the odds of survival from sudden cardiac arrest (SCA).[9-16] The few communities that have high bystander CPR rates have been effective in communicating the importance of CPR to the general public and have encouraged the whole population to learn CPR, but they have also directed their training efforts toward those people who are most likely to encounter SCA, and have made training readily available through both traditional and innovative means. Offering a variety of CPR courses, using different methods, in different settings, and of variable lengths provides the greatest chance of success in involving the many and diverse individuals who comprise any community.

Whom to teach

The chance that any particular individual in a community will have an opportunity to perform CPR is very small, unless that individual lives or works in a high-risk area or with a high-risk population. Thus, the primary target population for CPR education should be those people who are most likely to encounter a cardiac arrest.[17] This group includes the families of high-risk patients, people who live in retirement communities and people who work in large office buildings, shopping malls, airports, and other similar venues.[18] Nevertheless, even though other individuals are unlikely to encounter SCA, the greater the proportion of the population capable of performing CPR, the greater the chance that SCA victims will receive bystander CPR, so it is important to attract the general public to CPR courses. If there is a social climate of expectation that people should know how to perform CPR, people are more likely to seek out and attend CPR courses. The media has an important role to play in creating this climate of expectation and they should be encouraged to do so with the offer of newsworthy stories of successful resuscitations and the role that bystanders play in the process.[19,20] Public

Cardiac Arrest: The Science and Practice of Resuscitation Medicine. 2nd edn., ed. Norman Paradis, Henry Halperin, Karl Kern, Volker Wenzel, Douglas Chamberlain. Published by Cambridge University Press. © Cambridge University Press, 2007.

events and celebrity participation are often helpful as well.[21] CPR awareness campaigns can often reach people through the workplace and through community groups: a co-worker or group member who is a proponent may interest others in participating. Government can assist in creating a climate of expectation and in encouraging CPR proficiency in the general population.

At first glance, instructing schoolchildren in CPR seems like misdirected energy since the likelihood of a schoolchild encountering a cardiac arrest is very small indeed. Instruction of schoolchildren is expected to pay large dividends in future years, however, because it exposes children to the concept and practice of CPR at a stage in their lives when they are best equipped to learn and retain knowledge and skills.[22–27] Research has shown that many adults are reluctant and unprepared to act in an emergency.[28] Teaching children to act in an emergency, before they have been socialized to fear and avoid such situations, makes it more likely that they will be prepared and willing to do so when they become adults.[29] Many communities have successfully incorporated CPR instruction into the standard school curriculum.[22,30,31]

What to teach and how to teach it

Since their inception in the 1960s, CPR courses have undergone regular updates in content, as well as changes in format and scope. Despite this regular renewal, available research suggests that courses are not particularly successful. Learners perform CPR poorly even immediately following their training and, when they are assessed 3 or 6 months later, their performance has further declined. This relative failure of CPR instruction may be due to the structure and content of the CPR courses themselves, teaching methods that are not appropriate to lay persons, the quality of instruction, or inadequate practice time.[32–40]

CPR courses were initially designed by clinicians and, until recently, have not been evaluated to determine how well they accomplish their intended goal of producing CPR proficiency. Feedback over the years has suggested that learners are intimidated by the skill requirements and have often left courses unwilling to perform CPR for fear of doing it incorrectly. This feedback has led to changes in course requirements (learners no longer have to produce a perfect strip on a recording manikin) and to the presentation of material – but courses have not been redesigned completely. Course development should be led by educational specialists and should be evidence-based. The course should be thoroughly tested for educational efficiency prior to its widespread use. A model for new course development is presented later in this chapter.

CPR courses were traditionally led by instructors, beginning with a lecture on theory, followed by a demonstration, and concluding with manikin practice. The ineffectiveness of this model was documented in 1985 and led to video-based skill instruction *(watch-then-practise)* where students were presented with standardized, accurate, and on-message information from an instructional video, with the instructor serving as a facilitator.[41,42] By 1999, *watch-then-practise* was the primary CPR instructional method in the USA. *Video self-instruction* (VSI), or *practise along with the video while you watch,* was developed during 1993–1997 because of limitations in *watch-then-practise* video instruction to produce competent CPR performance.[43–47] VSI is expected to be adopted by the leading US training organizations in 2006. An advantage of the video-based model is that the information and CPR technique that is presented can be standardized and optimized. Regardless of whether the instructor leads or facilitates, immediate hands-on practice (watch-then-practise or practise-while-you-watch) helps to reduce anxiety about skill performance and increases the relevance of oral information, in that answers follow rather than precede questions.

Instruction is always most effective when it is provided in a manner that meets the learner's personal objectives.[48] It is counterproductive to insist on a course duration of 4 hours when many learners want and/or need only an hour or less to learn CPR. Educational principles direct that the course be structured to suit the age and learning style of the group being taught.

Other CPR instructional programs that were video-, television-, CD-software-, and Internet-based were developed during the 1990s for specific populations at risk and were designed to be used at times and locations that were convenient and non-threatening to their target audiences.[36,39,43–47,49–52] The disadvantage of self-instruction is that the learner is unable to ask questions or receive correction of faulty technique, although approaches such as VSI uniformly produce competent CPR technique approaches without intervention from an instructor. For special target audiences, such as the spouses of heart attack patients, specially trained on-scene instructors are needed to address learner fears and to prepare the learner for what to expect. For this reason, families or caregivers of persons at high risk should not rely solely on self-instruction.[36,49,50,53,54]

Some automated external defibrillators (AEDs) include real-time CPR prompting to assist laypersons during training and during actual cardiac arrest situations. The prompting component is currently being evaluated. One obvious question is whether people who follow real-time instructions can act independently to provide CPR in situations when there is no machine on scene to prompt them – which is the usual real-life situation.

Assessment of a learner's ability to perform CPR is a critical step in determining program success in producing competent CPR performance. Skill assessments performed by instructors of the major US training organizations have traditionally been unreliable, with instructors coaching and cueing learners during testing and/or passing all students, regardless of the quality of CPR performance. Reliable and valid research instruments used for assessing CPR performance should be adapted for use by instructors.[55] Confidence to perform CPR is not a reliable and valid measure of CPR competence, because most learners express confidence at the conclusion of their CPR course, regardless of the quality of their CPR performance. Moreover, learners should understand that they need to review and practise their CPR skills at regular intervals in order to maintain their ability and confidence to perform CPR in real life.[56–60] Training agencies should also understand the importance of reinforcement of skills and knowledge and must work with learners, employers, and the media to ensure that this message is heard.

Summary

The provision of bystander CPR contributes to higher survival rates among victims of sudden cardiac arrest. While proven methods for teaching CPR have been developed, we have not yet succeeded in training a large proportion of the general public to be ready and able to perform CPR proficiently in an emergency.

Lay persons with a duty to respond

A lay person with a duty to respond (hereafter called a "lay responder") is any non-healthcare professional who is responsible for providing CPR or basic first aid skills in a given interior or outdoor environment as part of day-to-day responsibilities. Lay responders range from office workers to flight attendants to security guards to emergency first responders, such as lifeguards, police, and firefighters.

Lay responders face their own set of challenges. They must be prepared to perform CPR on coworkers (people they know and interact with on a daily basis) and on strangers. Since lay responders do not have the knowledge and experience, and hence neither the confidence nor comfort level, of healthcare professionals, it is critical to provide sufficient training and regular reinforcement to build the confidence needed to respond effectively. Feelings of reluctance or embarrassment in dealing intimately with co-workers, and feelings of repulsion or appre-

hension, or fear of being exposed to disease may be partly addressed by training and can be further reduced by the use of mouth-to-mask devices. Training should include precourse preparation, generous skill practice during the course, and reinforcement exercises after the program to assure long-term retention of core skills. The overall training program and response protocols should systematically integrate the specialized knowledge and skills that are peculiar to the work environments within which lay responders will be functioning.

Training lay responders represents one of the most successful strategies for increasing survival from sudden cardiac arrest. Public access defibrillation programs in airports,[61] with police first responders,[62,63] and in casinos[64] have resulted in out-of-hospital survival rates of 49%–60%.

In designing the course curricula to train lay responders, the following questions should be addressed.

1. What is the nature of the environment in which they will respond?
2. What skills do they need to respond effectively in the environment in which they work and what devices or adjuncts, if any, will they be expected to use as part of their response?
3. What is the probable frequency of skill use?
4. What safety issues are important in the environment?

The nature of the environment

The response environments of different categories of lay responders differ dramatically. In any educational program for lay responders, the challenges of their respective environments must be addressed in the training program. For example, flight attendants work in a very compact environment where formal medical back-up may not be available for a long period of time. In an emergency, flight attendants may have to deal with logistical barriers, such as difficult access to the patient (e.g., obese victim in a window seat of an aircraft). In this environment the responder will be faced with some very challenging decisions (e.g., whether to ask that the aircraft be landed urgently) and complicating factors (e.g., CPR may not be possible during the landing of the aircraft). All of these and other issues must be anticipated and addressed during training so that problems do not prevent effective interventions during a real-life emergency. Protocols should be established that clearly delineate the expected actions when an emergency situation arises.

Police and firefighters, on the other hand, work in highly diverse, complex, and sometimes dangerous environments. They confront a great variety of emergencies, including trauma, poisoning, burns, and a host of other life-threatening (to both the victims and themselves) situations. During training, emphasis on scene safety is critical.

The challenges described in these two examples illustrate the need for a systematic analysis of the lay responders' job and the circumstances they will encounter, as part of the planning of an educational program for the selected group. Such analysis can be adequately undertaken only by an individual or team with expertise in the specific environment, as well as expertise in the field of emergency medical education.

Group-specific scenarios should be used to practise the events most likely to be encountered. A sample scenario for a police first responder is illustrated in Box 70.1. This scenario integrates the primary police function of scene safety with the role of CPR/AED responder. Job-specific scenarios are invaluable for illustrating the context in which response takes place; they should be set in the environment of the target audience and simulated through role-playing with hands-on practice.

Box 70.1

Example scenario for police responder
Summary of Scenario: Potentially unsafe scene, VF, 1 Shock conversion
Case History: A 52-year-old male teller collapses following a hold-up at a bank. The dispatcher indicates that the situation is ongoing.
Scene safety: Check the scene before entering bank. The security guard advises you that the suspect has left the scene but the teller has collapsed. Notify dispatch of the status of the scene and respond to the teller.
Victim: Unresponsive, no breathing and no signs of circulation.
Expected Actions: Determine unresponsiveness, notify dispatch that you need an ambulance, apply the AED and leave AED attached.
Outcome: After first shock victim returns regains normal breathing and consciousness.

Skills for lay responders

The skills taught to lay responders can range from CPR and the use of barrier devices to comprehensive CPR, AED, and first aid training for adult and/or pediatric victims. The target population and environment should determine the selection of skills. For example, in a small business where the incidence of trauma is low (i.e., store or office), CPR and use of barrier devices may be sufficient to deal with common medical emergencies such as fainting, stroke, and cardiac arrest. In an industrial environment, additional skills, such as first aid and use of an AED, may be needed. In addition, there may be national standards that dictate the type of training that is required. In the United States, the US Department of Transportation provides a National Standard Curriculum for Certified First Responders that is routinely used by police and fire organizations.

There are many national programs that can lay the foundation for a well-organized course of instruction. The American Heart Association, the American Red Cross, The National Safety Council, the Heart and Stroke Foundation of Canada, and the American Safety and Health Institute are examples of organizations that provide training and certification in CPR and/or first aid. Before such a program is implemented, emergency medical educators should collaborate with experts from the specific target environment to evaluate the needs of the responders and develop specific objectives, learning activities, skills, and protocols most appropriate to a given training program.

Frequency of skill use and retention of Skills

The retention of skills may well be the most important issue for the lay responder, because most lay responders use these skills infrequently. To this end, the initial training course should be structured to allow the student multiple opportunities to learn, practise skills, and apply critical information. For example, materials such as manuals, reminder cards, interactive CD ROMS, videos, and others, should be provided to the participant well in advance of training to encourage independent acquisition of baseline knowledge. These materials should remain available to the student, so that independent review can be undertaken at any time. A formal strategy for regular reinforcement of skills and review of core knowledge should be included as part of the training program.

An important function of the course itself is to provide maximum opportunity to practise the core skills of CPR, AED, and the use of barrier devices so that the student becomes completely comfortable with the skills. The practice scenarios that use rescuer-specific case examples are critical to the learning process.

Drills can be invaluable for reinforcing skills and knowledge. A properly planned drill can identify flaws in the response system and allow for significant quality improvement. The optimal interval between drills has not been established, but many programs conduct short drills at 6- to 12-month intervals. Complete refresher training should be provided approximately every 2 years or according to local or national standards.

Safety issues

Every response environment represents some risk to the responder. Infection, for example, is a universal risk.

Clearly, issues of safety become more important in response environments that pose greater danger, such as construction sites, industrial settings, at a crime scene or a fire. Scene safety is paramount in these environments and should be emphasized in every aspect of training and protocol development. In some environments, safety protocols may be dictated by national or local standards.

Stress must also be considered. Lay responders who have never dealt with life-threatening emergencies may experience significant stress, both during the emergency and afterward, especially if the outcome is poor. When the victim is a close friend or co-worker of the responder, stress may be intensified. Post-event debriefing by a healthcare professional can reduce inappropriate feelings of guilt or inadequacy and should be routinely arranged as part of the response program. During initial training, it is also important, to set realistic expectations for the responder. Since the survival rate from SCA is only around 5%, responders should understand that positive outcomes in cardiac arrest are the exception rather than the rule.

Summary

The well-trained lay person with a duty to respond represents one of the most successful strategies for increasing survival from cardiac arrest and other life-threatening emergencies.

A training program for this target population should take into account all aspects of the response environment, including specific safety issues, and should provide responders with the skills, knowledge, and confidence they will need to carry out their duties effectively.

Healthcare professionals

Basic life support

Numerous studies have shown that doctors, nurses, and ambulance personnel are generally not proficient in basic life support (BLS) skills, and that their skill retention, while variable, is generally poor.[8,35,65–74] Moreover, many healthcare professionals are reluctant to attend BLS courses, and even more reluctant to attend a refresher course.

BLS training requirements for healthcare professionals vary significantly among countries. Some national organizations, such as the Irish Heart Foundation and the Resuscitation Council of Southern Africa, require formal BLS certification as an entry requirement for advanced life support training (ACLS or pediatric advanced life support, PALS), whereas others, such as the American Heart Association, require only a brief "demonstration of proficiency" in BLS skills at the start of an ALS course. In the UK, hospitals employ dedicated "Resuscitation Officers," who

are responsible for the ongoing training and competency of their healthcare professional and auxiliary staff members. Unfortunately, many hospitals do not require their staff to maintain or demonstrate their BLS skills, and many do not provide formal in-service BLS training.

The training of healthcare providers should be tailored to their professional work environment. Performing CPR in the outdoors in all weather, or indoors in limited space hampered by bulky furniture and poor lighting is quite different from performing CPR on a patient lying on an elevated hospital bed, surrounded by monitors and adjunctive equipment. Healthcare professionals must? should? be proficient in performing CPR in a variety of roles: as a single rescuer, as a team member, and as a team leader.

The educational background and personal experiences and responsibilities of doctors, nurses, and ambulance personnel differ significantly. During BLS training, paramedics employed by a busy emergency service or staff based in a large emergency department may demonstrate greater confidence than personnel working in an out-patient or small community facility. Trainers and facilitators (should be aware that) participants may feel intimidated or humiliated by their more confident colleagues. Similarly, sensitivities among different professions, such as the participation of doctors and nurses in the same class, may lead to withdrawal or inhibited behaviour. It takes a skilled educator to maintain a non-threatening and relaxed atmosphere for all participants.

BLS course format, content, and style should be tailored to specific groups of healthcare providers, but core objectives, cognitive and psychomotor skill acquisition should remain constant. The use of computer and video self-instruction is increasing, and may be useful, provided that practical competence is evaluated. Peer instruction (e.g., doctor-to-doctor or nurse-to-nurse) may improve acceptance of BLS training in some environments. Course design and implementation should be based on validated educational principles.[57,75–78]

BLS training should include skills and equipment that the healthcare professional would generally use or have available, including adjunctive equipment such as barrier devices, pocket masks, self-inflating bags, and proficiency in the use of automated external defibrillators (AEDs). Role-plays should involve single and multiple-rescuer settings, with and without adjunctive equipment, and include a variety of special resuscitation situations such as trauma, submersion, and pregnancy. Use of realistic scenarios enhances contextual learning, relevance, and retention when the scenarios are simple in design.

All healthcare providers, undergraduate and post-graduate, should be able to demonstrate practical competence in the skills of BLS. Refresher programs that evaluate only knowledge retention do not ensure practical ability. Regular re-evaluation of competency is required to asses and reinforce the knowledge and skill retention of healthcare professionals, which have been shown to deteriorate within a few months of initial training.[79]

Advanced life support

As with BLS, knowledge and skill retention after advanced life support (ALS) training is poor.[33,38,80–85] Nevertheless, ALS training has been shown to improve clinical outcomes.[86] A study of anesthetists' management of VF in the operating room showed that ALS training led to significantly better adherence to resuscitation protocols.[87] Before formal ALS training had commenced, the BRESUS study reported overall survival to hospital discharge at 21% for patients requiring defibrillation.[88] At the time of the UK national audit of 1997, when more than 50,000 people had been trained in ALS skills, survival to discharge had increased to 43% for patients requiring defibrillation.[89]

Training programs in ALS skills are well established in many countries.[90] Initially these courses were didactic and lecture-based but, more recently, the emphasis has changed to hands-on, role-playing, and scenario-based learning. Many courses provide combined training of BLS and ALS skills in which CPR is integrated with defibrillation and the use of AEDs.

There are significant international differences in the approaches to teaching advanced skills, ranging from large group lectures to small group skill stations, open and closed group discussions, workshops, tutorials, role-plays, video presentations, and multidisciplinary teamwork training in mock arrest situations ("mega-codes").

Large-group lecture-based teaching is relatively ineffective in changing practice and behavior. Small-group training has many advantages, being more interactive, more personal, and more hands-on, but it is also more time-consuming and instructor-intensive. The optimal size of small groups will depend on the skill being taught, but groups should generally comprise four to eight participants.

Scenario-based teaching allows for useful repetition of sequences and variations on themes, but requires thoughtful preparation, planning and supervision. Although this approach is time-consuming, the value of realism and relevance for healthcare professionals should not be underestimated.

Compared with instructor-directed training, high-fidelity simulation-directed instruction has the advantage of less personal interaction with the instructor and more with the "patient," providing accurate and relevant situations, real-time physiological measurements which add to the realism, and training that can be adapted to individual participant needs.[91–94] The value of sophisticated simulation is well recognized in aviation and military training programs, although the high cost and time required for this training may well restrict its utility.

Most ALS courses worldwide conclude with written and practical evaluations. An interesting innovation, extensively used by the Resuscitation Council of Southern Africa, is to start each course with the final written evaluation. If candidates fail to achieve 84% for the written test at the start, they may reattempt the test at the end of the course. This method has several educational benefits.

- Instructors know who the weak participants are, and can provide extra attention right from the start. Similarly, instructors immediately know who the knowledgable candidates are, and can ask them more challenging questions, while the weaker participants are given less challenging questions and tasks, building up their confidence as the course progresses.
- The more advanced candidates can be asked to help weaker participants where appropriate, allowing weaker participants to ask questions and read about their uncertainties before the course is completed.
- All those who have passed the test can relax and concentrate on the practical side of the course, knowing that there is no "threat" of a further written test, while those who have failed tend to listen particularly attentively.
- The course does not end in a negative environment (waiting to be tested, waiting for results, wondering if they have passed, upset if they failed, walking out "tail between legs").

In a survey of 3530 participants undertaking PALS Provider courses over a 3-year period (June 2002 to May 2005) at an AHA Training Centre in Johannesburg, South Africa, only 51 participants (1.4%) achieved an initial score of less than 84% on the PALS "final" written evaluation when the evaluation was written at the start of the PALS course. Before starting the course, none of the participants were given, or had access to, any preparatory written evaluations besides the prescribed AHA PALS Provider Manual.[95]

Summary

While healthcare professionals are a natural target audience for BLS and ALS training, course planning for these individuals must be as carefully thought out and organized as it is for the general public and lay responders. Many of the same issues should be addressed: making appropriate courses available, meeting the specific educational needs of the individual learner, and establishing a mechanism to encourage retention of skills.

Simulation in CPR training

Simulation is the use of an artificial environment to mimic appearances and/or behaviours encountered in real life. Simulators and simulation have been used in health care education, if only sporadically, for almost two decades. In acute medicine, most notably in resuscitation and anesthesiology, full-scale simulators (macrosimulators) have been used for many years for problem-based training and education.[91,96–103] Full-scale simulators contribute verisimilitude and standardization to megacode (practice resuscitation) cases, and are also valuable tools for team training, management of crew resources, leadership, and communication.[93,104–106] Smaller scale simulators that run on a personal computer (microsimulators) have extended simulation into a wide variety of problem-based learning areas, and have been successfully sharpened the participants' diagnostic acumen and skills.[107]

Strengths and weaknesses of current simulators

Simulators are either macrosimulators or microsimulators, and each of these can be classified as either simple or complex.[108] Macrosimulators have a physical component, usually a manikin or a part thereof, whereas microsimulators are purely computer-based. Simulators are classified as "simple" or "part-task simulators" if they teach simple algorithms or procedures, involving only a few aspects of a problem. Complex simulators target more complex issues that integrate several aspects of a problem. Note that the classification "simple" or "complex" refers to the complexity of the educational task, and not to the technical complexity of the simulator. There are several technically complex, but educationally simple, macro- and microsimulators. (These four types of simulators have characteristic advantages and disadvantages)

Macrosimulators

Simple macrosimulators range from advanced virtual reality simulators with haptic "force" feedback* for various endoscopic procedures (available from Immersion Medical, Simbionix, Medical Simulation Corporation and others),[109,110] through advanced manikins for difficult airway management (Laerdal AirMan™), to mechanical manikins for the training of chest compression and ventilation (e.g., Ambu® Man or Laerdal™ Resusci®Anne, or the inflatable Laerdal MiniAnne

Complex macrosimulators are typically used for anesthesia and for resuscitation training. This category of macrosimulators includes the "Megacode" simulators for Advanced Life Support training (e.g., Ambu Megacode or Laerdal HeartSim 4000) to more complex simulators for trauma and anesthesia/intensive care simulation. (e.g., Meti Human Patient Simulator™ or Laerdal SimMan™). They combine an advanced manikin with a PC or workstation. The manikins simulate palpable pulses, electrocardiograms, spontaneous breathing, airways that can be configured electromechanically to mimic airway problems, and many other clinically relevant responses. In some of the simulators, computer models are used to simulate human physiology/pathophysiology and pharmacokinetics/dynamics, but an operator is required to run the simulator, and several trained participants are needed to complete the elements of a realistic scenario. The main differences between the various macrosimulators are the number of mechanical features in the manikins and differing approaches to the simulation software. Whereas METI is based on physiological models, with particular emphasis on the correct physiological response, the Laerdal SimMan™ models focus on supporting the instructor in running a specific pathophysiological scenario.

Macrosimulators provide the learner with an opportunity to perform manual procedures with or without complex problem-solving activity. They are used for training in specific psychomotor procedures, such as difficult airway management (including intubation, cricoid pressure, tracheotomy, suction and others), insertion of IV lines and chest drains, chest compression and ventilation, defibrillation, drug administration, palpation of pulses and auscultation. Macrosimulators can also reproduce complex situations where several team members have to cooperate to solve the problem. Complex simulators offer a reproducible opportunity for teaching behavioral and interpersonal aspects of performance. They are typically operated by instructors who run both the scenarios and the subsequent debriefing.

Microsimulators

Microsimulators (which run on personal computers and are also called PC simulators) support autonomous, cognitive training. They differ fundamentally from

---

* Roughly speaking, haptics and force feedback are distinct in the use of what is essentially the same technology. A haptic device applies a force in such a way as to allow the user to discern geometry and texture. A force feedback device applies a force to a user holding it, representing the sensation of impact and vibration.

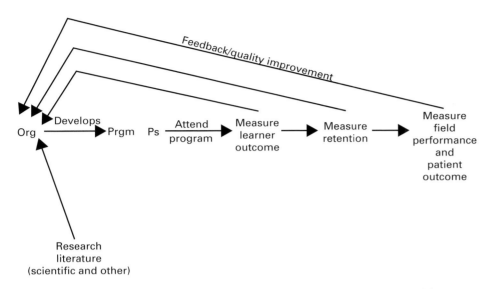

Org = training organization; Prgm = educational program; Ps = program participants

Fig. 70.1. Illustration of educational R&D/QA process

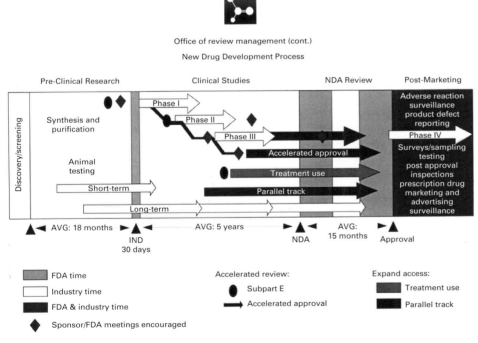

Office of review management (cont.)

New Drug Development Process

Fig. 70.2. FDA model

macrosimulators in that they do not have a physical component and do not require an operator to run the simulations and to provide educational feedback.

Microsimulators have the clear advantage over macrosimulators of accessibility, as most people have a PC either at work or at home. The programs are relatively inexpensive (US $80–280 for single-user licenses) and can be used informally. Whereas microsimulators cannot address issues at quite the same level of complexity as macrosimulators can, and they cannot train in crew resource management, leadership, or communication, microsimulators can be used to provide systematic learning and practice of a wide range of cognitive issues and problem-solving strategies in many different clinical circumstances. For example, trainees can use simple microsimulators, such as KinView Opioids or GasMan, to experiment with the pharmacokinetics and pharmacodynamics of drugs, or complex microsimulators to run scenarios.

Because microsimulators systematically provide multiple feedback opportunities (high quantity and focus of training) and, since they are easier to access than macrosimulators, they may train the user at a higher level of cognitive complexity than would be achieved with macrosimulator training. It must be emphasized, however, that whereas microsimulation can confidently be used to develop knowledge and problem-solving strategies, it cannot provide practice in manual skills or active role-playing. Moreover, the stress of real-life situations cannot be reproduced in microsimulations.

The ideal complex microsimulator provides credible simulations, followed by intelligent, context-specific evaluation of the user's decision-making during a simulation. Simulation training comes close to the educational principle of "practise by doing" in that well-made simulators give the user a feeling of actively solving the problem. Other training techniques, even if they involve the use of a PC, should not be confused with simulation. Multimedia programs, video teaching, lectures, and printed text tend to stimulate passive acquisition of knowledge and are primarily based on one-way communication of knowledge from the source to the user. The two approaches differ fundamentally in the extent to which the user is involved in the problem solving.

Applied microsimulation

Although the idea of algorithm training on computers is not new, few microsimulators are available for training in advanced life support in anesthesia, intensive care, or emergency medicine either for education of professionals or in basic life support for lay people. A few early microsimulators for anesthesia simulation were made during the late 1980s and 1990s. The ResusSim 98 project was the first to combine advanced PC simulation with elaborate feedback technology.[106] This approach were endorsed by several international authorities, including the European Resuscitation Council, the Australian Resuscitation Council, and the Resuscitation Council of Southern Africa. In 2003, the American Heart Association adopted microsimulation as the basis for their self-directed learning ACLS programme, HeartCode ACLS Anywhere. Successful completion of this programme, including a skills test, qualifies users for renewal of their AHA ACLS provider card (the user interface from HeartCode ACLS Anywhere appears in Fig. 70.4). Since 2000, Red Cross national societies in a number of European countries have used microsimulation as a tool for first aid education. (The user interface from the British Red Cross first aid simulator appears in Fig. 70.3.)

Feedback and debriefing in medical simulation

Macrosimulation and microsimulation differ significantly when it comes to debriefing – the heart of all simulation. In complex full-scale macrosimulation, the participants are typically debriefed by the instructor who has been guiding the scenario, using video and/or printed recordings of the sessions. The major challenge lies in enabling instructors to use a wide range of skills in interpersonal and educational, as well as medical, areas. In microsimulation, the major challenge is to achieve reliable, autonomous performance by the software.

In simple microsimulation, standardized feedback is generated by subtracting the actual performance from a given set of recommendations, producing a banal "error signal." In a more complex microsimulation, focused feedback would optimally evaluate the learner and analyze the entire performance, with reference to timeliness, sequencing, and appropriateness of actions, and indicating whether variances were minor or significant. Focused feedback should assist the trainee in improving subsequent performance.

The technical difficulties in autonomously evaluating individual performance are significant, however. The user often addresses more than one issue concurrently. For example, advanced airway management may be performed concurrently with a specific algorithm for a cardiac condition. Simultaneous approaches present a problem in evaluation, as the user does not clearly mark which action belongs to which strategy. Moreover, several actions may be relevant, but not crucial, to solving the problem, further

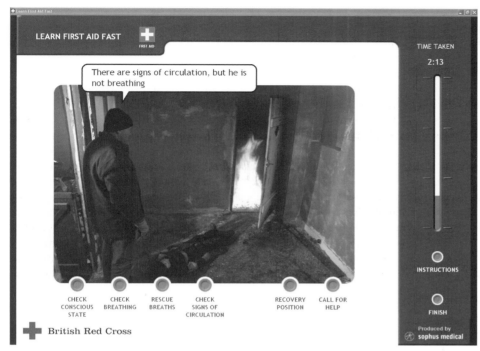

Fig. 70.3. In a number of countries, the Red Cross has used microsimulation for first aid education. This example is the Learn First Aid simulator used by British Red Cross.

complicating the debriefing. Optimal feedback technology distinguishes between important and less important actions and mistakes.

In the MicroSim programs (AHA's Heartcode is based on MicroSim), a debriefing technology – artificial intelligence debriefing (AID) – has been used. On the basis of modern research in pattern recognition and educational theory, AID has become an umbrella name for a range of technologies aimed at intelligent debriefing. It is capable, for instance, of detecting different algorithms mixed in a sequence of actions and can assign weight to actions and mistakes. AID can provide feedback on parts of the treatment (e.g., the cardiac treatment algorithm) without being "disturbed" by other actions performed in tandem. The feedback can be presented either in different visual formats or in text.

The relatively low reliance on microsimulators as a training technology may be due to current limitations in feedback technology. As technologies like AID develop and improve, more advanced and relevant microcomputers may play a greater part in resuscitation training

Summary

Simulation provides a uniquely safe and standardized, yet realistic, setting for research into human error. Many of the breaches in protocol made during clinical care result from the practitioner's doubts about which algorithms to follow, errors in drug dosage, and faulty clinical reasoning,[111] and most of these gaps in knowledge and logic can be identified and addressed by the use of simulators.

Simulation achieves interaction with a variety of critical scenarios quickly and allows rare, but time-critical, conditions to be practised and re-played by the user.[112] Simulation should always include a debriefing based on what the learner does during the simulation, to give instant feedback and highlight deficiencies in knowledge. Simulators can also evaluate the knowledge and performance of healthcare personnel, thus completing the educational feedback loop and improving the quality of the education.

CPR course development

Educational research and development/quality assurance model

The following educational R&D/QA model, is based on science-based educational curriculum development, instructional design, and related learning theories (See

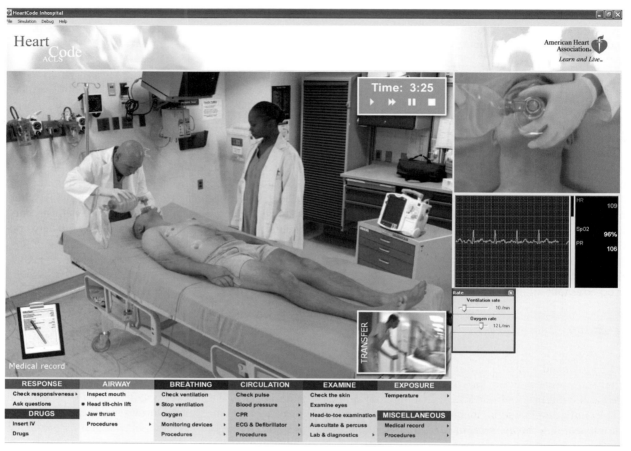

Fig. 70.4. Heartcode ACLS interface.

Fig. 70.1).[113–117] The model described in this section is analogous to the US Food and Drug Administration (FDA) process of drug development and testing to determine if a drug is "safe and effective" before approving its entry into the market (see Fig. 70.2). It is a logical model to use for the development of BLS and ACLS programs (and redevelopment/improvement of existing programs) for both providers and instructors. In contrast to many current programs that focus on what the instructor must teach, the design of educational R&D is focused on an in-depth understanding of the target audience and how best to help the audience to achieve specific outcomes related to patient survival.

The model is designed to be used to develop provider and instructor programs. With each program, learner audiences will have different instructional needs and learning styles, and will require unique programs tailored to their specific needs. For example, in BLS or AED training there may be separate R&D processes for school students by age group-

ing, adults by age, paraprofessional providers by level of training and exposure to cardiac emergencies, and professional providers by specialty and exposure to cardiac emergencies. There may also be different instructor materials (and programs) for different BLS or AED instructor audiences, such as teachers, EMS providers who are not credentialed teachers, and community volunteers with no formal training as teachers. The R&D model inventories the learning needs of providers and instructors early in the process.

Programs developed with this model focus on learner competence immediately following training, at a later date, and in actual (or realistically simulated) situations. Ideally, to show full compliance with a training organization's mission, training of significant populations should lead to decreased rates of morbidity and mortality. The model is iterative and linear, with completion of one step before the next; however, it allows for parallel development tracks (e.g., provider level program, testing/evaluation, and instructor program).

Attention to learner outcomes ensures establishment of the first link of the overall public health objectives of BLS and ALS programs (producing competent providers). Positive learner outcomes may not necessarily coincide with traditional indicators of program success, such as the satisfaction of end-users, clients, and instructors. This model ensures that programs meet the learning needs of the participant population. Mismatch of the learner needs and program design occur for a variety of reasons, including repackaging of programs designed for one audience for another (or other) audiences, and development of one program for more than one target-specific audience. Although the use of programs that attempt to meet the needs of multiple audiences with different learning needs may seem efficient, it can seriously undermine program effectiveness.

A scientifically sound development process for all educational programs (providers and instructors) would proceed as follows.

Select R&D team

Because this is an educational development process, the team should primarily comprise education specialists. The team would typically include a project manager, as well as specialists in education research and evaluation, curriculum development, instructional design, media design, learning theory, program evaluation, and public health.

If medical practice guidelines are already established, medical personnel generally should serve as outside consultants as necessary. If development of medical practice guidelines is required, this is not a direct education R&D process and should be completed as a separate process. In developing medical guidelines, education experts should serve as consultants to the medical guidelines committee in order to determine the feasibility of teaching (the "teachability") of various practices for specific target audiences, both professional and lay.

Discussion

The most important and fundamental change to the current process of program development, which will result in the greatest improvement in quality of programs, will be to assign the development of components of the educational agenda to appropriate experts. Educational research and development is a specialized field dedicated to development and delivery of educational interventions that bring about specific learner outcomes. In the cases of BLS and ALS, these specific learner outcomes are directly related to provider behaviors that are associated with saving human lives. The specialty of educational research and development, like specialties in medicine, can only be properly executed by properly trained experts.

Each training organization's BLS and ACLS committee should be made up of two separate committees with different responsibilities and expertise: medical and educational. These are essentially separate teams with separate missions While initial recommendations for changes in medical or educational program development could be generated from either subcommittee, substantive educational recommendations should be formulated only by experts in education. Homogeneous groupings (for example, committees made up of medical scientists, curriculum experts, representatives of the training network, and so on) are inefficient and reduce the quality of any program because they place committee members in a position of influencing work beyond their own expertise.

Conduct a needs assessment and establish the instructional goal

A needs assessment is a critical first step for every program and every major target audience. It documents the need for the program, potential benefits, and probability for success. Then, learning characteristics of the target audience must be ascertained, as well as their existing knowledge and skill sets.

Relevant public health statistics and literature are examined, as well as the success of similar or existing programs, and public health cost-effectiveness, consistent with the mission statement of the training organization (e.g., will AED training or traditional CPR training save more lives?). The process includes identification of a public health problem, specific target audiences that can intercede, and possible programmatic solutions.

The needs assessment is the product of a dynamic process, which begins with discussions and debate by advocates (and also dissenters), followed by several writing and discussion sessions to work towards consensus on the feasibility and justification for moving forward; in other words, the information required to make a "go/no go" decision. If a "go" decision to continue is made, the program's Instructional Goal is outlined. The Instructional Goal is the R&D team's collaborative opinion of what the program will actually accomplish – that is, in general terms what the target audience will be expected to do following exposure to the training program. A question generally asked is "Is the instructional goal feasible for the target audience, and to what extent?" This is answered as part of the target audience analysis.

Conduct a target audience analysis

With the identification of the target audience(s) for the program, the R&D team conducts the in-depth social and learning analysis of the audience. This comprehensive analysis may first study whether or not, or to what extent, members of the target audience are aware of the problem, their perceptions, as well as their potential role in addressing the problem, including their perceptions of participating in such a role, and their motivations for participating in the program. The learning characteristics of the target audiences must be ascertained (e.g., typical methods for self-learning), as well as their existing knowledge and skill sets. This step generally uses several methods including: review of education and psychosocial literature, focus groups, field and case studies, and review of effective educational programs for similar target audiences. The findings of the target audience analysis may also conclude with a "no-go" decision.

Discussion

The target audience analysis is a critical step and is often omitted, directly contributing to inaccurate assumptions about the target audience, and subsequent selection of inappropriate instructional strategies and materials, all contributing to poor learner outcomes.

Many public health papers have been written justifying the need for BLS and ALS in the general population, and suggesting a segment of the population to intercede. For example, public health analyses have suggested that spouses (and other family members) of heart disease patients be taught CPR, because of their obvious likely proximity to these patients if they experience a heart attack or a cardiac arrest. Thus far, however, this strategy remains problematic. The Needs Assessment and Target Audience Analysis are important because they go a step farther by examining the feasibility of utilizing particular audiences to intercede. In order to prioritize options for addressing a public health problem, definitive statements on the rationale for selecting a specific audience, balanced against threats to success, are necessary.

What happens if the Educational Needs Assessment determines that an educational intervention is not feasible or advantageous (e.g., no additional lives will be saved) leading to a "no-go" decision, but the Market Research leads to "go" decision? There are the following possibilities.

- The process is stopped at this phase, or
- An alternative program using a different target audience or technology as a substitute for the target audience is used (e.g., implantable defibrillators), or

- Because the training organization may need revenues to support other programs, the program may proceed (regardless of the program's utility in saving lives).

Develop learning objectives and evaluation instruments

With knowledge of the target audience's characteristics and abilities, the R&D team determines the competencies needed by learners to achieve the program goals efficiently and effectively. The R&D team translates these goals into precise observable learning objectives for the program, and they are also the basis for the development of assessment tools.

The instructional goals are converted into behavioral objectives, and the skills derived from analysis of the instructional goals above are converted into subordinate objectives. The objectives guide the R&D team in the design and development of instruction, especially with selecting content and developing the instructional strategies. Specific, finite, behavioral objectives are formulated from knowledge and understanding of the target audience's learning characteristics and abilities. Requisite entry characteristics and behaviors are also developed (i.e., what competencies participants must already possess before entry into the program).

These learning objectives are also used to construct measures of the learner's accomplishment of the task. Development of assessment tools (e.g., written tests, skill assessments) generally begin at this point and should be performed as a separate and concurrent process by a team of educators with expertise in evaluation. Initially, the assessment tools are tested without participant involvement (e.g., content validity, reading level, expert review), and are "piloted" using subjects with a broad range of the included abilities from novice to expert. Then, like the program itself, the tools are further developed and modified depending on the results of pilot testing, either independently or as part of the pilot testing of the overall program.

The valid and reliable assessment tools serve two purposes: assessment of individual participants during the program and of overall program effectiveness. During the formative stage of program development (i.e., during pilot testing), assessment tools are necessary for providing information about the effectiveness of the instruction (See Step 7, Pilot test program and revise instructional materials). Pretesting of knowledge and experience as entry criteria is important in many programs (in particular, instructor training and advanced classes such as ACLS) to assure that all learners have basic qualifications and understanding to participate effectively and efficiently in the program and achieve the desired learner outcomes.

Discussion

Learning objectives are the driving force for curriculum development, instructional design, and valid and reliable testing. Historically, developers have not completely recognized the purpose and importance of learning objectives and have assigned this task a low priority to be completed later in the process by a backwards-type logic (i.e., reasoning from the content of the program what the objectives might be), contributing to poor educational programs and poor assessment tools.

Well articulated learning objectives are the key to development of valid tests and measures. Good measures require adequate time for construction. With completion of the learning objectives, test development should begin. Often, test construction is delayed while the precise wordings of final provider materials are awaited. Such delays are not justified, because the structure and content of the test items themselves can be derived from the objectives alone, while wording changes can be made at any point in the process to reflect ongoing development of other materials.

Develop instructional outline (instructional script)

The learning objectives are organized into a logical presentation sequence specifically designed for the target audience. The instructional outline is based on the target audience's experience relative to the subject matter, their learning abilities and motivation, and the required competencies. The instructional outline or script becomes the basic foundation map and script for the program and will be enhanced as other components of the program are developed. The instructional script will also serve a key role in the development of instructor materials.

Select and develop instructional strategies and materials

With the detailed knowledge of the target audience, the specification of learning objectives, and an instructional outline, the R&D team can select and develop instructional strategies and materials. The most appropriate strategies are determined for accomplishing each objective. An instructional strategy is a method or set of methods used to assist a specific target learner audience master a learning objective.

Once the strategy is selected (or conceived), the material (or media) that will best communicate the specific strategy is selected (e.g., video, e-learning, book, instructor, among others). For example, if a visual model is selected as an instructional strategy, specifications for the visual model are first developed, followed by selection of the appropriate material to communicate the instructional strategy to the target learners (e.g., video, instructor demonstration, CD-ROM/DVD, slides, e-learning, interactive simulation, or a combination of materials).

To assist the instructional designer in understanding all the information and concepts that must be communicated through the instructional strategy and materials, traditional developers often begin by producing a self-instructional prototype of the program for themselves. According to Dick and Carey, this activity of putting oneself in the position of the learner forces the instructional designer to confront all the elements of the program that the student must face in mastering the program objectives.[113] When using the self-instructional prototype, the materials alone should permit the participant to acquire the competencies without intervention from an instructor. Once the detailed self-instructional materials are completed, other types of instructional media, specific to the instructional strategies, are considered.

Depending on the types and scope of instructional materials selected, several teams may be needed to complete the development of the instructional materials. Each team needs specific expertise in the (1) type of instructional material (e.g., book or video), (2) content, and (3) specific audience.

Discussion

Selection of instructional strategies as well as instructional materials (media) before fully addressing Steps 1–3 has historically contributed to program development and delivery problems and failures.

The traditional practice of including the instructor as part of the instructional strategy before consideration of other instructional strategies is often used to fill gaps in the materials; this may lead to incoherent program presentation and confusion. This practice allows the designer to avoid having to confront all the learner's challenges, which leads to an incomplete understanding and articulation of the instructional information and strategies, and undermines learning and efforts to control program quality. At the least, in the case of materials developed for a lay audience, research has shown that when considerable latitude is given to instructors, on the theory that they can best tailor the course to the learners, learner outcomes may be less successful. Well-trained educators may have this ability to adapt to learner needs, but the BLS and ALS instructor corps is largely made up of individuals without the appropriate background to do this.

Pilot test program (formative evaluation) and revise instructional materials

Instructional strategies and materials cannot be developed in a vacuum; it is only when materials are tested with learners that informed revisions can be made. The process of pilot testing and revision is ongoing and iterative (i.e., each pilot test brings the R&D team a step closer to an effective instructional program).

Pilot testing takes place at various stages of the ongoing development of instructional materials, often on a small scale with "mini-pilots" involving a few small convenient samples. Revisions are also ongoing, based on the findings of the pilot testing. During initial development of strategies and materials, small numbers of representative learners are asked to respond to sections or components of verbal (written and/or spoken) and visual materials. Findings from pilot tests are used to make decisions, such as program duration, class size, or the need for instructional supplies or equipment. Meaningful data are therefore used to make these decisions versus the tradition of arbitrary decision making.

Before pilot testing, the educational interventions are untested and therefore may be limited in their ability to bring about the expected learning behaviors (e.g., competent CPR performance) because the interventions are based primarily on expert opinion and conjecture and *not* on actual in-class evaluations with the target audiences. Pilot testing typically identifies communications and other instructional problems, and major modifications are often necessary. This trial and error iterative approach is key to the model and can contribute to the success of the final program. Time must be built into the development process for repeated trials and complete redrafting of the program, or sections, if necessary.

Qualitative methods used during pilot testing include videotaping and/or detailed observation of the pilot program, and interviews with all participants, including instructors, if applicable. Prototype learner outcome measures (i.e., assessment tools) are used to determine the extent to which learners are mastering behavioral objectives. In this way, the assessment tools themselves may also be piloted and revised.

Once a prototype instructional program is completed, more formal larger scale formative and summative evaluation, in as realistic a setting as possible, is performed, with learner outcomes as the primary measure of program success. Learner and instructor behaviors are still observed during the final phase of pilot testing. Instructional strategies and materials are modified in accordance with the results of pilot tests and are retested until the course participants master the learning objectives and related competencies.

Discussion

It is during pilot testing that the education developers determine how long it takes participants to master the objectives (i.e., determine program duration). Traditionally, pilot testing has been used to determine how long it takes the instructors to present the material, with lesser regard for how long it actually takes participants to master the objectives. Course length has most often been an arbitrary computation based on course administrative constraints, such as cost or consumer expectations.

External regulations often cause instructional developers to tailor programs to a specific length of time. In such cases, learner competence (i.e., learner outcome) must drive decisions concerning number of course objectives that can realistically be accomplished by learners. Only objectives that can be successfully accomplished within the mandated time frame should be part of the program.

Field test program and modify if necessary

After completion of pilot testing, the program is ready for field-testing (i.e., implementing the program on a limited scale but simulating a full roll-out). The program is tested as it would be delivered in the field.

In a field test setting, as opposed to a pilot test, the delivery simulates program roll-out and uses realistic materials; real-world instructors and participants are involved, who may be unaware that the product is not finalized. This step of product testing is typically focused on the testing of program *delivery*, rather than the *instructional materials* (i.e., what happens when the program reaches the end user). Field testing may uncover the need to change some aspects of the instructional system, such as with noncompliance of instructors. It may also indicate that the user audience does not match the intended target audience. Possible program revisions range from small modifications to comprehensive changes in program design and delivery.

Roll-out program

Following field testing, the program is disseminated to and implemented in the broader target population. Ideally, field testing activities continue throughout the roll-out and implementation of the program.

Establish and implement quality assurance monitoring team and system

The quality assurance monitoring team evaluates the program throughout its life cycle. Their findings, in part, guide the development of the next version of the program, and may inform the development of other BLS and ALS programs. The findings also inform online (i.e., immediate) revisions to the program, if needed.

Quality assurance is a dynamic, ongoing process of monitoring learner outcomes, retention, and field performance after program release, in which findings are used to inform revisions of existing programs and/or the development of new programs. The quality assurance monitoring team is a permanent group composed of experts in education and evaluation who design and monitor the QA system and work with the training organization's field staff and outside evaluators to provide regular evaluation of existing programs. The QA team may become involved with the program during field-testing. The team monitors the progress of the program through its life cycle.

Figure 70.1 presents the cycle of program R&D and QA. Data related to learner outcomes are collected at different time points after instruction, and findings are fed back to the R&D team to inform course revisions.

Monitoring of ongoing courses includes collecting objective, quantitative data, as well as qualitative feedback about the programs, often using the valid and reliable assessment instruments developed earlier by the R&D assessment team. Quantitative data are collected regarding learner outcomes (e.g., skill competencies). Qualitative data can include feedback collected from focus groups and systematic observations of programs. Programs sampled should represent a variety of geographic locales and typical target audiences.

A centralized system for collecting and analyzing data from evaluations should be developed. A reliable feedback mechanism (e.g., reporting of findings) should be in place so that the products of ongoing evaluation are fed back to the R&D group for continual program improvement.

Discussion

Early selection and involvement of the QA team, ideally during the R&D steps, permits QA team members to become familiar with the program and assessment tools and to pilot test aspects of the QA system (e.g., data management, analysis and feedback (to R&D).

REFERENCES

1. Eckstein, M., Stratton, S. & Chan, L. Cardiac arrest resuscitation evaluation in Los Angeles: CARE-LA. *Ann. Emerg. Med.* 2005; **45**(5): 504–509.

2. Hollenberg, J., Bang, A., Lindqvist, J. *et al.* Difference in survival after out-of-hospital cardiac arrest between the two largest cities in Sweden: a matter of time? *J. Intern. Med.* 2005; **257**(3): 247–254.

3. Herlitz, J., Engdahl, J., Svensson, L., Angquist, K., Young, M. & Holmberg, S. Factors associated with an increased chance of survival among patients suffering from an out-of-hospital cardiac arrest in a national perspective in Sweden. *Am. Heart. J.* 2005; **149**(1): 61–66.

4. Lerner, E., Fairbanks, R. & Shah, M. Identification of out-of-hospital cardiac arrest clusters using a geographic information system. *Acad. Emerg. Med.* 2005; **12**(1): 81–84.

5. Vaillancourt, C. & Stiell, I. Cardiac arrest care and emergency medical services in Canada. *Can. J. Cardiol.* 2004; **20**(11): 1081–1090.

6. Dowie, R., Campbell, H., Donohoe, R. & Clarke, P. "Event tree" analysis of out-of-hospital cardiac arrest data: confirming the importance of bystander CPR. *Resuscitation* 2003; **56**(2): 173–181.

7. Gallagher, E., Lombardi, G. & Gennis, P. Effectiveness of bystander cardiopulmonary resuscitation and survival following out-of-hospital cardiac arrest. *J. Am. Med. Assoc.* 1995; **274**(24): 1922–1925.

8. Abella, B.S., Alvarado, J.P., Myklebust, H. *et al.* Quality of cardiopulmonary resuscitation during in-hospital cardiac arrest. *J. Am. Med. Assoc.* 2005; **293**(3): 305–310.

9. Sedgwick, M.L., Dalziel, K., Watson, J., Carrington, D.J. & Cobbe, S.M. Performance of an established system of first responder out-of-hospital defibrillation. The results of the second year of the Heartstart Scotland Project in the "Utstein Style." *Resuscitation* 1993; **26**(1): 75–88.

10. Holmberg, M., Holmberg, S. & Herlitz, J. Effect of bystander cardiopulmonary resuscitation in out-of-hospital cardiac arrest patients in Sweden. *Resuscitation* 2000; **47**(1): 59–70.

11. Cummins, R.O., Ornato, J.P., Thies, W.H. & Pepe, P.E. Improving survival from sudden cardiac arrest: the "chain of survival" concept. A statement for health professionals from the Advanced Cardiac Life Support Subcommittee and the Emergency Cardiac Care Committee, American Heart Association. *Circulation* 1991; **83**(5): 1832–1847.

12. Engdahl, J., Bang, A., Lindqvist, J. & Herlitz, J. Factors affecting short- and long-term prognosis among 1069 patients with out-of-hospital cardiac arrest and pulseless electrical activity. *Resuscitation* 2001; **51**(1): 17–25.

13. Lateef, F. & Anantharaman, V. Bystander cardiopulmonary resuscitation in prehospital cardiac arrest patients in Singapore. *Prehosp. Emerg. Care.* 2001; **5**(4): 387–390.

14. Stiell, I.G., Wells, G.A., DeMaio, V.J., *et al.* Modifiable factors associated with improved cardiac arrest survival in a multi-

center basic life support/defibrillation system: OPALS Study Phase I results. Ontario Prehospital Advanced Life Support. *Ann. Emerg. Med.* 1999; **33**(1): 44–50.

15. Waalewijn, R.A., de Vos, R. & Koster, R.W. Out-of-hospital cardiac arrests in Amsterdam and its surrounding areas: results from the Amsterdam resuscitation study (ARREST) in "Utstein" style. *Resuscitation* 1998; **38**(3): 157–167.

16. Swor, R.A., Jackson, R.E., Cynar, M. *et al.* Bystander CPR, ventricular fibrillation, and survival in witnessed, unmonitored out-of-hospital cardiac arrest. *Ann. Emerg. Med.* 1995; **25**(6): 780–784.

17. Brennan, R. & Braslow, A. Are we training the right people yet? A survey of participants in public cardiopulmonary resuscitation classes. *Resuscitation* 1998; **37**(1): 21–25.

18. Becker, L., Eisenberg, M., Fahrenbruch, C. & Cobb, L. Public locations of cardiac arrest: implications for public access defibrillation. *Circulation* 1998; **97**(21): 2106–2109.

19. Meischke, H., Finnegan, J. & Eisenberg, M. What can you teach about cardiopulmonary resuscitation (CPR) in 30 seconds? Evaluation of a television campaign. *Eval. Health Prof.* 1999; **22**(1): 44–59.

20. Becker, L., Vath, J., Eisenberg, M. & Meischke, H. The impact of television public service announcements on the rate of bystander CPR. *Prehosp. Emerg. Care.* 1999; **3**(4): 353–356.

21. Fong, Y., Anantharaman, V., Lim, S., Leong, K. & Pokkan, G. Mass cardiopulmonary resuscitation 99 – survey results of a multi-organisational effort in public education in cardiopulmonary resuscitation. *Resuscitation* 2001; **49**(2): 201–205.

22. Lewis, R.M., Fulstow, R. & Smith, G.B. The teaching of cardiopulmonary resuscitation in schools in Hampshire. *Resuscitation* 1997; **35**(1): 27–31.

23. Moore, P.J., Plotnikoff, R.C. & Preston, G.D. A study of school students' long term retention of expired air resuscitation knowledge and skills. *Resuscitation* 1992; **24**(1): 17–25.

24. Plotnikoff, R. & Moore, P.J. Retention of cardiopulmonary resuscitation knowledge and skills by 11- and 12-year-old children. *Med. J. Aust.* 1989; **150**(6): 296, 298–299, 302.

25. Heath, J. & Nielsen, D. Teaching school children cardiopulmonary resuscitation. *Resuscitation* 1996; **32**(2): 159–160.

26. Lyttle, J. Mandatory CPR training for students may improve cardiac-arrest survival rate, MDs say. *Can. Med. Assoc. J.* 1996; **155**(8): 1172–1174.

27. Liberman, M., Golberg, N., Mulder, D. & Sampalis, J. Teaching cardiopulmonary resuscitation to CEGEP students in Quebec – a pilot project. *Resuscitation* 2000; **47**(3): 249–257.

28. Rowe, B., Shuster, M., Zambon, S. *et al.* Preparation, attitudes and behaviour in nonhospital cardiac emergencies: evaluating a community's readiness to act. *Can. J. Cardiol.* 1998; **14**(3): 371–377.

29. Lester, C.A., Weston, C.F., Donnelly, P.D., Assar, D. & Morgan, M.J. The need for wider dissemination of CPR skills: are schools the answer? *Resuscitation* 1994; **28**(3): 233–237.

30. Reder, S. & Quan, L. Cardiopulmonary resuscitation training in Washington state public high schools. *Resuscitation* 2003; **56**(3): 283–288.

31. Lafferty, C., Larsen, P.D. & Galletly, D. Resuscitation teaching in New Zealand schools. *N Z Med. J.* 2003; **116**(1181): U582.

32. Chamberlain, D., Smith, A., Woollard, M. *et al.* Trials of teaching methods in basic life support (3): comparison of simulated CPR performance after first training and at 6 months, with a note on the value of re-training. *Resuscitation* 2002; **53**(2): 179–187.

33. Kaye, W. Research on ACLS training – which methods improve skill and knowledge retention? *Respir. Care.* 1995; **40**(5): 538–546; discussion 546–549.

34. Ward, P., Johnson, L.A., Mulligan, N.W., Ward, M.C. & Jones, D.L. Improving cardiopulmonary resuscitation skills retention: effect of two checklists designed to prompt correct performance. *Resuscitation* 1997; **34**(3): 221–225.

35. Broomfield, R. A quasi-experimental research to investigate the retention of basic cardiopulmonary resuscitation skills and knowledge by qualified nurses following a course in professional development. *J. Adv. Nurs.* 1996; **23**(5): 1016–1023.

36. Dracup, K., Moser, D.K., Doering, L.V. & Guzy, P.M. Comparison of cardiopulmonary resuscitation training methods for parents of infants at high risk for cardiopulmonary arrest. *Ann. Emerg. Med.* 1998; **32**(2): 170–177.

37. Handley, J.A. & Handley, A.J. Four-step CPR – improving skill retention. *Resuscitation* 1998; **36**(1): 3–8.

38. Hammond, F., Saba, M., Simes, T. & Cross, R. Advanced life support: retention of registered nurses' knowledge 18 months after initial training. *Aust. Crit. care* 2000; **13**(3): 99–104.

39. Nolan, R.P., Wilson, E., Shuster, M., Rowe, B.H., Stewart, D. & Zambon, S. Readiness to perform cardiopulmonary resuscitation. an emerging strategy against sudden cardiac death. *Psychosomatic Med.* 1999; **61**(4): 546–551.

40. Amith, G. Revising educational requirements: challenging four hours for both basic life support and automated external defibrillators. *New Horiz.* 1997; **5**(2): 167–172.

41. Braslow, A. An evaluation of the knowledge and practices of basic cardiac life support instructors. In *University of Illinois.* Urbana-Champaign, IL, 1985.

42. Cross, A.R. ed. *Adult CPR*, Washington, DC: American National Red Cross, 1987.

43. Braslow, A., Brennan, R.T., Newman, M.M., Bircher, N.G., Batcheller, A.M. & Kaye, W. CPR training without an instructor: development and evaluation of a video self-instructional system for effective performance of cardiopulmonary resuscitation. *Resuscitation* 1997; **34**(3): 207–220.

44. Todd, K.H., Braslow, A., Brennan, R.T. *et al.* Randomized, controlled trial of video self-instruction versus traditional CPR training. *Ann. Emerg. Med.* 1998; **31**(3): 364–369.

45. Todd, K.H., Heron, S.L., Thompson, M., Dennis, R., O'Connor, J. & Kellermann, A.L. Simple CPR: a randomized, controlled trial of video self-instructional cardiopulmonary resuscitation training in an African American church congregation. *Ann. Emerg. Med.* 1999; **34**(6): 730–737.

46. Batcheller, A.M., Brennan, R.T., Braslow, A., Urrutia, A. & Kaye, W. Cardiopulmonary resuscitation performance of subjects over forty is better following half-hour video self-instruction compared to traditional four-hour classroom training. *Resuscitation* 2000; **43**(2): 101–110.

47. Brennan, R. *A Question of Life and Death: An Investigation of CPR Instruction Using Hierarchical Linear Modeling.* Harvard University: Cambridge, MA, 1989.

48. Lester, C., Donnelly, P. & Assar, D. Community life support training: does it attract the right people? *Public Health* 1997; **111**(5): 293–296.

49. Eisenburger, P. & Safar, P. Life supporting first aid training of the public – review and recommendations. *Resuscitation* 1999; **41**(1): 3–18.

50. Eisenberg, M., Damon, S., Mandel, L. *et al.* CPR instruction by videotape: results of a community project. *Ann. Emerg. Med.* 1995; **25**(2): 198–202.

51. Capone, P.L., Lane, J.C., Kerr, C.S. & Safar, P. Life supporting first aid (LSFA) teaching to Brazilians by television spots. *Resuscitation* 2000; **47**(3): 259–265.

52. Monsieurs, K., Vogels, C., Bossaert, L. *et al.* Learning effect of a novel interactive basic life support CD: the JUST system. *Resuscitation* 2004; **62**(2): 159–165.

53. Doherty, A., Damon, S., Hein, K. & Cummins, R.O. Evaluation of CPR prompt and home learning system for teaching CPR to lay rescuers. *Circulation* 1998; **98**(Suppl I): I–410.

54. Messmer, P., Meehan, R., Gilliam, N., White, S. & Donaldson, P. Teaching infant CPR to mothers of cocaine-positive infants. *Journal of continuing education in nursing*, 1993; **24**(5): 217–220.

55. Chamberlain, D. & Hazinski, M. Education in resuscitation. *Resuscitation* 2003; **59**(1): 11–43.

56. Morgan, C.L., Donnelly, P.D., Lester, C.A. & Assar, D.H. Effectiveness of the BBC's 999 training roadshows on cardiopulmonary resuscitation: video performance of cohort of unforewarned participants at home six months afterwards. *Br. Med. J.* 1996; **313**(7062): 912–916.

57. Brennan, R. & Braslow, A. Skill mastery in cardiopulmonary resuscitation training classes. *Am. J. Emerg. Med.* 1995; **13**: 505–508.

58. Donnelly, P., Assar, D. & Lester, C. A comparison of manikin CPR performance by lay persons trained in three variations of basic life support guidelines. *Resuscitation* 2000; **45**(3): 195–199.

59. Berden, H.J., Bierens, J.J., Willems, F.F., Hendrick, J.M., Pijls, N.H. & Knape, J.T. Resuscitation skills of lay public after recent training. *Ann. Emerg. Med.* 1994; **23**(5): 1003–1008.

60. Lester, C.A., Donnelly, P.D. & Assar, D. Lay CPR trainees: retraining, confidence and willingness to attempt resuscitation 4 years after training. *Resuscitation* 2000; **45**(2): 77–82.

61. Caffrey, S. Feasibility of public access to defibrillation. *Curr. Opin. Crit. Care* 2002; **8**(3): 195–198.

62. Bunch, T.J., White, R.D., Gersh, B.J., Shen, W.K., Hammill, S.C. & Packer, D.L. Outcomes and in-hospital treatment of out-of-hospital cardiac arrest patients resuscitated from ventricular

63. fibrillation by early defibrillation. *Mayo Clin. Proc.* 2004; **79**(5): 613–619.

63. White, R.D., Bunch, T.J. & Hankins, D.G. Evolution of a community-wide early defibrillation programme experience over 13 years using police/fire personnel and paramedics as responders. *Resuscitation* 2005; **65**(3): 279–283.

64. Valenzuela, T.D., Roe, D.J., Nichol, G., Clark, L.L., Spaite, D.W. & Hardman, R.G. Outcomes of rapid defibrillation by security officers after cardiac arrest in casinos. *N. Engl. J. Med.* 2000; **343**(17): 1206–1209.

65. Goucke, C.R. & Dobb, G.J. Cardiopulmonary resuscitation skills of hospital medical and nursing staff members. *Med. J. Aust.* 1986; **145**(10): 496–497.

66. Wynne, G., Marteau, T.M., Johnston, M., Whiteley, C.A. & Evans, T.R. Inability of trained nurses to perform basic life support. *Br. Med. J. (Clin. Res. Ed.)*, 1987; **294**(6581): 1198–1199.

67. Flint, L.S., Jr., Billi, J.E., Kelly, K., Mandel, L., Newell, L. & Stapleton, E.R. Education in adult basic life support training programs. *Ann. Emerg. Med.* 1993; **22**(pt 2)(2): 468–474.

68. Jansen, J.J., Berden, H.J., van der Vleuten, C.P., Grol, R.P., Rethans, J. & Verhoeff, C.P. Evaluation of cardiopulmonary resuscitation skills of general practitioners using different scoring methods. *Resuscitation* 1997; **34**(1): 35–41.

69. David, J. & Prior-Willeard, P. Resuscitation skills of MRCP candidates. *Br. Med. J. (Clin. Res. Ed.)*, 1993; **306**: 1578–1579.

70. Chin, D., Morphet, J., Coady, E. & Davidson, C. Assessment of cardiopulmonary resuscitation in the membership examination of the Royal College of Physicians. *J. Roy. Coll. Phys. Lond.* 1997; **31**: 198–201.

71. Nyman, J. & Sihvonen, M. Cardiopulmonary resuscitation skills in nurses and nursing students. *Resuscitation* 2000; **47**(2): 179–184.

72. Ragavan, S., Schneider, H. & Kloeck, W.G.J. Basic resuscitation – knowledge and skills of full-time medical practitioners at public hospitals in Northern Province. *S. Afr. Med. J.* 2000; **90**(5I): 504–508.

73. Hollis, S., Gillespie, N. An audit of basic life support skills amongst general practitioner principals: is there a need for regular training? *Resuscitation* 2000; **44**(3): 171–175.

74. Wik, L., Kramer-Johansen, J., Myklebust, H. *et al.* Quality of cardiopulmonary resuscitation during out-of-hospital cardiac arrest. *J. Am. Med. Assoc.* 2005; **293**(3): 299–304.

75. Kaye, W., Rallis, S.F., Mancini, M.E. *et al.* The problem of poor retention of cardiopulmonary resuscitation skills may lie with the instructor, not the learner or the curriculum. *Resuscitation* 1991; **21**(1): 67–87.

76. Cummins, R.O. & Hazinski, M.F. Cardiopulmonary resuscitation techniques and instruction: when does evidence justify revision? *Ann. Emerg. Med.* 1999; **34**(6): 780–784.

77. Whyte, S.D. & Wyllie, J.P. Paediatric basic life support: a practical assessment. *Resuscitation* 1999; **41**(2): 153–157.

78. Wik, L., Brennan, R. & Braslow, A. A peer training model for basic cardiac life-support. *Resuscitation* 1995; **29**(2): 119–128.

79. Berden, H.J., Willems, F.F., Hendrick, J.M., Pijls, N.H. & Knape, J.T. How frequently should basic cardiopulmonary resuscita-

tion training be repeated to maintain adequate skills? *Br. Med. J.* 1993; **306**(6892): 1576–1577.

80. Anthonypillai, F. Retention of advanced cardiopulmonary resuscitation knowledge by intensive care trained nurses. *Inten. Crit. Care Nurs.* 1992; **8**(3): 180–184.

81. Billi, J.E. & Membrino, G.E. Education in adult advanced cardiac life support training programs: changing the paradigm. Members of the Advanced Cardiac Life Support Education Panel. *Ann. Emerg. Med.* 1993; **22**(2 Pt 2): 475–483.

82. Young, R. & King, L. An evaluation of knowledge and skill retention following an in-house advanced life support course. *Nurs. Crit. Care* 2000; **5**(1): 7–14.

83. Gausche-Hill, M. Pediatric continuing education for out-of-hospital providers: is it time to mandate review of pediatric knowledge and skills? *Ann. Emerg. Med.* 2000; **36**(1): 72–74.

84. Su, E., Schmidt, T.A., Mann, N.C. & Zechnich, A.D. A randomized controlled trial to assess decay in acquired knowledge among paramedics completing a pediatric resuscitation course. *Acad. Emerg. Med.* 2000; 7(7): 779–786.

85. Azcona, L.A., Gutierrez, G.E., Fernandez, C.J., Natera, O.M., Ruiz-Speare, O. & Ali, J. Attrition of advanced trauma life support (ATLS) skills among ATLS instructors and providers in Mexico. *J Am. Coll. Surg.* 2002; **195**(3): 372–377.

86. Sanders, A.B., Berg, R.A., Burress, M., Genova, R.T., Kern, K.B. & Ewy, G.A. The efficacy of an ACLS training program for resuscitation from cardiac arrest in a rural community. *Ann. Emerg. Med.* 1994; **23**(1): 56–59.

87. Kurrek, M.M., Devitt, J.H. & Cohen, M. Cardiac arrest in the OR: how are our ACLS skills? *Can. J. Anaesth.* 1998; **45**(2): 130–132.

88. Tunstall-Pedoe, H., Bailey, L., Chamberlain, D.A., Marsden, A.K., Ward, M.E. & Zideman, D.A. Survey of 3765 cardiopulmonary resuscitations in British hospitals (the BRESUS Study): methods and overall results. *Br. Med. J.* 1992; **304**(6838): 1347–1351.

89. Gwinnutt, C.L., Columb, M. & Harris, R. Outcome after cardiac arrest in adults in UK hospitals: effect of the 1997 guidelines. *Resuscitation* 2000; **47**(2): 125–135.

90. Nolan, J. Advanced life support training. *Resuscitation* 2001; **50**(1): 9–11.

91. Chopra, V., Gesink, B.J., de Jong, J., Bovill, J.G., Spierdijk, J. & Brand, R. Does training on an anaesthesia simulator lead to improvement in performance? *Br. J. Anaesth.* 1994; **73**(3): 293–297.

92. Devitt, J.H., Kurrek, M.M., Cohen, M.M. *et al.* Testing internal consistency and construct validity during evaluation of performance in a patient simulator. *Anesth. Analg.* 1998; **86**(6): 1160–1164.

93. Small, S.D., Wuerz, R.C., Simon, R., Shapiro, N., Conn, A. & Setnik, G. Demonstration of high-fidelity simulation team training for emergency medicine. *Acad. Emerg. Med.* 1999; **6**(4): 312–323.

94. Reznek, M., Harter, P. & Krummel, T. Virtual reality and simulation: training the future emergency physician. *Acad. Emerg. Med.* 2002; **9**(1): 78–87.

95. Statistics of the Resuscitation Council of Southern Africa. 2005: Personal communication.

96. Abrahamson, S., Denson, J.S. & Wolf, R.M. Effectiveness of a simulator in training anesthesiology residents. *J. Med. Educ.* 1969; **44**(6): 515–519.

97. Euliano, T. & Good, M.L. Simulator training in anesthesia growing rapidly; LORAL model born in Florida. *J. Clin. Monit.* 1997; **13**(1): 53–57.

98. Gaba, D.M. & DeAnda, A. A comprehensive anesthesia simulation environment: re-creating the operating room for research and training. *Anesthesiology* 1988; **69**(3): 387–394.

99. Rettedal, A., Freier, S., Ragna, K. & Petter, L. PatSim – simulator for practising anesthesia and intensive care. Development and observations. *Int. J. Clin. Monit. Comp.* 1996; **13**(3): 147–52.

100. Lippert, A., Østergaard, H., White, J., Skagen, K. & Østergaard, D. The knowledge and performance of the cardiopulmonary resuscitation team. In *ASA Annual Meeting Anesthesiology 2000.* San Franscico, USA, 2000.

101. Christensen, U.J., Andersen, S.F., Jensen, P.F., Jacobsen, J. & Ørding H. The Sophus Anaesthesia Simulator v. 2.0. *Int. J. Clin. Monit. Comput.* 1997; **14**: 11–16.

102. Brennan, R.T., Braslow, A., Batcheller, A.M. & Kaye, W. A reliable and valid method for evaluating cardiopulmonary resuscitation training outcomes. *Resuscitation* 1996; **32**(2): 85–93.

103. Quiney, N.F., Gardner, J. & Brampton, W. Resuscitation skills amongst anaesthetists. *Resuscitation* 1995; **29**(3): 215–218.

104. Marsch, S. Team oriented medical simulation. In Henson, L. & Lee, A., eds. *Simulators in Anesthesiology Education.* Plenum Press: New York, 1998.

105. Holzman, R.S., Cooper, J.B., Gaba, D.M., Philip, J.H., Small, S.D. & Feinstein, D. Anesthesia crisis resource management: real-life simulation training in operating room crises. *J. Clin. Anesth.* 1995; **7**(8): 675–687.

106. Howard, S.K., Gaba, D.M., Fish, K.J., Yang, G. & Sarnquist, F.H. Anesthesia crisis resource management training: teaching anesthesiologists to handle critical incidents. *Aviat. Space Environ. Med.* 1992; **63**(9): 763–770.

107. Christensen, U.J., Heffernan, D., Andersen, S.F. & Jensen, P.F. ResusSim 98 – a PC advanced life support trainer. *Resuscitation* 1998; **39**(1–2): 81–4.

108. Christensen, U., Heffernan, D. & Barach, P. Microsimulators in medical education: an overview. *Simulation Gaming* 2001; **32**: 250–262.

109. Ursino, M., Tasto, J.L., Nguyen, B.H., Cunningham, R. & Merril, G.L. CathSim: an intravascular catheterization simulator on a PC. *Stud. Health Technol. Inform.* 1999; **62**: 360–366.

110. Bro-Nielsen, M., Tasto, J.L., Cunningham, R. & Merril, G.L. PreOp endoscopic simulator: a PC-based immersive training system for bronchoscopy. *Stud. Health Technol. Inform.* 1999; **62**: 76–82.

111. Jensen, P. Development of a methodology for cognitive analysis of critical incidents in anesthesia – a Ph.D. thesis. 1997, University of Copenhagen: Copenhagen.

112. Gaba, D.M. Anaesthesiology as a model for patient safety in health care. *Br. Med. J.* 2000; **320**(7237): 785–788.

113. Dick, W., Carey, L. & Carey, J. The systematic design of instruction. 5th edn. New York: Longman, 2001.

114. Gagné, R., Briggs, L. & Wager, W. *Principles of Instructional Design.* 4th edn. Fort Worth: Harcourt Brace Jovanovich College Publishers, 1992.

115. Keirns, J. *Designs for Self-Instruction: Principles, Processes.* San Jose, Calif: VIP Graphics, 1998.

116. Kemp, J. & Smellie, D. Planning, producing, and using instructional technologies. 7th ed. ed. 1994, New York, NY: HarperCollins College Publishers.

117. Reiser, R. & Dick, W. *Instructional Planning: A guide for Teachers.* 2nd edn. Boston: Allyn and Bacon, 1996.

71

Consensus development in resuscitation: the growing movement towards international emergency cardiovascular care guidelines

Jerry P. Nolan[1], Douglas Chamberlain[2], William H. Montgomery[3] and Vinay M. Nadkarni[4]

[1] Department of Anaesthesia and Intensive Care Medicine, Royal United Hospital, Bath BA1 3NG, UK
[2] Department of Resuscitation Medicine, School of Medicine, Cardiff University, Wales, UK
[3] Department of Anesthesiology, Straub Clinic and Hospital, University of Hawaii School of Medicine, Honolulu, Hawaii, USA
[4] Departments of Anesthesia, Critical Care and Pediatrics, University of Pennsylvania School of Medicine, Philadelphia, Pennsylvania, USA

Introduction

Clinical guidelines are defined by the Institute of Medicine in the United States as "systematically developed statements to assist practitioner and patient decisions about appropriate health care for specific clinical circumstances."[1] The main objective of guidelines is to improve the quality of care received by patients by closing the gap between what clinicians do and what scientific evidence supports. Guidelines provide a point of reference for auditing performance of clinicians or hospitals and may improve effectiveness and efficiency. The development of guidelines requires appropriate resources: expert clinicians, group process leaders, and financial support.[2] All these statements refer to guideline development in general, but they are particularly relevant to the development of resuscitation guidelines that have existed for at least 40 years. The steps involved in the process for developing evidence-based guidelines have been outlined by the Grades of Recommendation Assessment, Development and Evaluation (GRADE) Working Group (Table 71.1).[3]

This chapter will review the history of consensus development in resuscitation, the role of the International Liaison Committee on Resuscitation (ILCOR), the process involved in undertaking a systematic review of resuscitation science, and the writing of clinical guidelines based on a consensus of the science.

The history of international CPR consensus and guideline development

The modern approach to cardiopulmonary resuscitation (CPR) was described in the late 1950s and early 1960s.

Although this was undoubtedly the birth of CPR, it was immediately realized that the challenge was to spread the word and educate healthcare workers and laypeople throughout the world. This same challenge faces us today whenever CPR guidelines are modified and updated.

One of the earliest "consensus" decisions on CPR was to agree on the terminology for this new technique (extensive discussions on terminology in resuscitation continue today). The term "cardiopulmonary resuscitation" and the abbreviation "CPR" were proposed first by the American Heart Association (AHA) Ad Hoc Committee on Closed Chest Cardiac Resuscitation in February 1962.[4] Initially, after considerable debate and concern about the risks, the AHA recommended that only doctors should be trained in CPR. It was recommended for rescue groups in April 1962.

In 1966 the National Academy of Sciences' National Research Council convened an ad hoc conference on CPR. This was the first conference to review specifically the evidence and recommend standard CPR techniques; more than 30 national organizations were represented.[5] International awareness was enhanced in the following year, when an International Symposium on Emergency Resuscitation was held in Oslo, Norway; recommendations from this conference were published in 1968.[6] The American Heart Association sponsored subsequent conferences in 1973 and 1979.[7,8] Parallel efforts occurred internationally as other resuscitation organizations faced a growing demand for CPR training.[9,10] Inevitably, variations in resuscitation techniques and training methods began to emerge from individual countries and regions of the world.

Increasing awareness of international variations in resuscitation practices generated interest in the possibility of gathering international experts at a single location with the aim of achieving consensus in resuscitation tech-

Table 71.1. The GRADE Working Group sequence for developing guidelines[3]

First steps

1. Establishing the process, e.g., prioritizing problems, selecting a panel, declaring conflicts of interest, agreeing on group processes.

Preparatory steps

2. Systematic review – identify and critically appraise or prepare systematic reviews of the best available evidence for all important outcomes.

3. Prepare evidence profile for important outcomes – profiles are needed for each subpopulation or risk group, based on the results of systematic reviews, and should include a quality assessment and summary of findings.

Grading quality of evidence and strength of recommendations

4. Quality of evidence for each outcome – judged on information summarized in the evidence profile and based on predefined criteria.

5. Relative importance of outcomes – only important outcomes should be included in the evidence profiles.

6. Overall quality of evidence – judged across outcomes based on the lowest quality of evidence for any of the critical outcomes.

7. Balance of benefits and harms – classified as net benefits, trade-offs, uncertain trade-offs, or no net benefits based on the important health benefits and harms.

8. Balance of net benefits and costs – are incremental benefits worth the costs? Because resources are always limited, it is important to consider costs (resource utilization) when making a recommendation.

9. Strength of recommendation – recommendations should be formulated to reflect their strength – that is, the extent to which one can be confident that adherence will do more good than harm.

Subsequent steps

10. Implementation and evaluation, e.g., using effective implementation strategies that address barriers to change, evaluation of implementation, and keeping up to date.

niques. With this in mind, in 1985, the AHA invited resuscitation leaders from many countries to observe its review of standards and guidelines for CPR and emergency cardiovascular care (ECC).[11] By all accounts, the international guests played a very active role in the discussions![10]

In June 1990, representatives from the AHA, European Resuscitation Council (ERC), Heart and Stroke Foundation of Canada (HSFC), and the Australian Resuscitation Council (ARC) attended a meeting, hosted by the Laerdal Foundation, at Utstein Abbey on the island of Mosteroy, Norway. The purpose of this meeting was to discuss the problems of resuscitation nomenclature and the lack of standardized terminology in reports relating to adult out-of-hospital cardiac arrest. This was the first major collaborative venture involving resuscitation councils from around the world. A follow-up meeting was held in December 1990 in Surrey, England, where the decision was made to adopt the term "Utstein-style" for the uniform reporting of data from out-of-hospital cardiac arrests.[12] Many other 'Utstein-style' international consensus statements have been published over the last 15 years, including the uniform reporting of pediatric advanced life support,[13] laboratory CPR research,[14] in-hospital resuscitation,[15] neonatal life support,[16] drowning,[17] and CPR registers.[18]

The Fifth National Conference on CPR and ECC was held in Dallas, Texas, USA in 1992. More than 40% of the participants were from outside the United States, representing 25 countries and 53 international organizations.[19,20] Three international issues were addressed: the desirability of international support for countries to develop effective ECC; the creation of a permanent infrastructure for international cooperation; the desirability of common international guidelines and an international conference on CPR and ECC. An international CPR and ECC panel discussion, cochaired by Richard Cummins and Douglas Chamberlain, endorsed the need for international cooperation. This would have several advantages: the world's leading experts would achieve constructive communication and cooperation; advice for guidelines would be less likely to be dominated by tradition or peer pressure; guidelines generated in this way would be accepted widely within existing organizations; similar or identical guidelines would be produced by different groups and the potential would exist for eventual universal guidelines.

The International Liaison Committee on Resuscitation (ILCOR)

The first international conference held by the ERC took place in Brighton, England in 1992. At the end of the conference, representatives from the guidelines-producing organizations (AHA, ERC, HSFC, ARC, and the Resuscitation Council of Southern Africa (RCSA)) held the first meeting of the International Liaison Committee.[20] The founding cochairs of this organization were Douglas Chamberlain and Richard Cummins. At its second meeting, held in 1993 in Vienna, Austria, the International Liaison Committee adopted a formal mission statement:

To provide a consensus mechanism by which the international science and knowledge relevant to emergency cardiac care can be identified and reviewed. This consensus mechanism will be used to provide consistent international guidelines on emergency cardiac care for Basic Life Support (BLS), Paediatric Life Support (PLS) and Advanced Life Support (ALS). While the major focus will be upon treatment guidelines, the steering committee will also address the effectiveness of educational and training approaches and topics related to the organisation and implementation of emergency cardiac care. The Committee will also encourage coordination of dates for guidelines development and conferences by various national resuscitation councils. These international guidelines will aim for a commonality supported by science for BLS, ALS and PLS.

Formal BLS, ALS, and PLS working groups were established and tasked with reviewing scientific data in their respective area of expertise. The name "International Liaison Committee on Resuscitation (ILCOR)" was suggested by Walter Kloeck, the chairman of RCSA, and adopted formally in 1996.[20] The founding organizations were joined in 1997 by the Consejo Latino-Americano de Resuscitación (which now forms part of the Inter-American Heart Foundation) and in 1998 by the New Zealand Resuscitation Council (joining with the ARC to form the Australia and New Zealand Committee on Resuscitation (ANZCOR)). Since 1999, representatives from Japan, China, Taiwan, Thailand, Malaysia, and Singapore have joined some ILCOR meetings as observers. In 2006, the Resuscitation Council of Asia, which includes representatives from Japan, Korea, Singapore and Taiwan, formally joined ILCOR.

The mission statement of ILCOR was updated in 2005:

The International Liaison Committee on Resuscitation (ILCOR) will provide a mechanism by which the international science and knowledge relevant to cardiopulmonary resuscitation (CPR) and emergency cardiovascular care (ECC) is identified and reviewed. ILCOR will periodically develop and publish a consensus on resuscitation science. When possible, ILCOR will publish treatment recommendations applicable to all member organisations. This consensus mechanism may be used by member organisations to provide consistent guidelines on resuscitation. ILCOR will encourage co-ordination of guideline development and publication by its member organisations. While the major focus will be on evaluation of cardiopulmonary resuscitation and emergency cardiovascular care science, ILCOR will also address the effectiveness of education and training, and approaches to the organisation and implementation of emergency cardiovascular care.

The activities undertaken by ILCOR to achieve the objectives set out in its mission statement are listed in Table 71.2.

By 2005, ILCOR had convened 22 official meetings culminating in the 2005 International Consensus Conference on Cardiopulmonary Resuscitation and Emergency Cardiovascular Care Science with Treatment Recommendations, held in Dallas, Texas.[20,21] With the benefit of international cooperation, ILCOR has assessed systematically the evidence supporting resuscitation standards and guidelines. Initially, ILCOR experts identified numerous

Table 71.2. The activities undertaken by the International Liaison Committee on Resuscitation

- Provide a forum for discussion and for co-ordination of cardiopulmonary and cerebral resuscitation worldwide.
- Facilitate a process for collecting, reviewing and sharing international scientific data on resuscitation.
- Provide a channel for scientific review and guidance to enable a process of international consensus to be achieved.
- Produce appropriate statements on specific issues related to resuscitation that reflect international consensus.
- Foster scientific research in areas of resuscitation where there is a lack of data or where there is controversy.
- Facilitate a process for dissemination of information on training and education in resuscitation.

national differences in the practices of BLS, ALS, and pediatric and newborn resuscitation. ILCOR has published 18 scientific advisory statements with the goal of explaining, eliminating, or reducing these international variations while endorsing mainly evidence-based resuscitation guidelines.[20,22–29]

The Guidelines 2000 Conference and the goal of universal CPR and ECC guidelines

Early ILCOR meetings were driven by the belief that evaluation of international science by a common group of experts should lead to universal evidence-based resuscitation guidelines and practices. This view was particularly strong leading up to the Guidelines 2000 Conference, the world's first international conference assembled to produce international resuscitation guidelines.[30,31] This was the first major conference to be held under the auspices of ILCOR and it incorporated a sophisticated process for gathering and assessing evidence; this process evolved further in 2005 (see below).[32] Although the output from the Guidelines 2000 Conference was published in both *Circulation*[33] and *Resuscitation*[30] and was subtitled "An International Consensus on Science," the ERC subsequently published its own resuscitation guidelines.[34–39] These included some differences from the "International Guidelines" – the most significant being simpler algorithms and minor differences in recommendations for drug therapy.

What were the reasons for failing to achieve truly universal guidelines? Guidelines cannot be based on data alone – judgment is unavoidable.[40] If our clinical practice was supported entirely by indisputable level 1 evidence, there would be considerably less scope for differences among councils and regions in the translation of science into guidelines. In reality, much resuscitation practice is supported by lower level evidence or conflicting evidence. This situation can easily be summarized in a consensus on science statement by stating simply that there is no clear evidence for or against a specific therapy or intervention. Nevertheless, clinical guidelines have to be simple and relatively dogmatic – one has to commit to a treatment or technique in preference to another. It will be difficult to reach consensus on the extent to which evidence obtained from selected populations of patients or animal studies can be extrapolated to the general population.[41] The specific endpoint of a given resuscitation intervention that is most relevant (e.g., return of spontaneous circulation, survival to hospital admission, survival to hospital discharge, intact neurological survival, quality of life) will continue to be controversial. By the time educational, cultural, financial, and organizational factors, and differences in drug availability are taken into account, despite consensus on the science, differences in guidelines from one country to another are inevitable.[42] Many problems in resuscitation require local modifications and solutions. The common goals of the resuscitation community are ultimately reducing rates of morbidity and mortality from cardiac arrest.

The Evidence Evaluation Process for the 2005 International Consensus on Cardiopulmonary Resuscitation and Emergency Cardiovascular Care Science

Evidence-based medicine is now a fundamental component of clinical practice and its principles are well established.[43] The evidence evaluation process used in preparation for the 2005 International Consensus on CPR and ECC Science (C2005) has been described in detail by Morley and Zaritsky, who took the lead in ensuring a high-quality review of the evidence supporting resuscitation.[32] Clinical research in resuscitation is challenging – cardiac arrest is generally an unpredictable event and there are increasing ethical problems associated with enrolling unconscious patients in trials.[44] Inevitably, this means that there are relatively few controlled human studies and in many cases we must rely on animal and manikin studies.

In 2003 and 2004, international experts (worksheet reviewers) were assigned questions to evaluate. With use of a hybrid of a nominal group technique and Delphi survey,[42] the questions for systematic review were refined by each of six ILCOR specialty task forces (BLS, ALS, acute coronary syndromes, PLS, Neonatal Life Support, and interdisciplinary) and from the ILCOR member resuscitation councils and their training networks. Use of the Cochrane

Collaboration PICO system for structuring the question for systematic review was encouraged but was not adopted universally, partly because it applies only to clinical studies. The PICO system structures the question into four components: the patient, population, or problem (P); the intervention or independent variable (I); the comparison (C); and the independent variables or outcome(s) of interest (O).[45] Each structured, evidence-based review was entered onto a standardized worksheet developed specifically for the C2005 Conference (Appendix 1). Two worksheet experts (Morley and Zaritsky) reviewed all submitted worksheets. The steps involved in preparing these worksheets are outlined below.[32]

Step 1. Gathering and selection of the evidence

Reviewers documented their search strategies to ensure reproducibility of the search. The minimum electronic databases to be searched included the Cochrane database for systematic reviews and the Central Register of Controlled Trials [http://www.cochrane.org/], MEDLINE [http://www.ncbi.nlm.nih.gov/PubMed/], EMBASE (www.embase.com), and the EndNote (www.endnote.com) reference library collated by the AHA.

Step 2. Assessing the quality of the evidence

Reviewers determined the level of evidence of relevant studies and assessed their quality. The quality of evidence indicates the extent to which one can be confident that an estimate of effect is correct.[3] There are many established systems for grading the quality of evidence.[3,46] The levels of evidence used for the 2005 consensus process were modified from those used in 2000 (Table 71.3).[30,33] Using predefined criteria, the reviewers assessed the quality of research design and methods and allocated each study to one of five categories: excellent, good, fair, poor, or unsatisfactory. Studies graded as poor or unsatisfactory were excluded from further analysis.

Step 3. Class of recommendation

The strength of recommendation indicates the extent to which one can be confident that adherence to a recommendation will do more good than harm.[3] Unfortunately, there are many systems for grading evidence-based guidelines. The class of recommendation system used in the 2005 AHA Guidelines for CPR and ECC is outlined in Table 71.4.[47] Many of the experts outside the United States did not want to use these classes of recommendation and they

Table 71.3. Levels of evidence used in the C2005 process[52]

Evidence	Definition
Level 1	Randomized clinical trials or meta-analyses of multiple clinical trials with substantial treatment effects
Level 2	Randomized clinical trials with smaller or less significant treatment effects
Level 3	Prospective, controlled, non-randomized cohort studies
Level 4	Historic, non-randomized cohort or case-control studies
Level 5	Case series; patients compiled in serial fashion, control group lacking
Level 6	Animal studies or mechanical model studies
Level 7	Extrapolations from existing data collected for other purposes, theoretical analyses
Level 8	Rational conjecture (common sense); common practices accepted before evidence-based guidelines

do not appear in the ILCOR 2005 Consensus on CPR and ECC Science publication or in the ERC guidelines.[48]

Step 4. Management of conflict of interest

Experts in resuscitation science establish their expertise by undertaking and publishing research and participating in scientific conferences. This work creates potential financial and intellectual conflicts of interest (COI) for the expert.[49,50] Intellectual conflicts of interest include intellectual collaboration or intellectual investment in personal ideas, and long-term research agendas in which investigators have invested a substantial time. A robust COI policy was developed to ensure full disclosure of potential conflicts and to protect the objectivity and credibility of the evidence evaluation and consensus development process.[51]

Step 5. Summary of the science

Worksheet reviewers summarized the science, providing a detailed discussion of the evidence, including the outcomes evaluated and the strengths and limitations of the data.

Consensus on science statements and treatment recommendations were drafted using standardized templates.

Step 6. References

Worksheet reviewers provided an EndNote database file containing the references that were used and these were added to the master reference library collated by the AHA.

Step 7. Posting on the Internet

In December 2004 the completed worksheets, blinded to authorship, were posted on an Internet site (www.C2005.org) that could be accessed by the public for further review and feedback before the 2005 Consensus Conference in Dallas. All individuals making responses or suggestions were required to submit potential or perceived conflict of interest statements.

The 2005 Consensus Conference

A total of 281 experts completed 403 worksheets on 276 topics; 380 people from 18 countries attended the 2005 Consensus Conference (C2005) in January 2005. All C2005 participants received a copy of the worksheets on CD-ROM. Internet access was available to all conference participants during the conference to facilitate real-time verification of the literature.[52] Expert reviewers presented topics in plenary, concurrent, and poster conference sessions. Presenters and participants then debated the evidence, conclusions, and draft summary statements. Each day the most controversial topics from the previous day were presented and debated in one or more additional

Table 71.4. The American Heart Association classes of recommendation[47]

Class 1 Benefit >>> risk	Class IIa Benefit >> risk	Class IIb Benefit ≥ risk	Class III Risk ≥ benefit
Procedure/treatment or diagnostic test/ assessment should be performed/ administered.	It is reasonable to perform procedure/ administer treatment or perform diagnostic test/ assessment.	Procedure/treatment or diagnostic test/ assessment may be considered.	Procedure/treatment or diagnostic test/ assessment should not be performed/ administered. It is not helpful and may be harmful.

sessions. Science statements were drafted to summarize the experts' interpretation of all the relevant data on a specific topic. Draft treatment recommendations were added if a consensus was reached. The 2005 International Consensus on CPR and ECC Science with Treatment Recommendations (CoSTR) was published simultaneously in Resuscitation[21] and Circulation.[53] This consensus on science has provided the evidence from which the latest resuscitation guidelines were derived.

From science to guidelines

The resuscitation organizations forming ILCOR have published individual resuscitation guidelines that are consistent with the science in the 2005 Consensus Conference document. These guidelines are broadly similar, but consideration of geographic, economic, and system differences in practice, and the availability of medical devices and drugs, has inevitably forced some differences. All ILCOR member organizations strive to minimize these international differences in resuscitation practice and to optimize the effectiveness of instructional methods, teaching aids, and training networks.

The recommendations of the 2005 Consensus Conference confirmed the safety, feasibility, and efficacy of some current approaches, acknowledged that other approaches were not optimal, and introduced new treatments resulting from evidence-based evaluation. Whenever guidelines are updated, healthcare providers and laypeople must be assured that it takes time for these changes to permeate down to frontline clinical practice and that, in the meantime, their existing techniques are reasonable and safe. The introduction to the 2005 Consensus Conference document included the statement: "New and revised treatment recommendations do not imply that clinical care that involves the use of previously published guidelines is unsafe."[52] Members of ILCOR considered these new recommendations to be the most effective and easily learned interventions that could be supported by existing knowledge, research, and experience, including the emerging science of ECC education. Treatment changes, such as the compression:ventilation ratio of 30:2 and the single- versus three-shock defibrillation strategy, which were adopted to minimize interruptions to compressions, were often based upon feasibility and teachability, and not on randomized controlled trials. Implications for education and retention were considered carefully when developing the final treatment recommendations.

The 2005 Universal Algorithm

The 2005 Consensus Conference document includes an updated ILCOR Universal Cardiac Arrest Algorithm (Fig. 71.1), which incorporates many of the new treatment recommendations. The algorithm is applicable to attempted resuscitation of infant, child, and adult victims of cardiac arrest (excluding newborns). Every effort was made to keep the algorithm simple yet widely applicable. Resuscitation organizations subsequently based their guidelines on the ILCOR algorithm, although a comparison of the ERC (Fig. 71.2) and AHA ALS (Fig. 71.3) algorithms reveals differences in style.

Implementing guidelines

Failure to translate research findings into daily practice is a well recognized problem.[54] The development of good guidelines does not ensure that they will be adopted in clinical practice and passive methods of disseminating and implementing guidelines (e.g., publication in journals) are unlikely to change professional behavior.[55] Resuscitation organizations have a primary responsibility for disseminating and implementing resuscitation guidelines; this will require significant resources. Summary booklets to supplement the full guidelines will be helpful for busy healthcare personnel. Full use of the Internet to make guidelines freely and easily downloadable is essential: the ERC and the AHA guidelines can be downloaded at www.erc.edu and http://circ.ahajournals.org/content/vol112/24_suppl/, respectively. Resuscitation guidelines can be disseminated effectively through national scientific meetings and by local meetings held in hospitals and in the community. Resuscitation training materials should be updated as rapidly as possible to reflect the new guidelines. The updating of training materials also requires considerable resources and often involves many of the individuals who have been involved in the guideline process. Standardized courses such as the ERC Advanced Life Support Course and the AHA Advanced Cardiac Life Support Course play a crucial role in disseminating resuscitation guidelines. Evaluation and verification of the implementation of new guidelines is achieved through audit.

The future for consensus development in resuscitation

The science of resuscitation is evolving rapidly. It would not be in the best interests of patients if resuscitation

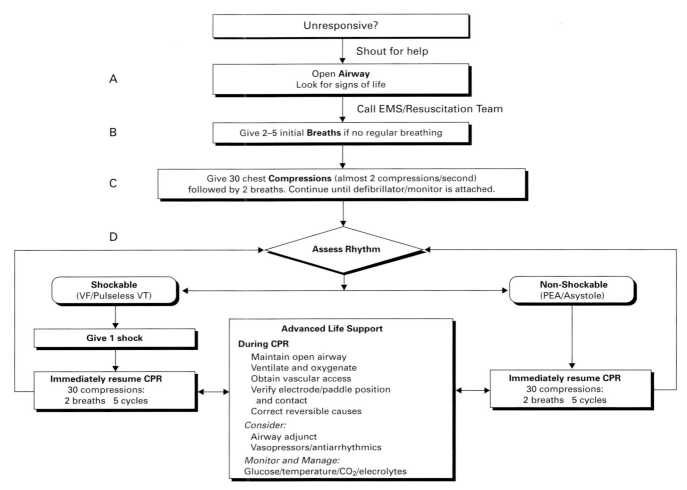

Fig. 71.1. The 2005 ILCOR Universal Algorithm.

experts were to wait five or more years to inform healthcare professionals of therapeutic advances in this field. Some groups have advocated reviewing guidelines as frequently as every two years.[42] Frequent changes in recommendations that do not have a major impact on outcome might undermine the process, however, because teaching and learning new guidelines takes time and resources. New science must be reviewed continually; if major new research evidence is published, groups such as ILCOR should publish interim consensus advisory statements to update treatment guidelines. Large multicentre registries that use Utstein-style consensus definitions of the process of care and outcomes following resuscitation will track the dissemination of new techniques and interventions from science to guidelines and to practice, and lead to further refinements in the guidelines.[18,56,57] Ideally, important interventions and practices could be taught and reviewed rapidly, giving feedback on quality

of performance for all healthcare providers. The interface between resuscitation research and continuous quality improvement (audit) is becoming more blurred. Innovative strategies to improve the process and outcomes of evidence evaluation and resuscitation are being incorporated into the planning for a consensus conference on resuscitation in 2010. Whether this 2010 consensus conference will result in truly universal guidelines has yet to be determined.

Summary

International consensus development in resuscitation has evolved over the last 40 years. Major international reviews of resuscitation science occur every 5 years under the auspices of ILCOR; the result is that CPR guidelines around the world are now broadly similar. Standardized training materials and courses help to disseminate the guidelines and change the practice of healthcare professionals and first responders.

REFERENCES

1. Woolf, S.H., Grol, R., Hutchinson, A., Eccles, M. & Grimshaw, J. Clinical guidelines: potential benefits, limitations, and harms of clinical guidelines. *Br. Med. J.* 1999; **318**: 527–530.

2. Shekelle, P.G., Woolf, S.H., Eccles, M., Grimshaw, J. Clinical guidelines: developing guidelines. *Br. Med. J.* 1999; **318**: 593–596.

3. Atkins, D., Best, D., Briss, P.A. *et al.* Grading quality of evidence and strength of recommendations. *Br. Med. J.* 2004; **328**: 1490.

4. Eisenberg, M.S. The birth of CPR. In Eisenberg, M.S., ed. *Life in the Balance Emergency Medicine and the Quest to Reverse Sudden Death.* Oxford: Oxford University Press, 1997: 130–136.

5. Cardiopulmonary resuscitation: statement by the Ad Hoc Committee on Cardiopulmonary Resuscitation, of the Division of Medical Sciences, National Academy of Sciences, National Research Council. *J. Am. Med. Assoc.* 1966; **198**: 372–379.

6. Anonymous. Recommendations of the Second International Symposium on Emergency Resuscitation. *Acta Anaesthesiol. Scand.* 1968; **29**: 383–384.

7. Standards for cardiopulmonary resuscitation (CPR) and emergency cardiac care (ECC). *J. Am. Med. Assoc.* 1974; **227**(Suppl.): 833–868.

8. Standards and guidelines for cardiopulmonary resuscitation (CPR) and emergency cardiac care (ECC). *J. Am. Med. Assoc.* 1980; **244**: 453–509.

9. Chamberlain, D. Editorial introducing ERC Guidelines. *Resuscitation* 1992; **24**: 99–101.

10. Chamberlain, D., Cummins, R.O., Montgomery, W.H., Kloeck, W.G. & Nadkarni, V.M. International collaboration in resuscitation medicine. *Resuscitation* 2005; **67**: 163–165.

11. Anonymous. Standards and guidelines for Cardiopulmonary Resuscitation (CPR) and Emergency Cardiac Care (ECC). National Academy of Sciences – National Research Council. [erratum appears in *J. Am. Med. Assoc.* 1986 Oct 3; 256(13): 1727]. *J. Am. Med. Assoc.* 1986; **255**: 2905–2989.

12. Cummins, R.O., Chamberlain, D.A., Abramson, N.S. *et al.* Recommended guidelines for uniform reporting of data from out-of-hospital cardiac arrest: the Utstein style. A statement for health professionals from a task force of the American Heart Association, the European Resuscitation Council, the Heart and Stroke Foundation of Canada, and the Australian Resuscitation Council. *Circulation* 1991; **84**: 960–975.

13. Zaritsky, A., Nadkarni, V., Hazinski, M.F. *et al.* Recommended guidelines for uniform reporting of pediatric advanced life support: the Pediatric Utstein Style. A statement for healthcare professionals from a task force of the American Academy of Pediatrics, the American Heart Association, and the European Resuscitation Council. *Resuscitation* 1995; **30**: 95–115.

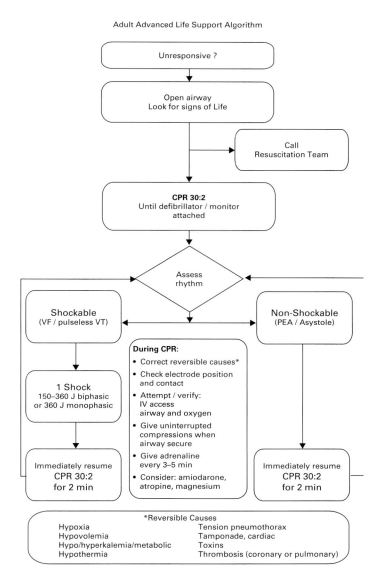

Adult Advanced Life Support Algorithm

Unresponsive ?

Open airway
Look for signs of Life

Call
Resuscitation Team

CPR 30:2
Until defibrillator / monitor attached

Assess rhythm

Shockable
(VF / pulseless VT)

Non-Shockable
(PEA / Asystole)

1 Shock
150–360 J biphasic
or 360 J monophasic

During CPR:
- Correct reversible causes*
- Check electrode position and contact
- Attempt / verify:
  IV access
  airway and oxygen
- Give uninterrupted compressions when airway secure
- Give adrenaline every 3–5 min
- Consider: amiodarone, atropine, magnesium

Immediately resume
CPR 30:2
for 2 min

Immediately resume
CPR 30:2
for 2 min

*Reversible Causes
Hypoxia   Tension pneumothorax
Hypovolemia   Tamponade, cardiac
Hypo/hyperkalemia/metabolic   Toxins
Hypothermia   Thrombosis (coronary or pulmonary)

Fig. 71.2. The 2005 European Resuscitation Council advanced life support algorithm.

14. Idris, A.H., Becker, L.B., Ornato, J.P. *et al.* Utstein-style guidelines for uniform reporting of laboratory CPR research. A statement for healthcare professionals from a Task Force of the American Heart Association, the American College of Emergency Physicians, the American College of Cardiology, the European Resuscitation Council, the Heart and Stroke Foundation of Canada, the Institute of Critical Care Medicine, the Safar Center for Resuscitation Research, and the Society for Academic Emergency Medicine. *Resuscitation* 1996; **33**: 69–84.

15. Cummins, R.O., Chamberlain, D., Hazinski, M.F. *et al.* Recommended guidelines for reviewing, reporting, and conducting research on in-hospital resuscitation: the in-hospital

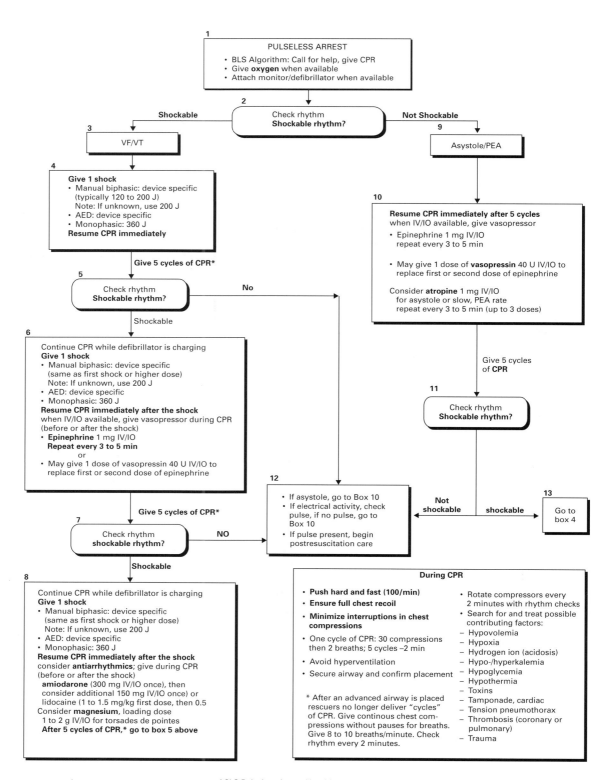

ACLS Pulseless Arrest Algorithm.

Fig. 71.3. The 2005 American Heart Association advanced cardiac life support algorithm.

'Utstein style'. A statement for healthcare professionals from the American Heart Association, the European Resuscitation Council, the Heart and Stroke Foundation of Canada, the Australian Resuscitation Council, and the Resuscitation Councils of Southern Africa. *Resuscitation* 1997; **34**: 151–183.

16. Kattwinkel, J., Niermeyer, S., Nadkarni, V. *et al.* Resuscitation of the newly born infant: an advisory statement from the Pediatric Working Group of the International Liaison Committee on Resuscitation. *Resuscitation* 1999; **40**: 71–88.

17. Idris, A.H., Berg, R.A., Bierens, J. *et al.* Recommended guidelines for uniform reporting of data from drowning: The "Utstein style". *Resuscitation* 2003; **59**: 45–57.

18. Jacobs, I., Nadkarni, V., Bahr, J. *et al.* Cardiac arrest and cardiopulmonary resuscitation outcome reports: update and simplification of the Utstein templates for resuscitation registries. A statement for healthcare professionals from a task force of the international liaison committee on resuscitation (American Heart Association, European Resuscitation Council, Australian Resuscitation Council, New Zealand Resuscitation Council, Heart and Stroke Foundation of Canada, InterAmerican Heart Foundation, Resuscitation Council of Southern Africa). *Resuscitation* 2004; **63**: 233–249.

19. Guidelines for cardiopulmonary resuscitation (CPR) and emergency cardiac care (ECC). *J. Am. Med. Assoc.* 1992; **286**: 2135–2302.

20. Chamberlain, D. The International Liaison Committee on Resuscitation (ILCOR)-Past and present Compiled by the Founding Members of the International Liaison Committee on Resuscitation. *Resuscitation* 2005; **67**: 157–161.

21. International Liaison Committee on Resuscitation. 2005 International Consensus on Cardiopulmonary Resuscitation and Emergency Cardiovascular Care Science with Treatment Recommendations. *Resuscitation* 2005; **67**: 157–341.

22. Handley, A.J., Becker, L.B., Allen, M., van Drenth, A., Kramer, E.B. & Montgomery, W.H. Single rescuer adult basic life support. An advisory statement from the Basic Life Support Working Group of the International Liaison Committee on Resuscitation (ILCOR). *Resuscitation* 1997; **34**: 101–108.

23. Kloeck, W., Cummins, R., Chamberlain, D. *et al.* The Universal ALS algorithm. An advisory statement by the Advanced Life Support Working Group of the International Liaison Committee on Resuscitation. *Resuscitation* 1997; **34**: 109–111.

24. Kloeck, W., Cummins, R.O., Chamberlain, D. *et al.* Early defibrillation: an advisory statement from the Advanced Life Support Working Group of the International Liaison Committee on Resuscitation. *Circulation* 1997; **95**: 2183–2184.

25. Nadkarni, V., Hazinski, M.F., Zideman, D. *et al.* Paediatric life support: an advisory statement by the Paediatric Life Support Working Group of the International Liaison Committee on Resuscitation. *Resuscitation* 1997; **34**: 115–127.

26. Kloeck, W., Cummins, R.O., Chamberlain, D. *et al.* Special resuscitation situations: an advisory statement from the International Liaison Committee on Resuscitation. *Circulation* 1997; **95**: 2196–2210.

27. Chamberlain, D.A. & Hazinski, M.F. Education in resuscitation. *Resuscitation* 2003; **59**: 11–43.

28. Nolan, J.P., Morley, P.T., Vanden Hoek, T.L. & Hickey, R.W. Therapeutic hypothermia after cardiac arrest. An advisory statement by the Advancement Life support Task Force of the International Liaison committee on Resuscitation. *Resuscitation* 2003; **57**: 231–235.

29. Samson, R., Berg, R. & Bingham, R. Pediatric Advanced Life Support Task Force ILCoR. Use of automated external defibrillators for children: an update. An advisory statement from the Pediatric Advanced Life Support Task Force, International Liaison Committee on Resuscitation. *Resuscitation* 2003; **57**: 237–243.

30. American Heart Association in collaboration with International Liaison Committee on Resuscitation. Guidelines for Cardiopulmonary Resuscitation and Emergency Cardiovascular Care – An International Consensus on Science. *Resuscitation* 2000; **46**: 3–430.

31. Proceedings of the Guidelines 2000 Conference for Cardiopulmonary Resuscitation and Emergency Cardiovascular Care: An International Consensus on Science. *Ann. Emerg. Med.* 2001; **37**: S1–S200.

32. Morley, P. & Zaritsky, A. The evidence evaluation process for the 2005 International Consensus on Cardiopulmonary Resuscitation and Emergency Cardiovascular Care Science With Treatment Recommendations. *Resuscitation* 2005; **67**: 167–170.

33. American Heart Association in collaboration with International Liaison Committee on Resuscitation. Guidelines 2000 for Cardiopulmonary Resuscitation and Emergency Cardiovascular Care. *Circulation* 2000; **102**(Suppl.): I1–I384.

34. de Latorre, F., Nolan, J., Robertson, C., Chamberlain, D. & Baskett, P. European Resuscitation Council Guidelines 2000 for Adult Advanced Life Support. A statement from the Advanced Life Support Working Group(1) and approved by the Executive Committee of the European Resuscitation Council. *Resuscitation* 2001; **48**: 211–221.

35. Handley, A.J., Monsieurs, K.G. & Bossaert, L.L. European Resuscitation Council Guidelines 2000 for Adult Basic Life Support. A statement from the Basic Life Support and Automated External Defibrillation Working Group(1) and approved by the Executive Committee of the European Resuscitation Council. *Resuscitation* 2001; **48**: 199–205.

36. Monsieurs, K.G., Handley, A.J. & Bossaert, L.L. European Resuscitation Council Guidelines 2000 for Automated External Defibrillation. A statement from the Basic Life Support and Automated External Defibrillation Working Group(1) and approved by the Executive Committee of the European Resuscitation Council. *Resuscitation* 2001; **48**: 207–209.

37. Phillips, B., Zideman, D., Garcia-Castrillo, L., Felix, M. & Shwarz-Schwierin, U. European Resuscitation Council Guidelines 2000 for Basic Paediatric Life Support. A statement from the Paediatric Life Support Working Group and approved by the Executive Committee of the European Resuscitation Council. *Resuscitation* 2001; **48**: 223–229.

38. Phillips, B., Zideman, D., Garcia-Castrillo, L., Felix, M. & Shwarz-Schwierin, V. European Resuscitation Council Guidelines 2000 for Advanced Paediatric Life Support. A state-

ment from Paediatric Life Support Working Group and approved by the Executive Committee of the European Resuscitation Council. *Resuscitation* 2001; **48**: 231–234.

39. Phillips, B., Zideman, D., Wyllie, J., Richmond, S. & van Reempts, P. European Resuscitation Council Guidelines 2000 for Newly Born Life Support. A statement from the Paediatric Life Support Working Group and approved by the Executive Committee of the European Resuscitation Council. *Resuscitation* 2001; **48**: 235–239.

40. Raine, R., Sanderson, C., Hutchings, A., Carter, S., Larkin, K. & Black, N. An experimental study of determinants of group judgments in clinical guideline development. *Lancet* 2004; **364**: 429–437.

41. Burgers, J.S. & van Everdingen, J.J. Beyond the evidence in clinical guidelines. *Lancet* 2004; **364**: 392–393.

42. Raine, R., Sanderson, C. & Black, N. Developing clinical guidelines: a challenge to current methods. *Br. Med. J.* 2005; **331**: 631–633.

43. Sackett, D., Richardson, W., Rosenberg, W. & Haynes, R. *Evidence-based Medicine. How to Practise and Teach EBM.* London: Churchill Livingstone; 1997.

44. Lemaire, F., Bion, J., Blanco, J. *et al.* The European Union Directive on Clinical Research: present status of implementation in EU member states' legislations with regard to the incompetent patient. *Intensive Care Med* 2005; **31**: 476–479.

45. Stone, P.W. Popping the (PICO) question in research and evidence-based practice. *Appl. Nurs. Res.* 2002; **15**: 197–198.

46. Harbour, R. & Miller, J. A new system for grading recommendations in evidence based guidelines. *Br. Med. J.* 2001; **323**: 334–336.

47. 2005 American Heart Association Guidelines for Cardiopulmonary Resuscitation and Emergency Cardiovascular Care. *Circulation* 2005; **112**: IV1–203.

48. Nolan, J.P. & Baskett P.J.F. *European Resuscitation Council Guidelines for Resuscitation 2005.* Amsterdam: Elsevier; 2005.

49. Davidoff, F., DeAngelis, C.D., Drazen, J.M. *et al.* Sponsorship, authorship, and accountability. *Lancet* 2001; **358**: 854–856.

50. Choudhry, N.K., Stelfox, H.T. & Detsky, A.S. Relationships between authors of clinical practice guidelines and the pharmaceutical industry. *J. Am. Med. Assoc.* 2002; **287**: 612–617.

51. Billi, J.E., Eigel, B., Zideman, D., Nolan, J.P., Montgomery, W. & Nadkarni, V. Conflict of interest management before, during and after the 2005 International Consensus Conference on Cardiopulmonary Resuscitation and Emergency Cardiovascular Care Science With Treatment Recommendations. *Resuscitation* 2005; **67**: 171–173.

52. International Liaison Committee on Resuscitation. Part 1. Introduction. 2005 International Consensus on Cardiopulmonary Resuscitation and Emergency Cardiovascular Care Science with Treatment Recommendations. *Resuscitation* 2005; **67**: 181–186.

53. International Liaison Committee on Resuscitation. 2005 International Consensus on Cardiopulmonary Resuscitation and Emergency Cardiovascular Care Science with Treatment Recommendations. *Circulation* 2005; **112**: III-1–III-136.

54. Grimshaw, J., Eccles, M. & Tetroe, J. Implementing clinical guidelines: current evidence and future implications. *J. Contin. Educ. Health Prof.* 2004; **24** Suppl. 1: S31–S37.

55. Feder, G., Eccles, M., Grol, R., Griffiths, C. & Grimshaw, J. Clinical guidelines: using clinical guidelines. *Br. Med. J.* 1999; **318**: 728–730.

56. Herlitz, J., Engdahl, J., Svensson, L., Angquist, K.A., Young, M. & Holmberg, S. Factors associated with an increased chance of survival among patients suffering from an out-of-hospital cardiac arrest in a national perspective in Sweden. *Am. Heart J.* 2005; **149**: 61–66.

57. Nadkarni, V.M., Larkin, G.L., Peberdy, M.A. *et al.* First documented rhythm and clinical outcome from in-hospital cardiac arrest among children and adults. *J. Am. Med. Assoc.* 2006; **295**: 50–57.

Index

Note: page numbers in *italics* refer to figures and tables. Plates are indicated by Plate number.